Inflammation

Basic Principles and
Clinical Correlates

Inflammation

Basic Principles and Clinical Correlates

Editors

John I. Gallin, M.D.
Director, Intramural Research Program
National Institute of Allergy and Infectious Diseases
National Institutes of Health
Bethesda, Maryland

Ira M. Goldstein, M.D.
Professor of Medicine
University of California, San Francisco
San Francisco, California
Director, Rosalind Russell Arthritis Research Laboratory
Head, Division of Rheumatology
San Francisco General Hospital
San Francisco, California

Ralph Snyderman, M.D.
Vice President—Medical Research and Development
Genentech Inc.
San Francisco, California
Adjunct Professor of Medicine
Duke University
Durham, North Carolina
Adjunct Professor of Medicine
University of California at San Francisco
San Francisco, California

Raven Press 🐦 New York

Raven Press, 1185 Avenue of the Americas, New York, New York 10036

Made in the United States of America

Library of Congress Cataloging-in-Publication Data

Inflammation: basic principles and clinical correlates.
    Includes bibliographies and index.
    1. Inflammation.   I. Gallin, John I.   II. Goldstein,
Ira M.   III. Snyderman, Ralph.   [DNLM: 1. Inflammation—
immunology.   2. Inflammation—physiopathology.
QZ 150 I435]
RB131.I519   1988   616'.0473   87-23334
ISBN 0-88167-344-7

_66492_

9 8 7 6 5 4 3 2

_66492_

Preface

The inflammatory process is vital to the survival of all complex organisms and its functions play a profound role in health and disease. Despite its importance to diverse areas of research and clinical medicine, there are, at best, few comprehensive resource books that encompass the entire subject in a contemporary manner. This volume was assembled to fill this void. It is an advanced text that is designed to be of use to students, fellows, and physicians of differing backgrounds, as well as to senior scientists to use as a reference. As such, it should appeal to medical and graduate students and research fellows as well as to primary investigators and clinical subspecialists interested in infectious diseases, rheumatology, dermatology, pathology, and hematology–oncology.

The Overview and Historical Perspective provide an introduction to the field. The sections on soluble and cellular components of inflammation offer those with little prior knowledge of inflammation a sophisticated exposure to the elements of the inflammatory process. The section on clinical correlates is designed to provide vivid examples of the various ways in which disorders of the inflammatory process are manifested clinically, and serves to fortify and expand concepts presented in the earlier sections. The final section on pharmacologic modulation of inflammation reviews the current approaches to therapy while pointing out potential new ways to manipulate the inflammatory process.

This volume will be important to many research and clinical subspecialties. Each chapter is written by an individual actively engaged in research reviewed in the chapter. Some areas are controversial, and varying opinions may be represented here. These discussions reflect the rapidly evolving nature of the field and we urge the reader to view these topics with a critical eye. Like many other areas of biomedical research, the field of inflammation has undergone explosive growth in the past few years. Our hope is that this volume will reflect this exciting new understanding of the inflammatory process. It is our intention that the book will not only teach the reader the basic principles of inflammation, but will also prepare him for the rapid changes that will occur in the future.

John I. Gallin
Ira M. Goldstein
Ralph Snyderman

Acknowledgments

We extend special thanks to our secretaries Patricia Runyon, Cathryn Roseberry, and Jodi Telander, without whose help this book would not have been possible.

Contents

PHARMACOLOGIC MODULATION OF INFLAMMATION

Contributors

Dolph O. Adams, M.D., Ph.D. *Professor, Department of Pathology, Duke University Medical Center, Box 3712, Durham, North Carolina 27710*

K. Frank Austen, M.D. *Robert Brigham Division, Brigham and Women's Hospital, Sealy G. Mudd Bldg., Room 604, 250 Longwood Avenue, Boston, Massachusetts 02115*

Dorothy Ford Bainton, M.D. *Professor and Chairman, Department of Pathology, University of California School of Medicine, HSW 501, Box 0506, Third and Parnassus Avenues, San Francisco, California 94143*

Timothy D. Bigby, M.D. *Cardiovascular Research Institute, Box 0130, University of California at San Francisco, San Francisco, California 94143-0130*

Debra L. Bowen, M.D. *Senior Staff Fellow, Laboratory of Immunoregulation, NIAID–National Institutes of Health, Bethesda, Maryland 20892*

Donna L. Bratton, M.D. *National Jewish Center for Immunology and Respiratory Medicine, 1400 Jackson Avenue, Denver, Colorado 80206*

Ward E. Bullock, M.D. *MSB-7168, ML 560, University of Cincinnati Medical Center, 231 Bethesda Avenue, Cincinnati, Ohio 45267*

George J. Cianciolo, Ph.D. *Pharmacological Sciences, Genentech, Inc., 460 Point San Bruno Boulevard, South San Francisco, California 94080*

Charles G. Cochrane, M.D. *Department of Immunology, IMM12, Scripps Clinic and Research Foundation, 10666 North Torrey Pines Road, La Jolla, California 92037*

Harvey R. Colten, M.D. *Professor and Chairman, Department of Pediatrics, Washington University School of Medicine, 400 South Kingshighway, St. Louis, Missouri 63110*

George S. Deepe, Jr., M.D. *Assistant Professor of Medicine, University of Cincinnati Medical Center, 231 Bethesda Avenue, Cincinnati, Ohio 45267*

Charles A. Dinarello, M.D. *Associate Professor of Medicine, Division of Geographic Medicine and Infectious Diseases, New England Medical Center Hospitals, NEMCH Box 68, 750 Washington Street, Boston, Massachusetts 02111*

Peter Elsbach, M.D. *Professor, Department of Medicine, New York University School of Medicine, 550 First Avenue, New York, New York 10016*

Anthony S. Fauci, M.D. *Director, NIAID–National Institutes of Health, Bldg. 31, Room 7A03, Bethesda, Maryland 20892*

Michael M. Frank, M.D. *Chief, Laboratory of Clinical Investigation, and Clinical Director, NIAID–National Institutes of Health, Bldg. 10, Room 11N228, Bethesda, Maryland 20892*

Claus Fittschen, M.D. *National Jewish Center for Immunology and Respiratory Medicine, 1400 Jackson Avenue, Denver, Colorado 80206*

Louis F. Fries, M.D. *Laboratory of Clinical Investigation, NIAID–National Institutes of Health, Bethesda, Maryland 20892*

Elaine K. Gallin, Ph.D. *Department of Physiology, Armed Forces Radiobiology, Research Institute, Naval Medical Center, Bethesda, Maryland 20814*

John I. Gallin, M.D. *Director, Intramural Research Program, NIAID–National Institutes of Health, Bldg. 10, Room 11C103, Bethesda, Maryland 20892*

Marvin R. Garovoy, M.D. *Associate Professor, Immunogenetics and Transplantation Laboratory, HSE520, Department of Medicine and Surgery, University of California, San Francisco, Third and Parnassus Avenues, San Francisco, California 94143*

Judith C. Gasson, M.D. *Department of Medicine, UCLA School of Medicine, Los Angeles, California 90024*

Mark H. Ginsberg, M.D. *Department of Immunology, Scripps Clinic and Research Foundation, 10666 North Torrey Pines Road, La Jolla, California 92037*

David W. Golde, M.D. *Division of Hematology/Oncology, Department of Medicine, UCLA School of Medicine, Los Angeles, California 90024*

Ira M. Goldstein, M.D. *Department of Medicine, University of California, San Francisco, Third and Parnassus Avenues, San Francisco, California 94143-0868*

Thomas P. Gordon, M.D. *Division of Immunology, Scripps Clinic and Research Foundation, 10666 North Torrey Pines Road, La Jolla, California 92037*

Warner C. Greene, M.D., Ph.D. *Professor of Medicine, Duke University School of Medicine, 487 Carl Bldg., Research Drive, P.O. Box 3705, Durham, North Carolina 27710*

T. A. Hamilton, M.D. *Department of Pathology, Duke University Medical Center, Box 3712, Durham, North Carolina 27710*

Edward D. Harris, Jr., M.D. *Professor and Chairman, Department of Medicine, UNDMJ–Robert Wood Johnson Medical School, Academic Health Sciences Center, CN19, One Robert Wood Johnson Place, New Brunswick, New Jersey 08903-0019*

Koji Hashimoto, M.D. *Department of Dermatology, University of Pennsylvania, Philadelphia, Pennsylvania 19104*

Barton F. Haynes, M.D. *Professor of Medicine, Chief, Division of Rheumatology and Immunology, Duke University School of Medicine, P.O. Box 3258, Durham, North Carolina 27710*

Janet E. Henson, M.D. *National Jewish Center for Immunology and Respiratory Medicine, 1400 Jackson Avenue, Denver, Colorado 80206*

Peter M. Henson, M.D. *Executive Vice President, Biomedical Affairs, National Jewish Center for Immunology and Respiratory Medicine, 1400 Jackson Avenue, Denver, Colorado 80206*

Ronald B. Herberman, M.D. *Director, Pittsburgh Cancer Institute, 230 Lothrop Street, Suite 706, Pittsburgh, Pennsylvania 15213*

Eric A. Jaffe, M.D. *Associate Professor, Department of Medicine, Cornell University Medical College, 1300 York Avenue, New York, New York 10021*

Aaron Janoff, Ph.D. *Professor of Pathology, Health Sciences Center, State University of New York, Stony Brook, New York 11794*

Pamela J. Jensen, M.D. *Department of Dermatology, University of Pennsylvania, Philadelphia, Pennsylvania 19104*

Joseph L. Jorizzo, M.D. *Professor and Chairman, Department of Dermatology, Bowman-Gray School of Medicine, 300 South Hawthorne Road, Winston-Salem, North Carolina 27103*

Paula Kadison, M.D. *Department of Medicine, Duke University Medical Center, P.O. Box 3258, Durham, North Carolina 27710*

Michael A. Kaliner, M.D. *Head, Allergic Diseases Section, Laboratory of Clinical Investigation, NIAID–National Institutes of Health, Bldg. 10, Room 11C205, Bethesda, Maryland 20892*

Andrew H. Kang, M.D. *Professor and Chairman, Department of Medicine, University of Tennessee Center for Health Sciences, 1030 Jefferson Avenue, Memphis, Tennessee 38163*

Allen P. Kaplan, M.D. *Chairman, Department of Medicine, Health Sciences Center, T-16, Room 040, State University of New York, Stony Brook, New York 11794*

Gachuhi Kimani, M.D. *National Jewish Center for Immunology and Respiratory Medicine, 1400 Jackson Avenue, Denver, Colorado 80206*

Seymour J. Klebanoff, M.D., Ph.D. *Professor of Medicine, University of Washington School of Medicine, Seattle, Washington 98195*

Franklin Kozin, M.D. *Department of Immunology, Scripps Clinic and Research Foundation, 10666 North Torrey Pines Road, La Jolla, California 92037*

Gerald S. Lazarus, M.D. *Chairman, Department of Dermatology, University of Pennsylvania Hospital, 3400 Spruce Street, Philadelphia, Pennsylvania 19104*

Robert A. Lewis, M.D. *Departments of Immunology and Rheumatology, Brigham and Women's Hospital, Boston, Massachusetts and Syntex Research, 3401 Hill View Avenue, P.O. Box 10850, Palo Alto, California 94303*

Peter E. Lipsky, M.D. *Department of Internal Medicine, University of Texas Health Sciences Center, 5323 Harry Hines Boulevard, Dallas, Texas 75235*

Janet C. Ludwig, M.D. *Department of Pathology, The University of Texas Health Science Center, 7703 Floyd Curl Drive, San Antonio, Texas 78284*

Harry L. Malech, M.D. *Head, Bacterial Diseases Section, Laboratory of Clinical Investigation, NIAID–National Institutes of Health, Bldg. 10, Room 11N112, Bethesda, Maryland 20892*

Aaron J. Marcus, M.D. *Department of Hematology and Oncology, New York Veterans Administration Medical Center, 408 First Avenue, New York, New York 10010*

Linda M. McManus, M.D. *Department of Pathology, The University of Texas Health Science Center, 7703 Floyd Curl Drive, San Antonio, Texas 78284*

Shinji Morioka, M.D. *Department of Dermatology, Juntendo University School of Medicine, Hongo, Tokyo, Japan*

Hans J. Müller-Eberhard, M.D. *Department of Immunology, Scripps Clinic and Research Foundation, 10666 North Torrey Pines Road, La Jolla, California 92037*

Jay A. Nadel, M.D. *Cardiovascular Research Institute, Box 0130, University of California at San Francisco, San Francisco, California 94143-0130*

Carl Nathan, M.D. *Department of Medicine, Division of Hematology/Oncology, Cornell University Medical College, 1300 York Avenue, New York, New York 10021*

David H. Perlmutter, M.D. *Department of Pediatrics, Washington University School of Medicine, St. Louis Children's Hospital, 400 South Kingshighway, St. Louis, Missouri 63110*

R. Neal Pinckard, Ph.D. *Department of Pathology, The University of Texas Health Science Center, 7703 Floyd Curl Drive, San Antonio, Texas 78284*

Arnold E. Postlethwaite, M.D. *Professor, Department of Medicine, University of Tennessee Center for Health Sciences and Veterans Administration Medical Center, 1030 Jefferson Avenue, Memphis, Tennessee 38163*

David W. H. Riches, M.D.   *National Jewish Center for Immunology and Respiratory Medicine, 1400 Jackson Avenue, Denver, Colorado 80206*

Alan S. Rosenthal, M.D.   *Research and Development Laboratories, Boehringer-Ingelheim Pharmaceuticals, Ridgefield, Connecticut 06877*

Michael F. Seldin, M.D., Ph.D.   *Arthritis Branch, NIAMS–National Institutes of Health, Bethesda, Maryland 20892*

Paul A. Sheehy, Ph.D.   *Laboratory of Neurophysiology, NINDS–National Institutes of Health, Bethesda, Maryland 20892*

John N. Sheagren, M.D.   *Chief of Staff, Veterans Administration Medical Center, 2215 Fuller Road, Ann Arbor, Michigan 48105*

Richard H. Simon, M.D.   *Division of Pulmonary and Critical Care Medicine, 3916 Taubman Center, University of Michigan Medical Center, Ann Arbor, Michigan 48109*

Kay H. Singer, M.D.   *Department of Medicine, Division of Rheumatology and Immunology, Duke University Medical Center, Durham, North Carolina 27710*

Reuben P. Siraganian, M.D., Ph.D.   *Chief, Clinical Immunology Section, LMI, National Institute of Dental Research, National Institutes of Health, Bldg. 10, Room 1A-26, Bethesda, Maryland 20892*

Ralph Snyderman, M.D.   *Vice President of Medical Research and Development, Genentech, Inc., 460 Point San Bruno Blvd., South San Francisco, California 94080*

Hans L. Spiegelberg, M.D.   *Department of Immunopathology, Scripps Clinic and Research Foundation, 10666 North Torrey Pines Road, La Jolla, California 92037*

Alfred D. Steinberg, M.D.   *NIADDK–National Institutes of Health, Bldg. 10, Room 8D19, Bethesda, Maryland 20892*

John D. Stobo, M.D.   *Professor and Chairman, Department of Medicine, Johns Hopkins University, Baltimore, Maryland 21218*

Thomas P. Stossel, M.D.   *Hematology–Oncology Unit, Department of Medicine, Massachusetts General Hospital, Fruit Street, Boston, Massachusetts 02114*

Robert Terkeltaub, M.D.   *Division of Rheumatology, Veterans Administration Medical Center, University of California, San Diego, California 92161*

Harley Y. Tse, M.D.   *Department of Immunology and Microbiology, Wayne State University School of Medicine, Detroit, Michigan 48201*

Ronald J. Uhing, M.D.   *Division of Rheumatology and Immunology, Department of Medicine, Duke University Medical Center, Durham, North Carolina 27710*

Jay C. Unkeless, Ph.D.   *Associate Professor, Department of Biochemistry, Mount Sinai School of Medicine, 1 Gustave Levy Place, New York, New York 10021*

Ralph van Furth, M.D.   *Department of Infectious Diseases, University Hospital, Rijnsburgerweg 10, 2333 AA Leiden, The Netherlands*

Julio C. Voltarelli, M.D., Ph.D.   *Department of Clinical Medicine, School of Medicine of Ribeirao Preto, University of São Paulo, Brazil*

Sharon M. Wahl, Ph.D.   *Head, Cellular Immunology Section, Laboratory of Microbiology and Immunity, National Institute of Dental Research, National Institutes of Health, Bldg. 30, Room 326, Bethesda, Maryland 20892*

Peter A. Ward, M.D. *Professor and Chairman, Department of Pathology, University of Michigan Medical School, M5240 Medical Sciences I, Box 0602, 1301 Catherine Road, Ann Arbor, Michigan 48109-0602*

Jerrold Weiss, Ph.D. *Department of Medicine, New York University School of Medicine, 550 First Avenue, New York, New York 10016*

Gerald Weissmann, M.D. *Department of Medicine, New York University School of Medicine, 550 First Avenue, New York, New York 10016*

Babette B. Weksler, M.D. *Department of Medicine, C-608, Division of Hematology/Oncology, New York Hospital–Cornell University Medical College, 1300 York Avenue, New York, New York 10021*

Martha V. White, M.D. *Laboratory of Clinical Investigation, NIAID–National Institutes of Health, Bldg. 10, Room 11C207, Bethesda, Maryland 20892*

Samuel D. Wright, M.D. *Laboratory of Cellular Physiology and Immunology, The Rockefeller University, New York, New York 10021*

Ryotaro Yoshida, M.D. *Department of Medicine, Division of Hematology/Oncology, Cornell University Medical College, 1300 York Avenue, New York, New York 10021*

Inflammation
Basic Principles and
Clinical Correlates

Overview

Inflammation is a localized protective response elicited by injury or destruction of tissues, which serves to destroy, dilute, or wall-off both the injurious agent and the injured tissue. It is characterized in the acute form by the classical signs of pain (dolor), heat (calor), redness (rubor), swelling (tumor), and loss of function (functio laesa). Microscopically it involves a complex series of events, including (a) dilation of arterioles, capillaries, and venules, with increased permeability and blood flow; (b) exudation of fluids, including plasma proteins; and (c) leukocytic migration into the inflammatory focus.

Diseases characterized by inflammation are an important cause of morbidity and mortality in humans. With the possible exception of some reactions to toxins and mechanical trauma, inflammation occurs in an attempt by leukocytes to defend the host from "foreign invaders." The accumulation and subsequent activation of leukocytes are central events in the pathogenesis of virtually all forms of inflammation. Absence of inflammation leads to a compromised host. Excessive inflammation, either secondary to abnormal recognition of host tissue as "foreign" or abnormal turn-off of an otherwise normal inflammatory process, leads to inflammatory diseases. Information concerning the mechanisms whereby inflammatory cells accumulate in tissues, as well as the mechanisms whereby such cells are stimulated to damage tissues, should provide better insights into the pathogenesis of human diseases and also should provide clues for developing more rational forms of therapy.

Regardless of their etiology, most forms of acute and chronic inflammation are amplified as well as propagated as a result of the recruitment of humoral and cellular components of the immune system. Immunologically mediated elimination of foreign material proceeds through a series of integrated steps. First, the material to be eliminated (i.e., antigen) is recognized as being "foreign" by immunoglobulins (i.e., antibodies) or by receptors on T lymphocytes that bind to specific determinants (epitopes). Binding of a recognition component of the immune system to an antigen generally leads to activation of an amplification system, initiating production of proinflammatory substances. These mediators alter blood flow, increase vascular permeability, augment adherence of circulating leukocytes to vascular endothelium, promote migration of leukocytes into tissues, and stimulate leukocytes to destroy the inciting agent. The actual destruction of antigens by immune mechanisms is mediated by phagocytic cells. Such cells may migrate freely or may exist at fixed tissue sites as components of the mononuclear phagocyte system. Macrophages and related cells (e.g., Kupffer cells, type-A synovial lining cells) are central components of this system. Destruction of antigens outside of the mononuclear phagocyte system generally takes place in tissue spaces and is mediated by polymorphonuclear leukocytes (neutrophils) or monocytes, which are recruited from circulating blood.

It is important to note that immune processes are probably ongoing and, in most instances, lead to the elimination of antigens without producing clinically detectable inflammation. The development of clinically apparent inflammation indicates that the immune system has encountered either an unusually large amount of antigen, antigen in an unusual location, or antigen that was difficult to digest. In some diseases (e.g., rheumatoid arthritis), the inciting agent is unknown or may be related to normal host tissue components. In others (e.g., systemic lupus erythematosus), inherent or acquired immunoregulatory abnormalities may contribute to the sustained nature of the inflammatory process.

Inflammation and tissue injury on an immune basis characterize a wide variety of human diseases. Although little is known concerning the etiologies of these disorders,

TABLE 1. *Immunopathologic processes*[a]

Type of inflammation	Immune recognition component	Soluble mediator	Inflammatory response	Disease/example
Reagenic/allergic	IgE	Basophil and mast cell products (i.e., histamine, arachidonate metabolites)	Immediate flare and wheal; smooth muscle constriction	Atopy; anaphylaxis
Cytotoxic antibody	IgG, IgM	Complement	Lysis or phagocytosis of circulating antigens; acute inflammation in tissues	Autoimmune hemolytic anemia; thrombocytopenia associated with lupus erythematosus
Immune complex	IgG, IgM	Complement	Accumulation of PMNs and macrophages	Rheumatoid arthritis; lupus erythematosus
Delayed hypersensitivity	T lymphocytes	Cytokines	Mononuclear cell infiltrate	Tuberculosis; sarcoidosis; polymyositis; granulomatosis; vasculitis

[a] Adapted from Snyderman, R. (1985): Mechanisms of inflammation and tissue destruction in the rheumatic diseases. In: *Cecil Textbook of Medicine,* 17th edition, edited by J. B. Wyngaarden and L. H. Smith, Jr., pp. 1898–1906. W. B. Saunders, Philadelphia.

considerable progress has been made toward understanding their pathogenesis. A convenient way of classifying immunologically induced inflammation is shown in Table 1.

ALLERGIC (REAGINIC) INFLAMMATION

Certain types of antigens have a propensity for stimulating production of IgE antibodies in genetically susceptible individuals. IgE antibodies bind nonspecifically, via their Fc regions, to receptors on basophils and mast cells. Subsequent attachment of antigens to the Fab portions of such cell-bound IgE antibodies causes mast cells and basophils to secrete contents of their cytoplasmic granules (e.g., histamine), as well as to synthesize and secrete biologically active products of arachidonic acid (e.g., leukotrienes). These mediators alter blood flow, increase vascular permeability, and constrict bronchial smooth muscle. Reaginic reactions are responsible for such allergic phenomena as urticaria, seasonal rhinitis, asthma, and, in situations where large amounts of allergens gain access to the circulation, systemic anaphylaxis.

INFLAMMATION MEDIATED BY CYTOTOXIC ANTIBODIES

Severe tissue injury can result from the binding of complement-fixing antibodies to cells. Recognition, by antibodies, of antigens on circulating erythrocytes, platelets, or leukocytes can lead to complement activation and deposition of complement fragments (e.g., C3b) on the sur-

faces of these cells. Macrophages of the mononuclear phagocyte system express plasma membrane receptors for the Fc portion of IgG as well as for C3b; these macrophages also eliminate, from the circulation, particles coated with these proteins. Extravascularly, binding of complement-fixing antibodies to cells or to extracellular structures (e.g., basement membrane) also activates the complement cascade and leads to binding of complement fragments to the antigen, as well as to generation of mediators of inflammation. Cleavage products derived from C4, C3, and C5 (i.e., C4a, C3a, and C5a) increase vascular permeability and induce vascular stasis. C5a is a potent chemotactic factor that attracts granulocytes and macrophages. The accumulation of inflammatory cells as well as direct complement-mediated lysis causes the destruction of tissues coated with antibody. Goodpasture's syndrome is a dramatic example of a human disease that results from the deposition of antibodies onto glomerular and pulmonary basement membranes. Many common rheumatologic disorders also are characterized by the development of antibodies to cells. Systemic lupus erythematosus, for example, frequently is accompanied by autoimmune hemolytic anemia as well as immune-mediated thrombocytopenia.

INFLAMMATION MEDIATED BY IMMUNE COMPLEXES

Inflammation due to the deposition of immune complexes in tissues is a common feature of numerous rheumatic disorders. The following is an overview of how inflammation results after formation or deposition of immune complexes in tissues.

The combination of IgM or IgG antibodies with antigen is followed by activation of complement and the generation of several complement-derived peptides with proinflammatory activity. C3a and C5a, for example, enhance vascular permeability, contract smooth muscle, and degranulate mast cells. C5a, in addition, is a potent chemotactic factor and leads to the accumulation of inflammatory cells at sites of immune complex formation or deposition.

Polymorphonuclear leukocytes and mononuclear phagocytes recognize immune complexes via their surface receptors for C3b and IgG. Suitable ligand-receptor interactions ultimately lead to phagocytosis. When the amount of immune complexes deposited locally is not great, phagocytic cells ingest and degrade the complexes without causing tissue destruction. However, if the amount of immune complexes is great or if they are enmeshed in the basement membrane of blood vessels, leukocytes are incapable of completely ingesting and digesting the inflammatory stimulus. Rather, they adhere to immune complexes and degranulate, that is, release a portion of their lysosomal contents. Binding of immune complexes to phagocytes also activates a respiratory burst and causes the cells to release toxic oxygen metabolites. These events frequently cause disruption of the integrity of blood vessels and lead to hemorrhagic necrosis as well as to local tissue destruction.

When a large amount of antigen gains access to the circulation (as after administration of heterologous serum), it can initiate a serum sickness reaction. As antibody is produced, antigen-antibody complexes form in great antigen excess. Such complexes do not activate complement efficiently and may circulate harmlessly. As antibody production increases, however, immune complexes develop a lower ratio of antigen to antibody and thereby increase their ability to activate complement. Such complexes may deposit in the walls of small blood vessels, where they initiate inflammatory reactions via the mechanisms described above. Deposition of antigen in glomerular basement membrane can lead to the formation of immune complexes at that site. Alternatively, certain complexes may be phagocytosed by mesangial cells in the glomerulus. In either case, complement is deposited and inflammation ensues. Associated with immune complex-mediated inflammation are leukocytic vasculitis (palpable purpuric skin lesions), arthritis, glomerulitis, and fever. Rheumatoid arthritis has many characteristics of a local immune complex reaction, whereas systemic erythematosus has many clinical features of serum sickness.

DELAYED-TYPE HYPERSENSITIVITY REACTIONS (INFLAMMATION MEDIATED BY MONONUCLEAR LEUKOCYTES)

When antigen is recognized by receptors on T lymphocytes, a delayed-type hypersensitivity reaction may be stimulated. The term "delayed-type hypersensitivity" is based on the kinetics of the inflammation that follows deposition of antigen in the skin. Whereas allergic reactions occur within seconds to minutes and immune-complex-mediated reactions occur within several hours to 24 hr, delayed-type hypersensitivity reactions peak at 48 to 72 hr after deposition of antigen. In delayed hypersensitivity reactions, antigen is encountered and processed by macrophages. The processed form of antigen is "presented" to T lymphocytes that contain receptors for the antigen as well as for Ia antigens on the macrophage. Binding of the processed antigen to T lymphocytes leads to the production of lymphokines (e.g., interleukin-2, gamma-interferon, lymphocyte-derived chemotactic factor) as well as monokines (e.g., interleukin-1). Lymphokines and monokines (cytokines) are important mediators of inflammatory responses by virtue of their ability to attract and activate macrophages as well as other lymphocytes. Macrophages ingest and degrade antigen in most cases. Delayed-type hypersensitivity reactions appear to be particularly important for the destruction of many intracellular parasites, tumor cells, and viruses. Lesions typical of delayed-type hypersensitivity reactions are seen in such human diseases as tuberculosis, sarcoidosis, and polymyositis.

The importance of the inflammatory response for host defense has been recognized for well over a century. During the past decade, however, dramatic advances have been made in understanding the precise biochemical and cellular mechanisms that regulate this process. Inflammatory processes play a central role in mediating immune host defense and wound healing but also participate in the pathogenesis of many diseases. Better control of this complex inflammatory system offers a great challenge and opportunity for medical research. The following chapters summarize our current understanding of inflammation and its clinical consequences.

The Editors

Inflammation: Basic Principles and Clinical Correlates.
Edited by J. I. Gallin, I. M. Goldstein, and R. Snyderman.
Raven Press, Ltd., New York © 1988.

CHAPTER 1

Inflammation: Historical Perspective

Gerald Weissmann

Redness and swelling with heat and pain—*rubor et tumor cum calore et dolore*—have been recognized as the four cardinal signs of inflammation since the writings of Cornelius Celsus in the first century of the common era (30 BC to AD 38). And Celsus—who is sometimes mistaken for Celsius of thermometry—was describing the typical reaction of flesh to microbes. Although all sorts of injuries to humans and beasts will elicit inflammation, it seems clear that our extensive arsenal of host defenses has not been stocked by evolution against such recent threats as ionizing radiation, Saturday night specials, overturned tractor-trailers, and free-based cocaine. No, the drab Darwinism of biology suggests that, whereas inflammation may help the individual cope with cuts and bruises, most of the redness and swelling with heat and pain is there to make sure that the species is not wiped out by epidemics.

It seems to me that the more we learn about inflammation, the simpler its message becomes: Our cells and humors defend the self against invisible armies of the other. We call our losses "infection" and our victories "immunity." It has also occurred to me that the language we use to describe this conflict owes less to biology than to the temper of our times.

This warfare between humans and bacteria was not appreciated as an order of battle until the "microbe hunters" of the nineteenth century recognized the opposing forces and the territory in dispute. By 1908, when the Nobel prize was given to Paul Ehrlich for his work on humoral immunity (antibodies) and to Elie Metchnikoff for his work on cellular immunity (phagocytosis), it was clear that the body uses these two strategies in concert to identify and destroy invaders. The discourse that announced the discovery was that of Darwinian survival:

> When the aggressor in this struggle is much smaller than its adversary the result is that the former introduces itself into the body of the latter and destroys it by means of infection. . . . But infection also has its counter. The attacked organism defends itself against the little aggressor. It protects itself by interposing a resistant membrane, or it uses all the means at its disposal to destroy the invader (5).

The tendency to couch descriptions of inflammation in terms of nineteenth-century battle has proved irresistible. Indeed, the assumptions of the microbe hunters were based not only on models of Darwinian zoology but also on the military legend of empire. Here the distinguished pathologist Joseph McFarland (4) sums up the field of inflammation from Rudolf Virchow to Valy Menkin:

> To many, the situation here encountered resembles a battlefield on which the leukocytes meet the invading bacteria and contest their further increase and invasion until they triumph, and, the infection overcome, the inflammation subsides.

The microbe hunters drew their images of battle from romantic accounts of skirmishes waged more often than not by British troops against "lesser breeds." Those imperial campaigns were directed by astute generals who viewed the destruction of foreigners through the lenses of binoculars. One catches the whiff of inflammation in this account, by John Bowle (1), of Kitchener's revenge (1896) for the uprising in the Sudan that killed the noble Gordon:

> The campaign culminated in the battle of Omdurman . . . when some 60,000 of the Khalifa's horde flung themselves with superb courage against Kitchener's line, to be mowed down by machine guns, rifles and artillery. . . . By 11:30 a.m. Kitchener handed his binoculars to an aide de camp, remarked that the enemy had had a "thorough dusting" and ordered the advance on Omdurman and Khartoum. The victory had cost 48 killed, including 3 British officers and 25 other ranks and 434 wounded, as against over 11,000 "dervish" dead and about 16,000 wounded and prisoner. Gordon had been more than avenged: the British and Egyptian flags again floated over Khartoum, and when, at the service of thanksgiving the troops sang "Abide with me," Gordon's favorite hymn, even Kitchener was seen to weep.

Substitute "endothelium" for "line," replace "machine guns, rifles and artillery" with "macrophages, leukocytes and fixatives (antibodies)," and we can appreciate the language in which the nineteenth century learned how higher organisms deal with the dervishes of microbes. Metchnikoff, Ehrlich, Cohnheim, and Adami peered through the lenses of microscopes to watch battalions of white cells avenge the revolt of bacilli. Caught in the Victorian structures of hierarchy, Metchnikoff, the gentle scholar, taught the lesson of Darwinian phylogeny from the evidence of phagocytosis:

> The diapedesis of the white corpuscles, their migration through the vessel wall . . . is one of the principal means of defense possessed by an animal. As soon as the infective agents have penetrated into the body, a whole army of white corpuscles proceed towards the menaced spot, there entering into a struggle with the micro-organisms. The leukocytes, having arrived at the spot where the intruders are found, seize them after the manner of the Amoeba and within their bodies subject them to intracellular digestion (6).

Metchnikoff was not the only champion of white corpuscles; we owe their classification as basophils, eosinophils, and neutrophils to Ehrlich's doctoral thesis on aniline dyes. Blue, red, and white colors depended on the way in which positive or negative charges lined up in the granules of the phagocytes; aniline dyes marked the combatants as clearly as red or blue tunics identified cavalry units in the Franco-Prussian War of 1870. Indeed, aniline dyes were the response of German synthetic chemistry to French control of the colonies that yielded natural dyestuffs. Ehrlich's studies with dyes—which introduced the language of colors and fixation—helped Germany to become the arsenal of chemotherapy and had the happy side effect of launching immunochemistry. Ehrlich's dictum, *Corpora non agunt nisi fixata* ("Bodies that do not attach do not act" was the basis not only for the first treatment of syphilis—Salvarsan—but also for modern ligand–receptor theory. It might be argued that Ehrlich's doctrine also applies directly to the means whereby cells—white cells and platelets—stick to vessel walls and to each other in the course of inflammation.

Central to the humoral theories of Ehrlich and the cellular ones of Metchnikoff was the late Victorian conviction that the body would not injure itself wittingly. As the nation-states of Europe placed their faith in the social doctrine of Darwinian survival, so the microbe hunters were sure that the body had a *horror autotoxicus*—an incapacity to turn defensive weapons into tools of self-destruction. Time and events have overturned that nineteenth-century conviction. The bad news of the twentieth century—from Flanders' fields to the fall of Paris, from the siege of Madrid to the Berlin Wall, from the battle of Algiers to the mess in Beirut—has added anxiety to the orderly prose of biology. Nowadays when we speak of inflammation, we speak of unplanned mischief, as Lewis Thomas does here (9):

> I suspect that the host is caught up in mistaken, inappropriate, and unquestionably self-destructive mechanisms by the very multiplicity of defenses available to him, defenses which do not seem to have been designed to operate in net coordination with each other. The end result is not defense, it is an agitated, committee-directed, harum-scarum effort to make war, with results that are remarkably like those sometimes observed in human affairs when war-making institutions pretend to be engaged in defense. If, to push the analogy, there were no limit to the number of people who could set off for northern Minnesota at the season of the great flyover of geese and no limit on the type and power of the weapons to be used by each, we would undoubtedly observe . . . with M-16's, howitzers, SAM missiles, lasers and perhaps tactical nuclear rockets, considerably more destruction of people than geese, of host than invader.

One might trace that sea change in our opinion of all that redness and swelling with heat and pain, that change in our notion that inflammation is benign, to the first great war of this century. It may not be a complete coincidence that the terms "allergy," "anaphylaxis," and "serum sickness" began to crowd the clinical literature while the medical profession was prepping the national armies of Europe for slaughter in the trenches of 1914. The immunologists of Europe were prepared to believe that cells could respond to inflammation as readily by revolt as by enlistment. World War I succeeded not only in trimming the rhetoric of battle of its operatic glamor but also in striking the set of nationalism. "Class struggle" began to dissolve the ties of patriotism as the effects of that war of attrition spread over Europe. It soon became apparent that World War I had dismantled the ceremonies of class upon which the Victorian nation-state had relied. The captains and the kings had killed each other, leaving corporals to rule a diminished world. Ford Madox Ford recognized the changing of the guard in *Parade's End* (2):

> He was devising the ceremonial for the disbanding of a Kitchener battalion. . . . Well the end of the show was to be; the adjutant would stand the battalion at ease; the band would play *Land of Hope and Glory,* and then the adjutant would say: There will be no more parades. . . . For there won't. . . . No more Hope, no more Glory, no more parades for you and me any more. Not for the country . . . nor for the world, I dare say . . . None . . . Gone . . . No . . . More . . . parades!

Carrying forward the analogy we have drawn between the discourse of politics and the discourse of biology, we might say that science in the 1920s and 1930s learned about histamine, serotonin, enzymes, and peptides—widely diffused mediators of inflammation—as the nations learned about other mediators of inflammation: fascism, Stalinism, and the Nazis. Biologists were taught by

Sir Henry Dale and Sir Thomas Lewis that human cells can synthesize and release chemicals as disabling to the organism as any toxin released by microbes. That unpleasant lesson coincided with one of the few points of doctrine agreed upon by parties of both right and left: that the body politic carries the seeds of its own destruction. No longer were human differences drawn by national borders alone; to the separations of class were added the divisions of ideology. Again, it may be no accident that we learned about shock lung and the crush syndrome (now attributed at least in part to activation of anaphylatoxins in the circulation) from Loyalist surgeons in the Spanish civil war. That rehearsal for the world war against fascism reached a stalemate at the medical school in Madrid in November of 1936 (8):

> Hours of artillery and aerial bombardment, in which neither side gave way, were succeeded by hand-to-hand battles for single rooms or floors of buildings. In the Clinical Hospital, the Thaelmann Battalion (of the Republican International Brigades) placed bombs in the lifts to be sent up to explode in the faces of the Moroccans (of the Franco forces) on the next floor. And, in the next building, the Moroccans suffered losses by eating inoculated animals kept for experimental purposes.

Nevertheless, until the civil warfare in Madrid, it had been clear on which side of the battle line each soldier stood. It was in Madrid that the fascists boasted of a "fifth column"—secret right-wing partisans who would join with the four regular columns of Franco troops to conquer the republic. "Right" and "left," "communist" and "fascist," these terms had a generally accepted meaning, of sorts. But when World War II came and the Germans occupied most of Europe, even those boundaries became blurred. Distinctions among classes, ideologies, nationalities, religions, and genders became most confused in the colonies of France occupied by the Germans. A model of this confused state was Andre Gide in 1943—Gide the obscure—in Tunis. Gide—the gay ex-communist litterateur, friend of De Gaulle and Malraux on the one hand and of cultivated Germans on the other—here records in his journal the advance of Eisenhower's troops on the German-occupied town (3):

> Several trustworthy farmers confirm the lamentable, absurd retreat of the American forces before the semblance of German opposition. The sudden appearance of a handful of resolute men forced the withdrawal of those who, very superior in numbers and equipment, would have had only to continue their advance to become masters of their objective . . . Tunis.
> Germans everywhere. Well turned-out, in becoming uniforms, young, vigorous, strapping, jolly, clean-shaven, with pink cheeks. . . . Can there be a more wretched humanity than the one I see here? One wonders what God could ever possibly come forth from these sordid creatures, bent over toward the most immediate satisfactions, tattered, dusty, abject and forsaken by the future. Walking

among them in the heart of the Arab town, I looked in vain for a likable face on which to pin some hope: Jews, Moslems, South Italians, Sicilians, or Maltese, accumulated scum as if it were thrown up along the current of clear waters.

From a similar matrix of "accumulated scum" and "jolly" Germans, Hollywood distilled *Casablanca.* That tough tearjerker set the measure of language for my generation. Redness and swelling with heat and pain seemed to be the cardinal emotions of *Casablanca,* and since Bogey was the last hero we could trust, we were sure that all its passions were worthwhile. But in the dreary half-century since the film, we have learned to distrust our leaders, our heroes, and our wars. We have gotten very good only at rounding up the usual suspects.

In science, we have isolated and defined the components of complement, the kinins, and the prostaglandins but have been disappointed to find that our own cells and fluids collaborate with hostile invaders to provoke inflammation. Sometimes these Quislings and Lavals turn on us in the absence of an enemy. In exposing the treasons of lymphocytes, we have come to view them as a cast of Levantine characters. In our film-derived discourse Peter Lorre launders the money for the contrasuppressor T cell, and Sydney Greenstreet cashes in the loot at the bursa of Fabricius. Controlled by a network of codes—could we call the signs of genetics anything else?—the alliances of inflammatory cells shift, their affinities wane; wounds heal but scars remain.

The new synthesis makes only superficial sense. Like the "Marseillaise" in the film, the humors of immunity flood our spirit. Our psyches are lifted or depressed by the products of inflammation; we have learned that the battle cries of injury (interleukins, interferons, tumor necrosis factor) make us febrile, debilitated, sleepy, and cross even as they arouse battalions of lymphocytes. Related molecules activate the troops of defense: phagocytes, which wear receptors on their sleeves as if they were the arm bands of local resistance. Paul Henried leads the forces of that interior.

But in this postbacterial world, the phagocytes fail, white cells do damage, and our antibodies form complexes (the very coin of neuroses) and plug our kidneys. In the course of these confused responses, much harm is done and resolution is not invariable achieved. Every few years we add a new felon to the list of usual suspects: substance P, anti-idiotypes, leukotrienes, lipoxins, and the appropriately named free radicals. Since the days of the cold war we speak neither the language of war nor that of peace; we can no longer decide if our tissues are entirely inflamed or partially immune. In the discourse of politics and of science, we have replaced defined suspects with uncertain suspicions. In that sense, the high sentiment of *Casablanca* has yielded to the flat affect of the spy story, such as Elliot West's *The Night Is a Time for Listening* (10):

> A courier gets hit on the head—not by the opposition, but by some cheap crook who never saw him before and is just after his wallet. The goods you've waited for never get there and a whole mission is scratched. . . .
> "You want it to work, don't you? What could be better than if she's part of the cover? That's one they'll really never dream of."
> "To be an agent," Disa said to herself sadly.
> "On the other side this time," Darsos said, turning to her.
> "Bear that in mind."

The affect of new molecular biology is—like Norfolk—very flat. We have just learned that the hierarchy of genes is controlled by runs of DNA (called homeoboxes) which do not set us apart from fruit flies. All the signals of chromosomes seem to be able to work "on the other side this time." Every codon has an anticodon: Every strand of DNA can be read for sense in one direction and perhaps even greater sense in the other. We have been assured (by L. R. Smith et al.) (7) that:

> assuming each individual has a proteinaceous receptor for all ligands (both peptide and nonpeptide), then the complementarity of nucleic acids and the aforementioned pattern in the genetic code dictates the potential for an endogenous peptide recognition unit. These peptide recognition units in turn may be thought of as endogenous homologues of all ligands or antigens. Individuals, then, are a composite and reflection of all universal shapes represented in the ligand or antigen repertoire to which they respond.

In other words, we recognize the invader—call him antigen or Ishmael—and recognize him because we have his template in our genes, but "on the other side this time."

We are told that we have seen the enemy and he is coded, in language a fruit fly can understand, in our genetic strands. Structures of language, structures of nucleic acids—capable of transcription, translation, and betrayal. On either side, in any direction.

But stop! I'm not quite ready for that kind of diminished script just yet. No, I'm ready to cheer again for that last shot of Bogart and Raines walking off on their way to Brazzaville to join the free French. I want to hear the swelling music that plays at what could be the start of a beautiful friendship. I want to believe that all that redness and swelling with heat and pain is up to some good. Ingrid Bergman will be there, waiting to heal the wound. And still on the same side—our side this time.

REFERENCES

1. Bowle, J. (1974): *The Imperial Achievement,* p. 313, Little, Brown and Co., Boston.
2. Ford, F. M. (1961, original 1922): *Parade's End,* p. 193, Alfred Knopf, New York.
3. Gide, A. (1951): *Journals, Vol. IV, 1939–1949,* translated by J. O'Brien, pp. 159–206, Alfred Knopf, New York.
4. McFarland, J. (1941): In: *Cyclopedia of Medicine—Surgery and Specialties, Vol. VII,* edited by G. M. Persol and E. L. Bortz, p. 806, F. A. Davis and Co., Philadelphia.
5. Metchnikoff, E. (1968, original 1905): *Immunity in Infective Diseases,* p. 545, Johnson Reprint Corp., New York.
6. Metchnikoff, E. (1968, original 1905): *Immunity in Infective Diseases,* p. 548, Johnson Reprint Corp., New York.
7. Smith, L. R., Bost, K. L., and Blalock, J. E. (1987): Generation of idiotypic and anti-idiotypic antibodies by immunization with peptides encoded by complementary RNA: A possible molecular basis for the network theory. *J. Immunol.,* 138:7–9.
8. Thomas, H. (1961): *The Spanish Civil War,* p. 328, Harper & Row, New York.
9. Thomas, L. (1971): In: *Immunopathology of Inflammation,* edited by B. K. Forscher and J. C. Houck, p. 2, Excerpta Medica, Amsterdam.
10. West, E. (1967): *The Night Is a Time for Listening,* p. 241, Victor Gollanca, London.

Soluble Components of Inflammation

Inflammation: Basic Principles and Clinical Correlates.
Edited by J. I. Gallin, I. M. Goldstein, and R. Snyderman.
Raven Press, Ltd., New York © 1988.

CHAPTER 2

Immunoglobulins

Hans L. Spiegelberg

STRUCTURE OF IMMUNOGLOBULINS (ANTIBODIES)

Basic Structure of Antibodies

All antibodies or immunoglobulins (Ig) are composed of two types of polypeptide chains, called heavy and light chains, which are linked by disulfide bonds (Fig. 1) (18,23). The amino acid sequences at the NH-terminal end of the heavy and light chains vary from antibody to antibody to provide the diversity necessary to form antibodies of different specificities for different antigens (56,62). In contrast, the structures of the COOH-terminal portions of the heavy and light chains are constant except for minor genetically determined variations which do not appear to affect the function of antibodies. The polypeptide chains can be divided into segments of approximately 110 amino acids showing homology with each other, suggesting that they evolved by gene duplication (17). These segments are called domains. The light chains have one variable and one constant domain, whereas heavy chains have one variable and three or four constant domains.

Antibody Classes and Subclasses

Antibodies are divided into classes and subclasses on the basis of antigenic and amino acid sequence differences

in the constant region of the heavy chain (58). In humans, nine; and in rodents, eight different constant regions of the heavy chains are recognized. Antisera to five of these constant regions do not cross-react with each other, and the amino acid sequence of these five different constant regions of heavy chains show only approximately 30% homology with each other. Based on these observations, antibodies are divided into five classes called IgG, IgA, IgM, IgD, and IgE. IgG antibodies can be further subdivided into four subclasses and, in humans, IgA into two subclasses on the basis of minor antigenic and amino acid sequence differences in the constant region of the heavy chain. IgA subclasses are not found in mice and rats. In humans, the IgG subclasses are called IgG1, IgG2, IgG3, and IgG4 based on the order of their concentration in the serum, IgG1 having the highest concentration (70). Murine IgG subclasses are named IgG1, IgG2a, IgG2b, and IgG3, and rat IgG subclasses IgG1, IgG2a, IgG2b, and IgG2c (4). IgG, IgD, and IgE antibodies all have the basic four-chain structure. In contrast, IgA antibodies also form dimers having the basic structure (25,77). Human serum IgA is almost 100% monomeric IgA, whereas IgA found in secretions such as saliva, tears, etc., is dimeric and attached to a polypeptide called secretory component (76). In contrast to human serum IgA, rodent serum IgA consists of approximately 50% monomeric and dimeric IgA. The dimers are formed through COOH-terminal disulfide

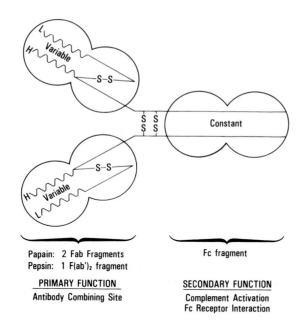

Papain: 2 Fab Fragments
Pepsin: 1 F(ab')₂ fragment

Fc fragment

PRIMARY FUNCTION

SECONDARY FUNCTION

Antibody Combining Site

Complement Activation
Fc Receptor Interaction

FIG. 1. Basic structure of Ig and localization of submolecular sites mediating the primary and secondary or (effector) functions of antibodies.

bonds of the heavy chains and involve a third polypeptide chain called J, for joining chain (27,43,53). All IgM antibodies consist of covalent pentamers having the basic four-chain structure that are linked by disulfide bonds and a J chain. The molecular weights of the antibodies of the five classes are approximately 150,000 for IgG, 160,000 for IgD, 180,000 for IgE, 160 and 320,000 for IgA monomers and dimers, and 900,000 for IgM. The heavy chains of IgG, IgD, and IgA antibodies have one variable and three constant domains, and those of IgM and IgE one variable and four constant domains. All heavy chains have carbohydrate side chains attached to them. IgG heavy chains (γ chains) have one carbohydrate chain, and the total carbohydrate of IgG is approximately 3% of the molecular weight. In contrast, the heavy chains of the other four classes have multiple carbohydrate side chains, the carbohydrate representing approximately 10% of the molecular weight. The function of the carbohydrate side chains of antibodies is unknown. The κ and λ chains have one variable and one constant domain. Heavy chains are combined with either two κ or two λ chains. It does not appear that the κ or λ constant domain is associated with a particular function of a class of antibodies.

Concentration of Antibodies in Body Fluids

The concentration of the different classes of Ig varies greatly. IgG has the highest concentration, followed in decreasing order by IgA > IgM ≫ IgD > IgE (70). In

secretions such as saliva, tears, bile, etc., IgA is the predominant class (76,77). In humans, the IgG subclasses are numbered according to relative concentration, IgG1 having the highest concentration and making up 65% of all IgG, followed by IgG2 (25%), IgG3 (7%), and IgG4 (3%). In other species, the numbering of the IgG subclasses is according to electrophoretic mobility in serum electrophoresis. IgG1 has anodal mobility, and IgG2 cathodal mobility. Whereas the serum concentrations of the two major IgG subclasses are relatively constant, there are wide variations in normal humans in the concentration of IgG3 and IgG4 (57,79). In sheep and goat, the two minor subclasses are not yet defined because of lack of monoclonal Ig; therefore, IgG is divided into only IgG1 and IgG2 based on electrophoretic mobility.

Fab, F(ab')₂, and Fc Fragments of Antibodies

IgG antibodies are fragmented by papain into three fragments, two Fab fragments consisting of a light chain and the NH-terminal domain of the heavy chain (Fd fragment), and one Fc fragment containing the COOH-terminal domains of the heavy chain (63). Digestion of IgG with pepsin destroys the Fc fragment and leaves a fragment consisting of two Fab fragments linked by the disulfide bonds between heavy chains, which is called the F(ab')₂ fragment (59). The biological activities of antibodies are divided into two categories, namely, primary and secondary functions (Fig. 1) (70). The primary function is localized to the Fab fragment and consists of specific binding to antigen. The secondary or effector functions are mediated by the constant portion of the heavy chain, particularly the Fc fragment. Because the structure of the Fc fragment is identical (except for minor genetically controlled amino acid substitutions) in antibodies of a given class, the secondary functions are shared by all antibodies of the same class. It has clearly been shown that the Fc fragment determines the biological half-life of an antibody class, whether the antibodies are secreted in saliva, tears, etc., or whether they activate the complement system and bind to and cross-link cell membrane receptors (Fc receptors, FcR) (70). By activating the complement system and cross-linking FcR on leukocytes to induce these cells to release mediators, antibodies can cause inflammation.

Heterogeneity of Fc Fragment Functions of Monoclonal Proteins

Because the effector functions of antibodies are mediated by the constant portion of the heavy chains, one would expect that they would be identical from molecule to molecule within a given class or subclass. However, when individual myeloma proteins were studied for effector functions, significant differences within a class or subclass were observed (70). The structural basis for this heterogeneity is unexplained. Since most effector functions are elicited only by aggregated Ig, it is possible that the variation reflects the ability of a monoclonal Ig to form aggregates, and this property could depend on the variable region. However, significant differences between myeloma proteins of the same class were also found when their half-lives (73) and the binding of monomeric proteins to FcR were studied (44,75). Therefore, there must be additional reasons for the heterogeneity among effector functions. Our efforts to correlate the differences with genetic variants or carbohydrate differences in the constant portion of the heavy chains did not show a correlation (73). In the future, studies on monoclonal antibodies will perhaps resolve the unexplained variation in effector functions of myeloma proteins of the same class. As will be described below for activation of the complement system, the variations in effector functions of myeloma proteins within a given class may explain discrepancies reported from different laboratories concerning the effector functions of a class or subclass of Ig.

The precise structures on the Fc fragment that mediate the effector functions are not well understood, and conflicting data regarding the submolecular sites have been reported. The main reason for this is that peptides, and even single domains, show only very low (<10%) activity compared to that of the intact Fc fragment (16,40). This makes it difficult to interpret the significance of the low residual activity of individual domains or enzymatically or synthetically produced peptides of the constant region of the heavy chain. The reason for the low activity of the Fc subfragments could be conformational changes in the active sites and/or the possibility that the functional sites involve more than one domain of the Fc fragment (3,71). The evidence available to date indicates that the site(s) responsible for activation of the complement system are located in the second domain of IgG (32,40) and that binding sites for FcR may be present in both domains. However, more work, such as blocking the effector site with monoclonal antibodies to defined surface structures on the Fc fragment, will be necessary to elucidate the configurations responsible for the effector functions. Also, there is one exception to the rule that all effector functions are mediated by the Fc fragment. This is the activation of the alternative complement pathway, which is mediated by site(s) located on the $F(ab')_2$ fragment (67).

Distribution of Antibodies in Different Ig Classes and Subclasses

IgM antibodies are produced first after immunization, followed by antibodies of the other classes. Complex pro-

tein antigens usually elicit antibodies of most classes. In contrast, carbohydrate antigens of the T-lymphocyte-independent variety elicit predominantly antibodies of one IgG subclass, human IgG2 (78), murine IgG3 (60), and rat IgG2c (15). Certain parasitic infections (37), as well as "allergens," induce a predominant IgE response. The mechanism determining the class of antibodies to a given antigen is not well understood and is most likely complex. It depends on the nature of the antigen and the mode of immunization (13). Recent evidence suggests that subtypes of helper T lymphocytes exist that produce different lymphokines which either affect the switch from IgM to another class or induce expansion of B cells that have switched from IgM to another class (45,75).

EFFECTOR FUNCTIONS OF IMMUNOGLOBULINS OF DIFFERENT CLASSES AND SUBCLASSES

Activation of Complement

Classical Pathway

The complement system can be activated by two mechanisms, called the classical and the alternative pathways, which are described in detail in Chapter 3. Activation of the classical pathway by different Ig classes has been studied systematically by Ishizaka et al. (34). These investigators aggregated human myeloma proteins chemically with bis-diazotized benzidine and measured the ability of the aggregates to consume hemolytic units of complement. As summarized in Table 1, human IgM, IgG1, and IgG3 were most capable of activating the classical pathway, IgG2 was quantitatively less active, and no activation was observed with aggregated IgG4, IgA, IgE, and IgD. Similar findings were made in other species, in that IgM and three of the four IgG subclasses were able to bind and activate the first complement component, which leads to activation of the classical pathway. In mice, IgG2a, IgG2b, and IgG3 (26), and in rats, IgG2a, IgG2b, and IgG2c (49), activate the classical pathway. The two quantitatively minor IgG subclasses are not characterized in many species because of lack of monoclonal antibodies or myeloma proteins. However, usually the IgG having cathodal mobility, IgG2, activates C1, whereas the IgG with anodal mobility, IgG1, does not. There is no clear-cut functional correlation between human and animal IgG subclasses. Presumably, human IgG1 and IgG3 correlate with rodent IgG2a and IgG2b, human IgG4 with rodent IgG1, and IgG2 with mouse IgG3 and rat IgG2c.

Although the initial findings of Ishizaka et al. (34) concerning activation of the classical complement pathway were confirmed by many investigators, exceptions to the rule have been reported. First, activation of complement

TABLE 1. *Activation of complement by Ig of different classes and subclasses*

	Activation of complement								
	Human Ig[a]								
Pathway	IgM	IgG1	IgG2	IgG3	IgG4	IgA1	IgA2	IgD	IgE
Classical	++	++	+	++	−	−	−	−	−
Alternative	−	−	−	−	−	++	++	+	+
	Mouse Ig								
	IgM	IgG1	IgG2a	IgG2b	IgG3	IgA	IgD	IgE	
Classical	++	−	+	+	+	−	−	−	
	Rat Ig								
	IgM	IgG1	IgG2a	IgG2b	IgG2c	IgA	IgD	IgE	
Classical	++	+	+	+	−	−	−	−	

[a] −, No activation; ++, a significantly smaller quantity of aggregated proteins is necessary to fix the same amount of complement as compared to that needed for + proteins.

through the classical pathway by certain IgA (31) and IgE (65) myeloma proteins has been reported. Also, it was shown that human IgG4 bound C1 weakly (68) and that the Fc fragment of IgG4, but not intact IgG4 myeloma proteins (32), activated the classical pathway. The reasons for these discrepant findings are unknown. Because the site interacting with C1 is located on the constant portion of the heavy chain, one would expect that all antibodies or myeloma proteins of the same class would activate complement similarly. However, this is not the case. First, aggregated myeloma proteins of the same class or subclass consume greatly different quantities of hemolytic units per microgram of aggregated Ig (34). Although this could be the result of differences in the ability of a myeloma protein to form chemical aggregates, it seems unlikely. Significant differences in the half-lives of monomeric human myeloma proteins of the same IgG subclass (71) and differences in binding to FcR (44,75) have also been observed. No correlation between variation in the half-life and genetic variants or between variations in the carbohydrate moiety and half-life could be demonstrated. It is conceivable that the variations in effector functions within a class of Ig are responsible for the discrepant reports of complement activation. Although the reason for the different behavior of aggregated myeloma proteins is unclear, it is important to know that exceptions to the rule with respect to effector functions of a given class of antibodies exist. Therefore, when a monoclonal antibody is used for a biological test, its effector function has to be examined because it cannot be predicted with certainty whether a monoclonal antibody of a given immunoglobin class will behave like the majority of that class.

Alternative Pathway

In 1971, Sandberg and co-workers (66,67) were the first to demonstrate that complement could be activated by a mechanism other than activation of C1. These authors showed that guinea pig IgG1 induced activation of C3 through C9 in the absence of consumption of C1, C4, and C2. Subsequently, it was shown that guinea pig IgG1 induced cleavage of C3 proactivator, now called factor B, of the alternative complement pathway. Because C3 activated through the classical pathway also induces cleavage of factor B (1), we studied conversion of the C3 proactivator (factor B) by aggregated myeloma proteins of different classes in C2-deficient sera (74). As shown in Table 1, we found that aggregated human myeloma proteins or their Fc fragments of classes IgA1 and IgA2, and to a lesser extent of classes IgE and IgD, cleaved factor B in C2-deficient sera. Using different experimental systems, other investigators also found that IgA (5,61), IgE (35), and IgD (42) could activate the alternative complement pathway. Evidence for activation of the alternative pathway by IgA *in vivo* has also been obtained. By immunofluorescence, IgA and factor B were detected in lesions of patients with dermatitis herpetiformis (38) and in kidney biopsies of patients with mesangial IgA nephropathy (46) in the absence of the early components of the classical pathway, C1, C4, and C2. As in activation of the classical pathway, exceptions involving the activation of the alternative pathway have been reported; e.g., Colten and Bienenstock (14) did not observe activation of the alternative pathway by IgA anti-blood group A antibodies. Guinea pig IgG F(ab')$_2$ fragments activate the alternative pathway

(64,67). The submolecular site(s) on IgA, IgE, and IgD responsible for activation of the alternative pathway are unknown. Because certain polysaccharides activate the alternative pathway, the carbohydrate moieties of IgA, IgE, and IgD may be responsible (8).

In summary, antigen–antibody complexes of almost all classes and subclasses of Ig activate the complement system in one way or another. This leads to the formation of peptides, such as the C3a and C5a fragments, that have potent anaphylactic and chemotactic properties. Therefore, antibodies of all classes play an important role in inducing inflammation through activation of the complement system.

Release of Mediators from Leukocytes by Cross-linking of FcR

All white blood cells and many other cells have receptors on their cell membrane that bind the Fc fragment of Ig (FcR). Although there are exceptions, FcR usually bind specifically one class of Ig. One cell type can have different FcR for different Ig classes. Although the affinity with which FcR bind Ig varies, they usually can be divided into high- and low-affinity FcR which function differently. High-affinity FcR for IgE, for example, are found only on mast cells and basophilic granulocytes (55); they bind monomeric IgE with a K_a of 10^9 M^{-1}. FcR for IgE on all other cell types and IgG and IgA FcR have relatively low affinity; they bind monomeric Ig with a K_a of 10^6–10^8 M^{-1}. In the case of high-affinity FcR, monomeric IgE binds to the mast cells and remains on the cell for long periods of time. Interaction of cell-bound IgE with antigen results in cross-linking of the FcR, which induces the release of mediators of inflammation from the mast cells and basophils. In contrast, monomeric IgE does not persist on low-affinity FcR for long periods of time (2) and presumably does not sensitize the cells for interaction with antigen analogous to IgE on mast cells. Most likely, low-affinity FcR interact functionally only with preformed immune aggregates. Because antigen–antibody complexes contain many antibodies, they offer multiple Fc fragment–FcR interactions, thus increasing the binding affinity of immune complexes to the FcR-bearing cells. Furthermore, they cause cross-linking of FcR, which activates the cells. The two major functions of low-affinity FcR are promotion of phagocytosis and, like that of high-affinity FcR for IgE on mast cells, induction of release of mediators of inflammation.

For many years it has been debated whether a configurational change in the Fc fragment resulting from antigen–antibody interaction is necessary to induce the FcR function. However, such configurational changes have never been convincingly demonstrated. Furthermore, because cross-linking of FcR on basophils with antireceptor antibodies induces mediator release in the absence of IgE, it is now generally believed that no signal by a configurationally changed Fc fragment is involved in the activation of FcR functions (55).

The presence of FcR on cells can be determined by measuring the binding of radiolabeled or fluoresceinated Ig, rosette formation, and functional assays. Rosette formation is often used to demonstrate FcR because the result is obtained in a short period of time. In this assay, erythrocytes are sensitized with antierythrocyte antibodies (47) or erythrocytes are coated with myeloma proteins (24). In both cases, the Ig-coated erythrocytes bind to the FcR on the white cells. A white cell surrounded by erythrocytes is called a rosette. Functional assays include phagocytosis of antibody-coated erythrocytes and measurement of mediators of inflammation in the supernatant of cells incubated with antigen–antibody complexes or chemically aggregated myeloma proteins. The FcR specific for the different Ig classes and subclasses demonstrated on white cells by these methods are summarized in Table 2.

Basophils and Mast Cells

The "classical" FcR is that for IgE on basophils and tissue mast cells. Of all known FcR, it has the highest affinity for its ligand. IgE binds to the FcR with a K_a of 10^9 to 10^{10} M^{-1}; in particular, it dissociates very slowly from the cells (55). Cross-linking of cell-bound IgE by antigen induces the release of histamine, leukotrienes, and other mediators of inflammation from the cells (33). Murine IgG1 and rat IgG2a cross-react with the IgE FcR (69). However, the binding of these IgG antibody subclasses is weak, and they dissociate rapidly from the FcR. Therefore, mast cells in the skin can be passively sensitized with IgG antibodies for histamine release for only 4 to 6 hr. In contrast, IgE bound to mast cells dissociates from the cells with a half-life of approximately 2 weeks. Whether antibodies of one of the human IgG subclasses also cross-react with IgE FcR on mast cells is controversial. It is possible that some IgG4 antibodies induce histamine release (19), but attempts to induce histamine release with IgG antibodies usually fail, or histamine release appears to be the result of IgE contamination of the IgG preparation, because a large portion of IgE elutes from DEAE-cellulose columns together with IgG.

Using IgG-sensitized erythrocytes, we could not demonstrate FcR for IgG on human basophils. In contrast, Ishizaka et al. (36) demonstrated that human basophils bound heat-aggregated human IgG; however, interaction of basophils with the aggregated IgG did not induce histamine release. Similarly, aggregated IgA or IgM did not induce histamine release from basophils. From these data

TABLE 2. *Presence of Fc receptors for different Ig classes on different human white blood cell types*[a]

White cell	IgM	IgG1	IgG2	IgG3	IgG4	IgA1	IgA2	IgD	IgE
Basophil	−	−?	−	−	−	−	−	−	+
Neutrophil	−	+	+	+	+	+	+	−	−
Eosinophil	−	+	?	?	?	?	?	?	+
Monocyte	−	+	+	+	+	+	+	−	+
Platelet	−	+	+	+	+	−	−	−	+

[a] −, Absent; +, present; ?, unknown.

it can be concluded that basophils and mast cells carry only one type of functionally important FcR, high-affinity FcR for IgE. Because IgE antibodies bind with high affinity to these FcR, only minute amounts of antibody are necessary to sensitize the mast cells. Therefore, even at the low serum concentrations of IgE, 20 to 200 ng/ml in normal humans and 400 to 10,000 ng/ml in allergic patients, sufficient IgE molecules are bound to the mast cells to fully sensitize the cells for histamine release. This system of mast cell sensitization is highly efficient and unique among the different FcR–cell interactions (54).

Neutrophils

FcR on neutrophils promote phagocytosis of antibody-coated particles and induce the release of lysosomal constituents (28). By studying both binding of radiolabeled myeloma proteins (44) and measurement of the release of the granule enzyme β-glucuronidase (28), it was demonstrated that neutrophils had FcR for IgG and IgA. As shown in Fig. 2, aggregated IgG and IgA of all subclasses induced β-glucuronidase release from neutrophils in a similar manner. In contrast, monomeric IgG1 and IgG3

bound better to neutrophils than IgG1 and IgG4 (44). No evidence for FcR specific for IgG or IgA subclasses was found on human neutrophils (44) by inhibition analyses. In contrast, rodents have two IgG receptors for IgG2a and IgG2b. Large, insoluble aggregates were most effective inducers of β-glucuronidase release from neutrophils when mixed with cells in suspension. Soluble, presumably small, aggregates of myeloma proteins, induced either no or only a small β-glucuronidase release. However, when the soluble aggregates were adhered to Millipore membranes and the neutrophils added to the membranes, they were as active as the insoluble aggregates (28). These experiments suggest that particular antigens coated with antibodies or soluble immune complexes adherent to membranes such as glomerular basement membranes, synovial membranes, and blood vessel walls might be especially potent in activating neutrophils to release mediators of inflammation.

Eosinophils

Interaction of eosinophils with Ig of different classes and subclasses has, to our knowledge, not been studied systematically. However, IgG and recently IgE (11,72) have been shown to bind to eosinophils and to induce release of mediators of inflammation (12). IgE FcR differ structurally from those on mast cells. They bind IgE with a low affinity similar to the binding of IgG to IgG FcR. The number of FcR for IgG and IgE per cell appears to vary depending on the stage of differentiation of the cells and whether blood or tissue eosinophils are examined. Activated blood eosinophils, which have a low density, and tissue eosinophils express more IgE and fewer IgG receptors than the majority of "normodense" blood eosinophils (11). The function of IgE FcR is release of mediators of inflammation that are presumably important in allergic reactions and killing of IgE-inducing parasites such as schistosomes. Whether the IgE and/or IgG FcR induce formation of leukotriene C4 and contribute by this pathway to bronchoconstriction and asthma is unknown. Because eosinophils have FcR for IgG, IgG antibodies presumably induce the release of mediators from

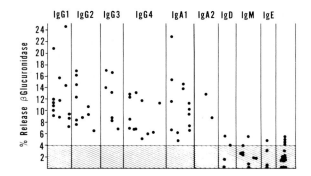

NEUTROPHILS IN SUSPENSION

FIG. 2. Release of β-glucuronidase from human neutrophils stimulated with aggregated myeloma proteins of different classes and subclasses. Each dot represents an experiment with neutrophils of an individual cell donor, and each column of dots, aggregates of the same myeloma protein. The shaded area represents nonspecific release.

eosinophils, thus contributing to the induction of inflammatory processes.

Monocytes and Macrophages

Almost all blood monocytes and alveolar and peritoneal macrophages express FcR for IgG (7,47,72). Smaller fractions of monocytes or macrophages also bind IgA (20) and IgE (10,50,51), whereas binding of IgM and IgD usually cannot be demonstrated. The percent of macrophages expressing FcR for IgA and IgE determined by rosette formation varies depending on the differentiation of the macrophages and on the anatomical location (7,48). The fraction of cells expressing FcR for IgE also depends on the activity of the IgE system. Patients with severe allergic disease and high IgE serum levels have a higher percentage of IgE FcR-positive monocytes (52). Macrophages of rats infected with parasites also express more IgE FcR per cell (6). The number of IgA receptors per cell may also depend on anatomical location and environmental factors, because large variations in IgA FcR-positive cells are observed (20,48). The function of the FcR on macrophages is promotion of phagocytosis and induction of release of granule enzymes (21,39). Furthermore, FcR activate the arachidonic acid cascade. As shown in Table 3, when chemically aggregated human myeloma proteins were mixed with blood monocytes, they induced formation of leukotrienes C_4 and B_4 and prostaglandin E_2 (22). The order of activity of the three Ig classes was IgG > IgA > IgE, which correlated with the percentage of cells that formed rosettes with IgG, IgA-, and IgE-coated erythrocytes.

Platelets

Binding of Ig to platelets has been studied using binding of radioiodinated Ig (9) and activation of platelets with

PLATELETS

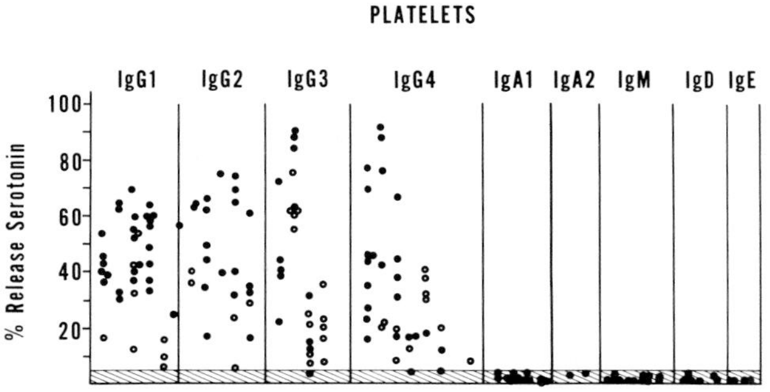

FIG. 3. Release of ^{3}H-labeled serotonin from human platelets stimulated with aggregated myeloma proteins of different classes and subclasses. Each dot represents an experiment with platelets of an individual donor, and each column of dots, aggregates of the same myeloma protein. The shaded area represents nonspecific release.

aggregated Ig to release serotonin (29) and produce chemiluminescence (9). It has been shown that IgG binds to most platelets and that aggregated IgG of all human subclasses induces the release of serotonin (Fig. 3). Aggregated Ig of the other classes did not release serotonin. In contrast, aggregated IgE induced chemiluminescence of platelets, and labeled monomeric IgE bound to a subpopulation of platelets (9). It is not clear at this time why aggregated IgE induces platelets to produce chemiluminescence but not to release serotonin. Whether IgG and/or IgE induces arachidonic acid metabolism, particularly thromboxane formation by platelets, has not been investigated.

Killer and Natural Killer Cells

Most lymphocytes bearing FcR are large, granular lymphocytes (75) that kill antibody-coated target cells (killer cells) (75) or allogeneic cells (natural killer cells) (41). FcR for IgG are typical for killer lymphocytes, and they have been shown to induce lysis of IgG-coated target cells. Although killing of IgM-coated target cells has also been reported, the presence of IgM FcR on natural killer cells remains controversial because IgM-induced killing cannot easily be reproduced in all laboratories. The role of IgG FcR on natural killer cells is unclear but does not appear to be important in the killing by the cells because IgG antibodies are not needed for that process (30).

CONCLUSIONS

Ig play an important role both in initiating and perpetuating inflammatory reactions. The main pathways for fulfilling this function involve activation of the complement system and activation of leukocytes by antigen–antibody complexes. Depending on the class of antibodies,

TABLE 3. *Release of leukotrienes B_4, C_4, and prostaglandin E_2 from normal human monocytes stimulated with aggregated human myeloma proteins of different classes[a]*

Stimulus	Nanograms per 10^6 cells		
	LTB_4	LTC_4	PGE_2
None	<0.01	<0.02	<0.2
IgG1	1.9 ± 0.8	1.4 ± 0.8	0.4 ± 0.4
IgA1	1.5 ± 0.1	1.0 ± 0.4	0.3 ± 0.3
IgE	0.4 ± 0.3	0.6 ± 0.4	0.4 ± 0.2
IgM	<0.01	<0.02	<0.2

[a] Monocytes (2×10^6) were incubated in a final volume of 0.2 ml with 250 μg aggregated immunoglobulins per milliliter for 30 min at 37°C before extraction of the arachidonic acid metabolites released into the supernatant. The values represent the mean $\pm$ SD of five experiments.

complement is activated either by the classical or the alternative pathway. Granulocytes and mononuclear phagocytes express receptors that react specifically with the Fc fragment of antibodies. Antigen–antibody complexes cross-link these FcR, which induces the cells to release mediators of inflammation such as histamine from basophils and mast cells and lysosomal enzymes from neutrophils and macrophages. In addition, cross-linking of FcR induces the metabolism of arachidonic acid. Depending on the cell type, different leukotrienes and prostaglandins are formed and released into the cells' environment after interaction with immune complexes. Because at least one, but usually more than one, class of antibodies can activate a specific type of leukocyte, antibodies are very important participants in inflammatory reactions involved in the host's defense mechanisms.

ACKNOWLEDGMENTS

This is publication no. 4550 IMM from the Research Institute of Scripps Clinic, La Jolla, California. This work was supported by NIH grants AI-10734 and AI-10386.

REFERENCES

1. Abramson, N., Alper, C. A., Lachmann, P. J., Rosen, F. S., and Jandl, J. H. (1971): Deficiency of C3 inactivator in man. *J. Immunol.,* 107:19.
2. Anderson, C. L., and Spiegelberg, H. L. (1981): Macrophage receptors for IgE: Binding of IgE to specific IgE Fc receptors on a human macrophage cell line, U937. *J. Immunol.,* 126:2470.
3. Barnett-Foster, D. E., Dorrington, K. J., and Painter, R. H. (1980): Structure and function of immunoglobulin domains. VIII. An analysis of the structural requirements in human IgG1 for binding to the Fc receptor of human monocytes. *J. Immunol.,* 124:2186.
4. Bazin, H., Beckers, A., and Querinjean, P. (1974): Three classes and four subclasses of rat immunoglobulins: IgM, IgA, IgE and IgG1, IgG2a, IgG2b, IgG2c. *Eur. J. Immunol.,* 4:44.
5. Boackle, R. J., Pruitt, K. M., and Mestecky, J. (1974): The interaction of human complement with interfacially aggregated preparations of human secretory IgA. *Immunochemistry,* 11:543.
6. Boltz, G., Plummer, J. M., and Spiegelberg, H. L. (1984): Increased expression of the IgE Fc receptors on rat macrophages induced by elevated serum IgE levels. *Immunology,* 53:9.
7. Boltz-Nitulescu, G., Bazin, H., and Spiegelberg, H. L. (1981): The specificity of Fc receptors for IgG2a, IgG1/IgG2b, and IgE on rat macrophages. *J. Exp. Med.,* 154:374.
8. Capel, P. J. A., Groeneboer, O., Grosvald, G., and Pondman, K. W. (1978): The binding of activated C3 to polysaccharides and immunoglobulins. *J. Immunol.,* 121:2566.
9. Capron, A., Ameisen, J. C., Joseph, M., Auriault, C., Tonnel, A. B., and Caen, J. (1985): New functions for platelets and their pathological implications. *Int. Arch. Allergy Appl. Immunol.,* 77:107.
10. Capron, A., Dessaint, J.-P., Joseph, M., Rousseaux, R., Capron, M., and Bazin, H. (1977): Interaction between IgE complexes and macrophages in the rat: A new mechanism of macrophage activation. *Eur. J. Immunol.,* 315:7.
11. Capron, M., Kusnierz, J. P., Prin, L., Spiegelberg, H. L., Gosset, P., Tonnel, A. B., and Capron, A. (1984): Cytophilic IgE on human blood and tissue eosinophils: Detection by flow microfluorometry and relation to serum IgE. *J. Immunol.,* 134:3013.
12. Capron, M., Kusnierz, J. P., Prin, L., Spiegelberg, H. L., Khalife,
13. Cebra, J. J., Komisar, J. L., and Schweitzer, P. A. (1984): CH isotype "switching" during normal B-lymphocyte development. *Annu. Rev. Immunol.,* 2:493.
14. Colten, H. R., and Bienenstock, J. (1976): Lack of C3 activation through classical and alternate pathways by human secretory IgA anti-blood group A antibody. *Adv. Exp. Med. Biol.,* 45:305–308.
15. Der Balian, G. P., Slack, J., Clevinger, B. L., Bazin, H., and Davie, J. M. (1980): Subclass restriction of murine antibodies. III. Antigens that stimulate IgG3 in mice stimulate IgG2c in rats. *J. Exp. Med.,* 152:209.
16. Dorrington, K. J., and Painter, R. H. (1977): Biological activities of the constant region. In: *Progress in Immunology III,* p. 288, North-Holland, New York.
17. Edelman, G. M., Cunningham, B. A., Gall, W. E., Gottlieb, P. B., Rutishauser, H., and Waxdal, M. J. (1969): The covalent structure of an entire γG immunoglobulin molecule. *Proc. Natl. Acad. Sci. USA,* 63:78.
18. Edelman, G. M., and Poulik. (1961): Studies on structural units of γ-globulin. *J. Exp. Med.,* 113:861.
19. Fagan, D. L., Slaughter, C. A., Capra, J. D., and Sullivan, T. J. (1982): Monoclonal antibodies to immunoglobulin G4 induce histamine release from human basophils in vitro. *J. Allergy Clin. Immunol.,* 70:399.
20. Fanger, M. W., Shen, L., Pugh, J., and Bernier, G. M. (1980): Subpopulations of human peripheral granulocytes and monocytes express receptors for IgA. *Proc. Natl. Acad. Sci. USA,* 77:3640.
21. Ferreri, N. R., Beck, L., and Spiegelberg, H. L. (1986): β-Glucuronidase release from human monocytes induced with aggregated immunoglobulins of different classes. *Cell. Immunol.,* 98:57.
22. Ferreri, N. R., Howland, W. C., and Spiegelberg, H. L. (1986): Release of leukotrienes C4 and B4 and prostaglandin E2 from human monocytes stimulated with aggregated IgG, IgA and IgE. *J. Immunol.,* 136:4188.
23. Fleischman, J. B., Porter, R. R., and Press, E. M. (1963): The arrangement of peptide chains in gamma globulin. *Biochem. J.,* 88:220.
24. Gonzalez-Molina, A., and Spiegelberg, H. L. (1977): A subpopulation of normal human peripheral B lymphocytes that bind IgE. *J. Clin. Invest.,* 59:616.
25. Grey, H. M., Abel, C. A., and Yount, W. M. (1968): A subclass of human A-globulins (A2) which lacks the disulfide bonds linking heavy and light chains. *J. Exp. Med.,* 128:1223.
26. Grey, H. M., Hirst, J. W., and Cohn, M. (1971): A new mouse immunoglobulin: IgG3. *J. Exp. Med.,* 133:289.
27. Halpern, M. S., and Koshland, M. E. (1970): Novel subunit in secretory IgA. *Nature,* 228:1276.
28. Henson, P. M., Johnson, H. B., and Spiegelberg, H. L. (1972): Release of granule enzymes from human neutrophils stimulated by aggregated immunoglobulins of different classes and subclasses. *J. Immunol.,* 109:1182.
29. Henson, P. M., and Spiegelberg, H. L. (1973): Release of serotonin from human platelets induced by aggregated immunoglobulins of different classes and subclasses. *J. Clin. Invest.,* 52:1282.
30. Herberman, R. B., Reynolds, C. W., and Ortaldo, J. (1986): Mechanisms of cytotoxicity by natural killer (NK) cells. *Annu. Rev. Immunol.,* 4:651.
31. Iida, K., Fujita, T., Imai, S., Sasaki, M., Kato, T., and Kobayashi, K. (1976): Complement fixing abilities of IgA myeloma proteins and their fragments. The activation of complement through the classical pathway. *Immunochemistry,* 13:747.
32. Isenman, D. E., Ellerson, J. R., Painter, R. H., and Dorrington, K. J. (1977): Correlation between the exposure and aromatic chronophores at the surface of the Fc domains of immunoglobulin G and their ability to bind complement. *Biochemistry,* 16:233.
33. Ishizaka, T., and Ishizaka, K. (1975): Biology of immunoglobulin E: Molecular basis of reaginic hypersensitivity. *Prog. Allergy,* 19:60.
34. Ishizaka, T., Ishizaka, K., Salmon, S., and Fudenberg, H. (1967): Biologic activities of aggregated γ-globulin. VIII. Aggregated immunoglobulins of different classes. *J. Immunol.,* 99:82.

J., Tonnel, A. B., and Capron, A. (1985): Cytophilic IgE on human blood and tissue eosinophils. *Int. Arch. Allergy Appl. Immunol.,* 77:246.

35. Ishizaka, T., Siau, C. M., and Ishizaka, K. (1972): Complement fixation by aggregated IgE through alternate pathway. *J. Immunol.*, 108:848.

36. Ishizaka, T., Sterk, A. R., and Ishizaka, K. (1979): Demonstration of Fc γ receptors on human basophil granulocytes. *J. Immunol.*, 123:578.

37. Jarrett, E. E. E. (1978): Stimuli for the production and control of IgE in rats. *Immunol. Rev.*, 41:52.

38. Katz, S. S., and Strober, W. (1978): The pathogenesis of dermatitis herpetiformis. *J. Invest. Dermatol.*, 70:63.

39. Keeling, P. J., and Henson, P. M. (1982): Lysosomal enzyme release from human monocytes in response to particulate stimuli. *J. Immunol.*, 128:563.

40. Kehoe, J. M., and Fougereau, M. (1969): Immunoglobulin peptide with complement fixing activity. *Nature*, 224:1212.

41. Kishimoto, T. (1985): Factors affecting B-cell growth and differentiation. *Annu. Rev. Immunol.*, 3:133.

42. Konno, T., Hirai, H., and Inai, S. (1975): Studies in IgD. I. Complement fixing activities of IgD myeloma proteins. *Immunochemistry*, 12:773.

43. Koshland, M. E. (1985): The coming of age of the immunoglobulin J chain. *Annu. Rev. Immunol.*, 3:425.

44. Lawrence, D. A., Weigle, W. O., and Spiegelberg, H. L. (1975): Immunoglobulins cytophilic for human lymphcoytes, monocytes and neutrophils. *J. Clin. Invest.*, 55:368.

45. Layton, J. E., Vitetta, E. S., Uhr, J. W., and Krammer, P. H. (1984): Clonal analysis of B cells induced to secrete IgG by T cell-derived lymphokine(s). *J. Exp. Med.*, 160:1850.

46. Lewis, E. H., and Lowenthal, D. J. (1977): IgA nephropathy. In: *Kidney Biopsy Interpretation*, pp. 114–124, F. A. Davis and Co., Philadelphia.

47. LoBuglio, A. F., Cotran, R. S., and Jandl, J. H. (1967): Red cells coated with immunoglobulin G: Binding sphering by mononuclear cells in man. *Science*, 158:1582.

48. Maliszewski, C. R., Shen, L., and Fanger, M. W. (1985): The expression of receptors for IgA on human monocytes and calcitriol-treated HL-60 cells. *J. Immunol.*, 135:3878.

49. Medgyesi, G. A., Fust, G., Gergely, J., and Bazin, H. (1978): Classes and subclasses of rat immunoglobulins: Interaction with the complement system and with staphylococcal protein A. *Immunochemistry*, 15:125.

50. Melewicz, F. M., Kline, L. E., Cohen, A., and Spiegelberg, H. L. (1982): Characterization of Fc receptors for IgE on human alveolar macrophages. *Clin. Exp. Immunol.*, 49:364.

51. Melewicz, F. M., and Spiegelberg, H. L. (1980): Fc receptors for IgE on a subpopulation of human peripheral blood monocytes. *J. Immunol.*, 125:1026.

52. Melewicz, F. M., Zeiger, R. S., Mellon, M. H., O'Connor, R. D., and Spiegelberg, H. L. (1981): Increased peripheral blood monocytes with Fc receptors for IgE in patients with severe allergic disorders. *J. Immunol.*, 126:1592.

53. Mestecky, J., Zikan, J., and Butler, W. T. (1971): Immunoglobulin M and secretory immunoglobulin A: Presence of a common polypeptide chain different from light chains. *Science*, 171:1163.

54. Metzger, H. (1978): The IgE-mast cell system as a paradigm for the study of antibody mechanisms. *Immunol. Rev.*, 41:186.

55. Metzger, H., Alcaraz, G., Hohman, R., Kinet, J.-P., Pribluda, V., and Quarto, R. (1986): The receptor with high affinity for immunoglobulin E. *Annu. Rev. Immunol.*, 4:389.

56. Metzger, H., and Davies, D. R. (1983): Structural basis of antibody function. *Annu. Rev. Immunol.*, 1:87.

57. Morrell, A., Skvaril, F., and Barandum, S. (1976): Serum concentrations of IgG subclasses. *Clin. Immunobiol.*, 3:37.

58. Natvig, J. B., and Kunkel, H. G. (1973): Human immunoglobulins: Classes, subclasses, genetic variants and idiotypes. *Adv. Immunol.*, 16:1.

59. Nisonoff, A., Wissler, F. C., Lipman, L. N., and Woernly, D. L. (1960): Separation of univalent fragments from bivalent rabbit antibody by reduction of disulfide bonds. *Arch. Biochem. Biophys.*, 89:230.

60. Perlmutter, R. M., Hansburg, D., Briles, D. E., Nicolotti, R. A., and Davie, J. M. (1978): Subclass restriction of murine anti-carbohydrate antibodies. *J. Immunol.*, 121:566.

61. Pfaffenbach, G., Lamm, M. E., and Gigli, I. (1982): Activation of guinea pig alternative complement pathway by mouse IgA immune complexes. *J. Exp. Med.*, 155:231.

62. Porter, R. R. (1972): The antigen-binding sites of immunoglobulins. *Contemp. Top. Immunochem.*, 1:145.

63. Porter, R. R. (1959): The hydrolysis of rabbit gamma globulin and antibodies with crystalline papain. *Biochem. J.*, 73:119.

64. Ratnoff, W. D., Fearon, D. R., and Austen, K. F. (1983): The role of antibody in the activation of the alternative complement pathway. *Springer Semin. Immunopathol.*, 6:361–371.

65. Saint-Remy, J.-M. R. (1984): Mechanism of activation of the classical pathway of complement by monoclonal IgE (DES). Restricted regulation of C4b by C4b-binding protein. *Eur. J. Immunol.*, 14:254–259.

66. Sandberg, A. L., Götze, O., Müller-Eberhard, H. J., and Osler, A. G. (1971): Complement utilization by guinea pig gamma-1 and gamma-2 immunoglobulins through the C3 activator system. *J. Immunol.*, 107:920.

67. Sandberg, A. L., Oliveira, B., and Osler, A. G. (1971): Two complement interaction sites in guinea pig immunoglobulins. *J. Immunol.*, 106:282.

68. Schumaker, V. N., Calcott, M. A., Spiegelberg, H. L., and Müller-Eberhard, H. J. (1976): Ultracentrifuge studies of the binding of IgG of different subclasses to the C1q subunit of the first component of complement. *Biochemistry*, 15:5175.

69. Segal, D. M., Sharrow, S. O., Jones, J. F., and Siraganian, R. P. (1981): Fc (IgG) receptors on rat basophilic leukemia cells. *J. Immunol.*, 126:138.

70. Spiegelberg, H. L. (1974): Biological activities of immunoglobulins of different classes and subclasses. *Adv. Immunol.*, 19:259.

71. Spiegelberg, H. L. (1975): Human myeloma IgG half-molecules. Catabolism and biological properties. *J. Clin. Invest.*, 56:588.

72. Spiegelberg, H. L. (1984): Structure and function of Fc receptors for IgE on lymphocytes, monocytes and macrophages. *Adv. Immunol.*, 35:61.

73. Spiegelberg, H. L., Fishkin, B. G., and Grey, H. M. (1968): The catabolism of human γG immunoglobulins of different subclasses. I. The catabolism of γG myeloma proteins in man. *J. Clin. Invest.*, 47:2327.

74. Spiegelberg, H. L., and Götze, O. (1972): Conversion of C3 proactivator and activation of the alternate pathway of complement activation by different classes and subclasses of human immunoglobulins. *Fed. Proc.*, 31:655.

75. Spiegelberg, H. L., Perlmann, H., and Perlmann, P. (1976): Interaction of K lymphocytes with myeloma proteins of different IgG subclasses. *J. Immunol.*, 117:1464.

76. Tomasi, T. (1972): Secretory immunoglobulins. *N. Engl. J. Med.*, 287:500.

77. Underdown, B. J., and Schiff, J. M. (1986): Immunoglobulin A: Strategic defense initiative at the mucosal surface. *Annu. Rev. Immunol.*, 4:389.

78. Yount, W. J., Dorner, M. M., Kunkel, H. G., and Kabat, E. A. (1968): Studies on human antibodies. VI. Selective variations in subgroup composition and genetic markers. *J. Exp. Med.*, 127:633.

79. Yount, W. J., Hong, R., Seligman, M., Good, R. A., and Kunkel, H. G. (1970): Imbalances of gamma globulin subgroups and gene defects in patients with primary hypogammaglobulinemia. *J. Clin. Invest.*, 49:1957, 1970.

Inflammation: Basic Principles and Clinical Correlates.
Edited by J. I. Gallin, I. M. Goldstein, and R. Snyderman.
Raven Press, Ltd., New York © 1988.

CHAPTER 3

Complement: Chemistry and Pathways

Hans J. Müller-Eberhard

Complement constitutes an integral component of host defense against infections and of the inflammatory process. The activities in both processes derive from proteolytic fragments of inert precursor proteins and from the fusion of multiple-protein molecules into supramolecular organizations. Complement is composed of 20 plasma proteins. In addition, there are multiple distinct cell surface receptors that exhibit ligand specificity for complement reaction products and occur on inflammatory cells and cells of the immune system. Also, there are several regulatory membrane proteins that protect host cells from accidental complement attack. The role of complement in host defense was established through genetic deficiencies that manifest life-threatening recurrent infections. Its role in inflammation and tissue injury became apparent through clinical investigations and the finding that the pathogenesis of certain experimental disease models is complement dependent.

The system is organized into two activation pathways and the common pathway of membrane attack (Fig. 1). The classical activation pathway is initiated by the binding of C1 to antigen-antibody complexes. C1 consists of two reversibly interacting subunits, C1q and C1r$_2$s$_2$. The complex tends to undergo spontaneous activation by an intramolecular autocatalytic mechanism that is controlled by the C1 inhibitor (C1-In). On binding to immune complexes through C1q, the subunits of C1 become firmly associated, and autoactivation commences even in the presence of C1-In. The initial enzyme of the pathway constitutes conformationally activated pro-C1r$_2$, which acts upon itself. Cleaved C1r$_2$ then activates C1s$_2$, which catalyzes the assembly of the C3 convertase, C4b,2a, from C2 and C4. The enzyme is either formed in the fluid phase or becomes covalently attached to the surface of a target particle. The catalytic site is located in the C2a subunit. Control at this stage is exerted by the C4-binding protein (C4bp) and factor I (I) in plasma and by the cell-surface proteins C3b receptor (CR1) and decay-accelerating factor (DAF). The target-bound C3 convertase becomes the C5 convertase, C4b,2a,3b, on activation of C3 and binding of C3b, which modulates C5 for cleavage by C4b,2a.

The alternative pathway is initiated spontaneously by

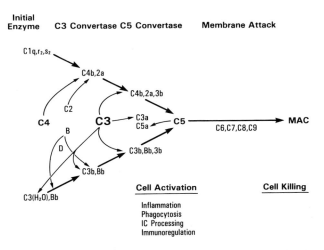

Initial
Enzyme   C3 Convertase C5 Convertase   Membrane Attack

FIG. 1. Schematic representation of the molecular organization of the complement pathways. The upper left segment of the scheme represents the classical pathway; the lower left segment represents the alternative pathway. C3 occupies a central position in both pathways. Regulatory proteins have been omitted.

the reaction of native C3 with a molecule of water, i.e., by hydrolysis of its internal thioester. C3 so modified ($C3(H_2O)$) becomes a subunit of the initial C3 convertase, $C3(H_2O)$,Bb, when it binds factor B (B) for activation by factor D (D). The initial enzyme of the alternative pathway is D, which is always present in plasma in active and uninhibited form but which cannot act on its substrate, B, unless it is bound to $C3(H_2O)$ or C3b. $C3(H_2O)$,Bb is a fluid-phase enzyme, and its active site resides in subunit Bb. In acting on native C3, the enzyme produces metastable C3b, which can covalently attach to the surface of nearby biological particles. D then catalyzes the formation of the particle-bound C3 convertase, C3b,Bb, by cleaving and activating B. The enzyme is under positive regulation by properdin and negative regulation by factor H (H), I, CR1, and DAF. With the addition of a molecule of C3b the enzyme becomes capable of acting on C5. Although polysaccharides are thought to be critical in the activation of the alternative pathway, antibodies may play an important part in this process.

Both pathways eventuate in cleavage and activation of C5 and, thus, in assembly of the membrane-attack complex (MAC). Through its metastable membrane-binding site, the MAC binds firmly to target membranes owing to hydrophobic interaction with the lipid bilayer. The final events are unfolding, namely oligomerization or polymerization of C9, which cause weakening of membrane structure and formation of transmembrane channels. MAC assembly is regulated by the S-protein of plasma and by the homologous restriction factor (HRF) of host cell membranes.

C3 is pivotal in the organization and function of the complement system (Fig. 1). It is the precursor of a number of biologically active fragments that function by binding to cell-surface complement receptors or by associating with other complement proteins. The molecule harbors at least 10 distinct binding sites, namely those for CR1, CR2 (C3dg receptor), CR3 (C3bi receptor), C3a receptor, B, properdin (P), H, C5, conglutinin, and for covalent attachment to membranes or other surfaces.

Cell-surface complement receptors have assumed increasing importance, particularly those with specificity for fragments of C3. The structure of CR1 and CR2 is being elucidated. CR2 has been identified with the Epstein-Barr virus receptor on B lymphocytes, and CR3 has been shown to belong structurally to the LFA-1 family of leukocyte surface antigens. By and large, C3 receptors aid in the removal of potentially harmful substances, including immune complexes from the tissues or the circulation.

The anaphylatoxins C3a, C4a, and C5a are derived from C3, C4, and C5. C5a, in particular, is a highly potent mediator of inflammation. These peptides are hormone-like messenger molecules inasmuch as they bind to specific cell-surface receptors with high affinity. Cells endowed with such receptors and capable of responding to the stimuli imparted by the anaphylatoxins include: polymorphs, monocytes, macrophages, mast cells, and smooth muscle cells. The cellular responses to the anaphylatoxins include: release of histamine, serotonin, hydrolytic enzymes, platelet-activating factor, interleukin 1 (IL-1), arachidonic acid metabolites, and active oxygen species; chemotactic migration; cell adhesion; smooth muscle contraction; and enhanced expression of CR1. C3a and C5a may also function as regulators of the immune response, with C3a suppressing the antibody response *in vitro* and C5a enhancing it. For these lymphocyte effects, macrophages are required.

The large number of seemingly different proteins comprising this complex biological system may be bewildering for the uninitiated. Recent genetic and structural analyses have uncovered the existence of remarkable relationships among these proteins. Both C3 convertases are genetically linked to the major histocompatibility complex (MHC), with C2, B, and C4 being products of the class III MHC genes. C2 and B are genetically linked and homologous in structure. C3, C4, and C5 exhibit extensive structural homology and are considered evolutionary relatives. C1r and C1s have a very similar primary structure. And whereas a close genetic linkage has been established for H, C4bp, and CR1, it has now become apparent that structural homologies are shared by all C3b/C4b-binding proteins. Thus, similar repeating homology regions of about 60 amino acids have been found in H, C4bp, DAF, CR1, CR2, C2, and B. C1r and C1s also possess two such regions. Furthermore, four proteins of the MAC, namely

C6, C7, C8, and C9, cross-react immunochemically, and a definite structural relationship has been established to date between C8α, C8β, and C9. HRF, the membrane-bound inhibitor of MAC channel formation, also belongs to this group of proteins.

Another important member of the latter group is the C9-related protein (C9RP), which is the cytolytic protein of cytotoxic lymphocytes. Electron microscopic studies had revealed that killer lymphocytes insert MAC-like structures into their target membranes. The precursor protein of these cyclic structures has been isolated and shown to share antigenic properties with C9 and other MAC precursor proteins. Thus, this intricate system involves interrelated proteins of plasma, lymphocytes, and cell membranes.

THE ALTERNATIVE PATHWAY

Overview

The alternative pathway constitutes a humoral component of natural defense against infections which can operate without antibody participation. By themselves, the six proteins C3, B, D, H, I, and P perform the functions of initiation, recognition, and activation of the pathway, resulting in formation of the activator-bound C3/C5 convertase (168,186).

Activators are certain particulate polysaccharides, fungi, bacteria, and viruses but are also certain mammalian cells and aggregates of immunoglobulins (118). It is not known which structures activators have in common that are recognized by the pathway. But it is clear that recognition involves C3b (193,239). The microenvironment of particle-bound C3b determines whether C3b prefers binding of B, which causes activation of the pathway, or of H, which abrogates progression of the reaction (52,53,183). Since C3b becomes covalently bound to receptive surfaces, interaction between the putative recognition site in C3b and the recognized structure in its immediate environment may be quite weak. This strategy would allow a wide spectrum of different, but related, substances to be recognized by C3b. Obviously the degree of specificity of the pathway is low, but it is by no means nonspecific. For example, rabbit erythrocytes are strong activators of the human alternative pathway, but they do not activate the alternative pathway of the rabbit, although the rabbit, like the human pathway, recognizes zymosan and similar particulate polysaccharides (85).

Some unusual, in fact novel, biochemical properties of proteins and enzymes have come to light during the course of the molecular exploration of the pathway. For example, C3 was shown to contain a thioester (265), the spontaneous slow hydrolysis of which converts inactive native C3 to a functionally C3b-like molecule (190). This form of C3, referred to as C3(H$_2$O), constitutes a subunit of the initial C3 convertase, and its continuous production is the chemical basis of what has been called phenomenologically the "tick-over" (177). The thioester bond also came to be recognized as the chemical basis of another unique property, the metastable membrane-binding site of C3 (169). Still another example is that C3b, the product of the reaction catalyzed by the C3 convertase, forms a subunit of the enzyme itself. This circumstance, obviously, is the cause of the positive feedback (164), which is the driving force of amplification of the pathway, a property the classical pathway lacks. Other unusual features will be pointed out during the description of the reaction mechanism.

That the six proteins are indeed sufficient to generate all known biological activities ascribed to the pathway was shown with the mixture of the six isolated proteins: It behaved qualitatively and quantitatively like the alternative pathway in whole human serum. Incubation of rabbit erythrocytes or zymosan with this mixture in the presence of Mg^{2+} resulted in efficient deposition of functionally active C3b on the surface of these particles (239). This did not occur with human erythrocytes, which are not activators. Also, immune precipitates were readily solubilized upon incubation with the isolated protein mixture (64). Addition of the five precursor proteins of the MAC to the six proteins reconstituted the cytolytic and bactericidal alternative pathway, as evidenced by lysis of rabbit erythrocytes (236) and killing of Raji cells (240) or gram-negative bacteria (238).

At an earlier stage of understanding of the alternative pathway, this pathway was called the *properdin system* (197), in part because P was historically the first of the six proteins recognized and thought to be of paramount importance for natural resistance to infections. Today, C3 is seen as the preeminent protein because it is involved in each of the reaction steps of the pathway (Fig. 1).

The Proteins

C3

Human C3 (167) is a 190-kilodalton (kDa) protein that is composed of two chains, the ~110-kDa α chain and the ~75-kDa β chain. The normal serum concentration ranges between 1,000 and 1,600 μg/ml. The complete primary structure for human (39) and murine C3 (136,287) has been derived from complementary DNA (cDNA) sequence analysis. The α chain of human C3 consists of 992 amino acid residues and has a carbohydrate moiety attached to the asparagine residue in position 939, whereas the β chain contains 645 amino acid residues and a carbohydrate group linked to asparagine in position 85 (39,82). Both carbohydrate moieties are N-linked high-mannose oligosaccharides (81,262). There are 27 cysteine residues in the molecule but apparently only one inter-chain disulfide bond that links the N-terminal region (22.5 kDa) of the α' chain to the C-terminal portion of the β chain (97,143) (Fig. 2). C3 is synthesized as a single chain and processed after translation. It begins with a 22-residue signal peptide that is followed by the residues of the β chain, four arginine residues, and then the α-chain sequence (39). The mature two-chain protein is sensitive to treatment with dilute hydrazine (159) or chaotropic agents (31), which was shown to abolish the ability of the molecule to bind to surface acceptors. This binding potential is now known to reside in the thioester located in the α chain.

A β-cysteinyl-γ-glutaminyl thioester bond is present in the d-domain of the α chain (Fig. 2) within the sequence -Gly-Cys-Gly-Glu-Glu-Asn (265,266). The bond involves the sulfur of the Cys (position 1010) and the carbonyl of the second Glu (position 1013). Treatment of native C3 with radiolabeled methylamine (CH_3NH_2) resulted in incorporation of 1 mole of the nitrogen nucleophile into the protein. Concomitantly, 1 mole of SH became detectable in the treated C3 (129,184,251,266). Both the free SH and the CH_3NH_2-binding site were found in the 35-kDa C3d domain, and it was then shown that the responsible Cys and the CH_3NH_2-reactive Glu were separated only by two amino acid residues, which was consistent with the concept of the existence of an internal thioester. The hexapeptide referred to above was synthesized and the thioester formed, producing a 15-membered thiolactone, which underwent rearrangement to form a pyroglutamyl structure (106). It was suggested, therefore, that in C3, the thioester exists in an equilibrium between the thiolactone and the five-membered lactam (107).

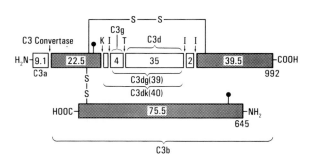

FIG. 2. Schematic representation of the human C3 molecule. The numbers indicate molecular mass in kilodaltons, except for the number at the C-terminus of the α chain and that at the N-terminus of the β chain, which indicate the number of amino acid residues in each chain. The information was derived from cDNA sequence analysis (39). The shaded bars together represent C3c. (I) Factor-I cleavage sites; (K) kallikrein cleavage site in C3bi. K and the adjacent I are mutually exclusive.

B

B is the single-chain zymogen (90 kDa) of the serine protease Bb (60 kDa) (73,74). It occurs in serum at a concentration of $\sim$210 μg/ml. The primary sequence has been derived from the structural analysis of the protein (20,156) and its cDNA (156,228), as well as of genomic DNA (12,13). B is composed of 739 amino acid residues: Ba, its activation fragment, consists of 234 residues; Bb consists of 505. Ba (30 kDa) constitutes the N-terminal portion of B, and the bond cleaved by D to generate Ba and Bb is an Arg-Lys bond (132). Ba contains three $\sim$60-residue repeat sequences that are homologous to those in H (115), suggesting that the initial contact of B with C3b is made through its Ba domain. Direct binding of the Ba fragment to C3b has been demonstrated (214). Transmission electron microscopy studies have shown that B consists of three globular domains of about equal size and that Bb has the appearance of a dumbbell consisting of two globular domains, each about 40 Å in diameter, which are connected by a short linker segment (254). The structural homology with other serine proteases and the active site of the enzyme reside in the C-terminal half of Bb, whereas the N-terminal half is unrelated and may represent the binding domain for interaction with C3b.

Although Bb is active within the alternative pathway only when it is in complex with C3b, decayed Bb possessed metal-dependent hemolytic activity in B-depleted serum which was $\sim$1% that of B (57). It also retained C3 and C5 cleaving activity, which required the presence of cobra venom factor and metal ions. Attempts to separate the two domains of Bb enzymatically for further functional studies have not been successful. However, limited degradation of native B with porcine elastase yielded several fragments, one of which (33 kDa) expressed metal-dependent affinity for C3b. Limited sequence analysis established that the 33-kDa fragment was produced by cleavage of an Ile-Asp bond and that it comprised the entire C-terminal half of Bb (120). In addition to the C3b-binding activity, this fragment exhibited esterolytic activity and residual hemolytic activity, which was 60-fold less than that of B. These observations indicate that there is a C3b-binding site in the catalytic domain of Bb; however, it is not clear whether this site is identical with the physiological binding site of Bb.

D

D (24 kDa), being the activating enzyme of the C3/C5 convertase, occurs in serum and plasma always in active form (131). It is not inhibited by the protease inhibitors of serum. An inactive zymogen of D has not been described. The enzyme is a serine protease of very high substrate specificity. It attacks exclusively a single Arg-Lys bond of B, which becomes susceptible to D only when B is in complex with C3b (132). The sequence of the single-chain protein has been elucidated at the protein level (100,178). It contains 222 amino acid residues and exhibits structural homology with plasmin (40%), trypsin (35%), and thrombin (30%) but very little with Bb (20%) (178). D is a trace constituent of serum, its concentration being ~1 μg/ml (131).

H

H (160 kDa) is one of the C3b/C4b-binding proteins. The amino acid sequence has been derived from cDNA analysis for murine H (113) and partially also for human H (114,222). The single-chain protein consists of ~1,216 amino acid residues and contains 20 contiguous repeating homology sequences of about 60 residues each. Similar homology units occur also in C4bp, CR1, CR2, C2, B, and DAF, as well as in C1r, C1s, and some other proteins not related to complement (115). Trypsin cleaves H into two fragments that are disulfide linked. After reduction and separation, only the 38-kDa N-terminal fragment displayed C3b-binding activity (2). Preliminary electron microscopic analysis of H revealed images of a highly elongated (280 Å) filamentous and flexible molecule (255). Cell-surface H receptors occur on B lymphocytes, lymphoblastoid cells, monocytes, and polymorphs. The H-binding structure appears to be composed of two components of 50 and 100 kDa. Engagement of the receptor elicits three distinct responses: (i) release of endogenous I, (ii) increased DNA synthesis and blastogenesis of B cells, and (iii) a respiratory burst in human monocytes (121,234). The serum concentration of H varies between 360 and 550 μg/ml.

I

I (88 kDa) is a two-chain (38 kDa and 50 kDa) serine protease of high substrate specificity which occurs in serum and plasma as an active enzyme (47,189). Its serum concentration is ~35 μg/ml. For its action on C3b it requires H (189,282,288) or CR1 (49,147,150,225) as a cofactor; for its action on C4b, it requires the C4bp (63,71,172,231) or CR1 (92). The primary structure has been derived from cDNA sequence analysis (16,72). The active site resides in the 38-kDa chain, which exhibits homology with other serine proteases (34). The 50-kDa chain has a mosaic structure (16), including low-density-lipoprotein(LDL)-receptor repeating sequences that also occur in C8α, C8β, and C9. The two chains are disulfide linked, and both contain carbohydrate.

Properdin

Electron microscopy of P (subunit ~53 kDa) (155) revealed polydispersity of the protein, which consisted of cyclic dimers, trimers, tetramers, and higher oligomers (256). Monomers could not be detected. Specific activity increased with oligomer size. The protomer was visualized within the polymers as a flexible elongated structure 260 Å in length and 25 Å in diameter, with thickening at each end. It is bivalent with respect to binding to other P monomers, and the binding sites involved the thickened ends. All molecular species are characterized by a beaded repeating substructure. The amino acid composition shows that glutamic acid, proline, glycine, and cysteine account for 46% of the residues (155). Limited sequencing of P-derived peptides revealed no evidence for the occurrence of repeating sequences (220). Its function in the alternative pathway is to bind to cell-bound C3b and to stabilize the C3/C5 convertase (50,146). Considering its variable cyclic polymer structure, it is conceivable that P functions as a flexible cross-linking agent within clusters of C3/C5 convertase molecules on the surface of alternative pathway activating cells.

Activation and Physiological Degradation of C3

Fragmentation Sequence

The physiological fragmentation of C3 is schematically depicted in Fig. 3. Activation of C3 is caused by C3 convertase, which cleaves an Arg-Ser bond in the N-terminal segment of the α chain and produces the fragments C3a (9.1 kDa) and C3b (~180 kDa) (161). Nascent C3b undergoes a rapid conformational change during which the metastable membrane-binding site is transiently exposed and then inactivated (95,169). C3b is converted to C3bi by removal of C3f (2 kDa) from the α chain (36). This requires cleavage of two Arg-Ser bonds (positions 1303-1304 and 1320-1321), which is accomplished by H and I (39). With the excision of C3f, which is composed of 17 residues, the α chain of C3bi consists of an N-terminal piece of 62.5 kDa and a C-terminal piece of 39.5 kDa. C3bi is further cleaved by I, with CR1 acting as cofactor and involving an Arg-Glu bond (positions 954-955) which is located in the 62.5-kDa fragment of the α chain. This reaction creates two dissociable molecules, C3c (137 kDa) and C3dg (39 kDa) (147,150,225). C3dg consists of a single chain; C3c consists of three chains. These fragments are relatively stable in serum; however, under certain conditions, serine proteases such as those released by inflammatory cells may cause further degradation: C3dg is cleaved into C3d (35 kDa) and C3g (4 kDa) (119), and an acidic fragment called C3e (~10 kDa) is split off C3c

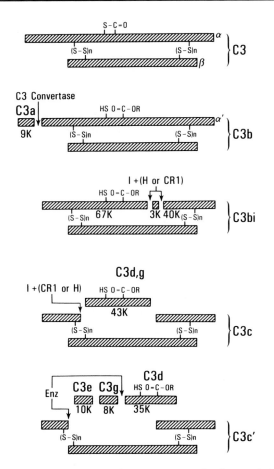

FIG. 3. Fragmentation sequence upon activation and degradation of human C3.

dent phagocytosis. C3bi interacts with CR3 and enhances antibody-dependent cellular cytotoxicity (ADCC) and phagocytosis (234). C3dg is a ligand for CR2 on B lymphocytes and has been shown to affect B-cell activation (93,153,226). C3d on the surface of target cells was found to enhance ADCC (196). C3e induces lysosomal enzyme release from neutrophils (69) and causes leukocytosis (70). C3dk inhibits T-cell proliferative responses (154) and, like C3e, causes leukocytosis when injected into rabbits. A synthetic nonapeptide corresponding to the N-terminal sequence of C3dk was active in inducing leukocytosis but had no effect on T cells (83). C3dk and C3e probably share this sequence. No biological activity has been attributed to C3c and C3f.

Multiple Binding Sites in C3 for Physiological Ligands

Concealed within the C3 molecule are at least 10 binding sites for different kinds of interactions that underlie the biological activities of C3. As the C3 molecule is processed by C3 convertase and then by I and its cofactors, sites appear and disappear. Work is being conducted to identify the chemical structure of binding regions, partly to gather information for the rational design of inhibitors of complement. Some of these sites may consist of simple linear amino acid sequences that can be mimicked by synthetic peptides. Others may be composed of two or more noncontiguous sequences and may therefore depend on the tertiary structure of the protein. In the following, several examples will be cited.

Active Site of C3a

The observation that removal of the C-terminal Arg residue abolished the biological activity of C3a focused attention on the C-terminal sequence of the molecule. To probe the essential structural basis for C3a activity, synthetic peptide analogues were constructed (90). The smallest peptide synthesized according to the C3a sequence, which expressed C3a activity, was the pentapeptide Leu-Gly-Leu-Ala-Arg (C3a 73-77). Whereas the activity was qualitatively C3a-like, it was quantitatively only 0.2% to 0.5% of that displayed by the natural 77-residue peptide. Single-residue substitutions in this prototypic synthetic peptide generally resulted in major loss of activity. The arginyl residue was found to be particularly essential. Even amidation of its carboxyl group caused inactivation. The only substitutions that led to enhancement of biological activity were phenylalanine in position 73 and alanine in position 74. It was concluded that multiple and precise interactions between this five-residue active site of C3a and the C3a receptor are required to evoke a cellular response. Further explorations showed that the

(70). Also, the action of kallikrein on C3bi produces C3dk (40 kDa), which is comprised of C3dg with an N-terminal extension of nine amino acid residues (154).

Biological Functions of C3 Fragments

The 77-residue C3a, one of the anaphylatoxins (90), is a ligand for a receptor that occurs on mast cells, neutrophils, eosinophils, basophils, and macrophages. Ligand-receptor interaction elicits release of histamine, stimulates the cyclooxygenase pathway of arachidonic acid metabolism, and causes smooth muscle contraction. C3a also suppresses antibody formation *in vitro*, presumably via an effect on macrophages (281). The active site of C3a is represented by a linear sequence at the C-terminus of the molecule. All activities of the peptide are abrogated by removal of the C-terminal arginine residue (90).

C3b has recognition function in the alternative pathway, is a subunit of the C3/C5 convertase, and is a ligand for CR1 (168,186,234). As such it enhances antibody-depen-

specific biological activity increased with peptide length and that the 21-residue peptide C3a 57-77 (C-N-Y-I-T-E-L-R-R-Q-H-A-R-A-S-H-L-G-L-A-R) exhibited nearly 100% of C3a activity. It was proposed that the N-terminal extension confers a critical orientation or restriction in flexibility upon the pentapeptide active-site portion of C3a (90). This was the first example showing that an active entity of complement can be reduced to a simple synthetic peptide.

Membrane-Binding Site of C3b: Thioester

Upon proteolytic removal of C3a, C3b undergoes a rapid conformational rearrangement (95) allowing the thioester in the d-domain to become reactive (129,184,251,266). Its carbonyl group can now form an ester bond with a hydroxyl group (86,126,128,130) on the target membrane or an amide bond with amino groups (251). C3b thus becomes covalently bound to the attacked target. The half-life of the reactive site in metastable C3b has been estimated to be 60 μsec (251). Metastable C3b that fails to react with the target surface reacts with water and remains in the fluid phase as a conformationally stable molecule that has lost its activated binding site.

The concept of the metastable binding site evolved from early observations: It emerged that C3 had to become physically bound to the target cell to be cytolytically active. It was then realized that C3 binding was mediated by an enzyme, subsequently called *C3 convertase,* which effected the binding of a large multiplicity of C3 molecules. In addition, many more C3 molecules accumulated in the fluid phase in an inactive and physicochemically altered form. A labile intermediate state was therefore postulated in which the molecule was endowed with a metastable binding site enabling it to attach to targets, but failing to achieve this within a very short time period, the site would decay (169). This concept was entirely new in protein chemistry and envisaged unique properties for C3 that were without precedent. The chemical analysis of the binding reaction began with the demonstration that the linkage between C3b and zymosan resembled an ester bond with respect to its sensitivity to nucleophiles. Hydroxylamine treatment of C3b-zymosan released C3b that contained a hydroxamate group, suggesting that the bond was zymosan-O-CO-C3b (126,128). The hydroxamate group was located in the d-domain, and these and other observations led to the description of the internal thioester.

The H-Binding Site

Studies conducted to date suggest that this site may be complex, involving a secondary or orientation region located in the 22.5-kDa segment of the α chain (Fig. 2) and a primary binding region in the 35-kDa C3d portion. A synthetic peptide spanning the 21 N-terminal amino acid residues of the 22.5-kDa sequence (749-789) inhibited H binding to C3b-coated sheep erythrocytes (EC3b) (66). Twelve other peptides synthesized according to sequences of the C3 α chain had no inhibitory effect. These sequences were chosen on the basis of predicted hydrophilicity and probability of β-turn content. The Fab fragment of purified rabbit antibody to peptide 749-789 also inhibited H binding to EC3b. These findings suggest that the corresponding sequence of the α chain has a definite function in the interaction of H with C3b.

However, another study (122) indicates that a sequence of the α chain (1244-1271) that is located much farther toward the C-terminus is a strong candidate for the H-binding site. This work originated with the description of the H receptor on lymphocytes employing anti-idiotype antibody to anti-human H (aaH) (121). This antibody detected an H-binding structure on lymphocytes that was distinct from C3b with regard to molecular size and chain composition. However, aaH also reacted with C3b, indicating that the H receptor and C3b share H-binding structures. Like H, aaH bound to EC3b but not to EC3d. When the C3 fragments were fixed to microtiter plates, possibly altering their conformation, aaH and H not only bound to C3b, but also to C3d. Subsequently, it was determined that both ligands interacted selectively with one of the CNBr fragments of C3d (8.6 kDa; positions 1200–1274). H also bound to a synthetic peptide (J28) spanning residues 1244–1271 but did not bind with other synthetic peptides that did not contain this sequence (122). One interpretation is that the site detected by aaH is the main H-binding site and that the other site facilitates H binding by conferring on this elongated asymmetrical molecule a fitting orientation. The interaction of H with C3b may be even more complex in view of recent evidence indicating that there are H-binding domains also within the 39.5-kDa segment of the α chain (179).

The Properdin and Conglutinin Sites

By ultracentrifugation, P was found to bind reversibly to C3c but not to C3d (18). Using enzyme-linked immunosorbent assay (ELISA) and plastic plates coated with C3 fragments, P bound to C3b, C3c, α chain, and the 39.5-kDa C-terminal fragment of the α chain but not to other α chain fragments or to the β chain (123). It has now been determined that the linear sequence from residues 1422–1458 of C3 contains the P-binding site (33).

Conglutinin was shown to bind to C3b, C3bi, C3c, the α chain, and the 22.5-kDa N-terminal piece of the α chain of C3b but not to C3d, the C-terminal 39.5-kDa segment of the α chain or the β chain (82). Since removal of the carbohydrate moieties by *endo-β-N*-acetylglucosaminidase H abolished binding of conglutinin, it was concluded that conglutinin binds to the carbohydrate group located on the 22.5-kDa segment of the α chain. Apparently this group becomes fully available for interaction with conglutinin only upon conversion of C3b to C3bi.

Conglutinin is a bovine plasma protein, of unknown physiologic function, that binds to yeast cell walls and to solid-phase C3bi. It is a collagen-like protein containing hydroxylysine and hydroxyproline (35). Visualized in the electron microscope, the molecule consists of four rigid ~410-Å-long and 20-Å-wide arms that have thickened peripheral ends (heads) and are held together in a common center (hub) (260). Since the molecule is composed of identical 33-kDa polypeptide chains, the following organizational model was proposed. Three chains form one monomer subunit with interchain disulfide linkages within the C-terminal noncollagenous regions that become the head portion (consisting of a triple-helical collagen-like stem and a non-collagen-like N-terminal portion), which interacts noncovalently with three other subunits to form the hub of intact conglutinin (260).

The CR2 Site

CR2, constituting the C3d receptor (224,226) and Epstein-Barr virus (EBV) receptor (55,60,173) on human B lymphocytes, has a mass of 140 kDa. The receptor has immunoregulatory functions. Limited peptide sequencing and nucleotide sequencing of two cDNA clones indicate that CR2 contains internal repeating units that are homologous with those of CR1 and the other C3b/C4b-binding proteins (283). CR2 differs from the other proteins of this family because it has specificity for C3dg, C3d, and C3bi, rather than for C3b, and because it lacks C3 convertase regulatory function (224).

To identify the CR2-binding site in C3d, this fragment was treated with CNBr, which generated two major fragments of molecular weight 12.5 kDa and 8.6 kDa. Only the 8.6-kDa fragment was capable of binding to CR2. Amino-terminal sequence analysis of the fragment showed it to consist of residues 1200–1274 of the C3 sequence (39). Computer analyses predicted hydrophilicity and high probability for the occurrence of a strong β-turn within the sequence 1209–1236. The synthetic peptide constructed accordingly exhibited CR2-binding activity (124). Two of three smaller synthetic peptides representing different portions of this sequence also were active. The sequence that the three CR2 reactive peptides had in common was LYNVEA (residues 1227–1232), suggesting that the binding site comprises these six or fewer amino acid residues. Binding of the active peptides was inhibited by mAb OKB7, which also inhibits the binding of C3d and

EBV to the receptor (173). Thus, the CR2 site in C3 is only a few residues removed from the sequence (1244–1271) harboring one of the H-binding sites (122) and is immediately adjacent to the neoantigenic site recognized by mAb 130 (124,267).

Although it is not known whether C3d and EBV react with the same site on CR2, it was explored whether C3d and gp350, the CR2 ligand of EBV, share any homology regions in their primary structure. Two regions of significant primary sequence homology were identified, one involving the thioester region of C3d and the other involving its Leu-Tyr-Asn-Val-Glu-Ala (LYNVEA) sequence (174). Particularly the latter homology region appears to be a strong candidate for the CR2-binding site in the viral coat protein.

Molecular Dynamics of Activation and Amplification

Formation and Function of the Initial C3 Convertase

Spontaneous generation of C3(H₂O)

Activation and progression of the alternative pathway depend on the continuous supply of C3b. Because C3b is not available initially, the essential modifier of B for activation by D is lacking. It now appears that in the assembly of the initial C3 convertase, $C3(H_2O)$ serves as a B modifier and acceptor of Bb (186,190).

Early studies showed that C3 hemolytic activity decays spontaneously in aqueous solution (167) and that chaotropic agents enhance this process (31). The rate of spontaneous decay was 0.005%/min at 37°C and pH 7.0, and it increased to 6.25%/min in the presence of $0.33\,M$ KSCN (190). Inactivation of C3 was accompanied by the appearance of a free sulfhydryl group, which has also been observed upon treatment of native C3 with CH_3NH_2 (98,190). These observations led to the conclusion that the product of spontaneous decay or exposure to chaotropic agents is uncleaved C3 in which the thioester has undergone hydrolysis (190,279). Subsequently, it was shown that C3 modified at the thioester site either by water or by CH_3NH_2 possessed all the functional properties of C3b: Together with B, D, and Mg^{2+} it forms a fluid-phase C3 convertase, and it is cleaved and inactivated by H and I (95,190,279).

The conformational changes caused by CH_3NH_2 binding were monitored by circular dichroism spectroscopy and ANS (1-anilino-8-naphthalene sulfonate) fluorescence (95). The spectra resembled those of C3b; however, the rate of conformational rearrangement and of appearance of functional sites was much slower than the rate of CH_3NH_2 uptake. Also, the acquisition of H-binding capacity was slower than the acquisition of B-binding sites. For instance, at a given CH_3NH_2 concentration, CH_3NH_2 uptake was essentially complete at 5 min, whereas 50%

B- and H-binding activity became expressed at 25 and 35 min, respectively. These kinetics suggest that C3 modified at the thioester site has a temporarily greater chance to form the fluid-phase C3 convertase than to become enzymatically degraded by H and I.

Although $C3(H_2O)$ is structurally indistinguishable from native C3 by its appearance on sodium dodecylsulfate–polyacrylamide gel electrophoresis (SDS-PAGE), its α chain is susceptible to cleavage by I. H and I cleave the α chain of $C3(H_2O)$ into a 76-kDa and a 40-kDa fragment. The 76-kDa fragment contains the 67-kDa piece of the α chain of C3bi plus the covalently linked C3a domain (95,190,279).

The initial C3 convertase, C3(H₂O),Bb

Entirely without participation of enzymes, initiation of the alternative pathway is safeguarded by spontaneous low-rate hydrolysis of the thioester in C3 and the resultant continuous supply of $C3(H_2O)$. Upon Mg^{2+}-dependent binding of B, $C3(H_2O)$ triggers activation of the proenzyme complex by D. Cleavage of B results in the release of the 30-kDa fragment Ba and formation of $C3(H_2O)$, Bb(Mg), which is the initial C3 convertase that is necessarily confined to the fluid phase (190). The enzymatically active complex has a short half-life, and its physicochemical demonstration and characterization has therefore been difficult. When it was found that Ni^{2+} could replace Mg^{2+} in C3 convertase formation and produce a considerably more stable complex, physicochemical studies of the enzyme became feasible (56). The $C3(H_2O)$,Bb(Ni) complex had a sedimentation coefficient of 10.7S, was resistant to ethylenediaminetetraacetic acid (EDTA), and contained Ni^{2+}, Bb, and $C3(H_2O)$ in equimolar amounts (59). The metal content was determined using $^{63}Ni^{2+}$, which was retained by the complex even in the presence of EDTA, suggesting that the metal is concealed or completely coordinated by the proteins. The specific enzymatic activity (k_{cat}/K_m) of $C3(H_2O)$,Bb made with Mg or Ni was nearly identical ($\sim 1.6 \times 10^5$ M^{-1} sec^{-1}), but the Ni-containing enzyme was six times more stable (186,187).

Formation of the Target-Cell-Bound C3/C5 Convertase

C3b deposition

It is the function of the initial C3 convertase to produce metastable C3b ($t_{1/2} \sim 60$ μsec) and to deposit C3b on the surface of surrounding particles. Compared to the thioester in native C3, which has a half-life of 231 hr at 37°C, the thioester in metastable C3b is 10^{10} times more reactive. Its reactive carbonyl group exhibits preference for certain carbohydrates but appears to be as reactive with hydroxyl groups as with amines (130,251).

Because C3b deposition is catalyzed by a fluid-phase enzyme, it is expected to be a random process. The hypothesis of spontaneous initiation suggests that if these C3b molecules fall randomly onto surfaces, then at early times during the reaction, activation will have begun on some particles but not on others (191). Using fluorescein-isothiocyanate-labeled C3 (FITC-C3), C7-depleted human serum, and rabbit erythrocytes, the extent of activation at 37°C that had occurred on individual cells was determined by fluorescence-activated cell sorting (186). Deposition of FITC-C3b exhibited a lag of ~ 1 min. After 1.2 min the cells showed distinct heterogeneity, some cells being highly fluorescent, whereas most of the cells had little or no FITC-C3b. At 1.4 min, activation had begun on the majority of cells, but the heterogeneity of the amount of C3b deposited had greatly increased. Two minutes after initiation of the reaction the cells assumed a normal distribution with respect to FITC-C3b fluorescence. This experiment was interpreted to indicate randomness of initial C3b deposition.

The C3 convertase C3b,Bb

The proenzyme C3b,B(Mg) is a reversible trimolecular complex that is activated by D. C3b serves as substrate modifier enabling D to cleave B and as acceptor for Bb. The activated C3 convertase is covalently linked to the surface of target cells through C3b. Its function is to increase the number of target-cell-bound C3b molecules in its immediate environment. The decay-dissociation half-time for C3b,Bb(Mg) is 90 sec at physiological ionic strength, pH, and temperature (51,146,187,191). The activation energy for dissociation of the trimolecular complex is 19.5 kcal/mole (187).

Transmission electron microscopy studies have shown that Bb consists of two domains, each ~ 40 Å in diameter, which are connected by a short (~ 10 Å) linker segment. Within the C3 convertase complex, Bb binds to C3b through only one domain, indicating that this is the binding domain and suggesting that the other may be the catalytic domain (254). If the freely projecting domain of Bb contains the catalytic site, then it would represent the C-terminal half of Bb because that portion of the molecule is homologous to other serine proteases, and the binding domain would constitute the N-terminal half.

In the formation of the enzyme, Ni^{2+} can substitute Mg^{2+}, yielding an active and more stable complex. Ni^{2+} was also found to be more efficient in enzyme formation than Mg^{2+}. Up to nine times more B was specifically bound to EC3b in the presence of Ni^{2+} than in the presence of Mg^{2+}. To form one effective hemolytic site per EC3b with Ni^{2+}, three times less B, 12 times less D, and 66 times less metal ion were required than when using Mg^{2+} (56). C3b,Bb(Ni) was sevenfold more stable than the Mg^{2+}-containing enzyme, and its enzymatic activity was slightly lower (k_{cat}/K_m was 2.5×10^5 instead of $3.1 \times 10^5 M^{-1} sec^{-1}$) (187). As in the case of the initial C3 convertase, the enhanced stability of C3b,Bb(Ni) has permitted the physicochemical characterization of the enzyme. The complex sediments at 10.7S and is composed of one molecule of Ni^{2+}, Bb, and C3b (58). The metal is released on decay-dissociation of the enzyme.

The C3 convertase can function as a C5 convertase provided an additional C3b molecule is available in close proximity (27,146). The role of the second C3b molecule is to bind C5 and to modify it for cleavage by Bb (94,160,278). The interaction between C3b and C5 has a stoichiometry of 1:1 and an association constant of $5.7 \times 10^6 M^{-1}$ for bound C3b and $4.8 \times 10^5 M^{-1}$ for fluid-phase C3b. Cleavage of C5 releases the anaphylatoxin C5a; it also creates labile C5b, which initiates assembly of the membrane attack complex.

The role of P

P is a protein with a cyclic subunit structure (256). Its function is to increase the stability of the C3/C5 convertase by physically associating with it (51,146). Native P does not bind to C3b-bearing particles, nor does it induce C3 convertase formation in serum (146). Its interaction with C3 convertase is nonenzymatic, and binding to the enzyme complex may involve a conformational rearrangement of the molecule. P is not an essential component for the activation of the alternative pathway, but its presence does result in more rapid amplification of bound C3b (236). However, in certain cases, such as measles-virus-infected cells, P needs to participate in order that activation of the pathway may progress to lysis of the cells (253). Native P has been contrasted with activated P, which binds to C3b-bearing cells and, when added to serum, activates the alternative pathway. Recently, this form of P has been shown to represent denatured protein with a noncyclic ultrastructure resembling protein aggregates (46).

Amplification

The C3b-dependent positive feedback is a unique feature of the alternative pathway: C3b, the product of the reaction between C3 convertase and its substrate C3, forms a subunit of the C3 convertase itself (164). Each newly produced C3b molecule has the potential to form the enzyme together with B, D, and Mg^{2+} and thus to produce more C3b and more enzyme. This process occurs rapidly in solution upon mixing purified C3, B, and D, or it occurs on the surface of C3b-bearing cells when these proteins are present (239). In the latter case, cells become covered with C3b. Progression of amplification is controlled by H

and I, both in the fluid phase and on nonactivating particles. C3b, instead of binding B, binds H and is subsequently cleaved to C3bi. But on an activator of the alternative pathway, C3b is relatively resistant to inactivation by H and I, and binding of B to C3b is favored. This competition between progression and C3b breakdown permits the pathway to amplify only those few molecules of C3b that were deposited on activating particles.

Discrimination and Regulation

Little is known about the specificity and recognition of the alternative pathway. Unknown are the chemical structures that are recognized and that activators must have in common. This diverse group of particles includes polysaccharides, immunoglobulin aggregates, certain viruses, fungi, bacteria, mammalian tumor cells, and parasites. Uncertain is the molecular mechanism by which the pathway discriminates between host cells and activating particles. However, it has been established that discrimination involves the interaction between particle-bound C3b and the regulatory proteins. The original observation was that C3 convertase on activating particles such as zymosan or rabbit erythrocytes was relatively resistant to the regulatory action of H and I (52,53). It was subsequently shown that it is the interaction between bound C3b and H that is reduced on activators, while the binding of B, I, and P to C3b was unaffected by the type of particle to which C3b was attached (183).

It is the normal function of H and I to prevent the spontaneous activation and progression of the alternative pathway. H restricts formation of C3 convertase and accelerates decay-dissociation of C3b,Bb, even when stabilized by P (183,282,288). The action of I on C3b requires that C3b is in complex with H so that the actual substrate for I is C3b,H (185). Since the serum concentration of H ($3.7 \times 10^{-6} M$) is considerably greater than the dissociation constant of C3b,H ($0.62 \times 10^{-6} M$), C3b, when occurring in serum at low concentration, will be virtually all in complex with H. The second-order rate constant, k_{cat}/K_m ($5.2 \times 10^6 M^{-1} sec^{-1}$ at 37°C), indicates that I is a very efficient protease, and its unusually low k_m for C3b,H ($2.5 \times 10^{-7} M$), which is similar to the serum concentration of I ($3.9 \times 10^{-7} M$), permits it to act on C3b even when this is present at very low concentrations (185). Thus, H and I together constitute a very efficient scavenger system for C3b and also for C3(H_2O).

Recognition of an activator of the alternative pathway is expressed on the molecular level by reduction in binding affinity of surface-bound C3b for H. On potent activators such as rabbit erythrocytes or zymosan, H-C3b interaction is only one-tenth of the interaction that is characteristic for the nonactivating sheep erythrocytes. Some nonactivators can be converted to activators by several defined modifications. One involves enzymatic removal or chemical modification of cell-surface sialic acid. In the case of sheep erythrocytes, this treatment reduced the relative binding affinity of C3b for H to less than one-third (48,183). However, it is wrong to assume that all particles low or deficient in sialic acid are activators. For example, pronase treatment of human erythrocytes removes over 90% of the sialic acid so that the treated cells retain less of it than is present on untreated rabbit erythrocytes. Nevertheless, pronase-treated human erythrocytes are not activators, and the relative binding affinity of cell-bound C3b for H is almost twice that of sheep erythrocytes (192). Another modification involves attachment of chemically defined molecules. Incorporation of LPS of *E. coli* 04 into the membrane of C3b-bearing sheep erythrocytes reduced drastically the affinity of C3b for H and induced lysis of the cells via the alternative pathway (193). In yet another example, liposomes composed of cholesterol and dimyristoylphosphatidylcholine did not activate the guinea-pig alternative pathway. Upon incorporation of trinitrophenyl phosphatidylethanolamine, the liposomes became efficient activators (181).

A systematic study was conducted to determine whether the recognition mechanism established for the human pathway held true also for the alternative pathway of another species. The rabbit was chosen because rabbit erythrocytes are potent activators of the human pathway but do not activate the rabbit pathway. Therefore, the key proteins C3, B, and H were isolated from rabbit serum, and the binding affinity of B and H for particle-bound C3b was measured and compared with the corresponding values of the human proteins (84). In both species the average affinity of H for bound C3b on homologous cells (nonactivators) was 8 to 10 times higher than that on zymosan (activator) (85). Rabbit H bound strongly to rabbit C3b on rabbit erythrocytes; it also bound on human erythrocytes, which are nonactivators for the rabbit alternative pathway. These results indicated that the molecular mechanism of recognition in both species is analogous and species-specific.

Role of Antibody

Evidence has accumulated showing that antibody, independent of its classical pathway role, can have a function in the alternative pathway (218). A number of examples may be cited: (a) Incubation of immune precipitates containing the F(ab')$_2$ fragment of guinea-pig antibody with guinea-pig serum caused consumption of B but not of C2 (230). (b) Solubilization of immune precipitates by serum required B and Mg^{2+} but not C4 or Ca^{2+} (26). In fact, a mixture of isolated C3, B, D, H, I, and P was sufficient

to solubilize immune complexes (64). After a 10-min incubation at 37°C, C3 was bound in an equimolar ratio with IgG. (c) Activators such as zymosan showed increased C3 and B uptake in the presence of antibody (232); measles-virus-infected HeLa cells activated the isolated alternative pathway as evidenced by C3 uptake, but cell lysis required specific antibody (253). (d) Antibody reactive with sialic acid epitopes on certain bacteria converted these cells from nonactivators to activators of the pathway (44). By covering sialic acid the antibody appeared to decrease C3b-H interaction.

Metastable C3b is capable of binding directly to IgG. The Fd portion of the heavy chain appears to be the preferred binding site, and both ester and amide bonds have been demonstrated (65). Important for the role of immunoglobulin in alternative pathway function is that C3b covalently bound to IgG displays relative resistance to inactivation by H and I when compared to free C3b or C3b bound to ceruloplasmin. Resistance was entirely due to reduced affinity of C3b-IgG for H, and this conferred on the complex an enhanced capacity to activate C3 in serum relative to C3b (61). The complex of C3b with bactericidal IgG was found markedly more effective than IgG in the killing of *E. coli* by serum (101).

There is yet another antibody-involving mechanism of alternative pathway activation; however, this mechanism is dependent on C1. Originally described as the "C1-bypass activation pathway" for the lysis of heavily sensitized sheep erythrocytes by C4-deficient guinea-pig serum (144), this mechanism may indeed have physiological significance: Lysis of *Giardia lamblia* trophozoites by human serum was found to require antibody, C1q, C1r, C1s, and an intact alternative pathway as well as Ca^{2+} and Mg^{2+} but did not require C2 or C4 (40).

THE CLASSICAL PATHWAY

Overview

The classical pathway of complement activation is a mediator of the specific antibody response. With few exceptions, it is triggered by antigen-bound antibody molecules. It is as elaborately controlled as the alternative pathway, but it lacks that pathway's spontaneous initiation, antibody-independent recognition function, and feedback amplification mechanism.

The initial enzyme C1 is a metalloprotein complex of two reversibly interacting subunits C1q and C1r$_2$s$_2$ (22,23,241,301). C1 occurs in serum as a proenzyme which tends to undergo autoactivation (299) but which is strictly controlled by C1 inhibitor (C1-In) (300). Upon binding of C1 to immune complexes by virtue of the affinity of C1q for immunoglobulins (242), the controlling action of C1-In is overcome (300) and C1q effects activation of $C1r_2s_2$. First, the zymogen is activated by a conformational change of C1r, then proteolytic activation occurs, resulting in cleavage of all four polypeptide chains of $C1r_2s_2$ (303). The two activated C1s subunits are then able to catalyze the assembly of the C3 convertase C4b-2a. In the process, nascent C4b expresses a metastable binding site owing to its internal thioester through which it can covalently attach to a receptive surface. Action of the C3 convertase on C3 forms metastable C3b, and its binding to an acceptor in the immediate environment of C4b,2a generates the classical C3/C5 convertase. Formation of the enzyme is rigidly controlled by fluid-phase and membrane-regulatory proteins, and there is no positive regulator corresponding to properdin of the alternative pathway. C1 turnover by immune complexes is inhibited by both nascent C3b and C4b (302). Activated C1 is inactivated by binding of C1-In to $C1r_2s_2$ and dissociation from C1q (249,303,305). The C3 convertase undergoes spontaneous decay-dissociation and thereby inactivation. It is actively dissociated by the C4bp (71,172) in serum and by decay-accelerating factor (DAF) (175) on the surface of blood cells. Also, C4b is degraded by C4bp and I (71,172) or by CR1 and I (92).

The Proteins

C1q

This protein was recognized through its ability to precipitate soluble IgG aggregates (165). It was found early to be a collagen-like protein containing hydroxylysine, hydroxyproline, a large proportion of glycine residues, and glucose-galactose disaccharide units linked to the hydroxyl groups of hydroxylysine (11). Its normal serum concentration is ~ 70 μg/ml. C1q (~ 410 kDa) is composed of three kinds of chains, namely A, B, and C, each being represented in the molecule with six copies. The primary sequence of the entire A and B chains, as well as the sequence of $\sim 50\%$ of the C chain, has been worked out on the protein level (221). Recently, cDNA and genomic DNA were isolated for the B chain (219). Each chain consists of 226 amino acid residues, including a stretch of 78 to 81 residues located toward the N-terminus, which is collagen-like (221).

The unusual structure of C1q became apparent by electron microscopic analysis (109). Each of six globular head domains (50 × 70 Å) is linked to a central portion (45 × 112 Å) by a 115-Å-long connecting strand that is somewhat flexible. The image was described to be reminiscent of a bouquet of flowers. Each of the ultrastructural subunits contains three chains: an A-B heterodimer with an interchain disulfide bond near the N-termini and one C chain. The C chains of adjacent subunits are linked by a disulfide bond located also in the N-terminal region. The head portions are composed of the C-terminal globular structure, and the strands have collagen-like triple helical structures (reviewed in ref. 23).

C1r and C1s

C1r (~ 85 kDa) and C1s (~ 85 kDa) (reviewed in refs. 23 and 301) are homologous single-chain zymogens, and the complete sequence of both has been deduced from the analysis of cDNA clones (103,269). The sequence of C1r had previously been obtained by protein sequence analysis. In isolated form, C1r occurs as a noncovalently linked dimer, with C1s occurring as a monomer. Together they form the tetrameric Ca^{2+}-dependent $C1r_2s_2$ complex (304). On activation, the 688-residue-containing chains are cleaved at an Arg-Ile bond which produces disulfide bridged fragments of 57 kDa (A chain) and 28 kDa (B chain). The latter subunits contain the serine protease active site. Two homology regions located in tandem in the A chain of activated C1r (residues 292 to 354 and 359 to 430) are related to the conserved cysteine-containing repeating sequences found in C3b/C4b-binding proteins. Two such repeats are similarly located in the A chain of activated C1s. The serum concentration is ~ 35 μg/ml for both proteins.

C2

The protein is a single-chain zymogen (~ 102 kDa) with considerable similarity to B. The concentration of C2 in normal human serum is 20 to 30 μg/ml. Its primary structure was deduced from cDNA sequence analysis (5). The overall homology with B is 39%. On activation, the 732-residue chain is cleaved into two fragments: (i) the N-terminal C2b consisting of 223 amino acids and (ii) the C-terminal C2a consisting of 509 amino acid residues. C2b consists of three repeating sequences that are homologous to the repeats in Ba-, H-, and other C3b/C4b-binding proteins. C2a is homologous to Bb and contains the serine protease site.

Both C2 and B contain a free sulfhydryl group that is located near the N-terminus of C2a and Bb (194). Treatment of C2 with iodine results in chemical modification of the free sulfhydryl group and a 10- to 20-fold increase in C2 hemolytic activity (209). Treatment of C2 with certain sulfhydryl blocking reagents abrogated its hemolytic activity. Neither of these treatments affected the hemolytic activity of B.

C4

C4 (~ 200 kDa) is a three-chain protein consisting of α (~ 93 kDa), β (~ 75 kDa), and γ chains (~ 33 kDa) (235). Its serum concentration ranges from 450 to 750

μg/ml. The molecule is synthesized as a single chain of 1,722 amino acid residues containing the chains of the mature protein in the order β-α-γ. The complete amino acid sequence of pro-C4 was deduced from cDNA sequence analysis (4). C4, like C3, possesses an internal thioester (265) in its α chain which, upon enzymatic removal of C4a ($\sim$9 kDa), becomes the metastable binding site of nascent C4b (166). C4 occurs in the form of two structurally and functionally distinct isotypes, C4A and C4B (15). The thioester of C4A reacts with amino groups, but little with hydroxyl groups, whereas C4B, which is three times more hemolytically active than C4A, reacts preferentially with hydroxyl groups (127). Gene duplication may thus have conferred on C4 the ability to react with a wide range of different substances.

The large fragment C4b is under the control of I and C4bp or CR1 (63,92). The C4d piece is cleaved out of the α chain of C4b, which converts it to the four-chain fragment C4c (189). An N-terminal 25-kDa segment of the α chain and a 12-kDa C-terminal piece remain disulfide-bonded to the β-γ chains.

C1-In

The protein ($\sim$104 kDa) is the only inhibitor of activated C1r and C1s in plasma. The normal serum concentration of the inhibitor is $\sim$200 μg/ml. It contains 35% carbohydrate and is a highly asymmetrical rod-shaped molecule (180). The complete primary structure has been deduced from cDNA sequencing (10,37). It is a single-chain molecule composed of 478 amino acid residues. It has been identified as a member of the plasma serine protease inhibitor superfamily. The interaction of C1-In with activated C1s results in formation of a covalent complex. In the course of this reaction, a peptide bond near the C-terminus of the inhibitor is cleaved by C1s (229).

C4bp

This protein ($\sim$570 kDa) is a regulator of the C3 convertase of the classical pathway (172,231). By binding to C4b, C4bp accelerates the decay-dissociation of the enzyme (71) and renders C4b susceptible to degradation by I (63). Human C4bp is composed of seven identical chains (70 kDa each) that are linked by disulfide bonds at their C-termini (29). Visualized by electron microscopy, the molecule was found to have a spider-like structure consisting of seven thin (30 Å), elongated (330 Å), and flexible subunits (tentacles) that are linked to a small central body (30). In complex with C4b, the peripheral ends of the tentacles were seen to be in direct contact with C4b, suggesting seven C4b-binding sites per C4bp. Limited proteolysis by chymotrypsin produced fragments of $\sim$50 kDa

and $\sim$160 kDa (28). The latter fragment is composed of disulfide-linked 25-kDa polypeptides and constitutes the central body of C4bp, which appeared as a ring-like structure with an inner and outer diameter of 13 Å and 60 Å, respectively. The liberated 50-kDa fragment represents the major portion (290 Å) of the tentacles. Kinetic analysis of chymotrypsin digestion monitored by SDS-PAGE also indicated the number of peripheral subunits to be seven.

The primary structure of C4bp showed that one chain consists of 549 amino acid residues grouped in eight conserved repeating domains starting from the N-terminus, each about 60 residues long and homologous to the repeating sequences in the C3b/C4b-binding proteins (21). The C-terminal region is unrelated, contains cysteine residues, probably participating in interchain disulfide bridging, and forms the central body of the spider. By ultracentrifugation at physiological ionic strength, C4bp exhibited four binding sites for C4b, each having an association constant of 1.2×10^7 M^{-1} (306). At reduced ionic strength, two additional sites were detected, suggesting that after four C4b molecules have bound to C4bp, the binding of additional C4b molecules is sterically hindered. C4bp weakly bound C4c but did not bind C4 or C4d. It exhibited a low affinity for C3b which was specific, since C4bp mediated the cleavage of C3b by I with concomitant dissociation of the complex (306).

Activation and Control of C1

Structure of C1

Under physiological conditions C1 ($\sim$750 kDa) exists in the form of two reversibly interacting subunits, namely C1q and the C1r$_2$s$_2$ tetramer (245,304). Considering the serum concentration of C1 (1.8×10^7 M) and the association constant for the reaction between C1q and the tetramer ($\sim$5 $\times$ 10^7 M^{-1}), it is estimated that $\sim$70% of C1 is at all times present as a complex (244,304). The C1r$_2$s$_2$ tetramer ($\sim$340 kDa) has been visualized by electron microscopy as a linear chain of subcomponents (277). Each C1r and C1s monomer was found to consist of two globular domains connected by a thin linker filament, one domain being the catalytic domain and the other being the contact domain. The sequence of the subunits within the C1r$_2$s$_2$ chain is C1s-C1r-C1r-C1s, where the catalytic domains of the two C1s subunits are located at the very ends of the chain and where the catalytic domains of the two C1r subunits are located at the very center (285).

The model proposed for the architecture of the C1 complex envisions the tetrameric chain inserted between the collagenous strands of C1q. The two protruding ends are wrapped around the outside of the C1q cone in such a fashion that the distal catalytic domains of C1s are brought in contact with the centrally located catalytic domains of the C1r dimer. This arrangement places the C1r-C1s contact domains outside the C1q cone and the four catalytic domains inside the cone. It also implies that the tetramer imposes constraints on the freedom of movement of the C1q strands (22,241,285).

Two conformationally distinct forms of unactivated C1 have been hypothesized (241): (i) the "closed" complex, in which the two C1s terminal domains are in contact with complementary sites on C1r and which is incapable of autoactivation; and (ii) the "open" complex or transitional state of C1, in which the catalytic sites of unactivated C1r are exposed.

Activation of C1

Activated C1 contains cleaved C1r and C1s, i.e., each subunit of the tetramer consists of two disulfide-bridged chains, A (57 kDa) and B (28 kDa) (250,303). The B chains exhibit serine protease activity. Activation results from an intramolecular autocatalytic mechanism. It proceeds spontaneously, is inhibited by C1-In, and is enhanced by interaction of C1 with immune complexes.

In isolated form, unactivated C1 has a half-life of 4 min at 37°C, i.e., 50% of the molecules convert to activated C1 during this period (299). It has been proposed that in the transitional or open complex state of C1, C1r is released from inhibitory contact with C1s, and its catalytic site is thereby enabled to cleave the neighboring C1r chain. After reciprocal cleavage and activation of the two C1r chains, activated C1r then cleaves and activates C1s (303). Activation of the tetramer results in ∼10-fold reduction in the association constant for the interaction of $C1r_2s_2$ with C1q. Decreased interaction with C1q might allow the tetramer to unfold and to extend its C1s ends outside the C1q cone for interaction with C4 and C2 (241).

Upon binding of unactivated C1 to immune complexes, the association constant for the interaction of C1q with $C1r_2s_2$ is increased by an order of magnitude, and the rate of activation becomes ∼5 times greater than that of spontaneous C1 activation (in absence of C1-In) (89). It is thought that the binding of C1q to clustered antibody molecules leads to distortion of the C1q strands. Distortion results in a conformational change of the tetramer (located 50–100 Å from the C1q heads), favoring the transitional or open complex state and thus enhancing activation (118,241).

Binding to immune complexes takes place through the globular heads of C1q, which interact with specific C1q-binding sites in the Fc region of IgG and IgM. At least two heads of a C1q molecule must be engaged in order to bind C1 firmly enough for activation (88; reviewed in ref. 118). The single-site association constant for the binding of C1q to monomeric IgG is ∼5×10^4 M^{-1}. The average duration of this bond is less than 1 sec, which is too short to effect C1 activation. Binding of C1q via two or more heads, as it occurs with immune complexes, has association constants of 5×10^7 M^{-1} to 1×10^{10} M^{-1}. The affinity of C1q for IgG decreased in the order IgG3, IgG1, IgG2, IgG4 (242). C1q does not bind to IgA, IgD, or IgE. Certain nonimmune substances may also function as activators of C1 in the total absence of antibody. One example is murine leukemia virus, which binds C1 via its coat protein p15E (3).

Control of C1 Activation by C1-In

C1-In blocks the spontaneous activation of C1, but it does not significantly affect C1 activation by immune complexes (300). At physiological concentrations there is a sevenfold molar excess of C1-In over C1. It is thought that C1-In reversibly binds to C1 when it is in the transitional or open complex state, in which the C1r pro-catalytic sites are exposed. Presumably, two molecules of C1-In bind to the two C1r sites, thus preventing autocatalytic activation. Binding of C1-In to unactivated C1 was demonstrable on immune complexes at reduced temperatures, at which C1-In is capable of blocking even immune activator-induced C1 activation (300).

Upon binding of C1 to immune complexes the C1-In is displaced and sterically hindered to re-enter the C1q cone to gain access to C1r (241). The association between the C1 subunits becomes firmer, and the intramolecular autocatalytic activation proceeds rapidly as described above.

Control of Activated C1

After proteolytic activation, the subunit association within the C1 complex is weakened. The structure of the tetramer is loosened, and activated C1s is exposed and enabled to efficiently turn over substrate. Under physiological conditions, its active state has a half-life of only 13 sec because C1-In rapidly enters into covalent interaction with C1s abrogating its enzymatic activity (301). C1-In also gains access to activated C1r at this stage, resulting in the disassembly of immune complex bound C1. Two molecules of $C1rC1s(C1-In)_2$ (∼380 kDa) are released into the fluid phase, whereas C1q remains bound to the activator (125,305).

Immune-complex-activated C1 is further controlled by feedback inhibition involving nascent C3b and C4b (302). In a purified protein mixture of C1 and C1-In, limited amounts of immune complexes can consume all the C1 available. However, in the presence of C2, C3, and C4, C1 consumption is drastically reduced, presumably due to covalent attachment of nascent C3b and C4b to the immune complexes with concomitant modification of activator. Thus, excessive complement activation by low concentrations of immune complexes is prevented.

Formation, Structure, and Function of C3/C5 Convertase

Assembly of the C3 Convertase

Formation of this enzyme is catalyzed by activated C1, specifically by the serine protease sites of the two C1s subunits. C2 and C4 are the natural substrates for activated C1s and the precursors of the C3 convertase of the classical pathway. Because the K_m for C4 activation is 0.96×10^{-6} M and the physiological concentration of C4 in serum is 2.0×10^{-6} M, activation proceeds at a high rate. The turnover rate is 303 C4/C1 min^{-1}. This rate affords ~35 C4 molecules to be activated during the life-span of a single activated C1 molecule (298). Primarily because the molar concentration of C2 is about one-twentieth that of C4, only an average of four C2 molecules are activated during that same period.

Cleavage of peptide bond 74-75 of the α chain of C4 by C1s removes the activation peptide C4a and generates metastable C4b. In metastable C4b the internal thioester is activated and is enabled to form amide or ester bonds with respective groups on the target surface or to react with water. C4A reacts preferentially with amino groups, and C4B reacts preferentially with hydroxyl groups (127). A large number of C4b molecules react with water and remain unbound in the fluid phase (166). But a significant percentage of molecules becomes covalently bound to the surface of activators (24). On the surface of antibody-coated cells, these C4b molecules cluster around an antibody-C1 complex or, in part, bind directly to the antibody.

C2 enters into reversible metal-dependent interaction with C4b, thus forming the proenzyme C4b,C2(Mg). Upon cleavage of C2 by C1s the C2a fragment (70 kDa) becomes firmly associated with C4b, and the C3 convertase C4b,2a is generated (170,210). The inactive fragment C2b (34 kDa) slowly dissociates from the complex. Whereas C2 by itself can be cleaved by C1s, this reaction does not result in activation. On the target cell surface, only those C2 molecules can become activated that are bound to C4b molecules located within reach of C1. Because the length of the unfolded C1r$_2$s$_2$ tetramer is 640 Å, the activatable area around a C1 molecule may have a radius of ~360 Å. The classical C3 convertase appears to be somewhat less efficient than its analog in the alternative pathway. The K_m for C3 cleavage is 1.8×10^{-6} M. The enzyme undergoes decay-dissociation with a half-life of 3 min at 37°C. When Ni^{2+} was used instead of Mg^{2+},

enzyme formation was more efficient and the resultant C4b,2a(Ni) complex exhibited enhanced stability, its half-life at 37°C being 6 min (56).

The Structure of C3 Convertase

The enzyme may be generated in solution by incubation of C2, C4, and Mg^{2+} with C1s. However, because of its intrinsic lability it was originally not possible to subject it to physical examination. This became possible when the enzyme was produced with iodine-treated C2, because the stability of the enzyme was thereby enhanced 10- to 20-fold (209). Using zone ultracentrifugation, molecular sieve chromatography, and radiolabeled proteins, it was shown that C3 convertase activity resided in a bimolecular complex of C4b and C2a (170,210). By electron microscopy the classical C3 convertase appeared strikingly similar in structure to its analog of the alternative pathway (254). C2a consists of two globular domains, one measuring 42 Å in diameter and the other being 47 Å, which are connected by a thin 10-Å-long linker segment. It is bound to C4b through the larger of the two domains, suggesting that the freely projecting domain bears the catalytic site. C4b, like C3b, has a globular appearance and an irregular multiple-domain substructure. The dimensions are ~125 Å × 75 Å × 65 Å. The zymogen, C2, appears globular with a diameter of ~85 Å and a three-lobed substructure, each lobe measuring ~40 Å in diameter. If the freely projecting domain of the catalytic subunit of the C3 convertase contains the catalytic site, then this domain would represent the C-terminal half of C2a, which is known to contain the critical serine protease residues (5), and the binding domain would constitute the N-terminal portion.

Generation of C5 Convertase

The classical C5 convertase is generated upon addition of a molecule of C3b to the C4b,2a complex (25). The change in substrate specificity of C4b,2a is accomplished by "activation" of C5 by C3b, not by modulation of the enzyme. This molecular strategy applies also to the C5 convertase of the alternative pathway. The helper molecule does not bind directly to the C3 convertase complex, although theoretically this should be possible. The efficiency of the C5 convertase is maximized therefore when multiple C3b molecules are grouped in dense clusters around the enzyme. Such membrane-bound C3b clusters have been visualized by electron microscopy (139), and binding studies with radiolabeled proteins have shown that as many as 200 C3b molecules can be deposited on a cell surface by a single-membrane-bound C4b,2a complex (169). In fact, these observations were the first to reveal that C4b,2a is an enzyme, and hence the term *C3 convertase* was coined.

It had been assumed that C5 convertase can occur only in particle-bound form, or that at least C3b must be surface bound in order to function as a helper molecule for the C5 convertase (278). However, fluid-phase C5 consumption by C4b,2a in the presence of C3 could be demonstrated, provided the enzyme was produced with iodine oxidized C2 (160). The phenomenon of fluid-phase C5 convertase activity was explained by the finding that C3b and C5 interact reversibly in solution, with the association constant for this reaction being $2 \times 10^6 \ M^{-1}$ at ionic strength 0.06 (94). Thus, if the concentrations of C3b and C5 are sufficiently high, complex formation will occur and cleavage of C5 by the C3 convertase will proceed.

Control of the C3/C5 Convertase

C4bp binds to C4b and allows I to degrade it to C4c and C4d (63). The normal concentration of C4bp in serum ($4 \times 10^{-7} \ M$) is greater than the single-site dissociation constant of the C4bp-C4 interaction ($0.8 \times 10^{-7} \ M$) (306). Under most conditions the concentration of C4bp greatly exceeds the small amounts of C4b generated by the activation of the classical pathway, and C4b is therefore readily bound and inactivated. The same applies to spontaneously formed C4(H_2O), in which the internal thioester is hydrolyzed. C4bp also dissociates C4b,C2 and enhances the spontaneous decay of C4b,2a (71). Activation of C1 by small amounts of immune complexes may lead to some consumption of C2 and C4, but it leads to very little turnover of C3. However, in serum depleted of C4bp, C3 consumption may go to completion under otherwise identical conditions. C4bp also controls the cell-bound C3 convertase, causing C2a to dissociate and displaying a much higher affinity for clustered cell-surface C4b than for fluid-phase C4b (62).

C4bp also may bind to C3b and serve as cofactor for I in its conversion to C3bi. However, the affinity of C4bp for C3b ($\sim 10^5 \ M^{-1}$) is much lower than that of H ($4.4 \times 10^6 \ M^{-1}$) (306). Conversely, H has been shown to have weak cofactor activity for the cleavage of C4b by I (189).

MEMBRANE-REGULATORY PROTEINS OF BOTH ACTIVATION PATHWAYS

Overview

CR1 (long known as the *immune adherence receptor*) and DAF control both C3/C5 convertases. Together they exercise vital functions in the protection of cellular elements of the blood against accidental attack by autologous complement. DAF inhibits C3 convertase formation (149)

and accelerates the decay of the assembled enzymes (175). CR1 serves as cofactor in the cleavage of C3b, C3bi, and C4b by I (92,147,150,225). Although DAF exhibits only negligible affinity for C3b and C4b (182), it does belong, on the basis of its chemical structure, to the family of C3b/C4b-binding proteins (14,152). CR1 and DAF differ not only in function, but also membrane orientation. CR1 is a transmembrane protein (108), whereas DAF is anchored in the lipid bilayer via phosphatidyl inositol (38,151). CR1 deficiency, limited to erythrocytes, has been observed in one individual and is not associated with apparent disease (227). However, DAF deficiency involving all types of blood cells constitutes one of the molecular defects underlying paroxysmal nocturnal hemoglobinuria (PNH) (176,192).

CR1

CR1 is a single-chain integral membrane glycoprotein that occurs as four different allotypes (160–250 kDa) (234). The partial primary structure of the F allotype deduced from cDNA sequences indicates that this protein may contain 30 short consensus repeats (SCR) (each 60–70 residues long), of which 23 have been sequenced (108). The SCR resemble similar sequences of other C3b/C4b-binding proteins. The only nonrepetitive sequences identified are located at the C-terminal region of the chain. This region contains a 25-residue membrane-spanning segment, which is followed by a 43-residue cytoplasmic sequence (108).

CR1 is present on erythrocytes, granulocytes, B lymphocytes, monocytes, macrophages, and dendritic reticulum cells. The number of CR1 molecules per erythrocyte ranges from 50 to 1,500 and is genetically determined. On leukocytes, this number may vary between 3,000 and 30,000, depending on the cell type and state of activation (224,234).

On erythrocytes, CR1 serves two important functions. It is the essential cofactor for I in the cleavage of C3bi to C3c and C3dg. It also is operative in the transport of circulating immune complexes by erythrocytes to liver macrophages and, thus, in the clearance of such complexes from the blood. The function of CR1 on white cells is described in Chapters 4 and 23.

DAF

The protein (~ 70 kDa) consists of a single chain that has a membrane-anchoring glycophospholipid attached to the C-terminal residue (38,151). The primary structure was deduced from cloned DAF cDNA that encodes a polypeptide consisting of 347 amino acid residues (14,152). Beginning at the N-terminus, the protein possesses four ~60-residue repeating units that are homologous to the repeating sequences in the C3b/C4b-binding proteins. This is followed by a serine- and threonine-rich region of ~70 residues and a concluding C-terminal stretch of 23 residues, constituting a hydrophobic transmembrane anchor sequence. This hydrophobic C-terminal domain appears to be removed during posttranslational processing and replaced with a phosphatidylinositol anchor (14).

DAF cDNA analysis revealed two classes of DAF mRNA, one probably derived from the other by a splicing event that induced a coding frame shift near the C-terminus (14). It was assumed that the spliced DAF mRNA, which accounts for 90% of DAF mRNA, encodes membrane DAF and the unspliced cDNA secreted DAF. Cells transfected with spliced or unspliced DAF cDNA produced DAF, but only those transfected with spliced DAF cDNA expressed DAF protein on the cell surface. A hydrophilic form of DAF has been described to occur in normal human urine.

The only activity DAF expresses is directed toward C3b,Bb and C4b,2a: It prevents assembly of the complexes, and it disassembles the formed enzymes. It has no cofactor activity for I action on C3b or C4b, and it does not function as a receptor, although DAF possesses a measurable affinity for C3b (but not for C4b) (182). It is not inhibitable on the human erythrocyte (E_H) surface by fluid-phase C3b dimer or C3b,Bb(Ni^{2+}), nor is DAF on E_H capable of controlling C3 convertase bound to another particle (188). This is in contradistinction to CR1, which binds fluid-phase C3b and can act as I-cofactor on C3b bound to another cell (148). However, DAF can be inhibited by C3b located on the same cell where just a few thousand molecules per cell have a significant effect. The regulatory efficiency of DAF on E_H is limited. The maximum velocity of enzyme inactivation was estimated to be 1,075 ± 103 (±SE) C3b,Bb(Mg^{2+})/E_H min^{-1} (188).

DAF provides more than 95% of the decay-accelerating activity on E_H, as experiments with anti-DAF and anti-CR1 have shown (192). Anti-DAF extended the half-life of C3b,Bb(Mg^{2+}) on E_H from 2 to 9 min at 22°C, which is the half-life of the enzyme in solution; it also extended the half-life of C3b,Bb(Mg^{2+}) on pronase-treated E_H's that have lost the DAF and CR1 function. Anti-CR1 had no such effect. However, in detergent solubilized E_H membranes, 40% of the decay-accelerating activity was due to CR1, and 60% was due to DAF (188). It is conceivable that the lack of expression of CR1 decay-accelerating activity in the intact E_H membrane is caused by restricted lateral mobility of CR1 relative to DAF.

The relative role of DAF and H in controlling C3b,Bb on E_H and other blood cells is puzzling. H at one-thousandth its concentration in serum was as effective as membrane-bound DAF in controlling C3b,Bb(Mg^{2+}) on

E_H (188). C3b,Bb(Mg^{2+}) on pronase-treated E_H had a half-life of 10 min at 22°C. To reduce it to 2 min, which is the half-life of the enzyme on untreated E_H, 0.4 μg/ml of H was sufficient.

THE MEMBRANE-ATTACK COMPLEX

Overview

Cell injury by complement occurs as a consequence of activation of either the classical or the alternative pathway on the surface of a cell. The "killer molecule" is the membrane-attack complex (MAC) (6,162,163,171). It constitutes a supramolecular organization that is composed of ~20 protein molecules and has a molecular weight of about 1.7 million. The complex has five precursors, namely C5, C6, C7, C8, and C9, which are hydrophilic glycoproteins with molecular weights ranging from 71,000 to 191,000. When C5 is cleaved by C5 convertase and nascent C5b (5b*) is produced, self-assembly of the MAC ensues: C5b* and C6 form a soluble and stable bimolecular complex that binds to C7 and induces it to express a metastable site through which the nascent complex (C5b-7*) can insert itself into membranes. Membrane-bound C5b-7 commits MAC assembly to a membrane site and constitutes the receptor for C8. The C5b-8 complex binds and polymerizes C9. During the assembly process the proteins undergo hydrophilic-amphiphilic transition. The fully assembled MAC contains one molecule each of C5b, C6, C7, and C8, with one or more molecules of C9. The end-product consists of the tetramolecular C5b-8 complex (~550 kDa) and tubular poly-C9 (~1,100 kDa) (Fig. 4).

The MAC forms transmembrane channels that vary in size, depending on the number of C9 molecules incorporated into the channel structure. In the absence of C9, C5b-8 forms a small functional channel of ~30-Å diameter. Tubular poly-C9, for which at least 12 C9 molecules are required, has a functional channel diameter of ~100 Å (290). Whereas poly-C9 is not essential for the lysis of erythrocytes or nucleated cells (140), it may be

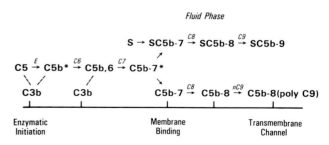

FIG. 4. Schematic representation of the assembly of the MAC at the surface of a target membrane and its control in the fluid phase by S-protein. (*) Metastable binding sites.

necessary for the killing of bacteria (102). In the electron microscope the MAC is visualized as a hollow cylinder and, inserted into a target membrane, it evokes the image of a 100-Å-wide circular membrane hole that is surrounded by a 50-Å-wide rim (91). These characteristic and well-known images of the MAC and the membrane lesions are by and large due to the tubular poly-C9 contained in the MAC (274).

Evidence has accumulated, strongly suggesting that the proteins participating in transmembrane channel formation are structurally interrelated. The notion of a complement supergene was first proposed in this context when a close linkage between the loci for C6 and C7 was demonstrated through family studies of their genetic polymorphism (117) and when C6 and C7 were described as similar proteins (208). Subsequently, antibodies directed to neoantigens on the MAC (110) were shown to detect apparently cross-reacting antigens on human killer lymphocytes in contact with target cells (263). Conversely, monoclonal antibodies specifically detecting target cells killed by lymphocytes cross-reacted with erythrocytes lysed by complement (280). It was logical to attempt the isolation of the cytolytic protein from human cytotoxic lymphocytes using anti-human C9 immunoadsorbent chromatography. Isolation was accomplished in this manner, and the protein was found to be immunochemically related to C9 (C9-related protein, C9RP) and to C8 (292,295).

Further exploration of these relationships disclosed that an antibody raised to a synthetic peptide corresponding to a limited sequence in C9 (residues 101–111) not only reacted with C9, but also reacted with the α chain of C8 (272). In fact, at the cDNA level, strong homologies have been established for the sequences of C9, C8α, and C8β (216). It has now become clear that the five proteins C6, C7, C8, C9, and C9RP (also called cytolysin, perforin, or pore-forming protein) share certain antigenic properties (273,289). Information on how extensive the sequence similarity is between these proteins will have to await the complete structural elucidation of C6, C7, and C9RP.

The Proteins

C5

The protein ($\sim$191 kDa) consists of two disulfide-linked chains, α ($\sim$115 kDa) and β ($\sim$75 kDa). The complete primary structure for murine C5 has been derived from cDNA sequence analysis (286). Pro-C5, which, like C3 and C4, has a β-α chain orientation, spans 1,640 amino acid residues. In the mature protein, the α chain comprises 1,001 residues, including 26 cysteine residues. The β chain contains three cysteine residues, and the exact total num-

ber of amino acid residues is not known because the N-terminus is blocked and therefore has not been sequenced. Extensive sequence homology was shown with C3 and C4 even in the domain corresponding to the thioester region. However, C5 lacks the critical cysteine and glutamine residues required for thioester formation (265). These residues have been replaced by serine and alanine, respectively (286). The same replacements were found in human C5. A human cDNA clone was isolated and found to contain coding sequence for the C-terminal 262-amino-acid residues of the β chain, the entire C5a sequence, and the N-terminal 98 residues of the α' chain (137). Human recombinant C5a has been expressed in *E. coli* and was found to be biologically active (54,138). C5a (11.2 kDa) and C5b ($\sim$180 kDa) arise physiologically when C5 convertase selectively cleaves the arginyl-leucine bond at position 74-75 of the α chain. C5a is one of the three anaphylatoxins and is a potent leukocyte chemotactic factor (90). C5b, in its nascent state, constitutes the nucleus in the assembly of the MAC. The concentration of C5 in normal serum is $\sim$70 μg/ml.

C6 and C7

C6 and C7 have similar physical and chemical properties (208), and a close linkage between the loci for both proteins has been demonstrated (117). Both are single-chain glycoproteins, and the reported molecular weights for C6 range from 104,800 to 128,000, with those for C7 ranging from 92,400 to 121,000 (208). Both proteins differ decisively in their reaction with 1% deoxycholate. Whereas the hemolytic activity and molecular properties of C6 are unaffected by treatment with this detergent for 1 hr at 37°C, C7 forms an amphiphilic dimer ($\sim$230 kDa) that is hemolytically inactive (212). This behavior of C7 has implications for the interaction of metastable C5b-7 with membranes. It has been claimed previously that C6 is a serine protease and that the enzyme activity is essential for C6 hemolytic activity (112). The enzyme hypothesis was supported by the observation that the α chain of C5 is cleaved within the acid-induced C(5,6)^a complex (76). It was subsequently shown that the C6-associated protease activity is due to thrombin and that it can be inactivated without impairment of C6 hemolytic activity. C(5,6)^a formed with protease-free C6 contains uncleaved C5 (17). The serum concentration of C6 and C7 is 50 to 70 μg/ml each.

C8

C8 (151 kDa) consists of three nonidentical chains; the α (64 kDa) and γ (22 kDa) chains are disulfide-linked, and the α-γ subunit is noncovalently associated with the β chain (64 kDa) (111). Both subunits are encoded by separate loci (1). The β chain possesses a specific recognition site for C5 (258), and the α chain possesses one for C9 (259). Serum contains $\sim$55 μg/ml of C8.

The amino acid sequence of C8 was established through isolation and sequencing of cDNA clones encoding C8α and C8β (216,217). Both exhibit considerable homology to each other and to C9. Both chains contain clusters of cysteine residues in the N- and C-terminal regions. The central portion of each chain features a stretch of $\sim$170 residues devoid of cysteine, which therefore is probably quite flexible. Within this region of the α chain, but not β chain, are two potential transmembrane segments of 10 to 11 amino acid residues (216,217).

C9

C9 ($\sim$71 kDa) is a single-chain glycoprotein with an amphiphilic organization of its primary structure (42,257). The structure has been derived from the sequence of C9 cDNA. The N-terminal half of the 537-amino-acid residue protein is predominantly hydrophilic, and the C-terminal half is considerably more hydrophobic. α-Thrombin cleaves C9 at a His-Gly bond in position 244-245, producing the hydrophilic C9a fragment ($\sim$34 kDa) and the hydrophobic C9b fragment ($\sim$37 kDa) (8). Both fragments remain noncovalently associated, and the cleaved molecule retains full cytolytic activity. When cleaved C9 was employed in MAC assembly on phospholipid vesicles containing membrane-restricted photoactivatable probes, photoactivation labeled C9b but not C9a, showing that the C-terminal half of C9 is involved in membrane insertion (96). However, epitope analysis using immuno-electron microscopy indicated no clear segregation of C9a and C9b in poly-C9 (41). The N-terminal half of C9 contains a 39-residue segment (76–116) that is homologous with the major repeat unit of the low-density lipoprotein receptor (257). This domain is cysteine-rich and is also homologous to cysteine-rich sequences in C8α and C8β (216,217). The concentration of C9 in serum is 50 to 60 μg/ml.

S-Protein

S-protein ($\sim$80 kDa) is the primary MAC inhibitor of serum (K_i = 39 μg/ml) (200,213). It binds to the metastable membrane-binding site of C5b-7 and allows binding of C8 and C9, but it prevents C9 polymerization (204). The protein was shown to be identical with vitronectin, which promotes cell attachment and binds glucosaminoglycans and proteoglycans (99,264). The serum concentration is $\sim$500 μg/ml.

Assembly of the MAC

Formation of Metastable C5b-7 and of the C8 Receptor

Proteolytic activation of C5 leads to generation of metastable C5b (C5b*), the labile binding site of which has specificity for C6. Bimolecular C5b,6 remains loosely bound to C3b on the target cell surface until it reacts with C7. The trimolecular complex then undergoes hydrophilic-amphiphilic transition (211), leaves the C3b holding position, and transfers to the surface of the membrane. It overcomes the charge barrier of the membrane by ionic interactions that probably involve its C5b,6 portion, and then it anchors itself firmly in the lipid bilayer by hydrophobic interactions primarily through its C7 subunit. The ability of C5b-7 to anchor itself in the membrane is a result of the acquisition of high-affinity phospholipid-binding sites (202). C5b-7 does not compromise membrane function as evidenced by lack of leakiness of lipid vesicles or erythrocytes. The lifetime of the transient binding site of C5b-7* has been estimated to be less than 10 msec (207).

Bound to single-bilayer phospholipid vesicles of 200- to 400-Å diameter, C5b-7 predominantly appeared as a V-shaped two-leaflet structure on electron microscopy, which extends $\sim$210 Å above the vesicle surface and is associated with the membrane through an $\sim$40-Å-long stalk (211). This structure is thought to be the dimer of C5b-7 because occasionally a single leaflet structure is visualized on the smallest vesicles, with this structure likely being the monomer. When C5b-7* is formed in the fluid phase, self-aggregation occurs and its cytolytic activity is lost. Soluble protein micelles are formed which exhibit a sedimentation rate of $\sim$36S. In the electron microscope the aggregates are imaged as flower-like structures in which the C5b-7 monomers remain clearly distinguishable and terminate in a pedicle at the center of the flower, indicating that the pedicellar regions are the sites of hydrophobic interactions (211).

The rate-limiting process in the binding of C5b-7 to phospholipid vesicles was the interaction of C5b,6 and C7, which displayed an activation energy of 37 kcal/mole (248). C5b-7 interacted with a variety of phospholipids tested. It showed a preference for small unilamellar phospholipid vesicles instead of large vesicles and also preferred vesicles with a high negative charge density. Considering that the major barrier for C5b-7 insertion may be penetration through the polar head groups of a lipid bilayer, selectivity might be explained by increased separation of head groups as a result of surface curvature and charge-charge repulsion. Vesicle-bound C5b-7 behaved like an integral membrane protein in that its dissociation from vesicles was <6.2 $\times$ 10^{-5} sec^{-1}.

Evidence has been reported showing that it is primarily

activated C7 that confers amphiphilicity on C5b-7*. Isolated C7, but not C5 or C6, has the propensity to undergo hydrophilic-amphiphilic transition, to aggregate, and to incorporate itself into lipid bilayers (212). Treatment of isolated C7 with 1% deoxycholate (DOC) at 37°C for 10 min resulted in complete loss of hemolytic activity and dimerization of the protein. The dimer possessed hydrophobic surface domains, as evidenced by its ability to bind ~82 moles of DOC per mole of dimer and by its prompt precipitation from solution on removal of the detergent. The most direct demonstration of the role of C7 as the donor of the binding site for C5b-7 was obtained by electron microscopy using colloidal gold particles coated with either C5b,6 or C7. When gold–C7 conjugates were treated with C5b,6, they showed finger-like protein structures protruding from their surface. However, when gold–C5b,6 conjugates were treated with C7, clusters of gold particles were visualized in which the individual particles were linked by proteinaceous material. This experiment was interpreted to indicate that C7, upon binding to C5b,6, becomes amphiphilic and interacts with other C7 molecules, thus aggregating C5b,6-coated particles (211).

The available information suggests that C5b,6 acts on C7 in the manner DOC does; i.e., it converts C7 to an activated state in which it expresses binding sites that are concealed in the native molecule. This leads to C5b-7 insertion into the membrane, which commits MAC assembly to a discrete membrane site. Insertion consists of nonspecific hydrophobic interaction between C7 and the hydrocarbon core of the membrane. Inserted C5b-7 constitutes an integral membrane protein that functions as a receptor for C8.

Structure and Function of C5b-8

Native C8 has no detectable affinity for membranes and is therefore entirely dependent on the mediating function of C5b-7, which determines the site of membrane attack. C8 binds to C5b-7 with its β chain, which possesses a specific recognition site for C5 (258). This initial contact probably brings a second site of the receptor into play which might be located on C7, enabling C8 to undergo the necessary conformational rearrangement to allow the α chain to penetrate into the hydrophobic core of the lipid bilayer.

The penetration of C5b-8 into the membrane and its influence on the order of the bilayer were measured on planar lipid bilayers doped with spin-labels using electron paramagnetic resonance spectroscopy (45). These studies showed that whereas C5b-7 interacted strongly with the ionic part of the bilayer and penetrated only slightly into the hydrophobic region, C5b-8 penetrated into the hydrophobic phase more deeply. Insertion caused an increase in disorder of the membrane lipids, i.e., the fatty acyl chains adopted a wider distribution of angles with respect to each other than they would in a normal bilayer structure. This reorientation of the ordered bilayer lipids into domains more micellar in nature is due to strong binding of phospholipid molecules to the inserted polypeptides of C5b-8.

The size of the C5b-8 channel was explored by performing kinetic sieving experiments with resealed erythrocyte ghosts using sucrose and inulin as markers (145). C5b-8 caused release of sucrose, which has a molecular diameter of 9 Å, but not of inulin, which has a diameter of 30 Å. Conductance changes across black lipid membranes suggested a channel diameter of 16 Å. Recently, the size of the C5b-8 channel was explored using the liposome swelling assay (290). The radius of the pore formed by C5b-8 assembled on liposomes was estimated to be between 11 and 15 Å. Solute flux could be inhibited by certain monoclonal anti-C8, as well as being slightly inhibited by one anti-C7, suggesting a channel composed of C8 with possible involvement of C7. Electron microscopy of C5b-8 bound to small phospholipid vesicles visualized monomeric C5b-8 as a 250-Å-long, 50- to 140-Å-wide, rod-like structure with a rather polymorphic appearance (162). Binding of C9 occurs via a recognition site of the α chain of C8 (259).

Structure and Function of C5b-9

The MAC is heterogeneous with respect to size and composition because of its variation in C9 content (205,276). The basic composition of the MAC is represented by the formula $C5b_1, C6_1, C7_1, C8_1, C9_n$, where n can vary between 1 and 18. Hence, the minimum molecular weight of the MAC ranges between 660,000 and 1,850,000.

Isolated C8 in solution has one C9 binding site, and C8-C9 association is reversible ($K_a \sim 10^7 M^{-1}$) (205); on the other hand, C5b-8 can mediate the binding of multiple C9 molecules, and that association is virtually irreversible ($K_a \sim 10^{11} M^{-1}$) (207). Light-scattering intensity measurements of the assembly of the MAC in the fluid phase (246) or on small unilamellar phospholipid vesicles (247) showed that one C9 molecule associated rapidly with each functional C5b-8 complex, which was followed by slower incorporation of the remaining C9 molecules. The activation energy for the slow phase of C9 association was 37 kcal/mole. The maximum ratio of C9:C5b-8 was 16 for the vesicle-bound MAC (247) and 14 for the fluid-phase complex (246). Thus, the mechanism of C5b-8-dependent C9 polymerization on vesicles is indistinguishable from that occurring in the fluid phase. Insertion of C9 into the membrane is therefore not a rate-limiting process. Binding of the first C9 molecule to C5b-8 might result in a slow conformational change of the bound C9 with exposure of hydrophobic regions that insert themselves into the membrane. The second C9 molecule binds directly to the activated first C9 molecule and is thereby induced to undergo the same conformational change. According to this model, C5b-8 behaves like activated C9, and C9 polymerization becomes independent of C5b-8 once the first C9 molecule has been activated (246).

The poly-C9 tubule of the membrane-bound MAC extends 120 Å above the surface of the membrane, it has an inner diameter of 100 Å, and it terminates at its upper hydrophilic end in a 30-Å-thick annulus that has an outer diameter of 200 Å (270,274). The C5b-8 subunit appears firmly attached to the poly-C9 tubule and extends 160 to 180 Å above its annulus as a 50- to 140-Å-wide elongated structure (275).

Because the structure of the MAC varies greatly with the C9/C5b-8 ratio, this ratio also determines the size of the transmembrane channel produced by C5b-9 as well as determining the electron microscopic appearance of the complex. As increasing numbers of C9 molecules are incorporated into the channel structure, its functional size increases from a diameter of ~30 Å (C5b-8) to ~100 Å (poly-C9) (290). When the MAC was assembled on vesicles or erythrocytes and the molar C9/C5b-8 ratio was 1 or 3, no poly-C9 was detectable by SDS-PAGE (276) and no complement membrane lesions were seen on electron microscopy (205). When this ratio was 6 or 12, the percentage of C9 present as poly-C9 was 35 and 72, respectively. At these ratios, discrete ring structures were observed on the cell surface by electron microscopy; these structures appeared unaggregated and well separated from each other. Obviously, SDS-resistant poly-C9 cannot be regarded as being an obligatory constituent of the MAC, and C5b-9 does not necessarily manifest itself as the typical ultrastructural membrane lesion.

C5b-8-Independent C9 Polymerization

Spontaneous poly-C9 formation is temperature- and metal-dependent and does not occur at 15°C, even at optimal environmental conditions (201,274). Examination of isolated C9 at 15°C by analytical ultracentrifugation revealed self-association of C9 which was metal-ion- and protein-concentration-dependent, ionic, and reversible (19). Because conditions promoting reversible C9-C9 interaction at 15°C allowed poly-C9 formation at 37°C, reversible oligomerization appears to be a prerequisite for tubular poly-C9 formation. C9 polymerization appears to involve constrained unfolding of the molecule, and unfolded C9 then associates laterally with itself; then

polymerization terminates with closure of the circular structure. Electron microscopy showed that the long axis of monomeric C9 is ~80 Å and that the height of the poly-C9 cylinder is 160 Å. To test the unfolding hypothesis, native C9 was treated with an excess of succinic anhydride at room temperature in order to substitute lysine residues with negatively charged, mutually repellent, succinyl groups. Native C9 and succinyl-C9 were then compared by analytical ultracentrifugation and molecular sieve chromatography on Sephacryl S-300. Succinylation reduced the sedimentation rate of C9 from 4.7S to 2.6S and increased the apparent molecular weight from 80,000 to 440,000. The pronounced increase in Stokes radius from 38 to 61 Å indicates a considerable increment in molecular asymmetry upon succinylation of C9 (19). This observation is consistent with the notion that C9 is capable of changing its conformation from globular to rod-like.

The assembling poly-C9 tubule is capable of inserting itself into the membrane of phospholipid vesicles and to render them leaky (274). To measure the size of the poly-C9 channel, the marker retention assay was used in which high-molecular-weight proteins of defined molecular diameter are entrapped in lipid vesicles (290). Preformed poly-C9 was incorporated into the membrane of the vesicles during their preparation. Alcohol dehydrogenase, which has a Stokes radius of 45 Å, escaped through the poly-C9 channel, whereas C3, which has a Stokes radius of 51 Å, did not. The functional diameter of the poly-C9 channel is therefore between 90 and 102 Å, which is in excellent agreement with the electron microscopic image. Whereas spontaneously forming poly-C9 is capable of inserting into lipid bilayer membranes, it appears unable to attack cell membranes. C5b-8 is required for such attack, and it allows polymerization in the absence of Me^{2+} and enhances the rate of poly-C9 formation 10,000-fold (276). However, the activation energy, derived from light-scattering intensity measurements, was found virtually identical for C5b-8-dependent and -independent poly-C9 formation (37 and 41 kcal/mole, respectively) (246). This finding suggests that the molecular mechanism of C9 polymerization is identical in the presence or absence of C5b-8.

Thrombin-cleaved C9 (C9a-b) was reported to be unable to form tubular poly-C9 but was found, instead, to polymerize to string-like aggregates (32). However, this claim was refuted by the demonstration that C9a-b, under defined conditions, does polymerize into the typical, SDS-resistant tubular structures (41).

Control of MAC Formation by S-Protein in Fluid Phase

The S-protein of plasma competes with membrane lipids for the metastable binding site of C5b-7; and by binding to the complex, it prevents its attachment to the cell surface. The inhibition constant, K_i, is 39 μg/ml, which is less than one-tenth of the plasma concentration of the protein (204). Its function appears to be to protect cells adjacent to the site of complement activation from accidental attack. The resultant SC5b-7 complex contains three molecules of S-protein and has a sedimentation rate of 18.5S and a molecular weight of 668,000. The hydrophilic complex binds C8 and three molecules of C9 to form SC5b-8 and SC5b-9, the molecular weight of the latter being 1,030,000 (203). All three complexes contain neoantigens that are not detectable in the precursor proteins and that are distinct from the neoantigens of poly-C9. In addition to blocking the membrane binding site, S-protein also prevents polymerization of C9 (204).

Control of MAC Channel Formation by Membrane-Bound Homologous Restriction Factor

It is known that complement is much more efficient in lysing heterologous erythrocytes than it is in lysing homologous or autologous red cells. The phenomenon has been referred to as *homologous restriction of complement-mediated hemolysis* and has been attributed variously to interference of an unknown erythrocyte membrane constituent with the action of C8 or C9 (77).

Recent work led to the isolation of a protein from membranes of human erythrocytes that exhibits marked affinity for C9 (293). It was capable of incorporating into the lipid bilayer of liposomes, and in this form it was active in inhibiting channel formation by C5b-8 and C5b-9 as well as in polymerizing C9. Antibody produced to this membrane protein caused a 20-fold increase in reactive lysis of human erythrocytes by isolated C5b,6, C7, C8, and C9. The antibody did not affect C5b-7 uptake but enhanced C9 binding to the target cell membrane. The antibody effect was not seen when C8 and C9 of other species were tested. The protein was therefore termed *homologous restriction factor* (HRF) (293).

HRF, as first isolated, was found to be a 38-kDa protein. Anti-38-kDa HRF, however, detected in immunoblots of fresh erythrocyte membranes primarily a 65-kDa protein (293). This observation suggested that the 38-kDa protein was an active fragment of the 65-kDa membrane HRF. It also related HRF to the C8-binding protein described by others (233). Subsequent preparations using rabbit anti-HRF immunoadsorbent columns consisted of the 65-kDa HRF. Being a membrane protein, HRF is not soluble in aqueous solvents, with at least 0.02% DOC being required to prevent precipitation. The protein is detectable also on human platelets, polymorphonuclear leukocytes, monocytes, and lymphocytes. A water-soluble form of HRF (65 kDa) has been isolated from human urine (291). Isolated

membrane HRF could be incorporated into sheep erythrocytes. Subsequent reactive lysis of HRF-bearing sheep erythrocytes could be almost completely suppressed by ~8500 HRF molecules per cell (294).

The abnormal erythrocytes of patients with paroxysmal nocturnal hemoglobinuria (PNH) are deficient in DAF, the cell-membrane-associated complement-regulatory protein that accelerates the spontaneous decay of the classical and the alternative C3 convertase and inhibits assembly of these enzymes (176,192). DAF deficiency explains the markedly extended half-life of C3 convertase on the surface of PNH cells, as compared to normal cells, and therefore, at least in part, explains the susceptibility of PNH erythrocytes to lysis in serum acidified to pH 6.4. However, DAF deficiency does not account for the enhanced sensitivity of PNH erythrocytes to reactive lysis by C5b-9 (87,223). Both C9 binding and C9 polymerization have been reported to be abnormally high on PNH erythrocytes (243). When abnormal PNH cell membranes were recently analyzed for HRF, the patients who were tested lacked HRF completely (297). Incubation of the abnormal cells with radiolabeled isolated HRF resulted in firm association of HRF with the cells. Approximately 1,000 molecules of HRF per cell reduced the characteristic susceptibility of these cells to reactive lysis by C5b-9 to nearly normal levels. These findings suggest that HRF deficiency constitutes an additional molecular defect in PNH (297).

Killing of Nucleated Cells by the MAC as a Function of Its Molecular Composition

Nucleated cells are capable of defense against attack by complement (157,215). The MAC causes a rapid increase in intracellular free calcium ion concentration long before cell lysis becomes detectable, thereby activating certain cellular functions. Cell defense has been attributed to enhanced cellular metabolic activity resulting in inactivation of complement channels by shedding and internalization. Studying recovery from complement attack employing human neutrophils, vesiculation was detected as early as 1 min after initiation of the reaction (157). The plasma membrane vesicles were covered with classical complement lesions, and the molar ratio of vesicle-associated C9 and C8 was 12:1. The irreversible phase of MAC-mediated nucleated cell damage may be due to activation of Ca^{2+}-dependent, membrane bound phospholipases leading to lethal disruption of cellular membranes (271).

Because there exists a spectrum of channels of different size as a result of variation of C9 multiplicity in the MAC, work was conducted to determine the molecular conditions that lead to complement-mediated killing of nucleated cells with respect to C8, C9, and poly-C9. The questions addressed were: (a) Is C5b-8 attack on nucleated cells sufficient for killing? (b) Is tubular poly-C9 essential for the killing of cells? (c) Which are the conditions of complement attack that allow cell recovery? Human M21 melanoma cells were employed as targets.

The following results were obtained (140): (a) C5b-8 was sufficient to cause functional transmembrane channel formation, as determined by ^{86}Rb release and propidium iodide (PI) uptake. Cell killing was effected at high C5b-8 density in the absence of C9 with more than 5×10^5 C5b-8 per cell, as evidenced by ^{51}Cr release; ~3 million bound C5b-8 per M21 cell caused 90% lysis in 90 min. (b) With nonlytic numbers of C5b-8 (4.7×10^5/cell), >90% killing ensued at a C9:C8 ratio of 2.8:1, at which ~9,000 poly-C9 per cell were formed; also, 50% killing ensued at a ratio of 1:1, at which ~1,000 SDS-resistant poly-C9 structures could be detected by SDS polyacrylamide gel electrophoresis. When the MAC was assembled on the M21 cells at 0°C, consisting of C5b-8$_1$9$_1$ (7), and unbound C9 was removed before incubation at 37°C, killing was similar to that observed when poly-C9 formation was allowed to occur (140). Thus, MAC lytic efficiency toward M21 cells may be enhanced by, but does not depend on, poly-C9 formation. (c) Although C8 binding and functional channel formation (PI uptake) were nearly simultaneous, C5b-8-dependent cytolysis showed a temporal lag, and a proportion of the channel bearing cells was capable of regaining membrane integrity. Membrane permeability for PI was maximal after 30 min of C5b-8 attack and markedly decreased thereafter and reached a constant level at 90 min of incubation, indicating channel elimination. Recovery by 90 min was between 55% and 64% under conditions at which 45% to 55% of cells were PI-permeable at 30 min (140).

These results indicate that M21 cells (and presumably other metabolically active cells) can be killed by C5b-8 and suggest that killing with nonlytic numbers of C8 molecules is optimized by amounts of C9 producing only few or no poly-C9 structures. Killing by C5b-8 has also been observed with human U937 histiocytes (158) and *Giardia lamblia* trophozoites (40). Thus, tubular poly-C9 is not an essential requirement for the killing of nucleated cells.

MOLECULAR MECHANISM OF LYMPHOCYTE-MEDIATED CYTOTOXICITY: THE CYTOLYTIC C9-RELATED PROTEIN

Overview

The molecular mechanism that cytotoxic lymphocytes utilize to kill target cells has not been fully elucidated. It was shown that cytotoxic lymphocytes produce discrete functional pores in the membranes of target cells (252). Also, antibodies directed to the neoantigens of the MAC were found to react with human lymphocytes that were in the process of killing their targets, suggesting antigenic cross-reactivity between the MAC and lymphocyte constituents possibly involved in the cytotoxic reaction (263). Subsequently, killing lymphocytes were shown to leave an electron microscopically detectable lesion on the membranes of target cells that resembled the MAC or poly-C9 (43). Such ultrastructural circular membrane lesions have been observed on cells killed by human (43,133,295), murine (198), and rat (9) lymphocytes. The pore-forming activity was located to the cytoplasmic granules of rat (79), murine (199), and human (295) lymphocytes. The protein responsible for pore formation was isolated from murine T cells and was shown to have a molecular weight of 66,000 and 72,000 to 75,000, respectively (142,206). The cytolytic protein was also isolated from human cytotoxic lymphocytes, in this case by anti-human C9 immunoadsorbence, and was found to be a 70-kDa protein (292,295). Because of its cross-reaction with C9, it was called *C9-related protein* (C9RP), a term obviously synonomous with lymphopore, cytolysin (78), perforin (198), and pore-forming protein (133). Using monoclonal antibodies to the "plug" protein of human lymphocytes, a cross-reaction with human complement was demonstrated (280).

Killing requires effector-target cell contact (78,80); after contact is achieved, the microtubule organizing center and the Golgi apparatus of cytotoxic T lymphocytes (CTL) and of natural killer cells (NK) are repositioned to face the contact area with the target cell (67,116). Cell polarization might serve to direct the cytoplasmic granules toward the contact site and to allow their contents to be secreted by exocytosis into the narrow spaces between effector and target cell. Under the influence of calcium, functional transmembrane channels are then formed in the target membrane as a result of insertion and polymerization of C9RP. The subsequent steps may involve calcium influx into the target cell or may involve its intracellular release with complex biochemical consequences possibly involving target cell excitation (268).

Although the channel produced by C9RP is sufficient to kill a target cell, the question has been asked as to whether killing lymphocytes introduce into the target cell a cytotoxin or enzyme that accelerates cell killing. Evidence has been presented showing that CTL-mediated lysis involves internal disintegration of the target cell with nuclear damage and DNA fragmentation and not simply colloid osmotic lysis. Using human Raji cells and mouse P815 mastocytoma cells as target cells and human or mouse cytotoxic lymphocytes, one study concluded that the pattern and extent of DNA degradation in lysed cells was determined by the target cell, suggesting that DNA degradation proceeds through activation of target cell endonucleases (75). It is not known whether recently described cytotoxic T-lymphocyte-specific serine proteases are involved in this activation process (68,135).

An overall similarity between the molecular mechanisms underlying complement- and lymphocyte-mediated cytotoxicity has become apparent. The spatial prerequisites in the case of complement are that the molecules of the recognition and activation units become physically, in part covalently, attached to the target cells. In the case of cytotoxic lymphocytes, close effector-cell–target-cell contact is required. The next step in complement cytotoxicity is generation of C5 convertase on the target cell surface, the enzyme that catalyzes the initiation of MAC self-assembly. The lymphocyte undergoes polarization within the cytoplasm, and it prepares the final attack by secretion of cytoplasmic granule contents into the intercellular space. Then, in both circumstances, transmembrane channels are formed in the target membrane by protein polymerization.

Although C9 and C9RP are similar (probably homologous proteins) and may be analogous in functional aspects, they differ in that isolated C9RP is cytotoxic by itself, whereas isolated C9 is not. Under conditions promoting homopolymerization, C9RP kills cells and C9 does not. To exert its cytotoxic effect, C9 requires target-cell-bound C5b-8. An important structural difference must be responsible for this differential behavior of the two proteins.

Isolation of the Cytolytic C9RP from Human Large Granular Lymphocytes

A 70-kDa protein was isolated from cytotoxic human large granular lymphocytes (LGL) and was shown to have cytolytic activity (292,295). In the presence of Ca^{2+}, the isolated protein efficiently killed, in 4 hr ^{51}Cr release-assay, K562 cells, human melanoma cells, Raji cells, and cells of a variety of human cancer cell lines. Usually 0.8 μg of protein was sufficient to effect 50% killing of 6.25×10^4 cells in a 200-μl reaction volume. The protein was demonstrated to be immunochemically related to C9, suggesting that C9RP and C9 share homology in primary structure and have a common evolutionary ancestry. Initially, C9RP was isolated by affinity chromatography employing anti-human C9-Sepharose, either from purified cytoplasmic granules of cultured human LGL or from whole cell lysates. The cells were isolated from healthy blood donors and maintained in IL-2-dependent cultures. The isolation procedure is now utilizing anti-C9RP immunoadsorbance. The immunochemical cross-reactivity of C9 with C9RP was 3% to 4% using a murine anti-C9RP antiserum. Early evidence suggested that C9RP is related also to C8 (295), and it is now clear that this relationship extends to C6, C7 (273,289), and HRF (291).

Certain murine monoclonal antibodies to C9RP and to C9 inhibited killing of K562 cells by human LGL (295). Killed target cells identified by PI staining and isolated by fluorescence-activated cell sorting exhibited clusters of circular membrane lesions that resembled poly-C9 in appearance. They differed from poly-C9 in that their size varied from 40 to 160 Å in diameter (Fig. 5). The inner diameter of the smaller circular structures ranged from 35 to 75 Å, with a maximum at 60 Å, and that of the larger ones ranged from 100 to 165 Å. Polymerized C9RP could be incorporated into liposomes and, as such, gave rise to channels of two different sizes. The smaller channel had a functional diameter of 50 to 90 Å, and the larger one had a functional diameter of more than 102 Å (295). Using ^{125}I-C9RP, it was found that a high multiplicity of specifically bound molecules per cell was required for effective killing of K562 cells or Raji cells. Considering the large number of C9RP molecules bound to the target cells, the circular lesions visualized by electron microscopy were sparse, suggesting that a large proportion of molecules was bound in oligomeric form.

Isolation of the Cytolytic C9RP from OKT3-Activated Human Peripheral Blood Mononuclear Cells

T lymphocytes of peripheral human blood are resting cells that are virtually noncytolytic. They can be stimulated by the anti-CD3 monoclonal antibody OKT3 to undergo proliferation (284). After 3 to 4 days of OKT3 stimulation, these cells become potent killer cells (CTL) (104,105). The cytotoxic potential of these CTL can be directed toward target cells by cell-bridging antibody conjugates with anti-target-cell and anti-CD3 specificity overcoming MHC restrictions (105,134,195). Peripheral blood mononuclear cells (PBMC) were depleted of $CD16^+$ cells so that they consisted largely of $CD4^+$ and $CD8^+$ cells and were activated with OKT3 for 3 days. Using antibody to C9RP isolated from LGL linked to Sepharose, a cytolytic 70-kDa protein was isolated from the CTL (296). By ELISA the isolated protein and C9RP of LGL reacted to the same extent with the anti-C9RP. The cytolytic activity of the CTL protein toward K562 or M21 human melanoma cells was comparable to that of C9RP of LGL. It was concluded that the cytolytic protein of OKT3-activated CTL is identical with C9RP of IL-2-stimulated LGL.

Induction of C9RP Synthesis and Cytotoxicity in Human Lymphocytes

After it was established that C9RP is the cytolytic protein of both types of human killer lymphocytes, it was possible to study induction of C9RP synthesis upon lymphocyte activation and to correlate C9RP content with

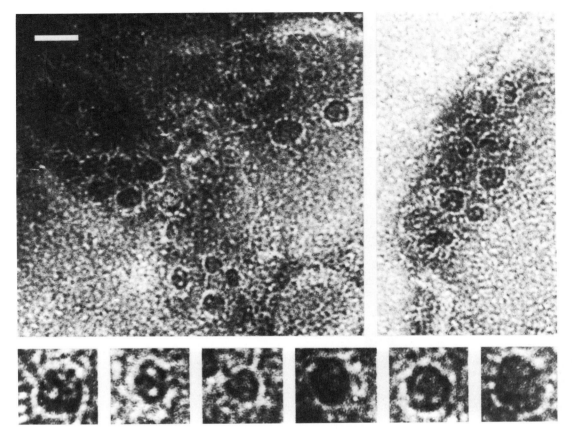

FIG. 5. Electron microscopic analysis of the circular lesions on the membranes of K562 cells killed by C9RP isolated from human LGL. The membranes were treated with trypsin and chymotrypsin and were stained with uranyl formate. The inner diameter of the circular structures ranged from 104 to 166 Å.

expression of cellular cytotoxicity in subpopulations of PBMC (141). Synthesis was induced in resting peripheral T lymphocytes by incubation of PBMC with OKT3 or IL-2 for several days. Resting CTL, which exhibit no cytotoxic activity, contained little or no C9RP. Comparison of cellular cytotoxicity and C9RP content at various time points during activation yielded a coefficient of correlation $r = 0.92$. Since isolated C9RP is cytolytic, these observations indicate that the cytotoxic potential of killer lymphocytes depends, at least in part, on C9RP. Unlike CTL, it was found that freshly isolated, unstimulated Leu 19+ NK cells had a high content of C9RP ($\sim 2.5 \times 10^6$ molecules per cell), which is consistent with their known cytotoxic activity. In OKT3-activated CD8+ cells, C9RP increased from barely detectable at day 0 to $\sim 3 \times 10^6$ molecules per cell at day 3, with a corresponding increase in lysis of human melanoma cells mediated by anti-CD3-anti-melanoma antibody conjugates. IL-2-stimulated CD8+ cells showed similar increases, but cytotoxicity was conjugate-independent. Activated CD4+ cells showed minimal increase in C9RP content (141).

Inhibition of C9RP Cytolytic Activity by HRF

Because of certain structural and functional similarities between C9RP and C9, it was tested whether HRF might affect the function of human killer lymphocytes. The antibody-dependent cellular cytotoxicity reaction (ADCC) was chosen with human LGL as effectors and erythrocytes as targets. Membrane HRF was found to bind readily to sheep erythrocytes as well as to PNH erythrocytes and to retain its activity. Using sensitized sheep erythrocytes bearing 1,000 to 3,000 HRF per cell, ADCC was reduced by 62% in a 4-hr cytotoxicity assay. Lysis of sensitized PNH erythrocytes by LGL was similarly suppressed by HRF incorporation (294). Further, lysis of sheep erythrocytes by isolated C9RP could be inhibited by cell-bound HRF (294). These findings suggest that HRF inhibits channel formation not only by C5b-9, but also by cytotoxic lymphocytes. They also suggest that HRF can interact directly with C9RP, as it does with C8 and C9. It is unknown at present whether this interaction is biologically significant. It is conceivable that HRF is operative in self-protection of cytotoxic lymphocytes.

ACKNOWLEDGMENTS

This chapter was formerly Publication No. 4847-IMM from the Department of Immunology, Research Institute of Scripps Clinic. This work was supported by Grants AI 17354, HL 07195, and HL 16411 from the National Institutes of Health.

REFERENCES

1. Alper, C. A., Marcus, D., Raum, D., Petersen, B. H., and Spira, T. J. (1983): Genetic polymorphism in C8 β-chains. Evidence for two unlinked genetic loci for the eighth component of human complement (C8). *J. Clin. Invest.,* 72:1526–1531.
2. Alsenz, J., Schulz, T. F., Lambris, J. D., Sim, R. B., and Dierich, M. P. (1985): Structural and functional analysis of the complement component factor H with the use of different enzymes and monoclonal antibodies to factor H. *Biochem. J.,* 232:841–850.
3. Bartholomew, R. M., Esser, A. F., and Müller-Eberhard, H. J. (1978): Lysis of oncornaviruses by human serum: Isolation of the viral complement (C1) receptor and identification as P15E. *J. Exp. Med.,* 147:844–853.
4. Belt, K. T., Carroll, M. C., and Porter, R. R. (1984): The structural basis of the multiple forms of human complement component C4. *Cell,* 36:907–914.
5. Bentley, D. R. (1986): The primary structure of human complement component C2. Homology to two unrelated protein families. *Biochem. J.,* 239:339–345.
6. Bhakdi, S., and Tranum-Jensen, J., (1983): Membrane damage by complement. *Biochim. Biophys. Acta,* 737:343–372.
7. Bhakdi, S., and Tranum-Jensen, J. (1986): C5b-9 assembly: Average binding of one C9 molecule to C5b-8 without poly-C9 formation generates a stable transmembrane pore. *J. Immunol.,* 136:2999–3005.
8. Biesecker, G., Gerard, C., and Hugli, T. E. (1981): An amphiphilic structure of the ninth component of human complement. Evidence from analysis of fragments produced by α-thrombin. *J. Biol. Chem.,* 257:2584–2590.
9. Blumenthal, R., Millard, P. J., Henkart, M. P., Reynolds, C. W., and Henkart, P. A. (1984): Liposomes as targets for granule cytolysin from cytotoxic large granular lymphocyte tumors. *Proc. Natl. Acad. Sci. USA,* 81:5551–5555.
10. Bock, S. C., Skriver, K., Nielsen, E., Thogersen, H.-C., Wiman, B., Donaldson, V. H., Eddy, R. L., Marrinan, J., Radziejewska, R., Huber, R., Shows, T. B., and Magnusson, S. (1986): Human C1 inhibitor: Primary structure, cDNA cloning and chromosomal localization. *Biochemistry,* 25:4292–4301.
11. Calcott, M. A., and Müller-Eberhard, H. J. (1972): C1q protein of human complement. *Biochemistry,* 11:3443–3450.
12. Campbell, R. D., and Porter, R. R. (1983): Molecular cloning and characterization of the gene coding for human complement protein factor B. *Proc. Natl. Acad. Sci. USA,* 80:4464–4468.
13. Campbell, R. D., Bentley, D. R., and Morley, B. J. (1984): The factor B and C2 genes. *Philos. Trans. R. Soc. Lond. (Biol.),* 306:367–378.
14. Caras, I. W., Davitz, M. A., Rhee, L., Weddell, G., Martin, D. W., Jr., and Nussenzweig, V. (1987): Cloning of decay-accelerating factor suggests novel use of splicing to generate two proteins. *Nature,* 325:545–549.
15. Carroll, M. C., Campbell, R. D., Bentley, D. R., and Porter, R. R. (1984): A molecular map of the human major histocompatibility complex class III region linking complement genes C4, C2 and factor B. *Nature,* 307:237–241.
16. Catterall, C. F., Lyons, A., Sim, R. B., Day, A. J., and Harris, J. R. (1986): Characterization of the primary amino acid sequence of human complement control protein factor I from an analysis of cDNA clones. Personal communication.
17. Chakravarti, D. N., and Müller-Eberhard, H. J. (1985): Purification of human C6 to homogeneity: Lack of evidence of serine protease nature. *Complement,* 2:16 (abstract).
18. Chapitis, J., and Lepow, I. H. (1976): Multiple sedimenting species of properdin in human serum and interaction of purified properdin with the third component of complement. *J. Exp. Med.,* 143:241–257.
19. Chiu, F. J., Ziccardi, R. J., and Müller-Eberhard, H. J. (1985): Reversible self-association of monomeric C9 preceding poly C9 formation and dissociation of poly C9 into monomeric C9. *Fed. Proc.,* 44(6):1874 (abstract).
20. Christie, D. L., and Gagnon, J. (1983): Amino acid sequence of the Bb fragment from complement factor B. Sequence of the major cytogen bromide-cleavage peptide (CB-II) and completion of the sequence of the Bb fragment. *Biochem. J.,* 209:61–70.
21. Chung, L. P., Bentley, D. R., and Reid, K. B. M. (1985): Molecular cloning and characterization of the cDNA coding for C4b-binding protein, a regulatory protein of the classical pathway of the human complement system. *Biochem. J.,* 230:133–141.
22. Colomb, M. G., Arlaud, G. J., and Villiers, C. L. (1984): Structure and activation of C1: Current concepts. *Complement,* 1:69–80.
23. Cooper, Neil R. (1985): The classical complement pathway: Activation and regulation of the first complement component. *Adv. Immunol.,* 37:151–216.
24. Cooper, N. R., and Müller-Eberhard, H. J. (1968): A comparison of methods for the molecular quantitation of the fourth component of human complement. *Immunochemistry,* 5:155–169.
25. Cooper, N. R., and Müller-Eberhard, H. J. (1970): The reaction mechanism of human C5 in immune hemolysis. *J. Exp. Med.,* 132:775–793.
26. Czop, J., and Nussenzweig, V. (1976): Studies on the mechanism of solubilization of immune precipitates by serum. *J. Exp. Med.,* 143:615–630.
27. Daha, M. R., Fearon, D. T., and Austen, K. F. (1976): Requirements for formation of alternative pathway C5 convertase. *J. Immunol.,* 117:630–634.
28. Dahlback, B., and Müller-Eberhard, H. J. (1984): Ultrastructure of C4b-binding protein fragments formed by limited proteolysis using chymotrypsin. *J. Biol. Chem.,* 259:11631–11634.
29. Dahlback, B., and Stenflo, J. (1981): High molecular weight complex in human plasma between vitamin K-dependent protein S and complement component C4b binding protein. *Proc. Natl. Acad. Sci. USA,* 78:2512–2516.
30. Dahlback, B., Smith, C. A., and Müller-Eberhard, H. J. (1983): Visualization of human C4b-binding protein and its complexes with vitamin K-dependent protein S and complement protein C4b. *Proc. Natl. Acad. Sci. USA,* 80:3461–3465.
31. Dalmasso, A. P., and Müller-Eberhard, H. J. (1966): Hemolytic activity of lipoprotein-depleted serum and effect of certain anions on complement. *J. Immunol.,* 97:680–685.
32. Dankert, J. R., and Esser, A. F. (1985): Proteolytic modification of human complement protein C9: Loss of poly (C9) and circular lesion formation without impairment of function. *Proc. Natl. Acad. Sci. USA,* 82:2128–2132.
33. Daoudaki, M. E., Becherer, J. D., and Lambris, J. D. (1984): Localization of the P and C5 binding sites on the third component of complement. *Fed. Proc.,* 46:1024 (abstract).
34. Davis, A. E. (1981): The C3b inactivator of the human complement system: Homology with serine proteases. *FEBS Lett.,* 134:147.
35. Davis, A. E., III, and Lachmann, P. J. (1984): Bovine conglutinin is a collagen-like protein. *Biochemistry,* 23:2139–2144.
36. Davis, A. E., Harrison, R. A., and Lachmann, P. J. (1984): Physiologic inactivation of fluid phase C3b: Isolation and structural analysis of C3c, C3dg (α2D), and C3g. *J. Immunol.,* 132:1960–1966.
37. Davis, A. E., Whitehead, A. S., Harrison, R. A., Dauphinais, A., Bruns, G. A. P., Cicardi, M., and Rosen, F. S. (1986): Human

inhibitor of the first component of complement C1: Characterization of cDNA clones and localization of the gene to chromosome II. *Proc. Natl. Acad. Sci. USA,* 83:3161–3165.

38. Davitz, M. A., Low, M. G., and Nussenzweig, V. (1986): Release of decay-accelerating factor (DAF) from the cell membrane by phosphatidylinositol-specific phospholipase C (PIPLC). *J. Exp. Med.,* 163:1150–1161.

39. deBruijn, M. H. L., and Fey, G. H. (1985): Human complement component C3: cDNA coding sequence and derived primary structure. *Proc. Natl. Acad. Sci. USA,* 82:708–712.

40. Deguchi, M., Gillin, F. D., and Gigli, I. (1987): Mechanism of killing of *Giardia lamblia* trophozoites by complement. *J. Clin. Invest. (in press).*

41. DiScipio, R. G., and Hugli, T. E. (1985): The architecture of complement component C9 and poly (C9). *J. Biol. Chem.,* 260:14802–14809.

42. DiScipio, R. G., Gehring, M. R., Podack, E. R., Kan, C. C., Hugli, T. E., and Fey, G. H. (1984): Nucleotide sequence of cDNA and derived amino acid sequence of human complement component C9. *Proc. Natl. Acad. Sci. USA,* 81:7298–7302.

43. Dourmashkin, R. R., Deteix, P., Simone, C. B., and Henkart, P. (1980): Electron microscopic demonstration of lesions in target cell membranes associated with antibody-dependent cellular cytotoxicity. *Clin. Exp. Immunol.,* 42:554–560.

44. Edwards, M. S., Nicholson-Weller, A., Baker, C. J., and Kasper, D. L. (1980): The role of specific antibody in alternative complement pathway-mediated opsonophagocytosis of type III, group B streptococcus. *J. Exp. Med.,* 151:1275–1287.

45. Esser, A. F., Kolb, W. P., and Podack, E. R. (1979): Reorganization of lipid bilayers by complement: A possible mechanism for membranolysis. *Proc. Natl. Acad. Sci. USA,* 76:1410–1414.

46. Farries, T. C., Finch, J. T., Lachmann, P. J., and Harrison, R. A. (1987): Resolution and analysis of "native" and "activated" properdin. *Biochem. J. (in press).*

47. Fearon, D. T. (1977): Purification of C3b inactivator and demonstration of its two polypeptide chain structure. *J. Immunol.,* 119:1248–1252.

48. Fearon, D. T. (1978): Regulation by membrane sialic acid of β1H-dependent decay-dissociation of amplification C3 convertase of the alternative complement pathway. *Proc. Natl. Acad. Sci. USA,* 75:1971–1975.

49. Fearon, D. T. (1979): Regulation of the amplification C3 convertase of human complement by an inhibitory protein isolated from human erythrocyte membrane. *Proc. Natl. Acad. Sci. USA,* 76:5867–5871.

50. Fearon, D. T., and Austen, K. F. (1975): Properdin: Binding to C3b and stabilization of the C3b-dependent C3 convertase. *J. Exp. Med.,* 142:856–863.

51. Fearon, D. T., and Austen, K. F. (1975): Properdin: Binding to C3b and stabilization of the C3b-dependent C3 convertase. *J. Exp. Med.,* 142:856–863.

52. Fearon, D. T., and Austen, K. F. (1977): Activation of the alternative complement pathway with rabbit erythrocytes by circumvention of the regulatory action of endogenous control proteins. *J. Exp. Med.,* 146:22–33.

53. Fearon, D. T., and Austen, K. F. (1977): Activation of the alternative complement pathway due to resistance of zymosan-bound amplification convertase to endogenous regulatory mechanisms. *Proc. Natl. Acad. Sci. USA,* 74:1683–1687.

54. Fey, G. H., Kan, C. C., Fukuoka, Y., and Hugli, T. E. (1985): Expression of recombinant human C5a anaphylatoxins in *Escherichia coli. Complement,* 2:24–25.

55. Fingeroth, J. D., Wells, J. J., Tedder, T. F., Strominger, J. L., Bird, P. A., and Fearon, D. T. (1984): Epstein-Barr virus receptor of human B lymphocytes is the C3d receptor CR2. *Proc. Natl. Acad. Sci. USA,* 81:4510–4516.

56. Fishelson, Z., and Müller-Eberhard, H. J. (1982): C3 convertase of human complement: Enhanced formation and stability of the enzyme generated with nickel instead of magnesium. *J. Immunol.,* 129:2603–2607.

57. Fishelson, Z., and Müller-Eberhard, H. J. (1984): Residual he-

molytic and proteolytic activity expressed by Bb after decay-dissociation of C3b,Bb. *J. Immunol.,* 132:1425–1429.

58. Fishelson, Z., Pangburn, M. K., and Müller-Eberhard, H. J. (1983): C3 convertase of the alternative complement pathway: Demonstration of an active, stable C3b,Bb(Ni) complex. *J. Biol. Chem.,* 258:7411–7415.

59. Fishelson, Z., Pangburn, M. K., and Müller-Eberhard, H. J. (1984): Characterization of the initial C3 convertase of the alternative pathway of human complement. *J. Immunol.,* 132:1430–1434.

60. Frade, R., Barel, M., Ehlin-Henriksson, B., and Klein, G. (1985): gp140, the C3d receptor of human B lymphocytes, is also the Epstein-Barr virus receptor. *Proc. Natl. Acad. Sci. USA,* 82:1490–1493.

61. Fries, L. F., Gaither, T. A., Hammer, C. H., and Frank, M. M. (1984): C3b covalently bound to IgG demonstrates a reduced rate of inactivation by factors H and I. *J. Exp. Med.,* 160:1640–1655.

62. Fujita, T., and Tamura, N. (1983): Interaction of C4-binding protein with cell-bound C4b. A quantitative analysis of binding and the role of C4-binding protein in proteolysis of cell-bound C4b. *J. Exp. Med.,* 157:1239–1251.

63. Fujita, T., Gigli, I., and Nussenzweig, V. (1978): Human C4-binding protein. II. Role in proteolysis of C4b by C3b-inactivator. *J. Exp. Med.,* 148:1044–1051.

64. Fujita, T., Takata, Y., and Tamura, N. (1981): Solubilization of immune precipitates by six isolated alternative pathway proteins. *J. Exp. Med.,* 154:1743–1751.

65. Gadd, K. J., and Reid, K. B. M. (1981): The binding of complement component C3 to antibody-antigen aggregates after activation of the alternative pathway in human serum. *Biochem. J.,* 195:471–480.

66. Ganu, V. S., and Müller-Eberhard, H. J. (1985): Inhibition of factor B and factor H binding to C3b by a synthetic peptide corresponding to residues 749–789. *Complement,* 2:27 (abstract).

67. Geiger, B., Rosen, D., and Berke, G. (1982): Spatial relationships of microtubule-organizing centers and the contact area of cytotoxic T lymphocytes and target cells. *J. Cell Biol.,* 95:137–143.

68. Gershenfeld, H. K., and Weissman, I. L. (1986): Cloning of cDNA for a T cell-specific serine protease from a cytotoxic T lymphocyte. *Science,* 232:854–858.

69. Ghebrehiwet, B. (1982): C3e induced lysosomal enzyme release from polymorphonuclear leukocytes. *Fed. Proc.,* 41:966 (abstract).

70. Ghebrehiwet, B., and Müller-Eberhard, H. J. (1979): C3e: An acidic fragment of human C3 with leukocytosis-inducing activity. *J. Immunol.,* 123:616–621.

71. Gigli, I., Fujita, T., and Nussenzweig, V. (1979): Modulation of the classical pathway C3 convertase by plasma proteins C4 binding protein and C3b inactivator. *Science USA,* 76:6596–6600.

72. Goldberger, G., Rits, M., Kwiatkowski, D. J., and Edge, M. D. (1987): Nucleotide sequence analysis of human factor I cDNA. Personal communication.

73. Götze, O. (1975): Proteases of the properdin system. In: *Proteases and Biological Control,* edited by E. Reich, D. B. Rifkin, and E. Shaw, pp. 155–272. Cold Spring Harbor Laboratory, Cold Spring Harbor, N.Y.

74. Götze, O., and Müller-Eberhard, H. J. (1971): The C3 activator system: An alternate pathway of complement activation. *J. Exp. Med.,* 134:90s–108s.

75. Gromkowski, S. H., Brown, T. C., Cerutti, P. A., and Cerottini, J.-C. (1986): DNA of human Raji target cells is damaged upon lymphocyte-mediated lysis. *J. Immunol.,* 136:752–756.

76. Hammer, C. H., Hansch, G., Gresham, D., and Shin, M. L. (1983): Activation of the fifth and sixth components of the human complement system: C6-dependent cleavage of C5 in acid and the formation of a bimolecular lytic complex, C5b,6a. *J. Immunol.,* 131:892–898.

77. Hansch, G. M., Hammer, C. H., Vanguri, P., and Shin, M. L. (1981): Homologous species restriction in lysis of erythrocytes by terminal complement proteins. *Proc. Natl. Acad. Sci. USA,* 78:5118–5121.

78. Henkart, P. A. (1985): Mechanism of lymphocyte mediated cytotoxicity. *Annu. Rev. Immunol.,* 3:31–58.

79. Henkart, P. A., Millard, P. J., Reynolds, C. W., and Henkart, M. P. (1984): Cytolytic activity of purified cytoplasmic granules from cytotoxic rat large granular lymphocyte tumors. *J. Exp. Med.,* 160:75–93.

80. Herberman, R. B., Reynolds, C. W., and Ortaldo, J. (1986): Mechanism of cytotoxicity by natural killer (NK) cells. *Annu. Rev. Immunol.,* 4:651–680.

81. Hirani, S., Lambris, J. D., and Müller-Eberhard, H. J. (1985): Structural analysis of asparagine linked oligosaccharides of human C3. *Biochem. J.,* 233:613–616.

82. Hirani, S., Lambris, J. D., and Müller-Eberhard, H. J. (1985): Localization of the conglutinin binding site on the third component of human complement. *J. Immunol.,* 134:1105–1109.

83. Hoeprich, P. D., Jr., Dahinden, C. A., Lachmann, P. J., Davis, A. E., III, and Hugli, T. E. (1985): A synthetic nonapeptide corresponding to NH_2-terminal sequence of C3d-K causes leukocytosis in rabbits. *J. Biol. Chem.,* 260:2597–2600.

84. Horstmann, R. D., and Müller-Eberhard, H. J. (1985): Isolation of rabbit C3, factor B and factor H and comparison of their properties with those of the human analogues. *J. Immunol.,* 134:1094–1100.

85. Horstmann, R. D., Pangburn, M. K., Müller-Eberhard, H. J. (1985): Species specificity of recognition by the alternative pathway of complement. *J. Immunol.,* 134:1101–1104.

86. Hostetter, M. K., Thomas, M. L., Rosen, F. S., and Tack, B. F. (1982): Binding of C3b proceeds by a transesterification reaction at the thiolester site. *Nature,* 298:72–75.

87. Hu, V. W., and Nicholson-Weller, A. (1985): Enhanced complement-mediated lysis of type III paroxysmal nocturnal hemoglobinuria erythrocytes involves increased C9 binding and polymerization. *Proc. Natl. Acad. Sci. USA,* 82:5520–5524.

88. Hughes-Jones, N. C. (1977): Functional affinity constants of the reaction between ^{125}I-labelled C1q and C1q binders. *Immunology,* 32:191–198.

89. Hughes-Jones, N. C., and Gorick, B. D. (1982): The binding and activation of the C1r-C1s subunit of the first component of human complement. *Mol. Immunol.,* 19:1105–1112.

90. Hugli, T. E. (1984): Structure and function of the anaphylatoxins. *Springer Sem. Immunopathol.,* 7:193–219.

91. Humphrey, J. H., and Dourmashkin, R. R. (1969): The lesions in cell membranes caused by complement. *Adv. Immunol.,* 11:75–115.

92. Iida, K., and Nussenzweig, V. (1983): Functional properties of membrane-associated complement receptor CR1. *J. Immunol.,* 130:1876–1880.

93. Iida, K., Nadler, L., and Nussenzweig, V. (1983): Identification of the membrane receptor for the complement fragment C3d by means of a monoclonal antibody. *J. Exp. Med.,* 158:1021–1033.

94. Isenman, D. E., Podack, E. R., and Cooper, N. R. (1980): The interaction of C5 with C3b in free solution: A sufficient condition for cleavage by fluid phase C3/C5 convertase. *J. Immunol.,* 124:326–331.

95. Isenmann, D. E., Kells, D. I. C., Cooper, N. R., Müller-Eberhard, H. J., and Pangburn, M. K. (1981): Nucleophilic modification of human complement protein C3: Correlation of conformational changes with acquisition of C3b-like functional properties. *Biochemistry,* 20:4458–4467.

96. Ishida, B., Wisnieski, B. J., Lavine, C. H., and Esser, A. F. (1982): Photolabeling of a hydrophobic domain of the ninth component of human complement. *J. Biol. Chem.,* 257:10551–10553.

97. Janatova, J. (1986): Detection of disulfide bonds and localization of interchain linkages in the third (C3) and the fourth (C4) components of human complement. *Biochem. J.,* 233:819–825.

98. Janatova, J., Lorenz, P. E., Schechter, A. N., Prahl, J. W., and Tack, B. F. (1980): Third component of human complement: appearance of a sulfhydryl group following chemical or enzymatic inactivation. *Biochemistry,* 19:4471–4478.

99. Jenne, D., and Stanley, K. K. (1985): Molecular cloning of S-protein, a link between complement, coagulation and cell-substrate adhesion. *Eur. Mol. Biol. Org. J.,* 4:3153–3157.

100. Johnson, D. M. A., Gagnon, J., and Reid, K. B. M. (1984): Amino acid sequence of human factor D of the complement system. Similarity in sequence between factor D and proteases of nonplasma origin. *FEBS Lett.,* 166:347–351.

101. Joiner, K. A., Fries, L. F., Schmetz, M. A., and Frank, M. M. (1985): IgG bearing covalently bound C3b has enhanced bactericidal activity for *Escherichia coli* 0111. *J. Exp. Med.,* 162:877–889.

102. Joiner, K. A., Schmetz, M. A., Sanders, M. E., Murray, T. G., and Hammer, C. H. (1985): Multimeric complement component C9 is necessary for killing of *Escherichia coli* J5 by terminal attack complex C5b-9. *Proc. Natl. Acad. Sci. USA,* 82:4808–4812.

103. Journet, A., and Tosi, M. (1986): Cloning and sequencing of full-length cDNA encoding the precursor of human complement component C1r. *Biochem. J.,* 240:783–787.

104. Jung, G., Ledbetter, J. A., and Müller-Eberhard, H. J. (1987): Induction of cytotoxicity in resting human T lymphocytes bound to tumor cells by antibody heteroconjugates. *Proc. Natl. Acad. Sci. USA,* 84 (*in press*).

105. Jung, G., Honsik, C. J., Reisfeld, R. A., and Müller-Eberhard, H. J.: Activation of human peripheral blood mononuclear cells by anti-T3: Killing of tumor target cells coated with anti-target-anti-T3 conjugates. *Proc. Natl. Acad. Sci. USA,* 83:4479–4483.

106. Khan, S. A., and Erickson, B. W. (1981): Synthesis of macrocyclic peptide tiolactones as models of the metastable binding sites of α_2-macroglobulin and complement proteins C3b. *J. Am. Chem. Soc.,* 103:7374–7376.

107. Khan, S. A., and Erickson, B. W. (1982): An equilibrium model of the metastable binding sites of α_2-macroglobulin and complement proteins C3 and C4. *J. Biol. Chem.,* 257:11864–11867.

108. Klickstein, L. B., Wong, W. W., Smith, J. A., Weis, J. H., Wilson, J. G., and Fearon, D. T. (1987): Human C3b/C4b receptor (CR1). Demonstration of long homologous repeating domains that are composed of the short consensus repeats characteristic of C3/C4 binding proteins. *J. Exp. Med.,* 165:1095–1112.

109. Knobel, H. R., Villiger, W., and Isliker, H. (1975): Chemical analysis and electron microscopy studies of human C1q prepared by different methods. *Eur. J. Immunol.,* 5:78–82.

110. Kolb, W. P., and Müller-Eberhard, H. J. (1975): Neoantigens of the membrane attack complex of human complement. *Proc. Natl. Acad. Sci. USA,* 72:1687–1689.

111. Kolb, W. P., and Müller-Eberhard, H. J. (1976): The membrane attack mechanism of complement: The three polypeptide chain structure of the eighth component (C8). *J. Exp. Med.,* 143:1131–1139.

112. Kolb, W. P., Kolb, L., and Savary, J. R. (1982): Biochemical characterization of sixth component (C6) of human complement. *Biochemistry,* 21:294–301.

113. Kristensen, T., and Tack, B. F. (1986): Murine protein H is comprised of 20 repeating units, 61 amino acids in length. *Proc. Natl. Acad. Sci. USA,* 83:3963–3967.

114. Kristensen, T., Wetsel, R. A., and Tack, B. F. (1986): Structural analysis of human complement protein H: Homology with C4b binding protein, β_2-glycoprotein I, and the Ba fragment of B. *J. Immunol.,* 136:3407–3411.

115. Kristensen, T., D'Eustachio, P., Ogata, R., Chung, L. P., Reid, K. B. M., and Tack, B. F. (1987): The superfamily of C3b/C4b binding proteins. *Fed. Proc.,* 46 (*in press*).

116. Kupfer, A., Dennert, G., and Singer, S. J. (1983): Polarization of the Golgi apparatus and the microtubule-organizing center within cloned natural killer cells bound to their targets. *Proc. Natl. Acad. Sci. USA,* 80:7224–7228.

117. Lachmann, P. J., and Hobart, M. J. (1978): C6-C7: A further "complement supergene." *J. Immunol.,* 120:1781 (abstract).

118. Lachmann, P. J., and Hughes-Jones, N. C. (1984): Initiation of complement activation. *Springer Sem. Immunopathol.,* 7:143–162.

119. Lachmann, P. J., Pangburn, M. K., and Oldroyd, R. G. (1982): Breakdown of C3 after complement activation. Identification of a new fragment, C3g, using monoclonal antibodies. *J. Exp. Med.,* 156:205–216.

120. Lambris, J. D., and Müller-Eberhard, H. J. (1984): Isolation and characterization of a 33,000 dalton fragment of complement factor B with catalytic and C3b binding activity. *J. Biol. Chem.,* 259:12685–12690.

121. Lambris, J. D., and Ross, G. D. (1982): Characterization of the

lymphocyte membrane receptor for factor H (β_1H-globulin) with an antibody to anti-factor H idiotype. *J. Exp. Med.*, 155:1400–1411.

122. Lambris, J. D., Becherer, D., and Müller-Eberhard, H. J. (1985): Localization of the factor H binding site on the third component of complement. *Complement*, 2:48 (abstract).

123. Lambris, J. D., Alsenz, J., Schulz, T. F., and Dierich, M. P. (1984): Mapping of the properdin-binding site in the third component of complement. *Biochem. J.*, 217:323–326.

124. Lambris, J. D., Ganu, V., Hirani, S., and Müller-Eberhard, H. J. (1985): Mapping of the C3d receptor (CR$_2$) binding site and a neoantigenic site in the C3d domain of the third component of complement. *Proc. Natl. Acad. Sci. USA*, 82:4235–4239.

125. Laurell, A.-B., Johnson, U., Martensson, U., and Sjoholm, A. G. (1978): Formation of complexes composed of C1r, C1s and C1 inactivator in human serum on activation of C1. *Acta Pathol. Microbiol. Scand.*, 86:299–306.

126. Law, S. K., and Levine, R. P. (1977): Interaction between the third complement protein and cell surface macromolecules. *Proc. Natl. Acad. Sci. USA*, 74:2701–2705.

127. Law, S. K., Dodds, A. W., and Porter, R. R. (1984): A comparison of the properties of two classes, C4A and C4B, of the human complement component C4. *Eur. Mol. Biol. Org. J.*, 3:1819–1823.

128. Law, S. K., Lichtenberg, N. A., and Levine, R. P. (1979): Evidence for an ester linkage between the labile binding site of C3b and receptive surfaces. *J. Immunol.*, 123:1388–1394.

129. Law, S. K., Lichtenberg, N. A., and Levine, R. P. (1980): Covalent binding and hemolytic activity of complement proteins. *Proc. Natl. Acad. Sci. USA*, 77:7194–7198.

130. Law, S. A., Minich, T. M., and Levine, R. P. (1981): Binding reaction between the third human complement protein and small molecules. *Biochemistry*, 20:7457–7463.

131. Lesavre, P., and Müller-Eberhard, H. J. (1978): Mechanism of action of factor D of the alternative complement pathway. *J. Exp. Med.*, 148:1498–1509.

132. Lesavre, P. H., Hugli, T. E., Esser, A. F., and Müller-Eberhard, H. J. (1979): The alternative pathway C3/C5 convertase: Chemical basis of factor B activation. *J. Immunol.*, 123:529–534.

133. Liu, C.-C., Perussia, B., Cohn, Z. A., and Young, J. D.-E. (1986): Identification and characterization of a pore-forming protein of human peripheral blood natural killer cells. *J. Exp. Med.*, 164:2061–2076.

134. Liu, M. A., Kranz, D. M., Kurnick, J. T., Boyle, L. A., Levy, R., and Eisen, H. N. (1985): Heteroantibody duplexes target cells for lysis by cytotoxic T lymphocytes. *Proc. Natl. Acad. Sci. USA*, 82:8648–8652.

135. Lobe, C. G., Finlay, B. B., Paranchych, W., Paetkau, V. H., and Bleackley, R. C. (1986): Novel serine proteases encoded by two cytotoxic T lymphocyte-specific genes. *Science*, 232:858–861.

136. Lundwall, A., Wetsel, R. A., Domdey, H., Tack, B. F., and Fey, G. H. (1984): Structure of murine complement component C3. I. Nucleotide sequence of cloned complementary and genomic DNA coding for the β chain. *J. Biol. Chem.*, 259:13851–13856.

137. Lundwall, A. B., Wetsel, R. A., Kristensen, T., Whitehead, A. S., Woods, D. E., Ogden, R. C., Colten, H. R., and Tack, B. F. (1985): Isolation and sequence analysis of a cDNA clone encoding the fifth complement component. *J. Biol. Chem.*, 260:2108–2112.

138. Mandecki, W., Mollison, K. W., Bolling, T. J., Powell, B. S., Carter, G. W., and Fox, J. L. (1985): Chemical synthesis of a gene encoding the human complement fragment C5a and its expression in *Escherichia coli. Proc. Natl. Acad. Sci. USA*, 82:3543–3547.

139. Mardiney, M. R., Müller-Eberhard, H. J., and Feldman, J. D. (1968): Ultrastructural localization of the third and fourth components of complement on complement-cell complexes. *Am. J. Pathol.*, 53:253–262.

140. Martin, D. E., Chiu, F. J., Gigli, I., and Müller-Eberhard, H. J. (1987): Killing of human melanoma cells by the membrane attack complex of human complement as a function of its molecular composition. *J. Clin. Invest. (in press)*.

141. Martin, D. E., Zalman, L. S., Jung, G., and Müller-Eberhard, H. J. (1987): Induction of synthesis of the cytolytic C9 related protein in human peripheral mononuclear cells by monoclonal anti-

142. Masson, D., and Tschopp, J. (1985): Isolation of a lytic, pore forming protein (perforin) from cytolytic T lymphocytes. *J. Biol. Chem.*, 260:9069–9072.

143. Matsuda, T., Seya, T., and Nagasawa, S. (1985): Location of the interchain disulfide bonds of the third component of human complement. *Biochem. Biophys. Res. Commun.*, 127:264–269.

144. May, J. E., and Frank, M. M. (1973): A new complement-mediated cytolytic mechanism—the C1-bypass activation pathway. *Proc. Natl. Acad. Sci. USA*, 70:649–652.

145. Mayer, M. M. (1982): Membrane attack by complement (with comments on cell-mediated cytotoxicity). In: *Mechanisms of Cell-Mediated Cytotoxicity*, edited by W. R. Clark and P. Golstein, pp. 193–216. Plenum Press, New York.

146. Medicus, R. G., Götze, O., and Müller-Eberhard, H. J. (1976): Alternative pathway of complement: Recruitment of precursor properdin by the labile C3/C5 convertase and the potentiation of the pathway. *J. Exp. Med.*, 144:1076–1093.

147. Medicus, R. G., Melamed, J., and Arnaout, M. A. (1983): The role of human factor I and C3b receptor in the cleavage of surface-bound C3bi molecules. *Eur. J. Immunol.*, 13:465–470.

148. Medof, M. E., and Nussenzweig, V. (1984): Control of the function of substrate-bound C4b-C3b by the complement receptor CR1. *J. Exp. Med.*, 159:1669–1685.

149. Medof, M. E., Kinoshita, T., and Nussenzweig, V. (1984): Inhibition of complement activation on the surface of cells after incorporation of decay-accelerating factor (DAF) into their membranes. *J. Exp. Med.*, 160:1558–1578.

150. Medof, M. E., Iida, K., Mold, C., and Nussenzweig, V. (1982): Unique role of the complement receptor CR1 in the degradation of C3b associated with immune complexes. *J. Exp. Med.*, 156:1739–1754.

151. Medof, M. E., Walter, E. I., Roberts, W. L., Haas, R., and Rosenberry, T. L. (1986): Decay accelerating factor of complement is anchored to cells by a C-terminal glycolipid. *Biochemistry*, 25:6740–6747.

152. Medof, M. E., Lublin, D. M., Holers, V. M., Ayers, D. J., Getty, R. R., Leykam, J. F., Atkinson, J. P., and Tykocinski, M. L. (1987): Cloning and characterization of cDNAs encoding the complete sequence of decay-accelerating factor of human complement. *Proc. Natl. Acad. Sci. USA*, 84:2007–2011.

153. Melchers, F., Erdei, A., Schulz, T., and Dierich, M. D. (1985): Growth control of activated synchronized murine B cells by the C3d fragments of human complement. *Nature*, 318:264–267.

154. Meuth, J. L., Morgan, E. L., DiScipio, R. G., and Hugli, T. E. (1983): Suppression of lymphocyte functions by human C3 fragments. I. Inhibition of human T cell proliferative responses by a kallikrein cleavage fragment of human C3b. *J. Immunol.*, 130:2605–2611.

155. Minta, J. O., and Lepow, I. H. (1974): Studies on the subunit structure of human properdin. *Immunochemistry*, 11:361–368.

156. Mole, J. E., Anderson, J. K., Davison, E. A., and Woods, D. E. (1984): Complete primary structure for the zymogen of human complement factor B. *J. Biol. Chem.*, 259:3407–3412.

157. Morgan, B. P., Dankert, J. R., and Esser, A. F. (1987): Recovery of human neutrophils from complement attack: Removal of the membrane attack complex by endocytosis and exocytosis. *J. Immunol.*, 138:246–253.

158. Morgan, B. P., Imagawa, D. K., Dankert, J. R., and Ramm, L. E. (1986): Complement lysis of U937, a nucleated mammalian cell line in the absence of C9: Effect of C9 on C5b-8 mediated cell lysis. *J. Immunol.*, 136:3402–3406.

159. Müller-Eberhard, H. J. (1961): Isolation and description of proteins related to the human complement system. *Acta Soc. Med. Upsala*, 66:152–170.

160. Müller-Eberhard, H. J. (1975): Initiation of membrane attack by complement: Assembly and control of C3 and C5 convertase. In: *Proteases and Biological Control*, edited by E. Reich, D. B. Rifkin, and E. Shaw, pp. 229–241. Cold Spring Harbor Laboratory, Cold Spring Harbor, N.Y.

161. Müller-Eberhard, H. J. (1981): Human complement protein C3:

Its unusual functional and structural versatility in host defense and inflammation. *Advances in Immunopathology*, 141–160. Elsevier/North-Holland, Amsterdam.

162. Müller-Eberhard, H. J. (1984): The membrane attack complex. *Springer Semin. Immunopathol.*, 7:93–141.

163. Müller-Eberhard, H. J. (1986): The membrane attack complex of complement. *Annu. Rev. Immunol.*, 4:503–528.

164. Müller-Eberhard, H. J., and Götze, O. (1972): C3 proactivator convertase and its mode of action. *J. Exp. Med.*, 135:1003–1008.

165. Müller-Eberhard, H. J., and Kunkel, H. G. (1961): Isolation of a thermolabile serum protein which precipitates γ-globulin aggregates and participates in immune hemolysis. *Proc. Soc. Exp. Biol. Med.*, 106:291–295.

166. Müller-Eberhard, H. J., and Lepow, I. H. (1965): C'1 esterase effect on activity and physicochemical properties of the fourth component of complement. *J. Exp. Med.*, 121:819–833.

167. Müller-Eberhard, H. J., and Nilsson, U. (1960): Relation of a β_1-glycoprotein of human serum to the complement system. *J. Exp. Med.*, 111:217–234.

168. Müller-Eberhard, H. J., and Schreiber, R. D. (1980): Molecular biology and chemistry of the alternative pathway of complement. *Adv. Immunol.*, 29:1–53.

169. Müller-Eberhard, H. J., Dalmasso, A. P., and Calcott, M. A. (1966): The reaction mechanism of β1C-globulin (C'3) in immune hemolysis. *J. Exp. Med.*, 122:33–54.

170. Müller-Eberhard, H. J., Polley, M. J., and Calcott, M. A. (1967): Formation and functional significance of a molecular complex derived from the second and the fourth component of human complement. *J. Exp. Med.*, 125:359–380.

171. Müller-Eberhard, H. J., Zalman, L. S., Chiu, F. J., Jung, G., and Martin, D. E. (1986): Molecular mechanisms of cytotoxicity: Comparison of complement and killer lymphocytes. In: *Progress in Immunology VI*, edited by B. Cinader and R. G. Miller, pp. 268–281. Academic Press, New York.

172. Nagasawa, S., Ischihara, C., and Stroud, R. M. (1980): Cleavage of C4b inactivator: Production of a nicked form of C4b, C4b', as an intermediate cleavage product of C4b by C3b inactivator. *J. Immunol.*, 125:578–582.

173. Nemerow, G. R., Wolfert, R., McNaughton, M. E., and Cooper, N. R. (1985): Identification and characterization of the Epstein-Barr virus receptor on human B lymphocytes and its relationship to the C3d complement receptor (CR2). *J. Virol.*, 55:347–351.

174. Nemerow, G. R., Mold, C., Keivens-Schwend, V., Tollefson, V., and Cooper, N. R. (1987): Identification of gp350 as the viral glycoprotein mediating attachment of Epstein-Barr virus (EBV) to the EBV/C3d receptor of B cells: Sequence homology of gp350 and the C3 complement fragment C3d. *J. Virol.*, 61 (*in press*).

175. Nicholson-Weller, A., Burge, J., Fearon, D. T., Weller, P. F., and Austen, K. F. (1982): Isolation of a human erythrocyte membrane glycoprotein with decay-accelerating activity for C3 convertases of the complement system. *J. Immunol.*, 129:184–189.

176. Nicholson-Weller, A., March, J. P., Rosenfeld, S. I., and Austen, K. F. (1983): Affected erythrocytes of patients with paroxysmal nocturnal hemoglobinuria are deficient in the complement regulatory protein, decay-accelerating factor. *Proc. Natl. Acad. Sci. USA*, 80:5066–5070.

177. Nicol, P. A. E., and Lachmann, P. J. (1973): The alternative pathway of complement activation. The role of C3 and its inactivator (KAF). *Immunology*, 24:259–275.

178. Niemann, M. A., Bhown, A., Bennett, J. C., and Volanakis, J. E. (1984): Amino acid sequence of human D of the alternative complement pathway. *Biochemistry*, 23:2482–2486.

179. Nilsson, B., and Nilsson, U. R. Anti-idiotypic antibodies in antisera against human C3 and factor H and their application in the enrichment of antibodies specific for H-binding domains of C3. *J. Immunol.*, 138:1858–1863.

180. Odermatt, E., Berger, H., and Sano, Y. (1981): Size and shape of human C1-inhibitor. *FEBS Lett.*, 131:283–285.

181. Okada, N., Yasuda, T., Tsumita, T., and Okada, H. (1982): Activation of the alternative complement pathway of guinea pig by liposomes incorporated with trinitrophenylated phosphatidylethanolamine. *Immunology*, 45:115–124.

182. Pangburn, M. K. (1986): Differences between the binding sites of the complement regulatory proteins DAF, CR1 and factor H on C3 convertases. *J. Immunol.*, 136:2216–2221.

183. Pangburn, M. K., and Müller-Eberhard, H. J. (1978): Complement C3 convertase: Cell surface restriction of β1H control and generation of restriction on neuraminidase treated cells. *Proc. Natl. Acad. Sci. USA*, 75:2416–2420.

184. Pangburn, M. K., and Müller-Eberhard, H. J. (1980): Relation of a putative thioester bond in C3 to activation of the alternative pathway and the binding of C3b to biological targets of complement. *J. Exp. Med.*, 152:1102–1114.

185. Pangburn, M. K., and Müller-Eberhard, H. J. (1983): Kinetic and thermodynamic analysis of the control of C3b by the complement regulatory proteins factor H and factor I. *Biochemistry*, 22:178–185.

186. Pangburn, M. K., and Müller-Eberhard, H. J. (1984): The alternative pathway of complement. *Springer Semin. Immunopathol.*, 7:163–192.

187. Pangburn, M. K., and Müller-Eberhard, H. J. (1986): The C3 convertase of the alternative pathway of human complement. Enzymic properties of the bimolecular proteinase. *Biochem. J.*, 235:723–730.

188. Pangburn, M. K., and Müller-Eberhard, H. J. (1987): To be submitted.

189. Pangburn, M. K., Schreiber, R. D., and Müller-Eberhard, H. J. (1977): Human complement C3b inactivator: Isolation, characterization, and demonstration of an absolute requirement for the serum protein β1H for cleavage of C3b and C4b in solution. *J. Exp. Med.*, 146:257–270.

190. Pangburn, M. K., Schreiber, R. D., and Müller-Eberhard, H. J. (1981): Formation of the initial C3 convertase of the alternative complement pathway. Acquisition of C3b-like activities by spontaneous hydrolysis of the putative thioester in native C3. *J. Exp. Med.*, 154:856–867.

191. Pangburn, M. K., Schreiber, R. D., and Müller-Eberhard, H. J. (1983): C3b deposition during activation of the alternative complement pathway and the effect of deposition on the activating surface. *J. Immunol.*, 131:1930–1935.

192. Pangburn, M. K., Schreiber, R. D., and Müller-Eberhard, H. J. (1983): Deficiency of an erythrocyte membrane protein with complement regulatory activity in paroxysmal nocturnal hemoglobinuria. *Proc. Natl. Acad. Sci. USA*, 80:5430–5434.

193. Pangburn, M. K., Morrison, D. C., Schreiber, R. D., and Müller-Eberhard, H. J. (1980): Activation of the alternative complement pathway: Recognition of surface structures on activators by bound C3b. *J. Immunol.*, 124:977–982.

194. Parker, C., Gagnon, J., and Keii, M. A. (1983): The reaction of iodine- and thiol-blocking reagents with human complement components C2 and factor B. Purification and *N*-terminal amino acid sequence of a peptide from C2a containing a free thiol group. *Biochem. J.*, 213:201–209.

195. Perez, P., Hoffman, R. W., Shaw, S., Bluestone, J. A., and Segal, D. M. (1985): Specific targeting of cytotoxic T cells by anti-T3 linked to anti-target cell antibody. *Nature*, 316:354–356.

196. Perlmann, H., Perlmann, P., Schreiber, R. D., and Müller-Eberhard, H. J. (1981): Interaction of target cell-bound C3bi and C3d with human lymphocyte receptors. Enhancement of antibody-mediated cellular cytotoxicity. *J. Exp. Med.*, 153:1592–1603.

197. Pillemer, L., Blum, L., Lepow, I. H., Ross, O. A., Todd, E. W., and Wardlaw, A. C. (1954): The properdin system and immunity. I. Demonstration and isolation of a new serum protein, properdin, and its role in immune phenomena. *Science*, 120:279–285.

198. Podack, E. R., and Dennert, G. (1983): Assembly of two types of tubules with putative cytolytic function by cloned natural killer cells. *Nature*, 302:442–445.

199. Podack, E. R., and Konigsberg, P. J. (1984): Cytolytic T cell granules. Isolation, structural, biochemical and functional characterization. *J. Exp. Med.*, 160:695–710.

200. Podack, E. R., and Müller-Eberhard, H. J. (1979): Isolation from human serum of an inhibitor of the membrane attack complex of complement. *J. Biol. Chem.*, 254:9908–9914.

201. Podack, E. R., and Tschopp, J. (1982): Polymerization of the ninth

component of complement (C9): Formation of poly C9 with a tubular ultrastructure resembling the membrane attack complex of complement. *Proc. Natl. Acad. Sci. USA*, 79:574–578.

202. Podack, E. R., Biesecker, G., and Müller-Eberhard, H. J. (1979): Membrane attack complex of complement: Generation of high affinity phospholipid binding sites by fusion of five hydrophilic plasma proteins. *Proc. Natl. Acad. Sci. USA*, 76:897–901.

203. Podack, E. R., Kolb, W. P., and Müller-Eberhard, H. J. (1978): The C5b-6 complex: Formation, isolation and inhibition of its activity by lipoprotein and the S-protein of human serum. *J. Immunol.*, 120:1841–1848.

204. Podack, E. R., Preissner, K. T., and Müller-Eberhard, H. J. (1984): Inhibition of C9 polymerization within the SC5b-9 complex of complement by S-protein. *Acta Pathol. Microbiol. Immunol. Scand. (Suppl. C)*, 284:89–96.

205. Podack, E. R., Tschopp, J., and Müller-Eberhard, H. J. (1982): Molecular organization of C9 within the membrane attack complex of complement: Induction of circular C9 polymerization by the C5b-8 assembly. *J. Exp. Med.*, 156:268–282.

206. Podack, E. R., Young, J. D.-E., and Cohn, Z. A. (1985): Isolation and biochemical and functional characterization of perforin 1 from cytolytic T cell granules. *Proc. Natl. Acad. Sci. USA*, 82:8629–8633.

207. Podack, E. R., Biesecker, G., Kolb, W. P., and Müller-Eberhard, H. J. (1978): The C5b,6 complex: Reaction with C7, C8, C9. *J. Immunol.*, 121:484–490.

208. Podack, E. R., Kolb, W. P., Esser, A. F., and Müller-Eberhard, H. J. (1979): Structural similarities between C6 and C7 of human complement. *J. Immunol.*, 123:1071–1077.

209. Polley, M. J., and Müller-Eberhard, H. J. (1967): Enhancement of the hemolytic activity of the second component of human complement by oxidation. *J. Exp. Med.*, 126:1013–1025.

210. Polley, M. J., and Müller-Eberhard, H. J. (1968): The second component of human complement: Its isolation, fragmentation by C'1 esterase and incorporation into C'3 convertase. *J. Exp. Med.*, 128:533–551.

211. Preissner, K. T., Podack, E. R., and Müller-Eberhard, H. J. (1985): The membrane attack complex of complement: Relation of C7 to the metastable membrane binding site of the intermediate complex C5b-7. *J. Immunol.*, 135:445–451.

212. Preissner, K. T., Podack, E. R., and Müller-Eberhard, H. J. (1985): Self-association of the seventh component of human complement (C7): Dimerization and polymerization. *J. Immunol.*, 135:452–458.

213. Preissner, K. T., Wassmuth, R., and Muller-Berghaus, G. (1985): Physicochemical characterization of human S-protein and its function in the blood coagulation system. *Biochem. J.*, 231:349–355.

214. Pryzdial, E. L. G., and Isenman, D. E. (1987): Alternative complement pathway activation fragment Ba binds to C3b. *J. Biol. Chem.*, 262:1519–1525.

215. Ramm, L. E., Whitlow, M. B., Koski, C. L., Shin, M. L., and Mayer, M. M. (1983): Elimination of complement channels from the plasma membranes of U937, a nucleated mammalian cell line: Temperature dependence of the elimination rate. *J. Immunol.*, 131:1411–1415.

216. Rao, A. G., Howard, M. Z., Ng, S. N., Snider, J. V., Whitehead, A. S., Colten, H. R., and Sodetz, J. M. (1986): Characterization of a cDNA clone encoding the α subunit of the eighth component of human complement (C8). *6th Int. Congr. Immunol.*, Toronto, p. 197 (abstract).

217. Rao, A. G., Howard, O. M. Z., Ng, S. N., Whitehead, A. S., Colten, H. F., and Sodetz, J. M. cDNA and amino acid sequence of the a and b subunits of human C8. Evidence for the existence of separate mRNA's and identification of structural homologies. Personal communication.

218. Ratnoff, W. D., Fearon, D. T., and Austen, K. F. (1983): The role of antibody in the activation of the alternative complement pathway. *Springer Semin. Immunopathol.*, 6:361–372.

219. Reid, K. B. M. (1985): Molecular cloning and characterization of the complementary DNA and gene coding for the β-chain of sub-

component C1q of the human complement system. *Biochem. J.*, 231:729–735.

220. Reid, K. B. M., and Gagnon, J. (1981): Amino acid sequence studies of human properdin-N-terminal sequence analysis and alignment of the fragments produced by limited proteolysis with trypsin and the peptides produced by cyanogen bromide treatment. *Mol. Immunol.*, 18:949–959.

221. Reid, K. B. M., Gagnon, J., and Frampton, J. (1982): Completion of the amino acid sequences of the A and B chains of subcomponent C1q of the first component of human complement. *Biochem. J.*, 203:559–569.

222. Ripoche, J., Day, A. J., Willis, A. C., Belt, K. T., Campbell, R. D., and Sim, R. B. (1986): Partial characterization of human complement factor H by protein and cDNA sequencing: Homology with other complement and noncomplement proteins. *Biosci. Rep.*, 6:65–72.

223. Rosenfeld, S. I., Jenkins, D. E., and Leddy, J. P. (1985): Enchanced reactive lysis of paroxysmal nocturnal hemoglobinuria erythrocytes by C5b-9 does not involve increased C7 binding on cell-bound C3b. *J. Immunol.*, 134:506–511.

224. Ross, G. D., and Medof, M. E. (1985): Membrane complement receptors specific for bound fragments of C3. *Adv. Immunol.*, 37:217–267.

225. Ross, G. D., Lambris, J. D., Cain, J. A., and Newman, S. L. (1982): Generation of three different fragments of bound C3 with purified factor I or serum. I. Requirements for factor H vs. CR₁ cofactor activity. *J. Immunol.*, 129:2051–2060.

226. Ross, G. D., Polley, M. J., Rabellino, E. M., and Grey, H. M. (1973): Two different complement receptors on human lymphocytes, one specific for C3b and one specific for C3b inactivator-cleaved C3b. *J. Exp. Med.*, 138:798–811.

227. Rothman, I. K., Gelfand, J. A., Fauci, A. S., and Frank, M. M. (1975): The immune adherence receptor: Dissociation between the expression of erythrocyte and mononuclear cell C3b receptors. *J. Immunol.*, 115:1312–1315.

228. Sackstein, R., Colten, H. R., and Woods, D. E. (1983): Phylogenetic conservation of a class III major histocompatibility complex antigen, factor B. Isolation and nucleotide sequencing of mouse factor B cDNA clones. *J. Biol. Chem.*, 258:14693–14697.

229. Salvesen, G. S., Catanese, J. J., Kress, L. F., and Travis, J. (1985): Primary structure of the reactive site of human C1-inhibitor. *J. Biol. Chem.*, 260:2432–2436.

230. Sandberg, A. L., Götze, O., Müller-Eberhard, H. J., and Osler, A. G. (1971): Complement utilization by guinea pig gamma-1 and gamma-2 immunoglobulins through the C3 activator system. *J. Immunol.*, 107:920–923.

231. Scharfstein, J., Ferreira, A., Gigli, I., and Nussenzweig, V. (1978): Human C4-binding protein. I. Isolation and characterization. *J. Exp. Med.*, 148:207–222.

232. Schenkein, H. A., and Ruddy, S. (1981): The role of immunoglobulins in alternative complement pathway activation by zymosan. I. Human IgG with specificity for zymosan enhances alternative pathway activation by zymosan. *J. Immunol.*, 126:7–10.

233. Schonermark, S., Rauterberg, E. W., Shin, M. L., Loke, S., Roelcke, D., and Hansch, G. M. (1986): Homologous species restriction in lysis of human erythrocytes: A membrane-derived protein with C8-binding capacity functions as an inhibitor. *J. Immunol.*, 136:1772–1776.

234. Schreiber, R. D. (1984): The chemistry and biology of complement receptors. *Springer Semin. Immunopathol.*, 7:221–249.

235. Schreiber, R. D., and Müller-Eberhard, H. J. (1974): Fourth component of human complement: Description of a three polypeptide chain structure. *J. Exp. Med.*, 140:1324–1335.

236. Schreiber, R. D., and Müller-Eberhard, H. J. (1978): Assembly of the cytolytic alternative pathway of complement from 11 isolated plasma proteins. *J. Exp. Med.*, 148:1722–1727.

237. Schreiber, R. D., Medicus, R. G., Götze, O., and Müller-Eberhard, H. J. (1975): Properdin- and nephritic factor-dependent C3 convertases: Requirement of native C3 for enzyme formation and the function of bound C3b as properdin receptor. *J. Exp. Med.*, 142:760–772.

238. Schreiber, R. D., Morrison, D. C., Podack, E. R., and Müller-Eber-

hard, H. J. (1979): Bactericidal activity of the alternative complement pathway generated from eleven isolated plasma proteins. *J. Exp. Med.*, 149:870–882.

239. Schreiber, R. D., Pangburn, M. K., Lesavre, P., and Müller-Eberhard, H. J. (1978): Initiation of the alternative pathway of complement: Recognition of activators by bound C3b and assembly of the entire pathway from six isolated proteins. *Proc. Natl. Acad. Sci. USA*, 75:3948–3952.

240. Schreiber, R. D., Pangburn, M. K., Medicus, R. G., and Müller-Eberhard, H. J. (1980): Raji cell injury and subsequent lysis by the purified cytolytic alternative pathway of human complement. *Clin. Immunol. Immunopathol.*, 15:384–396.

241. Schumaker, V. N., Zavodszky, P., and Poon, P. H. (1987): Activation of the first component of complement. *Annu. Rev. Immunol.*, 5:21–42.

242. Schumaker, V. N., Calcott, M. A., Speigelberg, H. L., and Müller-Eberhard, H. J. (1976): Ultracentrifuge studies of the binding of IgG of different subclasses to the C1q subunit of the first component of complement. *Biochemistry*, 15:5175–5181.

243. Shin, M. L., Hansch, G., Hu, V. W., and Nicholson-Weller, A. (1986): Membrane factors responsible for homologous species restriction of complement-1-mediated lysis: Evidence for a factor other than DAF operating at the stage of C8 and C9. *J. Immunol.*, 136:1777–1783.

244. Siegel, R. C., and Schumaker, V. N. (1983): Measurement of the association constants of the complexes formed between intact C1q or pepsin-treated C1q stalks and the unactivated or activated C1r₂s₂ tetramers. *Mol. Immunol.*, 20:53–66.

245. Siegel, R. C., Schumaker, V. N., and Poon, P. K. (1981): Stoichiometry and sedimentation properties of the complex formed between C1q and C1r₂s₂ subcomponent of the first component of complement. *J. Immunol.*, 127:2447–2452.

246. Silversmith, R. E., and Nelsestuen, G. L. (1986): Fluid-phase assembly of the membrane attack complex of complement. *Biochemistry*, 25:841–851.

247. Silversmith, R. E., and Nelsestuen, G. L. (1986): Assembly of the membrane attack complex of complement on small unilamellar phospholipid vesicles. *Biochemistry*, 25:852–860.

248. Silversmith, R. E., and Nelsestuen, G. L. (1986): Interaction of complement proteins C5b-6 and C5b-7 with phospholipid vesicles: Effects of phospholipid structural features. *Biochemistry*, 25:7717–7725.

249. Sim, R. B., Arlaud, G. J., and Colomb, M. G. (1979): C1-inhibitor dependent dissociation of human complement C1 bound to immune complexes. *Biochem. J.*, 179:449–457.

250. Sim, R. B., Porter, R. R., Reid, K. B. M., and Gigli, I. (1977): The structure and enzymatic activities of the C1r and C1s subcomponents of C1, the first component of human serum complement. *Biochem. J.*, 163:219–227.

251. Sim, R. B., Twose, T. M., Paterson, D. S., and Sim, E. (1981): The covalent-binding reaction of complement component C3. *Biochem. J.*, 193:115–128.

252. Simone, C. B., and Henkart, P. A. (1980): Permeability changes induced in erythrocyte ghost targets by antibody-dependent cytotoxic effector cells: Evidence for membrane pores. *J. Immunol.*, 124:954–963.

253. Sissons, J. G. P., Oldstone, M. B. A., and Schreiber, R. D. (1980): Antibody-independent activation of the alternative complement pathway by measles virus-infected cells. *Proc. Natl. Acad. Sci. USA*, 77:559–562.

254. Smith, C. A., Vogel, C.-W., and Müller-Eberhard, H. J. (1984): MHC class III products: An electron microscope study of the C3 convertases of human complement. *J. Exp. Med.*, 159:324–329.

255. Smith, C. A., Pangburn, M. K., Vogel, C. W., and Müller-Eberhard, H. J. (1983): Structural investigations of properdin and factor H of human complement. *Immunobiology*, 164:298 (abstract).

256. Smith, C. A., Pangburn, M. K., Vogel, C. W., and Müller-Eberhard, H. J. (1984): Molecular architecture of human properdin, a positive regulator of the alternative pathway of complement. *J. Biol. Chem.*, 259:4582–4588.

257. Stanley, K. K., Kocher, H. P., Luzio, J. P., Jackson, P., and Tschopp, J. (1985): The sequence and topology of human complement component C9. *EMBO J.*, 4:375–382.

258. Stewart, J. L., and Sodetz, J. M. (1985): Existence of a specific C5 recognition site on the β subunit of human C8. *Complement*, 2:76.

259. Stewart, J. L., and Sodetz, J. M. (1985): Analysis of the specific association of the eighth and ninth components of human complement: Identification of a direct role for the alpha-subunit of C8. *Biochemistry*, 24:4598–4602.

260. Strang, C. J., Slayter, H. S., Lachmann, P. J., and Davis, A. E., III (1986): Ultrastructure and composition of bovine conglutinin. *Biochem. J.*, 234:381–389.

261. Strang, C. J., Siegel, R. C., Phillips, M. L., Poon, P. H., and Schumaker, V. N. (1982): Ultrastructure of the first component of human complement: Electron microscopy of the crosslinked complex. *Proc. Natl. Acad. Sci. USA*, 79:586–590.

262. Sumihiro, H., Kikuchi, N., Ikenaka, T., and Inoue, K. (1985): Structures of sugar chains of the third component of human complement. *J. Biochem.*, 98:863–874.

263. Sundsmo, J. S., and Müller-Eberhard, H. J. (1979): Neoantigen of the complement membrane attack complex on cytotoxic human peripheral blood lymphocytes. *J. Immunol.*, 122:2371–2378.

264. Suzuki, S., Oldberg, A., Hayman, E. G., Pierschbacher, M. D., and Ruoslahti, E. (1985): Complete amino acid sequence of human vitronectin deduced from cDNA. Similarity of cell attachment sites in vitronectin and fibronectin. *Eur. Mol. Biol. Org. J.*, 4:2519–2524.

265. Tack, B. F. (1983): The β-Cys-γ-Glu thiolester bond in human C3, C4, and α₂-macroglobulin. *Springer Semin. Immunopathol.*, 6:259–282.

266. Tack, B. F., Harrison, R. A., Janatova, J., Thomas, M. L., and Prahl, J. W. (1980): Evidence for presence of an internal thiolester bond in third component of human complement. *Proc. Natl. Acad. Sci. USA*, 77:5764–5768.

267. Tamerius, J. D., Pangburn, M. K., and Müller-Eberhard, H. J. (1985): Detection of a neoantigen on human C3bi and C3d by monoclonal antibody. *J. Immunol.*, 135:2015–2019.

268. Tirosh, R., and Berke, G. (1985): T-lymphocyte-mediated cytolysis as an excitatory process of the target. I. Evidence that the target cell may be the site of Ca²⁺ action. *Cell. Immunol.*, 95:113–123.

269. Tosi, M., Colomb, M., and Meo, T. (1986): Molecular genetics of the complement serine proteases C1r and C1s and their inhibitor C1-INH. *6th Int. Congr. Immunol.*, p. 198 (abstract).

270. Tranum-Jensen, J., Bhakdi, S., Bhakdi-Lehnen, B., Bjerrum, O. J., and Speth, V. (1978): Complement lysis: The ultrastructure and orientation of the C5b-9 complex on target sheep erythrocyte membranes. *Scand. J. Immunol.*, 7:45–56.

271. Trump, B. F., Berezesky, I. K., and Osornio-Vargas, A. R. (1981): In: *Cell Death in Biology and Pathology*, edited by I. D. Bowen and R. A. Lockshin, p. 209. Chapman and Hall, London.

272. Tschopp, J. and Mollnes, T.-E. (1986): Antigenic crossreactivity of the α subunit of complement component C8 with the cysteine-rich domain shared by complement component C9 and low density lipoprotein receptor. *Proc. Natl. Acad. Sci. USA*, 83:4223–4227.

273. Tschopp, J., Masson, D., and Stanley, K. K. (1986): Structural/functional similarity between proteins involved in complement- and cytotoxic T-lymphocyte-mediated cytolysis. *Nature*, 322:831–834.

274. Tschopp, J., Müller-Eberhard, H. J., and Podack, E. R. (1982): Formation of transmembrane tubules by spontaneous polymerization of hydrophilic complement protein C9. *Nature*, 298:534–538.

275. Tschopp, J., Podack, E. R., and Müller-Eberhard, H. J. (1982): Ultrastructure of the membrane attack complex of complement: Detection of the tetramolecular C9 polymerizing complex C5b-8. *Proc. Natl. Acad. Sci. USA*, 79:7474–7478.

276. Tschopp, J., Podack, E. R., and Müller-Eberhard, H. J. (1985): The membrane attack complex of complement: C5b-8 complex as accelerator of C9 polymerization. *J. Immunol.*, 134:495–499.

277. Tschopp, J., Villiger, W., Fuchs, H., Kilchherr, E., and Engel, J. (1980): Assembly of subcomponents C1r and C1s of first component

of complement: Electron microscopic and ultracentrifugal studies. *Proc. Natl. Acad. Sci. USA*, 77:7014–7018.

278. Vogt, W., Schmidt, G., von Buttlar, B., and Dieminger, L. (1978): A new function of the activated third component of complement: Binding to C5, an essential step for C5 activation. *Immunology*, 34:29–40.

279. VonZabern, I., Nolte, R., and Vogt, W. (1981): Treatment of human complement components C4 and C3 with amines or chaotropic ions. *Scand. J. Immunol.*, 13:413–431.

280. Ward, R. H. R., and Lachmann, P. J. (1985): Monoclonal antibodies which react with lymphocyte-lysed target cells and which cross-react with complement-lysed ghosts. *Immunology*, 56:179–188.

281. Weigle, W. O., Goodman, M. G., Morgan, E. L., and Hugli, T. E. (1983): Regulation of immune response by components of the complement cascade and their activated fragments. *Springer Semin. Immunopathol.*, 6:173–194.

282. Weiler, J. M., Daha, M. R., Austen, K. F., and Fearon, D. T. (1976): Control of the amplification convertase of complement by the plasma protein β1H. *Proc. Natl. Acad. Sci. USA*, 73:3268–3272.

283. Weis, J. J., Toothaker, L. E., Richards, S. A., Weis, J. H., and Fearon, D. T. (1987): cDNA sequence analysis and genomic organization of human CR2. *Fed. Proc.*, 46:1024 (abstract).

284. Weiss, A., Imboden, J., Hardy, K., Manger, B., Terhorst, C., and Stobo, J. (1986): The role of the T3/antigen receptor complex in T-cell activation. *Annu. Rev. Immunol.*, 4:593–619.

285. Weiss, V., Fauser, C., and Engel, J. (1986): Functional model of subcomponent C1 of human complement. *J. Mol. Biol.*, 189:573–581.

286. Wetsel, R. A., Ogata, R. T., and Tack, B. F. (1987): Primary structure of the fifth component of murine complement. *Biochemistry*, 26:737–743.

287. Wetsel, R. A., Lundwall, A., Davidson, F., Gibson, T., Tack, B. F., and Fey, G. H. (1984): Structure of murine complement component C3. II. Nucleotide sequence of cloned complementary DNA coding for the α chain. *J. Biol. Chem.*, 259:13857–13862.

288. Whaley, K., and Ruddy, S. (1976): Modulation of the alternative complement pathway by β1H globulin. *J. Exp. Med.*, 144:1147–1163.

289. Young, J. D.-E., Liu, C.-C., Leong, L. G., and Cohn, Z. A. (1986): The pore-forming protein (perforin) of cytolytic T lymphocytes is immunologically related to the components of membrane attack complex of complement through cysteine-rich domains. *J. Exp. Med.*, 164:2077–2082.

290. Zalman, L. S., and Müller-Eberhard, H. J. (1985): Comparison of channels formed by poly C9, C5b-8 and the membrane attack complex using the liposome swelling assay. *Fed. Proc.*, 44:551 (abstract).

291. Zalman, L. S., and Müller-Eberhard, H. J. (1987): To be published.

292. Zalman, L. S., Brothers, M. A., and Müller-Eberhard, H. J. (1985): A C9 related channel forming protein in the cytoplasmic granules of human large granular lymphocytes. *Biosci. Rep.*, 5:1093–1100.

293. Zalman, L. S., Wood, L. M., and Müller-Eberhard, H. J. (1986): Isolation of a human erythrocyte membrane protein capable of inhibiting expression of homologous complement transmembrane channels. *Proc. Natl. Acad. Sci. USA*, 83:6975–6979.

294. Zalman, L. S., Wood, L. M., and Müller-Eberhard, H. J. (1987): Inhibition of antibody dependent lymphocyte cytotoxicity by homologous restriction factor incorporated into target cell membranes. *J. Exp. Med.* (in press).

295. Zalman, L. S., Brothers, M. A., Chiu, F. J., and Müller-Eberhard, H. J. (1986): Mechanism of cytotoxicity of human large granular lymphocytes: Relationship of the cytotoxic lymphocyte protein to C8 and C9 of human complement. *Proc. Natl. Acad. Sci. USA*, 83: 5262–5266.

296. Zalman, L. S., Martin, D. E., Jung, G., and Müller-Eberhard, H. J. (1987): The cytolytic protein of human lymphocytes related to the ninth component (C9) of human complement: Isolation from anti-CD3-activated peripheral blood mononuclear cells. *Proc. Natl. Acad. Sci. USA*, 84:2426–2429.

297. Zalman, L. S., Wood, L. M., Frank, M. M., and Müller-Eberhard, H. J. (1987): Deficiency of the homologous restriction factor in paroxysmal nocturnal hemoglobinuria. *J. Exp. Med.*, 165:572–577.

298. Ziccardi, R. J. (1981): Activation of the early components of the classical complement pathway under physiologic conditions. *J. Immunol.*, 126:1769–1773.

299. Ziccardi, R. J. (1982): Spontaneous activation of the first component of human complement (C1) by an intramolecular autocatalytic mechanism. *J. Immunol.*, 128:2500–2504.

300. Ziccardi, R. J. (1982): A new role for C1-inhibitor in homeostasis: Control of activation of the first component of human complement. *J. Immunol.*, 128:2505–2508.

301. Ziccardi, R. J. (1983): The first component of human complement (C1): activation and control. *Springer Sem. Immunopath.*, 6:213–230.

302. Ziccardi, R. J. (1986): Control of C1 activation by nascent C3b and C4b: A mechanism of feedback inhibition. *J. Immunol.*, 136: 3378–3383.

303. Ziccardi, R. J., and Cooper, N. R. (1976): Activation of C1r by proteolytic cleavage. *J. Immunol.*, 116:504–509.

304. Ziccardi, R. J., and Cooper, N. R. (1977): The subunit composition and sedimentation properties of human C1. *J. Immunol.*, 118:2047–2052.

305. Ziccardi, R. J., and Cooper, N. R. (1979): Active disassembly of the first complement component, C1, by C1-inactivator. *J. Immunol.*, 123:788–792.

306. Ziccardi, R. J., Dahlback, B., and Müller-Eberhard, H. J. (1984): Characterization of the interaction of human C4b-binding protein (C4BP) with physiological ligands. *J. Biol. Chem.*, 259:13674–13678.

Inflammation: Basic Principles and Clinical Correlates.
Edited by J. I. Gallin, I. M. Goldstein, and R. Snyderman.
Raven Press, Ltd., New York © 1988.

CHAPTER 4

Complement: Biologically Active Products

Ira M. Goldstein

Activation of complement, by either the classical or alternative pathway, leads to the generation of products that not only help to maintain normal host defenses but also mediate inflammation and tissue injury. With respect to host defenses and inflammation, the most important products of complement include large fragments of C3 (e.g., C3b, C3bi) with opsonic activity, as well as low-molecular-weight peptides (derived from C3 and C5) that exhibit anaphylatoxin activity and directly stimulate leukocytes. These and other biologically active products of complement activation are the subject of this review. The sections that follow include descriptions of certain chemical properties of these biologically active complement components, discussions concerning the mechanisms by which they exert their effects on cells and tissues, and examples of their relevance to human diseases.

FRAGMENTS OF C3 WITH OPSONIC ACTIVITY

As described in detail in Chapter 3, activation of both the classical and alternative complement pathways leads to the assembly of enzymes (i.e., C3 convertases) that cleave the alpha chain of native C3 between amino acid residues 77 and 78 to yield two fragments. The smaller of these fragments (C3a), which represents the amino-terminal portion of the alpha chain, has a molecular weight of approximately 9,000 and is active in the fluid phase as an anaphylatoxin (see below). The larger fragment (nascent C3b), with a molecular weight of approximately 170,000, rapidly undergoes a conformational change which activates a thiolester bond in the alpha chain (167). The activated thiolester bond, or "labile binding site," either can be hydrolyzed or can react nonspecifically with a hydroxyl or amino group to form an ester or amide bond. Hydrolysis leads to inactivation of C3b, whereas reactions between a glutamyl residue in the labile binding site and a hydroxyl or amino group permit biologically active C3b to become covalently attached to a variety of surfaces.

The biologic activities of surface-bound C3b are regulated by factor H and factor I. Factor H attaches to C3b and renders it susceptible to the action of factor I (a serine proteinase). Factor I initially cleaves the alpha chain of C3b at two sites to yield fragments with molecular weights of 67,000, 40,000, and 3,000. Because disulfide bonds between the two larger fragments and the beta chain of C3b remain intact, the product formed by the initial action of factor I has a molecular weight (167,000) very similar to that of C3b. This product (C3bi) is unable to participate in the assembly of a C5 convertase but remains surface-bound and is recognized by phagocytic leukocytes. Factor I can cleave a third bond in the 67,000-dalton alpha-chain fragment of C3bi to yield two additional products. One of these products (C3d,g), a single-chain polypeptide with a molecular weight of 41,000, contains the labile binding site and therefore remains bound to surfaces. The other fragment (C3c), consisting of three polypeptide chains, is released into the fluid phase. Surface-bound C3d,g can be cleaved further by a variety of serine proteinases (e.g., plasmin, elastase) to yield C3d (molecular weight 35,000). In contrast to C3b and C3bi, surface-bound C3d is not recognized by phagocytic cells.

Wright and Douglas (189) originated the term "opsonize," meaning (from the Greek) "to prepare for dining." They observed that fresh human serum greatly enhanced ingestion and killing of bacteria by peripheral blood polymorphonuclear leukocytes (neutrophils). It is now known that there are two major components of serum (opsonins) that act on certain bacteria, fungi, and other particles to facilitate their ingestion by phagocytic cells. One is heat-stable (56°C for 30 min) and present only in serum from animals previously exposed to the test particle (i.e., immune serum); the other is heat-labile and present in fresh normal serum. The heat-stable component is immunoglobulin (i.e., antibody) of the IgG class (particularly subclasses IgG$_1$ and IgG$_3$). The Fc regions of IgG that have attached to antigens are recognized by structurally specific receptors (i.e., Fc receptors) on the surfaces of phagocytic leukocytes. Phagocytes, therefore, bind specifically to particles (including bacteria and fungi) sensitized with IgG antibody.

Heat-labile opsonic activity is attributable to fragments of the third component of complement (e.g., C3b, C3bi) that bind to the surfaces of particles as a consequence of complement activation by either the classical or alternative pathway. C3b and C3bi render particles to which they are attached recognizable by phagocytic leukocytes as a consequence of binding to structurally specific receptors and mediate firm particle–cell adherence. Particles to which C4b is bound also are recognized by C3 receptors on human neutrophils and monocytes. However, the extent to which C4b promotes attachment of phagocytic leukocytes to sensitized particles and stimulates phagocytosis is not known. Most evidence indicates that these important functions are mediated primarily by C3b and C3bi.

Whereas polymorphonuclear and mononuclear leukocytes appear to be capable of ingesting seemingly inert particles (e.g., polystyrene latex beads), particularly under conditions where particle–cell contact is maximized, opsonins such as IgG, C3b, and C3bi clearly increase the rate and extent of phagocytosis. Mechanisms by which IgG and fragments of C3 promote particle recognition and phagocytosis, as well as specific receptors for these opsonins, are discussed in detail elsewhere in this volume (Chapter 21).

C3b and C3bi not only promote ingestion of particles by neutrophils but also stimulate these cells to generate potentially toxic products of molecular oxygen (53,155) and to secrete histaminase (116). C3b also stimulates human monocytes to increase their oxidative metabolism (154). Finally, there is ample evidence that fragments of human C3 influence both cellular and humoral immune responses. C3 fragments, for example, have been reported to be mitogenic for B and T lymphocytes, to inhibit mitogen- and alloantigen-induced lymphocyte proliferation, to suppress specific and nonspecific antibody responses, to block generation of cytotoxic T lymphocytes, and to localize antigen (39,184).

ANAPHYLATOXINS—PEPTIDES DERIVED FROM C3, C4, AND C5

Anaphylatoxins are low-molecular-weight, biologically active peptides that are defined functionally by their actions on small blood vessels, smooth muscle, mast cells, and peripheral blood leukocytes (81,84) (Table 1). Osler et al. (133) provided the first direct experimental evidence that anaphylatoxin activity was derived from complement. Subsequently, studies in several laboratories established conclusively that low-molecular-weight peptides with anaphylatoxin activity could be generated enzymatically from C3, C4, and C5 (i.e., C3a, C4a, and C5a, respectively) (11,25,57).

Considerable progress has been made recently in elucidating the primary structures of individual anaphylatoxins. Furthermore, a great deal of information has accumulated concerning structure–activity relationships. For example, analyses of the complete amino acid sequences of C3a, C4a, and C5a from humans and from a

TABLE 1. *Biologic activities of human anaphylatoxins*[a]

Target cells or tissue	Response
Small blood vessels	Increased permeability
Smooth muscle	Contraction
Mast cells, basophils	Release of histamine
Polymorphonuclear leukocytes	Polarization, directed migration, secretion of lysosomal enzymes, increased oxidative metabolism, increased adherence to surfaces, aggregation, increased expression of C3 receptors
Monocytes and macrophages	Polarization, directed migration, secretion of lysosomal enzymes, increased oxidative metabolism, increased expression of C3 and IgG receptors, generation of interleukin-1

[a] Small blood vessels, smooth muscle, mast cells, and basophils respond to C3a, C4a, and C5a. Polymorphonuclear leukocytes, monocytes, and macrophages respond only to C5a.

variety of animal species have revealed striking similarities among these peptides, suggesting a common evolutionary origin. In addition, circular dichroism measurements, X-ray diffraction studies, and studies with synthetic peptides have provided information concerning the three-dimensional structures of anaphylatoxins, as well as information concerning their active sites.

Human C3a was the first biologically active component of complement for which a complete primary structure was elucidated (80,83). Human C3a is a highly cationic polypeptide with a molecular weight of approximately 9,000 (Table 2). Human C3a is composed of 77 amino acid residues in a single polypeptide chain. It contains two cysteinylcysteine sequences, a total of six half-cystine residues, and three internal disulfide linkages. Circular dichroism measurements, as well as crystallographic analyses, have confirmed that large portions of the C3a molecule have an alpha-helical conformation (77,82). The carboxy-terminal arginine of C3a is absolutely essential

for anaphylatoxin activity, as is the carboxy-terminal pentapeptide leu-gly-leu-ala-arg (15). Indeed, the pentapeptide alone exhibits spasmogenic activity and enhances vascular permeability. A synthetic polypeptide corresponding to the 21 carboxy-terminal amino acids of human C3a, which spontaneously assumes an alpha-helical conformation under certain solvent conditions, exhibits anaphylatoxin activity nearly equivalent to that exhibited by the native molecule (73).

Based on detailed chemical and biologic characterization, C4a also has been identified as an anaphylatoxin (57,58). Human C4a is a highly cationic polypeptide with a molecular weight of 9,000 and a primary structure quite similar to that of C3a (58,119). Like C3a, human C4a is composed of 77 amino acids in a single polypeptide chain. Human C4a also resembles C3a with respect to its content of six half-cystine residues. Finally, C4a resembles C3a in that its minimal effective structure appears to be a carboxy-terminal pentapeptide (ala-gly-leu-gln-arg) (86). Although this pentapeptide contracts smooth muscle (i.e., guinea pig ileum), it is approximately 500-fold less active in this respect than the C3a pentapeptide.

The first detailed description of the anaphylatoxin activity of isolated human C5a was provided by Cochrane and Müller-Eberhard (25). These investigators demonstrated that incubation of purified human C5 with trypsin, or with the classical complement pathway C5 convertase, yielded a low-molecular-weight peptide that increased capillary permeability when injected into guinea pig skin and contracted atropinized guinea pig ileum. The C5a anaphylatoxin isolated from activated human serum by Vallota and Müller-Eberhard (172) also contracted guinea pig ileum (at a concentration of 0.1 nM) and produced complete desensitization to subsequent exposure of the smooth muscle preparation to C5a obtained by trypsin treatment of isolated C5 (see following).

Human C5a is a cationic glycopeptide with a molecular weight of approximately 16,000 (as estimated by gel filtration and by sodium dodecyl sulfate polyacrylamide gel electrophoresis) (40,42). The polypeptide portion of C5a contains 74 amino acids, accounting for a molecular

TABLE 2. *Physicochemical properties of human anaphylatoxins*

	C3a	C4a	C5a
Molecular weight	9,000	9,000	11,200
Amino acid residues	77	77	74
Cysteinylcysteine sequences	2	2	2
Half-cystine residues	6	6	6
Internal disulfide linkages	3	3	3
Alpha-helical conformation	41–43%	54%	48–50%
Carboxyl-terminus	leu-gly-leu-ala-arg	ala-gly-leu-gln-arg	met-gln-leu-gly-arg
Carbohydrate	No	No	Yes
Isoelectric point	9.0–9.5	9.0–9.5	8.5

weight of 8,200, whereas the carbohydrate portion accounts for approximately 3,000 daltons. Thus, the protein and carbohydrate portions together have an actual molecular weight (approximately 11,200) considerably less than that determined by physical measurements. This discrepancy has been attributed to the high carbohydrate content of the C5a molecule. The carbohydrate portion of C5a exists as a single complex oligosaccharide (containing 4 moles of glucosamine, 3 to 4 moles of sialic acid, 4 moles of mannose, and 2 moles of galactose) attached to an asparagine residue at position 64 (40,42). The oligosaccharide moiety of human C5a readily distinguishes this molecule from rat and porcine C5a, as well as from human C3a and human C4a, all of which are devoid of carbohydrate (80,84,119).

Human C5a resembles C3a and C4a with respect to its large content of half-cystine residues. C5a also contains three disulfide bridges, and approximately 40% of its amino acid residues are in an alpha-helical conformation (126). Consequently, human C5a (like human C3a and C4a) is functionally stable over a wide range of pH conditions and resists heating at 56°C for 30 min (81,84). Human C5a, however, is susceptible to attack by a variety of enzymes that alter or destroy its biologic activities (see following).

Analysis of the complete amino acid sequence in human C5a has revealed a carboxy-terminal arginine which is essential for the expression of maximal anaphylatoxin activity (42,172). As is the case with the carboxy-terminal pentapeptide portions of human C3a and C4a, the carboxy-terminal pentapeptide portion of human C5a (met-gln-leu-gly-arg) also is essential for biologic activity (19). Unlike C3a and C4a, however, synthetic peptides corresponding to the carboxy-terminal portion of C5a do not exhibit anaphylatoxin activity. The amino-terminal 69 residues of C5a also are inactive, either alone or in combination with the carboxy-terminal pentapeptide. Nevertheless, C5a 1–69 competes with native C5a 1–74 for binding to the C5a receptor on the surface membranes of neutrophils (20). It appears, therefore, that multiple sites on the native C5a molecule are required to induce cellular responses.

Before discussing the biologic activities of anaphylatoxins further, it should be pointed out that cellular responses to these molecules frequently are stimulus-specific, tissue-specific, and species-specific. For example, among human anaphylatoxins, the rank order of potency with respect to causing contraction of guinea pig ileum is C5a > C3a ≫ C4a (relative activities are approximately 3,000, 200, and 1, respectively) (85). In contrast, although the rank order of potency is the same, the relative activities of human C5a, C3a, and C4a in enhancing vascular permeability in human skin are approximately 25,000, 100,

and 1, respectively (81). Similarly, although porcine C3a and human C3a are indistinguishable with respect to their effects on vascular permeability in guinea pig skin, porcine C5a is approximately 10-fold more active than human C5a (81).

The capacity of human C5a and human C3a to contract guinea pig ileum diminishes markedly with repeated applications and is inhibited completely by pretreatment of a smooth muscle preparation with antihistamines. The tachyphylaxis produced by anaphylatoxins is quite specific (25). Repeated exposure of smooth muscle to C5a is followed by a state of unresponsiveness to subsequent stimulation by C5a. The same phenomenon occurs with C3a. C5a, however, will stimulate smooth muscle rendered unresponsive to C3a, and vice versa. Smooth muscle stimulated repeatedly with C4a, however, becomes unresponsive to both C4a and C3a (57). Similarly, stimulation with C3a renders smooth muscle unresponsive to C4a. These observations are consistent with the suggestion that C3a and C4a are recognized by the same cell surface receptors and that these receptors are distinct from those that recognize C5a (81).

Receptor–ligand interactions alone are insufficient to account for the heterogeneous cellular and tissue responses to anaphylatoxins. The mechanisms whereby C3a and C5a provoke contraction of smooth muscle and enhance vascular permeability appear to be quite complex. For example, whereas contractile responses of guinea pig ileum to C5a and C3a can be inhibited by prior exposure to antihistamines (particularly H_1-type antagonists), responses of other tissues appear to be only partially mediated by, or dependent on, histamine release. In particular, anaphylatoxin-mediated contractions of guinea pig lung strips and guinea pig trachea appear to be histamine-independent. Stimler et al. (163,165), for example, found that contractions of guinea pig lung parenchymal strips induced by human or porcine C3a were unaffected by antihistamines but were inhibited significantly by agents that interfere with the metabolism of arachidonic acid by the cyclooxygenase pathway (e.g., aspirin, indomethacin). C3a-induced contractions were reduced maximally by combinations of antihistamines and cyclooxygenase inhibitors. Regal and Pickering (147) found that contractions of isolated guinea pig tracheal strips induced by guinea pig C5a also were unaffected by antihistamines. Interestingly, C5a-induced contractions of tracheal smooth muscle were unaffected by aspirin but were inhibited significantly by agents that interfere either with the metabolism of arachidonic acid by lipoxygenases or with the actions of the leukotrienes C_4 and D_4. Leukotriene antagonists, but not antihistamines, also inhibit human C5a-induced contraction of enzymatically dispersed smooth muscle cells from toad stomach (153), human C3a-induced contraction of guinea pig portal vein (107), and the positive inotropic effects induced by human C3a and C5a on guinea pig atria (78). These observations, as well as the findings that C3a and C5a provoke selective release from lung tissue of prostaglandins and leukotrienes, respectively (81,164), suggest that anaphylatoxins mediate some of their effects on tissues by stimulating cells to generate biologically active products of arachidonic acid. Support for this suggestion has come from Hartung et al. (69), who found C3a capable of directly stimulating guinea pig peritoneal macrophages to synthesize and release thromboxane A_2.

Although the role that histamine plays in the smooth muscle-contracting activities of human C3a and C5a is not at all clear, there is ample evidence that C3a and C5a provoke release of histamine in a variety of tissues. For example, C3a and C5a provoke histamine release in guinea pig lung and mesentery (25,32), as well as in human skin (192,193). Human C5a produces immediate wheal and flare reactions in human skin at doses as low as 0.1 pmole (193) and causes release of histamine from isolated rat mast cells at concentrations ranging from 0.4 to 8.0 μM (88).

Human C3a and C5a also have been found capable of provoking release of histamine from human peripheral blood basophils (60,68,143,157). Although complement-induced histamine release from human basophils is similar in some respects to that provoked by IgE and antigen, C5a-induced release occurs more rapidly than IgE-induced release and is optimal at lower temperatures (25 to 30°C) (157). Human basophils can be desensitized to the C5a-induced reaction by pretreatment with C5a in the presence of agents that chelate divalent cations. Such treated cells respond normally to IgE. Similarly, basophils desensitized for IgE-mediated reactions release histamine normally upon exposure to C5a (143). These observations suggest that C5a and IgE utilize separate pathways to provoke release of histamine from basophils.

Regulation of Anaphylatoxin Activity— Anaphylatoxin Inactivator

The ease with which complement-derived anaphylatoxin activity could be demonstrated in sera from rats, guinea pigs, pigs, and dogs—but not from humans—suggested to some investigators that anaphylatoxins were not generated in human serum as a consequence of complement activation (32,133). Bokisch et al. (11) subsequently provided an alternative explanation by demonstrating that the anaphylatoxin activity of isolated human C3a was destroyed completely when this peptide was incubated briefly with human serum. The substance in human serum

that was responsible for this phenomenon subsequently was identified as a carboxypeptidase B-like enzyme and was termed "anaphylatoxin inactivator" (12).

Anaphylatoxin inactivator is a 300,000-dalton α-globulin which is present in human serum (and plasma) in its active form at a concentration of 5 mg/dl. It rapidly abolishes the anaphylatoxin activities of both C3a and C5a by removing argininyl residues from the carboxy-terminal ends of these polypeptides (12,42). Anaphylatoxin inactivator also hydrolyzes bradykinin, as well as the synthetic substrates hippuryl-L-arginine and hippuryl-L-lysine. It is heat-labile (56°C for 30 min) and is inhibited by ethylenediaminetetraacetic acid and ϵ-aminocaproic acid. Anaphylatoxin inactivator appears to be identical with plasma carboxypeptidase N (144).

Anaphylatoxin inactivator activity has been demonstrated in serum from guinea pigs, rats, and rabbits (12). Although sera from these species destroy the activities of human anaphylatoxins, they have little or no effect on the activities of anaphylatoxins generated in autologous or other heterologous sera. The physical and/or chemical properties of human C3a and C5a that render these polypeptides so susceptible to the action of anaphylatoxin inactivator are unknown. These properties, however, account for the unsuccessful attempts by several investigators to demonstrate anaphylatoxin activity in whole human serum after complement activation.

Vallota and Müller-Eberhard (172) were the first to demonstrate that anaphylatoxin activity could be formed in whole human serum. They took advantage of the fact that ϵ-aminocaproic acid effectively inhibits the anaphylatoxin inactivator in human serum but allows complement activation to proceed. Biologically active C3a and C5a were obtained by treating whole human serum with a variety of substances (e.g., antigen–antibody complexes, inulin, endotoxin) after inhibiting the anaphylatoxin inactivator with 1.0 M ϵ-aminocaproic acid. Fernandez and Hugli (42) subsequently demonstrated that, when serum lacking ϵ-aminocaproic acid was used as starting material, only the des Arg form of C5a was recovered after complement activation. C5a des Arg is identical to C5a except that it lacks the carboxy-terminal arginyl residue. Human C5a des Arg, whether isolated from human serum after complement activation or formed from isolated human C5a with pancreatic carboxypeptidase B, completely lacks smooth muscle-contracting activity (41,42). Human C5a des Arg, however, does enhance vascular permeability in guinea pig, human, and rabbit skin (81,92). The effects of human C5a des Arg on vascular permeability, as well as the effects of rabbit C5a des Arg and, to some extent, human and rabbit C5a, appear to be mediated by neutrophils and vasodilatory prostaglandins (10,87,92,182). Since C3a and C5a have been found capable of activating platelets (117,146), it is possible that platelet products also play a role in the pathogenesis of anaphylatoxin-induced increases in vascular permeability.

C5-DERIVED PEPTIDES WITH CHEMOTACTIC ACTIVITY TOWARD NEUTROPHILS

Leber (98) provided one of the earliest descriptions of leukocyte chemotaxis. He suggested that the direction of migrating cells was determined by chemical substances in their environment and concluded that extravascular migration of leukocytes was caused by gradients of chemical attractants between inflamed tissues and blood vessels. There is now abundant evidence that chemotaxis of leukocytes plays an important role in the mediation of inflammation and in the maintenance of normal host defenses against infection.

Perhaps the earliest evidence of a role for complement in attracting neutrophils was provided by Boyden (13), who found that a heat-stable chemotactic substance was generated when antigen–antibody complexes were incubated in medium containing rabbit serum. Ward et al. (174) subsequently confirmed that complement activation resulted in the formation of chemoattractants and suggested that a trimolecular complex of C5, C6, and C7 was responsible for this activity. Snyderman et al. (160a), however, showed that the major chemoattractant generated after complement activation in serum was a low-molecular-weight (approximately 15,000) peptide presumed to be a cleavage product of C5. Shin et al. (156) also found that activation of complement in guinea pig serum (by sensitized erythrocytes coated with C1 to C4) resulted in the formation of a low-molecular-weight peptide with anaphylatoxin activity and chemotactic activity toward rabbit neutrophils. Subsequent studies (176) documented that fragments of human C5 also exhibited chemotactic activity. Exposure of purified human C5 to either trypsin or sensitized sheep erythrocytes (coated with C1 to C4) resulted in the generation of low-molecular-weight, C5-derived peptides capable of attracting rabbit neutrophils.

Interestingly, incubation of isolated human C5 with low concentrations of either trypsin or α-thrombin for brief durations yields a chemotactically active product with a molecular weight (210,000) identical to that of native C5 (186). Low concentrations of trypsin and α-thrombin cleave the alpha chain of native C5 at a single site to yield two fragments (molecular weights of 25,000 and 95,000) that remain attached to an intact beta chain by disulfide bonds. Cleavage of the alpha chain alone, therefore, appears sufficient to convert native C5 to a biologically active molecule.

It is now quite clear that human C5-derived peptides with chemotactic activity toward neutrophils (41), eosinophils (94), basophils (100), and monocytes (34; and see below) can be generated as a result of activating both the classical and alternative complement pathways, as well as by the action of various proteinases on native C5. It also is clear that of the various peptides that can be cleaved from native human C5, C5a anaphylatoxin is the most potent chemoattractant. Highly purified human C5a exhibits chemotactic activity toward human neutrophils at concentrations as low as 0.1 nM (17,41,139,181). Higher concentrations (e.g., >1.0–5.0 nM) result in decreased neutrophil migration, a phenomenon termed "deactivation" or "desensitization" (175). Whereas C3a, C4a, and C5a cause contraction of smooth muscle, increases in vascular permeability, and release of histamine from mast cells, only C5a exhibits potent chemotactic activity toward neutrophils and monocytes.

C5a des Arg Cochemotaxin

It is unlikely that C5a accounts for the bulk of chemotactic activity generated in human serum as a consequence of complement activation. This is because human serum contains anaphylatoxin inactivator (carboxypeptidase N) which rapidly converts C5a to C5a des Arg (12). Consequently, the des Arg form of C5a is the predominant C5-derived peptide found in whole human serum after complement activation. Highly purified human C5a des Arg lacks smooth muscle-contracting activity and, at low concentrations, also lacks chemotactic activity (41,139,181). Highly purified human C5a des Arg is 10- to 20-fold less potent than C5a as a chemoattractant for human neutrophils. Nevertheless, normal human serum and plasma contain a heat-stable anionic polypeptide with a molecular weight of approximately 60,000 (termed "cochemotaxin") that permits low concentrations of C5a des Arg to exhibit significant chemotactic activity toward human neutrophils (138,139). Purified cochemotaxin acts in a concentration-dependent manner to permit low concentrations of C5a des Arg to attract neutrophils. The profile of chemotactic activity exhibited by C5a des Arg and its cochemotaxin closely resembles that exhibited by dilutions of zymosan-activated serum and by highly purified C5a (139). Thus C5a des Arg and its cochemotaxin probably account for most of the chemotactic activity generated in human serum after limited complement activation.

The precise mechanism by which cochemotaxin augments the chemotactic activity of C5a des Arg is unknown. However, a mechanism was described recently whereby the biologic activities of human C5-derived peptides can be modulated. Gerard and Hugli (44) found that human C5a des Arg "regained" anaphylatoxin activity when the single oligosaccharide chain was removed by glycosidases, leaving a single glucosamine residue attached to asparagine-64. Deglycosylated C5a des Arg contracted guinea pig ileum and enhanced vascular permeability in guinea pig skin. Gerard et al. (43) subsequently demonstrated that deglycosylated human C5a des Arg was approximately 10-fold more active than native C5a des Arg with respect to its ability to promote neutrophil chemotaxis. In contrast, native C5a and deglycosylated C5a behaved identically. These findings suggest that the oligosaccharide moiety does not influence the biologic activities of human C5a but does modulate the biologic activities of C5a des Arg.

Perez et al. (141) recently confirmed that deglycosylated human C5a des Arg was significantly more potent than native human C5a des Arg as a chemoattractant for human neutrophils and found that the chemotactic activity of deglycosylated C5a des Arg was not affected at all by purified cochemotaxin. In light of these findings, the possibility was considered that cochemotaxin interacts directly with the oligosaccharide chain of native C5a des Arg. Indeed, evidence (albeit indirect) had already been obtained that cochemotaxin interacted with sugar moieties. The apparent molecular weight of cochemotaxin, as determined by sodium dodecyl sulfate polyacrylamide gel electrophoresis (60,000), differed substantially from that estimated by molecular sieve chromatography on Sephadex G-75 (20,000–30,000) (139). Moreover, the elution profile of cochemotaxin activity observed after Sephadex G-75 chromatography of heat-inactivated human serum was similar to the elution profile of low-molecular-weight C5-derived chemotactic activity observed when zymosan-activated serum was chromatographed under identical conditions (138). It seemed likely, therefore, that binding of cochemotaxin to Sephadex (agarose) gels accounted for its retarded elution and, consequently, for its coelution with low-molecular-weight C5-derived peptides (predominantly C5a des Arg). Such binding was not observed with polyacrylamide gels. Purified cochemotaxin eluted from columns of Bio-Gel P-150 with an apparent molecular weight of 60,000.

To determine whether cochemotaxin interacts with components of the oligosaccharide chain of C5a des Arg, Perez et al. (141) measured the chemotactic activity expressed by mixtures of these two polypeptides in the presence and absence of various monosaccharides. Of the monosaccharides known to be components of the oligosaccharide chain of C5a des Arg, only sialic acid prevented enhancement by cochemotaxin of the chemotactic activity exhibited by low concentrations of C5a des Arg. In contrast, sialic acid did not influence directed migration of

neutrophils toward either high concentrations of C5a des Arg alone or low concentrations of C5a. These findings suggested that cochemotaxin formed a physical "complex" with native C5a des Arg, possibly by attaching to a sialic acid residue on the oligosaccharide chain.

More direct evidence that cochemotaxin attaches to the oligosaccharide chain of native C5a des Arg was obtained in three ways. First, electrophoretic migration of radiolabeled C5a des Arg into acid polyacrylamide gels was retarded significantly by cochemotaxin, an effect that was reversed by sialic acid. Second, when examined by molecular sieve chromatography on polyacrylamide gels, cochemotaxin markedly altered the elution profile of radiolabeled C5a des Arg (the peak of radioactivity eluted with an apparent molecular weight of 85,000), an effect that also was prevented by sialic acid. Finally, sucrose density gradient ultracentrifugation of radiolabeled C5a des Arg and purified cochemotaxin revealed that the two polypeptides formed a physical complex with an apparent molecular weight of 85,000 (141). Indirect evidence that C5a des Arg complexes with other components in serum was provided previously by Beebe et al. (6), who isolated from zymosan-activated human serum an anionic C5-derived chemotactic factor with an apparent molecular weight of 65,000.

Obviously, more work must be done to confirm that cochemotaxin exhibits "lectinlike" activity and attaches to a sialic residue on the oligosaccharide chain of native C5a des Arg. Much more work must also be done to determine the precise mechanism(s) by which cochemotaxin augments the chemotactic activity of native C5a des Arg. For example, it is possible that cochemotaxin enhances the chemotactic activity of native C5a des Arg by "masking" the oligosaccharide chain in such a manner as to make the molecule resemble deglycosylated C5a des Arg.

It should be noted that C5a des Arg cochemotaxin differs significantly from the "cocytotaxin" described previously by Wissler et al. (188). Cocytotaxin is a cationic peptide with an apparent molecular weight of 8,500 that is generated as a consequence of complement activation in guinea pig, rat, and hog serum. It exhibits neither smooth muscle-contracting activity nor chemotactic activity, but it does permit the "classical complement-derived anaphylatoxin" formed in guinea pig, rat, and hog serum to provoke directed migration of neutrophils. A factor resembling cocytotaxin has not been detected in human serum.

Receptors for C5-Derived Peptides on Neutrophils

The ability of human C5a and C5a des Arg to promote directed migration of neutrophils appears to be mediated by binding of these peptides to specific cell surface receptors. Webster et al. (181), for example, demonstrated that both C5a and C5a des Arg desensitized human neutrophils to subsequent stimulation by C5a; however, 25- to 50-fold more C5a des Arg than C5a was required to induce desensitization. These findings suggested that C5a des Arg binds to the same receptor as does C5a, but with a lower binding affinity. Experiments using radiolabeled C5a have delineated characteristics of ligand–cell surface interactions consistent with the presence of a specific receptor for C5a on neutrophils. Chenoweth and Hugli (18) demonstrated specific, rapid, and saturable binding of radiolabeled C5a to human neutrophils. Binding of C5a was inhibited to some extent by structural analogs of this peptide (e.g., C5a des Arg) but was unaffected either by other components of complement (e.g., C3a) or by structurally unrelated synthetic chemotactic peptides. Half-saturation of C5a binding occurred at a concentration of 3.0 to 7.0 nM, and the number of binding sites per cell was estimated to be 100,000 to 300,000. C5a did not bind to human erythrocytes or to cultured human lymphoblastoid cell lines. Similar studies by Huey and Hugli (79) have confirmed that binding of radiolabeled C5a to human neutrophils is specific, saturable, and reversible. Comparison of the concentration-dependent uptake of C5a by neutrophils with the biologic activity of this peptide revealed that nearly identical concentrations of ligand were required for binding and for eliciting chemotaxis. Finally, recent studies with photoactivatable cross-linking reagents have identified the C5a receptor on the surface of human neutrophils as a polypeptide with a molecular weight of approximately 42,000–48,000 (79,90,149).

Obviously, much more needs to be learned of the interactions between C5-derived peptides and their specific receptors on the surface membranes of leukocytes. For example, the distribution of receptors, their disposition following ligand binding, and the precise mechanisms whereby ligand–receptor interactions promote leukocyte migration are all unknown. Similarly, there is much more to be learned of the chemical structure–activity relationships of C5-derived peptides. While it is apparent that the carboxy-terminal arginine of C5a enhances chemotactic activity (41,139,181), and that the carbohydrate moiety of C5a des Arg reduces chemotactic activity (43,141), much less is known of other components in these molecules. For example, Clark et al. (24) have shown that myeloperoxidase-mediated oxidation of methionine inactivates several chemotactic factors, including human C5a. It is likely, therefore, that the methionyl residue at position 70 in C5a plays an important role in the expression of chemotactic activity. A tyrosine at position 23 in human C5a also may be important for the expression of chemotactic activity (91). Further elucidation of the three-dimensional structure of C5a (62), as well as site-specific

mutagenesis of synthetic genes that encode for human C5a (106), likely will provide additional information concerning structure–activity relationships. More information about the mechanisms whereby ligand–receptor interactions promote leukocyte migration and other cellular responses is presented in Chapter 19.

C5-DERIVED PEPTIDES WITH CHEMOTACTIC ACTIVITY FOR MONOCYTES

Although it had been demonstrated that human peripheral blood monocytes responded chemotactically to C5-derived peptides (34,161), it was not until recently that information became available concerning the relative potencies of C5a and C5a des Arg as chemoattractants for these cells. Marder et al. (108) found that human monocytes, unlike human neutrophils, responded identically to C5a and C5a des Arg when these peptides were used as chemoattractants. Both peptides acted at identical concentrations to stimulate suboptimal and optimal migration of monocytes. Furthermore, the chemotactic activity of C5a des Arg toward monocytes was unaffected by cochemotaxin. These results could not be accounted for simply by differences between the assay conditions used to measure neutrophil and monocyte chemotaxis. Even under conditions in which migration of monocytes was compared directly with migration of neutrophils (i.e., under agarose), monocytes responded identically to C5a and C5a des Arg. These results also could not be accounted for by the presence of carboxypeptidase-like activity in mononuclear leukocyte suspensions (which could convert C5a to C5a des Arg). Such activity was not detected.

C5a and C5a des Arg also were equipotent with respect to their ability to induce suspended monocytes to acquire a polarized morphology (i.e., a "head" and a "tail"). The concentrations of peptides required to induce maximum monocyte polarization were identical with those required to provoke maximum monocyte chemotaxis. Furthermore, approximately half of the total number of monocytes in suspension assumed a polarized shape, confirming that only a subpopulation of these cells was capable of recognizing C5a and C5a des Arg (23,34,173).

To determine directly whether C5a and C5a des Arg bind to the same receptor on monocytes, Marder et al. (108) performed experiments using biologically active radiolabeled peptides. Binding of radiolabeled human C5a to human monocytes was specific and saturable. Half-maximal uptake of C5a occurred at a concentration of 1.8 nM, similar to the concentration (1.0–1.2 nM) required to induce half-maximal chemotaxis and polarization. In contrast, specific binding of radiolabeled human C5a des Arg to monocytes reached saturation at a peptide concentration of 500 nM. Furthermore, whereas 0.3 nM

unlabeled C5a inhibited binding of 5.0 nM radiolabeled C5a des Arg by 50%, 250 nM unlabeled C5a des Arg was required to inhibit binding of 1.0 nM radiolabeled C5a to a similar extent. C5a des Arg, therefore, binds to monocytes much less avidly than does C5a. Thus, certain leukocyte responses to C5a and C5a des Arg vary depending on the target cell type and cannot be accounted for simply on the basis of primary ligand–receptor interactions.

C5-DERIVED PEPTIDES WITH CHEMOTACTIC ACTIVITY TOWARD TUMOR CELLS

Peptides derived from human C5 have been found capable of stimulating directed locomotion of various cultured tumor cells (129,150). Chemotactic activity for tumor cells can be generated from isolated native human C5 either by treatment with trypsin (129,151) or by treatment with leukocyte proteinases (i.e., elastase and cathepsin G) (131). Interestingly, during proteolysis of purified human C5, chemotactic activity toward leukocytes is generated first. As digestion is continued, however, chemotactic activity toward leukocytes declines and is replaced by chemotactic activity toward tumor cells. These observations, as well as physicochemical data, suggest that C5-derived peptides chemotactic for leukocytes are not identical to C5-derived peptides chemotactic for tumor cells. There is evidence, however, that the tumor cell chemotactic factor originates from the same region of native C5 as the leukotactic peptides. Cleavage of either purified human C5a or purified C5a des Arg with trypsin, for example, yields a 6,000-dalton peptide with chemotactic activity toward tumor cells (130). It appears likely, therefore, that the tumor cell chemotactic factor is resident, but "hidden" in the amino-terminal region of the alpha chain of native C5. This C5-derived peptide attracts some, but not all, cultured tumor cells. The most responsive cells include those from transmissible ascites tumors (e.g., Walker carcinosarcoma, Novikoff hepatoma) and murine myeloid leukemias (C-1498). Cells from a murine malignant lymphoma (EL-4), however, do not respond to this factor (129). Studies *in vivo* by Ozaki et al. (134) and by Lam et al. (97) have documented that circulating malignant cells localize to tissue sites injected with tumor cell chemotactic factors but not to tissue sites injected with either vasopermeability factors or substances chemotactic for leukocytes. Furthermore, C5-derived chemotactic factors for tumor cells have been recovered from inflammatory and neoplastic effusions (132). Thus, established patterns of metastatic growth, which are characteristic of various tumors, may be the consequence of responses of specific tumor cell types to chemotactic factors generated by different means in different tissues.

INACTIVATORS AND INHIBITORS OF C5-DERIVED CHEMOTACTIC ACTIVITY

The chemotactic activity of C5a and related polypeptides can be modulated by a variety of factors. For example, a neutral endoproteinase on the surface of virulent group A streptococci inactivates C5a by cleaving a six-residue peptide from the carboxy-terminal portion of the molecule (187). Lysosomal lysates obtained from human neutrophils also inactivate C5-derived chemotactic peptides at neutral pH (190). The inactivating enzymes have been localized to the azurophil granules of neutrophils (191) and have been identified as elastase and cathepsin G (14). The fact that these enzymes are inhibited so readily by α_1-antiproteinase and α_2-macroglobulin (128) makes it difficult to assess the roles they play in modulating inflammatory reactions *in vivo*.

The chemotactic activity of C5-derived peptides can be regulated by factors other than neutral proteinases. For example, Berenberg and Ward (8) described the presence in normal human serum of chemotactic factor inactivator activity. Two distinct chemotactic factor inactivators have been described in human serum: an α-globulin that specifically and irreversibly inactivates C5-derived chemotactic fragments, and a β-globulin that inactivates bacterial chemotactic factor(s) as well as the chemotactic activity of some synthetic peptides (95,169). Chemotactic factor inactivator activity is heat-labile (56°C for 30 min), is time- and temperature-dependent, and can be distinguished from the activity of anaphylatoxin inactivator. The mechanism whereby the chemotactic factor inactivator affects C5-derived peptides has not been elucidated. It not only inactivates the chemotactic activity of C5-derived peptides but also abrogates their ability to provoke selective release of lysosomal enzymes from neutrophils (35; and see below).

Reduced levels of chemotactic factor inactivator activity have been found in serum from some patients with a deficiency in α_1-antiproteinase (178). In contrast, increased levels have been demonstrated in patients with Hodgkin's disease (179), sarcoidosis (105), hepatic cirrhosis (104), and lepromatous leprosy (180). The presence of elevated levels of chemotactic factor inactivator activity in these patients is associated with defects in the mobilization of inflammatory cells in both acute and chronic inflammatory reactions. In fact, it has been suggested that chemotactic factor inactivators may function as endogenous regulators of inflammatory responses. Simultaneous injection of chemotactic factor inactivators and specific antibody resulted in complete suppression of the reverse passive Arthus reaction and acute immune complex-induced alveolitis in rats (89). Although naturally occurring inhibitors or inactivators of C5-derived peptides might be valuable adjuncts for the therapy of immunologically mediated inflammation, it must not be forgotten that inflammation is an important host defense mechanism. Thus, by specifically blocking the activities of C5-derived peptides, natural defenses against infection may be affected adversely.

Evidence that an inhibitor of C5-derived chemotactic activity can adversely affect host defenses has come from studies in patients with systemic lupus erythematosus. Perez et al. (136) demonstrated that sera from some patients with systemic lupus erythematosus contained a heat-stable (56°C for 30 min) cationic protein that reversibly inhibited the chemotactic activity of C5-derived peptides in a manner quite distinct from that of anaphylatoxin inactivator or chemotactic factor inactivators. The presence of this inhibitor in serum correlated with disease activity in patients with lupus and, perhaps more importantly, with increased susceptibility of such patients to severe bacterial infections (137). This inhibitor, which is chemically and antigenically similar to the Bb fragment of factor B, has no effect on the chemotactic activity of highly purified C5a but abolishes the chemotactic activity exhibited by mixtures of C5a des Arg and cochemotaxin (138,142).

Another specific inhibitor of C5-derived chemotactic activity has been found in normal human synovial fluid (109) and in normal human peritoneal fluid (110). This inhibitor, which acts directly on human C5a, has been characterized as a heat-stable (56°C for 30 min) protein with a molecular weight of approximately 40,000. Interestingly, levels of this inhibitor in synovial and peritoneal fluids from patients with familial Mediterranean fever appear to be markedly reduced (111,112). Because these patients suffer from frequent episodes of sterile arthritis and peritonitis, it has been proposed that the C5a inhibitor is an endogenous antiinflammatory protein.

Yet another inhibitor of complement-derived chemotactic activity has been found in sera from some patients undergoing hemodialysis (48). The inhibitor has a sedimentation coefficient of 4 S, is heat-stable (56°C for 30 min), and inhibits in a nonspecific fashion the migration of normal neutrophils toward C5-derived peptides, as well as toward chemotactic factors derived from *Escherichia coli*. Thus, several complex mechanisms appear to be operative in health and disease to regulate the chemotactic activity of complement (C5)-derived peptides.

EFFECTS OF C5-DERIVED PEPTIDES ON LEUKOCYTE DEGRANULATION

Phagocytosis by neutrophils entails recognition of the particles to be ingested, attachment of the particles to the cell surface, and finally, engulfment of the particles within vacuoles and closure of the plasma membrane. Shortly after, or coincident with these events, cytoplasmic (lysosomal) granules fuse with those portions of the plasma membrane that constitute phagocytic vacuoles (phagosomes). Membrane fusion leads to the discharge of lysosomal enzymes and other granule constituents into newly formed, or forming, phagosomes. This process, termed "degranulation," leads to the formation of phagolysosomes within which ingested material is digested. Degranulation and phagolysosome formation in neutrophils that engulf bacteria or fungi are essential for normal killing of ingested microorganisms (see Chapters 23 and 24).

Phagocytosis is not an absolute prerequisite for degranulation by neutrophils. In fact, a substantial amount of evidence has accumulated indicating that degranulation by neutrophils can be provoked by a wide variety of ligand–surface membrane receptor interactions (50). When neutrophils encounter appropriate soluble stimuli, for example, cytoplasmic granules fuse directly with the plasma membrane, and granule constituents are discharged into the surrounding medium. Granule exocytosis in response to soluble stimuli is enhanced significantly when neutrophils are treated with the fungal metabolite cytochalasin B. Cytochalasin B-treated neutrophils are unable to ingest particles, but nevertheless release, or secrete, lysosomal but not cytoplasmic constituents (i.e., degranulate) when appropriate particles or soluble stimuli come in contact with their surfaces (195).

Studies in several laboratories have documented that partially purified C5-derived peptides are capable of provoking cytochalasin B-treated human neutrophils to release lysosomal enzymes (4,5,51). Lysosomal enzyme release in response to C5-derived peptides occurs in the absence of phagocytosis and is selective in that it is not accompanied by release of cytoplasmic enzymes. Highly purified human C5a and C5a des Arg also stimulate cytochalasin B-treated human neutrophils to selectively discharge lysosomal enzymes (18,181). Concentrations of these complement fragments that produce half-maximal responses are 1.0–5.0 nM and 100–800 nM, respectively. Interestingly, human C5a and C5a des Arg have been found to be equipotent with respect to their ability to provoke lysosomal enzyme secretion by rabbit and human alveolar macrophages (114). These findings are in accord with the observation that C5a and C5a des Arg act at identical concentrations to stimulate directed migration of human peripheral blood monocytes (108).

In addition to stimulating secretion of lysosomal constituents from cytochalasin B-treated neutrophils, C5a and C5a des Arg appear to be capable of provoking a similar response in untreated cells (7), especially in cells that are adherent to suitable surfaces (e.g., micropore filters) (5). Ultrastructural studies on neutrophils exposed to C5-derived peptides have revealed fusion of lysosomal granules with each other and with the plasma membrane (51). Extensive degranulation of cytochalasin B-treated human neutrophils occurs within the first minute of exposure to human C5a. A striking feature of cells stimulated with C5a is the immediate appearance of large numbers of cytoplasmic microtubules radiating from the centriolar region. C5a appears to stimulate assembly of microtubules almost immediately on contact with neutrophils, an effect which is quite reversible and which, after 5 min, leaves the cells degranulated but otherwise structurally intact.

The precise mechanism whereby C5a stimulates intracellular membrane fusion and transient assembly of cytoplasmic microtubules in neutrophils is unknown. The almost instantaneous change in the cell profile observed after an encounter with C5a (and its prompt reversal), however, suggests that this peptide affects processes common to chemotaxis and membrane fusion. Furthermore, both chemotaxis and lysosomal enzyme release closely parallel uptake by neutrophils of C5a (18), suggesting that the same ligand–receptor interaction leads to stimulation of both of these cellular responses. A more detailed discussion of stimulus–response coupling in neutrophils appears in Chapter 19.

As indicated above, both human C5a and C5a des Arg provoke lysosomal enzyme secretion by alveolar macrophages. Only C5a des Arg, however, has been found capable of inducing secretion by rabbit alveolar macrophages of a complement-independent chemotactic factor for neutrophils (114). In accord with this finding, human C5a des Arg administered intratracheally to rabbits proved to be far more effective than C5a in provoking exudation of neutrophils into alveoli (70). Thus, the naturally occurring fragment of C5 formed as a consequence of complement activation exhibits biologic activities in vivo that are quite relevant to host defenses and inflammation.

In both hamsters and rabbits, complement-induced intraalveolar accumulation of neutrophils is accompanied by moderate perivascular edema, intravascular margination of leukocytes, and deposition of fibrin within alveolar spaces. Fibrin deposition also may result from interactions between C5-derived peptides and either neutrophils or alveolar macrophages. Human C5a and C5a des Arg have been found capable of stimulating production by both human neutrophils and rabbit alveolar macrophages of procoagulant (i.e., tissue factor) activity (127,158).

EFFECTS OF C5-DERIVED PEPTIDES ON LEUKOCYTE OXIDATIVE METABOLISM

Marked changes in oxidative metabolism ordinarily accompany ingestion of a variety of particles by neutro-

phils. The cells consume increased amounts of oxygen (by a mechanism that is insensitive to cyanide) to produce hydrogen peroxide, as well as several highly reactive, unstable intermediates such as superoxide anion radicals, hydroxyl radicals, and possibly, singlet oxygen. Concomitantly, there is stimulation of the hexose monophosphate shunt pathway of glucose oxidation and iodination of protein (mediated by the granule enzyme myeloperoxidase). The increased ability of phagocytosing neutrophils to reduce nitroblue tetrazolium dye is a reflection of enhanced generation of superoxide anion radicals. These metabolic events and their importance in relation to microbial killing and inflammation are described in Chapter 23.

As is the case with degranulation, there is considerable evidence that oxidative metabolism in neutrophils can be stimulated in the absence of phagocytosis. The first evidence that C5-derived peptides are capable of stimulating neutrophil oxidative metabolism was provided by Goetzl and Austen (47), who showed that purified human C5a (generated by treating isolated C5 with trypsin) increased, in a concentration-dependent fashion, the rate of aerobic glycolysis and hexose monophosphate shunt activity in human neutrophils. Subsequently, Goldstein et al. (52,53) demonstrated enhancement of nitroblue tetrazolium dye reduction by partially purified C5-derived peptides and enhancement of superoxide anion production by human neutrophils. These metabolic responses to C5-derived peptides occurred in the absence of cytochalasin B but were enhanced by prior treatment of cells with this agent (53). The concentrations of C5a and C5a des Arg required to stimulate half-maximal superoxide anion production by normal human neutrophils are in the range 30–60 nM and 1.0–3.0 μM, respectively (181). The generation of superoxide anion radicals by cells exposed to C5a and C5a des Arg is extremely rapid, reaching maximum values within 2 min at 37°C. C5a and C5a des Arg also stimulate carrier-mediated transport of glucose into human neutrophils (113), which may be a source of energy for motility and degranulation.

IMMUNOREGULATORY EFFECTS OF ANAPHYLATOXINS

In addition to stimulating effector functions of neutrophils and monocytes, human anaphylatoxins exhibit immunoregulatory activities. When added to lymphocytes and macrophages in vitro, C3a, C5a, and C5a des Arg can influence both humoral and cell-mediated immune responses (123,183). Human C3a, for example, but not C3a des Arg, suppresses antigen-specific as well as polyclonal antibody responses of both mouse spleen cells and human peripheral blood leukocytes. Similar effects have been observed in experiments using synthetic peptides corresponding to the carboxy-terminal portion of human C3a (122) and have been attributed to C3a-mediated generation of suppressor T lymphocytes (120,124,125). Synthetic peptides corresponding to the carboxy-terminal portion of human C3a also have been found capable of inhibiting human T-lymphocyte migration and generation of lymphokines by T lymphocytes (135).

Human C5a and C5a des Arg, on the other hand, have been found capable of augmenting antigen-specific as well as nonspecific humoral immune responses of both mouse spleen cells and human peripheral blood leukocytes (55,121). Human C5a and C5a des Arg also potentiate antigen- and alloantigen-induced human T-lymphocyte proliferative responses, as well as human T-lymphocyte-mediated cytotoxic reactions. Although helper T cells are required for C5a-mediated potentiation of polyclonal antibody responses, C5a may not act directly on lymphocytes. Rather, evidence has been presented that C5a enhances humoral immune reactions *in vitro* by binding to macrophages and by stimulating production of interleukin-1 (56). Chenoweth et al. (22) found that radiolabeled human C5a bound to murine peritoneal macrophages in a temperature- and concentration-dependent fashion. Binding was saturable, and Scatchard analysis revealed the presence of a single class of receptors with an apparent dissociation constant of approximately 3.0 nM. Incubation of macrophages with increasing amounts of unlabeled C5a progressively diminished binding of radiolabeled C5a, with half-maximal inhibition at 3.0–5.0 nM. In contrast, 1.6 μM unlabeled C5a des Arg was required to inhibit binding of radiolabeled C5a by 50%. Thus, although C5a and C5a des Arg were equipotent with respect to their ability to stimulate production of interleukin-1 by murine macrophages, competitive binding studies demonstrated that C5a bound much more avidly to the C5a receptor on the plasma membrane of these cells than did C5a des Arg. These results are quite similar to those reported by Marder et al. (108) from studies performed with human peripheral blood monocytes.

EFFECTS OF C5-DERIVED PEPTIDES ON LEUKOCYTE ADHESIVENESS

Adherence of circulating neutrophils to the walls of small blood vessels is an early event in nearly all forms of acute inflammation (61). Adherence is a prerequisite for subsequent diapedesis into the extravascular compartment. Factors responsible for provoking adherence of neutrophils to endothelial surfaces are largely unknown. It has been suggested, however, that the same factors that stimulate directed migration (i.e., chemotaxis) of neutrophils toward sites of inflammation also enhance attachment of neutrophils to endothelial cells (74,75).

Several investigators have reported that complement (C5)-derived peptides, as well as other chemotactic factors, increase adherence of human neutrophils to cultured endothelial cells (16,17,74,75,160,171). Hoover et al. (74,75), for example, reported that adherence of human neutrophils to bovine aortic endothelial cells was enhanced by trypsinized human C5, zymosan-activated human serum, or the formylated peptides N-formyl-met-ala and N-formyl-met-leu-phe. Using isolated C5-derived peptides, Tonnesen et al. (171) reported recently that both C5a and C5a des Arg augmented the adherence of human neutrophils to cultured human umbilical vein endothelial cells. It should be noted, however, that this phenomenon has not been observed by all investigators (17,160). Furthermore, evidence has been presented that effects of chemotactic factors on the adhesiveness of neutrophils vary depending on concentration (17,93,159). Finally, it has been suggested that C5a des Arg may not influence the adhesiveness of neutrophils at all (38).

Charo et al. (17) recently demonstrated that highly purified human C5a influences directed migration of human neutrophils as well as adherence of human neutrophils to monolayers of cultured human umbilical vein endothelial cells in a concentration-dependent, reciprocal fashion. Low concentrations of C5a (0.1 nM) significantly reduced adherence and stimulated directed migration of neutrophils, whereas higher concentrations (>1.0 nM) significantly augmented adherence and reduced directed migration. As expected, highly purified C5a des Arg was considerably less potent than C5a with respect to its ability to stimulate directed migration of neutrophils. Nevertheless, as in the experiments with C5a, concentrations of C5a des Arg that stimulated directed migration of neutrophils (>5.0 nM) also reduced adherence of neutrophils to endothelial monolayers. However, in contrast to what was observed in experiments with C5a, high concentrations of C5a des Arg (up to 80 nM) neither decreased neutrophil migration nor augmented adherence.

C5a des Arg generated by incubating fresh human serum with either zymosan or purified C5a also reduced adherence of neutrophils. In contrast, adherence of neutrophils was augmented significantly by C5a generated by incubating fresh serum with zymosan in the presence of the carboxypeptidase inhibitor ε-aminocaproic acid and by C5a added to serum in which carboxypeptidase N had been inactivated by heating. Thus, the effects on neutrophil adherence of zymosan-activated serum alone and zymosan-activated serum containing ε-aminocaproic acid could be accounted for entirely by the effects of C5a des Arg and C5a, respectively. Furthermore, there did not appear to be a protein in serum that permitted C5a des Arg to augment adherence of neutrophils, such as cochemotaxin, which permits low concentrations of C5a des Arg to exhibit chemotactic activity for neutrophils (139).

Similar biphasic and reciprocal effects of chemotactic factors on the motility and adherence of neutrophils have been observed by others. Smith et al. (160), for example, found that low chemotactic concentrations of N-formyl-met-leu-phe (0.1–1.0 nM) decreased adherence of rabbit peritoneal neutrophils to cultured porcine aortic endothelial cells. Higher concentrations of N-formyl-met-leu-phe (>10 nM), which decreased directed migration of rabbit neutrophils, augmented adherence. Keller et al. (93), as well as Fehr and Dahinden (37), also observed that human neutrophils adhered more avidly to glass and to plastic when exposed to concentrations of N-formyl-met-leu-phe (>100 nM) that reduced both directed and random migration. Finally, Smith et al. (159) reported that high concentrations of chemotactic factors enhanced adherence of human neutrophils to glass and simultaneously reduced motility. Based on these observations, it has been suggested that the rate of neutrophil locomotion is inversely related to how avidly these cells adhere to surfaces (e.g., plastic) (93), and that the phenomenon of "deactivation" (i.e., high-dose inhibition of neutrophil migration) is a consequence, at least in part, of increased adhesiveness (37).

Others have found C5a des Arg incapable of augmenting adherence of neutrophils to artificial surfaces. Keller et al. (93), for example, found that high concentrations of porcine C5a des Arg (>100 nM) neither decreased locomotion of neutrophils nor enhanced adherence of these cells to glass. Fehr and Huber (38) also found that high concentrations of human C5a des Arg (50–500 nM) failed to increase adherence of human neutrophils to plastic. However, Tonnesen et al. (171) reported recently that human C5a and human C5a des Arg were equipotent with respect to their ability to enhance adherence of neutrophils to human umbilical vein endothelial cells. Furthermore, several investigators have reported that zymosan-activated serum and zymosan-activated plasma (which contain primarily C5a des Arg) increase the adhesiveness of neutrophils (74,75,171).

One possible explanation for the differences between the results reported by Charo et al. (17) (with C5a des Arg and zymosan-activated serum) and results reported by some other investigators involves the phenomenon of neutrophil aggregation. It has been demonstrated previously that C5-derived peptides cause neutrophils in suspension to aggregate (detectable *in vitro* using standard nephelometric techniques) (29,30,64). Almost immediately after cells are exposed to C5-derived peptides, pseudopod formation is enhanced with resultant cell–cell association (29). Well-defined aggregates consisting of 5–30 cells are seen within 3–5 min. Cell–cell attachment (aggregation) clearly can influence measurements of cell–substrate attachment. McGillen and Phair (115), for example, observed that "augmented adherence" of neutro-

phils to columns of packed nylon fibers in response to zymosan-activated plasma could be accounted for by trapping of neutrophil aggregates. Similarly, the formation of microaggregates could lead to misleading results in experiments designed to measure adherence of individual neutrophils to endothelial monolayers. Charo et al. (17) confirmed that C5a des Arg and zymosan-activated serum, at concentrations that do not augment adherence of neutrophils to endothelial monolayers, provoke changes in light transmission through concentrated suspensions of neutrophils. Fehr and Huber (38) made similar observations and concluded that aggregation of neutrophils and enhanced adherence of neutrophils to substrates were dissociable phenomena that could occur simultaneously in response to some (but not all) chemotactic factors. It is possible, therefore, that aggregation of neutrophils (i.e., cell–cell attachment) accounted for the apparent increase in neutrophil adherence to substrates observed by some investigators when cells (at high density) were exposed to zymosan-activated serum (and C5a des Arg).

The precise mechanism by which high concentrations of C5a augment the adhesiveness of neutrophils is unknown. Whereas altered surface charge may be an important factor, roles for neutrophil granule constituents, oxygenation products of arachidonic acid, and plasma membrane proteins also have to be considered. Concerning the latter, evidence has been presented recently that C5-derived peptides augment adherence of neutrophils by provoking translocation of "adhesive glycoproteins" (with C3bi receptor activity) from an intracellular pool (in specific granules) to the cell surface (2,3,9). Interestingly, C5-derived peptides also cause increased expression of C3b receptors on the surfaces of human neutrophils (36), as well as increased expression of Fc and C3b receptors on the surfaces of human peripheral blood monocytes (194).

It is less easy to account for the phenomenon of decreased adherence observed when neutrophils were exposed to chemotactic concentrations of C5a and C5a des Arg. It is possible, however, that changes in the morphology of neutrophils provoked by low concentrations of chemotactic factors interfere with firm attachment of these cells to endothelial monolayers. Chemotactic concentrations of C5a, for example, cause neutrophils in suspension to assume a polarized morphology (i.e., to acquire a head and a tail). Higher concentrations of C5a (i.e., concentrations that inhibit directed migration and enhance adherence) do not cause these morphologic changes (108).

Whatever the mechanisms may be, the observations summarized above support the suggestion that C5-derived peptides modulate adhesive interactions between human neutrophils and the walls of blood vessels *in vivo*. It is intriguing to speculate that C5a causes localized adherence (and immobilization) of neutrophils along endothelial surfaces immediately adjacent to sites of inflammation (and sites of complement activation), whereas carboxypeptidase-mediated conversion of C5a to C5a des Arg serves to limit attachment (and immobilization) of neutrophils along the walls of blood vessels at more remote sites. By reducing tight adherence of neutrophils to endothelial surfaces, C5a des Arg may facilitate neutrophil chemotaxis and emigration.

OTHER BIOLOGICALLY ACTIVE PRODUCTS OF COMPLEMENT ACTIVATION

C3e: Leukocytosis-Promoting Factor

Observations that immunologic reactions *in vivo* often are accompanied by a leukocytosis prompted a search for complement-derived factors that might be responsible for provoking release of neutrophils from the bone marrow compartment. Rother (152) was the first to report that an anionic C3-derived peptide provoked release of leukocytes from perfused guinea pig and rat femora *in vitro* and caused prompt leukocytosis when injected intravenously into intact animals. Ghebrehiwet and Müller-Eberhard (46) also isolated an acidic fragment of human C3 (C3e) that was capable of mobilizing leukocytes *in vitro* and *in vivo*. C3e has a molecular weight of 10,000 to 12,000 and is generated either by incubating isolated human C3 with trypsin at 37°C for 120 min or by incubating whole human serum at 37°C for 5 days. Based on immunologic cross-reactivity, it was concluded that C3e was distinct from C3a and derived from a portion of the alpha chain of native C3 that is part of the C3c fragment. Purified C3e mobilizes leukocytes from rat bone marrow and causes a two- to three-fold increase in the number of circulating leukocytes when injected intravenously into rabbits. Although devoid of chemotactic activity and smooth muscle-contracting activity, C3e does increase vascular permeability when injected intradermally into rabbit skin. C3e also provokes selective release of lysosomal enzymes from cytochalasin B-treated human neutrophils (45).

Meuth et al. (118) described another fragment of C3 that causes leukocytosis when injected intravenously into rabbits. This fragment, termed "C3d-K," is a polypeptide with a molecular weight of 41,000 that is generated from the alpha chain of human C3bi by limited proteolysis with kallikrein. In addition to causing leukocytosis in rabbits, C3d-K suppresses mitogen- and antigen-induced proliferation of human T lymphocytes. Hoeprich et al. (72) recently demonstrated that a synthetic nonapeptide (thr-leu-asp-pro-glu-arg-leu-gly-arg), corresponding to the amino-terminal sequence of C3d-K, shared with native C3d-K and with C3e the ability to induce leukocytosis in

rabbits. These investigators concluded that the nonapeptide represents the active site of both C3d-K and C3e.

Fragments of Factor B

During activation of the alternative complement pathway, factor B is cleaved into two fragments. The larger of these fragments (Bb) participates in assembly of the alternative pathway C3 convertase, whereas the smaller fragment (Ba) is released into the fluid phase. Although specific cellular receptors for these fragments of factor B have not been identified, guinea pig Ba has been reported to be chemotactic for guinea pig peritoneal polymorphonuclear leukocytes (66), and human Bb has been found capable of inducing the spreading of mouse peritoneal macrophages and human peripheral blood monocytes (59,166). Enzymatically inactive human Bb does not induce spreading of macrophages or monocytes, and the spreading response appears to be dependent on C5, C6, and C7. Human Bb also augments monocyte-mediated cytotoxicity (63,99) and has been found capable of stimulating murine peritoneal exudate macrophages to secrete lysosomal enzymes (71). Finally, evidence has been reported recently that human Bb inhibits the chemotactic activity exhibited by mixtures of human C5a des Arg and its cochemotaxin (142).

The Membrane Attack Complex (C5b-9)

Whether bound to surfaces or in the fluid phase, C5b forms a stable macromolecular complex with the "terminal" complement components, C6 to C9. This hydrophobic complex inserts into lipid bilayers and forms transmembrane channels that permit bidirectional flow of ions and macromolecules (see Chapter 3). It is by this mechanism that complement causes lysis of cells. It should be noted that stable complexes of C5b, C6, and C7 can bind nonspecifically to cell membranes and, together with C8 and C9, provoke lysis. Such "reactive lysis" or "bystander lysis" can account for injury to cells not recognized by specific antibodies (49,96).

The complement membrane attack complex has been implicated recently in the pathogenesis of antiglomerular basement membrane antibody-induced glomerulonephritis in rats and in the pathogenesis of various forms of renal disease in humans (26,31). Although the lytic activity of the complex undoubtedly plays a role in producing renal injury, evidence has appeared recently indicating that the complex also can act in a nonlytic fashion to stimulate production of inflammatory mediators by cells. For example, the complement membrane attack complex stimulates metabolism of arachidonic acid by platelets (145) and macrophages (67) and also stimulates cultured rat mesangial cells to produce reactive oxygen metabolites (1). Although it has been reported that fluid phase C5b67 is chemotactic for neutrophils and eosinophils (96), important physiologic or pathologic roles for this activity have not been demonstrated.

CLINICAL CORRELATES

Complement and Anaphylaxis

It is unclear whether the smooth muscle-contracting and histamine-releasing activities of human anaphylatoxins play any significant role in the pathogenesis of inflammation or tissue injury in humans. As discussed earlier, the anaphylatoxin activities of human C3a and C5a are abolished rapidly by a naturally occurring serum enzyme (12). Nevertheless, when large amounts of C3a and C5a are generated *in vivo*, the anaphylatoxin activities of these peptides may be expressed clinically. Possible examples of this phenomenon are the untoward reactions observed in some patients during intravenous infusions of iodinated radiographic contrast media. These reactions, which often are accompanied by urticaria, angioedema, and/or asthma, resemble anaphylaxis and may be mediated by histamine released from mast cells and basophils (101). Iodinated radiographic contrast media have been found capable of activating complement in human serum (with the generation of C5a-like activity) (170). However, radiographic contrast media also appear to have serum-independent effects on peripheral blood leukocytes (148). This finding, and the apparent lack of any correlation between clinical responses to radiographic contrast media and effects on either serum complement components or cells (102), make it difficult to assign a primary role for anaphylatoxins in mediating untoward reactions to these agents.

Complement and Host Defenses

All the functions of neutrophils that are relevant to host defenses can be influenced or mediated by products of complement activation. For example, some microorganisms, even in the absence of specific antibody, call initial attention to themselves as a consequence of activating the alternative complement pathway. In the presence of antibody, of course, activation of the classical pathway also may occur. Following either or both of these events, peptides (i.e., C3e, C5a, C5a des Arg) are generated which increase the number of circulating neutrophils, promote adherence of neutrophils to vascular endothelium, and attract neutrophils to sites of microbial invasion. Having arrived at foci of infection, neutrophils then recognize, ingest, and kill the invaders. Fragments of C3 (C3b, C3bi)

promote recognition of particles and phagocytosis. Fragments of C3 also promote degranulation of neutrophils and cause these cells to increase their oxidative metabolism (C5a and C5a des Arg produce similar effects). The important roles played by lysosomal enzymes (e.g., myeloperoxidase) and products of oxidative metabolism (e.g., hydrogen peroxide) in microbial killing are discussed in Chapters 23 and 24. In some instances, killing may not even require the action of phagocytes. Certain microorganisms are very susceptible to lysis by the membrane attack complex and may be killed by the action of complement alone. It is not surprising, therefore, that in certain clinical situations where specific complement components are totally absent (as the result of a congenital defect), host defenses are severely compromised. Consequences of complement deficiencies are discussed in Chapter 6.

Complement and Inflammation

The same biologically active complement components that help to maintain normal host defenses against infection also are capable of mediating inflammation and tissue injury. C5-derived peptides, for example, have been detected in synovial fluids from patients with inflammatory arthritides (177), as well as in dermal scales of patients with psoriasis and inflammatory pustular dermatoses (168). C5-derived peptides also have been implicated in the pathogenesis of phototoxic skin reactions in patients with erythropoietic protoporphyria and porphyria cutanea tarda (103). Finally, it has been proposed that C5-derived peptides are involved in the pathogenesis of certain forms of microvascular injury in the lung that lead to increased-permeability pulmonary edema (i.e., the adult respiratory distress syndrome) (see Chapter 44).

As discussed above, C5-derived peptides augment the adhesiveness of neutrophils. This is manifested *in vitro* either by increased adherence of neutrophils to substrates such as plastic and cultured endothelial cells or by aggregation of neutrophils in suspension. When infused intravenously into experimental animals, C5-derived peptides cause neutropenia, markedly increased margination of neutrophils, and pulmonary vascular leukostasis (27,28). The possibility that similar phenomena occur in humans has been suggested by studies in patients with diverse clinical disorders that lead to lung injury.

Among the disorders known to be associated with the development of increased-permeability pulmonary edema, circulating C5-derived peptides have been detected (by radioimmunoassay and/or by bioassay) in patients with sepsis (33,65,162,185), acute pancreatitis (76,140,162), and multisystem trauma (65,162). Circulating C5-derived peptides also have been detected in patients undergoing hemodialysis (3) and in patients during cardiopulmonary bypass (21).

REFERENCES

1. Adler, S., Baker, P. J., Johnson, R. J., Ochi, R. F., Pritzl, P., and Couser, W. G. (1986): Complement membrane attack complex stimulates production of reactive oxygen metabolites by cultured rat mesangial cells. *J. Clin. Invest.*, 77:762–767.
2. Arnaout, M. A., Spits, H., Terhost, C., Pitt, J., and Todd, R. F., III (1984): Deficiency of a leukocyte surface glycoprotein (LFA-1) in two patients with Mol deficiency: Effects of cell activation on Mol/LFA-1 surface expression in normal and deficient leukocytes. *J. Clin. Invest.*, 74:1291–1300.
3. Arnaout, M. A., Hakim, R. M., Todd, R. F., III, Dana, N., and Colten, H. R. (1985): Increased expression of an adhesion-promoting surface glycoprotein in the granulocytopenia of hemodialysis. *N. Engl. J. Med.*, 312:457–462.
4. Becker, E. L., and Showell, H. J. (1974): The ability of chemotactic factors to induce lysosomal enzyme release. II. The mechanism of release. *J. Immunol.*, 112:2055–2062.
5. Becker, E. L., Showell, H. J., Henson, P. M., and Hsu, L. S. (1974): The ability of chemotactic factors to induce lysosomal enzyme release. I. The characteristics of the release, the importance of surfaces and the relation of enzyme release to chemotactic responsiveness. *J. Immunol.*, 112:2047–2054.
6. Beebe, D. P., Ward, P. A., and Spitznagel, J. K. (1980): Isolation and characterization of an acidic chemotactic factor from complement-activated human serum. *Clin. Immunol. Immunopathol.*, 15:88–105.
7. Bentwood, B. J., and Henson, P. M. (1980): The sequential release of granule constituents from human neutrophils. *J. Immunol.*, 124:855–862.
8. Berenberg, J. L., and Ward, P. A. (1973): The chemotactic factor inactivator in normal human serum. *J. Clin. Invest.*, 52:1200–1206.
9. Berger, M., O'Shea, J., Cross, A. S., Folks, T. M., Chused, T. M., Brown, E. J., and Frank, M. M. (1984): Human neutrophils increase expression of C3bi as well as C3b receptors upon activation. *J. Clin. Invest.*, 74:1566–1571.
10. Björk, J., Hugli, T. E., and Smedegård, G. (1985): Microvascular effects of anaphylatoxins C3a and C5a. *J. Immunol.*, 134:1115–1119.
11. Bokisch, V. A., Müller-Eberhard, H. J., and Cochrane, C. G. (1969): Isolation of a fragment (C3a) of the third component of human complement containing anaphylatoxin and chemotactic activity and description of an anaphylatoxin inactivator of human serum. *J. Exp. Med.*, 129:1109–1130.
12. Bokisch, V. A., and Müller-Eberhard, H. J. (1970): Anaphylatoxin inactivator of human plasma: Its isolation and characterization as a carboxypeptidase. *J. Clin. Invest.*, 49:2427–2436.
13. Boyden, S. (1962): The chemotactic effect of mixtures of antibody and antigen on polymorphonuclear leukocytes. *J. Exp. Med.*, 115:453–466.
14. Brozna, J. P., Senior, R. M., Kreutzer, D. L., and Ward, P. A. (1977): Chemotactic factor inactivators of human granulocytes. *J. Clin. Invest.*, 60:1280–1288.
15. Caporale, L. H., Tippett, P. S., Erickson, B. W., and Hugli, T. E. (1980): The active site of C3a anaphylatoxin. *J. Biol. Chem.*, 255:10758–10763.
16. Charo, I. F., Yuen, C., and Goldstein, I. M. (1985): Adherence of human polymorphonuclear leukocytes to endothelial monolayers: Effects of temperature, divalent cations, and chemotactic factors on the strength of adherence measured with a new centrifugation assay. *Blood*, 65:473–479.
17. Charo, I. F., Yuen, C., Perez, H. D., and Goldstein, I. M. (1986): Chemotactic peptides modulate adherence of human polymorphonuclear leukocytes to monolayers of cultured endothelial cells. *J. Immunol.*, 136:3412–3419.
18. Chenoweth, D. E., and Hugli, T. E. (1978): Demonstration of specific C5a receptor on intact human polymorphonuclear leukocytes. *Proc. Natl. Acad. Sci. USA*, 75:3943–3947.
19. Chenoweth, D. E., Erickson, B. W., and Hugli, T. E. (1979): Human C5a-related synthetic peptides as neutrophil chemotactic factors. *Biochem. Biophys. Res. Commun.*, 68:227–231.
20. Chenoweth, D. E., and Hugli, T. E. (1980): Human C5a and C5a analogs as probes of the neutrophil C5a receptor. *Mol. Immunol.*, 17:151–161.
21. Chenoweth, D., Cooper, S. W., Hugli, T. E., Stewart, R. W., Blackstone, E. H., and Kirklin, J. W. (1981): Complement activation during cardiopulmonary bypass: Evidence for generation of C3 and C5a anaphylatoxins. *N. Engl. J. Med.*, 304:497–503.
22. Chenoweth, D. E., Goodman, M. G., and Weigle, W. O. (1982): Demonstration of a specific receptor for human C5a anaphylatoxin on murine macrophages. *J. Exp. Med.*, 156:68–78.
23. Cianciolo, G. J., and Snyderman, R. (1981): Monocyte responsiveness to chemotactic stimuli is a property of a subpopulation of cells that can respond to multiple chemoattractants. *J. Clin. Invest.*, 67:60–68.
24. Clark, R. A., Szot, S., Venkatasubramanian, K., and Schiffmann, E. (1980): Chemotactic factor inactivation by myeloperoxidase-mediated oxidation of methionine. *J. Immunol.*, 124:2020–2025.
25. Cochrane, C. G., and Müller-Eberhard, H. J. (1968): The derivation of two distinct anaphylatoxin activities from the third and fifth components of human complement. *J. Exp. Med.*, 127:371–386.
26. Couser, W. G., Baker, P. J., and Adler, S. (1985): Complement and the direct mediation of immune glomerular injury: A new perspective. *Kidney Int.*, 28:879–890.
27. Craddock, P. R., Fehr, J., Brigham, K. L., Kronenberg, R. S., and Jacob, H. S. (1977): Complement and leukocyte-mediated pulmonary dysfunction in hemodialysis. *N. Engl. J. Med.*, 296:769–774.
28. Craddock, P. R., Fehr, J., Dalmasso, A. P., Brigham, K. L., and Jacob, H. S. (1977): Hemodialysis leukopenia: Pulmonary vascular leukostasis resulting from complement activation by dialyzer cellophane membranes. *J. Clin. Invest.*, 59:879–888.
29. Craddock, P. R., Hammerschmidt, D., White, J. G., Dalmasso, A. P., and Jacob, H. S. (1977): Complement (C5a)-induced granulocyte aggregation in vitro: A possible mechanism of complement-mediated leukostasis and leukopenia. *J. Clin. Invest.*, 60:260–264.
30. Craddock, P. R., White, J. G., and Jacob, H. S. (1978): Potentiation of complement (C5a)-induced granulocyte aggregation by cytochalasin B. *J. Lab. Clin. Med.*, 91:490–499.
31. Cybulsky, A. V., Rennke, H. G., Feintzeig, I. D., and Salant, D. J. (1986): Complement-induced glomerular epithelial cell injury: Role of the membrane attack complex in rat membranous nephropathy. *J. Clin. Invest.*, 77:1096–1107.
32. Dias Da Silva, W., Eisele, J. W., and Lepow, I. H. (1967): Complement as a mediator of inflammation. III. Purification of the activity with anaphylatoxin properties generated by interaction of the first four components of complement and its identification as a cleavage product of C'3. *J. Exp. Med.*, 126:1027–1048.
33. Duchateau, J., Haas, M., Schreyen, H., Radoux, L., Sprangers, I., Noel, F. X., Braun, M., and Lamy, M. (1984): Complement activation in patients at risk of developing the adult respiratory distress syndrome. *Am. Rev. Resp. Dis.*, 130:1058–1064.
34. Falk, W., and Leonard, E. J. (1981): Specificity and reversibility of chemotactic deactivation of human monocytes. *Infect. Immun.*, 32:464–468.
35. Fantone, J., Senior, R. M., Kreutzer, D. L., Jones, M., and Ward, P. A. (1979): Biochemical quantitation of the chemotactic factor inactivator activity in human serum. *J. Lab. Clin. Med.*, 93:17–24.
36. Fearon, D. T., and Collins, L. A. (1983): Increased expression of C3b receptors on polymorphonuclear leukocytes induced by chemotactic factors and by purification procedures. *J. Immunol.*, 130:370–375.
37. Fehr, J., and Dahinden, C. (1979): Modulating influence of chemotactic factor-induced cell adhesiveness on granulocyte function. *J. Clin. Invest.*, 64:8–16.
38. Fehr, J., and Huber, A. (1984): Complement-induced granulocyte adhesion and aggregation are mediated by different factors: Evidence for non-equivalence of the two cell functions. *Immunology*, 53:583–593.
39. Feldbush, T. L., Hobbs, M. V., Severson, C. D., Ballas, Z. K., and Weiler, J. M. (1984): Role of complement in the immune response. *Fed. Proc.*, 43:2548–2552.

40. Fernandez, H. N., and Hugli, T. E. (1976): Partial characterization of human C5a anaphylatoxin. I. Chemical description of the carbohydrate and polypeptide portions of human C5a. *J. Immunol.,* 117:1688–1694.

41. Fernandez, H. N., Henson, P. M., Otani, A., and Hugli, T. E. (1978): Chemotactic response to human C3a and C5a anaphylatoxins. I. Evaluation of C3a and C5a leukotaxis *in vitro* and under simulated *in vivo* conditions. *J. Immunol.,* 120:109–115.

42. Fernandez, H. N., and Hugli, T. E. (1978): Primary structural analysis of the polypeptide portion of human C5a anaphylatoxin: Polypeptide sequence determination and assignment of the oligosaccharide attachment site in C5a. *J. Biol. Chem.,* 253:6955–6962.

43. Gerard, C., Chenoweth, D. E., and Hugli, T. E. (1981): Response of human neutrophils to C5a: A role for the oligosaccharide moiety of C5a des Arg-74 but not of C5a in biologic activity. *J. Immunol.,* 127:1978–1982.

44. Gerard, C., and Hugli, T. E. (1981): Identification of classical anaphylatoxin as the des-Arg form of the C5a molecule: Evidence of a modulator role for the oligosaccharide unit in human des-Arg^{74}-C5a. *Proc. Natl. Acad. Sci. USA,* 78:1833–1837.

45. Ghebrehewit, B. (1984): The release of lysosomal enzymes from human polymorphonuclear leukocytes by human C3e. *Clin. Immunol. Immunopathol.,* 30:321–329.

46. Ghebrehewit, B., and Müller-Eberhard, H. J. (1979): C3e: An acidic fragment of human C3 with leukocytosis-inducing activity. *J. Immunol.,* 123:616–621.

47. Goetzl, E. J., and Austen, K. F. (1974): Stimulation of human neutrophil leukocyte aerobic glucose metabolism by purified chemotactic factors. *J. Clin. Invest.,* 53:591–599.

48. Goldblum, S. E., Van Epps, D. E., and Reed, W. P. (1979): Serum inhibitor of C5 fragment-mediated polymorphonuclear leukocyte chemotaxis associated with chronic hemodialysis. *J. Clin. Invest.,* 64:255–264.

49. Goldman, J. M., Ruddy, S., and Austen, K. F. (1972): Reaction mechanisms of nascent C$\overline{567}$ (reactive lysis). I. Reaction characteristics for production of EC567 and lysis by C8 and C9. *J. Immunol.,* 109:353–359.

50. Goldstein, I. M. (1984): Neutrophil degranulation. *Contemp. Top. Immunobiol.,* 14:189–208.

51. Goldstein, I. M., Hoffstein, S., Gallin, J., and Weissmann, G. (1973): Mechanisms of lysosomal enzyme release from human leukocytes: Microtubule assembly and membrane fusion induced by a component of complement. *Proc. Natl. Acad. Sci. USA,* 70:2916–2920.

52. Goldstein, I. M., Feit, F., and Weissmann, G. (1975): Enhancement of nitroblue tetrazolium dye reduction by leukocytes exposed to a component of complement in the absence of phagocytosis. *J. Immunol.,* 114:516–518.

53. Goldstein, I. M., Roos, D., Weissmann, G., and Kaplan, H. (1975): Complement and immunoglobulins stimulate superoxide production by human leukocytes independently of phagocytosis. *J. Clin. Invest.,* 56:1155–1163.

54. Goldstein, I. M., Kaplan, H. B., Radin, A., and Frosch, M. (1976): Independent effects of IgG and complement upon human polymorphonuclear leukocyte function. *J. Immunol.,* 117:1282–1287.

55. Goodman, M. G., Chenoweth, D. E., and Weigle, W. O. (1982): Potentiation of the primary humoral immune response *in vitro* by C5a anaphylatoxin. *J. Immunol.,* 129:70–75.

56. Goodman, M. G., Chenoweth, D. E., and Weigle, W. O. (1982): Induction of interleukin 1 secretion and enhancement of humoral immunity by binding of human C5a to macrophage surface C5a receptors. *J. Exp. Med.,* 156:912–917.

57. Gorski, J. P., Hugli, T. E., and Müller-Eberhard, H. J. (1979): C4a: The third anaphylatoxin of the human complement system. *Proc. Natl. Acad. Sci. USA,* 76:5299–5302.

58. Gorski, J. P., Hugli, T. E., and Müller-Eberhard, H. J. (1981): Characterization of human C4a anaphylatoxin. *J. Biol. Chem.,* 256:2707–2711.

59. Götze, O., Bianco, C., and Cohn, Z. A. (1979): The induction of macrophage spreading by factor B of the properdin system. *J. Exp. Med.,* 149:372–386.

60. Grant, J. A., Settle, L., Whorton, E. B., and Dupree, E. (1976): Complement-mediated release of histamine from human basophils.

II. Biochemical characterization of the reaction. *J. Immunol.,* 117:450–456.

61. Grant, L. (1973): The sticking and emigration of white blood cells in inflammation. In: *The Inflammatory Process, Vol. II,* edited by B. W. Zweifach, L. Grant, and R. McCluskey, pp. 205–249. Academic Press, New York.

62. Greer, J. (1985): Model structure for the inflammatory protein C5a. *Science,* 228:1055–1060.

63. Hall, R. E., Blaese, R. M., Davis, A. E., III, Decker, J. M., Tack, B. F., Colten, H. R., and Muchmore, A. V. (1982): Cooperative interaction of factor B and other complement components with mononuclear cells in the antibody-independent lysis of xenogeneic erythrocytes. *J. Exp. Med.,* 156:834–843.

64. Hammerschmidt, D. E., Bowers, T. K., Lammi-Keefe, C. J., Jacob, H. S., and Craddock, P. R. (1980): Granulocyte aggregometry: A sensitive technique for the detection of C5a and complement activation. *Blood,* 55:898–902.

65. Hammerschmidt, D. E., Hudson, L. D., Weaver, L. J., Craddock, P. R., and Jacob, H. S. (1980): Association of complement activation and elevated plasma-C5a with adult respiratory distress syndrome: Pathophysiological relevance and possible prognostic value. *Lancet,* 1:947–949.

66. Hamuro, J., Hadding, U., and Bitter-Suermann, D. (1978): Fragments Ba and Bb derived from guinea pig factor B of the properdin system: Purification, characterization, and biologic activities. *J. Immunol.,* 120:438–444.

67. Hansch, G. M., Seitz, M., Martinotti, G., Betz, M., Rauterberg, E. W., and Gemsa, D. (1984): Macrophages release arachidonic acid, prostaglandin E$_2$, and thromboxane in response to late complement components. *J. Immunol.,* 133:2145–2150.

68. Hartman, C. T., Jr., and Glovsky, M. M. (1981): Complement activation requirements for histamine release from human leukocytes: Influence of purified C3a$_{hu}$ and C5a$_{hu}$ on histamine release. *Int. Arch. Allergy Appl. Immunol.,* 66:274–281.

69. Hartung, H.-P., Bitter-Suermann, D., and Hadding, U. (1983): Induction of thromboxane release from macrophages by anaphylatoxic peptide C3a of complement and synthetic hexapeptide C3a 72–77. *J. Immunol.,* 130:1345–1349.

70. Henson, P. M., McCarthy, K., Larsen, G. L., Webster, R. O., Giclas, P. C., Dreisin, R. B., King, T. E., and Shaw, J. O. (1979): Complement fragments, alveolar macrophages and alveolitis. *Am. J. Pathol.,* 97:93–105.

71. Hirani, S., Fair, D. S., Papin, R. A., and Sundsmo, J. S. (1985): Leukocyte complement: Interleukin-like properties of factor Bb. *Cell. Immunol.,* 92:235–246.

72. Hoeprich, P. D., Dahinden, C. A., Lachmann, P. J., Davis, A. E., III, and Hugli, T. E. (1985): A synthetic nonapeptide corresponding to the NH$_2$-terminal sequence of C3d-K causes leukocytosis in rabbits. *J. Biol. Chem.,* 260:2597–2600.

73. Hoeprich, P. D., Jr., and Hugli, T. E. (1986): Helical conformation at the carboxyl-terminal portion of human C3a is required for full activity. *Biochemistry,* 25:1945–1950.

74. Hoover, R. L., Briggs, R. T., and Karnovsky, M. J. (1978): The adhesive interaction between polymorphonuclear leukocytes and endothelial cells *in vitro. Cell,* 14:423–428.

75. Hoover, R. L., Folger, R., Haering, W. A., Ware, B. R., and Karnovsky, M. J. (1978): Adhesion of leukocytes to endothelium: Roles of divalent cations, surface charge, chemotactic agents and substrate. *J. Cell Sci.,* 45:73–86.

76. Horn, J. K., Ranson, J. H. C., Ong, R., Poulis, D., Perez, H. D., and Goldstein, I. M. (1982): Complement catabolism and chemotaxis in acute pancreatitis. *J. Surg. Res.,* 32:569–575.

77. Huber, R., Scholze, H., Pâques, E. P., and Deisenhofer, J. (1980): Crystal structure analysis and molecular model of human C3a anaphylatoxin. *Hoppe Seylers Z. Physiol. Chem.,* 361:1389–1399.

78. Huey, R., Bloor, C. M., and Hugli, T. E. (1984): Effects of human anaphylatoxins on guinea pig atria. *Immunopharmacology,* 8:147–154.

79. Huey, R., and Hugli, T. E. (1985): Characterization of a C5a receptor on human polymorphonuclear leukocytes (PMN). *J. Immunol.,* 135:2063–2068.

80. Hugli, T. E. (1975): Human anaphylatoxin (C3a) from the third

component of complement: Primary structure. *J. Biol. Chem.,* 250: 8293–8301.

81. Hugli, T. E. (1984): Structure and function of the anaphylatoxins. *Springer Semin. Immunopathol.,* 7:193–219.

82. Hugli, T. E., Morgan, W. T., and Müller-Eberhard, H. J. (1975): Circular dichroism of C3a anaphylatoxin: Effects of pH, heat, guanidinium chloride and mercaptoethanol on conformation and function. *J. Biol. Chem.,* 250:1479–1483.

83. Hugli, T. E., Vallota, E. H., and Müller-Eberhard, H. J. (1975): Purification and partial characterization of human and porcine C3a anaphylatoxin. *J. Biol. Chem.,* 250:1472–1478.

84. Hugli, T. E., and Müller-Eberhard, H. J. (1978): Anaphylatoxins: C3a and C5a. *Adv. Immunol.,* 26:1–53.

85. Hugli, T. E., Gerard, C., Kawahara, M., Scheetz, M. E., II, Barton, R., Briggs, S., Koppel, G., and Russell, S. (1981): Isolation of three separate anaphylatoxins from complement-activated human serum. *Mol. Cell Biochem.,* 41:59–66.

86. Hugli, T. E., Kawahara, M. S., Unson, C. G., Molinar-Rode, R., and Erickson, B. W. (1983): The active site of the human C4a anaphylatoxin. *Mol. Immunol.,* 20:637–645.

87. Issekutz, A. C., Movat, K. W., and Movat, H. Z. (1980): Enhanced vascular permeability and hemorrhage inducing activity of rabbit C5a des Arg: Probable role of PMN-leukocyte lysosomes. *Clin. Exp. Immunol.,* 41:512–520.

88. Johnson, A. R., Hugli, T. E., and Müller-Eberhard, H. J. (1975): Release of histamine from rat mast cells by the complement peptides C3a and C5a. *Immunology,* 28:1067–1080.

89. Johnson, K. J., Anderson, T. P., and Ward, P. A. (1977): Suppression of immune complex-induced inflammation by the chemotactic factor inactivator. *J. Clin. Invest.,* 59:951–958.

90. Johnson, R. J., and Chenoweth, D. E. (1985): Labeling the granulocyte C5a receptor with a unique photoreactive probe. *J. Biol. Chem.,* 260:7161–7164.

91. Johnson, R. J., and Chenoweth, D. E. (1985): Structure and function of human C5a anaphylatoxin: Selective modification of tyrosine 23 alters biologic activity but not antigenicity. *J. Biol. Chem.,* 260: 10339–10345.

92. Jose, P. J., Forrest, M. J., and Williams, T. J. (1981): Human C5a des Arg increases vascular permeability. *J. Immunol.,* 127:2376–2380.

93. Keller, H. U., Wissler, J. H., and Damerau, B. (1981): Diverging effects of chemotactic serum peptides and synthetic f-met-leu-phe on neutrophil locomotion and adhesion. *Immunology,* 42:379–383.

94. Klebanoff, S. J., Durack, D. T., Rosen, H., and Clark, R. A. (1977): Functional studies on human peritoneal eosinophils. *Infect. Immun.,* 17:167–173.

95. Kreutzer, D. L., Claypool, W. D., Jones, M. L., and Ward, P. A. (1979): Isolation by hydrophobic chromatography of the chemotactic factor inactivators from human serum. *Clin. Immunol. Immunopathol.,* 12:162–179.

96. Lachmann, P. J., Kay, A. B., and Thompson, R. A. (1970): The chemotactic activity for neutrophil and eosinophil leucocytes of the trimolecular complex of the fifth, sixth and seventh components of human complement (C̄567) prepared in free solution by the "reactive lysis" procedure. *Immunology,* 19:895–899.

97. Lam, W. C., Delikatny, E. J., Orr, F. W., Wass, J., Varani, J., and Ward, P. A. (1981): The chemotactic response of tumor cells: A model for cancer metastasis. *Am. J. Pathol.,* 104:69–76.

98. Leber, T. (1888): Über die entstehung der entzündung und die wirkung der entzündunserrengenden schädlichkeiten. *Fortschr. Med.,* 6:460–464.

99. Leijh, P. C. J., van den Barsellar, M. T., Daha, M. R., and van Furth, R. (1982): Stimulation of the intracellular killing of *Staphylococcus aureus* by monocytes: Regulation by immunoglobulin G and complement components C3/C3b and B/Bb. *J. Immunol.,* 129:332–337.

100. Lett-Brown, M. A., Boetcher, D. A., and Leonard, E. J. (1976): Chemotactic responses of normal human basophils to C5a and to lymphocyte-derived chemotactic factors. *J. Immunol.,* 117:246–252.

101. Lieberman, P., Siegle, R. L., and Taylor, W. W., Jr. (1978): Ana-

phylactoid reactions to iodinated contrast media. *J. Allergy Clin. Immunol.,* 62:174–180.

102. Lieberman, P., and Siegle, R. L. (1979): Complement activation following intravenous contrast material administration. *J. Allergy Clin. Immunol.,* 64:13–17.

103. Lim, H. W., Poh-Fitzpatrick, M. B., and Gigli, I. (1984): Activation of the complement system in patients with porphyrias after irradiation in vivo. *J. Clin. Invest.,* 74:1961–1965.

104. Maderazo, E. G., Ward, P. A., and Quintilliani, R. (1975): Defective regulation of chemotaxis in cirrhosis. *J. Lab. Clin. Med.,* 85:621–630.

105. Maderazo, E. G., Ward, P. A., Woronick, C. L., Kubik, J., and DeGraff, A. C. (1976): Leukotactic dysfunction in sarcoidosis. *Ann. Intern. Med.,* 84:414–419.

106. Mandecki, W., Mollison, K. W., Bolling, T. J., Powell, B. S., Carter, G. W., and Fox, J. L. (1985): Chemical synthesis of a gene encoding the human complement fragment C5a and its expression in *Escherichia coli. Proc. Natl. Acad. Sci. USA,* 82:3543–3547.

107. Marceau, F., and Hugli, T. E. (1984): Effect of C3a and C5a anaphylatoxins on guinea-pig isolated blood vessels. *J. Pharmacol. Exp. Ther.,* 230:749–754.

108. Marder, S. R., Chenoweth, D. E., Goldstein, I. M., and Perez, H. D. (1985): Chemotactic responses of human peripheral blood monocytes to the complement-derived peptides C5a and C5a des Arg. *J. Immunol.,* 134:3325–3331.

109. Matzner, Y., Partridge, R. E. H., and Babior, B. M. (1983): A chemotactic inhibitor in synovial fluid. *Immunology,* 49:131–138.

110. Matzner, Y., and Brzezinski, A. (1984): A C5a inhibitor in peritoneal fluid. *J. Lab. Clin. Med.,* 103:227–235.

111. Matzner, Y., and Brzezinski, A. (1984): C5a-inhibitor deficiency in peritoneal fluids from patients with familial Mediterranean fever. *N. Engl. J. Med.,* 311:287–290.

112. Matzner, Y., Partridge, R. E. H., Levy, M., and Babior, B. M. (1984): Diminished activity of a chemotactic inhibitor in synovial fluids from patients with familial Mediterranean fever. *Blood,* 63: 629–633.

113. McCall, C. E., Bass, D. A., Cousart, S., and DeChatelet, L. R. (1979): Enhancement of hexose uptake in human polymorphonuclear leukocytes by activated complement component C5a. *Proc. Natl. Acad. Sci. USA,* 76:5896–5900.

114. McCarthy, K., and Henson, P. M. (1979): Induction of lysosomal enzyme secretion by alveolar macrophages in response to the purified complement fragments C5a and C5a des-arg. *J. Immunol.,* 123:2511–2517.

115. McGillen, J. J., and Phair, J. P. (1979): Adherence, augmented adherence, and aggregation of polymorphonuclear leukocytes. *J. Infect. Dis.,* 139:69–73.

116. Melamed, J., Arnaout, M. A., and Colten, H. R. (1982): Complement (C3b) interaction with the human granulocyte receptor: Correlation of binding of fluid-phase radiolabeled ligand with histaminase release. *J. Immunol.,* 128:2313–2318.

117. Meuer, S., Ecker, U., Hadding, U., and Bitter-Suermann, D. (1981): Platelet-serotonin release by C3a and C5a: Two independent pathways of activation. *J. Immunol.,* 126:1506–1509.

118. Meuth, J. L., Morgan, E. L., DiScipio, R. G., and Hugli, T. E. (1983): Suppression of T lymphocyte function by human C3 fragments. I. Inhibition of human T cell proliferative responses by a kallikrein cleavage fragment of human iC3b. *J. Immunol.,* 130: 2605–2611.

119. Moon, K. E., Gorski, J. P., and Hugli, T. E. (1981): Complete primary structure of human C4a anaphylatoxin. *J. Biol. Chem.,* 256:8685–8692.

120. Morgan, E. L., Weigle, W. O., and Hugli, T. E. (1982): Anaphylatoxin-mediated regulation of the immune response. I. C3a-mediated suppression of human and murine humoral immune responses. *J. Exp. Med.,* 155:1412–1426.

121. Morgan, E. L., Thoman, M. L., Weigle, W. O., and Hugli, T. E. (1983): Anaphylatoxin-mediated regulation of the immune response. II. C5a-mediated enhancement of human humoral and T cell-mediated immune responses. *J. Immunol.,* 130:1257–1261.

122. Morgan, E. L., Weigle, W. O., Erickson, B. W., Fok, K.-F., and

Hugli, T. E. (1983): Suppression of humoral immune responses by synthetic C3a peptides. *J. Immunol.,* 131:2258–2261.

123. Morgan, E. L., Weigle, W. O., and Hugli, T. E. (1984): Anaphylatoxin-mediated regulation of human and murine immune responses. *Fed. Proc.,* 43:2543–2547.

124. Morgan, E. L., Thoman, M. L., Hobbs, M. V., Weigle, W. O., and Hugli, T. E. (1985): Human C3a-mediated suppression of the immune response. II. Suppression of human *in vitro* polyclonal antibody responses occurs through the generation of nonspecific OKT8⁺ suppressor T cells. *Clin. Immunol. Immunopathol.,* 37: 114–123.

125. Morgan, E. L., Thoman, M. L., Weigle, W. O., and Hugli, T. E. (1985): Human C3a-mediated suppression of the immune response. I. Suppression of murine *in vitro* antibody responses occurs through the generation of nonspecific Lyt-2⁺ suppressor T cell. *J. Immunol.,* 134:51–57.

126. Morgan, W. T., Vallota, E. H., and Müller-Eberhard, H. J. (1974): Circular dichroism of the C5a anaphylatoxin of porcine complement. *Biochem. Biophys. Res. Commun.,* 57:572–577.

127. Muhlfelder, T. W., Niemetz, J., Kreutzer, D., Beebe, D., Ward, P. A., and Rosenfeld, S. I. (1979): C5 chemotactic fragment induces leukocyte production of tissue factor activity. A link between complement and coagulation. *J. Clin. Invest.,* 63:147–150.

128. Ohlsson, K. (1971): Neutral leukocyte proteases and elastase inhibited by plasma alpha 1-antitrypsin. *Scand. J. Clin. Lab. Invest.,* 28:251–253.

129. Orr, W., Varani, J., and Ward, P. A. (1978): Characteristics of the chemotactic response of neoplastic cells to a factor derived from the fifth component of complement. *Am. J. Pathol.,* 93:405–422.

130. Orr, W., Phan, S. H., Varani, J., Ward, P. A., Kreutzer, D. L., Webster, R. O., and Henson, P. M. (1979): Chemotactic factor for tumor cells derived from the C5a fragment of complement component C5. *Proc. Natl. Acad. Sci. USA,* 76:1986–1989.

131. Orr, F. W., Varani, J., Kreutzer, D. L., Senior, R. M., and Ward, P. A. (1979): Digestion of the fifth component of complement by leukocyte enzymes: Sequential generation of chemotactic activities for leukocytes and for tumor cells. *Am. J. Pathol.,* 94:75–83.

132. Orr, F. W., Delikatny, E. J., Mokashi, S., Krepart, G. V., and Stiver, H. G. (1983): Detection of a complement-derived chemotactic factor for tumor cells in human inflammatory and neoplastic effusions. *Am. J. Pathol.,* 110:41–47.

133. Osler, A. G., Randall, G. H., Hill, B. M., and Ovary, Z. (1959): Studies on the mechanism of hypersensitivity phenomena. III. The participation of complement in the formation of anaphylatoxin. *J. Exp. Med.,* 110:311–339.

134. Ozaki, T., Yoshida, K., Ushijima, K., and Hayashi, H. (1971): Studies on the mechanisms of invasion in cancer. II. *In vivo* effects of a factor chemotactic for cancer cells. *Int. J. Cancer,* 7:93–100.

135. Payan, D. G., Trentham, D. E., and Goetzl, E. J. (1982): Modulation of human lymphocyte function by C3a and C3a(70–77). *J. Exp. Med.,* 156:756–765.

136. Perez, H. D., Lipton, M., and Goldstein, I. M. (1978): A specific inhibitor of complement (C5)-derived chemotactic activity in serum from patients with systemic lupus erythematosus. *J. Clin. Invest.,* 62:29–38.

137. Perez, H. D., Andron, R. I., and Goldstein, I. M. (1979): Infection in patients with systemic lupus erythematosus: Association with a serum inhibitor of complement (C5)-derived chemotactic activity. *Arthritis Rheum.,* 22:1326–1333.

138. Perez, H. D., Goldstein, I. M., Chernoff, D., Webster, R. O., and Henson, P. M. (1980): Chemotactic activity of C5a des Arg: Evidence of a requirement for an anionic peptide "helper factor" and inhibition by a cationic protein in serum from patients with systemic lupus erythematosus. *Mol. Immunol.,* 17:163–169.

139. Perez, H. D., Goldstein, I. M., Webster, R. O., and Henson, P. M. (1981): Enhancement of the chemotactic activity of human C5a des Arg by an anionic polypeptide ("cochemotaxin") in normal serum and plasma. *J. Immunol.,* 126:800–804.

140. Perez, H. D., Horn, J. K., Ong, R., and Goldstein, I. M. (1983): Complement (C5)-derived chemotactic activity in serum from patients with pancreatitis. *J. Lab. Clin. Med.,* 101:123–129.

141. Perez, H. D., Chenoweth, D. E., and Goldstein, I. M. (1986): At-

tachment of human C5a des Arg to its cochemotaxin is required for maximum expression of chemotactic activity. *J. Clin. Invest.,* 78:1589–1595.

142. Perez, H. D., and Hooper, C. (1986): A specific inhibitor of complement (C5)-derived chemotactic activity in patients with lupus is immunologically related to the Bb fragment of factor B. *Clin. Res.,* 34:621A.

143. Petersson, B.-A., Nilsson, A., and Stalenheim, G. (1975): Induction of histamine release and desensitization in human leukocytes: Effect of anaphylatoxin. *J. Immunol.,* 114:1581–1584.

144. Plummer, T. H., Jr., and Hurwitz, M. Y. (1978): Human plasma carboxypeptidase N: Isolation and characterization. *J. Biol. Chem.,* 253:3907–3912.

145. Polley, M. J., Nachman, R. L., and Weksler, B. B. (1981): Human complement in the arachidonic acid transformation pathway in platelets. *J. Exp. Med.,* 153:257–268.

146. Polley, M. J., and Nachman, R. L. (1983): Human platelet activation by C3a and C3a des-arg. *J. Exp. Med.,* 158:603–615.

147. Regal, J. F., and Pickering, R. J. (1981): C5a-induced tracheal contraction: Effect of an SRS-A antagonist and inhibitors of arachidonate metabolism. *J. Immunol.,* 126:313–316.

148. Ring, J., Arroyave, C. M., Fritzler, M. J., and Tan, E. M. (1978): *In vitro* histamine and serotonin release by radiographic contrast media (RCM): Complement-dependent and -independent release reaction and changes in ultrastructure of human blood cells. *Clin. Exp. Immunol.,* 32:105–118.

149. Rollins, T. E., and Springer, M. S. (1985): Identification of the polymorphonuclear leukocyte C5a receptor. *J. Biol. Chem.,* 260: 7157–7160.

150. Romualdez, A. G., Jr., and Ward, P. A. (1975): A unique complement derived chemotactic factor for tumor cells. *Proc. Natl. Acad. Sci. USA,* 72:4128–4132.

151. Romualdez, A. G., Jr., Ward, P. A., and Torikata, T. (1976): Relationship between the C5 peptides chemotactic for leukocytes and tumor cells. *J. Immunol.,* 117:1762–1766.

152. Rother, K. (1972): Leucocyte mobilizing factor: A new biological activity derived from the third component of complement. *Eur. J. Immunol.,* 2:550–558.

153. Scheid, C. R., Webster, R. O., Henson, P. M., and Findlay, S. R. (1983): Direct effect of complement factor C5a on the contractile state of isolated smooth muscle cells. *J. Immunol.,* 130:1997–1999.

154. Schopf, E., Hammann, K. P., Scheiner, O., Lemmel, E.-M., and Dierich, M. P. (1982): Activation of human monocytes by both human 1H and C3b. *Immunology,* 46:307–312.

155. Schreiber, R. D., Pangburn, M. K., Bjornson, A. B., Brothers, M. A., and Müller-Eberhard, H. J. (1982): The role of C3 fragments in endocytosis and extracellular cytotoxic reactions by polymorphonuclear leukocytes. *Clin. Immunol. Immunopathol.,* 23:335–357.

156. Shin, H. S., Snyderman, R., Friedman, E., Mellors, A., and Mayer, M. M. (1968): Chemotactic and anaphylatoxic fragment cleaved from the fifth component of guinea pig complement. *Science,* 162: 361–362.

157. Siraganian, R. P., and Hook, W. A. (1976): Complement-induced histamine release from human basophils. II. Mechanism of the histamine release reaction. *J. Immunol.,* 116:639–646.

158. Sitrin, R. G., Kaltreider, H. B., Ansfeld, M. J., and Webster, R. O. (1983): Procoagulant activity of rabbit alveolar macrophages. *Am. Rev. Resp. Dis.,* 128:282–287.

159. Smith, C. W., Hollers, J. C., Patrick, R. A., and Hassett, C. (1979): Motility and adhesiveness in human neutrophils: Effects of chemotactic factors. *J. Clin. Invest.,* 63:221–229.

160. Smith, R. P. C., Lackie, J. M., and Wilkinson, P. C. (1979): The effects of chemotactic factors on the adhesiveness of rabbit neutrophil granulocytes. *Exp. Cell Res.,* 122:169–177.

160a. Snyderman, R., Gewurz, H., and Mergenhagen, S. E. (1968): Interactions of the complement system with endotoxic lipopolysaccharide: Generation of a factor chemotactic for polymorphonuclear leukocytes. *J. Exp. Med.,* 128:259–275.

161. Snyderman, R., Altman, L. C., Hausman, M. S., and Mergenhagen, S. E. (1972): Human mononuclear leukocyte chemotaxis: A quan-

tititative assay for humoral and cellular chemotactic factors. *J. Immunol.*, 108:857–860.

162. Solomkin, J. S., Cotta, L. A., Satoh, P. S., Hurst, J. M., and Nelson, R. D. (1985): Complement activation and clearance in acute illness and injury: Evidence for C5a as a cell-directed mediator of the adult respiratory distress syndrome in man. *Surgery,* 97:668–678.

163. Stimler, N. P., Brocklehurst, W. E., Bloor, C. M., and Hugli, T. E. (1981): Anaphylatoxin-mediated contraction of guinea pig lung strips: A nonhistamine tissue response. *J. Immunol.*, 126:2258–2261.

164. Stimler, N. P., Bach, M. K., Bloor, C. M., and Hugli, T. E. (1982): Release of leukotrienes from guinea pig lung stimulated by C5a$_{des\ Arg}$ anaphylatoxin. *J. Immunol.*, 128:2247–2252.

165. Stimler, N. P., Bloor, C. M., and Hugli, T. E. (1983): C3a-induced contraction of guinea pig lung parenchyma: Role of cyclooxygenase metabolites. *Immunopharmacology,* 5:251–257.

166. Sundsmo, J. S., and Götze, O. (1983): Human monocyte spreading induced by activated factor B of the complement alternative pathway: Differential effects of Fab′ and F(ab′)$_2$ antibody fragments directed to C5, C6, and C7. *Cell Immunol.*, 77:176–186.

167. Tack, B. F. (1983): The β-cys-γ-glu thiolester bond in human C3 and C4. *Springer Semin. Immunopathol.*, 6:259–282.

168. Takematsu, H., Ohkohchi, K., and Tagami, H. (1986): Demonstration of anaphylatoxins C3a, C4a and C5a in the scales of psoriasis and inflammatory pustular dermatoses. *Br. J. Dermatol.*, 114:1–6.

169. Till, G., and Ward, P. A. (1975): Two distinct chemotactic factor inactivators in human serum. *J. Immunol.*, 114:843–847.

170. Till, G., Rother, U., and Gemsa, D. (1978): Activation of complement by radiographic contrast media: Generation of chemotactic and anaphylatoxin activities. *Int. Arch. Allergy Appl. Immunol.*, 56:543–550.

171. Tonnesen, M. G., Smedly, L. A., and Henson, P. M. (1984): Neutrophil-endothelial cell interactions: Modulation of neutrophil adhesiveness induced by complement fragments C5a and C5a des Arg and formyl-methionyl-leucyl-phenylalanine. *J. Clin. Invest.*, 74:1581–1592.

172. Vallota, E. H., and Müller-Eberhard, H. J. (1973): Formation of C3a and C5a anaphylatoxins in whole human serum after inhibition of the anaphylatoxin inactivator. *J. Exp. Med.*, 137:1109–1123.

173. Van Epps, D. E., and Chenoweth, D. E. (1984): Analysis of the binding of fluorescent C5a and C3a to human peripheral blood leukocytes. *J. Immunol.*, 132:2862–2867.

174. Ward, P. A., Cochrane, C. G., and Müller-Eberhard, H. J. (1965): The role of serum complement in chemotaxis of leukocytes in vitro. *J. Exp. Med.*, 122:327–346.

175. Ward, P. A., and Becker, E. L. (1968): The deactivation of rabbit neutrophils by chemotactic factor and the nature of the activable esterase. *J. Exp. Med.*, 127:693–709.

176. Ward, P. A., and Newman, L. J. (1969): A neutrophil chemotactic factor from human C′5. *J. Immunol.*, 102:93–99.

177. Ward, P. A., and Zvaifler, N. J. (1971): Complement-derived leukotactic factors in inflammatory synovial fluids of humans. *J. Clin. Invest.*, 50:606–616.

178. Ward, P. A., and Talamo, R. C. (1973): Deficiency of the chemotactic factor inactivator in human sera with alpha$_1$-antitrypsin deficiency. *J. Clin. Invest.*, 52:516–519.

179. Ward, P. A., and Berenberg, J. L. (1974): Defective regulation of inflammatory mediators in Hodgkin's disease: Supernormal levels of chemotactic-factor inactivator. *N. Engl. J. Med.*, 290:76–80.

180. Ward, P. A., Goralnick, S., and Bullock, W. E. (1976): Defective leukotaxis in patients with lepromatous leprosy. *J. Lab. Clin. Med.*, 87:1025–1032.

181. Webster, R. O., Hong, S. R., Johnston, R. B., Jr., and Henson, P. M. (1980): Biological effects of the human complement fragments C5a and C5a des Arg on neutrophil function. *Immunopharmacology,* 2:201–219.

182. Wedmore, C. V., and Williams, T. J. (1981): Control of vascular permeability by polymorphonuclear leukocytes in inflammation. *Nature,* 289:646–650.

183. Weigle, W. O., Morgan, E. L., Goodman, M. G., Chenoweth, D. E., and Hugli, T. E. (1982): Modulation of the immune response by anaphylatoxin in the microenvironment of the interacting cells. *Fed. Proc.*, 41:3099–3103.

184. Weigle, W. O., Goodman, M. G., Morgan, E. L., and Hugli, T. E. (1983): Regulation of immune response by components of the complement cascade and their activated fragments. *Springer Semin. Immunopathol.*, 6:173–194.

185. Weinberg, P. F., Matthay, M. A., Webster, R. O., Roskos, K. V., Goldstein, I. M., and Murray, J. F. (1984): Biologically active products of complement and acute lung injury in patients with the sepsis syndrome. *Am. Rev. Resp. Dis.*, 130:791–796.

186. Wetsel, R. A., and Kolb, W. P. (1983): Expression of C5a-like biological activities by the fifth component of human complement (C5) upon limited digestion with noncomplement enzymes without release of polypeptide fragments. *J. Exp. Med.*, 157:2029–2048.

187. Wexler, D. E., Chenoweth, D. E., and Cleary, P. P. (1985): Mechanism of action of the group A streptococcal C5a inactivator. *Proc. Natl. Acad. Sci. USA,* 82:8144–8148.

188. Wissler, J. H., Stecker, V. J., and Sorkin, E. (1972): Biochemistry and biology of a leucotactic binary serum peptide system related to anaphylatoxin. *Int. Arch. Allergy Appl. Immunol.*, 42:722–747.

189. Wright, A. E., and Douglas, S. R. (1903): An experimental investigation of the role of blood fluids in connection with phagocytosis. *Proc. R. Soc. Lond. [Biol.],* 72:357–362.

190. Wright, D. G., and Gallin, J. I. (1975): Modulation of the inflammatory response by products released from human polymorphonuclear leukocytes during phagocytosis: Generation and inactivation of the chemotactic factor C5a. *Inflammation,* 1:23–39.

191. Wright, D. G., and Gallin, J. I. (1977): A functional differentiation of human neutrophil granules: Generation of C5a by a specific (secondary) granule product and inactivation of C5a by azurophil (primary) granule products. *J. Immunol.*, 119:1068–1076.

192. Wuepper, K. D., Bokisch, V. A., Müller-Eberhard, H. J., and Stoughton, R. B. (1972): Cutaneous responses to human C3 anaphylatoxin in man. *Clin. Exp. Immunol.*, 11:13–20.

193. Yancey, K. B., Hammer, C. H., Harvath, L., Renfer, L., Frank, M. M., and Lawley, T. J. (1985): Studies of human C5a as a mediator of inflammation in normal human skin. *J. Clin. Invest.*, 75:486–495.

194. Yancey, K. B., O'Shea, J., Chused, T., Brown, E., Takahashi, T., Frank, M. M., and Lawley, T. J. (1985): Human C5a modulates monocyte Fc and C3 receptor expression. *J. Immunol.*, 135:465–470.

195. Zurier, R. B., Hoffstein, S., and Weissmann, G. (1973): Cytochalasin B: Effect of lysosomal enzyme release from human leucocytes. *Proc. Natl. Acad. Sci. USA,* 70:844–848.

Inflammation: Basic Principles and Clinical Correlates.
Edited by J. I. Gallin, I. M. Goldstein, and R. Snyderman.
Raven Press, Ltd., New York © 1988.

CHAPTER 5

Complement: Molecular Genetics

David H. Perlmutter and Harvey R. Colten

The complement system consists of 20 or more proteins, the biological activities of which include induction
of inflammatory responses and the promotion of ingestion, killing, and lysis of microorganisms (see Chapters 3
and 4). These proteins include components of a limited
proteolytic cascade (i.e., the classical and alternative activating pathways), the terminal components which assemble to form the membrane attack complex, regulatory
proteins, and cellular receptors. Complementary DNA
(cDNA) clones for more than 15 of the 20 complement
genes are now available. Application of these probes to
studies on the complement system has permitted the determination of primary structure and, in some cases,
chromosomal localization of complement genes. More
extensive knowledge of primary structure will allow predictions about higher-order structure, identification of
homologies with other complement and noncomplement
gene products, and a deeper understanding of the structural requirements for unique physiological functions.
Molecular genetic studies will also provide insights into
the basis of complement deficiency disorders and linkage
to other diseases. Finally, the application of molecular
genetic techniques permits more detailed studies on the
expression and regulation of complement production
during homeostasis and inflammation.

GENE FAMILIES

Genes have been grouped into families on the basis of
similarities in structure, function, or chromosomal localization. The description of gene families has provided new
insights into the structure, function, and evolution of existing genes, as well as the identification of new genes.
Several complement genes have been described as parts
of supergene families on the basis of clustering in specific
chromosomal regions. The genes encoding C2, factor B,
and C4 constitute the class III region of the major histocompatibility complex (MHC) on human chromosome
6 and on mouse chromosome 17 (Fig. 1). The organization
of these genes is also very similar in the two species
(27,28,31,32,92). The 3' terminus of the C2 gene is upstream of, and close to, the 5' terminus of the factor B
(BF) gene (<500 base pairs) (26). The two C4 genes [C4A
and C4B in humans, sex-limited protein (Slp) and C4 in
mice] lie approximately 30 kilobases (kb) downstream
from the C2 and factor B genes, separated by 10 kb, and
each has a cytochrome P-450 steroid 21-hydroxylase (21-
OH) gene within 1.5 kb of the 3' terminus (29,133). The
order of the genes in the direction of transcription is C2-
BF-C4A-21-OHA-C4B-21-OHB, and they have been
mapped within a 0.7-centimorgan region between HLA-

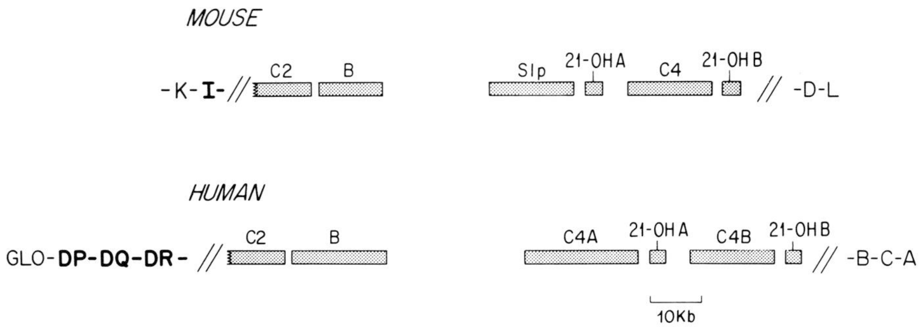

MOUSE

-K- **I**- // C2 B Slp 21-OHA C4 21-OHB // -D-L

HUMAN

GLO- **DP-DQ-DR** - // C2 B C4A 21-OHA C4B 21-OHB // -B-C-A

10Kb

FIG. 1. Organization of the murine and human MHCs. The 5' terminus of the C2 gene has not been determined, so it is represented by a jagged line. Class I genes are K, D, and L for the mouse MHC, and A, B, and C for the human MHC. Class II genes are I for the mouse MHC, and DP, DQ, and DR for the human MHC (boldface). GLO represents the locus for the glyoxylase gene. (From ref. 41.)

B and HLA-DR (84,137). The C2 and factor B genes are homologous in structure and function. The C4 genes have greater homology with C3, C5, and α_2-macroglobulin than with C2 and factor B.

The genes encoding the complement receptor for C3b/C4b (CR1) (62), C4-binding protein (C4BP), factor H (H) (111), and decay-accelerating factor (DAF) (D. Lublin, unpublished observations) are closely clustered on the long arm of chromosome 1 (Fig. 2). Because CR1, C4BP, H, and DAF are regulatory proteins with similar functional characteristics, they have been considered members of a distinct gene family. Detailed structural studies on genes within this family have recently demonstrated repeating homology units of approximately 60 residues which are also seen in the sequence of C2 (19), factor B (71,133), and C1r (63). One property common to all these proteins with highly conserved repeating homology units is the capacity to bind fragments of C3 and C4. Therefore, the complement regulatory genes on chromosome 1 and the genes encoded in the class III region of the MHC may be considered parts of a supergene family related by the common functional characteristic of interaction with the activation fragments of C3 and C4 (reviewed in 105). Since repeating homology units are also found in noncomplement proteins, i.e., the interleukin-2 (IL-2) receptor, β_2-

glycoprotein-1, haptoglobin alpha chain, and herpes simplex virus glycoprotein C, proteins which have not been shown to interact with C3 and C4, alternate gene taxonomy may be proposed. For example, the presence of these repeating homology sequences in herpes simplex virus glycoprotein C may reflect sequences arising either by fortuitous or directed insertion of the viral genome at one or several of these loci during evolution (Table 1), i.e., organization not based on divergence from an ancestral gene but on an encounter with an infectious agent.

The genes for complement proteins C3, C4, and C5 have been described as a family which shares primary structural and functional properties with α_2-macroglobulin and pregnancy zone protein (Table 1). These genes, however, do not appear to be clustered in a specific chromosomal region. The human C3 gene has been mapped to chromosome 19 (134), whereas that of the mouse is on chromosome 17, distant from the H-2 complex (75) (Fig. 2). The C5 gene has been localized to chromosome 2 in the mouse (60).

C1 inhibitor shares structural and functional characteristics with several serine proteinase inhibitors (SERPINS) and is often included in the SERPIN supergene family (see below). The chromosomal localization of several SERPIN genes has been determined. C1 inhibitor

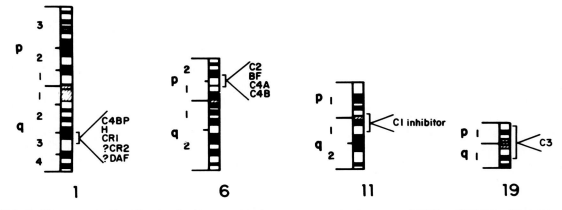

FIG. 2. Chromosomal localization for human complement genes. Assignment of CR2 and DAF to chromosome 1 has not yet been published. The orientation and order of the complement genes on chromosome 1 is not known.

TABLE 1. *Structural homologies*

Complement components			Noncomplement homologs
C2	Unique serine proteinase		
Factor B			
C4BP			IL-2 receptor
Factor H		Highly conserved tandem repeats	β_2-Glycoprotein-1
CR1			Haptoglobin alpha chain
CR2			Herpes simplex virus
DAF			glycoprotein C
Clr	Unique serine proteinase		
Cls			
C3			α_2-Macroglobulin
	Multichain disulfide-linked proteins	Thiolester bond	Pregnancy zone protein
C4			
C5			

maps to human chromosome 11 (44) (Fig. 2), whereas α_1-proteinase inhibitor is localized to chromosome 14.

GENE STRUCTURE AND POLYMORPHISM

C2 and Factor B Genes

Human (26–28) and murine (32) factor B are each encoded at single genetic loci. The human factor B gene is approximately 6 kb long and is divided into 18 exons (26). Three exons coding for regions within the Ba fragment show significant sequence homology with each other; i.e., they may be products of tandem duplication. These exons encode repeating homology units of 60 amino acids which are also found in C2, Clr, C4BP, CR1, factor H, IL-2 receptor, β_2-glycoprotein-1, and clotting factor XIII (105). With the exception of a single exon, the organization of the factor B gene in the region encoding the carboxy-terminus of the Bb fragment is similar to that observed in chymotrypsin, elastase, kallikrein, and trypsin. The amino-terminus of the Bb fragment is encoded by five exons which do not share any homology with other serine proteases. This is consistent with the observation that both factor B and C2 are unique among the serine proteases in having catalytic chains approximately twice the size of those in other serine proteases (26).

There is also a high degree of structural conservation of factor B between mice and humans (116). For the 477 amino acids determined in the Bb fragment of murine factor B, 83% of the residues are identical with the corresponding region of the human protein. There is also 59% sequence identity in the 3' untranslated region, and an unusual polyadenylation signal is found in both species. The functional significance of homology in noncoding sequences in the 3' flanking region is unknown. Conservation of structure in this region may reflect functional importance of the 3' untranslated region in the expression of factor B protein.

The fine details of C2 genomic structure have not been published, but preliminary data suggest many similarities between the C2 and factor B genes, even though there is only approximately 35% homology in the derived amino acid sequence (26,28). There is a significantly lower frequency of polymorphic variation in C2 and factor B than in C4 and the class I and class II MHC gene products. Nevertheless, several allelic forms of these two proteins have been defined by electrophoretic techniques (1) or by restriction endonuclease digestion (42,52,142). One recently identified restriction fragment length polymorphism is found in a previously recognized MHC extended haplotype associated with insulin-dependent diabetes (42). Further investigation of the structural basis of this polymorphism may provide important information about genetic susceptibility to diabetes and other MHC-linked disorders or may provide a marker for the identification of susceptible individuals.

In the mouse, a sexual dimorphism in the electrophoretic pattern of factor B has been described (113). More recently, restriction fragment length polymorphism analysis has indicated a total of five C2 and seven factor B alleles in a large number of inbred and wild mouse strains (52). In these mice, C2 and factor B variants usually correlate with the species or subspecies origin of the H-2 haplotypes tested. It is not known whether these polymorphic variants are associated with variations in C2 or factor B function.

C4 Genes

There are at least two genetic loci for C4 in humans, C4A and C4B. The complete nucleotide sequences of the C4A and C4B genes have been determined (17,18). The

C4A gene is 22 kb in size, and a variation in size of the C4B gene (16 kb in some individuals and 22 kb in others) is a result of the absence or presence of a 6.8-kb intron toward the 5′ terminus (30,96). There are only four amino acid differences between the two genes (145). This variation in sequence is clustered around the active site, the thiolester region of the C4 alpha chain, and is thought to explain the differences in functional activity of C4A and C4B gene products. C4B reacts more effectively with hydroxyl groups and is two- to four-fold more effective in complement activation. C4A reacts more readily with amino groups, such as those displayed by immune aggregates (16,59,66). The variation in sequence between C4A and C4B does not explain the apparent 2-kilodalton (kD) difference in alpha-chain size between the two isotypes (114). The complete nucleotide sequence of C4 also confirms previous predictions that clusters of basic amino acid residues are located at the junctions between beta, alpha, and gamma chains and that these peptides are proteolytically excised during conversion to the mature three-chain molecule (17,18).

There are also two C4-like genes in the mouse, C4 and Slp (reviewed in 122). These two genes are similar to C4A and C4B in chromosomal localization; i.e., they are encoded within the MHC and are in a similar orientation with respect to the direction of transcription (32). C4 and Slp are also characterized by differences in specific hemolytic activity; i.e., Slp has no detectable activity in conventional assays. C4 circulates in mouse plasma at much higher concentrations than Slp in some strains and at approximately equivalent concentrations in other strains, whereas C4A and C4B circulate in human plasma at approximately equivalent concentrations (1). Expression of the Slp gene in most haplotypes is regulated by androgens (89).

The cDNA and genomic structure of murine C4 and Slp has been reported (80,81,83). The two genes are similar in size and exon-intron organization. There is extensive sequence homology in coding regions (96% nucleotide, 94% amino acid), but divergence in the sequence of the 5′ flanking regions. A number of -CACA- repeats were demonstrated in the 5′ flanking region of C4 but not in that of Slp. The importance of this finding is unknown.

A relatively high frequency of duplications, deletions, and rearrangements lead to polymorphic variation in human C4 genes. Many of the variants and null alleles ascribed to these genes were based on electrophoretic mobility of the C4 protein and linkage with disease phenotypes. By direct analysis of gene structure, several additional polymorphic variations have been defined (119,136,145). Some of the variants have been associated with diseases of the immune system, including systemic lupus erythematosus, scleroderma, and subacute sclerosing panencephalitis (54,106,107).

Structural, functional, and regulatory variants of murine C4 and Slp genes have been demonstrated (122). Such genetic variation includes a 20-fold difference among mouse strains in the circulating plasma levels of C4. It now appears that the difference in C4 levels in C4-high and C4-low mice is due to a difference in steady-state concentrations of C4 messenger RNA (mRNA) (32,82,115). A difference in the rate of transcription is the likely explanation for this finding, but a change in C4 mRNA stability cannot be excluded. Tissue specificity also contributes to genetic variation, because macrophages from C4-high and C4-low strains synthesize similar amounts of C4 protein (77,117). Genetic variation in Slp expression appears to be even more complex. There are strains of mice which do not express Slp, strains in which Slp expression is androgen-regulated, and strains in which Slp expression is constitutive. Control of constitutive Slp expression is associated with H-2 haplotypes as well as non-H-2 loci. In the first case, duplications of the C4/Slp gene complex have been identified (23,57,67).

C3 and C5 Genes

The complete nucleotide sequences of human and murine C3 cDNA clones have been reported (45,53). The human C3 precursor contains a signal peptide of 22 amino acids, a region of 645 residues corresponding to the beta chain, and a 992-amino acid alpha chain. A region of four basic amino acids separating the beta and alpha chains is the intersubunit peptide cleaved during processing to the mature two-chain molecule. The murine C3 gene is 24 kb long and shares extensive homology with the human C3 gene. There is strong homology in the sequences of C3, C4, C5, and α_2-macroglobulin, suggesting a common evolutionary origin for these genes.

There are two common polymorphic variants of C3, designated C3F (fast) and C3S (slow) according to their relative electrophoretic mobilities, and several rare allelic variants have been described (2,6). A hypomorphic C3F variant is associated with C3 deficiency (5), and a similar variant has been found in an individual with hypocomplementemia and hematuria (65).

Most of the coding sequence of human and murine C5 has been determined (69,132). The sequence includes 4,920 base pairs specifying 1,640 amino acid residues. A four-residue basic sequence (Arg-Ser-Lys-Arg) was present toward the amino-terminal side of C5a, thereby specifying a beta-alpha chain orientation for pro-C5. Comparison of the derived murine C5 sequence with previously determined sequences for murine C3 and C4 revealed a high degree of primary structural homology, including the thiolester region. The cysteine and proximal glutamine which give rise to the intramolecular thiolester bond in

C3 and C4 were absent in C5, being replaced by serine and alanine, respectively. Human C5 is highly homologous to murine C5 in the sequence from positions 372 to 812.

As judged by electrophoretic mobilities, polymorphism of C5 has rarely been detected; i.e., C5 polymorphism has thus far been detected only in populations in the South Pacific region (58). Southern blot analysis using molecular probes should provide more detailed information about polymorphisms of C5.

C1 Genes

The C1q B-chain gene is 2.6 kb long and has a single 1.1-kb intron in its coding region (104). This intron is located in the middle of a region coding for the collagen-like moiety of the molecule, interrupting the collagen sequence exactly at the site at which the triple helix of C1q bends when viewed in the electron microscope. This is one of the characteristics that distinguishes C1q from human collagen proteins (34). Complementary DNA sequences for the A and C chains of C1q have not been reported. Further information about the structure of C1q may allow elucidation of the molecular mechanisms for several variants that have been described: a C1q deficiency associated with immune complex diseases and a C1q molecule with an apparent molecular mass of 155 kD as compared to the normal 460 kD (103); fibroblast C1q with an apparent molecular mass of 800 kD (102); a colostral C1q having an unusually large apparent molecular mass (143); and a form of C1q which functions as a Fc receptor in guinea pig peritoneal macrophages (68).

Isolation of cDNA clones for the C1 subcomponents, C1r and C1s, has been reported in abstract form (130). These two subcomponents are similar in chymotrypsin-like proteolytic activity, in the size of their subunits, and in their two-domain configuration, but differ markedly in autocatalytic and dimerizing properties (9,40). C1r and C1s also appear to be under distinct regulatory controls (74). The complete nucleotide sequence of these two subcomponents will allow further understanding of the structure–function relationships and regulation of C1r and C1s.

C8 Gene

The alpha and beta subunits of human C8 have been cloned (99). The alpha subunit is 1,659 bases long, with a leader sequence of 30 amino acids and a region of 10 amino acids followed by an arginine-rich tetrapeptide typical for a propeptide. A 2.5-kb mRNA in human hepatoma cells hybridizes with this cDNA probe. The beta subunit is 1,608 bases long. Considerable homology has been demonstrated between the alpha and beta subunits, C9, and the low-density lipoprotein (LDL) receptor. Three allelic variants of the C8 alpha-gamma subunit have been identified by isoelectric focusing (95,100,108). Family studies on one of these variants have suggested linkage with markers known to be localized to chromosome 1 (reviewed in 109).

C9 Gene

The primary amino acid sequence of C9 includes 573 residues as deduced from cDNA sequencing (46,123,124). The amino-terminal portion is hydrophilic, and the carboxy-terminus is hydrophobic in nature. This structure is consistent with previous studies suggesting that the carboxy-terminus of C9 is inserted into phospholipid membranes during the formation of complement-mediated membrane lesions. In the amino-terminal portion of the molecule there is a region with many cysteines which is highly homologous to a cysteine-rich domain in the LDL receptor. There is also structural homology between C9 and the pore-forming protein from cytotoxic lymphocytes known as perforin (144).

Complement Receptor Genes: CR1, CR2, and CR3

A partial cDNA sequence for the human C3b/C4b receptor (CR1) has been published (141), of which an estimated 78% of the coding sequence has now been determined. Three long, homologous repeats, each of 450 amino acids, are present in the extracellular domain. Within each long, homologous repeat are seven consensus repeats of 60 to 70 amino acids each. Invariant residues in these consensus repeats include four half-cystines, a tryptophan, and a glycine similar to those in factor H, C4BP, CR2, Ba, C2b, the IL-2 receptor, β_2-glycoprotein-1, C1r, factor XIIIb subunit, and haptoglobin alpha chain. Limited sequence analysis of CR1 genomic clones suggests that each repeat is encoded by a distinct exon, as is the case for the Ba fragment of factor B. A nonrepetitive sequence has been identified in the carboxy-terminal portion of CR1. A hydrophobic segment of 25 amino acids followed by four positively charged amino acids is probably the membrane-spanning segment, and 43 amino acids at the carboxy-terminus probably represent the cytoplasmic tail. There is a six-residue sequence in the cytoplasmic tail which bears 65% homology to the protein kinase C phosphorylation site in the epidermal growth factor (EGF) receptor and the *erb B* oncogene.

Several structural polymorphisms of CR1 have been identified. Three allotype variants, S, F, and F′, are associated with proteins of different apparent molecular mass (47–49,140). Another variant, resulting in a lower number of CR1 molecules per cell but without a change in structure (138), has recently been associated with a specific restriction fragment length polymorphism (139).

The C3d/Epstein–Barr virus receptor of human B lymphocytes (complement receptor CR2) has also been partially characterized by molecular cloning (131). CR2 is highly homologous to CR1, having repeating units of 60 amino acids each, with 10 to 14 conserved residues. Both genes have been localized to band 3.2 of human chromosome 1.

Partial sequence analysis of cDNA clones for the beta subunit and the p150,95 alpha subunit of complement receptor CR3 is now available (118; T. Springer, unpublished observations; S. K. A. Law, unpublished observations; M. A. Arnaout, unpublished observations). The beta subunit is 760 amino acids long, including a 22-amino acid signal sequence, a cystine-rich external domain with three or four tandem duplications, a single hydrophobic membrane-spanning region, and a 46-amino acid cytoplasmic tail. The beta subunit also appears to share homology with chicken fibronectin and laminin receptors. The p150,95 alpha subunit is homologous with the human vitronectin receptor and platelet surface glycoprotein IIbIIIa. A structural polymorphism of the beta subunit appears to be associated with CR3 receptor deficiency syndrome in one kindred (T. Springer, unpublished observations).

Regulatory Protein Genes: C4BP, H, I, DAF, and C1 Inhibitor

cDNA clones for human (35) and murine (63) C4-binding protein have allowed determination of the complete nucleotide sequence of these proteins. Human C4BP contains 549 amino acids with the amino-terminal 491 divided into eight 60-amino acid homologous repeating units with a characteristic framework of highly conserved residues. C4BP appears in the electron microscope as a spiderlike structure with "tentacles" connected at one end to a central "core" (43), making it likely that the repeating units are arranged as tentacles with the nonhomologous carboxy-terminal residues constituting the core (105). There is extensive homology between murine and human C4BP, i.e., 61% in the predicted amino acid sequence (T. Kristensen, unpublished observations). Murine C4BP has only six long, homologous repeats, accounting for the lesser number of amino acid residues and smaller apparent molecular mass. Residues corresponding to the four cysteines involved in interchain disulfide links in human C4BP are not found in murine C4BP, which may account for the lack of covalent association between the mouse C4BP polypeptide chains.

Several polymorphic variants of C4BP have been demonstrated by isoelectric focusing (110). Comparison of the derived amino acid sequence of human C4BP and the amino acid sequence determined for the protein purified from pooled human plasma suggests that there are at least two regions in which variability is likely to occur (101).

cDNA clones corresponding to murine (63) and human (64) factor H mRNA have also been isolated and sequenced. Factor H is composed of 20 homologous repeating units starting from the amino-terminus of the 160-kD processed protein and similar to those of the other functionally related and unrelated proteins mentioned above.

DAF is a glycoprotein which also regulates the complement pathway by accelerating the decay of C3 convertases. The complete nucleotide sequence of human DAF has been determined (D. M. Lublin, unpublished observations). This cDNA sequence codes for 347 amino acids beginning at the amino-terminus with four contiguous 61-amino acid consensus repeats similar to those described above. There is also a serine- and threonine-rich sequence similar to that of the LDL receptor. The carboxy-terminus consists of a hydrophobic sequence similar to that of most integral membrane proteins. There is also evidence of a distinct DAF mRNA which enters an alternative posttranscriptional splicing pathway and thereby encodes a secreted form of DAF (I. W. Caras, unpublished observations).

The human complement C3b/C4b inactivator, factor I (I), has also been cloned, but the cDNA sequence is not yet available (G. Goldberger, unpublished observations; C. F. Catterall, unpublished observations). It will be interesting to compare this sequence with the other serine proteinase-like complement proteins and other proteins that bind C3 and C4.

The primary sequence of the C1 inhibitor has been determined (20,44). C1 inhibitor shares approximately 20% homology with the serine protease inhibitors, α_1-proteinase inhibitor, α_1-antichymotrypsin, antithrombin III, and angiotensinogen. It differs from the other plasma proteinase inhibitors at only 14 of 41 invariant residues. It also has an amino-terminal domain that is not homologous to that of the other proteinase inhibitors. Preliminary data on the genomic structure of C1 inhibitor suggests an intron-exon structure similar to that of antithrombin III, α_1-proteinase inhibitor, and rat angiotensinogen. A restriction fragment length polymorphism which is informative in two families with type II C1 inhibitor deficiency (dysfunctional protein) has been identified.

GENETICS OF COMPLEMENT DEFICIENCIES

The clinical features of complement deficiency states are described in detail elsewhere in this volume (Chapter

6). Consequently, only information concerning the molecular mechanisms of complement deficiencies will be summarized here.

Homozygous C2 deficiency is the most common inherited complement deficiency state in Western European populations. It is inherited as an autosomal codominant trait and is found in linkage disequilibrium with several HLA haplotypes. Approximately 40% of individuals with C2 deficiency develop systemic autoimmune disease or a lupuslike syndrome. The molecular basis of this deficiency has not been completely determined but involves a failure of transcription of the C2 gene (38). Monocytes from deficient individuals do not contain detectable C2 mRNA or incorporate radiolabeled amino acid precursors into newly synthesized C2 protein. In several kindreds that have been examined, failure to express C2 is not due to a major deletion or rearrangement of the C2 gene.

Homozygous deficiency in C4 is rare, even though there are frequent deletions and duplications at the C4 loci. C4-deficient individuals often develop a lupuslike syndrome. This association may result from a linkage relationship between the C4 genes and other major histocompatibility loci which predispose to disorders of immune regulation, or from altered inflammation in the absence of C4 activity. Preliminary data obtained from characterization of the class III MHC genomic structure by Southern blot analysis suggests that 10% of lupus patients have a homozygous deletion of C4A and another 34% have a heterozygous deletion of C4A (D. D. Chaplin, unpublished observations). Deficiency in C4 in guinea pigs results from a failure to produce mature, functional C4 mRNA (135). This deficiency may not be an adequate model of human C4 deficiency, because there is only a single C4 locus in guinea pigs. Nevertheless, C4-deficient guinea pigs develop characteristics of immune complex disease (21).

Patients with C3 deficiency are more susceptible to bacterial infection than the general population. In monocytes from deficient individuals, the rate of C3 synthesis is 25% of that in monocytes from normal individuals. Plasma from these individuals contains less than 0.1% of the C3 found in normal individuals (50). A C3 deficiency in guinea pigs may provide an important model in which to study the human deficiency. In the C3-deficient guinea pig, serum C3 levels are low, but the rate of C3 synthesis and secretion in monocytes and hepatocytes is similar to that in normals. The C3 synthesized is structurally abnormal (14,24). In vivo catabolism of normal C3 has been measured in homozygous deficient animals, but no data on catabolism of the defective C3 protein have been reported. Preliminary data suggest that a complex defect affects the structural gene for C3 in the domain encoding its active site (H. S. Auerbach, unpublished observations).

C9 deficiency is common in Oriental populations but is not associated with clinical manifestations. Deficiencies in the other terminal complement components, C5, C6, C7, and C8, are more common in black than in white populations. These deficiencies result in an increased susceptibility to Neisserial infections, including meningitis and extragenital gonorrhea. In a mouse model of C5 deficiency, there appears to be a complex molecular mechanism that results in low circulating concentrations of C5 protein (128). Two forms of C5 mRNA are present in deficient cells, but there is a reduction in total C5 RNA to approximately 5% of that in normal cells. Similarly, the rate of C5 synthesis is 5% or less of that in normal cells. A genomic polymorphism of C5 detectable on Southern blot analysis is linked to C5 deficiency, but the relationship of this polymorphism to the defect in post-transcriptional processing is not known.

Autoimmune disorders are found in association with several genetically determined C1 deficiencies. These include codominantly inherited deficiencies in C1q and C1r. Preliminary studies on C1q-deficient kindreds by Southern blot analysis of genomic DNA suggest that a number of different mechanisms account for this deficiency state. A single restriction fragment length polymorphism within the coding region of the C1q B chain has been identified in a patient with a C1q deficiency and a lupuslike disorder (K. B. M. Reid and R. A. McAdam, unpublished observations).

As described above, a decrease in the number of CR1 molecules on red cells, neutrophils, and monocytes is associated with systemic lupus erythematosus and a specific restriction fragment length polymorphism (139), but the molecular mechanism for decreased receptor number has not been determined. Several types of CR3 deficiency have been described. These are associated with a defect primarily in leukocyte adherence, which results in recurrent bacterial infection (10,11,22). More information about the molecular basis of these deficiencies should become available in the near future with the application of DNA probes encoding the receptor subunits.

Paroxysmal nocturnal hemoglobinuria, a disorder characterized by intermittent hemolytic anemia, has been associated with a deficiency in DAF (78,87). This deficiency affects cells of the granulocytic, monocytic, erythrocytic, and megakaryocytic lineages, but does so in a clonal fashion (79). The molecular basis of this deficiency is not known. It is also not clear whether the deficiency is inherited or acquired. There is some evidence that other membrane proteins, such as the acetylcholine receptor, are affected in these individuals.

An inherited deficiency in factor I has also been described in individuals with recurrent bacterial infections (4,129). The absence of this protein, which controls the amplification loop for C3 activation, leads to hypercatabolism of C3 and components of the alternative complement pathway. These patients also have intermittent urticaria, which has been attributed to the liberation of C3a with anaphylatoxic consequences. The molecular basis of this disorder has not been reported.

C1 inhibitor deficiency, or hereditary angioedema, is inherited as a dominant trait. Two forms of C1 inhibitor deficiency have been recognized. In type I deficiency, the plasma concentration of the inhibitor is markedly reduced; in type II deficiency (approximately 15% of kindreds) a dysfunctional protein is found in normal or elevated concentrations. Treatment of individuals with type I C1 inhibitor deficiency with the synthetic androgen danazol increases serum levels of the inhibitor and reduces the frequency and severity of angioedema episodes, but the mechanism of this effect is unknown. Preliminary studies on C1 inhibitor synthesis in monocytes from deficient individuals suggest that several different mechanisms result in the deficient phenotype (M. Cicardi, unpublished observations).

An acquired form of C1 inhibitor deficiency has been described in individuals with angioedema (25,121). This disorder is frequently associated with lymphoma, especially B-cell lymphoma (25). In contrast to hereditary angioedema, the rate of synthesis of C1 inhibitor is normal in the acquired form of the disease. The entire deficit can be ascribed to an increased fractional catabolic rate in these individuals (120). Two mechanisms for the development of acquired C1 inhibitor deficiency have been suggested by recent studies. Geha et al. (55) isolated an anti-idiotypic IgG antibody to monoclonal immunoglobulins in this deficiency. Presumably, this antibody fixes complement and consumes C1 inhibitor. More recently, Jackson et al. (61) isolated an IgG autoantibody to C1 inhibitor in a patient with acquired C1 inhibitor deficiency but without lymphoproliferative disease.

EXPRESSION AND REGULATION OF COMPLEMENT GENES

Sites of Synthesis

Most of the complement proteins are synthesized in the liver, especially in hepatocytes. After orthotopic liver transplantation, isotypes of complement proteins C3, C6, C8, and factor B change to that of the donor liver (3,7). Furthermore, Morris et al. (73) demonstrated synthesis of complement proteins C1r, C1s, C2, C3, C4, C5, factor B, C1 inhibitor, C3b inactivator (factor I), C6, and C8 in human hepatoma HepG2 cells (Figs. 3 and 4). On closer examination in later studies, synthesis of several other complement proteins has been demonstrated in human liver (39).

Many complement proteins are also synthesized at extrahepatic sites. Mononuclear phagocytes synthesize C1, C2, C3, C4, C5, factor B, factor D, CR1, CR2, CR3, C1

inhibitor, and DAF (11,39). Synthesis of other complement components in mononuclear phagocytes has not been examined or, at best, examined with relatively insensitive techniques. Epithelial cells of the gastrointestinal and genitourinary tracts synthesize C1q and DAF (12,72). Several fibroblast cell lines synthesize C1, C2, C3, and C5 (39).

Regulation of Complement Synthesis Is Tissue Specific

Synthesis of complement proteins is regulated in a tissue-specific manner. The most striking examples are those that apply to human and guinea pig C2 and murine C4 and Slp. In extrahepatic mononuclear phagocytes, the proportion of C2-producing cells and rate of C2 synthesis per cell vary as a function of the tissue of origin. The proportion of C2-producing cells is zero in marrow, 10% in blood monocytes, and 45% in spleen and peritoneal cavity. Only 2.5% of bronchoalveolar macrophages produce C2, but the higher rate of synthesis of C2 per bronchoalveolar macrophage compensates for the lower proportion of C2-producing cells (8,36). The mechanism of this tissue-specific regulation is pretranslational (37).

There is tissue-specific regulation of C4 synthesis in murine hepatocytes and macrophages. Serum levels of C4 in different mouse strains reflect hepatic synthetic rates (115) and content of C4-specific mRNA (117), whereas macrophages from high- and low-serum-C4 strains syn-

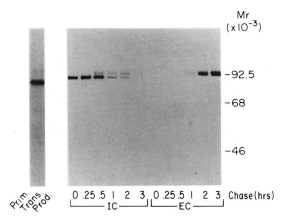

FIG. 3. Biosynthesis, posttranslational processing, and secretion of complement protein factor B. Total cellular RNA was isolated from fresh human adult liver using guanidine HCl extraction and ethanol precipitation (33). A rabbit reticulocyte lysate system was used for cell-free translation (90), and primary translation products (Prim. Trans. Prod.) were immunoprecipitated with polyclonal antiserum to factor B as previously described (91). Confluent monolayers of human hepatoma cells HepG2 were subjected to pulse-chase radiolabeling with analysis of intracellular (IC) and extracellular (EC) products performed by immunoprecipitation, sodium dodecyl sulfate polyacrylamide gel electrophoresis (SDS-PAGE) and fluorography (91). Molecular mass markers are indicated.

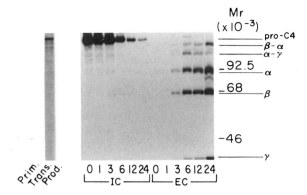

FIG. 4. Biosynthesis, posttranslational processing, and secretion of C4. Experiments were performed exactly as indicated in the legend for Fig. 3, except that polyclonal antiserum to C4 was used.

thesize similar amounts of C4 protein (77,117). Tissue specificity also affects the synthesis of Slp. For instance, Slp is expressed in hepatocytes, but not macrophages, of most Slp+ inbred strains. The notable exception is found in several strains designated H-2w (57,112).

Similar tissue-specific regulation of C2 and factor B synthesis has been demonstrated in mice (51,56,88). Serum concentrations of C2 and factor B vary among mouse strains of several H-2 types. Variations in the rates of C2 and factor B synthesis in liver, but not those in extrahepatic macrophages, correspond to variations in serum concentration. This tissue-specific regulation of C2 and factor B synthesis among mouse strains also involves a pretranslational mechanism.

Regulation of Complement Synthesis Involves Different Molecular Mechanisms

Increases or decreases in the rate of synthesis of complement proteins may involve pretranslational, translational, and posttranslational mechanisms. For example, mouse resident peritoneal macrophages synthesize C4, but in tissue culture the rate of secretion declines within the first few hours (76,77). The decrease is not due to limitations of the culture system, because total protein synthesis remains approximately constant and factor B synthesis increases severalfold. This change in C4 biosynthesis in culture is regulated at a pretranslational level, since the content of C4 mRNA changes in parallel and there is no difference in postsynthetic processing, rate of secretion, or stability of secreted C4 (117). Elicited murine macrophages in inflammatory exudates produce considerably less C4 than resident macrophages (76). This phenomenon is also under pretranslational control in that steady-state levels of C4 mRNA correspond to the amount of pro-C4 synthesis in the respective cell populations.

There are also examples of complement synthesis reg-

ulation at the translational level. In fact, the increase in the rate of synthesis of C3 and factor B in human monocytes mediated by bacterial lipopolysaccharide (LPS) involves distinct pretranslational and translational mechanisms. Steady-state levels of C3 and factor B mRNA and rates of C3 and factor B synthesis increase proportionally in LPS-treated adult monocytes. In cord blood monocytes, mRNA levels increase but the rates of synthesis of C3 and factor B remain unchanged in medium supplemented with LPS alone. However, if LPS-supplemented medium is incubated with adult monocytes and then transferred to cord blood monocytes, steady-state levels of C3 and factor B mRNA and rates of C3 and factor B synthesis increase together (125,126; F. S. Cole, unpublished observations). These results imply distinct pretranslational and translational effects, the latter requiring a change in the function of monocytes during development.

Posttranslational mechanisms are required for other types of regulation of complement synthesis. For instance, Ooi et al. (85,86) demonstrated that elicited mouse peritoneal macrophages synthesized five times more immunochemically detectable C5 than resident peritoneal macrophages, but the cell culture fluid of the elicited cells had four to five times less C5 hemolytic activity. Preliminary data suggest that posttranslational modification of C2 during inflammatory activation of macrophages increases the specific activity of locally synthesized C2, possibly by oxidation-dependent stabilization of the classical pathway C3 convertase (F. S. Cole, unpublished observations).

Regulation of Complement Synthesis Involves Specific Mediators

Interleukin-1 (IL-1) is a monokine which mediates many, if not all, of the changes in metabolism that constitute the host response to acute inflammation, the acute phase response (see Chapter 12). Since the plasma concentrations of many of the complement proteins increase during the acute phase response, we examined the possibility that IL-1 regulates the synthesis of these proteins. Recombinant-generated IL-1 mediated dose- and time-dependent increases in the rates of synthesis of factor B and C3, and decreases in the rate of albumin synthesis, but had no effect on the synthesis of C2 in human hepatoma cells (94). Similar results were observed in murine fibroblast L cells transfected with a cosmid DNA fragment bearing human C2 and factor B genes (Figs. 5 and 6) and in primary cultures of murine hepatocytes (98). In all cases, regulation involved a pretranslational mechanism as reflected by steady-state levels of specific mRNAs.

Cachectin/tumor necrosis factor (TNF) is a monokine that is structurally distinct but shares many of the biological activities of IL-1 (see Chapter 12). TNF also mediates dose- and time-dependent regulation of comple-

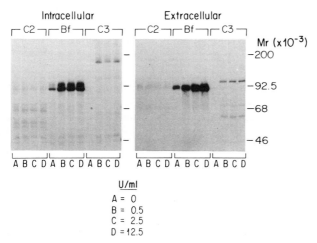

FIG. 5. Effect of IL-1 on the expression of complement proteins by transfected L cells. Murine fibroblast L cells transfected with cosmid DNA bearing the human C2 and factor B genes (92) were incubated for 18 hr in control medium (A, 0 U/ml) or in medium supplemented with different concentrations of purified human monocyte IL-1 (B, 0.5 U/ml; C, 2.5 U/ml; D, 12.5 U/ml). Cells were then biosynthetically labeled for 3 hr, and rates of synthesis and secretion of complement proteins ascertained by immunoprecipitation with polyclonal antisera to human C2, human factor B, and murine C3, followed by SDS-PAGE and fluorography (94). Molecular mass markers are indicated.

ment synthesis in human hepatoma cells and transfected mouse fibroblasts (93). The effects are similar to those produced by IL-1 and include increases in the rate of synthesis of factor B and C3 but no effect on the rate of synthesis of C2 and C4. All these effects correspond to changes in plasma levels of complement proteins during the acute phase response except for that of C4. Therefore, C4 is an example of IL-1- and TNF-unresponsive acute phase complement protein.

Recombinant IL-1 has also been administered parenterally into endotoxin-resistant C3H/Hej mice (97), resulting in an increase in factor B and C3 mRNA in liver, lung, kidney, intestine, spleen, heart, and peritoneal macrophages. In this study, then, it was clearly shown that the change in expression of acute phase complement proteins in hepatocytes during inflammation or following endotoxin administration could be accounted for by IL-1. It was not clear, however, whether extrahepatic complement gene expression was mediated directly by IL-1 in an autocrine or paracrine mechanism or indirectly through another mediator such as γ-interferon (see Chapter 14).

Synthesis of complement proteins is also regulated by γ-interferon. An increase in synthesis of C2 and factor B in human macrophages is mediated by recombinant-generated human interferon at concentrations lower that 50

pg/ml. The response is also elicited by recombinant-generated murine γ-interferon acting on mouse fibroblasts transfected with the human genes (127). This regulatory effect provides further evidence that these two closely linked, structurally and functionally similar complement proteins are selectively and independently regulated. Factor B expression is affected by both IL-1 and γ-interferon, while C2 is affected only by γ-interferon.

γ-Interferon also regulates the synthesis of C4. A dose- and time-dependent increase in synthesis of C4 in HepG2 cells and mouse fibroblasts transfected with cloned C4A and C4B DNA has recently been demonstrated (70). There were fivefold increases in steady-state levels of C4 mRNA and in the rate of C4 synthesis in C4A transfectants. There was also a fivefold increase in the rate of C4 synthesis in HepG2 cells which express both C4A and C4B gene products but predominantly that of C4A. A 1.5- to 2-fold increase in C4 mRNA was identified in the C4B transfectants. Since C4 synthesis is not responsive to IL-1 or TNF, it is possible that the acute phase response of this gene is predominantly mediated by interferon.

Bacterial LPS has direct and indirect effects on the synthesis of complement proteins. Indirect effects may be mediated through the release of IL-1, TNF, or γ-interferon. LPS also directly increases the synthesis of C2, factor B, and C3 in human mononuclear phagocytes by a tissue-specific, pretranslational, and translational effect (125,126). Informative variations in this effect have been mentioned above and are currently being studied in greater detail.

Recent studies suggest that complement synthesis may also be regulated by neuropeptides. Auerbach et al. (15) demonstrated a specific increase in the rate of synthesis

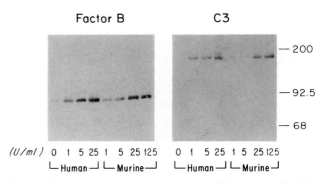

FIG. 6. Effect of varying concentrations (U/ml) of purified human monocyte and recombinant-generated murine IL-1 on the expression of complement proteins by transfected L cells. Transfectants were incubated with IL-1 for 18 hr and biosynthetically labeled for 30 min (94). Rates of synthesis of transferred human factor B and endogenous murine C3 were ascertained by subjecting cell lysates to the same analytical system described in the legend for Fig. 5. Molecular mass markers are indicated.

of C3 in guinea pig resident peritoneal macrophages mediated by substance P. This effect also involved an increase in steady-state levels of C3 mRNA. Substance P had no effect on C3 synthesis in elicited macrophages, but the latter may be a consequence of down-regulation of substance P receptors in the elicited cell population.

Finally, complement biosynthesis may be regulated by the complement proteins themselves. For instance, synthesis of C4 in guinea pig macrophages is inhibited by the presence of C4 in the extracellular medium (13). Addition of biologically active or methylamine-inactivated C4 to the cell culture fluid of guinea pig macrophages leads to the disappearance of C4 mRNA but not of factor B mRNA.

REFERENCES

1. Alper, C. A. (1981): Complement and the MHC. In: *The Role of the Major Histocompatibility Complex in Immunology,* edited by M. E. Dorf, pp. 173–220, Garland Press, New York.
2. Alper, C. A., and Propp, R. R. (1968): Genetic polymorphism of the third component of human complement (C3). *J. Clin. Invest.,* 47:2181–2191.
3. Alper, C. A., Johnson, A. M., Birtch, A. G., and Moore, R. D. (1969): Human C3: Evidence for the liver as the primary site of synthesis. *Science,* 163:286–288.
4. Alper, C. A., Abramson, N., Johnston, R. B. Jr., Jandl, J. H., and Rosen, F. S. (1970): Studies in vivo and in vitro on an abnormality in the metabolism of C3 in a patient with increased susceptibility to infection. *J. Clin. Invest.,* 49:1975–1985.
5. Alper, C. A., and Rosen, F. S. (1971): Studies of a hypomorphic variant of human C3. *J. Clin. Invest.,* 50:324–326.
6. Alper, C. A., Azen, E. A., Geserick, G., Guedde, H. W., Rittner, C., Teisberg, P., and Wieme, R. (1972): Statement on the polymorphism of the third component of complement in man (C3). *Vox Sang.,* 25:18–20.
7. Alper, C. A., Raum, D., Awdeh, Z., Petersen, B. H., Taylor, P. D., and Starzl, T. E. (1980): Studies of hepatic synthesis in vivo of plasma proteins including orosomucoid, transferrin, alpha-1-antitrypsin, C8 and factor B. *Clin. Immunol. Immunopathol.,* 16:84–91.
8. Alpert, S. E., Auerbach, H. S., Cole, F. S., and Colten, H. R. (1983): Macrophage maturation: Differences in complement secretion by marrow, monocyte and tissue macrophages detected with an improved hemolytic plaque assay. *J. Immunol.,* 130:102–107.
9. Arlaud, G. J., Gagnon, J., Villiers, C. L., and Colomb, M. G. (1986): Molecular characterization of the catalytic domains of human complement serine protease C1r. *Biochemistry,* 25:5177–5182.
10. Arnaout, M. A., Pitt, J., Cohen, H. J., Melamed, J., Rosen, F. S., and Colten, H. R. (1982): Deficiency of a granulocyte membrane glycoprotein (gp150) in a boy with recurrent bacterial infections. *N. Engl. J. Med.,* 306:693–699.
11. Arnaout, M. A., and Colten, H. R. (1984): Complement C3 receptors: Structure and function. *Mol. Immunol.,* 21:1191–1199.
12. Asch, A. S., Kinoshita, T., Jaffe, E. A., and Nussenzweig, V. (1986): Decay-accelerating factor is present on cultured human umbilical vein endothelial cells. *J. Exp. Med.,* 163:221–226.
13. Auerbach, H. S., Baker, R. D., Matthews, W. J., and Colten, H. R. (1984): Molecular mechanism for feedback regulation of C4 biosynthesis in guinea pig peritoneal macrophages. *J. Exp. Med.,* 159:1750–1768.
14. Auerbach, H. S., Burger, R., Bitter-Suermann, D., Goldberger, G., and Colten, H. R. (1985): C3-deficient guinea pig mRNA directs synthesis of a structurally abnormal protein. *Complement,* 2:5.
15. Auerbach, H. S., Pawlowski, N., and Ezekowitz, R. A. B. (1987): Down regulation of substance P receptors on newly recruited macrophages. Receptor occupation induces cellular response in resident but not elicited guinea pig peritoneal macrophages or monocytes. *J. Clin. Invest.* (in press).
16. Awdeh, Z. L., and Alper, C. A. (1980): Inherited structural polymorphism of the fourth component of human complement. *Proc. Natl. Acad. Sci. USA,* 77:3576–3580.
17. Belt, K. T., Carroll, M. C., and Porter, R. R. (1984): The structural bases of the multiple forms of human complement component C4. *Cell,* 36:907–914.
18. Belt, K. T., Yu, C. Y., Carroll, M. C., and Porter, R. R. (1985): Polymorphism of the human complement component C4. *Immunogenetics,* 21:173–180.
19. Bentley, D. R. (1986): Primary structure of human complement component C2. Homology to two unrelated protein families. *Biochem. J.,* 239:339–345.
20. Bock, S. C., Skriver, K., Neilson, E., Thogersen, H.-C., Wiman, B., Donaldson, V. H., Eddy, R. L., Muarinan, J., Rodziejewska, E., Huber, R., Shows, T. B., and Magnusson, S. (1986): Human C1 inhibitor: Primary structure, cDNA cloning and chromosomal localization. *Biochemistry,* 25:4292–4301.
21. Bottger, E. C., Hoffmann, T., Hadding, U., and Bitter-Suermann, D. (1986): Guinea pigs with inherited deficiencies of complement components C2 or C4 have characteristics of immune complex disease. *J. Clin. Invest.,* 78:689–695.
22. Bowen, T. J., Ochs, H. D., Altman, L. C., Price, T. H., van Epps, D. E., Brautigan, D. L., Rosin, R. E., Perkins, W. D., Babior, B. M., Klebanoff, S. J., and Wedgewood, R. J. (1982): Severe recurrent bacterial infections associated with defective adherence and chemotaxis in two patients with neutrophils deficient in a cell-associated glycoprotein. *J. Pediatr.,* 101:932–940.
23. Brown, L. J., and Shreffler, D. C. (1980): Female expression of H-2 linked sex-limited protein (Slp) due to non-H-2 genes. *Immunogenetics,* 10:19–29.
24. Burger, R., Gordon, J., Stevenson, J., Ramadori, G., Zankar, B., Hadding, U., and Bitter-Suermann, D. (1986): An inherited deficiency of the third component of complement C3 in guinea pigs. *Eur. J. Immunol.,* 16:7–13.
25. Caldwell, J. R., Ruddy, S., Schur, P. H., and Austen, K. F. (1982): Acquired C1 inhibitor deficiency in lymphosarcoma. *Clin. Immunol. Immunopathol.,* 1:39–47.
26. Campbell, R. D., Bentley, D. R., and Morley, B. J. (1984): The factor B and C2 genes. *Philos. Trans. R. Soc. Lond. [Biol.],* 306:367–378.
27. Carroll, M. C., Belt, T., Palsdottir, A., and Porter, R. R. (1984): Structure and organization of the C4 genes. *Philos. Trans. R. Soc. Lond. [Biol.],* 306:379–388.
28. Carroll, M. C., Campbell, R. D., Bentley, D. R., and Porter, R. R. (1984): A molecular map of the human major histocompatibility complex class III region linking complement genes C4, C2 and factor B. *Nature,* 307:237–241.
29. Carroll, M. C., Campbell, R. D., and Porter, R. R. (1985): Mapping of steroid 21-hydroxylase genes adjacent to complement component C4 genes, in HLA, the major histocompatibility complex in man. *Proc. Natl. Acad. Sci. USA,* 82:521–525.
30. Carroll, M. C., Palsdottir, A., Belt, K. T., and Porter, R. R. (1985): Deletion of complement C4 and steroid 21-hydroxylase genes in the HLA class III region. *EMBO J.,* 4:2547–2552.
31. Chaplin, D. D., Sackstein, R., Perlmutter, D. H., Weis, J. H., Kruse, A., Coligan, J., Colten, H. R., and Seidman, J. G. (1984): Expression of hemolytically active murine fourth component of complement in transfected L-cells. *Cell,* 37:569–576.
32. Chaplin, D. D., Woods, D. E., Whitehead, A. S., Goldberger, G., Colten, H. R., and Seidman, J. G. (1985): Molecular map of the murine S region. *Proc. Natl. Acad. Sci. USA,* 80:6947–6951.
33. Chirgwin, J. M., Przybyla, A. E., MacDonald, R. J., and Rutter, W. J. (1979): Isolation of biologically active ribonucleic acid from sources enriched in ribonuclease. *Biochemistry,* 18:5294–5299.
34. Chu, M.-L., DeWet, W., Bernard, M., Ding, J.-F., Mosabito, L. M., Meyers, J., Williams, C., and Ramirez, F. (1984): Human pro alpha-1 (1) collagen gene structure reveals evolutionary conservation of a pattern of introns and exons. *Nature,* 310:337–340.
35. Chung, L. P., Bentley, D. R., and Reid, K. B. M. (1985): Molecular

cloning and characterization of the cDNA coding for C4b-binding protein, a regulatory protein of the classical pathway of the human complement system. *Biochem. J.,* 230:133–141.

36. Cole, F. S., Matthews, W. J., Marino, J. T., Gash, D. J., and Colten, H. R. (1980): Control of complement synthesis and secretion in bronchoalveolar and peritoneal macrophages. *J. Immunol.,* 125: 1120–1124.

37. Cole, F. S., Auerbach, H. S., Goldberger, G., and Colten, H. R. (1985): Tissue-specific pre-translational regulation of complement production in human mononuclear phagocytes. *J. Immunol.,* 134: 2610–2616.

38. Cole, F. S., Whitehead, A. S., Auerbach, H. S., Lint, T., Zeitz, H. J., Kilbridge, P., and Colten, H. R. (1985): The molecular basis for genetic deficiency of the second component of human complement. *N. Engl. J. Med.,* 313:11–16.

39. Cole, F. S., and Colten, H. R. (1987): Complement biosynthesis. In: *The Complement System,* edited by K. D. Rother and G. O. Till, Springer-Verlag, Heidelberg (in press).

40. Colomb, M. G., Arlaud, G. J., and Villiers, C. L. (1984): Activation of C1. *Philos. Trans. R. Soc. Lond. [Biol.],* 306:283–292.

41. Colten, H. R., and Dowton, S. B. (1986): Regulation of complement gene expression. *Biochem. Soc. Symp.,* 51:37–46.

42. Cross, S. J., Edwards, J. M., Bentley, D. R., and Campbell, R. D. (1985): DNA polymorphism of the C2 and factor B genes. Detection of a restriction fragment length polymorphism which subdivides haplotypes carrying the C2C and factor B F alleles. *Immunogenetics,* 21:39–48.

43. Dahlback, B., Smith, C. A., and Müller-Eberhard, H. J. (1983): Visualization of C4b-binding protein and its complexes with vitamin K-dependent protein S and complement protein C4b. *Proc. Natl. Acad. Sci. USA,* 80:3461–3465.

44. Davis, A. E., Whitehead, A. S., Harrison, R. A., Dauphinais, A., Bruns, G. A. P., Cicardi, M., and Rosen, F. S. (1986): Human inhibitor of the first component of complement, C1: Characterization of cDNA clones and localization of the gene to chromosome 11. *Proc. Natl. Acad. Sci. USA,* 83:3161–3165.

45. de Bruijn, M. H. L., and Fey, G. (1985): Human complement component C3: cDNA coding sequence and derived primary structure. *Proc. Natl. Acad. Sci. USA,* 82:708–713.

46. DiScipio, R. G., Gehring, M. R., Podack, E. R., Kan, C. C., Hugli, T. E., and Fey, G. (1984): Nucleotide sequence of human complement component C9. *Proc. Natl. Acad. Sci. USA,* 81:7298–7302.

47. Dyckman, T. R., Cole, F. S., Iida, K., and Atkinson, J. P. (1983): Polymorphism of the human erythrocyte C3b/C4b receptor. *Proc. Natl. Acad. Sci. USA,* 80:1698–1702.

48. Dyckman, T. R., Hatch, J., and Atkinson, J. P. (1984): Polymorphism of the human C3b/C4b receptor: Identification of a third allele and analysis of receptor phenotypes in families and patients with systemic lupus erythematosus. *J. Exp. Med.,* 159:691–700.

49. Dyckman, T. R., Hatch, J. A., Aqua, M. S., and Atkinson, J. P. (1985): Polymorphism of the C3b/C4b receptor (CR1): Characterization of a fourth allele. *J. Immunol.,* 134:1787–1793.

50. Einstein, L. P., Hansen, P. J., Ballow, M., Davis, A. E., Davis, J. S., Alper, C. A., Rosen, F. S., and Colten, H. R. (1977): Biosynthesis of the third component of complement (C3) in vitro by monocytes from both normal and homozygous C3-deficient humans. *J. Clin. Invest.,* 60:963–969.

51. Falus, A., Beuscher, H. U., Auerbach, H. S., and Colten, H. R. (1987): Strain and tissue specific complement gene expression. *J. Immunol.* 138:856–860.

52. Falus, A., Wakeland, E. K., McConnell, T. J., Gitlin, J., Whitehead, A. S., and Colten, H. R. (1987): DNA polymorphism of MHC III genes in inbred and wild mouse strains. *Immunogenetics* 25:290–298.

53. Fey, G. H., Lundwall, A., Wetsel, R. A., Tack, B. F., de Bruijn, M. H. L., and Domdey, H. (1984): Nucleotide sequence of complementary DNA and derived amino acid sequence of murine complement component C3. *Philos. Trans. R. Soc. Lond. [Biol.],* 306:333–344.

54. Fielder, A. H. L., Walport, M. J., Batchelor, J. R., Rynes, R. I., Black, C. M., Dodi, I. A., and Hughes, G. R. V. (1983): A family study of the MHC of patients with SLE: Null alleles of C4A and C4B may determine disease. *Br. Med. J.,* 186:425–428.

55. Geha, R. S., Quinti, I., Austen, K. F., Cicardi, M., Sheffer, A., and Rosen, F. S. (1985): Acquired C1 inhibitor deficiency associated with anti-idiotypic antibody to monoclonal immunoglobulins. *N. Engl. J. Med.,* 312:534–538.

56. Gorman, J. C., Jackson, R., Desantola, J. R., Shreffler, D. C., and Atkinson, J. P. (1980): Development of a hemolytic assay for mouse C2 and determination of its genetic control. *J. Immunol.,* 125: 344–349.

57. Hansen, T. H., and Shreffler, D. C. (1976): Characterization of a constitutive variant of the murine serum protein allotype, Slp. *J. Immunol.,* 117:1507–1513.

58. Hobart, M. J., Vazquedes, M. A., and Lachmann, P. J. (1981): Polymorphism of human C5. *Am. J. Hum. Genet.,* 45:1–4.

59. Isenman, D. E., and Young, J. R. (1984): The molecular basis for the difference in immune hemolysis activity of the Chido and Rodgers isotypes of human complement component C4. *J. Immunol.,* 132:3019–3027.

60. Itakura, K., Hutton, J. J., Boyse, E. A., and Old, L. J. (1972): Genetic linkage relationships of loci specifying differentiation alloantigens in the mouse. *Transplantation,* 13:239–243.

61. Jackson, J., Sim, R. B., Whelan, A., and Feighery, C. (1986): An IgG auto antibody which inactivates C1 inhibitor. *Nature,* 323: 722–724.

62. Klickstein, L. B., Wong, W. W., Smith, J. A., Morton, C., Fearon, D. T., and Weis, J. H. (1985): Identification of long homologous repeats in human CR1. *Complement,* 2:44.

63. Kristensen, T., and Tack, B. F. (1986): Murine protein H is comprised of 20 repeating units, 61 amino acids in length. *Proc. Natl. Acad. Sci. USA,* 83:3963–3967.

64. Kristensen, T., Wetsel, R. A., and Tack, B. F. (1986): Structural analysis of human complement protein H: Homology with C4b-binding protein, beta-2-glycoprotein-1 and the Ba fragment of B. *J. Immunol.,* 136:3407–3411.

65. Lachmann, P. J., Hobart, M. J., and Aston, W. P. (1974): Complement technology. In: *Handbook of Experimental Immunology,* edited by D. M. Weir, pp. 5.1–5.17, Blackwell Scientific Publications, Oxford.

66. Law, S. K. A., Dodds, A. W., and Porter, R. R. (1984): A comparison of the properties of the two classes, C4A and C4B, of the human complement component C4. *EMBO J.,* 3:1819–1823.

67. Levi-Strauss, M., Tosi, M., Steinmetz, M., Klein, J., and Meo, T. (1985): Multiple duplications of complement C4 gene correlate with H2-controlled testosterone-independent expression of its sex-limited isoform. *Proc. Natl. Acad. Sci. USA,* 82:1746–1750.

68. Loos, M. (1983): Biosynthesis of the collagen-like C1q molecule and its receptor functions for Fc and polyanionic molecules on macrophages. *Curr. Top. Microbiol. Immunol.,* 102:1–56.

69. Lundwall, A. B., Wetsel, R. A., Kristensen, T., Whitehead, A. S., Woods, D. E., Ogden, R. L., Colten, H. R., and Tack, B. F. (1985): Isolation of a cDNA clone encoding the fifth component of human complement. *J. Biol. Chem.,* 260:2108–2112.

70. Miura, N., Prentice, H., Schneider, P. M., and Perlmutter, D. H. (1987): Synthesis and regulation of the two human complement C4 genes in stable transfected mouse fibroblasts. *J. Biol. Chem.* 262:7298–7305.

71. Morley, B. J., and Campbell, R. D. (1984): Internal homologies of the Ba fragment from human complement component factor B, a class III MHC antigen. *EMBO J.,* 3:153–157.

72. Morris, K. M., Colten, H. R., and Bing, D. H. (1978): The first component of complement: A quantitative comparison of its biosynthesis in culture by human epithelial and mesenchymal cells. *J. Exp. Med.,* 148:1007–1019.

73. Morris, K. M., Aden, D. P., Knowles, B., and Colten, H. R. (1982): Complement biosynthesis by the human hepatoma-derived cell line, HepG2. *J. Clin. Invest.,* 70:906–913.

74. Muller, W., Hanauske-Abel, H., and Loos, M. (1978): Biosynthesis of the first component of complement by human and guinea pig peritoneal macrophages: Evidence for independent production of the C1 subunits. *J. Immunol.,* 121:1578–1584.

75. Natsuume-Sakai, S., Hayarawa, J. I., and Takahashi, M. (1978): Genetic polymorphism of murine C3 controlled by a single codominant locus on chromosome 17. *J. Immunol.*, 121:491–498.

76. Newell, S. L., and Atkinson, J. P. (1983): Biosynthesis of C4 by mouse peritoneal macrophages. II. Comparison of C4 synthesis by resident and elicited populations. *J. Immunol.*, 130:834–838.

77. Newell, S. L., Shreffler, D. C., and Atkinson, J. P. (1983): Biosynthesis of C4 by mouse peritoneal macrophages. II. Comparison of C4 synthesis of "low" versus "high" C4 strains. *J. Immunol.*, 130: 834–838.

78. Nicholson-Weller, A., March, J. P., Rosenfeld, S. I., and Austen, K. F. (1983): Affected erythrocytes of patients with paroxysmal nocturnal hemoglobinuria are deficient in the complement regulatory protein, decay accelerating factor. *Proc. Natl. Acad. Sci. USA*, 80:5066–5070.

79. Nicholson-Weller, A., Spicer, D. B., and Austen, K. F. (1985): Deficiency of the complement regulatory protein, "decay-accelerating factor," on membranes of granulocytes, monocytes and platelets in paroxysmal nocturnal hemoglobinuria. *N. Engl. J. Med.*, 312: 1091–1097.

80. Nonaka, M., Takahashi, M., Natsuume-Sakai, S., Nonaka, M., Taraka, S., Shimizu, A., and Honjo, T. (1984): Isolation of cDNA clones specifying the fourth component of mouse complement and its isotype, sex-linked protein. *Proc. Natl. Acad. Sci. USA*, 81:6822–6826.

81. Nonaka, M., Nakayama, K., Yeul, Y. D., Shimizu, A., and Takahashi, M. (1985): A complete nucleotide and derived amino acid sequences of the fourth component of mouse complement (C4): Evolutionary aspects. *J. Biol. Chem.*, 260:10936–10943.

82. Ogata, R. T., Shreffler, D. C., Sepich, D. S., and Lilly, S. P. (1983): cDNA clone spanning the alpha-gamma subunit junction in the precursor of the murine fourth component of complement (C4). *Proc. Natl. Acad. Sci. USA*, 80:5061–5065.

83. Ogata, R. T., and Sepich, D. S. (1984): Genes for murine fourth complement component (C4) and sex-linked protein (Slp) identified by hybridization to C4- and Slp-specific cDNA. *Proc. Natl. Acad. Sci. USA*, 81:4908–4912.

84. Olaisen, B., Teisberg, R., Jonassen, R., Thorsby, E., and Gedde-Dahl, T. (1983): Gene order and gene distance in the HLA regions studied by the haplotype method. *Am. J. Hum. Genet.*, 47:285–292.

85. Ooi, Y. M., Harris, D. E., Edelson, P. J., and Colten, H. R. (1980): Post-translational control of complement (C5) production by resident and stimulated mouse macrophages. *J. Immunol.*, 124:2077–2081.

86. Ooi, Y. M., and Colten, H. R. (1982): Biosynthesis and post-synthetic modification of precursor (proC5) of the fifth component of complement (C5) by mouse peritoneal macrophages. *J. Immunol.*, 129:200–205.

87. Pangburn, M. K., Schreiber, R. D., and Müller-Eberhard, H. J. (1983): Deficiency of an erythrocyte membrane protein with complement regulatory activity in paroxysmal nocturnal hemoglobinuria. *Proc. Natl. Acad. Sci. USA*, 80:5430–5434.

88. Paolucci, E. S., and Shreffler, D. C. (1983): H-2 linked murine factor B phenotypes. *Immunogenetics*, 17:67–73.

89. Passmore, H. C., and Shreffler, D. C. (1970): A sex-linked serum protein variant in the mouse: Inheritance and association with the H-2 region. *Biochem. Genet.*, 4:351–365.

90. Pelham, H. R. B., and Jackson, R. J. (1976): An efficient mRNA-dependent translation system from reticulocyte lysates. *Eur. J. Biochem.*, 67:247–256.

91. Perlmutter, D. H., Cole, F. S., Goldberger, G., and Colten, H. R. (1984): Distinct primary translation products from human liver RNA give rise to secreted and cell-associated forms of complement protein C2. *J. Biol. Chem.*, 259:10380–10385.

92. Perlmutter, D. H., Colten, H. R., Grossberger, D., Strominger, J., Seidman, J. G., and Chaplin, D. D. (1985): Expression of complement proteins C2 and factor B in transfected L-cells. *J. Clin. Invest.*, 76:1449–1454.

93. Perlmutter, D. H., Dinarello, C. A., Punsal, P. I., and Colten, H. R. (1986): Cachectin/tumor necrosis factor regulates hepatic acute phase gene expression. *J. Clin. Invest.*, 78:1349–1355.

94. Perlmutter, D. H., Goldberger, G., Dinarello, C. A., Mizel, S. B., and Colten, H. R. (1986): Regulation of class III major histocompatibility complex (MHC) gene products by interleukin-1. *Science*, 232:850–852.

95. Petersen, B. H., Graham, J. A., and Brooks, G. F. (1976): Human deficiency of the eighth component of complement. The requirement of C8 for serum *Neisseria gonorrhoeae* bactericidal activity. *J. Clin. Invest.*, 57:283–290.

96. Prentice, H. L., Schneider, P. M., and Strominger, J. L. (1986): C4B gene polymorphism detected in human cosmid clone. *Immunogenetics*, 23:274–276.

97. Ramadori, G., Sipe, J. D., and Colten, H. R. (1985): Expression and regulation of the murine serum amyloid A (SAA) gene in extrahepatic sites. *J. Immunol.*, 135:3645–3647.

98. Ramadori, G., Sipe, J. D., Dinarello, C. A., Mizel, S. B., and Colten, H. R. (1985): Pre-translational modulation of acute phase hepatic protein synthesis by murine recombinant interleukin-1 (IL-1) and purified human IL-1. *J. Exp. Med.*, 162:930–939.

99. Rao, A. G., Howard, O. M. Z., Ng, S. C., Snyder, J. V., Whitehead, A. S., Colten, H. R., and Sodetz, J. M. (1986): Characterization of a cDNA clone encoding the alpha subunit of the eighth component of human complement. In: *Proceedings of the Sixth International Congress of Immunology*, edited by B. Cinader, pp. 197, National Research Council of Canada, Ottawa.

100. Raum, D., Spencer, M. A., Balavitch, D., Tidoman, S., Merritt, A. D., Taggart, R. T., Petersen, B. H., Day, N. R., and Alper, C. A. (1979): Genetic control of the eighth component of complement. *J. Clin. Invest.*, 64:858–865.

101. Reid, K. B. M. (1985): Application of molecular cloning to studies on the complement system. *Immunology*, 55:185–196.

102. Reid, K. B. M., and Soloman, E. (1977): Biosynthesis of the first component of complement by human fibroblasts. *Biochem. J.*, 167: 647–660.

103. Reid, K. B. M., and Thompson, R. A. (1983): Characterization of a nonfunctional form of C1q found in patients with a genetically linked deficiency of C1q activity. *Mol. Immunol.*, 20:117–125.

104. Reid, K. B. M., Bentley, D. R., and Wood, K. J. (1984): Cloning and characterization of the complementary DNA for the B chain of normal human serum C1q. *Philos. Trans. R. Soc. Lond. [Biol.]*, 306:345–354.

105. Reid, K. B. M., Bentley, D. R., Campbell, R. D., Chung, L. P., Sim, R. B., Kristensen, T., and Tack, B. F. (1986): Complement system proteins which interact with C3b or C4b. A superfamily of structurally related proteins. *Immunol. Today*, 7:230–234.

106. Rittner, C., Kuehnl, P., Black, C. M., Pereira, S., and Welsh, K. I. (1984): Scleroderma: Possible association with the C4 system—A progress report. In: *Histocompatibility Testing*, edited by E. D. Albert, pp. 394–397, Springer-Verlag, Berlin.

107. Rittner, C., Meier, E. M. M., Stradmann, B., Giles, C. M., Koechling, R., Mollenhauer, E., and Kreth, H. W. (1984): Partial C4 deficiency in subacute sclerosing panencephalitis. *Immunogenetics*, 20:407–415.

108. Rittner, C., Hargesheimer, W., Stradmann, B., Bertrams, J., Baur, M. P., and Petersen, B. H. (1986): Human C81 (alpha-gamma) polymorphism: Detection in the alpha-gamma subunit on SDS-PAGE, formal genetics and linkage relationship. *Am. J. Hum. Genet.*, 38:482–486.

109. Rittner, C., and Schneider, P. M. (1987): Genetics and polymorphism of the complement components. In: *The Complement System*, edited by K. D. Rother and G. O. Till, Springer-Verlag, Heidelberg (in press).

110. Rodriguez de Cordoba, S., Ferreira, A., Nussenzweig, V., and Rubinstein, P. (1983): Genetic polymorphism of human C4-binding protein. *J. Immunol.*, 131:1565–1569.

111. Rodriguez de Cordoba, S., Lublin, D. M., Rubinstein, P., and Atkinson, J. P. (1985): Human genes for 3 complement components that regulate the activation of C3 are tightly linked. *J. Exp. Med.*, 161:1189–1195.

112. Roos, M. H., Atkinson, J. P., and Shreffler, D. C. (1978): Molecular

characterization of the Ss(C4) and Slp proteins of the mouse H-2 complex: Subunit composition, chain size, polymorphism and an intracellular (pro-Ss) precursor. *J. Immunol.,* 121:1106–1115.

113. Roos, M., and Demant, P. (1982): Murine complement factor B (BF): Sexual dimorphism and H-2 linked polymorphism. *Immunogenetics,* 15:23–30.

114. Roos, M. H., Mollenhauer, E., Demant, P., and Rittner, C. (1982): A molecular basis for the two locus model of human complement component C4. *Nature,* 298:854–856.

115. Rosa, P. A., and Shreffler, D. C. (1982): Cultured hepatocytes from mouse strains expressing high and low levels of the fourth component of complement differ in rate of synthesis of the protein. *Proc. Natl. Acad. Sci. USA,* 80:2332–2336.

116. Sackstein, R., Colten, H. R., and Woods, D. E. (1983): Phylogenetic conservation of class III major histocompatibility complex antigen, factor B: Isolation and nucleotide sequence of mouse factor B cDNA clones. *J. Biol. Chem.,* 258:14693–14697.

117. Sackstein, R., and Colten, H. R. (1984): Molecular regulation of MHC class III (C4 and factor B) gene expression in mouse peritoneal macrophages. *J. Immunol.,* 129:653–659.

118. Sastre, L., Roman, J. M., Teplow, D. B., Dreyer, W. J., Gee, C. E., Larson, R. S., Roberts, T. M., and Springer, T. A. (1986): A partial genomic DNA clone for the alpha subunit of the mouse complement receptor type 3 and cellular adhesion molecule Mac-1. *Proc. Natl. Acad. Sci. USA,* 83:5644–5648.

119. Schneider, P. M., Carroll, M. C., Alper, C. A., Rittner, C., Whitehead, A. S., Yunis, E. J., and Colten, H. R. (1986): Polymorphism of the human complement C4 and steroid 21-hydroxylase genes: Restriction fragment length polymorphisms revealing structural deletions, homoduplications and size variants. *J. Clin. Invest.,* 78: 650–657.

120. Sheffer, A. L., Melamed, J., Fearon, D. T., and Austen, K. F. (1983): Clinical/biochemical assessment of acquired C1 inhibitor deficiency. *J. Allergy Clin. Immunol.,* 71:107.

121. Sheffer, A. L., Austen, K. F., Rosen, F. S., and Fearon, D. T. (1985): Acquired deficiency of the inhibitor of the first component of complement: Report of five additional cases with commentary on the syndrome. *J. Allergy Clin. Immunol.,* 75:640–646.

122. Shreffler, D. C., Atkinson, J. P., Chan, A. C., Karp, D. R., Killion, C. C., Ogata, R. T., and Rosa, P. A. (1984): The C4 and Slp genes of the complement region of the murine H-2 major histocompatibility complex. *Philos. Trans. R. Soc. Lond. [Biol.],* 306:395–403.

123. Stanley, K. K., and Luzio, J. P. (1984): Construction of a new family of high efficiency bacterial expression vectors: Identification of cDNA clones for human liver proteins. *EMBO J.,* 3:1429–1437.

124. Stanley, K. K., Kocher, H.-P., Luzio, J. P., Jackson, P., and Tschopp, J. (1985): The sequence and topology of human complement component C9. *EMBO J.,* 4:375–383.

125. St. John Sutton, M. B., Strunk, R. C., and Cole, F. S. (1986): Regulation of synthesis of the third component of complement and factor B in cord blood monocytes by lipopolysaccharide. *J. Immunol.,* 136:1366–1372.

126. Strunk, R. C., Whitehead, A. S., and Cole, F. S. (1985): Pretranslational regulation of the synthesis of the third component of complement in human mononuclear phagocytes by the lipid A portion of lipopolysaccharide. *J. Clin. Invest.,* 76:985–990.

127. Strunk, R. C., Cole, F. S., Perlmutter, D. H., and Colten, H. R. (1986): Gamma-interferon increases expression of class III complement genes C2 and factor B in human monocytes and in murine fibroblasts transfected with human C2 and factor B genes. *J. Biol. Chem.,* 260:15280–15285.

128. Strunk, R. C., Wheat, W. H., Wetsel, R. A., Falus, A., Ramadori, G., and Tack, B. F. (1986): The fifth component of complement (C5) in the mouse: Analysis of the molecular basis for deficiency. *Fed. Proc.,* 45:1102.

129. Thompson, R. A., and Lachmann, P. J. (1977): A second case of C3b inhibitor (KAF) deficiency. *Clin. Exp. Immunol.,* 27:23–29.

130. Tosi, M., Journet, A., Colomb, M., and Meo, T. (1985): Construction, isolation and characterization of cDNA clones encoding human C1r and C1s. *Complement,* 2:79.

131. Weis, J. J., Fearon, D. T., Klickstein, L. B., Wong, W. W., Richards, S. A., De Bruyn Kops, A., Smith, J. A., and Weis, J. H. (1986): Identification of a partial cDNA clone for the C3d/Epstein-Barr virus receptor of human B lymphocytes: Homology with the receptor for fragments C3b and C4b of the third and fourth components of complement. *Proc. Natl. Acad. Sci. USA,* 83:5639–5643.

132. Wetsel, R. A., Ogata, R. T., and Tack, B. F. (1987): Primary structure of the fifth component of murine complement. *Biochemistry* 26:737–743.

133. White, P. C., Grossberger, D., Onufer, B. J., Chaplin, D. D., New, M. I., Dupont, B., and Strominger, J. L. (1985): Two genes encoding 21-hydroxylase are located near the genes encoding the fourth component of complement in man. *Proc. Natl. Acad. Sci. USA,* 82:5111–5115.

134. Whitehead, A. S., Solomon, E., Chambers, S., Bodmer, W. F., Povey, S., and Fey, G. (1982): Assignment of the structural gene for the third component of human complement to chromosome 19. *Proc. Natl. Acad. Sci. USA,* 79:5021–5025.

135. Whitehead, A. S., Goldberger, G., Woods, D. E., Markham, A. F., and Colten, H. R. (1983): Use of cDNA clone for the fourth component of human complement (C4) for analysis of a genetic deficiency of C4 in guinea pigs. *Proc. Natl. Acad. Sci. USA,* 80:5387–5392.

136. Whitehead, A. S., Woods, D. E., Fleishnick, E., Chin, J. E., Katz, A. J., Gerald, P. S., Alper, C. A., and Colten, H. R. (1984): DNA polymorphism of the C4 gene: A new marker for analysis of the major histocompatibility complex. *N. Engl. J. Med.,* 310:88–91.

137. Whitehead, A. S., Colten, H. R., Chang, C. C., and Demars, R. (1985): Localization of MHC-linked complement genes between HLA-B and HLA-DR by using HLA mutant cell lines. *J. Immunol.,* 134:641–643.

138. Wilson, J. G., Wong, W. W., Schur, P. H., and Fearon, D. T. (1982): Mode of inheritance of decreased C3b receptors on erythrocytes of patients with systemic lupus erythematosus. *N. Engl. J. Med.,* 307:981–986.

139. Wilson, J. G., Murphy, E. F., Wong, W. W., Klickstein, L. B., Weis, J. H., and Fearon, D. T. (1986): Identification of a restriction fragment length polymorphism by a CR1 cDNA that correlates with the number of CR1 on erythrocytes. *J. Exp. Med.,* 164:50–59.

140. Wong, W. W., Wilson, J. G., and Fearon, D. T. (1983): Genetic regulation of a structural polymorphism of human C3b receptor. *J. Clin. Invest.,* 72:685–690.

141. Wong, W. W., Klickstein, L. B., Smith, J. A., Weis, J. H., and Fearon, D. T. (1985): Identification of a partial cDNA clone for the human receptor for complement fragments C3b/C4b. *Proc. Natl. Acad. Sci. USA,* 82:7711–7715.

142. Woods, D. E., Edge, M. D., and Colten, H. R. (1984): Isolation of a cDNA clone for the human complement protein C2 and its use in identification of restriction fragment length polymorphism. *J. Clin. Invest.,* 74:634–638.

143. Yonemasu, K., Kitajuma, H., Tanabe, S., Ochi, T., and Shinkai, H. (1979): Effect of age on C1q and C3 levels in human serum and their presence in colostrum. *Immunology,* 35:523–530.

144. Young, J. D.-E., Cohn, Z. A., and Podack, E. R. (1986): The ninth component of complement and the pore-forming protein (perforin 1) from cytotoxic T cells: Structural, immunological and functional similarities. *Science,* 233:184–190.

145. Yu, C. Y., Belt, K. T., Giles, C. M., Campbell, R. D., and Porter, R. R. (1986): Structural basis of the polymorphism of human complement components C4A and C4B: gene size, reactivity and antigenicity. *EMBO J.,* 5:2873–2881.

Inflammation: Basic Principles and Clinical Correlates.
Edited by J. I. Gallin, I. M. Goldstein, and R. Snyderman.
Raven Press, Ltd., New York © 1988.

CHAPTER 6

Complement and Related Proteins: Inherited Deficiencies

Louis F. Fries and Michael M. Frank

The human complement system is an important element of host defense which comprises over 25 plasma and membrane-bound glycoproteins that interact in a precise and highly regulated manner (see Chapters 3 and 4). Host defense processes that are dependent on or modified by complement activation include the opsonization and phagocytosis of microorganisms and foreign substances, recruitment and activation of immunologically active cells at sites of inflammation, processing and clearance of immune complexes, and direct lysis of many types of targets such as enveloped viruses, gram-negative bacteria, and eukaryotic cells recognized as foreign by the host. In addition, complement proteins appear to have as yet poorly understood immunoregulatory functions. A detailed discussion of the biologic activities of complement proteins and their activation fragments is provided in Chapter 4.

Given the multiple important functions of the complement proteins, it is not surprising that patients deficient in these proteins are at risk of developing both infectious diseases and a variety of autoimmune disorders. In this chapter we will briefly review some of the better documented roles of complement in host defense, immune complex handling, and inflammation. We will then explore the manifestations of disease in patients with genetically controlled, and certain acquired, deficiencies in the various complement proteins.

Many cell types active in the immune response display receptors for various complement proteins or fragments. The distribution and functions of these receptors have been reviewed in Chapters 3, 4, and 21. In addition, at least four cell membrane glycoproteins have been identified which function to regulate complement activation on the surface of normal cells. These proteins function to protect normal tissues from damage by autologous complement. Several congenital and/or acquired defects in complement-related cell surface proteins have been described. We will also review the disease manifestations associated with these deficiencies and discuss current understanding of the biochemical abnormalities which underlie these disorders.

INTERACTIONS OF COMPLEMENT PROTEINS WITH BACTERIA

The complement system is central in host defense against bacterial disease. Its function in this system has been studied extensively. Complement acts by direct lysis of bacteria, augmentation of the inflammatory response, recruitment of phagocytic cells, and facilitation of the phagocytosis of organisms through opsonization. Much progress has been made in the understanding of these interactions (14,40).

Both gram-positive and gram-negative organisms activate the alternative pathway in the absence of antibody. Specific antibodies bound to bacterial structures may also activate the classical pathway, usually mediating more rapid and more extensive bacterial damage. The complement-dependent killing of serum-sensitive gram-negative organisms is caused by insertion of the C5b-9 complex into the bacterial membrane, inducing cell death and, in the presence of lysozyme, lysis. In serum-resistant gram-negative bacilli, which usually have long polysaccharide chains attached to the lipid A core of their lipopolysaccharide, C5b-9 deposition is inefficient in producing lysis. This may be in part because deposition occurs at sites on the lipopolysaccharide too distant from vital outer membrane structures to allow killing of these organisms (41). Some *Neisseria* are also resistant to complement-mediated lysis, but the mechanism of this resistance has not been ascertained. Gram-positive bacteria have much thicker cell walls which act as a physical barrier to C5b-9 disruption of their cytoplasmic membrane.

In bacteria resistant to complement-mediated lysis, the primary mechanism of host defense is phagocytosis. Complement activation products, especially C3 fragments C3b and iC3b, deposited on bacterial surfaces can facilitate binding, ingestion, and killing of such organisms by phagocytic cells (13,33).

THE FUNCTION OF COMPLEMENT IN THE PROCESSING OF CIRCULATING IMMUNE COMPLEXES

The fate of circulating immune complexes is determined by multiple factors including the size and chemical nature of the antigen, the class and subclass of the interacting antibodies, the functional integrity of the mononuclear phagocyte system, and the action of complement.

For particulate antigens, complement activation appears to accelerate the rate of clearance of IgG-bearing complexes and, with heavy complement coating, progressively shifts the site of clearance from the spleen to the liver (28,69). IgM-bearing particles and alternative pathway-activating particles in the naive host are cleared primarily by the liver via a complement-dependent mechanism (28,69).

Soluble immune complexes are handled by mechanisms that are much less well understood. Factors such as charge, carbohydrate composition, and overall complex size may be of crucial importance. In primate blood it appears that complement-activating complexes, when formed, are rapidly bound by erythrocyte C3b receptors (CR1) (19). A substantial proportion of these bound complexes are then stripped from the red cells by Kupffer cells as they pass through the liver and are deposited there (19). In addition to serving as a transport mechanism, erythrocyte CR1 may have a major role as a cofactor in the enzymatic stepwise degradation of C3b to iC3b and C3dg (45). Covalent binding of complement fragments to antigen or antibody may also disrupt immune complex lattice structure, resulting in the fragmentation of large complexes into smaller, more soluble subunits (47).

COMPLEMENT AND INFLAMMATION

In addition to its roles in host defense and immune complex clearance, complement is an important element in the inflammatory response. Complement activation in tissue due to microbial pathogens or endogenous immune complexes results in the production of a series of activation peptides, anaphylatoxins, which increase vascular permeability and cause histamine release from mast cells (36,37). The most potent of these peptides, C5a, is also chemotactic for inflammatory cells and stimulates release of toxic oxygen products and lysosomal enzymes by neutrophils (36). Complement system proteases interact directly with the coagulation, fibrinolytic, and kinin-generating systems, and membrane attack complexes can promote platelet aggregation (72,77). Finally, the cytotoxic potential of complement may cause direct tissue damage in some instances, although the contribution of complement itself is frequently difficult to assess in the face of tissue infiltration by inflammatory cells (8,20).

COMPLEMENT RECEPTORS

Complement receptors are reviewed in Chapters 3 and 19 and in a more detailed fashion in several recent reviews (24,63).

In addition to receptors for the major C3 fragments, discussed below, cell surface proteins or carbohydrates that bind specifically a number of complement proteins or fragments have been identified. Complement proteins thought to serve as ligands for cell surface receptors include C1q, C3a, C4a, C4b, C5a, Bb, and factor H. In some cases (i.e., anaphylatoxins), the binding reactions and physiologic roles of these ligand–receptor systems have been extensively explored. The others listed are much less well studied at present.

Receptors for the target-bound fragments of C3 have been extensively studied and are designated CR1, CR2, and CR3. The first cleavage product of C3, C3b, is the primary ligand of CR1. CR1 is present on erythrocytes, neutrophils, monocytes, macrophages, B lymphocytes, some T lymphocytes, and glomerular podocytes. The function of CR1 on erythrocytes appears to be related primarily to its factor H-like activity, and erythrocyte-borne CR1 is thought to be a major processor of circulating immune complexes that have bound complement. The principal function of neutrophil and monocyte or macrophage CR1 is believed to be facilitation of phagocytosis of C3b-bearing particles. The function of lymphocyte CR1 is poorly understood.

The primary receptor for the second degradation product of C3, iC3b, is known as CR3. CR3 is a heterodimer related to a family of membrane glycoproteins, which includes LFA-1 and p150,95, by a common β chain. CR3 is present on neutrophils, monocytes, macrophages, and cytotoxic lymphocytes responsible for antibody-dependent cellular cytotoxicity and natural killer activity. It functions not only in the process of phagocytosis but may also be important in the adhesive properties of phagocytic cells (see also Chapter 24).

The final C3 degradation product, C3d-g (and/or the slightly smaller molecule termed C3d), is recognized by a receptor known as CR2 which is present on B lymphocytes. The physiologic function of this receptor is not well understood, although recent data suggest that ligation of this receptor, at least in murine systems, may have a role in promoting B-cell activation and proliferation (46).

GENETICS OF COMPLEMENT PROTEINS

The proteins of the complement system demonstrate a large number of genetic polymorphisms. Variants have been reported for C2, C3, C4, C6, C7, C8, factor B, factor D̄, factor H, C4-binding protein, C1 inhibitor, and CR1. In almost all cases these allotypic variants show autosomal codominant inheritance. In general, these variants function normally, except for variants of C1 inhibitor (see below).

Complement proteins C4, C2, and factor B, referred to as class III gene products, are coded for by genes within the major histocompatibility complex (MHC) on chromosome 6 in humans. C4 is encoded at two separate loci within the MHC, and these two genes give rise to products with subtle differences, as detailed below. Because of their proximity to class I and class II genes, linkage of C2, C4, and factor B allelic variants with particular histocompatibility phenotypes has been noted (3). Given the location of these complement genes, the association of deficiency in these proteins with autoimmune disorders is notable and has given rise to considerable speculation regarding its nature (see below). An additional linkage group of complement-related proteins has recently been identified. The genes encoding C4-binding protein, factor H, CR1, and the C3d/dg receptor (CR2) reside on chromosome 1 in humans (76). Interestingly, these C4b- and C3b-binding proteins show areas of strong sequence homology with C2 and factor B—suggesting the existence of a superfamily of structurally related proteins responsible for complement activation and control (59). Decay-accelerating factor (DAF) and gp 45–70, both cell membrane-bound complement regulatory proteins, have also been proposed for membership in this family (32). Recently published data confirm that DAF shares a homologous repeating sequence with the other C3b- and C4b-binding proteins listed (15).

INCIDENCE OF COMPLEMENT DEFICIENCY SYNDROMES

Genetic deficiencies in complement proteins are distinctly uncommon in the general population. An extensive review in 1984 that collected all reported cases up to that time was able to document only 244 individuals with genetically controlled total deficiencies (66). Heterozygosity for C2 deficiency is found in approximately 1.2% of the population, and it has been estimated that 1 in 28,000 to 40,000 individuals would be expected to be homozygous for C2 deficiency, thought to be the most common complement component deficiency in the white population. In populations defined by certain disease entities, the incidence of complement component deficiencies may be strikingly higher. In rheumatologic disorders such as systemic lupus erythematosus (SLE), the incidence of C2 deficiency may be as high as 5.9% (31). The rate of terminal component complement deficiencies in patients with recurrent disseminated neisserial infections has been estimated to be as high as 20%, and one study has demonstrated a surprising 15% incidence of late component deficiency in patients with even a single meningococcal infection (23). Table 1 summarizes the currently identified

TABLE 1. *Inherited complement and complement-related protein deficiency states*

Deficient protein	Observed pattern of inheritance at clinical level	Reported major clinical correlates[a]
C1q	Autosomal recessive	Glomerulonephritis, SLE
C1r	Probably autosomal recessive	SLE-like syndrome
C1s	?	SLE
C4	Probably autosomal recessive	SLE-like syndromes
C2	Autosomal recessive, HLA-linked	SLE, discoid lupus erythematosus, juvenile rheumatoid arthritis, glomerulonephritis
C3	Autosomal recessive	Recurrent pyogenic infections, glomerulonephritis
C5	Autosomal recessive	Recurrent disseminated neisserial infections, SLE
C6	Autosomal recessive	Recurrent disseminated neisserial infections
C7	Autosomal recessive	Recurrent disseminated neisserial infections, Raynaud's phenomenon
C8 β chain or C8 α-γ chains	Autosomal recessive?	Recurrent disseminated neisserial infections
C9	Autosomal recessive	None identified
Properdin	X-linked recessive	Recurrent pyogenic infections, fulminant meningococcemia
Factor D̄	?	Recurrent pyogenic infections
C1 inhibitor	Autosomal dominant	Hereditary angioedema, increased incidence of several autoimmune diseases[b]
Factor H	Autosomal recessive	Glomerulonephritis
Factor I	Autosomal recessive	Recurrent pyogenic infections
CR1	Autosomal recessive[c]	Association between low erythrocyte CR1 numbers and SLE
CR3	Autosomal recessive[d]	Leukocytosis, recurrent pyogenic infections, delayed umbilical cord separation

[a] Note that a significant number of individuals with complement deficiencies, especially C2 and terminal component deficiencies, are clinically well.

[b] Approximately 85% of these cases involved silent alleles and 15% involved alleles encoding for dysfunctional variant C1 inhibitor protein.

[c] Homozygosity for low (not absent) numerical expression of CR1 on erythrocytes is detectable *in vitro* and appears to be associated with SLE. An acquired defect in CR1 numbers may also be operative.

[d] Low but not absent leukocyte CR3 is detectable in both parents of most CR3-deficient children.

genetic complement and complement-related protein deficiencies.

DEFICIENCIES IN CLASSICAL PATHWAY PROTEINS

C1 Deficiency

As shown in Table 1, patients have been identified who lack each of the C1 subunits (C1q, C1r, and C1s). No patient has been found clearly lacking only C1s, but combined C1r and C1s deficiencies have been described (66). These individuals frequently develop discoid lupus erythematosus or SLE and/or renal disease, as well as meningitis. The majority of C1q-deficient individuals produce no identifiable C1q, but the elaboration of a dysfunctional variant protein has been noted in at least one family (74). Depressed levels of C1q have also been noted in patients with hypogammaglobulinemia (42). The synthetic rate of C1q is normal in these patients, but in the presence of reduced immunoglobulin concentrations there is accel-

erated removal of C1q from the intravascular pool. Patients with thymic hypoplasia also have low C1q levels, but the mechanism of this defect is not understood.

C4 Deficiency

As noted above, there are two separate C4 loci within the human MHC that give rise to two products: C4A and C4B. C4A and C4B differ in molecular weight, electrophoretic mobility, and hemolytic efficiency (16). Multiple allelic variants exist for both C4A and C4B. Thus, any one individual has four genes that code for C4 synthesis and may be heterozygous at either or both of the two loci, yielding up to four C4 variants in a given plasma. A deficiency-producing allele at either C4 locus is termed q0 (for "quantity 0") for the gene product in question, i.e., C4Aq0 or C4Bq0. An individual with a single silent allele can have a C4 titer which falls in the normal range as long as the other C4 loci encode production of normal proteins. The complete absence of one or both of the normal C4 gene products is highly associated with the development of autoimmune disease.

Among complement component-deficient patients, those lacking C4 completely have the highest incidence of SLE, and 62% to 85% of these extremely rare patients are reported to manifest some autoimmune disorder (1,66). Family members heterozygous for C4 deficiency also have an increased risk of autoimmunity (7). The relative risk of SLE is increased 16.6-fold for white individuals homozygous for the C4Aq0 allele, and the presence of even a single copy of the C4Aq0 allele correlates with an increased risk of SLE in both whites and blacks (35). A portion of this increased risk may be related to the autoimmune diathesis of the HLA B8, DR3 haplotype with which the C4Aq0 allele is in linkage disequilibrium. However, the C4Aq0 allele appears to represent an independent risk factor for SLE even in the setting of other HLA haplotypes (a situation common among blacks) (35). Other diseases reportedly associated with silent alleles at one or both C4 loci include Graves' disease, insulin-dependent diabetes mellitus, and chronic active hepatitis (60,75). Infectious complications have been described in three homozygous C4-deficient patients, one of whom died as a result of disseminated herpes simplex and cytomegalovirus infections (66). In addition, it has been suggested that partial C4 deficiency may predispose to the development of subacute sclerosing panencephalitis (61).

C2 Deficiency

Autoimmune disorders, and less commonly infectious complications, are also seen in C2-deficient patients. The infectious complications, including pneumonia, bacteremia, and meningitis, are generally caused by pyogenic bacteria that require opsonization and phagocytosis for adequate host defense. Autoimmune or rheumatic diseases have been reported to occur in approximately one-half of C2-deficient individuals (1,31,66). The most common disorder in this setting is SLE, but a variety of others have been reported. SLE in C2-deficient subjects tends to be characterized by early age of onset, modest anti-nuclear antibody titers, and relatively mild renal involvement (1,31). As in individuals with heterozygous C4 deficiency, increased risk for the development of autoimmune disorders has been reported in individuals heterozygous for C2 deficiency as well as in C2-sufficient first-degree relatives of C2-deficient patients (31). One interpretation of this finding is that the C2-deficient allele may in some way be associated with another disease susceptibility gene in these families. Molecular studies in C2-deficient humans suggest that the structural gene for C2 is present and grossly intact in these individuals but, for reasons not yet clear, is not transcribed into an RNA message (17). C2 deficiency may be associated with below-normal, but not absent, factor B levels in some individuals, which appears to be an acquired defect.

IMMUNOREGULATION, ANTIBODY RESPONSES, AND COMPLEMENT DEFICIENCY

As described above, autoimmune disease is perhaps the most prominent manifestation of classical pathway component deficiencies. The underlying mechanisms are unclear; aberrant immune complex catabolism, susceptibility to unusual (especially viral) infections, and linkage of complement deficiency-producing alleles to other disease susceptibility genes inside or outside the MHC have all been proposed. It is noteworthy that a number of animal models of classical pathway complement deficiency, especially C4- and C2-deficient guinea pigs, demonstrate serologic abnormalities (rheumatoid factors, etc.) suggestive of autoimmunity despite clinical good health (10). In addition, animals deficient in C4, C2, or C3 have repeatedly shown impaired antibody responses to prototypical test antigens and, in particular, failure of isotype switching from IgM to IgG. These abnormalities are at least partially correctable by infusion of the missing component (51). Similar abnormalities in the antibody response have been documented in classical pathway-deficient human subjects (51). The molecular mechanisms underlying these defects are the object of ongoing investigation (46). The increased incidence of autoimmunity in first-degree relatives of complement-deficient patients, despite normal complement function in these individuals, argues that defective complement activation may not be the sole mechanism operative.

DEFICIENCIES IN ALTERNATIVE PATHWAY COMPONENTS

Properdin Deficiency

Properdin deficiency is the only reported complement component deficiency that demonstrates sex-linked inheritance. The deficiency has been associated with fulminant and rapidly fatal meningococcal infections. Female carriers also appear to be at increased risk for overwhelming meningococcal infection (66).

Factor $\bar{D}$ Deficiency

Partial factor $\bar{D}$ deficiency has been reported in two adult twin sisters, both of whom suffered from recurrent upper and lower respiratory tract infections and unexplained infertility. Family studies failed to provide adequate data to suggest a mode of inheritance (43).

C3 Deficiency

Given the central role of C3 in both complement activation pathways and the multiple biologic roles that C3 fragments subserve, it is not surprising that C3 deficiency has among the most severe consequences of the various complement deficiency states. No homozygous C3-deficient patient thus far reported has been disease-free. Infectious complications predominate and have included meningitis, bacteremia, pneumonia, urinary tract infection, and peritonitis—all frequently recurrent (1,2,66). *Streptococcus pneumoniae* and *Neisseria meningitidis* have been the major reported pathogens. In addition, SLE, vasculitic syndromes, and glomerulonephritis have each been reported in 15% to 21% of C3-deficient patients (1,6,66). The exact molecular basis of human C3 deficiency is unknown, but at least some patients have detectable, albeit extremely low, amounts of C3 in plasma. In addition, mononuclear phagocytes from such persons synthesize reduced but readily detectable amounts of C3 *in vitro* (18). At least one individual with a highly dysfunctional structural variant of C3 has been reported (21).

TERMINAL COMPONENT DEFICIENCIES

Lysis by terminal complement components is a significant host defense mechanism against some gram-negative organisms, especially *Neisseria* species. Individuals lacking these components are at increased risk of acquiring such infections. Patients lacking any of the complement components C5 through C8 present a relatively homogeneous clinical picture with recurrent episodes of meningococcemia, meningococcal meningitis, and/or disseminated gonococcal infection. Fifty percent of such patients reported have had significant neisserial infections (66). In addition, other infectious complications, including brucellosis, toxoplasmosis, chronic pyelonephritis, and pneumonia, have been reported. Of the terminal component-deficient patients reported to date, 11% have had autoimmune disorders (often SLE-like syndromes or Raynaud's phenomenon) without infectious complications (66). In most cases these deficiencies have followed a simple Mendelian inheritance pattern.

C8 deficiency is a particularly interesting case. C8 is a three-chain molecule with α, β, and γ chains. The genetic locus encoding for the β chain is separate from the locus coding for the α and γ chains (58,73). Thus, two types of C8 deficiency are recognized: C8β deficiency and C8α-γ

deficiency. Whereas all reported C8β-deficient patients are white, those with a C8α-γ-deficiency have been largely black or Hispanic (66). Admixture of serum from α-γ- and β-chain-deficient patients permits the reassembly of functional C8 and restores complement activity (73).

Ross and Densen (66) have pointed out several issues regarding disseminated neisserial infections in patients with late component deficiency. Perhaps the most striking is that, although the relapse rate (6.3%) and recurrence rate (45%) of infection in these individuals are considerably greater than in the normal population (0.6% and 0%, respectively), the mortality rate is greater in the normal population (19%) than in late component-deficient patients (2.9%). Also of note is that fulminant onset of meningococcal disease is not characteristic of illness seen in late component-deficient patients (unlike other complement-deficient patients), and most such individuals have had prodromal symptoms. Other unusual aspects in the pattern of meningococcal disease in deficient patients include a higher male-to-female ratio, an increase in the incidence of infection with serogroup Y organisms, and a higher median age at onset of the first infection. It is interesting to speculate about possible reasons for these differences. While complement-mediated bactericidal activity is clearly important in dealing with these organisms, complement action is probably not the only mechanism that provides host defense. Given the figures quoted above, it is apparent that terminal component-deficient patients acquire systemic neisserial infections readily but are capable of at least partial containment of the organisms—presumably via phagocytic cells. It is reasonable to suspect that in older individuals antibody is present as a result of previous exposure to these or related organisms, which provides an additional measure of protection. It is also striking that the pattern of serum resistance seen in isolates from terminal component-deficient patients exactly parallels that seen in *Neisseria* isolated from apparently normal subjects with systemic disease. Thus, terminal component deficiency does not simply confer pathogenicity on a broad spectrum of innocuous neisserial strains that would otherwise have been killed by serum lytic activity. These complex issues have been carefully reviewed elsewhere (12,14,66).

Because killing of some bacteria may occur in the absence of C9, albeit slowly, it has been suggested that C9 deficiency may be of little consequence. Eighty percent of the patients reported to date have not had infectious complications. In Japan, screening studies have shown that C9 deficiency is the most common complement deficiency, with a gene frequency of approximately 3.5%, and is present in relatively large numbers of individuals (38). By and large it is a silent abnormality (38). C9 deficiency is found with identical frequency in healthy blood donors and hospitalized populations in Japan—suggesting no association with disease. However, there has been a single report in the American literature of a patient with C9 deficiency who developed meningococcal meningitis (25). Data are insufficient at present to determine whether this case represents a purely random association.

DEFICIENCIES IN REGULATORY PROTEINS

C1 Inhibitor Deficiency: Hereditary Angioedema

The clinical syndrome of C1 inhibitor deficiency, hereditary angioedema (HAE), is inherited as an autosomal dominant trait. A critical plasma level of C1 inhibitor, about one-third to one-half of normal, appears to be required for normal inhibitor function (70). Since the C1 inhibitor molecule is continuously consumed *in vivo* by interactions with many plasma protease systems, the output of one normal gene cannot maintain 50% of normal plasma levels in the face of normal (or increased) utilization in heterozygotes for C1 inhibitor deficiency (57). Plasma levels frequently fall below the critical threshold, and symptoms result. HAE is manifested by recurrent attacks of nonpruritic, nonurticarial swelling of the extremities, face, trunk, abdominal viscera, and most critically the airways (27). Bowel edema is manifested as bouts of abdominal pain which may mimic an acute abdomen but can usually be distinguished by the absence of fever, leukocytosis, or clear-cut signs of peritoneal irritation (27). Swelling typically lasts 24 to 72 hr and may occur spontaneously or in response to trauma, particularly dental manipulation. The biochemical mediator of this swelling has not been clearly elucidated as yet. C1 inhibitor is an important regulator of not only complement activation but also Hageman factor and its enzymatically active fragments, as well as clotting factor XIa, kallikrein, and plasmin (68). Thus, the mediators responsible for angioedema may arise from the coagulation, fibrinolytic, complement, or kinin-generating systems, or a combination of these. It is of interest that, while complement consumption is chronic in HAE, acute alterations of both prekallikrein and high-molecular-weight kininogen levels can be detected in temporal relation to swelling attacks (68). While activation of C1 is unregulated, the multiplicity of control mechanisms at the level of C4b and C3 are intact. Thus, HAE patients manifest depletion of the early classical pathway components (C4 and C2), but alternative pathway and terminal component functions remain unaffected (27).

HAE patients do not appear to be at increased risk for infection. However, detailed studies have suggested that, analogous to the effects of deficiencies in the classical pathway components, HAE patients have an immuno-regulatory abnormality and are at increased risk for developing autoimmune disorders such as SLE, Sjögren's syndrome, Crohn's disease, and scleroderma (11). Clinical symptoms of these autoimmune disorders are usually mild in this patient group.

Approximately 85% of individuals with HAE have one normal and one silent C1 inhibitor gene. The remaining 15% are heterozygous for one of several antigenically normal but functionless inhibitors (62). Thus, in a minority of patients, C1 inhibitor antigen levels may be normal, and functional testing is required if HAE is a strong diagnostic consideration. The C1 inhibitor gene maps to chromosome 11 in humans; molecular studies in a limited number of HAE patients have not revealed any gross deletions or rearrangements at the C1 inhibitor locus (9).

A clinically similar acquired form of C1 inhibitor deficiency is also known to exist in some patients. Low levels of C1, and sometimes C3, distinguish these patients from those with the hereditary form of C1 inhibitor deficiency. Acquired C1 inhibitor deficiency is associated with lymphoproliferative disorders in most reported cases but may also follow the spontaneous development of an autoantibody that binds to and neutralizes the C1 inhibitor (39).

Factor I Deficiency

Because factor I regulates the alternative pathway C3 convertase by inactivation of bound C3b, the absence of this protein leads to unrestrained consumption of C3 through spontaneous alternative pathway turnover. Thus, these patients are clinically similar to individuals with C3 deficiency. They suffer from recurrent infections due to pyogenic organisms, including meningococcal meningitis (66).

Factor H Deficiency

There are two reports of families with factor H-deficient siblings. Symptomatic individuals have had acute and/or chronic glomerulopathies, while one deficient patient has been clinically well. Surprisingly, no abnormal incidence of infection has been noted in these subjects despite depressed C3 levels (66).

DEFICIENCIES IN CELL SURFACE COMPLEMENT REGULATORY PROTEINS AND RECEPTORS

CR1 Deficiency

There is one report of a patient, apparently well, who has no detectable erythrocyte CR1 (67). It has been shown that in patients with SLE, as well as in patients with a number of other immunologically mediated diseases such as Sjögren's syndrome and autoimmune hemolytic anemia, the amount of CR1 displayed on the erythrocytes is below normal (65). The degree of CR1 depression correlates with disease activity. Interestingly, depressed levels of erythrocyte CR1 can also be seen in patients deficient in the C3 regulatory protein, factor I (56). Thus, C3 hypercatabolism, rather than autoimmunity *per se,* appears to be the central mechanism of CR1 depression. Clearly, these forms of partial CR1 deficiency are acquired. Nevertheless, it is also suggested that relative CR1 deficiency can be genetically determined, and it appears that both mechanisms may be operative in SLE (65,78). The role of this relative deficiency in the pathogenesis of SLE has not been definitely elucidated. It has been speculated that soluble immune complex handling may be altered in the face of low levels of CR1 in the blood.

Syndromes Related to CR3 Deficiency

A lack of CR3, the iC3b receptor, as determined by the failure of leukocytes to bind a variety of monoclonal antibodies directed against this cell surface molecule, has been reported in a small number of patients (5,64,71 and Chapter 24). Most of these individuals have also been shown to be lacking two other cell membrane glycoproteins, LFA-1 and p 150,95, which are related to CR3 by a common β subunit. These patients, mostly children, suffer from recurrent severe pyogenic bacterial infections. They have been shown to have defects in multiple neutrophil and mononuclear phagocyte microbicidal and adhesive functions. Lymphocyte functions related to adhesion are also impaired, especially cytotoxic activity. The clinical correlates of these *in vitro* findings are delayed separation of the umbilical cord, persistent leukocytosis, recurrent pyogenic infections (particularly of the skin and mucous membranes), and aggressive periodontal disease (4). Two phenotypic variants, moderate and severe, have been identified on the basis of severity of the recurrent infection problems. These appear to correlate with reduced (in the moderate phenotype) versus absent (in the severe phenotype) CR3 expression (4). The biochemical basis of this disorder appears to be an inability to synthesize the chromosome 21-encoded β subunit common to CR3, LFA-1, and p 150,95—resulting in failure to glycosylate these cellular adhesion proteins and insert them into cell membranes (44).

Paroxysmal Nocturnal Hemoglobinuria

Paroxysmal nocturnal hemoglobinuria (PNH) is an acquired bone marrow disorder characterized by chronic intravascular hemolysis. It is included here to exemplify the critical role of cell-borne complement-regulatory proteins in normal homeostasis. PNH is a clonal disorder of the myeloid series which frequently terminates in myelogenous leukemia or another myeloproliferative disease. Cells derived from the abnormal clone acquire varying degrees of exaggerated complement sensitivity during differentiation (48). Two groups have reported deficiency in a 70,000-dalton membrane glycoprotein, termed DAF, in PNH erythrocyte membranes (49,53). DAF normally regulates the lytic capacity of both the classical and alternative pathway C3 convertases by reducing their active half-life. Formation of either C3 convertase on PNH erythrocyte surfaces deficient in DAF may thus result in abnormally efficient C3 deposition onto the membrane of such cells and uncontrolled recruitment of the lytic terminal components (54). This in part explains the enhanced complement sensitivity of PNH erythrocytes. Chronic intravascular hemolysis presumably results from exposure of the abnormal erythrocytes to the slow, continuous turnover of the alternative pathway in plasma (52). It has more recently been demonstrated that affected erythrocytes of patients with PNH are lacking another membrane protein termed C8-binding protein or homologous restriction factor (79). This protein normally inhibits C9 polymerization at the site of C5b-8 complexes, thereby protecting homologous cells from complement lysis. Lack of this protein therefore renders PNH cells more susceptible to lysis by any late components deposited on their surface. DAF and acetylcholinesterase, which is also absent from PNH cell membranes, are linked to the membrane via a phosphatidylinositol-containing glycolipid tail (22). While homologous restriction factor has not yet been shown to require this linkage, it has been suggested that a defect in the biosynthetic pathways responsible for the glycolipid-anchoring mechanism may be the central lesion in PNH (22,79). This hypothesis is bolstered by the observation that cells of PNH patients can indeed produce DAF antigen, which is detectable in the intracellular compartment but not on the membrane. Leukocytes and platelets have been shown to share the DAF deficiency in PNH (50), which thus may also be related to the leukopenia, thrombocytopenia, and thrombotic disease often seen in these patients.

DIAGNOSIS OF COMPLEMENT DEFICIENCY

The complement deficiency states are an important, if uncommon, element of a differential diagnosis when a history of autoimmune disorder or recurrent bacterial infections is elicited. A history of recurrent, unexplained abdominal pain, laryngeal edema, or episodes of non-pruritic, nonurticarial peripheral swelling is suggestive of hereditary or acquired angioedema (C1 inhibitor deficiency). The family history is often, but not always, positive in inherited complement and complement-related protein deficiencies and may include both infectious and autoimmune elements. The characteristics of the CR3-deficient patient have been outlined in the preceding section.

The next step in the evaluation of patients suspected of having a complement deficiency is the determination of total hemolytic complement (CH_{50}). If any of the classical pathway or terminal components are absent, the CH_{50} value will be zero or extremely low. Upon finding a CH_{50} value that is below normal, one may then assay individual components. Selection of the most likely deficiencies, based on known gene frequencies and the clinical presentation, directs the initial investigation of individual components. Antigenic assays for C3 and C4 are widely available in hospital laboratories. The functional titrations of these and other components are exquisitely sensitive and specific but are largely confined to reference laboratories.

CH_{50} determinations in the diagnosis of HAE are unreliable. Because of the unregulated consumption of C4 in HAE, the functional titration of this component is a very useful screen in suspected cases of HAE, but antigenic and/or functional titration of the C1 inhibitor is required for definitive diagnosis.

Detection of alternative pathway component deficiency is more difficult and is best performed in research laboratories, although commercial kits for the assay of factor B and properdin antigens are available. Likewise, quantitative assessment of cellular CR1 and CR3 expression is best performed by specialized facilities at present, although reagents for such studies are theoretically widely available. A characteristic spectrum of neutrophil functional abnormalities has been described in CR3-deficient patients and may serve to raise diagnostic suspicion of this entity (4).

In inherited forms of complement deficiency, testing for individual components will reveal the deficient component to be essentially absent in homozygotes. On detailed testing for the component in question, heterozygotes will exhibit below-normal functional and antigenic levels that may not be readily apparent by CH_{50} assay. In acquired deficiencies in complement components, such as the complement consumption seen in active SLE or HAE, multiple components may be low, but are usually not zero. Simultaneous depression of more than one complement component argues strongly for a consumptive, rather than hereditary, etiology.

MANAGEMENT

The management of HAE has been the subject of considerable interest and study. In patients who are debilitated by their symptoms or have had life-threatening airway involvement, long-term prophylactic treatment with androgenic steroids is currently the treatment of choice (26,30). These agents appear to act by increasing synthesis of the C1 inhibitor directed by the one normal gene and are effective in patients with silent C1 inhibitor alleles and those who produce a dysfunctional protein (29). Antifibrinolytic agents (ϵ-aminocaproic acid and tranexamic acid) are also efficacious in many patients but are probably more hazardous (27). Adverse effects of androgen therapy have included virilization of women, weight gain, myalgias, headache, microscopic hematuria, abnormal liver function tests, anxiety, altered libido, and nausea (34). These effects are minimized by using impeded androgens such as danazol and titrating dosage to the minimum necessary to suppress symptoms (regardless of measurable changes in plasma complement titers) (30,34). Antifibrinolytic therapy may potentially be complicated by thrombotic episodes (not seen in our patients) and by myalgias, with or without elevation of muscle enzymes. Short-term prophylaxis of HAE attacks may be achieved by the infusion of purified C1 inhibitor or, more readily available, fresh frozen plasma 12 to 24 hr before anticipated surgery, endoscopy, or dental manipulation (26,27). Therapy of established attacks consists primarily of supportive care and analgesia; the use of plasma in this setting is unproven and controversial. There is anecdotal evidence that acute attacks may respond to epinephrine in certain patients, but antihistamines and glucocorticoids are without effect (26).

There has been far less study of the management of other complement deficiencies. Plasma infusion treatment has been attempted in a variety of patients. In several cases, the reversal of clinical or biochemical abnormalities has been of sufficient magnitude and duration to suggest the clinical utility of plasma infusion in the setting of acute infectious diseases (2,58). However, because the *in vivo* half-life of most complement proteins is short, plasma therapy requires evaluation on a case-by-case basis. For a variety of reasons, including inconvenience, sensitization to the replaced protein, and the attendant risks of plasma infusions, this approach cannot be recommended for long-term therapy. Vaccination with polyvalent meningococcal and pneumococcal vaccines has been recommended. Chronic administration of prophylactic antibiotics has also been suggested and, in some patients, has markedly reduced the incidence of clinically apparent infection (6,66). Given the failure of penicillin in the prophylaxis of meningococcal disease in the past, this approach may have only limited utility in individuals deficient in terminal components (66). While a considerable number of complement-deficient individuals may be clinically well, or have primarily autoimmune disease manifestations, both the literature and the authors' experience suggest that infection, usually bacterial, accounts for substantial morbidity and mortality in this setting. A persistent high index of suspicion for infection is thus appropriate in the long-term management of all complement component-deficient patients. Therapy of rheumatologic or other autoimmune conditions in complement-deficient individuals has not been extensively studied but does not appear to differ from optimal treatment of the same syndromes in complement-sufficient patients. The influence of replacement therapy (or aggressive androgen therapy to achieve normalization of C4 and C2 in HAE) on autoimmune disorders in this population has not been assessed in a controlled manner.

REFERENCES

1. Agnello, V. (1978): Complement deficiency states. *Medicine,* 57:1–23.
2. Alper, C. A., Abramson, N., Johnston, R. B., Jandl, J. H., and Rosen, F. S. (1970): Increased susceptibility to infection associated with abnormalities of complement-mediated functions and of the third component of complement (C3). *N. Engl. J. Med.,* 282:349–354.
3. Alper, C. A., Raum, D., Karp, S., Awdeh, Z. L., and Yunis, E. J. (1983): Serum complement "supergenes" of the major histocompatibility complex in man (complotypes). *Vox Sang.,* 45:62–67.
4. Anderson, D. C., Schmalsteig, F. C., Finegold, M. J., Hughes, B. J., Rothlein, R., Miller, L. J., Kohl, S., Tosi, M. F., Jacobs, R. L., Waldrop, T. C., Goldman, A. S., Shearer, W. T., and Springer, T. A. (1985): The severe and moderate phenotypes of heritable Mac-1, LFA-1 deficiency: Their quantitative definition and relation to leukocyte dysfunction and clinical features. *J. Infect. Dis.,* 152:668–689.
5. Arnaout, M. A., Dana, N., Pitt, J., and Todd, R. F., III (1985): Deficiency of two human leukocyte surface membrane glycoproteins (Mo1 and LFA-1). *Fed. Proc.,* 44:2664–2670.
6. Berger, M., Balow, J. E., Wilson, C. B., and Frank, M. M. (1983): Circulating immune complexes and glomerulonephritis in a patient with congenital absence of the third component of complement. *N. Engl. J. Med.,* 308:1009–1012.
7. Berliner, S., Weinberger, A., Zamir, R., Salomon, F., Joshua, H., and Pinkhas, J. (1981): Familial systemic lupus erythematosus and C4 deficiency. *Scand. J. Rheumatol.,* 10:280–282.
8. Biesecker, G., Lavin, L., Ziskind, M., and Koffler, D. (1982): Cutaneous localization of the membrane attack complex in discoid and systemic lupus erythematosus. *N. Engl. J. Med.,* 306:264–270.
9. Bock, S. C., Skriver, K., Nielson, E., Thogerson, H. C., Wiman, B., Donaldson, V., Eddy, R. L., Marrinan, J., Radziejewska, E., Huber, R., Shows, T. B., and Magnusson, S. (1986): Human C1 inhibitor: primary structure, cDNA cloning, and chromosomal localization. *Biochemistry,* 25:4292–4301.
10. Bottger, E. C., Hoffmann, T., Hadding, U., and Bitter-Suermann, D. (1986): Guinea pigs with inherited deficiencies of complement component C2 or C4 have characteristics of immune complex disease. *J. Clin. Invest.,* 78:689–695.
11. Brickman, C. M., Tsokos, G. C., Balow, J. E., Lawley, T. J., Santaella, M., Hammer, C. H., and Frank, M. M. (1986): Immunoregulatory disorders associated with hereditary angioedema. *J. Allergy Clin. Immunol.,* 77:749–757.
12. Britigan, B. E., Cohen, M. S., and Sparling, F. P. (1985): Gonococcal infection: A model of molecular pathogenesis. *N. Engl. J. Med.,* 312:1683–1694.
13. Brown, E. J., Hosea, S. W., Hammer, C. H., Burch, C. G., and Frank, M. M. (1982): A quantitative analysis of the interaction of antipneumococcal antibody and complement in experimental pneumococcal bacteremia. *J. Clin. Invest.,* 69:85–98.
14. Brown, E. J., Joiner, K. A., and Frank, M. M. (1983): The role of complement in host resistance to bacteria. *Springer Semin. Immunopathol.,* 6:349–360.
15. Carras, I. W., Davitz, M. A., Rhee, L., Weddell, G., Martin, D. W. Jr., and Nussenzweig, V. (1987): Cloning of decay-accelerating factor suggests novel use of splicing to generate two proteins. *Nature,* 325:545–549.
16. Chan, A. C., Karp, D. R., Shreffler, D. C., and Atkinson, J. P. (1984): The 20 faces of the fourth component of complement. *Immunol. Today,* 5:200–203.
17. Cole, F. S., Whitelead, A. S., Auerbach, H. S., Lint, T., Zeitz, H. J., Kelbridge, P., and Colten, H. R. (1985): The molecular basis for genetic deficiency of the second component of human complement. *N. Engl. J. Med.,* 313:11–15.
18. Colten, H. R. (1986): Genetics and synthesis of components of the complement system. In: *Immunobiology of the Complement System,* edited by G. D. Ross, pp. 163–181, Academic Press, Orlando, FL.
19. Cornacoff, J. B., Hebert, L. A., Smead, W. L., Van Aman, M. E., Birmingham, D. J., and Waxman, J. F. (1983): Primate erythrocyte-immune complex-clearing mechanism. *J. Clin. Invest.,* 71:236–247.
20. Couser, W. G., Baker, P. J., and Adler, S. (1985): Complement and the direct mediation of immune glomerular injury: A new perspective. *Kidney Int.,* 28:879–890.
21. Davis, A. E., Davis, J. S., Rabson, A. R., Osofsky, S. G., Colten, H. R., Rosen, F. S., and Alper, C. A. (1977): Homozygous C3 deficiency: Detection of C3 by radioimmunoassay. *Clin. Immunol. Immunopathol.,* 8:543–549.
22. Davitz, M. A., Low, M. G., and Nussenzweig, V. (1986): Release of decay accelerating factor (DAF) from the cell membrane by phosphatidylinositol-specific phospholipase C (PIPLC). *J. Exp. Med.,* 163:1150–1161.
23. Ellison, R. T., Kohler, P. F., Curd, J. G., Judson, F. N., and Beller, L. B. (1983): Prevalence of congenital or acquired complement deficiency in patients with sporadic meningococcal disease. *N. Engl. J. Med.,* 308:913–916.
24. Fearon, D. T., and Wong, W. W. (1983): Complement ligand-receptor interactions that mediate biological responses. *Annu. Rev. Immunol.,* 1:243–271.
25. Fine, D. P., Gewurz, H., Griffiss, M., and Lint, T. F. (1983): Meningococcal meningitis in a woman with inherited deficiency of the ninth component of complement. *Clin. Immunol. Immunopathol.,* 28:413–417.
26. Frank, M. M. (1985): Hereditary angioedema. In: *Current Therapy in Allergy Immunology, and Rheumatology,* edited by L. M. Lichtenstein and A. S. Fauci, pp. 54–57, B. C. Decker, Inc., Philadelphia.
27. Frank, M. M., Gelfand, J. A., and Atkinson, J. P. (1976): Hereditary angioedema: The clinical syndrome and its management. *Ann. Intern. Med.,* 84:580–593.
28. Frank, M. M., Schreiber, A. D., Atkinson, J. P., and Jaffe, C. J. (1977): Pathophysiology of immune hemolytic anemia. *Ann. Intern. Med.,* 87:210–222.
29. Gadek, J. E., Hosea, S. W., Gelfand, J. A., and Frank, M. M. (1979): Response of variant hereditary angioedema phenotypes to danazol therapy. *J. Clin. Invest.,* 64:280–286.
30. Gelfand, J. A., Sherins, R. J., Alling, D. W., and Frank, M. M. (1976): Treatment of hereditary angioedema with danazol: Reversal of clinical and biochemical abnormalities. *N. Engl. J. Med.,* 295:1444–1448.
31. Glass, D., Raum, D., Gibson, D., Stillman, J. S., and Schur, P. H. (1976): Inherited deficiency of the second component—Complement rheumatic disease association. *J. Clin. Invest.,* 58:853–861.
32. Holers, V. M., Cole, J. L., Lublin, D. M., Seya, T., and Atkinson, J. P. (1985): Human C3b and C4b-regulatory proteins: A new multigene family. *Immunol. Today,* 6:188–191.

33. Horwitz, M. A., and Silverstein, S. C. (1980): Influence of *Escherichia coli* capsule on complement fixation and on phagocytosis and killing by human phagocytes. *J. Clin. Invest.*, 65:82–94.

34. Hosea, S. W., Santaella, M. L., Brown, E. J., Berger, M., Katusha, K., and Frank, M. M. (1980): Long term therapy of hereditary angioedema with danazol. *Ann. Intern. Med.*, 93:809–912.

35. Howard, P. F., Hochberg, M. C., Bias, W. A., Arnett, F. C. Jr., and McLean, R. H. (1986): Relationship between C4 null genes, HLA-D region antigens, and genetic susceptibility to systemic lupus erythematosus in Caucasian and black Americans. *Am. J. Med.*, 81:187–193.

36. Hugli, T. E. (1981): The structural basis for anaphylatoxin and chemotactic function of C3a, C4a, and C5a. *CRC Crit. Rev. Immunol.*, 2:321–366.

37. Hugli, T. E., and Muller-Eberhard, H. J. (1987): Anaphylatoxins: C3a and C5a. *Adv. Immunol.*, 26:1–53.

38. Inai, S., Kitamura, H., Hiramatsu, S., and Nagaki, K. (1979): Deficiency of the ninth component of complement in man. *J. Clin. Lab. Immunol.*, 2:85–87.

39. Jackson, J., Sim, R. B., Whelan, A., and Feighery, C. (1986): An IgG autoantibody which inactivates C1-inhibitor. *Nature*, 323:722–724.

40. Joiner, K. A., Brown, E. J., and Frank, M. M. (1984): Complement and bacteria: Chemistry and biology in host defense. *Annu. Rev. Immunol.*, 2:461–491.

41. Joiner, K. A., and Frank, M. M. (1985): Mechanisms of bacterial resistance to complement-mediated killing. In: *Bayer-Symposium VIII: The Pathogenesis of Bacterial Infections*, pp. 122–136, Springer-Verlag, Berlin.

42. Kohler, P. F., and Müller-Eberhard, H. J. (1972): Metabolism of human C1q: Studies in hypogammaglobulinemia, myeloma, and systemic lupus erythematosus. *J. Clin. Invest.*, 51:868–875.

43. Kluin-Nelemans, H. C., van Velzen-Blad, H., van Helden, H. P. T., and Daha, M. R. (1984): Functional deficiency of complement factor D̄ in a monozygous twin. *Clin. Exp. Immunol.*, 58:724–730.

44. Marlin, S. D., Morton, C. C., Anderson, D. C., and Springer, T. A. (1986): LFA-1 immunodeficiency diseases: Definition of the genetic defect and chromosomal mapping of α and β subunits of the lymphocyte function-associated antigen 1 (LFA-1) by complementation in hybrid cells. *J. Exp. Med.*, 164:855–867.

45. Medof, M. E., Iida, K., Mold, C., and Nussenzweig, V. (1982): Unique role of the complement receptor CR1 in the degradation of C3b associated with immune complexes. *J. Exp. Med.*, 156:1739–1754.

46. Melchers, F., Erdei, A., Schultz, T., and Dierich, M. P. (1985): Growth control of activated, synchronized murine B cells by the C3d fragment of human complement. *Nature*, 317:264–267.

47. Miller, G. W., and Nussenzweig, V. (1975): A new complement function: Solubilization of antigen-antibody aggregates. *Proc. Natl. Acad. Sci. USA*, 72:418–422.

48. Moore, J. G., Humphries, R. K., Frank, M. M., and Young, N. (1986): Characterization of the hematopoetic defect in paroxysmal nocturnal hemoglobinuria. *Exp. Hematol.*, 14:222–229.

49. Nicholson-Weller, A., March, J. P., Rosenfeld, S. I., and Austen, K. F. (1983): Affected erythrocytes of patients with paroxysmal nocturnal hemoglobinuria are deficient in the complement regulatory protein, decay accelerating factor. *Proc. Natl. Acad. Sci. USA*, 80:5066–5070.

50. Nicholson-Weller, A., Spicer, D. B., and Austen, K. F. (1985): Deficiency of the complement regulatory protein, "decay-accelerating factor," on membranes of granulocytes, monocytes and platelets in paroxysmal nocturnal hemoglobinuria. *N. Engl. J. Med.*, 312:1019–1097.

51. Ochs, H. D., Wedgewood, R. J., Heller, S. R., and Beatty, P. G. (1986): Complement, membrane glycoproteins and complement receptors: Their role in regulation of the immune response. *Clin. Immunol. Immunopathol.*, 40:94–104.

52. Pangburn, M. K. (1983): Activation of complement via the alternative pathway. *Fed. Proc.*, 42:139–143.

53. Pangburn, M. K., Schreiber, R. D., and Müller-Eberhard, H. J. (1983): Deficiency of an erythrocyte membrane protein with complement regulatory activity in paroxysmal nocturnal hemoglobinuria. *Proc. Natl. Acad. Sci. USA*, 80:5430–5434.

54. Parker, C. J., Baker, P. J., and Rosse, W. F. (1982): Increased enzymatic activity of the alternative pathway convertase when bound to the erythrocytes of paroxysmal nocturnal hemoglobinuria. *J. Clin. Invest.*, 69:337–346.

55. Podak, E. R., and Tschopp, J. (1984): Membrane attack by complement. *Mol. Immunol.*, 21:589–603.

56. Porteu, F., Fischer, A., Deschamps-Latscha, B., and Halbwachs-Mecarelli, L. (1986): Defective complement receptors (CR1 and CR3) on erythrocytes and leukocytes of factor I (C3b-inactivator) deficiency patients. *Clin. Exp. Immunol.*, 66:463–471.

57. Quastel, M., Harrison, R., Cicardi, M., Alper, C. A., and Rosen, F. S. (1983): Behaviour in vivo of normal and dysfunctional C1 inhibitor in normal subjects and patients with hereditary angioneurotic edema. *J. Clin. Invest.*, 71:1041–1046.

58. Rao, C. P., Minta, J. O., Laski, B., Alper, C. A., and Gelfand, E. W. (1985): Inherited C8D subunit deficiency in a patient with recurrent meningococcal infections: In vivo functional kinetic analysis of C8. *Clin. Exp. Immunol.*, 60:183–190.

59. Reid, K. B. M., Bentley, D. R., Campbell, R. D., Chung, L. P., Sim, R. B., Kristensen, T., and Tack, B. F. (1986): Complement system proteins which interact with C3b or C4b. *Immunol. Today*, 7:230–234.

60. Rich, S., O'Neill, G., Dalmasso, A. P., Nerl, C., and Barbosa, J. (1985): Complement and HLA: Further definition of high-risk haplotypes in insulin dependent diabetes. *Diabetes*, 34:504–508.

61. Rittner, C., Neier, E. M. M., Stradman, B., Giles, C. M., Kochling, R., Mollengauer, E., and Kreth, H. W. (1984): Partial C4 deficiency in subacute sclerosing panencephalitis. *Immunogenetics*, 20:407–414.

62. Rosen, F. S., Alper, C. A., Pensky, J., Klemperer, M. R., and Donaldson, V. H. (1971): Genetically determined heterogeneity of the C1 esterase inhibitor in patients with hereditary angioneurotic edema. *J. Clin. Invest.*, 50:2143–2149.

63. Ross, G. D., and Medof, M. E. (1985): Membrane complement receptors specific for bound fragments of C3. *Adv. Immunol.*, 37:217–267.

64. Ross, G. D., Thompson, R. A., Walport, M. J., Springer, T. A., Watson, J. V., Ward, R. H. R., Lida, J., Newman, S. L., Harrison, R. A., and Lachmann, P. J. (1985): Characterization of patients with an increased susceptibility to bacterial infections and a genetic deficiency of leukocyte membrane complement receptor type 3 and the related membrane antigen LFA-1. *Blood*, 66:882–890.

65. Ross, G. D., Yount, W. J., Walport, M. J., Winfield, J. B., Parker, C. J., Fuller, C. R., Taylor, R. P., Myones, B. L., and Lachmann, P. J. (1985): Disease associated loss of erythrocyte complement receptors (CR1, C3b receptors) in patients with systemic lupus erythematosus and other diseases involving autoantibodies and/or complement activation. *J. Immunol.*, 135:2005–2014.

66. Ross, S. C., and Densen, P. (1984): Complement deficiency states and infection: Epidemiology, pathogenesis and consequences of neisserial and other infections in an immune deficiency. *Medicine*, 63:243–272.

67. Rothman, I. K., Gelfand, J. A., Fauci, A. S., and Frank, M. M. (1975): The immune adherence receptor: Dissociation between the expression of erythrocyte and mononuclear cell C3b receptors. *J. Immunol.*, 115:1312–1315.

68. Schapira, M., deAgostini, A., Schifferli, J. A., and Colman, R. W. (1985): Biochemistry and pathophysiology of human C1 inhibitor: Current issues. *Complement*, 2:111–126.

69. Schreiber, A. D., and Frank, M. M. (1972): The role of antibody and complement in the immune clearance and destruction of erythrocytes. I. In vivo effects of IgG and IgM complement-fixing sites. *J. Clin. Invest.*, 51:575–582.

70. Späth, P. J., Wüthrich, B., and Bütler, R. (1984): Quantification of C1-inhibitor functional activities by immunodiffusion assay in plasma of patients with hereditary angioedema—Evidence of a functionally critical level of C1-inhibitor concentration. *Complement*, 1:147–159.

71. Springer, T. A., and Anderson, D. C. (1986): The importance of the

MAC-1, LFA-1 glycoprotein family in monocyte and granulocyte adherence, chemotaxis and migration into inflammatory sites: Insights from an experiment of nature. *Ciba Found. Symp.,* 118:102–126.

72. Sundsmo, J. S., and Fair, D. S. (1983): Relationships among the complement, kinin, coagulation and fibrinolytic systems. *Springer Semin. Immunopathol.,* 6:231–258.

73. Tedesco, F., Densen, P., Villa, M. A., Petersen, B. H., and Sirchia, G. (1983): Two types of dysfunctional eighth component of complement (C8) molecules in C8 deficiency in man: Reconstitution of normal C8 from the mixture of two abnormal C8 molecules. *J. Clin. Invest.,* 71:183–191.

74. Thompson, R. A., Harney, M., Reid, K. B. M., Davies, J. G., White, R. H. R., and Cameron, A. H. (1980): A genetic defect of the C1q subcomponent of complement associated with childhood (immune complex) nephritis. *N. Engl. J. Med.,* 303:22–24.

75. Vergani, D., Larcher, V. F., Davies, E. T., Wells, L., Nasaruddin, B. A., Mieli-Vergani, G., and Mowat, A. P. (1985): Genetically determined low C4: A predisposing factor to autoimmune chronic active hepatitis. *Lancet,* 2:294–298.

76. Weis, J. H., Morton, C. C., Bruns, G. A. P., Weis, J. J., Klickstein, L. B., Wong, W. W., and Fearon, D. T. (1987): A complement receptor locus: Genes encoding C3b/4b receptor and C3d/Epstein-Barr virus receptor map to 1q32. *J. Immunol.,* 138:312–315.

77. Weidmer, T., Esmon, C. T., and Sims, P. J. (1986): Complement proteins C5b-9 stimulate procoagulant activity through platelet prothrombinase. *Blood,* 68:875–880.

78. Wilson, J. G., and Fearon, D. T. (1984): Altered expression of complement receptors as a pathogenetic factor in systemic lupus erythematosus. *Arthritis Rheum.,* 27:1321–1328.

79. Zalman, L. S., Wood, L. M., Frank, M. M., and Müller-Eberhard, H. J. (1987): Deficiency of the homologous restriction factor in paroxysmal nocturnal hemoglobinuria. *J. Exp. Med.,* 165:572–577.

Inflammation: Basic Principles and Clinical Correlates.
Edited by J. I. Gallin, I. M. Goldstein, and R. Snyderman.
Raven Press, Ltd., New York © 1988.

CHAPTER 7

The Contact Activation System of Plasma: Biochemistry and Pathophysiology

Franklin Kozin and Charles G. Cochrane

Components of the Contact System
  Hageman Factor (HF, Coagulation Factor XII) • Plasma Prekallikrein (PK) • High-Molecular-Weight Kininogen (HMWK) • Factor XI
Measuring Contact-System Proteins
Mechanisms of Contact Activation
  Initiation • Crystals • Collagen and Vascular Basement Membrane • Glycosaminoglycans and Glycoproteins • Bacterial Lipopolysaccharide (LPS) • Immune Complexes • Other Factors
Amplification
Dissemination
Regulation
  Inhibition of Surface Activation • Inhibition of Specific Activated Components • Other Inhibitors • Possible Role of HMWK

Cellular Activation of the Contact System
  Leukocytes • Endothelial Cells • Platelets
Cellular Effects of the Contact System
  Neutrophil Chemotaxis
Reactions with Other Plasma Proteins
  Complement System • Prostaglandins • Synovial Fluid Collagenase
Pathophysiologic Activities of Contact System
  Hageman Factor • High-Molecular-Weight Kininogen • Contact System and Renin Angiotensin System
Contact System in Human Disease
  Arthritis • Allergic and Anaphylactic Reactions • Bacteremic Shock • Hereditary Angioedema (HAE) • Renal Disorders and Blood Pressure Regulation • Other Disorders
References

The contact (Hageman factor or intrinsic clotting) system is one of four major plasma protein systems that contribute to the host's defense and, at times, participate in the development of inflammatory tissue injury. The other systems are: the coagulation, the fibrinolytic, and the complement systems. The contact system plays a central role in a complex series of reactions through which these systems interact. Progress in our understanding of these plasma protein pathways will be reviewed here.

The contact system consists of four primary proteins: Hageman factor (HF), prekallikrein (PK), high-molecular-weight kininogen (HMWK), and coagulation Factor XI (Table 1). Secondary reactions with plasminogen, Factor VII of the extrinsic coagulation system, and comple-ment proteins extend the physiologic effects of the contact system.

COMPONENTS OF THE CONTACT SYSTEM

Hageman Factor (HF, Coagulation Factor XII)

HF was initially recognized in 1955 by Ratnoff and Colopy in a patient (Hageman) who was found to have marked prolongation of his partial thromboplastin time (PTT) (169). HF is a β-globulin with a sedimentation coefficient of approximately 4.55 and molecular weight of 74 to 80 kilodaltons (see ref. 25). In normal plasma, HF has

TABLE 1. *Physical properties of contact-system proteins*

Protein	Molecular mass (kilodaltons)	Plasma concentration (μg/ml)	PI	Electrophoretic mobility
Hageman factor (Factor XII)	74–80	24–40	6.8	Beta-globulin
Prekallikrein (Fletcher factor)	80–88	50	8.5–9.0	Gamma-globulin
Factor XI (Plasma thromplastin antecedent)	160 (dimer)	4–8	8.5–9.0	Gamma-globulin
High-molecular-weight kininogen (Williams, Flaujac, or Fitzgerald factor)	110	70	4.5	Alpha-globulin

been measured at concentrations ranging from 23 to 40 μg/ml (171,181). HF exists as a single polypeptide chain containing 16.8% carbohydrate with 4.2% hexose, 4.7% hexosamine, and 7.9% *N*-acetylneuraminic acid. Amino acid sequence studies have shown that the amino terminal and active-site region of the light chain contain sequences common to a number of serine proteases that participate in coagulation (56).

Limited proteolysis of HF is necessary for its activation. The release of a fragment that acted as a prekallikrein-activating component was first recognized by Kaplan and Austen (97). Cleavage of HF may occur at two closely positioned sites, as illustrated in Fig. 1 (172). Cleavage at "site 1" within a disulfide loop generates an active enzyme, termed αHFa, which consists of disulfide-linked heavy (52,000 daltons) and light (28,000 daltons) chains. Cleavage at "site 2," just outside the disulfide bond, generates an active enzyme termed βHFa, a 28,000-dalton molecule derived from the carboxy-terminal portion of HF.

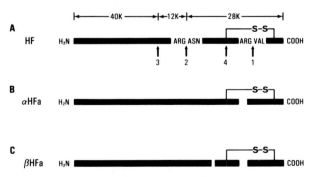

FIG. 1. Limited proteolytic cleavage of HF produces several different forms of activated HF (HFa). Two major forms of HFa exist: (i) αHFa produced by cleavage at site 1 within a disulfide loop, resulting in a molecule containing two polypeptide chains and 80,000 molecular weight; and (ii) βHFa produced by cleavage at site 2 outside the disulfide-linked segment in addition to that at site 1 and resulting in a single-chain molecule of 28,000 molecular weight. Cleavage at other sites may occur on further incubation with kallikrein.

The amino-terminal polypeptide of HF contains the binding site for negatively charged surfaces. Thus zymogen HF and αHFa (the two-chain active HF enzyme) are readily bound to negatively charged surfaces. In contrast, βHFa (the active HF enzyme derived from the carboxy terminus) is not surface bound (173). Data indicate that both αHFa and βHFa are potent activators of prekallikrein, whereas αHFa is at least 100 times more potent than βHFa in activating Factor XI (23,97,173). These features are summarized in Table 2.

HF cleavage results primarily from the action of plasma kallikrein (23,254). Plasmin (17,97,171), Factor IXa (171), and possibly leukocyte elastase may cleave HF *in vitro*, but these reactions are sufficiently weak as to make their significance doubtful. The basic mechanism of HF activation through limited proteolysis is probably identical to that for trypsinogen, chymotrypsinogen, and other coagulation zymogens (38). It is thought that formation of an ion pair between the newly formed amino-terminal residue of the light chain and the carboxy group of the aspartic acid residue adjacent to the active-site serine is required for this reaction (57).

HFa is capable of activating a number of plasma protein proenzymes. These reactions may be classified as major or minor, depending on their reaction rates and presence in normal plasma. Major reactions include the effect of HFa on PK and Factor XI; these demonstrate rapid reaction rates in plasma and with isolated components. The relatively weak action of HFa on plasminogen, Factor VII, and complement component C1 make the physiologic significance of these reactions uncertain.

HF, when bound to a negatively charged surface in sufficient concentration, undergoes a spontaneous autoactivation, yielding αHFa on the surface (248). The reaction is orders of magnitude slower than when prekallikrein and HMWK are present. Silverberg et al. (208) presented data suggesting that small amounts of HFa may be responsible for initiating this reaction.

αHFa also may cleave zymogen HF to yield additional

TABLE 2. *Characteristics of the different forms of Hageman factor*

Form	Molecular mass (kilodaltons)	Number of chains	Binding to negative surface	Activation of PK	Activation of Factor XI
HF	80	1	+	−	−
αHFa	80	2	+	+	+
βHFa	28	1	−	+	−

αHFa (217,218). This reaction does not occur when βHFa is incubated with HF, nor does it occur in the absence of a negatively charged surface (218), suggesting that both the enzyme HFa and substrate HF must be surface bound. This reaction has been observed with negatively charged surfaces such as kaolin, glass, dextran sulfate, sulfatides, and ellagic acid.

Plasma Prekallikrein (PK)

PK is a gamma-globulin single-chain glycoprotein of molecular weight 88,000 with an isoelectric point of 8.5 to 9.0 (253). Human plasma concentrations are approximately 50 μg/ml (15,182). PK is activated by limited proteolytic digestion by HFa, producing a two-chain disulfide-linked enzyme. A heavy chain of 52,000 molecular weight and a light chain of 35,000 molecular weight are produced with the active site contained on the light chain (14,84,119,216,224).

Plasma kallikrein has several potentially important actions, since it may interact with three different plasma substrates affecting coagulation, fibrinolysis, or kinin release. Kinetically, the most important reactions of plasma kallikrein are those with HF and HMWK, resulting in amplification of contact system activity and kinin release. Kallikrein cleaves HF at two sites, as discussed above. Kallikrein cleaves HMWK at two internal bonds, releasing bradykinin (141). Bovine kallikrein cleaves a third peptide bond in bovine HMWK, releasing a histidine-rich fragment (fragment 1-2) from the light chain (78). Less important reactions of kallikrein occur with plasminogen (25,26) and complement factors (35,245). The latter have been found to proceed with relatively slow reaction rates or only with isolated components. For example, little or no plasmin is found in whole plasma during the first 15 min of contact activation (26).

Recently, kallikrein was found to convert latent collagenase to active collagenase in rheumatoid synovial fluid (142). This may represent an important, major reaction of kallikrein.

High-Molecular-Weight Kininogen (HMWK)

Plasma kininogens are proteins that contain potent vasoactive peptides, the kinins, within their primary se-

quences (46,54,55). Human plasma contains at least two distinct kininogens: high- and low-molecular-weight kininogen (75,89). HMWK contains approximately 20% of total plasma kinin and exists as a single polypeptide chain of 110,000 molecular weight. Low-molecular-weight kininogen (LMWK), which contains the remaining 80% of plasma kinin, exists as a single polypeptide chain of 60,000 molecular weight. Kinins are released by limited proteolytic digestion of internal amino acid sequences by plasma or tissue kallikreins (Fig. 2). Tissue kallikrein is equally effective in liberating kinin from both HMWK and LMWK, whereas plasma kallikrein is about 40 times more active in releasing kinin from HMWK than from LMWK.

In a series of recent studies, Kitamura and colleagues have cloned and sequenced complementary DNAs (cDNAs) for bovine and human HMWK and LMWK (105,106,215). The signal-peptide, heavy-chain, and bradykinin moieties, which are common to the two kininogens, had virtually identical messenger RNAs (mRNAs), suggesting that these molecules are encoded by a single gene that is processed uniquely for each light chain.

The central role of HMWK in activating the contact system was recognized in 1975, when it was found that deficient plasmas exhibited abnormalities in contact activation (29,252). HMWK functions as a nonenzymatic cofactor in contact activation (72,127), whereas LMWK plays no apparent role in clotting or contact activation.

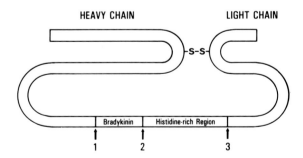

FIG. 2. Cleavage of human high-molecular-weight kininogen (HMWK) by kallikrein at two internal bonds, designated sites 1 and 2 in the figure, results in the release of bradykinin and formation of kinin-free HMWK. The latter is fully active in the contact-activation reaction. Cleavage at other internal bonds liberates fragment 1-2 in the bovine system.

HMWK antigen is not detectable in plasmas of patients with HMWK deficiency; LMWK is absent or present in reduced amount in these plasmas. In normal human plasma, the concentration of HMWK is 70 to 90 μg/ml (15,107,163). The carboxy terminus of HMWK functions as the cofactor in contact activation (103,213,219,233). This segment contains an unusual sequence of amino acids comprised of 30% histidine, 30% glycine, and 10% lysine (77,78). This positively charged segment is probably responsible for binding to negatively charged surfaces. It has been shown that kallikrein-induced cleavage of HMWK does not reduce its procoagulant activity (193).

Factor XI

Factor XI exhibits gamma electrophoretic mobility and is present in human plasma at a concentration of approximately 4 to 8 μg/ml (184,201). Patients deficient in this glycoprotein are asymptomatic or have a mild bleeding disorder (175).

Factor XI is composed of two similar or identical polypeptide chains linked by disulfide bonds. Each chain is approximately 80 kilodaltons, and activation depends on limited proteolytic cleavage by αHFa (16) at an internal peptide bond between Arg-369 and Ile-370 in each chain (59). Both of the 33-kilodalton light chains contain an active serine protease site, whereas the 48-kilodalton heavy chains contain the binding domain for HMWK (114,225). Amino acid sequence studies have shown considerable homology between bovine Factor XI and PK (113), suggesting a possible common origin for these proteins. Human Factor XI shows 58% identity with human plasma PK (59).

Factor XI plays an important role in the intrinsic pathway of blood coagulation. Its major known function is the proteolytic cleavage and activation of Factor IX (38). Other activities that have been reported are the proteolysis and activation of HF (23,71,127) and plasminogen (119), although the weak activity brings into question any biologic importance of these reactions.

MEASURING CONTACT-SYSTEM PROTEINS

Contact proteins may be quantitated by immunologic means or by functional assay.

Functional assays are extremely useful for identifying proteins of the contact system and for their rough quantification. These assays are based on measuring active products of the contact system.

·The most widely used method over recent years has been the activated partial thromboplastin time (PTT) assay (162), using plasmas deficient in the protein of interest. This assay is performed in two stages. In the first stage, a

deficient plasma (as a source of other coagulation proteins) is incubated with an unknown sample and kaolin (or other negatively charged surface) in the absence of calcium. During this stage, contact activation (which is not calcium-dependent) is allowed to proceed for a specific time period. Subsequently, calcium is added to initiate the second, or coagulation, stage of the assay. The rate of coagulation depends on the extent (quantity) of contact activation in the initial stage. Comparison of coagulation times with those of serially diluted normal plasmas allows quantification of the factor of interest. Plasmas deficient in HF or HMWK have extremely prolonged clotting times, whereas plasmas deficient in PK have moderately retarded ones (Fig. 3). Variation in the specific clotting activity of purified contact system proteins may occur, as discussed elsewhere (25).

Use of arginine oligopeptides for assay of contact system proteases has provided a method for accurately and specifically measuring active components (5). A chromogenic or fluorogenic moiety on the carboxyl terminus offers a convenient semiquantitative means of assay. The amino acid sequence of the peptide determines the sensitivity and specificity of the reaction, and the amount of chromophore/fluorophore released allows quantitation. These assays have supplanted similar approaches that measure the esterolytic capacity of the proteases with tosyl-Arg-methyl ester or benzoyl-Arg-ethyl esters (27,73,108).

Bioassays have been used to measure kinin and may be extended to measure PK, kallikrein, βHFa, and HMWK. Bradykinin may be readily measured in bioassays of rat uterus contractions. Although this assay is not quantitative, it appears to be highly specific (54,55).

Immunologic assays for contact proteins have grown in popularity and use in recent years. The radioimmu-

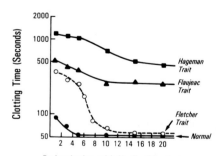

FIG. 3. The clotting times of plasmas deficient in different HF, PK, and HMWK related to the time of preincubation with a negatively charged surface (kaolin) prior to recalcification (stage 1) of the activated partial thromboplastin times. This allows cleavage of HF, and clotting occurs when Ca^{2+} is added to the incubation mixture (stage 2). Prolonged exposure of HMWK-deficient (Fletcher trait) plasma to kaolin completely corrected the clotting deficiency.

noassay (RIA) provides a specific and extremely sensitive assay for measuring proteins of the contact system. At present the RIA has not been effective in differentiating between activated and zymogen protein; however, monoclonal antibody methods undoubtedly will provide antibodies that uniquely recognize the activated components. Western blotting methods also provide a means for identifying activated components in biological fluids. We have used this approach in our laboratories successfully. Activated and cleaved HFa and kallikrein, as well as cleaved HMWK, migrate as heavy and light chains in reduced polyacrylamide gel electrophoresis, and these moieties may be recognized immunologically.

MECHANISMS OF CONTACT ACTIVATION

Four phases of the contact system will be considered in this section: initiation, amplification, propagation, and regulation.

Initiation

The initial phase of contact activation may be induced by negatively charged surfaces or possibly by cellular constituents. A variety of organic and inorganic substances may provide the surface negative charge required for contact activation, as shown in Table 3. Two series of studies have shown the importance of the surface negative charge in contact activation. First, binding of basic dyes to negatively charged surfaces was found to be proportional to the capacity of the surface to promote HF activation and clotting (121). Second, treatment of the negatively charged surface with positively charged compounds was found to inhibit contact activation (45,74,150). It is of interest that purified HF still binds to surfaces pretreated with posi-

TABLE 3. Surfaces responsible for contact activation

Organic substances	Inorganic substances
Monosodium urate crystals	Silica dioxide
Bacterial lipopolysaccharide	Glass
Ellagic acid	Kaolin, celite
Carageenan	Asbestos
Collagen	Calcium pyrophosphate
Vascular basement membrane	crystals
Articular cartilage	
Heparin	
Glycosaminoglycans and	
glycoproteins	
Dextran sulfate	
Skin	
Sulfatides	

tively charged hexadimethrine bromide or with silicone while its activation is inhibited, suggesting that the total amount or density of negative charge may be important (21).

The negatively charged surface appears to play a dual role in promoting contact activation. The four proteins of the contact system are brought into apposition on the surface, triggering their reciprocal activation (see below). HF binds to the surface through the positively charged amino acids of its heavy chain. PK and Factor XI are complexed to HMWK and attached to the surface through the histidine-rich positively charged segment of the light chain of HMWK. Surface binding also increases the susceptibility of HF to cleavage by kallikrein by 500-fold (71). Activation of 0.04% of plasma PK would be sufficient to produce significant activation of HF when the latter is surface bound. It has been proposed that this effect may be related to subtle conformational changes in HF structure. Thus surface binding acts to bring the molecules of the contact system in apposition and to make HF more susceptible to activation.

Crystals

A variety of crystals or particles may promote contact activation. Biologically important crystals such as silica (and silicates), monosodium urate (MSU), calcium pyrophosphate dihydrate (CPPD), and hypoxanthine (HX) have been shown to activate contact system factors. In a series of studies, Kellermeyer and Breckenridge (99–101) demonstrated the ability of MSU crystals to activate HF. Ginsberg et al. (65) provided a molecular understanding of this reaction, demonstrating the cleavage of [^{125}I]HF in joint fluids exposed to MSU crystals into the two activation products αHFa and βHFa.

Collagen and Vascular Basement Membrane

The extravascular space is a prime site for activation of the contact system because the connective tissues are rich in negatively charged components. Initial studies suggested that HF was bound to, and possibly activated by, human or bovine collagen (81,149,249), although other studies, utilizing highly purified triple-helical collagen failed to confirm these findings (58,70).

Preparations of vascular basement membrane bound and, after addition of PK, activated HF; this effect was blocked by addition of hexadimethrine bromide. Others have found that a variety of components of basement membrane, including type I, III, and IV collagen alone or mixed with proteoglycans, do not activate HF in normal plasma (70).

Glycosaminoglycans and Glycoproteins

Sulfated polysaccharides (such as dextran sulfate) and glycosaminoglycans have been reported to initiate activation of the contact system and release of kinins (43,102,129,196). Recently, Hojima and co-workers (87) tested a number of negatively charged macromolecules for their ability to activate the contact system *in vitro*, using highly purified materials. These investigators found that native connective tissue matrix glycosaminoglycans and proteoglycans were inactive; however, when chondroitin sulfate was further sulfated, it gained activity in their assay system. Naturally occurring heparin glycosaminoglycans from several sources, as well as chondroitin sulfate E, were effective in inducing activation of the contact system. Chemical modification by β-elimination of the heparin chains from the native proteoglycan macromolecule did not abrogate its activity, indicating that the 60- to 80-kilodalton glycosaminoglycan subunits were required for the interaction with HF.

Bacterial Lipopolysaccharide (LPS)

Several studies have suggested that LPS may activate HF in plasma (see, e.g., ref. 104). Morrison and Cochrane (136) studied LPS, which is comprised of polysaccharide and lipid-rich areas linked to a heptose backbone, and demonstrated the importance of the lipid-rich portion in HF activation. The lipid-rich area consists of two glucosamines linked to lipid side chains and phosphate groups; the latter appear to provide the negative charge required to bind and activate HF.

Immune Complexes

Early reports suggested that antibody-antigen complexes supported contact activation and kinin generation (see 2). However, extensive studies using highly purified components failed to confirm this finding (22).

Other Factors

A variety of particles or crystals have been found to support contact activation, including glass, kaolin, and celite. Soluble macromolecules also may lead to HF activation, including dextran sulfate and micelles of sulfatides (58,87,113). DNA does not support activation of HF or PK (87).

The *triggering event* in activation of HF has been the subject of intense study in several laboratories, and this will be discussed below.

AMPLIFICATION

Following the initial burst of HF activity, a series of events occur which serve to amplify the reaction and generate significantly increased amounts of active HF, kallikrein, and bradykinin (24). Studies of this phase of contact system activation have focused primarily on the molecular events leading to the assembly of contact system proenzymes on a negatively charged surface and their subsequent activation.

As noted above, HF binds to the surface through positively charged regions on its heavy chain. PK and Factor XI, linked noncovalently to HMWK in bimolecular complexes (118,220), are bound to the surface through the positively charged histidine-rich segment of HMWK. Surface binding serves to maintain the close spatial orientation of proenzyme PK, HF, and Factor XI and to augment activation probably via conformational changes in HF. HMWK functions as a nonenzymatic cofactor in this reaction, producing a 20- to 30-fold increase in the rate of HFa and kallikrein formation (72,246). HMWK also enhances βHFa-induced generation of kallikrein in fluid phase (117). The optimal concentration of HMWK required for such effects is equimolar to HF concentration (72,117), suggesting a stoichiometric relationship between these molecules on the surface.

Whereas HMWK readily binds to the negatively charged surface in normal plasma, binding is markedly reduced in HF-deficient plasma (199,214). It has been suggested that HMWK cleavage, possibly induced by HFa, may be necessary for surface binding of PK and Factor XI (32).

On the surface, HFa cleaves PK to kallikrein and Factor XI to Factor XIa. Kallikrein then reciprocally activates HF, as illustrated in Fig. 4. Recently it has been shown that Factor XIa is capable of cleaving HMWK, causing the release of bradykinin and formation of two chain HMWK (202). Factor XIa rapidly cleaves the light chain of HMWK which results in loss of biologic activity (202), leading to speculation that this reaction may liberate Factor XIa (from the HMWK complex) to activate Factor IX and the coagulation cascade (199,202).

The *initial or triggering* event in activation of the contact system has been the subject of considerable speculation. There is now ample evidence that surface-bound HF and PK in the presence of HMWK interact to produce a rapid burst of activity generating active HF and kallikrein. The nature of this burst is uncertain at this time (25). It is absent in PK- or HMWK-deficient plasma, although contact activation does proceed slowly in these plasmas (Fig. 3). Although it is possible that zymogen HF is itself weakly active, several investigators have suggested that autoactivation of surface-bound HF may occur (248), since single-chain HF, adsorbed to a surface at optimal

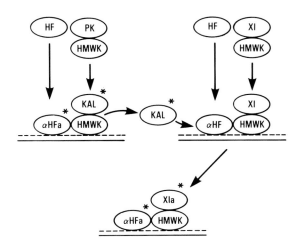

FIG. 4. Molecular model of the assembly of contact-system proteins on a negatively charged surface. HF binds to the surface through positively charged areas on its heavy chain. PK and Factor XI are noncovalently linked to HMWK in bimolecular complexes and are bound to the surface through the positively charged histidine-rich segment of HMWK. Binding of these factors to a surface brings them into apposition and enhances HF susceptibility to proteolysis. HF and PK are reciprocally activated (asterisk denotes presence of an active serine protease) on the surface. Kallikrein is released from the surface and may propagate activities of the contact system. HF may be cleaved to αHFa (which remains surface bound) or to βHFa (which also is released into the fluid phase, further disseminating certain activities of the contact system).

concentrations, slowly undergoes proteolytic cleavage (248). Silverberg et al. (208) confirmed this observation and suggested that small amounts of HF existed in the αHFa form. Alternatively the initial phase of contact activation may be due to a low level of PK (kallikrein) activity or another as-yet unidentified enzyme.

In a recent study, Rosing et al. (179) studied the surface-dependent activation of HF by kallikrein or by the light chain of kallikrein which bears its enzyme-active site. These authors found that fluid-phase kallikrein and the light chain of kallikrein were equally effective in activating HF. Surface binding greatly increased HFa formation by both kallikrein and its light chain, although kallikrein was found to be much more active than its light chain. Their data suggested that surface binding stimulates kallikrein-dependent HF activation through two mechanisms: (a) increased susceptibility to kallikrein and (b) enhanced formation of an enzyme-substrate complex.

DISSEMINATION

The question remained as to whether the active components of the contact system remained surface bound or could be propagated to other surface sites or released into fluid phase. Such dissemination of active products of the contact system into fluid phase is potentially important in mediating biologic reactions. Data have shown that surface-bound PK/kallikrein is released rapidly, since over 80% of formed kallikrein is found in the fluid phase within 5 min (26,173). In contrast only 20% of Factor XIa was released under identical conditions. Other studies, using PK-deficient (Fletcher trait) plasmas have demonstrated the importance of PK/kallikrein in the expression of contact system functions (90,241). Reconstitution of Fletcher trait plasma with PK or kallikrein restored its clotting, fibrinolytic, and kinin-generating activities. Addition of HFa, but not zymogen HF, restored the clotting and fibrinolytic activities but not the ability to liberate kinin from HMWK.

In the fluid phase, kallikrein has a number of substrates. However, the significance of these reactions is uncertain because the reaction rates are very slow and most have been demonstrated only with purified components. Kallikrein directly converts plasminogen to plasmin (31), although the reaction appears to be too slow to account for accelerated clot lysis. HFa and Factor XIa also convert plasminogen to plasmin, but the physiologic importance of these reactions is uncertain (133). Plasma kallikrein and HFa convert plasma prorenin to renin *in vitro* under conditions that suggest that this is not a physiologically important reaction (204). Conversion does not occur upon addition of kallikrein to whole plasma (166). Kallikrein cleaves C5 to C5a in the rabbit (244), producing chemotactic and secretagogue activity.

βHFa also is liberated from the negatively charged surface into the fluid phase during contact activation. βHFa may cleave HF to αHFa or βHFa, PK to kallikrein, and coagulation Factor VII to Factor VIIa. The effects of βHFa appear to be of lesser importance than kallikrein in the fluid phase (25).

REGULATION

Regulation of the contact system may occur at the negatively charged surface or following the generation of active enzymes.

Inhibition of Surface Activation

Surface activation may be inhibited or blocked by the presence of other plasma proteins or cationic molecules. Adsorption of these molecules to the surface, with resulting competition for binding with HF or HMWK, probably explains this effect. Purified IgG or albumin at plasma concentrations were about half as effective as whole plasma in inhibiting [¹²⁵I]HF binding to kaolin particles (22,23). Kozin and co-workers (111,112) studied adsorption of various serum proteins to MSU, CPPD, silica, and other crystals and demonstrated the relative efficiency of binding to these negatively charged surfaces.

Small positively charged molecules, such as hexadimethrine bromide, were found to prevent HF activation but did not prevent binding to a surface (21). Although this effect is not well understood, it has been hypothesized that the density of negative charge may be reduced to the extent that the conformational change(s) needed for activation cannot take place. Alternatively, the presence of adsorbed molecules may interfere with the assembly of the contact proteins on the surface.

Inhibition of Specific Activated Components (Table 4)

Activated HF (HFa)

C1 inhibitor (C1inh) is the primary inhibitor of HFa in normal human plasma. Evidence is available to show that C1inh inhibits both βHFa and αHFa (25). C1inh blocked βHFa("HF fragments" or HFf)-induced generation of kinin in plasma in a dose- and time-dependent manner (195). In addition, complexes of C1inh and βHFa have been found in a 1:1 stoichiometric relationship (174). C1inh appears to account for over 90% of the HFa inhibitory activity in plasma (39,160). This effect was not enhanced significantly by addition of heparin (161).

However, in C1inh-deficient plasma, HFa was complexed by antithrombin III in a reaction that was augmented by heparin (160,211). Both forms of HFa may be complexed to antithrombin III in a 1:1 stoichiometric reaction (211). Other plasma proteinase inhibitors, including α2-macroglobulin, α1-antitrypsin, and α2-antiplasmin, have been reported to possess little to no inhibitory activity toward HFa (19,183,195,211).

Kallikrein

C1 inhibitor and, to a lesser extent, α2-macroglobulin are the principal inhibitors of plasma kallikrein (80). C1inh and kallikrein form a 1:1 stoichiometric complex and follow second order kinetics (64). Interestingly, whereas α2-macroglobulin forms a complex with kallikrein and blocks its kinin generating activity, the esterolytic activity of kallikrein is only modestly (about 50%) reduced (80). It has been estimated that C1inh accounts for inhibition of over 50% of kallikrein activity in plasma (79,189,226), and α2-macroglobulin may account for 30% to 50% of the inhibitory activity, depending on assay conditions (79,189,226). At 4°C, 85% of kallikrein is bound to α2-macroglobulin (79).

Antithrombin III and α1-antitrypsin also inhibit kallikrein activity, although the importance of these reactions in whole plasma is uncertain.

Factor XIa

Factor XIa is inhibited by C1inh in a time- and dose-dependent manner (51), although C1inh accounts for only about 20% of the inhibitory activity of normal plasma (168). Factor XIa is the only contact-system serine protease that is not inhibited primarily by C1inh. It has been reported that α1-proteinase inhibitor is the major plasma inhibitor of Factor XIa, accounting for about 67% of plasma inhibitory activity (198). Antithrombin III, complexed with heparin, also has inhibitory activity toward Factor XIa, and although earlier studies suggested that it accounted for 40% of plasma inhibitory activity (37), more recent data question its significance (222).

Other Inhibitors

A number of protease inhibitors derived from plants, animal tissues, or microbial agents have been reported. These inhibitors, which may be quite specific and useful in laboratory experiments, are listed in Table 5.

Possible Role of HMWK

HMWK also may modulate inhibition of the active-contact protein enzymes by forming fluid-phase nonco-

TABLE 4. Plasma inhibition of contact-system proteases[a]

Inhibitor	Molecular weight (kilodaltons)	Factors inhibited			
		HFa	PKa	XIa	Plasmin
C1 inhibitor	96–105	+++	++	++	?
α2 Plasmin inhibitor (α2 antiplasmin)	65–70	+	−	−	+++
α2 Macroglobulin	725	+	++	−	?
Antithrombin III	58	+	+	+	?
α1 Antitrypsin inhibitor (α1 antiprotease)	53	−	+	+++	?

[a] Data from Cochrane and Griffin (25) and Travis and Salvesen (222).

TABLE 5. *Other inhibitor of contact-system proteases*[a]

Inhibitor	Molecular weight	Active-site sequence	Factors inhibited[b]			
			HFa	PKa	XIa	Plasmin
Plant inhibitors						
Soybean (SBTI)	21,500	Pro-Ser-Tyr-Chg[64]-Ile-Arg-Phe-Ile	−	+	+	+
Lima bean (LBTI)	8,000–10,000	Leu-Ala/Ser-Thy-Lys[Frommhagen (53)]-Ser-Ile-Pro-Pro	+	−	−	+
Corn	11,000–14,000	Ile-Pro-Gly-Arg[Fonnum and Walaas (50)]-Leu-Pro-Pro-Leu	+	−	−	−
Pumpkin	3,000–4,000		+	?	−	±
Microbial inhibitors						
Leupeptin	427	Ac-Leu-Leu-Arg	+	?	+	+
Antipain		Phe-Co-Arg-Val-Arg	?	?	−	±
Animal inhibitors						
Trasylol	6,000		±	+	+	+
Orosomucoid	28,000	X-X-X-Arg-Ala-X-X-X	−	−	−	−
Chemical inhibitors						
(DFP) Diisopropyl-phosphofluoridate 184			+	+	+	+
(PMSF) Phenyl-methyl-sulfonyl fluoride 174			+	?	−	?
(TLCK) Tosyl-lysine chloromethyl ketone 336			−	−	−	+

[a] Data from Cochrane and Griffin (25).
[b] ?, Not tested.

valent adducts with kallikrein and Factor XIa. It has been shown that HMWK reduces the rate of inactivation of kallikrein and Factor XIa by their primary plasma proteinase inhibitors (120,187,190). However, other studies failed to confirm these observations (227). HMWK has been found to reduce the rate of kallikrein inactivation by α2-macroglobulin (190,228).

CELLULAR ACTIVATION OF THE CONTACT SYSTEM

Leukocytes

Human neutrophils, and to a lesser extent eosinophils, are capable of generating kinin activity and concomitantly degrading kininogen from normal human plasma (131,132). Two pH optima were observed for this reaction: One is at neutral pH, and the other one is at pH 5 or below. This reaction is not supported by HF-deficient plasma, although a kininogenase activity was present in the media of cultured neutrophils. These observations have not been confirmed, however.

Lysosomal enzymes released from human neutrophils through antigen-antibody reactions reportedly cleave both high- and low-molecular-weight kininogen with the generation of kinin-like activity (138,139). Elastase was initially thought to be the responsible enzyme, although a series of recent studies (25) suggest the involvement of other enzymes. These studies also have not been confirmed.

In a series of experiments that will be discussed more fully below, Newball et al. (143–146) found that basophils release a kallikrein-like substance after stimulation with anti-IgE antibodies or specific antigens to which individuals were known to be allergic. Release of these enzymes paralleled histamine liberation. The kallikrein-like material had arginine-esterase kininogenase activity but differed from plasma kallikrein.

Endothelial Cells

Bovine and rabbit endothelial cells contain an enzyme, as yet unidentified, that cleaves and activates HF *in vitro* (243). Cleavage occurs within the disulfide loop (see Fig. 1), producing HFa capable of cleaving PK and Factor XI.

Platelets

The role of platelets in contact activation is based primarily on unconfirmed *in vitro* studies. Walsh (235) demonstrated that ADP-stimulated platelets could shorten the clotting of platelet-rich plasma in a contact-system-dependent reaction. Using washed human platelets and purified radiolabeled HF and Factor XI, platelets were found to promote the proteolytic cleavage of HF by kallikrein as well as the activation of Factor XI by both HF-dependent and independent mechanisms (237). However, recent studies by Kodama and Weerasinghe and their co-workers (109,239,240) failed to support these findings; they found that several cationic platelet proteins, including platelet factor 4, actually inhibited negatively charged surface-induced contact activation.

Specific high-affinity binding sites for Factor XI and Factor XIa have been identified on the surface of activated platelets (209). The sites for Factor XI and Factor XIa were distinct. HMWK was required for binding of these coagulation factors (209), and it has been shown that HMWK itself binds to specific receptors in a reaction potentiated by calcium or zinc (68). Walsh et al. (234) reported that platelet-bound Factor XIa was functionally and structurally identical to fluid-phase Factor XIa. However, others have found that platelets and platelet components inhibit Factor-XIa-induced activation of Factor IX (210).

Factor XI activity and Factor XI antigen (with a different molecular weight than in plasma) have been found in platelets (223). HMWK also was identified in platelets and was secreted after stimulation (194). It has been suggested that the binding of these factors to platelets may help localize procoagulant reactions and may protect activated factors from plasma proteinase inhibitors. These issues regarding the interaction of platelets and contact factors have recently been reviewed (236).

CELLULAR EFFECTS OF THE CONTACT SYSTEM

Neutrophil Chemotaxis

There have been several reports which show that human kallikrein induced chemotactic responses, superoxide anion generation, and lysosomal enzyme release in neutrophils (95,188,192,232). Recently, using highly purified preparations, Wiggins et al. (244) found that rabbit kallikrein did not induce neutrophil chemotaxis. Addition of complement C5 to the media restored the chemotactic effect, suggesting that a product of C5, possibly C5a, was responsible for this property. These data were obtained with purified rabbit components. In our laboratory, attempts to induce stimulation of neutrophils with human kallikrein have been uniformly unsuccessful. Aggregation, calcium translocation, and superoxide anion and lysosomal enzyme release could not be effected by kallikrein (or HFa). Kallikrein did not inhibit these functions induced by unrelated stimuli (e.g., formyl peptides). A resolution of these disparate results is not apparent.

REACTIONS WITH OTHER PLASMA PROTEINS

Complement System

Components of the contact system may react with complement proteins, generating additional phlogistic factors. It has been reported that βHFa, but not HF or αHFa, activates the classical complement pathway through C1 activation (62), although the significance of this *in-vitro* reaction has not been demonstrated. This reaction was found to be enzymatically mediated, since specific active-enzyme-site inhibitors blocked the effect of βHFa (63). The complement pathway also may be activated by kallikrein which generates a C5a-like chemotactic peptide from C5 (244). The interaction of the complement and contact systems may be of importance in hereditary angioedema and gouty arthritis (see following).

Prostaglandins

Bradykinin has been shown to augment arachidonic acid release from cells (125). In tissues, stimulation of bradykinin receptors may cause activation of phospholipases A2 and C (9,147), release of prostaglandins (88,125,135), and intracellular accumulation of cyclic adenosine monophosphate (cAMP) and cyclic guanosine monophosphate (cGMP) (6,212). Human fibroblasts and other cells (116) have specific bradykinin receptors (177), and binding leads to prostacyclin (PGI$_2$) (178) and prostaglandin E$_2$ (116) formation. Cultured human endothelial cells also synthesize prostacyclin and platelet-activating factor when stimulated with bradykinin (126).

Synovial Fluid Collagenase

Nagase has identified plasma kallikrein as a potentially important activator of latent collagenase in rheumatoid synovial fluid (142).

PATHOPHYSIOLOGIC ACTIVITIES OF CONTACT SYSTEM

Hageman Factor

Increased Vascular Permeability

For many years, it has been known that HF was required for generation of a permeability factor when plasma is exposed to glass (25). A number of studies suggested that HFa itself was this permeability factor. Purified HFa was shown to possess potent activity in increasing skin permeability in a guinea-pig model; it was found that HFa was 10- to 100-fold more active than bradykinin in this assay (256). HFa was shown to be identical to the permeability factor extracted from guinea-pig skin (255).

Hypotension

When intravenous infusions of albumin were found to result in hypotension or circulatory collapse (12,82,83), a study of the causative agent(s) was undertaken. Kallikrein and bradykinin were not found in these preparations, but the following evidence suggested the active factor to be βHFa: (a) its physical properties, (b) its ability to activate PK, and (c) its inhibition by anti-HF antibodies (3). Subsequently, immunoglobulin preparations were found to contain active contact system factors (4). However, Eibl (44) questioned the importance of these factors in producing systemic reactions.

Leukocyte Accumulation

Although extensive data are not available, studies by Graham (66) suggested that human HF may induce leukocyte margination.

High-Molecular-Weight Kininogen

Vascular Permeability

Bradykinin (BK) is a nonapeptide liberated from HMWK by the action of plasma kallikrein. This peptide has a number of biologic effects, including increases in vascular permeability, smooth muscle contraction, diminished arterial resistance and hypotension, leukocyte margination, increased intestinal motility, chloride secretion, and pain. These effects have been reviewed extensively elsewhere and will not be discussed in detail here (159,170).

Injection of BK into skin causes vasodilation and increased vascular permeability. These effects resemble those of histamine; however, there is no axon reflex so that the area of erythema is less and a burning pain is present rather than pruritis (96).

BK is rapidly inactivated by two proteases (kininases). Carboxypeptidase N (kininase I) cleaves the carboxy-terminal arginine from BK, yielding an inactive octapeptide (des-Arg-BK) (48). Carboxypeptidase N is the same enzyme that inactivates the anaphylatoxins C3a, C4a, and C5a generated through complement activation. The second enzyme, a dipeptidase (kininase II), cleaves the carboxy-terminal Phe-Arg to yield a septapeptide that is further degraded to a pentapeptide (257,258). This dipeptidase is identical to angiotensin-converting enzyme (257), and it appears to be most active in the pulmonary vascular bed (96).

Other kinins also exist in biological fluids. Action of tissue or glandular kallikrein (which is immunologically and chemically distinct from plasma kallikrein) on low-molecular-weight kininogen (LMWK) releases lysylbradykinin (kallidin or Lys-BK). The lysine is cleaved from this product by a plasma carboxypeptidase to yield BK. BK is degraded further by the kininases described above. However, carboxypeptidase N may remove the C-terminal arginine directly from Lys-BK, resulting in inactive des-Arg-Lys-BK (207).

Enhanced vascular permeability also may be produced by fragment 1-2 of HMWK. Fragment 1-2, the histidine-rich residue of HMWK, is liberated by the action of kallikrein on bovine, but not human, HMWK. Intradermal injection of fragment 1-2 or fragment 2 alone enhances vascular permeability, although this effect is about 100-fold less potent than that produced by bradykinin (123). Similar observations were made in rabbits (153).

Contact System and Renin Angiotensin System

The contact system and renin angiotensin system bear a number of interesting relationships. Bradykinin is hypotensive, whereas angiotensin II is hypertensive. The dipeptidase-converting enzyme inactivates bradykinin, whereas it converts the less active angiotensin I to the more active angiotensin II.

Angiotensin I is generated from angiotensinogen through the action of plasma renin. Renin circulates in plasma as a proenzyme, prorenin, which may be activated by trypsin, plasmin, urinary kallikrein, or plasma kallikrein (34,40,203). Prorenin also may be activated by cooling or acidifying plasma (203), conditions that result in activation of kallikrein.

It has been proposed that contact system proteins are essential for *in-vitro* activation of prorenin (41,134, 155,156,205). Addition of kallikrein to HF-deficient plasma restores its ability to activate prorenin, but addition of βHFa to PK-deficient plasma is not effective in activating prorenin (41,205). These data indicate that kallikrein is primarily responsible for prorenin activation, whereas HF probably acts through PK.

The pathophysiologic significance of these interactions is unknown. The recent observation of Blumberg et al. (13), demonstrating that kaolin-activated plasma does not necessarily lead to prorenin activation, indicates the lack of clarity in this area (13). These data suggest that the role of contact system proteases is minor and seen only under experimental conditions.

CONTACT SYSTEM IN HUMAN DISEASE

The pathogenic role of components of the contact system in human disorders may be difficult to recognize. The following criteria must be met in order to implicate these factors in disease:

1. Demonstration of changes in concentration of various contact-system proteins in plasma or biological fluids. These changes should be related to levels of reference proteins to avoid errors caused by hemoconcentration or dilution.

2. Evidence of activation of the components through functional assays of activity, proteolytic cleavage of components at specific sites, binding of activated components to inhibitor proteins, or other methods.
3. Localization of activated components at the site of inflammatory tissue injury.
4. Modification of the inflammatory reaction by removal of specific components of the contact system or by specific inhibition of the component (in experimental animals).

Arthritis

There is considerable evidence to suggest a role for the contact system in arthritis. Synovial fluid is known to contain components of the contact system required for full activity (99,101,186). Negatively charged factors that may activate the contact system are found in joint fluids, including chondroitin sulfate, articular cartilage components (137), or microcrystals. Synovial fluid from patients with arthritis contains elevated kinin levels (98,131), and synovial fluids from patients with active rheumatoid arthritis have reduced levels of HMWK (185).

Intra-articular infusion of bradykinin in dogs results in increased pain and warmth, reaching a peak in 10 min, but it does not produce an accumulation of leukocytes. Bradykinin was more potent in increasing synovial vascular permeability than were prostaglandin E_1 (10^{-1}) and histamine (10^{-2}) (69). Similar studies of other activated components of the contact system have not been reported. Injection of microcrystalline monosodium urate in a volunteer with gout resulted in a severe local arthritis and a rapid rise in bradykinin concentration (238). Injection of urate crystals in rat paws produced edema that slowly increased and peaked in 6 hr; pretreatment by intraperitoneal soybean trypsin inhibitor or infusion of carboxypeptidase B significantly reduced the edema formation (238). The importance of these observations has been questioned, because others found no decrease in intra-articular pressure or leukocyte accumulation by pretreatment with carboxypeptidase B, effective in inhibiting bradykinin-induced edema (157). In addition, spontaneous gouty arthritis may develop in chickens lacking contact factors (33), and gout and rheumatoid arthritis have been observed in HF-deficient subjects (42,67).

Allergic and Anaphylactic Reactions

Because of its inherent effects on smooth muscle and vascular permeability, bradykinin (BK) has long been suspected of playing a role in the pathogenesis of asthma and allergic reactions. This view was supported by studies, demonstrating that BK, administered by inhalation, provoked bronchospasm in asthmatic patients but not in normal subjects (60,85,230). Pinckard and co-workers (76,158) found that the whole-blood clotting time was initially shortened and then prolonged in rabbits immunized to produce IgE antibodies and then challenged with antigen. This was associated with a decrease in the functional activity of HF and Factors XI and IX.

Proud et al. (164) were the first to provide direct evidence of BK involvement in the local inflammatory response when they demonstrated elevated levels of kinins in nasal secretions of atopic subjects following challenge with allergen. In these experiments, the increased kinin levels correlated with the development of symptoms, release of histamine, appearance of esterolytic activity (164), and secretion of glandular kallikrein (7,8). Cold dry air and rhinovirus infection also were found to produce increased kinin concentrations in nasal lavage (140,221). Recently, Christiansen (20) identified a unique tissue kallikrein as well as lysyl-bradykinin in bronchoalveolar lavage (BAL) fluids of asthmatic patients. This enzyme releases lysyl-bradykinin from kininogen *in vitro*. Its only inhibitor in plasma and BAL fluid appears to be associated with α1-proteinase inhibitor, which produces only a slow inhibition.

In studies cited above, Newball and co-workers (143–146) found that lung fragments, lung mast cells, and circulating basophils released enzymes upon allergic challenge which were capable of cleaving HF, PK, and HMWK. Purified lung mast cells release a kininogenase on IgE stimulation (165), and Meier putatively identified the enzyme released from lung as a neutral serine protease (128).

Rothschild demonstrated that epinephrine-treated rat peritoneal mast cells released an enzyme which had arginine esterolytic activity and which depleted total kinin-releasing activity in plasma (180). Seppa (206) demonstrated a similar or identical enzyme in isolated rat mast cells immunohistochemically. In addition to enzyme activities generated by mast cells and basophils, these cells contain and release negatively charged sulfated glycosaminoglycans and proteoglycans (154,259), which may augment contact activation.

These observations suggest that the contact system may play a role in allergic and anaphylactic reactions. The majority of data have been obtained in *in vitro* experiments. In rabbits the data are indirect.

Bacteremic Shock

Diminished levels of PK have been observed in sepsis by a number of investigators (2,30,86,122,151,176) along with a fall in kallikrein inhibitory activity (2,122,151). In patients with typhoid fever, activation of PK has been suggested by the appearance of arginine esterase activity in plasma and C1inh-kallikrein complexes; however, there was no change in PK or HF levels, and HMWK concentration was increased (30). In patients with endotoxic shock, plasma levels of HF (122) and kininogen (2,86) were decreased, and free kinin was detected (2).

In experimental hypotensive shock, a fall in kininogen level and appearance of free kinin have been correlated with a fall in peripheral arterial resistance in rhesus monkeys (148) and in monkeys infected with *S. typhimurium* (250). Similar changes have been described in dogs (1,61). Whereas initial studies in rabbits reported a fall in kininogen in endotoxic shock (47), later studies failed to demonstrate a fall in human [^{125}I]kininogen or cleavage of circulating [^{125}I]kininogen despite severe shock (21). Purified HF and PK are readily activated through interaction with bacterial lipopolysaccharide (LPS) *in vitro* (92,136) or cell wall fractions (92), and this may be the mechanism of contact-system activation.

Another possible mechanism of contact-system activation is through the proteolytic activity of bacterial enzymes. Matsumoto (124) has shown that a 56-kilodalton protease produced by *Serratia maresceus* activated HF *in vitro*. This enzyme produced enhanced vascular permeability and edema in a guinea-pig model, and evidence suggests that this effect is mediated by bradykinin (94).

In summary, there is reason to suspect a role for the contact system in bacterial or LPS-induced hypotensive shock because edema, hypotension, and coagulopathy are features of this syndrome. In a recent study to assess the role of contact and complement components in bacteremia and bacteremic shock, Kalter et al. (93) measured the level of these proteins in patients' plasmas. They found no change in concentration in uncomplicated bacteremia but found a statistically significant fall in plasma levels in nonfatal (approximately 50–70%) or fatal (30–50%) bacteremic shock (93). Although plasma protein levels also were diminished, the authors found that contact-system proteins were reduced disproportionately. It was proposed that these findings represented consumption of the contact-system components, although no evidence of activated or cleaved factors was sought.

Hereditary Angioedema (HAE)

HAE, inherited as an autosomal dominant trait, is characterized by recurrent episodes of abdominal pain and mucocutaneous swelling which may be provoked by physical or emotional trauma (52). Patients lack functional C1 inhibitor, an important regulatory protein for control of the classical complement pathway and contact system as discussed above. C1inh inhibits HFa and kallikrein as well as C1. Curd et al. (36) induced suction blisters in subjects with HAE and in normal volunteers and found that blisters from HAE, but not normal, subjects contained large amounts of active kallikrein. Our

studies have shown that these blister fluids also contain large amounts of cleaved HMWK (110). Others have found that plasma levels of PK and HMWK, but not HF, Factor XI, or Factor IX, were reduced when patients with HAE were symptomatic (191). Circulating HMWK also was found to be cleaved during active angioedema, using sensitive immunoblotting techniques (11).

These findings suggest that there is contact-system activation during attacks in patients with HAE. The initiating event is unclear, although minor trauma may cause activation of HF, resulting in reciprocal activation of kallikrein. Recent studies have suggested that C1inh rapidly inactivates HFa produced through the "auto-activation" reaction but does not block initial surface-induced HF cleavage (242).

Renal Disorders and Blood Pressure Regulation

Diminished HF and PK concentrations and activation of the intrinsic coagulation and fibrinolytic systems have been found in subjects with nephrotic syndrome (91,115,229,231). In addition, HF has been identified on the glomerular basement membrane in subjects with membranous glomerulonephritis (10). Evidence of contact-system activation has been found in human renal allograft rejection (28) and in primate models of this reaction (18).

Wiggins (247) recently studied the role of contact activation in an experimental model in sensitized rabbits in which glomerulonephritis was induced by injection of guinea-pig IgG. [^{125}I]HF was found in Bowman's space, and cleaved [^{125}I]HF was present in the urine. Wiggins (247) suggested that HF passively crossed the damaged glomular basement membrane, became activated in Bowman's space, initiated the intrinsic coagulation cascade, and led to fibrin deposition.

These studies support, but provide little to no direct evidence of, a role for the contact system in renal glomerulopathy.

The importance of contact-system components in blood pressure regulation also remains controversial. Plasma prorenin may be converted to renin by neutral serine proteases after cooling or acidification (see above). However, kallikrein is able to cleave partially purified plasma prorenin (167). The renin-angiotensin and kallikrein-kinin interactions are complex and not well understood. These have been discussed more fully above and have been reviewed recently by Scicli and Carretero (197).

Other Disorders

Components of the contact system or activation of the contact system have been linked to a number of disorders. In the *postgastrectomy dumping syndrome,* increased plasma kinin levels and diminished kininogen concentrations have been found following oral ingestion of hypertonic glucose; similar findings are not present in control subjects (251). These biochemical changes corresponded with development of symptoms and fall in blood pressure. In the *carcinoid syndrome,* significant increases in hepatic venous blood kinin concentrations have been reported following catecholamine-induced flushes (130,152).

REFERENCES

1. Aasen, A. O., Frolish, W., Saugstad, O. D., and Amundsen, E. (1978): Plasma kallikrein activity and prekallikrein levels during endotoxic shock in dogs. *Eur. Surg. Res.,* 10:50.
2. Aasen, A. O., Gallimore, M. J., Lyngass, K., Larsbrasten, M., Amundsen, E., and Smith, N. (1979): In: *Proceedings of the VIIth International Congress on Thrombosis and Haemostasis,* p. 253.
3. Alving, B. M., Hojima, Y., Pisano, J. J., Mason, B. M., Buckingham, R. E., Mozen, M. M., and Finlayson, J. S. (1978): Hypotension associated with prekallikrein activator (Hageman-factor fragments) in plasma protein fraction. *N. Engl. J. Med.,* 299:66–70.
4. Alving, B. M., Tankersley, D. L., Mason, B. L., Rossi, F., Aronson, D. L., and Finlayson, J. S. (1980): Contact-activated factors: Contaminants of immunoglobulin preparations with coagulant and vasoactive properties. *J. Lab. Clin. Med.,* 96:334–346.
5. Amundsen, E., Svendsen, L., Vennerod, A. M., and Laake, K. (1974): Determination of plasma kallikrein with a new chromogenic tripeptide derivative. In: *Chemistry and Biology of the Kallikrein-Kinin in Health and Disease,* edited by J. J. Pisano and K. F. Austen, p. 215. DHEW Publication No. NIH 76-791.
6. Bareis, I. L., Manganiello, V. C., Hirato, F., Vaughan, M., and Axelrod, J. (1983): Bradykinin stimulates phospholipid methylation, calcium influx, prostaglandin formation and cAMP accumulation in human fibroblasts. *Proc. Natl. Acad. Sci. USA,* 80:2514–2518.
7. Baumgarten, C. R., Nichols, R. C., Naclerio, R. M., Lichtenstein, L. M., Norman, P. S., and Proud, D. (1986): Plasma kallikrein during experimentally induced allergic rhinitis: Role in kinin formation and contribution to TAME-esterase activity in nasal secretions. *J. Immunol.,* 137:977–982.
8. Baumgarten, C. R., Nichols, R. C., Naclerio, R. M., and Proud, D. (1986): Concentrations of glandular kallikrein in human nasal secretions increase during experimentally induced allergic rhinitis. *J. Immunol.,* 137:1323–1328.
9. Bell, R. J., Baenzinger, N. J., and Majerus, D. W. (1980): Bradykinin-stimulated release of arachidonate from phosphatidylinositol in mouse fibrosarcoma cells. *Prostaglandins,* 20:269–274.
10. Berger, J., and Yaneva, H. (1982): Hageman factor deposition in membranous glomerulopathy. *Transplant. Proc.,* 14:472–473.
11. Berrettini, M., Lammle, B., White, T., Heeb, M. J., Schwarz, H. P., Zuraw, B., Curd, J. G., and Griffin, J. H. (1986): Detection of *in vitro* and *in vivo* cleavage of high molecular weight kininogen in human plasma by immunoblotting with monoclonal antibodies. *Blood,* 68:455–462.
12. Bland, J. H. L., Lauer, M. D., and Lowenstein, F. (1973): Vasodilator effect of commercial 5% plasma protein fraction solutions. *JAMA,* 224:1721–1724.
13. Blumberg, J. H. L., Sealey, J. E., Atlas, S. A., Laragh, J. H., Dharingrongartama, B., and Kaplan, A. P. (1981): Contact activation of human plasma *in vitro. J. Lab. Clin. Med.,* 97:771–778.
14. Bouma, B. N., Miles, L. A., Baretta, G., and Griffin, J. H. (1980): Human plasma prekallikrein. Studies of its activation by activated Factor XII and of its inactivation by diasopropyl phosphofluoridate. *Biochemistry,* 19:1151–1160.
15. Bouma, B. N., Kerbiriou, D. M., Vlooswijk, R., and Griffin, J. H. (1980): Immunologic studies of prekallikrein, kallikrein and high molecular weight kininogen in normal and deficient plasmas and in normal plasma after cold-dependent activation. *J. Lab. Clin. Med.,* 96:693–709.

16. Bouma, B. N., and Griffin, J. H. (1977): Human blood coagulation Factor XI. Purification, properties, and mechanism of activation by activated Factor XII. *J. Biol. Chem.,* 252:6432–6437.
17. Burrowes, L. E., Movat, H. Z., and Soltay, M. J. (1972): The kinin system of human plasma. VI. The action of plasmin. *Proc. Soc. Exp. Biol. Med.,* 135:959–966.
18. Busch, G. J., Martinins, A. C. P., Hollenberg, N. K., Wilson, R. E., and Colman, R. W. (1975): A primate model of hyperacute renal allograft rejection. *Am. J. Pathol.,* 79:31–56.
19. Chan, J. Y. C., Burrowes, C. E., Habel, F. H., and Movat, H. Z. (1977): The inhibition of activated Factor XI (Hageman factor) by antithrombin III. The effect of other plasma proteinase inhibitors. *Biochem. Biophys. Res. Commun.,* 74:150–158.
20. Christiansen, S. R., Proud, D., and Cochrane, C. G. (1987): Detection of tissue kallikrein in the bronchoalveolar lavage fluids of asthmatic subjects. *J. Clin. Invest.,* 79:188–197.
21. Cochrane, C. G., Revak, S. D., Aiken, B. S., and Wuepper, K. D. (1972): The structural characteristics and activation of Hageman factor. In: *Inflammation: Mechanisms and Control,* edited by I. H. Lepow and P. A. Ward, p. 119. Academic Press, New York.
22. Cochrane, C. G., Wuepper, K. D., Aiken, B. S., Revak, S. D., and Spiegelberg, H. L. (1972): The interaction of Hageman factor and immune complexes. *J. Clin. Invest.,* 51:2736–2745.
23. Cochrane, C. G., Revak, S. D., and Wuepper, K. D. (1973): Activation of Hageman factor in solid and fluid phases. A critical role of kallikrein. *J. Exp. Med.,* 138:1564–1583.
24. Cochrane, C. G., and Griffin, J. H. (1979): Molecular assembly in the contact phase of the Hageman factor system. *Am. J. Med.,* 67: 657–664.
25. Cochrane, C. G., and Griffin, J. H. (1982): The biochemistry and pathophysiology of the contact system of plasma. *Adv. Immunol.,* 33:241–304.
26. Cochrane, C. G., and Revak, S. D. (1980): Dissemination of contact activation in plasma by plasma kallikrein. *J. Exp. Med.,* 152:608–619.
27. Colman, R. W., Mattler, L., and Sherry, S. (1969): Studies on the prekallikrein (kallikreinogen)-kallikrein enzyme system of human plasma. II. Evidence relating the kaolin-activated arginine esterase to plasma kallikreins. *J. Clin. Invest.,* 48:23–32.
28. Colman, R. W., Girey, G., Galvanek, E. G., and Busch, G. J. (1972): Human renal allografts: The protective effects of heparin, kallikrein activation and fibrinolysis during hyperacute reaction. In: *Symposium on Coagulation Problems in Transplanted Organs,* edited by K. V. Kaulla, p. 87. Charles C Thomas, Springfield, Ill.
29. Colman, R. W., Bagdasarian, A., Talamo, R. C., Scott, C. F., Seavey, M., Guimaroes, J. A., Pierce, J. V., and Kaplan, A. P. (1975): Williams trait: Human kininogen deficiency with diminished levels of plasminogen proactivator and prekallikrein associated with abnormalities of Hageman factor-dependent pathways. *J. Clin. Invest.,* 56:1650–1662.
30. Colman, R. W., Edelman, R., Scott, C. F., and Gilman, R. M. (1978): Plasma kallikrein activation and inhibition during typhoid fever. *J. Clin. Invest.,* 61:287–296.
31. Colman, R. W. (1969): Activation of plasminogen by human plasma kallikrein. *Biochem. Biophys. Res. Commun.,* 35:273–279.
32. Colman, R. W. (1984): Surface-mediated defense mechanisms. The plasma contact activation system. *J. Clin. Invest.,* 73:1249–1253.
33. Colman, R. W., and Wong, P. Y. (1977): Participation of Hageman factor pathways in human disease states. *Thromb. Haemost.,* 38: 751–775.
34. Cooper, R. M., Murray, G. E., and Osmond, D. H. (1977): Trypsin-induced activation of renin precursor in plasma of normal and anephric man. *Circ. Res.,* 40(Suppl I):171–179.
35. Cooper, N. R., Miles, L., and Griffin, J. H. (1980): Effects of plasma kallikrein and plasmin on the first component of complement. *J. Immunol.,* 124:1517–1524.
36. Curd, J. G., Prograis, L. J., Jr., and Cochrane, C. G. (1980): Detection of active kallikrein in induced blister fluids of hereditary angioedema patients. *J. Exp. Med.,* 152:742–747.
37. Damus, P. S., Hicks, M., and Rosenberg, R. D. (1973): Anticoagulant activity of heparin. *Nature,* 246:355–357.

38. Davie, E. W., Fujikawa, K., Kurachi, K., and Kesiel, W. (1979): The role of serine proteases in the blood coagulation cascade. *Adv. Enzymol.,* 48:227–318.

39. De Agostini, A., Lijnen, H. R., Pixley, R. A., Colman, R. W., and Schapira, M. (1984): Inactivation of Factor XII active fragment in normal plasma. Predominant role for C1-inhibitor. *J. Clin. Invest.,* 73:1542–1549.

40. Derkx, F. H. M., Tan-Tjiong, H. L., Man in't Veld, A. G., Schalekamp, M. P. A., and Schalekamp, M. A. D. H. (1979): Activation of inactive plasma renin by plasma and tissue kallikreins. *Clin. Sci.,* 57:351–357.

41. Derkx, F. H. M., Bouma, B. N., Schalekamp, M. P. A., and Schalekamp, M. A. D. H. (1979): An intrinsic Factor XII prekallikrein-dependent pathway activates the human renin-angiotensin system. *Nature,* 280:315–316.

42. Donaldson, V. H., Glueck, H. I., and Fleming, T. (1972): Rheumatoid arthritis in a patient with Hageman trait. *N. Engl. J. Med.,* 286:528–530.

43. Dos Santos, E., Rothschild, H. J., and Rocha e Silva, M. (1970): Studies of the activation of the pre-kininogenin-kininogenin (pre-kallikrein-kallikrein) system by sulfated polysaccharides and kaolin. In: *Advances in the Biosciences,* edited by G. L. Haberland and U. Homberg, Chapter 17, p. 145. Pergamon Press, Oxford.

44. Eibl, M. (1985): PKA contamination of immunoglobulin G (letter). *N. Engl. J. Med.,* 313:581.

45. Eisen, V. (1964): Effect of hexadimethrine bromide on plasma kinin formation, hydrolysis of *p*-tosyl-L-arginine methyl ester and fibrinolysis. *Br. J. Pharmacol.,* 22:87–103.

46. Erdos, E. (1979): *Advances in Experimental Medicine and Biology,* Springer-Verlag, Berlin.

47. Erdos, E. G., and Miwa, I. (1968): Effect of endotoxin shock on the plasma kallikrein-kinin system of the rabbit. *Fed. Proc.,* 27:92–95.

48. Erdos, E. G., and Sloane, E. M. (1962): An enzyme in human plasma that inactivated bradykinin and kallidins. *Biochem. Pharmacol.,* 11:585–592.

49. Espana, F., and Ratnoff, O. D. (1983): Activation of Hageman factor (Factor XII) by sulfatides and other agents in the absence of plasma proteases. *J. Lab. Clin. Med.,* 102:31–45.

50. Fonnum, F., and Walaas, I. (1981): Localization of neurotransmitters in nucleus accumbens. In: *The Neurobiology of the Nucleus Accumbens,* edited by R. B. Chronister and J. F. DeFrance, pp. 259–272. The Haer Institute, Brunswick, Maine.

51. Forbes, D. C., Pensky, J., and Ratnoff, O. D. (1970): Inhibition of activated Hageman factor and activated thromboplastin antecedent by purified C1-INH. *J. Lab. Clin. Med.,* 76:805–809.

52. Frank, M. M., Gelfand, J. A., and Atkinson, J. P. (1976): Hereditary angioedema: The clinical syndrome and its management. *Ann. Intern. Med.,* 84:580–593.

53. Frommhagen, L. (1965): The solubility and other physiochemical properties of human gamma globulin labeled with fluorescein isothiocyanate. *J. Immunol.,* 95:442–445.

54. Fujii, S., Moriya, H., and Suzuki, T. (1979): *Advances in Experimental Medicine and Biology,* p. 120A. Plenum Press, New York.

55. Fujii, S., Moriya, H., and Suzuki, T. (1979): *Advances in Experimental Medicine and Biology,* p. 120B. Plenum Press, New York.

56. Fujikawa, K., McMullen, B., Heimark, R. L., Kurachi, K., and Davie, E. W. (1980): The role of Factor XII (Hageman factor) in blood coagulation and a partial amino acid sequence of human Factor XII and its fragments. In: *Protides of the Biological Fluids,* edited by H. Peeters, pp. 193–196. Pergamon Press, New York.

57. Fujikawa, K., Kurachi, K., and Davie, E. W. (1977): Characterization of bovine Factor XIIa (activated Hageman factor). *Biochemistry,* 16:4182–4188.

58. Fujikawa, K., Heimark, R. L., Kurachi, K., and Daire, E. W. (1980): Activation of bovine Factor XII (Hageman factor) by plasma kallikrein. *Biochemistry,* 19:1322–1330.

59. Fujikawa, K., Chung, D. W., Hendrickson, L. E., and Davie, E. W. (1986): Amino acid sequence of human Factor XI, a blood coagulation factor with four tandem repeats that are highly homologous with plasma. *Biochemistry,* 25:2417–2424.

60. Fuller, R. W., Dixon, C. M. S., Dollery, C. T., and Barnes, P. J. (1986): Prostaglandin D-2 potentiates airway responsiveness to histamine and methacholine. *Am. Rev. Respir. Dis.,* 133:252–254.

61. Gallimore, M. J., Aasen, A. O., Lyngass, K. H. M., Larsbratten, M., and Amundsen, E. (1978): Falls in plasma levels of prekallikrein, high molecular weight kininogen, and kallikrein inhibitors during lethal endotoxin shock in dogs. *Thromb. Res.,* 12:307–318.

62. Ghebrehiwet, B., Silverberg, M., and Kaplan, A. P. (1981): Activation of the classical pathway of complement by Hageman factor fragment. *J. Exp. Med.,* 153:665–676.

63. Ghebrehiwet, B., Randazzo, B. P., Dunn, J. T., Silverberg, M., and Kaplan, A. P. (1983): Mechanisms of activation of the classical pathway of complement by Hageman factor fragment. *J. Clin. Invest.,* 71:1450–1456.

64. Gigli, I., Mason, J. W., Colman, R. W., and Austen, K. F. (1970): Interaction of plasma kallikrein with C1 inhibitor. *J. Immunol.,* 104:574–581.

65. Ginsberg, M. H., Jaques, B., Cochrane, C. G., and Griffin, J. H. (1980): Urate crystal-dependent cleavage of Hageman factor in human plasma and synovial fluid. *J. Lab. Clin. Med.,* 95:497–506.

66. Graham, R., Ebert, R. H., Ratnoff, O. D., and Moses, J. M. (1965): Pathogenesis of inflammation. II. *In vivo* observations of the inflammatory effects of activated Hageman factor and bradykinin. *J. Exp. Med.,* 121:807.

67. Green, D., Arseuer, C. L., Grumet, K. A., and Ratnoff, O. D. (1982): Classic gout in Hageman factor (Factor XII) deficiency. *Arch. Intern. Med.,* 142:1556–1557.

68. Greengard, J. S., and Griffin, J. H. (1984): Receptors for high molecular weight kininogen on stimulated washed human platelets. *Biochemistry,* 23:6863–6869.

69. Grennan, D. M., Mitchell, W., Miller, W., and Zeitlin, I. J. (1977): The effects of prostaglandin E1, bradykinin, and histamine on canine synovial vascular permeability. *Br. J. Pharmacol.,* 60:251–254.

70. Griffin, J. H., Harper, E., and Cochrane, C. G. (1975): Studies on the activation of human blood coagulation Factor XII (Hageman factor) by soluble collagen. *Fed. Proc.,* 34:860.

71. Griffin, J. H. (1978): The role of surface in surface-dependent activation of Hageman factor (Factor XII). *Proc. Natl. Acad. Sci. USA,* 75:1998–2002.

72. Griffin, J. H., and Cochrane, C. G. (1976): Mechanisms for the involvement of high molecular weight kininogen in surface-dependent reactions of Hageman factor. *Proc. Natl. Acad. Sci. USA,* 73:2554–2558.

73. Griffin, J. H., and Cochrane, C. G. (1976): Human Factor XII (Hageman factor). *Methods Enzymol.,* 45:56–65.

74. Haanan, C., Hommes, F., and Morselt, G. (1961): Some observations on the role of Hageman factor in blood coagulation. *Thromb. Diath. Haemorhag.,* 6:261–269.

75. Habal, F. M., Movat, H. Z., and Burrowes, C. E. (1974): Isolation of two functionally different kininogens from human plasma-separation from proteinase inhibitors and interaction with plasma kallikrein. *Biochem. Pharmacol.,* 23:2291–2303.

76. Halonen, M., and Pinckard, R. N. (1975): Intravascular effects of IgE antibody upon basophils, neutrophils, platelets, and blood coagulation in the rabbit. *J. Immunol.,* 115:519–524.

77. Han, Y. N., Komiya, M., Iwanga, S., and Suzuki, T. (1975): Studies on the primary structure of bovine high molecular weight kininogen. Amino acid sequence of a fragment ("histone rich peptide") released by kallikrein. *J. Biochem.,* 77:55–68.

78. Han, Y. N., Kato, H., Iwanaza, H., and Suzuki, T. (1976): Primary structure of bovine plasma high-molecular-weight kininogen. The amino acid sequence of a glycoprotein portion (fragment 1) following C-terminus of the bradykinin moiety. *J. Biochem.,* 79:1201–1222.

79. Harpel, P. C., Lewin, M. F., and Kaplan, A. P. (1985): Distribution of plasma kallikrein between C1 inactivator and alpha 2-macroglobulin in plasma utilizing a new assay for alpha 2-macroglobulin kallikrein complexes. *J. Biol. Chem.,* 260:4257–4263.

80. Harpel, P. C. (1970): Human plasma alpha-2-macroglobulin. An inhibitor of plasma kallikrein. *J. Exp. Med.,* 132:329–352.

81. Harpel, P. C. (1972): Studies on the interaction between collagen and a plasma kallikrein-like activity. *J. Clin. Invest.,* 51:1813–1822.

82. Harrison, G. A., Robinson, M., and Stacey, R. V. (1971): Hypotensive effects of stable plasma protein solution (SPPS): A preliminary communication. *Med. J. Aust.,* 2:1040–1041 (letter).

83. Harrison, G. A., Torda, J. A., and Schiff, P. (1971): Hypotensive effects of stable plasma protein solution (SPPS): A preliminary communication. *Med. J. Aust.,* 2:1308–1309 (letter).

84. Heimark, R. L., Kurachi, K., Fujikawa, K., and Davie, E. W. (1980): Surface activation of blood coagulation, fibrinolysis and kinin formation. *Nature,* 286:456–460.

85. Herxheimer, H., and Stresemann, E. (1961): The effect of bradykinin aerosol in guinea pigs and man. *J. Physiol.,* 158:38–39.

86. Hirsch, E. F., Nakayima, T., Oshima, G., Erdos, E. G., and Herman, C. M. (1974): Kinin system responses in sepsis after trauma in man. *J. Surg. Res.,* 17:147–153.

87. Hojima, Y., Cochrane, C. G., Wiggins, R. C., Austen, K. F., and Stevens, R. L. (1984): *In vitro* activation of the contact (Hageman factor) system of plasma by heparin and chondroitin sulfate E. *Blood,* 63:1453–1459.

88. Hong, S. C., and Levine, L. (1976): Stimulation of prostaglandin synthesis by bradykinin and thrombin and their mechanisms of action on MC5-5 fibroblasts. *J. Biol. Chem.,* 251:5814–5816.

89. Jacobsen, S., and Kriz, M. (1967): Some data on two purified kininogens from human plasma. *Br. J. Pharmacol. Chemother.,* 29: 25–36.

90. Johnston, A. R., Cochrane, C. G., and Revak, S. D. (1974): The relationship between PF/DIL and activated human Hageman factor. *J. Immunol.,* 113:103–109.

91. Kallen, R. J., and Soo-Kwang, L. (1975): A study of the plasma kinin-generating system in children with the minimal lesion, idiopathic nephrotic syndrome. *Pediatr. Res.,* 9:705.

92. Kalter, E. S., van Dijk, W. C., Timmerman, A., Verhoef, J., and Bouma, B. N. (1983): Activation of purified human plasma prekallikrein triggered by cell wall fractions of Escherichia coli and Staphylococcus aureus. *J. Infect. Dis.,* 148:682–691.

93. Kalter, E. S., Daha, M. R., ten Cate, J. W., Verhoef, J., and Bouma, B. N. (1985): Activation and inhibition of Hageman factor-dependent pathway and the complement system in uncomplicated bacteremia or bacterial shock. *J. Infect. Dis.,* 15:1019–1027.

94. Kamata, R., Yamamoto, T., Matsumoto, K., and Maeda, H. (1985): A serratial protease causes vascular permeability reaction by activation of the Hageman factor-dependent pathway in guinea pigs. *Infect. Immun.,* 48:747–753.

95. Kaplan, A. P., Kay, A. B., and Austen, K. F. (1972): A prealbumin activator of prekallikrein. III. Appearance of chemotactic activity for human neutrophils. *J. Exp. Med.,* 135:81–97.

96. Kaplan, A. P. (1983): Hageman factor-dependent pathways: Mechanism of initiation and bradykinin formation. *Fed. Proc.,* 42: 3123–3127.

97. Kaplan, A. P., and Austen, K. F. (1971): A prealbumin activator of prekallikrein. II. Derivation of activators of prekallikrein from active Hageman factor by digestion with plasmin. *J. Exp. Med.,* 133:696–712.

98. Keele, C. A., and Eisen, V. (1969): Plasma kinin formation in rheumatoid arthritis. In: *Bradykinin and Related Kinins,* edited by F. Sicuteri, M. Rocha e Silva, and N. Bach, p. 471. Plenum Press, New York.

99. Kellermeyer, R. W. (1967): The inflammatory process in acute gouty arthritis. III. Vascular permeability enhancing activity in normal human synovial fluid; induction by Hageman factor activators and inhibition by Hageman factor antiserum. *J. Lab. Clin. Med.,* 70:372–383.

100. Kellermeyer, R. W., and Breckenridge, R. T. (1965): The inflammatory process in acute gouty arthritis. I. Activation of Hageman factor by sodium urate crystals. *J. Lab. Clin. Med.,* 65:307–315.

101. Kellermeyer, R. W., and Breckenridge, R. T. (1966): The inflammatory process in acute gouty arthritis. II. The presence of Hageman factor and plasma thromboplastin antecedent in synovial fluid. *J. Lab. Clin. Med.,* 67:455–460.

102. Kellermeyer, W. F., Jr., and Kellermeyer, R. W. (1969): Hageman

103. Kerbiriou, D. M., Bouma, B. N., and Griffin, J. H. (1980): Immunochemical studies of human high molecular weight kininogen and of its complexes with plasma prekallikrein or kallikrein. *J. Biol. Chem.,* 255:3952–3958.

104. Kimball, H. R., Melmon, K. L., and Wolff, S. M. (1972): Endotoxin-induced kinin production in man. *Proc. Soc. Exp. Biol. Med.,* 139: 1078–1082.

105. Kitamura, N., Takagaki, Y., Furuto, S., Tanaka, T., Nawa, H., and Nakanishi, S. (1983): A single gene for bovine high molecular weight and low molecular weight kininogens. *Nature,* 305:545–549.

106. Kitamura, N., Kitagawa, H., Fukushima, D., Takagaki, Y., Miyata, T., and Nakanishi, S. (1985): Structural organization of the human kininogen gene and a model for its evolution. *J. Biol. Chem.,* 260: 8610–8617.

107. Kleniewski, J., and Donaldson, V. H. (1977): Quantification of human high-molecular-weight kininogen (HMW-KGN) by specific hemagglutination inhibition reaction. *Proc. Soc. Exp. Biol. Med.,* 156:113–117.

108. Kluft, C. (1978): Determination of human prekallikrein in human plasma: Optimal conditions for activating prekallikrein. *J. Lab. Clin. Med.,* 91:83–95.

109. Kodama, K., Kato, H., and Iwanago, S. (1985): Isolation of bovine platelet cationic proteins which inhibit the surface-mediated activation of Factor XII and prekallikrein. *J. Biochem.,* 97:139–151.

110. Kozin, F., Curd, J. G., Rickford, K., and Cochrane, C. G. Unpublished observations.

111. Kozin, F., Millstein, B. F., Mandel, G. S., and Mandel, N. S. (1982): Silica-induced membranolysis: A study of different structural forms of crystalline and amorphous silica and the effects of protein adsorption. *J. Colloid Interface Sci.,* 88:326–337.

112. Kozin, F., and McCarty, D. J. (1977): Protein binding to monosodium urate, calcium pyrophosphate dihydrate, and silica crystals. I. Physical characteristics. *J. Lab. Clin. Med.,* 89:1314–1325.

113. Kurachi, K., Fijikawa, K., and Davie, E. W. (1980): Mechanism of activation of bovine Factor XI by Factor XII and Factor XIIIa. *Biochemistry,* 19:1330–1338.

114. Kurachi, K., and Davie, E. W. (1977): Activation of human Factor XI (plasma thromboplastin antecedent) by Factor XIIa (activated Hageman factor). *Biochemistry,* 16:5831–5839.

115. Lange, L. G., Carvalho, A. C., Bagdasarian, A., Lahiri, B., and Colman, R. W. (1974): Activation of Hageman factor in the nephrotic syndrome. *Am. J. Med.,* 56:565–569.

116. Leikauf, G. D., Ueki, I. F., Nadel, J. A., and Widdicombe, J. H. (1985): Bradykinin stimulates Cl secretion and prostaglandin E2 release by canine tracheal epithelium. *Am. J. Physiol.,* 248:F48–F55.

117. Liu, C. Y., Scott, C. F., Bagdasarian, A., Pierce, T. V., Kaplan, A. P., and Colman, R. W. (1977): Potentiation of the function of Hageman factor fragments by high molecular weight kininogen. *J. Clin. Invest.,* 60:7–17.

118. Mandle, R., Jr., Colman, R. W., and Kaplan, A. P. (1976): Identification of prekallikrein and high molecular weight kininogen as a complex in plasma. *Proc. Natl. Acad. Sci. USA,* 73:4179–4183.

119. Mandle, R., and Kaplan, A. P. (1977): Hageman factor substrates. Human plasma prekallikrein: Mechanisms of activation by Hageman factor and participation in Hageman-factor-dependent fibrinolysis. *J. Biol. Chem.,* 252:6097–6104.

120. Mandle, R., Jr., and Kaplan, A. P. (1979): Hageman factor dependent fibrinolysis: Generation of fibrinolytic activity by the interaction of human activated Factor XI and plasminogen. *Blood,* 54: 850–862.

121. Margolis, J. (1963): The inter-relationship of coagulation of plasma and release of peptides. *Ann. NY Acad. Sci.,* 104:133–145.

122. Mason, J. M., Kleeberg, V., Dolan, P., and Colman, R. W. (1970): Plasma kallikrein and Hageman factor in gram-negative bacteremia. *Ann. Intern. Med.,* 73:545–551.

123. Matheson, R. T., Miller, D. R., Lacombe, M. J., Han, Y. N., Iwan-

factor activation and kinin formation in human plasma induced by cellulose sulfate solutions. *Proc. Soc. Exp. Biol. Med.,* 130:1310–1314.

ogo, S., Kato, H., and Wuepper, K. D. (1976): Flaujeac factor deficiency. Reconstruction with highly purified bovine high molecular weight kininogen and delineation of a new permeability-enhancing peptide released by plasma kallikrein from bovine high molecular weight kininogen. *J. Clin. Invest.*, 58:1395–1406.

124. Matsumoto, K., Yamamoto, T., Kamato, R., and Malda, H. (1984): Pathogenesis of serratial infection: Activation of the Hageman factor–prekallikrein cascade by serratial protease. *J. Biochem. (Tokyo),* 96:739–749.

125. McGiff, J. C., Itskovitz, H. D., Terragno, A., and Wong, P. Y-K. (1976): Modulation and mediation of the action of the renal kallikrein-kinin system by prostaglandins. *Fed. Proc.,* 35:175–180.

126. McIntyre, T. M., Zimmerman, G. A., Satoh, K., and Prescott, S. M. (1985): Cultured endothelial cells synthesize both platelet-activating factor and prostacyclin in response to histamine, bradykinin, and adenosine triphosphate. *J. Clin. Invest.,* 76:271–280.

127. Meier, H. L., Pierce, J. V., Colman, R. W., and Kaplan, A. P. (1977): Activation and function of human Hageman factor. The role of high molecular weight kininogen and prekallikrein. *J. Clin. Invest.,* 60:18–31.

128. Meier, H. L., Flowers, B., Silverberg, M., Kaplan, A. P., and Newball, H. H. (1986): The IgE-dependent release of a Hageman factor cleaving factor from human lung. *Am. J. Pathol.,* 123:146–154.

129. Meier, H. L., and Kaplan, A. P. (1978): Evaluation of potential initiation of the Hageman factor (HF) dependent pathways. *Fed. Proc.,* 37:1293.

130. Melmon, K. L., Louenberg, W., and Sjoerdsma, A. (1965): Characteristics of carcinoid tumor kallikrein: Identification of lysyl-bradykinin as a peptide it produces *in vitro. Clin. Chim. Acta,* 12:292–297.

131. Melmon, K. L., and Cline, M. J. (1967): Interaction of plasma kinins and granulocytes. *Nature,* 213:90–92.

132. Melmon, K. L., and Cline, M. J. (1968): The interaction of leukocytes and the kinin system. *Biochem. Pharmacol.,* 27(Suppl.): 271–281.

133. Miles, L. A., Greengard, J. S., and Griffin, J. H. (1983): A comparison of the abilities of plasma kallikrein, Beta-Factor XIIa, Factor XIa and urokinase to activate plasminogen. *Thromb. Res.,* 29:407–417.

134. Millar, J. A., Clappison, B. H., and Johnston, C. I. (1978): Kallikrein and plasmin as activators of inactive renin. *Lancet,* ii:1376 (letter).

135. Moncada, S., Mullane, K. M., and Vane, J. R. (1979): Prostacyclin release by bradykinin *in vivo. Br. J. Pharmacol.,* 66:969–979.

136. Morrison, D. C., and Cochrane, C. G. (1974): Direct evidence for Hageman factor (Factor XII) activation by bacterial lipopolysaccharides (endotoxins). *J. Exp. Med.,* 140:797–811.

137. Moskowitz, R. W., Schwartz, H. J., Michel, B., Ratnoff, O. D., and Astrup, T. (1970): Generation of kinin-like agents by chrondroitin sulfate, heparin, chitin sulfate, and human articular cartilage: Possible pathophysiologic implications. *J. Lab. Clin. Med.,* 76:790–798.

138. Movat, H. Z., Steinberg, S. G., Habal, F. M., and Ranadive, N. S. (1973): Demonstration of a kinin-generating enzyme in the lysosomes of human polymorphonuclear leukocytes. *Lab. Invest.,* 29: 669–684.

139. Movat, H. Z., Habal, F. M., and MacMorine, D. R. L. (1976): Neutral proteases of human PMN leukocytes with kininogenase activity. *Int. Arch. Allergy Appl. Immunol.,* 50:257–281.

140. Naclerio, R. M., Gwaltney, J. M., Hendley, J. O., Egglestrom, P., Baumgarten, C. R., Lichtenstein, L. M., and Proud, D. (1985): Kinins are generated during rhinovirus colds. *Clin. Res.,* 33:613A.

141. Nagasawa, S., and Nakayasu, T. (1973): Human plasma prekallikrein as a protein complex. *J. Biochem.,* 74:401–403.

142. Nagase, H., Cawston, T. E., DeSilva, M., and Barrett, A. J. (1982): Identification of plasma kallikrein as an activator of latent collagenase in rheumatoid synovial fluid. *Biochim. Biophys. Acta,* 702: 133–142.

143. Newball, H. H., Talamo, R., and Lichtenstein, L. (1975): Release of leukocyte kallikrein mediated by IgE. *Nature,* 25:635–636.

144. Newball, H. H., Meier, H. L., Kaplan, A. P., Cochrane, C. G., Revak, S. D., and Lichtenstein, L. (1978): Cleavage of Hageman

factor (HF) by a basophil kallikrein of anaphylaxis (BK-A). *Clin. Res.,* 26:519A.

145. Newball, H. H., Talamo, R. C., and Lichtenstein, L. M. (1979): Anaphylactic release of a basophil kallikrein-like activity. *J. Clin. Invest.,* 64:466–475.

146. Newball, H. H., Berninger, R., Talamo, R. C., and Lichtenstein, L. M. (1979): Anaphylactic release of a basophil kallikrein-like activity. *J. Clin. Invest.,* 64:457–465.

147. Newcombe, D. S., Fahey, J. V., and Ishikawa, Y. (1977): Hydrocortisone inhibition of the bradykinin activation of human synovial fibroblasts. *Prostaglandins,* 13:235–244.

148. Nies, A. S., Forsyth, R. P., Williams, H. E., and Melmon, K. L. (1968): Contribution of kinins to endotoxin shock in unanesthetized rhesus monkeys. *Circ. Res.,* 22:155–164.

149. Niewiarowski, S., Bankowski, E., and Ragowicka, I. (1965): Studies on the adsorption and activation of Hageman factor (Factor XII) by collagen and elastin. *Thromb. Diath. Haemorhag.,* 14:387–400.

150. Nossel, H. L., Rubin, H., Drillings, H., and Haich, R. (1968): Inhibition of Hageman factor activation. *J. Clin. Invest.,* 47:1172–1180.

151. O'Donnell, T. F., Clowes, G. H., Jr., and Talamo, R. C. (1976): Kinin activation in the blood of patients with sepsis. *Surg. Gynecol. Obstet.,* 143:539–545.

152. Oates, J. A., Melmon, K., Sjoerdsma, A., Gillespie, L., and Mason, D. T. (1964): Release of a kinin peptide in the carcinoid syndrome. *Lancet,* i:514–517.

153. Oh-Ishi, S., Tanaka, K., Katori, M., Han, Y. M., Kato, H., and Iwanago, S. (1977): Further studies on biological activities of new peptide fragments derived from high molecular weight kininogen: An enhancement of the vascular permeability increase of the fragments by prostaglandin E2. *Life Sci.,* 20:695–700.

154. Ornstein, N. S., Galli, S. J., Dvorak, A. M., Silbert, J. E., and Dronak, H. F. (1978): Sulfated glycoaminoglycans of guinea pig basophilic leukocytes. *J. Immunol.,* 121:586–592.

155. Osmond, D. H., Lo, E. K., Loh, A. Y., Zingg, E. A., and Hedlin, A. H. (1978): Kallikrein and plasmin as activators of inactive renin. *Lancet,* ii:1375 (letter).

156. Osmond, D. H., and Loh, A. Y. (1978): Protease as endogenous activator of inactive renin. *Lancet,* i:102 (letter).

157. Phillips, P., Prockop, D. J., and McCarty, D. J. (1966): Crystal induced inflammation in canine joints. III. Evidence against bradykinin as a mediator of inflammation. *J. Lab. Clin. Med.,* 68: 433–444.

158. Pinckard, R. N., Tanigawa, C., and Halonen, M. (1975): IgE-induced blood coagulation alterations in the rabbit: Consumption of coagulation Factors XII, XI, and IX *in vivo. J. Immunol.,* 115: 525–532.

159. J. J. Pisano and K. F. Austen, editors, *DHEW Publication No. (NIH) 76-791,* DHEW, Washington, D.C. (1976).

160. Pixley, R. A., Schapira, M., and Colman, R. W. (1985): The regulation of human factor XIIa by plasma proteinase inhibitors. *J. Biol. Chem.,* 260:1723–1729.

161. Pixley, R. A., and Colman, R. W. (1983): Inhibition of human Factor XIIa by plasma protease inhibitors. *Fed. Proc.,* 42:1031.

162. Proctor, R. R., and Rapaport, S. I. (1961): The partial thromboplastin time with kaolin: A simple screening test for first stage plasma clotting deficiencies. *Am. J. Clin. Pathol.,* 35:212–219.

163. Proud, D., Pierce, J. V., and Pisano, J. J. (1980): Radioimmunoassay of human high molecular weight kininogen in normal and deficient plasma. *J. Lab. Clin. Med.,* 95:563–574.

164. Proud, D., Togias, R. M., Naclerio, S., Crush, S. A., Norman, P. S., and Lichtenstein, L. M. (1983): Kinins are generated *in vivo* following nasal airways challenge of allergic individuals with allergen. *J. Clin. Invest.,* 72:1678–1685.

165. Proud, D., MacGlashan, D. W., Newball, H. N., Schulman, E. S., and Lichtenstein, C. M. (1985): Immunoglobulin E-mediated release of a kininogenase from purified human lung mast cells. *Am. Rev. Resp. Dis.,* 132:405–408.

166. Purdon, D., Schapira, M., De Agostini, A., and Colman, R. W. (1983): Prorenin activation by plasma kallikrein in inhibitor deficient plasma. *Thromb. Haemost.,* 50:30 (abstract).

167. Purdon, A. D., Schapira, M., De Agostini, A., and Colman, R. W. (1985): Plasma kallikrein and prorenin in patients with hereditary angioedema. *J. Lab. Clin. Med.*, 105:694–699.

168. Ratnoff, O. D., Pensky, J., Donaldson, V. H., and Amir, J. (1972): The inhibitory properties of plasma against activated plasma thromboplastin antecedent (Factor XIa) in hereditary angioneurotic edema. *J. Lab. Clin. Med.*, 80:803–809.

169. Ratnoff, O. D., and Colopy, J. E. (1955): A familial hemorrhagic tract associated with a deficiency of clot-promoting fraction of plasma. *J. Clin. Invest.*, 34:602–612.

170. Regoli, D., and Barabe, J. (1980): Pharmacology of bradykinin and related kinins. *J. Pharmacol. Rev.*, 32:1–45.

171. Revak, S. D., Cochrane, C. G., Johnston, A. R., and Hugli, T. H. (1974): Structural changes accompanying enzymatic activation of human Hageman factor. *J. Clin. Invest.*, 54:619–627.

172. Revak, S. D., Cochrane, C. G., and Griffin, J. H. (1977): The binding and cleavage characteristics of human Hageman factor during contact activation. A comparison of normal plasma with plasmas deficient in Factor XI, prekallikrein, or high molecular weight kininogen. *J. Clin. Invest.*, 59:1167–1175.

173. Revak, S. D., Cochrane, C. G., Bouma, B. N., and Griffin, J. H. (1978): Surface and fluid phase activities of two forms of activated Hageman factor produced during contact activation. *J. Exp. Med.*, 147:719–729.

174. Revak, S. D., and Cochrane, C. G. (1976): The relationship of structure and function in human Hageman factor. The association of enzymatic and binding activities with separate regions of the molecule. *J. Clin. Invest.*, 57:852–860.

175. Rimon, A., Schiffman, S., Feinstein, D. I., and Rapaport, S. J. (1976): Factor XI activity and Factor XI antigen in homozygous and heterozygous Factor XI deficiency. *Blood*, 48:165–174.

176. Robinson, J. A., Kloduycky, M. L., Lock, H. H., Racic, M. R., and Gunner, R. M. (1975): Endotoxin, prekallikrein, complement and systemic vascular resistance sequential measurements in man. *Am. J. Med.*, 59:61–67.

177. Roscher, A. A., Mangiello, V. C., Jelsema, C. L., and Moss, J. (1983): Receptors for bradykinin in intact cultured fibroblasts. Identification and characterization by direct binding study. *J. Clin. Invest.*, 72:626–635.

178. Roscher, A. A., Mangiello, V. C., Jelsema, C. L., and Moss, J. (1984): Autoregulation of bradykinin receptors and bradykinin-induced prostacyclin formation in human fibroblasts. *J. Clin. Invest.*, 74:552–558.

179. Rosing, J., Tans, G., and Griffin, J. H. (1985): Surface-dependent activation of human Factor XII (Hageman factor) by kallikrein and its light chain. *Eur. J. Biochem.*, 151:531–538.

180. Rothschild, A. M. (1981): Plasma kallikrein-generating activity evoked by rat peritoneal-fluid mast cells following treatment with epinephrine, gamma-bromo-cyclic 3′,5′ guanosine monophosphate or compound 48/80. *Biochem. Pharmacol.*, 30:481–487.

181. Saito, H., Ratnoff, O. D., and Pensky, J. (1976): Radioimmunoassay of human Hageman factor (Factor XII). *J. Lab. Clin. Med.*, 88:506–514.

182. Saito, H., Poon, M. G., Vicic, W., Goldsmith, G. H., and Menitore, J. E. (1978): Human plasma prekallikrein (Fletcher factor) clotting activity and antigen in health and disease. *J. Lab. Clin. Med.*, 92:84–94.

183. Saito, H., Scott, J. G., Movat, H. Z., and Scealla, S. J. (1979): Molecular heterogeneity of Hageman trait (Factor XII deficiency). Evidence that two of 49 subjects are crossreacting material positive (CRM+). *J. Lab. Clin. Med.*, 94:256–265.

184. Saito, H., and Goldsmith, G. H., Jr. (1977): Plasma thromboplastin antecedent (PTA, Factor XI): A specific and sensitive radioimmunoassay. *Blood*, 50:377–385.

185. Saito, H., and Ratnoff, O. D. (1974): Inhibition of normal clotting and Fletcher factor activity by rabbit anti-kallikrein antiserum. *Nature*, 248:597–598.

186. Sawai, K., Niwa, S., and Katori, M. (1980): The significant reduction of high molecular weight kininogen in synovial fluid of patients with active rheumatoid arthritis. In: *Proceedings of the International Conference on Kinins*, edited by T. Suzuki and H. Moringa, pp. 195–202. Plenum Press, New York.

187. Schapira, M., Scott, C. F., and Colman, R. W. (1981): Protection of human plasma kallikrein from inactivation by C1-inhibitor and other protease inhibitors. The role of high molecular weight kininogen. *Biochemistry*, 20:2738–2743.

188. Schapira, M., Despland, E., Scott, C. F., Boxer, L. A., and Colman, R. W. (1982): Purified human plasma kallikrein aggregates human blood neutrophils. *J. Clin. Invest.*, 69:1199–1201.

189. Schapira, M., Scott, C. F., and Colman, R. W. (1982): Contribution of plasma protease inhibitors to the inactivation of kallikrein in plasma. *J. Clin. Invest.*, 69:462–468.

190. Schapira, M., Scott, C. F., James, A., Silver, L., Kueppers, F., James, H. L., and Colman, R. W. (1982): High molecular weight kininogen or its light chain protects human plasma kallikrein from inactivation by plasma protease inhibition. *Biochemistry*, 21:567–572.

191. Schapira, M., Silver, L. D., Scott, C. F., Schmaier, A. H., Prograis, L. J., Jr., Curd, J. G., and Colman, R. W. (1983): Prekallikrein activation and high molecular weight kininogen consumption in hereditary angioedema attacks. *N. Engl. J. Med.*, 308:1050–1053.

192. Schapira, M., Henry, M. J., Wachtfogel, Y. T., Scott, C. F., and Colman, R. W. (1983): A role for plasma kallikrein in rheumatoid arthritis. *Clin. Res.*, 31:454A.

193. Schiffman, S., Mannhalter, C., and Tyner, K. D. (1980): Human high molecular weight kininogen. Effects of cleavage by kallikrein on protein structure and procoagulant activity. *J. Biol. Chem.*, 255:6433–6438.

194. Schmaier, A. H., Zuckerberg, A., Silverman, C., Kachibholta, J., Tuszynski, G. P., and Colman, R. W. (1983): High molecular weight kininogen. A secreted platelet protein. *J. Clin. Invest.*, 71:1477–1489.

195. Schreiber, A. D., Kaplan, A. P., and Austen, K. F. (1973): Inhibition of C1-INH of Hageman factor fragment activation of coagulation, fibrinolysis, and kinin generation. *J. Clin. Invest.*, 52:1402–1409.

196. Schwartz, H. J., and Kellermeyer, R. W. (1969): Carrageenen and delayed hypersensitivity. II. Activation of Hageman factor by carrageenan and its significance. *Proc. Soc. Exp. Biol. Med.*, 132:1021–1024.

197. Scicli, A. G., and Carretero, O. A. (1986): Renal kallikrein-kinin system. *Kidney Int.*, 29:120–130.

198. Scott, C. F., Schapira, M., James, H. L., Cohen, A. B., and Colman, R. W. (1982): Inactivation of Factor XIa by plasma protease inhibitors. Predominant role of alpha-1-protease inhibitor and the protective effect of high molecular weight kininogen. *J. Clin. Invest.*, 69:844–852.

199. Scott, C. F., Silver, L. D., Purdon, A. D., and Colman, R. W. (1984): Plasma Factor XIa regulates contact-activated coagulation. *Fed. Proc.*, 43:775.

200. Scott, C. F., Silver, L. D., Schapira, M., and Colman, R. W. (1984): Cleavage of high molecular weight kininogen enhances its coagulant activity. Evidence that this molecule exists as a procofactor. *J. Clin. Invest.*, 73:954–962.

201. Scott, C. F., Sinha, D., Seaman, F. S., Walsh, P. N., and Colman, R. W. (1984): Amidolytic assay of human Factor XI in plasma. Comparison with a coagulant assay and a new rapid radioimmunoassay. *Blood*, 63:43–50.

202. Scott, C. F., Purdon, A. D., Silver, L. D., and Colman, R. W. (1985): Cleavage of human high molecular weight kininogen by Factor XIa *in vitro*. Effect on structure and function. *J. Biol. Chem.*, 260:10856–10863.

203. Sealey, J., Atlas, S. A., Laragh, J. H., Oza, N. B., and Ryan, J. W. (1978): Human urinary kallikrein converts inactive to active renin and is a possible physiologic activation of renin. *Nature*, 275:144–145.

204. Sealey, J. E., Atlas, S. A., Laragh, J. H., Silverberg, M., and Kaplan, A. P. (1979): Initiation of plasma prorenin activation by Hageman factor-dependent conversion of plasma prekallikrein to kallikrein. *Proc. Natl. Acad. Sci. USA*, 76:5914–5918.

205. Sealey, J., Atlas, S. A., Laragh, J. H., Silverberg, M. J., and Kaplan, A. P. (1979): Initiation of plasma prorenin activation by Hageman

factor dependent conversion of plasma prekallikrein to kallikrein. *Proc. Natl. Acad. Sci. USA*, 76:5914–5918.

206. Seppa, H. (1980): The role of chymotrypsin-like protease of rat mast cells in inflammatory vasopermeability and fibrinolysis. *Inflammation*, 4:1–8.

207. Sheikh, I. A., and Kaplan, A. P. (1986): Studies of the digestion of bradykinin lysyl-bradykinin, and kinin degradation products by carboxypeptides A, B, and N. *Biochem. Pharmacol.*, 35:1957–1963.

208. Silverberg, M., Dunn, J. T., Garen, L., and Kaplan, A. P. (1980): Autoactivation of human Hageman factor. Demonstration utilizing a synthetic substrate. *J. Biol. Chem.*, 255:7281–7286.

209. Sinha, D., Seaman, F. S., Koshy, A., Knight, L. C., and Walsh, P. N. (1984): Blood coagulation Factor XIa bind specifically to a site on activated human platelets distinct from that for Factor XI. *J. Clin. Invest.*, 73:1550–1556.

210. Soons, H., Janssen-Classen, T., Hemker, H. C., and Tans, G. (1986): The effect of platelets in the activation of human blood coagulation Factor IX by Factor XIa. *Blood*, 68:140–148.

211. Stead, N., Kaplan, A. P., and Rosenberg, R. D. (1976): Inhibition of activated factor XII by antithrombin-heparin cofactor. *J. Biol. Chem.*, 251:6481–6488.

212. Stoner, J., Manganiello, V. C., and Vaughan, M. (1973): Effects of bradykinin on cyclic AMP and cyclic GMP in lung slices. *Proc. Natl. Acad. Sci. USA*, 70:3830–3833.

213. Sugo, T., Ikari, N., Kato, H., Iwanga, S., and Fujii, S. (1980): Functional sites of bovine high molecular weight kininogen as a cofactor in kaolin-mediated activation of Factor XII (Hageman factor). *Biochem. J.*, 19:3215–3220.

214. Sugo, T., Kato, H., Iwanaga, S., Tahada, K., and Sakakibara, S. (1985): Kinetic studies on surface-mediated activation of bovine Factor XII and prekallikrein. Effects of kaolin and high molecular weight kininogen on activation reactions. *Eur. J. Biochem.*, 146:43–50.

215. Takagaki, Y., Kitamura, N., and Nakanishi, S. (1985): Cloning and sequence analysis of cDNAs for human high molecular weight and low molecular weight prekininogens. Primary structures of two human prekininogens. *J. Biol. Chem.*, 260:8601–8609.

216. Takahashi, H., Nagasawa, S., and Suzuki, T. (1980): Studies on prekallikrein of bovine plasma. II. Activation of prekallikrein with proteinases and properties of kallikrein activated by bovine Hageman factor. *J. Biochem.*, 87:23–34.

217. Tankersley, D. L., and Finlayson, J. S. (1984): Kinetics of activation and autoactivation of human Factor XII. *Biochemistry*, 23:273–279.

218. Tans, G., Rosing, J., and Griffin, J. H. (1983): Sulfatide-dependent autoactivation of human blood coagulation Factor XII (Hageman factor). *J. Biol. Chem.*, 258:8215–8222.

219. Thompson, R. E., Mandle, R., and Kaplan, A. P. (1978): Characterization of human high molecular weight kininogen. Procoagulant activity associated with the light chain of kinin-free high molecular weight kininogen. *J. Exp. Med.*, 147:488–499.

220. Thompson, R. E., Mandle, R., Jr., and Kaplan, A. P. (1979): Studies of binding of prekallikrein and Factor XI to high molecular weight kininogen and its light chain. *Proc. Natl. Acad. Sci. USA*, 76:4862–4866.

221. Togias, A. G., Naclerio, R. M., Pround, D., Fish, J. E., Adkinson, N. F., Jr., Sobotka, A. K., Norman, P. S., and Lichtenstein, L. M. (1985): Nasal challenge with cold, dry air results in release of inflammatory mediators. Possible mast cell involvement. *J. Clin. Invest.*, 76:1375–1381.

222. Travis, J., and Salvesen, G. S. (1983): Human plasma proteinase inhibitors. *Annu. Rev. Biochem.*, 52:655–709.

223. Tuszynski, G. P., Bevacqua, S. J., Schmaier, A. H., Colman, R. W., and Walsh, P. N. (1982): Factor XI antigen and activity in human platelets. *Blood*, 59:1148–1156.

224. Ulevitch, R. J., Cochrane, C. G., and Johnston, A. R. (1980): Rabbit prekallikrein. Purification, biochemical characterization, and mechanism of activation. *Inflammation*, 4:9–25.

225. Van Der Graaf, F., Tans, G., Bouma, B. N., and Griffin, J. H. (1982): Isolation and functional properties of the heavy and light chains of human plasma kallikrein. *J. Biol. Chem.*, 257:14300–14305.

226. Van Der Graaf, F., Koedam, J. A., and Bouma, B. N. (1983): Inactivation of kallikrein in human plasma. *J. Clin. Invest.*, 71:149–158.

227. Van Der Graaf, F., Koedam, J. A., Griffin, J. H., and Bouma, B. N. (1983): Interaction of human plasma kallikrein and its light chain with C1 inhibitor. *Biochemistry*, 22:4860–4866.

228. Van Der Graaf, F., Reitveld, A., Keus, F. J. A., and Bouma, B. N. (1984): Interaction of human plasma kallikrein and its light chain with alpha-2-macroglobulin. *Biochemistry*, 23:1760–1766.

229. Van Royen, E. A., de Boer, J. E. G., Wilnunk, J. M., Jenkins, C. S. P., and ten Cate, J. W. (1979): Acquired Factor XII deficiency in a patient with nephrotic syndrome. *Acta Med. Scand.*, 205:535–539.

230. Varonier, H. S., and Panzani, R. (1968): The effect of inhalation of bradykinin on healthy and atopic (asthmatic) children. *Int. Arch. Allergy*, 34:293–296.

231. Vaziri, N. D., Ngo, J-L. T., Ibsen, K. H., Mahalwas, K., Roy, S., and Hung, E. S. (1982): Deficiency and urinary losses of Factor XII in adult nephrotic syndrome. *Nephron*, 32:342–346.

232. Wachtfogel, Y. T., Kucich, U., James, H. L., Scott, C. F., Schapira, M., Zimmerman, M., Cohen, A. B., and Colman, R. W. (1983): Human plasma kallikrein releases neutrophil elastase during blood coagulation. *J. Clin. Invest.*, 72:1672–1677.

233. Waldman, R., Scicli, A. G., Scicli, G. M., Guimaraes, J. A., Carretero, O. A., Kato, H., Han, Y. N., and Iwanga, S. (1977): Significant role of fragment 1-2 plus light chain of bovine high molecular weight kininogen in contact mediated coagulation. *Thromb. Haemost.*, 38:14 (abstract).

234. Walsh, P. N., Sinha, D., Koshy, A., Seaman, F. S., and Bradford, H. (1986): Functional characterization of platelet-bound Factor XIa: Retention of Factor XIa activity on the platelet surface. *Blood*, 68:225–230.

235. Walsh, P. N. (1972): The role of platelets in the contact phase of blood coagulation. *Br. J. Haematol.*, 22:237–254.

236. Walsh, P. N. (1987): Platelet-mediated trigger mechanisms in the contact phase of blood coagulation. *Semin. Thromb. Hemost.*, 13:86–94.

237. Walsh, P. N., and Griffin, J. H. (1981): Contributions of human platelets to the proteolytic activation of blood coagulation Factors XII and XI. *Blood*, 57:106–118.

238. Webster, M. E., and Maling, H. M. (1970): *Bradykinin and Related Kinins: Cardiovascular, Biochemical and Neural Actions*, edited by F. Sicuteri, M. Rocha e Silva, and N. Bach, p. 493. Plenum Press, New York.

239. Weerasinghe, K. M., Scully, M. F., and Kakkar, V. V. (1984): The effect of collagen mediated platelet release on plasma kallikrein activation. *Thromb. Haemost.*, 51:37–41.

240. Weerasinghe, K. M., Scully, M. F., and Kakkar, V. V. (1984): Inhibition of cerebroside sulphate (sulfatide)-induced contact activation reactions by platelet factor four. *Thromb. Res.*, 33:625–631.

241. Weiss, A. S., Gallin, J. I., and Kaplan, A. P. (1974): Fletcher factor deficiency. A diminished rate of Hageman factor activation caused by absence of prekallikrein with abnormalities of coagulation, fibrinolysis, chemotactic activity and generation. *J. Clin. Invest.*, 53:622–633.

242. Weiss, R., Silverberg, M., and Kaplan, A. P. (1986): The effect of C1 inhibitor upon Hageman factor autoactivation. *Blood*, 68:239–243.

243. Wiggins, R. C., Loskutoff, D., Cochrane, C. G., Griffin, J. C., and Edgington, T. E. (1980): Activation of rabbit Hageman factor by homogenates of cultured rabbit endothelial cells. *J. Clin. Invest.*, 75:197–206.

244. Wiggins, R. C., Giclas, P. C., and Henson, P. M. (1981): Chemotactic activity generated from the fifth component of complement by plasma kallikrein of the rabbit. *J. Exp. Med.*, 153:1391–1404.

245. Wiggins, R. C., Giclas, P. C., and Henson, P. N. (1981): Chemotactic

activity generated from the fifth component of complement by plasma kallikrein of the rabbit. *J. Exp. Med.,* 153:1391–1404.

246. Wiggins, R. C. (1983): Kinin release from high molecular weight kininogen in the absence of kallikrein. *J. Biol. Chem.,* 258:8963–8970.

247. Wiggins, R. C. (1985): Hageman factor in experimental nephrotoxic nephritis in the rabbit. *Lab. Invest.,* 53:335–348.

248. Wiggins, R. C., and Cochrane, C. G. (1979): The autoactivation of rabbit Hageman factor. *J. Exp. Med.,* 150:1122–1133.

249. Wilner, G. D., Nossel, H. L., and Leroy, E. C. (1968): Activation of Hageman factor by collagen. *J. Clin. Invest.,* 47:2608–2615.

250. Wing, D. A., Yamada, T., Hayley, H. B., and Pettit, G. W. (1978): Model for disseminated intravascular coagulation: Bacterial sepsis in rhesus monkeys. *J. Lab. Clin. Med.,* 92:239–246.

251. Wong, P. Y., Talamo, R. C., and Colman, R. W. (1974): Kallikrein-kinin system in postgastrectomy dumping syndrome. *Ann. Intern. Med.,* 80:577–581.

252. Wuepper, K. D., Miller, D. R., and Lacombe, M. J. (1975): Flaujeac trait. Deficiency of human plasma kininogen. *J. Clin. Invest.,* 56:1663–1672.

253. Wuepper, K. D., and Cochrane, C. G. (1972): Plasma prekallikrein: Isolation, characterization and mechanism of activation. *J. Exp. Med.,* 135:1–20.

254. Wuepper, K. D., and Cochrane, C. G. (1972): Effect of plasma kallikrein on coagulation *in vitro. Proc. Soc. Exp. Biol. Med.,* 141:271.

255. Yamamoto, T., Kozono, K., Okomoto, T., Kato, H., and Kambara, T. (1980): Purification of guinea pig plasma prekallikrein. Activation by prekallikrein activator derived from guinea pig skin. *Biochim. Biophys. Acta,* 614:511–525.

256. Yamamoto, T., and Cochrane, C. G. (1981): Guinea pig Hageman factor as a vascular permeability enhancement factor. *Am. J. Pathol.,* 105:164–175.

257. Yang, H. Y. T., Erdos, E. G., and Levin, Y. (1971): Characterization of a dipeptide hydrolase (kinase II: angiotensin converting enzyme). *J. Pharmacol. Exp. Ther.,* 177:291–300.

258. Yang, H. Y. T., and Erdos, E. G. (1967): Second kininase in human blood plasma. *Nature,* 215:1402–1403.

259. Yurt, R., and Austen, K. F. (1977): Preparative purification of the rat mast cell chymase. Characterization and interaction with granule components. *J. Exp. Med.,* 146:1405–1419.

Inflammation: Basic Principles and Clinical Correlates.
Edited by J. I. Gallin, I. M. Goldstein, and R. Snyderman.
Raven Press, Ltd., New York © 1988.

CHAPTER 8

Leukotrienes

Robert A. Lewis and K. Frank Austen

Enzymes and Products of the 5-Lipoxygenase Pathway
Receptors for 5-Lipoxygenase Products and Functional
   Responses

References

The metabolism of arachidonic acid by the 5-lipoxygenase pathway in a variety of leukocyte types generates several products, including a hydroperoxy fatty acid, a hydroxy fatty acid, and hydroxy- and sulfidopeptide leukotrienes. *In vitro,* under selected conditions of cell activation and substrate presentation and in combination with a 15-lipoxygenase, it is possible to also generate conjugated tetraene products, lipoxins. The direct products of the 5-lipoxygenase pathway possess significant biologic potency as proinflammatory factors, and some may also participate in homeostatic immunoregulation. This review is intended to provide an update of state-of-the-art information on the 5-lipoxygenase pathway and its products since our last perspective (48).

ENZYMES AND PRODUCTS OF THE 5-LIPOXYGENASE PATHWAY

The 5-lipoxygenase and subsequent enzymes of the cascade it initiates have been definitively shown to exist only in a small number of cell types, including neutrophilic polymorphonuclear leukocytes (PMNs), eosinophils, basophils, monocytes, macrophages, and mast cells (48,55); there is also a suggestion that a modest capacity for this pathway exists in some lymphocyte subsets (23,29). That the 5-lipoxygenase is recovered from supernatants of broken cell preparations after sedimentation at $>100,000 \times g$ (34,63,90) demonstrates that the enzyme is not an intrinsic membrane protein, but it does not indicate that it and/or its substrate are cytosolic in the intact cell; indeed, it seems more likely that this rather hydro-

phobic enzyme is membrane-associated. The demonstration that apparently full activity of 5-lipoxygenase purified from human PMNs requires the back addition of several fractions that were removed during the purification (80) is additionally compatible with the necessity for membrane association of enzyme, substrate, or both for optimal catalytic activity. The apparent K_m of the 5-lipoxygenase for arachidonic acid, which is 10 to 20 μM for purified enzymes derived from the rat basophilic leukemia cell (RBL-1), guinea pig PMNs, and human PMNs (22,80,96), is comparable to that of the cyclooxygenase (103) and lower than that of the 15-lipoxygenase (61,90) for the same substrate. Since virtually all cells possessing a 5-lipoxygenase also contain the cyclooxygenase and some contain a 15-lipoxygenase, the activated enzymes compete for the same substrate according to both their K_m and catalytic rate (velocity) values unless there is compartmentalization. A further complexity in this competition is introduced by the obligatory requirement of the 5-lipoxygenase for availability of ionic calcium (22,80,96). Even when calcium ion is provided to the 5-lipoxygenase, this enzyme, like the cyclooxygenase, proceeds through an activation phase during which it generates enough of its hydroperoxide product to produce feedback augmentation and then inactivation of its catalytic capacity (41,77).

The product of the action of the 5-lipoxygenase on arachidonic acid is 5-hydroperoxyeicosatetraenoic acid (5-HPETE), which is short-lived in physiologic buffers and can be degraded either spontaneously or catalytically via a peroxidase to the corresponding alcohol, 5-hydroxyeicosatetraenoic acid (5-HETE) (Fig. 1). In addition, the 5-lipoxygenase enzyme can carry out a second catalytic step and process 5-HPETE to the epoxide, leukotriene A₄ (LTA₄). This process is apparently facilitated by the initial interaction of arachidonic acid with the 5-lipoxygenase, because the *de novo* addition of 5-HPETE to the purified enzyme results in less effective conversion (79). The oxygenation of arachidonic acid is carried out by the enzyme in concert with extraction of a specific prechiral hydrogen from the seventh carbon (C-7), and conversion of the hydroperoxide to the epoxide likewise involves the extraction of one prechiral hydrogen from C-10 in order to allow closure of the epoxide ring (52,80). It thus seems likely that the K_m of the 5-lipoxygenase for arachidonic acid should be significantly lower that that for 5-HPETE. There is no evidence that a portion of 5-HPETE released from the 5-lipoxygenase is significantly transported out of the cell of origin before its conversion to 5-HETE, although

it is possible that some 5-HPETE is reacylated into lysophospholipids before being reduced to the alcohol. 5-HETE can be directly reacylated into lysophospholipids (92) and can also be exported from leukocytes (101). The exported molecule can be taken up into platelets which, via action of their 12-lipoxygenase and subsequent reduction of the 12-hydroperoxide domain, can convert it into 5(S),12(S)-dihydroxy-6,10-*trans*-8,14-*cis*-eicosatetraenoic acid (12-epi-6-*trans*-8-*cis*-LTB₄) (81); 5-HETE could also enter a cell containing a 15-lipoxygenase, for conversion to a 5,15-diol (57), but would not be an appropriate substrate for generation of the 5,6,15- or 5,14,15-triol conjugated tetraenes, lipoxins A and B (19,82,83). There is no suggestion that the uptake of 5-HETE needs to be, or ever is, a facilitated process.

The 5-lipoxygenase can accept other polyunsaturated

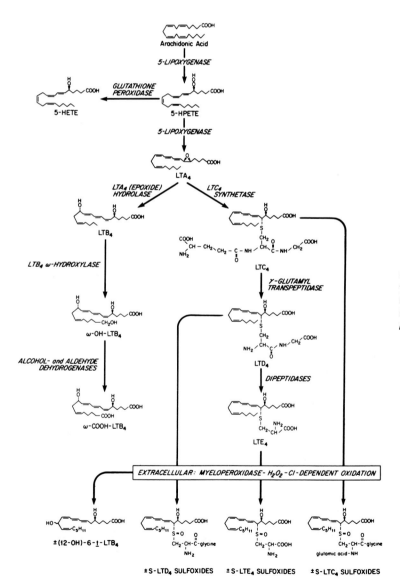

FIG. 1. Metabolism of arachidonic acid via the 5-lipoxygenase pathway and oxidative catabolism of the leukotriene products. [From Drazen, J. M., and Austen, K. F. (1987): Leukotrienes and airway responses. *Am. Rev. Respir. Dis.* (in press).]

fatty acids in addition to arachidonic acid, and these notably include the fish oil components eicosapentaenoic acid (EPA; 20:5, N-3) and docosahexaenoic acid (DCHA; 22:6, N-3). However, although EPA is converted to its C-5 hydroperoxide with an apparent K_m of 13 μM (63), which is comparable to that of the enzyme for arachidonic acid, it is inhibitory to the 5-lipoxygenase step when presented as an incorporated component of cell membrane phospholipids (45). Furthermore, DCHA is an exceedingly poor substrate with modest conversion to either the C-7 or C-4 hydroperoxide (16,46). Whereas 5-hydroperoxy-EPA (5-HPEPE) is readily converted to its epoxide leukotriene (LTA$_5$) by the 5-lipoxygenase in intact cells (45,46), the small quantities of 7- and 4-hydroperoxy-DCHAs are not metabolized to leukotrienes, presumably because of limitations imposed by the position of the methylene from which a proton would have to be extracted to allow epoxide ring closure.

Metabolism of LTA$_4$ to 5,12-dihydroxyleukotrienes can involve its catalytic conversion by a specific epoxide hydrolase (74,75) to LTB$_4$ in the cell containing the 5-lipoxygenase, export from the cell of origin and catalytic conversion by an epoxide hydrolase of another cell (10,18,58) or blood plasma (17), or nonenzymatic hydrolysis to 5(S),12(S)- and 5(S),12(R)-dihydroxy-6,8,10-*trans*-14-*cis*-eicosatetraenoic acids (the 12-epi-6-*trans*- and 6-*trans*-LTB$_4$ diastereoisomers). The epoxide hydrolase has a very favorable apparent K_m (20–30 μM) for LTA$_4$, which it readily converts to LTB$_4$ (75) while at the same time the enzyme becomes inactivated (62). LTA$_5$ is apparently an even more effective inactivator of the epoxide hydrolase (62).

The microsomal enzyme that preferentially metabolizes LTA$_4$ to LTC$_4$ (termed LTC$_4$ synthetase) is a unique member of the family of glutathione *S*-transferases and does not utilize conventional aromatic xenobiotics and aromatic chemical toxins as substrates, in contrast with the more classic glutathione *S*-transferases (2,104). Its apparent K_m for LTA$_4$ is approximately 5 to 10 μM, and for glutathione, 3 to 6 mM (104). Whereas this enzyme would compete with the epoxide hydrolase for substrate LTA$_4$ on the basis of relative K_m values, the relative apparent quantities of these enzymes in most cells containing the 5-lipoxygenase are grossly unequal. Eosinophils, which are highly competent for generation of LTC$_4$ in response to activation with the calcium ionophore A23187 or the synthetic chemotactic peptide *N*-formyl-met-leu-phe (fMLP) (5,32,66,86,98), produce little or no LTB$_4$. This is also the case for human pulmonary mast cells activated by A23187 or via IgE-dependent mechanisms (54,70). In contrast, human pulmonary macrophages produce relatively little LTC$_4$, although they generate large quantities of LTB$_4$ (15,21,53,56). Human PMNs selectively generate LTB$_4$ in response to activation with A23187. Only the

human monocyte has the capacity to generate approximately equal quantities of LTB$_4$ and LTC$_4$ in response to either the calcium ionophore or to transmembrane stimuli, including unopsonized zymosan and fMLP in the presence of cytochalasin B (9,28,100,102).

Further metabolism of LTB$_4$ has thus far been demonstrable only in PMNs and not in eosinophils, monocytes, or human alveolar macrophages during incubation periods of up to 30 min. The enzymes responsible for the processing of LTB$_4$ effect its ω-oxidation and inactivation. The LTB$_4$-20-hydroxylase, which oxidizes C-20 from a methyl group to an alcohol (35), is a unique enzyme which notably differs from prostaglandin ω-oxidases and fatty acid ω-oxidase (73,84,85,89) although each is a member of the cytochrome P-450 family and utilizes the same coupled P-450 reductase (91,99). Whereas it is possible that this enzyme can continue the oxidative process to produce the C-20 carboxylic acid, it has been demonstrated that oxidation of ω-hydroxy-LTB$_4$ can be effected by an NAD$^+$-dependent dehydrogenase (93). The K_m of the LTB$_4$-20-hydroxylase for its interaction with LTB$_4$ is 0.2 to 1.0 μM. Since LTB$_4$ is taken up into human PMNs via a specific receptor (26,27,37,51) and then becomes bioavailable for ω-oxidation, it seems that LTB$_4$ from cell sources other than PMN would be readily metabolized by this process, which does not require activation of the granulocytes. Some degree of sequestration of LTB$_4$ in human PMNs occurs when the leukotriene has been generated in response to a phagocytic stimulus by zymosan, and this too is metabolized to a large degree by ω-oxidation before it is secreted (101). It seems likely that ω-OH-LTB$_4$ can also be taken into PMNs, because it binds to the LTB$_4$ receptor (8).

Metabolism of LTC$_4$ has been shown to occur via two pathways, one of which is peptidolytic, and the other, oxidative. Peptide cleavage of LTC$_4$ occurs via the action of γ-glutamyl transpeptidase, with removal of glutamic acid, to leave LTD$_4$. This process probably does not occur to a significant extent in monocytes (100,102) and granulocytes (42). However, because a variety of nonleukocyte cell types also possess this exoenzyme activity (95), it is likely that the potential for peptidolytic cleavage of LTC$_4$ released by leukocytes would be significant in most tissues, including lung (31); certainly, γ-glutamyl transpeptidase is bioavailable for the conversion of LTC$_4$ to LTD$_4$ in blood plasma (49,67). The subsequent cleavage of LTD$_4$ to LTE$_4$, with the release of glycine, can be catalyzed by a variety of peptidases, including an activity from human PMN specific granules (42) and one in blood plasma (49,67). Oxidative metabolism of LTC$_4$, LTD$_4$, and LTE$_4$ occurs only in the extracellular environment of activated PMNs and eosinophils (43,44,98), leading to generation of the *S*-diastereoisomeric sulfoxides of each and the 6-*trans*-(C-12) diastereoisomers of LTB$_4$. The mechanism involves cellular production of hydrogen peroxide via the respiratory burst, secretion of the cell-specific peroxidase, and interaction of enzyme, peroxide, and chloride ion to produce hypochlorous acid as the moiety which attacks the sulfidopeptide leukotriene. The major biologic differences between the peptidolytic pathway and the oxidative one are that the former does not require activated cells and does not eliminate the biologic activities of LTC_4, whereas the latter requires activation and effects functional catabolism (43,44,98). It appears that in normal primates, as opposed to rodents, the metabolic fate of LTC_4 or LTD_4 is largely that of urinary excretion of LTE_4, without additional modification by *N*-acetylation (30,64,65). *In vivo* assessment for oxidative degradation of the sulfidopeptide leukotrienes during inflammation has not yet been carried out.

The utility of employing the calcium ionophore as an activating probe for the generation of leukotrienes is that, because the bioavailability of calcium to the 5-lipoxygenase is apparently limiting, the ionophore optimizes this process. However, since A23187 translocates calcium ion between all cellular and extracellular compartments, it activates biochemical processes in addition to those activated by receptor-dependent physiologic stimuli (59) and thus would make the assessment of physiologic regulation difficult at best. There are as yet still relatively few studies that have employed nonionophoric activating stimuli to elicit leukotriene generation. IgE Fc-dependent stimuli activate human mast cells and basophils for LTC_4 generation and release (54,55,70). Zymosan activates human PMNs, monocytes, and alveolar macrophages for generation of LTB_4, $LTB_4 + LTC_4$, and LTB_4, respectively (53,56,101). The peptide fMLP, acting on human monocytes and eosinophils after pretreatment with cytochalasin B, also elicits the production of $LTC_4 + LTB_4$ and LTC_4, respectively (66,102); most investigators would agree that fMLP does not effect biosynthesis of LTB_4 in PMN. It is likewise clear that phorbol myristate acetate (PMA), which interacts with and activates protein kinase C, leading to evolution of the respiratory burst in PMN (11,36), does not evoke LTB_4 generation, because calcium ion would not be presented by this stimulus for activation of the 5-lipoxygenase.

Modulation of leukotriene biosynthesis *in vitro* occurs via the actions of cytokines. In the limited setting of A23187-dependent activation of PMNs and eosinophils, pretreatment with an apparently related group of highly acidic monokines enhances generation of the predominant leukotriene of each cell by up to severalfold (12); this phenomenon is also demonstrable following preincubation of human eosinophils with recombinant granulocyte-macrophage colony stimulating factor before cell activation by the ionophore (87). Heat-aggregated IgG does not elicit the generation and release of LTB_4 when incubated

with otherwise untreated cells from bronchoalveolar lavage, but it becomes effective if the macrophages have been previously exposed for 24 hr to γ-interferon. The intervening events include at least the induction of an increased number of cell surface IgG Fc receptors in response to the γ-interferon (76), whether by decreased clearance, increased availability of already synthesized intracellular receptors or by increased transcription, translation, or posttranslational modification. Experiments carried out in order to differentiate human cord blood cells into basophils, and utilizing human lymphokine-conditioned media depleted of interleukin-1 and interleukin-2, produced cells with morphologic characteristics of basophils, high-affinity IgE Fc receptors, and immunologically releasable histamine-containing granules, but without the capacity of the mature basophil to generate and release LTC_4 in response to IgE-dependent activation or stimulation with the calcium ionophore (33). This indicates that some additional differentiation factor is required to establish this particular aspect of the biologic identity of the cell.

RECEPTORS FOR 5-LIPOXYGENASE PRODUCTS AND FUNCTIONAL RESPONSES

In the relatively short modern history of this field, rapid accumulation of information has occurred largely in response to the presumption that 5-lipoxygenase products are mediators of hypersensitivity and of various types of inflammation. It thus seems pertinent to focus on a sequence in which 5-lipoxygenase products are generated, released from the generating cell, and then interact with a target cell—possibly via a specific receptor—to elicit a biologic effect. In addition, however, it is not unlikely that certain 5-lipoxygenase products act as intracellular regulators in their cell of origin. It has been suggested that modest quantities of these products are all that is required for such intracellular regulatory events; for example, the barely detectable level of LTB_4 allegedly synthesized by 10^6 T cells (23,29) is held sufficient for its participation in the process of differentiating fully competent suppressor T cells (1,67,78). That a subpopulation of these cells is also believed to possess LTB_4 receptors (69) is consistent with the possibility of intracellular regulation or cell recruitment as well as self-initiation of the differentiation process. LTB_4-mediated cellular events, such as the activation of human PMNs for self-adherence (aggregation) (20), chemotactic deactivation (24), and granule secretion (88), may involve the receptor as a conduit—in the mode of an ion channel—or as an element in a transduction process. LTB_4 uptake in the human PMN is rapid, as monitored by evidence of ω-oxidation within 2 min of addition of the leukotriene to the cells (35), and thus occurs within the same time frame as the initiation of these biologic responses; this suggests but does not prove linkage of uptake with effect. LTB_4-mediated chemotaxis (25,50), like chemotaxis to any receptor-dependent stimulus, is a directional event and thus would not be stimulated by intracellular generation of the ligand. The molar dissociation constant (K_d) of the putative high-affinity LTB_4 receptor, 4 to 5×10^{-10} M, is clearly in the range of the minimal effective concentration for chemotaxis, whereas the K_d of the low-affinity LTB_4 receptor, 0.6 to 5×10^{-7} M, has been suggested to relate to secretion of PMN granules (27,51). These data do not, however, discriminate effector function related to receptor-mediated transduction from that related to ligand uptake, especially because radioligand binding studies must be carried out at subphysiologic temperatures to limit ligand uptake.

That neither of the 6-*trans*-LTB_4 diastereoisomers can effect any of the known responses to LTB_4 in a wide variety of assays strongly suggests that they are biologically inactive by-products when produced from either LTA_4 or from catabolism of the sulfidopeptide leukotrienes. There is additionally no evidence that either 6-*trans*-LTB_4 diastereoisomer is taken up into PMNs from the extracellular environment and, because LTA_4 has been shown to be secreted from ionophore-activated PMNs (58), it is clear that nonenzymatic hydrolysis of LTA_4 to these LTB_4 isomers can occur extracellularly. However, without strong evidence against nonenzymatic hydrolysis of intracellular LTA_4, it is not possible to rule out an intracellular function for either or both isomers.

Most of the known biologic responses to LTC_4, LTD_4, and LTE_4 are presumed to be receptor-mediated. These responses are mainly cellular and tissue contractile events, such as airway constriction via nonvascular smooth muscle, arterial and arteriolar vasoconstriction via vascular smooth muscle, and vasopermeability via contraction of endothelial cells. A number of other organ effects proceed indirectly through these same mechanisms, for example, negative inotropic effects on the heart via coronary arteriolar vasoconstriction (4,71) and decreased glomerular filtration via renovascular vaso- or glomeruloconstriction (3). The evidence for LTD_4 receptors on responding airway tissues includes ligand specificity and stereospecificity (47,72), regulation of the affinities of these receptors for their ligands by guanosine triphosphate (GTP), thus implying association with a GTP binding protein, and solubilization of the receptor–ligand complex (60).

The issue of distinct LTC_4 receptors is far more complicated and not yet resolved. A number of cells, including guinea pig ileal smooth muscle, a smooth muscle line derived from hamster ductus deferens (termed DDT_1 MF-2), and bovine aortic endothelium each have highly selective binding sites for LTC_4 over LTD_4, LTE_4, and less related ligands (6,38,39). For the ileum and the endothelium, these selective binding sites exist in association with

both plasma membrane and mitochondrial membranes. As for the LTD_4 receptors on guinea pig and human lung tissues (47,72), the cell surface LTC_4 binding sites meet the presumptive definition for receptors in that radioligand binding reaches equilibrium, is saturable, reversible, and specifically competed for by unlabeled ligands, and occurs in a concentration range similar to that needed for the biologic effects. It nonetheless remains possible that the specific cell membrane binding sites for LTC_4 that have been identified in radioligand binding studies are not identical with the receptors which transduce the ligand signal. To date, attempts to solubilize these binding sites from guinea pig ileal smooth muscle and endothelium have been unsuccessful with any combination of ionic and nonionic detergents, in that the binding sites remained largely associated with insoluble (presumably cytoskeletal) elements. It is suggested from functional data on guinea pig tissues that unique LTC_4 recognition exists, differing from that for LTD_4 or LTE_4 in its relative lack of antagonism by the classic slow-reacting substance antagonist FPL55712 versus the relative efficacy of the (voltage-regulated) calcium channel blocker diltiazem (13,14). Furthermore, the nearly full maintenance of the guinea pig ileal smooth muscle contractile response to LTC_4 in the presence of the γ-glutamyl transpeptidase inhibitor serine–borate complex suggests that the LTC_4 response does not require prior conversion of LTC_4 to LTD_4 for interaction with an LTD_4 receptor (40).

The existence of intracellular binding sites has a number of alternative explanations, for example, that they represent a portion of the same receptor population as that existing on the cell surface and recycle, that they represent separate receptors which require prior ligand uptake to mediate their unique effects on the cell, or that they are not receptors for LTC_4 but their interaction with this ligand is adventitious or mediates a noncontractile function. That a high-affinity interaction of LTC_4 can occur with a highly specific nonreceptor binding unit has been demonstrated for rat liver cytosolic glutathione *S*-transferase type 1-1 (94) and suggests that the demonstration of specific LTC_4 binding factors in homogenates of a great variety of tissues (7) should be reexamined. Because the catalytic function of the glutathione *S*-transferase isoenzyme is inhibited by LTC_4 and a semispecific inhibition of human eosinophil arylsulfatase B by sulfidopeptide leukotrienes also occurs at submicromolar concentrations (97), it is premature to assume that high-affinity interactions of LTC_4 with cellular elements are either receptor-specific or biologically relevant to spasmogenic responses.

REFERENCES

1. Atluru, D., and Goodwin, J. S. (1984): Control of polyclonal immunoglobulin production from human lymphocytes by leuko-

trienes: Leukotriene B_4 induces an OKT8(+), radiosensitive suppressor cell from resting human OKT8(−) T cells. *J. Clin. Invest.*, 74:1444–1450.

2. Bach, M. K., Brashler, J. R., and Morton, D. R., Jr. (1984): Solubilization and characterization of the leukotriene C_4 synthetase of rat basophil leukemia cells: A novel, particulate glutathione-*S*-transferase. *Arch. Biochem. Biophys.*, 230:455–465.

3. Badr, K. F., Baylis, C., Pfeffer, J. M., Pfeffer, M. A., Soberman, R. J., Lewis, R. A., Austen, K. F., Corey, E. J., and Brenner, B. M. (1984): Renal and systemic hemodynamic responses to intravenous infusion of leukotriene C_4 in the rat. *Circ. Res.*, 54:492–499.

4. Bittl, J. A., Pfeffer, M. A., Lewis, R. A., Mehrotra, M. M., Corey, E. J., and Austen, K. F. (1985): Mechanism of the negative inotropic action of leukotrienes C_4 and D_4 on isolated rat heart. *Cardiovasc. Res.*, XIX:426–432.

5. Borgeat, P., de Laclos, B. F., Rabinovich, H., Picard, S., Braquet, P., Hebert, J., and Laviolette, M. (1984): Eosinophil-rich human polymorphonuclear leukocyte preparations characteristically release leukotriene C_4 on ionophore A23187 challenge. *J. Allergy Clin. Immunol.*, 74:310–315.

6. Chau, L.-Y., Hoover, R. L., Austen, K. F., and Lewis, R. A. (1986): Subcellular distribution of leukotriene C_4 binding units in cultured bovine aortic endothelial cells. *J. Immunol.*, 137:1985–1992.

7. Cheng, J. B., Lang, D., Bewtra, A., and Townley, R. G. (1985): Tissue distribution and functional correlation of [^{3}H]leukotriene C_4 and [^{3}H]leukotriene D_4 binding sites in guinea-pig uterus and lung preparations. *J. Pharmacol. Exp. Ther.*, 232:80–87.

8. Clancy, R. M., Dahinden, C. A., and Hugli, T. E. (1984): Oxidation of leukotrienes at the omega end: Demonstration of a receptor for the 20-hydroxy derivative of leukotriene B_4 on human neutrophils and implications for the analysis of leukotriene receptors. *Proc. Natl. Acad. Sci. USA*, 81:5729–5733.

9. Czop, J. K., and Austen, K. F. (1985): Generation of leukotrienes by human monocytes upon stimulation of their β-glucan receptor during phagocytosis. *Proc. Natl. Acad. Sci. USA*, 82:2751–2755.

10. Dahinden, C. A., Clancy, R. M., Gross, M., Chiller, J. M., and Hugli, T. E. (1985): Leukotriene C_4 production by murine mast cells: Evidence for a role for extracellular leukotriene A_4. *Proc. Natl. Acad. Sci. USA*, 82:6632–6636.

11. DeChatelet, L. R., Shirley, P. S., Johnson, R. B., Jr. (1976): Effect of phorbol myristate acetate on the oxidative metabolism of human polymorphonuclear leukocytes. *Blood*, 47:545–554.

12. Dessein, A. J., Lee, T. H., Elsas, P., Ravalese, J. R., III, Silberstein, D., David, J. R., Austen, K. F., and Lewis, R. A. (1986): Enhancement by monokines of leukotriene generation by human eosinophils and neutrophils stimulated with calcium ionophore A23187. *J. Immunol.*, 136:3829–3838.

13. Drazen, J. M., Austen, K. F., Lewis, R. A., Clark, D. A., Goto, G., Marfat, A., and Corey, E. J. (1980): Comparative airway and vascular activities of leukotrienes C-1 and D *in vivo* and *in vitro*. *Proc. Natl. Acad. Sci. USA*, 77:4353–4358.

14. Drazen, J. M., Fanta, C. H., Lacouture, P., Corey, E. J. (1984): Physiologic evidence for leukotriene receptor heterogeneity in guinea pig pulmonary parenchymal strips *in vitro*. *Clin. Res.*, 32:528A (abstract).

15. Fels, A. O. S., Pawlowski, N. A., Cramer, E. B., King, T. K. C., Cohn, Z. A., and Smith, W. A. (1982): Human alveolar macrophages produce leukotriene B_4. *Proc. Natl. Acad. Sci. USA*, 79:7866–7870.

16. Fischer, S., Schacky, C. V., Siess, W., Strasser, T., and Weber, P. C. (1984): Uptake, release and metabolism of docosahexaenoic acid (DHA C22:6ω3) in human platelets and neutrophils. *Biochem. Biophys. Res. Commun.*, 120:907–918.

17. Fitzpatrick, F. A., Haeggström, J., Granström, E., and Samuelsson, B. (1983): Metabolism of leukotriene A_4 by an enzyme in blood plasma. *Proc. Natl. Acad. Sci. USA*, 80:5425–5429.

18. Fitzpatrick, F. A., Liggett, W., McGee, J., Bunting, S., Morton, D., and Samuelsson, B. (1985): Metabolism of leukotriene A_4 by human erythrocytes: A novel cellular source of leukotriene B_4. *J. Biol. Chem.*, 259:11403–11407.

19. Fitzsimmons, B. J., Adams, J., Evans, J. F., Leblanc, Y., and Rokach, J. (1985): The lipoxins: Stereochemical identification and determination of their biosynthesis. *J. Biol. Chem.*, 260:13008–13012.

20. Ford-Hutchinson, A. W., Bray, M. A., Doig, M. V., Shipley, N. E., and Smith, M. J. (1980): Leukotriene B, a potent chemokinetic and aggregating substance released from polymorphonuclear leukocytes. *Nature*, 286:264–265.

21. Godard, P., Damon, M., Michel, F.-B., Corey, E. J., Austen, K. F., and Lewis, R. A. (1983): Leukotriene B_4 production from human alveolar macrophages. *Clin. Res.*, 31:548 (abstract).

22. Goetze, A. M., Fayer, L., Bouska, J., Bornemeier, D., and Carter, G. W. (1985): Purification of a mammalian 5-lipoxygenase from rat basophilic leukemia cells. *Prostaglandins*, 29:689–701.

23. Goetzl, E. J. (1981): Selective feedback inhibition of the 5-lipoxygenation of arachidonic acid in human T lymphocytes. *Biochem. Biophys. Res. Commun.*, 101:344–350.

24. Goetzl, E. J., Boeynaems, J. M., Oates, J. A., and Hubbard, W. G. (1981): Stimulus-specificity of the chemotactic deactivation of human neutrophils by lipoxygenase products of arachidonic acid. *Prostaglandins*, 22:279–288.

25. Goetzl, E. J., and Pickett, W. C. (1981): Novel structural determinants of the human neutrophil chemotactic activity of leukotriene B. *J. Exp. Med.*, 153:482–487.

26. Goldman, D. W., and Goetzl, E. J. (1982): Specific binding of leukotriene B_4 to receptors on human polymorphonuclear leukocytes. *J. Immunol.*, 129:1600–1604.

27. Goldman, D. W., and Goetzl, E. J. (1984): Heterogeneity of human polymorphonuclear leukocyte receptors for leukotriene B_4: Identification of a subset of high affinity receptors that transduce the chemotactic response. *J. Exp. Med.*, 159:1027–1041.

28. Goldyne, M. E., Burrish, G. F., Poubelle, P., and Borgeat, P. (1984): Arachidonic acid metabolism among human mononuclear leukocytes: Lipoxygenase related pathways. *J. Biol. Chem.*, 259:8815–8819.

29. Goodwin, J. S., and Atluru, D. (1986): Mechanism of action of cocorticoid-induced immunoglobulin production: Role of lipoxygenase metabolites of arachidonic acid. *J. Immunol.*, 136:3455–3460.

30. Hammarström, S., Örning, L., Bernström, N., Gustafsson, B., Norin, E., and Kaijser, L. (1985): Metabolism of leukotriene C_4 in rats and humans. *Adv. Prostaglandin Thromboxane Leukotriene Res.*, 15:185–188.

31. Harper, T. W., Westcott, J. Y., Voelkel, N., and Murphy, R. C. (1984): Metabolism of leukotrienes B_4 and C_4 in the isolated perfused rat lung. *J. Biol. Chem.*, 259:14437–14440.

32. Henderson, W. R., Harley, J. B., and Fauci, A. S. (1984): Arachidonic acid metabolism in normal and hypereosinophilic syndrome human eosinophils: Generation of leukotriene B_4, C_4, D_4, and 15-lipoxygenase products. *Immunology*, 51:679–686.

33. Ishizaka, T., Conrad, D. H., Huff, T. F., Metcalfe, D. D., Stevens, R. L., and Lewis, R. A. (1985): Unique features of human basophilic granulocytes developed in *in vitro* culture. *Int. Arch. Allergy Appl. Immunol.*, 77:137–143.

34. Jakschik, B. A., and Lee, C. H. (1980): Enzymatic assembly of slow reacting substance. *Nature*, 287:51–52.

35. Jubiz, W., Rådmark, O., Malmsten, C., Hansson, G., Lindgren, J. A., Palmblad, J., Udén, A. M., and Samuelsson, B. (1982): A novel leukotriene produced by stimulation of leukocytes with formylmethionylleucylphenylalanine. *J. Biol. Chem.*, 257:6106–6110.

36. Kikkawa, W., Takai, Y., Tanaka, Y., Miyake, R., and Nishizuka, Y. (1983): Protein kinase C as a possible receptor protein of tumor-promoting phorbol esters. *J. Biol. Chem.*, 258:11442–11445.

37. Kreisle, R. A., and Parker, C. W. (1983): Specific binding of leukotriene B_4 to a receptor on human polymorphonuclear leukocytes. *J. Exp. Med.*, 157:628–641.

38. Krilis, S., Lewis, R. A., Corey, E. J., and Austen, K. F. (1983): Specific receptors for leukotriene C_4 on a smooth muscle cell line. *J. Clin. Invest.*, 72:1516–1519.

39. Krilis, S., Lewis, R. A., Corey, E. J., and Austen, K. F. (1984): Specific binding of leukotriene C_4 to ileal segments and subcellular

fractions of ileal smooth muscle cells. *Proc. Natl. Acad. Sci. USA,* 81:4529–4533.

40. Krilis, S., Lewis, R. A., Corey, E. J., and Austen, K. F. (1983): Bioconversion of C-6 sulfidopeptide leukotrienes by the responding guinea pig ileum determines the time course of its contraction. *J. Clin. Invest.,* 71:909–915.

41. Lands, W. E. M. (1985): Interactions of lipid hydroperoxides with eicosanoid biosynthesis. *J. Free Radicals Biol. Med.,* 1:97–101.

42. Lee, C. W., Lewis, R. A., Corey, E. J., and Austen, K. F. (1983): Conversion of leukotriene D_4 to leukotriene E_4 by a dipeptidase released from the specific granule of human polymorphonuclear leucocytes. *Immunology,* 48:27–35.

43. Lee, C. W., Lewis, R. A., Corey, E. J., Barton, A., Oh, H., Tauber, A. I., and Austen, K. F. (1982): Oxidative inactivation of leukotriene C_4 by stimulated human polymorphonuclear leukocytes. *Proc. Natl. Acad. Sci. USA,* 79:4166–4170.

44. Lee, C. W., Lewis, R. A., Tauber, A. I., Mehrotra, M. M., Corey, E. J., and Austen, K. F. (1983): The myeloperoxidase-dependent metabolism of leukotrienes C_4, D_4, and E_4 to 6-*trans*-leukotriene B_4 diastereoisomers and the subclass-specific *S*-diastereoisomeric sulfoxides. *J. Biol. Chem.,* 258:15004–15010.

45. Lee, T. H., Hoover, R. L., Williams, J. D., Sperling, R. I., Ravalese, J. R., III, Spur, B. W., Robinson, D. R., Corey, E. J., Lewis, R. A., and Austen, K. F. (1985): Effect of dietary enrichment with eicosapentaenoic and docosahexaenoic acids on *in vitro* neutrophil and monocyte leukotriene generation and neutrophil function. *N. Engl. J. Med.,* 312:1217–1223.

46. Lee, T. H., Mencia-Huerta, J.-M., Shih, C., Corey, E. J., Lewis, R. A., and Austen, K. F. (1984): Effects of exogenous arachidonic, eicosapentaenoic, and docosahexaenoic acids on the generation of 5-lipoxygenase pathway products by ionophore-activated human neutrophils. *J. Clin. Invest.,* 74:1922–1933.

47. Lewis, M. A., Mong, S., Vessella, R. L., and Crooke, S. T. (1985): Identification and characterization of leukotriene D_4 receptors in adult and fetal human lung. *Biochem. Pharmacol.,* 34:4311–4317.

48. Lewis, R. A., and Austen, K. F. (1984): The biologically active leukotrienes: Biosynthesis, metabolism, receptors, functions, and pharmacology. *J. Clin. Invest.,* 73:889–897.

49. Lewis, R. A., Drazen, J. M., Figueiredo, J., Corey, E. J., and Austen, K. F. (1982): A review of recent contributions on biologically active products of arachidonate conversion. *Int. J. Immunopharmacacol.,* 4:85–90.

50. Lewis, R. A., Goetzl, E. J., Drazen, J. M., Soter, N. A., Austen, K. F., and Corey, E. J. (1981): Functional characterization of synthetic leukotriene B and its stereochemical isomers. *J. Exp. Med.,* 154:1243–1248.

51. Lin, A. H., Ruppel, P. L., and Gorman, R. R. (1984): Leukotriene B_4 binding to human neutrophils. *Prostaglandins,* 28:837–849.

52. Maas, R. L., Ingram, C. D., Taber, D. F., Oates, J. A., and Brash, A. R. (1982): Stereospecific removal of the DR hydrogen atom at the 10-carbon of arachidonic acid in the biosynthesis of leukotriene A_4 by human leukocytes. *J. Biol. Chem.,* 257:13515–13519.

53. MacDermot, J., Kelsey, C. R., Waddell, K. A., Richmond, R., Knight, R. K., Cole, P. J., Dollery, C. T., London, D. N., and Blair, I. A. (1984): Synthesis of leukotriene B_4 and prostanoids by human alveolar macrophages: Analysis by gas chromatography/mass spectrometry. *Prostaglandins,* 27:163–179.

54. MacGlashan, D. W., Schleimer, R., Peters, S. P., Schulman, E. S., Adams, G. K., Newball, H. H., and Lichtenstein, L. M. (1982): Generation of leukotrienes by purified human lung mast cells. *J. Clin. Invest.,* 70:747–751.

55. MacGlashin, D. W., Jr., Peters, S. P., Warner, J., and Lichtenstein, L. M. (1986): Characteristics of human basophil sulfidopeptide leukotriene release: Releasability defined as the ability of the basophil to respond to dimeric cross-links. *J. Immunol.,* 136:2231–2239.

56. Martin, T. R., Altman, L. C., Albert, R. K., and Henderson, W. R. (1984): Leukotriene B_4 production by the human alveolar macrophage: A potential mechanism for amplifying inflammation in the lung. *Am. Rev. Respir. Dis.,* 129:106–111.

57. Maas, R. L., Turk, J., Oates, J. A., and Brash, A. (1982): Formation

of a novel dihydroxy acid from arachidonic acid by lipoxygenase-catalyzed double oxygenation in rat mononuclear cells and human leukocytes. *J. Biol. Chem.,* 257:7056–7067.

58. McGee, J. E., and Fitzpatrick, F. A. (1986): Erythrocyte-neutrophil interactions: Formation of leukotriene B_4 by transcellular biosynthesis. *Proc. Natl. Acad. Sci. USA,* 83:1349–1353.

59. McGivney, A., Morita, Y., Crews, F. T., Hirata, F., Axelrod, J., and Siraganian, R. P. (1981): Phospholipase activation to the IgE-mediated and Ca^{2+} ionophore A23187-induced release of histamine from rat basophilic leukemia cells. *Arch. Biochem. Biophys.,* 212:577–580.

60. Mong, S., Wu, H. L., Stadel, J. M., Clark, M. A., and Crook, S. T. (1986): Solubilization of [^{3}H]leukotriene D_4 receptor complex from guinea pig lung membranes. *Mol. Pharmacol.,* 29:235–243.

61. Narumiya, S., Salmon, J. A., Coltee, L. H., Weatherly, B. G., and Flower, R. J. (1981): Arachidonic acid 15-lipoxygenase from rabbit peritoneal polymorphonuclear leukocytes: Partial purification and properties. *J. Biol. Chem.,* 256:9583–9592.

62. Nathaniel, D. J., Evans, J. F., Leblanc, Y., Leveille, C., Fitzsimmons, B. J., and Ford-Hutchinson, A. W. (1985): Leukotriene A_5 is a substrate and an inhibitor of rat and human neutrophil LTA_4 hydrolase. *Biochem. Biophys. Res. Commun.,* 131:827–835.

63. Ochi, K., Yoshimoto, T., Yamamoto, S., Taniguchi, K., and Miyamoto, T. (1983): Arachidonate 5-lipoxygenase of guinea pig peritoneal polymorphonuclear leukocytes: Activation by adenosine-5′ triphosphate. *J. Biol. Chem.,* 258:5754–5758.

64. Örning, L., Kaijser, L., and Hammarström, S. (1985): *In vivo* metabolism of leukotriene C_4 in man: Urinary excretion of leukotriene E_4. *Biochem. Biophys. Res. Commun.,* 130:214–220.

65. Örning, L., Norin, E., Gustafsson, B., and Hammarström, S. (1986): *In vivo* metabolism of leukotriene C_4 in germ-free and conventional rats: Fecal excretion of *N*-acetyl leukotriene E_4. *J. Biol. Chem.,* 261:766–771.

66. Owen, W. F., Soberman, R. J., Yoshimoto, T., Sheffer, A. L., Lewis, R. A., and Austen, K. F. (1987): Synthesis and release of leukotriene C_4 by human eosinophils. *J. Immunol.,* 138:532–538.

67. Parker, C. W., Koch, D., Huber, M. M., and Falkenhein, S. F. (1980): Formation of the cysteinyl form of slow reacting substance (leukotriene E_4) in human plasma. *Biochem. Biophys. Res. Commun.,* 97:1038–1046.

68. Payan, D. G., and Goetzl, E. J. (1983): Specific suppression of human T lymphocyte function by leukotriene B_4. *J. Immunol.,* 131:551–553.

69. Payan, D. G., and Goetzl, E. J. (1984): Recognition of leukotriene B_4 by a unique subset of human T-lymphocytes. *J. Allergy Clin. Immunol.,* 74:403–406.

70. Peters, S. P., MacGlashan, D. W., Jr., Schulman, E. S., Schleimer, R., Hayes, E. C., Rokach, J., Adkinson, N. F., Jr., and Lichtenstein, L. M. (1984): Arachidonic acid metabolism in purified human lung mast cells. *J. Immunol.,* 132:1972–1979.

71. Pfeffer, M. A., Pfeffer, J. M., Lewis, R. A., Braunwald, E., Corey, E. J., and Austen, K. F. (1983): Systemic hemodynamic effects of leukotrienes C_4 and D_4 in the rat. *Am. J. Physiol.,* 244:H628–H633.

72. Pong, S.-S., and DeHaven, R. N. (1983): Characterization of a leukotriene D_4 receptor in guinea pig lung. *Proc. Natl. Acad. Sci. USA,* 80:7415–7419.

73. Powell, W. S. (1984): Properties of leukotriene B_4 20-hydroxylase from polymorphonuclear leukocytes. *J. Biol. Chem.,* 259:3082–3089.

74. Rådmark, O., Malmsten, C., Samuelsson, B., Clark, D. A., Goto, G., Marfat, A., and Corey, E. J. (1980): Leukotriene A: Stereochemistry and enzymatic conversion to leukotriene B. *Biochem. Biophys. Res. Commun.,* 92:954–961.

75. Rådmark, O., Shimizu, T., Jörnvall, M., and Samuelsson, B. (1984): Leukotriene A_4 hydrolase in human leukocytes: Purification and properties. *J. Biol. Chem.,* 259:12339–12345.

76. Rankin, J. A., Schrader, C. E., and Lewis, R. A. (1986): Leukotriene B_4 release from human alveolar macrophages incubated with IgG: Effect of γ-interferon. *Fed. Proc.,* 45:212 (abstract).

77. Reddy, C. C., Rao, M. K., Mastro, A. M., and Egan, R. W. (1984): Measurement of glutathione requiring enzymes involved in ara-

chidonic acid cascade of rat basophil leukemia cells. *Biochem. Int.,* 9:755–761.

78. Rola-Pleszczynski, M., Borgeat, P., and Sirois, P. (1982): Leukotriene B_4 induces human suppressor lymphocytes. *Biochem. Biophys. Res. Commun.,* 108:1531–1537.

79. Rouzer, C. A., Matsumoto, T., and Samuelsson, B. (1986): Single protein from human leukocytes possesses 5-lipoxygenase and leukotriene A_4 synthase activities. *Proc. Natl. Acad. Sci. USA,* 83:857–861.

80. Rouzer, C. A., and Samuelsson, B. (1985): On the nature of the 5-lipoxygenase reaction in human leukocytes: Enzyme purification and requirement for multiple stimulatory factors. *Proc. Natl. Acad. Sci. USA,* 82:6040–6044.

81. Samuelsson, B., Hammarström, S., Hamberg, M., and Serhan, C. N. (1985): Structural determination of leukotrienes and lipoxins. *Adv. Prostaglandin Thromboxane Leukotriene Res.,* 14:45–71.

82. Serhan, C. N., Hamberg, M., and Samuelsson, B. (1984): Trihydroxytetraenes: A novel series of compounds formed from arachidonic acid in human leukocytes. *Biochem. Biophys. Res. Commun.,* 118:943–949.

83. Serhan, C. N., Hamberg, M., Samuelsson, B., Morris, J., and Wishka, D. G. (1986): On the stereochemistry and biosynthesis of lipoxin B. *Proc. Natl. Acad. Sci. USA,* 83:1983–1987.

84. Shak, S., and Goldstein, I. M. (1985): Leukotriene B_4 ω-hydroxylase in human polymorphonuclear leukocytes. *J. Clin. Invest.,* 76:1218–1228.

85. Shak, S., and Goldstein, I. M. (1984): Omega-oxidation is the major pathway for the catabolism of leukotriene B_4 in human polymorphonuclear leukocytes. *J. Biol. Chem.,* 259:10181–10187.

86. Shaw, R. J., Cromwell, O., and Kay, A. B. (1984): Preferential generation of leukotriene C_4 by human eosinophils. *Clin. Exp. Immunol.,* 56:716–722.

87. Silberstein, D. S., Owen, W. F., Gasson, J. C., DiPersio, J., Golde, D. W., Bina, J. C., Soberman, R. J., Austen, K. F., and David, J. R. (1986): Enhancement of human eosinophil cytotoxicity and leukotriene synthesis by biosynthetic (recombinant) granulocyte-macrophage colony-stimulating factor. *J. Immunol.,* 137:3290–3294.

88. Smith, R. J., Iden, S. S., and Bowman, B. J. (1984): Activation of the human neutrophil secretory process with 5(S),12(R)-dihydroxy-6,14-cis-8,10-trans-eicosatetraenoic acid. *Inflammation,* 8:365–384.

89. Soberman, R. J., Harper, R. W., Murphy, R. C., and Austen, K. F. (1985): Identification and functional characterization of leukotriene B_4 20-hydroxylase of human polymorphonuclear leukocytes. *Proc. Natl. Acad. Sci. USA,* 82:2292–2295.

90. Soberman, R. J., Harper, T. W., Betteridge, D., Lewis, R. A., and Austen, K. F. (1985): Characterization and separation of the arachidonic acid 5-lipoxygenase and linoleic acid ω-6 lipoxygenase (arachidonic acid 15-lipoxygenase) of human polymorphonuclear leukocytes. *J. Biol. Chem.,* 260:4508–4515.

91. Soberman, R. J., Okita, R. T., Fitzsimmons, B., Rokach, J., Spur, B., and Austen, K. F. (1986): Stereochemical requirements for substrate specificity of LTB_4 20-hydroxylase. *J. Biol. Chem., (in press).*

92. Stenson, W. F., and Parker, C. W. (1979): Metabolism of arachidonic acid in ionophore-stimulated neutrophils: Esterification of a hydroxylated metabolite into phospholipids. *J. Clin. Invest.,* 64:1457–1465.

93. Sumimoto, H., Takeshige, K., and Minakami, S. (1985): NAD^+-dependent conversion of 20-OH-LTB_4 to 20-COOH-LTB_4 by a cell-free system of human polymorphonuclear leukocytes. *Biochem. Biophys. Res. Commun.,* 132:864–870.

94. Sun, F. F., Chau, L.-Y., Spur, B., Corey, E. J., Lewis, R. A., and Austen, K. F. (1986): Identification of a high affinity leukotriene C_4-binding protein in rat liver cytosol as glutathione S-transferase. *J. Biol. Chem.,* 261:8540–8546.

95. Tate, S. S., and Meister, A. (1981): Gamma-glutamyl transpeptidase: Catalytic, structural and functional aspects. *Monogr. Cell. Biochem.,* 39:357–368.

96. Ueda, N., Kaneko, S., Yoshimoto, T., and Yamamoto, S. (1986): Purification of arachidonate 5-lipoxygenase from porcine leukocytes and its reactivity with hydroperoxyeicosatetraenoic acids. *J. Biol. Chem.,* 261:7982–7988.

97. Weller, P. F., Corey, E. J., Austen, K. F., and Lewis, R. A. (1986): Inhibition of homogeneous human eosinophil arylsulfatase B by sulfidopeptide leukotrienes. *J. Biol. Chem.,* 261:1737–1744.

98. Weller, P. F., Lee, C. W., Foster, D. W., Corey, E. J., Austen, K. F., and Lewis, R. A. (1983): Generation and metabolism of 5-lipoxygenase pathway leukotrienes by human eosinophils: Predominant production of leukotriene C_4. *Proc. Natl. Acad. Sci. USA,* 80:7626–7630.

99. Williams, D. E., Hale, S. E., Okita, R. T., and Masters, B. S. (1984): A prostaglandin omega-hydroxylase cytochrome P-450 (P-450PG-omega) purified from lungs of pregnant rabbits. *J. Biol. Chem.,* 259:14600–14608.

100. Williams, J. D., Czop, J. K., and Austen, K. F. (1984): Release of leukotrienes by human monocytes on stimulation of their phagocytic receptor for particulate activators. *J. Immunol.,* 132:3034–3040.

101. Williams, J. D., Lee, T. H., Lewis, R. A., and Austen, K. F. (1985): Intracellular retention of the 5-lipoxygenase pathway product, leukotriene B_4, by human neutrophils activated with unopsonized zymosan. *J. Immunol.,* 134:2624–2630.

102. Williams, J. D., Robin, J.-L., Lewis, R. A., Lee, T. H., Austen, K. F. (1986): Generation of leukotrienes by human monocytes pretreated with cytochalasin B and stimulated with formyl-methionyl-leucyl-phenylalanine. *J. Immunol.,* 136:642–648.

103. Yamamoto, S. (1982): Purification and assay of PGH synthase from bovine seminal vesicles. *Methods Enzymol.,* 86:55–68.

104. Yoshimoto, T., Soberman, R. J., Lewis, R. A., and Austen, K. F. (1985): Isolation and characterization of leukotriene C_4 synthetase of rat basophilic leukemia cells. *Proc. Natl. Acad. Sci. USA,* 82:8399–8403.

Inflammation: Basic Principles and Clinical Correlates.
Edited by J. I. Gallin, I. M. Goldstein, and R. Snyderman.
Raven Press, Ltd., New York © 1988.

CHAPTER 9

Eicosanoids: Transcellular Metabolism

Aaron J. Marcus

HEMOSTASIS—A MULTICELLULAR PROCESS

Trauma, or any comparable interruption in the continuity of a blood vessel, initiates a physiological process known as primary and secondary hemostasis. The events involved in the hemostatic process culminate in the spontaneous arrest of bleeding. Major components of the hemostatic mechanism include local vasoconstriction, adhesion of blood platelets to the site of damage, cohesion (aggregation) of additional platelets in this local area, and coagulation, i.e., fibrin accumulation and fibrin admixture with accumulated platelets, leukocytes, and erythrocytes. Biological systems involved in hemostasis include blood vessels, platelets, and coagulation proteins of both the intrinsic and extrinsic pathways (24).

The immediate response to interruption of vascular continuity is known as *primary hemostasis*—a sequence of events involving platelets and the vessel surface. Proteins of the coagulation system are not involved in primary hemostasis. Injury to the vasculature is accompanied by vessel contraction and adhesion of platelets to exposed collagen in the subendothelial tissues. This is an adhesive process involving a glycoprotein in the platelet membrane (glycoprotein Ib) and is mediated by von Willebrand factor polymers in plasma which adsorb both to subendothelial collagen and to platelets. Collagen contact is stimulatory

for adherent platelets, and this results in physical and biochemical alterations which amplify the primary hemostatic process. Biologically active substances are secreted from intracellular platelet granules (the platelet release reaction), including platelet-derived von Willebrand factor, fibrinogen, serotonin (5-hydroxytryptamine), and adenosine diphosphate (ADP). Esterified arachidonic acid (eicosatetraenoic acid) is enzymatically liberated by phospholipase(s). Free arachidonate is oxygenated via the particulate cyclooxygenase pathway to form endoperoxides and subsequently thromboxane A_2, 12-hydroxyheptadecatrienoic acid (HHT), and malondialdehyde (MDA). Reactions leading to the formation of 12-hydroxyeicosatetraenoic acid (12-HETE) are catalyzed by the cytoplasmic lipoxygenase enzyme system. The events in primary hemostasis are depicted in Fig. 1 and also are discussed in Chapter 28.

As platelets continue to accumulate at the site of injury, platelet-to-platelet contact results in further stimulation and a shape change from disk to spiny sphere. This shape change, which occurs in the presence of all agonists except epinephrine, results in a rearrangement of platelet surface phospholipoprotein such that it develops procoagulant potential. Secreted factor V binds to the activated platelet surface and then interacts with factor Xa, generating a complex which catalyzes the formation of thrombin from

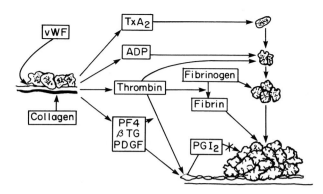

FIG. 1. Summary of reactions in primary and secondary hemostasis. Vessel wall injury is accompanied by adherence of platelets to endothelial surfaces in the presence of von Willebrand factor (vWF). Contact of platelets with collagen induces a release reaction wherein intracellular components such as adenosine diphosphate (ADP), serotonin, platelet factor 4 (PF4), β-thromboglobulin (βTG) and platelet-derived growth factor (PDGF) are secreted into the microenvironment. Formation of thrombin via interactions between clotting factors and the stimulated platelet surface initiates secondary hemostasis. Fibrinogen is converted to fibrin, which represents the "consolidation phase" of secondary hemostasis. Thrombin is a stimulus for the synthesis of eicosanoids by the vessel wall, including prostacyclin (PGI$_2$), which may limit the size of the platelet mass (or thrombus) via stimulation of adenylate cyclase and elevation of platelet cAMP with consequent blockage of calcium mobilization. Collagen and thrombin are agonists for platelet arachidonic acid mobilization and subsequent oxygenation to thromboxane A$_2$ (TxA$_2$), which is a vasoconstrictor substance and a stimulus for platelet aggregation. [Modified from Thompson, A. R., and Harker, L. A. (1983): *Manual of Hemostasis and Thrombosis*, 3rd ed. F. A. Davis and Co., Philadelphia.]

prothrombin by an order of magnitude of 300,000 times (12). In the older literature, this property of the stimulated platelet surface was known as platelet factor 3. No such factor exists as a biochemical entity, but rather the platelet contribution to coagulation is a property of the activated, shape-changed surface. Thrombin production, which culminates in the formation of fibrin from fibrinogen, represents the phase known as *secondary hemostasis*. Fibrin strands form a mesh in the interstices of the platelet aggregate and serve to consolidate and render it impermeable to cells or plasma.

The proteolytic enzyme *thrombin* is the keystone of secondary hemostasis. Thrombin is a strong agonist for platelet aggregation via release of ADP, formation of thromboxane A$_2$, release of serotonin, and further catalytic action on fibrinogen to form fibrin.

The *platelet secretory process* can be induced not only by thrombin, but also by collagen, ADP, and epinephrine. ADP induces the platelet secretory process indirectly in that it is a direct stimulus for platelet aggregation, and the

aggregating, physically interacting platelets themselves stimulate secretion. ADP, serotonin (a powerful vasoconstrictor substance), and calcium are secreted from platelet dense granules and recruit additional circulating platelets into the hemostatic plug. Alpha-granule constituents include platelet factor 4 (a protein which neutralizes heparin), β-thromboglobulin (a platelet-specific protein with no known function), and platelet-derived growth factor which promotes mitosis in smooth muscle and fibroblasts. Also secreted are factor V and the "adhesive" proteins, von Willebrand factor, thrombospondin, fibrinogen, and fibronectin. Although a given agonist may be capable of inducing a full aggregation response *in vitro*, each does so via different mechanisms. This is illustrated in Fig. 2. Thus, agents such as ADP and platelet activating factor (acetyl glyceryl ether phosphorylcholine) induce a modest release reaction and a modest production of thromboxane A$_2$. Collagen, thrombin, and arachidonate, however, stimulate a significantly greater release reaction and more thromboxane A$_2$ production when added to platelet-rich plasma *in vitro*.

Released platelet ADP promotes exposure of fibrinogen binding sites on the platelet surface. These platelet fibrinogen receptor moieties result from a rearrangement of platelet glycoprotein IIb (GPIIb) and glycoprotein IIIa (GPIIIa) during platelet activation. The heterodimer complex between GPIIb and GPIIIa represents the platelet fibrinogen receptor (24).

Microscopic observations of primary and secondary hemostasis indicate that, with the passage of time, cell components of the hemostatic plug increase in a heterogeneous, qualitative manner. Initially, only platelet–en-

PLATELET RESPONSES TO STIMULI

STIMULUS	AGGREGATION	RELEASE	O$_2$ BURST	TXB$_2$
ADP	++++	++	0	+
AGEPC	++++	++	0	+
COLLAGEN	++++	++++	+++	+++
ARACHIDONATE	++++	++++	++++	++++

FIG. 2. Platelet responses to various agonists as studied *in vitro* in platelet-rich plasma. Adenosine diphosphate (ADP) and platelet-activating factor (AGEPC) aggregate platelets directly and result in modest (++) (e.g., 28%) release of serotonin and only small amounts (+) of thromboxane B$_2$ (TxB$_2$) formation. Lack of an oxygen burst indicates little or no oxygenation of arachidonate by cyclooxygenase to endoperoxides. In contrast, collagen (or thrombin in suspensions of washed platelets) and arachidonate are strong (++++) releasing agents and stimuli of the eicosanoid pathway (+++ and ++++, respectively). Therefore, their action is probably less direct on the platelet *per se* and more indirect via release of ADP, serotonin, and eicosanoid formation.

dothelial cell contact is observed. Soon thereafter, polymorphonuclear leukocytes, mononuclear leukocytes, and erythrocytes accumulate adjacent to the platelet mass. Fibrin strands bring this heterogeneous mixture of cells into closer apposition as increasing quantities of thrombin form and the plug consolidates. Initially, participation of other cells in hemostasis was thought to be mainly a passive phenomenon. There is now biochemical evidence to suggest that other cell types such as polymorphonuclear leukocytes (neutrophils) enter the hemostatic plug via chemoattraction, possibly owing to substances released from platelets such as 12-HETE (7). As will be discussed, the close apposition of different cell types in hemostasis and thrombosis provides the opportunity for cell–cell interactions—particularly with regard to the eicosanoid pathway. This is why we have emphasized the multicellular aspects of hemostasis, thrombosis, and inflammation (22).

EICOSANOID PRECURSORS AND INTERMEDIATES IN HEMOSTASIS AND THROMBOSIS

As previously mentioned, platelet–collagen contact or platelet exposure to thrombin results in liberation of the n-6 essential fatty acid arachidonate, which is immediately oxygenated by two platelet enzymes. The first of these, cyclooxygenase, is particulate and is susceptible to inactivation by an acetylating agent such as aspirin. On cyclooxygenation, platelet arachidonate is converted to the endoperoxides, prostaglandin G_2 (PGG$_2$) and prostaglandin H_2 (PGH$_2$). The endoperoxides are transient intermediates which are then processed to several other products, the most important of which at present is thromboxane A_2 (Fig. 3). Thromboxane A_2 is quickly and entirely released into the surrounding medium where it induces vasoconstriction and further platelet aggregation.

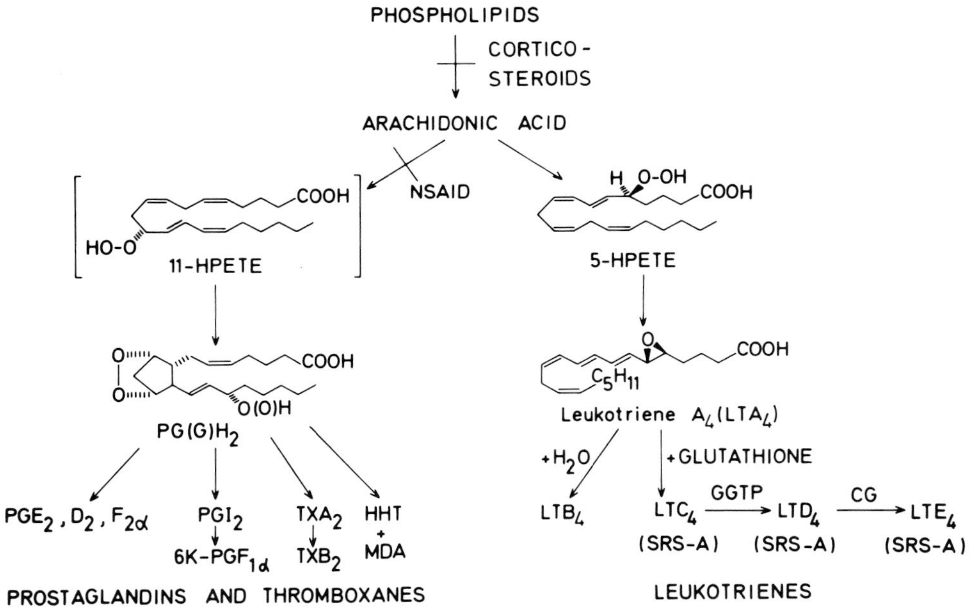

FIG. 3. Formation of eicosanoids from free arachidonic acid previously esterified in the cell phospholipid fraction. Hydrolysis of esterified arachidonate is the initial rate-limiting step and can be inhibited by corticosteroids. Cyclooxygenation of arachidonate (left) induces rearrangement and oxygenation of the molecule to the endoperoxides, prostaglandin G_2 (PGG$_2$) and prostaglandin H_2 (PGH$_2$). Nonsteroidal antiinflammatory drugs (NSAIDs) such as aspirin block cyclooxygenation of arachidonate. PGG$_2$ and PGH$_2$ are transient intermediates whose further conversion to eicosanoids is specific to a given cell or tissue. Thromboxane A_2 (TxA$_2$) (platelets) and prostacyclin (PGI$_2$) (endothelial cells) are formed enzymatically and measured as the end products, thromboxane B_2 (TxB$_2$) and 6-keto prostaglandin $F_{1\alpha}$ (6-keto-PGF$_{1\alpha}$), respectively. Shown on the right is the 5-lipoxygenase pathway, which is found mainly in cells involved in maintaining host defenses and in mediating inflammation. Platelets contain a 12-lipoxygenase, and eosinophils possess a 15-lipoxygenase pathway. The transient intermediate in the lipoxygenase pathway, leukotriene A_4 (LTA$_4$), is converted to leukotriene B_4 (LTB$_4$) in neutrophils or, in the presence of glutathione S-transferase, is metabolized to slow-reacting substances of anaphylaxis (SRS-A) (LTC$_4$, LTD$_4$, LTE$_4$) in leukocytes other than neutrophils. The ability of various cells to transform free arachidonate into a wide variety of eicosanoids with diverse biological properties provides a natural setting for cell–cell interactions. (Courtesy of Dr. Bengt Samuelsson.)

Thromboxane A$_2$ is inactivated to thromboxane B$_2$. Thromboxane A$_2$ is an inhibitor of platelet adenylate cyclase, and the resultant fall in platelet cyclic adenosine monophosphate (cAMP) levels enhances mobilization of calcium from intracellular stores. The level of free cytoplasmic calcium in platelets is a critical factor in platelet activation. This sequence is summarized in Fig. 4. Thrombin and collagen promote intracellular platelet calcium mobilization via stimulation of thromboxane A$_2$ formation plus additional mechanisms which remain to be defined (24). Thus, when thromboxane A$_2$ formation is blocked following aspirin ingestion, thrombin and collagen in appropriate doses are still capable of eliciting a full aggregation response and a normal platelet release reaction.

In contrast to the situation in platelets, human endothelial cell endoperoxides are converted to prostacyclin (prostaglandin I$_2$, PGI$_2$) and other eicosanoids. As shown in Fig. 4, prostacyclin is an inhibitor of platelet aggregation and the release reaction because it stimulates adenylate cyclase, which increases the level of cAMP in platelets, thereby inhibiting mobilization of calcium.

The second enzyme responsible for oxygenation of free arachidonate in platelets is a 12-lipoxygenase. Cytoplasmic lipoxygenase enzymes were originally characterized in plant cells, as exemplified by the 15-lipoxygenase in soybean. The initial catalytic step in lipoxygenation is similar to that of the cyclooxygenase system (Fig. 3). Arachidonate is derivatized to a hydroperoxy compound first, rapidly followed by formation of the hydroxy compound 12-

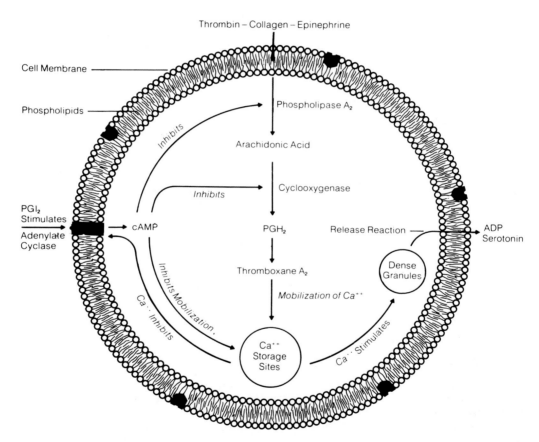

FIG. 4. Regulation of the platelet release reaction by thromboxane A$_2$, prostacyclin (PGI$_2$), and calcium. Thromboxane A$_2$ formed in the platelet stimulates calcium mobilization. Free intracellular calcium exerts an inhibitory effect on adenylate cyclase, thus lowering levels of cAMP, and may elicit a contractile response by the dense tubular system. These calcium-initiated reactions lead to platelet aggregation. PGI$_2$ is an agonist for adenylate cyclase, resulting in elevation of cAMP levels and inhibition of platelet aggregation by several mechanisms. First, elevations in the cAMP level favor calcium sequestration, which attenuates the release reaction. Elevations in cAMP levels also inhibit phospholipase and cyclooxygenase activities via unknown mechanisms. Therefore, all the actions of thromboxane A$_2$ are proaggregatory, and the effects of PGI$_2$ are antiaggregatory. [From Gorman, R. R., and Marcus, A. J. (1981): *Prostaglandins and Cardiovascular Disease*. Scope Publication, Upjohn Company, Kalamazoo, MI.]

HETE. In contrast to thromboxane A_2, which is rapidly formed and released, 12-HETE is synthesized in increasing amounts with time until all available free arachidonate is consumed. In the setting of aspirin ingestion, 12-HETE formation, as evaluated by time course studies *in vitro,* is further enhanced because of the availability of increased quantities of free arachidonate which were not cyclooxygenated.

The functional implications of 12-HETE formation with regard to platelets have not as yet been elucidated. The addition of 12-HETE to platelets *in vitro* does not elicit a discernible effect. It is known that unstimulated neutrophils further metabolize 12-HETE to 12(*S*),20-dihydroxyeicosatetraenoic acid (12,20-DiHETE) via an ω-hydroxylation reaction (28; and see following). The capacity for 12-HETE production is somewhat unique to platelets. In fact, whenever 12-HETE synthesis is described in a tissue, the presence of even minor platelet contamination may be responsible, especially if the platelets were perturbed when the tissue in question was processed. 12-HETE (in micromolar concentrations) is chemotactic for human neutrophils *in vitro* (7) and *in vivo* (5) and is chemokinetic for smooth muscle cells (30). 12-HETE is synthesized in increased quantities by the kidney in experimental animals following immune glomerular injury (17). Recently, we demonstrated that 12-HETE enhanced the procoagulant (tissue factor) activity of mononuclear leukocytes induced by endotoxin (19).

Current concepts of platelet eicosanoid metabolism and function may be summarized as follows: *In vitro,* platelets are exquisitely sensitive to free arachidonic acid, whether it is provided exogenously or released by agonists such as thrombin, collagen, and epinephrine. Thromboxane A_2, the major cyclooxygenase product, is a moderate stimulus for platelet aggregation and release (Fig. 2) and is a strong vasoconstrictor substance. The functions of HHT and MDA (if any) are not known. As will be discussed, endoperoxides and free arachidonate are actively or passively released from stimulated platelets and can interact with cells in the immediate microenvironment. Since the stimulated platelet synthesizes 12-HETE in rather significant quantities, one would imagine that it may play some heretofore undescribed functional role in hemostasis or thrombosis. In any case, it is important to accumulate more information concerning the metabolism of 12-HETE and concerning the interactions of 12-HETE with other cells.

CELL–CELL INTERACTIONS IN THE EICOSANOID PATHWAY

The concept that eicosanoid precursors and intermediates can be metabolized by different cell types stems from several of their unique biological properties: (a) They are not stored in tissues but are evanescent biological substances (autacoids) synthesized only in response to stimulation (4). (b) Production of eicosanoids is qualitatively tissue-specific, and these labile lipid autacoids exert their effects in the immediate microenvironment of the cell. (c) Eicosanoids probably enhance or synergize the inherent functional capacity of a tissue, but usually they are not the sole modulator of a given cell function. Evidence for the latter statement is that the functional integrity of a cell is not abolished by pharmacological eicosanoid inhibition; rather, cell responsiveness is mildly attenuated. Such properties include regulation of blood flow, smooth muscle contraction and/or relaxation, platelet stimulation or inhibition, and mineral metabolism, among others. It can therefore be appreciated that a physiological or pathological stimulus is potentially capable of eliciting responses from several cell types, either because the stimulus is "recognized" by multiple cells or because it induces release of eicosanoid precursors or intermediates which can be shared and metabolized simultaneously. In an inflammatory site or thrombus, this could include leukocytes, platelets, endothelial cells, or smooth muscle cells; i.e., we are dealing with multicellular events modulated at least in part by eicosanoids (23).

CLASSIFICATION OF CELL–CELL INTERACTIONS IN THE EICOSANOID PATHWAY

Type I: The Sharing of a Common Precursor by Two or More Cells in Close Proximity

Some cells are capable of synthesizing their own eicosanoid precursors, but they can also acquire these precursors from a neighboring cell in close physical proximity (Table 1). This results in the production of more endogenous end products than the cell could have produced individually (type IA) (23). An example of a type IA cell–cell interaction is utilization of platelet-derived endoperoxides by aspirin-treated endothelial cells for the production of prostacyclin (25,35). This phenomenon was demonstrated *in vitro* by labeling platelets with radioactive arachidonate and placing them in suspension with unla-

TABLE 1. *Cell–cell interactions in the eicosanoid pathway*

Type I: Different cells metabolize a common precursor
Type II: Eicosanoids from one cell are metabolized to a new product which neither cell can synthesize alone
Type III: An eicosanoid from one cell acts as an agonist or as an inhibitor for another

beled, aspirin-treated endothelial cells. Stimulation of these combined platelet–endothelial cell suspensions with thrombin, collagen, or ionophore resulted in the production of labeled prostacyclin and all other eicosanoids known to be synthesized by endothelial cells. The labeled endothelial cell eicosanoids could only have originated from labeled platelets. Also, platelets in these stimulated mixtures did not aggregate in the presence of aspirin-treated endothelial cells, presumably because of the prostacyclin which was generated. The platelet–endothelial cell interaction for prostacyclin production also could be demonstrated in unlabeled cell suspensions and quantified by radioimmunoassay (25), as illustrated in Table 2. It is also possible that endothelial cells produce other inhibitors of platelet aggregation which have not yet been defined. It would not be surprising to find that platelets can enhance eicosanoid formation by other hematological cell types in proximity when tested in *in vitro* systems.

Another example of a type 1A cell–cell interaction is utilization of platelet arachidonate by stimulated neutrophils for the production of leukotriene B_4 (26). Ionophore-stimulated suspensions of platelets labeled with radioactive arachidonate and unlabeled neutrophils produce radiolabeled leukotriene B_4 and 5-hydroxyeicosatetraenoic acid (5-HETE). These products cannot be produced by platelets alone, because these cells do not contain a 5-lipoxygenase. The clinical significance of this *in vitro* reaction is that aspirin-treated platelets can release free arachidonate, which can then interact with other cells such as stimulated neutrophils and serve as a source of proinflammatory eicosanoids such as leukotriene B_4 and 5-HETE.

TABLE 2. *Platelet contribution to prostacyclin formation by endothelial cells*[a]

Components	6-Keto-PGF$_{1\alpha}$ (ng)
Aspirin-treated endothelial cells plus thrombin	0
Aspirin-treated endothelial cells plus platelets plus thrombin	8.4
Endothelial cells plus thrombin	7.7
Endothelial cells plus platelets plus thrombin	19.2

[a] Endothelial cells stimulated by thrombin to produce PGI_2 from endogenous sources synthesized no more PGI_2 (measured as the stable end product 6-keto-PGF$_{1\alpha}$) than when aspirin-treated endothelial cells were combined with platelets as the sole source of endoperoxides. When a mixture of platelets and endothelial cells was stimulated by thrombin, approximately twice as much 6-keto-PGF$_{1\alpha}$ was formed as when platelets were omitted. Therefore, in the mixed-cell system, endothelial cells formed approximately one-half of their PGI_2 from platelet endoperoxides (cell–cell interaction type IA). Radioimmunoassays were performed by Dr. Babette Weksler (25).

A further example of a type 1A cell–cell interaction involves the production of leukotriene C_4 by mast cells (2,3). When human neutrophils are stimulated with ionophore A23187 and the released leukotriene A_4 trapped and complexed to albumin, this leukotriene A_4 is converted to leukotriene C_4 when added to unstimulated suspensions of mast cells. This also indicates that mast cells possess the glutathione S-transferase required for synthesis of leukotriene C_4 from leukotriene A_4 (Fig. 3). It is therefore clear that stimulated mixed-cell suspensions can synthesize more eicosanoids than can individual components of the suspensions alone (2,25).

There is a second form of type I cell–cell interaction in which a given cell type is unable to produce a precursor endogenously but possesses mechanisms for further processing the precursor if it can be obtained from another stimulated cell in the microenvironment (type IB). For example, erythrocytes cannot mobilize arachidonate when perturbed. Yet, if leukotriene A_4 at physiological concentrations is incubated with human erythrocytes, they have the capacity to transform leukotriene A_4 to leukotriene B_4 (6,29). A comparable phenomenon has recently been demonstrated in human platelets (32). Incubation of platelet suspensions with tritium-labeled leukotriene A_4 in the presence of reduced glutathione resulted in the production of radiolabeled leukotriene C_4. Since platelets contain glutathione S-transferase, the exogenously provided leukotriene A_4 was directly converted to leukotriene C_4. It is interesting that some cells are unable to initiate eicosanoid metabolism but have retained biosynthetic mechanisms for the further processing of an available eicosanoid intermediate to an end product of physiological significance.

Type II: The Capability of One Cell to Transform an Eicosanoid from Another Cell into a New Product Which Neither Cell Can Synthesize Alone

Type II cell–cell interactions can also be subdivided according to whether one or both cells have been stimulated (Table 1). In type IIA, both cells have been activated. Thus, if a suspension of [^{3}H]arachidonate-labeled platelets is stimulated by ionophore A23187 (a common agonist for both neutrophils and platelets), in the presence of unlabeled neutrophils, 5(S),12(S)-dihydroxyeicosatetraenoic acid [5(S),12(S)-DiHETE] is formed. This phenomenon occurs because 12-HETE released by platelets is converted to 5(S),12(S)-DiHETE by neutrophil 5-lipoxygenase which has been activated by the ionophore (1,26). In this reaction system, 12-HETE generated by platelets in the reaction mixtures can be replaced by purified 12-HETE and the same result obtained. Furthermore, addition of radiolabeled 5-HETE to activated platelets will result in formation of the same compound—$5(S),12(S)$-DiHETE (26). In a sense, these reactions are a variant of type IB, except that a new and previously known metabolite has been formed. The type IIB cell–cell interaction is exemplified by the *in vitro* situation where only one component of a two-cell system is activated. If cell suspensions containing [³H]arachidonate-labeled platelets and unlabeled neutrophils are stimulated with thrombin or collagen (two platelet stimuli which do not activate neutrophil eicosanoid metabolism), a labeled compound appears within 5 mins which can be identified as $12(S),20$-dihydroxyeicosatetraenoic acid (12,20-DiHETE), a novel eicosanoid which cannot be synthesized by platelets or neutrophils alone (27,37). In this cell–cell interaction, the unstimulated neutrophil hydroxylates released platelet 12-HETE to 12,20-DiHETE. This is in sharp contrast to the fully stimulated system (type IIA) wherein stimulated neutrophils did not process platelet 12-HETE to 12,20-DiHETE to a significant degree but rather transformed platelet 12-HETE to $5(S),12(S)$-DiHETE (27).

Type III: The Ability of an Eicosanoid Synthesized by One Cell to Act as an Agonist or as an Inhibitor for Another Cell

Under specific experimental circumstances, it can be shown that peptide containing leukotrienes, leukotrienes C_4, D_4, and E_4, can induce biological effects attributable to the induction of cyclooxygenase products in tissues and organs (33). Thus, intravenous infusion of leukotriene C_4 or leukotriene D_4 in guinea pigs produces bronchoconstriction which can be inhibited by pretreatment with indomethacin. In isolated, perfused lungs, leukotrienes C_4, D_4, and E_4 can induce release of thromboxane A_2 (33).

Another example of a type III cell–cell interaction is the inhibitory effect of 12-HETE on the production of prostacyclin (8). Exposure of human umbilical vein endothelial cells to 1.0 μM 12-HETE for 2 hr, followed by stimulation with thrombin, results in inhibition of the synthesis of prostacyclin and other eicosanoids ordinarily produced by these cells (e.g., prostaglandin $F_{2\alpha}$, prostaglandin E_2, and HHT). This inhibition probably occurs at the level of cyclooxygenase and, although it takes place only after a long incubation period, it nevertheless represents an instance where one eicosanoid inhibits the production of another (8). Furthermore, in a bovine endothelial cell system, 5-HETE and 15-hydroxyeicosatetraenoic acid (15-HETE) also reduced prostacyclin formation following exposure of the cells to arachidonic acid (8).

As a third example of a type III cell–cell interaction, biosynthesis of leukotriene B_4 by neutrophils on stimu-

lation with released platelet 12-hydroperoxyeicosatetraenoic acid (12-HPETE) has also been reported (20). However, it has recently been shown that 12-HETE-induced leukotriene B_4 formation requires the presence of endogenous or exogenous free arachidonic acid (14). Interestingly, lipoxygenase-deficient platelets from patients with myeloproliferative disorders do not adequately stimulate leukotriene B_4 synthesis during platelet–neutrophil interactions because they are defective with respect to the formation of 12-HETE (14). This defect might result in deficient responsiveness at sites of thrombosis or inflammation in patients with platelet lipoxygenase deficiency (15).

OBSERVATIONS ON THE MECHANISM OF ω-HYDROXYLATION OF PLATELET 12-HETE TO 12,20-DiHETE BY UNSTIMULATED NEUTROPHILS

As already mentioned, 12,20-DiHETE formation by unstimulated neutrophils can be classified as a type IIB cell–cell interaction in the eicosanoid pathway. Biosynthesis of this compound represents formation of a new product by two different circulating blood cells wherein only one of the cell types was stimulated. Total organic synthesis of 12,20-DiHETE has recently been accomplished by two laboratories (16,21). As already mentioned, platelets synthesize 12-HETE in significant quantities, and therefore it is important to determine its ultimate metabolic fate and also to discern whether it interacts with other cells in the circulation. Furthermore, production of 12-HETE by stimulated platelets continues, and may even be enhanced, in the setting of aspirin ingestion. This is in contrast to thromboxane production, which occurs rapidly following platelet activation and then ceases. On the other hand, 12-HETE production persists until available free arachidonate has been consumed in the process or is no longer available because of binding to albumin or reincorporation by the cell.

We recently devised an assay system utilizing reversed-phase high-performance liquid chromatography for studying *in vitro* interactions between neutrophils and eicosanoids such as 12-HETE (28). During a 5-min incubation period, 24–46% of 12-HETE was metabolized to 12,20-DiHETE. Formation of 12,20-DiHETE occurred via a cytochrome P-450 ω-hydroxylation mechanism (28). Neutrophil 12,20-DiHETE formation was inhibitable by known antagonists of cytochrome P-450 enzyme systems such as α-naphthoflavone, SKF 525-A, and imidazole. Inhibition was also observed with eicosatetraynoic acid, a phenomenon which has been previously reported for cytochrome P-450 oxidase systems. Interestingly, ω-hydroxylation of 12-HETE was also blocked by ethylenediaminetetraacetic acid despite addition of calcium to the assay system in quantities sufficient to compensate for the effects of this chelating agent. Exposure of neutrophils to carbon monoxide, which forms a complex with the ferrous ion of heme present in cytochrome P-450, inhibited 12,20-DiHETE formation by 94%. This inhibition was completely reversible on reoxygenation of the neutrophils.

In contrast to cytochrome P-450 enzyme components of other tissues such as kidney and liver, cell disruption by any technique resulted in loss of neutrophil 12-HETE ω-hydroxylase activity. This was due to release of neutrophil proteolytic enzymes and could be prevented by pretreatment of intact neutrophils with the protease inhibitor diisopropylfluorophosphate (DFP). When neutrophils pretreated with DFP were disrupted and fractionated, the capacity to convert 12-HETE to 12,20-DiHETE was localized solely to the microsomal fraction, a characteristic of cytochrome P-450 enzymes. In this context, we use the term "microsomal fraction" operationally, because it may contain both plasma and intracellular membranes. This possibility is considered because we have hypothesized that the neutrophil enzyme under study may be located at or in close proximity to the cell surface. In this situation it may be susceptible to degradation by proteases in the surrounding medium. Furthermore, the enzyme is quite readily available to externally added, purified 12-HETE. Finally, 12,20-DiHETE, the end product, was found almost exclusively in the supernatant of cell suspensions in which the reaction was carried out (27). The neutrophil microsomal 12-HETE ω-hydroxylating activity was also dependent on reduced nicotinamide adenine dinucleotide phosphate (NADPH), reaching a plateau of activity at 2.5 μM NADPH which was 33-fold greater than that observed in the absence of either exogenous NADPH or an NADPH-regenerating system.

Involvement of cytochrome P-450 enzymes in eicosanoid metabolism by cell types which function in hemostasis, thrombosis, and inflammation has been demonstrated in several laboratories (11,36). Furthermore, hydroxylation of eicosanoids, such as leukotriene B$_4$, is well documented in the literature (10,13,18,34). Thus, the neutrophil leukotriene B$_4$ ω-hydroxylase (36) and the recently described 12-HETE ω-hydroxylase (28) may be similar or even identical enzymes. Interestingly, exposure of neutrophils to leukotriene B$_4$, rapidly followed by addition of 12-HETE, resulted in the inhibition of 12,20-DiHETE formation. It appears, therefore, that leukotriene B$_4$ is actually a competitive inhibitor of 12,20-DiHETE formation. This inhibition correlates with the K_m value for ω-hydroxylation of leukotriene B$_4$ (0.6 μM) reported by Shak and Goldstein (36). If the hydroxylating enzymes for leukotriene B$_4$ and 12-HETE are identical, the apparent higher degree of affinity for leukotriene B$_4$ does not alter the possible significance of a cell–cell interaction between unstimulated neutrophils and 12-HETE. In hypothetical situations, wherein platelets alone have been stimulated (as with thrombin or collagen), neutrophils remain in the unstimulated form and leukotriene B$_4$ is not synthesized (27). In these instances, 12-HETE released from activated platelets is the primary substrate.

SUMMARY

Vascular and extravascular injury leads to activation of hemostasis, coagulation, and the inflammatory response. Cells involved in these processes, such as platelets, leukocytes, and endothelial cells, have the inherent capacity to mobilize arachidonic acid and to transform it into eicosanoids with a large variety of biological activities (31). It has now become apparent that precursors and intermediates of eicosanoids can be utilized by different cell types either for the production of new products or for enhancement of the biosynthesis of eicosanoids in the framework of the inherent capacity of the cell. Activated cells may also release materials, as yet incompletely identified, which in themselves can stimulate arachidonic acid metabolism (9). Interleukin-1 has been implicated as an eicosanoid-releasing factor in some tissues (31).

In this review, we have discussed the hemostatic and thrombotic processes as representing a multicellular response to hemorrhage, tissue injury, and inflammation. This concept may eventually lead to a possible therapeutic approach to modulating the inflammatory response and host defense mechanisms in vascular and extravascular tissues.

ACKNOWLEDGMENTS

Research cited was supported by grants from the Veterans Administration, the National Institutes of Health (HL 18828-11 SCOR), the Edward Gruenstein Fund, and the Sallie Wichman Fund. I thank Lenore B. Safier, Harris L. Ullman, Naziba Islam, and M. Johan Broekman for helpful discussions and suggestions. The expert editorial assistance of Ms. Evelyn Ludwig is also acknowledged.

Note Added in Proof

Inhibition of platelet aggregation by endothelial cells is also produced by the endothelium-derived relaxing factor (EDRF). This substance, thought to be nitric oxide (NO), is also a strong vasodilator and its production is not inhibited by aspirin (38).

REFERENCES

1. Borgeat, P., Fruteau de Laclos, B., Picard, S., Vallerand, P., and Sirois, P. (1982): Double dioxygenation of arachidonic acid in leukocytes by lipoxygenases. In: *Leukotrienes and Other Lipoxygenase*

Products, edited by B. Samuelsson and R. Paoletti, pp. 45–51. Raven Press, New York.

2. Clancy, R. M., Dahinden, D. A., and Hugli, T. E. (1985): Complement-mediated arachidonate metabolism. *Prog. Biochem. Pharmacol.,* 20:120–131.

3. Dahinden, C. A., Clancy, R. M., Gross, M., Chiller, J. M., and Hugli, T. E. (1985): Leukotriene C₄ production by murine mast cells. Evidence of a role for extracellular leukotriene A₄. *Proc. Natl. Acad. Sci. USA,* 82:6632–6636.

4. Douglas, W. W. (1985): Autocoids. In: *The Pharmacological Basis of Therapeutics,* edited by A. G. Gilman, L. S. Goodman, T. W. Rall, and F. Murad, pp. 604–659. Macmillan Publishing Co., New York.

5. Dowd, P. M., Black, A. K., Woollard, P. M., Camp, R. D. R., and Greaves, M. W. (1985): Cutaneous responses to 12-hydroxy-5,8,10,14-eicosatetraenoic acid (12-HETE). *J. Invest. Dermatol.,* 84:537–541.

6. Fitzpatrick, F., Liggett, W., McGee, J., Bunting, S., Morton, D., and Samuelsson, B. (1984): Metabolism of leukotriene A₄ by human erythrocytes. A novel cellular source of leukotriene B₄. *J. Biol. Chem.,* 259:11403–11407.

7. Goetzl, E. J., Brash, A. R., Tauber, A. I., Oates, J. A., and Hubbard, W. C. (1980): Modulation of human neutrophil function by monohydroxyeicosatetraenoic acids. *Immunology,* 39:491–501.

8. Hadjiagapiou, C., and Spector, A. A. (1986): 12-Hydroxyeicosatetraenoic acid reduces prostacyclin production by endothelial cells. *Prostaglandins,* 31:1135–1144.

9. Hajjar, D. P., Marcus, A. J., and Hajjar, K. A. (1987): Interactions of arterial cells. Studies on the mechanisms of endothelial cell modulation of cholesterol metabolism in co-cultured smooth muscle cells. *J. Biol. Chem.,* 262:6976–6981.

10. Hansson, G., Lindgren, J. A., Dahlén, S.-E., Hedqvist, P., and Samuelsson, B. (1981): Identification and biological activity of novel ω-oxidized metabolites of leukotriene B₄ from human leukocytes. *FEBS Lett.,* 130:107–112.

11. Haurand, M., and Ullrich, V. (1985): Isolation and characterization of thromboxane synthase from human platelets as a cytochrome P-450 enzyme. *J. Biol. Chem.,* 260:15059–15067.

12. Hawiger, J. (1987): Bleeding and thromboembolic complications of trauma and infection. In: *The Physiological Basis for Treatment of Trauma and Infection,* edited by G. H. A. Clowes. Marcel Dekker, New York (in press).

13. Jubiz, W., Rådmark, O., Malmsten, C., Hansson, G., Lindgren, J. A., Palmblad, J., Udén, A.-M., and Samuelsson, B. (1982): A novel leukotriene produced by stimulation of leukocytes with formylmethionylleucylphenylalanine. *J. Biol. Chem.,* 257:6106–6110.

14. Kanaji, K., Okuma, M., Sugiyama, T., Sensaki, S., Ushikubi, F., and Uchino, H. (1986): Requirement of free arachidonic acid for leukotriene B₄ biosynthesis by 12-hydroxyeicosatetraenoic acid-stimulated neutrophils. *Biochem. Biophys. Res. Commun.,* 138:589–595.

15. Kanaji, K., Okuma, M., and Uchino, H. (1986): Deficient induction of leukotriene synthesis in human neutrophils by lipoxygenase-deficient platelets. *Blood,* 67:903–908.

16. Leblanc, Y., Fitzsimmons, B. J., Adams, J., Perez, F., and Rokach, J. (1986): The total synthesis of 12-HETE and 12,20-DiHETE. *J. Org. Chem.,* 51:789–793.

17. Lianos, E. A., Rahman, M. A., and Dunn, M. J. (1985): Glomerular arachidonate lipoxygenation in rat nephrotic serum nephritis. *J. Clin. Invest.,* 76:1355–1359.

18. Lindgren, J. A., Hansson, G., and Samuelsson, B. (1981): Formation of novel hydroxylated eicosatetraenoic acids in preparations of human polymorphonuclear leukocytes. *FEBS Lett.,* 128:329–335.

19. Lorenzet, R., Niemetz, J., Marcus, A. J., and Broekman, M. J. (1986): Enhancement of mononuclear procoagulant activity by platelet 12-hydroxyeicosatetraenoic acid. *J. Clin. Invest.,* 78:418–423.

20. Maclouf, J., Fruteau de Laclos, B., and Borgeat, P. (1982): Stimulation of leukotriene biosynthesis in human blood leukocytes by platelet-derived 12-hydroperoxyeicosatetraenoic acid. *Proc. Natl. Acad. Sci. USA,* 79:6042–6046.

21. Manna, S., Viala, J., Yadagiri, P., and Falck, J. R. (1986): Synthesis of 12(*S*),20-, 12(*S*),19(*R*)- and 12(*S*),19(*S*)-dihydroxy-eicosa-*cis*-5,8,14-*trans*-10-tetraenoic acids, metabolites of 12(*S*)-HETE. *Tetrahedon Lett.,* 27:2679–2682.

22. Marcus, A. J. (1984): The eicosanoids in biology and medicine. *J. Lipid Res.,* 25:1511–1516.

23. Marcus, A. J. (1986): Transcellular metabolism of eicosanoids. *Prog. Hemost. Thromb.,* 8:127–142.

24. Marcus, A. J. (1988): Hemorrhagic disorders: Abnormalities of platelet and vascular function. In: *Cecil Textbook of Medicine,* 18th ed., edited by J. B. Wyngaarden and L. H. Smith, Jr. W. B. Saunders, Philadelphia (in press).

25. Marcus, A. J., Weksler, B. B., Jaffe, E. A., and Broekman, M. J. (1980): Synthesis of prostacyclin from platelet-derived endoperoxides by cultured human endothelial cells. *J. Clin. Invest.,* 66:979–986.

26. Marcus, A. J., Broekman, M. J., Safier, L. B., Ullman, H. L., Islam, N., Serhan, C. N., Rutherford, L. E., Korchak, H. M., and Weissmann, G. (1982): Formation of leukotrienes and other hydroxy acids during platelet-neutrophil interactions in vitro. *Biochem. Biophys. Res. Commun.,* 109:130–137.

27. Marcus, A. J., Safier, L. B., Ullman, H. L., Broekman, M. J., Islam, N., Oglesby, T. D., and Gorman, R. R. (1984): 12*S*,20-dihydroxyicosatetraenoic acid: A new icosanoid synthesized by neutrophils from 12*S*-hydroxyicosatetraenoic acid produced by thrombin- or collagen-stimulated platelets. *Proc. Natl. Acad. Sci. USA,* 81:903–907.

28. Marcus, A. J., Safier, L. B., Ullman, H. L., Islam, N., Broekman, M. J., and von Schacky, C. (1987): Studies on the mechanism of ω-hydroxylation of platelet 12-hydroxyeicosatetraenoic acid (12-HETE) by unstimulated neutrophils. *J. Clin. Invest.,* 79:179–187.

29. McGee, J. E., and Fitzpatrick, F. A. (1986): Erythrocyte-neutrophil interactions: Formation of leukotriene B₄ by transcellular biosynthesis. *Proc. Natl. Acad. Sci. USA,* 83:1349–1353.

30. Nakao, J., Ooyama, T., Chang, W.-C., Murota, S., and Orimo, H. (1982): Platelets stimulate aortic smooth muscle cell migration in vitro. Involvement of 12-L-hydroxy-5,8,10,14-eicosatetraenoic acid. *Atherosclerosis,* 43:143–150.

31. Needleman, P., Turk, J., Jakschik, B. A., Morrison, A. R., and Lefkowitz, J. B. (1986): Arachidonic acid metabolism. *Annu. Rev. Biochem.,* 55:69–102.

32. Pace-Asciak, C. R., Klein, J., and Spielberg, S. P. (1986): Metabolism of leukotriene A₄ into C₄ by human platelets. *Biochim. Biophys. Acta,* 877:68–74.

33. Piper, P. J. (1983): Pharmacology of leukotrienes. *Br. Med. Bull.,* 39:255–259.

34. Powell, W. S. (1984): Properties of leukotriene B₄ 20-hydroxylase from polymorphonuclear leukocytes. *J. Biol. Chem.,* 259:3082–3089.

35. Schafer, A. I., Crawford, D. D., and Gimbrone, M. A., Jr. (1984): Unidirectional transfer of prostaglandin endoperoxides between platelets and endothelial cells. *J. Clin. Invest.,* 73:1105–1112.

36. Shak, S., and Goldstein, I. M. (1985): Leukotriene B₄ ω-hydroxylase in human polymorphonuclear leukocytes: Partial purification and identification as a cytochrome P-450. *J. Clin. Invest.,* 76:1218–1228.

37. Wong, P. Y.-K., Westlund, P., Hamberg, M., Granström, E., Chao, P. H.-W., and Samuelsson, B. (1984): ω-Hydroxylation of 12-L-hydroxy-5,8,10,14-eicosatetraenoic acid in human polymorphonuclear leukocytes. *J. Biol. Chem.,* 259:2683–2686.

38. Moncada, S., Palmer, R. M. J., and Higgs, E. A. (1987): Prostacyclin and endothelium-derived relaxing factor: Biological interaction and significance. In: *Thrombosis and Haemostasis,* edited by M. Verstraete, J. Vermylen, H. R. Lijnen, and J. Arnout. Leuven University Press, Leuven, pp. 597–618.

Inflammation: Basic Principles and Clinical Correlates.
Edited by J. I. Gallin, I. M. Goldstein, and R. Snyderman.
Raven Press, Ltd., New York © 1988.

CHAPTER 10

Platelet-Activating Factors

R. Neal Pinckard, Janet C. Ludwig, and Linda M. McManus

Intrinsic to the biological events that constitute the inflammatory and repair process is a multiplicity of interacting mediators and autacoids (autopharmacologic substances that have potent local activity). Inflammatory autacoids have diverse chemical structures ranging from relatively simple molecules, such as histamine, to more complex polypeptides, such as the interleukins. The isolation and biochemical characterization of these diverse agents have provided the basis for much of our current concepts regarding the mechanisms that regulate this essential biological response.

Important to the modulation of inflammation are several classes of lipid autacoids which have the collective ability to orchestrate virtually every aspect of the inflammatory process via primary, secondary, and/or synergistic actions. These lipid autacoids, including the eicosanoids and platelet-activating factors, are not stored as preformed mediators but are rapidly generated after cell stimulation or perturbation. Inasmuch as a myriad of recent studies suggest that these lipid autacoids are indispensable to the regulation of inflammation, their potential contribution to tissue injury and disease is currently being intensively investigated. The following discussion will focus upon one of the most recently described lipid autacoids, i.e., the family of structurally related, acetylated phosphoglycerides known as the platelet-activating factors.

The historical name given to this autacoid family, "platelet-activating factor (PAF)," should not be construed to be indicative of a principal physiologic action inasmuch as many of the biological properties of PAF are platelet-independent (see below). Moreover, although PAF has been extensively studied with respect to its ability to induce acute allergic and inflammatory reactions, the overall role of this autacoid family in modulating normal as well as abnormal (patho)physiological processes should not be restricted in this context. Indeed, current evolving evidence strongly suggests that PAF is intimately involved in a variety of other (patho)biological phenomena, including the modulation of cardiovascular, pulmonary, renal and hepatic function, neurophysiology, tumor biology, and reproductive physiology (cf. refs. 15,16, 57,114,129,150,168,184, and 218). With this caveat, the present discussion will principally focus upon the potential role of PAF in modulating normal as well as abnormal acute and chronic inflammatory reactions.

HISTORICAL BACKGROUND

PAF was initially recognized in investigations designed to characterize the cell-cell interactions following antigen stimulation of rabbit buffy coat leukocytes containing IgE-sensitized basophils (18,187). During this immunologically initiated reaction, a fluid-phase intermediate was released as characterized by its ability to induce the aggregation of, and initiate the release reaction from, isolated rabbit platelets. Because its chemical nature was not known, the term "platelet-activating factor (PAF)" was coined to describe its functional activity (18). Subsequent studies demonstrated that hog leukocyte PAF was extractable into ethanol and chloroform, suggestive of a lipid-like molecule (19). In the latter studies, PAF activity eluted from silicic acid columns in phospholipid-rich fractions and migrated on thin-layer chromatography (TLC) between lysolecithin and sphingomyelin. Additional enzymatic studies demonstrated that PAF activity was susceptible to inactivation by phospholipase A_2, C, and D but not by an sn-1 specific lipase or sphingomyelinase. In other investigations, the PAF released from antigen-stimulated, rabbit buffy coat leukocytes containing IgE-sensitized basophils was characterized as a polar lipid that was clearly separable from any known phospholipid by TLC (166). The biological activity of this PAF was resistant to acid treatment and heating in the presence of atmospheric oxygen, thereby eliminating the possibilities that vinyl ether groupings ($-OCH=CH-$) or unsaturations in aliphatic side chains were important structural determinants. In addition, treatment of PAF with periodate, acetic acid anhydride, or sodium nitrite also did not affect biological activity, thus ruling out vicinal glycols, unmodified hydroxyls, amino groups, or glycosidic bonds as important structural components. However, an important observation, key to providing the structure of PAF, was that its biological activity was rapidly destroyed by base-catalyzed methanolysis (50,166).

The sensitivity of PAF to degradation by methanolic sodium hydroxide proved to be very important in the structural elucidation of PAF. Because a critical ester linkage (presumably fatty acyl) was a mandatory requirement for the biological activity of PAF, experiments were conducted to restore biological activity after base treatment of native PAF (50). Thus, after extraction into chloroform, the base-catalyzed degradation product(s) was first acylated with stearic acid anhydride; however, the product was not biologically active. In contrast, if acetic, proprionic, or butyric acid anhydrides were employed as the acylating agents, re-expression of PAF activity was realized. These latter observations facilitated the structural elucidation of PAF for the following reasons. First, only the acetylated product had TLC behavior identical to that of native PAF. Of equal importance, the base-catalyzed PAF degradation product was fully soluble in the chloroform-rich phase of a mixture of chloroform:methanol: water, 1:1:0.9, respectively; this indicated that PAF was not a diacyl phosphoglyceride but that it likely contained an alkyl linkage (an alk-1-enyl linkage had been previously

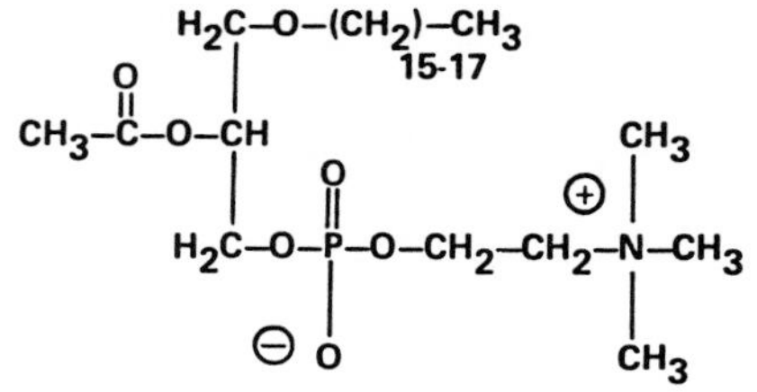

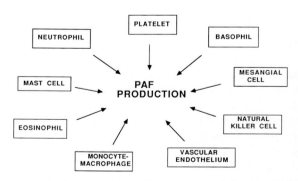

FIG. 1. 1-o-Hexadecyl/octadecyl-2-acetyl-sn-glycero-3-phosphocholine (AGEPC, PAF, PAF-acether). The C16:0- and C18: 0-AGEPC alkyl chain homologs are the principal PAFs synthesized and released from antigen-stimulated, IgE-sensitized rabbit basophils (78) and from rabbit and human PMN activated by various secretagogues and phagocytic stimuli (141,167). Additional PAF homologs and analogs also are synthesized by stimulated inflammatory cells; however, the precise chemical structures of many of these molecules await identification.

ruled out because PAF was stable to acid conditions). These findings, coupled with its TLC migratory properties and its susceptibility to PLA_2 degradation indicated that PAF was 1-O-alkyl-2-acetyl-sn-glycero-3-phosphocholine (AGEPC). Indeed, semisynthesis of such a compound was reported to result in a molecule with potent platelet stimulating and hypotensive actions (29,50). Moreover, the synthetic AGEPC molecule was shown to cross-desensitize rabbit platelets to native PAF, indicating that the native and synthetic molecules were interacting with the same receptor (50). Subsequently, gas-chromatographic–mass-spectrometric analyses identified the glyceryl ether, acetate, and phosphocholine components of rabbit basophil-derived PAF (78); i.e., the chemical structure of native PAF was 1-O-hexadecyl/octadecyl-2-acetyl-sn-glycero-3-phosphochline (AGEPC; Fig. 1).

SOURCES OF PAF

PAF is not a stored, preformed autacoid but is rapidly synthesized by a variety of cells after stimulation (Table 1 and Figs. 2 and 3). This diversity of cells that produce

FIG. 2. Cellular sources of PAF. PAF is not a preformed autacoid but is rapidly synthesized by inflammatory cells after activation by a variety of stimuli (see Table 1).

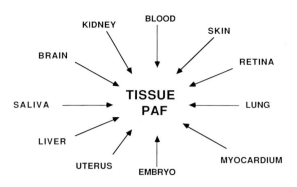

FIG. 3. Tissue sources of PAF. PAF has been isolated from various tissues under different physiologic conditions: e.g., following ischemic injury, immune complex and acute allergic reactions, or during endotoxemia, etc. The chemical structures, cell of origin, and the (patho)biological role of these PAFs remain to be established.

PAF explains, in part, why this phospholipid autacoid may be important in the modulation of normal, as well as abnormal, acute and chronic inflammatory processes. In most cases, the precise chemical structures of the PAFs produced by these cells have not been determined. Rather, most studies have physicochemically characterized the molecules, e.g., by TLC and normal or reverse phase high-performance liquid chromatographic (HPLC) behaviors, by susceptibility to phospholipases or acetylhydrolase, and/or by incorporation of radiolabeled substrates into the PAF derived from stimulated cells. Since we now recognize that multiple, heterogeneous PAF molecules are concurrently produced by stimulated cells (see below), more definitive qualitative and quantitative characterizations of these various cell-derived PAFs will have to be accomplished. As outlined below, the existence of extensive PAF molecular heterogeneity may be important in the modulation of the biological efficacy of this autacoid in the inflammatory process.

In view of the above, and for the remainder of this chapter, the term PAF will be used to describe the molecule(s) that is synthesized by various cells but whose structure(s) has not been determined. The term AGEPC will refer to those chemically defined molecules whose structures are that of 1-O-alkyl-2-acetyl-sn-glycero-3-phosphocholine. For completeness, PAF-acether is also commonly used in the literature to define such a molecule, employing the *acetyl* and *ether* suffixes to denote two important structural components for biological activity (21).

PATHWAYS FOR PAF SYNTHESIS AND DEGRADATION

The principal enzymatic pathway for the biosynthesis of PAF (or more specifically AGEPC) in inflammatory cells involves a two-step, enzymatic deacylation-reacety-lation reaction (Fig. 4) (1,139,220). In brief, upon cell stimulation and the resulting activation of phospholipase A_2, long-chain fatty acyl residues esterified in the 2 position are hydrolyzed from intracellular precursor pools of 1-O-alkyl-2-acyl-sn-glycero-3-phosphocholine. The lysophospholipid product, 1-O-alkyl-sn-glycero-3-phosphocholine (lyso-GEPC), is then acetylated by a specific acetyltransferase to form the biologically active molecule, 1-O-alkyl-2-acetyl-sn-glycero-3-phosphocholine (AGEPC). Metabolic degradation of AGEPC occurs via acetylhydrolase, an enzyme that rapidly hydrolyzes the acetyl group from AGEPC (31,214). The biologically inactive lyso-GEPC product (50) is then reacylated with a long-chain fatty acid by the action of acyltransferase (1,220), thereby completing the metabolic cycle (Fig. 4).

The essential role of lysophosphoglycerides and acetate in AGEPC biosynthesis has been suggested by a variety of studies. First, a temporal relationship exists between the production of lysophospholipids and PAF in stimulated polymorphonuclear leukocytes (PMN) (20). Supporting these findings were studies documenting that human neutrophilic PMN contain substantial amounts of the 1-O-alkyl-containing precursor molecules, constituting approximately one-half of the choline-containing phospholipids in these cells (140). Further evidence in the search for AGEPC biosynthetic substrates was provided by the findings that stimulated rabbit peritoneal PMN effectively incorporate exogenous [3H]acetate as well as [3H]lyso-GEPC into [3H]AGEPC (139). These findings indicate that PMN have a high capacity for acetylating endogenously produced lyso-phospholipids. Similarly, [3H]lyso-GEPC incorporated into the endogenous pools of 1-O-alkyl-2-acyl-sn-glycero-3-phosphocholine in cultured rat alveolar macrophages is converted into [3H]AGEPC after cell stimulation (1). Finally, the addition of acetate and acetyl CoA to macrophages enhances both PAF production and release upon cell stimulation (136). Thus, lyso-GEPC and acetate (i.e., acetyl CoA) are likely the principal, immediate precursors of AGEPC in stimulated inflammatory cells.

A second *de-novo* enzymatic pathway for AGEPC biosynthesis in various tissues has also been described and is catalyzed by cholinephosphotransferase, which utilizes CDP-choline and 1-O-alkyl-2-acetyl-sn-glycerol (173). This enzyme may, in part, provide the basis for the strong hypotensive property of alkylacetylglycerol since it provides a pathway for conversion of this acetylated diglyceride into AGEPC, which has potent antihypertensive properties (29,32). Nevertheless, the deacylation-reacetylation pathway for PAF biosynthesis described above likely predominates in stimulated inflammatory cells inasmuch as the activity of acetyltransferase significantly increases after cell stimulation while cholinephosphotransferase activity remains unchanged (3).

TABLE 1. *Cellular sources of PAF*[a]

Cell	Species	Stimulus	
PMN (peripheral blood)	Human	A23187	Immune complexes
		Aggregated IgG	Immune complex-coated beads
		C5a	or RBC
		C5a-des-Arg	NaF
		Cationic protein des-Arg	Opsonized zymosan
		FMLP	PMA
		IgG- or IgG/C3-coated RBC	PMN cationic protein
	Rabbit	A23187	
		C5a	
		Opsonized zymosan	
		Zymosan EDTA	
	Pig	Autolysis	
PMN (peritoneal)	Rat	A23187	
	Guinea pig	A23187	
Macrophage (peritoneal)	Rat	A23187	Bacteria
		Antibody-coated RBC	Immune complexes
		Autolysis	Opsonized zymosan
	Mouse	A23187	
		Autolysis	
Macrophage (alveolar)	Rat	A23187	
		Zymosan	
	Rabbit	A23187	
		Zymosan	
	Human	A23187	
	Monkey	A23187	
Monocyte	Human	A23187	C3b- and C3d-coated yeast
		Autolysis	spores
		Bacteria	Immune complexes
	Rabbit	Opsonized zymosan	
HL60 cells differentiated to macrophages	Human	Autolysis	
		C3b- and C3d-coated yeast spores	
Eosinophil	Human	A23187	
		C5a	
		Eosinophil chemotactic factor of anaphylaxis	
		FMLP	
Mast cell	Mouse (bone marrow)	Antigen	
	Human (pulmonary)	Anti-IgE	
		Antigen	
Endothelial cells	Human	A23187	Interleukin 1
		ADP	K235 endotoxin
		Angiotensin II	Leukotriene C_4 and D_4
		Anti-human factor VIII	Thrombin
		Bradykinin	Vasopressin
		Histamine	
	Rabbit	Goat anti-lung angiotensin converting enzyme	
	Bovine	K235 endotoxin	
Mesangial cells	Rat	A23187	
Natural killer lymphocyte	Human	Fc receptor	
Platelet	Rabbit	A23187	
		Collagen	
		Thrombin	
	Human	A23187	
		Thrombin	

Table 1. (*Continued*)

Cell	Species		Stimulus
Basophil	Rabbit	A23187	
		Anti-IgE	
		Antigen	
	Human	A23187	C5a
		Anti-IgE	PMN cationic protein
		Autolysis	Synacthen

[a] PAF, platelet-activating factor; PMN, polymorphonuclear leukocyte; FMLP, N'-formyl-methionyl-leucyl-phenylalanine; PMA, phorbol myristate acetate; RBC, red blood cell; EDTA, ethylenediaminetetraacetic acid; ADP, adenosine diphosphate.

Many of the biological activities of AGEPC may be modulated through synergistic interactions with various arachidonic acid metabolites derived from the lipoxygenase and cyclooxygenase pathways. This attractive relationship between two classes of potent, lipid inflammatory mediators is further strengthened by the findings that arachidonic acid metabolites and PAF, concomitantly produced by stimulated inflammatory cells, are likely derived from a common precursor, i.e., 1-*O*-alkyl-2-arachidonyl-*sn*-glycero-3-phosphocholine (43). Indeed, in many cells, the 1-*O*-alkyl-linked, choline-containing phosphoglycerides that serve as AGEPC precursors are enriched in arachidonic acid when compared to the diacyl phosphocholine pool (140). Furthermore, in resting human PMN, over 80% of exogenously added lyso-GEPC that is incorporated into the cell becomes acylated with arachidonic

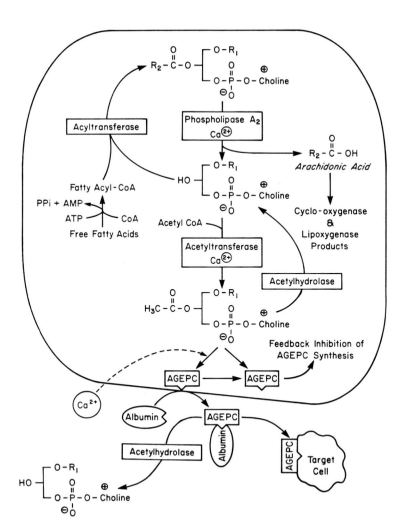

FIG. 4. Proposed biosynthetic pathway for AGEPC (PAF). The deacylation-reacetylation pathway is the principal route of PAF biosynthesis by stimulated inflammatory cells. Activation of phospholipase A_2 hydrolyzes the long-chain fatty acyl group (predominantly arachidonic acid) at the 2 position of PAF precursors, followed by reacetylation of this position by acetyltransferase. The mechanisms for PAF release are currently not known but may be coupled to sustained PAF synthesis. Degradation of PAF occurs via deacetylation of PAF by acetylhydrolase.

acid (45). More recent studies have shown that PMN from rats depleted of arachidonic acid (by dietary deficiency) produce only 10% of the AGEPC and 5S,12R-dihydroxy-5,8,11,14-eicosatetraenoic acid or leukotriene B$_4$ (LTB$_4$) in comparison to PMN from control rats fed a normal diet (172). The preceding strongly support a close inter-relationship between arachidonic acid metabolism and AGEPC formation in PMN and likely other inflammatory cells. Thus, it is tempting to speculate that inflammatory cells have an activatable phospholipase A$_2$, highly specific for 1-O-alkyl-2-arachidonyl-sn-glycero-3-phosphocholine, which plays a central role in the regulation of AGEPC biosynthesis.

The following will briefly describe the principal enzymes involved in the deacylation-reacetylation pathway of PAF biosynthesis. It should be noted, however, that many of the studies designed to characterize the synthesis and degradation of AGEPC have been conducted using exogenously supplied AGEPC or precursors. Thus, it is conceivable that alternative enzymatic pathways for the metabolism of endogenously generated PAF may exist and thus form the basis for many ongoing studies.

Phospholipase A$_2$

Phospholipase A$_2$ plays a central role in the biosynthesis of AGEPC, since it generates the immediate precursor molecule, lyso-GEPC (Fig. 4). Putative inhibitors of phospholipase A$_2$, such as mepacrine, bromophenacyl bromide, and hydrocortisone, concomitantly inhibit both lyso-GEPC and AGEPC formation (1,38,163). Although the specificities and intracellular targets of such inhibitory agents may be questioned, it is noteworthy that while bromophenacyl bromide inhibits PAF release from monocytes, it does not affect lysosomal enzyme release or phagocytosis by these cells (38). On the other hand, certain lipoxygenase products may potentiate phospholipase A$_2$ activity in stimulated human PMN (27). This observation provides an additional basis for the previously mentioned link between arachidonic acid metabolism and PAF biosynthesis. Thus, the addition of 5-hydroperoxy-eicosatetraenoic acid (5-L-HPETE), 5-L-HETE, or LTB$_4$ to stimulated human PMN not only augments the cellular release of arachidonic acid, but also augments AGEPC formation. Consistent with these findings, nordihydroguaiaretic acid (NDGA) and other dual lipoxygenase/cyclooxygenase inhibitors decrease both arachidonic acid release and PAF formation in these cells. In contrast, specific cyclooxygenase inhibitors do not inhibit, but slightly enhance, arachidonic acid release and PAF formation (27). Thus, the action of phospholipase A$_2$ likely modulates the availability of lysophospholipid precursors for subsequent utilization by acetyltransferase to generate PAF in stimulated inflammatory cells.

Acetyltransferase

Acetyltransferase catalyzes the transfer of acetate from acetyl CoA to the 2 position of lyso-GEPC and other lysophospholipids (Fig. 4). Since there is a temporal relationship between AGEPC formation and the level of acetyltransferase activation in stimulated PMN, it has been suggested that this enzyme may play a rate-limiting role in the biosynthesis of AGEPC (3). Similarly, in several other cell types, agents that stimulate or inhibit AGEPC production correspondingly affect acetyltransferase activity (114,220). Regarding the characteristics of this enzyme, its activity is increased by phosphorylation via a protein kinase (116). Acetyltransferase is distinct from the analogous acyltransferase that preferentially acylates with long-chain fatty acids (113). In human PMN, acetyltransferase activity is localized primarily in the plasma membrane and has a pH optimum between 7.5 and 8.0 (220). For PMN-derived acetyltransferase, exogenous Ca^{2+} is not necessary (220); however, in murine macrophages, this divalent cation is required (146). With respect to substrate specificity, rat spleen acetyltransferase can effectively acetylate a variety of lysophospholipids, including molecules with polar head groups other than choline (113). This is of particular interest since the PAF derived from activated inflammatory cells consists of several molecular species of PAF, i.e., PAF molecules having polar head groups other than choline (see below). Thus, it will be important to clearly define the substrate specificities of this enzyme(s) in inflammatory cells and to determine whether activation of acetyltransferase regulates, at least in part, the ultimate types and proportions of PAF molecules that are synthesized and released by these stimulated cells.

Acetylhydrolase

Acetylhydrolase catalyzes the hydrolysis of the acetyl group from AGEPC and other related acetylated phosphoglycerides (Fig. 4). In cells, the lipid product of this reaction (lyso-GEPC and other lysophospholipids) is rapidly reacylated at the 2 position with a long-chain fatty acid (45,114). Of interest is that both an intracellular and a plasma form of acetylhydrolase have been identified (31,166). Intracellular acetylhydrolase in rat tissues is distinct from phospholipase A$_2$ in that it is Ca^{2+}-independent, is specific for short-chain fatty acyl residues at the 2 position, and is located predominantly in the cytosol (31). The pH optimum of kidney-derived acetylhydrolase is between 7.5 and 8.5, with an apparent K_m and V_{max} of 3.1 μM and 1.1 μmole/hr/mg protein, respectively (31). Human PMN acetylhydrolase has similar characteristics (220). Additional studies are clearly necessary to characterize the role of intracellular acetylhydrolase as a potential regulating step in PAF metabolism by stimulated inflammatory cells.

Similar to the above, plasma-derived acetylhydrolase has profound implications relative to the potent phlogistic and physiologic properties of fluid-phase AGEPC. Indeed, the half-life of exogenously added AGEPC in whole human blood is identical to its half-life in cell-free plasma (194). Plasma acetylhydrolase, which is associated with the low-density lipoprotein fraction, is Ca^{2+}-independent, is specific only for short-chain fatty acyl-linked groups at the 2 position, and is inhibited by diisopropylfluorophosphate (214). Recent purification of this enzyme has revealed an apparent K_m of 13.7 μM and a V_{max} of 568 μmole/hr/mg protein utilizing a micellar form of AGEPC as substrate (195). Plasma acetylhydrolase effectively hydrolyzes the acetyl group from PAF analogs with an acyl linkage (rather than an alkyl linkage) at the 1 position (195,214). Furthermore, and of importance, ethanolamine-containing PAF analogs competitively inhibit AGEPC hydrolysis by plasma-derived acetylhydrolase (195); moreover, this acetylhydrolase cannot cleave the acetyl group from an ethanolamine PAF analog (214). These latter observations may be critical to bioregulation of PAF activities *in vivo*.

Acyltransferase

Intracellular acyltransferase catalyzes the transfer of a long-chain fatty acid to the 2 position of lyso-GEPC (Fig. 4). This enzyme likely is responsible for the rapid metabolism of AGEPC to 1-*O*-alkyl-2-acyl-*sn*-glycero-3-phosphocholine after its addition to various cell types and tissues or after the *in vivo* administration of AGEPC (45,126,220). In human PMN and platelets, acyltransferase is located primarily in the plasma membrane and does not require acyl-CoA, ATP, or Mg^{2+} (108,148). As mentioned previously, the link between arachidonic acid metabolism and PAF biosynthesis in PMN by way of a common precursor is further strengthened by the finding that lyso-GEPC is predominantly acylated with arachidonic acid (42,45). This reaction (determined by pulse-labeling PMN with [^{3}H]arachidonic acid) is time-dependent in that arachidonic acid is rapidly incorporated into ester-linked phospholipid pools with subsequent incorporation into ether-linked phosphoglycerides (42). Human platelets exhibit similar reactions, i.e., AGEPC is specifically reacylated with arachidonic acid via an acyl-CoA-independent

reaction (108,126). In both PMN and platelets, this activity is inhibited by *N*-ethylmaleimide and detergents (108,220). Thus, the exclusive reacylation of lyso-GEPC with arachidonic acid appears to be catalyzed by a CoA-independent acyltransferase (42,220).

PAF SYNTHESIS-RELEASE COUPLING

Despite the relatively abundant efforts to characterize the metabolism of PAF outlined above, only a few investigations have attempted to address the mechanisms that regulate the *release* of this autacoid from stimulated cells. In this regard, although cell-associated PAF likely is involved in cell-cell communication (e.g., leukocyte-endothelium, leukocyte-platelet, platelet-endothelium), the release of fluid-phase PAF would allow the full expression of its potent phlogistic and physiologic properties. Further, while increases in the activities of phospholipase A_2 and acetyltransferase are undoubtedly important in the regulation of PAF biosynthesis, the release of newly synthesized PAF also is critical in this regard. Thus, the release of newly synthesized AGEPC is tightly linked to augmented and sustained PAF synthesis (124). However, not all of the PAF that is synthesized by stimulated cells is subsequently released; i.e., human endothelial cells (128), pulmonary mast cells (168), and basophils (25) release little, if any, PAF. With human PMN, the release of PAF occurs only after a critical, intracellular concentration of PAF has been synthesized (122,123). Although the extent of PAF release appears to be related to the degree of lysosomal enzyme secretion, these PMN events are kinetically dissociated (24,123). In brief, in the absence of extracellular Ca^{2+}, endogenous stores of intracellular Ca^{2+} support up to 40% to 50% of maximal lysosomal enzyme secretion in *N'*-formyl-methionyl-leucyl-phenylalanine-(FMLP)-stimulated PMN (in the presence of cytochalasin B); however, PAF synthesis is significantly depressed, and no PAF is released. In contrast, extracellular Ca^{2+} (>0.01 mM), in a dose-dependent manner, not only significantly enhances PAF synthesis, but also initiates PAF release in concert with an augmentation in lysosomal enzyme secretion. These findings suggest that there are two mechanisms regulating PAF synthesis and release in stimulated human PMN. The first allows the initial synthesis of PAF after cell stimulation and requires only intracellular Ca^{2+}; the second requires extracellular Ca^{2+} and modulates both PAF release and sustained PAF synthesis.

PAF synthesis-release coupling also is modulated by the concentration of extracellular albumin (122). In brief, in the absence of albumin, FMLP-stimulated PMN synthesize only small amounts of PAF (which attain maximum levels within 1 to 2 min after stimulation); however,

PAF release does not occur, and further PAF synthesis is abrogated. In contrast, the presence of 0.25% albumin results in a profound increase in total PAF biosynthesis and initiates the release of 30% to 40% of the newly synthesized PAF within 5 min after stimulation. Moreover, in the presence of 5% albumin, there is an additional sevenfold increase in PAF synthesis and release which is sustained for 30 min. Thus, like extracellular Ca^{2+}, the presence of albumin during PMN stimulation induces a dose-dependent increase in PAF release and significantly augments and sustains the synthesis of PAF.

The albumin-dependent regulation of PAF synthesis and release from stimulated PMN may operationally reflect the ability of albumin to solubilize and maintain PAF in aqueous solution, particularly at PAF concentrations below its critical micellar concentration (CMC; 1.1–1.3 μM AGEPC, ref. 109). Thus, because of its insolubility in the absence of extracellular albumin, PAF expressed on the surface of the stimulated PMN could not be released because the maximum concentration of PAF synthesized by the PMN (10 nM, assuming that PAF is C16:0-AGEPC) is two orders of magnitude below its CMC. In the absence of release, the cell-bound PAF likely would be rapidly metabolized by the PMN and reincorporated into the membrane phospholipid pool (108,148). In addition, if PAF release were reduced or abrogated, newly synthesized PAF could interact with a regulatory PAF receptor on the PMN surface causing cessation of further PAF synthesis. The regulatory role of extracellular Ca^{2+} upon PAF release and sustained PAF synthesis, described above, is also consistent with this hypothesis. That is, in the presence of both albumin and Ca^{2+}, newly synthesized PAF would be rapidly released from the PMN, thereby preventing it from interacting with such a putative PAF regulatory receptor, and would preclude its metabolic reincorporation into the cell. Thus, although the mechanisms that regulate the biosynthesis and release of AGEPC by stimulated cells have not been fully elucidated, further investigations in this area may lead to a better understanding of the role of this unique lipid autacoid in normal and abnormal inflammatory reactions.

PAF MOLECULAR HETEROGENEITY

The PAF synthesized by the stimulated human PMN is now known to be comprised of multiple molecular species, including both saturated and unsaturated 1-*O*-alkyl homologs of AGEPC, 1-*O*-acyl analogs, and acetylated phosphoglycerides having polar head groups other than choline (121,141,159,167,171,180,215). However, the majority of knowledge relating to the (patho)biological activities and metabolism of PAF has been derived from

studies utilizing only C16:0- and/or C18:0-AGEPC. In view of the above, the *in vivo* and *in vitro* consequences of PAF must now be reconsidered because the concomitant generation of multiple, structurally related phosphoglycerides may modify subsequent bioresponses. For example, structure-activity relationship studies (utilizing synthetic molecules) have shown that even minor structural alterations in AGEPC have significant effects upon both biological activities (Table 2) and metabolic breakdown (195,214). Furthermore, while the major pathway for the metabolism of PMN-derived AGEPC is through the deacylation-reacetylation pathway, the biosynthesis and degradation of other acetylated phosphoglycerides derived from endogenous phospholipid substrates has not been fully addressed. Thus, modulation of metabolism/distribution of the molecular species of PAF produced by activated inflammatory cells *in vivo* may alter the biological events that regulate inflammation or lead to tissue injury.

The first indication that PMN-derived PAF was more than C16:0- and C18:0-AGEPC was facilitated by the application of HPLC analytical procedures to phospholipid separation. As detected by rabbit platelet stimulation, the PAF synthesized by FMLP- or A23187-stimulated PMN and fractionated by reverse-phase HPLC consisted of various alkyl-chain homologs of AGEPC; fast atom bombardment–mass spectrometry (FAB-MS) identified several of these molecules to be C16:0-, C17:0-, C18:0-, C18:1-, C15:0-, and C22:2-AGEPC (121,215). Similarly, using reverse-phase HPLC with detection of PAF by substrate incorporation ([^{3}H]acetate), stimulated human PMN generated multiple alkyl-chain homologs of AGEPC including C16:0 (40%), C17:0 (two isomers of 8% and 5%), C18:0 (16%), and C18:1 (18%) (141). More recently, gas chromatography–mass spectrometry (negative-ion chemical ionization) has identified molecular species of AGEPC with alkyl chain lengths from C14:0- to C19:0- (171). Interestingly, the distribution of PAF molecular heterogeneity varies as a function of cell type, i.e., the PAF obtained from rat PMN is 96% C16:0-AGEPC, whereas PAF from guinea-pig PMN contains several 1-*O*-alkyl chain AGEPC homologs, including C16:0 (35%), C17:0 (35%), C18:1 (8%), and C18:0 (3%). Moreover, the quantitative distribution of the PAF molecular species does not correlate with the putative alkyl-chain precursor, 1-*O*-alkyl-2-acyl-*sn*-glycero-3-phosphocholine, within the cell (140). These latter observations suggest that there is either selectivity in endogenous PMN phospholipid substrates that are available for PAF biosynthesis or an alternative biosynthetic pathway for PAF generation.

In addition to variation in the chain length and degree of unsaturation in position 1 of PAF, changes in the linkage at this position also occur; i.e., 1-*O*-acyl PAF is pro-

TABLE 2. *Biological activities of acetylated AGEPC homologs and analogs*[a]

Carbon 1		Carbon 3	Platelet stimulation ED_{50} (nM)[b]	PMN lysozyme secretion ED_{10} (nM)[b]	Vascular permeability endpoint (pmole)[c]
Chain length	Linkage	Polar head group			
12:0	Ether	Phosphocholine	1.80	ND[d]	ND
14:0	Ether	Phosphocholine	1.30	26.0	ND
15:0	Ether	Phosphocholine	0.14	ND	ND
16:0	Ether	Phosphocholine	0.14	8.9	1.0
18:0	Ether	Phosphocholine	0.52	340.0	10.0
18:1	Ether	Phosphocholine	0.28	3.7	ND
12:0	Ester	Phosphocholine	700.00	ND	ND
16:0	Ester	Phosphocholine	46.00	Inactive	ND
18:0	Ester	Phosphocholine	700.00	Inactive	ND
16:0 + 18:0	Ether	Phosphodimethylethanolamine	0.40	18.0	10.0
16:0 + 18:0	Ether	Phosphomonomethylethanolamine	3.50	340.0	10.0[e]
16:0	Ether	Phosphoethanolamine	1,020.00	Inactive	Inactive
18:0	Ether	Phosphoethanolamine	9,940.00	ND	ND
18:1	Ether	Phosphoethanolamine	10,700.00	ND	ND
16:0 + 18:0	Ether	Phosphatidic acid	2.80[f]	Inactive	100.0

[a] Taken, in part, from refs. 50, 65, 92, 109, 179, 181, and 203.

[b] Final concentration required to cause 50% secretion of serotonin from washed rabbit platelets (within 60 sec) or 10% secretion of lysozyme from isolated human PMN (within 5 min) (inactive = no secretion at 1,000 nM).

[c] Minimum dose required to produce intracutaneous blueing >5 mm in diameter in rabbit skin (inactive = no blueing at 1,000 pmole).

[d] Not determined.

[e] Only 50% animals responded.

[f] Platelet response to AGEPA did not occur until 1–5 min after addition to platelets.

duced concomitantly with 1-*O*-alkyl PAF from stimulated PMN (141,180,215). In one study (141), 13% of the [³H]acetate-labeled PAF derived from stimulated human PMN was in the form of 1-*O*-acyl-2-acetyl-*sn*-glycero-3-phosphocholine. Such a 1-*O*-acyl molecular species of PAF was anticipated because acetyltransferase can acetylate 1-*O*-acyl-linked lysophospholipids (113). Further, in A23187-stimulated PMN, the release of arachidonic acid, which is associated with PAF biosynthesis, occurs from both the alkylacyl and diacyl pools of choline-containing phosphoglycerides (220). The occurrence of PAF molecular species with an acyl linkage at the 1 position could be of biological consequence, since these molecular species are far less active than their alkyl-linked counterparts.

Platelet-stimulating molecules with a polar head group other than choline are also synthesized by stimulated cells (121,139,202). Thus, activated human PMN produce non-choline-containing PAF-like molecules that have platelet-stimulating activity and are labeled with [³H]acetate; based upon HPLC behavior, this likely represents an alkyl-ethanolamine-containing phosphoglyceride (121,202). Again, these findings are not surprising because PMN have abundant quantities of 1-*O*-alkyl- and alk-1-enyl-ethanolamine-containing phosphoglycerides that could function as precursor molecules in the deacylation-reacetylation pathway (140). Indeed, evidence has been presented

that acetyltransferase can effectively acetylate 1-*O*-alkyl-*sn*-glycero-3-phosphoethanolamine (113).

In view of the above, our current understanding of the type, quantity, and biological importance of PAF synthesized by stimulated inflammatory cells in modulating normal and/or abnormal inflammatory reactions are currently inconclusive. First, the overall (patho)biological role of PAF is unknown because the majority of studies characterizing its biological activities (i.e., platelet stimulation, smooth muscle contraction, etc.) utilized only one or possibly two AGEPC derivatives. In this regard, synergistic or antagonistic actions of other PAF molecules have not been studied. Second, differences in the rates of synthesis and degradation of the various molecular species of PAF could be anticipated and expected to dramatically influence their beneficial or (patho)biological potentials. Finally, competition between PAF molecules for target cell receptors or for the active site on acetylhydrolase could have a profound impact upon subsequent (patho)biological events. Thus, each individual molecular species of PAF must be structurally identified and synthesized for investigations to rigorously characterize its biological activities and pathological potentials both alone and in combination with other PAF molecules. Then, the full (patho)biological significance of this important class of acetylated phospholipid autacoid will be realized.

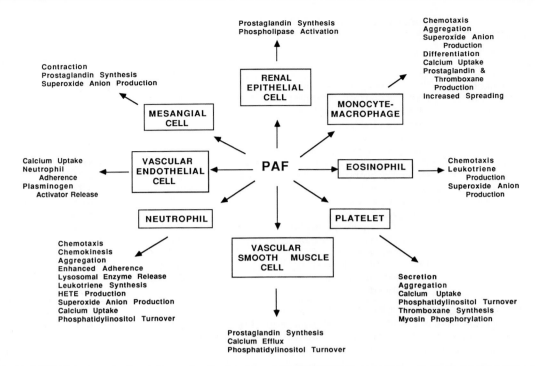

FIG. 5. AGEPC-induced stimulation of cells *in vitro*. AGEPC initiates a variety of diverse biological effects associated with modulation of inflammation, including the production of a variety of other phlogistic autacoids. AGEPC-induced cell stimulation is thought to involve AGEPC-receptor activation of phosphatidylinositol-specific phospholipase C and mobilization of intracellular and extracellular Ca^{2+}. The AGEPC receptor is most likely associated with guanine nucleotide regulatory proteins that are involved in transmembrane signal transduction.

INFLAMMATORY EFFECTS OF AGEPC *IN VITRO*

As mentioned previously, intravenous administration of AGEPC induced the development of thrombocytopenia, granulocytopenia, and monocytopenia. These early observations suggested that AGEPC might have agonist effects on multiple inflammatory cells. Indeed, subsequent studies have documented that AGEPC is a potent agonist not only for most inflammatory cells, but also for vascular smooth muscle and endothelial cells as well as renal mesangial and epithelial cells (Fig. 5). The following discussion will focus upon AGEPC-induced inflammatory cell activation *in vitro*.

Platelet Stimulation

Historically, the platelet aggregatory and secretory inflammatomimetic properties of PAF led to its identification as a fluid-phase mediator; however, until the structure of PAF was elucidated and AGEPC was synthesized, its relative potency and mode of action as a platelet agonist were not known. AGEPC is a potent agonist for platelets of most species (26,50,134,144,182); the notable ex-

ception is that murine platelets do not respond to AGEPC because they lack AGEPC receptors (177). With respect to rabbit and human platelets, AGEPC is now recognized to be a relatively potent platelet agonist, provided the platelets are isolated and stimulated under optimum conditions (106,132).

In rabbit platelets, AGEPC induces extracellular Ca^{2+}-independent shape change (0.01 n*M*) and extracellular Ca^{2+}-dependent irreversible aggregation concomitant with maximal secretion (0.1 n*M*) of dense body contents ([³H]serotonin, histamine), α-granule contents (platelet factor 4), and production of thromboxane B_2 (TxB_2) (0.5 n*M*) (50,132). These aggregatory and secretory responses are complete within 60 sec after AGEPC addition. ADP scavengers (creatine phosphate-creatine kinase, CPCK) slightly reduce rabbit platelet aggregation at lower AGEPC concentrations, but irreversible aggregation still occurs at 0.1 n*M* AGEPC; CPCK has no effect on AGEPC-induced secretion of dense body contents or α-granule contents. Cyclooxygenase inhibition with indomethacin or aspirin is also without effect on AGEPC-induced aggregation or secretion in rabbit platelets. Specific desensitization to AGEPC develops in platelets exposed to suboptimal concentrations of AGEPC or under nonstimulating conditions, i.e., in the absence of extracellular Ca^{2+}; although these platelets do not subsequently respond to AGEPC, they respond normally to thrombin or opsonized (C3b)-zymosan (50).

The relative potency of AGEPC-induced stimulation of human platelets was unclear until recently because of disparate findings of various investigators (82,106,112,127,134,144,162,200,207). While some studies employed citrated platelet-rich plasma, others utilized isolated, washed platelets prepared by different procedures and stimulated under varying conditions, e.g., in the presence or absence of fibrinogen and differing concentrations of extracellular Ca^{2+} and Mg^{2+}. Further, platelet responsiveness to AGEPC decreases with time after human platelet preparation (134), and platelets obtained from fasting subjects are more responsive (106). In any event, in the presence of fibrinogen and optimal extracellular $[Ca^{2+}]$ and $[Mg^{2+}]$, AGEPC induces a dose-dependent stimulation of isolated human platelets prepared by gel filtration (106). At lower concentrations (0.2–10 nM), AGEPC induces only a primary wave of platelet aggregation without initiating the secretory process; at higher concentrations (10–100 nM), primary wave aggregation occurs during the first 2 min and is followed by a second wave of platelet aggregation associated with secretion of the contents of dense bodies, α-granules, and acid-hydrolase-containing (lysosomal) granules. At 300 nM, AGEPC induces almost immediate platelet secretion, the expression of both high- and low-affinity fibrinogen receptors, and monophasic, irreversible platelet aggregation. The presence of ethylenediaminetetraacetic acid (EDTA) completely abolishes both AGEPC-induced aggregation of, and secretion by, human platelets in plasma (134) or platelets isolated by gel filtration (106); the latter also requires stirring to maximize the response. At lower AGEPC concentrations, CPCK and/or indomethacin or aspirin blocks the second wave of platelet aggregation and significantly reduces or abrogates the secretory response; however, platelet aggregation and secretion still occur at elevated concentrations of AGEPC (>500 nM) (134).

Finally, AGEPC-induced activation of platelets in their natural milieu (i.e., in plasma) requires 10- to 100-fold more AGEPC than is necessary to comparably stimulate isolated, washed platelets. This likely reflects the presence of (a) the AGEPC-degrading enzyme, i.e., acetylhydrolase, and (b) albumin, which binds AGEPC and interferes with its receptor interaction. Nevertheless, the concentrations of AGEPC necessary to effect platelet stimulation under these conditions are within the range of those that could be generated *in vivo*. In addition, the biological potencies of AGEPC can be greatly accentuated through synergistic interactions with other platelet agonists, e.g., epinephrine, ADP, and aggregated IgG (see following). Indeed, intra-

venous administration of physiologically relevant concentrations of AGEPC into experimental animals reproduces all of the AGEPC-induced platelet responses that occur *in vitro* (see following).

PMN Stimulation

Until the structure of PAF was elucidated and AGEPC was synthesized, the biological effects of this mediator were thought to be promoted solely through its potent platelet-stimulating actions. However, studies assessing the *in vivo* biological activity of AGEPC suggested that this phospholipid might have PMN-stimulating properties as well (133). In brief, within 60 sec after the intravenous infusion, submicrogram quantities of AGEPC not only induce acute platelet effects (i.e., intravascular platelet aggregation, thrombocytopenia, and platelet factor 4 release), but also initiate profound, but reversible, neutropenia. This acute, AGEPC-induced neutropenia is very reminiscent of the neutropenia that occurs following the intravenous injection of PMN chemotactic factors. Thus, preliminary *in vitro* studies demonstrated that AGEPC induces aggregation, chemotaxis and chemokinesis, and secretion of lysozyme and β-glucuronidase from isolated human PMN (169). AGEPC modulation of most aspects of PMN activation are now recognized and suggests that this unusual phospholipid may play an important role in the inflammatory process.

When added to stirred suspensions of human or rabbit PMN, AGEPC induces dose-dependent (1–1,000 nM) PMN aggregation (69,111,120,151,155,186). Although cytochalasin B greatly enhances AGEPC-induced PMN aggregation, this response is not dependent upon the presence of this fungal metabolite. AGEPC-induced PMN aggregation is highly dependent upon the presence of extracellular Ca^{2+} and Mg^{2+}, occurs within 60 sec after the addition of AGEPC, and, with time, is fully reversible (151,155,186). For human PMN, AGEPC-induced PMN aggregation is most likely mediated through stimulation of the 5-lipoxygenase pathway of arachidonate metabolism. Both ETYA (5,8,11,14-eicosatetraynoic acid, which blocks both lipoxygenase and cyclooxygenase) and NDGA (nordihydroguaiaretic acid, which blocks lipoxygenase) significantly reduce AGEPC-induced PMN aggregation in a dose-dependent fashion (120); in contrast, indomethacin inhibition of cyclooxygenase activity has no effect. Moreover, AGEPC stimulates the release of [^{3}H]arachidonate from PMN, with its subsequent metabolism through the lipoxygenase pathway to 5-, 11-, and 15-HETE (hydroxyeicosatetraenoic acid) and LTB_4, the latter product being 10 to 100 times more potent than AGEPC in inducing PMN aggregation (69,120). The amounts of LTB$_4$ synthesized by AGEPC-stimulated human PMN are within the concentration range required to induce PMN aggregation by this lipoxygenase product (44,69,120). Nevertheless, specific desensitization of PMN to LTB$_4$ (by prior exposure of the PMN to LTB$_4$ in the absence of extracellular Ca^{2+} and Mg^{2+}) significantly reduces, but does not abrogate, subsequent AGEPC-induced aggregation (120,151). Therefore, AGEPC-induced aggregation of human PMN is mediated, in part, through its ability to stimulate the endogenous synthesis of LTB$_4$. However, as is the case for many other AGEPC effects, species differences exist since AGEPC-induced aggregation of rat PMN is independent of LTB$_4$ synthesis (61). Lastly, because AGEPC has been shown to decrease electrophoretic mobility of isolated human PMN (99), this decrease in the net negative charge of the cell surface would also be expected to contribute to its proaggregatory actions. Such cell-surface charge alterations also could account for the AGEPC-induced increase in the adherence of PMN to endothelial cells (99).

AGEPC also effects the release of both specific and azurophil granule contents, including lysozyme, lactoferrin, β-glucuronidase, and myeloperoxidase, from isolated rabbit and human PMN (65,152,154,155,186,191). In the presence of cytochalasin B, AGEPC induces a rapid ($T_{1/2}$ = 20–30 sec), dose-dependent (1–1,000 nM) secretion of lysosomal enzymes, with maximal release occurring within 60 to 90 sec (186,193). Although it has generally been accepted that PMN secretion of lysosomal enzymes requires the presence of cytochalasin B, closer inspection of most studies reveals that AGEPC can induce a small, but significant, secretion of these enzymes in its absence; however, the concentrations of AGEPC required to release lysosomal enzymes are relatively high (1 μM or greater) and approach or exceed the critical micellar concentration (CMC) of AGEPC. These high AGEPC concentrations may induce nonspecific alterations in PMN (and other cells), as reflected both by the reduction in lysosomal enzyme secretion and by the release of lactate dehydrogenase (LDH). Thus, any biological response requiring these relatively high concentrations of lipid should be interpreted with some degree of caution. Nevertheless, more recent studies have demonstrated that, with human PMN, AGEPC induces a dose-dependent (10–1,000 nM) release of both gelatinase and vitamin-B-binding protein from secretory vesicles and specific granules, respectively, in the absence of cytochalasin B (12,52). On a molar basis, AGEPC was more effective than LTB$_4$ and as effective as FMLP, although the PMN secretory response to AGEPC was more rapid than that to FMLP. In contrast to PMN aggregation, extracellular Ca^{2+} is not a prerequisite for AGEPC-induced secretion of lysosomal enzymes from human PMN, although the presence of extracellular Ca^{2+} augments this response (154,186,191). As for other PMN

secretagogues, AGEPC-induced lysosomal enzyme secretion requires glycolysis (186,193). Further, inhibition of the lipoxygenase pathway of arachidonate metabolism by either NDGA or ETYA significantly inhibits AGEPC-induced lysosomal enzyme release in a dose-dependent fashion (154,191); however, indomethacin, ibuprofen, or flurbiprofen inhibition of the cyclooxygenase pathway are without effect. In contrast to PMN aggregation (see above), the synthesis of LTB$_4$ does not appear to be an important modulating factor in AGEPC-induced lysosomal enzyme secretion. Thus, PMN specifically desensitized to LTB$_4$-induced aggregation and lysosomal enzyme secretion respond normally to AGEPC-stimulated lysosomal enzyme secretion (157).

In addition to inducing PMN aggregation and the secretion of lysosomal enzymes, AGEPC also has been shown to initiate the respiratory burst (i.e., the production of superoxide anion, O$_2^-$) in human PMN, as reflected by the superoxide dismutase inhibitable reduction of ferricytochrome c (186,192). The kinetics of O$_2^-$ production are slower than the kinetics of lysosomal enzyme secretion and, in general, parallel the rate of PMN aggregation, $T_{1/2}$ = 30 to 90 sec (186). Most studies have found that cytochalasin B is a prerequisite for the initiation of AGEPC-induced O$_2^-$ production (99,186), although a few have reported O$_2^-$ production by human PMN in its absence (12,52,192). Of note, the concentrations of AGEPC necessary to initiate O$_2^-$ production are orders of magnitude greater than are required to effect either PMN aggregation or the secretion of lysosomal enzymes; e.g., even in the presence of cytochalasin B, 0.1 to 10 μM AGEPC was required. As previously mentioned, these high concentrations of AGEPC not only elicit LDH release, but also reduce PMN aggregation and lysosomal enzyme secretion (186).

Monocyte/Macrophage Stimulation

AGEPC initiates dose-dependent (0.1–1,000 nM) aggregation of stirred suspensions of isolated human blood monocytes (221). This potency in effecting monocyte aggregation may explain the acute monocytopenia after the intravenous administration of AGEPC into rabbits (Pinckard, *unpublished observations*). Human blood monocyte aggregation is dependent upon divalent cations (both Ca^{2+} and Mg^{2+}) and upon glycolysis. On a molar basis, AGEPC is slightly more active than FMLP in effecting monocyte aggregation and initiates the response more rapidly, i.e., within 8 sec after addition of AGEPC as opposed to 20 sec after FMLP. Whereas cytochalasin B decreases the lag time of monocyte aggregation to FMLP, it or its dihydroxy analog significantly reduces AGEPC-induced monocyte aggregation, suggesting a microfilament role in this response. As in the human PMN, prior exposure of monocytes to either AGEPC or FMLP desensitizes these cells to further aggregation to the homologous agonist, but cross-desensitization does not occur (221). These data are in keeping with the existence of specific receptors for both AGEPC and FMLP on human blood monocytes. In contrast to its aggregating properties, AGEPC does not effect the secretion of lysozyme and induces little, if any, O_2^- production in human monocytes (221). With respect to monocyte chemotactic properties, AGEPC is a relatively weak agonist, even at concentrations of 1 μM or greater (49). Of interest relative to possible mediator synergism (see below), the blood monocytes from patients with certain inflammatory dermatoses have augmented chemotactic responses to both AGEPC and LTB$_4$ (49).

In *Corynebacterium parvum*-elicited guinea-pig peritoneal macrophages, AGEPC induces a dose-dependent (1–1,000 nM) oxidative burst, as reflected by an increase in luminol-dependent chemiluminescence and H_2O_2 production (79,80). The production of H_2O_2 occurs within 10 min after the addition of AGEPC, maximizes by 30 min, and is not affected by the presence of indomethacin. In contrast, nonelicited guinea-pig peritoneal macrophages do not manifest an AGEPC-induced respiratory burst unless the cells are preincubated with gelatin. AGEPC also mobilizes arachidonic acid in guinea-pig alveolar macrophages (11) and induces the synthesis of PGE and TxB$_2$ from albumin-elicited guinea-pig peritoneal macrophage monolayers (79). The production of these eicosanoids is AGEPC dose-dependent (1–1,000 nM) and occurs over a 3-hr period. In this same system, AGEPC also enhances macrophage spreading, but only at the higher concentrations. As would be expected by its ability to initiate the respiratory burst, AGEPC increases glucose utilization in mineral-oil-elicited guinea-pig peritoneal macrophages in culture (83). Interestingly, when AGEPC is incorporated into phosphatidylcholine-cholesterol liposomes, the AGEPC concentrations (1–100 nM) required to stimulate these macrophages are lower than those of fluid-phase AGEPC (84). One explanation for this enhanced AGEPC responsiveness is that AGEPC incorporated into liposomes is more slowly metabolized to lyso-GEPC than is fluid-phase AGEPC. Alternatively, the physical state of AGEPC in liposomes could serve to facilitate cell stimulation. Indeed, in these studies, significantly enhanced activity of fluid-phase AGEPC was observed at concentrations where it would be present in a micellar form, i.e., >1 μM.

Stimulation of Other Cells

The eosinophil and vascular endothelial cell are two other inflammatory cells stimulated by AGEPC. As discussed below, AGEPC-induced increases in vascular permeability strongly suggest AGEPC targeting of postcapillary venular endothelial cell activation. Recent studies have shown that physiologically relevant concentrations of AGEPC can initiate rapid alterations in Ca^{2+} homeostasis in cultured human umbilical vein, baboon cephalic vein, and bovine aortic endothelial cells (34,37). In preloaded bovine aortic endothelial cells, AGEPC induces a dose-dependent (0.1–100 nM) efflux of $^{45}Ca^{2+}$ within 30 sec, with an EC$_{50}$ of 0.1 nM AGEPC (34). In quin-2-loaded endothelial cells, AGEPC increases free cytosolic Ca^{2+} ($[Ca^{2+}]_i$) to maximal levels within 30 to 60 sec. Efflux of $^{45}Ca^{2+}$ also occurs in cultured human-umbilical-vein endothelial cells, with an associated net increase of intracellular Ca^{2+} in the absence of increases in the levels of 6-keto-PGF$_{1\alpha}$ (37). Relative to a putative AGEPC receptor, Ca^{2+} fluxes are inhibited in a dose-dependent manner by a specific PAF receptor antagonist (34,37). Moreover, prior exposure of the cells to AGEPC significantly reduces Ca^{2+} fluxes during subsequent stimulation with AGEPC, whereas bradykinin-induced Ca^{2+} efflux is not affected (34). Finally, AGEPC induces the release of plasminogen activator from the isolated, perfused, rat hind limb by a calcium- and lipoxygenase-dependent process; this suggests a direct effect on the vascular endothelium (55).

Several *in vivo* studies have provided evidence that AGEPC may also be an important mediator in eosinophil activation. For example, after the intravenous administration of AGEPC, pulmonary periarterial accumulation of eosinophils subsequently develops in rabbits (130). Moreover, 24 hr after the intracutaneous injection of AGEPC into atopic subjects, significant numbers of eosinophils are observed in Rebuck skin windows, with many of these cells appearing degranulated (86). With isolated human eosinophils, AGEPC (1 μM) induces little, if any, LTC$_4$ production or increases in luminol-dependent chemiluminescence (35); however, AGEPC enhances the production of LTC$_4$ following opsonized zymosan stimulation of these cells.

Mechanisms of PAF-Induced Inflammatory Cell Activation

Like other Ca^{2+}-mobilizing autacoids, AGEPC-induced cell activation is initiated by its interaction with a specific membrane receptor(s) now thought to be associated with a guanine-nucleotide(GTP)-binding protein. AGEPC receptor occupancy effects transmembrane signal transduction, initiating the rapid metabolic turnover of polyphosphoinositides, alterations in Ca^{2+} homeostasis, and subsequent functional cellular responses. The existence of a specific AGEPC membrane receptor was first suggested by observations that prior exposure of various cells or tissues to AGEPC specifically desensitizes them to subsequent stimulation with AGEPC, even though these cells respond normally to other agonists (34,50,59, 186,197,221). Further, structure-activity relationship studies revealed that rather stringent structural and stereochemical requirements are necessary to maintain biological potency of various AGEPC homologs and analogs (30,92,179,181,219). Subsequently, high-affinity AGEPC receptors were identified on platelet, PMN, and other cell membranes (94–97,105,205), and several structurally related and unrelated AGEPC receptor antagonists were identified and characterized (182).

As with many other cell stimuli, the rapid turnover of polyphosphoinositides, the mobilization of intracellular Ca^{2+}, and the influx of extracellular Ca^{2+} immediately after AGEPC-receptor occupancy play a central role in inflammatory cell activation (22,188,217); particularly important in this regard are the guanine nucleotide regulatory proteins that modulate transmembrane autacoid-receptor transduction signaling (14,64,68,189,217; see Chapter 19 by Snyderman, this volume). In brief, the GTP-binding proteins were first recognized in a variety of different cells by their role in stimulating (G_s or N_s) or inhibiting (G_i or N_i) receptor-coupled activation of adenylate cyclase. Both the GTP-binding G_s and G_i proteins are heterotrimers composed of α, β, and γ subunits; the β and γ subunits appear to be similar in G_s and G_i, whereas the α subunits are different. In unstimulated cells, GDP is bound to the inactive α subunits of G_s and G_i; upon autacoid occupancy of the respective G_s- or G_i-coupled receptors, GTP replaces GDP, thus initiating the dissociation of the GTP-α_s or GTP-α_i subunits from G_s and G_i, respectively. In the case of G_s, the activated GTP-α_s subunit then associates with, as well as activates, adenylate cyclase; on the other hand, the GTP-α_i subunit and/or β/γ subunits inactivate adenylate cyclase through as-yet undefined mechanisms. This may, in part, involve dissociation of the GTP-α_s subunit from adenylate cyclase by free β/γ subunits; alternatively, receptor stimulation of intrinsic, high-affinity GTPase activities of the active GTP-α subunits may convert the GTP-α_s to GDP-α_s, with the dissociation of the latter inactive subunit from adenylate cyclase thereby inactivating the enzyme. Importantly, the islet-activating protein (IAP) component of *Bordetella pertussis* toxin effects the ADP ribosylation of the α subunit of G_i, thereby abrogating its inhibitory properties; cholera toxin, on the other hand, ADP-ribosylates the α subunit of G_s, thus facilitating its activation and stabilization by reducing receptor-stimulated GTPase activity. These actions of pertussis toxin and cholera toxin on G_i and G_s, respectively, have been widely exploited as probes to assess whether or not the GTP-binding proteins are involved in transmembrane autacoid-receptor transduction signaling.

In addition to modulating adenylate cyclase activity, the GTP-binding proteins also play a role in the autacoid-receptor signal transduction of the activation of phosphatidylinositol-specific phospholipase C (PI-PLC) and the modulation of Ca^{2+} and other ion fluxes. In many inflammatory cells, including the platelet (70,71, 115,158,175), PMN (110,143,213), monocyte/macrophage (47), and endothelial cell (34,37), one of the first physiologic events to occur after AGEPC stimulation is a rapid increase in free cytosolic Ca^{2+} ($[Ca^{2+}]_i$). This occurs in concert with the rapid metabolism of phosphatidylinositol, i.e., significant, but reversible, decreases in phosphatidylinositol 4,5-bisphosphate (PIP_2) and a rapid influx of extracellular Ca^{2+}. In the PMN, the specific receptors for certain secretagogues, such as FMLP, LTB_4, C5a, and AGEPC, seem to be associated with G_i-like GTP-binding proteins (13,56,67,107,110,111,137,142, 143,145,160,161,189,190); similar GTP-binding-protein-linked receptors have been identified on platelets (81,82,88,89,95,216) and monocytes (210). Following stimulus-receptor occupancy, the activated GTP-binding protein associates with, and allows the activation of, PI-PLC in the presence of low concentrations of ambient $[Ca^{2+}]_i$. The activated phosphodiesterase then hydrolyzes PIP_2, resulting in the intracellular release of inositol 1,4,5-triphosphate (IP_3) and diacylglycerol (DAG). The ionophoric actions of IP_3 increase $[Ca^{2+}]_i$ by modulating the mobilization of endogenous, membranous stores of intracellular Ca^{2+} (22,158). The other phosphodiesterase product, DAG, would effect the translocation of cytosolic protein kinase C to the plasma membrane, thus facilitating its activation. The DAG could also be phosphorylated by DAG kinase, thus producing phosphatidic acid, which also may be involved in intracellular Ca^{2+} mobilization. Alternatively, diglyceride lipase could hydrolyze the arachidonate esterified in the 2 position of DAG, and arachidonate release could occur as a result of phosphatidic-acid-specific phospholipase A_2 acting on the phosphatidic acid produced in the PI cycle. The released arachidonic acid could then be metabolized through the cyclooxygenase and/or lipoxygenase pathways or stimulate the production of cyclic GMP by activation of guanylate cyclase. In view of the preceding, the release of these second messengers derived directly or indirectly from the autacoid-receptor GTP-binding-protein-coupled activation of PI-PLC can account for many aspects of inflammatory cell activation.

PMN Stimulation

As previously discussed, extracellular Ca^{2+} is either mandatory for (rabbit PMN), or enhances (human PMN), most (but not all) AGEPC-induced PMN responses. In both rabbit and human PMN, AGEPC (0.01–100 nM) mobilizes intracellular membrane-associated Ca^{2+} stores within seconds, as indicated by the rapid decrease in fluorescence of the preloaded chlortetracycline (CTC) Ca^{2+} chelate probe (110,143). Other fluorescent Ca^{2+} probes (quin-2 and fura-2) also indicate significant increases in $[Ca^{2+}]_i$ in AGEPC-stimulated rabbit (142,143) and human PMN (110,213) responses, which are maximal within 20 to 30 sec. Because increases in the quin-2 signals are significantly reduced when PMN are stimulated with AGEPC in the absence of extracellular Ca^{2+}, most of the AGEPC-induced increase in $[Ca^{2+}]_i$ is due to the influx of extracellular Ca^{2+}, particularly at higher AGEPC concentrations (>1 nM).

Current evidence suggests that both PI-PLC-dependent and -independent mechanisms are operative in the mobilization of Ca^{2+} in AGEPC-stimulated PMN. First, AGEPC rapidly induces transient, but significant, decreases in PIP_2 in both human and rabbit PMN (110,142,143); in the rabbit PMN, decreases in phosphatidylinositol 4-monophosphate (PIP) and increases in phosphatidic acid also occur (143). Second, pretreatment with pertussis toxin obliterates AGEPC-induced PIP_2 turnover (143) and mobilization of intracellular Ca^{2+} stores in both human and rabbit PMN (110,143). In human PMN, the influx of extracellular Ca^{2+} is also significantly reduced but not abrogated by pertussis toxin (110). In contrast, pertussis toxin does not affect AGEPC-induced influx of extracellular Ca^{2+} in rabbit PMN (143). Finally, pretreatment in both rabbit and human PMN with the co-carcinogen phorbol myristate acetate (PMA) abrogates subsequent AGEPC-induced increases in $[Ca^{2+}]_i$ and lysosomal enzyme secretion in rabbit and human PMN (110,142). Although not yet established, this PMA effect could be due to the activation of protein kinase C, which subsequently phosphorylates and inactivates the α subunit of G_i-coupled adenylate cyclase and/or PI-PLC-coupled receptors (101,125). Regarding the former possibility, elevations in platelet cAMP have been shown to abrogate both Ca^{2+} mobilization and PIP_2 turnover (176). Further, pretreatment of rabbit PMN with cholera toxin, which activates G_s, significantly reduces AGEPC-induced lysosomal enzyme secretion (143). Direct activation of adenylate cyclase by the diterpene forskolin, in the presence of the phosphodiesterase inhibitor, 3-isobutyl-1-methylxanthine (IMBX), significantly inhibits AGEPC-induced lysosomal enzyme secretion from human PMN, as does PGE_1-receptor G_s-coupled activation of adenylate cyclase (147).

In view of the above, it would appear that AGEPC mobilizes increases in $[Ca^{2+}]_i$ through pertussis toxin-insensitive PI-PLC-independent mechanisms as well as through pertussis toxin-sensitive PI-PLC-dependent ones, thus suggesting the existence of at least two PAF receptors (110,143,148). The first receptor is associated with an apparent preexisting calcium channel and is not linked to a G_i-like GTP-binding protein because it is resistant to pertussis toxin. The second receptor is pertussis toxin-sensitive and is therefore coupled to a G_i-like GTP-binding protein. AGEPC occupancy of the latter receptor initiates signal transduction, causing rapid PIP_2 turnover and increases in $[Ca^{2+}]_i$ from intracellular Ca^{2+} stores, with subsequent enhancement in Na^+/H^+-antiport transient cell depolarization, increases in cytoskeletal actin, and secretion of N-acetyl β-glucosaminidase in the rabbit PMN (142,143). An analogous pertussis toxin-sensitive AGEPC receptor in the human PMN similarly modulates (a) PIP_2 turnover and initial mobilization of intracellular Ca^{2+} stores, (b) a major portion of extracellular Ca^{2+} influx, (c) production of O_2^-, secretion of lysozyme, and (d) PMN aggregation and chemotaxis (110,111). Further evidence that this AGEPC receptor is linked to a GTP-binding protein, other than its inactivation by pertussis toxin, derives from recent observations that GTP, GDP, and their analogs decrease the binding affinity of AGEPC for its receptor on isolated human PMN membranes (145). The pertussis toxin-sensitive AGEPC receptor in human PMN probably is not coupled to G_i, since even high (1 μM) concentrations of AGEPC only slightly enhance the stimulation of PGE_1-G_s-coupled cAMP production (110); this small enhancement, however, most likely is additive, since AGEPC-induced cAMP production occurs secondary to the synthesis of LTB_4 (69,87). These observations support the existence of a G_i-like GTP-binding protein that is coupled to the AGEPC receptor(s) involved in signal transduction as well as activation of PI-PLC and Ca^{2+} mobilization. In this regard, the FMLP, LTB_4, and C5a receptors on human PMN are also likely linked to a similar GTP-binding protein.

In summary, the mechanisms modulating AGEPC-induced responses in rabbit and human PMN may not be identical. In the rabbit PMN, extracellular Ca^{2+} is a mandatory requirement for lysosomal enzyme secretion in response to AGEPC but not to other secretagogues (13,14,137,142,143). Thus, in the rabbit PMN, it is likely that both the pertussis toxin-insensitive and pertussis toxin-sensitive AGEPC receptors must be occupied to effect lysosomal enzyme secretion; the latter receptor induces Ca^{2+} influx, whereas the former activates PI-PLC, thus providing second messengers. In contrast, because extracellular Ca^{2+} only slightly enhances AGEPC-induced lysosomal enzyme secretion in human PMN (see above), AGEPC occupancy only of the pertussis toxin-sensitive G_i-like receptor is required to initiate stimulus secretion coupling.

Platelet Stimulation

The mechanisms modulating AGEPC-induced platelet activation are, in many ways, similar in nature to PMN activation; however, as with the PMN, there are many unanswered questions requiring further study (cf. ref. 174). Like other platelet stimuli (i.e., thrombin) (178), AGEPC induces an immediate increase in $[Ca^{2+}]_i$ as a result of both mobilization of intracellular stores and a rapid influx of extracellular Ca^{2+}, the latter accounting for the majority of the increases in $[Ca^{2+}]_i$ (71). Concomitantly, there is a rapid turnover of PIP_2, with the production of DAG, IP_3, and phosphatidic acid (26,112). These events are associated with an increase in fibrinogen receptors, platelet aggregation, secretion of dense body and α-granule contents, and the production of TxB_2.

The first functional response of platelets after stimulation with AGEPC and other agonists is an almost instantaneous shape change that is independent of extracellular Ca^{2+}. AGEPC-induced shape change in washed human platelets is correlated with the production of phosphatidic acid and the phosphorylation of a 40,000-molecular-weight protein (112); while these responses are independent of arachidonic acid release and metabolism, they are inhibited by prostacyclin, presumably through elevations of cAMP. Thus, AGEPC-induced platelet shape change likely involves the activation of PI-PLC, with the production of DAG; however, these events (which are inhibited by cAMP), in the absence of extracellular Ca^{2+}, do not effect subsequent platelet aggregation and the release reaction.

Although the precise mechanisms modulating AGEPC-induced platelet aggregation and secretion remain to be clearly established, both of these functional platelet responses are highly dependent upon the influx of extracellular Ca^{2+} (106,134). In the absence of extracellular Ca^{2+}, AGEPC induces only a platelet shape change, with aggregatory and secretory responses being virtually obliterated. In the presence of extracellular Ca^{2+}, AGEPC induces almost an instantaneous increase in quin-2 fluorescence; however, in the absence of extracellular Ca^{2+}, the quin-2 signals are significantly suppressed but not abrogated (71,174). Thus, like the PMN, most of the AGEPC-induced increases in $[Ca^{2+}]_i$ in the platelet are due to an influx of extracellular Ca^{2+} through the opening of a voltage-independent Ca^{2+} channel (175). The opening of this Ca^{2+} channel by AGEPC is transient and apparently closes within 3 to 5 min (71,206). Furthermore, this Ca^{2+} channel cannot reopen after a second addition of AGEPC 2 to 3 min later, although stimulation of these same platelets with thrombin results in increases in quin-2 fluorescence (71). Since both platelet aggregation and secretion are dependent upon the influx of extracellular Ca^{2+}, the preceding observations may, in part, explain the mechanisms of specific AGEPC-induced desensitization (206).

Increasing evidence has suggested that the AGEPC receptor on platelets is also coupled to a G_i-like GTP-binding protein. Thus, AGEPC significantly reduces PGE_1-G_s-coupled activation of adenylate cyclase in rabbit platelets (81). AGEPC-induced inhibition of adenylate cyclase is not due to the secondary effects of ADP or TxA_2, since neither CPCK nor indomethacin alter this inhibitory response. In contrast, AGEPC does not affect G_i-coupled inhibition of adenylate cyclase in intact human platelets; however, AGEPC can modulate inhibition of adenylate cyclase in disrupted human platelet particulate fractions, especially in the presence of Na^+ and GTP (82,216). The reason for these apparent disparate results between intact and disrupted platelets is currently not known. Further, permeabilized human platelets equilibrated with Ca^{2+} and GTP at 0°C subsequently release $[^3H]$serotonin when incubated at 25°C. Notably, when AGEPC is added to these equilibrated cells, a marked synergistic release of $[^3H]$serotonin occurs in concert with an enhanced production of DAG (82). Taken together, these data suggest that AGEPC-induces a G_i-like coupled receptor activation of PI-PLC and a platelet-release reaction, even at ambient, 0.1 to 1.0 μM, $[Ca^{2+}]_i$. Further, AGEPC also stimulates GTPase activity in human platelets and platelet membranes, an activity that is not affected by cholera toxin and only slightly reduced by pertussis toxin, demonstrating that the AGEPC receptor is linked to a GTP-binding protein other than G_s or G_i (88,89).

INFLAMMATORY EFFECTS OF AGEPC *IN VIVO*

Assignment of a biologically important modulatory role for a putative, inflammatory autacoid requires documentation of *in vivo* phlogistic activities utilizing physiologically relevant concentrations of the mediator in question. Indeed, under *in vitro* conditions, some of the intrinsic agonist actions of an autacoid may be overestimated because of the lack of naturally occurring inhibitors and/or autacoid degradation processes. For example, AGEPC has far more potent actions in stimulating washed platelets as opposed to platelets in plasma. Two explanations could account for this disparate platelet reactivity. First, plasma contains acetylhydrolase, which rapidly deacetylates AGEPC to the biologically inactive product lyso-GEPC (see above). Second, plasma albumin significantly impairs AGEPC-induced platelet and PMN stimulation (124); this effect most likely is due to the ability of albumin to bind AGEPC, thereby preventing its interaction with target cell receptor(s). In contrast to possible overestimation of biological activity *in vitro,* the phlogistic potencies of a given autacoid could also be underestimated if important or essential synergistic interactions with other autacoids *in vivo* were precluded (see below). Thus, definition of the consequences of *in vivo* administration of putative autacoids is essential in the consideration of their possible role in tissue injury or disease.

Relative to the above, it is of paramount importance to ascertain what constitutes a physiologically relevant concentration of an autacoid when objectively appraising its *in vivo* (patho)biological potential(s). Presently, little information is available to accurately estimate how much, if any, PAF is generated during inflammatory events. As an exception to this general conclusion, the peak levels of PAF released intravascularly during the extreme biological events associated with systemic, IgE-mediated allergic reactions in the rabbit (166) have been calculated to be equivalent to a fluid-phase concentration of 10 nM C16:0-AGEPC (10 pmole/ml or 5 ng/ml). Interestingly, this concentration also approximates the amounts of PAF released from optimally stimulated human PMN *in vitro* (122,123). Taken together, these observations suggest that fluid-phase concentrations of PAF released during various other settings of inflammation will be well below the CMC of the autacoid (i.e., <1 μM C16:0-AGEPC).

It may appear that the terms PAF and AGEPC have been utilized interchangeably here; however, they have not. Only one of the PAFs synthesized by activated inflammatory cells is C16:0-AGEPC (see above), and although this phospholipid appears to be the most biologically potent member of the PAF autacoid family, many other PAF molecules are also synthesized and released by these same cells. Nevertheless, physiologic and phlogistic actions of "PAF" have been derived from studies utilizing only C16:0- and/or C18:0-AGEPC. In view of the above, the ultimate (patho)biological potentials of the multiple PAFs that are synthesized and released *in situ* during inflammatory reactions remain to be clearly established.

AGEPC-Induced Intravascular Alterations

A variety of acute intravascular events occur following the intravenous infusion of C16:0-AGEPC. In brief, and consistent with its potent *in vitro* effects on platelets, immediately after the intravenous infusion, AGEPC initiates intravascular platelet aggregation, with subsequent thrombocytopenia in rabbits, guinea pigs, dogs, pigs, hamsters, and baboons (23,28,133,135,208). During their absence from the circulation, platelets are sequestered in the pulmonary microvasculature (131,133). Of importance in this regard, AGEPC dose-dependent platelet activation accompanies these acute events, as estimated by the intravascular accumulation of platelet factor 4 (PF4) (133); while intravascular levels of TxB$_2$ are also increased in parallel with PF4, the platelet origin of this arachidonate metabolite remains to be documented (132). Concomitant with these platelet alterations, significant neutropenia and basopenia also occur (133,135). Despite the extent of these profound intravascular alterations following AGEPC infusion, in nonlethal reactions most parameters rapidly reverse and return to preinfusion levels within 60 min.

Indeed, the platelets that return to the circulation are the same cells that were sequestered in the pulmonary microvasculature (133).

AGEPC-Induced Vascular Permeability

The intracutaneous administration of AGEPC results in dramatic and potent inflammatory actions. Shortly after the structural identification and synthesis of AGEPC, profound vasoactive activity in human skin induced by this acetylated alkyl phosphoglyceride was reported (169). Immediately after the intracutaneous administration of as little as 0.1 pmole of AGEPC dissolved in pyrogen-free saline containing human albumin, blanching of the skin was noted, indicative of vasoconstriction; pain and pruritis often were experienced by the volunteers. This was followed by the development of erythema and edema, which maximized within 10 to 15 min; these skin reactions subsided within 60 min, and no late-phase skin reactions were noted. The erythema and pruritis were subsequently reported to be histamine-dependent (60). Similar AGEPC-induced vasoactivity occurs in rabbits, rats, guinea pigs, hamsters, and nonhuman primates (7,9,28,91,92,93,165). In the guinea pig, the potency of AGEPC is similar to that reported in humans, i.e., 0.1 pmole; rats and rabbits require 10 times this amount to consistently induce increases in vascular permeability (91,92). Nevertheless, in all species tested, AGEPC (on a molar basis) appears to be from 1,000 to 10,000 times more potent than histamine.

With respect to the mechanisms of its vasoactivity, AGEPC induces contraction of endothelial cells in postcapillary venules similar to other vasoactive autacoids (91). AGEPC-induced vasoactivity appears to be platelet-independent, since rat platelets are unresponsive to AGEPC (177). In rats, rabbits, and hamsters, depletion of circulating PMN does not alter the vasoactive potency of AGEPC (28,91); these observations are of importance because AGEPC initiates leukocyte infiltrates after incutaneous administration (see following). In rabbits, rats, and humans, the vasoactive properties of AGEPC are not effected by H$_1$ antagonists or indomethacin, thereby ruling out the possible involvement of either histamine or cyclooxygenase-derived arachidonate products (7,92,93).

AGEPC-induced increased vascular permeability is of short duration, i.e., 15 to 30 min. However, when greater amounts of AGEPC are employed (100–200 pmole), the vasoactive effects of AGEPC are prolonged to 60 to 80 min in guinea pigs and rabbits (92); also, in humans, a late-phase reaction, consisting of erythema and hyperalgesia, is noted (8,9). Some reservation should be made regarding the utilization of high concentrations of AGEPC, i.e., 100 pmole/0.1 ml or greater. These concentrations approach or exceed the CMC of AGEPC, and thus its altered physical state could effect adverse, possibly detergent-induced, responses. Indeed, when 100 pmole of AGEPC is injected intracutaneously into guinea pigs, hemorrhagic skin lesions develop within 60 min (92). Similarly, severe necrotizing vasculitis occurs after the intracutaneous injection of 800 pmole of AGEPC into humans (8). Finally, AGEPC-induced increases in vascular permeability are not limited to the cutaneous microcirculation, since intraarticular injection of AGEPC induces rat paw edema (66,98). Moreover, in the guinea pig, rat, dog, and nonhuman primate, the intravascular administration of AGEPC induces hemoconcentration and generalized vascular leakage of plasma proteins (182).

AGEPC-Induced Leukocyte Infiltration

In addition to its potent cutaneous vasoactive activity, the intracutaneous administration of as little as 5 to 50 pmole of AGEPC into rabbits and rats induces PMN margination and plugging within venules within 5 to 15 min (90,91). At this time, PMN are commonly found under the vascular endothelium and in the vascular adventitia. Perivascular PMN infiltration subsequently develops, with maximal accumulation occurring at 3 hr (90). PMN accumulation occurs predominantly in venules in the deep dermis near the panniculus carnosus, most likely in the deep portion of the cutaneous venous plexus. Interestingly, this is the same anatomic location where AGEPC also induces vascular labeling with colloidal carbon, which demarcates both the endothelial cell contraction in postcapillary venules and the location of increased vascular permeability (91). In humans, the intracutaneous administration of AGEPC in a micellar form (200 pmole) induces a biphasic inflammatory response (8). The perivascular infiltrate at 4 and 12 hr consists principally of PMN, followed subsequently at 24 hr by lymphocyte and mononuclear infiltration. Severe vasculitis characterized by overt vessel destruction, endothelial swelling, and perivascular infiltration of PMN, mononuclear cells, and eosinophils occurs within 32 hr after the intracutaneous injection of 800 pmole of AGEPC. Leukocyte accumulation also occurs in normal human subjects within 24 hr after intracutaneous AGEPC administration; 70% to 80% of the cells recovered in Rebuck skin windows are PMN, and the remainder are mononuclear cells (86).

Pulmonary leukocytic infiltrates also occur after the intravenous or transtracheal administration of AGEPC into rabbits and dogs (46,118,131). In the rabbit, the intravenous infusion of AGEPC (0.5 μg/kg) induces profound platelet and PMN accumulation in the pulmonary circulation within 30 sec (131). Five minutes after AGEPC

infusion, pulmonary platelet aggregates are no longer present, although the pulmonary PMN sequestration persists; at this time, large mononuclear cells, as well as focal vascular endothelial cell damage, are widespread throughout the pulmonary microvasculature. These latter changes, together with continued PMN sequestration, persist for up to 60 min, and discrete areas of interstitial hemorrhage develop around small and medium-sized pulmonary arteries (130,131). Interestingly, within 6 hr after AGEPC infusion, eosinophils accumulate subendothelially in medium-sized pulmonary arteries in rabbits. Subsequently, focal accumulation of these cells in the vascular media and adventitia occurs, an infiltration that is maximal at 24 to 48 hr (130).

PAF SYNERGISM WITH OTHER AUTACOIDS

A very important and biologically relevant synergism exists between AGEPC and other inflammatory autacoids, including certain lipoxygenase and cyclooxygenase products of arachidonate metabolism. By design and implication in most *in vitro* experiments, a single mediator concept of inflammatory cell activation has emerged; however, during inflammatory responses *in vivo*, several classes of inflammatory mediators are simultaneously produced and may collectively initiate either additive or synergistic effects. Indeed, while the singular potency of AGEPC in some inflammatomimetic actions could well be questioned, the synergistic interactions of AGEPC and other autacoids more clearly establish an *in vivo* relevance and physiological import for AGEPC in modulating the inflammatory process, as follows.

Several platelet agonists at subthreshold concentrations have been shown to significantly enhance the release reaction from, and/or the aggregation of, human platelets in response to subsequent suboptimal concentrations of AGEPC. These agents include ADP, arachidonic acid, epinephrine, collagen, calcium ionophore A23187, thrombin, and aggregated human IgG (4,162,200,204, 207). With the exception of aggregated IgG (204), reverse synergism is operative in the human platelet, i.e., subthreshold concentrations of AGEPC augment platelet responses to suboptimal concentrations of the other agonists and vice versa. In contrast, one-way synergism is operative in the case of aggregated IgG, which potentiates AGEPC-induced platelet aggregation (but not secretion), whereas AGEPC does not potentiate platelet stimulation by aggregated IgG (204). The synergistic priming of platelets for subsequent AGEPC-induced enhanced stimulation lasts for minutes; in contrast, AGEPC-induced synergistic priming is transient, lasting less than 60 sec.

The mechanisms underlying the synergism between

platelet agonists remain to be clearly established. Utilizing citrated human platelet-rich plasma, the synergism between AGEPC and other platelet agonists is significantly reduced or abrogated by cyclooxygenase blockade and/or ATP and ADP scavengers (200). In contrast, with washed human platelets in the presence of extracellular Ca^{2+}, this synergism occurs independently of arachidonate metabolism or ADP release (207). In the case with aggregated IgG, AGEPC synergism occurs via an apparent cyclooxygenase-dependent release of ADP (204). Further, aggregated IgG-augmented AGEPC-induced platelet aggregation is not due to enhanced AGEPC receptor expression. Apparent discrepancies in the mechanisms modulating platelet autacoid synergism may, in part, be explained by both the different methods of platelet preparation and the concentrations of AGEPC utilized. Nevertheless, that AGEPC synergizes with other platelet agonists which are often released prior to, or simultaneously with, AGEPC strengthens the (patho)biological significance of this phospholipid, since such synergistic events could potentiate platelet activation *in vivo*.

Profound synergism between AGEPC and other autacoids also potentiate leukocyte activation (149,156). For example, although 5-L-HETE and its racemate, 5-*rac*-HPETE, alone induce little or no secretory responses in human PMN, they significantly augment (up to 30–100-fold) AGEPC-induced lysosomal enzyme secretion (153). Indeed, and of *in vivo* relevance, 5-L-HETE synergizes with AGEPC in the absence of cytochalasin B. Interestingly, this synergistic relationship between 5-L-HETE and AGEPC would appear to be unique, since this 5-lipoxygenase product does not act synergistically with other inflammatory autacoids (including FMLP or the complement fragment, C5a) and only modestly synergizes with LTB_4. In addition, AGEPC synergizes with 5-L-HETE, whereas it does not synergize with either 15-L-HETE or LTB_4 in modulating the PMN secretory process (156).

As previously discussed, relatively high concentrations of AGEPC are required to induce significant O_2^- production in the PMN. However, through its synergistic interaction with other inflammatory autacoids, AGEPC more effectively initiates the respiratory burst in human PMN. For example, prior or simultaneous exposure of human PMN to AGEPC (which by itself does not induce O_2^- production) significantly enhances both the rate and total production of O_2^- induced by adding FMLP or PMA to human PMN (62,99). Moreover, although in the absence of extracellular Ca^{2+} the amounts of O_2^- produced by the FMLP-stimulated human PMN are reduced, the synergistic action of AGEPC still augments this response (99). Thus, it is tempting to speculate that this priming effect of very low concentrations of AGEPC to augment O_2^- production might be operative through its ability to rap-

idly mobilize intracellular Ca^{2+} stores. Of interest, reverse synergism between FMLP and AGEPC also occurs, since pretreatment of the human PMN with FMLP allows the subsequent expression of O_2^- production in response to AGEPC (99). Although LTB_4 can initiate O_2^- production and is also synergistic during FMLP-induced O_2^- generation by human PMN, it is postulated that AGEPC-synergized, FMLP-induced O_2^- production is likely not dependent upon AGEPC-induced LTB_4 production, i.e., ETYA has no effect on AGEPC-enhanced production of O_2^-, either by FMLP- or PMA-stimulated human PMN (99). Thus, unlike other human PMN responses to AGEPC, both extracellular Ca^{2+} and stimulation of the lipoxygenase pathway of arachidonate metabolism are not required for its priming or synergistic effects in up-regulating O_2^- production induced by other inflammatory autacoids. Again, it is interesting to note that the synergizing actions of AGEPC appear to be somewhat stimulus-specific, since little, if any, AGEPC-induced augmentation in O_2^- production occurs in PMN stimulated with LTB_4 or opsonized zymosan (53,99).

As mentioned previously, one of the potent phlogistic properties of AGEPC is its ability to increase vascular permeability. Indeed, on a molar basis, AGEPC is two to four orders of magnitude more potent than any other currently known vasoactive autacoid. This (patho)physiologic action of AGEPC takes on even greater significance in view of its synergism with other autacoids. It is well known that autacoids that increase blood flow in the microcirculation significantly enhance vascular permeability in response to other vasoactive mediators that initiate contraction of endothelial cells in postcapillary venules. Thus, AGEPC potency for increasing vascular permeability is significantly enhanced by certain vasodilatory prostaglandins (e.g., PGE_1 and PGE_2) and by the vasodilatory calcitonin gene-related peptide, which by themselves do not increase vascular permeability (9,33,93). In addition, under certain circumstances, PGE_2 allows expression of AGEPC vasoactivity, which normally is absent. Thus, whereas AGEPC has potent vasoactive properties in the adult, 3-month-old rabbit, it does not induce increases in vascular permeability in perinatal, 3- and 4-week-old rabbits (5). Although it was initially felt that postcapillary endothelial cells in the 4-week-old rabbits lacked specific PAF receptors, co-injection of PGE_2 with AGEPC allows the full expression of its vasoactive activity. Further, AGEPC-induced intracutaneous PMN accumulation is also significantly reduced in the 4-week-old rabbit (5). Nevertheless, this also is not due to a lack of PAF receptors on the PMN, since co-injection of PGE_2 with AGEPC restores the PMN infiltrative response to levels comparable to the adult animal. Whether or not this synergism of PGE_2 and AGEPC in modulating leukocyte infiltration is indirect, through the ability of the vasodilatory prostaglandin to increase blood flow (hence microcirculation surface area) or through its ability to augment AGEPC-induced increases in vascular permeability, is currently not known.

Other, as-yet unexplained, enhanced leukocyte responses to AGEPC also might involve synergistic interactions with various autacoids. For example, the AGEPC-induced production of O_2^- is virtually absent in resident, guinea-pig peritoneal macrophages; however, significant AGEPC-induced O_2^- production occurs in *Corynebacterium-parvum*-elicited peritoneal macrophages (79,80). Whether the recruitment of monocyte/macrophages into the peritoneal cavity, presumably by the generation of a chemotactic factor(s), primes these cells for enhanced O_2^- production by AGEPC is unclear but is suggested. Perhaps analogously, monocytes from normal human subjects exhibit poor chemotactic responses to AGEPC *in vitro,* but the monocytes from patients with certain active dermatoses, i.e., psoriasis and atopic eczema, express significantly greater chemotactic responses toward AGEPC. Of interest, following treatment and disease remission, the monocyte chemotactic responses to AGEPC return to the levels of normal subjects (49). Finally, whereas normal and atopic, presumably asthmatic, subjects develop comparable wheal and flare reactions after intradermal AGEPC injection, only the atopic patients develop subsequent eosinophil accumulation in Rebuck skin windows 24 hr later (86). Thus, underlying inflammatory disease processes may result in leukocyte priming by certain inflammatory autacoids, thereby expressing enhanced responsiveness to other autacoids such as AGEPC.

OTHER AGEPC-INDUCED (PATHO)PHYSIOLOGIC EFFECTS

As summarized above, AGEPC initiates several phlogistic actions *in vitro* and *in vivo,* suggesting that similar effects may contribute to acute and chronic inflammatory reactions in humans. In addition to this proinflammatory potential, AGEPC also promotes a variety of other physiologic actions which, while similarly profound, are less directly related to inflammatory reactions per se (Fig. 6). The following is a brief description of other AGEPC-induced physiologic effects.

In vitro, AGEPC induces smooth muscle contraction, i.e., guinea-pig and rat ileal contraction (59,198). This activity is not affected by the presence of antagonists of

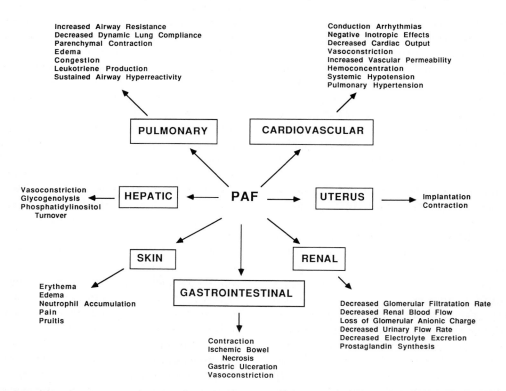

FIG. 6. (Patho)physiologic effects of AGEPC *in vivo.* Through its ability to contract smooth muscle and endothelial cells and to stimulate the release of other autacoids, AGEPC initiates a variety of physiologic responses, with their consequential beneficial or detrimental effects.

histamine, leukotrienes, and acetylcholine or by cyclooxygenase inhibition. Not unlike other cells and tissues, this AGEPC-induced response is specifically reduced by prior exposure to AGEPC (i.e., tachyphylaxis), suggesting the presence of AGEPC receptors on intestinal smooth muscle cells. In this regard, AGEPC promotes Na^+-dependent Ca^{2+} influx with concomitant polyphosphoinositide turnover in plasmalemmal vesicles isolated from the rat ileum (104). In addition, with cultured smooth muscle cells of vascular origin, AGEPC stimulates phospholipase A_2 and C and associated prostaglandin production as well as mobilizes intracellular Ca^{2+} (54,102). Because smooth muscle contraction plays an important role in cardiovascular and airway dynamics in allergy and inflammation, additional studies are required to assess the *in vivo* significance of AGEPC-induced smooth muscle contraction as it may relate to the pathogenesis of these disorders.

AGEPC also contracts isolated parenchymal strips of lung obtained from guinea pigs, rabbits, rats, and humans (39,197–199). Similar to the ileum, AGEPC-induced parenchymal lung contraction is unaffected by antihistamines or antagonists of arachidonate metabolites; further, AGEPC-specific tachyphylaxis also develops in parenchymal lung strips. Of interest, AGEPC-induced guinea-pig lung parenchymal contraction is blocked by parasympathetic inhibition with the neurotoxin, tetrodotoxin (199). This suggests that AGEPC stimulates neural pathways, resulting in neurotransmitter release and leading to subsequent smooth muscle contraction (199). Whether or not comparable AGEPC-induced contracting actions also develop *in vivo* remains to be established; however, profound pulmonary physiological alterations do occur following both intravascular and transtracheal AGEPC administration (see following).

The effects of AGEPC on isolated perfused lungs of rabbits, rats, and guinea pigs have been evaluated. Thus, AGEPC initiates increases in pulmonary airway pressures in concert with pulmonary hypertension and edema formation (40,63,77,85,119,212). In isolated rat lungs, which also develop tachyphylaxis to AGEPC, a bolus intra-arterial injection of AGEPC (1–5 μg in 0.1 ml) promotes leukotriene synthesis; interestingly, both pulmonary hypertension and edema are abrogated by inhibition of leukotriene production (212). Although AGEPC promotes leukotriene-dependent pulmonary hypertension in isolated perfused rat lungs, it (0.1–1.0 μg) also causes acute vasodilatation of preconstricted pulmonary vessels in this same model (63). Thus, AGEPC can promote opposite vascular effects under varying circumstances. Thromboxane A_2 generation also appears to play a role in all AGEPC-induced pulmonary alterations in isolated perfused lungs from guinea pigs (1 μg AGEPC) and rabbits (20 μg AGEPC); however, the platelet as a source of TxA_2

in these systems remains controversial (77,85). In summary, it is clear that, *in vitro*, AGEPC can promote substantial alterations in the lung, an important target organ in allergic and inflammatory diseases.

AGEPC also has potent negative inotropic effects in isolated perfused guinea-pig and rat hearts (17,117,196). In brief, AGEPC (0.01–1,000 pmole) induces dose-related decreases in left ventricular contractile force and coronary flow and impairs atrioventricular conduction in the guinea pig (17,103,117). These potent AGEPC-induced cardiac alterations are not affected by the presence of leukotriene antagonists or cyclooxygenase inhibitors (117). In contrast, inhibition of leukotriene production markedly attenuates AGEPC-induced coronary flow reduction in rat hearts (196). Further, the isolated perfused rabbit heart does not develop negative inotropic responses when AGEPC is administered unless the hearts are perfused with blood (103). Thus, species variation in cardiac responsiveness to AGEPC (or secondary mediators generated following its administration) exists *in vitro*.

Negative inotropic effects also develop in the electrically paced left atrium and right ventricular papillary muscle from the guinea pig (117). In contrast and of interest, AGEPC initiates a transient, positive inotropic effect in preparations of human papillary muscles, a response that is blocked by propranolol; this initial response is followed by a prolonged negative inotropism, which is significantly reduced by indomethacin (2). Because AGEPC restores electrical responses in partially depolarized guinea-pig papillary muscles (an effect inhibited by verapamil), AGEPC effects on this muscle are likely via Ca^{2+} influx across the membrane through enhancement of the slow inward current (201). In combination and because similar AGEPC-induced cardiovascular alterations develop *in vivo* (see following), the above suggests that PAF (AGEPC) may contribute to contractile failure, reduced coronary flow, or conduction arrhythmias that develop during cardiac anaphylaxis or myocardial inflammation.

The intravenous infusion of physiologically relevant amounts of AGEPC (i.e., <1 μg/kg) reproduces the entire physiologic and inflammatory sequelae of IgE-induced systemic anaphylaxis in the rabbit (72–74). In brief, within seconds of AGEPC infusion, significant increases in right ventricular and pulmonary artery pressures are followed by a biphasic development of profound systemic hypotension. In concert with the cardiovascular alterations, equally profound and reversible changes also occur in ventilation and lung mechanics (75,76). Initially, there are decreases in respiratory frequency, which often result in respiratory arrest; in nonlethal responses and with resumption of breathing, significant decreases in dynamic lung compliance and increases in total pulmonary resistance develop (76). These significant physiological events occur while intravascular platelets and leukocytes are sequestered in the pulmonary microvasculature (118,131). In the rabbit and guinea pig, AGEPC-induced lung mechanical changes appear to be platelet-dependent and prevented by antihistamines; in contrast, the cardiovascular responses are platelet-independent (74,75,209). Comparable, profound physiological events develop following the intravascular infusion of AGEPC into dogs (0.4–4.7 μg/kg), sheep (1 μg/kg), and guinea pigs (16–132 ng/kg) (23,36,58,103,209). In sheep, AGEPC-induced pulmonary vasoconstriction is mediated, in part, by cyclooxygenase metabolites (36). Further, the hemodynamic changes following AGEPC infusion in dogs are blocked by diethylcarbamazine (103).

The intracoronary infusion of AGEPC also promotes significant alterations in coronary functions in pigs and dogs (6,58,100). In the pig, intracoronary AGEPC (0.05–5 μg) stimulates an initial transient increase in coronary blood flow (within 8–12 sec), followed immediately (within 25–30 sec) by a decrease in this hemodynamic parameter; AGEPC-induced decreased coronary flow persists for approximately 60 sec and is attenuated by cyclooxygenase inhibition (58). In contrast to the pig, only increased coronary flow occurs following intracoronary AGEPC infusion into the dog (1.48 μg) (100). This coronary vascular response is platelet-dependent and appears to be the result of a platelet-derived factor that is released following AGEPC-induced platelet activation (100). In a stenosed canine coronary artery, however, the intracoronary infusion of AGEPC (5 μg/min) induces cyclic flow variations, i.e., spontaneous decreases in coronary blood flow interrupted by restorations of blood flow (6). In summary, the combined results of studies designed to evaluate cardiovascular and pulmonary alterations following the intravascular infusion of AGEPC indicate that this phospholipid either directly or indirectly initiates significant physiological responses which may be of import if comparable events occur in allergic or inflammatory responses in humans.

Similar to the bronchoconstriction that develops following the intravascular infusion of AGEPC, the transtracheal instillation of AGEPC in dogs, nonhuman primates, and humans also induces immediate bronchoconstriction (46,48,51,164). In baboons, AGEPC (60 μg/kg) initiates an immediate increase in airway resistance and heart rate, which are unaffected by aspirin but attenuated by albuterol (51). Interestingly, both thrombocytopenia and leukopenia develop in these animals. When rhesus monkeys are aerosol-challenged with AGEPC (10 μg/ml), similar airway responses are observed; of interest, the animals challenged with AGEPC subsequently display enhanced airway reactivity to other stimuli, i.e., LTD$_4$ (164). Similar bronchoconstriction and airway hyperresponsiveness follow AGEPC aerosolization (1 mg) in dogs;

this effect is maximal within 3 hr and sustained for at least 6 hr, although it is largely dependent upon thromboxane generation (46). Further, inhalation of AGEPC results in increased leukocyte (primarily PMN) recovery in pulmonary lavage specimens in dogs, an effect that is independent of thromboxane production (46). When inhaled by normal humans, AGEPC also causes dose-dependent (6.25–400 μg) bronchoconstriction and, of importance, sustained airway hyperreactivity (48). Tachyphylaxis to AGEPC-induced bronchoconstriction occurs rapidly in humans; in contrast, AGEPC-induced airway hyperresponsiveness is maximal for several days followed by a gradual return to normal within several weeks (48). Current studies are in progress to expand our understanding of this AGEPC bioactivity inasmuch as airway hyperreactivity is a characteristic abnormality in asthma.

Systemic AGEPC infusion into dogs also causes decreases in renal blood flow, glomerular filtration, and fluid and electrolyte excretion, which are likely a reflection of AGEPC-induced systemic conditions, i.e., profound hypotension (184). Further, the infusion of AGEPC directly into the renal artery of dogs results in similar renal alterations; indomethacin pretreatment increases these effects (183). Nevertheless, aortic infusion of AGEPC into rabbits (1.5 μg/kg) results in proteinuria and loss of glomerular anionic charge (41). *In vitro*, AGEPC stimulates prostaglandin production both in isolated kidneys and in cultured glomerular mesangial cells (185). Further, cultured rat mesangial cells undergo contraction when exposed to AGEPC (1 nM to 1 μM), an effect that is enhanced in the presence of indomethacin (185). Thus, a potential role for this autacoid in the pathophysiology of renal alterations is suggested.

CONCLUDING REMARKS: ROLE OF PAF AND DISEASE

The rapid advances in our understanding of the chemistry and biology of PAF, or, more appropriately, the family of acetylated phosphoglycerides, have provided the basis for speculation that these autacoids may participate in the etiology of various diseases (see Fig. 7). Indeed, the pioneering efforts to define the molecular/cellular mechanisms involved in the onset of antigen-induced systemic IgE anaphylaxis led to the biochemical and structural identification of this potent, unique phospholipid family. Recent and continuing investigations are directed toward defining the extent to which PAF may influence tissue injury during acute or chronic allergic and inflammatory conditions. To this end, several approaches have been undertaken. First, both *in vivo* and *in vitro* targets of PAF have been evaluated, and putative PAF receptors on var-

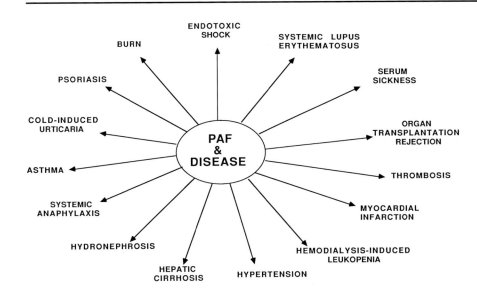

FIG. 7. PAF association to disease. Because of its potent phlogistic and physiologic actions and its isolation from various tissues and body fluids during pathologic processes, PAF has been implicated in the pathogenesis of human disease. Final documentation of its potential detrimental effects must await clear demonstration that specific PAF receptor antagonists and/or inhibition of PAF synthesis reduces or abrogates these pathologic conditions.

ious target cells have been described. Second, the isolation and characterization of PAF from diseased tissues have been initiated in an attempt to define a possible causative link between the presence of PAF and the initiation of tissue injury. And finally, several PAF antagonists have been produced and are widely available. This latter development is a logical extension of endeavors to probe the molecular mechanisms that account for PAFs' actions on target cells (94,182,211). Of even greater import, these PAF receptor antagonists are, and will continue to be, invaluable in studies designed to assess the potential contributions of PAF to the biological events leading to the development of various experimental models of disease (182). Hopefully, application of the combined results of these studies will be useful in defining a role and possible intervention or prevention of PAF-mediated effects that may contribute to tissue injury and disease in humans.

ACKNOWLEDGMENTS

The authors gratefully acknowledge the long-standing technical support from a cast of thousands, including Richard Castillo, Carol Hoppens, Cindy Lear, and Patricia Padilla. The preparation of this manuscript by Adelaida Garcia is also greatly appreciated. This work was supported, in part, by USPHS Grants HL-22555, HL-28724, and AI-21818 as well as by the American Heart Association, Texas Affiliate.

REFERENCES

1. Albert, D. H., and Snyder, F. (1983): Biosynthesis of 1-alkyl-2-acetyl-*sn*-glycero-3-phosphocholine by rat alveolar macrophages. Phospholipase A_2 and acetyltransferase activities during phagocytosis and ionophore stimulation. *J. Biol. Chem.*, 258:97–102.

2. Alloatti, G., Montrucchio, G., Mariano, F., Tetta, C., De Paulis, R., Morea, M., Emmanuelli, G., and Camussi, G. (1986): Effect of platelet-activating factor (PAF) on human cardiac muscle. *Int. Arch. Allergy Appl. Immunol.*, 79:108–112.

3. Alonso, F., Gil, M., Sanchez-Crespo, M., and Mato, J. (1982): Activation of 1-alkyl-2-lyso-glycero-3-phosphocholine: Acetyl-CoA transferase during phogocytosis in human polymorphonuclear leukocytes. *J. Biol. Chem.*, 257:3376–3378.

4. Altman, R., and Scazziota, A. (1986): Synergistic actions of paf-acether and sodium arachidonate in human platelet aggregation. 2. Unexpected results after aspirin intake. *Thromb. Res.*, 43:113–120.

5. Angle, M. J., McManus, L. M., and Pinckard, R. N. (1986): Age-dependent differential development of leukotactic and vasoactive responsiveness to acute inflammatory mediators. *Lab. Invest.*, 55:616–621.

6. Apprill, P., Schmitz, J. M., Campbell, W. B., Tilton, G., Ashton, J., Raheja, S., Buja, L. M., and Willerson, J. T. (1985): Cyclic blood flow variations induced by platelet-activating factor in stenosed canine coronary arteries despite inhibition of thromboxane synthetase, serotonin receptors, and α-adrenergic receptors. *Circulation*, 72:397–405.

7. Archer, C. B., MacDonald, D. M., Morley, J., Page, C. P., Paul, W., and Sanjar, S. (1985): Effects of serum albumin, indomethacin and histamine H_1-antagonists on PAF-acether-induced inflammatory responses in the skin of experimental animals and man. *Br. J. Pharmacol.*, 85:109–113.

8. Archer, C. B., Page, C. P., Morley, J., and MacDonald, D. M. (1985): Accumulation of inflammatory cells in response to intracutaneous platelet activating factor (PAF-acether) in man. *Br. J. Dermatol.*, 112:285–290.

9. Archer, C. B., Page, C. P., Paul, W., Morley, J., and MacDonald, D. M. (1984): Inflammatory characteristics of platelet activating factor (PAF-acether) in human skin. *Br. J. Dermatol.*, 110:45–50.

10. Arnoux, B., Duval, B., and Benveniste, J. (1980): Release of platelet-activating factor (PAF-acether) from alveolar macrophages by the calcium ionophore A23187 and phagocytosis. *Eur. J. Clin. Invest.*, 10:437–441.

11. Bachelet, M., Masliah, J., Vargaftig, B. B., Bereziat, G., and Colard, O. (1986): Changes induced by PAF-acether in diacyl and ether phospholipids from guinea-pig alveolar macrophages. *Biochim. Biophys. Acta*, 878:177–183.

12. Baggiolini, M., and Dewald, B. (1986): Stimulus amplification by PAF and LTB_4 in human neutrophils. *Pharmacol. Res. Commun.*, 18:51–59.

13. Becker, E. L., Kermode, J. C., Naccache, P. H., Yassin, R., Marsh,

M. L., Munoz, J. J., and Sha'afi, R. I. (1985): The inhibition of neutrophil granule enzyme secretion and chemotaxis by pertussis toxin. *J. Cell Biol.*, 100:1641–1646.

14. Becker, E. L., Kermode, J. C., Naccache, P. H., Yassin, R., Munoz, J. J., Marsh, M. L., Huang C., and Sha'afi, R. (1986): Pertussis toxin as a probe of neutrophil activation. *Fed. Proc.*, 45:2151–2155.
15. Benveniste, J., and Pretolani, M. (1986): PAF-acether (platelet-activating factor): Its role in inflammation. *Adv. Inflam. Res.*, 10:7–19.
16. Benveniste, J., and Vargaftig, B. B. (1983): Platelet-activating factor: An ether lipid with biological activity. In: *Ether Lipids,* edited by H. D. Mangold and F. Paltauf, pp. 355–376. Academic Press, New York.
17. Benveniste, J., Boullet, C., Brink, C., and Labat, C. (1983): The actions of PAF-acether (platelet-activating factor) on guinea-pig isolated heart preparations. *Br. J. Pharmacol.*, 80:81–83.
18. Benveniste, J., Henson, P. M., and Cochrane, C. G. (1972): Leukocyte-dependent histamine release from rabbit platelets, The role of IgE, basophils, and a platelet activating factor. *J. Exp. Med.*, 136:1356–1377.
19. Benveniste, J., Le Couedic, J. P., Polonsky, J., and Tence, M. (1977): Structural analysis of purified platelet-activating factor by lipases. *Nature,* 269:170–171.
20. Benveniste, J., Roubin, R., Chignard, M., Jouvin-Marche, E., and LeCouedic J.-P. (1982): Release of platelet-activating factor (PAF-acether) and 2-lyso PAF-acether from three cell types. *Agents Actions,* 12:711–713.
21. Benveniste, J., Tence, M., Varenne, P., Bidault, J., Boullet, C., and Polonsky J. (1979): Semi-synthèse et structure proposée du facteur activant les plaquettes (P.A.F.): PAF-acether, un alkyl ether analogue de la lysophosphatidylcholine. *C. R. Acad. Sci. (Paris),* 289:1037–1040.
22. Berridge, M. J. (1984): Inositol trisphosphate and diacylglycerol as second messengers. *Biochem. J.,* 220:345–360.
23. Bessin, P., Bonnet, J., Apffel, D., Soulard, C., Desgroux, L., Pelas, I., and Benveniste, J. (1983): Acute circulatory collapse caused by platelet-activating factor (PAF-acether) in dogs. *Eur. J. Pharmacol.,* 86:403–413.
24. Betz, S. J., and Henson, P. M. (1980): Production and release of platelet-activating factor (PAF); dissociation from degranulation and superoxide production in the human neutrophil. *J. Immunol.,* 125:2756–2763.
25. Betz, S. J., Lotner, G. Z., and Henson, P. M. (1980): Generation and release of platelet-activating factor (PAF) from enriched preparations of rabbit basophils; failure of human basophils to release PAF. *J. Immunol.,* 125:2749–2755.
26. Billah, M. M., and Lapetina, E. G. (1983): Platelet-activating factor stimulates metabolism of phosphoinositides in horse platelets: Possible relationship to Ca^{++} mobilization during stimulation. *Proc. Natl. Acad. Sci. USA,* 80:965–968.
27. Billah, M. M., Bryant, R. W., and Siegel, M. I. (1985): Lipoxygenase products of arachidonic acid modulate biosynthesis of platelet-activating factor (1-*O*-alkyl-2-acetyl-*sn*-glycero-3-phosphocholine) by human neutrophils via phospholipase A$_2$. *J. Biol. Chem.,* 260:6899–6906.
28. Bjork, J., and Smedegard, G. (1983): Acute microvascular effects of PAF-acether, as studied by intravital microscopy. *Eur. J. Pharmacol.,* 96:87–94.
29. Blank, M. L., Cress, E. A., and Snyder, F. (1984): A new class of antihypertensive neutral lipids: 1-Alkyl-2-acetyl-*sn*-glycerols. *Biochem. Biophys. Res. Commun.,* 118:344–350.
30. Blank, M. L., Cress, E. A., Lee, T.-C., Malone, B., Surles, J. R., Piantadosi, C., Hajdu, M., and Snyder, F. (1982): Structural features of platelet activating factor (1-alkyl-2-acetyl-*sn*-glycero-3-phosphocholine) required for hypotensive and platelet serotonin responses. *Res. Commun. Chem. Pathol. Pharmacol.,* 38:3–20.
31. Blank, M. L., Lee, T.-C., Fitzgerald, V., and Snyder, F. (1981): A specific acetylhydrolase for 1-alkyl-2-acetyl-*sn*-glycero-3-phosphocholine (a hypotensive and platelet-activating lipid). *J. Biol. Chem.,* 256:175–178.

32. Blank, M. L., Snyder, F., Byers, L. W., Brooks, B., Muirhead, E. E. (1979): Antihypertensive activity of an alkyl ether analogue of phosphatidylcholine. *Biochem. Biophys. Res. Commun.,* 90:1194–1200.
33. Brain, S. D., and Williams, T. J. (1985): Inflammatory oedema induced by synergism between calcitonin gene-related peptide (CGRP) and mediators of increased vascular permeability. *Br. J. Pharmacol.,* 86:855–860.
34. Brock, T. A., and Gimbrone, M. A., Jr. (1986): Platelet activating factor alters calcium homeostasis in cultured vascular endothelial cells. *Am. J. Physiol.,* 252:H1086–H1092.
35. Brunynzeel, P. L. B., Koenderman, L., Kok, P. T. M., Hameling, M. L., and Verhagen, J. (1986): Platelet-activating factor (PAF-acether) induced leukotriene C$_4$ formation and luminol dependent chemiluminescence by human eosinophils. *Pharmacol. Res. Commun.,* 18:61–69.
36. Burhop, K. E., van der Zee, H., Bizios, R., Kaplan, J. E., and Malik, A. B. (1986): Pulmonary vascular response to platelet-activating factor in awake sheep and the role of cyclooxygenase metabolites. *Am. Rev. Resp. Dis.,* 134:548–554.
37. Bussolino, F., Aglietta, M., Sanavio, R., Stacchini, A., Lauri, D., and Camussi, G. (1985): Alkyl-ether phosphoglycerides influence calcium fluxes into human endothelial cells. *J. Immunol.,* 135:2748–2753.
38. Camussi, G., Bussolino, F., Tetta, C., Piacibello, W., and Agleitta, M. (1983): Biosynthesis and release of platelet-activating factor from human monocytes. *Int. Arch. Allergy Appl. Immunol.,* 70:245–251.
39. Camussi, G., Montrucchio, G., Antro, C., Bussolino, F., Tetta, C., and Emanuelli, G. (1983): Platelet-activating factor-mediated contraction of rabbit lung strips: Pharmacologic modulation. *Immunopharmacology,* 6:87–96.
40. Camussi, G., Pawlowski, I., Tetta, C., Roffinello, C., Alberton, M., Brentjens, J., and Andres, G. (1983): Acute lung inflammation induced in the rabbit by local instillation of 1-*O*-octadecyl-2-acetyl-*sn*-glyceryl-3-phosphorylcholine or of native platelet-activating factor. *Am. J. Pathol.,* 112:78–88.
41. Camussi, G., Tetta, C., Coda, R., Segoloni, G. P., and Vercellone, A. (1984): Platelet-activating factor-induced loss of glomerular anionic charges. *Kidney Int.,* 25:73–81.
42. Chilton, F. H., and Murphy, R. C. (1986): Remodeling of arachidonate-containing phosphoglycerides within the human neutrophil. *J. Biol. Chem.,* 261:7771–7777.
43. Chilton, F. H., Ellis, J. M., Olson, S. C., and Wykle, R. L. (1984): 1-*O*-Alkyl-2-arachidonoyl-*sn*-glycero-3-phosphocholine. A common source of platelet-activating factor and arachidonate in human polymorphonuclear leukocytes. *J. Biol. Chem.,* 259:12014–12019.
44. Chilton, F. H., O'Flaherty, J. T., Walsh, C. E., Thomas, M. J., Wykle, R. L., DeChatelet, L. R., and Waite, B. M. (1982): Platelet-activating factor. Stimulation of the lipoxygenase pathway in polymorphonuclear leukocytes by 1-*O*-alkyl-2-*O*-acetyl-*sn*-glycero-3-phosphorylcholine. *J. Biol. Chem.,* 257:5402–5407.
45. Chilton, F. H., O'Flaherty, J. T., Ellis, J. M., Swendsen, C. L., and Wykle, R. L. (1983): Metabolic fate of platelet-activating factor in neutrophils. *J. Biol. Chem.,* 258:6357–6361.
46. Chung, K. F., Aizawa, H., Leikauf, G. D., Ueki, I. F., Evans, T. W., and Nadel, J. A. (1986): Airway hyperresponsiveness induced by platelet-activating factor: Role of thromboxane generation. *J. Pharmacol. Exp. Ther.,* 236:580–584.
47. Conrad, G. W., and Rink, T. J. (1986): Platelet activating factor raises intracellular calcium ion concentration in macrophages. *J. Cell Biol.,* 103:439–450.
48. Cuss, F. M., Dixon, C. M., and Barnes, P. J. (1986): Effects of inhaled platelet activating factor on pulmonary function and bronchial responsiveness in man. *Lancet,* 2:189–192.
49. Czarnetzki, G. (1983): Increased monocyte chemotaxis towards leukotriene B$_4$ and platelet activating factor in patients with inflammatory dermatoses. *Clin. Exp. Immunol.,* 54:486–492.
50. Demopoulos, C. A., Pinckard, R. N., and Hanahan, D. J. (1979): Platelet-activating factor. Evidence for 1-*O*-alkyl-2-acetyl-*sn*-glyceryl-3-phosphorylcholine as the active component (a new class of lipid chemical mediators). *J. Biol. Chem.,* 254:9355–9358.

51. Denjean, A., Arnoux, B., Masse, R., Lockhart, A., and Benveniste, J. (1983): Acute effects of intratracheal administration of platelet-activating factor in baboons. *J. Appl. Physiol.*, 55:799–804.

52. Dewald, B., and Baggiolini, M. (1986): Platelet-activating factor as a stimulus of exocytosis in human neutrophils. *Biochim. Biophys. Acta*, 888:42–48.

53. Dewald, B., and Baggiolini, M. (1985): Activation of NADPH oxidase in human neutrophils. Synergism between FMLP and the neutrophil products PAF and LTB_4. *Biochem. Biophys. Res. Commun.*, 128:297–304.

54. Doyle, V. M., Creba, J. A., and Ruegg, U. T. (1986): Platelet-activating factor mobilizes intracellular calcium in vascular smooth muscle cells. *FEBS Lett.*, 197:13–16.

55. Emeis, J. J., and Kluft, C. (1985): PAF-acether-induced release of tissue-type plasminogen activator from vessel walls. *Blood*, 66:86–91.

56. Feltner, D. E., Smith, R. H., and Marasco, W. A. (1986): Characterization of the plasma membrane bound GTPase from rabbit neutrophils. I. Evidence for an N_f-like protein coupled to the formyl peptide C5a, and leukotriene B_4 chemotaxis receptors. *J. Immunol.*, 137:1961–1970.

57. Feuerstein, G., and Hallenbeck, J. M. (1987): Prostaglandins, leukotrienes, and platelet-activating factor in shock. *Annu. Rev. Pharmacol. Toxicol.*, 27:301–313.

58. Feuerstein, G., Boyd, L. M., Ezra, D., and Goldstein, R. E. (1984): Effect of platelet-activating factor on coronary circulation of the domestic pig. *Am. J. Physiol.*, 246:H466–H471.

59. Findlay, S. R., Lichtenstein, L. M., Hanahan, D. J., and Pinckard, R. N. (1981): The contraction of guinea pig ileal smooth muscle by acetyl glyceryl ether phosphorylcholine. *Am. J. Physiol.*, 241:C130–C134.

60. Fjellner, B., and Hagermark O. (1985): Experimental pruritus evoked by platelet-activating factor (PAF-acether) in human skin. *Acta Derm. Venereol. (Stockh.)*, 65:409–412.

61. Ford-Hutchinson, A. W. (1983): Neutrophil aggregating properties of PAF-acether and leukotriene B_4. *Int. J. Immunopharmacol.*, 5:17–21.

62. Gay, J. C., Beckman, J. K., Zaboy, K. A., and Lukens, J. N. (1986): Modulation of neutrophil oxidative responses to soluble stimuli by platelet-activating factor. *Blood*, 67:931–936.

63. Gillespie, M. N., and Bowdy, B. D. (1986): Impact of platelet activating factor on vascular responsiveness in isolated rat lungs. *J. Pharmacol. Exp. Ther.*, 236:396–402.

64. Gilman, A. G. (1984): G proteins and dual control of adenylate cyclase. *Cell*, 36:577–579.

65. Goetzl, E. J., Derian, C. K., Tauber, A. I., and Valone, F. H. (1980): Novel effects of 1-*O*-hexadecyl-2-acyl-*sn*-glycero-3-phosphorylcholine mediators on human leukocyte function: Delineation of the specific roles of the acyl substituents. *Biochem. Biophys. Res. Commun.*, 94:881–888.

66. Goldenberg, M. M., and Meurer, R. D. (1984): A pharmacologic analysis of the action of platelet-activating factor in the induction of hindpaw edema in the rat. *Prostaglandins*, 28:271–278.

67. Goldman, D. W., Chang, F.-H., Gifford, L. A., Goetzl, E. J., and Bourne, H. R. (1985). Pertussis toxin inhibition of chemotactic factor-induced calcium mobilization and function in human polymorphonuclear leukocytes. *J. Exp. Med.*, 162:145–156.

68. Gomperts, B. D., Barrowman, M. M., and Cockcroft, S. (1986): Dual role for guanine nucleotides in stimulus-secretion coupling. *Fed. Proc.*, 45:2156–2161.

69. Gorman, R. R., Morton, D. R., Hopkins, N. K., and Lin, A. H. (1983): Acetyl glyceryl ether phosphorylcholine stimulates leukotriene B_4 synthesis and cyclic AMP accumulation in human polymorphonuclear leukocytes. *Adv. Prostaglandin Thromboxane Leukotriene Res.*, 12:57–63.

70. Hallam, T. J., and Rink, T. J. (1985): Agonists stimulate divalent cation channels in the plasma membrane of human platelets. *FEBS Lett.*, 186:175–179.

71. Hallam, T. J., Sanchez, A., and Rink, T. J. (1984): Stimulus-response coupling in human platelets. Changes evoked by platelet-

72. Halonen, M., and Pinckard, R. N. (1975): Intravascular effects of IgE antibody upon basophils, neutrophils, platelets and blood coagulation in the rabbit. *J. Immunol.*, 115:519–524.

73. Halonen, M., Fisher, H. K., Blair, C., Butler, C., and Pinckard, R. N. (1976): IgE-induced respiratory and circulatory changes during systemic anaphylaxis in the rabbit. *Am. Rev. Resp. Dis.*, 114:961–969.

74. Halonen, M., Lohman, I. D., Dunn, A. M., McManus, L. M., and Palmer, J. D. (1985): Participation of platelets in the physiological alterations of the AGEPC response and of IgE anaphylaxis in the rabbit. Effects of PGI_2 inhibition of platelet function. *Am. Rev. Resp. Dis.*, 131:11–17.

75. Halonen, M., Palmer, J. D., Lohman, C., McManus, L. M., and Pinckard, R. N. (1981): Differential effects of platelet depletion on the cardiovascular and pulmonary alterations of IgE anaphylaxis and AGEPC infusion in the rabbit. *Am. Rev. Resp. Dis.*, 124:416–421.

76. Halonen, M., Palmer, J. D., Lohman, I. C., McManus, L. M., and Pinckard, R. N. (1980): Respiratory and circulatory alterations induced by acetyl glyceryl ether phosphorylcholine (AGEPC), a mediator of IgE anaphylaxis in the rabbit. *Am. Rev. Resp. Dis.*, 122:915–924.

77. Hamasaki, Y., Mojarad, M., Saga, T., Tai, H., and Said, S. I. (1984): Platelet-activating factor raises airway and vascular pressures and induces edema in lungs perfused with platelet-free solution. *Am. Rev. Resp. Dis.*, 129:742–746.

78. Hanahan, D. J., Demopoulos, C. A., Liehr, J., and Pinckard, R. N. (1980): Identification of platelet-activating factor isolated from rabbit basophils as acetyl glyceryl ether phosphorylcholine. *J. Biol. Chem.*, 255:5514–5516.

79. Hartung, H.-P. (1983): Acetyl glyceryl ether phosphorylcholine (platelet-activating factor) mediates heightened metabolic activity in macrophages. *FEBS Lett.*, 160:209–212.

80. Hartung, H.-P., Parnham, M. J., Winkelmann, J., Englberger W., and Hadding, U. (1983): Platelet activating factor (PAF) induces the oxidative burst in macrophages. *Int. J. Immunopharmacol.*, 5:115–121.

81. Haslam, R. J., and Vanderwel, M. (1982): Inhibition of platelet adenylate cyclase by 1-*O*-alkyl-2-*O*-acetyl-*sn*-glyceryl-3-phosphorylcholine (platelet-activating factor). *J. Biol. Chem.*, 257:6879–6885.

82. Haslam, R. J., Williams, K. A., and Davidson, M. M. L. (1985): Receptor-effector coupling in platelets: Roles of guanine nucleotides. *Adv. Exp. Med. Biol.*, 192:265–280.

83. Hayashi, H., Kudo, I., Inoue, K., Onozaki, K., Tsushima, S., Nomura H., and Nojima, S. (1985): Activation of guinea pig peritoneal macrophages by platelet activating factor (PAF) and its agonists. *J. Biochem.*, 97:1737–1745.

84. Hayashi, H., Kudo, I., Inoue, K., Nomura, H., and Nojima, S. (1985): Macrophage activation by PAF incorporated into dipalmitoylphosphatidylcholine-cholesterol liposomes. *J. Biochem.*, 97:1255–1258.

85. Heffner, J. E., Shoemaker, S. A., Canham, E. M., Patel, M., McMurtry, I. F., Morris, H. G., and Repine, J. E. (1983): Acetyl glyceryl ether phosphorylcholine stimulated human platelets cause pulmonary hypertension and edema in isolated rabbit lungs. Role of thromboxane A_2. *J. Clin. Invest.*, 71:351–357.

86. Henocq, E., and Vargaftig, B. B. (1986): Accumulation of eosinophils in response to intracutaneous PAF-acether and allergens in man. *Lancet*, 1378–1379.

87. Hopkins, N. K., Lin, A. H., and Gorman, R. R. (1983): Evidence for mediation of acetyl glyceryl ether phosphorylcholine stimulation of adenosine 3′,5′-(cyclic)monophosphate levels in human polymorphonuclear leukocytes by leukotriene B_4. *Biochim. Biophys. Acta*, 763:276–283.

88. Houslay, M. D., Bojanic, D., Gawler, D., O'Hagan, S., and Wilson, A. (1986): Thrombin, unlike vasopressin, appears to stimulate two distinct guanine nucleotide regulatory proteins in human platelets. *Biochem. J.*, 238:109–113.

89. Houslay, M. D., Bojanic, D., and Wilson, A. (1986): Platelet ac-

tivating factor and U44069 stimulate a GTPase activity in human platelets which is distinct from the guanine nucleotide regulatory proteins, N$_s$ and N$_i$. *Biochem. J.,* 234:737–740.

90. Humphrey, D. M., Hanahan, D. J., and Pinckard, R. N. (1982): Induction of leucocytic infiltrates in rabbit skin by acetyl glyceryl ether phosphorylcholine (AGEPC). *Lab. Invest.,* 47:227–234.

91. Humphrey, D. M., McManus, L. M., Hanahan, D. J., and Pinckard, R. N. (1984): Morphologic basis of increased vascular permeability induced by acetyl glyceryl ether phosphorylcholine. *Lab. Invest.,* 50:16–25.

92. Humphrey, D. M., McManus, L. M., Satouchi, K., Hanahan, D. J., and Pinckard, R. N. (1982): Vasoactive properties of acetyl glyceryl ether phosphorylcholine (AGEPC) and AGEPC analogues. *Lab. Invest.,* 46:422–427.

93. Hwang, S.-B., Chang-Ling, L., Lam, M.-H., and Shen, T. Y. (1985): Characterization of cutaneous vascular permeability induced by platelet activating factor (PAF) in guinea pigs and rats and its inhibition by a PAF receptor antagonist. *Lab. Invest.,* 52:617–630.

94. Hwang, S.-B., and Lam, M.-H. (1986): Species differences in the specific receptors of platelet activating factor. *Biochem. Pharmacol.,* 35:4511–4518.

95. Hwang, S.-B., Lam, M.-H., and Pong, S.-S. (1986): Ionic and GTP regulation of binding of platelet-activating factor to receptors and platelet-activating factor-induced activation of GTPase in rabbit platelet membranes. *J. Biol. Chem.,* 261:532–537.

96. Hwang, S.-B., Lam, M.-H., and Shen, T. Y. (1985): Specific binding sites for platelet activating factor in human lung tissues. *Biochem. Biophys. Res. Commun.,* 128:972–979.

97. Hwang, S.-B., Lee, C.-S. C., Cheah, M. J., and Shen, T. Y. (1983): Specific receptor sites for 1-*O*-alkyl-2-*O*-acetyl-*sn*-glycero-3-phosphocholine (platelet activating factor) on rabbit platelet and guinea pig smooth muscle membranes. *Biochemistry,* 22:4756–4763.

98. Hwang, S. B., Lam, M. H., Li, C. L., and Shen, T. Y. (1986): Release of platelet activating factor and its involvement in the first phase of carrageenin-induced rat foot edema. *Eur. J. Pharmacol.,* 120:33–41.

99. Ingraham, L. M., Coates, T. D., Allen, J. M., Higgins, C. P., Baehner, R. L., and Boxer, L. A. (1982): Metabolic, membrane, and functional responses of human polymorphonuclear leukocytes to platelet-activating factor. *Blood,* 59:1259–1266.

100. Jackson, C. V., Schumacher, W. A., Kunkel, S. L., Driscoll, E. M., and Lucchesi, B. R. (1986): Platelet-activating factor and the release of a platelet-derived coronary artery vasodilator substance in the canine. *Circ. Res.,* 58:218–229.

101. Katada, T., Gilman, A. G., Watanabe, Y., Bauer, S., and Jakobs, K. H. (1985): Protein kinase C phosphorylates the inhibitory guanine-nucleotide-binding regulatory component and apparently suppresses its function in hormonal inhibition of adenylate cyclase. *Eur. J. Biochem.,* 151:431–437.

102. Kawaguchi, H., and Yasuda, H. (1986): Platelet-activating factor stimulates prostaglandin synthesis in cultured cells. *Hypertension,* 8:192–197.

103. Kenzora, J. L., Perez, J. E., Bergmann, S. R., and Lange, L. G. (1984): Effects of acetyl glyceryl ether of phosphorylcholine (platelet-activating factor) on ventricular preload, afterload, and contractility in dogs. *J. Clin. Invest.,* 74:1193–1203.

104. Kester, M., Kumar, R., and Hanahan, D. J. (1986): Alkylacetyl-glycerophosphocholine stimulates Na$^+$-Ca^{2+} exchange, protein phosphorylation and polyphosphoinositide turnover in rat ileal plasmalemmal vesicles. *Biochem. Biophys. Acta,* 888:306–315.

105. Kloprogge, E., and Akkerman, J. W. N. (1984): Binding kinetics of PAF-acether (1-*O*-alkyl-2-acetyl-*sn*-glycero-3-phosphocholine) to intact human platelets. *Biochem. J.,* 223:901–909.

106. Kloprogge, E., Haas de, G. H., Gorter, G., and Akkerman, J. W. N. (1983): Properties of PAF-acether-induced platelet aggregation and secretion. Studies in gel-filtered human platelets. *Thromb. Res.,* 29:595–608.

107. Koo, C., Lefkowitz, R. J., and Snyderman R. (1983): Guanine nucleotides modulate the binding affinity of the oligopeptide chemoattractant: Receptor on human polymorphonuclear leukocytes. *J. Clin. Invest.,* 72:748–753.

108. Kramer, R. M., Patton, G. M., Pritzker, C. R., and Deykin, D. (1984): Metabolism of platelet-activating factor in human platelets. Transacylase-mediated synthesis of 1-*O*-alkyl-2-arachidonoyl-*sn*-glycero-3-phosphocholine. *J. Biol. Chem.,* 259:13316–13320.

109. Kramp, W., Pieroni, G., Pinckard, R. N., and Hanahan, D. J. (1984): Observations on the critical micellar concentration of 1-*O*-alkyl-2-acetyl-*sn*-glyceryl-3-phosphorylcholine (PAF) and a series of its homologs and analogs. *Chem. Phys. Lipids,* 35:49–62.

110. Lad, P. M., Olson, C. V., Grewal, I. S., Scott, S. J., Learn, D. B., Smiley, P. A., and Lafrance-Flolich, M. (1987): Molecular mechanisms in the action of platelet activating factor and other mediators of inflammation. In: *New Horizons in Platelet Activating Factor Research,* edited by C. M. Winslow and J. L. Lee, pp. 103–122. John Wiley & Sons, New York.

111. Lad, P. M., Olson, C. V., and Grewall, I. S. (1985): Platelet-activating factor mediated effects on human neutrophil function are inhibited by pertussis toxin. *Biochem. Biophys. Res. Commun.,* 129:632–638.

112. Lapetina, E. G., and Siegel, F. L. (1983): Shape change induced in human platelets by platelet-activating factor. Correlation with the formation of phosphatidic acid and phosphorylation of a 40,000 dalton protein. *J. Biol. Chem.,* 258:7241–7244.

113. Lee, T.-C. (1985): Biosynthesis of platelet activating factor substrate specificity of 1-alkyl-2-lyso-*sn*-glycero-3-phosphorylcholine:acetyl-CoA acetyltransferase in rat spleen microsomes. *J. Biol. Chem.,* 260:10952–10955.

114. Lee, T.-C., and Snyder, F. (1985): Function, metabolism, and regulation of platelet activating factor and related ether lipids. In: *Phospholipids and Cellular Regulation,* edited by J. F. Kuo, pp. 1–39. CRC Press, Boca Raton, Fl.

115. Lee, T.-C., Malone, B., Blank, M. L., and Snyder, F. (1981): 1-Alkyl-2-acetyl-*sn*-glycero-3-phosphocholine (platelet-activating factor) stimulates calcium influx in rabbit platelets. *Biochem. Biophys. Res. Commun.,* 102:1262–1268.

116. Lenihan, D. J., and Lee, T.-C. (1984): Regulation of platelet activating factor synthesis: Modulation of 1-alkyl-2-lyso-*sn*-glycero-3-phosphocholine:acetyl-CoA acetyltransferase by phosphorylation and dephosphorylation in rat spleen microsomes. *Biochem. Biophys. Res. Commun.,* 120:834–839.

117. Levi, R., Burke, J. A., Guo, Z.-G., Hattori, Y., Hoppens, C. M., McManus, L. M., Hanahan, D. J., and Pinckard, R. N. (1984): Acetyl glyceryl ether phosphorylcholine (AGEPC): A putative mediator of cardiac anaphylaxis in the guinea pig. *Circ. Res.,* 54:117–124.

118. Lewis, J. C., O'Flaherty, J. T., McCall, C. E., Wykle, R. L., and Bond, M. G. (1983): Platelet-activating factor effects on pulmonary ultrastructure in rabbits. *Exp. Mol. Pathol.,* 38:100–108.

119. Lichey, J., Friedrich, T., Franke, J., Nigam, S., Priesnitz, M., and Oeff, K. (1984): Pressure effects and uptake of platelet-activating factor in isolated rat lung. *J. Appl. Physiol.,* 57:1039–1044.

120. Lin, A. H., Morton, D. R., and Gorman, R. R. (1982): Acetyl glyceryl ether phosphorylcholine stimulates leukotriene B$_4$ synthesis in human polymorphonuclear leukocytes. *J. Clin. Invest.,* 70:1058–1065.

121. Ludwig, J. C., and Pinckard, R. N. (1987): Diversity in the chemical structures of neutrophil-derived platelet-activating factors. In: *New Horizons in Platelet Activating Factor Research,* edited by C. M. Winslow and J. L. Lee, pp. 59–71. John Wiley & Sons, New York.

122. Ludwig, J. C., Hoppens, C., McManus, L. M., Mott, G. E., and Pinckard, R. N. (1985): Modulation of platelet-activating factor (PAF) synthesis and release from human polymorphonuclear leukocytes (PMN): Role of extracellular albumin. *Arch. Biochem. Biophys.,* 241:337–247.

123. Ludwig, J. C., McManus, L. M., Clark, P. O., Hanahan, D. J., and Pinckard, R. N. (1984): Modulation of platelet-activating factor (PAF) synthesis and release from human polymorphonuclear leukocytes (PMN): Role of extracellular calcium. *Arch. Biochem. Biophys.,* 232:102–110.

124. Ludwig, J. C., McManus, L. M., and Pinckard, R. N. (1986): Synthesis-release coupling of platelet activating factors (PAF) from stimulated human neutrophils. *Adv. Inflam. Res.,* 11:111–125.

125. MacIntyre, D. E., McNicol, A., and Drummond, A. H. (1985): Tumour-promoting phorbol esters inhibit agonist-induced phosphatidate formation and Ca²⁺ flux in human platelets. *FEBS Lett.,* 180:160–164.

126. Malone, B., Lee, T.-C., and Snyder, F. (1985): Inactivation of platelet activating factor by rabbit platelets. Lyso-platelet activating factor as a key intermediate with phosphatidylcholine as the source of arachidonic acid in its conversion to a tetraenoic acylated product. *J. Biol. Chem.,* 260:1531–1534.

127. Marcus, A. J., Safier, L. B., Ullman, H. L., Wong, K. T. H., Broekman, M. J., Weksler, B. B., and Kaplan, K. L. (1981): Effects of acetyl glyceryl ether phosphorylcholine on human platelet function *in vitro. Blood,* 58:1027–1031.

128. McIntyre, T. M., Zimmerman, G. A., and Prescott, S. A. (1986): Leukotrienes C₄ and D₄ stimulate human endothelial cells to synthesize platelet-activating factor and bind neutrophils. *Proc. Natl. Acad. Sci. (USA),* 83:2204–2208.

129. McManus, L. M. (1986): Pathobiology of platelet-activating factor. *Pathol. Immunopathol. Res.,* 5:104–117.

130. McManus, L. M. (1987): Acute lung injury induced by intravascular platelet activating factor. In: *New Horizons in Platelet Activating Factor Research,* edited by C. M. Winslow and M. L. Lee, pp. 233–244. John Wiley & Sons, New York.

131. McManus, L. M., and Pinckard, R. N. (1985): Kinetics of acetyl glyceryl ether phosphorylcholine (AGEPC)-induced acute lung injury in the rabbit. *Am. J. Pathol.,* 121:55–68.

132. McManus, L. M., Fitzpatrick, F. A., Hanahan, D. J., and Pinckard, R. N. (1983): Thromboxane B₂ release following acetyl glyceryl ether phosphorylcholine (AGEPC) infusion in the rabbit. *Immunopharmacology,* 5:197–207.

133. McManus, L. M., Hanahan, D. J., Demopoulos, C. A., and Pinckard, R. N. (1980): Pathobiology of the intravenous infusion of acetyl glyceryl ether phosphorylcholine (AGPEC), a synthetic platelet-activating factor (PAF), in the rabbit. *J. Immunol.,* 124:2919–2924.

134. McManus, L. M., Hanahan, D. J., and Pinckard, R. N. (1981): Human platelet stimulation by acetyl glyceryl ether phosphorylcholine (AGEPC). *J. Clin. Invest.,* 67:903–906.

135. McManus, L. M., Pinckard, R. N., Fitzpatrick, F. A., O'Rourke, R. A., Crawford, H., and Hanahan, D. J. (1981): Acetyl glyceryl ether phosphorylcholine (AGEPC): Intravascular alterations following intravenous infusion in the baboon. *Lab. Invest.,* 45:303–307.

136. Mencia-Huerta, J. M., Roubin, R., and Benveniste, J. (1981): Acetyl coenzyme A (Ac-CoA) and sodium acetate enhance the release of platelet-activating factor (PAF-acether) from murine peritoneal cells. *Int. Arch. Allergy Appl. Immunol.,* 66:178–179.

137. Molski, T. F. P., Naccache, P. H., Marsh, M. L., Kermode, J., Becker, E. L., and Sha'afi. (1984): Pertussis toxin inhibits the rise in the intracellular concentration of free calcium that is induced by chemotactic factors in rabbit neutrophils: Possible role of the "G Proteins" in calcium mobilization. *Biochem. Biophys. Res. Commun.,* 124:644–650.

138. Mossmann, H., Bamberger U., Velev, B. A., Gehrung, M., and Hammer, D. K. (1986): Effect of platelet-activating factor on human polymorphonuclear leukocyte enhancement of chemiluminescence and antibody-dependent cellular cytotoxicity. *J. Leukocyte Biol.,* 39:153–165.

139. Mueller, H. W., O'Flaherty, J. T., and Wykle, R. L. (1983): Biosynthesis of platelet-activating factor in rabbit polymorphonuclear neutrophils. *J. Biol. Chem.,* 258:6213–6218.

140. Mueller, H. W., O'Flaherty, J. T., Greene, D. G., Samuel, M. P., and Wykle, R. L. (1984): 1-*O*-alkyl-linked glycerophospholipids of human neutrophils: Distribution of arachidonate and other acyl residues in the ether-linked and diacyl species. *J. Lipid Res.,* 25:383–388.

141. Mueller, H. W., O'Flaherty, J. T., and Wykle, R. L. (1984): The molecular species distribution of platelet-activating factor synthesized by rabbit and human neutrophils. *J. Biol. Chem.,* 259:14554–14559.

142. Naccache, P. H., Molski, M. M., Volpi, M., Becker, E. L., and Sha'afi, R. I. (1985): Unique inhibitory profile of platelet activating factor induced calcium mobilization, polyphosphoinositide turnover and granule enzyme secretion in rabbit neutrophils towards pertussis toxin and phorbol ester. *Biochem. Biophys. Res. Commun.,* 130:677–684.

143. Naccache, P. H., Molski, M. M., Volpi, M., Shefcyk, J., Molski, T. F. P., Loew, L., Becker, E. L., and Sha'afi, R. I. (1986): Biochemical events associated with the stimulation of rabbit neutrophils by platelet-activating factor. *J. Leukocyte Biol.,* 40:533–548.

144. Namm, D. H., Tadepalli, A. S., and High, J. A. (1982): Species specificity of the platelet responses to 1-*O*-alkyl-2-acetyl-*sn*-glycero-3-phosphorylcholine. *Thromb. Res.,* 25:341–350.

145. Ng, D. S., and Wong, K. (1986): GTP regulation of platelet-activating factor binding to human neutrophil membranes. *Biochem. Biophys. Res. Commun.,* 141:353–359.

146. Ninio, E., Mencia-Huerta, J. M., Heymans, F., and Benveniste, J. (1982): Biosynthesis of platelet-activating factor. 1. Evidence for an acetyltransferase activity in murine macrophages. *Biochim. Biophys. Acta,* 710:23–31.

147. Nourshargh, S., and Hoult, J. R. S. (1986): Inhibition of human neutrophil degranulation by forskolin in the presence of phosphodiesterase inhibitors. *Eur. J. Pharmacol.,* 122:205–212.

148. O'Flaherty, J. L., Surles, J. R., Redman, J., Jacobson, D., Piantadosi, C., and Wykle, R. (1986): Binding and metabolism of platelet-activating factor by human neutrophils. *J. Clin. Invest.,* 78:381–388.

149. O'Flaherty, J. T. (1985): Neutrophil degranulation: Evidence pertaining to its mediation by the combined effects of leukotriene B₄, platelet-activating factor, and 5-HETE. *J. Cell. Physiol.,* 122:229–239.

150. O'Flaherty, J. T., and Wykle, R. L. (1983): Biology and biochemistry of platelet-activating factor. *Clin. Rev. Allergy,* 1:353–367.

151. O'Flaherty, J. T., Hammett, M. J., Shewmake, T. B., Wykle, R. L., Love, S. H., McCall, C. E., and Thomas, M. J. (1981): Evidence for 5,12-dihydroxy-6,8,10,14-eicosatetraenoate as a mediator of human neutrophil aggregation. *Biochem. Biophys. Res. Commun.,* 103:552–558.

152. O'Flaherty, J. T., Swendsen, C. L., Lees, C. J., and McCall, C. E. (1981): Role of extracellular calcium in neutrophil degranulation responses to 1-*O*-alkyl-2-acetyl-*sn*-glycero-3-phosphocholine. *Am. J. Pathol.,* 105:107–113.

153. O'Flaherty, J. T., Thomas, M. J., Hammett, M. J., Carroll, C., McCall, C. E., and Wykle, R. L. (1983): 5-L-Hydroxy-6,8,11,14-eicosatetraenoate potentiates the human neutrophil degranulating action of platelet-activating factor. *Biochem. Biophys. Res. Commun.,* 111:1–7.

154. O'Flaherty, J. T., Wykle, R. L., Lees, C. J., Shewmake, T., McCall, C. E., and Thomas, M. J. (1981): Neutrophil-degranulating action of 5,12-dihydroxy-6,8,10,14-eicosatetraenoic acid and 1-*O*-alkyl-2-acetyl-*sn*-glycero-3-phosphocholine. Comparison with other degranulating agents. *Am. J. Pathol.,* 105:264–269.

155. O'Flaherty, J. T., Wykle, R. L., Miller, C. H., Lewis, J. C., Waite, M., Bass, D. A., McCall, C. E., and DeChatelet, L. R. (1981): 1-*O*-alkyl-*sn*-glyceryl-3-phosphorylcholines. A novel class of neutrophil stimulants. *Am. J. Pathol.,* 103:70–78.

156. O'Flaherty, J. T., Wykle, R. L., Thomas, M. J., and McCall, C. E. (1984): Neutrophil degranulation responses to combinations of arachidonate metabolites and platelet-activating factor. *Res. Commun. Chem. Pathol. Pharmacol.,* 43:3–23.

157. O'Flaherty, J. T., Wykle, R. L., McCall, C. E., Shewmake, T. B., Lees, C. J., and Thomas, M. (1981): Desensitization of the human neutrophil degranulation response: Studies with 5,12-dihydroxy-6,8,10,14-eicosatetraenoic acid. *Biochem. Biophys. Res. Commun.,* 101:1290–1296.

158. O'Rourke, F. A., Halenda, S. P., Zavoico, G. B., and Feinstein, M. B. (1985): Inositol 1,4,5-trisphosphate releases Ca²⁺ from a Ca²⁺-transporting membrane vesicle fraction derived from human platelets. *J. Biol. Chem.,* 260:956–962.

159. Oda, M., Satouchi, K., Yasunaga, K., and Saito, K. (1985): Molecular species of platelet-activating factor generated by human neutrophils challenged with ionophore A23187. *J. Immunol.,* 134:1090–1093.

160. Okajima, F., and Ui, M. (1984): ADP-ribosylation of the specific membrane protein by islet-activating protein, pertussin toxin, associated with inhibition of a chemotactic peptide-induced arachidonate release in neutrophils. A possible role of the toxin substrate in Ca^{2+}-mobilizing biosignaling. *J. Biol. Chem.*, 259:13863–13871.

161. Okajima, F., Katada, T. and Ui, M. (1985): Coupling of the guanine nucleotide regulatory protein to chemotactic peptide receptors in neutrophil membranes and its uncoupling by islet-activating protein, pertussis toxin. A possible role of the toxin substrate in Ca^{2+}-mobilizing receptor-mediated signal transduction. *J. Biol. Chem.*, 260:6761–6768.

162. Ostermann, G., Till, U., and Thielmann, K. (1983): Studies on the stimulation of human blood platelets by semi-synthetic platelet-activating factor. *Thromb. Res.*, 30:127–136.

163. Parente, L., and Flower, R. J. (1985): Hydrocortisone and 'macrocortin' inhibit the zymosan-induced release of lyso-PAF from rat peritoneal leucocytes. *Life Sci.*, 36:1225–1231.

164. Patterson, R., Bernstein, P. R., Harris, K. E., and Krell, R. D. (1984): Airway responses to sequential challenges with platelet-activating factor and leukotriene D_4 in rhesus monkeys. *J. Lab. Clin. Med.*, 104:340–345.

165. Patterson, R., Harris, K. E., Lee, M. L. and Houlihan, W. J. (1986): Inhibition of rhesus monkey airway and cutaneous responses to platelet-activating factor (PAF) (AGEPC) with the anti-PAF agent SRI 63-072. *Int. Arch. Allergy Appl. Immunol.*, 81:265–268.

166. Pinckard, R. N., Farr, R. S., and Hanahan, D. J. (1979): Physicochemical and functional identity of platelet-activating factor (PAF) released *in vivo* during IgE anaphylaxis with PAF released *in vitro* from IgE sensitized basophils. *J. Immunol.*, 123:1847–1857.

167. Pinckard, R. N., Jackson, E. M., Hoppens, C., Weintraub, S. T., Ludwig, J. C., McManus, L. M., and Mott, G. E. (1984): Molecular heterogeneity of platelet-activating factor produced by stimulated human polymorphonuclear leukocytes. *Biochem. Biophys. Res. Commun.*, 122:325–332.

168. Pinckard, R. N. (1985): Platelet-activating factor. In: *Allergy*, edited by A. P. Kaplan, pp. 165–174. Churchill Livingstone, New York.

169. Pinckard, R. N., McManus, L. M., Demopoulos, C. A., Halonen, M., Clark, P. O., Shaw, J. O., Kniker, W. T., and Hanahan, D. J. (1980): Molecular pathobiology of acetyl glyceryl ether phosphorylcholine (AGEPC): Evidence for the structural identity with platelet-activating factor (PAF). *J. Reticuloendothel. Soc.*, 28:95s–103s.

170. Pirotzky, E., Ninio, E., Bidault, J., Pfister, A., and Benveniste, J. (1984): Biosynthesis of platelet-activating factor. VI. Precursor of platelet-activating factor and acetyltransferase in isolated rat kidney cells. *Lab. Invest.*, 51:567–572.

171. Ramesha, C. S., and Pickett, W. C. (1987): Species-specific variations in the molecular heterogeneity of the platelet-activating factor. *J. Immunol.*, 138:1559–1563.

172. Ramesha, C. S., and Pickett, W. C. (1986): Platelet-activating factor and leukotriene biosynthesis is inhibited in polymorphonuclear leukocytes depleted of arachidonic acid. *J. Biol. Chem.*, 261:7592–7595.

173. Renooij, W., and Snyder, R. (1981): Biosynthesis of 1-alkyl-2-acetyl-*sn*-glycero-3-phosphocholine (platelet activating factor and a hypotensive lipid) by cholinephosphotransferase in various rat tissues. *Biochim. Biophys. Acta*, 663:545–556.

174. Rink, T. J., and Hallam, T. J. (1984): What turns platelets on? *Trends Biochem. Sci.*, 9:215–219.

175. Sage, S. O., and Rink, T. J. (1986): Effects of ionic substitution on $[Ca^{2+}]_i$ rises evoked by thrombin and PAF in human platelets. *Eur. J. Pharmacol.*, 128:99–107.

176. Sage, S. O., and Rink, T. J. (1985): Inhibition by forskolin of cytosolic calcium rise, shape change and aggregation in quin-2-loaded human platelets. *FEBS Lett.*, 188:135–140.

177. Sanchez-Crespo, M., Alonso, F., Inarrea, P., Alvarez, V., and Egido, J. (1982): Vascular actions of synthetic PAF-acether (a synthetic platelet-activating factor) in the rat: Evidence for a platelet independent mechanism. *Immunopharmacology*, 4:173–185.

178. Sano, K., Takai, Y., Yamanishi. J., and Nishizuka, Y. (1983): A role of calcium-activated phospholipid-dependent protein kinase in human platelet activation. Comparison of thrombin and collagen actions. *J. Biol. Chem.*, 258:2010–2013.

179. Satouchi, J., Pinckard, R. N., McManus, L. M., and Hanahan, D. J. (1981): Modification of the polar head group of acetyl glyceryl ether phosphorylcholine and subsequent effects upon platelet activation. *J. Biol. Chem.*, 256:4425–4432.

180. Satouchi, K., Oda, M., Yasunaga, K., and Saito, K. (1985): Evidence for the production of 1-acyl-2-acetyl-*sn*-glyceryl-3-phosphorylcholine concomitantly with platelet-activating factor. *Biochem. Biophys. Res. Commun.*, 128:1409–1417.

181. Satouchi, K., Pinckard, R. N., and Hanahan, D. J. (1981): Influence of alkyl ether chain length of acetyl glyceryl ether phosphorylcholine and its ethanolamine analog on biological activity towards rabbit platelets. *Arch. Biochem. Biophys.*, 211:683–688.

182. Saunders, R. N., and Handley, D. A. (1987): Platelet-activating factor antagonists. *Annu. Rev. Pharmacol. Toxicol.*, 27:237–255.

183. Scherf, H., Nies, A. S., Schwertschlag, U., Hughes, M., and Gerber, J. G. (1986): Hemodynamic effects of platelet activating factor in the dog kidney *in vivo*. *Hypertension*, 8:737–741.

184. Schlondorff, D., and Neuwirth, R. (1986): Platelet-activating factor and the kidney. *Am. J. Physiol.*, 251:F1–F11.

185. Schlondorff, D., Satriano, J. A., Hagege, J., Perez, J., and Baud, L. (1984): Effect of platelet-activating factor and serum-treated zymosan on prostaglandin E_2 synthesis, arachidonic acid release, and contraction of cultured rat mesangial cells. *J. Clin. Invest.*, 73:1227–1231.

186. Shaw, J. O., Pinckard, R. N., Ferrigni, K. S., McManus, L. M., and Hanahan, D. J. (1981): Activation of human neutrophils with 1-*O*-hexadecyl/octadecyl-2-acetyl-*sn*-glyceryl-3-phosphorylcholine (platelet-activating factor). *J. Immunol.*, 127:1250–1255.

187. Siraganian, R. P., and Osler, A. G. (1971): Destruction of rabbit platelets in the allergic response of sensitized leukocytes. I. Demonstration of a fluid phase intermediate. *J. Immunol.*, 106:1244–1251.

188. Sklar, L. A. (1986): Ligand-receptor dynamics and signal amplification in the neutrophil. *Adv. Immunol.*, 39:95–143.

189. Smith, C. D., Cox, C. C., and Snyderman, R. (1986): Receptor-coupled activation of phosphoinositide-specific phospholipase C by an N protein. *Science*, 232:97–100.

190. Smith, C. D., Lane, B. C., Kusaka I., Verghese, M. W., and Snyderman, R. (1985): Chemoattractant receptor-induced hydrolysis of phosphatidylinositol 4,5-bisphosphate in human polymorphonuclear leukocyte membranes. Requirement for a guanine nucleotide regulatory protein. *J. Biol. Chem.*, 260:5875–5878.

191. Smith, R. J., and Bowman, B. J. (1982): Stimulation of human neutrophil degranulation with 1-*O*-octadecyl-2-*O*-acetyl-*sn*-glyceryl-3-phosphorylcholine: Modulation by inhibitors of arachidonic acid metabolism. *Biochem. Biophys. Res. Commun.*, 104:1495–1501.

192. Smith, R. J., Bowman, B. J., and Iden, S. S. (1984): Stimulation of the human neutrophil superoxide anion-generating system with 1-*O*-hexadecyl/octadecyl-2-acetyl-*sn*-glyceryl-3-phosphorylcholine. *Biochem. Pharmacol.*, 33:973–978.

193. Smith, R. J., Bowman, B. J., and Iden, S. S. (1983): Characteristics of 1-*O*-hexadecyl- and 1-*O*-octadecyl-2-*O*-acetyl-*sn*-glycerol-3-phosphorylcholine-stimulated granule enzyme release from human neutrophils. *Clin. Immunol. Immunopathol.*, 28:13–38.

194. Stafforini, D. M., McIntyre, T., Carter, M. E., and Prescott, S. M. (1987): Human plasma platelet activating factor acetylhydrolase, association with lipoprotein and role in the degradation of platelet-activating factor. *J. Biol. Chem.*, 62:4215–4222.

195. Stafforini, D. M., Prescott, S., and McIntyre, T. (1987): Human plasma platelet-activating factor acetylhydrolase, Purification and Properties. *J. Biol. Chem.*, 262:4223–4230.

196. Stewart, A. G., and Piper, P. J. (1986): Platelet-activating factor-induced vasoconstriction in rat isolated, perfused hearts: Contribution of cyclo-oxygenase and lipoxygenase arachidonic acid metabolites. *Pharmacol. Res. Commun.*, 18:163–172.

197. Stimler, N. P., and O'Flaherty, J. T. (1983): Spasmogenic properties of platelet-activating factor: Evidence for a direct mechanism in the contractile response of pulmonary tissues. *Am. J. Pathol.*, 113:75–84.

198. Stimler, N. P., Bloor, C. M., Hugli, T. E., Wykle, R. L., McCall, C. E., and O'Flaherty, J. T. (1981): Anaphylactic actions of platelet-activating factor. *Am. J. Pathol.*, 105:64–69.

199. Stimler-Gerard, N. P. (1986): Parasympathetic stimulation as a mechanism for platelet-activating factor-induced contractile responses in the lung. *J. Pharmacol. Exp. Ther.*, 237:209–213.

200. Sturk, A., Asyee, G. M., Schaap, M. C., van Maanen, M., and ten Cate, J. W. (1985): Synergistic effects of platelet-activating factor and other platelet agonists in human platelet aggregation and release: The role of ADP and products of the cyclooxygenase pathway. *Thromb. Res.*, 40:359–372.

201. Tamargo, J., Tejerina, T., Delgado, C., and Barrigon, S. (1985): Electrophysiological effects of platelet-activating factor (PAF-acether) in guinea-pig papillary muscles. *Eur. J. Pharmacol.*, 109:219–227.

202. Tessner, T., and Wykle, R. (1987): Stimulated human neutrophils synthesize an ethanolamine plasmologen analog of platelet-activating factor. *Fed. Proc.* 46:2033.

203. Tokumura, A., Homma, H., and Hanahan, D. J. (1985): Structural analogs of alkylacetylglycerophosphocholine inhibitory behavior on platelet activation. *J. Biol. Chem.*, 260:12710–12714.

204. Valone, F. H. (1986): Synergistic platelet activation by aggregates of IgG and the phospholipid platelet-activating factor 1-*O*-alkyl-2-acetyl-*sn*-glycero-3-phosphorylcholine. *J. Clin. Immunol.*, 6:57–64.

205. Valone, F. H., and Goetzl, E. J. (1983): Specific binding by human polymorphonuclear leucocytes of the immunological mediator 1-*O*-hexadecyl/octadecyl-2-acetyl-*sn*-glycero-3-phosphorylcholine. *Immunology*, 48:141–149.

206. Valone, F. H., and Johnson, B. (1985): Decay of the activating signal after platelet stimulation with 1-*O*-alkyl-2-acetyl-*sn*-glycero-3-phosphorylcholine: Changes in calcium permeability. *Thromb. Res.*, 40:385–392.

207. Vargaftig, B. B., Fouque, F., Benveniste, J., and Odiot, J. (1982): Adrenaline and PAF-acether synergize to trigger cyclooxygenase-independent activation of plasma-free platelets. *Thromb. Res.*, 28:557–573.

208. Vargaftig, B. B., Lefort, J., Wal, F., Chignard, M., and Medeiros, M. C. (1982): Non-steroidal anti-inflammatory drugs if combined with anti-histamine and anti-serotonin agents interfere with the bronchial and platelet effects of "platelet-activating factor" (PAF-acether). *Eur. J. Pharmacol.*, 82:121–130.

209. Vargaftig, B. B., Lefort, J., Chignard, M., and Benveniste, J. (1980): Platelet-activating factor induces a platelet-dependent broncho-constriction unrelated to the formation of prostaglandin derivatives. *Eur. J. Pharmacol.* 65:185–192.

210. Verghese, M. W., Smith, C. D., Charles, L. A., Jakoi, L., and Snyderman, R. (1986): A guanine nucleotide regulatory protein controls polyphosphoinositide metabolism, Ca^{2+} mobilization, and cellular responses to chemoattractants in human monocytes. *J. Immunol.*, 137:271–275.

211. Voelkel, N. F., Chang, S.-W., Pfeffer, K. D., Worthen, S. G., McMurtry, I. F., and Henson, P. M. (1986): PAF antagonists: Different effects on platelets, neutrophils, guinea pig ileum and PAF-induced vasodilation in isolated rat lung. *Prostaglandins*, 32:359–372.

212. Voelkel, N. F., Worthen, S., Reeves, J. T., Henson, P. M., and Murphy, R. C. (1982): Nonimmunological production of leukotrienes induced by platelet-activating factor. *Science*, 218:286–288.

213. von Tscharner, V., Prodhom, B., Baggiolini, M., and Reuter, H. (1986): Ion channels in human neutrophils activated by a rise in free cytosolic calcium concentration. *Nature*, 324:369–372.

214. Wardlow, M. L., Cox, C. P., Meng, K. E., Greene, D. E., and Farr, R. S. (1986): Substrate specificity and partial characterization of the PAF-acylhydrolase in human serum that rapidly inactivates platelet-activating factor. *J. Immunol.*, 136:3441–3446.

215. Weintraub, S. T., Ludwig, J. C., Mott, G. E., McManus, L. M., Lear, C., and Pinckard, R. N. (1985): Fast atom bombardment-mass spectrometric identification of molecular species of platelet-activating factor produced by stimulated human polymorphonuclear leukocytes. *Biochem. Biophys. Res. Commun.*, 129:868–876.

216. Williams, K. A., and Haslam, R. J. (1984): Effects of NaCl and GTP on the inhibition of platelet adenylate cyclase by 1-*O*-octadecyl-2-*O*-acetyl-*sn*-glyceryl-3-phosphorylcholine (synthetic platelet-activating factor). *Biochim. Biophys. Acta*, 770:216–223.

217. Williamson, J. R. (1986): Role of inositol lipid breakdown in the generation of intracellular signals. State of the art lecture. *Hypertension*, 8:140–156.

218. Winslow, C. M., and Lee, M., editors (1987): *New Horizons in Platelet Activating Factor Research*. John Wiley & Sons, New York.

219. Wykle, R. L., Miller, C. H., Lewis, J. C., Schmitt, J. D., Smith, J. A., Surles, J. R., Piantadosi, C., and O'Flaherty, J. T. (1981): Stereospecific activity of 1-*O*-alkyl-2-*O*-acetyl-*sn*-glycero-3-phosphocholine and comparison of analogs in the degranulation of platelets and neutrophils. *Biochem. Biophys. Res. Commun.*, 100:1651–1658.

220. Wykle, R. L., Olson, S. C., and O'Flaherty, J. T. (1986): Biochemical pathways of platelet-activating factor synthesis and breakdown. *Adv. Inflam. Res.*, 11:71–81.

221. Yasaka, T., Boxer, L. A., and Baehner, R. L. (1982): Monocyte aggregation and superoxide anion release in response to formyl-methionyl-leucyl-phenylalanine (FMLP) and platelet-activating factor (PAF). *J. Immunol.*, 128:1939–1944.

Inflammation: Basic Principles and Clinical Correlates.
Edited by J. I. Gallin, I. M. Goldstein, and R. Snyderman.
Raven Press, Ltd., New York © 1988.

CHAPTER 11

Histamine

Martha V. White and Michael A. Kaliner

Histamine was first observed to be a potent vasoactive substance by Dale and Laidlaw in 1911 (43) but was not conclusively associated with tissue mast cells until 1953 (156). Over the past 75 years, histamine has been studied extensively, particularly in the past decade since the appreciation of its actions through H-1 and H-2 receptors has become clear. In this chapter, we will focus on current concepts of the biosynthesis and biodegradation of histamine, the physiology of its release from mast cells and basophils, and its actions on target cells. In the course of this discussion, we will consider the role of histamine in inflammation and the mechanisms by which it may contribute to the physiologic alterations seen in inflammatory processes.

HISTAMINE SYNTHESIS AND METABOLISM

Histamine, 2-(4-imidazolyl)ethylamine or 5β-amino-ethylimidazole, is formed by decarboxylation of the amino acid histidine by the pyridoxal phosphate-dependent enzyme L-histidine decarboxylase (Fig. 1) (146). Most histamine is stored preformed in cytoplasmic granules of mast cells and basophils in close association with the an-

ionic side chains of proteoglycans comprising the granule matrix. The predominant proteoglycan found varies with cell type: heparin in human connective tissue mast cells (125), chondroitin sulfates di-B and E in rodent mucosal mast cells, and chondroitin 4-sulfate in human blood basophils (55,84,127,151,152,193).

In humans, the mast cell is found in the loose connective tissue of all organs, especially around blood vessels, nerves, and lymphatics. Mast cells are most abundant in the skin and in the mucosa of the upper and lower respiratory tract, gastrointestinal tract, and reproductive mucosa (125). In the lung, they occur in concentrations of 1 to 7×10^6 cells per gram of lung tissue (212), comprise up to 2% of alveolar cells (59), and are found in the connective tissue beneath the airway basement membrane, near the submucosal blood vessels and glands, throughout the muscle bundles, and in the interalveolar septa as well as the bronchial lumen.

Activation of human mast cells by antigen bridging of membrane-bound IgE, thereby aggregating IgE receptors, initiates a cascade of membrane lipid metabolic events leading to the opening of calcium channels, cleavage of arachidonic acid from phosphatidylcholine, and release

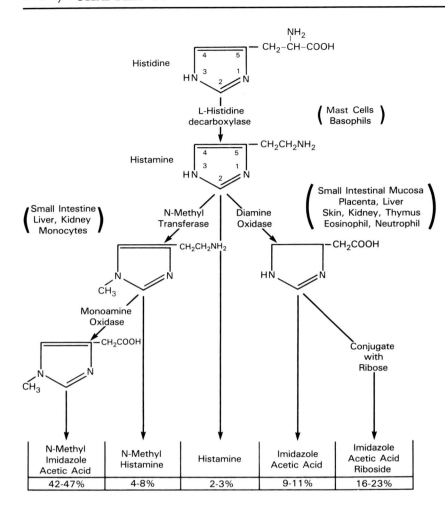

FIG. 1. Synthesis and catabolism of histamine. Percent recovery of histamine and its metabolites in the urine in the 12 hr following intradermal [^{14}C]histamine in human males. (From ref. 220.)

N-Methyl Imidazole Acetic Acid	N-Methyl Histamine	Histamine	Imidazole Acetic Acid	Imidazole Acetic Acid Riboside
42-47%	4-8%	2-3%	9-11%	16-23%

of secretory granules containing preformed granule constituents such as histamine. The morphologic changes accompanying histamine release have been reviewed by Friedman and Kaliner (61). Briefly, human skin mast cells release into the extracellular milieu intact granules, some of which can be subsequently phagocytosed by connective tissue fibroblasts (226). In contrast, degranulation of human lung and nasal mucosal mast cells involves intracellular solubilization of granule contents and fusion of granular membranes with each other and with the cell membrane to form channels to the outside through which the solubilized granule contents are secreted (36,60).

Numerous other substances also cause mast cells or basophils to release histamine (Table 1). Among these mast cell secretagogues are the by-products of complement activation, C3a and C5a, which are both potent mast cell degranulators and are prevalent in areas of inflammation. Certain neurohormones, such as substance P, and neurotensin and other substances which may be released during inflammatory reactions such as interleukin-1 (IL-1) and adenosine triphosphate are also capable of inducing mast cell degranulation (126, 222). Several inflammatory cells, including neutrophils, mononuclear cells, platelets, endothelial cells, and eosinophils, make histamine releasing factors (112,138,206,219-221,228). The histamine releasing activity (HRA) derived from neutrophils, termed HRA-N, is released spontaneously within minutes after incubation (220,221), whereas the mononuclear cell-derived factor, HRA, is synthesized and released over hours (206). The endothelial cell-, platelet-, and macrophage-derived factors bind IgE and are dependent on IgE

TABLE 1. *Mast cell secretagogues*

IgE
C3a
C5a
Substance P
Morphine
Physical stimuli: vibration, heat, cold
Adenosine triphosphate
Neurotensin
Histamine releasing activities from lymphocytes (HRA), neutrophils (HRA-N), platelets, endothelial cells, human lung macrophages, eosinophils

activation for their function (138), whereas the neutrophil- and mononuclear cell-derived factors function independently of IgE. All four factors induce rapid histamine release. Thus, numerous biologic substances capable of causing histamine release, including neuropeptides, complement components, and inflammatory cell products, are present during inflammatory reactions.

Once released, histamine diffuses rapidly into the surrounding tissues and appears in draining blood within minutes. Following ice water challenge of the hand of patients with cold urticaria, elevations of plasma histamine can be found in the venous effluent by $2\frac{1}{2}$ min, peak at 5 min, and return to baseline values by 15 to 30 min (89). Plasma histamine levels as low as 100 pg/ml (normal, 200–300 pg/ml) can be measured by a radioenzymatic assay in which the histamine-specific enzyme N-methyltransferase, isolated from rat kidney, transfers a radiolabeled methyl group from S-[methyl]-adenosyl-L-methionine onto histamine. The labeled 1-methylhistamine is then organically extracted and isolated by thin-layer chromatography, and the radioactivity quantitated (53).

The fluorometric assay for histamine, which is sensitive to 1 to 5 ng/ml, is based on the ability of o-phthalaldehyde to couple with histamine at alkaline pH to form a fluorescent complex which is then acidified to increase stability and intensity. To obtain maximum sensitivity with this method, which has been fully automated, samples are first dialyzed or acid-treated to remove protein. Other interfering compounds are removed in two organic extraction steps before condensation with o-phthalaldehyde (190). While this method is used primarily for research purposes, a variation employing cation exchange before organic extraction and o-phthalaldehyde condensation has been developed for the measurement of urine histamine (133). Normal urine histamine levels are 13 ± 8 ng/ml, 14 ± 9 µg/24 hr, or 14 ± 12 ng/mg creatinine/ml urine. Spot urine tests give the same information as 24-hr urine collections (133). Urine histamine assays offer the advantage of being less expensive than plasma radioenzyme assays, and because urinary histamine elevations are more prolonged than plasma elevations, abnormalities are more easily detected with the former. However, the assay for urine histamine is more labor-intensive than the plasma assay.

Elevations in plasma or tissue histamine levels have been found following experimental provocation with physical stimuli in a variety of physical urticarias, in antigen- and exercise-induced anaphylaxis (213) and bronchospasm (52,104), and in patients with mastocytosis (62,168). The urinary histamine level is increased in mastocytosis, as well as in a subgroup of patients with idiopathic hypereosinophilic syndrome and allergic disease, some patients with Zollinger–Ellison syndrome, and occasionally in pregnancy.

Only 2% to 3% of histamine is excreted unchanged in the urine. The rest is metabolized by two major enzymatic pathways (16,50,227) (Fig. 1). Fifty to seventy percent of histamine is metabolized by N-methyltransferase, located in the small intestine, liver, kidney, other tissues, and leukocytes, into N-methylhistamine, and 4% to 10% of histamine is excreted in this form. The rest of the histamine entering the N-methyltransferase pathway is further metabolized by monoamine oxidase to N-methylimidazoleacetic acid and excreted in the urine. The remaining 30% to 45% of histamine is metabolized by diamine oxidase, also called histaminase and located in small-intestinal mucosa, placenta, liver, skin, kidney, thymus, eosinophils, and neutrophils, to imidazoleacetic acid. Approximately one-third of the histamine entering this pathway is excreted in this form. The rest is conjugated with ribose and excreted in the urine as imidazoleacetic acid riboside.

HISTAMINE RECEPTORS

The presence of more than one histamine receptor was suggested by Ash and Schild (8) who initially noted that the classic antihistamine mepyramine could block histamine-induced contractions of guinea pig ileum but not histamine-induced gastric acid secretion. The presence of a histamine H-2 receptor was later confirmed by Black (26), who introduced burimimide, the first effective H-2 antagonist. Thus, the actions of histamine are mediated through two distinct receptors defined pharmacologically by the actions of their respective agonists and antagonists. Histamine H-1 receptor-mediated activities are stimulated by the H-1 agonists 2-methylhistamine, 2-[2-pyridyl]-ethylamine, and 2-[2-thiazolyl]ethylamine and are inhibited by "classic" H-1 antihistamines such as diphenhydramine, chlorpheniramine, and mepyramine. Histamine H-2 receptor-mediated activities are stimulated by the H-2 agonists 4-methylhistamine and dimaprit (26) and are inhibited by the H-2 receptor antagonists cimetidine, burimimide, and ranitidine (Table 2).

In early work, the distribution of histamine receptors

TABLE 2. *Histamine agonists and antagonists*

H-1 Agonists	H-2 Agonists
2-Methylhistamine	4-Methylhistamine
2-[Pyridyl]ethylamine (2PEA)	Dimaprit
2-[2-Thiazolyl]ethylamine	
H-1 Antagonists	H-2 Antagonists
Mepyramine	Burimimide
Diphenhydramine	Cimetidine
Chlorpheniramine	Ranitidine
Pyrilamine	
Promethazine	

on blood cells was determined by a histamine rosette assay (3,12,95,121,139,140,173). One-third of peripheral blood B lymphocytes, 10% of peripheral blood T cells, and macrophages were histamine rosette-positive. Immature B cells did not rosette with histamine. More recent work has focused on distinguishing between histamine H-1 and H-2 receptors on various blood cells (Table 3). The binding of [3H]pyrilamine has been employed to characterize the distribution of histamine H-1 receptors on human neutrophils and mononuclear cells (34,35,217). Neutrophils contain 2.6×10^5 H-1 receptors per cell with a single dissociation constant (K_D) of 52 nM (217), whereas unfractionated mononuclear cells contain two distinct classes of H-1 binding sites with K_D values of 4 nM and 55 μM and binding capacities of 21 fmole and 117 pmole, respectively (35). When human mononuclear cells were fractionated and binding of [3H]pyrilamine studied, additional H-1 receptors were noted (34). Resting monocytes had the highest affinity for [3H]pyrilamine ($K_D = 3.8$ nM), followed by helper T cells ($K_D = 5$ nM), B cells ($K_D = 14$ nM), and suppressor T cells ($K_D = 45$ nM). The rank order of the number of receptors per cell was opposite that of receptor affinity. Suppressor T cells expressed the greatest number of H-1 receptors per cell (3×10^5), followed by B cells (10^5), helper T cells (9×10^4), and monocytes (7×10^4). T cells stimulated with conconavalin A (Con A) or phytohemagglutinin (PHA) increased the receptor number by greater than fourfold without changing receptor affinity for [3H]pyrilamine.

The distribution and binding characteristics of H-2 receptors is less clear. Histamine conjugated to rabbit serum albumin (RSA) has been bound to Sepharose beads and used either in columns or in rosetting assays to detect histamine receptors (12). These histamine–albumin conjugates were 500 times more effective in binding leukocytes than unconjugated histamine (215) and have since been shown to bind nonspecifically (41). Other investigators have attempted to quantify H-2 receptors employing histamine conjugated to fluoresceinated human albumin (139), however, these conjugates also bind nonspecifically (132). Functional assays have demonstrated the presence of H-2 receptors on helper T cells (97), suppressor T cells (189), cytotoxic T cells (147,174), monocytes (102), eosinophils (39), neutrophils (4,182), and basophils (109,110).

TABLE 3. H-1 receptors on various blood cells

Cell	Receptors per cell	K_D (nM)
Monocyte	7×10^4	3.8
Helper T	9×10^4	5
B	10^5	14
Polymorphonuclear leukocyte	2.6×10^5	52
Suppressor T	3×10^5	45

TABLE 4. Pathogenic processes induced by histamine in various diseases

Process[a]	Relevant disease(s)
Vascular permeability	Rhinitis, asthma, urticaria, anaphylaxis
Smooth muscle contraction	Asthma
Pruritus	Urticaria, eczema, rhinitis
Vasodilation, flushing	Urticaria, anaphylaxis
Mucus secretion	Asthma, rhinitis
Gastric acid secretion	Peptic ulcer disease
Hypotension, shock	Anaphylaxis
Tachycardia	Anaphylaxis
Inhibition of T-cell function	Acquired agammaglobulinemia
Increases in cGMP, cAMP	—
Prostaglandin formation	Asthma, rhinitis

[a] cAMP, Cyclic adenosine monophosphate; cGMP, cyclic guanosine monophosphate.

Thus, H-1 receptors can be found (in order of number of receptors per cell) on suppressor T cells, neutrophils, B cells, helper T cells, and monocytes, as well as on basophils (196), mast cells (218), and eosinophils (39). H-2 receptors are defined functionally on helper T cells, suppressor T cells, cytotoxic T cells, monocytes, eosinophils, neutrophils, and basophils (144). A summary of some relevant H-1- and H-2-mediated actions of histamine is presented in Tables 4 to 8. Histamine H-1 and H-2 effects

TABLE 5. Activities mediated through histamine H-1 and H-2 receptors in humans

Receptor	Action[a]
H-1	Smooth muscle contraction
	Increase vascular permeability
	Increase in cGMP
	Pruritis
	Prostaglandin generation
	Decrease in arterioventricular node conduction time
	Activation of airway vagal afferent nerves
H-2	Gastric acid secretion
	Increase in airway mucus secretion
	Increase in cAMP
	Bronchial dilation (sheep and rabbit, possibly human)
	Esophageal contraction
H-1 + H-2	Hypotension
	Flushing
	Headache
	Tachycardia

[a] cAMP, Cyclic adenosine monophosphate; cGMP, cyclic guanosine monophosphate.

TABLE 6. *Effects of histamine on human granulocytes*

Cell type and effect[a]	H-1	H-2
Basophils		
↓ Antigen-induced histamine release		
Basophils	−	+
Skin mast cells	−	+
Lung mast cells	−	−
↑ Basophil cAMP level	−	+
↓ C5a-directed chemotaxis	−	+
↑ Basophil histamine production	+	−
Eosinophil		
Directly chemotactic	+	+
↓ C5a-mediated chemotaxis	−	+
↑ Chemotaxis	+	−
↑ cAMP level	−	+
↑ C3b receptors	+	−
↑ Parasite killing	+	−
Neutrophil		
↑ Chemokinesis	+	+
↓ Chemotaxis	−	+
↑ cAMP level	−	+
↓ FMLP-induced degranulation	−	+
↓ Degranulation	−	+

[a] ↑, Increases; ↓, decreases; cAMP, cyclic adenosine monophosphate; FMLP, N-formyl-met-leu-phe.

TABLE 7. *Effect of histamine on human mononuclear cells*

Cell type and effect[a]	H-1	H-2
Suppressor T cells		
Induction of contrasuppressor cells	+	−
Induction of suppressor T cells	−	+
Production of histamine suppressive factor	−	+
Cytotoxic T cells		
↓ Effector function	−	+
Helper T cells		
↑ cAMP level	−	+
↑ IL-2 production[b]	?	?
B cells		
↓ Ab synthesis	+	−
Monocytes		
↓ Complement production	−	+
↑ cGMP level	+	−
↑ O_2^- generation[c]	+	−
Lymphokine production		
↓ Production of MIF-like activity	−	+
Lymphocyte chemoattractant factor	−	+
LyMIF$_{35K+75K}$	+	−
Histamine suppressive factor	−	+

[a] ↑, Increases; ↓, decreases; cAMP, cyclic adenosine monophosphate; cGMP, cyclic guanosine monophosphate; IL-2, interleukin-2; MIF, migration inhibitory factor; LyMIF, lymphocyte migration inhibiting factor.
[b] Mouse only.
[c] Guinea pig only.

TABLE 8. *Histamine effects mediated by suppressor T cells*

Effect[a]	Mechanism[b]
↓ Lymphocyte proliferation	HSF
↓ Natural killer activity	HSF
↓ Production or release of immunoglobulins	Direct
↓ Helper T-cell generation	HSF
↓ Response of B cells to helper T factors	HSF

[a] ↓, Decreases.
[b] HSF, Histamine suppressive factor.

on inflammatory cells will be discussed in detail later in this chapter. Other effects relevant to inflammation, increases in cyclic nucleotides, prostaglandin generation, tachycardia, vasodilation, increased vascular permeability, and neural reflexes will be discussed briefly.

HISTAMINE AND VASODILATION

Erythema, secondary to vasodilation, is one of the cardinal signs of inflammation. The vasodilation-associated symptoms—flushing, headache, and hypotension—as well as some components of tachycardia can be caused by combined H-1 and H-2 stimulation. Histamine-induced tachycardia is due partly to H-1-induced decreased arterioventricular node conduction time (107) and probably is also influenced by vasodilation and adrenal catecholamine secretion. When histamine was infused into normal volunteers, plasma histamine elevations from the resting 300 pg/ml to between 1.5 and 2.5 ng/ml were associated with a 30% increase in heart rate, significant flush and headache, and a 30% increase in pulse pressure, primarily reflecting diastolic hypotension. Pretreatment with a H-2 antagonist alone had no effect on these actions, although pretreatment with a H-1 antagonist increased the histamine level required to elicit tachycardia but not the other symptoms. Pretreatment with combined H-1 and H-2 antagonists increased the histamine level required to induce the vasodilation-related symptoms and further increased the threshold for tachycardia (88). These results suggest that the treatment of hypotension associated with anaphylaxis which is unresponsive to epinephrine should include intravenous administration of both H-1 and H-2 antihistamines. (*Caution:* Intravenous H-2 antagonists must be administered slowly to avoid bradycardia or asystole.)

HISTAMINE AND EDEMA

Another important feature of inflammation is edema. Local or systemic administration of histamine causes increased microvascular permeability with edema formation in both connective tissue and mucosal surfaces (128,222).

Ultrastructural studies on rat skin have suggested that this is a consequence of the contraction of endothelial actin-myosin filaments in postcapillary venules, which leads to the formation of intercellular gaps (17,116). Plasma proteins larger than 135 Å (93) extravasate through these gaps which are estimated to be at least 12 nm in diameter (94). The presence of plasma proteins in connective tissue alters the normal colloid osmotic gradient, and fluid efflux rapidly ensues. The familiar wheal formation at allergy skin test sites is the clinical correlate of this phenomenon. Marks and Greaves (116) evaluated the wheal and flare responses to injected histamine and compound 48/80 in healthy volunteers pretreated with placebo, chlorpheniramine, and/or cimetidine. They found that cimetidine alone decreased both the wheal (19%) and flare (21%) responses to histamine, but not to 48/80. Chlorpheniramine also inhibited both histamine responses (each by 30%), as well as responses to 48/80. While a small, additive inhibition was noted when both chlorpheniramine and cimetidine were used, it was not statistically significant. Smith et al. (191) studied the effect of oral cimetidine on antigen skin test responses in eight atopic patients. The area of the wheals formed both before and during cimetidine treatment were essentially unchanged for each individual patient as well as for the group as a whole. Summers et al. (197) was unable to confirm any H-2 actions of histamine on human cutaneous whealing responses to histamine, compound 48/80, or antigen, whereas H-1 antagonists effectively reversed each reaction. Thus, evidence for H-2 receptor influence on vascular permeability is weak and not reproducible, suggesting that increased vascular permeability is largely H-1-mediated.

HISTAMINE AND NEURAL INTERACTIONS

Histamine can also influence certain neural reflexes, and these interactions have been best studied in the lung. The interaction of histamine with the parasympathetic nervous system has been well studied in canine models of asthma. Vagotomized dogs were administered histamine or antigen with or without atropine, and parasympathetic discharge, dynamic compliance, and total lung resistance measured. Histamine caused discharge of irritant receptors, triggering both local and central vagal reflexes with resultant bronchoconstriction (46,67,188). The vagal reflexes were more important in low-dose compared to high-dose histamine-induced bronchostriction and were inhibitable by H-1 but not H-2 antagonists, thus suggesting H-1 receptor mediation.

Evidence for the importance of histamine–vagus interactions in human airway constriction stems from inflammatory models of airway reactivity. When compared to healthy controls, normal subjects develop increased his-

tamine responsiveness after upper respiratory tract infections with pathogens capable of denuding airway epithelium. This increased responsiveness can be reversed or prevented by atropine inhalation, suggesting that histamine is acting by stimulating irritant receptors exposed by the infection (54). Similarly, a 2-hr exposure to 0.6 ppm of ozone causes increased airway reactivity to inhaled histamine in about 50% of healthy nonsmoking adults. The response to histamine can be blocked with atropine inhalation, suggesting that the histamine-induced bronchospasm in ozone-exposed subjects may be secondary to vagal reflexes (68).

There is some evidence to suggest that histamine may also act to "prime" α-adrenergic responses in the lung. Tracheal smooth muscle preparations from normal human subjects or from canines do not respond *in vitro* to exogenous norepinephrine. However, the same tissue pretreated with histamine contracts on subsequent exposure to norepinephrine. This response is inhibited by the α-adrenergic blocking agent phentolamine. Tracheal and bronchial tissues obtained from patients with a variety of respiratory diseases contract in response to norepinephrine without requiring histamine pretreatment; however, histamine augments the contractile response. In both normal and diseased tissues, phentolamine prevents the contractile response, suggesting that histamine is capable of increasing airway α-adrenergic responsiveness *in vitro* (99).

In addition to interacting with the cholinergic and adrenergic nervous systems, histamine can also interact with neuropeptides, a class of neurotransmitters found in endocrine glands and coexisting in nerve fibers and ganglia with other neurotransmitters. The best studied neuropeptides are vasoactive intestinal peptide (VIP), the possible mediator of the nonadrenergic, noncholinergic inhibitory system, and substance P. Much of our knowledge to date stems from nonhuman primate studies from which inferences can be drawn to human models.

Cholinergic, adrenergic, and motor nerve fibers have been demonstrated to contain VIP in various organ systems (170). Animal gut and airways undergoing vagal or electrical field stimulation release VIP, and this can be inhibited by hexamethonium or by the neurotoxin tetrodotoxin, but not by cholinergic or adrenergic blockage (47). Thus, VIP is released directly from cholinergic, adrenergic, and motor nerve endings. Since histamine is capable of causing vagal stimulation with release of acetylcholine, histamine stimulation would theoretically also be expected to result in VIP release. This has not yet been demonstrated in the human, however.

VIP in the airway causes relaxation of tracheobronchial smooth muscle, vasodilation, increased ion transport into the airway lumen, and in the human, a decrease in secretion of sulfated macromolecules (136). It can inhibit antigen-induced release of histamine from guinea pig lung *in vitro* (210) and also inhibits the bronchoconstrictive effects of a prostaglandin (PGF$_{2\alpha}$), histamine (171), and a leukotriene (LTD$_4$) in the guinea pig (74). Several investigators found that VIP inhalation caused bronchodilation in some but not all human asthmatic subjects (13,129,130). Overall, the data suggest that histamine, probably acting through cholinergic stimulation, may induce release of VIP. This neuropeptide might be capable of inhibiting further histamine release from mast cells and may counteract some of the direct and indirect bronchoobstructive effects of histamine in the large airways.

Substance P is located in the C fibers of afferent sensory nerves innervating human connective tissue, smooth muscle, and blood vessels (113). Substance P in nanomolar concentrations induces histamine release from rat mucosal and peritoneal mast cells (184). In human skin, substance P injected intradermally in picomolar concentrations causes a wheal and flare reaction inhibitable by the mast cell stabilizer doxantrazole, by the histamine H-1 antagonists diphenhydramine (86) and chlorcyclizine, or by mast cell histamine depletion with compound 48/80 (73). Pretreatment of human skin with capsaicin, which depletes C fibers of substance P and other neurotransmitters, inhibits the flare, but not the wheal, response to histamine injected intradermally (114). These data taken together suggest that substance P causes release of histamine from human mast cells, that histamine is capable of causing release of substance P from sensory nerve fibers, and that both histamine and substance P contribute to histamine-induced vasodilation.

Thus, histamine is capable of stimulating cholinergic discharge, increasing α-adrenergic responsiveness, and stimulating substance P release. A negative feedback loop may exist in which histamine causes release of VIP, which could reduce further release of histamine. Interactions with the cholinergic system involve direct activation of irritant receptors via H-1 receptors with resultant vagal reflexes. The mechanism by which histamine interacts with the α-adrenergic system is less clear; however, data suggest that increasing α-adrenergic responsiveness is probably involved. The neurologic mechanism by which histamine causes liberation of VIP and substance P is not known.

HISTAMINE AND PROSTAGLANDIN GENERATION

Histamine-induced generation of PGs is also of interest. Platshon and Kaliner (142) showed that antigen-induced anaphylaxis of human lung resulted in release of histamine as well as PGF$_{2\alpha}$, PGE$_2$, and thromboxane B$_2$. Release of PGF$_{2\alpha}$ could also be induced by treatment with exogenous histamine or the H-1 agonist 2-methylhistamine,

but not by the H-2 agonist dimaprit. Further, the generation of PGF$_{2\alpha}$ could be blocked by pretreatment with H-1, but not H-2, antagonists. Thus, H-1 receptor stimulation of human lung results in PGF$_{2\alpha}$ generation (142).

This work was extended to animal models in order to delineate mechanisms by which histamine stimulation of lung tissue lead to PG formation (195). It was found that histamine H-1 stimulation of airways led to the formation of PGE$_2$, whereas peripheral guinea pig lung produced PGF$_{2\alpha}$ as well as PGE$_2$. Although other studies have shown lung tissue to additionally produce thromboxane A$_2$, PGI$_2$, 5-, 12-, and 15-hydroxyeicosatetraenoic acids, and leukotrienes (2,75,157,175,176,222), the mechanisms observed for histamine-induced PG release in guinea pig lung may be illustrative of the mechanisms responsible for the generation of these other eicosanoids as well. In peripheral lung, histamine's actions, prevented by H-1 antagonists, are not reproduced by either muscarinic stimulation or depolarizing concentrations of KCl, indicating that prostaglandin generation is unrelated to muscle contraction. Thus, it appears that histamine stimulation of nonmuscle cells accounts for PGF$_{2\alpha}$ generation. Airway stimulation by histamine also causes PG generation, but this tissue responds equally well to muscarinic stimulation and KCl, indicating that PG formation in airways probably reflects muscle contraction. Thus, the likely source of PGE$_2$ and PGI$_2$ from airways stimulated with histamine is the contracting muscle fiber itself.

HISTAMINE EFFECTS ON BASOPHILS

Histamine, released locally during inflammation, is capable of affecting cells recruited into the inflammatory response. Histamine in low concentrations (10^{-6}–$10^{-7}M$) inhibits antigen-induced histamine release from human basophils (27,207) and human skin mast cells (207), but does not affect histamine release from human lung cells (87) or calcium ionophore A23187-induced histamine release from human basophils (108). Antigen-induced basophil histamine release is inhibited 80% to 90% if basophils are exposed to antigen and histamine together, compared to 20% to 40% inhibition if histamine is introduced 2 min after basophil exposure to antigen (27). Thus, exogenous histamine inhibits antigen-induced histamine release from human basophils and skin mast cells, but not from human lung mast cells, and this inhibitory effect in the basophil occurs during the activation stage of IgE-mediated histamine release rather than during the mediator releasing stage.

When basophils were exposed to exogenous histamine, inhibition of antigen-induced histamine release was proportional to the rise in basophil intracellular cyclic adenosine monophosphate (cAMP) levels. Both effects were blocked maximally by the histamine receptor H-2 antagonist burimimide (10^{-5}–10^{-6} M), but not by the histamine H-1 receptor antagonists pyrilamine, promethazine, and chlorpheniramine (10^{-4} M) (109). Further, the effect of histamine on basophil cAMP and histamine release could be mimicked by the histamine H-2 receptor agonists 4-methylhistamine and dimaprit, but not by the histamine H-1 receptor agonist 2-methylhistamine (110). The histamine H-2 antagonist cimetidine alone enhanced antigen-induced basophil histamine release by blocking the inhibitory effect of released histamine (208). Thus, inhibition of human basophil histamine release is mediated through H-2 receptors and correlates with increases in basophil intracellular cAMP levels.

Histamine in low concentrations (10^{-8} M) also inhibits the chemotactic response of human basophils to C5a but not to a lymphokine-derived chemotactic factor or to *N*-formyl-met-leu-phe (FMLP) (107). The histamine H-2 receptor antagonist metiamide (10^{-4} M) blocked histamine-induced inhibition of chemotaxis to C5a. Pyrilamine alone, an H-1 receptor antagonist, inhibited C5a-induced basophil chemotaxis and had no further effect on histamine-induced inhibition of basophil chemotaxis. Thus, histamine, acting through H-2 receptors, inhibits basophil recruitment into complement but not lymphocyte-mediated inflammatory foci.

Stuart and Kay (196) showed that histamine in high concentrations (10^{-3} M) caused increased histidine uptake by human basophils with subsequent increased histamine production. Relatively low concentrations of histamine H-1 antagonists (10^{-5} M), but not histamine H-2 antagonists, blocked this response. Thus, the data taken together suggest that histamine in low concentrations, acting via its H-2 receptor, inhibits human basophil recruitment into complement-mediated inflammatory foci and inhibits antigen-induced histamine release from human basophils and skin but not lung mast cells. In contrast, histamine in high concentrations acting via its H-1 receptor increases histidine uptake and histamine synthesis by human basophils, thus increasing the basophils' capacity to participate in inflammatory reactions.

HISTAMINE AND EOSINOPHILS

Histamine, in a concentration of 10^{-5} to 10^{-4} M, is directly chemotactic for human eosinophils (40). Histamine-induced chemotaxis is not blocked by either H-1 or H-2 antagonists given alone, but is effectively blocked by the combination of histamine H-1 and H-2 antagonists (29,40,209). Similar results have been found in a guinea pig model of *in vivo* antigen-induced cutaneous anaphylaxis. The H-1 antagonist pyrilamine (2 mg/kg) and the H-2 antagonist cimetidine (120 mg/kg) given alone had

no effect on eosinophil infiltration. The two antagonists given in combination before antigen challenge, however, caused a 75% reduction in eosinophil infiltration measured 6 hr after antigen challenge (224). Thus, histamine-induced eosinophil chemotaxis can occur through stimulation of either histamine H-1 or H-2 receptors.

The effect of histamine on C5a-induced human eosinophil chemotaxis is concentration-dependent. Clark et al. (39) found that, at concentrations of at least 10^{-5} M, histamine caused an increase in eosinophil intracellular cAMP levels and a decrease in C5a-directed chemotaxis, whereas at lower concentrations, C5a-directed eosinophil chemotaxis was enhanced. The histamine-induced inhibition of C5a-directed chemotaxis correlated with the rise in cAMP levels and could be inhibited by the histamine H-2 antagonist metiamide (10^{-4} M) but not by the histamine H-1 antagonist pyrilamine. In contrast, the histamine-induced enhancement of C5a-directed eosinophil chemotaxis was inhibited by pyrilamine but not by metiamide. Thus, at low concentrations, histamine, acting through stimulation of its H-1 receptor, enhances C5a-directed chemotaxis, whereas at higher concentrations, histamine causes an increase in cAMP levels and a decrease in C5a-directed chemotaxis through stimulation of the histamine H-2 receptor.

Histamine also influences the expression of complement receptors on human eosinophils. Exogenous histamine (10^{-6}–10^{-4} M) added to human eosinophils caused a dose-dependent increase in the expression of C3b receptors as measured by a rosetting response (5). The effect on C3b receptor expression could be mimicked by the histamine H-1 receptor agonist 2-aminoethylthiazole, but not by the histamine H-2 receptor agonists dimaprit and 4-methylhistamine. Further, the histamine-induced increase in the expression of eosinophil C3b receptors could be blocked by the histamine H-1 antagonists chlorpheniramine and mepyramine (10^{-5} M), but not by the histamine H-2 antagonists burimimide and metiamide (6). When histamine-treated eosinophils were exposed to Schistosomula and Trichinella, parasite killing was enhanced (7). The enhanced killing correlated with enhanced C3b receptor expression and could be blocked by histamine H-1 but not H-2 receptor antagonists. Thus, histamine H-1 receptor stimulation causes increased expression of eosinophil C3b receptor expression and enhanced parasite killing.

The data, taken together, suggest that histamine is capable of enhancing the recruitment of human eosinophils into inflammatory lesions, as well as enhancing the killing efficiency of recruited eosinophils. Enhanced recruitment is achieved through a direct chemotactic effect of histamine on eosinophils mediated by both H-1 and H-2 receptor stimulation, as well as by H-1-mediated enhancement of complement-directed chemotaxis. H-2 receptor stimulation by high concentrations of histamine, however, causes decreased complement-directed eosinophil chemotaxis. Histamine-induced augmentation of parasite killing is closely associated with increased eosinophil C3b receptor expression and is mediated through stimulation of H-1 receptors. Thus, eosinophil H-1 receptor stimulation, particularly at low concentrations of histamine, has a proinflammatory effect through enhancement of chemotaxis, C3b receptor expression, and killing, whereas H-2 receptor stimulation inhibits complement-directed chemotaxis.

HISTAMINE AND NEUTROPHILS

Histamine is also capable of altering the function of human neutrophils. At concentrations between 10^{-4} and 10^{-6} M, histamine enhanced chemokinesis stimulated by casein, zymosan-activated serum (5), and the peptide FMLP (182). At concentrations between 10^{-3} and 10^{-6} M, histamine also inhibited stimulated chemotaxis to all three agents, but by itself had no effect on motility (4). The effect of histamine on enhancing chemokinesis and inhibiting chemotaxis was associated with an increase in cAMP levels (4) and could be mimicked by either H-1 or H-2 agonists (182). The inhibitory effect of histamine on stimulated chemotaxis could be blocked by pretreatment with levamisol, an agent which increased cyclic guanosine monophosphate (cGMP) levels, or by pretreatment with the H-2 antagonist metiamide, but not by pretreatment with the H-1 antagonists diphenhydramine and pyrilamine (4,182). Thus, histamine nonspecifically enhances neutrophil chemokinesis, and it inhibits chemotaxis through histamine H-2 receptors. The mechanism by which histamine exerts this dual effect is unclear but may involve inhibiting the detection of a gradient of chemotactic factor without altering the stimulation of motility by chemoattractants (182).

Histamine also influences various aspects of neutrophil activation. Pretreatment with histamine (10^{-7}–10^{-2} M) decreased FMLP- but not phorbol myristate acetate- or A23187-induced alterations in neutrophil membrane potential (182), superoxide anion production, and hydrogen peroxide production (141,150) without blocking FMLP binding or internalization. Release of the primary granule enzyme β-glucuronidase in response to cytochalasin B plus serum-treated zymosan (30,229) or FMLP (182) was also inhibited by histamine and paralleled a rise in cAMP levels (30). All four effects could be mimicked by the H-2 agonist dimaprit (30,182) and, at high concentrations only, by the H-1 agonists 2-pyridylethylamine (2PEA) and pyrilamine, which is consistent with their weak H-2 agonist properties (182). The effect could be blocked only by the H-2 antagonist metiamide and not by the H-1 antagonist

chlorpheniramine. Thus, histamine-induced inhibition of neutrophil activation and degranulation is mediated through the H-2 receptor.

Seligman et al. (182) demonstrated that histamine inhibited release of lysozyme, found in both primary and secondary neutrophil granules, to a lesser degree than β-glucuronidase, which is found only in primary neutrophil granules (182). This suggests that the inhibitory effect of histamine on neutrophil degranulation is specific for primary granules only. The inhibitory effect of histamine on degranulation was more potent on neutrophils from normal subjects, compared to neutrophils from subjects with asthma (18,31) or atopic eczema (32), and paralleled a relative decrease in histamine-induced cAMP production. The decreased sensitivity of neutrophils to histamine-induced inhibition of stimulated degranulation was unrelated to the intrinsic ability of the neutrophils to degranulate, as neutrophils from all three groups degranulated equally in response to cytochalasin B plus serum-treated zymosan. Thus, the data indicate that neutrophils of atopic and asthmatic subjects have an impairment in histamine H-2 receptor-mediated regulatory processes.

A relative insensitivity to histamine-induced inhibition of stimulated degranulation was also found in normal neutrophils incubated with viruses. This defect was not specific for histamine, however, as the cells also responded suboptimally to isoproterenol and PGE, suggesting a postreceptor defect (33). The possibility of β blockage contributing to histamine insensitivity in neutrophils incubated with virus and neutrophils from atopic and asthmatic patients was investigated. Pretreatment of normal neutrophils with the β-adrenergic antagonist propranolol did not alter the inhibitory effect of histamine on neutrophil degranulation. Thus, the decreased sensitivity of neutrophils incubated with virus and neutrophils from atopic and asthmatic individuals to histamine H-2 stimulation is unrelated to responsiveness to β agonists.

HISTAMINE AND SUPPRESSOR T CELLS

Most of histamine's actions on lymphocytes are mediated by suppressor T cells either directly or through a soluble suppressor factor, histamine-induced suppressor factor (HSF). The role of histamine in suppressor T-cell induction was initially characterized in animal models.

Mozes et al. (131) observed that *in vitro* exposure of mouse spleen cells to antigen resulted in induction of suppressor T cells which, when transferred into irradiated recipients, suppressed the immune response to subsequent antigen challenge. If the spleen cells were first exposed to antigen in the presence of histamine (10^{-4} M) or other cAMP active agents such as PGs or cholera enterotoxin, the induction of suppressor T cells was abrogated. This effect was blocked by addition to the mixture of the H-1 antagonist diphenhydramine, thus implicating the H-1 receptor in suppressing antigen induction of suppressor T cells.

Schwartz et al. (180) reported similar observations. Histamine (10^{-3} M) inhibited Con A induction of murine suppressor T cells. However, in this system the effect of histamine was mimicked by the H-2 agonist dimaprit (5×10^{-4} M) but not by the H-1 agonist 2PEA (10^{-4}–10^{-5} M). Similar results were found in the guinea pig. Histamine-induced inhibition of antigen-stimulated blastogenesis was inhibited by the H-2 antagonist burimimide but not by the H-1 antagonist chlorpheniramine (22,158). Thus, in contrast to Mozes' findings, histamine inhibition of Con A and antigen induction of suppressor T cells seemed to be H-2-mediated.

A series of cell mixing experiments helped explain these apparently contradictory results (189). Spleen cells from BGAF mice treated *in vivo* with the toleragen trinitrobenzenesulfonic acid (TNBS cells) exert no regulatory effect on *in vitro* primary generation of antitrinitrophenyl self-cytotoxic cells and do not themselves develop cytotoxic activity. When TNBS cells were incubated *in vitro* with histamine (10^{-4} M) for 30 to 60 min before coincubation with effector cells, suppressor activity could be induced in the TNBS cells. However, these results were found inconsistently. TNBS-treated spleen cells preincubated with the H-2 agonist dimaprit consistently suppressed primary induction of cytotoxicity, whereas cells preincubated with the H-1 agonist 2PEA alone, or in combination with dimaprit, exerted no regulatory effect. Thus, suppression was induced by histamine H-2 receptor stimulation, but this could be inhibited or reversed by H-1 receptor stimulation.

When TNBS cells preincubated with 2PEA were added to dimaprit-induced suppressor T cells, the suppressor activity was markedly reduced, suggesting that H-2 stimulation induces suppressor T cells, whereas H-1 stimulation induces a separate contrasuppressor cell population (189). Similar bidirectional findings were reported by Gershon et al. (64) and Yamauchi et al. (225) who uncovered substantial suppressor activity after treating 2PEA-induced (I^-J^+) contrasuppressor cells with anti-I-J antibody plus complement, thus removing the contrasuppressor population.

The mechanism by which histamine induces suppression of lymphocyte functions was investigated employing a guinea pig model. Lymph node cells from both immune and nonimmune strain-2 guinea pigs, when incubated with histamine (10^{-5}–10^{-3} M), elaborate a nondialyzable 23,000- to 40,000-molecular-weight factor (HSF). This factor, when added to sensitized lymphocytes, reversibly inhibited release of migration inhibitory factors (MIFs) and the proliferative response to antigen (159). HSF was made by macrophage-depleted and T-cell-enriched, but not B-cell-enriched (162), populations of lymph node cells, implicating the T lymphocyte as the source of HSF.

HSF activity was detectable in spleen and lymph nodes, but not in blood or thymic cells, before immunization. Activity increased, peaking 2 weeks following immunization, concomitant with the appearance of HSF activity in blood and thymic lymphocytes. The passage of lymphocytes over a histamine affinity column removed the HSF producing cells and rendered the nonadherent cells refractory to histamine (163).

Both H-1 (2-methylhistamine) and H-2 (4-methylhistamine) agonists in high (10^{-3} M) concentrations induced the production of HSF, but only the H-2 agonist was effective at low (10^{-5} M) concentrations (163). Further, only a H-2 antagonist (burimimide) and not an H-1 antagonist (chlorpheniramine) blocked the production of HSF (159). Thus, HSF production is mediated through the histamine H-2 receptor.

HSF activity was also found in a mouse model (202) in which spleen cells incubated with histamine (10^{-4} M) elaborated a 45,000- to 68,000-molecular-weight factor which inhibited the response of syngeneic spleen cells to PHA. The suppressive activity in the spleen cell supernatants was removed by passage over a histamine-RSA-Sepharose (H-RSA-S) column but not by passage over a rabbit anti-mouse Ig column. Suppressive activity was also blocked by prostaglandin synthetase inhibitors, suggesting that prostaglandin formation is required for expression of HSF activity.

Similar results have been found in the human (11,45,69,164,211). Human suppressor T cells activated by histamine elaborate a suppressive factor also termed HSF. Human HSF has been characterized (165); it is stable at pH 3 to 10, but sensitive to temperatures greater than 80°C. HSF is a glycoprotein, as it is sensitive to chymotrypsin, trypsin, sodium periodate, and neuraminidase. Its biologic activity remained intact following reduction and alkylation and following treatment with phenylmethylsulfonyl fluoride, an irreversible serine esterase inhibitor. Thus, HSF activity is not dependent on intact disulfide bonds or reactive serine groups. When supernatants from antigen-specific and nonspecifically stimulated lymphocytes were applied to Sephadex G100, two fractions that eluted with molecules with molecular weights of 25,000 to 40,000 had HSF activity (as measured by inhibition of [^{3}H]thymidine incorporation). When this material was subjected to polyacrylamide gel electrophoresis (pH 8.7) under nonreducing conditions, two peaks of HSF activity were found, one emerging with albumin and the other anodal to albumin. Thus, the data suggest that HSF is probably a family of molecules rather than a single molecule. Generation of HSF can be elicited by stimulation of a variety of lymphocyte receptors, including the histamine H-2 receptor.

However, Meretry (124) observed that the chemiluminescence of human mononuclear cells exposed to PHA was increased by low concentrations of histamine (10^{-8}–10^{-10} M) and inhibited by higher concentrations. When mononuclear cells were incubated with the H-2 antagonist cimetidine plus low concentrations of histamine, chemiluminescence was further augmented. 2PEA alone had no effect, but when cimetidine was added, augmentation of PHA-induced chemiluminescence occurred. Thus, there is evidence for bidirectional effects of histamine on human mononuclear cells similar to that seen in rodents where H-2 receptor stimulation activates suppressor T cells, whereas H-1 stimulation activates contrasuppressor cells. In most systems, however, the net effect of histamine has been activation of suppressor T cells with resultant immunosuppression.

Brostoff et al. (28) observed that histamine (10^{-4} M) incubated with human peripheral blood lymphocytes and Con A inhibited thymidine incorporation into the cells. These findings were confirmed by Rocklin and Haberek-Davidson (160), who found that human blood mononuclear cells incubated 24 hr with histamine suppressed PHA-induced thymidine incorporation into normal autologous cells under coculture conditions. The suppressive effect of histamine was dose-dependent (10^{-8}–10^{-3} M). The precursors of the cells mediating histamine-induced suppression bore histamine receptors, as cells not removed by passage over a histamine Sepharose column normally exerted no regulatory effect after incubation with histamine. A minimum of 2 hr incubation with histamine was required to activate suppressor cells, and maximum suppression was achieved by 18 to 24 hr.

The metabolic requirements for activation of suppressor T cells have been examined. Human blood mononuclear cells were incubated 24 hr with histamine (10^{-3}–10^{-5} M), with and without various metabolic inhibitors, washed, and added to lectin-stimulated autologous mononuclear cells, and the suppression of thymidine uptake was measured. Suppressor activity was abrogated by inhibitors of transcription (actinomycin D), translation (puromycin or cycloheximide), oxidative phosphorylation (sodium azide), glycolysis (2-deoxyglucose) and cytoskeletal function (cytochalasin B or colchicine) (161). Thus, active cell metabolism and protein production are necessary for the induction of suppressor T cells, but DNA synthesis and cell proliferation are not necessary, as suppression was unaffected by mitomycin (161) or irradiation (172).

HISTAMINE-INDUCED SUPPRESSOR T CELLS AND MONOCYTES

Hebert et al. (77) observed that mononuclear cells incubated 24 hr with histamine, mitomycin-treated, and subsequently cocultured with normal autologous mononuclear cells suppressed the blastogenic response to mitogen (Con A or PHA) and antigen. In order to delineate

which cell was responsible for histamine-induced inhibition of mitogen-induced proliferation, fractionated lymphocytes were studied separately. Enriched B lymphocytes incubated with histamine exerted no regulatory effects, while partially purified T cells caused a reduced amount of inhibition. When T cells were further purified by depletion of glass-adherent cells, suppression was markedly reduced. Suppressor activity could be restored by the addition of monocytes. Thus, monocytes or their products are a necessary component in histamine-induced suppressor T-cell induction and/or expression.

To delineate the role of monocytes in histamine-induced suppression, monocytes were selectively eliminated from the induction and/or the effector stage of T-cell-mediated suppression (21). Cells depleted of glass-adherent cells during incubation with histamine (10^{-3}–10^{-4} M) could not exert suppression. When autologous adherent cells or supernatants from autologous monocytes stimulated by phagocytosis of heat-killed *Staphylococcus albus* were added during the generation phase, suppressor T-cell activity was restored. If, however, intact monocytes were removed and replaced by supernatants of stimulated monocytes during both the generation and effector stages, suppression was markedly reduced. Suppression was also reduced if indomethacin was added with intact monocytes during the effector stage, but not during the generation phase. Thus, monocytes or their products are required during both the generation and effector stages of histamine-induced T-cell-mediated suppression, but the accessory product is different for each phase.

Insights into the role of monocytes in histamine activation of suppressor T cells was gained by the observation that supernatants from human mononuclear cells caused monocytes but not lymphocytes to increase production of PGE$_2$, PGF$_{2\alpha}$, and thromboxane B$_2$. These same supernatants mimicked histamine-activated suppressor T cells in inhibiting mitogen-induced lymphocyte proliferation, and there was a chromatographic overlap of the factor which inhibited proliferation (24,000–40,000 molecular weight) and that which induced prostaglandin production (25,000 molecular weight) (166). Thus, histamine-induced suppressor T cells release a soluble factor, HSF, which inhibits mitogen-induced lymphocyte proliferation and may also induce prostaglandin production by monocytes. To better understand the role of prostaglandins in histamine-induced suppression, histamine-treated mononuclear cells were cocultured with normal autologous cells and mitogen in the presence of indomethacin with or without exogenous PGE$_2$ (166). In the absence of PGE$_2$, inhibition was suppressed. However, when the indomethacin-treated mononuclear cells were reconstituted with PGE$_2$, the suppressor T cells were able to exert an inhibitory effect. Thus, monocyte-derived PGE$_2$ is necessary for the expression of histamine-induced suppression.

The nature of the factor in activated monocyte supernatants required during the generation phase of histamine-induced suppressor T cells was also investigated. Sequential purification and separation of crude monocyte supernatants using gel filtration, immunoadsorption, and isoelectric focusing demonstrated that only those fractions containing leukocyte pyrogen and lymphocyte activating factor, now collectively known as IL-1, were capable of reconstituting histamine or Con A-induced suppressor activity in T lymphocytes depleted of glass-adherent monocytes (19). Thus, these studies suggest that the accessory role of activated monocyte supernatants in generating histamine- or mitogen-induced suppressor T cells is mediated by IL-1. Taking the data as a whole, histamine, in the presence of monocytes or IL-1, induces the generation of suppressor T cells. These suppressor cells release HSF, which causes elaboration from monocytes of PGE_2 as well as $PGF_{2\alpha}$ and thromboxane B_2. It is unclear whether PGE_2 directly mediates the inhibition of mitogen-induced blastogenesis or whether it acts as an accessory to suppressor T cells (Fig. 2).

There are several observations suggesting that atopic individuals have a defect in histamine-induced suppressor function (18,20,117,118,197,198). Martinez et al. (117) and Staszak et al. (194) reported that peripheral blood mononuclear cells of atopic and HLA-B12 individuals, respectively, contained a normal number of histamine receptor bearing cells but required a higher-than-normal concentration of histamine to induce suppression *in vitro* (10^{-3} M compared to 10^{-5} M in normal controls). There was no difference in Con A-induced suppression between the normal and the atopic subjects.

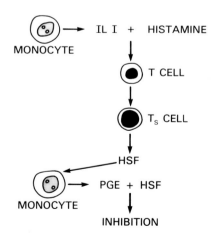

FIG. 2. Proposed mechanism of HSF-induced suppression. Histamine in the presence of monocytes or exogenous IL-1 induces differentiation of T cells into suppressor T cells with elaboration of a suppressor factor, HSF. HSF then stimulates monocyte PGE_2 production which, acting with HSF, causes suppression. IL-1, Interleukin-1; HSF, histamine suppressive factor; PGE, prostaglandin E.

When the distribution of H-1 and H-2 receptors was studied, the percentage of T cells bearing H-2 receptors was found to be reduced in atopic subjects, whereas the percentage of cells bearing H-1 receptors was unchanged (20). This reduction in the expression of H-2 receptors correlated positively with abnormal histamine-induced T suppression. Nonatopic controls with mastocytosis expressed normal numbers and function of lymphocyte H-2 receptors. Thus, the defect in histamine-induced suppression seen in atopic patients is not due to a down-regulation of H-2 receptors by chemically elevated plasma histamine.

Further investigation revealed a defect in the interaction of lymphocytes and monocytes in producing histamine-induced suppression (118). Atopic subjects had normal numbers of helper and suppressor cells, but their lymphocytes generated less suppressor activity as well as less HSF than did normal lymphocytes, and the defects were not corrected by exogenous IL-1. Thus, the defect in histamine-induced HSF production is not secondary to decreased monocyte IL-1 production or to reduced numbers of suppressor T cells. PGE_2 production stimulated by HSF was, however, reduced in atopic monocytes compared to normals. Thus, decreased suppressor activity in atopic individuals is due both to decreased production of HSF and to decreased monocyte response to native as well as exogenous HSF.

HISTAMINE-INDUCED SUPPRESSOR T CELLS AND HELPER T CELLS

The role of helper T cells in T-cell-mediated suppression is poorly characterized. Khan et al. (97) observed that histamine (10^{-3}–10^{-2} M) induced elevations in cAMP levels in Leu 2^+ 9.3^- human suppressor T cells, and to a lesser degree in Leu 3^+ helper T cells and Leu 2^+ 9.3^+ cytotoxic T cells. The effect was inhibited by the H-2 antagonist cimetidine (10^{-5} M), but not by the H-1 antagonist mepyramine 10^{-6} M, suggesting that the cAMP response in all three cell types was mediated through functional H-2 receptors. Following stimulation with PHA or with Con A plus monocytes, responsiveness to histamine (10^{-4} M) increased in helper and cytotoxic T cells, but not in suppressor T cells. Thus, resting suppressor T cells are responsive to physiologic concentrations of histamine, whereas cytotoxic and helper T cells are responsive only when activated or when in the presence of activated suppressor T cells.

This work was extended in a murine model (96). Alloreactive helper T cells were cocultured with allogeneic stimulator cells, and interleukin-2 (IL-2) production was measured. If the helper cells were preincubated with histamine before exposure to alloantigen, IL-2 production was enhanced. Conversely, if histamine was added together with helper and stimulator cells, IL-2 production, but not helper T-cell proliferation, was suppressed. Thus, the effect of histamine on helper T-cell function is dependent on the conditions. It is not clear in the human, however, whether helper T cells are necessary for the generation or expression of histamine-induced suppressor T cells.

HISTAMINE-INDUCED T SUPPRESSION AND NATURAL KILLER CELLS

Histamine also inhibits natural killer (NK) cell activity in the mouse (167) and human (134,135). Nair and Schwartz (134) observed that both the H-1 antagonist clemastine fumarate and the H-2 antagonist cimetidine, but not histamine, inhibited the NK activity (^{51}Cr release assay) of peripheral blood lymphocytes, T cells, and NK-enriched cells when added directly to mixtures of effector and target cells. Interestingly, histamine reversed the inhibitory effect of H-1 and H-2 antagonists. Histamine antagonists decreased target–effector cell binding, although histamine alone had no effect on binding.

When histamine (10^{-3}–10^{-7} M) was added to peripheral blood mononuclear cells together with target cells, NK activity was enhanced. This effect was dependent on the presence of monocytes and was not ascribable to interferon (IFN) (79). However, peripheral blood lymphocytes precultured for 24 hr with histamine (10^{-4}–10^{-3} M) showed a significant decrease in NK activity. Further, adherent cell-depleted lymphocytes precultured with histamine contained increased numbers of OKT8$^+$ cells and suppressed the NK activity of fresh autologous effector lymphocytes (134). Thus, the data suggest that histamine is capable of acting with monocytes to enhance NK activity, as well as to inhibit NK activity through activation of suppressor T cells.

To determine whether suppressor T-cell inhibition of NK activity could be mediated by HSF, lymphocytes were precultured with supernatants from histamine-activated lymphocytes and cocultured with K562 target cells, and NK activity was measured by ^{51}Cr release assay. HSF caused a dose-dependent suppression of NK activity throughout a wide range of target/effector cell ratios. Production of HSF was elicited by histamine, but not by H-1 or H-2 antagonists, and was blocked by the H-2 antagonist cimetidine. Although HSF inhibited the activity of large granular lymphocytes (LGLs), it was not produced by LGLs. Further, the inhibition of NK activity could be reversed by treating effector lymphocytes with interferon-α (IFN-α) for 1 or 2 hr or by culturing them with IL-2 for 36 hr (135).

Thus, histamine inhibition of NK activity is mediated through HSF, which is elaborated by histamine-induced suppressor T cells. Further, the effects of HSF on NK activity can be overcome by treating effector cells with IFN-α for 1 or 2 hr or with IL-2 for 36 hr. The exact mechanism through which HSF exerts its inhibitory effect on NK cells has not been studied, however, several possibilities exist. HSF is known to interfere with DR expression on human lymphocytes (63), and several investigators have observed that IFN-α can increase lymphocyte DR expression (14,120). Thus, HSF may interfere with DR expression on NK cells, and the reversal of inhibition caused by IFN-α could be secondary to restoration of DR expression.

HSF can decrease murine IL-2 production (96), and there is evidence to suggest a critical role of IL-2 in IFN-α production (90,91). Thus, HSF may interfere with IFN-α production, and IL-2 would be expected to reverse this effect. These and other possible mechanisms need to be examined.

HISTAMINE-INDUCED SUPPRESSOR T CELLS AND B CELLS

Histamine-induced suppressor T cells also regulate B-cell function. Segal et al. (181) rendered BalbC mice immune to sheep red blood cells by repetitive injection of lysed red blood cells in high doses. Suppression of T-cell-dependent IgG production was transferable by adoptive cell transfer into irradiated syngeneic recipients. However, transfer was blocked if spleen or peripheral blood immune cells were first passed over a histamine affinity column and the adherent cells removed. Suppression was restored by reconstitution with adherent cells. Further, suppression could be blocked by treating immune cells with complement and anti-φ (anti-T-cell antibody) before the transfer. Thus, the cell responsible for transferring suppression of IgG production was a T cell with a histamine receptor. Histamine-adherent cells from antigen-exposed mice, but not from unexposed mice, could cause suppression of antibody production. Thus, generation of antigen-specific suppressor T cells required antigen exposure. Since the suppressor cells had no effect on IgM (T-cell-independent) production, the target cell for suppression was a helper T cell rather than a B cell.

The role of histamine-induced suppressor cells in inhibiting antibody production was further studied *in vitro* in the human (111). Histamine (10^{-6}–10^{-4} M) added to human mononuclear cells caused a dose-dependent inhibition of pokeweed-induced, but not spontaneous, IgG production. The suppressive effect was observed 7 days after pokeweed stimulation and was found when histamine was added up to but not after 72 hr following pokeweed exposure. The cell responsible for causing inhibition was an E rosette$^+$, OKT8$^+$, OKT4$^-$ cell sensitive to irradiation and activated by histamine. To determine the type of histamine receptor responsible for activation, T cells were incubated with histamine in the presence or absence of H-1 or H-2 agonists or antagonists for 24 hr, washed, and added together with pokeweed to B cells, and IgG production was measured. The H-1 antagonist diphenhydramine (10^{-4} M) was slightly more effective than histamine 10^{-4} M in inhibiting IgG production, but the effect of histamine plus diphenhydramine was not additive. The H-2 antagonist cimetidine (10^{-4} M) had no effect alone and did not inhibit the effect of histamine. Both the H-1 agonist 2PEA (10^{-4} M) and the H-2 agonist dimaprit (10^{-6} M) caused equal inhibition of IgG synthesis (112). Thus, the mechanism by which histamine induces suppressor T-cell-mediated inhibition of IgG synthesis is unclear from these experiments but appeared to involve activation of either H-1 or H-2 receptors or both.

These results were partially explained by experiments in which human peripheral blood T lymphocytes were fractionated according to their ability to bind sheep red blood cells after exposure to theophylline (24,25). Cells which retained the ability to bind sheep red blood cells were termed theophylline-resistant, and those which lost the ability were termed theophylline-sensitive. Resting theophylline-sensitive T cells bore receptors for the Fc portion of IgG (RFcγ) and caused radiosensitive inhibition of pokeweed mitogen-induced B-cell differentiation. Theophylline-resistant T cells were depleted of RFcγ and enhanced pokeweed mitogen-induced B-cell differentiation. Brief exposure of theophylline-resistant cells to the H-2 agonist impromidine caused a rapid increase in the number of cells bearing RFcγ, β_2-microglobulin, and the surface antigen recognized by OKT8, whereas the proportion of cells bearing the OKT4 antigen decreased. There was no change in the expression of OKT3, OKT5, or Ia antigens, C1q, surface immunoglobulin, or sheep erythrocyte receptors. Impromidine treatment of theophylline-resistant T lymphocytes also induced a radioresistant suppression of pokeweed mitogen-induced B-cell differentiation. Conversely, exposure of theophylline-sensitive T cells to the H-1 agonist 2PEA caused a marked decrease in radiosensitive suppressor activity, as well as a decrease in the number of RFcγ expressed on theophylline-sensitive cells. Thus, histamine, acting through its H-1 receptor, causes differentiation of a theophylline-resistant subset of T cells into cells which suppress polyclonal B-cell activation. Conversely, H-2 stimulation enhances polyclonal B-cell activation by down-regulating a separate subset of theophylline-sensitive cells which normally suppress polyclonal B-cell activation.

The mechanism by which suppressor T cells inhibit IgG production was also studied. Histamine- or Con A-induced suppressor T cells, generated *in vitro* and then irradiated with 3000 rads, were added to fresh lymphocytes either at the beginning of culture or after 7 days in culture with pokeweed mitogen, and IgG was measured by a re-

verse hemolytic plaque assay (78). Con A-induced suppressor cells caused inhibition of IgG production when added at the beginning or at the end of culture (40% and 8% inhibition, respectively), whereas histamine-induced suppressor cells caused inhibition only if added at the end of culture (43%). Thus, histamine-induced suppressor cells are different than Con A-induced suppressor cells and function by directly inhibiting either the production or release of IgG without affecting the proliferation and maturation of B lymphocytes. This effect was not due to HSF, as low-dose irradiation (1200 rads) abrogates the release of HSF (160,205).

Garovoy et al. (63) studied the role of HSF in the inhibition of immunoglobulin production. Polyclonal B-cell activation was assessed by measuring plaque forming cells generated during a primary mixed-lymphocyte culture in the presence or absence of HSF. The addition of HSF on day 0 of culture reduced IgG, IgM, and IgA production equally (60–80%). To study the effect of HSF on the helper T component of immunoglobulin synthesis, purified T cells were activated in a unidirectional mixed-lymphocyte culture and then combined with unprimed B cells to induce a polyclonal plaque forming cell response. HSF added either during the generation phase of helper T cells or during the coculture phase inhibited the plaque forming cell response equally (83% and 76%). Further, the expression of Ia and autologous DR antigens detectable on 50% to 60% of control activated T cells was reduced to 20%, suggesting that HSF prevented the activation as well as the functioning of helper T cells. HSF also reduced the polyclonal B-cell response to preformed mixed-lymphocyte culture-derived helper T factors. Thus, HSF inhibits immunoglobulin production by interfering with the generation and functioning of human helper T cells as well as the B-cell response to helper T factors.

As a whole, the data indicate that histamine modulates immunoglobulin synthesis through several different T-cell-dependent mechanisms. H-2 receptor stimulation decreases radiosensitive suppression of polyclonal B-cell activation caused by a theophylline-sensitive subset of suppressor T cells. It also activates suppressor T cells to elaborate HSF, which then interferes with helper T-cell maturation as well as the response of B cells to preformed helper factors. H-1 receptor stimulation causes maturation of a theophylline-resistant subset of T cells into suppressor cells which exert radioresistant suppression on polyclonal B-cell activation. Thus, the effect of histamine-induced T cells on immunoglobulin synthesis depends on the balance of these three effects.

HISTAMINE AND CYTOTOXIC T CELLS

Histamine directly inhibits the effector function of cytotoxic T lymphocytes. Henney et al. (80) demonstrated that the activity of cytotoxic T lymphocytes obtained from the spleen of C57BL/6 mice immunized with mastocytoma DBA/2 cells was inhibited by histamine (10^{-5}–10^{-3} M). The maximal inhibition obtainable was 50% and paralleled a rise in cAMP levels (80). This inhibition of cytotoxic T-cell effector function is mediated through the histamine H-2 receptor, as both the inhibitory effect (147,148) and the rise in cAMP levels (179) are competitively inhibited by the H-2 antagonists cimetidine (147,148,179), burimimide, and metiamide but not by the H-1 antagonists diphenhydramine and pyrilamine (147,148). Further, cytotoxic T-cell inhibition is induced by the H-2 agonists 4-methylhistamine, dimaprit, and impromidine, whereas the H-1 receptor agonists 2-PEA and 2-methylhistamine mimic the effect only at high concentrations (145), reflecting their weak H-2 agonist properties.

Cytotoxic T cells can be desensitized to H-2 receptor stimulation. A 5-min incubation with histamine reduced by 50% the ability of cloned mouse cytotoxic T cells to raise their cAMP level following subsequent histamine challenge. The receptors were completely desensitized after a 60-min incubation with histamine and remained desensitized over 24 hr. The dose of histamine causing a 50% maximal response was unaltered by preincubation with histamine, suggesting that desensitization does not affect the receptor number (179). Similarly, cells could be desensitized *in vivo* by intraperitoneal injection of histamine 1 to 3 hr before a histamine challenge. Full activity was restored if cells were maintained *in vivo* for several days (145).

If histamine or a H-2 agonist is present during immunization, induction of cytotoxic T cells specific for the immunizing alloantigen is inhibited (179). Following induction of cytotoxic T cells, *in vivo* sensitized spleen cells are refractory to modulation by histamine or other cAMP-active agents until the seventh day after immunization when stimulation of H-2 receptors causes inhibition of cytotoxic activity (149). The cytotoxic activity of spleen cells sensitized *in vitro* is not inhibitable by histamine or other cAMP-active drugs (149). This seems to be an effect of the culture conditions, because cells sensitized *in vivo* lose their histamine responsiveness within 3 hr when maintained in culture (146).

Histamine receptor bearing cells are essential for the development of cytotoxicity. When spleen cells from balb/c mice were passed over a H-RSA-S column before sensitization with irradiated C57B/6 cells, the cytotoxic response was markedly diminished. The response was completely restored by repleting the culture with H-RSA-S-adherent cells, but was unaffected by varying the concentrations of macrophages or suppressor T cells (177). Thus, either precursors or amplifiers of cytotoxic T cells bear histamine receptors.

These findings raise the interesting question of whether histamine effects on cytotoxic T lymphocytes may be mediated through suppressor T cells or some other cell type. To investigate this possibility, C57BL/6 mice were immunized with PT18 cells intraperitoneally, or their spleen cells were sensitized in culture. Cytotoxic T cells generated *in vivo* but not *in vitro* were inhibitable by histamine. Histamine inhibition of cytotoxic T-cell activity from mixed populations of *in vivo* and *in vitro* spleen cells was only additive—not augmented—suggesting that the lack of histamine responsiveness in cultured cells is not due to the absence of suppressor cells. Further, the histamine responsiveness of *in vivo* generated cytotoxic T cells was lost if the cells were restimulated *in vitro* within 24 hr (143).

To ascertain that histamine acts directly on the cytotoxic T cells rather than through a soluble factor, such as HSF, immunized spleen cells were exposed to histamine in the presence of target cells, and the resulting supernatants were then added to fresh immunized spleen cells plus target cells. The supernatant-induced inhibition of cytotoxic T-cell function was abolished by the addition of histaminase, supporting a direct action of histamine on cytotoxic T cells (145).

Thus, histamine acting through a H-2 receptor inhibits induction of specific cytotoxic T lymphocytes and directly inhibits cytotoxic activity after induction. Histamine H-2 receptors on cytotoxic T cells can be desensitized *in vivo* but regain full function within 24 hr. Histamine refractoriness in cultured cytotoxic T lymphocytes results from a loss of functional H-2 receptors secondary to the culture conditions.

HELPER T CELLS

Relatively little is known about the effect of histamine on helper T cells. Histamine (10^{-3}–10^{-2} M) causes a mild increase in cAMP accumulation in resting Leu 3$^+$ human helper T cells. Pretreatment of unfractionated T cells with PHA for 72 hr augments only slightly the cAMP response to histamine (10^{-4}). However, purified helper T cells activated with PHA showed a marked enhancement in their ability to respond to histamine. The effect of histamine on helper T cells was totally blocked by the H-2 antagonist cimetidine (10^{-5} M) but not by the H-1 antagonist mepyramine (10^{-6} M) (97). Thus, although resting human helper T cells respond only minimally to histamine, activated helper T cells dramatically increase cAMP accumulation following histamine challenge. This effect is mediated through H-2 receptor stimulation and is inhibited by other T-lymphocyte subsets, presumably suppressor T cells.

The effects of histamine on helper T cells were further studied in a murine model (96). Alloreactive helper T cells were cocultured with allogeneic stimulator cells, and IL-2 production was measured. When cloned helper T cells were preincubated with histamine (10^{-4} M) for 1 hr, washed, and subsequently added to stimulator cells, IL-2 production was enhanced. This effect was due to a shift in the kinetics (a 6- to 10-hr peak in the treated and an 18-hr peak in the untreated group), as well as an increase in the amount of IL-2 released.

In contrast, when histamine was added to the helper-stimulator T-cell culture, the time course of IL-2 release was unchanged, but the amount of activity released was significantly diminished. The receptor specificity for these effects is unknown (96). Thus, histamine is capable of activating and enhancing IL-2 release from isolated helper T cells, but this effect is negated in the presence of other lymphocytes. It is probable that the effect of histamine on helper T cells is regulated by suppressor T cells.

HISTAMINE AND B CELLS

In addition to the effects described previously, histamine also inhibits immunoglobulin synthesis in mice by non-T suppressor-mediated mechanisms. Melmon et al. (122) noted that histamine (10^{-5}–10^{-3} M) and other agents which increase cAMP inhibited plaque formation by spleen cells of *in vivo* immunized mice. The effect was enhanced by theophylline (which inhibits phosphodiesterase) and inhibited by cholera toxin (which activates adenylate cyclase), suggesting mediation through cAMP. However, several histamine antagonists, pyribenzamine, pyrilamine, diphenhydramine, and antazolidine, also cause inhibition of plaque formation without raising cAMP levels. Thus, the receptor specificity of the histamine effect could not be determined, and the association of inhibition with increased cAMP was not clear. Histamine receptor bearing cells are an important component in plaque formation, however, as immune spleen cells not binding to an immobilized histamine column have a greatly reduced capacity to make anti-sheep red blood cell antibodies (123).

LAF$_1$ mice pretreated with intravenous histamine (5 × 10^{-6} M) 1 day before immunization with trinitrophenol (TNP) also had a reduced capacity to mount an IgG antibody response (203). Inhibition of antibody production was transferable by serum, but not by spleen cells, from histamine-treated immunized mice. The factors responsible for inhibition were IgG$_1$ and IgG$_{2a}$ antibodies against the Fab$_2$ portion of LAF$_1$-derived anti-TNP. Thus, the data suggest that histamine treatment before antigen exposure induced the formation of auto antiidiotype antibodies which then inhibit *in vitro* antibody production.

Experiments in which mice were treated with histamine after Con A exposure suggest that histamine may interfere with the induction phase of antibody synthesis, either at the level of macrophage processing or at the level of the helper T cell (10). Mice were injected with Con A 24 hr

before administration of high-dose histamine, and the antibody response to sheep red blood cells (T-cell-dependent) or polyvinylpyrrolidone (PVP-T-independent) given 2 hr later was measured. Histamine inhibited the antibody response to the T-dependent, but not the T-independent, antigen. Immune suppression was not due to suppressor T cells, as it was not transferable with treated spleen cells nor was it reversed by adoptive transfer of normal syngeneic spleen cells at the time of antigen administration. Because fresh cells could not reverse the effect, inhibition was at the level of the induction phase. The effect was mimicked by the H-1 agonist 2-methylhistamine and by adrenocorticotropic hormone and corticosterone, but not by the H-2 agonist dimaprit. Thus, the data suggest that H-1 receptor stimulation causes release of glucocorticoids which then inhibit either helper T function or antigen processing.

The data taken together suggest that H-1 receptor stimulation causes inhibition of the induction of antibody synthesis, and that this effect is mediated by glucocorticoids. Further, histamine stimulation can induce the formation of auto antiidiotype antibodies which interfere with antibody production. It is possible that H-1 receptor stimulation, acting through glucocorticoids, induces helper T cells which enhance auto antiidiotype antibody production.

HISTAMINE AND MONOCYTES AND MACROPHAGES

The effects of histamine on human monocytes and macrophages are limited. Lappin and Whaley (102) found that histamine caused an irreversible, dose-dependent (10^{-7}–10^{-4} M) inhibition of the production of the second component of complement (C2) by cultured human monocytes. The inhibition was prevented by the H-2 antagonist cimetidine but not by the H-1 antagonist chlorpheniramine, and was simulated by the H-2 agonists dimaprit and 4-methylhistamine but not by the H-1 agonist 2(2-aminoethylthiazole). Thus, the inhibition of C2 production is mediated through H-2 receptors.

In further work, Lappin et al. (103) studied the effect of histamine on monocyte production and release of various components of the complement cascade. Histamine (10^{-7}–10^{-3} M) cultured 7 days with human monocytes inhibited the release of newly synthesized C2, C4, C3, factor B, and β1H-globulin. Immunofluorescent staining demonstrated the presence of the five complement components in all monocytes cultured with histamine. However, synthesis of complement was decreased as assessed by measuring the uptake of ^{3}H-labeled amino acids into complement components. Taken together, the data suggest a negative feedback loop mediated through the H-2 receptor. Histamine released from mast cells or basophils following stimulation by C5a and C3a inhibits synthesis and release of several components of complement necessary to form the C3 ($\overline{C42}$) and C5 ($\overline{C423b}$) convertases.

Histamine also causes accumulation of intracellular cGMP in guinea pig alveolar macrophages (183) but has no effect on adenylate cyclase activity from guinea pig peritoneal macrophages (154). To determine the receptor specificity of the cGMP effect, guinea pig lung was exposed to histamine and treated with an immunofluorescent probe for cGMP (183). Alveolar macrophages were one of the earliest cells to demonstrate a rise in cGMP levels. The results could be simulated by the H-1 agonist 2-methylhistamine but not by the H-2 agonist dimaprit. Thus, increased cGMP accumulation is mediated by H-1 receptors.

Histamine conjugated to serum-treated zymosan also caused an increase in guinea pig alveolar macrophage production of superoxide anion radicals (O_2^-) (48). This effect could be blocked by the H-1 antagonists chlorpheniramine and mepyramine, but not by the H-2 antagonists burimimide and metiamide (49). Thus, H-1 stimulation appears to cause production of O_2^- in guinea pig alveolar macrophages. The receptor specificity data must be viewed with caution, however, since histamine–protein conjugates can bind nonspecifically (41).

Overall, the data indicate that histamine, acting through its H-1 receptor, is proinflammatory, causing accumulation of intracellular cGMP and O_2^- generation. In contrast, stimulation of H-2 receptors decreases inflammation by inhibiting the synthesis and release of several complement components necessary to form C3 and C5 convertases.

HISTAMINE AND LYMPHOKINES

In addition to HSF, histamine causes elaboration by lymphocytes of a factor chemotactic for eosinophil (100) and also effects the production of MIF-like activity (153,155). Histamine caused a 40% to 60% suppression of delayed-type hypersensitivity (DTH) responses of guinea pigs immunized with *o*-chlorobenzene–bovine γ-globulin (OCB-BGG) in complete Freund's adjuvant when given intradermally together with the OCB-BGG (158,178,216). Inhibition of DTH was completely reversed with the H-2 antagonist burimimide, but only partially reversed with the H-1 antagonist chlorpheniramine. Exogenous histamine (10^{-5}–10^{-3} *M*) inhibited the production of MIF by T cells in a mixed T cell–macrophage culture when given within 1 hr of antigen sensitization. The *in vitro* effect was inhibited by H-2 antagonists, but unlike the situation in the *in vivo* DTH model, H-1 antagonists had no effect on *in vitro* inhibition of MIF production (158). When histamine-adherent mononuclear cells were removed, MIF production in response to antigen was normal (162). Thus, MIF producing cells are regulated

by histamine receptor bearing cells, although they do not themselves express histamine receptors.

The putative agent responsible for inhibiting MIF production is a 23,000- to 40,000-dalton molecule elaborated by human T cells (155). This factor is poorly characterized but is distinct from cAMP, as its activity is unaffected by phosphodiesterase (159).

Histamine also causes elaboration of chemoattractant lymphokines. Foon et al. (58) found that histamine in combination with serotonin, but not alone, caused lymphocytes to secrete a factor chemotactic for monocytes. A second factor, lymphocyte chemoattractant factor (LCF), is produced by human mononuclear cells (37,38) and is chemokinetic for human lymphocytes but not for neutrophils or monocytes. LCF is a 56,000-dalton cationic factor with an isoelectric point of 9. It is stable to heat, sensitive to trypsin and neuraminidase, and has no HSF activity. The production of LCF is blocked by the H-2 antagonist cimetidine, but not by the H-1 antagonist diphenhydramine. Thus, LCF production is H-2-mediated.

Histamine also causes elaboration of two noncytotoxic inhibitors of T-cell migration, lymphocyte migration inhibiting factors (LyMIFs) (38). LyMIF$_{35K}$ is a 35,000-dalton cationic glycoprotein with an isoelectric point of 8.5, which is susceptible to heat and neuraminidase but not to trypsin. LyMIF$_{75K}$ is a 75,000-dalton molecule with an isoelectric point of 7.5, which is sensitive to trypsin but not to heat or neuraminidase. Elaboration of both LyMIF$_{35K}$ and LyMIF$_{75K}$ is inhibited by H-1 but not by H-2 antagonists. Further, cells not adherent to histamine-albumin-Sepharose columns do not make LyMIFs or LCF (23). Thus, LyMIF production is mediated through H-1 receptors, whereas LCF production is H-2-mediated.

On the whole the data suggest that histamine causes elaboration of several lymphokines. HSF made by suppressor T cells inhibits lymphocyte proliferation, NK activity, and antibody production, and a second T-cell factor inhibits MIF production. Both factors are under H-2 receptor control. Four other factors exist. One is a poorly defined monocyte chemotactic factor made by lymphocytes stimulated concomitantly by both serotonin and histamine. LCF, chemotactic for lymphocytes, is made by H-2-stimulated mononuclear cells, whereas LyMIF$_{35K}$ and LyMIF$_{75K}$, made by H-1-stimulated mononuclear cells, inhibit lymphocyte mobility. Thus, the influence of histamine on the accumulation of mononuclear cells at sites of inflammation is dependent on the combined effects of these six lymphokines.

CLINICAL CORRELATES

The role of histamine in clinical inflammation has been evaluated in several diseases. Late phase allergic reactions (LPRs) are characterized by burning induration beginning approximately 4 hr after antigen challenge in susceptible allergic subjects and last for 24 hr or longer. They are characterized by early neutrophil and eosinophil infiltration, followed by a predominately round-cell infiltrate as the lesion matures. Mast cell degranulation detected by the presence of histamine and neutrophil chemotactic factor of anaphylaxis occurs early during LPRs.

Intradermal histamine alone will not elicit LPRs (204). Antihistamines, however, have been noted to inhibit LPRs, suggesting that histamine may contribute. Lemanske et al. (105) evaluated the intensity of the inflammatory and blueing responses during LPRs in rats injected intradermally with anti-IgE or with mast cell granules. Pretreatment with the H-1 antihistamine diphenhydramine partially inhibited the intensity of inflammation 24 hr after challenge. The H-2 antihistamine cimetidine had no effect alone but potentiated the effect of diphenhydramine when the two were used in combination. The inhibitory effect was lost when a LPR was elicited by mast cell granules washed free of histamine, suggesting that H-1 antihistamines alone or in combination with H-2 antihistamines inhibited LPR by specifically antagonizing the effects of histamine.

Similar results have been found in the human. Aas (1) studied the effect of the H-1 antagonist clemastine on the LPR elicited by local antigen challenge following passive cutaneous sensitization. When given daily for 3 days before the challenge, the H-1 antagonist mildly suppressed the LPR. Smith et al. (192) examined the effect of H-2 as well as H-1 antagonists on the immediate wheal and flare reaction and the LPR responses to cutaneous antigen challenge with timothy grass and ragweed. The H-1 antagonist alone (clemastine) given the day of and 1 day before the challenge inhibited the immediate but not the late response, whereas the H-2 antagonist alone (cimetidine) had no effect on either response. When the H-2 antagonist was given in combination with the H-1 antagonist, inhibition of the immediate response was augmented and the LPR was completely inhibited in most subjects.

The effect of local administration of the H-1 antagonist mepyramine on cutaneous LPRs has also been studied. Gronneberg et al. (72) found that the LPR caused by intradermal anti-IgE (1:40) was inhibited by administration of 30 μg mepyramine mixed with the anti-IgE. A lower dose of mepyramine (3 μg) was ineffective.

Thus, H-1 antagonists partially inhibit cutaneous LPRs, and the intensity of the inhibitory effect is related to the dose and time of administration of the H-1 antagonist. H-2 antagonists given alone have no effect on cutaneous LPRs, but the combination of H-1 and H-2 antagonists causes moderate to strong inhibition of cutaneous LPRs in both the rat and the human. Thus, the data, taken as a whole, suggest that histamine is at least partially responsible for causing cutaneous LPRs and that this effect is mediated through both H-1 and H-2 receptors.

Histamine has also been evaluated in hyper IgE (HIE or Job's) syndrome, a disease characterized by recurrent cutaneous Staphylococcus aureus infections, eczema, soft-tissue pyogenic infections, and hyper IgE, much of which is directed against S. aureus. As noted above, histamine has been demonstrated in vitro to interfere with neutrophil chemotaxis, and H-2 receptor antagonists have been reported to be effective in reversing the neutrophil chemotactic defect in HIE both in vitro (81) and in vivo (119). Dreskin et al. (51), however, were unable to find a correlation between 24-hr urinary histamine concentrations and either the presence of infection or the level of total or S. aureus-directed IgE. However, urinary histamine but not plasma histamine was elevated in a subgroup of HIE patients with chronic eczematous dermatitis compared to HIE patients with no skin manifestations, normal controls, and patients with chronic granulomatous disease. Thus, the data indicate that histamine is not involved in the pathogenesis of recurrent infections but may play a role in chronic eczematoid dermatitis in HIE patients.

The knowledge that histamine exerts an immunosuppressive effect largely through H-2 receptor stimulation has led to the use of H-2 antagonists in several disease states characterized by immune suppression. Jorizzo et al. (85) studied four patients with chronic mucocutaneous candidiasis with absent cell-mediated responses to candida as assessed by absent DTH skin tests, MIF production, and lymphocyte transformation to candida antigen for 4 to 8 weeks. Cimetidine therapy reversibly corrected the defect in MIF production and DTH, but not lymphocyte transformation. Cimetidine has also been reported to increase the DTH response to a variety of antigens in duodenal ulcer patients (9) and to cause increased immunoglobulin production in patients with common variable hypogammaglobulinemia and elevated suppressor T function (223). Cimetidine has also been found to reverse immune suppression commonly found following cholecystectomy (76) and in malignant disorders such as ovarian carcinoma (98), melanoma, and colorectal cancer (57).

The exact mechanism by which cimetidine enhances immunity is unclear. Certainly in clinical situations of increased histamine-induced suppression cimetidine could exert its immunostimulatory effect as an H-2 antagonist. However, there are conflicting reports suggesting that cimetidine may also have intrinsic immunomodulary function. Gifford and Schmidtke (65,66) reported that cimetidine exposure in vitro augmented bacterial antigen-, mitogen-, and alloantigen-induced blastogenesis of human peripheral blood lymphocytes. However, Festen et al. (56) was unable to confirm these findings and reported that cimetidine had no effect on human DTH, lymphocyte counts, or blastogenic responses to either mitogen or antigen.

The effect of cimetidine on NK activity has been better studied. Láng et al. (101) reported that cimetidine inhibited NK activity in normal subjects in a dose-dependent fashion. These findings were confirmed by Ruiz-Argüelles et al. (169) who found a biphasic dose response of cimetidine inhibition of NK activity. Subsequently, Flodrgen and Sjögren (57) reported that cimetidine enhanced NK activity in normal subjects as well as in patients with malignant melanoma and colorectal cancer.

These conflicting results were explained by the finding that cimetidine pretreatment enhanced the IFN-α augmentation of NK activity but also decreased IFN-α production (83). Further studies showed that cimetidine enhanced the antiviral properties of IFN-α. When effector cells were pretreated with cimetidine for 16 hr, both NK activity and IFN-α production were decreased (82). Thus, although cimetidine inhibits NK activity by inhibiting IFN-α production, it can also enhance the efficacy of IFN-α. Thus, the net effect of cimetidine on NK activity is a balance of decreased production and increased efficacy of IFN-α.

Cimetidine has also been found to decrease *in vivo* activity of dinitrofluorobenzenesulfonic acid (DNFB)-induced mouse Lyt 2^+ suppressor T cells in a model of contact sensitivity (70). Both the expression and, to a lesser extent, the induction of suppressor T cells was inhibited. In contrast, Lyt 1^+ suppressor T cells induced by ultraviolet irradiation were not affected by cimetidine (71), suggesting that at least two classes of suppressor T cells exist that differ in susceptibility to down-regulation by cimetidine.

In contrast to these findings, Mekori et al. (120) found that cimetidine reversed the nonspecific immunosuppression of contact sensitivity caused by burns, but not that caused by DNFB. The reasons for these conflicting results are not clear, but may be due to variations in the murine subjects used or treatment protocols. Clearly, more work needs to be done to establish the mechanisms by which cimetidine exerts its immunomodulatory functions.

CONCLUSIONS

The cardinal signs of inflammation are erythema, fever, edema, and pain. Histamine, released in response to antigen stimulation, certain inflammatory cell factors, opioids, and physical stimuli, is capable of causing vasodilation, increased vascular permeability, and pain. Thus, histamine is capable of causing three of the four cardinal signs of inflammation and, by triggering increased vascular permeability, it is capable of augmenting the infiltration of leukocytes into inflammatory foci. H-1 stimulation of leukocytes tends to be proinflammatory, whereas H-2 stimulation suppresses inflammation in most tissues. Many of the immunosuppressive actions of histamine are mediated through a soluble factor, HSF, elaborated by suppressor T cells. The role of histamine in human disease is best documented in atopic eczema, peptic ulcer disease, late phase allergic reactions, and some cases of acquired hypogammaglobulinemia. It is likely that histamine is important in other immunosuppressed states as well.

ACKNOWLEDGMENTS

The authors would like to thank Vickie Zabel for technical assistance.

REFERENCES

1. Aas, K. (1979): Effects of ketotifen and clemastine on passive transfer of reaginic reaction. *Allergy,* 34:121–124.
2. Adkinson, N. F., Jr., Newball, H. H., Findlay, S., Adams, K., and Lichtenstein, L. M. (1980): Anaphylactic release of prostaglandins from human lung *in vitro. Am. Rev. Respir. Dis.,* 121:911–920.
3. Alvares, J. M. N. (1980): Characterization of human peripheral blood lymphocyte cells on the basis of surface properties. *Allergol. Immunopathol. (Madr.),* 8:679–684.
4. Anderson, R., Glover, A., and Rabson, A. Z. (1977): The *in vitro* effects of histamine and metiamide on neutrophil motility and their relationship to intracellular cyclic nucleotide levels. *J. Immunol.,* 118:1690–1697.
5. Anwar, A. R. E., and Kay, A. B. (1977): The ECF-A tetrapeptides and histamine selectively enhance human eosinophil complement receptors. *Nature,* 269:522–524.
6. Anwar, A. R. E., and Kay, A. B. (1978): Enhancement of human eosinophil complement receptors by pharmacologic mediators. *J. Immunol.,* 121:1245–1250.
7. Anwar, A. R. E., and Kay, A. B. (1980): H1-receptor dependence of histamine-induced enhancement of human eosinophil C3b rosettes. *Clin. Exp. Immunol.,* 42:196–199.
8. Ash, A. S., and Schild, H. O. (1966): Receptors mediating some actions of histamine. *Br. J. Pharmacol.,* 27:427–439.
9. Avella, J., Madsen, J. E., Binder, H. J., and Askenase, P. W. (1978): Effect of histamine H2-receptor antagonists on delayed hypersensitivity. *Lancet,* 1:624–626.
10. Badger, A. M., Griswold, D. E., DiMartino, M. J., and Poste, G. (1982): Inhibition of antibody synthesis by histamine in concanavalin A-treated mice: The possible role of glucocorticosteroids. *J. Immunol.,* 129:1017–1022.
11. Badger, A. M., Young, J., and Poste, G. (1984): Reversal of histamine-mediated immunosuppression by structurally diverse histamine type II (H₂) receptor antagonists. *Int. J. Immunopharmacol.,* 6:467–473.
12. Ballet, J. J., and Merler, E. (1976): The separation and reactivity *in vitro* of a subpopulation of human lymphocytes which bind histamine: Correlation of histamine reactivity with cellular maturation. *Cell. Immunol.,* 24:250–269.
13. Barnes, P. J., and Dixon, C. M. S. (1984): The effect of inhaled vasoactive intestinal peptide on bronchial reactivity to histamine in humans. *Am. Rev. Respir. Dis.,* 130:162–166.
14. Basham, T. Y., and Merigan, T. C. (1983): Recombinant interferon increases HLA-DR synthesis and expression. *J. Immunol.,* 130:1492–1494.
15. Bealieu, L., Beaudoin, J., Jobie, M., and Hébert, J. (1986): Effects of H₁ and H₂ receptor agonists on nonspecific proliferative response of human peripheral blood lymphocytes. *Int. Arch. Allergy Appl. Immunol.,* 79:249–252.
16. Beavens, M. A. (1978): Histamine: Its role in physiologic and pathologic processes. *Monogr. Allergy,* 13:1–20.
17. Becker, C. G., and Nachman, R. L. (1973): Contractile proteins of endothelial cells, platelets and smooth muscle. *Am. J. Pathol.,* 71:1–22.

18. Beer, D. J. (1984): Abnormalities in the histamine-induced suppressor cell network in atopic subjects. *N.E.R. Allergy Proc.*, 5: 318–323.

19. Beer, D. J., Dinarello, C. A., Rosenwasser, L. J., and Rocklin, R. E. (1982): Human monocyte-derived soluble product(s) has an accessory function in the generation of histamine- and concanavalin A-induced suppressor T cells. *J. Clin. Invest.*, 70:393–400.

20. Beer, D. J., Osband, M. E., McCaffrey, R. P., Soter, N. A., and Rocklin, R. E. (1982): Abnormal histamine-induced suppressor-cell function in atopic subjects. *N. Engl. J. Med.*, 306:454–458.

21. Beer, D. J., Rosenwasser, L. J., Dinarello, C. A., and Rocklin, R. E. (1982): Cellular interactions in the generation and expression of histamine-induced suppressor activity. *Cell. Immunol.*, 69:101–112.

22. Beets, J. L., and Dale, M. M. (1979): Inhibition of guinea-pig lymphocyte activation by histamine and histamine analogues. *Br. J. Pharmacol.*, 66:365–372.

23. Berman, J. S., McFadden, R. G., Cruikshank, W. W., Center, D. M., and Beer, D. J. (1984): Functional characteristics of histamine receptor-bearing mononuclear cells. II. Identification and characterization of two histamine-induced human lymphokines that inhibit lymphocyte migration. *J. Immunol.*, 133:1495–1504.

24. Birch, R. E., and Polmar, S. H. (1982): Pharmacological modification of immunoregulatory T lymphocytes. I. Effect of adenosine, H_1 and H_2 histamine agonists upon T lymphocyte regulation of B lymphocyte differentiation *in vitro*. *Clin. Exp. Immunol.*, 48:218–230.

25. Birch, R. E., Rosenthal, A. K., and Polmar, S. H. (1982): Pharmacological modification of immunoregulatory T lymphocytes. II. Modulation of T lymphocyte cell surface characteristics. *Clin. Exp. Immunol.*, 48:231–238.

26. Black, J. W., Duncan, W. A. M., Durant, C. J., Ganellin, R., and Parsons, E. M. (1972): Definitions and antagonism of histamine H-2 receptors. *Nature*, 236:385–390.

27. Bourne, H. R., Melmon, K. L., and Lichtenstein, L. M. (1971): Histamine augments leukocyte adenosine 3′,5′-monophosphate and blocks antigenic histamine release. *Science*, 173:743–745.

28. Brostoff, J., Pack, S., and Lydyard, P. M. (1980): Histamine suppression of lymphocyte activation. *Clin. Exp. Immunol.*, 39: 739–745.

29. Bryant, D. H., and Kay, A. B. (1977): Cutaneous eosinophil accumulation in atopic and non-atopic individuals: The effects of an ECF-A tetrapeptide and histamine. *Clin. Allergy*, 7:211–217.

30. Busse, W. W., and Sosman, J. (1976): Histamine inhibition of neutrophil lysosomal enzyme release: An H2 histamine receptor response. *Science*, 194:737–738.

31. Busse, W. W., and Sosman, J. (1977): Decreased H2 histamine response of granulocytes of asthmatic patients. *J. Clin. Invest.*, 59: 1080–1087.

32. Busse, W. W., and Lantis, S. D. H. (1979): Impaired H2 histamine granulocyte response in active atopic eczema. *J. Invest. Dermatol.*, 73:184–187.

33. Busse, W. W., Cooper, W., Warshauer, D. M., Dick, E. C., Wallow, I. H. L., and Albrecht, R. (1979): Impairment of isoproterenol, H2 histamine, and prostaglandin E: Response of human granulocytes after incubation *in vitro* with live influenza vaccines. *Am. Rev. Respir. Dis.*, 119:561–569.

34. Cameron, W., Doyle, K., and Rocklin, R. E. (1986): Histamine type I (H_1) receptor radioligand binding studies on normal T cell subsets, B cells, and monocytes. *J. Immunol.*, 136:2116–2120.

35. Casale, T. B., Wescott, S., Rodbard, D., and Kaliner, M. (1985): Characterization of histamine H-1 receptors on human mononuclear cells. *Int. J. Immunopharmacol.*, 7:639–645.

36. Caulfield, J. P., Lewis, R. A., Hein, A., and Austen, K. F. (1980): Secretion in dissociated human pulmonary mast cells. *J. Cell. Biol.*, 85:299–311.

37. Center, D. M., and Cruikshank, W. (1982): Modulation of lymphocyte migration by human lymphokines. I. Identification and characterization of chemoattractant activity for lymphocytes from mitogen-stimulated mononuclear cells. *J. Immunol.*, 128:2563–2568.

38. Center, D. M., Cruikshank, W. W., Berman, J. S., and Beer, D. J. (1983): Functional characteristics of histamine receptor-bearing mononuclear cells. I. Selective production of lymphocyte chemoattractant lymphokines with histamine used as a ligand. *J. Immunol.*, 131:1854–1859.

39. Clark, R. A. F., Gallin, J. I., and Kaplan, A. P. (1975): The selective eosinophil chemotactic activity of histamine. *J. Exp. Med.*, 142: 1462–1476.

40. Clark, R. A. F., Sandler, J. A., Gallin, J. I., and Kaplan, A. P. (1977): Histamine modulation of eosinophil migration. *J. Immunol.*, 118:137–145.

41. Cohen, M. G., Munro, A. J., Dracott, B. M., Ife, R. J., and Vickers, M. R. (1985): Histamine receptors on leukocytes: The binding of histamine serum albumin conjugates is non-specific. *Int. Arch. Allergy Appl. Immunol.*, 76:9–15.

42. Cruikshank, W., and Center, D. M. (1982): Modulation of lymphocyte migration by human lymphokines. II. Purification of a lymphotactic factor (LCF). *J. Immunol.*, 128:2569–2574.

43. Dale, H. H., and Laidlaw, P. P. (1911): The physiologic action of β-imidazolylethylamine. *J. Physiol.*, 41:318–344.

44. Daly, J. W., McNeal, E. T., and Creveling, C. R. (1977): Accumulation of cyclic AMP in brain tissue: Role of H_1- and H_2-histamine receptors. In: *Proceedings of the A. N. Richards Symposium, Philadelphia, Pennsylvania, March 21–22, 1977*, edited by T. O. Yellin, pp. 299–323. S.P. Medical and Scientific Books, New York.

45. Damle, N. K., and Gupta, S. (1981): Autologous mixed lymphocyte reaction in man. II. Histamine-induced suppression of the autologous mixed lymphocyte reaction by T-cell subsets defined with monoclonal antibodies. *J. Clin. Immunol.*, 1:241–249.

46. DeKock, M. A., Nadel, J. A., Zwi, S., Colebatch, H. J. H., and Olsen, C. R. (1966): New method for perfusing bronchial arteries: Histamine bronchoconstriction and apnea. *J. Appl. Physiol.*, 21: 185–194.

47. Diamond, L., Szarek, J. L., Gillespie, M. N., Altiere, R. J. (1983): *In vivo* bronchodilator activity of vasoactive intestinal peptide in the cat. *Am. Rev. Respir. Dis.*, 128:827–832.

48. Diaz, P., Jones, D. G., and Kay, A. B. (1979): Histamine-coated particles generate superoxide (O_2^-) and chemiluminescence in alveolar macrophages. *Nature*, 278:454–456.

49. Diaz, P., Jones, D. G., and Kay, A. B. (1979): Histamine receptors on guinea-pig alveolar macrophages: Chemical specificity and the effects of H1- and H2-receptor agonists and antagonists. *Clin. Exp. Immunol.*, 35:462–469.

50. Douglas, W. W. (1980): Histamine and 5-hydroxytryptamine (serotonin) and their antagonists. In: *The Pharmacologic Basis of Therapeutics*, 6th ed., edited by A. G. Gilman, L. S. Goodman, and A. Gilman, pp. 609–646. Macmillan Publishing Co., New York.

51. Dreskin, S. C., Kaliner, M. A., and Gallin, J. I. (1987): Elevated urinary histamine in the hyperimmunoglobulin E and recurrent infection (Job's) syndrome: Association with eczematoid dermatitis and not with infection. *J. Allergy Clin. Immunol.* (in press).

52. Durham, S. R., Lee, T. H., Cromwell, O., Shaw, R. J., Merrett, T. G., Merrett, J., Cooper, P., and Kay, A. B. (1984): Immunologic studies in allergen-induced late-phase asthmatic reactions. *J. Allergy Clin. Immunol.*, 74:49–60.

53. Dyer, J., Warren, K., Merlin, S., Metcalfe, D. D., and Kaliner, M. (1982): Measurement of plasma histamine: Description of an improved method and normal values. *J. Allergy Clin. Immunol.*, 70: 82–87.

54. Empy, D. W., Laitnen, L. A., Jacobs, L., Gold, W. M., and Nadel, J. A. (1976): Mechanisms of bronchial hyperreactivity in normal subjects after upper respiratory tract infection. *Am. Rev. Respir. Dis.*, 113:131–139.

55. Enerback, L., Kolset, S. O., Kusche, M., Hjerpe, A., and Lindahl, U. (1985): Glycosaminoglycans in rat mucosal mast cells. *Biochem. J.*, 227:661–668.

56. Festen, H. P. M., de Pauw, B. E., Smeulders, J., and Wagener, D. J. T. (1981): Cimetidine does not influence immunological parameters in man. *Clin. Immunol. Immunopathol.*, 21:33–38.

57. Flodgren, P., and Sjögren, H. O. (1985): Influence *in vitro* on NK

and K cell activities by cimetidine and indomethacin with and without simultaneous exposure to interferon. *Cancer Immunol. Immunother.*, 19:28–34.

58. Foon, K. A., Wahl, S. M., Oppenheim, J. J., and Rosenstreich, D. L. (1976): Serotonin-induced production of a monocyte chemotactic factor by human peripheral blood leukocytes. *J. Immunol.*, 117:1545–1552.

59. Fox, B., Bull, T. B., and Guz, A. (1981): Mast cells in the human alveolar wall: An electron microscopic study. *J. Clin. Pathol.*, 34:1333–1342.

60. Friedman, M. M., and Kaliner, M. A. (1985): *In situ* degranulation of human nasal mucosal mast cells: Ultrastructural features and cell-cell association. *J. Allergy Clin. Immunol.*, 76:70–82.

61. Friedman, M. M., and Kaliner, M. (1987): The human lung mast cell and asthma. *Am. Rev. Respir. Dis.*, 135:1157–1164.

62. Frieri, M., Alling, D. W., and Metcalfe, D. D. (1985): Comparison of the therapeutic efficacy of cromolyn sodium with that of combined chlorpheneramine and cimetidine in systemic mastocytosis: Results in a double-blind clinical trial. *Am. J. Med.*, 78:9–14.

63. Garovoy, M. R., Reddish, M. A., and Rocklin, R. E. (1983): Histamine-induced suppressor factor (HSF): Inhibition of helper T cell generation and function. *J. Immunol.*, 130:357–361.

64. Gershon, R. K., Eardley, D. D., Duram, S., Green, D. R., Shen, F.-W., Yamauchi, K., Cantor, H., and Murphy, D. B. (1981): Contrasuppression: A novel immunoregulatory activity. *J. Exp. Med.*, 153:1533–1546.

65. Gifford, R. R. M., Sr., and Schmidtke, J. R. (1979): Cimetidine-induced augmentation of human lymphocyte blastogenesis: Comparison with levamisole in mitogen stimulation. *Surg. Forum*, 30:113–115.

66. Gifford, R. R. M., Sr., Hatfield, S. M., and Schmidtke, J. R. (1980): Cimetidine-induced augmentation of human lymphocyte blastogenesis by mitogen, bacterial antigen, and alloantigen. *Transplantation*, 29:143–148.

67. Gold, W. M., Kessler, G. F., and Yu, D. Y. (1972): Role of vagus nerves in experimental asthma in dogs. *J. Appl. Physiol.*, 33:719–725.

68. Golden, J. A., Nadel, J. A., and Boushey, H. A. (1978): Bronchial hyperirritability in healthy subjects after exposure to ozone. *Am. Rev. Respir. Dis.*, 118:287–294.

69. Goodwin, J. S., Messner, R. P., and Williams, R. C., Jr. (1979): Inhibitors of T-cell mitogenesis: Effect of mitogen dose. *Cell Immunol.*, 45:303–308.

70. Griswold, D. E., Alessi, S., Badger, A. M., Poste, G., and Hanna, N. (1984): Inhibition of T suppressor cell expression by histamine type 2 (H_2) receptor antagonists. *J. Immunol.*, 132:3054–3057.

71. Griswold, D. E., Alessi, S., Badger, A. M., Poste, G., and Hanna, N. (1986): Differential sensitivity of T suppressor cell expression to inhibition by histamine type 2 receptor antagonists. *J. Immunol.*, 137:1811–1815.

72. Gronneberg, R., Strandberg, K., Stalenheim, G., and Zetterstrom, O. (1981): Effect in man of anti-allergic drugs on the immediate and late phase cutaneous allergic reactions induced by anti-IgE. *Allergy*, 36:201–208.

73. Hägermark, Ö., Hökfelt, T., and Pernow, B. (1978): Flare and itch induced by substance P in human skin. *J. Invest. Dermatol.*, 71:233–235.

74. Hamasaki, Y., Saga, T., Mojarad, M., and Said, S. I. (1983): VIP counteracts leukotriene D_4-induced contractions of guinea pig trachea, lung and pulmonary artery. *Trans. Assoc. Am. Physicians*, 96:406–411.

75. Hamberg, M., Hedquist, P., and Radegran, K. (1980): Identification of 15-hydroxy-5,8,11,13-eicosatetraenoic acid (15-HETE) as a major metabolite of arachadonic acid in human lung. *Acta Physiol. Scand.*, 110:219–221.

76. Hansbrough, J. F., Zapata-Sirvent, R. L., and Bender, E. M. (1986): Prevention of alterations in postoperative lymphocyte subpopulations by cimetidine and ibuprofen. *Am. J. Surg.*, 151:249–255.

77. Hébert, J., Beaudoin, R., Aubin, M., and Fontaine, M. (1980): The regulatory effect of histamine on the immune response: Characterization of the cells involved. *Cell. Immunol.*, 54:49–57.

78. Hébert, J., Beaudoin, R., Fontaine, M., and Fradet, G. (1981): The regulatory effect of histamine on the immune response. II. Effect on the *in vitro* IgG synthesis. *Cell. Immunol.*, 58:366–371.

79. Hellstrand, K., and Hermodsson, S. (1986): Histamine H_2-receptor-mediated regulation of human natural killer cell activity. *J. Immunol.*, 137:656–660.

80. Henney, C. S., Bourne, H. R., and Licktenstein, L. M. (1972): The role of cyclic 3′,5′ adenosine monophosphate in the specific cytolytic activity of lymphocytes. *J. Immunol.*, 108:1526–1534.

81. Hill, H. R., Estensen, R. D., Hogan, N. A., and Quie, P. G. (1976): Severe staphylococcal disease associated with allergic manifestations, hyperimmunoglobulinemia E, and defective neutrophil chemotaxis. *J. Lab. Clin. Med.*, 88:796–806.

82. Hirai, N., Hahori, N., Hill, N. P., and Osther, K. (1985): Effects of cimetidine on various biological activities of human leukocyte interferon and on interferon production in lymphocytes. *Tohoku J. Exp. Med.*, 147:199–212.

83. Hirai, N., Hill, H. O., Motoo, Y., and Osther, K. (1985): Cimetidine enhances interferon induced augmentation of NK cell activity and suppresses interferon production. *Acta Pathol. Microbiol. Immunol. Scand.*, 93:153–159.

84. Ishizaka, T., Conrad, D. H., Hugg, T. E., Metcalfe, D. D., Stevens, R. L., and Lewis, R. A. (1985): Unique features of human basophilic granulocytes developed *in vitro* culture. *Int. Arch. Allergy Appl. Immunol.*, 77:137–143.

85. Jorizzo, J. L., Sams, W. M., Jr., Jegasothy, B. V., and Olansky, A. J. (1980): Cimetidine as an immunomodulator: Chronic mucocutaneous candidiasis as a model. *Ann. Int. Med.*, 92:192–195.

86. Jorizzo, J. L., Coutts, A. A., Eady, R. A. J., and Greaves, M. W. (1983): Vascular responses of human skin to injection of substance P and mechanisms of action. *Eur. J. Pharmacol.*, 87:67–76.

87. Kaliner, M. (1978): Human lung tissue and anaphylaxis: The effects of histamine on the immunologic release of mediators. *Am. Rev. Respir. Dis.*, 118:1015–1022.

88. Kaliner, M., Shelhamer, J. H., and Ottesen, E. A. (1982): Effects of infused histamine: Correlation of plasma histamine levels and symptoms. *J. Allergy Clin. Immunol.*, 69:283–289.

89. Kaplan, A. P., Beaven, M. A. (1976): *In vivo* studies of the pathogenesis of cold urticaria, cholinergic urticaria and vibration-induced swelling. *J. Invest. Dermatol.*, 67:327–332.

90. Kasahara, T., Hooks, J. J., Dougherty, S. F., and Oppenheim, J. J. (1983): Interleukin 2-mediated immune interferon (IFN) production by human T cells and T cell subsets. *J. Immunol.*, 130:1784–1789.

91. Kawase, I., Brooks, C. G., Kuribayashi, K., Olabuenaga, S., Newman, W., Gillis, S., and Henney, C. S. (1983): Interleukin 2 induces interferon production: Participation of macrophages and NK-like cells. *J. Immunol.*, 131:288–292.

92. Kay, A. B. (1979): The role of the eosinophil. *J. Allergy Clin. Immunol.*, 64:90–104.

93. Keahey, T. M., Indrisano, J., and Kaliner, M. A. (1984): Delayed vibratory angioedema. *J. Allergy Clin. Immunol.*, 73:183.

94. Keahey, T. B., Indrisano, J., and Kaliner, M. A. (1985): Measurement of cutaneous vascular permeability. *J. Allergy Clin. Immunol.*, 75:129.

95. Kedar, E., and Bonavida, B. (1974): Histamine receptor-bearing leukocytes (HRL). I. Detection of histamine receptor-bearing cells by rosette formation with histamine-coated erythrocytes. *J. Immunol.*, 113:1544–1552.

96. Khan, M. M., Melmon, K. L., Fathman, C. G., Hertel-Wulff, B., and Strober, S. (1985): The effects of autacoids on cloned murine lymphoid cells: Modulation of IL 2 secretion and the activity of natural suppressor cells. *J. Immunol.*, 134:4100–4106.

97. Khan, M. M., Sansoni, P., Engleman, E. G., and Melmon, K. L. (1985): Pharmacologic effects of autacoids on subsets of T cells: Regulation of expression/function of histamine-2 receptors by a subset of suppressor cells. *J. Clin. Invest.*, 75:1578–1583.

98. Kikuchi, Y., Oomori, K., Kizawa, I., and Kato, K. (1985): The effect of cimetidine on natural killer activity of peripheral blood lymphocytes of patients with ovarian carcinoma. *Jpn. J. Clin. Oncol.*, 15:377–383.

99. Kneussl, M. P., and Richardson, J. B. (1978): Alpha-adrenergic receptors in human and canine tracheal and bronchial smooth muscle. *J. Appl. Physiol.*, 45:307–311.

100. Kownatzki, E., Till, G., Gagelmann, M., Terwort, G., and Gemsa, D. (1977): Histamine induces release of an eosinophil immobilizing factor from mononuclear cells. *Nature*, 270:67–69.

101. Láng, I, Gergely, P., and Petrányi, G. (1981): Effect of histamine-receptor blocking on human spontaneous lymphocyte-mediated cytotoxicity. *Scand. J. Immunol.*, 14:573.

102. Lappin, D., and Whaley, K. (1980): Effects of histamine on monocyte complement production. I. Inhibition of C2 production mediated by its action on H2 receptors. *Clin. Exp. Immunol.*, 41:497–504.

103. Lappin, D., Moseley, H. L., and Whaley, K. (1980): Effect of histamine on monocyte complement production. II. Modulation of protein secretion, degradation and synthesis. *Clin. Exp. Immunol.*, 42:515–522.

104. Lee, T. H., Nagakura, T., Papgeorgiou, N., Iikura, Y., and Kay, A. B. (1983): Exercise-induced late asthmatic reactions with neutrophil chemotactic activity. *N. Engl. J. Med.*, 308:1502–1505.

105. Lemanske, R. F., Barr, L., and Kaliner, M. (1983): The biologic activity of mast cell granules. V. The effects of antihistamine treatment on rat cutaneous early- and late-phase allergic reactions. *J. Allergy Clin. Immunol.*, 72:94–99.

106. Lett-Brown, M. A., and Leonard, E. J. (1977): Histamine-induced inhibition of normal human basophil chemotaxis to C5a. *J. Immunol.*, 118:815–818.

107. Levi, R., Owen, D. D. A., and Trzeciakowski, J. (1982): Actions of histamine on the heart and vasculature. In: *Pharmacology of Histamine Receptors*, edited by C. R. Ganellin and M. E. Parsons, pp. 236–297. Wright and PSG, Boston.

108. Lichtenstein, L. M. (1975): The mechanism of basophil histamine release induced by antigen and by the calcium ionophore A23187. *J. Immunol.*, 114:1692–1699.

109. Lichtenstein, L. M., and Gillespie, E. (1973): Inhibition of histamine release by histamine controlled by H2 receptor. *Nature*, 244:287–288.

110. Lichtenstein, L. M., and Gillespie, E. (1975): The effects of the H1 and H2 antihistamines on "allergic" histamine release and its inhibition by histamine. *J. Pharmacol. Exp. Ther.*, 192:441–450.

111. Lima, M., and Rocklin, R. E. (1981): Histamine modulates *in vitro* IgG production by pokeweed mitogen-stimulated human mononuclear cells. *Cell. Immunol.*, 64:324–336.

112. Liu, M. C., Proud, D., Lichtenstein, L. M., MacGlashan, D. W., Jr., Schleimer, R. P., Adkinson, N. F., Jr., Kagey-Sobotka, A., Schulman, E. S., and Plaut, M. (1986): Human lung macrophage-derived histamine-releasing activity is due to IgE-dependent factors. *J. Immunol.*, 136:2588–2595.

113. Lundberg, J. M. (1987): Airway responses to tachykinins. In: *The Airways in Health and Disease*, edited by M. Kaliner and P. J. Barnes. Marcel Dekker, New York (in press).

114. Lundblad, L., Lundberg, J. M., Änggärd, A., Zetterström, O. (1985): Capsaicin pretreatment inhibits the flare component of the cutaneous allergic reaction in man. *Eur. J. Pharmacol.*, 113:461–462.

115. Majno, G., and Palade, G. E. (1961): Studies on inflammation. I. The effect of histamine and serotonin on vascular permeability: An electron microscopic study. *J. Biophys. Bioch. Cytol.*, 11:571–606.

116. Marks, R., and Greaves, M. W. (1977): Vascular reactions to histamine and compound 48/80 in human skin: Suppression by a histamine H2-receptor blocking agent. *Br. J. Clin. Pharmacol.*, 4:367–369.

117. Martinez, J. D., Santos, J., Stechschulte, D. J., and Abdou, N. I. (1979): Nonspecific suppressor cell function in atopic subjects. *J. Allergy Clin. Immunol.*, 64:485–490.

118. Matloff, S. M., Kiselis, I. K., and Rocklin, R. E. (1983): Reduced production of histamine-induced suppressor factor (HSF) by atopic mononuclear cells and decreased prostaglandin E2 output by HSF-stimulated atopic monocytes. *J. Allergy Clin. Immunol.*, 72:359–364.

119. Mawhinney, H. M., Killen, M., Fleming, W. A., and Roy, A. D. (1980): The hyperimmunoglobulin E syndrome: A neutrophil chemotactic defect reversible by histamine H2 receptor blockade? *Clin. Immunol. Immunopathol.*, 17:483–491.

120. Mekori, Y. A., Bender, E. M., Zapata-Sirvent, R., Hansbrough, J. F., and Claman, H. N. (1985): The effect of histamine receptor antagonists on specific and nonspecific suppression of experimental contact sensitivity. *J. Allergy Clin. Immunol.*, 76:90–96.

121. Melmon, K. L., Bourne, H. R., Weinstein, J., and Sela, M. (1972): Receptors for histamine can be detected on the surface of selected leukocytes. *Science*, 177:707–709.

122. Melmon, K. L., Bourne, H. R., Weinstein, Y., Shearer, G. M., Kram, J., and Bauminger, S. (1974): Hemolytic plaque formation by leukocytes *in vitro*: Control by vasoactive hormones. *J. Clin. Invest.*, 53:13–21.

123. Melmon, K. L., Weinstein, Y., Shearer, G. M., Bourne, H. R., and Bauminger, S. (1974): Separation of specific antibody-forming mouse cells by their adherence to insolubilized endogenous hormones. *J. Clin. Invest.*, 53:22–30.

124. Meretey, K., Fekete, M. I., Bohm, U., and Falus, A. (1985): Effect of H1 and H2 agonists on the chemiluminescence of human blood mononuclear cells induced by phytohemagglutinin. *Immunopharmacology*, 9(3):175–180.

125. Metcalfe, D. D., Lewis, R. A., Silbert, J. E., Rosenberg, R. D., Wasserman, S. I., and Asuten, K. F. (1979): Isolation and characterization of heparin from human lung. *J. Clin. Invest.*, 4:1537–1543.

126. Metcalfe, D. D., Kaliner, M. A., and Donlon, M. A. (1981): The mast cell. *CRC Crit. Rev. Immunol.*, 3:23–74.

127. Metcalfe, D. D., Bland, C. E., and Wasserman, S. I. (1984): Biochemical and functional characteristics of proteoglycans isolated from basophils of patients with chronic myelogenous leukemia. *J. Immunol.*, 130:1943–1950.

128. Metzger, W. J., Hunninghake, G. W., and Ticherson, H. B. (1985): Late asthmatic responses: Inquiry into mechanisms and significance. *Clin. Rev. Allergy*, 3:145–165.

129. Mojarad, T. L., Grode, C., Cox, C., Kimmel, G., and Said, S. I. (1985): Differential responses of human asthmatics to inhaled vasoactive intestinal peptide (VIP). *Am. Rev. Respir. Dis.*, 131:A281.

130. Morice, A. H., Unwin, R. J., and Sever, P. S. (1984): Vasoactive intestinal peptide as a bronchodilator in asthmatic subjects. *Peptides*, 5:439–440.

131. Mozes, E., Weinstein, Y., Bourne, H. R., Melmon, K. L., and Shearer, G. M. (1974): *In vitro* correction of antigen-induced immune suppression: Effects of histamine, dibutyryl cyclic AMP and cholera enterotoxin. *Cell. Immunol.*, 11:57–63.

132. Muirhead, K., Bender, P., Hanna, N., and Poste, G. (1985): Binding of histamine and histamine analogs to lymphocyte subsets analyzed by flow cytometry. *J. Immunol.*, 135:4120–4128.

133. Myers, G., Donlon, M., and Kaliner, M. (1981): Measurement of urinary histamine: Development of methodology and normal values. *J. Allergy Clin. Immunol.*, 67:305–311.

134. Nair, M. R. N., and Schwartz, S. A. (1983): Effect of histamine and histamine antagonists on natural and antibody-dependent cellular cytotoxicity of human lymphocytes *in vitro*. *Cell. Immunol.*, 81:45–60.

135. Nair, M. P. N., Cilik, J. M., and Schwartz, S. A. (1986): Histamine-induced suppressor factor inhibition of NK cells: Reversal with interferon and interleukin 2. *J. Immunol.*, 136:2456–2462.

136. Nathanson, I., Widdicombe, J. H., and Barnes, P. J. (1983): Effect of vasoactive intestinal peptide on ion transport across dog tracheal epithelium. *J. Appl. Physiol.*, 55:1844–1848.

137. Norrby, K. (1980): Mast cell histamine, a local mitogen acting via H2-receptors in nearby tissue cells. *Virchows Arch. [Cell Pathol.]*, 34:13–20.

138. Orchard, M. A., Kagey-Sobotka, A., Proud, D., and Lichtenstein, L. M. (1986): Basophil histamine release induced by a substance from stimulated human platelets. *J. Immunol.*, 136:2240–2244.

139. Osband, M. E., Cohen, E. B., McCaffrey, R. P., and Shapiro,

H. M. (1980): A technique for the flow cytometric analysis of lymphocytes bearing histamine receptors. *Blood,* 56:923–925.

140. Osband, M. E., Cohen, E. B., Miller, B. R., Shen, Y.-J., Cohen, L., Flescher, L., Brown, A. E., and McCaffrey, R. P. (1981): Biochemical analysis of specific histamine H1 and H2 receptors on lymphocytes. *Blood,* 58:87–90.

141. Ozaki, Y., Kume, S., and Ohashi, T. (1984): Effects of histamine agonists and antagonists on luminol-dependent chemiluminescence of granulocytes. *Agents Actions,* 15:182–188.

142. Platshon, L. F., and Kaliner, M. A. (1978): The effects of the immunologic release of histamine upon human lung cyclic nucleotide levels and prostaglandin generation. *J. Clin. Invest.,* 62:1113–1121.

143. Plaut, M. (1979): The role of cyclic AMP in modulating cytotoxic T lymphocytes. I. *In vivo*-generated cytotoxic lymphocytes, but not *in vitro*-generated cytotoxic lymphocytes, are inhibited by cyclic AMP-active agents. *J. Immunol.,* 123:692–701.

144. Plaut, M., and Berman, I. J. (1978): Histamine receptors on human and mouse lymphocytes. *J. Allergy Clin. Immunol.,* 61:132–133.

145. Plaut, M., and Lichtenstein, L. M. (1982): Histamine and immune responses. In: *Pharmacology of Histamine Receptors,* edited by C. R. Ganellin and M. E. Parsons, pp. 392–435. Wright and PSG, Bristol, England.

146. Plaut, M., and Lichtenstein, L. M. (1983): Cellular and chemical basis of the allergic inflammatory response. In: *Allergy Principles and Practice,* 2nd ed., edited by E. Middleton, C. E. Reed, and E. F. Ellis, pp. 119–146. C. V. Mosby Co., St. Louis.

147. Plaut, M., Lichtenstein, L. M., Gillespie, E., and Henney, C. S. (1973): Studies on the mechanism of lymphocyte-mediated cytolysis. IV. Specificity of the histamine receptor on effector T cells. *J. Immunol.,* 111:389–394.

148. Plaut, M., Lichtenstein, L. M., and Henney, C. S. (1973): Increase in histamine receptors on thymus-derived effector lymphocytes during the primary immune response to alloantigens. *Nature,* 244: 284–286.

149. Plaut, M., Lichtenstein, L. M., and Henney, C. S. (1975): Properties of a subpopulation of T cells bearing histamine receptors. *J. Clin. Invest.,* 55:856–874.

150. Puustinen, T., and Uotila, P. (1984): Thromboxane formation in human neutrophils is inhibited by prednisone and stimulated by leukotrienes B_4, C_4, D_4, and histamine. *Prostaglandins Leukotrienes Med.,* 14(2):161–167.

151. Razin, E., Stevens, R. L., Akiyama, F., Schmidt, K., and Austen, K. F. (1982): Culture from mouse bone marrow of a subclass of mast cells possessing a distinct chondroitin sulfate proteoglycan with glycosaminoglycans rich in *N*-acetyl galactosamine-4,6-disulfate. *J. Biol. Chem.,* 257:7729–7736.

152. Razin, E., Stevens, R. L., Austen, K. F., Caufield, J. P., Hein, A., Liu, F. T., Clabby, M., Nabel, H., Cantor, H., and Friedman, S. (1984): Cloned mouse mast cells derived from immunized lymph node cells and from foetal liver cells exhibit characteristics of bone marrow-derived mast cells containing chondroitin sulfate E proteoglycan. *Immunology,* 52:563–575.

153. Reichman, B. L., Handzel, Z. T., Segal, S., Weinstein, Y., and Levin, S. (1979): Participation of a histamine-Sepharose-adherent subpopulation of human mononuclear cells in the production of leukocyte migration inhibition factor (LIF) in healthy children. *Clin. Exp. Immunol.,* 37:562–566.

154. Remold-O'Donnell, E. (1974): Stimulation and desensitization of macrophage adenylate cyclase by prostaglandins and catecholamines. *J. Biol. Chem.,* 249:3615–3621.

155. Rigal, D., Monier, J. C., and Souweine, G. (1979): The effect of histamine on leukocyte migration test in man. I. Demonstration of a LIF production inhibitor (LIF-PI). *Cell. Immunol.,* 46:360–372.

156. Riley, J. F., and West, D. B. (1953): Histamine and tissue mast cells. *J. Physiol.,* 120:528–537.

157. Robert, R. J., Lewis, R. A., Oates, J. A., and Asuten, K. F. (1979): Prostaglandin, thromboxane, and 12-hydroxy-5,8,10,14-eicosatetraenoic acid production by ionophore stimulated rat serosal mast cells. *Biochem. Biophys. Acta,* 575:185–192.

158. Rocklin, R. E. (1976): Modulation of cellular-immune responses *in vivo* and *in vitro* by histamine receptor-bearing lymphocytes. *J. Clin. Invest.,* 57:1051–1058.

159. Rocklin, R. E. (1977): Histamine-induced suppressor factor (HSF): Effect on migration inhibitory factor (MIF) production and proliferation. *J. Immunol.,* 118:1734–1738.

160. Rocklin, R. E., and Haberek-Davidson, A. (1981): Histamine activates suppressor cells *in vitro* using a coculture technique. *J. Clin. Immunol.,* 1:73–79.

161. Rocklin, R. E., and Habarek-Davidson, A. (1984): Pharmacologic modulation *in vitro* of human histamine-induced suppressor cell activity. *Int. J. Immunopharmacol.,* 6:179–186.

162. Rocklin, R. E., Greineder, D., Littman, B. H., and Melmon, K. L. (1978): Modulation of cellular immune function *in vitro* by histamine receptor-bearing lymphocytes: Mechanism of action. *Cell. Immunol.,* 37:162–173.

163. Rocklin, R. E., Greineder, D. K., and Melmon, K. L. (1979): Histamine-induced suppressor factor (HSF): Further studies on the nature of the stimulus and the cell which produces it. *Cell. Immunol.,* 44:404–415.

164. Rocklin, R. E., Breard, J., Gupta, S., Good, R. A., and Melmon, K. L. (1980): Characterization of the human blood lymphocytes that produce a histamine-induced suppressor factor (HSF). *Cell. Immunol.,* 51:226–237.

165. Rocklin, R. E., Blidy, A., and Kamal, M. (1983): Physiochemical characterization of human histamine-induced suppressor factor. *Cell. Immunol.,* 76:243–252.

166. Rocklin, R. E., Kiselis, I., Beer, D. J., Rossi, P., Maggi, F., and Bellanti, J. A. (1983): Augmentation of prostaglandin and thromboxane production *in vitro* by monocytes exposed to histamine-induced suppressor factor (HSF). *Cell. Immunol.,* 77:92–98.

167. Roder, J. C., and Klein, M. (1979): Target-effector interaction in the natural killer cell system. IV. Modulation by cyclic nucleotides. *J. Immunol.,* 123:2785–2790.

168. Rosenbaum, R. C., Frieri, M., and Melcalfe, D. D. (1984): Patterns of skeletal scintigraphy and their relationship to plasma and urinary histamine levels in systemic mastocytosis. *J. Nucl. Med.,* 25:859–864.

169. Ruiz-Argüelles, A., Seroogy, K. B., and Ritts, R. E., Jr. (1982): *In vitro* effect of cimetidine on human cell-mediated cytotoxicity. I. Inhibition of natural killer cell activity. *Cell. Immunol.,* 69:1–12.

170. Said, S. I. (1987): Vasoactive intestinal peptide. *Adv. Metab. Res.* (in press).

171. Said, S. I., Geumei, A., and Hara, N. (1982): Bronchodilator effect of VIP *in vivo:* Protection against bronchoconstriction induced by histamine or prostaglandin $F_{2\alpha}$. In: *Vasoactive Intestinal Peptide,* edited by D. I. Said, pp. 185–192. Raven Press, New York.

172. Sansoni, P., Silverman, E. D., Khan, M. M., Melmon, K. L., and Engelman, E. G. (1985): Immunoregulatory T cells in man: Histamine-induced suppressor T cells are derived from a Leu 2^+ ($T8^+$) subpopulation distinct from that which gives rise to cytotoxic T cells. *J. Clin. Invest.,* 75:650–656.

173. Saxon, A., Morledge, V. D., and Bonavida, B. (1977): Histamide receptor leucocytes (HRL): Organ and lymphoid subpopulation distribution in man. *Clin. Exp. Immunol.,* 28:394–399.

174. Schreurs, J., Dailey, M. O., and Schulman, H. (1984): Pharmacological characterization of histamine H_2 receptors on clonal cytolytic T lymphocytes. *Biochem. Pharmacol.,* 1713:3375–3382.

175. Schulman, E. S., Newball, H. H., Demers, L. M., Fitzpatrick, F. A., Adkinson, N. F., Jr. (1981): Anaphylactic release of thromboxane A_2, prostaglandin D_2 and prostacyclin from human lung parenchyma. *Am. Rev. Respir. Dis.,* 124:402–406.

176. Schulman, E. S., Adkinson, N. F., Jr., and Newball, H. H. (1982): Cyclooxygenase metabolites in human lung anaphylaxis: Airway vs. parenchyma. *J. Appl. Physiol.,* 53:589–595.

177. Schulman, E. S., Liu, M. C., Proud, D., MacGlashan, D. W., Jr., Lichtenstein, L. M., and Plaut, M. (1985): Human lung macrophages induce histamine release from basophils and mast cells. *Am. Rev. Respir. Dis.,* 131:230–235.

178. Schwartz, A., Askenase, P. W., and Gershon, R. K. (1977): The effect of locally injected vasoactive amines on the elicitation of delayed-type hypersensitivity. *J. Immunol.*, 118:159–165.

179. Schwartz, A., Askenase, P. W., and Gershon, R. K. (1980): Histamine inhibition of the *in vitro* induction of cytotoxic T-cell responses. *Immunopharmacology*, 2:179–190.

180. Schwartz, A., Sutton, S. L., Askenase, P. W., and Gershon, R. K. (1981): Histamine inhibition of concanavalin A-induced suppressor T-cell activation. *Cell. Immunol.*, 60:426–439.

181. Segal, S., Melmon, K. L., and Weinstein, Y. (1981): Isolation of suppressor T-lymphocytes adherent to histamine conjugated albumin and their role in suppression of IgG response to SRBC. *Cell. Immunol.*, 59:171–180.

182. Seligman, B. E., Fletcher, M. P., and Gallin, J. I. (1983): Histamine modulation of human neutrophil exodative metabolism, locomotion, degranulation, and membrane potential changes. *J. Immunol.*, 130:1902–1909.

183. Sertl, K., Casale, T., Wescott, S., and Kaliner, M. (1985): Immunohistochemical localization of histamine stimulated increases in cyclic GMP in guinea pig lung. *Am. Rev. Respir. Dis.*, 131:A7.

184. Shanahan, J. I., Denburg, J. A., Fox, J., Bienenstock, J., and Befus, D. (1985): Mast cell heterogeneity: effects of neuroenteric peptides on histamine release. *J. Immunol.*, 1331–1337.

185. Shearer, G. M., Melmon, K. L., Weinstein, Y., and Sela, M. (1972): Regulation of antibody response by cells expressing histamine receptors. *J. Exp. Med.*, 136:1302–1307.

186. Shearer, G. M., Weinstein, Y., and Melmon, K. L. (1974): Enhancement of immune response potential of mouse lymphoid cells fractionated over insolubilized conjugated histamine columns. *J. Immunol.*, 113:597–607.

187. Shearer, G. M., Simpson, E., Weinstein, Y., and Melmon, K. L. (1977): Fractionation of lymphocytes involved in the generation of cell-mediated cycotoxicity over insolubilized conjugated histamine columns. *J. Immunol.*, 118:756–761.

188. Shore, S. A., Bai, T. R., Wang, C. G., and Martin, J. G. (1985): Central and local cholinergic components of histamine-induced bronchoconstriction in dogs. *J. Appl. Physiol.*, 58:533–551.

189. Siegel, J. N., Schwartz, A., Askenase, P. W., and Gershon, R. K. (1982): T-cell suppression and contrasuppression induced by histamine H_2 and H_1 receptor agonists, respectively. *Proc. Natl. Acad. Sci. USA*, 79:5052–5056.

190. Siraganian, R. P. (1976): Histamine release and assay methods for the study of human allergy. In: *Manual of Clinical Immunology*, edited by N. R. Rose, and H. Friedman, pp. 603–614. American Society for Microbiology, Washington, D.C.

191. Smith, J. A., Mansfield, L. E., and Nelson, H. S. (1979): The effect of cimetidine on the immediate cutaneous response to allergens. *Ann. Allergy*, 42:353–354.

192. Smith, J. A., Mansfield, L. E., deShazo, R. D., and Nelson, H. S. (1980): An evaluation of the pharmacologic inhibition of the immediate and late cutaneous reaction to allergen. *J. Allergy Clin. Immunol.*, 65:118–121.

193. Sredni, B., Friedman, M. M., Bland, C. E., and Metcalfe, D. D. (1983): Ultrastructural, biochemical and functional characteristics of histamine-containing cells cloned from mouse bone marrow: Tentative identification as mucosal mast cells. *J. Immunol.*, 131: 915–922.

194. Staszak, C., Goodwin, J. S., Troup, G. M., Pathak, D. R., and Williams, R. C., Jr. (1980): Decreased sensitivity to prostaglandin and histamine in lymphocytes from normal MLA-B12 individuals: A possible role in autoimmunity. *J. Immunol.*, 125:181–185.

195. Steel, L., Platshon, L., and Kaliner, M. (1979): Prostaglandin generation by human and guinea pig lung tissue: Comparison of parenchymal and airway responses. *J. Allergy Clin. Immunol.*, 64: 287–293.

196. Stuart, J., and Kay, A. B. (1980): Histamine increases histadine uptake by basophils. *Clin. Exp. Immunol.*, 40:423–426.

197. Strannegård, I.-L., and Strannegård, Ö. (1977): Increased sensitivity of lymphocytes from atopic individuals to histamine-induced suppression. *Scand. J. Immunol.*, 6:1225–1231.

198. Strannegård, I.-L., and Strannegård, Ö. (1979): Stimulatory and inhibitory effects of cyclic AMP on lymphocytes from atopic children. *Int. Arch. Allergy Appl. Immunol.*, 58:167–174.

199. Summers, R., Sigler, R., Shelhamer, J. H., and Kaliner, M. (1981): Effects of infused histamine on asthmatic and normal subjects: Comparison of skin test responses. *J. Allergy Clin. Immunol.*, 67: 456–464.

200. Sutherland, J., Mannoni, P., Rosa, F., Huyat, D., Turner, A. R., and Fellows, M. (1985): Induction of the expression of HLA class I antigens in K562 by interferons and sodium butyrate. *Hum. Immunol.*, 12:65–73.

201. Suzuki, S., and Huchet, R. (1981): Mechanism of histamine-induced inhibition of lymphocyte response to mitogens in mice. *Cell. Immunol.*, 62:396–405.

202. Suzuki, S., and Huchet, R. (1982): Properties of histamine-induced suppressor factor in the regulation of lymphocyte response to PHA in mice. *Cell. Immunol.*, 68:349–358.

203. Szewczuk, M. R., Campbell, R. J., and Smith, J. W. (1981): Evidence for histamine-induced auto-anti-idiotypic antibody immunoregulation *in vivo. Cell. Immunol.*, 65:152–165.

204. Tannenbaum, S., Oertel, H., Henderson, W., and Kaliner, M. (1980): The biologic activity of mast cell granules. I. Elicitation of inflammatory responses in rat skin. *J. Immunol.*, 125:325–335.

205. Thomas, Y., Huchet, R., and Granjon, D. (1981): Histamine-induced suppressor cells of lymphocyte mitogenic response. *Cell. Immunol.*, 59:268–275.

206. Thueson, D. O., Speck, L. S., Lett-Brown, M. A., and Grant, J. A. (1979): Histamine-releasing activity (HRA). I. Production by mitogen- or antigen-stimulated human mononuclear cells. *J. Immunol.*, 626–632.

207. Ting, S., Dunsky, E. N., and Zweiman, B. (1980): Histamine suppression of eosinophiltaxis and histamine release *in vivo. J. Allergy Clin. Immunol.*, 65:196–197.

208. Tung, R., Kagey-Soboyka, A., Plaut, M., and Lichtenstein, L. M. (1982): H_2 antihistamines augment antigen-induced histamine release from human basophils *in vitro. J. Immunol.*, 129:2113–2115.

209. Turnbull, L. W., and Kay, A. B. (1976): Eosinophils and mediators of anaphylaxis: Histamine and imidazole acetic acid as chemotactic agents for human eosinophil leukocytes. *Immunology*, 31:797–802.

210. Undem, B. J., Dick, E. C., and Buckner, C. K. (1983): Inhibition by vasoactive intestinal peptide of antigen-induced histamine release from guinea pig minced lung. *Eur. J. Pharmacol.*, 88:247–249.

211. Wang, S. R., and Zweiman, B. (1978): Histamine suppression of human lymphocyte responses to mitogens. *Cell. Immunol.*, 36:28–36.

212. Wasserman, S. I. (1980): The lung mast cells: Its physiology and potential relevance to defense of the lung. *Environ. Health Perspect.*, 35:153–164.

213. Wasserman, S. I. (1983): Mediators of immediate hypersensitivity. *J. Allergy Clin. Immunol.*, 72:101–115.

214. Weinstein, Y., and Melmon, K. L. (1976): Control of immune responses by cyclic AMP and lymphocytes that adhere to histamine columns. *Immunol. Commun.*, 5:401–416.

215. Weinstein, Y., Melmon, K. L., Bourne, H., and Sela, M. (1973): Specific leukocyte receptors for small endogenous hormones: Detection by cell binding to insolubilized hormone preparation. *J. Clin. Invest.*, 52:1349–1361.

216. Weinstock, J. V., Chensue, S. W., and Boros, D. L. (1983): Modulation of granulomatous hypersensitivity. V. Participation of histamine receptor positive and negative lymphocytes in the granulomatous response of *Schistosoma mansoni*-infected mice. *J. Immunol.*, 130:423–427.

217. Wescott, S., and Kaliner, M. (1983): Histamine H-1 binding site on human polymorphonuclear leukocytes. *Inflammation*, 7:291–300.

218. Wescott, S. L., Hunt, W. A., and Kaliner, M. (1982): Histamine H-1 receptors on rat peritoneal mast cells. *Life Sci.*, 31:1911–1919.

219. White, M. V., and Kaliner, M. A. (1985): Neutrophil induced mast cell degranulation. *J. Allergy Clin. Immunol.*, 75:175.

220. White, M. V., Baer, H., and Kaliner, M. A. (1985): Neutrophil-derived histamine releasing activity. *Ann. Allergy,* 55:273.
221. White, M. V., Kaliner, M. A., and Baer, H. (1986): Stimulated neutrophils release a histamine releasing factor. *J. Allergy Clin. Immunol.,* 77:132.
222. White, M. V., Slater, J., and Kaliner, M. (1987): Histamine and asthma. *Am. Rev. Resp. Dis.* (in press).
223. White, W. B., and Ballow, M. (1985): Modulation of suppressor-cell activity by cimetidine in patients with common variable hypogammaglobulinemia. *N. Engl. J. Med.,* 312:198–203.
224. Woodward, D. F., Spade, C. S., Hawley, S. B., and Nieves, A. L. (1985): Histamine H1 and H2-receptor involvement in eosinophil infiltration and the microvascular changes associated with cutaneous anaphylaxis. *Agents Actions,* 17(2):121–125.
225. Yamauchi, K., Green, D. R., Eardley, D. D., and Gershon, R. (1981): Immunoregulatory circuits that modulate responsiveness to suppressor cell signals: Failure of B10 mice to respond to suppressor factors can be overcome by quenching the contrasuppression circuit. *J. Exp. Med.,* 152:1547–1561.
226. Yasunori, T. (1985): Phagocytosis of mast cell granules by fibroblasts in the human gingiva. *Virchows Arch.* [*A*], 406:197–201.
227. Zeiger, R. S., Yurdin, D. L., and Colten, H. R. (1976): Histamine metabolism. II. Cellular and subcellular localization of the catabolic enzymes, histaminase and histamine methyl transferase in human leukocytes. *J. Allergy Clin. Immunol.,* 58:172–179.
228. Zheutlin, L. M., Ackerman, S. J., Gleich, G. J., and Thomas, L. L. (1984): Stimulation of basophil and rat mast cell histamine release by eosinophil granule-derived cationic proteins. *J. Immunol.,* 133:2180–2185.
229. Zuier, R. B., Weissmann, N. G., Hoffstein, S., Kammerman, S., and Tai, H. H. (1974): Mechanisms of lysosomal enzyme release from human leukocytes. II. Effects of cAMP and cGMP, autonomic agonists, and agents which affect microtubule functions. *J. Clin. Invest.,* 53:297–309.

Inflammation: Basic Principles and Clinical Correlates.
Edited by J. I. Gallin, I. M. Goldstein, and R. Snyderman.
Raven Press, Ltd., New York © 1988.

CHAPTER 12

Cytokines: Interleukin-1 and Tumor Necrosis Factor (Cachectin)

Charles A. Dinarello

HISTORICAL OVERVIEW

Throughout the animal kingdom, one observes the elaborate strategies various species have developed in order to fight life-threatening microbial invasion or localize tissue injury. Mammals have developed a large number of varied responses which signal the onset of disease and trigger appropriate defensive measures. The responses are called "acute phase responses" because they are often observed within hours following the injury or initiation of infection. Some of the responses include behavioral changes; for example, animals often stop eating, reduce activity, conserve energy expenditure, and increase sleep time. The metabolic and hematological responses can be substantial and are frequently costly to the host, especially when they persist and become chronic components of the disease. In this chapter, one of the interleukins, interleukin-1 (IL-1), will be discussed as the body's key mediator of acute responses to microbial invasion, inflammation, immunological reaction, and tissue injury. Evidence will be presented which implicates IL-1 as one of the first and most prominent molecules synthesized during the acute phase response and indicates that its biological effects are manifested in nearly every tissue and organ system.

The story of IL-1 began in the 1940s when researchers described a substance in acute exudate fluid which, when injected into animals or humans, produced fever (reviewed in 11 and 14). This material was a small protein (10,000–20,000 daltons) and was called "endogenous pyrogen." It was later shown that endogenous pyrogen was not preformed in cells but rather was synthesized *de novo* when phagocytic cells, primarily macrophages, were stimulated with small (picogram/milliliter) concentrations of endotoxins or by phagocytosis of a few (three to five) bacteria. Attempts to purify the endogenous pyrogen activity in inflammatory fluids or stimulated macrophage culture supernates proved difficult. Submicrogram amounts of protein seemingly possessed potent biological activity, and loss of activity was common during multiple purification steps. Nevertheless, purification procedures were established in the 1970s (15,47), and it was shown that 30 to 50 ng/kg of homogeneous endogenous pyrogen produced monophasic fever in rabbits. No amino acid sequence for endogenous pyrogen was known at that time.

As a consequence of improved purification methods, it was demonstrated that endogenous pyrogen did more than cause fever. Kampschmidt and co-workers (31) showed that endogenous pyrogen activity copurified with a substance called "leukocytic endogenous mediator." When this material was injected into animals, it induced hepatic acute phase protein synthesis, caused decreases in plasma iron and zinc levels, and produced neutrophilia. Purified human endogenous pyrogen stimulated serum amyloid A protein synthesis when injected into mice (44). Immunologists had also become interested in macrophage products, and a substance called "lymphocyte activating factor" was described; it was a 10,000- to 20,000-dalton protein which augmented T-cell responses to mitogens and antigens (23). Early observations on the chemical characteristics of lymphocyte activating factor suggested several similarities to endogenous pyrogen, and in 1979 and 1980 the first reports were published on the ability of purified endogenous pyrogen to act as lymphocyte activating factor (48,56). As more data confirmed these findings, the name "lymphocyte activating factor" was changed to "interleukin-1," which now includes the originally described endogenous pyrogen and leukocytic endogenous mediator activities as well as lymphocyte activating factor, mononuclear cell factor (33), and catabolin (58).

The concept that a molecule which acts on the brain to produce fever, in the liver to induce acute phase protein synthesis, and on the bone marrow to release neutrophils is, in fact, the same molecule that stimulates T and B cells was not initially accepted. However, preparations of endogenous pyrogens which were homogeneous by sodium dodecyl sulfate polyacrylamide gel electrophoresis (SDS-PAGE) induced T-cell proliferation (16,27). The dilemma was resolved by the molecular cloning of IL-1. Two IL-1 forms have been cloned, IL-1β from human monocytes (1) and IL-1α from a murine macrophage line (41). The two forms had originally been identified as pI 7 (IL-1β) and pI 5 (IL-1α) on isoelectric focusing. Homologs of IL-1β and -α have been found in other species. The two forms of IL-1 are initially synthesized as 31,000-dalton precursor polypeptides and share only small stretches of amino acid homology (26% in the case of human IL-1). Neither form contains a signal peptide sequence indicating a cleavage site for the N-terminus. This fact makes IL-1 a highly unique substance; the biological significance of lacking a signal peptide will be discussed below. Generation of complementary DNAs (cDNAs) for IL-1 resulted in two important advances: (a) entire amino acid sequences were deduced from nucleotide sequences, and (b) expression of cDNAs resulted in ample quantities of recombinant IL-1 for biological experimentation. For the most part, recombinant IL-1 has confirmed previous studies demonstrating the widespread multiple biological properties of IL-1.

The results of studies employing recombinant IL-1β or -α led to the conclusion that most acute phase responses could be explained by the action of IL-1 on a variety of organs and tissues. However, another macrophage product, tumor necrosis factor (TNF), was cloned and shown to be identical to a substance called "cachectin" which mediated hemodynamic shock and cachexia associated with various diseases (4). TNF (cachectin) shares only 3% amino acid homology with IL-1β and less with IL-1α; in addition, TNF has a receptor which is independent of the putative receptor for IL-1 (4,6,20,32,43). However, many of the biological properties of TNF and IL-1 overlap, particularly those involved in acute phase responses. Moreover, IL-1 and TNF often act synergistically. Therefore, for the host, acute phase changes which herald the onset of disease and participate in the inflammatory process to combat infection and injury are, in fact, the net result of the biological activities of IL-1 and TNF.

AMINO ACID SEQUENCES OF IL-1 AND RELATED POLYPEPTIDES

Before molecular cloning was possible, IL-1 was described more in terms of biological activity than molecular structure. Adherent human blood monocytes were used as a source of RNA for IL-1β (1), and the murine macrophage cell line P388D was used as the source of RNA for IL-1α (41). Identification of messenger RNA (mRNA) coding for IL-1 was made by immunoprecipitation of reticulocyte translation products; however, it was necessary to confirm polyadenylated RNA coding for IL-1 by biological activity following injection of RNA into frog oocytes. The results indicated that IL-1 mRNA coded for a precursor protein which was processed by oocytes into biologically active smaller peptides. This concept was consistent with previous reports that human IL-1 activity existed at molecular weights (as estimated following gel filtration) of 38, 15, 4, and 2 kilodaltons (kD). A cDNA library was made from human mRNA enriched for IL-1. cDNA clones were eliminated based on their presence in unstimulated, nonadherent human blood mononuclear cells. With the use of an appropriate probe for IL-1 it was found that mRNA for IL-1 was not detectable until adherence to a glass surface or activation by endotoxin. Polyadenylated RNA coding for the IL-1 precursor polypeptide rose from an undetectable level to approximately 5% of the total poly A-extracted RNA after adherence to glass and stimulation by endotoxin (1,64). The sequences of both IL-1β and -α cDNAs revealed that the processed mRNA coded for a 31-kD precursor polypeptide, but on SDS-PAGE this polypeptide appeared to have a relative molecular mass of 35 kD (1,41).

The amino acid sequences of IL-1 precursors are unique because there are no clear signal peptide sequences indicating a likely cleavage site for the precursor yielding a mature peptide. Van Damme, Billiau, and their co-workers reported the N-terminal sequence of purified human blood IL-1 at position 117 (alanine) of the IL-1β precursor (61), and an N-terminus at position 113 (serine) was reported for human IL-1α (21). Despite their dissimilarities (only 26% amino acid homology), both IL-1 forms had similar precursor sizes, potential glycosylation sites, and polybasic regions. Whereas human IL-1β mRNA represented as much as 5% of the total polyadenylated pool following stimulation of human monocytes (1,64), the amount of IL-1α mRNA in the superinduced P388D cell line was estimated at 0.005% (41), and that of human IL-1α, 0.1%.

To date, IL-1β has been cloned in mice (26) and humans, and IL-1α in humans, mice, and rabbits (21). The IL-1β sequences have a conserved amino acid homology of 78%, whereas that of the IL-1α sequences is in the range 60% to 70%; between the IL-1β and -α within a species, conserved amino acid homology is about 25%. The human genes for each IL-1 form have been cloned (8,22). Each gene contains seven exons coding for IL-1 mRNA and raise the possibility that alternate RNA processing is possible. The gene for human IL-1β is located on the long arm of chromosome 2 (63).

When the two IL-1 forms are compared, only five small stretches of amino acid homology exist. These have been identified and are called regions A, B, C, D, and E (2); as regions A and B are contained in the precursor sequence, which is missing in the mature IL-1 form, the significant regions of homology for the two IL-1 forms are located in the carboxyl C, D, and E regions. These regions may actually represent a likely "active site" of the IL-1 molecule, which would explain the observation that, although the two forms are structurally distinct, they share the multiple biological properties of IL-1. The concept of other IL-1 forms (as separate gene products or the result of processed mRNA) has recently been introduced in studies using IL-1 from human B cells and human keratinocytes. However, it remains to be shown that these latter cells produce a different IL-1 gene product or that posttranslational processing may result in IL-1 of different molecular weight and charge. This may be the result of unique processing of the IL-1 precursor polypeptide. In fact, historically, descriptions of macrophage IL-1 sizes and charges have varied greatly.

IL-1 stimulates fibroblast proliferation and collagen synthesis (7). A brain-derived polypeptide, termed "fibroblast growth factor" (or endothelial cell growth factor) has been shown to stimulate fibroblast proliferation and endothelial cell growth. Similar to IL-1, these brain-derived molecules exist in two forms, acidic (pI 5) and basic (pI 7). Bovine brain-derived acidic and basic fibroblast growth factors have significant amino acid homology with IL-1β and to a lesser degree with IL-1α (25). The stretches of IL-1 and brain-derived fibroblast growth factor amino acid

homology are distributed throughout the sequences. However, analysis of the IL-1 sequence in the C and D regions with that of the brain-derived growth factors does not reveal any particular homology. Nevertheless, the amino acid sequence similarities between the two IL-1 forms and the two forms of bovine brain-derived growth factor suggest that other biological properties of these molecules may be shared. From a structural point of view, these sequence homologies may indicate the existence of a family of IL-1-related molecules.

MULTIPLE BIOLOGICAL PROPERTIES OF IL-1

The expression of IL-1α and -β has been accomplished by several groups and, in general, there does not seem to be any difference in the spectrum of biological activities of either form (12). However, IL-1β is vulnerable to oxidation, and thus its biological specific activities can be lower than those of IL-1α which is highly stable. This observation is supported by experiments on naturally occurring IL-1 pI 7 (β) or IL-1 pI 5 (α). If care is taken to express and purify recombinant IL-1β under nonoxidative conditions, the IL-1β form will be equipotent with the α form in a variety of in vivo and in vitro assays. Both recombinant human IL-1β and -α augment T-cell responses to antigens or mitogens and cause fever in rabbits and other species (17). Both forms induce hepatic acute phase protein synthesis and cause sleep. However, some biological properties reported for natural IL-1 have not been confirmed with either recombinant form. These include the ability of IL-1 to cause neutrophil degranulation and muscle proteolysis in vitro. It appears that these apparent biological properties of IL-1 may have been due to contaminating protein(s) or to the ability of IL-1 to augment the biological property of another protein. One likely candidate for contaminating protein is TNF. Recombinant IL-1 induces histamine release from human blood basophils and eosinophil degranulation of arylsulfatase and β-glucuronidase (54). Synergism between IL-1 and TNF may explain the effects formerly attributed to IL-1 alone.

The multiple biological activities of IL-1 have been studied in terms of in vivo and in vitro effects. In patients with bacterial infection, injury, or chronic inflammatory disease, the multiple biological activities of IL-1 account for a majority of the observed acute phase changes. It is difficult to study such subjective symptoms as headache, myalgias, arthralgias, and lassitude in animal models, but the potency (10^{-12}–10^{-15} M) of IL-1 in inducing the release of prostaglandin E_2 (PGE_2) from fibroblasts, synovial cells, and other cells suggests that these symptoms are likely mediated by increased levels of IL-1. Certainly, the vast majority of such clinical complaints, including fever, are ameliorated by cyclooxygenase inhibitors. Sleep disturbances have been reported in a variety of patients during various disease states, and IL-1 increases slow-wave sleep in rabbits (34).

Effects of IL-1 on Hepatic Protein Synthesis

One of the more dramatic effects of IL-1 is its ability to induce hepatocytes to synthesize a spectrum of acute phase proteins; these include serum amyloid A (SAA), C-reactive protein (CRP), complement components, and various clotting factors. At the same time, albumin levels appear to decrease. Recent studies have demonstrated that recombinant IL-1 regulates the synthesis of these proteins at the level of mRNA transcription (55). In isolated hepatocytes, IL-1 decreases the transcription of RNA coding for albumin, increases transcription of factor B, and initiates SAA mRNA synthesis, but has no effect on gene expression of a control protein, actin. Other proteins have been studied in hepatic cell line cultures (HepG2 and Hep3B), and in picomolar ranges IL-1 stimulates the biosynthesis of complement protein C3 and α_1-antichymotrypsin. There is also a modest stimulation of α_1-acid glycoprotein and inter-α_1-trypsin inhibitor synthesis. In addition to decreased albumin transcription, hepatic cells exposed to IL-1 synthesize less transferrin (53). In hepatic cells lines, IL-1 does not increase the expression of CRP, although intravenous injection of recombinant IL-1 results in elevated CRP levels after 24 hr. In murine fibroblasts transfected with cosmid DNA bearing the genes for C2 and factor B, IL-1 stimulated the expression of factor B but did not affect the synthesis of C2 (52).

IL-1 has other effects on liver metabolism. It depresses the activity of liver cytochrome P-450-dependent drug metabolism in mice (24), and this observation may explain the impaired drug clearance and excretion in patients with infections and fever. The liver's response to IL-1 also includes the synthesis of metalloproteins which bind serum iron and zinc and account for the hypozincemia and hypoferremia induced by IL-1. The ability of IL-1 to reduce serum iron and zinc levels has important implications for the role of IL-1 in nonspecific resistance to infection. Bacteria and tumor cells require large amounts of iron for cell growth, particularly during fever, and the ability of the host to remove iron from tissue fluids seems to be a fundamental host defense mechanism.

Effects of IL-1 on Endothelial Cells

Of its many biological properties, IL-1-induced changes in endothelial cells relate directly to the initiation and progression of pathological lesions in vascular tissue. From a physiological viewpoint, IL-1 activates human endo-thelial cells *in vitro* to synthesize and release PGI_2 and PGE_2, both potent vasodilators. A 10-fold increase in PGI_2 release was observed with one IL-1 unit per milliliter (57), and these results have recently been confirmed using recombinant IL-1 (10). Although these two arachidonate metabolites increase blood flow, at the same time, IL-1 also orchestrates a cascade of cellular and biochemical events that lead to vascular congestion, clot formation, and cellular infiltration. One of these initiating steps involves the ability of IL-1 to alter endothelial cell plasma membranes so that neutrophils, monocytes, and lymphocytes adhere avidly (5). As in PGI_2 and PGE_2 induction, IL-1 activates cultured vascular endothelial cells at relatively low concentrations. Endothelial cells need to be exposed to IL-1 for 1 hr or less in order to increase their adhesiveness. The action of IL-1 in this process appears to be related to interaction of the leukocyte glycoprotein complex called "leukocyte function antigen" with a cell surface molecule called "intercellular adhesion molecule-1." Patients with defective leukocyte function antigen expression have repeated bouts of bacterial infection. Within 1 hr following IL-1 exposure, endothelial cells increase the expression of intercellular adhesion molecule-1. In addition to activating endothelial cell–leukocyte adhesion, IL-1 also increases the binding and lysis by natural killer (NK) cells to a variety of tumor targets (28) and is chemotactic for monocytes and lymphocytes (30). Consistent with the effects of IL-1 on leukocyte chemotaxis and adherence to endothelial cells, IL-1 injected intradermally causes the accumulation of neutrophils (45), and IL-1 can substitute for endotoxin in either limb of the local Schwartzman reaction. This latter property is most apparent using a combination of IL-1 and TNF.

IL-1 dramatically increases endothelial cell surface procoagulant activity (10) which serves as a tissue factor in coagulation. There is also evidence that IL-1 induces the production of a plasminogen activator inhibitor (50). These events lead to activation of factor VII and thrombin in the initiation of clotting. Thrombin production may also act directly on endothelial cells. Taken together, these effects decrease blood flow in vessels and increase the accumulation of leukocytes and platelets. As IL-1 is a potent stimulator of neutrophil thromboxane release (9), activated neutrophils adhering to endothelial cells may increase platelet aggregation. Recombinant IL-1 stimulates endothelial cell release of platelet activating factor (10). Finally, IL-1 has angiogenic properties in the rabbit eye anterior chamber model, and this may be related to the fact that IL-1 and the related brain-derived growth factor share significant amino acid homology. In general, the effects of IL-1 on endothelial cells represent a well-coordinated effort to localize tissue inflammation and contribute to the initiation of pathological lesions leading to vasculitic-like changes.

The effects of IL-1 stimulation of endothelial cell functions should be considered in light of the fact that endothelial cells produce their own IL-1. Several investigators have shown that nanogram/milliliter concentrations of bacterial endotoxins or TNF induce cultured endothelial cells to release IL-1 (37). In addition, thrombin stimulates endothelial cell IL-1 production. The IL-1 derived from human endothelial cells is either the same as monocyte IL-1β or a closely related molecule. For example, antibody directed against human monocyte pI 7 IL-1 neutralizes and binds endothelial cell-derived IL-1. Northern hybridization of endothelial cell mRNA supports a close relationship between the predominant IL-1β and endothelial cell-derived IL-1. Thus, the induction of endothelial cell IL-1 by two clinically relevant stimulators (endotoxin and thrombin) may initiate a cascade of events further leading to the development of vasculitic processes. Although immune complexes stimulate monocyte IL-1 production, there are no reported studies as yet demonstrating that immune complexes stimulate endothelial cell IL-1 synthesis. Recent studies demonstrated that arterial smooth muscle produced IL-1 (38).

Catabolic Effects of IL-1

The catabolic properties of IL-1 are usually considered in terms of either local or systemic effects. For example, IL-1 produced locally acts in a paracrine-like fashion in destructive joint and bone disease and local tumor invasion. On the other hand, IL-1 in the systemic circulation exerts its catabolic effects on liver, fat, and connective tissue. IL-1 is a potent inducer of collagenase production in synovial cells (33); in addition, IL-1 induces the release of metalloproteinases from chondrocytes (60). In fact, because of its local catabolic biological activities, pig IL-1 was previously known as "catabolin" (58). Recombinant IL-1 added to bone cultures *in vitro* induces dramatic resorptive processes and shrinkage of bone matrix. Just as catabolin was the name first given to pig IL-1, osteoclast activating factor (OAF) has now been identified as having the same amino acid sequence as human IL-1β. Thus, it is presently considered that the catabolic properties of IL-1 in cartilage and bone contribute to the tissue destruction and matrix loss occurring in a variety of joint diseases.

Effects of IL-1 on Fibroblasts and Fibrosis

In contrast to its catabolic activities, IL-1 increases fibroblast proliferation and collagen synthesis. IL-1 is mitogenic for fibroblasts, although it is presently unclear whether this represents a true growth factor function of IL-1 or rather that IL-1 acts to increase the production of receptors for endogenous growth factors such as epi-dermal growth factor and transforming growth factor. IL-1 was shown to stimulate the production of PGE₂ and granulocyte-monocyte colony stimulating factor by fibroblasts. Nevertheless, IL-1 directly increases the transcription of type I and type III collagen (7) and type IV (basement membrane) collagen (42). Therefore, fibrosis and deposition of abnormal proteins in tissues appear to be, in part, mediated by IL-1. In rheumatoid joint disease, IL-1 is thought to contribute to pannus formation (33).

Effect of IL-1 on Immunocompetent Cells

Recombinant human IL-1 has been used to confirm the importance of IL-1 in the mechanism of T-cell activation. Initial studies involved human peripheral blood T cells. In order to help elucidate early events in initiating T-cell proliferation, an antibody directed against the CD3 protein complex was used to stimulate the T cells to produce a mitogenic response (the uptake of labeled thymidine). Activation was also assessed by measuring RNA and DNA synthesis rates, as well as the appearance of IL-2 receptors (65). In such experiments, human T cells are activated by antibodies directed against the CD3 cell surface protein complex, resulting in a mitogenic response; adding IL-1 to T cells in the presence of macrophages does not enhance the response. However, in the absence of macrophages, there is no cell activation, and it cannot be restored by the addition of purified human monocyte pI 7 IL-1. Thus the response to soluble CD3 requires the presence of macrophages, and these cells provide something more than IL-1. Immobilizing anti-CD3 on Sepharose provides a physical structure for cross-linking the CD3 complex. When the experiment is repeated using immobilized anti-CD3 with T cells depleted of macrophages, the addition of exogenous IL-1 results in a proliferative response. Experiments with recombinant IL-1 have confirmed these findings.

Under these experimental conditions, human T cells depleted of macrophages were stimulated by immobilized anti-CD3, and in the presence of recombinant IL-1, increased RNA synthesis was observed. This stimulation also resulted in increased synthesis of IL-2 and expression of the IL-2 receptor. Increased DNA synthesis followed these events. Thus, human T-cell activation requires a cross-linking mechanism for the CD3 complex and the T-cell antigen receptor (Ti) complex. Under normal conditions, the macrophage provides this cross-linking, as well as a source of IL-1. In the absence of macrophage membranes, T-cell activation takes place when cross-linking is accomplished by immobilized anti-CD3 or large macromolecular lectin mitogens; however, because there are no macrophages to provide a source of IL-1 under these conditions, soluble IL-1 is required. The interpretation of these findings suggests that macrophages provide two signals to the T cell: a cross-linking step and a source of IL-1.

Many investigators have shown that B cells and other cells serve as accessory cells in antigen recognition but have failed to demonstrate a role for IL-1 because it cannot be detected in B-cell supernatants. This issue may have been resolved by studies demonstrating that B cells produced IL-1 (59) and B cells expressed membrane-bound IL-1 (35). In fact, nearly all cells which can act as accessory cells produce IL-1. These include astrocytes, mesangial cells, keratinocytes, and endothelial cells. The lack of a signal peptide for IL-1 is consistent with the view that IL-1 can easily be trapped in the plasma membrane. Some cells may have a greater ability to process the IL-1 precursor polypeptide, resulting in detectable IL-1 in the extracellular fluid, whereas others may have a limited ability to process the precursor, resulting in a considerable amount remaining in the membrane or intracellular compartments (36). These observations are supported by the unique lack of a clear signal peptide in both forms of IL-1. Figure 1 illustrates the production of IL-1 by cell activation—through transcription and the synthesis of precursor IL-1 (pro-IL-1). Also depicted are the postulated events which lead to membrane IL-1 (22 kD) (35) and processed mature IL-1 (17 kD) (16) with its proteolytic cleavage products.

The effects of IL-1 on B cells and immunoglobulin production have recently been reviewed (40,46). The function of IL-1 in these cells seems to be similar to that shown in T cells; that is, IL-1 acts as a helper or cofactor during the activation process, particularly with IL-4, also known as B-cell stimulating factor-1 (BSF-1). IL-1 activates B cells and contributes to the formation of antibody. The first experiments to show the critical role of IL-1 in B-cell activation were performed with anti-IL-1 (38). Early addition of this antibody to human peripheral blood mononuclear cells stimulated with pokeweed mitogen completely prevented B-cell activation and subsequent antibody formation. Other studies demonstrated that IL-1 synergized with various B-cell growth and differentiation factors, leading to increased proliferation and antibody formation (46). The ability of IL-1 to induce other B-cell stimulating factors, including interferon-γ (IFN-γ) and IL-2, must also be considered, because these substances activate B cells.

Recent evidence demonstrates that IL-1 induces the production of another B-cell stimulating factor. This factor was originally described as a 26-kD protein from IL-1-stimulated fibroblasts which had hybridoma growth factor activity. The 26-kD protein also had the ability to stimulate plasmacytoma cell growth. The N-terminus of the homogeneous 26-kD factor matches that of an IFN-β_2 (62). Others have also reported a B-cell stimulating factor

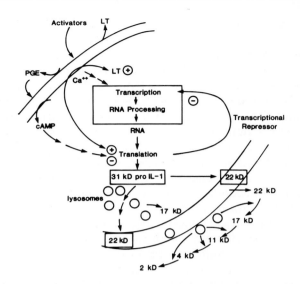

FIG. 1. Steps leading to the production and processing of IL-1. Activation of the cell stimulates generation of arachidonic acid metabolites such as the leukotrienes (LT) and prostaglandins (PG). PGs are not necessary for IL-1 production and, in fact, reduce production. PGE$_2$ buildup, following cell activation, stimulates the generation of cyclic adenosine monophophate (cAMP) which acts as a negative signal for translation. LTs that are formed seem to participate in IL-1 production, as inhibitors of the 5-lipoxygenase pathway reduce IL-1 production. Transcription begins within 15 min of cell activation. For human blood monocytes, mRNA can be detected 15 min after cells are exposed to glass with any exogenous stimulus; however, no protein is made. Once translation begins, there is a strong transcriptional repressor synthesized which can be demonstrated with the addition of cycloheximide. Translation requires a positive signal, and this is usually provided by substances such as endotoxin in very low concentrations. The primary translation product is the 31-kD IL-1 precursor molecule, termed "pro-IL-1." Pro-IL-1 has weak biological activity and no signal peptide sequence, and it is unclear how it is processed to a 22- or 17-kD active molecule. Processing may take place in the lysosomal fraction or elsewhere. A significant amount of translated pro-IL-1 is found in the cell membrane as a 22-kD molecule. The primary extracellular form of IL-1 is 17 kD and is vulnerable to extracellular proteases which yield biologically active IL-1 peptides with molecular weights of 11-, 4-, and 2-kD IL-1. ACTH, Adrenocorticotrophic hormone; TxA$_2$, thromboxane A$_2$; plt, platelet.

(BSF-2) which is the same molecule as the 26-kD IFN-β_2 (29). It seems that the role of IL-1 in augmenting B-cell function, and ultimately leading to the production of protective antibodies, may involve its ability to induce the synthesis of B-cell stimulating factors and/or up-regulating their receptors.

IL-1 also plays a role in host defense against tumor cells. There is evidence that IL-1 increases the binding of NK cells to tumor targets and that tumor cells induce the synthesis of IL-1 by NK cells (28). In addition, NK cells from patients with large tumor burdens produce significantly less IL-1 and have decreased killing ability compared to cells from healthy individuals. When incubated with exogenous IL-1, impaired NK function is restored. IL-1 also augments the binding of NK cells from healthy donors to tumor targets. Because IL-1 induces interferon (62) and because interferon synergizes with IL-1 with respect to its actions on NK cells, one could view both mechanisms as an efficient aspect of host defense against tumors. However, unlike the augmentation of T- and B-cell responses by IL-1, which is enhanced at febrile temperatures (49), the effect of IL-1 on NK cells is reduced at such temperatures (19).

SYSTEMIC VERSUS LOCAL EFFECTS OF IL-1

Table 1 and Fig. 2 illustrate the systemic effects of IL-1 as determined by experiments with either recombinant IL-1β or -α. These studies were carried out by injecting IL-1 either intravenously or intraperitoneally into experimental animals. In many cases, IL-1-induced changes mimic the animal's response to an injection of endotoxin or other microbial toxin or product. To date, these include fever as well as increased levels of adenocorticotrophic hormone (ACTH), corticosterone, insulin, a variety of hepatic acute phase proteins, and blood neutrophils, as well as slow-wave sleep. *In vivo,* IL-1 decreases the number of circulating neutrophils within a few minutes of a systemic injection, and this reflects the activation of endothelial surfaces and the adherence of leukocytes; after several hours, there is an increase in the number of circulating neutrophils, particularly new forms released from the marrow. IL-1 causes a decrease in systemic arterial pressure, systemic vascular resistance, cytochrome P-450 enzyme activity and serum albumin, iron, and zinc levels. The systemic changes may be related to local events; for example, 45 min after an intravenous injection of IL-1, which results in a 1°C fever, plasma levels are approximately 100 pg/ml, and this concentration is similar to the *in vitro* concentration for one half-maximal lymphocyte activating unit per milliliter.

Compared to the number of whole-animal studies, there have been considerably more studies on the *in vitro* effects of IL-1. However, some of the *in vitro* effects are probably relevant to systemic responses. The effects of IL-1 on endothelial cell arachidonic acid metabolism and procoagulant activity *in vitro* likely explain the shocklike state that IL-1 produces *in vivo* (51). In addition, the ability of IL-1 to induce various lymphokines *in vitro* probably occurs *in vivo,* but it is difficult to demonstrate circulating levels of interferons (IFN-β or -γ) and interleukins (IL-2 and -3) unless large doses are given. Some human studies, however, have employed large amounts of recombinant IL-2 and IFN-γ, and some of the systemic effects of these therapies may be due to IL-1 production.

TABLE 1. *Systemic effects of recombinant human IL-1*[a]

Central nervous system	Metabolic
Fever	Hypozincemia, hypoferremia
Brain PGE$_2$ synthesis	Decreased cytochrome P-450 enzyme
Increased ACTH levels	Increased acute phase proteins
Increased corticosteroid levels	Decreased albumin synthesis
Increased slow-wave sleep	Increased survival rate in mice
Decreased appetite[b]	Increased bacterial clearance
	Increased (high dose decreased) insulin
	Lipoprotein lipase inhibition
	Increased sodium excretion
Hematological	Vascular wall
Neutrophilia	Increased leukocyte adherence
Lymphopenia	Increased PGI and PGE synthesis
Neutrophil TbxA generation	Increased platelet activating factor
Tumor necrosis	Increased procoagulant activity
Bone marrow release	Increased plasminogen activator
Inhibitor	

Hemodynamic effects
Hypotension
Decreased systemic vascular resistance
Decreased central venous pressure
Increased cardiac output
Increased heart rate
Decreased blood pH

[a] PG, Prostaglandin; ACTH, adrenocorticotrophic hormone; TbxA, thromboxane A.
[b] Indirect mechanism.

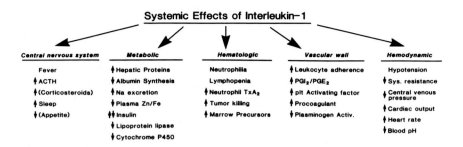

FIG. 2. Multiple systemic effects of IL-1.

However, one approach to interpreting the large body of evidence for multiple biological effects of IL-1 is to view local production and action as the "autocrine or paracrine" action of IL-1, and these effects are listed in Table 2. In contrast, the systemic effects of IL-1 can be considered related to the "hormonal" property. At present, it seems that autocrine or paracrine effects of IL-1 predominate in some diseases, whereas systemic effects are characteristic of IL-1 produced as a result of toxemia, septicemia, widespread tissue damage, or intravenous antigen challenge. What seems increasingly clear is that tissues that produce IL-1 either are themselves the targets of local IL-1 effects or are capable of acting on adjacent tissues. For example, IL-1 produced by macrophages in lymph nodes likely induces IL-2, IL-2 receptors, IL-3, hybridoma growth factor, and IFN-γ which exert their effects on nearby T, B, and NK cells. In addition, in a dense cellular response, even low concentrations of IL-1 probably synergize with IL-2 and -4 for enhancement of lymphocyte responses. Table 3 summarizes some immunological properties of IL-1.

IL-1 produced by microglia and astrocytes in the brain has its effect on local gliosis but may induce no systemic responses. A similar case can be made for the ability of IL-1 to stimulate production of fibroblast granulocyte-macrophage colony stimulating factor, IFN-β, and hybridoma growth factor. However, local production and biological activity of IL-1 in the joint space has attracted considerable attention because of a potential role for IL-1 in the pathogenesis of various joint diseases such as rheumatoid arthritis and osteoarthritis. The joint macrophage has been shown to produce IL-1, and IL-1 has been measured in synovial fluid from patients with a variety of arthritides. Special dendritic fibroblasts cultured from human arthritis synovia produce large amounts of collagenase and PGE₂ in response to IL-1, and this local property of IL-1 likely contributes to pain and destructive disease (33). In addition, IL-1 is a direct stimulator of *de novo* collagen synthesis and induces fibroblast proliferation. Thus, there is also a role for IL-1 in the process of synovial membrane thickening. IL-1 has been shown to stimulate chondrocyte metalloproteinases and PGE₂ production (60), and IL-1 induces the resorption of bone in its role as an OAF. Thus, the autocrine or paracrine effects

---

TABLE 2. *Autocrine effects of interleukin-1*[a]

Attraction of neutrophils, lymphocytes, monocytes (*in vivo*)
Basophil histamine release
Eosinophil degranulation
Proliferation of dermal fibroblasts
Increased collagen synthesis
Increased collagenase production
Chondrocyte protease release
Induction of fibroblast and endothelial GM-CSF activity
Production of PGE₂ in dermal and synovial fibroblasts
Increased neutrophil and monocyte thromboxane synthesis
Cytotoxic for human melanoma cells
Cytotoxic for human β islet cells (insulin producing)
Cytotoxic for thyrocytes
Increased bone resorption (osteoclast activating factor)
Stimulation of fibroblast interferon-β synthesis
Stimulation of fibroblast hybridoma growth factor synthesis
Keratinocyte proliferation
Mesangial cell proliferation
Gliosis

[a] PGE₂, Prostaglandin E₂; GM-CSF, granulocyte-monocyte colony stimulating factor.

TABLE 3. *Immunological effects of IL-1*[a]

T-cell activation
  IL-2 production, increased IL-2 receptor number or
    binding

B-cell activation
  Synergism with B-cell growth factor (BSF-1/IL-4)
  Induction of interferon-β₂/hybridoma growth factor/BSF-2

Natural killer cells
  Synergism with IL-2 and interferon for tumor killing
  Increased natural killer cell–tumor binding
  Production of IL-1 from natural killer cells

Increased lymphokine production
  IL-2, IL-3, GM-CSF, interferon-β₁, interferon-β₂
  Interferon-γ, leukocyte inhibitory migration factor

Macrophage cytotoxicity
  Increased IL-1 production

[a] IL, Interleukin; BSF, B-cell stimulating factor; GM-CSF, granulocyte-monocyte colony stimulating factor.

of IL-1 may play a major role in the pathogenesis of several disease processes in addition to being a prominent response to local infection and injury.

HOW IL-1 MEDIATES HOST DEFENSE MECHANISMS

From the preceding discussion, it seems clear that IL-1 affects many tissues and organ systems. Are these effects beneficial to the host in the struggle to overcome microbial invasion? IL-1-mediated responses appear to fall into two types: (a) acute phase changes such as fever, sleep, ACTH release, effects on vascular tissue, hepatic acute phase protein synthesis, decreased plasma iron and zinc levels, increased numbers of neutrophils, and increased interferon and colony stimulating factor production; and (b) general immunological stimulation leading to the development of specific antibodies or specific cytotoxic T cells involved in ultimate eradication of the invader.

Acute phase changes are produced within hours of the onset of infection. Fever may play various roles. An elevated body temperature itself reduces the replication rate of some bacteria and several viruses. Moreover, several studies have demonstrated that immunological responses such as helper T-cell activation, the generation of cytotoxic T cells, B-cell activation, and antibody synthesis are augmented by an elevated temperature (49). Considering the fact that most lymph nodes are located close to the surface of the skin and are at 34 to 36°C, the rise in temperature due to the pyrogenic effect of IL-1 may play a direct role in host defense. There is also evidence that neutrophil phagocytosis and some oxidative processes are enhanced by elevated temperatures. *In vivo* studies have also provided substantial evidence that elevated temperatures in fish, reptiles, and mammals augment various host defense mechanisms, resulting in increased survival (3).

IL-1 increases the synthesis of several normally produced hepatic proteins including various antiproteases, several complement components, fibrinogen, haptoglobin, ceruloplasmin, and others. However, IL-1 also initiates gene expression of new products, generally proteins not synthesized in health but in association with infection or injury or other pathological processes. IL-1-induced increases in normal hepatic proteins are usually in the range of 2- to 3-fold, but IL-1-initiated synthesis of pathological proteins can be 100- to 1,000-fold. Two such proteins, SAA protein and CRP, are classic "acute phase reactants" and serve as markers of disease. SAA contributes to the development of secondary amyloidosis. Other pathological acute phase proteins include α-macroglobulin and acid-l-glycoprotein.

Do these hepatic proteins play a role in host defense mechanisms? The strongest implication that they serve an important function comes from data showing the presence of acute phase reactants such as the pentaxins SAA and CRP in the invertebrate horseshoe crab *Limulus*. Not only is their presence for 400 million years of evolution an indication of their importance to the host, but, in addition, their structure has been amazingly conserved in that the primary structure of *Limulus* pentaxin is nearly identical to that of human pentaxin. The overwhelming physical property of CRP and SAA is their ability to bind to lipids. In addition, other proteins such as α_1-macroglobulin and ceruloplasmin act as oxygen scavengers. Because many acute phase proteins are large glycoproteins, they bind to bacterial surfaces, and this physical property allows them to act as all-purpose, nonspecific opsonins. Acute phase proteins also include a series of antiproteases, and these may play a role in offsetting the action of some bacterial proteases. Finally, the liver is the source of other proteins which bind divalent cations such as iron and zinc. These metalloproteins are usually not secreted but bind plasma iron and zinc and localize these elements in the liver, spleen, and bone marrow. One major benefit to the host is that the lowered tissue levels of iron and zinc result in reduced microbial replication, particularly at febrile temperatures. It appears that acute phase proteins have served evolution and host defense well enough so that many species survive without T cells, B cells, or the ability to make specific antibodies.

The clinical association of increased sleepiness with infectious disease has received clarification and new information has been provided by studies on IL-1. "Sleep factor," isolated from the urine of sleep-deprived humans and the cerebrospinal fluid of animals, has been chemically identified as an N-acetylated muramic acid linked to a tetrapeptide structure, similar to the peptidoglycan units of muramic acid tetrapeptide found in all bacterial cell walls (34). Sleep factor purified from either human urine or peritoneal dialysis fluid is, like other muramyl peptides, an inducer of IL-1 (13). Like sleep factor, both natural and recombinant IL-1 induce increased slow-wave sleep when injected either intravenously or intracerebroventricularly. The onset of IL-1-mediated increases in slow-wave sleep is considerably faster than that for sleep factor, and there is evidence that sleep factor induces slow-wave sleep via the production of IL-1 either peripherally or by astrocytes and microglia within the central nervous system. The benefit to the host of increased sleep may be conservation of energy and metabolic resources at a time when they are needed to fight infection. Therefore, sleep and decreased appetite, also an IL-1-induced change associated with acute phase responses, may be considered part of the behavioral alterations serving a host defense mechanism. A decrease in appetite reduces the desire to seek food with its attendant dangers for much of the animal world. It is unclear how effective reduced food intake is to specific host defense mechanisms. Nevertheless, we are reminded of Pasteur's comment that, during infection, the host attempts to "starve out" the microbe as a mechanism of resistance.

COMPARISON BETWEEN IL-1 AND TUMOR NECROSIS FACTOR (CACHECTIN)

Another monocyte or macrophage product, synthesized and released as a consequence of microbial stimulation and tissue injury, is TNF. The biological properties of TNF are remarkably similar to those of IL-1 with the notable exception that TNF, at concentrations which induce acute phase changes in many tissues, has no immunostimulatory effects. However, nearly every biological property of IL-1 has been observed with TNF. These include fever (18), the induction of PGE_2 and collagenase synthesis in a variety of tissues (4), bone resorption, inhibition of lipoprotein lipase, increases in hepatic acute phase reactants, and a decrease in albumin synthesis (53). Slow-wave sleep is also observed following the injection of TNF or IL-1. Both molecules also induce fibroblast proliferation and new collagen synthesis. The cytotoxic activity of TNF differs from that of IL-1. For example, IL-1 is cytotoxic for the β cells of the pancreatic islets of Langerhans and also for human melanoma cells, but in the same assays TNF has no effect. Likewise, IL-1 is inactive on a variety of tumor targets for which TNF is a potent cytotoxin. In fact, the cells most often used in assays of TNF cytotoxic activity, L929 fibroblasts, are unaffected by IL-1.

In vivo, IL-1 and TNF induce fever through their direct ability to induce hypothalamic PGE_2 synthesis. In addition to fever, these cytokines cause hypotension, leukopenia, and local tissue necrosis. On a weight basis, rabbits are equally sensitive to the shock inducing properties of IL-1 (51) and TNF/cachectin (4). These responses likely reflect the effects of these two cytokines on the vascular endothelium. Both IL-1 and TNF/cachectin stimulate PGI_2, PGE_2, and platelet activating factor production by cultured endothelium. In addition, both cytokines stimulate procoagulant activity, leukocyte adherence, and plasminogen activator inhibitor on these cells. Despite these similarities, receptors for TNF have been shown to be specific and distinct, and receptor binding is unaffected by IL-1. Thus, the most likely explanation is that TNF and IL-1 stimulate similar intracellular messages and alter cellular metabolism in a similar way. Table 4 lists the biological similarities between TNF and IL-1. As noted, both TNF and IL-1 stimulate the production of more IL-1. This can be shown *in vivo* and *in vitro* with human monocytes and human endothelium.

At present, there are no data suggesting that IL-1α or

TABLE 4. *Comparison of biological properties of IL-1 and TNF (cachectin)[a]*

Biological property	IL-1	TNF
Endogenous pyrogen fever	+	+
Slow-wave sleep	+	+
Hemodynamic shock	+	+
Increased hepatic acute phase protein synthesis	+	+
Decreased albumin synthesis	+	+
Activation of endothelium	+	+
Decreased lipoprotein lipase level	+	+
Decreased cytochrome P-450 level	+	+
Decreased plasma levels of iron and zinc	+	+
Increased fibroblast proliferation	+	+
Increased synovial cell collagenase and PGE_2 levels	+	+
Induction of IL-1	+	+
T- and B-cell activation	+	−

[a] IL-1, Interleukin-1; TNF, tumor necrosis factor; PGE_2, prostaglandin E_2.

-β and TNF are related at the amino acid level or even at the secondary or tertiary structural level. However, it seems clear that cytokines are biologically related molecules. One can only speculate that acute phase responses such as fever, hepatic protein synthesis, decreases in plasma iron or zinc levels, etc., are of such importance to host survival that nature imparted these responses to more than a single molecule.

SOURCES OF IL-1

Fixed Macrophages

These cells are often located in strategic blood filtering organs and are involved in primary phagocytic defense mechanisms against invading microorganisms. For example, there are fixed macrophages lining the alveolar space, in the lamina propria, in the dermis, in the lining of blood filtering organs, and in lymph nodes. Peritoneal macrophages are also part of the primary phagocytic defense mechanism, because these cells would be involved with microorganisms derived from intestinal perforations. Most studies involving IL-1 production by peritoneal cells employ an agent such as oil or thioglycollate, and this agent may not only raise the total number of macrophages in the peritoneal cavity but also "prime" the macrophages for subsequent stimulation *in vitro*. Several biologically active molecules such as tuftsin, while not an IL-1 inducer, lower the threshold of peritoneal macrophages to exogenous stimuli like endotoxin. Such priming may also be part of the mechanism by which pretreatment of blood monocytes with interferons increases endotoxin-induced

IL-1 production. Langerhans' cells isolated from the skin can be separated from keratinocytes by adherence techniques and, when stimulated, these cells produce IL-1. With the use of a similar method, dendritic cells from human synovium can also be separated from other synovial cells and produce IL-1 upon stimulation.

Keratinocytes

Several keratinocyte lines of human or mouse origin produce IL-1 without any apparent stimulant but increase production when incubated with endotoxin or toxic shock syndrome toxin-1. Keratinocyte IL-1 also shares biological activities with monocyte-derived IL-1, for example, fever induction. Keratinocyte-derived IL-1 is the source of IL-1 found in cornified epidermis. Rabbits irradiated with ultraviolet light have circulating levels of IL-1, and it seems probable that it is keratinocyte-derived. It has also been speculated that keratinocyte IL-1 production may be involved in a variety of skin lesions, including acute sunburn and lesions which result from treatment with ultraviolet B-wave phototherapy for certain skin diseases.

Large Granular Lymphocytes

These cells are also known as NK cells and have been purified from human blood and shown to release IL-1 upon stimulation with endotoxin or tumor cell targets. Patients with large tumor burdens have circulating NK cells which produce little IL-1 and have markedly reduced ability to bind and lyse tumor targets (28).

Mesangial Cells

Rat mesangial cell lines produce IL-1 which is active in both thymocyte and fever assays. Rat IL-1 derived from mesangial cells has been subjected to several purification procedures and has multiple molecular-weight and charged forms. In addition to stimulating thymocytes and the thermoregulatory center, mesangial cell IL-1 has also been shown to act as a growth factor for mesangial cells.

Astroglia and Microglia

Brain astrocytes present antigen and express major histocompatibility complex (MHC) class II antigens on their cell surface. In addition, these neural cells produce IL-1. Human glioma cell lines produce an IL-1 which is antigenically related to human monocyte IL-1. Mice injected with endotoxin intraperitoneally develop fever for several hours, and astrocytes separated from other neural tissue contain large amounts of intracellular IL-1. In fact, astro-cyte IL-1 may play an important role in fever induction. IL-1 also stimulates glial cell proliferation, and locally produced IL-1 may be involved in central nervous system tissue scarring, also known as "gliosis." Recent studies have also focused on other central nervous system cells, microglia, as a potent source of IL-1. The relative production of IL-1 by microglia seems to be 10 to 50 times greater than that by astrocytes. This is not surprising, because microglia are considered brain tissue macrophages.

IL-1 Production by Blood Vessel Cells

The two major blood vessel cells, endothelium and smooth muscle, both produce IL-1. Endothelial cell IL-1 has been reported by several groups to produce IL-1 and recently shown at the level of gene expression (37). In general, IL-1 production by endothelial cells is an inducible event, and endotoxin is particularly effective when compared to other well-known inducers of monocyte IL-1. Smooth muscle cell lines of human origin produce IL-1 which is similar to monocyte IL-1 based on immunoprecipitation and mRNA hybridization (38). The finding that both blood vessel-derived cells produce IL-1 is important to the understanding of pathological processes in vasculitis, as endothelial cells are activated by IL-1 to increase their adhesiveness for leukocytes and their procoagulant activity. Therefore, in disease processes in which antigen–antibody complexes mediate tissue injury and vessel disruption, endothelial and/or smooth muscle IL-1 likely acts as an autacoid and contributes to progression of the lesion.

Epithelial Cells

Epithelial cell IL-1 production has been reported in two studies involving (a) IL-1 from the gingival epithelial cell and (b) IL-1 produced by corneal epithelium. In the gingiva, local IL-1 production clearly plays an important role, as IL-1 stimulates bone resorption and OAF has been shown to have the same amino acid sequence as IL-1β. IL-1 production by corneal epithelium is also of considerable clinical significance, because IL-1 is chemotactic for neutrophils, monocytes, and lymphocytes *in vivo*.

MECHANISMS OF ACTION

The multiple biological properties of IL-1 seem to fall into two categories: (a) abrupt changes such as fever, hemodynamic shock, increased slow-wave sleep, sodium excretion, ACTH and insulin release, and degranulation of eosinophils and basophils; and (b) slow-onset changes such as hepatic protein synthesis, production of growth factors, cell proliferation, cytotoxicity (β cells of the islets of Langerhans, some tumors), and induction of synthesis of a variety of enzymes and structural proteins. The lymphokines IL-2, interferons, IL-4, and IFN-β_2 (also known as BSF-2) are in the latter category.

Are these responses related? Does the same mechanism(s) of action account for both the acute as well as the late-onset changes? In general, tissue injury represents a good example of the biology of IL-1. One can observe this most dramatically in rabbit skin injected with IL-1 (45). There is an acute period of marked inflammation associated with vasodilation (cyclooxygenation of arachidonic acid and histamine release), infiltration and adherence of neutrophils and lymphocytes (lipoxygenation of arachidonate), and destructive lesions (release of preformed enzymes); this is followed by a later phase associated with protein synthesis, cell growth, and repair. One hypothesis is that the entire spectrum of IL-1 multiple biological properties is due to rapid activation of the phosphoinositide pathway whereby phosphoinositol is liberated by receptor binding to stimulatory G protein and activation of phosphodiesterase. The phosphodiesterase converts phosphotidylinositol 4,5,-biphosphate into diacylglycerol and free inositol triphosphate. Subsequent activation of phospholipases by inositol triphosphate and calcium would lead to the release of free arachidonic acid, the rate-limiting step in conversion to cyclooxygenase products. Can this pathway explain the rapid increase in PGE$_2$ which occurs during the induction of fever? Another hypothesis is that the action of IL-1 leads to a direct and rapid increase in phospholipase A$_2$ activity which liberates membrane arachidonate. This arachidonate is rapidly converted by cyclooxygenation to PGE$_2$ which gains access to the extracellular compartment and causes fever and other acute changes.

The mechanism by which IL-1 accomplishes the release of arachidonate must be fast in order to account for the rapid onset of fever and other systemic changes observed with IL-1. The ability of IL-1 to act as an inducer of hemodynamic shock and fever within minutes following intravenous injection is linked to the cyclooxygenase products, but the concept that IL-1 induces the generation of free arachidonic acid associated with an increase in phospholipase A$_2$ requires experimental data. Cell lines such as fibroblasts or neuroblastomas and cultured synovial cells and chondrocytes are used by many investigators. The time course of PGE$_2$ production following IL-1 stimulation of cultured chondocytes, synovial cells, and neuroblastoma cells or fibroblasts, even at high concentrations of IL-1, is at least 4 hr and reaches a maximum at 24 hr. Similar results have been reported for IL-1-induced endothelial PGI$_2$ synthesis. Cultured rabbit chondrocyte phospholipase A$_2$ production induced by IL-1 is not detected until after 60 min and reaches a maximum after 24 hr. In contrast, fever production starts at 10 min and begins to decline after 45 to 55 min.

The proinflammatory action of IL-1 is to be contrasted with its growth promoting effect. It is possible that the events taking place in the first minutes of the proinflammatory response involve second messengers distinct from those participating in the progrowth response. It seems that the choice of the type of target cell rather than the type of second messenger pathway explains the time course difference. One striking difference is that growth promoting responses are observed in cultured cells, whereas proinflammatory properties are usually detected in freshly isolated cells. However, one cannot attribute this difference to deprivation of arachidonic acid precursors in cultured cells, because adding excess arachidonic acid to cultured cells does not shorten the time course of IL-1-induced PGE$_2$ production. It is likely that many of the growth promoting effects of IL-1 are mediated through leukotrienes. A role for the lipoxygenase pathway in mediating the effects of IL-1 on T lymphocytes and B cells is supported by considerable evidence. Studies indicate that specific 5-lipoxygenase inhibitors reduce the effects of IL-1 on immunocompetent cells.

ACKNOWLEDGMENTS

The studies described in this chapter were supported by NIH grant AI 15614. The author wishes to thank Dr. Sheldon M. Wolff for his support.

REFERENCES

1. Auron, P. E., Webb, A. C., Rosenwasser, L. J., Mucci, S. F., Rich, A., Wolff, S. M., and Dinarello, C. A. (1984): Nucleotide sequence of human monocyte interleukin-1 precursor cDNA. *Proc. Natl. Acad. Sci. USA*, 81:7907–7911.
2. Auron, P. E., Rosenwasser, L. J., Matsushima, K., Copeland, T., Dinarello, C. A., Oppenheim, J. J., and Webb, A. C. (1985): Human and murine interleukin-1 share sequence similarities. *J. Mol. Immunol.*, 2:231–239.
3. Bernheim, H. A., Bodel, P. T., Askenase, P. W., and Atkins, E. (1978): Effects of fever on host defense mechanisms after infection in the lizard. *Br. J. Exp. Pathol.*, 59:76–84.
4. Beutler, B., and Cerami, A. (1986): Cachectin and tumor necrosis factor: Two sides of the same biological coin. *Nature*, 320:584–588.
5. Bevilacqua, M. P., Pober, J. S., Wheeler, M. E., Mendrick, D., Cotran, R. S., and Gibrone, M. A., Jr. (1985): Interleukin-1 acts on cultured human vascular endothelial cells to increase the adhesion of polymorphonuclear leukocytes, monocytes and related leukocyte cell lines. *J. Clin. Invest.*, 76:2003–2011.
6. Bird, T. A., and Saklatvala, J. (1986): Identification of a common class of high affinity receptors for both types of porcine interleukin-1 on connective tissue cells. *Nature*, 324:263–265.
7. Canalis, E. (1986): Interleukin-1 has independent effects on DNA and collagen synthesis in cultures of rat calvariae. *Endocrinology*, 118:74–81.
8. Clark, B. D., Collins, K. L., Gandy, M. S., Webb, A. C., and Auron, P. E. (1986): Genomic sequence for human prointerleukin-1 beta: Possible evolution from a reverse transcribed prointerleukin-1 alpha gene. *Nucleic Acids Res.*, 14:7897–7905.

9. Conti, P., Cifone, M. G., Alesse, E., Reale, M., Fieschi, C., and Dinarello, C. A. (1986): In vitro enhanced thromboxane B2 release by polymorphonuclear leukocytes and macrophages after treatment with human recombinant interleukin-1. *Prostaglandins*, 32:111–115.

10. Dejana, E., Brevario, F., Erroi, A., Bussolino, F., Mussoni, L., Gramse, M., Pintucci, G., Casali, B., Dinarello, C. A., Van Damme, J., and Mantovani, A. (1987): Modulation of endothelial cell function by different molecular species of interleukin-1. *Blood*, 69:695–699.

11. Dinarello, C. A. (1984): Interleukin-1. *Rev. Infect. Dis.*, 6:51–95.

12. Dinarello, C. A. (1986): Interleukin-1: Amino acid sequences, multiple biological activities and comparison with tumor necrosis factor (cachectin). *Year Immunol.*, 2:68–89.

13. Dinarello, C. A., and Krueger, J. M. (1986): Induction of interleukin-1 by synthetic and naturally occurring muramyl peptides. *Fed. Proc.*, 45:2545–2548.

14. Dinarello, C. A., and Wolff, S. M. (1982): Molecular basis of fever in humans. *Am. J. Med.*, 72:799–819.

15. Dinarello, C. A., Renfer, L., and Wolff, S. M. (1977): Human leukocytic pyrogen: Purification and development of a radioimmunoassay. *Proc. Natl. Acad. Sci. USA*, 74:4624–4627.

16. Dinarello, C. A., Bernheim, H. A., Cannon, J. G., LoPreste, G., Warner, S. J. C., Webb, A. C., and Auron, P. E. (1985): Purified, ^{35}S-met, ^{3}H-leu-labeled human monocyte interleukin-1 with endogenous pyrogen activity. *Br. J. Rheumatol.*, 24:(suppl)59–64.

17. Dinarello, C. A., Cannon, J. G., Mier, J. W., Bernheim, H. A., LoPreste, G., Lynn, D. L., Love, R. N., Webb, A. C., Auron, P. E., Reuben, R. C., Rich, A., Wolff, S. M., and Putney, S. D. (1986): Multiple biological activities of human recombinant interleukin-1. *J. Clin. Invest.*, 77:1734–1739.

18. Dinarello, C. A., Cannon, J. G., Wolff, S. M., Bernheim, H. A., Beutler, B., Cerami, A., Figari, I. S., Palladino, M. A., Jr., and O'Connor, J. V. (1986): Tumor necrosis factor (cachectin) is an endogenous pyrogen and induces interleukin-1. *J. Exp. Med.*, 163: 1433–1450.

19. Dinarello, C. A., Dempsey, R. A., Allegretta, M., LoPreste, G., Dainiak, N., Parkinson, D. R., and Mier, J. W. (1986): Inhibitory effects of elevated temperature on cytokine production and natural killer activity. *Cancer Res.*, 46:6235–6241.

20. Dower, S. K., Kronheim, S. R., March, C. J., Colon, P. J., Hopp, T. P., Gillis, S., and Urdal, D. L. (1985): Detection and characterization of high affinity receptors for human interleukin-1. *J. Exp. Med.*, 162:501–515.

21. Furutani, Y., Notake, M., Yamayoshi, M., Yamagishi, J., Nomura, H., Ohue, M., Fukui, T., Yamada, M., and Nakamura, S. (1985): Cloning and characterization of the cDNAs for human and rabbit interleukin-1 precursor. *Nucleic Acids Res.*, 13:5869–5882.

22. Furutani, Y., Notake, M., Fuki, T., Ohue, M., Nomura, H., Yamada, M., and Nakamura, S. (1986): Complete nucleotide sequence of the gene for human interleukin-1-alpha. *Nucleic Acids Res.*, 14:3167–3179.

23. Gery, I., and Waksman, B. H. (1972): Potentiation of the T-lymphocyte response to mitogens. II. The cellular source of potentiating mediator(s). *J. Exp. Med.*, 136:143–155.

24. Ghezzi, P., Saccardo, B., Villa, P., Rossi, V., Bianchi, M., and Dinarello, C. A. (1986): Role of interleukin-1 in the depression of liver drug metabolism by endotoxin. *Infect. Immun.*, 54:837–840.

25. Gimenez-Gallego, G., Rodkey, J., Bennett, C., Rios-Candelore, M., DiSalvo, J., and Thomas, K. (1985): Brain-derived acidic fibroblast growth factor: Complete amino acid sequence and homologies. *Science*, 230:1385–1388.

26. Gray, P. W., Glaister, D., Chen, E., Goeddel, D. V., and Pennica, D. (1986): Two interleukin-1 genes in the mouse: Cloning and expression of the cDNA for murine interleukin-1-beta. *J. Immunol.*, 137:3644–3648.

27. Hanson, D. F., and Murphy, P. A. (1984): Demonstration of interleukin-1 activity in apparently homogeneous specimens of the pI 5 form of rabbit endogenous pyrogen. *Infect. Immun.*, 45:483–490.

28. Herman, J., Dinarello, C. A., Kew, M. C., and Rabson, A. R. (1985): The role of interleukin-1 in tumor NK cell interactions: Correction of defective NK cell activity in cancer patients by treating target cells with IL-1. *J. Immunol.*, 135:2882–2886.

29. Hirano, T., Yasukawa, K., Harada, H., Taga, T., Wantanabe, Y., Matsuda, T., Kashiwamura, S., Nakajima, K., Koyama, K., Iwasmatsu, A., Tsunasawa, S., Sakiyama, F., Matsui, H., Takahara, Y., Taniguchi, T., and Kishimoto, T. (1986): Complementary DNA for a novel human interleukin (BSF-2) that induces B lymphocytes to produce immunoglobulin. *Nature*, 324:73–76.

30. Hunninghake, G. W., Glazier, A. J., Monick, M. M., and Dinarello, C. A. (1986): Interleukin-1 is a chemotactic factor for human T-lymphocytes. *Am. Rev. Respir. Dis.*, 135:66–71.

31. Kampschmidt, R. F. (1981): Leukocytic endogenous mediator/endogenous pyrogen. In: *Physiologic and Metabolic Responses of the Host*, edited by M. C. Powanda and P. G. Canonico, pp. 55–74. Elsevier/North-Holland, Amsterdam.

32. Kilian, P. L., Kaffka, K. L., Stern, A. S., Woehle, D., Benjamin, W. R., DeChiara, T. M., Gubler, U., Farrar, J. J., Mizel, S. B., and Lomedico, P. T. (1986): Interleukin-1-alpha and interleukin-1-beta bind to the same receptor on T-cells. *J. Immunol.*, 136:4509–4514.

33. Krane, S. M., Dayer, J.-M., Simon, L. S., and Byrne, S. (1985): Mononuclear cell-conditioned medium containing mononuclear cell factor (MCF), homologous with interleukin-1, stimulates collagen and fibronectin synthesis by adherent rheumatoid synovial cells: Effects of prostaglandin E$_2$ and indomethacin. *Collagen Related Res.*, 5:99–117.

34. Kreuger, J. M., Walter, J., Dinarello, C. A., Wolff, S. M., and Chedid, L. (1984): Sleep-promoting effects of endogenous pyrogen (interleukin-1). *Am. J. Physiol.*, 246:R994–R999.

35. Kurt-Jones, E. A., Kiely, J. M., and Unanue, E. R. (1985): Conditions required for expression of membrane IL-1 on B-cells. *J. Immunol.*, 135:1548–1550.

36. Lepe-Zuniga, B., and Gery, I. (1984): Production of intracellular and extracellular interleukin-1 (IL-1) by human monocytes. *Clin. Immunol. Immunopathol.*, 31:222–230.

37. Libby, P., Ordovas, J. M., Auger, K. R., Robbins, A. H., Birinyi, L. K., and Dinarello, C. A. (1986): Endotoxin and tumor necrosis factor induce interleukin-1 gene expression in adult human vascular endothelial cells. *Am. J. Pathol.*, 124:179–186.

38. Libby, P., Ordovas, J. M., Auger, K. R., Robbins, A. H., Birinyi, L. K., and Dinarello, C. A. (1986): Inducible interleukin-1 gene expression in vascular smooth muscle cells. *J. Clin. Invest.*, 78:1432–1438.

39. Lipsky, P. E., Thompson, P. A., Rosenwasser, L. J., and Dinarello, C. A. (1983): The role of interleukin-1 in human B cell activation: Inhibition of B cell proliferation and the generation of immunoglobulin secreting cells by an antibody against human leukocytic pyrogen. *J. Immunol.*, 130:2708–2714.

40. Lipsky, P. E. (1985): Role of interleukin-1 in human B-cell activation. *Contemp. Top. Mol. Immunol.*, 10:195–217.

41. Lomedico, P. T., Gubler, U., Hellman, C. P., Dukovich, M., Giri, J. G., Pan, Y. E., Collier, K., Semionow, R., Chua, A. O., and Mizel, S. B. (1984): Cloning and expression of murine interleukin-1 in *Escherichia coli. Nature*, 312:458–462.

42. Matsushima, K., Bano, M., Kidwell, W. R., and Oppenheim, J. J. (1985): Interleukin 1 increases collagen type IV production by murine mammary epithelial cells. *J. Immunol.*, 134:904–909.

43. Matsushima, K., Yodoi, J., Tagaya, Y., and Oppenheim, J. J. (1986): Down regulation of interleukin-1 receptor expression by IL-1 and fate of internalized 125-I-labeled IL-1-beta in a human large granular lymphocyte cell line. *J. Immunol.*, 137:3183–3188.

44. McAdam, K. P. W. J., and Dinarello, C. A. (1980): Induction of serum amyloid A synthesis by human leukocytic pyrogen. In: *Bacterial Endotoxins and Host Response*, edited by M. K. Agawal, pp. 167–178. Elsevier/North Holland Press, Amsterdam.

45. Movat, H. Z., Cybulsky, M. I., Colditz, I. G., Chan, M. K. W., and Dinarello, C. A. (1987): Acute inflammation in Gram negative infection: Endotoxin, interleukin-1, tumor necrosis factor, and neutrophils. *Fed. Proc.*, 46:97–104.

46. Muraguchi, A., Kehrl, J. H., Butler, J. L., and Fauci, A. S. (1984): Regulation of human B-cell activation, proliferation, and differentiation by soluble factors. *J. Clin. Immunol.*, 4:337–347.

47. Murphy, P. A., Chesney, J., and Wood, W. B., Jr. (1974): Further purification of rabbit leukocyte pyrogen. *J. Lab. Clin. Med.*, 83: 310–322.

48. Murphy, P. A., Simon, P. L., and Willoughby, W. F. (1980): Endogenous pyrogens made by rabbit peritoneal exudate cells are identical with lymphocyte activating factors made by rabbit alveolar macrophages. *J. Immunol.*, 124:2498–2501.

49. Murphy, P. A., Hanson, D. F., Guo, Y. N., and Angster, D. E., (1985): The effects of variations in pH and temperature on the activation of mouse thymocytes by both forms of rabbit interleukin-1. *Yale J. Biol. Med.*, 58:115–122.

50. Nachman, R. L., Hajjar, K. A., Silverstein, R. L., and Dinarello, C. A. (1986): Interleukin-1 induces endothelial cell synthesis of plasminogen activator inhibitor. *J. Exp. Med.*, 163:1545–1547.

51. Okusawa, S., Gelfand, J. A., Connolly, R. A., and Dinarello, C. A. (1987): Interleukin-1 induces hemodynamic shock: Reversal by a cyclooxygenase inhibitor. *Fed. Proc.* (in press).

52. Perlmutter, D., Goldberger, G., Dinarello, C. A., Mizel, S. B., and Colten, H. R. (1986): Regulation of class III major histocompatability complex gene products by interleukin-1. *Science*, 232:850–852.

53. Perlmutter, D. H., Dinarello, C. A., Punsal, P., and Colten, H. R. (1986): Cachectin/tumor necrosis factor regulates hepatic acute phase gene expression. *J. Clin. Invest.*, 78:1349–1354.

54. Pincus, S. H., Whitcomb, E. A., and Dinarello, C. A. (1986): Interaction of interleukin-1 and TPA in modulation of eosinophil function. *J. Immunol.*, 137:3509–3514.

55. Ramadori, G., Sipe, J. D., Dinarello, C. A., Mizel, S. B., and Colten, H. R. (1985): Pretranslational modulation of acute phase hepatic protein synthesis by murine recombinant interleukin-1 and purified human IL-1. *J. Exp. Med.*, 162:930–942.

56. Rosenwasser, L. J., Dinarello, C. A., and Rosenthal, A. (1979): Adherent cell function in murine T-lymphocyte antigen recognition. IV. Enhancement of murine T-cell antigen recognition by human leukocytic pyrogen. *J. Exp. Med.*, 150:709–714.

57. Rossi, V., Breviario, F., Ghezzi, P., Dejana, E., and Mantovani, A. (1985): Interleukin-1 induces prostacyclin in vascular cells. *Science*, 229:1174–1176.

58. Saklatvala, J., Sarsfield, S. J., and Townsend, Y. (1985): Pig interleukin-1: Purification of two immunologically different leukocyte proteins that cause cartilage resorption, lymphocyte activation, and fever. *J. Exp. Med.*, 162:1208–1222.

59. Scala, G., Kuang, Y. D., Hall, R. E., Muhmore, A. V., and Oppenheim, J. J. (1984): Acessory cell function of human B cells: Production of both interleukin-1-like activity and an interleukin-1 inhibitory factor by an EBV-transformed human B cell line. *J. Exp. Med.*, 159:1637–1652.

60. Schnyder, J., Payne, T., and Dinarello, C. A. (1987): Human monocyte or recombinant interleukin-1s are specific for the secretion of a metalloproteinase from chondrocytes. *J. Immunol.*, 138:496–503.

61. Van Damme, J., De Ley, M., Opdenakker, G., Billiau, A., and De Somer, P. (1985): Homogeneous interferon-inducing 22K factor is related to endogenous pyrogen and interleukin-1. *Nature*, 314:266–268.

62. Van Damme, J., and Billiau, A. (1987): Interferon beta-2 and plasmacytoma growth factor are identical to B-cell stimulating factor-2. *J. Exp. Med.* (in press).

63. Webb, A. C., Collins, K. L., Auron, P. E., Eddy, R. L., Nakai, H., Byers, M. G., Haley, L. L., Henry, W. M., and Shows, T. B. (1986): Interleukin-1 gene (IL-1) assigned to long arm of human chromosome 2. *Lymphokine Res.* 5:77–85.

64. Webb, A. C., Auron, P. E., Rosenwasser, L. J., Mucci, S. F., Rich, A., Wolff, S. M., and Dinarello, C. A. (1985): Isolation and characterization of human interleukin-1 mRNA by molecular cloning. *Br. J. Rheumatol.*, 24:(suppl)82–86.

65. Williams, J. M., DeLoria, D., Hansen, J. A., Dinarello, C. A., Loertscher, R., Shapiro, H. M., and Strom, T. B. (1985): The events of primary T cell activation can be staged by use of Sepharose-bound anti-T3 (64.1) monoclonal antibody and purified interleukin-1. *J. Immunol.*, 135:2249–2255.

Inflammation: Basic Principles and Clinical Correlates.
Edited by J. I. Gallin, I. M. Goldstein, and R. Snyderman.
Raven Press, Ltd., New York © 1988.

CHAPTER 13

Cytokines: Interleukin-2 and Its Receptor

Warner C. Greene

OVERVIEW

In 1976, a factor capable of promoting the *in vitro* growth of activated human T cells was first identified by Morgan et al. (1). Over the ensuing 10 years, considerable progress has been made in defining the functional, biochemical, and molecular properties of this T-cell growth factor now referred to as interleukin-2 (IL-2) (2,3). The availability of supernatants containing IL-2 made possible the successful cloning and long-term culture of human and mouse T cells. IL-2 also played an important role in the isolation and characterization of the first pathogenic human retrovirus, human T lymphotrophic virus I (HTLV-I), subsequently linked with the cause of adult T-cell leukemia (ATL) (4,5). Human IL-2 has been purified to homogeneity (6–10), cDNAs encoding this lymphokine have been isolated and the primary sequence elucidated (11,12), and the IL-2 gene has been cloned (13,14) and localized to chromosome 4q bands 26 to 28 (15). Recently, crystals of recombinant IL-2 have been isolated, which should soon permit determination of its three-dimensional

structure. Recombinant IL-2 has also been rapidly introduced into clinical medicine and is presently being used to treat patients with different neoplasms and immunodeficiencies. The regression of several well-advanced solid tumors has been reported by Rosenberg and colleagues (16) following the combined administration of this lymphokine and peripheral blood leukocytes activated *in vitro* with IL-2 (lymphokine-activated killer cells).

Like other polypeptide hormones, IL-2 exerts its action through binding to specific membrane receptors (17–20). However, unlike most other growth factor receptors, functional receptors for IL-2 are not expressed on the surface of resting T cells (17) (Fig. 1). Rather, antigen or mitogen activation is required for IL-2 receptor gene expression as well as for IL-2 production. Some, but perhaps not all, T cells are capable of both synthesizing IL-2 and expressing IL-2 receptors. The subsequent binding of IL-2 with newly synthesized high-affinity membrane receptors stimulates T-cell proliferation, producing an expansion of the clone of cells activated by antigen, and culminates in the emergence of effector T cells mediating

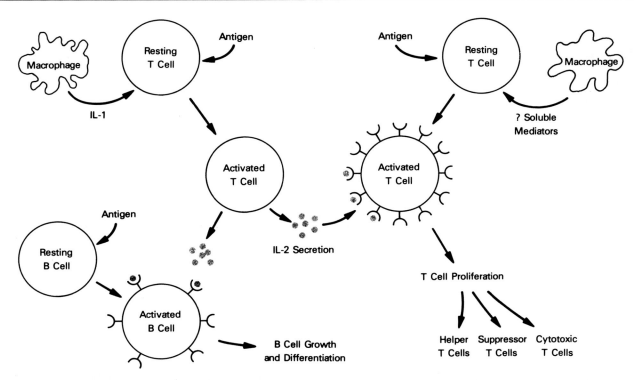

FIG. 1. Schematic model illustrating the role of interleukin-2 (IL-2) in human T- and B-cell growth. At least some activated T lymphocytes both secrete IL-2 and express IL-2 receptors and thus presumably proliferate by an autocrine mechanism.

helper, suppressor, and cytotoxic T-cell functions (18–20). With the use of monoclonal antibodies which recognize a subunit of the human (21–25), mouse (26), or rat (27) IL-2 receptor (Tac antigen), this surface structure has been biochemically characterized (28–32) and purified to homogeneity. The availability of receptor protein has made possible the isolation, sequencing, and expression of IL-2 receptor cDNAs (33–37). The gene encoding this IL-2 receptor subunit has been cloned (38,39) and mapped to chromosome 10p bands 14 and 15 (40). IL-2 receptor expression occurs in a dynamic fashion during T-cell activation. Early after antigen stimulation, IL-2 receptor expression rapidly increases; however, later, gene expression declines and the surface receptor number decreases (41–46). This rise and fall in receptor expression is paralleled by similar changes in T-cell proliferation. These findings suggest that the level of IL-2 receptor expression plays an important regulatory role in governing both the magnitude and duration of the normal T-cell immune response. In addition, the production of IL-2 may in turn lead to or facilitate the production of other lymphokines, such as γ-interferon, which play an important role in the inflammatory response. In the following sections, the molecular biology, biochemistry, and function of IL-2 and its cellular receptor in the human immune response will be considered.

IL-2: HISTORICAL CONSIDERATIONS

Following the initial identification of T-cell growth promoting activity in the supernatants of activated T-cell cultures, several laboratories initiated studies to investigate the biological and biochemical properties of this unique lymphokine. Progress in the purification of IL-2, however, was hampered both by the lack of rich cellular sources of IL-2 and the hydrophobic nature of the molecule, which produced large absorptive losses in most purification protocols. The limitation of a high-producing cell line was largely circumvented by Gillis and Watson (47) who demonstrated that the human leukemic T-cell line Jurkat produced very large quantities of IL-2 following stimulation with phytohemagglutinin (PHA) and phorbol myristate acetate (PMA). Gillis and associates (48) also developed a specific and sensitive bioassay for IL-2 based on the ability of this lymphokine to promote prompt proliferation of murine cytotoxic T-cell lines which stably express high-affinity IL-2 receptors when cultured in the presence of IL-2. This assay provided a rapid and reproducible method for quantitating IL-2. Jurkat-derived IL-2, as well as IL-2 from other cell sources, was purified to homogeneity using a variety of classic chromatographic approaches, often exploiting the hydrophobic nature of the molecule (6–10). Monoclonal antibodies specific for

IL-2 were also prepared (10,49–51) and then used as immunoaffinity supports for more efficient purification of this lymphokine (8). IL-2 was also biosynthetically labeled with radioactive amino acids and used to identify and quantitate cellular receptors for IL-2 (15,52). A major advance in the study of this lymphokine occurred with the molecular cloning of IL-2 cDNAs (11,12). With the cDNA in hand, large-scale production of recombinant IL-2 in prokaryotic hosts rapidly followed. Milligram amounts of purified recombinant IL-2 are now routinely produced by commercial laboratories. Furthermore, within only 2 years after cloning, recombinant IL-2 was introduced into clinical trials for patients with different immunodeficiencies and neoplasms.

THE MOLECULAR BIOLOGY OF IL-2

Using activated Jurkat T cells as a source of mRNA, Taniguchi and colleagues (11) first succeeded in cloning and expressing cDNAs for IL-2. Devos and associates (12) also isolated IL-2 cDNA from normal activated human splenocytes. The amino acid sequence deduced by DNA sequencing indicated that IL-2 was synthesized as a pre-protein composed of 153 amino acids (17,632 daltons). The mature IL-2 protein is produced by cleavage of a 20-residue signal peptide, yielding a 15,420-dalton peptide composed of 133 amino acids (Fig. 2). Consensus sequences for N-linked glycosylation (Asn-X-Ser, Asn-X-Thr) were not detected within the IL-2 protein sequence, and a neutral isoelectric point of the unmodified protein was predicted by the presence of equal numbers of basic and acidic amino acid residues. Furthermore, the mature protein contained three cysteine residues, two of which could participate in intramolecular disulfide bonding. A disulfide bond between residues 58 and 105 is critical for function of the protein, as reduced and alkylated IL-2 is biologically inactive (10). No significant homologies of IL-2 with other known protein or DNA sequences have been noted.

Following the identification and expression of cDNAs for IL-2, attention next focused on the structure of the IL-2 gene. Fujita and colleagues (13) and Holbrook and co-workers (14) succeeded in isolating the IL-2 gene from genomic DNA libraries as two *Eco*RI fragments spanning 8,000 base pairs (bp). Sequence analysis indicated that

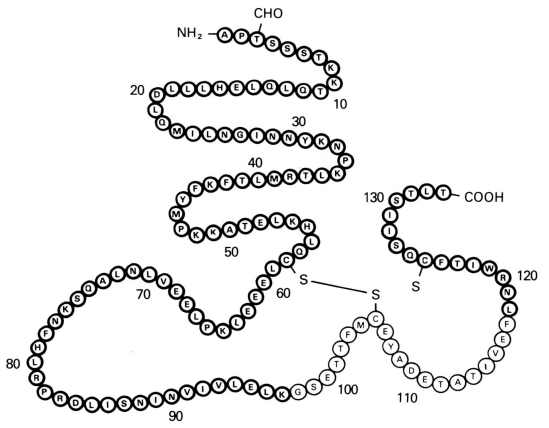

FIG. 2. Primary amino acid sequence of human IL-2 folded in an arbitrary manner. Posttranslational modifications including glycosylation at threonine-3 and disulfide bonding between cysteine-58 and -105 are shown.

the IL-2 gene was organized as four exons and three introns. The first exon comprised the 5′ untranslated region (47 bases) and the initial 49 amino acids, including the 20-residue signal peptide. The first intron contained only 91 bp, while the second exon was composed of 60 nucleotides encoding the next 20 amino acids. The second intron proved quite large, being composed of 2,292 bp. This intron was noted to contain the sequence GGTGTGTAAAG, which is homologous to the core sequence of viral enhancer elements. Similarly, Holbrook et al. (14) detected four additional enhancer-like homologies within this intron. The third exon encodes the next 48 amino acids and is followed by the third intron composed of 1,364 bp. The fourth and final exon encodes the carboxy 36 amino acids and contains the 261-nucleotide 3′ untranslated region. Thus, the gene encoding the 133 amino acids of this growth factor is distributed over more than 5 kilobases (kb) of DNA sequence.

Salient features of the upstream regulatory region controlling expression of the IL-2 gene include a classic TATA box at positions −32 to −26 and a CAT homology region at position −104 (13,14). Furthermore, within the 5′ flanking region, two blocks of sequence exist which share homology with upstream sequences within the interferon-γ gene (13). The sequence within one of these blocks (positions −69 to −51) could potentially form a stem-loop structure with a corresponding upstream sequence at positions −175 to −161. Although intriguing, the biological significance of this homology, as well as the potential stem-loop structure in lymphokine gene expression, remains unknown.

Recently, Fujita and co-workers (53) have identified upstream regulatory regions of the IL-2 gene which control sensitivity to concanavalin A activation in Jurkat T cells and PMA activation in EL-4 cells. These sequences are contained within a 200-bp region located about 40 bp upstream from the promoter (position −81). Some homology of this regulatory region is found in the upstream control segments of the human interferon-γ and IL-2 receptor (Tac) genes, as well as within the long terminal repeat (LTR) of the human immunodeficiency virus (HIV). This latter homology of the HIV LTR and the IL-2 control region is particularly intriguing in view of the observation that HIV replication is markedly increased when infected T cells are activated with mitogens.

Using Southern blot analysis, Holbrook et al. (14) found no evidence for IL-2 gene rearrangement or amplification in varying human T and B lymphoid malignancies, including the HUT 102 T-cell line known to secrete an aberrant form of this growth factor (54). In contrast, Chen et al. (55) have noted a different restriction enzyme protein of the IL-2 gene in Gibbon ape leukemia virus-infected MLA-144 cells. This cell line constitutively produces IL-2 (9) that appears to be related to insertion of the leukemia virus near the IL-2 gene.

Using Southern blot analysis of rodent–human somatic cell hybrids which retain select human chromosomes, along with *in situ* hybridization, Siegel and colleagues (15) localized the human IL-2 gene to chromosome 4q bands 26 to 28 in both normal cells and HTLV-I-infected HUT 102 cells. Translocation of this region of chromosome 4 has not been detected in cases of lymphoid leukemia. In addition, polymorphisms of the IL-2 gene in normal individuals have not been defined.

IL-2 AT THE PROTEIN LEVEL

Human IL-2 is secreted from activated T cells as a single-chain polypeptide with a molecular size of 15,000–17,000 daltons (3,6,7,10,50). Under dissociating conditions, murine IL-2 has a similar size; however, this molecule *in vivo* has a greater propensity to form 30,000-dalton dimers. As noted earlier, the IL-2 protein is markedly hydrophobic. Circular dichroism studies suggest that approximately 50% of the protein is in an alpha-helical conformation (W. F. Delgrade, unpublished data). The IL-2 protein isolated from Jurkat cells has been sequenced as a series of tryptic peptides by Robb and associates (10). These sequence data completely agree with the deduced primary structure determined by cDNA sequencing (11,12). Thus far, none of the isolated tryptic peptides has been found to contain IL-2 biological activity (R. J. Robb, unpublished data). Amino acid sequencing of the mature protein confirmed that the signal peptide for this protein is 20 residues in length (10). As noted earlier, the secreted protein contains 133 amino acids with a single disulfide bond formed by the cysteines at positions 58 and 105 (3). Disruption of this disulfide bridge is associated with a marked loss of biological activity. In *Escherichia coli,* inappropriate disulfide bonding of recombinant IL-2 involving the cysteine residue at position 125 has been circumvented by site-directed mutagenesis of this amino acid (56). In addition to disulfide bonding, the only other form of posttranslational processing identified for IL-2 involves O-linked sugar addition to the threonine residue at position 3 (10,51,57). Fast atom bombardment and mass spectroscopy of the tryptic peptide composed of amino acids 1 to 8 indicated that this threonine either was not glycosylated or, alternatively, was initially modified with *N*-acetylgalactosamine and subsequently with galactose and sialic acid. These findings provide an explanation for the previously recognized microheterogeneity of isoelectric points for IL-2 (7,51). IL-2 molecules containing either no carbohydrate or only *N*-acetylgalactosamine display alkaline isoelectric points, whereas those containing galactose and sialic acid have more acidic isoelectric points. The biological activity of these various glycosylated forms of IL-2 appears to be identical. Furthermore, nonglycosylated recombinant IL-2 produced in *E. coli* has full biological activity, suggesting that carbohydrate addition is not a prerequisite for function.

Considerable investigative effort has focused on defining the regions of the IL-2 molecule that interact with its cell surface receptor. Using antibodies against synthetic IL-2 peptide fragments, Kuo and Robb (58) have demonstrated that residues 8 to 27 and 33 to 54 appear important in IL-2 binding to its receptor. These residues may either serve as contact points with the receptor or be important in maintaining the appropriate conformation of the IL-2 protein (see the discussion of high-affinity IL-2 receptor). Site-specific mutagenesis has also implicated important contributions of residues located near the carboxy end of the molecule. The recent crystallization of IL-2 should yield more definitive three-dimensional structural information regarding this molecule and its interaction with its receptor.

REGULATION OF IL-2 GENE EXPRESSION

In normal T cells two discrete activation signals appear to be required for optimal induction of IL-2 production (2,59). One signal is produced by the interaction of antigen or mitogen with the specific T-cell antigen receptor–T3 complex. The second signal is provided by interleukin-1 (IL-1) derived from macrophages. In the Jurkat T-cell model of activation, dual signals are also required. Stimulation with PHA (or OKT3) or PMA alone results in little or no IL-2 production; however, combined addition of PHA and PMA results in marked induction of IL-2 production in these cells (60). Weiss et al. (61,62) have suggested that the interaction of ligand with the antigen receptor results in an increase in cytoplasmic free calcium levels; however, this signal alone appears insufficient to activate IL-2 production. Mutants of the Jurkat T-cell line lacking one chain of the T-cell antigen heterodimeric receptor cannot be induced with combinations of OKT3 monoclonal antibody or clonotypic reagents and PMA to secrete IL-2 (63). However, IL-2 production will occur if calcium ionophores (A23187, ionomycin) are added with PMA, thus bypassing the requirement for signaling through the antigen receptor (63). Presumably, PMA acts through activating protein kinase C (64,65); however, it is presently unknown whether this is also the mechanism of action of IL-1 in normal T cells.

Using nuclear runoff assays, Krönke et al. (66) have studied IL-2 gene transcription in peripheral blood T lymphocytes activated with PHA. These investigators have observed that IL-2 transcription begins 6 to 9 hr after activation and peaks at 20 to 24 hr. Thereafter, a marked decline in IL-2 gene expression occurs. Neither the rise nor the fall in IL-2 gene transcription is altered by pretreatment of the cells with cycloheximide, indicating that protein synthesis is not required for these changes in IL-2 gene expression. Transcription of the c-*myc,* interferon-γ, and IL-2 receptor genes slightly precedes IL-2 gene expression and is also transient and similarly unaltered by the addition of protein synthesis inhibitors.

Cyclosporin A and corticosteroids have been reported to inhibit IL-2 production. These agents have been widely used as immunosuppressive agents (67–70). Krönke et al. (71) have demonstrated that cyclosporin A markedly inhibits IL-2 gene transcription, which may in part explain its utility in the prevention of graft rejection. Interference with IL-2 production may block the expansion of cytotoxic T cells which mediate graft rejection. Recent interest has focused on the possibility that cyclosporin A may interfere with the function of calmodulin (72). Similarly, corticosteroids inhibit IL-2 production by T cells; however, the mechanism by which these agents act has not been clearly delineated but appears different from that of cyclosporin A.

Using an oocyte RNA injection assay, Efrat and Kaempfer (73) have proposed the existence of a regulatory protein that inhibits the normal transport or processing of IL-2 nuclear RNA into cytoplasmic mRNA. This protein is produced after cellular activation but not in cycloheximide-treated cells. As is the case with many regulatory proteins, this regulatory protein is characterized by a very short half-life. Nuclear runoff studies suggest a posttranscriptional level of action of this protein, as transcription of the IL-2 gene is not altered. It is possible that this protein is importantly involved in the transient nature of IL-2 production, but additional regulatory mechanisms must exist, as the level of IL-2 gene transcription also changes (71).

BIOLOGICAL PROPERTIES OF IL-2

As will be discussed in greater detail in a later section, a principal action of IL-2 is to promote the growth of T cells expressing receptors for this lymphokine. However, recent studies in several systems indicate that the spectrum of IL-2 activity may involve more than function solely as a growth factor for T cells. For example, IL-2 has been demonstrated to promote the proliferation and differentiation of certain activated B cells (73–79). Furthermore, IL-2 can stimulate T-cell production of B-cell growth factor (80) and interferon-γ (81) independently of its effects on T-cell proliferation. IL-2 has also been implicated in the activation of natural killer (NK) cell function. At least in part, this effect is mediated through the induction of interferon-γ production (82), which also augments cytolytic function of these cells. However, direct activation of cytolytic activity by IL-2, independently of interferon-γ, also occurs when large amounts of the lymphokine are added (80). Interestingly, the NK cell does not appear to express the Tac antigen, and anti-Tac, an anti-IL-2 receptor antibody, does not block IL-2 induction of cytolytic activity in these cells (83). These data raise the interesting possibility that IL-2 may promote differentiation in these cells through interactions with receptors distinct from those present on activated T cells (see the discussion of high-affinity IL-2 receptor). Finally, IL-2 has recently been demonstrated to promote proliferation of oligodendrocytes (84). Thus, the biological effects of IL-2 are not solely confined to cells of the T-cell lineage.

IL-2 also has the capacity to activate potent killer cell activity in non-T cells directed at a wide array of solid tumor cells (85–88). Rosenberg and colleagues have termed these cells lymphokine-activated killer (LAK) cells. LAK precursor cells do not contain T-cell markers; however, after activation with large quantities of IL-2, the cells express IL-2 receptors. The spectrum of cell killing appears to differ from that characteristic of NK cells, although these cells may be related. Recently, LAK cells have been successfully used in the therapy of patients with widely metastatic solid cancers (16). Approximately one-third of these patients have had dramatic therapeutic responses, with renal cell carcinomas and melanomas forming a group of tumors particularly susceptible to this form of adoptive immunotherapy. Unfortunately, this mode of therapy has been complicated by rather severe toxicity manifested as a widespread capillary-leak syndrome.

RECEPTORS FOR IL-2

IL-2 exerts its biological effects through binding to specific receptors present on the surface of activated T cells. Recently, considerable progress has been made in defining the structure of this critical membrane receptor. In the following sections, the molecular biology, biochemistry, and function of the human IL-2 receptor will be discussed.

Detection of IL-2 Receptors

The presence of inducible receptors for IL-2 was first implied by the observation that activated but not resting T-cell populations removed IL-2 from conditioned medium (89–91). The cell-absorbed IL-2 could also be recovered by mild acid (pH 4) treatment (54). These data were consistent with the possibility that IL-2 receptors are expressed on activated but not resting T cells.

Direct demonstration of specific IL-2 binding sites on activated T cells was made possible by the preparation of highly purified, biosynthetically radiolabeled IL-2 by Robb and colleagues (17). Using this material, these investigators were able to demonstrate specific, saturable, high-affinity binding sites (K_d = 2–20 pM) on IL-2-dependent T-cell lines, mitogen- and alloantigen-activated T cells, and HUT 102B2 cells, an IL-2-independent T-cell line derived from a patient with HTLV-I-induced ATL. Significant numbers of receptors were not detectable on resting T or B cells or macrophages. Human IL-2 was found to react not only with activated human T cells but also with activated mouse T cells. In contrast, mouse IL-2 did not bind to the human IL-2 receptor, indicating an interesting phylogenetic restriction of IL-2 action.

Further biochemical characterization of the human IL-2 receptor was made possible by the production of monoclonal antireceptor antibodies. The first such antibody, termed anti-Tac, was prepared by Uchiyama et al. (21) and proven to react with activated T cells. Leonard and colleagues (22), Miyawaki and co-workers (23), and Robb and Greene (24) subsequently provided several lines of evidence demonstrating that anti-Tac recognized the human IL-2 receptor, including the following: (a) Anti-Tac inhibits >80% of IL-2-induced [³H]thymidine incorporation in IL-2-dependent continuous T-cell lines but does not alter DNA synthesis in IL-2-independent T-cell lines (22); (b) anti-Tac, but not control antibodies, blocks >95% of [³H]IL-2 binding to HUT 102B2 cells (22), as well as IL-2 absorption to activated T cells (23); (c) IL-2 inhibits the binding of [³H]anti-Tac to PHA-activated lymphoblasts (24); (d) IL-2 immobilized on Affigel beads and used as an affinity column is able to bind a protein identical in size to that identified by anti-Tac coupled to Sepharose (24); and (e) both anti-Tac and anti-IL-2 monoclonal antibodies precipitate the same protein complex produced by covalent cross-linking of IL-2 to its receptor with disuccinimidyl suberate (28).

Distribution of IL-2 Receptors

T Lymphocytes

As noted above, specific binding of [³H]IL-2 initially was found on activated T cells but not on resting T cells, B cells, or macrophages (17). Multiple investigations employing monoclonal anti-IL-2 receptor antibodies have extended these findings (22,24–27,92,93). Zero to fifteen percent (mean of <5%) of freshly isolated, unstimulated human peripheral blood lymphocytes react with anti-Tac, presumably reflecting *in vivo* activation of cells. The majority of T lymphocytes display IL-2 receptors 24 to 48 hr after mitogenic lectin activation. A transient rise in Tac-positive cells has been detected 12 hr after *in vivo* immunization with tetanus toxoid (94). Long-term IL-2-

dependent T-cell clones mediating helper and cytotoxic functions are uniformly IL-2 receptor-positive, and both purified T4 and T8 subsets activated with mitogen express IL-2 receptors (95). Histological evaluation of human lymphoid tissue with anti-Tac showed localization of Tac-positive cells in paracortical and interfollicular regions of lymph nodes and tonsils. By dual fluorescent staining, 80% of these cells were Leu 3 (helper or inducer) and 20% Leu 2 (suppressor or cytotoxic) (96). While thymocytes do not normally display IL-2 receptors, these cells could be induced to express receptors with mitogens (97,98). Moreover, stimulation of thymocytes with monoclonal antibodies directed at certain epitopes associated with the sheep erythrocyte receptor (T11 determinant) resulted in IL-2 receptor display preceding expression of the T3 antigen or the secretion of IL-2. These findings suggest a possible antigen-independent role for IL-2 receptor display in normal thymic maturation (93).

IL-2 Receptors on B Lymphocytes

A survey of leukemic B-cell populations revealed that a limited number of Burkitt's lymphoma B-cell lines bound low levels of [^{3}H]anti-Tac antibody (J. M. Depper and W. C. Greene, unpublished observations). Korsmeyer and colleagues (74) subsequently demonstrated nearly uniform specific binding of the anti-Tac antibody to hairy-cell leukemia cells. These leukemic cells represented cells committed to the B-lymphocyte lineage based on the presence of productive heavy- and light-chain immunoglobulin gene rearrangements. Although resting B cells do not express IL-2 receptors, many laboratories have now demonstrated specific binding of IL-2 or anti-IL-2 receptor monoclonals to activated human or murine B lymphocytes (75–78). Functionally, purified IL-2 may support the proliferation of activated B cells, induce secretion of immunoglobulin, and increase the expression of IL-2 receptors. Although high-affinity IL-2 receptor sites on a cloned activated B-cell line have been demonstrated (76), Ralph et al. (79) provided evidence that large amounts of IL-2 stimulated immunoglobulin synthesis and secretion in a cloned Epstein–Barr virus (EBV)-transformed B-cell line lacking the Tac antigen. This finding was most curious and suggested the possible existence of a second IL-2 binding protein that did not react with anti-Tac (see the high-affinity receptor discussion).

IL-2 Receptors on Nonlymphoid Cells

Recent evidence indicates that macrophages activated with interferon-γ or lipopolysaccharide also express IL-2 receptors (99). The function of these receptors in macrophage physiology, however, remains undefined. IL-2

receptor display has also been reported on various granulocyte leukemic cells (100) and IL-3-activated hematopoietic cells (101). Thus, the spectrum of IL-2 receptor (Tac antigen) display appears considerably broader than that originally appreciated.

Biochemical Characterization of the Human IL-2 Receptor (Tac Antigen)

The first biochemical description of the human IL-2 receptor defined by the anti-Tac antibody stemmed from studies on HTLV-I-infected HUT 102B2 cells (4,5). These cells constitutively express large numbers (300,000–600,000 per cell) of IL-2 receptors (54,102,103). After biosynthetic labeling with [^{35}S]methionine or D-[^{3}H]glucosamine or surface labeling with Na^{125}I and lactoperoxidase, cellular proteins were solubilized in nonionic detergent and immunoprecipitated with anti-Tac. These experiments demonstrated that the Tac antigen was a glycoprotein with an apparent molecular size of 50,000 daltons when electrophoresed in the presence of reducing agents (22,28–31). Under nonreducing conditions, the receptor migrated with an apparent size of 45,000 daltons, suggesting the presence of intramolecular disulfide bonding. In addition, nonreducing analysis revealed a larger band (100,000–115,000 daltons) which subsequently was shown to represent a disulfide-linked homodimer (K. A. Smith et al., unpublished observations).

The IL-2 receptor on normal activated T cells differs slightly in size from the receptor on HUT 102B2 cells (28,29). The normal IL-2 receptor migrated more slowly, with an apparent size of 55,000 daltons (p55), and had a pI of 5.4 to 5.7 compared with a pI of 5.5 to 6.0 for the HUT 102B2 receptor.

In view of the size difference in IL-2 receptors on HUT 102B2 cells and normal activated T cells, several additional HTLV-I-infected T-cell lines were studied to determine whether retroviral infection was uniformly associated with "aberrant" IL-2 receptor size. Both HTLV-I-infected tumor cells and cord blood cells transformed with HTLV-I *in vitro* were evaluated. These studies demonstrated that, while occasional HTLV-I-infected T-cell lines expressed IL-2 receptors differing slightly in size from those in normal activated T cells, most such cell lines had normal sized receptors (29,30,103). Thus, HTLV-I infection does not appear to confer uniform differences in IL-2 receptor size. The molecular basis for the size heterogeneity, when present, appears to be produced by alterations in Golgi-associated posttranslational processing, including, at least in part, diminished addition of sialic acid and sulfate (30).

Pulse-chase radiolabeling studies and experiments employing tunicamycin, endoglycosidase F, and neuraminidase have provided considerable insight into the biosynthesis and posttranslational processing of the Tac protein (28–30) (Fig. 3). Translation of HUT 102 or PHA blast mRNA in a cell-free system and immunoprecipitation of sodium dodecyl sulfate-denatured protein with a Tac-specific heteroantiserum permitted identification of the primary translation product as a 34,500-dalton peptide (33). Pulse-chase labeling in the presence of tunicamycin, which blocks N-linked glycosylation, revealed a single 33,000-dalton protein at early time points. This protein presumably represents the unmodified receptor peptide backbone which is slightly smaller than the primary translation product as a result of cleavage of a signal peptide. In the absence of tunicamycin, at 0 to 30 min of chase, two protein bands with apparent sizes of 35,000 and 37,000 daltons were detected, which were produced by cotranslational addition of N-linked sugar to the 33,000-dalton peptide backbone. After 60 min of chase, the 55,000-dalton mature form of the receptor appeared concomitantly with the disappearance of the N-glycosylated precursors. Identically sized precursor forms (p34.5, p33, p35, p37) were found in HUT 102 cells, supporting a role for alterations in late Golgi-associated processing in the apparent size differences of these and normal receptors. Experiments with endoglycosidase F, which cleaves all N-linked carbohydrate structures in HUT 102 and normal activated T-cell IL-2 receptors, recapitulated the findings obtained in the tunicamycin experiments. Both the 35,000- and 37,000-dalton precursors were converted to the 33,000-dalton form. The large saltatory increase in size that occurs between the N-glycosylated precursor and mature forms suggests that O-linked carbohydrate is added to the IL-2 receptor. Digestion with neuraminidase confirmed that sialic acid was also added. When neuraminidase digestion was performed after N-linked sugars were removed with endoglycosidase F, a further decrease in receptor size was detected. These findings suggest that at least a portion of the sialic acid residues

is not involved in N-linked carbohydrate side groups. Both the protein backbone and N-glycosylated precursor forms were precipitated by IL-2 conjugated to Affigel beads. Thus, while extensive posttranslational processing occurs with this receptor, these events do not appear obligately required for ligand binding to the receptor. However, it is unknown whether these posttranslational processing events alter the affinity of the receptor for its ligand. Other studies have indicated that the Tac protein is constitutively sulfated (30) and phosphorylated (31,32). The principal site of phosphorylation appears to be a serine residue located within the intracytoplasmic domain (32). In contrast to many other receptors, no tyrosine-specific phosphorylation of the Tac protein has been identified. Furthermore, convincing evidence for IL-2-induced phosphorylation of its receptor in normal activated T cells is lacking but not yet excluded. The site(s) of sulfate addition is unknown, and the role of this form of posttranslational modification is unclear.

Molecular Biology of the Tac Protein

Isolation of IL-2 Receptor cDNAs

Three groups independently initiated efforts to and succeeded in molecularly cloning cDNAs for the Tac protein (33–35). Receptor protein was purified using monoclonal antireceptor antibodies which permitted determination of the N-terminal amino acid sequence. The N-terminal sequence obtained by sequential Edman degradation was as follows: H_2N-glu-leu-cys-asp-asp-asp-pro-pro-glu-ile-pro-his-ala-thr-phe-lys-ala-met-ala-tyr-lys-glu-gly-thr-met-leu-asn-cys-glu. Appropriate oligonucleotide probes were then synthesized and used to screen appropriate cDNA libraries.

The isolated IL-2 receptor cDNAs contained a long open reading frame encoding a 251-amino acid polypep-

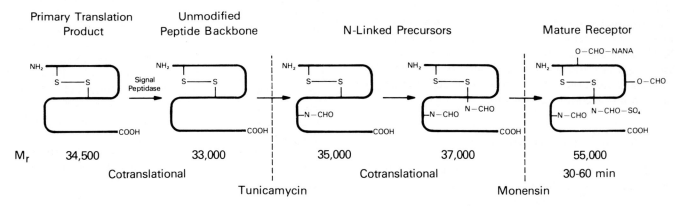

FIG. 3. Schematic of steps in the posttranslational processing of the Tac protein.

tide that included the N-terminal sequence indicated above. In addition, cDNA clones lacking a 216-base segment present within the midportion of the protein coding region were also identified (33,35). These aberrant cDNAs corresponded to mRNAs generated by alternate mRNA splicing. RNA hybridization experiments demonstrated that both forms of cDNA selectively hybridized to IL-2 receptor mRNA which, when translated in a wheat germ lysate cell-free translation system and the translation products then immunoprecipitated with an anti-IL-2 receptor heteroantiserum, yielded the 34,500-dalton primary translation product for the IL-2 receptor (33).

To more fully characterize the spliced and unspliced forms of the IL-2 receptor cDNA, these inserts were ligated in the correct orientation into SV40 expression vectors and transfected into COS-1 cells. Analysis of the COS-1 cell membranes indicated that only the unspliced form of the receptor cDNA directed the synthesis of an IL-2 receptor protein capable of binding IL-2 and anti-Tac (33). These findings were also confirmed in a stable expression system utilizing murine L cells (104). S1 nuclease protection assays demonstrated that the spliced cDNA corresponded to a mature mRNA species present in normal activated T cells and ATL cells and was not the result of

a cloning artifact (105). Thus far, the protein product of the spliced cDNA remains undefined in eukaryotic cells.

Structure of the Tac Protein

The primary amino acid sequence of the Tac protein was deduced by sequencing full-length Tac cDNAs (33–35) (Fig. 4). The receptor contains 272 amino acids, including a 21-residue leader peptide that is cotranslationally cleaved by signal peptidase. Multiple cysteine residues are present, some of which participate in the formation of intramolecular disulfide bonds required for IL-2 and anti-Tac binding. Interchain disulfide bonding may also occur, producing homodimers of the receptor (K. A. Smith et al., unpublished data). The receptor contains two sites for N-linked glycosylation and multiple potential sites for O-linked sugar addition. Nineteen hydrophobic amino acids are present near the C-terminus of the protein. This region probably forms the transmembrane domain of the receptor. In view of the position of the signal peptide and N-linked carbohydrate addition sites, the receptor likely is an "NH₂ terminus out, COOH terminus in" transmembrane structure. In this orientation, the intracytoplasmic

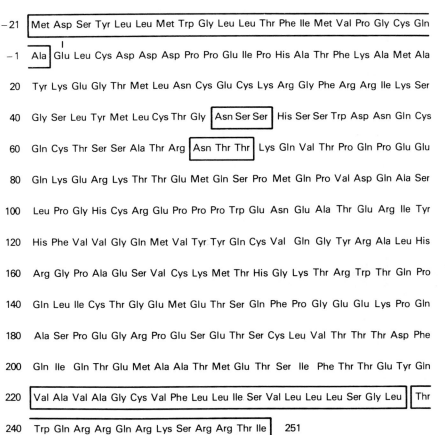

−21	Met Asp Ser Tyr Leu Leu Met Trp Gly Leu Leu Thr Phe Ile Met Val Pro Gly Cys Gln
−1	Ala Glu Leu Cys Asp Asp Asp Pro Pro Glu Ile Pro His Ala Thr Phe Lys Ala Met Ala
20	Tyr Lys Glu Gly Thr Met Leu Asn Cys Glu Cys Lys Arg Gly Phe Arg Arg Ile Lys Ser
40	Gly Ser Leu Tyr Met Leu Cys Thr Gly Asn Ser Ser His Ser Ser Trp Asp Asn Gln Cys
60	Gln Cys Thr Ser Ser Ala Thr Arg Asn Thr Thr Lys Gln Val Thr Pro Gln Pro Glu Glu
80	Gln Lys Glu Arg Lys Thr Thr Glu Met Gln Ser Pro Met Gln Pro Val Asp Gln Ala Ser
100	Leu Pro Gly His Cys Arg Glu Pro Pro Pro Trp Glu Asn Glu Ala Thr Glu Arg Ile Tyr
120	His Phe Val Val Gly Gln Met Val Tyr Tyr Gln Cys Val Gln Gly Tyr Arg Ala Leu His
160	Arg Gly Pro Ala Glu Ser Val Cys Lys Met Thr His Gly Lys Thr Arg Trp Thr Gln Pro
140	Gln Leu Ile Cys Thr Gly Glu Met Glu Thr Ser Gln Phe Pro Gly Glu Glu Lys Pro Gln
180	Ala Ser Pro Glu Gly Arg Pro Glu Ser Glu Thr Ser Cys Leu Val Thr Thr Thr Asp Phe
200	Gln Ile Gln Thr Glu Met Ala Ala Thr Met Glu Thr Ser Ile Phe Thr Thr Glu Tyr Gln
220	Val Ala Val Ala Gly Cys Val Phe Leu Leu Ile Ser Val Leu Leu Leu Ser Gly Leu Thr
240	Trp Gln Arg Arg Gln Arg Lys Ser Arg Arg Thr Ile 251

FIG. 4. Deduced primary amino acid sequence of the Tac protein. The signal peptide, N-glycosylation consensus sequences, hydrophobic transmembrane domain, and 13-residue intracytoplasmic domain are individually boxed.

domain of the receptor consists of only 13 residues. Thus, in contrast to many other growth factor receptors which contain tyrosine kinase enzymatic activity within their intracytoplasmic domains, the intracellular tail of the Tac protein is too short to encode such an activity. This is a particularly relevant issue with regard to both the existence of high- and low-affinity forms of the IL-2 receptor and the mechanism by which growth signals are transduced through the receptor. The cytoplasmic tail, however, does contain six positively charged amino acids which presumably are involved in anchoring the receptor protein within the plasma membrane. Recently, an "anchor minus" Tac cDNA was prepared by introducing a stop codon following the fourth residue of the transmembrane domain (106). When expressed in mouse fibroblasts, this truncated receptor cDNA exclusively directed the synthesis of a secreted form of the receptor which retained the capacity to bind both IL-2 and anti-Tac. Furthermore, in contrast to some truncated forms of membrane proteins, the rate of biosynthesis and intracellular transport was not altered by removal of the C-terminal 28 residues of this protein.

Multiple IL-2 Receptor mRNAs

Northern blotting analysis of activated T-cell mRNA demonstrated the presence of three discrete bands hybridizing to the radiolabeled Tac cDNA (107). The use of 3′ probes and S1 nuclease protection studies demonstrated that these different sized mRNAs were produced by the use of different polyadenylation sites. The most 3′ polyadenylation signal is preferentially utilized in certain cases; for example, normal T cells activated with PHA or PMA alone predominantly use this distal poly A site. However, when cells are maximally activated with combinations of PHA and PMA, increased polyadenylation occurs at the two proximal sites. The protein produced,

of course, is not altered by the polyadenylation signal used; thus, the biological significance of different polyadenylation signal site utilization is unclear. It is possible that certain forms of IL-2 receptor mRNA may be more stable or more efficiently translated than others.

In addition to variability in the length of the 3′ untranslated region and alternate splicing of a 216-bp region within the protein coding region, the 5′ end of the Tac mRNAs may also vary (38). Primer extension and S1 nuclease protection analyses of this region have demonstrated that transcription is initiated at at least two different sites separated by 58 bp in normal activated T cells. An additional further 5′ transcription initiation site has also been identified in HTLV-I-infected ATL cells (38). TA-TAA-like promoter regions are present 25 to 30 bases upstream from the two principal start sites. Thus, at least 12 different IL-2 receptor mRNAs are produced in normal activated T cells corresponding to two different transcription initiation sites, variable splicing of the coding region segment, and the use of at least three different 3′ polyadenylation sites.

THE TAC GENE

Despite the presence of multiple mRNAs, the Tac protein is encoded by a single gene (38,39). Genomic phage DNA libraries were screened with the Tac cDNA to isolate this receptor gene. Sequence analysis of the inserts of these phages indicated that the gene was composed of eight exons and seven introns spanning a minimum distance of 25 kb (16) (Fig. 5). *In situ* hybridization studies have localized the receptor gene to chromosome 10p band 14 → 15 (40). Thus far, karyotypic abnormalities of this region of chromosome 10 have not been found in lymphoid malignancies. Exon 1 of the receptor gene encodes the 5′ untranslated region as well as the 21-amino acid signal peptide required for transport of the protein into the en-

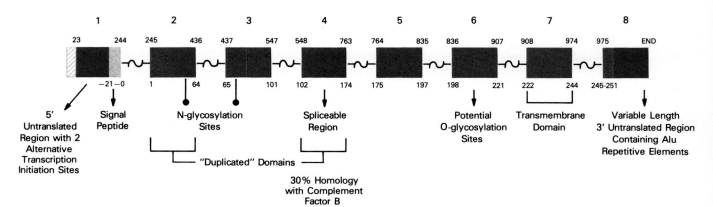

FIG. 5. Schematic of the genomic organization of the human Tac gene.

doplasmic reticulum. The first intron is quite large, encompassing at least 15 kb. Thus far, genomic phage clones completely bridging this intron have not been isolated; thus, the exact size of the receptor gene is unknown and may be considerably greater than the minimal estimate of 25 kb provided. Exon 2 encodes the N-terminal 66 amino acids of the mature receptor protein and includes one of the two N-glycosylation sites (consensus sequence Asn-X-Ser or Thr). Exon 3 contains the next 35 amino acids and the second N-glycosylation site. Exon 4 encodes 72 amino acids which share unexpected homology with exon 2. These data suggest that these exons were derived from an internal gene duplication event. Similar homology is present in the mouse IL-2 receptor cDNA (37), suggesting that this internal duplication occurred at least 50 million years ago, before the genetic radiation of mice and humans. The presence of this internal duplication raises the interesting, but unproven, possibility that the IL-2 receptor contains two ligand binding sites. ^{125}I-labeled IL-2 cross-linking studies and tryptic digestion have clearly implicated the N-terminal 83 amino acids (exon 2 and part of exon 3) as one contact point for IL-2 binding to the receptor (108). Exon 4 is also homologous to the recognition domain of human complement factor B (Ba fragment) (38). The significance of this finding is also unclear, but it suggests that these two proteins share a common ancestral exon. Exon 4 also precisely corresponds to the 216 bp lacking in the aberrantly spliced form of receptor mRNA. As noted earlier, expression of cDNA corresponding to this aberrantly spliced mRNA in murine fibroblasts does not result in the display of functional membrane IL-2 receptors. The sixth exon contains multiple potential sites for O-linked glycosylation and, topographically, is situated immediately extracytoplasmic to the plasma membrane. A similarly positioned exon rich in O-linked glycosylation sites has been described in the low-density lipoprotein (LDL) and platelet-derived growth factor (PDGF) receptors. The seventh exon encodes the majority of the 19 residue hydrophobic transmembrane domain, and the eighth exon encodes part of the 13 amino acids comprising the intracytoplasmic domain as well as the 3' untranslated region of the IL-2 receptor. As noted earlier, this 3' untranslated region contains at least three functional polyadenylation signal sequences, and unexpected multiple Alu repetitive elements are found between the second and third poly A sites.

HIGH- AND LOW-AFFINITY RECEPTORS FOR IL-2

The initial receptor studies of Robb and associates (17) performed with purified radiolabeled IL-2 demonstrated that PHA-activated T cells contained 2,000 to 4,000 IL-2 receptors per cell. The K_d for IL-2 binding to these receptors was 2 to 20 pM, indicating an unexpectedly high affinity interaction. In contrast, binding studies performed with radiolabeled anti-Tac antibody indicated 30,000 to 60,000 IL-2 receptors per cell (42). Scatchard analysis of the anti-Tac binding data suggested a single affinity class of receptors. This discrepancy in receptor number in the two assays was proven not to be the result of inadvertent Fc receptor binding by anti-Tac nor due to partial occupancy of receptor sites by endogenously produced IL-2. These data raised the interesting possibility that two different affinity forms of the IL-2 receptor might exist and that the IL-2 binding assay, as previously performed, detected only one form of the receptor. To test this hypothesis, the IL-2 binding studies were repeated using much greater quantities of ligand (52,109). These assays, in fact, revealed a previously undetected large pool of IL-2 binding sites displaying a 1,000- to 10,000-fold lower apparent affinity for ligand. The total number of high- and low-affinity IL-2 binding sites was nearly equivalent (within a factor of 2) to the number of sites measured with anti-Tac (52,109). These data indicate that anti-Tac binding does not distinguish between the high- and low-affinity forms of the IL-2 receptor. The high-affinity receptors comprise only 2% to 10% of the membrane IL-2 receptors, however, these high-affinity sites appear to mediate the growth promoting response to physiological concentrations of IL-2 (17,52). The function of the far more numerous low-affinity IL-2 receptors presently remains unknown. Studies on the postbinding fate of IL-2 have recently shown that high-affinity, but not low-affinity, IL-2 receptors mediate internalization of membrane-bound ligand (110,111). These differences in receptor-mediated endocytosis further underscore a basic functional and structural difference in these receptor classes (Table 1).

To begin to explore the molecular differences in the high- and low-affinity forms of the IL-2 receptor, the Tac cDNA was stably expressed in murine fibroblasts (104,112,113). These transfected fibroblasts were found to display the Tac antigen; however, only low-affinity binding sites were detected in ^{125}I-labeled IL-2 binding assays. These findings raised the possibility that a second

TABLE 1. *Comparison of high- and low-affinity IL-2 receptors*[a]

Characteristic	High affinity	Low affinity
Apparent K_d for IL-2	2–50 pM	10–30 nM
Sites per PHA lymphoblast	2,000–4,000	30,000–60,000
Reactivity with anti-Tac	Yes	Yes
Internalization of IL-2	Yes	No
Function	T-cell growth	?

[a] IL-2, Interleukin-2; PHA, phytohemagglutinin.

gene encoded the high-affinity IL-2 receptor, while the Tac cDNA corresponded only to the low-affinity form of the receptor. This "two-gene" model for receptor affinity classes, however, became untenable with the demonstration that the Tac cDNA encoded both high- and low-affinity forms of the receptor when expressed in mouse T cells (112,114). Furthermore, Robb (115) demonstrated that a fraction of the low-affinity mouse IL-2 receptors present on fibroblasts transfected with the murine IL-2 receptor cDNA could be converted to high-affinity receptors by fusion with human T-cell lines displaying high-affinity human IL-2 receptors. These studies took advantage of the capacity of anti-Tac to block IL-2 binding to human receptors but not mouse receptors. Together these findings suggested that an additional component(s) present within T cells was involved in the formation of high-affinity IL-2 receptors. The potential assembly of a high-affinity receptor complex was an attractive model in terms of the mechanism of growth signal transduction by the high-affinity IL-2 receptor. Since the intracytoplasmic domain of the Tac antigen was only 13 residues in length, it was difficult to envision how this domain mediated signal transduction. If a receptor complex is formed, the other components of the complex might play a key role in signaling.

Recently, evidence for a high-affinity IL-2 receptor membrane complex has been obtained. Utilizing ^{125}I-labeled IL-2 for chemical cross-linking to high-affinity IL-2 receptors, two principal proteins have been identified (108,116). These proteins include the Tac antigen and a second 70,000- to 75,000-dalton protein [the cross-linked molecular complex including IL-2 (15,500 daltons) migrates as 85,000–90,000 daltons, hence this indirect estimate of size]. Endoglycosidase cleavage and metabolic labeling with [^{3}H]mannose have demonstrated that the p70 polypeptide is glycosylated (116,117). Furthermore, peptide mapping of proteolytic fragments has clearly confirmed that the Tac and p70 proteins are structurally different (116,117). In other studies, Tsudo and Waldmann (118) were the first to provide evidence that the p70 protein was capable of binding IL-2. This finding has been confirmed in other laboratories (117,119,120). This previously unrecognized IL-2 receptor appears to bind IL-2 with intermediate affinity (0.6–1.2 nM) compared with the recognized high- and low-affinity forms of the IL-2 receptor. The p70 protein also lacks reactivity with the anti-Tac antibody (117–120). This novel IL-2 binding protein has been identified, in the absence of Tac antigen, on the surface of resting T cells, large granular lymphocytes (NK cells), and some B cells, including the SKW6.4 B-cell line; however, these cells lack high-affinity IL-2 receptors.

As noted, the selective cross-linking of radiolabeled IL-2 to high-affinity IL-2 receptors revealed labeling of both Tac and p70 proteins. Furthermore, the cross-linking of IL-2 to both these proteins was blocked by the anti-Tac antibody. In contrast, anti-Tac did not inhibit IL-2 cross-linking to cells containing only the p70 protein. Together, these data suggested that the high-affinity IL-2 receptor might correspond to a receptor complex involving the Tac antigen and the p70 protein. Such a high-affinity receptor complex model has recently been strengthened by studies involving the expression of Tac cDNA in a T-cell line (MLA-144) that displays only the p70 protein (120). In these cells, high-affinity IL-2 receptors (K_d = 35–70 pM) were reconstituted by transfection of plasmids containing Tac cDNA but not by transfection of control plasmids. Furthermore, the reconstituted high-affinity receptors appeared to involve the Tac antigen, as addition of the anti-Tac antibody blocked detection of the high-affinity, but not the intermediate-affinity, binding sites (120). Similarly, high-affinity IL-2 receptors have been reconstituted in the "NK-like" YT cell line by the activation of endogenous Tac gene expression (117,119). These YT cells express the p70 protein in the virtual absence of the Tac antigen; however, stimulation with forskolin, IL-1, or adult T-cell leukemia-derived factor (ADF) promotes Tac gene activation and leads to the display of large numbers of high-affinity IL-2 receptors (117,119). Addition of anti-Tac blocks the high-affinity component of binding and reveals the reappearance of intermediate-affinity (K_d = 810 pM) binding sites (117).

Recent studies have provided evidence that the p70 and Tac proteins interact with different epitopes on the IL-2 molecule. As noted earlier, Kuo and Robb (58) had demonstrated that residues 8 to 27 and 33 to 54 within the primary sequence of IL-2 appeared to be importantly involved in high-affinity receptor interactions. With the use of antibodies specific for these peptide regions, evidence has been assembled suggesting that amino acids 8 to 27 interact with the p70 protein, whereas residues 33 to 54 may preferentially interact with the Tac antigen (117). Certainly, the identification of a receptor complex which interacts with IL-2 at two distinct sites provides a plausible mechanism explaining high-affinity ligand binding.

The capacity of IL-2 to activate cytolytic activity in NK cells and immunoglobulin production in SKW6.4 B cells suggests that the p70 protein may be capable of signal transduction. This supposition is further supported by the recent finding that the p70 protein mediates rapid endocytosis of cell-bound IL-2 (121). Using lymphoid cell lines that express p70 but lack high-affinity receptors, Robb and Greene (121) have demonstrated that IL-2 bound to the p70 protein is internalized with kinetics essentially identical to that observed for the high-affinity receptor ($t_{1/2}$ = 10–15 min). In contrast, the Tac antigen alone failed to promote internalization of IL-2. This finding predicts that the intracytoplasmic domain of the p70 protein may be larger than that present in the Tac protein and that the endocytotic properties of the high-affinity IL-2 receptor are imparted to it by the p70 protein.

Other studies have revealed a role for the p70 protein in direct activation by IL-2 of resting T-cell proliferation in the absence of other mitogenic stimuli (122). This response appears to involve two discrete stages mediated by the interaction of IL-2 with two different forms of IL-2 receptors. Some, and perhaps all, resting T cells constitutively display the p70 protein (400–600 sites per cell assuming uniform distribution on all resting T cells) (120,122). Data currently available suggest a model for IL-2 activation of resting T cells involving an initial binding of IL-2 to the intermediate-affinity p70 receptors. This binding event leads to the generation of "competence" which is associated with the rapid expression of several T-cell activation genes, including c-*myc,* c-*myb,* and Tac. The production of Tac antigen, in the presence of the p70 protein, then permits the assembly of high-affinity IL-2 receptors that in turn bind IL-2 and generate the second stage "progression" signals leading to T-cell proliferation. This "two-step" model for IL-2 activation of T-cell growth involving the intermediate- and high-affinity forms of the IL-2 receptor is supported by the finding that the anti-Tac antibody inhibits events associated with progression but does not block the early metabolic changes associated with competence.

At present, the p70 protein has not been purified, nor have specific monoclonal antibodies been prepared. In addition, formal proof for the high-affinity ternary complex of p70, Tac, and IL-2 has not yet been obtained, perhaps because of the inherent inefficiency of the cross-linking reactions and the requirement for two internal cross-links to stabilize the putative ternary complex. Clearly, a more complete biochemical and molecular description of the p70 protein should provide important insights into the structure and function of the high-affinity IL-2 receptor. It remains possible that other, yet unidentified, proteins also participate with Tac and p70 in formation of the high-affinity IL-2 receptor complex. It seems likely that the total number of high-affinity IL-2 receptors expressed during T-cell activation may be limited by the level of the p70 receptors. In contrast, the constitutive nature of p70 expression on many lymphoid cells underscores the important role played by the inducible expression of the Tac gene in the control of high-affinity receptor expression.

REGULATION OF TAC GENE EXPRESSION IN NORMAL T CELLS

Tac protein is normally detectable on the surface of T cells within 4 to 6 hr after PHA activation. Peak expression, measured by anti-Tac binding (30,000–60,000 receptors per cell), occurs 48 to 72 hr after stimulation (42). The induction of receptor display is inhibited by actinomycin D and cycloheximide, but not by mitomycin C or X-irradiation, indicating requirements for *de novo* RNA and protein synthesis but not DNA synthesis. Analysis of cytoplasmic RNA and nuclear transcription have confirmed rapid induction (2–4 hr) of Tac gene expression following mitogen addition (107). These results are also consistent with the cytofluorometric detection of Tac positivity at least 8 hr before the entry of T cells into the S phase of the cell cycle (92).

The signal requirements for IL-2 receptor (Tac) expression remain controversial. Accessory cells appear to be strictly required for IL-2 receptor appearance following lectin activation, a function not fully replaced by IL-1 (123,124). In contrast, an absolute requirement for IL-1 has been reported for IL-2 receptor expression in an antigen-specific murine T-cell line (125). An increase in intracellular calcium may also be involved in IL-2 receptor expression, as the calcium ionophore A23187 is capable of inducing receptor expression in human peripheral blood lymphocytes (126). In Jurkat cells and normal T lymphocytes, PMA alone is also capable of inducing IL-2 receptor expression (127). These effects of PMA suggest the possibility that protein kinase C may be involved in IL-2 receptor expression (42). Finally, recent studies have suggested that IL-2 may also play an important regulatory role in the expression of its own receptor. Reem and Yeh (128), using Con A, and Welte et al. (129), using anti-T3 antibodies, demonstrated that IL-2 receptor expression was inhibited when cells were activated in the presence of dexamethasone at concentrations sufficient to block IL-2 production. IL-2 receptor expression was restored in the studies by the addition of IL-2. Similarly, Smith and Cantrell (130) and Depper and co-workers (131) have shown that IL-2 modulates production of its own receptor.

Reinduction of Transient Tac Antigen Expression

As noted, the number of high- and low-affinity IL-2 receptors reaches a maximum 2 to 3 days after activation with mitogenic lectins. Thereafter, a progressive decline in receptor number occurs over time such that after 7 to 12 days in culture receptor levels are 10% to 20% of those occurring at peak expression. A similar rise and fall in receptor number occurs with antigen stimulation (43–45,132,133). It was unclear whether T cells that had lost IL-2 receptors could be reactivated to grow. It was found, however, that IL-2 receptor expression could be readily reinduced by addition of the initial stimulus, including either mitogenic lectin or antigen. This rise and fall in IL-2 receptor number is paralleled by changes in the proliferation of T cells. It is likely that both the number of IL-2 receptors and the availability of IL-2 contribute first to the development of the T-cell immune response and then to its termination.

The reexpression of IL-2 receptors on long-term cutured PHA lymphoblasts has been examined carefully by Depper and co-workers (131). These investigators found that receptor number was augmented 2- to 10-fold by reexposure to stimulating mitogen. Mitogen-induced receptor reexpression was inhibited by actinomycin D and cycloheximide, indicating that the mobilization of preformed intracellular receptors back to the cell surface was not entirely responsible for the receptor up-regulation phenomenon. Moreover, cytofluorometric analyses with anti-Tac indicated that the majority of such cells expressed small numbers of Tac receptors before restimulation and that activation resulted in an increase in the Tac receptor number in virtually the entire cell population.

Phorbol diesters, including PMA, also augmented IL-2 receptor expression. Recent evidence suggests that protein kinase C may serve as a cellular receptor for PMA (64,65). A role for protein kinase C activation in IL-2 receptor expression was further suggested by the finding that phospholipase C, which indirectly activates protein kinase C by cleaving phosphatidylinositol biphosphate into inositol triphosphate and diacylglycerol, also augmented Tac antigen expression (42). Moreover, experiments employing a synthetic diacylglycerol congener (syn-1,2-dioctanoyl glycerol), which directly activates protein kinase C, also revealed increases in Tac receptor display.

Tac expression in this restimulation system also was directly increased by exposure of the cells to recombinant IL-2 (76,130,131). In Northern blotting studies, IL-2 also augmented levels of IL-2 receptor mRNA with maximal increases noted 12 hr after stimulation. The increase in IL-2 receptor mRNA was, at least in part, due to an increase in IL-2 receptor gene transcription as assessed in nuclear runoff assays (131). Recent experiments by Farrar and Anderson (134) demonstrating that IL-2 produced translocation of cytosolic protein kinase C to a tightly membrane-associated form may explain the similar effects observed with PMA and IL-2 in this receptor reexpression system.

Finally, Tac receptor expression has been found to increase following the treatment of activated cells with 5-azacytidine (46), suggesting a possible role for DNA methylation in the regulation of Tac gene expression. However, hydroxyurea also increased the receptor number, presumably by blocking the transition of these cells out of the S phase of the cell cycle. Because 5-azacytidine may produce similar alterations in cell cycle progression, the mechanism of action of this drug in Tac gene expression is unclear.

While multiple signals may be involved in the initial Tac receptor expression and subsequent reexpression, the display of these receptors is transient in all the systems thus far examined. Therefore, regardless of the stimulus, after the peak in expression, receptor number progressively declines despite the continuous presence of antigen or mitogen, IL-2, or PMA. The transient nature of Tac receptor expression, like that of IL-2 secretion, is mirrored by similar changes in IL-2 receptor mRNA levels and Tac gene transcription. The cellular mechanisms controlling IL-2 receptor gene expression remain poorly defined.

ALTERED IL-2 RECEPTOR EXPRESSION IN HTLV-I-INDUCED T-CELL LEUKEMIAS

HTLV-I infection of human T4+ lymphocytes may lead to development of ATL (4,5,135). This aggressive and usually fatal leukemia is clinically associated with hypercalcemia, dermal or epidermal leukemic infiltrates, and increased susceptibility of the patient to opportunistic infections (136,137). ATL occurs in geographically clustered areas where the virus is endemic, including the southwestern region of Japan, the Caribbean basin, the southeastern United States, and sub-Saharan Africa. Thus far, effective therapy for HTLV-I-induced leukemia has not been defined. Cultured ATL cell lines are characterized by a uniform display of large numbers of membrane IL-2 receptors (54,102,103). Both high- and low-affinity binding sites are present; however, most of these leukemic cell lines do not produce IL-2 (138) or require IL-2 for growth. Thus, an autocrine mechanism of leukemic cell growth does not appear likely in these cells; however, as discussed below, autocrine growth may play an important role during the early stages of HTLV-I-induced transformation.

The constitutive expression of Tac receptors in ATL cell lines does not appear to be the result of chromosomal translocation, rearrangement, or amplification of the Tac gene (105). Furthermore, the primary amino acid sequences of the normal and HUT 102B2 leukemic receptor protein are identical (38,39). ATL cell lines constitutively express large quantities of Tac mRNA, and each of the three known poly A addition sites are used. As with normal T cells, posttranscriptional splicing of the fourth exon also occurs in HTLV-I-infected T cells. Nuclear runoff assays confirm high-level Tac gene transcription in ATL cells (105).

A comparison of Tac receptor promoter structure in normal and ATL cells also revealed an intriguing difference. As noted above, in normal activated T cells IL-2 receptor gene transcription is primarily initiated at two discrete sites. In contrast, although these two sites were also utilized in ATL cells, transcription was mediated from a third additional site located further upstream as well (38). The presence of unique transcription start sites in these HTLV-I-infected T cells is interesting in view of the high-level constitutive expression of receptors; however, this third promoter appears to be considerably weaker than the two promoters shared by normal and ATL cells and has recently been detected in normal lymphoid populations. While it is conceivable that mRNA generated from the third transcription initiation site is more stable or more efficiently translated, it seems unlikely that the third extra promoter provides a full explanation for the deregulated expression of IL-2 receptors encountered in this leukemia.

HTLV-I and HTLV-II retroviruses are able to acutely transform human cord blood T cells in culture (139). Despite this capacity, neither virus contains a recognized oncogene characteristic of other acutely transforming animal retroviruses. Furthermore, these viruses do not appear to transform T cells by promoter-enhancer insertion with cis-activation of an endogenous cellular oncogene, because the sites of proviral integration vary markedly from tumor to tumor (140). Clues to the mechanism of HTLV transformation have stemmed from sequence analysis of the virus (141). Like other retroviruses, HTLV-I and HTLV-II contain flanking LTRs as well as *gag, pol,* and *env* genes. However, an extra region, termed pX, was found near the 3′ end of the virus (142–145). Sodroski et al. (146) subsequently demonstrated that, following a unique double-splicing event, the pX region encoded a subgenomic mRNA and corresponding protein capable of trans-activation of the transcription of genes controlled by the viral LTR. This trans-activator gene was originally termed LOR or X-LOR, but more recently *tat* (*trans-activator of transcription), given its function. It has been suggested that the *tat* protein may, in addition to augmenting viral transcription and viral replication, also activate the expression of select cellular genes involved in T-cell growth.

Inoue and colleagues (147) demonstrated that the *tat*-I cDNA cloned into an expression vector was able to activate transient expression of the cellular genes encoding Tac and IL-2 when transfected into Jurkat or HSB-2 T cells. In parallel studies, Siekevitz et al. (148) prepared a *tat*-I cDNA expression vector containing the HTLV-I LTR as the promoter. This vector transactivates its own production of the *tat*-I gene product, leading to high-level production. This plasmid was shown to make a functional trans-activator gene product in cotransfection assays in Jurkat T cells, as evidenced by marked stimulation of the HTLV-I LTR linked to the reporter gene, chloramphenicol acetyltransferase (CAT). (Activity of a promoter can be quantitated by examining the degree of acetylation of radiolabeled chloramphenicol catalyzed by the CAT enzyme.) In contrast, a control cDNA corresponding to a

21,000-dalton protein also produced by the pX region had no trans-activating properties (M. Siekevitz, M. Feinberg, and W. C. Greene, unpublished data).

To examine potential effects on cellular gene expression, the *tat*-I expression vector was cotransfected into Jurkat T cells with a plasmid containing the IL-2 receptor promoter linked to the CAT gene. These studies revealed that the *tat*-I gene product markedly increased the activity of the IL-2 receptor promoter while not altering the expression of several other cellular promoters (148). These findings thus provided a link between the deregulated display of IL-2 receptors encountered in HTLV-I-infected T cells and the *tat* gene product produced by these viruses. Similar results regarding the capacity of the *tat*-I gene product to activate the *tat* promoter have been reported by Maruyama et al. (152) and Cross et al. (153).

Potential effects of the *tat*-I gene on IL-2 gene expression were also evaluated. In contrast to the IL-2 receptor promoter, the *tat*-I gene product alone had little or no effect on the IL-2 promoter (148). However, in the Jurkat T-cell model, two signals (PHA and PMA) are required both for the activation of IL-2 production (60) and IL-2 promoter CAT expression. It was observed that the *tat*-I gene product was able to replace the requirement for either of these activation signals. Thus, *tat*-I and PHA or PMA stimulated high-level IL-2 promoter CAT activity essentially identical in magnitude to that obtained with combinations of PHA and PMA. Thus, the *tat*-I gene product appears able to mediate partial activation of IL-2 gene expression.

In contrast to PHA and PMA stimulation, PMA and *tat*-I-induced IL-2 promoter activity was found to be entirely resistant to the inhibitory effects of cyclosporin A. These findings suggest that the *tat*-I gene product exerts its effects on IL-2 gene expression at a point distal to the site of inhibition produced by cyclosporin A.

Retrovirus-induced transformation has now been associated with the introduction of oncogenes resembling growth factors (v-*sis* → β chain of PDGF) or growth factor receptors (v-*erb*-B → truncated epidermal growth factor receptor). Alternatively, retroviruses may produce leukemia by cis-activation of an endogenous cellular oncogene via promoter-enhancer insertion (e.g., avian leukosis virus activation of c-*myc* expression). The findings presented above suggest that the HTLV-I retrovirus employs a third strategy involving its trans-activator gene product, which results in the induced expression of the Tac gene and partial activation of the IL-2 gene (Fig. 6). The activation of these genes involved in T-cell growth may well play an important role in HTLV-I-mediated leukemogenesis, particularly at stages occurring soon after viral infection.

As noted earlier, no effective treatment for patients with ATL has yet been identified. The presence of the Tac

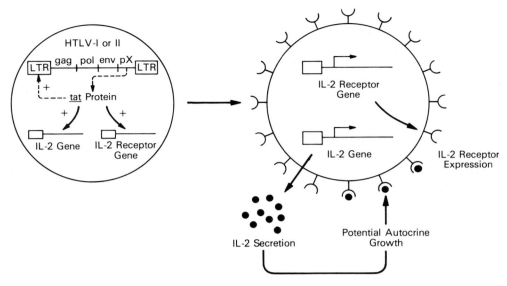

FIG. 6. Possible model for the action of the *tat*-I gene product in HTLV-I-induced T-cell transformation. These events may occur early in the transformation process, facilitating the occurrence of second-stage events which result in the outgrowth of interleukin-2 (IL-2)-independent clonal populations of fully transformed T cells.

antigen on the surface of these cells forms a relatively tumor-specific marker, as most resting T and B cells do not express this gene product. Krönke and colleagues (149) and FitzGerald et al. (150) have demonstrated that anti-Tac antibody conjugated to the A chain of the ricin toxin or to the *Pseudomonas* exotoxin, respectively, forms an effective cytotoxic agent capable of killing HTLV-I-infected T cells *in vitro*. Furthermore, immunotoxin killing of ATL cells can be accentuated by the addition of lysosomotropic agents (e.g., chloroquine, monensin) which presumably facilitate entry of the immunotoxin into the cytoplasm (151). Though *in vitro* successes with immunotoxins do not necessarily predict *in vivo* utility, the clinical efficacy of anti-Tac–*Pseudomonas* exotoxin conjugates is presently under study at the National Cancer Institute.

SUMMARY

IL-2 and one subunit of its high-affinity cellular receptor have now been characterized at the gene, mRNA, and protein levels. It is clear from these studies that expression of these genes forms critical events required for full development of the normal immune response. The availability of cloned genes for both the Tac antigen and IL-2 makes this experimental system attractive for further study. Dominant questions which will form the focus of future research involve (a) the further study of the second IL-2 receptor, p70, and the structure of the high-affinity IL-2 receptor, (b) the regulatory mechanisms which govern IL-2 and IL-2 receptor gene expression, (c) the mechanism of IL-2 growth signal transduction through its high-affinity

receptor, (d) the trans-activator genes of HTLV-I and HTLV-II and their relationship to the activation of IL-2 and IL-2 receptor gene expression and the potential role played by these genes in leukemic transformation, (e) the three-dimensional structure of the growth factor and its receptor, and (f) the use of IL-2, IL-2-activated cytolytic cells, and antireceptor antibodies in the therapy of certain diseases.

REFERENCES

1. Morgan, D. A., Ruscetti, F. W., and Gallo, R. C. (1976): Selective *in vitro* growth of T lymphocytes from normal human bone marrows. *Science,* 193:1007–1008.
2. Smith, K. A. (1980): T-cell growth factor. *Immunol. Rev.,* 51:337–357.
3. Robb, R. J. (1984): Interleukin 2: The molecule and its function. *Immunol. Today,* 5:203–209.
4. Poiesz, B. J., Ruscetti, F. W., Gazdar, A. F., Bunn, P. A., Minna, J. D., and Gallo, R. C. (1980): Detection and isolation of type-C retrovirus particles from fresh and cultured lymphocytes of a patient with cutaneous T-cell lymphoma. *Proc. Natl. Acad. Sci. USA,* 77: 7415–7419.
5. Poiesz, B. J., Ruscetti, F. W., Reitz, M. S., Kalyanaraman, V. S., and Gallo, R. C. (1981): Isolation of a new type-C retrovirus (HTLV) in primary uncultured cells of a patient with Sezary T-cell leukemia. *Nature,* 294:268–271.
6. Mier, J. W., and Gallo, R. C. (1980): Purification and some characterisics of human T-cell growth factor from phytohemagglutinin stimulated lymphocyte conditioned media. *Proc. Natl. Acad. Sci. USA,* 77:6134–6138.
7. Welte, K., Wang, C. Y., Mertelsman, R., Venuta, S., Feldman, S. P., and Moore, M. A. S. (1982): Purification of human interleukin 2 to apparent homogeneity and its molecular heterogeneity. *J. Exp. Med.,* 156:454–464.
8. Riendeau, D., Harnish, D. G., Bleackley, R. C., and Paetkau, V. (1983): Purification of mouse interleukin 2 to apparent homogeneity. *J. Biol. Chem.,* 258:12114–12117.

9. Henderson, L. E., Hewetson, J. F., Hopkins, R. F., III, Sowder, R. C., Neubauer, R. H., and Rabin, H. (1983): A rapid, large scale purification procedure for gibbon interleukin 2. *J. Immunol.,* 131: 810–815.

10. Robb, R. J., Kutny, R. M., and Chowdhry, V. (1983): Purification and partial sequence analysis of human T cell growth factor. *Proc. Natl. Acad. Sci. USA,* 80:5990–5994.

11. Taniguchi, T., Matsui, H., Fujita, T., Takaoka, C., Kashima, N., Yoshimoto, R., and Hamuro, J. (1983): Structure and expression of a cloned cDNA for human interleukin 2. *Nature,* 302:305–310.

12. Devos, R., Plaetinck, G., Cheroutre, H., Simons, G., Degrave, W., Tavernier, J., Remaut, E., and Fiero, W. (1983): Molecular cloning of human interleukin 2 cDNA and its expression in *E. coli. Nucleic Acids Res.,* 11:4307–4323.

13. Fujita, T., Takaoka, C., Matsui, H., and Taniguchi, T. (1983): Structure of the human interleukin 2 gene. *Proc. Natl. Acad. Sci. USA,* 80:7437–7441.

14. Holbrook, N. J., Smith, K. A., Fornace, A. J., Jr., Comeau, C. H., Wiskocil, R. L., and Crabtree, G. R. (1984): T-cell growth factor: Complete nucleotide sequence and organization of the gene in normal and malignant cells. *Proc. Natl. Acad. Sci. USA,* 81:1634–1638.

15. Siegel, L. J., Harper, M. E., Wong-Staal, F., Gallo, R. C., Nash, W. G., and O'Brien, S. J. (1984): Gene for T-cell growth factor: Location on human chromosome 4q and feline chromosome B1. *Science,* 223:175–178.

16. Rosenberg, S. A., Lotze, M. T., Muul, L. M., Leitman, S., Chang, A. E., Ettinghausen, S. E., Matory, Y. L., Skibber, J. M., Shiloni, E., and Vetto, J. T. (1985): Observations on the systemic administration of autologous lymphokine-activated killer cells and recombinant interleukin-2 to patients with metastatic cancer. *N. Engl. J. Med.,* 313:1485–1492.

17. Robb, R. J., Munck, A., and Smith, K. A. (1981): T-cell growth factor receptors: Quantification, specificity, and biological relevance. *J. Exp. Med.,* 154:1455–1474.

18. Greene, W. C., and Robb, R. J. (1985): Receptors for T-cell growth factor: Structure, function and expression on normal and neoplastic cells. *Contemp. Top. Mol. Immunol.,* 10:1–34.

19. Greene, W. C., Leonard, W. J., and Depper, J. M. (1986): Growth of human T lymphocytes: An analysis of interleukin-2 and its cellular receptor. *Prog. Hematol.,* 14:283–301.

20. Greene, W. C., and Leonard, W. J. (1986): The human interleukin-2 receptor. *Annu. Rev. Immunol.,* 4:69–95.

21. Uchiyama, T., Broder, S., and Waldmann, T. A. (1981): A monoclonal antibody (anti-Tac) reactive with activated and functionally mature human T cells. *J. Immunol.,* 126:1293–1297.

22. Leonard, W. J., Depper, J. M., Uchiyama, T., Smith, K. A., Waldmann, T. A., and Greene, W. C. (1982): A monoclonal antibody that appears to recognize the receptor for human T cell growth factor: Partial characterization of the receptor. *Nature,* 300:267–269.

23. Miyawaki, T. A., Yachie, A., Uwandana, N., Ohzeki, S., Nagaoki, T., and Taniguchi, N. (1982): Functional significance of Tac antigen expressed on activated human T lymphocytes: Tac antigen interacts with T cell growth factor in cellular proliferation. *J. Immunol.,* 129:2474–2478.

24. Robb, R. J., and Greene, W. C. (1983): Direct demonstration of the identity of T cell growth factor binding protein and the Tac antigen. *J. Exp. Med.,* 158:1332–1337.

25. Rubin, L. A., Kurman, C. L., Biddison, W. E., Goldman, N. D., and Nelson, D. L. (1985): A monoclonal antibody, 7G7/B6, binds to an epitope on the human IL-2 receptor that is distinct from that recognized by IL-2 or anti-Tac. *Hybridoma,* 4:91–102.

26. Ortega, R. G., Robb, R. J., Shevach, E. M., and Malek, T. R. (1984): The murine IL-2 receptor. I. Monoclonal antibodies that define distinct functional epitopes on activated T-cells and react with activated B-cells. *J. Immunol.,* 133:1970–1975.

27. Osawa, H., and Diamantstein, T. (1983): The characterization of a monoclonal antibody that binds specifically to rat T lymphoblasts and inhibits IL-2 receptor functions. *J. Immunol.,* 130:51–55.

28. Leonard, W. J., Depper, J. M., Robb, R. J., Waldmann, T. A., and Green, W. C. (1983): Characterization of the human receptor for T cell growth factor. *Proc. Natl. Acad. Sci. USA,* 80:6957–6961.

29. Wano, Y., Uchiyama, T., Fukui, K., Maeda, M., Uchino, H., and Yodoi, J. (1984): Characterization of human interleukin 2 receptor (Tac expression) in normal and leukemic T-cells: Coexpression of normal and aberrant receptors in HUT 102 cells. *J. Immunol.,* 132:3005–3010.

30. Leonard, W. J., Depper, J. M., Kronke, M., Robb, R. J., Waldmann, T. A., and Greene, W. C. (1985): The human receptor for T-cell growth factor: Evidence for variable post-translational processing, phosphorylation, sulfation, and the ability of precursor forms of the receptor to bind TCGF. *J. Biol. Chem.,* 260:1872–1880.

31. Urdal, D. L., March, C. J., Gillis, S., Larsen, A., and Dower, S. K. (1984): Purification and chemical characterization of the receptor for interleukin-2 from activated human T lymphocytes and from a human T-cell lymphoma cell-line. *Proc. Natl. Acad. Sci. USA,* 81:6481–6485.

32. Shackelford, D. A., and Trowbridge, I. S. (1984): Induction of expression and phosphorylation of the human interleukin 2 receptor by a phorbol diester. *J. Biol. Chem.,* 259:11706–11712.

33. Leonard, W. J., Depper, J. M., Crabtree, G. R., Rudikoff, S., Pumphrey, J., Robb, R. J., Krönke, M., Svetlik, P. B., Peffer, N. J., Waldmann, T. A., and Greene, W. C. (1984): Molecular cloning and expression of cDNAs for the human interleukin-2 receptor. *Nature,* 311:626–631.

34. Nikaido, T., Shimizu, N., Ishida, N., Sabe, H., Teshigawara, K., Maeda, M., Uchiyama, T., Yodoi, J., and Honjo, T. (1984): Molecular cloning of cDNA encoding human interleukin-2 receptor. *Nature,* 311:631–635.

35. Cosman, D., Cerretti, D. P., Larsen, A., Park, L., March, C., Dower, S., Gillis, S., and Urdal, D. (1984): Cloning, sequence and expression of human interleukin-2 receptor. *Nature,* 312:768–771.

36. Shimizu, A., Kondo, S., Takada, S., Yodoi, J., Ishida, N., Sabe, N., Osawa, H., Diamantstein, T., Nikaido, T., and Honjo, T. (1985): Nucleotide sequence of mouse IL-2 receptor cDNA and its comparison with the human IL-2 receptor sequence. *Nucleic Acids Res.,* 13:1505–1516.

37. Miller, J., Malek, T. R., Leonard, W. J., Greene, W. C., Shevach, E. M., and Germain, R. N. (1985): Nucleotide sequence and expression of a mouse interleukin-2 receptor cDNA. *J. Immunol.,* 134:4212–4217.

38. Leonard, W. J., Depper, J. M., Kronke, M., Peffer, N. J., Svetlik, P. B., Kanehisa, M., Sullivan, M., and Greene, W. C. (1985): Structure of the human interleukin-2 receptor gene. *Science,* 230:633–639.

39. Ishida, N., Kanamori, H., Noma, T., Nikaido, T., Sabe, H., Suzuki, N., Shimizu, A., and Honjo, T. (1985): Molecular cloning and structure of the human interleukin-2 gene. *Nucleic Acids Res.,* 13: 7579–7589.

40. Leonard, W. J., Donlon, T. A., Lebo, R. V., and Greene, W. C. (1985): Localization of the gene encoding the human interleukin-2 receptor on chromosome 10. *Science,* 228:1547–1549.

41. Cantrell, D. A., and Smith, K. A. (1983): Transient expression of interleukin-2 receptors: Consequences for T-cell growth. *J. Exp. Med.,* 158:1895–1911.

42. Depper, J. M., Leonard, W. J., Krönke, M., Noguchi, P. D., Cunningham, R. E., Waldmann, T. A., and Greene, W. C. (1984): Regulation of interleukin-2 receptor expression: Effects of phorbol diester, phospholipase-c, and reexposure to lectin and antigen. *J. Immunol.,* 133:3054–3061.

43. Hemler, M. D., Brenner, M. B., McLean, J. M., and Strominger, J. L. (1984): Antigen stimulation regulates the level of expression of IL-2 receptors on human T-cells. *Proc. Natl. Acad. Sci. USA,* 81:2172–2175.

44. Reske-Kunz, A. B., von Steldern, D., Rude, E., Osawa, H., and Diamantstein, T. (1984): Interleukin-2 receptors on an insulin specific T-cell line: Dynamics of receptor expression. *J. Immunol.,* 133:1356–1361.

45. Kaplan, D. R., Braciale, V. L., and Braciale, T. J. (1984): Antigen dependent regulation of interleukin-2 receptor expression on cloned human cytotoxic T lymphocytes. *J. Immunol.,* 133:1966–1969.

46. Depper, J. M., Leonard, W. J., Krönke, M., Drogula, C., Waldmann, T. A., and Greene, W. C. (1985): Activators of protein kinase C and 5-azacytidine induce IL-2 receptor expression in human T lymphocytes. *J. Cell. Biochem.,* 27:267–276.

47. Gillis, S., and Watson, J. (1980): Biochemical and biological characterization of lymphocyte regulatory molecules. V. Identification of an interleukin 2-producing human leukemia T cell line. *J. Exp. Med.,* 152:1709–1719.

48. Gillis, S., Ferm, M. M., Ou, W., and Smith, K. A. (1978): T-cell growth factor: Parameters of production and a quantitative microassay for activity. *J. Immunol.,* 120:2027–2032.

49. Stadler, B. M., Berenstein, E. H., Siraganian, R. P., and Oppenheim, J. J. (1982): Monoclonal antibody against human interleukin (IL-2). I. Purification of IL-2 for the production of monoclonal antibodies. *J. Immunol.,* 128:1620–1624.

50. Robb, R. J., and Lin, Y. (1983): T-cell growth factor: Purification, interaction with a cellular receptor, and *in vitro* synthesis. In: *Thymic Hormones and Lymphokines,* edited by A. L. Goldstein, pp. 247–256. Plenum Publishing Co., New York.

51. Robb, R. J., and Smith, K. A. (1981): Heterogeneity of human T cell growth factor(s) due to variable glycosylation. *Mol. Immunol.,* 18:1087–1094.

52. Robb, R. J., Greene, W. C., and Rusk, C. M. (1984): Low and high affinity cellular receptors for interleukin 2. Implications for the level of Tac antigen. *J. Exp. Med.,* 160:1126–1146.

53. Fujita, T., Shibuya, H., Ohashi, T., Yamanishi, K., and Taniguchi, T. (1986): Regulation of human interleukin-2 gene: Functional DNA sequences in the 5′ flanking region for the gene expression in activated T lymphocytes. *Cell,* 46:401–405.

54. Gootenberg, J. E., Ruscetti, F. W., Mier, J. W., Gazdar, A., and Gallo, R. C. (1981): Human cutaneous T-cell lymphoma and leukemia-cell lines produced and respond to T-cell growth factor. *J. Exp. Med.,* 154:1403–1417.

55. Chen, S. J., Holbrook, N. J., Mitchell, K. F., Vallone, C. A., Greengard, J. S., Crabtree, G. R., and Cin, Y. (1985): A viral long terminal repeat in the interleukin-2 gene of a cell line that constitutively produces interleukin-2. *Proc. Natl. Acad. Sci. USA,* 82:7284–7288.

56. Wang, A., Lu, S.-D., and Mark, D. F. (1984): Site specific mutagenesis of the human interleukin-2 gene: Structure-function analysis of the cysteine residues. *Science,* 224:1431–1433.

57. Robb, R. J., Kutny, R. M., Panico, M., Morris, H., De Grado, W. F., and Chowdhry, V. (1983): Post-translational modification of human T-cell growth factor. *Biochem. Biophys. Res. Commun.,* 116:1049–1055.

58. Kuo, L. M., and Robb, R. J. (1986): Structure-function relationships for the IL 2-receptor system. I. Localization of a receptor binding site on IL 2. *J. Immunol.,* 137:1538–1543.

59. Larsson, E. L., Iscove, N., and Coutinho, A. (1980): Two distinct factors are required for induction of T cell growth. *Nature,* 283:664–666.

60. Wiskocil, R., Weiss, A., Imboden, J., Kamin-Lewis, R., and Stobo, J. (1985): Activation of a human T cell line: A two-stimulus requirement in the pretranslational events involved in the coordinate expression of interleukin 2 and gamma-interferon genes. *J. Immunol.,* 134:1599–1603.

61. Weiss, A., Imboden, J., Shoback, D., and Stobo, J. (1984): Role of T3 surface molecules in human T-cell activation: T3-dependent activation results in an increase in cytoplasmic free calcium. *Proc. Natl. Acad. Sci. USA,* 81:4169–4173.

62. Imboden, J. B., Weiss, A., and Stobo, J. D. (1985): The antigen receptor on a human T cell line initiates activation by increasing cytoplasmic free calcium. *J. Immunol.,* 134:663–665.

63. Weiss, A., and Stobo, J. D. (1984): Requirement for the coexpression of T3 and the T cell antigen receptor on a malignant human T cell line. *J. Exp. Med.,* 160:1284–1299.

64. Nishizuka, Y. (1984): The role of protein kinase C in cell surface signal transduction and tumour promotion. *Nature,* 308:693–698.

65. Kikkawa, U., Takai, Y., Tanaka, Y., Miyake, R., and Nishizuka, Y. (1983): Protein kinase C as a possible receptor protein of tumor-promoting phorbol esters. *J. Biol. Chem.,* 258:11442–11445.

66. Krönke, M., Leonard, W. J., Depper, J. M., and Greene, W. C. (1985): Sequential expression of genes involved in human T cell growth and differentiation. *J. Exp. Med.,* 161:1593–1598.

67. Shevach, E. M. (1985): The effects of cyclosporin A on the immune system. *Annu. Rev. Immunol.,* 3:397–423.

68. Carpenter, C. B., and Strom, T. B. (1984): Immunosuppressive therapy for renal transplantation. *Springer Semin. Immunopathol.,* 7:43–57.

69. Arya, S. K., Wong-Staal, F., and Gallo, R. C. (1984): Dexamethasone-mediated inhibition of human T cell growth factor and gamma-interferon messenger RNA. *J. Immunol.,* 133:273–276.

70. Lillehoj, H., and Shevach, E. M. (1985): A comparison of the effects of cyclosporin A, dexamethasone, and ouabain on the interleukin-2 cascade. *J. Immunopharmacol.,* 7:267–284.

71. Krönke, M., Leonard, W. J., Depper, J. M., Arya, S. K., Wong-Staal, F., Gallo, R. C., Waldmann, T. A., and Greene, W. C. (1984): Cyclosporin A inhibits T-cell growth factor gene expression at the level of mRNA transcription. *Proc. Natl. Acad. Sci. USA,* 81:5214–5218.

72. LeGrue, S. J., Turner, R., Weisbrodt, N., and Dedman, J. R. (1986): Does the binding of cyclosporine to calmodulin result in immunosuppression? *Science,* 234:68–71.

73. Efrat, S., and Kaempfer, R. (1984): Control of biologically active interleukin 2 messenger RNA formation in induced human lymphocytes. *Proc. Natl. Acad. Sci. USA,* 81:2601–2605.

74. Korsmeyer, S. J., Greene, W. C., Cossman, J., Hsu, S., Jensen, J. P., Neckers, L. M., Marshall, S. L., Bakhshi, A., Depper, J. M., Leonard, W. J., Jaffe, E. S., and Waldmann, T. A. (1983): Rearrangement and expression of immunoglobulin genes and expression of Tac antigen in hairy cell leukemia. *Proc. Natl. Acad. Aci. USA,* 80:4522–4526.

75. Tsudo, M., Uchiyama, T., and Uchino, H. (1984): Expression of Tac antigen on activated normal human B-cells. *J. Exp. Med.,* 160:612–617.

76. Waldmann, T. A., Goldman, C. K., Robb, R. J., Depper, J. M., Leonard, W. J., Sharrow, S. O., Bongiovanni, K. F., Korsmeyer, S. J., and Greene, W. C. (1984): Expression of interleukin-2 receptors on activated human B-cells. *J. Exp. Med.,* 160:1450–1466.

77. Nakanishi, K., Malek, T. R., Smith, K. A., Hamaoka, T., Shevach, E. M., and Paul, W. E. (1984): Both interleukin-2 and a second T-cell derived factor in EL-4 supernatants have activity as differentiation factors in IgM synthesis. *J. Exp. Med.,* 160:1605–1621.

78. Mittler, R., Rao, P., Olini, G., Westberg, E., Newman, W., Hoffmann, M., and Golstein, G. (1985): Activated human B-cells display a functional IL-2 receptor. *J. Immunol.,* 134:2393–2399.

79. Ralph, P., Jeong, G., Welte, K., Mertlesman, R., Rabin, H., Henderson, L. E., Souza, L. M., Boone, T. C., and Robb, R. J. (1984): Stimulation of immunoglobulin secretion in human B lymphocytes as a direct effect of high concentrations of IL-2. *J. Immunol.,* 133:2442–2445.

80. Howard, M., Matis, L., Malek, T. R., Shevach, E., Kell, W., Cohen, D., Nakanishi, K., and Paul, W. E. (1983): Interleukin 2 induces antigen reactive T cell lines to secrete BCGF-1. *J. Exp. Med.,* 158:2024–2039.

81. Farrar, J. J., Benjamin, W. R., Hilfiker, M. L., Howard, M., Farrar, W. L., and Fuller-Farrar, J. (1982): The biochemistry, biology, and role of interleukin 2 in the induction of cytotoxic T cell and antibody forming B cell responses. *Immunol. Rev.,* 63:129–166.

82. Brooks, C. G., and Henney, C. S. (1985): Interleukin-2 and regulation of natural killer activity in cultured cell populations. *Contemp. Top. Mol. Immunol.* 10:63–92.

83. Ortaldo, J. R., Mason, A. T., Gerard, J. P., Henderson, L. E., Farrar, W., Hopkins, R. F., III, Herberman, R. B., and Rabin, H. (1984): Effects of natural and recombinant IL 2 on regulation of IFN gamma production and natural killer activity: Lack of involvement of the Tac antigen for these immunoregulatory effects. *J. Immunol.,* 133:779–783.

84. Benveniste, E. N., and Merrill, J. E. (1986): Stimulation of oligodendroglial proliferation and maturation by interleukin-2. *Nature,* 321:610–613.

85. Rosenberg, S. A., Spiess, P. J., and Schwarz, S. (1983): *In vivo*

administration of interleukin-2 enhances specific alloimmune responses. *Transplantation*, 35:631–634.

86. Lotze, M. T., Grimm, E. A., Mazumder, A., Strausser, J. L., and Rosenberg, S. A. (1981): *In vitro* growth of cytotoxic T lymphocytes: Lysis of fresh and cultured autologous tumor by human lymphocytes cultured in T-cell growth factor. *Cancer Res.*, 41:4420–4425.

87. Grimm, E. A., Ramsey, K., Mazumder, A., Wilson, D. J., Djeu, J. Y., and Rosenberg, S. A. (1983): Lymphokine activated killer cell phenomenon. II. Precursor phenotype is serologically distinct from peripheral T lymphocytes, memory cytotoxic thymus-derived lymphocytes, and natural killer cells. *J. Exp. Med.*, 157:884–897.

88. Grimm, E. A., Robb, R. J., Roth, J. A., Neckers, L. M., Lachman, L. B., Wilson, O. J., and Rosenberg, S. A. (1983): Lymphokine activated killer cell phenomenon: III. Evidence that IL-2 is sufficient for direct activation of peripheral blood lymphocytes into lymphokine activated killer cells. *J. Exp. Med.*, 158:1356–1561.

89. Bonnard, G. D., Yasaka, D., and Jacobson, D. (1979): Ligand-activated T cell growth factor induced proliferation: Absorption of T cell growth factor by activated T cells. *J. Immunol.*, 123:2704–2708.

90. Coutinho, A., Larsson, E. L., Gronvik, K. O., and Andersson, J. (1979): Studies on T lymphocyte activation. II. The target cells for concanavalin A induced growth factors. *Eur. J. Immunol.*, 9:587–592.

91. Smith, K. A., Gillis, S., Baker, P. E., McKenzie, D., and Ruscetti, F. W. (1979): T-cell growth factor mediated T-cell proliferation. *Ann. NY Acad. Sci.*, 332:423–432.

92. Cotner, T., Williams, J. M., Christenson, L., Shapiro, H. M., Strom, T. B., and Strominger, J. (1983): Simultaneous flow cytometric analysis of human T cell activation antigen expression and DNA content. *J. Exp. Med.*, 157:461–472.

93. Fox, D. A., Hussey, R. E., Fitzgerald, K. A., Bensussan, A., Daley, J. F., Schlossman, S. F., and Reinherz, E. L. (1984): Activation of human thymocytes via the 50KD T11 sheep erythrocyte binding protein induces the expression of interleukin 2 receptors on both T3⁺ and T3⁻ populations. *J. Immunol.*, 134:330–335.

94. Yachie, A., Miyawaki, T., Uwadana, N., Ohzeki, S., and Taniguchi, N. (1983): Sequential expression of T cell activation (Tac) antigen and Ia determinants on circulating human T cells after immunization with tetanus toxoid. *J. Immunol.*, 131:731–735.

95. Lane, H. C., Depper, J. M., Greene, W. C., Whalen, G., Waldmann, T. A., and Fauci, A. S. (1985): Qualitative analysis of immune function in patients with the acquired immunodeficiency syndrome: Evidence for a selective defect in soluble antigen recognition. *N. Engl. J. Med.*, 313:79–84.

96. Miyawaki, T., Ohzeki, S., Ikuta, N., Seki, H., Taga, K., and Taniguchi, N. (1984): Immunohistologic localization and immune phenotypes of lymphocytes expressing Tac antigen in human lymphoid tissues. *J. Immunol.*, 133:2996–3000.

97. Ceredig, R., Lowenthal, J. W., Nabholz, M., and MacDonald, H. R. (1985): Expression of interleukin-2 receptors as a differentiation marker on intrathymic stem-cells. *Nature*, 314:98–100.

98. Raulet, D. H. (1985): Expression and function of interleukin-2 receptors on immature thymocytes. *Nature*, 314:101–103.

99. Herrmann, F., Cannistra, S. A., Levine, H., and Griffin, J. D. (1985): Expression of interleukin 2 receptors and binding of interleukin 2 by gamma interferon-induced human leukemic and normal monocytic cells. *J. Exp. Med.*, 162:1111–1116.

100. Yamamoto, S., Hattori, T., Matsuoka, M., Ishii, T., Asou, N., Okada, M., Tagaya, Y., Yodoi, J., and Takatsuki, K. (1986): Induction of Tac antigen and proliferation of myeloid leukemic cells by ATL-derived factor: Comparison with other agents that promote differentiation of human myeloid or monocytic leukemic cells. *Blood*, 67:1714–1720.

101. Birchenall-Sparks, M. C., Farrar, W. L., Rennick, D., Kilian, P. L., and Ruscetti, F. W. (1986): Regulation of expression of the interleukin-2 receptor on hematopoietic cells by interleukin-3. *Science*, 233:455–458.

102. Waldmann, T. A., Greene, W. C., Sarin, P. S., Saxinger, C., Blayney, D. W., Blattner, W. A., Goldman, C. K., Bongiovanni, K., Sharrow, S., Depper, J. M., Leonard, W. J., and Gallo, R. C. (1984): Func-

tional and phenotypic comparison of human T cell leukemia/lymphoma virus positive adult T cell leukemia with human T cell leukemia/lymphoma virus negative Sezary leukemia. *J. Clin. Invest.*, 73:1711–1718.

103. Depper, J. M., Leonard, W. J., Kronke, M., Waldmann, T. A., and Greene, W. C. (1984): Augmented T-cell growth-factor receptor expression in HTLV-1 infected human leukemic T-cells. *J. Immunol.*, 133:1691–1695.

104. Greene, W. C., Robb, R. J., Svetlik, P. B., Rusk, C. M., Depper, J. M., and Leonard W. J. (1985): Stable expression of cDNA encoding the human interleukin receptor in eukaryotic cells. *J. Exp. Med.*, 162:363–368.

105. Krönke, M., Leonard, W. J., Depper, J. M., and Greene, W. C. (1985): Deregulation of interleukin receptor gene expression in HTLV-1 induced adult T cell leukemia. *Science*, 228:1215–1217.

106. Treiger, B. F., Leonard, W. J., Svetlik, P., Rubin, L., Nelson, D. L., and Greene, W. C. (1986): A secreted form of the human interleukin-2 receptor encoded by an "anchor minus" cDNA. *J. Immunol.*, 136:4099–4105.

107. Leonard, W. J., Krönke, M., Peffer, N. J., Depper, J. M., and Greene, W. C. (1985): Interleukin-2 receptor gene expression in normal human T lymphocytes. *Proc. Natl. Acad. Sci. USA*, 82: 6281–6285.

108. Kuo, L. M., Rusk, C. M., and Robb, R. J. (1986): Structure-function relationships for the IL 2-receptor system. II. Localization of an IL 2 binding site on high and low affinity receptors. *J. Immunol.*, 137:1544–1551.

109. Lowenthal, J. W., Zubler, R. H., Nabholz, M., and MacDonald, H. R. (1985): Similarities between interleukin-2 receptor number and affinity on activated B and T lymphocytes. *Nature*, 315:669–672.

110. Weissman, A. M., Harford, J. B., Svetlik, P. B., Leonard, W. J., Depper, J. M., Waldmann, T. A., Greene, W. C., and Klausner, R. D. (1986): Only high affinity receptors for interleukin-2 mediate internalization of ligand. *Proc. Natl. Acad. Sci. USA*, 83:1463–1466.

111. Fujii, M., Sugamura, K., Sano, K., Nakai, M., Sugita, K., and Hinuma, Y. (1986): High-affinity receptor-mediated internalization and degradation of interleukin 2 in human T cells. *J. Exp. Med.*, 163:550–562.

112. Hatakeyama, M., Minamoto, S., Uchiyama, T., Hardy, R. R., Yamada, G., and Taniguchi, T. (1985): Reconstitution of functional receptor for human interleukin-2 in mouse cells. *Nature*, 318:467–470.

113. Sabe, H., Kondo, S., Shimizu, A., Tagaya, Y., Yodoi, J., Kobayashi, N., Hatanaka, M., Matsunami, N., Maeda, M., Noma, T., and Honjo, T. (1984): Properties of human interleukin-2 receptors expressed on nonlymphoid cells by cDNA transfection. *Mol. Biol. Med.*, 2:379–396.

114. Kondo, S., Shimizu, A., Maeda, M., Tagaya, Y., Yodoi, J., and Honjo, T. (1986): Expression of functional human interleukin-2 receptor in mouse T cells by cDNA transfection. *Nature*, 320:75–77.

115. Robb, R. J. (1986): Conversion of low-affinity interleukin 2 receptors to a high-affinity state following fusion of cell membranes. *Proc. Natl. Acad. Sci. USA*, 83:3992–3996.

116. Sharon, M., Klausner, R. D., Cullen, B. R., Chizzonite, R., and Leonard, W. J. (1986): Novel interleukin-2 receptor subunit detected by cross-linking under high affinity conditions. *Science*, 234:859–863.

117. Robb, R. J., Rusk, C. M., Yodoi, J., and Greene, W. C. (1987): An interleukin-2 binding molecule distinct from the Tac protein: Analysis of its role in formation of high affinity receptors. *Proc. Natl. Acad. Sci. USA*, 84:2002–2006.

118. Tsudo, M., Kozak, R. W., Goldman, C. K., and Waldmann, T. A. (1986): Demonstration of a non-Tac peptide that binds interleukin-2: A potential participant in a multichain interleukin-2 receptor complex. *Proc. Natl. Acad. Sci. USA*, 83:9694–9698.

119. Teshigawara, K., Wang, H.-M., Kato, K., and Smith, K. A. (1987): Interleukin-2 high affinity receptor expression requires two distinct binding proteins. *J. Exp. Med.*, 165:223–238.

120. Dukovich, M., Yano, Y., Thuy, L. T. B., Katz, P., Cullin, B. R., Kehrl, J. H., and Greene, W. C. (1987): Identification of a second human IL-2 binding protein and its possible role in the assembly of the high affinity IL-2 receptor complex. *Nature, 327*:518–522.

121. Robb, R. J., and Greene, W. C. (1987): Internalization of IL-2 is mediated by the beta chain of the high affinity IL-2 receptor. *J. Exp. Med.* (in press).

122. Thuy, L. T. B., Dukovich, M., Peffer, N. J., Fauci, A. S., Kehrl, J. H., and Greene, W. C. (1987): Direct activation of human T cells by IL-2: The role of an IL-2 receptor distinct from the Tac protein. *J. Exp. Med., 165*:1201–1206.

123. Hunig, T., Loos, M., and Schimpl, A. (1983): The role of accessory cells in polyclonal T cell activation. I. Both induction of interleukin 2 production and of interleukin 2 responsiveness by concanavalin A are accessory cell dependent. *Eur. J. Immunol., 13*:1–6.

124. Williams, J. M., Ransil, B. J., Shapiro, H. M., and Strom, T. B. (1984): Accessory cell requirement for activation of antigen expression and cell cycle progression by human T lymphocytes. *J. Immunol., 133*:2986–2994.

125. Kaye, J., Gillis, S., Mizel, S. B., Shevach, E. M., Malek, T. R., Dinarello, C. A., Lachman, L. B., and Janeway, C. A. (1984): Growth of a cloned helper T cell line induced by a monoclonal antibody specific for the antigen receptor: Interleukin 1 is required for the expression of receptors for interleukin 2. *J. Immunol., 133*: 1339–1345.

126. Koretsky, G. A., Daniele, R. P., Greene, W. C., and Nowell, P. C. (1983): Evidence for an interleukin-independent pathway for human lymphocyte activation. *Proc. Natl. Acad. Sci. USA, 80*:3444–3447.

127. Greene, W. C., Robb, R. J., Depper, J. M., Leonard, W. J., Drogula, C., Svetlik, P., Wong-Staal, F., Gallo, R. C., and Waldman, T. A. (1984): Phorbol diester induction of Tac antigen expression in human acute lymphocyte leukemic T-cells. *J. Immunol., 133*:1042–1047.

128. Reem, G., and Yeh, N.-H. (1984): Interleukin 2 regulates expression of its receptor and synthesis of gamma interferon by human T lymphocytes. *Science, 225*:429–430.

129. Welte, K., Andreef, M., Platzer, E., Holloway, K., Rubin, B. Y., Moore, M. A., and Mertlesmann, R. (1984): Interleukin 2 regulates the expression of Tac antigen in peripheral blood T lymphocytes. *J. Exp. Med., 160*:1390–1403.

130. Smith, K. A., and Cantrell, D. A. (1985): Interleukin-2 regulates its own receptor. *Proc. Natl. Acad. Sci. USA, 82*:864–868.

131. Depper, J. M., Leonard, W. J., Drogula, C., Krönke, M., Waldmann, T. A., and Greene, W. C. (1985): Interleukin-2 (IL-2) augments transcription of the interleukin-2 receptor gene. *Proc. Natl. Acad. Sci. USA, 82*:4230–4234.

132. Andrew, M. E., Churilla, A. M., Malek, T. R., Braciale, V. L., and Braciale, T. J. (1985): Activation of virus specific CTL clones: Antigen dependent regulation of interleukin 2 receptor expression. *J. Immunol., 134*:920–925.

133. Lowenthal, J. W., Tougne, C., MacDonald, H. R., Smith, K. A., and Nabholz, M. (1985): Antigenic stimulation regulates the expression of IL-2 receptors in a cytolytic T lymphocyte clone. *J. Immunol., 134*:931–939.

134. Farrar, W. J., and Anderson, W. (1985): Interleukin-2 stimulates association of protein kinase C with plasma membrane. *Nature, 315*:233–236.

135. Yoshida, M., Miyoshi, I., and Hinuma, Y. (1982): Isolation and characterization of retrovirus from cell lines of human adult T cell leukemia and its implication in disease. *Proc. Natl. Acad. Sci. USA, 78*:6476–6480.

136. Uchiyama, T., Yodoi, J., Sagawa, K., Takatsuki, K., and Uchino, H. (1977): Adult T cell leukemia: Clinical and hematologic features of 16 cases. *Blood, 50*:481–489.

137. Bunn, P. A., Schechter, G. P., Jaffe, E., Blayney, D., Young, R. C., Matthews, M. J., Blattner, W., Broder, S., Robert-Guroff, M., and Gallo, R. C. (1983): Clinical course of retrovirus associated adult T cell lymphoma in the United States. *N. Engl. J. Med., 309*: 257–262.

138. Arya, S. K., Wong-Staal, F., and Gallo, R. C. (1984): T-cell growth factor gene: Lack of expression on human T-cell leukemia lymphoma virus infected cells. *Science, 223*:1086–1087.

139. Wong-Staal, F., and Gallo, R. C. (1985): Human T lymphotropic retroviruses. *Nature, 317*:395–403.

140. Seiki, M., Eddy, R., Shows, T., and Yoshida, M. (1984): Nonspecific integration of HTLV provirus genome into adult T-cell leukemia cells. *Nature, 309*:640–642.

141. Seiki, M., Hattori, S., Hirayama, Y., and Yoshida, M. (1983): Human adult T-cell leukemia virus: Complete nucleotide sequence of the provirus genome integrated in leukemia cell DNA. *Proc. Natl. Acad. Sci. USA, 80*:3618–3622.

142. Haseltine, W. A., Sodroski, J., Patarca, R., Briggs, D., Perkins, D., and Wong-Staal, F. (1984): Structure of the 3′ terminal repeat region of type-II human T-lymphotropic virus: Evidence for a new coding region. *Science, 225*:419–421.

143. Kiyokawa, T., Seiki, M., Imagawa, K., Shimizu, F., and Yoshida, M. (1984): Identification of a protein (p40^x) encoded by a unique sequence pX of human T-cell leukemia-virus type-I. *Gann, 75*: 747–751.

144. Shimotohno, K., Miwa, M., Slamon, D. J., Chen, I. S. Y., Hoshino, H. O., Takano, M., Fujino, M., and Sugimura, T. (1985): Identification of new gene-products encoded from X-regions of human T-cell leukemia viruses. *Proc. Natl. Acad. Sci. USA, 82*:302–306.

145. Seiki, M., Hikikoshi, A., Taniguchi, T., and Yoshida, M. (1985): Expression of the pX gene of HTLV-I: General splicing mechanism in the HTLV family. *Science, 228*:1532–1534.

146. Sodroski, J. G., Rosen, C. A., and Haseltine, W. A. (1984): Trans-acting transcriptional activation of the long terminal repeat of human T-lymphotropic viruses in infected cells. *Science, 225*:381–385.

147. Inoue, J., Seiki, M., Taniguchi, T., Tsuru, S., and Yoshida, M. (1986): Induction of interleukin-2 receptor gene expression by p40^x encoded by human T cell leukemia virus-type 1. *EMBO J., 5*: 2883–2888.

148. Siekevitz, M., Feinberg, M. B., Holbrook, N., Yodoi, J., Wong-Staal, F., Gallo, R. C., and Greene, W. C. (1987): Activation of interleukin-2 and interleukin-2 receptor promoter expression by the transactivator (tat) gene product of HTLV-I. *Proc. Natl. Acad. Sci. USA, 84*:5389–5393.

149. Krönke, M., Depper, J. M., Leonard, W. J., Vitetta, E. S., Waldmann, T. A., and Greene, W. C. (1985): Adult T cell leukemia: A potential target for ricin A chain immunotoxins. *Blood, 65*:1416–1421.

150. FitzGerald, D. J. P., Waldmann, T. A., Willingham, M. C., and Pastan, I. (1984): Pseudomonas exotoxin-anti-Tac cell specific immunotoxin active against cells expressing the human T-cell growth factor receptor. *J. Clin. Invest., 74*:966–971.

151. Krönke, M., Schlick, E., Waldmann, T. A., Vitetta, E. S., and Greene, W. C. (1986): Selective killing of human T lymphotropic virus-I infected leukemic T cells by monoclonal anti-interleukin-2 receptor antibody-ricin A chain conjugates: Potentiation by ammonium chloride and monensin. *Cancer Res., 46*:3295–3298.

152. Maruyama, M., Shibuya, H., Harada, H., Hatakeyama, M., Seiki, M. Fujita, T., Inoue, J., Yoshida, M. and Taniguchi, T. (1987): Evidence for aberrant activation of the interleukin-2 autocrine loop by HTLV-I encoded p40 and T3/Ti complex triggering. *Cell, 48*: 343–350.

153. Cross, S. L., Feinberg, M. B., Wolf, J. B., Holbrook, N. J., Wong-Staal, F., and Leonard, W. J. (1987): Regulation of the human interleukin-2 receptor-α chain promoter: activation of a non-functional promoter by the transactivator gene of HTLV-I. *Cell, 49*: 47–56.

Inflammation: Basic Principles and Clinical Correlates.
Edited by J. I. Gallin, I. M. Goldstein, and R. Snyderman.
Raven Press, Ltd., New York © 1988.

CHAPTER 14

Cytokines: Interferon-γ

Carl Nathan and Ryotaro Yoshida

Cytokines are nonimmunoglobulin, nonendocrine (glyco)proteins, released by cells, that affect the functional properties of other cells of the same organism. Interferons, discovered in the 1950s (88,145), were probably the first cytokines to be well characterized. Interferon-γ, the first secretory product of T cells to be discovered (239) and cloned (63), has one of the longest and richest histories of investigation of any cytokine. Its story illustrates principles that apply to other cytokines of importance in inflammation that are not discussed in this book.

A combination of reductionist and integrationist approaches is rapidly expanding and revising our understanding of the role of interferon-γ and other cytokines. Of the two approaches, reductionism has made the most progress so far. Advances in the purification and sequencing of macromolecules, and in the cloning of antibody producing cells and DNA, have rewarded years of effort to isolate pure cytokines and pure target cells from complex mixtures and to study their interactions *in vitro*. Reductionists have handed integrationists the first highly specific tools with which to analyze the role of cytokines in the intact organism: monoclonal antibodies, complementary DNA (cDNA) probes, and pure recombinant cytokines. With these, integrationists have recently begun *in vivo* experiments in detection, deletion, and reconstitution. Naturally occurring states of cytokine deficiency or excess are being characterized and correlated with features of disease. Specific cytokines are being identified or neutralized *in situ* or injected in pure form.

It should come as no surprise that these two experimental approaches are yielding conflicting results. Some of the effects of injecting interferon-γ, for example, are the opposite of what *in vitro* assays predict. Cytokines introduced into an ongoing inflammatory response enter networks and trigger cascades. Thus, as matters seem to be coming clear in the test tube, they grow more complex in the host. The following discussion of interferon-γ in the inflammatory response emphasizes both our extensive information and our incomplete understanding.

BACKGROUND AND BIOCHEMISTRY

Discovery of Interferon-γ

Interferons are a family of proteins and glycoproteins produced by all nucleated cells in response to infection with viruses, and by some cells on exposure to a diverse array of other agents. Inducing agents vary with the cell type. Of primary physiologic importance among the nonviral interferon inducers are bacteria, protozoa, and some of their subcellular constituents, such as the lipopolysaccharide of the outer membrane of Gram-negative microbes. As was once customary in cytokine research, the first bioactivity of interferons to be discovered became the basis for naming them: "interferon" because of their interference with the replication of viruses (88,145).

About a decade after the discovery of interferon, more and more factors released from lymphocytes, and later from other cells, began to be discovered through the demonstration of bioactivities. These were first called "lymphocyte mediators," then "lymphokines," and more generally "cytokines." At first, it was assumed that each such bioactivity might correspond to a distinct molecule. Today, there is probably no purified cytokine that has not been shown to have more than one bioactivity. Obviously, the historical order in which the bioactivities of a cytokine are discovered need not reflect their relative physiologic importance. Nonetheless, many workers assume that a cytokine's name connotes its chief function. This assumption is now being challenged for several cytokines, including interferon-γ.

Virus-induced proteins, released from host cells, that induce an antiviral state in other host cells are serologically diverse. Initially, two antigenic types were discerned, interferon-α and -β (occasionally still collectively called type I). We will follow the convention of referring to each of these interferons in the singular, although there are multiple members of each type. There is a correlation between the antigenic type of interferon and the cell of origin, which is sometimes still reflected in the nomenclature (interferon-α used to be called "leukocyte interferon," and interferon-β, "fibroblast interferon"). However, this is misleading. For example, leukocytes as a group produce both interferon-α and -β, as well as an interferon of the third antigenic type to be discovered, interferon-γ. Still other interferons continue to be discovered, such as tumor necrosis factors (130,244), as will be discussed below.

The idea that there was a type of interferon distinct from interferon-α and -β stemmed from three interrelated discoveries. First was the appreciation of a special cell source (T lymphocytes) and set of eliciting stimuli (T-cell mitogens and any structure recognized by T cells as a specific antigen, including foreign cells). Thus, Wheelock's (239) discovery of antiviral activity from mitogen-stimulated lymphocytes was followed by evidence that lymphocytes from immune donors responded to a specific antigen by releasing an activity similar to that produced in response to mitogens (59,64). Second, an important new bioactivity was recognized that appeared to be associated with interferon arising from mitogen- or antigen-

stimulated T cells: enhancement of host cell resistance to *nonviral* pathogens (reviewed in 154). Antimicrobial effects associated with the presence of the new interferon were demonstrated on protozoa such as toxoplasma and malaria, and on bacteria such as rickettsia, shigella, salmonella, staphylococci, and mycobacteria. For years, this novel bioactivity could not be attributed definitively to the new interferon, because the latter proved extremely difficult to purify to homogeneity. Third, the appearance of this novel interferon in the circulation, or in the medium of lymphocytes incubated with microbial products, was correlated with the development of delayed-type hypersensitivity and cell-mediated immunity to the same obligate or facultative intracellular microbial pathogens (59,64,76,189). For all three reasons, the new cytokine was named "immune interferon" (189). Later, the term "type II interferon" was introduced. Currently, the standard designation is "interferon-γ."

Characterization of the Molecule

Interferon-γ was quickly recognized to have physicochemical properties fundamentally different from those of interferon-α and -β (168). Interferon-γ is inactivated on exposure to pH 2 or sodium dodecyl sulfate (SDS), unlike interferon-β and most interferon-α. Interferon-γ and -β are glycosylated, while interferon-α is not. Estimates of the molecular weight of interferon-γ by gel filtration ranged from 40,000 to 70,000 (41,107), although on reducing SDS polyacrylamide gel electrophoresis (SDS-PAGE) two forms were observed at 20 and 25 kilodaltons (kD) (249). The values from gel filtration were at least twice as high as the values obtained under similar conditions with interferon-α.

Recently, there has been great progress in the definitive characterization of interferon-γ. Results of cDNA cloning for interferon-γ were first reported in 1982 (62,63). The relative molecular mass of the mature protein was predicted to be 17,347 daltons. The difference from SDS-PAGE results with natural interferon-γ could be accounted for by the presence of carbohydrate. It was only after interferon-γ cDNA had been cloned and the recombinant molecule expressed in *Escherichia coli* that complete purification of natural human interferon-γ from peripheral blood lymphocytes was finally achieved (180). Two forms were isolated, with apparent molecular masses of 25 and 20 kD on reducing SDS-PAGE. The 25-kD interferon-γ is glycosylated on both possible N-linked sites (Asn-28 and -100), whereas the 20-kD interferon-γ is glycosylated only on Asn-28. Each of these peptides elutes in more than a single peak, suggesting that they are heterogeneous in their carbohydrate content. In the absence of detergent, natural interferon-γ elutes from sizing columns largely as a mixture of dimers (20 kD + 20 kD, 20 kD + 25 kD, and 25 kD + 25 kD). A further source of heterogeneity is the presence of six alternate COOH-termini on both the 20- and 25-kD glycoproteins, resulting from variable proteolytic processing. Finally, analysis of purified natural interferon-γ revealed a discrepancy from the NH$_2$-terminal sequence predicted from the cDNA. The natural molecule has an NH$_2$-terminal pyroglutamate corresponding to the fourth residue predicted from the cDNA. The first three predicted residues (Cys-Tyr-Cys) are absent. In fact, natural interferon-γ lacks Cys altogether. By this time, clinical trials were getting underway using recombinant interferon-γ with the nonnatural sequence. This historic episode illustrates the principle that definition of the primary sequence of a protein requires purification of the natural protein; it can be complemented by, but not supplanted by, deduction from the genetic sequence.

At present, recombinant interferon-γs of both NH$_2$-terminal structures are in clinical use. The possibility of effects due to disulfide bonding with Cys must be kept in mind. Moreover, the differences between *E. coli*-derived recombinant interferon-γ and the natural molecules (lack of glycosylation, preponderance of given COOH-termini) are potentially important. As yet, however, there has been no firm evidence linking any differential biological effect to one or another of these isoforms of interferon-γ.

In the case of human interferon-α, a multigene family has been detected, and the structures of at least a dozen genes and cDNAs have been elucidated. These genes and cDNAs are closely related structurally, and their deduced amino acid sequences are about 85% homologous (7). Double-stranded RNA, or poly I:poly C, induces only interferon-β in human fibroblasts, and 90% of this activity can be isolated as one protein, interferon-β_1. About 10% seems to represent other forms of interferon-β, including interferon-β_2. It is of interest that the various interferon-α genes and the interferon-β_1 gene on chromosome 9 have no introns. In contrast, there are three introns in the single interferon-γ gene (63), which is located on chromosome 12 (219). There are also introns in the interferon-β_2 gene, which is located on chromosome 6 (83).

Cellular Sources

Initially, interferon-γ was considered a product exclusively of T lymphocytes, especially of helper T cells. Both interpretations are now known to be too restrictive. Interferon-γ is one of the commonest products of T-cell clones, of both helper and suppressor or cytotoxic phenotypes. For example, a survey of 64 alloreactive T-cell clones, of which about half were helper and about half cytotoxic, revealed that 90% produced detectable inter-

feron-γ (96). Of the lymphokines tested, interferon-γ was the one most frequently secreted, by far exceeding interleukin-2. It is noteworthy that many cytolytic T cells release interferon-γ on contact with specific targets, such as virally infected syngeneic cells (99,135). Another important observation emerging from clonal surveys is that most T cells produce more than one lymphokine simultaneously (96,174). Thus, during a physiologic (polyclonal) immune response involving T cells, it can be anticipated that interferon-γ will almost always be released and will not be released alone. These circumstances have greatly complicated the identification of non-interferon-γ factors that may share some of interferon-γs actions (e.g., macrophage activation) and the recognition of actions of interferon-γ that are quantitatively or qualitatively affected by interactions with other lymphokines (e.g., myelosuppression).

More recently, natural killer (NK) cells have been recognized as a source of interferon-γ. So far, only two stimuli have been identified that lead to secretion of interferon-γ by NK cells: interleukin-2 (220) and hydrogen peroxide (136). The latter is of interest because it suggests a means by which an early response of macrophages to microbes (phagocytosis and production of reactive oxygen intermediates) might trigger the release of a factor from neighboring cells, which in turn is known to enhance the capacity of macrophages to undergo the respiratory burst (154). In theory, this positive feedback system might come into play before T cells reactive with an invading microorganism have had time to undergo clonal expansion.

More controversial is whether macrophages themselves can release interferon-γ. Reports of interferon-γ production by pulmonary alveolar macrophages from patients with sarcoidosis (e.g., 181) require confirmation at the single-cell level, simultaneously using probes for interferon-γ mRNA and for macrophage markers. It must be further established whether the production of interferon-γ by macrophages is limited to human pulmonary alveolar cells, and what stimuli elicit and suppress its release. If interferon-γ is indeed a macrophage product, it could drive an autocrine pathway for macrophage activation.

Cellular Receptors

Direct interaction of interferon with a receptor was first suggested by Friedman's observation (57) that trypsin treatment of cells previously exposed to interferon-α or -β at 4°C abolished the induction of an antiviral state on further incubation at 37°C. Direct binding studies rely on the availability of highly purified ligand labeled without loss of biologic activity. Accordingly, specific binding of interferon to cellular binding sites was demonstrated for the first time when highly purified mouse or human interferon-α, -β, and -γ preparations became available: about 1981 for interferon-α and -β and about 1982 for interferon-γ.

It has been repeatedly demonstrated that interferon-γ binds to a receptor different from that for interferon-α and -β (4,22,119,177,191), although several groups reported that there was some cross-reactivity with interferon-β for the binding site for interferon-γ (8,23,75,215). Interferon-γ may share more homology with interferon-β_1 than with interferon-α (38). Human interferon-α/β and human interferon-γ receptors have been tentatively identified by chemical cross-linking of ^{125}I-labeled interferon-α-A and -γ bound to human cells, yielding complexes of 140 to 150 kD (53,93) and 100 to 110 kD (191), respectively. Attempts to isolate the interferon-γ receptor, reconstitute receptor activity with the isolated material, and clone its DNA, are underway in several laboratories.

The presence of two kinds of receptors for human interferon-α (75) or -β (8) has been suggested. Recently, it has been clearly established that primary human macrophages display two distinct classes of receptors for interferon-γ (255). This was not apparent in earlier studies on mononuclear phagocytes employing monocytes or transformed macrophage-like cell lines (e.g., 32). H_2O_2-releasing capacity and antitoxoplasma activity could be induced in human macrophages derived by culture of blood monocytes for ≥ 5 days when pure natural or recombinant interferon-α or -β was added for a further 3-day period. No such response was detectable using monocytes. In contrast to the activating effects of high concentrations of interferon-α or -β, low concentrations of the same cytokines (50% inhibitory concentration of approximately 80 fM) blocked induction of the H_2O_2-releasing capacity by low concentrations (approximately 10 pM) of recombinant interferon-γ. Binding experiments were carried out to investigate the mechanism of this unexpected inhibitory effect. In contrast to the results obtained with monocytes or young macrophages, Scatchard plots of the binding of human ^{125}I-labeled recombinant interferon-γ to mature human macrophages indicated the presence of two classes of interferon-γ receptors [K_{d1} = $(4.3 \pm 0.3) \times 10^{-10}$ M and $K_{d2} = (6.4 \pm 1.1) \times 10^{-9}$ M]. The binding of approximately 0.5 nM ^{125}I-labeled recombinant interferon-γ to the high-affinity but not the low-affinity sites was blocked by simultaneously added interferon-α or -β, or reversed by subsequently added interferon-α or -β, with a 50% inhibitory concentration of approximately 2 pM. On the other hand, there appears to be a single class of interferon-γ receptors at the monocyte stage in the cell's maturation, with a K_d of approximately 1×10^{-9} M and approximately 1,600 sites per cell (reviewed in 255).

These observations suggest the developmentally regulated emergence on macrophages of an unusual type of receptor, namely, one with high affinity for an agonist (interferon-γ) but with even higher affinity for antagonists of interferon-γ action (interferon-α and -β) active at ultralow concentrations. Simultaneously, the maturing macrophage retains a receptor for interferon-γ with intermediate affinity, whose engagement by moderate to high concentrations of interferon-γ can override the antagonist effect of low-dose interferon-α and -β. Finally, as the macrophage matures, there emerges a low-affinity receptor for interferon-α and -β, which mediates an agonist response to high concentrations of the latter agents.

We speculate that this complex pattern may play an important regulatory role, namely, the ability to dampen systemic macrophage activation in response to low concentrations of interferon-γ circulating or diffusing from an inflammatory focus, while preserving the ability to activate macrophages vigorously at the site of inflammation itself. According to this view, traces of interferon-α or -β derived from stromal or parenchymal cells may tonically prevent activation of mature tissue macrophages by small amounts of interferon-γ. On the other hand, monocytes and early macrophages, the cells recruited to inflammatory sites, are resistant to the interferon-γ antagonizing action of low-dose interferon-α or -β, and can respond vigorously to interferon-γ even in low doses. At sites of interferon-γ production, where concentrations of 30 to 300 pM (100–1,000 U/ml) may well be attained, even mature resident tissue macrophages would be resistant to this antagonism. Moreover, high concentrations of interferon-α or -β could be produced at the same site and at these levels would act as agonists.

At this time, almost nothing is known about the signal transduction mechanisms that intervene between binding of interferon-γ to its receptor and induction of its biologic effects.

Mechanisms of Inhibition of Viral and Host Cell Proliferation by Interferons

Despite intensive study, it is not clear how interferons exert their two best known effects—the one for which they are named (antiviral activity) and the one for which they have been cloned and rushed into clinical trials (antiproliferative activity). Current understanding will be surveyed first for interferon-α and -β, and then for interferon-γ.

Treatment of cells with interferons does not affect the early steps of virus replication: adsorption to cells, penetration into cells, and partial uncoating of the virions. However, it does impair the accumulation of virus-specific messenger RNAs (mRNAs), double-stranded RNAs, and proteins. The development of this resistance can be prevented by the treatment of cells with inhibitors of transcription (e.g., actinomycin D) or translation (e.g., cycloheximide) when they are added simultaneously with interferon (120,214).

Although the predominant effect of interferons on host cell protein metabolism is suppression, many individual proteins are induced. Because of the evidence noted above that inhibitors of transcription and translation block interferon's ability to induce an antiviral state, investigation of the mechanism of interferon actions has focused on induced cellular proteins rather than on those whose production is suppressed. From neuroblastoma cells, for example, 18 cDNAs have been cloned corresponding to mRNAs whose levels were increased up to 40-fold by interferon-α, including metallothionein II and class I HLA (58). However, of the many interferon-induced proteins, only a handful have been analyzed to the point where an argument can be made for their contribution to the molecular mechanisms of interferon's antiviral and antiproliferative activities (112).

. Thus, type I interferons induce protein kinase(s) which, in the presence of adenosine 5'-triphosphate (ATP) and double-stranded RNA, phosphorylates two proteins of 67 and 35 kD (68,108). The latter appears to be the small subunit of the elongation initiation factor, eIF-2. The 67-kD moiety, also called P_1, is a ribosome-associated protein with guanylate binding activity in L_{929} cells. Another induced enzyme is 2'-5'-oligoadenylate synthetase. This catalyzes the synthesis of 2'-5'-linked oligoadenylates with the structure $ppp(A2'p5')_nA$ from ATP in the presence of double-stranded RNA (97). The oligoadenylates enhance mRNA degradation by activating a specific endoribonuclease already present in untreated cells. Third, a 2'-PD$_i$ phosphodiesterase is induced, which degrades 2'-5'-oligoadenylates into ATP and adenosine 5'-monophosphate (5'-AMP) (193). Fourth, indoleamine 2,3-dioxygenase is induced (251,252,254). This enzyme degrades the essential amino acid tryptophan to yield N-formylkynurenine, kynurenine, and further breakdown products. In tissue culture or in confined environments in vivo, tryptophan depletion can ensue and may contribute to the inhibition of protein synthesis (248).

However, there are situations which demonstrate that the interferon-induced antiviral state can exist in the absence of the specific enzymes listed above (such as 2'-5'-oligoadenylate synthetase and protein kinase) (131), that the enzyme levels do not always correlate with the degree of antiviral protection (84,245), and that certain cells with constitutively high enzyme levels do not exhibit the antiviral effects of interferons (227). Therefore, it now seems likely that there is no universal mechanism responsible for the antiviral action of type I interferons against all classes of animal viruses, nor for their antiproliferative effects. Alternatively, if there is such a mechanism, it has yet to be discovered.

Even less is known about the molecular basis of the antiviral and antiproliferative effects of interferon-γ. As a generalization, the antiviral activity of interferon-γ is considerably weaker than that of interferon-α or -β_1; it has been demonstrated in vivo for very few viruses (196). As with interferon-α, interferon-γ induces an antiviral state in human amniotic U cells without affecting the amount of vesicular stomatitis virus (VSV) bound to or internalized by the cells (225). The observation (225) that, at saturating interferon concentrations, molecularly cloned interferon-γ induced an antiviral state more slowly than did molecularly cloned interferon-α against VSV in human U cells confirms the original observations reported for the antiviral action of natural interferon preparations in diploid human fibroblast cells measured against Sindbis virus (43). Moreover, there was no significant alteration in the specific infectivity or the polypeptide composition of progeny virions produced by interferon-γ treated U cells as compared to untreated cells (225). Interferon-γ is much less effective than interferon-α or -β in inducing oligoadenylate synthetase in SV80 cells, WISH cells, or the lymphoblastoid line Ramos; even at 200 U/ml, the induction rate was only 1.3-fold over that of the medium control (235). In addition, interferon-γ does not induce the P_1/eIF-2 protein kinase in U cells in a manner that correlates with antiviral activity against VSV (190).

Comparison of two-dimensional gel electrophoregrams after treatment of the same cell types with interferon-γ, -α, or -β reveals partially overlapping sets of newly induced polypeptides (237). Similarly, Sedmak et al. (194) and Mackay and Russell (124) detected a set of polypeptides whose synthesis was uniquely induced by interferon-γ. In most instances, it is unknown whether there is a relationship between induction of particular polypeptides demonstrable by such techniques and the individual phenotypic changes induced by interferons. Certain interferon actions are likely to depend on the induction of polypeptides not sufficiently abundant to be conspicuous on such gels, not resolved from irrelevant polypeptides, or induced with kinetics not favoring their detection at the time when the majority of newly induced proteins are best demonstrated.

Mechanisms of Interferon Action: A Rethinking

Recently, three new ideas have been proposed to help explain the antiproliferative actions of interferon-γ, which are generally considered to exceed those of other interferons (187). First, interferon-γ induces differentiation in some cell types. Perhaps the best example is the human myelocyte, which is driven toward the monocytic lineage (167). The inhibition of replication of certain myelogenous leukemia cells can probably be understood as a counterpart to the induction of their differentiation (167). However, the mechanism of induction of differentiation by interferon-γ remains unexplained, nor is it understood precisely how differentiation leads to suppression of replication.

Second, indoleamine 2,3-dioxygenase was induced approximately 100-fold after interferon-γ treatment in human lung slices. Interferon-γ was much more potent than interferon-α or -β for induction of this enzyme (248). If depletion of tryptophan in response to interferon-γ occurs *in vivo,* as well as *in vitro,* it may represent an important element in the antiproliferative state.

Third, in some cell types, there is a correlation between the antiproliferative action of interferon-γ and its ability to reduce the number and affinity of receptors for other growth factors, such as epidermal growth factor (EGF) (256). Interferon-α had no such effect. Since EGF shares the same receptor with transforming growth factor-α (TGF-α), interferon-γ would be expected to interfere with the actions of TGF-α as well, although this has not yet been studied. Interferon-γ did not bind to the EGF receptor. The mechanism by which interferon-γ affects the expression of the EGF receptor remains to be explored.

Another unresolved issue involving the mechanism of antiviral and antiproliferative actions of interferons is the reported observation that such effects can be transferred from interferon-treated cells to other cells in the absence of exogenous or endogenous interferon (18). This has been most readily demonstrated using cells of a species responsive to a given exogenous interferon and transferring their conditioned medium to cells of a species not responsive to either the original interferon or to any interferon that the first set of cells may have made. The recent demonstration that interferon-γ can augment the secretion of tumor necrosis factor-α and -β (TNF-α and -β) (lymphotoxin) from some cells (160) may represent a partial explanation. TNF-α (130,244) and TNF-β (244) have antiviral as well as antiproliferative activities (211) but lack the species specificity exhibited by interferon-γ.

The foregoing discussion introduces a rapidly growing set of unexpected findings that collectively appear to call into question some of the current understanding of the antiviral and antiproliferative actions of interferons, and even the criteria for designating a cytokine as interferon. These observations include (a) the ability of interferon-γ to promote, rather than inhibit, the growth of some cell types, notably certain fibroblasts (25), an action shared by TNFs (211,229), and the remarkable potency of interferon-β_2 as a plasmacytoma growth factor (226); (b) the ability of interferon-γ to augment release of TNFs, noted above; (c) the ability of TNF-α to induce the release of at least one type of interferon, interferon-β_2 (102); (d) the antiviral actions of TNFs, also noted above; (e) the ability of interferon-γ to inhibit the synthesis of lipoprotein lipase in a mouse preadipocyte cell line (165), a bioactivity previously regarded as the cardinal characteristic of cachectin (TNF-α) (218), as well as the ability of interferon-γ to cause type IV hyperlipidemia in humans, suggesting that it may inhibit synthesis of lipoprotein lipase by nontransformed human adipocytes (105); (f) the contamination of even highly purified natural interferon-γ by TNF-β (206); and (g) the remarkably powerful synergy in antiproliferative effects between interferon-γ on the one hand and TNF-α or -β on the other hand (110).

Thus, among these cytokines, there may be (a) overlap in the spectrum of actions, (b) cross-contamination of the natural products with each other, (c) cross-induction of the cytokines from cell types contaminating the indicator cells on which bioactivity is measured, (d) cross-induction from the indicator cells themselves, and (e) synergistic interactions. It becomes extremely complex to sort out how much of the actions ascribed to interferons are due solely to interferons.

These considerations are among those contributing to an emerging view of interferons as members of a larger family of factors that promote cell differentiation. In varying degrees, these cytokines may share antiviral, other antimicrobial, growth inhibiting, and growth promoting activities, depending on the type of cell, its stage of differentiation at the time of assay, and other circumstances. The larger family may include interleukins-1, -2, -3, -4, and -5 (these include T-cell, B-cell, mast cell, and eosinophil growth factors); other myeloid colony stimulating factors (CSFs), such as CSF-1, CSF-G, and CSF-G/M; and other growth factors commonly regarded as directed chiefly toward cells of nonlymphohematopoietic origin, such as platelet-derived growth factor, epidermal growth factor, fibroblast or endothelial growth factors, and TGF-α and -β. Within this larger family, interferon-γ may be a closer functional relative of TNF-α, TNF-β, and interferon-β_2 than of interferon-α and -β. The specialized function of interferon-γ may be the induction and coordination of host cell resistance to protozoal and bacterial pathogens (see following). According to this view, the emphasis on antiviral activity implicit in the name "interferon-γ" may be more historic than heuristic.

EFFECTS ON INDIVIDUAL CELL TYPES

Macrophages

The effects of interferon-γ on macrophages seem to be more numerous, more marked, and more central to the chief physiologic functions of these cells than for almost any other cell type.

Macrophage Activation and Other Complex Functional Effects

Macrophage activation is one of the cardinal manifestations of cell-mediated immunity. Hosts unable to activate their macrophages often die of infection with obligate or facultative intracellular microbial pathogens (139). Although "macrophage activation" has many meanings for immunologists, the definition arising from the work of Metchnikoff, Lurie, Middlebrook, and Mackaness (reviewed in 148,149,153) can claim not only historic but also functional precedence because it focuses on the only feature of macrophage activation understood to be essential to host survival: the induction of enhanced antimicrobial activity.

We now recognize two distinct mechanisms of activation, paracrine and autocrine. In the paracrine pathway, immune lymphocytes, encountering specific antigen, release soluble glycoproteins that activate macrophages. This is in accord with the classic formulation by Mackaness (123) that induction of macrophage activation, like induction of cell-mediated immunity to intracellular bacterial pathogens, is adoptively transferrable by lymphocytes, whereas its expression is an attribute of macrophages; and that macrophage activation is immunologically specific in its induction but immunologically nonspecific in its expression. Defects in this paracrine pathway are associated with some of the most prevalent of the serious, chronic infectious diseases, such as acquired immune deficiency syndrome (139), lepromatous leprosy (158), visceral leishmaniasis (30), and possibly tuberculosis (228). There is a related defect in A/J strain mice, which display increased susceptibility to infection by rickettsia and schistosomes (73).

It is also possible for microbial products to activate macrophages in the absence of T lymphocytes. This may come about through the recently described autocrine pathway (42,197) in which microbial products induce the production by macrophages of the monokine TNF-α and the latter induces activation. A defect in this pathway has not yet been associated with disease.

Another attribute of the activated macrophage that has aroused intense interest is its relative (but not absolute) ability to discriminate neoplastic from nonneoplastic cells *in vitro* and to kill the former more readily than the latter (6,78,95). Antitumor activity is frequently but not always associated with enhanced antimicrobial activity. However, the literature contains many exaggerations regarding the putative inability of macrophages to destroy nonneoplastic cells. On the contrary, the foremost function of the macrophage in physiology and pathology is probably the scavenging or destruction of senescent, damaged, or bystander host cells, such as erythrocytes, neutrophils, fibroblasts,

and parenchymal elements in tissues that are remodeling, wounded, or inflamed. The ability of macrophages to damage normal host cells is enhanced during immunologic activation.

Finally, there are dozens of functional, phenotypic, and biochemical properties of macrophages that change during activation and serve as correlates with greater or lesser fidelity (1). Perhaps the closest correlate has been the ability of macrophages to secrete reactive oxygen intermediates such as hydrogen peroxide (159).

Thus, since the first discovery of lymphokines (19,36,239), one of the chief challenges in cellular immunology has been to identify the factors from lymphocytes that activate macrophages. In 1983–1984, the predominant macrophage activating factor from normal lymphocytes stimulated with antigens or mitogens was identified as interferon-γ (138,154,185,203,212). With reference to enhanced antimicrobial activity and production of reactive oxygen intermediates, the evidence for this factor *in vitro* has been of three types (reviewed in 150; the *in vivo* evidence will be discussed below).

First, neutralizing monoclonal anti-interferon-γ antibodies removed all detectable macrophage activating factor from media conditioned by polyclonally or oligoclonally activated, unselected populations of normal lymphocytes from blood or spleen. This has been demonstrated with both mouse and human cells, using at least six monoclonal antibodies derived in different laboratories and monitoring activation by the ability of macrophages to inhibit at least two protozoal and two bacterial pathogens. Second, macrophage activating factor copurified from such media with the antiviral activity of interferon-γ. Third, pure recombinant interferon-γ by itself was a potent macrophage activating factor by the same criteria, often acting in the picomolar range. Indeed, the ability of macrophages to kill at least 16 different pathogens has been shown to be enhanced by recombinant interferon-γ (Table 1).

Thus, interferon-γ fulfills the criteria for a macrophage activation factor working in the paracrine mode; i.e., its release is an immunologically specific function of lymphocytes, and it endows macrophages with enhanced antimicrobial activity in an immunologically nonspecific manner.

Evidence of the same three types has been obtained for interferon-γ as the predominant factor from polyclonally activated, unselected lymphocytes that enhances macrophage antitumor activity (203,212). In addition, among products of T-cell clones, a nearly perfect correlation has been noted between the secreted amount of interferon-γ and the secreted amount of macrophage activating factor for tumor cytotoxicity (96).

Other complex functions of macrophages induced with

TABLE 1. *Enhancement by interferon-γ of host cell resistance to nonviral pathogens*[a]

Cell	Pathogens
Endothelial cells	Rickettsia (91,243), chlamydia (186)
Fibroblasts	Toxoplasma (170)
Epithelial cells	Rickettsia (222,243), coxiella, chlamydia (186)
Hepatocytes	Plasmodia (55)
Macrophages	Toxoplasma (154,240), leishmania (81,138,144), plasmodia (163),[b] trypanosoma (171,242), rickettsia (243), chlamydia (185), listeria (166), mycobacteria (atypicals) (49), salmonella (192),[c] legionella (17), histoplasma (247), candida (27), blastomyces (27), schistosoma (90)

[a] This is not an exhaustive list. The references include original and confirmatory reports.

[b] Plasmodia killed within infected erythrocytes after contact of the latter with macrophages.

[c] Reversal of corticosteroid-induced suppression.

interferon-γ include inhibition of migration (216) and the formation of giant cells (238). Thus, interferon-γ released by T cells or natural killer (NK) cells might retain macrophages at the site of an immune response and drive their differentiation into the polykaryons that are a hallmark of granulomas in a wide variety of pathologic states.

Various features of macrophage activation can be induced by proteins not neutralized or immunoprecipitated by antibodies to interferon-γ. In no case is it yet known whether such a non-interferon-γ macrophage activating factor induces the full range of phenotypic changes ascribed to interferon-γ. Some of these factors are physicochemically defined (e.g., TNF-α, TNF-β). The effects of some others (e.g., CSF-1) are not consistently observed, for reasons that are not clear (155,241). Most are not yet characterized in detail either functionally or physicochemically; they arise from transformed lymphocyte cell lines or T-cell clones (e.g., 81,100,103,109). In these situations, it is not yet known whether or to what extent the factors are produced by nontransformed lymphocytes during polyclonal responses to physiologic antigens.

Secretion of Mediators of Inflammation

We do not understand how interferon-γ induces complex functional changes in macrophages. However, part of the explanation for enhanced antimicrobial and cytotoxic activities lies in the induction of an increased capacity to secrete cytotoxic molecules.

Macrophages are known to secrete almost 100 different molecular products (152). Many of these can profoundly affect the inflammatory response. Table 2 lists the products whose secretion is known to be affected by interferon-γ (a larger number are known to be affected by macrophage activation, but the changes have not yet been ascribed specifically to interferon-γ).

To consider the potential impact of altered secretion of these products, one must appreciate the enormous spectrum of actions attributed to some of them, especially interleukin-1 and TNF-α (152; and see Chapter 12). For example, TNF-α inhibits myeloid cell progenitors and promotes differentiation toward the monocytic lineage, actions it shares with interferon-γ. As already noted, TNF-α can enhance the ability of mature macrophages to secrete reactive oxygen intermediates and to kill at least one pathogen, *Trypanosoma cruzi*. Acting on mature myeloid cells, TNF-α promotes degranulation, triggers the release of reactive oxygen intermediates, and enhances phagocytosis as well as adherence of the cells to endothelium. Acting on endothelium, it exerts multiple actions that convert the usual antithrombogenic surface to a thrombogenic one, and the usual nonsticky surface to one that binds neutrophils, monocytes, and lymphocytes. TNF-α also promotes secretion by endothelial cells of IL-1 and colony stimulating factors. Acting on fibroblasts and synoviocytes, TNF-α promotes proliferation as well as the release of collagenase and prostaglandin E$_2$ (PGE$_2$). Similarly, TNF-α-treated chondrocytes release increased amounts of collagenase, PGE$_2$, and proteoglycanase, while synthesizing less proteoglycans. Osteoclasts and osteoblasts proliferate in response to TNF-α, synthesize less bone, and resorb bone faster. Skeletal muscle cells show membrane depolarization, sodium and water uptake, potassium release, protein breakdown, and PGE$_2$ secretion. Hepatocytes synthesize a variety of acute phase reactants in response to TNF-α. Renal mesangial cells proliferate

TABLE 2. *Macrophage products whose secretion is affected by interferon-γ*[a]

Product	Change
Interleukin-1	Increase (10), decrease (24)
Tumor necrosis factor-alpha	Increase (34,160)
C2 and factor B	Increase (208)
Plasminogen activator	Increase (34)
Prostanoids	Increase/decrease (21), increase (72)
1-α,25-Dihydroxyvitamin D3	Increase (2)
Neopterin	Increase (85,151)
Reactive oxygen intermediates	Increase (31,138,141,154)
Reactive nitrogen intermediates	Increase (210)
γ-Induced protein-10	Increase (122)

[a] The secretion of additional products is affected by macrophage activation, in many cases via lymphokines, but interferon-γ has not yet been directly implicated.

and secrete neutral proteases, and astroglia proliferate in response to TNF-α. On the other hand, pancreatic islet cells and many tumor cells respond to TNF-α with diminished cell growth or even cytolysis. *In vivo,* injection of TNF-α induces fever and the accumulation of neutrophils. At higher doses, neutrophilic infiltration and hemorrhagic necrosis of the lungs and gastrointestinal tract have been observed in rats. Thus, interleukin-1 and TNF-α can act at multiple phases of the inflammatory process: acute (fever, shock, altered hormone levels, coagulopathies, adherence of leukocytes to endothelium), subacute (tumor cell injury, muscle breakdown, augmentation of immune responses), and chronic (wound healing, fibrosis, erosion of cartilage, resorption of bone).

Interferon-γ induces a 1α-sterol hydroxylase in human pulmonary alveolar macrophages (2,101). The enzyme acts on 25-hydroxyvitamin D3 to produce the calcium elevating dihydroxy derivative. In sarcoidosis, the lung contains an abnormally large number of T cells secreting lymphokines, including interferon-γ (181). Macrophages from the lungs of some patients with sarcoidosis show elevated 1α-sterol hydroxylase activity, and it is these patients who have hypercalcemia (2).

Enhancement of plasminogen activator release may be a powerful inflammatory action of interferon-γ. Known substrates of plasminogen activator and its product, plasmin, include fibrin, C1, C3, activated Hageman factor (forming subunits that promote kallikrein formation), and fibronectin, whose proteolytic fragments are chemotactic for macrophages and fibroblasts (reviewed in 156).

Among the classes of macrophage products whose secretion is most markedly augmented by prior exposure to interferon-γ are the reactive metabolites arising from the sequential, one-electron reduction of oxygen to water (159), and from the sequential, one-electron oxidation of ammonia to nitrate (209). Both the reactive oxygen intermediates and the reactive nitrogen intermediates can be carcinogenic. The reactive oxygen intermediates also exert potent anti-tumor cell activity (12); this is likely to prove true for the reactive nitrogen intermediates when they are studied further. Of special interest in the present context are the potent pro- and antiinflammatory actions of the reactive oxygen intermediates, actions which have not yet been studied for the nitrogen metabolites.

Thus, we can speculate that a T lymphocyte, responding to an invading organism, releases interferon-γ, which enables macrophages to kill the organism more efficiently and to secrete large amounts of neutral proteases and oxidants. The latter inactivate α_1-antiprotease, while activating chemotactic lipids that attract neutrophils whose oxidants further inactivate antiprotease. Leukocyte-derived proteases and oxidants together appear to account for considerable tissue damage in many inflammatory settings (33).

Intracellular Processes

The above emphasis on secreted macrophage products reflects, in part, the fact that it has been easier to document the impact of macrophage activating factors on secretory responses than on intracellular events. However, the enhancement of macrophage antimicrobial activity by interferon-γ is expressed chiefly within phagosomes and phagolysosomes, where important processes may be affected by macrophage activating factors not mirrored in secretory processes. For example, immunologic activation enhances the ability of macrophages to acidify phagosomes containing ingested toxoplasmas (198). As *Trypanosoma gondii* trophozoites are sensitive to low pH, this may contribute to the toxoplasmacidal activity of interferon-γ-treated macrophages.

Perhaps central to many interferon-γ actions on macrophages is its ability to enhance the activity of protein kinase C. Interferon-γ neither triggers the enzyme nor appears to increase its content within mouse macrophages, but instead augments about fivefold its ability to phosphorylate exogenous substrates, an effect not shared by interferon-α or -β or bacterial lipopolysaccharide (71). In the study cited, this effect peaked at 3 hr and was gone by 12 hr, whereas many of the other effects of interferon-γ on macrophage cytotoxic function, secretory activity, or antigen expression require 24 to 72 hr for full expression.

Exposure of mouse macrophages to interferon-γ leads to an increase in the intracellular content of *S*-adenosylmethionine, which participates in methylation reactions and polyamine synthesis (20). However, the increase is less than twofold and has not yet been directly implicated in any functional effects.

Expression of Plasma Membrane Receptors and Antigens

The structure and function of macrophage plasma membrane glycoproteins change markedly in response to interferon-γ (Table 3). Two effects have received the most emphasis. First is the enhanced binding of opsonized particles via increased numbers of Fc receptors. However, such particles are generally ingested less well by interferon-γ-treated macrophages than by controls (44,52,69,167). One speculation is that interferon-γ converts the macrophage from a primarily phagocytic cell to one more competent to carry out antibody-dependent, cell-mediated cytotoxicity against extracellular targets coated with antibody. However, this seems counterproductive during infection with potentially phagocytizable microorganisms not known to be killed by macrophages extracellularly. In fact, we have no idea of the physiologic significance of

TABLE 3. *Alterations of macrophage surface receptors and antigens by interferon-γ*

Surface component	Response to interferon-γ
Ia antigens	Increased (204)
Fc receptors	Increased (52,69,167)
Lymphocyte function-associated antigen	Increased (129,207,246)
Mannosyl-fucosyl receptor	Decreased (51)
F4/80 (gp 160)	Decreased (51)
Transferrin receptor	Decreased (70)
C3bi receptor	No change in level, but decreased binding; reversed on contact with fibronectin (246)
C3b receptor	Decreased (50,246)
Interleukin-2 receptor	Induced (77)
Lipopolysaccharide binding sites	Increased (5)

the increased expression of Fc receptors by macrophages and their decreased ability to promote ingestion.

Second, exposure to interferon-γ improves the function of macrophages as accessory cells (14,204) for T-cell responses to antigens via increased expression of Ia molecules. In the mouse, it has been questioned whether increased expression of Ia antigens is induced directly by interferon-γ or via as yet unidentified mediators secreted in response to interferon-γ (234). Interferon-α and -β have little effect on murine or human Ia antigen expression under conditions where they modulate other important macrophage functions (e.g., Fc receptor expression) analogously to interferon-γ (231). With mouse macrophages, antagonism of interferon-γ-induced Ia expression by high concentrations of interferon-α or -β has been reported (87,118). The mechanisms underlying these interactions are unknown. Paradoxically, the interferon-γ-treated macrophage also tends to be more immunosuppressive via enhanced secretion of eicosanoids and oxidants, and possibly via enhanced oxidation of soluble immune response suppressor (SIRS) to its active form (236).

Among the other changes listed in Table 3, some are quantitatively quite minor (lymphocyte function-associated antigen, transferrin receptor, C3b receptor) and some have unknown functional consequences (interleukin-2 receptor).

Polymorphonuclear Leukocytes and Erythrocytes

Myelosuppression

In 1983, Broxmeyer and colleagues (26) demonstrated that highly purified natural interferon-γ exerted a potent suppressive activity *in vitro* on human multipotential colony forming cells, as well as on colony forming units (CFU) for granulocytes and macrophages (CFU-GM) and for erythrocytes. The effects appeared to be direct, in that depletion of T cells, B cells, and macrophages from the marrow had no effect. Complete inhibition was observed with as little as 100 antiviral units per culture, within the range of concentrations of interferon-γ observed in serum in various clinical states.

These studies were later confirmed with regard to erythroid suppression, using pure recombinant interferon-γ (125). However, in the latter study, lymphocytes and macrophages in the marrow appeared to mediate some of the suppression. A mechanism for a contributory role of macrophage and lymphocyte products in conjunction with interferon-γ was provided by the elegant experiments of Trinchieri and colleagues (37,137). These workers demonstrated powerful synergistic myelosuppressive effects involving interferon-γ on the one hand, and either TNF-α or -β on the other hand. Low concentrations of both cytokines together were suppressive when either alone had no detectable effect. In mixtures of the two cytokines, antibodies to either abrogated the effect of both.

Zoumbos et al. (257) presented evidence that myelosuppression by interferon-γ may be of clinical importance. They detected interferon-γ at levels above 10 antiviral units/ml in the circulation of 10 of 24 patients with aplastic anemia, compared to none of 34 controls (transfused patients and normal subjects). Bone marrow serum from the aplastic anemia patients showed particularly high levels of interferon (a mixture of interferon-γ and -α), averaging 200 antiviral units/ml, whereas no interferon-γ was detected in bone marrow serum from normal donors. The blood lymphocytes of the aplastic anemia patients not only released more interferon-γ *in vitro* than did controls in response to a mitogen, but released interferon-γ *spontaneously,* which was not observed with lymphocytes from normal donors. When bone marrow from the patients was cultured in the presence of antibody to interferon-γ, the number of CFUs nearly tripled, while normal bone marrow showed no response.

When recombinant interferon-γ is infused into cancer patients, however, the fall in counts of formed elements of the blood is not marked (104). A drop in the number of circulating neutrophils is observed but is so transient that it is not likely to reflect diminished proliferation of early precursors.

Taken together, these results suggest that in clinical states with intensive or extensive T-cell activation (such as chronic infections or autoimmune diseases), anemia and/or leukopenia may be due in part to the concerted actions of interferon-γ and other cytokines such as TNF-α and -β.

Monocytoid Differentiation of Neutrophils

In vitro, interferon-γ induces monocyte-like Fc receptors on mature human neutrophils and influences CFU-GM to differentiate in the direction of monocytes (167). Even the transformed neutrophil precursors in chronic myelogenous leukemia may be susceptible to this form of differentiation, which is accompanied by inhibition of proliferation (167).

Augmentation of the Function of Mature Neutrophils

Enhanced Fc receptor expression on neutrophils in response to interferon-γ is accompanied, as expected, by an increased capacity for antibody-dependent cytotoxicity (167,195). In addition, small increases have been described in the capacity of interferon-γ-treated neutrophils to phagocytize particles not coated with IgG (195) and to display a respiratory burst (16). These changes are similar to, but much less marked than, those that follow exposure to granulocyte-monocyte colony stimulating factor (121; and see Chapter 15).

T Cells

Two clear-cut differentiative effects of interferon-γ on T cells have been described. Since T cells are the primary source of interferon-γ, these can be considered examples of autocrine effects. First, endogenous interferon-γ may be an essential cofactor in the differentiation of precursors into cytolytic T cells (106,200). Thus, monoclonal antibody to interferon-γ blocked the formation of cytolytic cells in cultures of pure mouse Lyt 2⁺ lymph node cells responding to mitogen or alloantigen plus IL-2. In the absence of the antibody, production of interferon-γ could be demonstrated in such cultures. A nonspecific inhibitory effect of the antibody was ruled out by reversing its action with exogenous interferon-γ. The inhibitory effect of the monoclonal antibody was demonstrable even in cultures initially containing a single cell. Thus, one and the same T cell can produce interferon-γ and respond to it, and apparently must do so to acquire cytolytic capacity. Second, the production of TNF-β (lymphotoxin) by human blood T cells in response to IL-2 is enhanced by interferon-γ (160).

There are numerous but contradictory reports of other effects of interferon-γ on T-cell function. The apparent dependence of these effects on seemingly minor variables in the experimental conditions suggests that some of these actions may be indirect, weak, and/or artifactual.

B Cells

Early reports of "immunomodulating" activity stressed the inhibitory action of interferon-γ on antibody formation (202,230). However, these studies used impure materials. Results with recombinant interferon-γ have been quite the opposite, emphasizing the increase in polyclonal (199) or antigen-specific (111) plaque forming cells when mouse spleen B cells were exposed to interferon-γ alone or in addition to other cytokines. In fact, one component of "T-cell replacing factor" in antigen-specific mouse B-cell responses appears to be a material that induces the production of endogenous interferon-γ from the NK cells that contaminate even highly purified preparations of mouse B cells (28). In close analogy to the situation described above for differentiation of cytolytic T cells, the differentiation of antibody forming B cells is ablated by monoclonal antibody to interferon-γ. However, there continue to be seemingly contradictory observations, such as that interferon-γ blocks the ability of B cells to respond to B-cell stimulatory factor-1 (BSF-1) (175).

Work with human tonsillar B cells (many of which may be partly activated *in vivo*) has confirmed the role of interferon-γ as a B-cell differentiation factor, indicating a synergistic effect of interferon-γ with IL-2 and/or stimuli such as anti-mu chain for proliferation and immunoglobulin production (114,146,183). Thus, although interferon-γ alone does not suffice for B-cell differentiation, it appears to be an obligatory, late acting factor that synergizes with earlier acting stimuli.

For almost all cell types on which Ia antigens can be induced, interferon-γ functions as a potent inducer. B cells, which express Ia antigens constitutively, may represent something of an exception. BSF-1 increases B-cell Ia antigen expression severalfold, but such an effect has apparently not been reported with interferon-γ (182).

NK Cells

The differentiative effects of interferon-γ noted above for T cells and B cells extend also to NK cells. Again, interferon-γ appears to act as a cofactor, in this case together with interleukin-2 in promoting NK cell cytolytic capacity (220). Interferon-γ alone has small stimulatory effects on NK activity (172).

Endothelial Cells

Interferon-γ is a potent inducer of Ia antigens on human endothelial cells (173). In theory, this might endow endothelium in inflammatory sites with the capacity to present antigen to primed T cells. Interferon-γ-treated endothelium may also participate in the binding of Leu 3⁺ T cells (126).

Other, less well-defined antigens are also induced on endothelium by interferon-γ, including one that leads to complement-dependent cytolysis by an IgM that appears in the serum of patients with Kawasaki syndrome vasculitis (115). Although the role of this autoantibody in the etiology of the vasculitis is unclear, this report establishes a precedent for the reactivity of autoantibodies with antigens induced by interferon-γ.

Of particular interest is an antigen normally present only on the high cuboidal endothelium of postcapillary venules in lymph nodes. This is the barrier normally traversed by lymphocytes crossing from blood to lymph. The same antigen is induced on noncuboidal endothelium from other nonlymphoid sites, such as lung and marrow, by interferon-γ, but not by interferon-β, interleukin-1, or endothelial growth factors (46). Thus, local secretion of interferon-γ may facilitate the emigration of blood-borne lymphocytes to an inflammatory site. This concept leaves unexplained how the first antigen-specific T cells, which presumably supply the interferon-γ, gain access to antigen in extravascular nonlymphoid deposits.

More systematic studies on the effects of interferon-γ on endothelial cell physiology are at an early stage. One such effect is stimulation of the rate at which endothelial cells secrete an organized matrix of glycosaminoglycans (134), which may play a role in wound healing. Also of interest is the induction by interferon-γ of an early-response gene whose predicted protein product has extensive homology with platelet-derived chemotactic factors (122).

Several bacterial pathogens, such as rickettsia and chlamydia, can proliferate in endothelial cells. Treatment of endothelial cells with interferon-γ retards or ablates the proliferation of some of these organisms (186,243). These important observations were among the first to establish definitively that the antiinfective action of interferon-γ against nonviral pathogens is not limited to macrophages. On the contrary, interferon-γ may be able to confer antimicrobial activity on most cell types capable of harboring nonviral pathogens long enough to respond to the cytokine (typically, 1–3 days).

Fibroblasts and Chondrocytes

Except for the induction of a limited set of proteins, interferon-γ is generally considered to suppress overall host cell protein synthesis. However, its actions on human skin fibroblasts are quite different, i.e., selective suppression of collagen synthesis with little or no general suppression of overall protein synthesis (47,92,205). Interferon-α was far less effective. The collagen suppressing effect of interferon-γ was manifest at the level of procollagen mRNA (205). Effects of interferon-γ on collagen synthesis by synovial chondrocytes are similar (60).

Interferon-γ reportedly inhibits (47), stimulates (25), or has no effect (40) on the proliferation of primary human or mouse fibroblasts. The variables responsible for these divergent results are unknown. An "intercellular adhesion molecule" is induced on fibroblasts by interferon-γ (48). It physiologic functions have not yet been characterized.

Several bacterial and protozoal pathogens proliferate in fibroblasts. These include rickettsia, coxiella, chlamydia, and toxoplasma. Treatment of fibroblasts with interferon-γ inhibits the replication of each of these organisms (40,91,170,222,223). The mechanism in the case of *T. gondii* appears to be the induction of indoleamine dioxygenase in the fibroblast, with consequent depletion of tryptophan on which the parasite depends (170). However, tryptophan depletion does not appear to account either for the antibacterial effect of interferon-γ on fibroblasts (40,224) or for the antitoxoplasma effect of interferon-γ on macrophages (E. Pfefferkorn, personal communication). These observations emphasize both the multitude of cells on which interferon-γ exerts nonspecific, nonviral, antimicrobial effects and the fact that these effects are exerted through a variety of mechanisms, most of them unknown.

Osteoblasts and Osteoclasts

The release of calcium from mouse calvaria *in vitro* is stimulated by parathormone, interleukin-1 and factors that trigger arachidonic acid release. The action of each of these stimuli is blocked *in vitro* by interferon-γ, whose action in this regard resembles that of calcitonin (61,169). The mechanism of this effect is unknown. It is unclear whether interferon-γ exerts a similar antiresorptive action on other bones, especially in subarticular zones afflicted by erosive inflammatory or degenerative arthritides. *In vivo*, it is possible that counteractive effects of interferon-γ, such as enhancement of interleukin-1 and TNF-α release from macrophages and inhibition of collagen synthesis by chrondrocytes, might, on balance, promote rather than inhibit bone resorption.

Epithelial Cells

In normal human epidermis, the only Ia-positive cells are a subset of the dendritic Langerhans cells that comprise about 2% of the epidermal population. However, in a variety of pathologic states, almost all Langerhans cells and most keratinocytes express Ia, at least focally. Examples are psoriasis, lichen planus, mycosis fungoides, graft-versus-host disease, iatrogenic delayed-type hypersensitivity reactions, and cell-mediated antimicrobial immune reactions such as tuberculoid leprosy and cutaneous leishmaniasis (94). In all these conditions, T cells infiltrate the underlying dermis. T-cell products have thus been suspected of inducing Ia antigens. Indeed, interferon-γ is a potent inducer of Ia antigens *in vitro* on keratinocytes (13,232), Langerhans cells (15), and melanocytes (82). The elegant study of Houghton et al. (82) emphasizes the specificity of the response in the case of melanocytes. None of 14 other potential inducing agents (including interferon-α or -β) were effective. Of 38 antigenic systems expressed by melanocytes, interferon-γ induced only the major histocompatibility complex antigens HLA-DR, HLA-DC, HLA-A, HLA-B, and HLA-C, and β_2-microglobulin.

Pretreatment of transformed epithelial cell lines with interferon-γ blocks penetration of the cells by shigella or salmonella, by an unknown mechanism (161). It has not yet been studied whether such an effect is also manifested with nontransformed gastrointestinal epithelium, where it might represent a physiologic mechanism of host defense. Interferon-γ treatment of HeLa cells, a transformed cell line of epithelial origin, induces antichlamydia activity (185).

Hepatocytes

The antiinfective, nonviral effects of interferon-γ apply to hepatocytes as well as to macrophages, endothelial cells, and fibroblasts. Thus, replication of the exoerythrocytic stages of *Plasmodium berghei* and *P. vivax,* protozoan agents of malaria, is markedly suppressed in hepatocytes both *in vivo* and *in vitro* by very small amounts of interferon-γ (55). The effect is so marked that trials involving recombinant interferon-γ in patients with malaria are underway.

Reports of the induction of hepatic cytochrome P-450 by interferon-γ have not been confirmed in studies with the recombinant molecule (56).

Marked hepatotoxic effects of interferon-α/β in newborn mice account for the lethality of certain infections (65). In this setting, it appears to be the host response to the virus, rather than cytopathic effects of the virus itself, that is responsible for the lethal pathologic effects. The mechanism of the hepatotoxicity of interferon-α/β is unknown. Analogous studies with interferon-γ in neonates have not yet been reported. In adult humans the administration of high doses of recombinant interferon-γ is sometimes associated with mild, transient abnormalities of liver function (104).

Tumor Cells

After antiviral activity, the next effect of interferon-α/β to be discovered was its antiproliferative action on transformed cells (66). This generated intense interest, which was heightened by reports (e.g., 187) that the antiproliferative action of natural interferon-γ was much more marked than that of interferon-α or -β. Widespread hopes arose that interferons would provide an effective treatment for cancer through their antiproliferative effects.

However, as discussed earlier, mechanisms of the antiproliferative action of interferons remain poorly understood. Gresser and colleagues (personal communication, 1984) found that interferon-α/β inhibited the growth in mice of tumor cells that lacked receptors for interferon-α/β and were insensitive to their actions *in vitro*. Yet, no interferon-α/β-induced host response has yet been identified that seems to account for the inhibition of tumor growth. The relatively greater antiproliferative action of natural interferon-γ may be due in part to its synergistic interaction with TNF-β, which extensively copurifies with it (206). Pure recombinant interferon-γ displays antiproliferative activity in direct clonogenic assays, although only with certain tumors (188). The basis of synergistic cytotoxic effects between interferon-γ on the one hand and TNF-α or -β on the other hand (e.g., 110) is only partly explained by the fact that interferon-γ induces a two- to threefold increase in the expression of TNF receptors on some tumor cells (3,221). In addition, interferon-γ interacts synergistically with interferon-α or -β to inhibit the growth of some tumors (35). The mechanism of this interaction is likewise not understood.

Many types of tumors, like their normal cellular counterparts, express Ia antigens after exposure to interferon-γ. Examples are melanomas, astrocytomas, and carcinomas of the breast, colon, pancreas, bladder, kidney, and ovary (82). Induction of Ia antigens on tumors may favor the evolution and expression of an antitumor immune response on the part of the host. With many human tumors, only HLA-DR is induced. A non-interferon-γ polypeptide of 32 kD is elaborated during mixed leukocyte cultures which induces both HLA-DR and HLA-DQ on a variety of human tumors as well as on nontransformed cell lines and which interacts synergistically with interferon-γ in doing so (67).

In some patients with cancer, interferons have produced marked clinical benefit, but not in as many cases as would be predicted from *in vitro* studies if their primary action were direct and antiproliferative. Promotion of differentiation, augmentation of host immune responses, direct actions in synergy with cytokines supplied by the host, and effects on nonimmune host elements such as tumor vasculature, may all play a role, to different extents, with different tumors in different patients. It is likely that lack of a basic understanding of the mechanisms of interferon action has restricted their potential in the treatment of cancer.

EVIDENCE FOR A PATHOPHYSIOLOGIC ROLE *IN VIVO*

Detection of Interferon-γ and Interferon-γ-Induced Effects

Despite the short half-life of recombinant interferon-γ in humans (104), interferon-γ has been detected at relatively high concentrations in the serum of patients with autoimmune diseases. For example, in the study by Hooks et al. (80), interferon-γ titers equal to or greater than 16 antiviral units/ml were reported in serum from 71% of patients with active systemic lupus erythematosus (SLE) and about half of those with rheumatoid arthritis or scleroderma, compared to 1 of 34 controls. In the SLE patients, elevations in the titers of interferon-γ appeared to correlate with exacerbations of glomerulonephritis, arthritis, or hemolytic anemia. By present criteria, evidence that the antiviral activity detected in this early study was interferon-γ in all patients cannot be considered adequate. Several recent studies have not confirmed these findings, at least in rheumatoid arthritis (e.g., 39). On the other hand, interferon-γ has been detected in a substantial proportion of synovial fluids from such patients (39,86). Another possibly autoimmune disease in which interferon-γ has been detected in body fluids is multiple sclerosis, where cerebrospinal fluid was positive in each of 30 subjects (79).

During attacks of malaria in humans, interferon-α predominates in the serum during the first 48 hr, to be replaced by substantial levels of interferon-γ at later time points (179). Similar findings have been noted during murine listeriosis (147). This may be a general pattern for a variety of nonviral infectious diseases. Interferon-γ has also been demonstrated in body fluids during viral diseases (217).

An alternative investigative approach has been to remove lymphoid cells from patients with certain diseases and study their release of interferon-γ *in vitro*. Thus, pulmonary cells lavaged from patients with sarcoidosis secrete interferon-γ spontaneously *in vitro* (181), and blood lymphocytes of multiple sclerosis patients release much more interferon-γ than those from normal subjects in response to standard mitogens (79).

The above studies have relied on bioactivity or immunoassay for the detection of interferon-γ in fluids. More recently, investigators have employed monoclonal anti-interferon-γ antibodies to demonstrate interferon-γ

in pathologic specimens by immunocytology. For example, interferon-γ has been demonstrated in this way in association with epithelioid cells and multinucleated giant cells in sarcoid and tuberculous granulomata (74), and in the lesions of polymyositis (89).

Yet another approach to the detection of interferon-γ *in vivo* has been to infer its presence from observing some of its effects. Thus, many investigators have considered Ia expression by cells which are normally Ia-negative to reflect the action of endogenous interferon-γ, although, as noted above, other cytokines can also induce Ia antigen expression. Situations in which massive induction of Ia antigens is observed include transplant rejection (132), graft-versus-host disease, delayed-type hypersensitivity responses, and cell-mediated immune reactions.

Another marker presumed to indicate the action of endogenous interferon-γ is elevated urinary excretion of neopterin. The only known cellular source of this pteridine is the macrophage; its only known inducing agents are interferon-γ and, in one study, also interferon-α (85,151). Neopterin secretion is markedly elevated in patients with transplant rejection, tuberculosis, toxoplasmosis, malaria, leprosy, cytomegalovirus infection, various cancers, and acquired immune deficiency syndrome (233). Since the latter condition is believed to be associated with a marked reduction in the ability of T cells to secrete interferon-γ (140), at least in the late stages of the disease, the specificity of neopterin as a marker for endogenous interferon-γ secretion must be questioned.

Consequences of Endogenous Deficiency

As discussed above with regard to macrophage activation, marked and sustained impairment in the ability of lymphocytes to secrete interferon-γ on encountering most antigens is generally incompatible with life. The host usually succumbs to infection, often with viruses or opportunistic pathogens, which in many cases are held in check in the normal host by activated macrophages. Acquired immune deficiency syndrome dramatically illustrates this point (140).

Moderate temporary impairment in the ability of lymphocytes to secrete interferon-γ may be associated with an increased incidence and severity of infections. For example, T cells of the human neonate display a relative selective defect in their ability to transcribe the interferon-γ gene (116). It is likely that a similar defect appears with advanced malignancy.

Some of the world's most prevalent chronic bacterial infections are associated with selective deficiencies in interferon-γ production—selective in the sense that the deficiency is manifest mostly or only in response to the antigens of the infecting organism. Such deficiencies are characteristic of patients with lepromatous leprosy (162), visceral leishmaniasis (30), and possibly advanced tuberculosis (228). In most of these subjects, there is little or no evidence of host resistance to the pathogen in question, although resistance to other pathogens is usually normal, at least until late in the course of the primary disease.

Consequences of Endogenous Excess

The T cells which infiltrate the alveolar spaces in pulmonary sarcoidosis release interferon-γ spontaneously *in vitro* (181). Of course, release may not truly be spontaneous, but if there is an eliciting antigen, it has not yet been identified. Perhaps as a consequence, the pulmonary alveolar macrophages of sarcoidosis patients release substantially more reactive oxygen intermediates *in vitro* than those from normal subjects (54). Elevated production of interferon-γ by lymphocytes of patients with aplastic anemia has been implicated in myelosuppression, as reviewed above. In the rheumatoid joint, interferon-γ may promote the release of interleukin-1, neutral proteases, and immunoglobulin, while inhibiting the replacement of collagen. If interferon-γ serves a protective function in these settings, it is not apparent.

Effects of Administration

In mice, injection of recombinant interferon-γ results in massive and widespread induction of both class I and class II histocompatibility antigens (133,201). However, there is some selectivity among cell types in a manner for which no underlying principle is yet apparent.

Of great interest is the ability of pure recombinant interferon-γ to protect rodents and/or primates from a wide spectrum of protozoal and bacterial diseases, including toxoplasmosis (128), listeriosis (98), atypical tuberculosis (49), malaria (55), and leishmaniasis (143). Consistent with these observations, injection of mice with recombinant interferon-γ activates their peritoneal macrophages, as judged by the enhanced oxidative metabolism and antiprotozoal activity of explanted cells (141).

On administration to humans, recombinant interferon-γ also enhances the oxidative metabolism (142,157,158) and antiprotozoal activity (142) of explanted monocytes. *In situ*, there is preliminary evidence for human macrophage activation by recombinant interferon-γ, as assessed by an apparent decrease in the number of intracellular mycobacteria in dermal macrophages of patients with lepromatous leprosy (158).

The latter study also provided the first demonstration that interferon-γ induces HLA-DR antigens *in situ* in humans (the cells on which the class II antigens were induced included keratinocytes and fibroblasts) (Fig. 1). Keratin-

ocytes proliferated in the epidermis overlying lepromatous leprosy lesions injected with interferon-γ, Langerhans cells were markedly decreased in number in the epidermis, and helper T cells and monocytes were recruited into the lesions (158). Accompanying these cellular changes was induration of the injection sites. The foregoing constellation of responses to small doses of interferon-γ (1 or 10 μg daily for 3 days) closely mimics findings in typical delayed-type hypersensitivity reactions (such as to tuberculin), as well as in sites of successful cell-mediated immune reactions (94). The doses of recombinant interferon-γ used in the study by Nathan et al. (158) were lower than those used in any previous study in humans and constitute part of the argument that the responses observed may be physiologic.

Effects of Neutralizing Endogenous Interferon-γ *In Vivo*

Complementary to the administration of pure recombinant product has been the administration of monoclonal antibodies to interferon-γ with potent neutralizing activity. Thus, the ability of mice to recover from sublethal listeriosis (29) or rickettsiosis (117) was abolished by anti-interferon-γ antibody, as was their rejection of allogeneic tumors (107). This has been a powerful tool for assessing the physiologic role of endogenous interferon-γ, although its use in subjects with infections or malignancies is limited to experimental animals.

Thus, initial studies with both the administration and neutralization of interferon-γ strongly support the proposition that interferon-γ is a key mediator of delayed-type hypersensitivity and cell-mediated immunity.

Effects of Pharmacologic Inhibitors of Interferon-γ

Certain drugs widely used for immunosuppressive therapy block the release or action of interferon-γ *in vivo*. This has been observed for both cyclosporin (178) and glucocorticoids (113). Specific interferon-γ inhibitors, such as interferon-γ receptor antagonists, have not yet been described.

CONCLUSIONS

The physiologic role of interferon-γ has not yet emerged unmistakably from the plethora of its bioactivities *in vitro* or from the few early studies on its detection, administration, and neutralization *in vivo*. However, the evidence to date makes it reasonable to view interferon-γ as a molecule chiefly serving the interests of the host in defense against infection. The antiinfectious role of interferon-γ is broad—both in the spectrum of pathogens against which

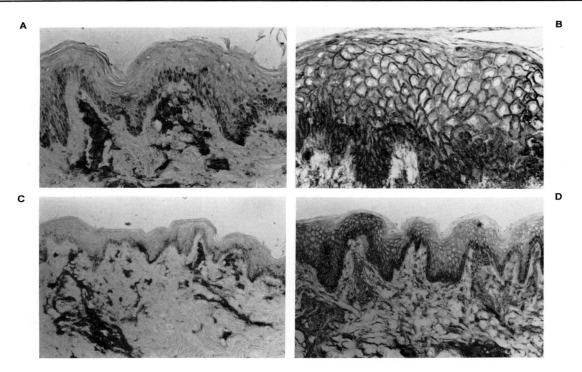

FIG. 1. Immunoperoxidase stain for revealing specific binding of a monoclonal antibody reactive with HLA-DR antigens in the skin of a patient with lepromatous leprosy. **(A,C)** Frozen sections of a biopsy taken 3 days after the last of three daily injections of excipient alone (control biopsy). Some pigmented melanocytes are evident in the lower epidermis (A), as well as some HLA-DR-positive inflammatory cells in the dermis (C). **(B, D)** Biopsy taken 3 days after the last of three daily injections of 10 μg recombinant interferon-γ. Massive induction of HLA-DR is apparent on virtually all cells in the epidermis, which is thickened through proliferation of keratinocytes (B), and in the dermis, which is heavily infiltrated by T cells and mononuclear phagocytes (D). For details, see ref. 158. The photomicrographs were taken by Gilla Kaplan.

resistance is manifest and in the range of host cells whose resistance is enhanced. The microbes include not just viruses, but also pathogens from almost every phylogenetic class. The host cells include not just macrophages, but many of the diverse cell types capable of sustaining prolonged infection, such as endothelial cells, fibroblasts, and hepatocytes.

The biochemical mechanisms of interferon-γ-induced antimicrobial activity are probably correspondingly diverse. They seem to depend on the combination of host cell type and pathogen. The few currently known or suspected biochemical mechanisms of interferon-γ-induced antimicrobial activity (enhanced production of reactive oxygen intermediates, reactive nitrogen intermediates, hydrogen ions, and the tryptophan degrading enzyme indoleamine 2,3-dioxygenase) are probably a fraction of those that will be discovered.

Most of the complex immunomodulatory and inflammatory effects of interferon-γ can be viewed as subserving the antiinfectious role described above. For example, induction of class II and class I antigens of the major his-tocompatibility complex is probably critical in promoting the afferent and efferent limbs, respectively, of the immune response to microbial pathogens including viruses. The same can be said of enhancement of differentiation of T and B cells.

The physiologic role of the antiproliferative action of interferon-γ is less apparent. The antiproliferative action of pure interferon-γ in isolation is not one of its most pronounced biologic effects and may be an incidental by-product of its induction of differentiation of host cells toward an antimicrobial state.

Many and eventually perhaps all the individual bioactivities of interferon-γ have been or will be found to be shared by other cytokines. Yet, no single cytokine to date has been shown to express the full range of actions of interferon-γ relevant to the defense of the host. When recombinant interferon-γ was injected into anergic inflammatory sites in humans, it entrained a complex constellation of responses typical of delayed-type hypersensitivity and cell-mediated immunity (158). The participation of other cytokines seems highly likely.

Nonetheless, it is remarkable that brief exposure to small amounts of a single molecule could orchestrate these reactions.

ACKNOWLEDGMENTS

We gratefully acknowledge the excellent editorial assistance of Christine Sinclair-Prince, and the gift of photomicrographs by Gilla Kaplan. This work was supported in part by grant CA 43610 from the National Institutes of Health.

REFERENCES

1. Adams, D. O., and Hamilton, T. A. (1984): The cell biology of macrophage activation. *Annu. Rev. Immunol.,* 2:283–318.
2. Adams, J. S., and Gacod, M. A. (1985): Characterization of 1-α-hydroxylation of vitamin D3 sterols by cultured alveolar macrophages from patients with sarcoidosis. *J. Exp. Med.,* 161:755–765.
3. Aggarwal, B. B., Eessalu, T. E., and Hass, P. E. (1985): Characterization of receptors for human tumour necrosis factor and their regulation by gamma-interferon. *Nature,* 318:665–667.
4. Aguet, M. (1980): High-affinity binding of ^{125}I-labeled mouse interferon to a specific cell surface receptor. *Nature,* 284:459–461.
5. Akagawa, K. S., and Tokunaga, T. (1985): Lack of binding of bacterial lipopolysaccharide to mouse lung macrophages and restoration of binding by gamma interferon. *J. Exp. Med.,* 162:1444–1459.
6. Alexander, P., and Evans, R. (1971): Endotoxin and double stranded RNA render macrophages cytotoxic. *Nature New Biol.,* 232:76–78.
7. Allen, G., and Fantes, K. H. (1980): A family of structural genes for human lymphoblastoid (leukocyte-type) interferon. *Nature,* 287:408–411.
8. Anderson, P., Yip, Y. K., and Vilček, J. (1982): Specific binding of ^{125}I-human interferon-γ to high affinity receptors on human fibroblasts. *J. Biol. Chem.,* 257:11301–11304.
9. Anderson, P., Yip, Y. K., and Vilček, J. (1983): Human interferon-γ is internalized and degraded by cultured fibroblasts. *J. Biol. Chem.,* 258:6497–6502.
10. Arenzana-Seisdedos, F., Virelizier, J. L., and Fiers, W. (1985): Interferons as macrophage activating factors. III. Preferential effect of interferon-γ on the interleukin 1 secretory potential of fresh or aged human monocytes. *J. Immunol.,* 134:2444–2448.
11. Aune, T. M., and Pierce, C. W. (1982): Activation of a suppressor T cell pathway by interferon. *Proc. Natl. Acad. Sci. USA,* 79:3808–3812.
12. Badwey, J. A., and Karnovsky, M. L. (1980): Active oxygen species and the functions of phagocytic leukocytes. *Annu. Rev. Biochem.,* 49:695–726.
13. Basham, T. Y., Nickoloff, B. J., Merigan, T. C., and Morhenn, V. B. (1984): Recombinant gamma interferon induces HLA-DR expression on cultured human keratinocytes. *J. Invest. Dermatol.,* 83:88–90.
14. Beller, D. I., and Unanue, E. R. (1982): Regulation of macrophage Ia expression in vivo and in vitro. *Adv. Exp. Med. Biol.,* 155:591–599.
15. Berman, B., Duncan, M. R., Smith, B., Ziboh, V. A., and Palladino, M. (1985): Interferon enhancement of HLA-DR antigen expression on epidermal Langerhans cells. *J. Invest. Dermatol.,* 84:54–58.
16. Berton, G., Zeni, L., Cassatella, M. A., and Rossi, F. (1986): Gamma interferon is able to enhance the oxidative metabolism of human neutrophils. *Biochem. Biophys. Res. Commun.,* 138:1276–1282.
17. Bhardwaj, N., Nash, T. W., and Horwitz, M. A. (1986): Interferon-γ activated human monocytes inhibit the intracellular multiplication of *Legionella pneumophila. J. Immunol.,* 137:2662–2669.
18. Blalock, J. E., Baron, S., Johnson, H. M., and Stanton, G. J. (1982): Transmission of IFN-induced activities by cell to cell communication. *Tex. Rep. Biol. Med.,* 41:344–349.
19. Bloom, B. R., and Bennett, B. (1966): Mechanism of a reaction in vitro associated with delayed-type hypersensitivity. *Science,* 153:80–82.
20. Bonvini, E., Hoffman, T., Herberman, R. B., and Varesio, L. (1986): Selective augmentation by recombinant interferon-gamma of the intracellular content of *S*-adenosylmethionine in murine macrophages. *J. Immunol.,* 136:2596–2604.
21. Boraschi, D., Censini, S., Bartalini, M., and Tagliabue, A. (1985): Regulation of arachidonic acid metabolism in macrophages by immune and nonimmune interferons. *J. Immunol.,* 135:502–505.
22. Branca, A. A., and Baglioni, C. (1981): Evidence that type I and type II interferons have different receptors. *Nature,* 294:768–770.
23. Branca, A. A., Faltynek, C. R., D'Alessandro, S. B., and Baglioni, C. (1982): Interaction of interferon with cellular receptors: Internalization and degradation of cell-bound interferon. *J. Biol. Chem.,* 257:13291–13296.
24. Brandwein, S. R. (1986): Regulation of interleukin 1 production by mouse peritoneal macrophages: Effects of arachidonic acid metabolites, cyclic nucleotides, and interferons. *J. Biol. Chem.,* 261:8624–8632.
25. Brinckerhoff, C. E., and Guyre, P. M. (1985): Increased proliferation of human synovial fibroblasts treated with recombinant immune interferon. *J. Immunol.,* 134:3142–3146.
26. Broxmeyer, H., Lu, L., Platzer, E., Feit, C., Juliano, L., and Rubin, B. Y. (1983): Comparative analysis of the influences of human gamma, alpha and beta interferons on human multipotential (CFU-GEMM), erythroid (BFU-E), and granulocyte-macrophage (CFU-GM) progenitor cells. *J. Immunol.,* 131:1300–1305.
27. Brummer, E., Morrison, C. J., and Stevens, D. A. (1985): Recombinant and natural gamma-interferon activation of macrophages in vitro: Different dose requirements for induction of killing activity against phagocytizable and nonphagocytizable fungi. *Infect. Immun.,* 49:724–730.
28. Brunswick, M., and Lake, P. (1985): Obligatory role of gamma interferon in T cell-replacing factor-dependent, antigen-specific murine B cell responses. *J. Exp. Med.,* 161:953–971.
29. Buchmeier, N. A., and Schreiber, R. D. (1985): Requirement of endogenous interferon-gamma production for resolution of *Listeria monocytogenes* infection. *Proc. Natl. Acad. Sci. USA,* 82:7404–7408.
30. Carvalho, E. M., Badaro, R., Reed, S. G., Jones, T. C., and Johnson, W. D., Jr. (1985): Absence of gamma interferon and interleukin 2 production during active visceral leishmaniasis. *J. Clin. Invest.,* 76:2066–2069.
31. Cassatella, M. A., Della-Bianca, V., Berton, G., and Rossi, F. (1985): Activation by gamma interferon of human macrophage capability to produce toxic oxygen molecules is accompanied by decreased K_m of the superoxide-generating NADPH oxidase. *Biochem. Biophys. Res. Commun.,* 132:908–914.
32. Celada, A., Allen, A., Esparza, I., Gray, P. W., and Schreiber, R. D. (1986): Demonstration and partial characterization of the interferon-gamma receptor on human monocytes and human monocyte-like cell lines. *J. Clin. Invest.,* 76:2196–2205.
33. Cochrane, C. G., Spragg, R., and Revak, S. D. (1983): Pathogenesis of adult respiratory distress syndrome: Evidence of oxidant activity in bronchoalveolar lavage fluid. *J. Clin. Invest.,* 71:754–761.
34. Collart, M. A., Belin, D., Vassali, J.-D., de Kossodo, S., and Vassali, P. (1986): γ Interferon enhances macrophage transcription of the tumor necrosis factor/cachectin, interleukin 1, and urokinase genes, which are controlled by short lived repressors. *J. Exp. Med.,* 164:2113–2118.
35. Czarniecki, C., Fennie, C. W., Powers, D. B., and Estell, D. A. (1984): Synergistic antiviral and antiproliferative activities of *Escherichia coli*-derived human alpha, beta, and gamma interferons. *J. Virol.,* 49:490–496.

36. David, J. R. (1966): Delayed hypersensitivity in vitro: Its mediation by cell-free substances formed by lymphoid cell-antigen interaction. *Proc. Natl. Acad. Sci. USA,* 56:72–77.

37. Degliantoni, G., Murphy, M., Kobayashi, M., Francis, M. K., Perussia, B., and Trinchieri, G. (1985). Natural killer (NK) cell-derived hematopoietic colony-inhibiting activity and NK cytotoxic factor: Relationship with tumor necrosis factor and synergism with immune interferon. *J. Exp. Med.,* 162:1512–1530.

38. De Grado, W. F., Wasserman, Z. R., and Chowdhry, V. (1982). Sequence and structural homologies among type I and type II interferons. *Nature,* 300:379–381.

39. Degre, M., Mellbye, O. J., and Clarke-Jenssen, O. (1983): Immune interferon in serum and synovial fluid in rheumatoid arthritis and related disorders. *Ann. Rheum. Dis.,* 42:672–676.

40. de la Maza, L. M., Peterson, E. M., Fennie, C. W., and Czarniecki, C. W. (1985): The anti-chlamydial and anti-proliferative activities of recombinant murine interferon-gamma are not dependent on tryptophan concentrations. *J. Immunol.,* 135:198–200.

41. Deley, M., Van Damme, J., Claeys, H., Weening, H., Heine, J. W., Billian A., Verylen, C., and de Somer, P. (1980): Interferon induced in human leukocytes by mitogens: Production, partial purification and characterization. *Eur. J. Immunol.,* 10:877–883.

42. de Titto, E. H., Catterall, J. R., and Remington, J. S. (1986): Activity of recombinant tumor necrosis factor on *Toxoplasma gondii* and *Trypanosoma cruzi. J. Immunol.,* 137:1342–1345.

43. Dianzani, F., Salter, F., Fleischman, W. R., Jr., and Zucca, A. (1978): Immune interferon activates cells more slowly than does virus-induced interferon. *Proc. Soc. Exp. Biol. Med.,* 159:94–97.

44. Ding, a., Wright, S. D., and Nathan, C. (1987): Activation of mouse peritoneal macrophages by monoclonal antibodies to Mac-1 (complement receptor type 3). *J. Exp. Med.,* 765:733–749.

45. Domke, I., Straub, P., Jacobsen, H., Kirchner, H., and Panet, A. (1985): Inhibition of replication of herpes simplex virus in mouse macrophages by interferons. *J. Gen. Virol.,* 66:2231–2236.

46. Duijvestijn, A. M., Schreiber, A. B., and Butcher, E. C. (1986): Interferon-γ regulates an antigen specific for endothelial cells involved in lymphocyte traffic. *Proc. Natl. Acad. Sci. USA,* 83:9114–9118.

47. Duncan, M. R., and Berman, B. (1985). Gamma interferon is the lymphokine and beta interferon the monokine responsible for inhibition of fibroblast collagen production and late but not early fibroblast proliferation. *J. Exp. Med.,* 162:516–527.

48. Dustin, M. L., Rothlein, R., Bhan, A. K., Dinarello, C. A., and Springer, T. A. (1986): Induction by IL 1 and interferon-gamma: Tissue distribution, biochemistry, and function of a natural adherence molecule (ICAM-1). *J. Immunol.* 137:245–254.

49. Edwards, C. K., 3rd, Hedegaard, H. B., Zlotnik, A., Gangadharam, P. R., Johnston, R. B., Jr., and Pabst, M. J. (1986). Chronic infection due to *Mycobacterium intracellulare* in mice: Association with macrophage release of prostaglandin E2 and reversal by injection of indomethacin, muramyl dipeptide, or interferon-gamma. *J. Immunol.,* 136:1820–1827.

50. Esparza, I., Fox, R. I., and Schreiber, R. D. (1986). Interferon-gamma-dependent modulation of C3b receptors (CR1) on human peripheral blood monocytes. *J. Immunol.,* 136:1360–1365.

51. Ezekowitz, R. A. B., and Gordon, S. (1982): Down regulation of mannosyl receptor mediated endocytosis and antigen F4/80 in bacillus Calmette-Guerin activated mouse macrophages: Role of T lymphocytes and lymphokines. *J. Exp. Med.,* 155:1623–1637.

52. Ezekowitz, R. A. B., Bampton, M., and Gordon, S. (1983): Macrophage activation selectively enhances expression of Fc receptors for IgG2a. *J. Exp. Med.,* 157:807–812.

53. Faltynek, C. R., Branca, A. A., McCandless, S., and Baglioni, C. (1983): Characterization of interferon receptor on human lymphoblastoid cells. *Proc. Natl. Acad. Sci. USA,* 80:3269–3273.

54. Fels, A. O. S., Nathan, C. F., and Cohn, Z. A. (1987): H₂O₂ release by alveolar macrophages from sarcoid patients and by alveolar macrophages from normals after exposure to recombinant interferons αA, β, γ and 1,25-dihydroxyvitamin D3. *J. Clin. Invest.,* 139:381–386.

55. Ferreira, A., Schofield, L., Enea, V., Schellekens, H., van der Meide, P., Collins, W. E., Nussenzweig, R. S., and Nussenzweig, V. (1986). Inhibition of development of exoerythrocytic forms of malaria parasites by gamma-interferon. *Science,* 232:881–884.

56. Franklin, M. R., and Finkle, B. S. (1985). Effect of murine gamma-interferon on the mouse liver and its drug-metabolizing enzymes: Comparison with human hybrid alpha-interferon. *J. Interferon Res.,* 5:265–272.

57. Friedman, R. M. (1967): Interferon binding: The first step in establishment of antiviral activity. *Science,* 156:1760–1761.

58. Friedman, R. L., Manly, S. P., McMahon, M., Kerr, I. M., and Stark, G. R. (1984): Transcriptional and posttranscriptional regulation of interferon-induced gene expression in human cells. *Cell,* 38:745–755.

59. Glasgow, L. A. (1966): Leukocytes and interferon in the host response to viral infections. II. Enhanced interferon response of leukocytes from immune animals. *J. Bacteriol.,* 91:2185–2191.

60. Goldring, M. B., Sandell, J. J., Stephenson, M. L., and Krane, S. M. (1986): Immune interferon suppresses levels of procollagen mRNA and type II collagen synthesis in cultured human articular and costal chondrocytes. *J. Biol. Chem.,* 261:9049–9055.

61. Gowen, M., and Mundy, G. R. (1986): Actions of recombinant interleukin 1, interleukin 2, and interferon-gamma on bone resorption in vitro. *J. Immunol.,* 136:2478–2482.

62. Gray, P. W., Leung, D. W., Derynck, R., Sherwood, P. J., Wallace, D. M., Berger, S. L., Levinson, A. D., and Goeddel, D. V. (1982): Expression of human immune interferon cDNA in *E. coli* and monkey cells. *Nature,* 295:503–508.

63. Gray, P., and Goeddel, D. V. (1982): Structure of the human immune interferon gene. *Nature,* 298:859–863.

64. Green, J. A., Cooperband, S. R., and Kibrick, S. (1969): Immune specific induction of interferon production in cultures of human blood lymphocytes. *Science,* 164:1415–1417.

65. Gresser, I. (1982): Can interferon induce disease? In: *Interferon 1982, Vol. 4,* edited by I. Gresser, pp. 95–128. Academic Press, New York.

66. Gresser, I., and Bourali, C. (1970): Antitumor effects of IFN preparations. *J. Natl. Cancer Inst.,* 45:365–376.

67. Groenewegen, G., de Ley, M., Jeunhomme, G. M., and Buurman, W. A. (1986): Supernatants of human leukocytes contain mediator, different from interferon gamma, which induces expression of MHC class II antigens. *J. Exp. Med.,* 164:131–143.

68. Gupta, S. L. (1979). Specific protein phosphorylation in interferon-treated uninfected and virus-infected mouse L929 cells: Enhancement by double-stranded RNA. *J. Virol.,* 29:301–311.

69. Guyre, P. M., Morganelli, P. M., and Miller, R. (1983): Recombinant interferon gamma increases immunoglobulin G Fc receptors on cultured human mononuclear phagocytes. *J. Clin. Invest.,* 72:393–397.

70. Hamilton, T. A., Gray, P. W., and Adams, D. O. (1984): Expression of the transferrin receptor on murine peritoneal macrophages is modulated by in vitro treatment with interferon-γ. *Cell. Immunol.,* 89:478–488.

71. Hamilton, T. A., Becton, D. L., Somers, S. D., Gray, P. W., and Adams, D. O. (1985): Interferon-gamma modulates protein kinase C activity in murine peritoneal macrophages. *J. Biol. Chem.,* 260:1378–1381.

72. Hamilton, T. A., Ribsbee, J. E., Scott, W. A., and Adams, D. O. (1985): Gamma-interferon enhances the secretion of arachidonic acid metabolites from murine peritoneal macrophages stimulated with phorbol diesters. *J. Immunol.,* 134:2631–2636.

73. Hamilton, T. A., Somers, S. D., Becton, D. L., Celada, A., Schreiber, R. D., and Adams, D. O. (1986): Analysis of deficiencies in IFN-γ-mediated priming for tumor cytotoxicity in peritoneal macrophages from A/J mice. *J. Immunol.,* 137:3367–3371.

74. Hancock, W. W., Kobzik, L., Colby, A. J., O'Hara, C. J., Cooper, A. G., and Godleski, J. J. (1986): Detection of lymphokines and lymphokine receptors in pulmonary sarcoidosis: Immunohistologic evidence that inflammatory macrophages express IL-2 receptors. *Am. J. Pathol.,* 123:1–8.

75. Hannigan, G. E., Gewert, D. R., and Williams, B. R. G. (1984): Characterization and regulation of α-interferon receptor expression in interferon-sensitive and -resistant human lymphoblastoid cells. *J. Biol. Chem.,* 259:9456–9460.

76. Havell, E. A., Spitalny, G. L., and Patel, P. J. (1982): Enhanced production of murine interferon-γ by T cells generated in response to bacterial infection. *J. Exp. Med.*, 156:112–127.

77. Herrmann, F., Cannistra, S. A., Levine, H., and Griffin, J. D. (1985): Expression of interleukin 2 receptors and binding of interleukin 2 by gamma interferon-induced human leukemic and normal monocytic cells. *J. Exp. Med.*, 162:1111–1116.

78. Hibbs, J. B., Jr., Lambert, L. H., Jr., and Remington, J. S. (1972): Possible role of macrophage mediated nonspecific cytotoxicity in tumor resistance. *Nature New Biol.*, 235:48–50.

79. Hirsch, R. L., Panitch, H. S., and Johnson, K. P. (1985): Lymphocytes from multiple sclerosis patients produce elevated levels of gamma interferon in vitro. *J. Clin. Immunol.*, 5:386–389.

80. Hooks, J. J., Moutsopoulos, H. M., Geis, S. A., Stahl, N., Decker, J. L., and Notkins, A. L. (1979): Immune interferon in the circulation of patients with autoimmune disease. *N. Engl. J. Med.*, 301:5–8.

81. Hoover, D. L., Nacy, C. A., and Meltzer, M. S. (1985): Human monocyte activation for cytotoxicity against intracellular *Leishmania donovani* amastigotes: Induction of microbicidal activity by interferon-gamma. *Cell. Immunol.*, 94:500–511.

82. Houghton, A. N., Thomson, T. M., Gross, D., Oettgen, H. F., and Old, L. J. (1984): Surface antigens of melanoma and melanocytes: Specificity of induction of Ia antigens by human γ-interferon. *J. Exp. Med.*, 160:255–269.

83. Houghton, M. M., Eaton, A. W., Stewart, A. G., Smith, J. C., and Doel, M. (1980): The complete amino acid sequence of human fibroblast interferon as deduced using synthetic oligodeoxyribonucleotide primers of reverse transcriptase. *Nucleic Acids Res.*, 8:2885–2893.

84. Hovanessian, A. G., Meurs, E., and Montagnier, L. (1981): Lack of systemic correlation between the interferon-mediated antiviral state and the level of 2-5A synthetase and protein kinase in three different types of murine cells. *J. Interferon Res.*, 1:179–190.

85. Huber, C., Batchelor, J. R., Fuchs, D., Hausen, A., Lang, A., Niederwieser, D., Reibnegger, G., Swetly, P., Troppmair, J., and Wachter, H. (1984): Immune response-associated production of neopterin release from macrophages primarily under control of interferon-γ. *J. Exp. Med.*, 160:310–316.

86. Husby, G., and Williams, R. C., Jr. (1985): Immunohistochemical studies of interleukin-2 and gamma-interferon in rheumatoid arthritis. *Arthritis Rheum.*, 28:174–181.

87. Inaba, K., Kitaura, M., Kato, T., Watanabe, Y., and Muramatsu, S. (1986): Contrasting effect of α/β- and γ-interferons on expression of macrophage Ia antigens. *J. Exp. Med.*, 163:1030–1035.

88. Isaacs, A., and Lindemann, J. (1957): Virus interference. I. The interferon. *Proc. R. Soc. Lond. [Biol.]*, 147:258–267.

89. Isenberg, D. A., Rowe, D., Shearer, M., Novick, D., and Beverley, P. C. (1986): Localization of interferons and interleukin 2 in polymyositis and muscular dystrophy. *Clin. Exp. Immunol.*, 63:450–458.

90. James, S. L., Natovitz, P. C., Farrar, W. L., and Leonard, E. J. (1984): Macrophages as effector cells of protective immunity in murine schistosomiasis: Macrophage activation in mice vaccinated with radiation-attenuated cercariae. *Infect. Immun.*, 44:569–575.

91. Jerrells, T. R., Turco, J., Winkler, H. H., and Spitalny, G. L. (1986): Neutralization of lymphokine-mediated antirickettsial activity of fibroblasts and macrophages with monoclonal antibody specific for murine interferon gamma. *Infect. Immun.*, 51:355–359.

92. Jimenez, S. A., Freundlich, B., and Rosenbloom, J. (1984): Selective inhibition of human diploid fibroblast collagen synthesis by interferons. *J. Clin. Invest.*, 74:1112–1116.

93. Joshi, A. R., Sarkar, F. H., and Gupta, S. L. (1982): Interferon receptors: Cross-linking of human leukocyte interferon-α₂ to its receptor on human cells. *J. Biol. Chem.*, 257:13884–13887.

94. Kaplan, G., Witmer, M. D., Nath, I., Steinman, R. M., Laal, S., Prasad, H. K., Sarno, E. N., Elvers, U., and Cohn, Z. A. (1986): Influence of delayed immune reactions on human epidermal keratinocytes. *Proc. Natl. Acad. Sci. USA*, 83:3469–3473.

95. Keller, R. (1973): Cytostatic elimination of syngeneic rat tumor cells in vitro by nonspecifically activated macrophages. *J. Exp. Med.*, 138:625–644.

96. Kelso, A., and Glasebrook, A. L. (1984): Secretion of interleukin 2, macrophage-activating factor, interferons, and colony-stimulating factor by alloreactive T lymphocyte clones. *J. Immunol.*, 132:2924–2931.

97. Kerr, I. M., and Brown, R. E. (1978): An inhibitor of protein synthesis synthesized with an enzyme fraction from interferon-treated cells. *Proc. Natl. Acad. Sci. USA*, 75:256–260.

98. Kiderlen, A. F., Kaufmann, S. H. E., and Lohmann-Matthes, M.-L. (1984): Protection of mice against the intracellular bacterium *Listeria monocytogenes* by recombinant immune interferon. *Eur. J. Immunol.*, 14:964–967.

99. Klein, J. R., Raulet, D. H., Pasternack, M. S., and Bevan, M. J. (1982): Cytotoxic T lymphocytes produce immune interferon in response to antigen or mitogen. *J. Exp. Med.*, 155:1198–1203.

100. Kleinerman, E. W., Zicht, R., Sarin, P. S., Gallo, R. C., and Fidler, I. J. (1984): Constitutive production and release of a lymphokine with macrophage activating factor activity distinct from γ-interferon by a human T cell leukemia virus-positive cell line. *Cancer Res.* 44:4470–4475.

101. Koeffler, H. P., Reichel, H., Bishop, J. E., and Norman, A. W. (1985): Gamma-interferon stimulates production of 1,25-dihydroxyvitamin D3 by normal human macrophages. *Biochem. Biophys. Res. Commun.*, 127:596–603.

102. Kohase, M., Henriksen-DeStefano, D., May, L. T., Vilček, J., and Sehgal, P. B. (1986): Induction of β₂-interferon by tumor necrosis factor: A homeostatic mechanism in the control of cell proliferation. *Cell*, 45:659–666.

103. Krammer, P. H., Kubelka, G. F., Falk, W., and Ruppel, A. (1985): Priming and triggering of tumoricidal and schistosomulicidal macrophages by two sequential lymphokine signals: Interferon-γ and macrophage cytotoxicity inducing factor 2. *J. Immunol.*, 135:3258–3263.

104. Kurzrock, R., Rosenblum, M. G., Sherwin, S. A., Rios, A., Talpaz, M., Quesada, J. R., and Gutterman, J. U. (1985): Pharmacokinetics, single-dose tolerance, and biological activity of recombinant γ-interferon in cancer patients. *Cancer Res.*, 45:2866–2872.

105. Kurzrock, R., Rohde, M. F., Quesada, J. R., Gianturco, S. H., Bradley, W. A., Sherwin, S. A., and Gutterman, J. U. (1986): Recombinant gamma interferon induces hypertriglyceridemia and inhibits post-heparin lipase activity. *J. Exp. Med.*, 164:1093–1101.

106. Landolfo, S., Cofano, F., Giovarelli, M., Prat, M., Cavallo, G., and Forni, G. (1985): Inhibition of interferon-gamma may suppress allograft reactivity by T lymphocytes in vitro and in vivo. *Science*, 229:176–179.

107. Langford, M. P., Georgiades, J. A., Stanton, G. J., Dianzani, F., and Johnson, H. M. (1979): Large-scale production and physicochemical characterization of human immune interferon. *Infect. Immun.*, 26:36–41.

108. Lebleu, B., Sen, G. C., Shaila, S., Cabrer, B., and Lengyel, P. (1976): Interferon, double-stranded RNA, and protein phosphorylation. *Proc. Natl. Acad. Sci. USA*, 73:3107–3111.

109. Lee, J. C., Rebar, L., Young, P., Ruscetti, F. W., Hanna, N., and Poste, G. (1986): Identification and characterization of a human T cell line-derived lymphokine with MAF-like activity distinct from interferon-gamma. *J. Immunol.*, 136:1322–1328.

110. Lee, S. H., Aggarwal, B. B., Rinderknecht, E., Assisi, F., and Chiu, H. (1984): The synergistic antiproliferative effect of γ-interferon and human lymphotoxin. *J. Immunol.*, 133:1083–1086.

111. Leisbon, H. J., Gefter, M., Zlotnik, A., Marrack, P., and Kappler, J. W. (1984): Role of γ-interferon in antibody-producing responses. *Nature*, 309:799–801.

112. Lengyel, P. (1982): Biochemistry of interferons and their actions. *Annu. Rev. Biochem.*, 51:251–282.

113. Leszczynski, D., Ferry, B., Schellekens, H., Meide, P. H. V. D., and Hayry, P. (1986): Antagonistic effects of γ interferon and steroids on tissue antigenicity. *J. Exp. Med.*, 164:1470–1477.

114. Le-thi, B.-T., and Fauci, A. S. (1986): Recombinant interleukin 2 and gamma-interferon act synergistically on distinct steps of in vitro terminal human B cell maturation. *J. Clin. Invest.*, 77:1173–1179.

115. Leung, D. Y., Collins, T., Lapierre, L. A., Geha, R. S., and Pober, J. S. (1986): Immunoglobulin M antibodies present in the acute

phase of Kawasaki syndrome lyse cultured vascular endothelial cells stimulated by gamma interferon. *J. Clin. Invest.*, 77:1428–1435.

116. Lewis, D. B., Larsen, A., and Wilson, C. B. (1986): Reduced interferon-gamma mRNA levels in human neonates: Evidence for an intrinsic T cell deficiency independent of other genes. *J. Exp. Med.*, 163:1018–1023.

117. Li, H., Jerrells, T., and Walker, D. H. (1986): In vivo evidence for γ-interferon in host defenses against *Rickettsia conorii*. Conference on Host Defenses and Immunomodulation to Intracellular Pathogens, Philadelphia, abstract 19.

118. Ling, P. D., Warren, M. K., and Vogel, S. N. (1985): Antagonistic effect of interferon-β on the interferon-γ-induced expression of Ia antigen on murine macrophages. *J. Immunol.*, 135:1857–1863.

119. Littman, S. J., Faltynek, C. K., and Baglioni, C. (1985): Binding of human recombinant ^{125}I-interferon-γ to receptors on human cells. *J. Biol. Chem.*, 260:1191–1195.

120. Lockart, R. Z., Jr. (1964): The necessity for cellular RNA and protein synthesis for viral inhibition resulting from interferon. *Biochem. Biophys. Res. Commun.*, 15:513–518.

121. Lopez, A. F., Williamson, D. J., Gamble, J. R., Begley, C. G., Harlan, J. M., Klebanoff, S. J., Waltersdorph, A., Wong, G., Clark, S. C., and Vadas, M. A. (1986): Recombinant human granulocyte-macrophage colony-stimulating factor stimulates in vitro mature human neutrophil and eosinophil function, surface receptor expression, and survival. *J. Clin. Invest.*, 78:1220–1228.

122. Luster, A. D., Unkeless, J. C., and Ravetch, J. V. (1985): Gamma-interferon transcriptionally regulates an early-response gene containing homology to platelet proteins. *Nature*, 315:672–676.

123. Mackaness, G. B. (1970): The mechanisms of macrophage activation: In: *Infectious Agents and Host Reactions*, edited by S. Mudd, pp. 61–75. W. B. Saunders Co., Philadelphia.

124. MacKay, R. J., and Russell, S. W. (1986): Protein changes associated with stages of activation of mouse macrophages for tumor cell killing. *J. Immunol.*, 137:1392–1398.

125. Mamus, S. W., Beck-Schroeder, S., and Zanjani, E. D. (1985): Suppression of normal human erythropoiesis by gamma interferon in vitro: Role of monocytes and T lymphocytes. *J. Clin. Invest.*, 75:1496–1503.

126. Masuyama, J., Minato, N., and Kano, S. (1986): Mechanisms of lymphocyte adhesion to human vascular endothelial cells in culture: T lymphocyte adhesion to endothelial cells through endothelial HLA-DR antigens induced by gamma interferon. *J. Clin. Invest.*, 77:1596–1605.

127. May, L. T., Helfgott, D. C., and Sehgal, B. (1986): Anti-β-interferon antibodies inhibit the increased expression of HLA-B7 mRNA in tumor necrosis factor-treated human fibroblasts: Structural studies of the β2 interferon involved. *Proc. Natl. Acad. Sci. USA*, 83:8957–8961.

128. McCabe, R. E., Luft, B. J., and Remington, J. S. (1984): Effect of murine interferon-γ on murine toxoplasmosis. *J. Infect. Dis.*, 150:961–962.

129. Mentzer, S. J., Faller, D. V., and Burakoff, S. J. (1986): Interferon-gamma induction of LFA-1-mediated homotypic adhesion of human monocytes. *J. Immunol.*, 137:108–113.

130. Mestan, J., Digel, W., Mittnacht, S., Hillen, H., Blohn, D., Moller, A., Jacobsen, H., and Kirchner, H. (1986): Antiviral effects of recombinant tumour necrosis factor in vitro. *Nature*, 323:816–819.

131. Meurs, E., Hovanessian, A. G., and Montagnier, L. (1981): Interferon-mediated antiviral state in human MRC5 cells in the absence of detectable levels of 2-5A synthetase and protein kinase. *J. Interferon Res.*, 1:219–232.

132. Milton, A. D., and Fabre, J. W. (1985): Massive induction of donor type class I and class II major histocompatibility complex antigens in rejecting cardiac allografts in the rat. *J. Exp. Med.*, 161:98–112.

133. Momburg, F., Koch, N., Moller, P., Moldenhauer, G., and Hammerling, G. J. (1986): In vivo induction of H-2K/D antigens by recombinant interferon-gamma. *Eur. J. Immunol.*, 16:551–557.

134. Montesano, R., Mossez, A., Ryser, J.-E., Orci, L., and Vassali, P. (1984): Leukocyte interleukins induce cultured endothelial cells to produce a highly organized glycosaminoglycan-rich pericellular matrix. *J. Cell Biol.*, 99:1706–1715.

135. Morris, A. G., Lin, Y. L., and Askonas, B. A. (1982): Immune interferon release when a cloned cytotoxic T cell line meets its correct influenza infected target cell. *Nature*, 295:150–152.

136. Munakata, T., Semba, U., Shibaya, Y., Kuwano, K., Akagi, M., and Arai, S. (1985): Induction of interferon-γ production by human natural killer cells stimulated by hydrogen peroxide. *J. Immunol.*, 134:2449–2455.

137. Murphy, M., Loudon, R., Kobayashi, M., and Trinchieri, G. (1986): Gamma interferon and lymphotoxin, released by activated T cells, synergize to inhibit granulocyte/monocyte colony formation. *J. Exp. Med.*, 164:263–279.

138. Murray, H. W., Rubin, B. Y., and Rothermel, C. D. (1983): Killing of intracellular *Leishmania donovani* by lymphokine-stimulated human mononuclear phagocytes: Evidence that interferon-γ is the activating lymphokine. *J. Clin. Invest.*, 72:1506–1510.

139. Murray, H. W. (1986): Macrophage activation in the acquired immunodeficiency syndrome. In: *Mechanisms of Host Resistance to Infectious Agents, Tumors, and Allografts*, edited by R. M. Steinman and R. J. North, pp. 321–333. Rockefeller University Press, New York.

140. Murray, H. W., Hillman, J. K., Rubin, B. Y., Kelly, C. D., Jacobs, J. L., Tyler, L. W., Donelly, D. M., Carriero, S. M., Godbold, J. H., and Roberts, R. B. (1985): Patients at risk for AIDS-related opportunistic infections: Clinical manifestations and impaired gamma-interferon production. *N. Engl. J. Med.*, 313:1504–1510.

141. Murray, H. W., Spitalny, G. W., and Nathan, C. F. (1985): Activation of mouse peritoneal macrophages in vitro and in vivo by interferon-gamma. *J. Immunol.*, 134:1619–1622.

142. Murray, H. W., Scavuzzo, D., Jacobs, J. L., Kaplan, M. H., Libby, D. M., and Roberts, R. B. (1987): In vitro and in vivo activation of human mononuclear phagocytes by gamma interferon: Studies with normal and AIDS monocytes. *J. Immunol.* (in press).

143. Murray, H. W., Stern, J. J., Welte, K., Rubin, B. Y., Carriero, S., and Nathan, C. F. (1987): Experimental visceral leishmaniasis: Production of interleukin 2 and interferon-γ, tissue immune reaction, and response to treatment with interleukin 2 and interferon-γ. *J. Immunol.*, 138:2290–2297.

144. Nacy, C. A., Fortier, A. H., Meltzer, M. S., Buchmeier, N., and Schreiber, R. D. (1985): Macrophage activation to kill *Leishmania major*: Activation of macrophages for intracellular destruction of amastigotes can be induced by both recombinant interferon-γ and non-interferon lymphokines. *J. Immunol.*, 135:3505–3511.

145. Nagano, Y., and Kojima, Y. (1954): Pouvoir immunisant du virus vaccinal inactive par des rayons ultraviolets. *C. R. Soc. Biol. (Paris)*, 148:1700–1702.

146. Nakagawa, T., Hirano, T., Nakagawa, N., Yoshizaki, K., and Kishimoto, T. (1985): Effect of recombinant IL-2 and γ-IFN on proliferation and differentiation on human B cells. *J. Immunol.*, 134:959–966.

147. Nakane, A., and Minagawa, T. (1984): The significance of alpha/beta interferons and gamma interferon produced in mice infected with *Listeria monocytogenes*. *Cell. Immunol.*, 88:29–40.

148. Nathan, C. F. (1983): Mechanisms of macrophage antimicrobial activity. *Trans. R. Soc. Trop. Med. Hyg.*, 77:620–630.

149. Nathan, C. (1986): Macrophage activation: Some questions. *Ann. Inst. Pasteur*, 137C:345–351.

150. Nathan, C. (1986): Interferon-gamma and macrophage activation in cell-mediated immunity. In: *Mechanisms of Host Resistance to Infectious Agents, Tumors, and Allografts*, edited by R. M. Steinman and R. J. North, pp. 165–184. Rockefeller University Press, New York.

151. Nathan, C. F. (1986): Peroxide and pteridine: A hypothesis on the regulation of macrophage antimicrobial activity by interferon γ. In: *Interferon 7*, edited by I. Gresser, pp. 125–143. Academic Press, London.

152. Nathan, C. (1987): Macrophage secretory products. *J. Clin. Invest.*, 79:319–326.

153. Nathan, C., Nogueira, N., Juangbhanich, C., Ellis, J., and Cohn, Z. (1979): Activation of macrophages in vivo and in vitro: Correlation between hydrogen peroxide release and killing of *Trypanosoma cruzi*. *J. Exp. Med.*, 149:1056–1068.

154. Nathan, C. F., Murray, H. W., Wiebe, M. E., and Rubin, B. Y.

(1983): Identification of interferon-γ as the lymphokine that activates human macrophage oxidative metabolism and antimicrobial activity. *J. Exp. Med.,* 158:670–689.

155. Nathan, C. F., Prendergast, T. J., Wiebe, M. E., Stanley, E. R., Platzer, E., Remold, H. G., Welte, K., Rubin, B. Y., and Murray, H. W. (1984): Activation of human macrophages: Comparison of other cytokines with interferon-γ. *J. Exp. Med.,* 160:600–605.

156. Nathan, C. F., and Cohn, Z. A. (1985): Cellular components of inflammation: Monocytes and macrophages. In: *Textbook of Rheumatology,* 2nd ed., edited by W. N. Kelley, E. D. Harris, Jr., S. Ruddy, and C. B. Sledge, pp. 144–168. W. B. Saunders Co., Philadelphia.

157. Nathan, C. F., Horowitz, C. R., de la Harpe, J., Vadhan-Raj, S., Sherwin, S. A., Oettgen, H. F., and Krown, S. E. (1985): Administration of recombinant interferon γ to cancer patients enhances monocyte secretion of hydrogen peroxide. *Proc. Natl. Acad. Sci. USA,* 82:8686–8690.

158. Nathan, C. F., Kaplan, G., Levis, W. R., Nusrat, A., Witmer, M. D., Sherwin, S. A., Job, C. K., Horowitz, C. R., Steinman, R. M., and Cohn, Z. A. (1986): Local and systemic effects of intradermal recombinant interferon-γ in patients with lepromatous leprosy. *N. Engl. J. Med.,* 315:6–15.

159. Nathan, C. F., and Tsunawaki, S. (1986): Secretion of toxic oxygen products by macrophages: Regulatory cytokines and their effects on the oxidase. *Ciba Found. Symp.,* 118:211–230.

160. Nedwin, G. E., Svedersky, L. P., Bringman, T. S., Palladino, M. A., Jr., and Goeddel, D. V. (1985): Effect of interleukin 2, interferon-gamma, and mitogens on the production of tumor necrosis factors alpha and beta. *J. Immunol.,* 135:2492–2497.

161. Niesel, D. W., Hess, C. B., Cho, Y. J., Klimpel, K. D., and Klimpel, G. R. (1986): Natural and recombinant interferons inhibit epithelial cell invasion by *Shigella* spp. *Infect. Immun.,* 52:828–833.

162. Nogueira, N., Kaplan, G., Levy, E., et al. (1983): Defective γ interferon production in leprosy: Reversal with antigen and interleukin 2. *J. Exp. Med.,* 158:2165–2170.

163. Ockenhouse, C. F., Schulman, S., and Shear, H. L. (1984): Induction of crisis forms in the human malaria parasite *Plasmodium falciparum* by γ-interferon-activated, monocyte-derived macrophages. *J. Immunol.,* 133:1601–1608.

164. Passwell, J. H., Schor, R., and Shoham, J. (1986): The enhancing effect of interferon-beta and -gamma on the killing of *Leishmania tropica major* in human mononuclear phagocytes in vitro. *J. Immunol.,* 136:3062–3066.

165. Patton, J. S., Shepard, H. M., Wilking, H., Lewis, G., Aggarwal, B. B., Eessalu, T. E., Gavin, L. A., and Grunfeld, C. (1986): Interferons and tumor necrosis factors have similar catabolic effects on 3T3 L1 cells. *Proc. Natl. Acad. Sci. USA,* 83:8313–8317.

166. Peck, R. (1985): A one-plate assay for macrophage bactericidal activity. *J. Immunol. Methods,* 82:131–140.

167. Perussia, B., Dayton, E. T., Lazarus, R., Fanning, V., and Trinchieri, G. (1983): Immune interferon induces the receptor for monomeric IgG1 on human monocytic and myeloid cells. *J. Exp. Med.,* 158:1092.

168. Pestka, S., and Baron, S. (1981): Definition and classification of the interferons. *Methods Enzymol.,* 78A:3–14.

169. Peterlik, M., Hoffman, O., Swetly, P., Klaushofer, K., and Koller, K. (1985): Recombinant gamma-interferon inhibits prostaglandin-mediated and parathyroid hormone-induced bone resorption in cultured neonatal mouse calvaria. *FEBS Lett.,* 185:287–290.

170. Pfefferkorn, E. R. (1984): Interferon gamma blocks the growth of *Toxoplasma gondii* in human fibroblasts by inducing the host cells to degrade tryptophan. *Proc. Natl. Acad. Sci. USA,* 81:908–912.

171. Plata, F., Wietzerbin, J., Pons, F. G., Falcoff, E., and Eisen, H. (1984): Synergistic protection by specific antibodies and interferon against infection by *Trypansoma cruzi* in vitro. *Eur. J. Immunol.,* 14:930–935.

172. Platsoucas, C. D. (1986): Regulation of natural killer cytotoxicity by *Escherichia coli*-derived human interferon gamma. *Scand. J. Immunol.,* 24:93–108.

173. Pober, J. S., Gimbrone, M. A., Jr., Cotran, R. S., Reiss, C. S., Burakoff, S. J., Fiers, W., and Ault, K. A. (1983): Ia expression by vascular endothelium is inducible by activated T cells and human γ interferon. *J. Exp. Med.,* 157:1339–1353.

174. Prystowski, M. B., Ely, M. M., Beller, D., Eisenberg, L., Goldman, J., Goldman, M., Goldwasser, E., Ihle, J., Quintans, J., Remold, H., Vogel, S. N., and Fitch, F. W. (1982): Alloreactive cloned T cell lines. VI. Multiple lymphokine activities secreted by helper and cytolytic cloned T cells. *J. Immunol.,* 129:2337–2344.

175. Rabin, E. M., Mond, J. J., Ohara, J., and Paul, W. E. (1986): Interferon-γ inhibits the action of B cell stimulatory factor (BSF-1) on resting B cells. *J. Immunol.,* 137:1573–1576.

176. Rashidbaigi, A., Kung, H., and Pestka, S. (1985): Characterization of receptors for immune interferon in U937 cells with ^{32}P-labeled human recombinant immune interferon. *J. Biol. Chem.,* 260:8514–8519.

177. Rashidbaigi, A., Langer, J. A., Jung, V., Jones, C., Morse, H. G., Tischfield, J. A., Trill, J. J., Kung, H. F., and Pestka, S. (1986): The gene for the human immune interferon receptor is located on chromosome 6. *Proc. Natl. Acad. Sci. USA,* 83:384–388.

178. Reems, G. H., Cook, L. A., and Vilček, J. (1983): Gamma interferon synthesis by human thymocytes and T lymphocytes inhibited by cyclosporin A. *Science,* 221:63–65.

179. Rhodes-Feuillette, A., Bellosguardo, M., Druilhe, P., Ballet, J. J., Chousterman, S., Canivet, M., and Peries, J. (1985): The interferon compartment of the immune response in human malaria. II. Presence of serum-interferon gamma following the acute attack. *J. Interferon Res.,* 5:169–178.

180. Rinderknecht, E., O'Connor, B. H., and Rodriguez, H. (1984): Natural human interferon-γ: Complete amino acid sequence and determination of sites of glycosylation. *J. Biol. Chem.,* 259:6790–6797.

181. Robinson, B. W., McLemore, T. L., and Crystal, R. G. (1985): Gamma interferon is spontaneously released by alveolar macrophages and lung T lymphocytes in patients with pulmonary sarcoidosis. *J. Clin. Invest.,* 75:1488–1495.

182. Roehm, N. W., Leibson, H. J., Zlotnick, A., Kappler, J., Marrack, P., and Cambier, J. C. (1984): Interleukin-induced increase in Ia expression by normal mouse B cells. *J. Exp. Med.,* 160:679–694.

183. Romagnani, S., Giudizi, M. G., Biagiotti, R., Almerigogna, F., Mingari, C., Maggi, E., Liang, C. M., and Moretta, L. (1986): B cell growth factor activity of interferon-gamma: Recombinant human interferon-gamma promotes proliferation of anti-mu activated human B lymphocytes. *J. Immunol.,* 136:3513–3516.

184. Romeo, G., Affabris, E., Federico, M., Mechti, N., Coccia, E. M., Jemma, C., and Rossi, G. B. (1985): Establishment of the antiviral state in alpha, beta-interferon-resistant Friend cells treated with gamma-interferon. *J. Biol. Chem.,* 260:3833–3838.

185. Rothermel, C. D., Rubin, B. Y., and Murray, H. W. (1983): γ-Interferon is the factor in lymphokine that activates human macrophages to inhibit intracellular *Chlamydia psittaci* replication. *J. Immunol.,* 131:2542–2544.

186. Rothermel, C. D., Rubin, B. Y., Jaffe, E. A., and Murray, H. W. (1986): Oxygen-independent inhibition of intracellular *Chlamydia psittaci* growth by human monocytes and interferon-γ-activated macrophages. *J. Immunol.,* 137:689–692.

187. Rubin, B. R., and Gupta, S. L. (1980). Differential efficacies of human type I and type II interferons as antiviral and antiproliferative agents. *Proc. Natl. Acad. Sci. USA,* 77:5928–5932.

188. Saito, T., Berens, M. E., and Welander, C. E. (1986): Direct and indirect effects of human recombinant gamma-interferon on tumor cells in a clonogenic assay. *Cancer Res.,* 46:1142–1147.

189. Salvin, S. B., Youngner, J. S., and Lederer, W. H. (1973): Migration inhibitory factor and interferon in the circulation of mice with delayed hypersensitivity. *Infect. Immun.,* 7:68–75.

190. Samuel, C. E., and Knutson, G. S. (1983): Mechanism of interferon action: Human leukocyte and immune interferons regulate the expression of different genes and induce different antiviral states in human amnion U cells. *Virology,* 130:474–484.

191. Sarkar, F. H., and Gupta, S. L. (1984): Receptors for human γ interferon: Binding and cross-linking of ^{125}I-labeled human recombinant γ interferon to receptors on WISH cells. *Proc. Natl. Acad. Sci. USA,* 81:5160–5164.

192. Schaffner, A. (1985): Therapeutic concentrations of glucocorticoids

suppress the antimicrobial activity of human macrophages without impairing their responsiveness to gamma interferon. *J. Clin. Invest.,* 76:1755–1764.

193. Schmit, A., Zilberstein, A., Shulman, L., Federman, P., Berissi, H., and Revel, M. (1978): Interferon action: Isolation of nuclease F, a translation inhibitor activated by interferon-induced (2'-5')oligo-isoadenylate. *FEBS Lett.,* 95:257–264.

194. Sedmak, J. J., Sabran, J. L., and Grossberg, S. E. (1983): A unique set of polypeptides is induced by γ interferon in addition to those induced in common with α and β interferons. *Nature,* 301:437–439.

195. Shalaby, M. R., Aggarwal, B. B., Rinderknecht, E., Svedersky, L. P., Finkle, B. S., and Palladino, M. A., Jr. (1985): Activation of human polymorphonuclear neutrophil functions by interferon-gamma and tumor necrosis factors. *J. Immunol.,* 135:2069–2073.

196. Shalaby, M. R., Hamilton, E. G., Benninger, A. H., and Marafino, B. J., Jr. (1985): In vivo antiviral activity of recombinant murine gamma interferon. *J. Interferon Res.,* 5:339–345.

197. Shparber, M., and Nathan, C. F. (1986): Autocrine activation of macrophages by recombinant tumor necrosis factor but not recombinant interleukin-1. *Blood,* 68:suppl. 86a (abstract).

198. Sibley, L. D., Weidner, E., and Krahenbuhl, J. L. (1985): Phagosome acidification blocked by intracellular *Toxoplasma gondii. Nature,* 315:416–419.

199. Sidman, C. L., Marshall, J. D., Shultz, L. D., Gray, P. W., and Johnson, H. M. (1984): γ-Interferon is one of several direct B cell maturing lymphokines. *Nature,* 309:801–804.

200. Simon, M. M., Hochgeschwender, U., Brugger, U., and Landolfo, S. (1986): Monoclonal antibodies to interferon-gamma inhibit interleukin 2-dependent induction of growth and maturation in lectin/antigen-reactive cytolytic T lymphocyte precursors. *J. Immunol.,* 136:2755–2762.

201. Skoskiewicz, M. J., Colvin, R. B., Scheeberger, E. E., and Russell, P. S. (1985): Widespread and selective induction of major histo-compatibility complex-determined antigens in vivo by gamma interferon. *J. Exp. Med.,* 162:1645–1664.

202. Sonnenfeld, G., Mandels, A., and Merigan, T. C. (1977): The immunosuppressive effect of type II mouse interferon preparations on antibody production. *Cell. Immunol.,* 34:193–206.

203. Spitalny, G. L., and Havell, E. A. (1984): Monoclonal antibody to murine gamma interferon inhibits lymphokine-induced antiviral and macrophage tumoricidal activities. *J. Exp. Med.,* 159:1560.

204. Steeg, P. S., Moore, R. N., Johnson, M., and Oppenheim, J. J. (1982): Regulation of murine macrophage Ia antigen expression by a lymphokine with immune interferon activity. *J. Exp. Med.,* 156:1780–1793.

205. Stephenson, M. L., Krane, S. M., Amento, E. P., McCroskery, P. A., and Byrne, M. (1985): Immune interferon inhibits collagen synthesis by rheumatoid synovial cells associated with decreased levels of the procollagen mRNAs. *FEBS Lett.,* 180:43–50.

206. Stone-Wolff, D. S., Yip, Y. K., Kelker, H. C., Junming, L. E., Henriksen-DeStefano, D., Rubin, B. Y., Rinderknecht, E., Aggarwal, B. B., and Vilček, J. (1984): Interrelationships of human interferon-γ with lymphotoxin and monocyte cytotoxin. *J. Exp. Med.,* 159:828–843.

207. Strassmann, G., Springer, T. A., and Adams, D. O. (1985): Studies on antigens associated with the activation of murine mononuclear phagocytes: Kinetics of and requirements for induction of lymphocyte function-associated (LFA)-1 antigen in vitro. *J. Immunol.,* 135:147–151.

208. Strunk, R. C., Cole, F. S., Perlmutter, D. H., and Colten, H. R. (1985): γ-Interferon increases expression of class III complement genes C2 and factor B in human monocytes and in murine fibroblasts. *J. Biol. Chem.,* 260:15280–15285.

209. Stuehr, D. J., and Marletta, M. A. (1985): Mammalian nitrate biosynthesis: Mouse macrophages produce nitrite and nitrate in response to *Escherichia coli* lipopolysaccharide. *Proc. Natl. Acad. Sci. USA,* 82:7738–7742.

210. Stuehr, D. J., and Marletta, M. A. (1987): Induction of nitrate/nitrate synthesis in murine macrophages by BCG infection lymphokines, or interferon-γ. *J. Immunol.,* 139:518–525.

211. Sugarman, B. J., Aggarwal, B. B., Hass, P. E., Figari, I. S., Palladino, M. A., and Shepard, H. M. (1985): Recombinant human tumor necrosis factor-α: Effects on proliferation of normal and transformed cells in vitro. *Science,* 230:943–945.

212. Svedersky, L. P., Benton, C. V., Berger, W. H., Rinderknecht, E., Harkins, R. N., and Palladino, M. A. (1984): Biological and antigenic similarities of murine interferon-γ and macrophage-activating factor. *J. Exp. Med.,* 159:812–827.

213. Svedersky, L. P., Nedwin, G. E., Goeddel, D. V., and Palladino, M. A., Jr. (1985): Interferon-gamma enhances induction of lymphotoxin in recombinant interleukin 2-stimulated peripheral blood mononuclear cells. *J. Immunol.,* 134:1604–1608.

214. Taylor, J. (1964): Inhibition of interferon action by actinomycin. *Biochem. Biophys. Res. Commun.,* 14:447–451.

215. Thompson, M. R., Zhang, Z., Fournier, A., and Tan, Y. H. (1985): Characterization of human β-interferon-binding sites on human cells. *J. Biol. Chem.,* 260:563–567.

216. Thurman, G. B., Braude, I. A., Gray, P. W., Oldham, R. K., and Stevenson, H. C. (1985): MIF-like activity of natural and recombinant human interferon-gamma and their neutralization by monoclonal antibody. *J. Immunol.,* 134:305–309.

217. Torseth, J. W., and Merigan, T. C. (1986): Significance of local gamma interferon in recurrent herpes simplex infection. *J. Infect. Dis.,* 153:979–984.

218. Torti, F. M., Dieckmann, B., Beutler, B., Cerami, A., and Ringold, B. J. (1985): A macrophage factor inhibits adipocyte gene expression: An in vitro model of cachexia. *Science,* 229:867–869.

219. Trent, J. M., Olson, S., and Cawn, R. M. (1982): Chromosomal localization of human leukocyte, fibroblast, and immune interferon genes by means of in situ hybridization. *Proc. Natl. Acad. Sci. USA,* 79:7809–7813.

220. Trinchieri, G., Matsumoto-Kobayashi, M., Clark, S. V., Sheera, J., London, L., and Perussia, B. (1984): Response of resting human peripheral blood natural killer cells to interleukin 2. *J. Exp. Med.,* 160:1147–1169.

221. Tsujimoto, M., and Vilček, J. (1986): Tumor necrosis factor receptors in HeLa cells and their regulation by interferon-gamma. *J. Biol. Chem.,* 261:5384–5388.

222. Turco, J., and Winkler, H. H. (1983): Cloned mouse interferon-γ inhibits the growth of *Rickettsia prowazekii* in cultured mouse fibroblasts. *J. Exp. Med.,* 158:2159–2164.

223. Turco, J., Thompson, H. A., and Winkler, H. H. (1984): Interferon-γ inhibits growth of *Coxiella burnetti* in mouse fibroblasts. *Infect. Immun.* 45:781–783.

224. Turco, J., and Winkler, H. H. (1986): Gamma-interferon induced inhibition of the growth of *Rickettsia prowazekii* in fibroblasts cannot be explained by the degradation of tryptophan or other amino acids. *Infect. Immun.,* 53:38–46.

225. Ulker, N., and Samuel, C. E. (1985): Mechanism of interferon action: Inhibition of vesicular stomatitis virus replication in human amnion U cells by cloned human γ-interferon. *J. Biol. Chem.,* 260: 4319–4323.

226. Van Damme, J., Opdenakker, G., Simpson, R. J., Rubira, M. R., Cayphas, S., Vink, A., Billiau, A., and Van Snick, J. (1987): Identification of the human 26K protein (IFN-β₂) as a B-cell hybridoma/plasmacytoma growth factor induced by interleukin-1 and tumor necrosis factor. *J. Exp. Med.,* 165:914–919.

227. Verhagen, M., Divizia, M., Vendenbussche, P., Kuwata, T., and Content, J. (1980): Abnormal behavior of interferon-induced enzymatic activities in an interferon-resistant cell line. *Proc. Natl. Acad. Sci. USA,* 77:4479–4483.

228. Vilček, J., Klion, A., Henriksen-DeStefano, D., Zemtsov, A., Davidson, D. M., Davidson, M., Friedman-Kien, A. E., and Le, J. (1986): Defective gamma-interferon production in peripheral blood leukocytes of patients with acute tuberculosis. *J. Clin. Immunol.,* 6:146–151.

229. Vilček, J., Palombella, V. J., Henriksen-DeStefano, D., Swenson, C., Feinman, R., Hirai, M., and Tsujimoto, M. (1986): Fibroblast growth enhancing activity of tumor necrosis factor and its relationship to other polypeptide growth factors. *J. Exp. Med.,* 163: 632–643.

230. Virelizer, J. L., Chan, E. L., and Allison, A. C. (1977): Immunosuppressive effects of lymphocyte (type II) and leukocyte (type I) interferon on primary antibody responses in vivo and in vitro. *Clin. Exp. Immunol.*, 30:299–304.

231. Vogel, S. N., English, K. E., Fertsch, D., and Fultz, M. J. (1983): Differential modulation of macrophage membrane markers by interferon: Analysis of Fc and C3b receptors, Mac-1 and Ia antigen expression. *J. Interferon Res.*, 3:153–160.

232. Volc-Platzer, B., Leibl, H., Luger, T., Zahn, G., and Stingl, G. (1985): Human epidermal cells synthesize HLA-DR alloantigens in vitro upon stimulation with gamma-interferon. *J. Invest. Dermatol.*, 85:16–19.

233. Wachter, H., Curtius, H. C., and Pfleiderer, W., Eds. (1982): *Biochemical and Clinical Aspects of Pteridines, Vol. 1*, pp. 1–372. Walter de Gruyter, Berlin.

234. Walker, E. B., Maino, V., Sanchez-Lanier, M., Warner, N., and Stewart, C. (1984): Murine gamma-interferon activates the release of a macrophage-derived Ia-inducing factor that transfers Ia inductive capacity. *J. Exp. Med.*, 159:1532–1547.

235. Wallach, D., Fellous, M., and Revel, M. (1982): Preferential effect of γ interferon on the synthesis of HLA antigens and their mRNAs in human cells. *Nature*, 299:833–836.

236. Webb, D. R., Mason, K., Semenuk, G., Aune, T. M., and Pierce, C. W. (1985): Purification and analysis of isoforms of soluble immune response suppressor (SIRS). *J. Immunol.*, 135:3238–3242.

237. Weil, J., Epstein, C. J., and Epstein, L. B. (1983): A unique set of polypeptides is induced by γ interferon in addition to those induced in common with α and β interferon. *Nature*, 301:437–439.

238. Weinberg, J. B., Hobbs, M. M., and Misukonis, M. A. (1985): Phenotypic characterization of gamma interferon-induced human monocyte polykaryons. *Blood*, 66:1241–1246.

239. Wheelock, E. F. (1965): Interferon-like virus inhibitor induced in human leukocytes by phytohemagglutinin. *Science*, 149:310–311.

240. Wilson, C. B., and Westall, J. (1985): Activation of neonatal and adult human macrophages by alpha, beta, and gamma interferons. *Infect. Immun.*, 49:351–356.

241. Wing, E. J., Ampel, N. M., Waheed, A., and Shadduck, R. K. (1985): Macrophage colony-stimulating factor (M-CSF) enhances the capacity of murine macrophages to secrete oxygen reduction products. *J. Immunol.*, 135:2052–2056.

242. Wirth, J. J., Kierszenbaum, F., Sonnenfeld, G., and Zlotnik, A. (1985): Enhancing effects of gamma interferon on phagocytic cell association with and killing of *Trypanosoma cruzi. Infect. Immun.*, 49:61–66.

243. Wisseman, C. L., Jr., and Waddell, A. (1983): Interferonlike factors from antigen- and mitogen-stimulated human leukocytes with antirickettsial and cytolytic actions on *Rickettsia prowazekii* infected human endothelial cells, fibroblasts, and macrophages. *J. Exp. Med.*, 157:1780–1793.

244. Wong, H. W., and Goeddel, D. V. (1986): Tumour necrosis factors α and β inhibit virus replication and synergize with interferons. *Nature*, 323:819–822.

245. Wood, J. N., and Hovanessian, A. G. (1979): Interferon enhances 2-5A synthetase in embryonal carcinoma cells. *Nature*, 282:74–76.

246. Wright, S. D., Detmers, P. A., Jong, M. T., and Meyer, B. C. (1986): Interferon-gamma depresses binding of ligand by C3b and C3bi receptors on cultured human monocytes, an effect reversed by fibronectin. *J. Exp. Med.*, 163:1245–1259.

247. Wu-Hsieh, B., Zlotnik, A., and Howard, D. H. (1984): T-cell hybridoma-produced lymphokine that activates macrophages to suppress intracellular growth of *Histoplasma capsulatum. Infect. Immun.*, 43:380–385.

248. Yasui, H., Takai, K., Yoshida, R., and Hayaishi, O. (1986): Interferon enhances tryptophan metabolism by inducing pulmonary indoleamine 2,3-dioxygenase: Its possible occurrence in cancer patients. *Proc. Natl. Acad. Sci. USA*, 83:6622–6626.

249. Yip, Y. K., and Vilček, J. (1982): Molecular weight of human gamma interferon is similar to that of other human interferons. *Science*, 215:411–413.

250. Yoshida, R., and Hayaishi, O. (1978): Induction of indoleamine 2,3-dioxygenase by intraperitoneal injection of bacterial lipopolysaccharide. *Proc. Natl. Acad. Sci. USA*, 75:3998–4000.

251. Yoshida, R., Urade, Y., Tokuda, M., and Hayaishi, O. (1979): Induction of indoleamine 2,3-dioxygenase in mouse lung during virus infection. *Proc. Natl. Acad. Sci. USA*, 76:4084–4086.

252. Yoshida, R., Imanishi, J., Oku, T., Kishida, T., and Hayaishi, O. (1981): Induction of pulmonary indoleamine 2,3-dioxygenase by interferon. *Proc. Natl. Acad. Sci. USA*, 28:129–132.

253. Yoshida, R., and Nathan, C. F. (1986): Agonist and antagonist effects of interferon-α and interferon-β on interferon-γ-stimulated release of H₂O₂ from human macrophages. *Clin. Res.*, 34:674 (abstract).

254. Yoshida, R., Oku, T., Imanishi, J., Kishida, T., and Hayaishi, O. (1986): Interferon: A mediator of indoleamine 2,3-dioxygenase induction by lipopolysaccharide, poly I:poly C and pokeweed mitogen in mouse lung. *Arch. Biochem. Biophys.*, 249:596–604.

255. Yoshida, R., Murray, H., and Nathan, C. F. (1987): Two classes of interferon-γ receptors on human macrophages: Blockade of the high-affinity sites by interferons-α or -β (in press).

256. Zoon, K. C., Karasaki, Y., zur Nedden, D. L., Hu, R., and Arnheiter, H. (1986): Modulation of epidermal growth factor receptors by human α interferon. *Proc. Natl. Acad. Sci. USA*, 83:8226–8230.

257. Zoumbos, N. C., Gascon, P., Djeu, J. Y., and Young, N. S. (1985): Interferon is a mediator of hematopoietic suppression in aplastic anemia in vitro and possibly in vivo. *Proc. Natl. Acad. Sci. USA*, 82:188–192.

Inflammation: Basic Principles and Clinical Correlates.
Edited by J. I. Gallin, I. M. Goldstein, and R. Snyderman.
Raven Press, Ltd., New York © 1988.

CHAPTER 15

Cytokines: Myeloid Growth Factors

David W. Golde and Judith C. Gasson

Stem Cells and Hematopoiesis
Humoral Regulation of Myelopoiesis
   GM-CSF • M-CSF • G-CSF

Role of CSF in Inflammation and Host Defense
   Host Defense
Clinical Prospects for Therapeutic Use of CSF
References

The production of granulocytes and mononuclear phagocytes from bone marrow progenitors is tightly regulated in the adult to maintain a relatively constant circulating level of effector cells in the peripheral blood. In the steady state it is estimated that the average production of neutrophils is 0.85×10^9/kg/day. The average person has about 2×10^9 circulating monocytes, and 4×10^8 leave the circulation each day. Unlike erythropoiesis, there is no theoretical limit to the expansion of myelopoiesis, and in disease states there may be more than a tenfold increase in circulating granulocytes. This chapter describes the known human myelopoietic growth factors and discusses their role in inflammation and host defense. Other features of myelopoiesis are discussed in Chapter 16.

STEM CELLS AND HEMATOPOIESIS

A multipotent stem cell is known to exist with the capability of giving rise to all of the formed blood elements (32). Like other stem cells, this multipotent stem cell has the capability to reproduce itself (self-renewal) and to differentiate along several lineages. The process of differentiation may be viewed as one of progressive lineage restriction; thus a myeloid stem cell exists that can give rise to granulocytes, monocytes, erythrocytes, and platelets but is no longer capable of lymphoid differentiation. With progressive differentiation, there is decreasing self-renewal capability. It is believed that when a stem cell becomes restricted to a single lineage, it no longer has extensive self-renewing capability and is frequently referred to as a

progenitor cell. A progenitor cell capable of giving rise to granulocytes and monocytes has been identified, and similar erythroid lineage-restricted precursors have been defined. Although the steps in hematopoietic cell differentiation can be roughly diagramed as in Fig. 1, it should be appreciated that lineage restriction is a progressive event in stem cell differentiation, and many intermediary stem cell levels have not been defined.

What regulates stem cell proliferation and differentiation? There is no simple answer to this question, although the weight of evidence suggests that the "decision" for a stem cell to self-renew or differentiate is a random or stochastic event (32). On the molecular level, differentiation may be viewed as a process in which lineage restriction is evidenced by the expression of specific cell surface receptor proteins and the absence of expression of others. Thus lineage-restricted responsiveness to growth factors is determined by the expression of specific hormone receptors. In this view, expansion of the granulocytic compartment would be accomplished by a rise in granulocyte-specific growth factors, leading to an expansion of progenitor cells with these receptors, ultimately causing increased production of mature effector cells. Thus the levels of circulating granulocytes and monocytes are regulated by specific hormones referred to as hemopoietins or colony-stimulating factors (20,21,39). Because the physiological function of erythrocytes is to transport oxygen, it is logical that erythropoiesis should be tied to the need for oxygen-carrying capacity. In fact, the hormone erythropoietin is regulated by "oxygen sensors" in the kidney. The "sensing" mechanisms for myelopoiesis are

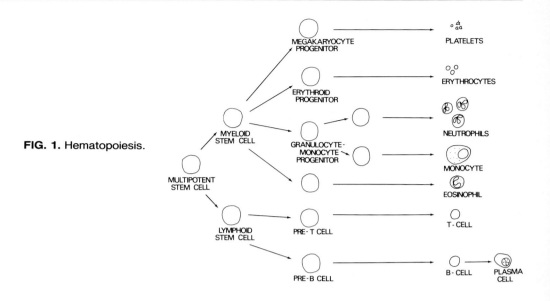

FIG. 1. Hematopoiesis.

not well defined, although mediators involved in host defense against microorganisms and in inflammation likely play an important role.

Although the regulation of stem cell development at the earliest levels is poorly understood, it is known that environmental factors are important (46). Thus in the adult normal hematopoiesis occurs only in the bone marrow, where the microenvironment is believed to be suitable for stem cell development. Although these microenvironmental influences are critical, the specifics of this system have not been delineated. Certain structural proteins such as fibronectin appear to be important, as are various stromal cells, including endothelial and fibroblast-like cells. These stromal cells may function in a number of ways with regard to hematopoiesis. They may produce structural proteins such as fibronectin, collagen, and laminin, which are stem cell permissive, and they may also produce hormones locally that are either permissive or directive with regard to stem cell development. Moreover, lymphocytes and macrophages in the bone marrow may produce hemopoietins *in situ* (4,19). The local production and action of such hormones may constitute an important paracrine system in hematopoiesis.

The factors that regulate stem cell replication and differentiation are not well understood. Interleukin-3 (IL-3) is a hemopoietin produced by activated T-lymphocytes that stimulates replication of pluripotent stem cells and precursor cells of all lineages, including basophils/mast cells (7). The human equivalent of IL-3 has been defined (50), and a hormone (hemopoietin-1) with no direct growth factor activity has been identified that enhances stem cell responsiveness to other hematopoietic growth factors. Evidence suggests that hemopoietin-1 is molecularly identical to interleukin-1 (IL-1).

As with any homeostatic system, there must be mechanisms for dampening a positive response to a growth stimulus. Although many inhibitors of myelopoiesis have been described, their physiological role has not been convincingly demonstrated. Although inhibitors may be significant in modulating hematopoiesis, it is also possible that dampening of the system may occur simply by withdrawal of positive stimuli.

HUMORAL REGULATION OF MYELOPOIESIS

The humoral regulators involved in myelopoiesis have been defined by *in vitro* culture systems (20). In 1965 and 1966 techniques for establishing the clonal growth of hematopoietic cells *in vitro* were described (1,33). These systems were later refined, but all have used a semisolid matrix to grow and analyze colonies of hematopoietic cells. Thus the humoral regulators of hematopoiesis defined by these systems have been referred to as colony-stimulating factors (CSFs) (20,21).

Humoral regulation of myelopoiesis has been extensively studied in murine systems; this chapter emphasizes the human regulators. Granulocyte–monocyte colony formation from human bone marrow cells was known to be stimulated by conditioned medium from peripheral blood leukocytes. Because it was found early that mononuclear phagocytes and stimulated T-lymphocytes produced potent colony-stimulating activities, much attention focused on these cells as producers or regulators of human myelopoiesis (4,19). In the mouse all tissues were found to produce some type of colony-stimulating activity, but ultimately four distinct CSFs were purified and characterized. These factors are granulocyte–macrophage CSF

(GM-CSF), G-CSF, M-CSF (macrophage CSF or CSF-1), and multi-CSF, referred to as IL-3 (7,22). The human analogs for GM-, M-, and G-CSF have been identified and analyzed at the molecular level (Table 1). The human equivalent for IL-3 has been identified, and the information available regarding its biology suggests close concordance with activities so critical to murine IL-3.

GM-CSF

Human GM-CSF was first purified from a human T-cell leukemia virus (HTLV)-II-infected human T-lymphoblastoid cell line known as Mo (10). The purified hormone is a glycoprotein of 22,000 molecular weight and was found to be identical with a previously described lymphokine referred to as neutrophil-migration inhibitory factor from T-cells (NIF-T) (43). This finding was consistent with previous evidence from both murine and human studies indicating that CSFs had direct effects on mature effector cells.

The complementary DNA (cDNA) encoding the human GM-CSF protein was first molecularly cloned by Wong and co-workers (48) and later by others (3,18). Initial cloning employed an expression system in monkey COS cells and screening of conditioned medium with a human myeloid leukemia cell line, KG-1, which responds to CSF (15). Analysis of the full-length cDNA for human GM-CSF revealed an open reading frame of 432 nucleotides encoding 144 amino acids. The mature protein has 127 amino acid residues after cleavage of a 17-amino acid leader sequence characteristic of secreted proteins. The human GM-CSF cDNA has significant homology only with the mouse GM-CSF, and there is approximately 60% amino acid homology throughout the molecule. The positioning of four cysteine residues is preserved between the mouse and human protein, suggesting important disulfide bridges in the structure of GM-CSF. There is both *N*- and *O*-linked glycosylation. Despite the homologies, human GM-CSF has no activity on mouse bone marrow.

Biosynthetic GM-CSF is produced in monkey COS cells or Chinese hamster ovary (CHO) cells using mammalian expression vectors; it also has been expressed in yeast and in bacteria in an unglycosylated form. The biosynthetic GM-CSF stimulates the production of neutrophil and monocyte colonies, pure neutrophil colonies, and eosinophil colonies in semisolid gel culture (24,40). Thus GM-CSF appears to be a human eosinophilopoietin, as well as a stimulator of granulocytes and monocytes. GM-CSF also augments the *in vitro* growth of erythroid progenitors known as burst-forming units (BFUs), although it is not clear that this effect is a direct one on erythroid precursors (24,36).

The activity of GM-CSF is seen in a concentration range between 1 and 100 pM. Half-maximal activity is usually seen at about 10 pM, and the purified biosynthetic material has a specific activity of 2×10^8 units/mg of protein. Thus human GM-CSF, like other human polypeptide hormones, acts in the low picomolar range. Specific receptors for human GM-CSF have been found on the leukemic myeloid cell lines HL-60 and KG-1, and on mature neutrophils, monocytes, and eosinophils (9). A high-affinity binding site has been defined, with a dissociation constant (Kd) of 10 to 30 pM. All biologic effects of human GM-CSF appear to occur in a range of concentrations suggesting interaction with this high-affinity receptor. No receptors have been identified on human erythroid cell lines or, thus far, on nonhematopoietic cells.

The human gene for GM-CSF has been molecularly cloned using cDNA as a probe (13). The GM-CSF gene exists as a single copy and is about 2.5 kilobases (kb) in length, comprising four exons and three introns. The gene has been localized to the long arm of chromosome 5 at bands q23–q31. This region is deleted in the 5q⁻ syndrome, a disorder characterized by refractory anemia in elderly women (17). Expression of the gene for human GM-CSF appears to be tightly regulated. Constitutive production has not been defined in any human cell, although it is produced by a number of HTLV-infected human T-lymphoblastoid cell lines and by a bladder carcinoma cell line referred to as 5637 (8,45). Messenger RNA (mRNA) for human GM-CSF and bioactive, immunoreactive protein are produced by normal T-lymphocytes responding to antigen or lectin, and endothelial

TABLE 1. *Human colony-stimulating factors*

Factor	Other names	MW of glycoprotein	Deduced MW of protein	Colonies stimulated[a]
GM-CSF	CSF-α, NIF-T, pluripoietin	22,000 (major form)	14,300	N, M, NM, BFU-E, eosinophils
G-CSF	CSF-β, pluripoietin	19,600	18,800	N, BFU-E
M-CSF	CSF-1, urinary CSF	70,000–90,000 (dimer)	21,000 (subunit)	M
IL-3	Multi-CSF	~20,000	14,600	Stem cells, NM, BFU-E, Meg

[a] N = neutrophil. M = monocyte/macrophage. NM = mixed neutrophil/monocyte. BFU-E = erythroid progenitor ("burst-forming unit"). Meg = megakaryocyte.

and some fibroblast cells responding to tumor necrosis factor, IL-1, or endotoxin. Thus it appears that the hormone is not produced constitutively by normal cells but can be induced in T-lymphocytes, endothelial cells, and certain fibroblastic cells when they are appropriately stimulated (2,27,48,51).

Human GM-CSF has a number of demonstrable effects on functions of mature neutrophils. It markedly inhibits the migration of neutrophils in vitro after a period of augmenting chemotactic responses to chemoattractants such as the N-formylated oligopeptide f-met-leu-phe. An important action of human GM-CSF on neutrophils is cellular priming for enhanced oxidative metabolism (42). Thus GM-CSF, although having no direct effect on neutrophil oxidative metabolism, causes a pronounced increase of superoxide production in response to f-met-leu-phe and other stimuli such as C5a and leukotriene B_4 (44). GM-CSF also augments neutrophil antibody-dependent cell-mediated cytotoxicity (ADCC) and increases the capacity of neutrophils to phagocytose opsonized staphylococci (6). GM-CSF causes eosinophils to augment their production of leukotriene C_4 in response to calcium ionophore and to enhance ADCC killing of schistosome larvae (37). The mature mononuclear phagocyte is also a target for GM-CSF action. GM-CSF induces macrophage tumoricidal activity (11) and causes U937 cells (a monocyte-like cell) to become functionally more active. Thus it has become clear that GM-CSF has effects on the proliferation of precursor cells and multiple effects regulating the activity of mature myeloid effector cells.

GM-CSF administration to monkeys leads to a prominent, dose-dependent increase in circulating leukocytes (5). When GM-CSF, with a specific activity of 1×10^7 to 2×10^7 units/mg, was infused at 50 units/hr/kg for 10 days, the white blood cell count reached a peak of about $60,000/\mu l$ at 8 days, with a prominent increase in neutrophils and eosinophils and a lesser augmentation in monocytes and some increase in lymphocytes. GM-CSF produced in Escherichia coli (unglycosylated) is also effective in stimulating myelopoiesis in monkeys, and it primes neutrophils in vivo for augmented oxidative metabolism when they are subsequently stimulated in vitro. Thus the effectiveness of GM-CSF as a granulopoietic hormone has been confirmed in vivo.

M-CSF

Macrophage CSF, or CSF-1, is a macrophage-specific growth factor that was initially purified from mouse L-cells and human urine (20,21,39). Human M-CSF is a glycosylated homodimer with a molecular size of about 70,000 to 90,000 daltons. Specific immuno- and radioreceptor assays have been developed for this hormone, and high-affinity receptors have been identified on cells of the mononuclear phagocyte lineage and, curiously, on choriocarcinoma cell lines (33). There appears to be a single gene encoding human M-CSF located on the long arm of chromosome 5, and M-CSF cDNAs have been isolated that when expressed in mammalian cells in vitro yield an active protein (14,47). There are multiple forms of M-CSF mRNA, and many tissues express the gene. A reported cDNA from a 1.5- to 2.0-kb message encodes a protein of 224 amino acids, including a putative leader sequence of 32 amino acids. The deduced molecular weight of the mature M-CSF protein is 26 kilodaltons (kD), which is much larger than the deglycosylated subunit (14.5 kD) of the human dimeric M-CSF. An M-CSF cDNA clone has been isolated from the 4.5-kb mRNA (47). This cDNA encodes a 61-kD precursor protein. When expressed in mammalian cells, this cDNA directs synthesis of M-CSF, which is identical in sequence with the purified urinary M-CSF.

The receptor for M-CSF has been shown to be highly related, if not identical, to the product of the c-fms proto-oncogene (34,35). The c-fms gene is also localized to the long arm of chromosome 5, distal to the genes encoding GM-CSF and M-CSF (17). The c-fms gene is induced in cells undergoing mononuclear phagocytic differentiation (12).

Like GM-CSF, M-CSF has prominent effects on the mature mononuclear phagocyte (25). It appears to stimulate activity of the cells as measured by RNA synthesis, protein synthesis, and activation of antibody-dependent cell-mediated cytotoxicity. Exposure of macrophages to M-CSF results in prostaglandin E (PGE) release, increased synthesis of proteinases, and release of tumor necrosis factor and IL-1. M-CSF also activates direct tumoricidal activity of macrophages. M-CSF stimulates proliferation of macrophages and was therefore originally known as macrophage growth factor.

G-CSF

G-CSF is a neutrophil-specific hemopoietin that was originally purified from mouse tissues (30). The human G-CSF has been purified from a bladder carcinoma cell line known as 5637 and a squamous carcinoma cell line, CHU-2 (31,45). This hemopoietin was previously known as CSF-beta, or human pluripotent hematopoietic CSF. cDNAs encoding human G-CSF have been isolated by two groups using oligonucleotide screening with probes constructed on the basis of amino acid sequence of the mature protein (28,38). These groups cloned the cDNA from mRNA obtained from cell lines used to purify the protein. G-CSF has a molecular weight of approximately 19,600, and it stimulates the growth of pure neutrophil colonies. There are no asparagine residues in the G-CSF molecule and hence no *N*-glycosylation; however, *O*-glycosylation is present. The gene encoding G-CSF is located on human chromosome 17.

Unlike human GM-CSF, human G-CSF has activity on mouse tissues and prominently causes differentiation of a murine myelomonocytic leukemic cell line known as WEHI-3B. G-CSF is also a potent inducer of differentiation of the human HL-60 promyelocytic leukemia cell line. The target cells for G-CSF activity appear to be limited to the neutrophilic myelocyte series. G-CSF stimulates ADCC by human neutrophils, and specific receptors for G-CSF have been identified on various murine monomyelocytic cell lines and mature neutrophils (29). The purified protein induces increased oxidative metabolism by neutrophils exposed to f-met-leu-phe. G-CSF, like GM-CSF, has half-maximal activity at approximately 24 pM and maximal effects at about 100 pM. G-CSF also causes an increase in neutrophil alkaline phosphatase and binds specifically to the human granulocytic leukemic cell lines KG-1 and HL-60. The G-CSF receptor on KG-1 cells appears to have a molecular weight of about 50,000.

When G-CSF is administered to mice, there is marked neutrophilia but no apparent effect on red blood cells or lymphocytes. There also appears to be an increase in splenic stem cells (CFU-S) but no increase in eosinophils. Treatment of monkeys with G-CSF in doses from 1 to 100 μg/kg leads to dose-dependent neutrophilia. The cellular sources of G-CSF in man are not yet defined, although the administration of endotoxin appears to result in the release of G-CSF into serum. G-CSF, GM-CSF, and M-CSF are structurally unrelated but apparently play an important and coordinated role in the regulation of myelopoiesis. A summary of the properties of these CSFs is provided in Table 1.

ROLE OF CSF IN INFLAMMATION AND HOST DEFENSE

Host Defense

Strong evidence has accumulated indicating that the CSFs are the specific hemopoietins responsible for regulating the circulating concentrations of granulocytes and mononuclear phagocytes. Thus the most direct role of the CSFs in host defense relates to control of the number of effector cells. The other major action of the CSFs is to modulate the functional state of mature effector cells, including their motility, metabolism, and cytotoxic capacity. When dissecting the physiology of the CSFs in host defense, it is critical to have knowledge regarding the cell producing the hormone and the conditions under which the hormone is elaborated. Unfortunately, information

in this regard is incomplete. Many tissues produce M-CSF; however, the production of GM-CSF appears to be restricted to activated T-lymphocytes, endothelial cells, and some fibroblast cells responding to specific inducers. Tumor necrosis factor, endotoxin, and IL-1 appear to induce GM-CF in endothelium and some fibroblasts. The cellular sources of G-CSF are incompletely defined. Because constitutive production of CSF is not well documented in man, the mechanisms regulating day-to-day granulopoiesis are uncertain. GM-CSF and G-CSF are not present in measurable quantities in normal serum. The circulating level of M-CSF has been reported to be approximately 40 pM, and M-CSF is excreted in the urine. Local hormonal control of hematopoiesis in the bone marrow therefore may be of major importance.

In terms of appropriately augmenting host defense, it is likely that a number of signals such as endotoxin, bacterial chemoattractants, activated complement components, and various inflammatory mediators may play a role in regulating CSF production. Thus it can be envisioned that bacterial invasion leads to the release of signals (e.g., endotoxin), causing the release of CSFs from several cell types and resulting in an augmentation of effector cells for host defense (Fig. 2).

The priming of various effector cells for increased function appears to be a common property of the CSFs. Exposure of neutrophils to GM-CSF leads to increased cellular chemotaxis toward various chemoattractants. This effect is seen over the first 15 min of exposure. Subsequently, there is neutrophil immobilization corresponding to the neutrophil migration-inhibitory factor activity (NIF-T). By 2 hr maximal priming for oxidative metabolism has occurred. These sequential effects on neutrophil activity may be correlated with concomitant changes in receptors for the *N*-formylated oligopeptides such as f-met-leu-phe. Thus after initial exposure to GM-CSF, f-met-leu-phe receptors rapidly increase in number to more than twofold the basal level. This increase in receptors corresponds to the period of increased chemotaxis; how-

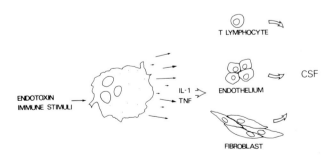

FIG. 2. Macrophage-regulated production of GM-CSF by T-lymphocytes, endothelium, and mesenchymal cells. *IL-1* = interleukin-1. *TNF* = tumor necrosis factor. *CSF* = colony-stimulating factor.

ever, the number of receptors then decreases over time and by 2 hr has returned to basal levels but with a much higher Kd, indicating lower affinity. The presence of low affinity f-met-leu-phe receptors may correspond to the higher levels of ligand found at specific sites of inflammation. Thus one can tentatively construct an outline of mechanisms whereby granulocytes and monocytes may be recruited and primed for activity in host defense (Fig. 3).

The CSFs likely play an important role in the localized inflammatory response (Fig. 4). Cell-mediated immune reactions are initiated by the encounter of specific antigen by sensitized T-lymphocytes. Interaction of the antigen with the specific T-cell receptor leads to T-cell activation and the release of various lymphokines, including GM-CSF. GM-CSF may then stimulate the production of effector cells, including local proliferation of mononuclear phagocytes. The GM-CSF would also facilitate chemotaxis toward the site of inflammation and prime granulocytes, mononuclear phagocytes, and eosinophils for heightened cytotoxic activity. The production of tumor necrosis factor and IL-1 by activated mononuclear phagocytes would lead to the release of CSFs from endothelium and other mesenchymal cells. These types of humoral interaction are likely important in granuloma development (sarcoid, histiocytosis, tuberculosis), and they may also play an important role in the pathophysiology of neoplastic disorders such as Hodgkin's disease.

Whereas the humoral mechanisms involved in the production of effector cells and their activation are important in host defense, conditions may exist whereby these growth factors are inappropriately released when autoimmunity is stimulated (Fig. 3). Under these circumstances it can be envisioned that T-lymphocytes responding to autoantigens are activated and release lymphokines including GM-CSF. In this situation, there would be a recruitment of effector cells and priming as in the physiological situ-

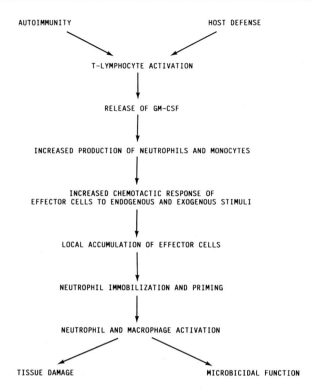

FIG. 4. Role of GM-CSF in the inflammatory response.

ation; however, inappropriate activation of effector cell function might be stimulated by activated complement components or other endogenous mediators. The inappropriate recruitment and activation of neutrophils and mononuclear phagocytes would then result in local tissue damage owing to the release of proteolytic enzymes and toxic moieties resulting from increased oxidative metabolism by these effector cells. It can be predicted that the target tissues sustaining damage in this scenario would be tissues expressing the antigen recognized in the autoimmune reaction.

CLINICAL PROSPECTS FOR THERAPEUTIC USE OF CSF

As previously noted, three human CSFs and IL-3 have been molecularly cloned and can now be produced in sufficient quantity for preclinical testing and human clinical trials. Initial results of testing GM-CSF in monkeys suggest low toxicity and marked efficacy in terms of stimulating myelopoiesis. The bacterially produced, unglycosylated GM-CSF appears to be as effective as the glycosylated protein produced in mammalian cells by recombinant technology. The pharmacokinetics of the

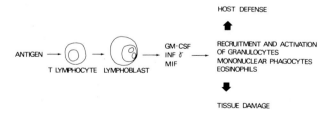

FIG. 3. T-lymphocyte activation leads to GM-CSF release coordinately with other lymphokines, causing recruitment and activation of effector cells. Activated macrophages, in turn, induce GM-CSF production by nonhematopoietic cells. *GM-CSF* = granulocyte-macrophage colony-stimulating factor. *INF* = interferon. *MIF* = macrophage migration-inhibiting factor.

various glycosylated and unglycosylated forms of the CSFs have not been completely worked out. The initial half-life of GM-CSF produced in CHO cells is 7 min (the alpha-phase), and the beta-phase shows an apparent half-life of 80 to 90 min. After 2 hr approximately 10% of a radiolabeled dose of GM-CSF remains in the circulation (5). GM-CSF clearly stimulates neutrophil, monocyte, and eosinophil production, but its *in vivo* effects on erythropoiesis and lymphopoiesis are uncertain. The material has been effective in monkeys when given by continuous intravenous infusion as well as subcutaneously.

G-CSF has also been tested in primates, and because it is active on murine tissues (unlike GM-CSF) it may also be tested *in vivo* in various subprimate species. As previously noted, G-CSF is active *in vivo* with the most prominent effect being an induction of neutrophilia. The effects of both G-CSF and GM-CSF with regard to stem cell activation and effects on the erythroid compartment need to be evaluated in detail in preclinical trials.

The role of M-CSF *in vivo* is not yet clear. The urinary M-CSF has been purified and studied in mice as well as in preliminary human trials (16,23,26,49). Injection of human urinary M-CSF into normal C57 black/6N mice (400,000 units/kg/day for 5 days) resulted in an increase in myeloid progenitors in the femur and spleen without granulocytosis or monocytosis. In previous studies injections of partially purified material led to leukocytosis in mice. Preliminary studies with purified human urinary CSF have been performed in patients undergoing chemotherapy for solid tumors. The CSF was given after chemotherapy and the recovery of neutrophil and monocyte counts measured. The period of granulocytopenia was shortened in treated patients, but the effects were not dramatic. The stimulation of granulocyte production may have been an indirect effect of the urinary CSF acting primarily on macrophages.

Future studies should clarify the potential therapeutic role of the CSFs, and the prospects for their application in human therapeutics is bright. Table 2 provides a list of possible therapeutic uses for various CSFs. It seems that the CSFs will have a major use in treating immunocompromised patients and perhaps may be useful in

cancer chemotherapy under circumstances of inducing an ADCC reaction *in vivo*. Such therapy might involve the use of human monoclonal antibodies or hybrid monoclonal antibodies with a human Fc receptor in which the Fab fragment is directed at a tumor-specific antigen. Such an antibody could be used to target neutrophils and monocytes (via the Fc receptor) for tumoricidal activity. CSFs can also induce direct tumoricidal activity mediated by mononuclear phagocytes. The CSFs also might find prominent use in ameliorating the granulocytopenia associated with chemotherapy or radiation therapy. Treatment of parasitic and other infectious diseases may be facilitated by CSFs. It is possible that a means of blocking CSF action may be developed and may be useful in modifying inflammatory reactions associated with autoimmune disease. It is clear, however, that development of the hematopoietic growth factors as therapeutic agents will herald a new era of medical therapeutics whereby the numbers and activity of host defense cells may be directly regulated by hormonal modulators.

ACKNOWLEDGMENTS

This work was supported by USPHS grants CA 30388, CA 40163, and CA 32737. The authors thank Wendy Aft for preparation of the manuscript.

TABLE 2. *CSFs: potential therapeutic applications*

Prevent/mitigate chemotherapy- and radiation-induced leukopenia
Induce anti-tumor activity *in vivo* (direct cytotoxicity and ADCC)
Improve host defense in immunocompromised patients
Treat infections and parasitic diseases
Facilitate recovery from autologous and allogeneic transplantation

REFERENCES

1. Bradley, T. R., and Metcalf, D. (1966): The growth of mouse bone marrow cells in vitro. *Aust. J. Exp. Biol. Med. Sci.,* 44:287–300.
2. Broudy, V. C., Kaushansky, K., Segal, G. M., Harlan, J. M., and Adamson, J. W. (1987): Tumor necrosis factor type stimulates human endothelial cells to produce granulocyte/macrophage colony-stimulating factor. *Proc. Natl. Acad. Sci. USA,* 83:7467–7471.
3. Cantrell, M. A., Anderson, D., Cerretti, D. P., Price, V., McKereghan, K., Tushinski, R. J., Mochizuki, D. Y., Larsen, A., Grabstein, K., Gillis, S., and Cosman, D. (1985): Cloning, sequence, and expression of a human granulocyte/macrophage colony-stimulating factor. *Proc. Natl. Acad. Sci. USA,* 82:6250–6254.
4. Cline, M. J., and Golde, D. W. (1979): Cellular interactions in haematopoiesis. *Nature,* 277:177–181.
5. Donahue, R. E., Wang, E. A., Stone, D. K., Kamen, R., Wong, G. G., Sehgal, P. K., Nathan, D. G., and Clark, S. C. (1986): Stimulation of hematopoiesis in primates by continuous infusion of recombinant human GM-CSF. *Nature,* 321:872–875.
6. Fleischmann, J., Golde, D. W., Weisbart, R. H., and Gasson, J. C. (1986): Granulocyte-macrophage colony-stimulating factor enhances phagocytosis of bacteria by human neutrophils. *Blood,* 68:708–711.
7. Fung, M. C., Hapel, A. J., Ymer, S., Cohen, D. R., Johnson, R. M., Campbell, H. D., and Young, I. G. (1984): Molecular cloning of cDNA for murine interleukin-3. *Nature,* 307:233–236.
8. Gabrilove, J. L., Welte, K., Harris, P., Platzer, E., Lu, L., Levi, E., Mertelsmann, R., and Moore, M. A. S. (1986): Pluripoietin α: a second human hematopoietic colony-stimulating factor produced by the human bladder carcinoma cell line 5637. *Proc. Natl. Acad. Sci. USA,* 83:2478–2482.
9. Gasson, J. C., Kaufman, S. E., Weisbart, R. H., Tomonaga, M., and Golde, D. W. (1986): High affinity binding of granulocyte-macro-

phage colony-stimulating factor to normal and leukemic human myeloid cells. *Proc. Natl. Acad. Sci. USA,* 83:669–673.

10. Gasson, J. C., Weisbart, R. H., Kaufman, S. E., Clark, S. C., Hewick, R. M., Wong, G. G., and Golde, D. W. (1984): Purified human granulocyte-macrophage colony-stimulating factor: direct action on neutrophils. *Science,* 226:1339–1342.

11. Grabstein, K. H., Urdal, D. L., Tushinski, R. J., Mochizuki, D. Y., Price, V. L., Cantrell, M. A., Gillis, S., and Conlon, P. J. (1986): Induction of macrophage tumoricidal activity by granulocyte-macrophage colony-stimulating factor. *Science,* 232:506–508.

12. Guilbert, L. J., and Stanley, E. R. (1986): The interaction of ^{125}-I-colony-stimulating factor-1 with bone marrow-derived macrophages. *J. Biol. Chem.,* 261:4024–4032.

13. Huebner, K., Isobe, M., Croce, C. M., Golde, D. W., Kaufman, S. E., and Gasson, J. C. (1985): The human gene encoding GM-CSF is at 5q21–q32, the chromosome region deleted in the 5q-anomaly. *Science,* 230:1282–1285.

14. Kawasaki, E. S., Ladner, M. B., Wang, A. M., Van Arsdell, J., Warren, M. K., Coyne, M. Y., Schweickart, V. L., Lee, M-T., Wilson, K. J., Boosman, A., Stanley, E. R., Ralph, P., and Mark, D. F. (1985): Molecular cloning of a complementary DNA encoding human macrophage-specific colony-stimulating factor (CSF-1). *Science,* 230: 291–296.

15. Koeffler, H. P., and Golde, D. W. (1978): Acute myelogenous leukemia: a human cell line responsive to colony-stimulating activity. *Science,* 200:1153–1154.

16. Kohsaki, M., Noguchi, K., Araki, K., Horikoshi, A., Sloman, J. C., Miyake, T., and Murphy, M. J. (1983): In vitro stimulation of murine granulopoiesis by human urinary extract of patients with aplastic anemia. *Proc. Natl. Acad. Sci. USA,* 80:3802–3806.

17. Le Beau, M. M., Westbrook, C. A., Diaz, M. O., Larson, R. A., Rowley, J. D., Gasson, J. C., Golde, D. W., and Sherr, C. J. (1986): Evidence for the involvement of GM-CSF and c-fms in the deletion (5q) in myeloid disorders. *Science,* 231:984–987.

18. Lee, F., Yokota, T., Otsuka, T., Gemmell, L., Larson, N., Luh, J., Arai, K-I., and Rennick, D. (1985): Isolation of cDNA for a human granuloctye-macrophage colony-stimulating factor by functional expression in mammalian cells. *Proc. Natl. Acad. Sci. USA,* 82:4360–4364.

19. Lipton, J. M., and Nathan, D. G. (1985): Interaction between lymphocytes and macrophages in hematopoiesis. In: *Hematopoietic Stem Cells,* edited by D. W. Golde and F. Takaku, pp. 145–202. Marcel Dekker, New York.

20. Metcalf, D. (1984): *The Hematopoietic Colony Stimulated Factors.* Elsevier, Amsterdam.

21. Metcalf, D. (1985): The granulocyte-macrophage colony-stimulating factors. *Science,* 229:16–22.

22. Metcalf, D. (1986): The molecular biology and functions of the granulocyte-macrophage colony-stimulating factors. *Blood,* 67:257–267.

23. Metcalf, D., and Stanley, E. R. (1971): Haematological effects in mice of partially purified colony-stimulating factor (CSF) prepared from human urine. *Br. J. Haematol.,* 21:481–492.

24. Metcalf, D., Begley, C. G., Johnson, G. R., Nicola, N. A., Vadas, M. A., Lopez, A. F., Williamson, D. J., Wong, G. G., Clark, S. C., and Wang, E. A. (1986): Biologic properties in vitro of a recombinant human granulocyte-macrophage colony-stimulating factor. *Blood,* 67:37–45.

25. Moore, R. N., Hoffeld, J. T., Farrar, J. J., Mergenhagen, S. E., Oppenheim, J. J., and Shadduck, R. K. (1981): Role of colony-stimulating factors as primary regulators of macrophage functions. In: *Lymphokines,* Vol. 3, pp. 119–148. Academic Press, New York.

26. Motoyoshi, K., Takaku, F., Kusumoto, K., Miura, Y., Yamanaka, T., and Kimura, K. (1982): Phase I and early phase II studies on human urinary colony-stimulating factor. *Jpn. J. Med.,* 21:187–191.

27. Munker, R., Gasson, J., Ogawa, M., and Koeffler, H. P. (1986): Recombinant human tumor necrosis factor induces production of granulocyte-monocyte colony stimulating factor mRNA and protein from lung fibroblasts and vascular endothelial cells in vitro. *Nature,* 323:79–82.

28. Nagata, S., Tsuchiya, M., Asano, S., Kaziro, Y., Yamazaki, T., Yamamoto, O., Hirata, Y., Kubota, N., Oheda, M., Nomura, H., and Ono, M. (1986): Molecular cloning and expression of cDNA for human granulocyte colony-stimulating factor. *Nature,* 319:415–418.

29. Nicola, N. A., and Metcalf, D. (1984): Binding of the differentiation-inducer, granulocyte-colony-stimulating factor, to responsive but not unresponsive leukemic cell lines. *Proc. Natl. Acad. Sci. USA,* 81: 3765–3769.

30. Nicola, N. A., Begley, C. G., and Metcalf, D. (1985): Identification of the human analogue of a regulator that induces differentiation in murine leukaemic cells. *Nature,* 314:625–628.

31. Nomura, H., Imazeki, I., Oheda, M., Kubota, N., Tamura, M., Ono, M., Ueyama, Y., and Asano, S. (1986): Purification and characterization of human granulocyte colony-stimulating factor (G-CSF). *EMBO J.,* 5:871–876.

32. Pharr, P. P., and Ogawa, M. (1985): Pluripotent stem cells. In: *Hematopoietic Stem Cells,* edited by D. W. Golde and F. Takaku, pp. 3–18. Marcel Dekker, New York.

33. Pluznick, D. H., and Sachs, L. (1965): The cloning of normal "mast" cells in tissue culture. *J. Cell. Physiol.,* 66:319–324.

34. Rettenmier, C. W., Sacca, R., Furman, W. L., Roussel, M. F., Holt, J. T., Nienhuis, A. W., Stanley, E. R., and Sherr, C. J. (1986): Expression of the human c-fms proto-oncogene product (colony-stimulating factor-1 receptor) on peripheral blood mononuclear cells and choriocarcinoma cell line. *J. Clin. Invest.,* 77:1740–1746.

35. Sherr, C. J., Rettenmier, C. W., Sacca, R., Roussel, M. F., Look, A. T., and Stanley, E. R. (1985): The c-fms proto-oncogene product is related to the receptor for the mononuclear phagocyte growth factor, CSF-1. *Cell,* 41:665–676.

36. Sieff, C. A., Emerson, S. G., Donahue, R. E., and Nathan, D. G. (1985): Human recombinant granulocyte-macrophage colony-stimulating factor: a multilineage hematopoietin. *Science,* 230:1171–1173.

37. Silberstein, D. S., Owen, W. F., Gasson, J. C., DiPersio, J. F., Golde, D. W., Bina, J. C., Soberman, R., Austen, K. F., and David, J. R. (1986): Regulation of human eosinophil function by granulocyte-macrophage colony-stimulating factor. *J. Immunol.,* 137:3290–3294.

38. Souza, L. M., Boone, T. C., Gabrilove, J., Lai, P. H., Zsebo, K. M., Murdock, D. C., Chazin, V. R., Bruszewski, J., Lu, H., Chen, K. K., Barendt, J., Platzer, E., Moore, M. A. S., Mertelsmann, R., and Welte, K. (1986): Recombinant human granulocyte colony-stimulating factor: effects on normal and leukemic myeloid cells. *Science,* 232:61–65.

39. Stanley, E. R. (1984): Hemopoietic growth factors. In: *Hematopoiesis: Methods in Hematology,* edited by D. W. Golde, pp. 319–332. Churchill Livingstone, New York.

40. Tomonaga, M., Golde, D. W., and Gasson, J. C. (1986): Biosynthetic (recombinant) human granulocyte-macrophage colony-stimulating factor: effect on normal bone marrow and leukemia cell lines. *Blood,* 67:31–36.

41. Weisbart, R. H., Golde, D. W., and Gasson, J. C. (1986): Biosynthetic human GM-CSF modulates the number and affinity of neutrophil f-met-leu-phe-receptors. *J. Immunol.,* 137:3584–3587.

42. Weisbart, R. H., Golde, D. W., Clark, S. C., Wong, G. G., and Gasson, J. C. (1985): Human granulocyte-macrophage colony-stimulating factor is a neutrophil activator. *Nature,* 314:361–363.

43. Weisbart, R. H., Golde, D. W., Spolter, L., Eggena, P., and Rinderknecht, H. (1979): Neutrophil migration inhibition factor from T-lymphocytes (NIF-T): a new lymphokine. *Clin. Immunol. Immunopathol.,* 14:441–448.

44. Weisbart, R. H., Kwan, L., Golde, D. W., and Gasson, J. C. (1987): Human GM-CSF primes neutrophils for enhanced oxidative metabolism in response to the major physiologic chemoattractants. *Blood,* 69:18–21.

45. Welte, K., Platzer, E., Lu, L., Gabrilove, J. L., Levi, E., Mertelsmann, R., and Moore, M. A. S. (1985): Purification and biochemical characterization of human pluripotent hematopoietic colony-stimulating factor. *Proc. Natl. Acad. Sci. USA,* 82:1526–1530.

46. Wolf, N. (1979): The haemopoietic microenvironment. *Clin. Haematol.,* 8:469–500.

47. Wong, G. G., Temple, P. A., Leary, A. C., Witek-Giannotti, J. S., Yang, Y-C., Ciarletta, A. B., Chung, M., Murtha, P., Kriz, R., Kaufman, R. J., Ferenz, C. R., Sibley, B. S., Turner, K. S., Hewick, R. M., and Clark, S. C. (1987): Human CSF-1: molecular cloning and expression of a 4 kb cDNA encoding the hematopoietin and determination of the complete amino acid sequence of the human urinary protein. *Science,* 235:1504–1508.

48. Wong, G. G., Witek, J. S., Temple, P. A., Wilkens, K. M., Leary, A. C., Luxenburg, D. P., Jones, S. S., Brown, E. L., Kay, R. M., Orr, E. C., Shoemaker, C., Golde, D. W., Kaufman, R. J., Hewick, R. M., Wang, E. A., and Clark, S. C. (1985): Human GM-CSF: molecular cloning of the complementary DNA and purification of the natural and recombinant proteins. *Science,* 228:810–815.

49. Yanai, N., Yamada, M., Watanabe, Y., Saito, M., Kuboyama, M., Motoyoshi, K., Takaku, F., Funakoshi, S., and Watanabe, M. (1983): The granulopoietic effect of human urinary colony stimulating factor on normal and cyclophosphamide treated mice. *Exp. Hematol.,* 11: 1027–1036.

50. Yang, Y-C., Ciarletta, A. B., Temple, P. A., Chung, M. P., Kovacic, S., Witek-Giannotti, J. S., Leary, A. C., Kriz, R., Donahue, R. E., Wong, G. G., and Clark, S. C. (1986): Human IL-3 (multi-CSF): Identification by expression cloning of a novel hematopoietic growth factor related to murine IL-3. *Cell,* 47:3–10.

51. Zucali, J. R., Dinarello, C. A., Oblon, D. J., Gross, M. A., Anderson, L., and Weiner, R. S. (1986): Interleukin 1 stimulates fibroblasts to produce granulocyte-macrophage colony-stimulating activity and prostaglandin E_2. *J. Clin. Invest.,* 77:1857–1863.

Cellular Components
of Inflammation

Inflammation: Basic Principles and Clinical Correlates.
Edited by J. I. Gallin, I. M. Goldstein, and R. Snyderman.
Raven Press, Ltd., New York © 1988.

CHAPTER 16

Phagocytic Cells: Developmental Biology of Neutrophils and Eosinophils

Dorothy Ford Bainton

Neutrophils

Light Microscopy and Peroxidase Histochemistry of Neutrophils in Bone Marrow and Blood Smears • Stages of Neutrophil Differentiation Observed by Electron Microscopy and Peroxidase Cytochemistry • Contents of Neutrophil Granules • Granule Abnormalities • *In Vitro* Experiments on Neutrophil Maturation • Distribution of the Mature Cell in Blood and Tissues

Eosinophils

Light Microscopy of Eosinophils in Bone Marrow and Blood Smears • Electron Microscopy and Cytochemistry • Granule Contents • Granule Abnormalities • *In Vitro* Experiments on Eosinophilic Differentiation • Distribution of the Mature Eosinophil in Blood and Tissues
References

The ability of each type of leukocyte to perform its special function depends on the synthesis of particular chemical substances during its maturation. Certain leukocytes, e.g., neutrophils and eosinophils, synthesize proteins at regular intervals early in their maturation in bone marrow and store them for days as large cytoplasmic granules. When appropriately stimulated these cells move from blood to tissues, and within seconds the granules may release their contents into an endocytic vacuole or, by fusion with the plasma membrane, to the exterior of the cell.

The bone marrow of a normal adult person weighs about 2,600 g, which is about 4.5% of body weight. Although widely distributed within the various bones, the marrow is a larger organ than even the liver, which weighs about 1,500 g. About 55 to 60% of bone marrow is dedicated to the production of one cell type, the neutrophil. The normal ratio of neutrophils to erythroid cells is 2:1. Developing eosinophils constitute about 3% of the bone marrow. The cellularity of bone marrow varies greatly with age; cells constitute 75% of the marrow in the young, 50% in young adults, and 25% in the elderly, although

there is great variability between individuals of a given age (47). Bone marrow is a highly proliferative tissue, and mitoses are observed in 10 to 25 cells per 1,000 nucleated cells (101).

Three major compartments of differentiation in the bone marrow have been distinguished. The most primitive compartment is characterized by pluripotent cells. These cells may properly be called stem cells, as each has enough proliferative potential, including the potential for self-renewal, to serve as the cellular basis for a self-maintaining hemopoietic clone containing multiple lineages. Such independent clones are the functional units of hemopoietic regulation. Several models of stem cell renewal and commitment have been formulated and are reviewed by Ogawa et al. (69). The favored model proposes that stem cell commitment is governed by progressive and stochastic restriction in the differentiation potentials of stem cells.

The second major compartment of differentiation in the marrow consists of progenitor cells committed to a single hemopoietic lineage. Although these cells have great proliferative potential and have acquired sensitivity to the regulatory mechanisms of their lineage, they are not self-renewing. When triggered by specific stimuli, they undergo terminal differentiation and become effector cells with various functions.

Stem cells can be detected in two ways. Till and McCulloch (92) developed the first assay system, in which stem cells are identified by their ability to form hemopoietic colonies in the spleens of lethally irradiated mice. This method, known as the spleen colony method, demonstrated the existence of a pluripotent stem cell capable of forming erythroid, granulocytic, thrombocytic, or mixed colonies in the spleen. This cell was called the colony-forming unit in the spleen (CFUs). In the second system, stem cells are detected by their ability to form granulocytic colonies in human cell cultures. Cell populations are placed in gel media that permit the descendants of single cells to remain localized as clonal colonies. The number of such colonies formed provides an estimate of progenitor cell frequency. These progenitor cells, called CFUc (colony-forming units in culture), proliferate *in vitro* only in the presence of a variety of colony-stimulating factors and have been reviewed by Metcalf (63). A number of these factors, now called cytokines, have been purified and cloned (see Chapter 15). They show similarities in the amino acid sequence at their *N*-terminus or in the putative signal peptide near the *N*-terminus. Granulocyte-macrophage colony-stimulating factor (GM-CSF) and interleukin-2 have the most extensive homology, about 25% of residues being identical in three regions comprising about 70% of the molecules. Although its evolutionary origin is uncertain, the homology around the *N*-terminus may provide a structural marker for a group of cytokines that act on the pluripotent hemopoietic stem cell and its derivatives (87).

The third and most familiar stage of hemopoiesis consists in cells identifiable by morphologic features, e.g., a characteristic nuclear configuration and the presence of obvious cytoplasmic granules. These cells are either fully mature leukocytes or those undergoing the last few divisions leading to maturity. It is on this third stage of development of neutrophils and eosinophils that this chapter dwells.

NEUTROPHILS

In the normal adult human, the life of polymorphonuclear neutrophils (PMNs) is spent in three environments: bone marrow, blood, and tissues. Bone marrow is the site of the important processes of proliferation and terminal maturation of neutrophilic granulocytes (myeloblast → PMN). Proliferation, consisting in approximately five divisions, takes place only during the first three stages of neutrophil maturation (blast, promyelocyte, and myelocyte). After the myelocyte stage, the cells become

"end cells" (cells no longer capable of mitosis) and enter a large storage pool. About 5 days later they are released into the blood, where they circulate for about 10 hr. Their fate after they have migrated to tissues is unknown, but they probably live for only 1 to 2 days.

Light Microscopy and Peroxidase Histochemistry of Neutrophils in Bone Marrow and Blood Smears

Figure 1 shows the stages of neutrophil maturation. The myeloblast is a relatively undifferentiated cell with a large oval nucleus, sizable nucleoli, and few or no granules. It originates from a precursor pool of stem cells and is followed by the promyelocyte and myelocyte stages, during which two distinct types of granules are formed. The first type, the azurophil or primary granule, is formed during the promyelocyte stage and contains peroxidase. The second type, the specific or secondary granule, is formed later, during the myelocyte stage, and is peroxidase-negative. (In the figure, the azurophil is shown as a solid black granule and the specific granule as a light granule.) The metamyelocyte and band forms are nonsecretory, nonproliferating stages leading to the mature PMN, which contains both types of granule in the proportion 33% azurophils and 67% specifics. The figures in the diagram indicating the time spent in the various stages were determined by isotope-labeling techniques (29). Note that no mitoses occur after the myelocyte stage.

At this point a few comments are necessary to clarify the relation between azurophil and specific granules. Around the turn of the century, it was proposed that the granules produced during the promyelocyte stage, which stain azurophilic (reddish-purple), change, "ripen," or differentiate into specific granules. Such a change would explain why the large, metachromatic reddish-purple azurophils, so prominent in the early neutrophil precursors in Wright-stained smears of normal bone marrow, are no longer observed after the myelocyte stage. It is now known, however, that a loss of metachromasia during maturation accounts for the change in appearance of the azurophils. Increasing concentration of their contents at the myelocyte stage may lead to decreased absorption of dye molecules and lessening metachromasia, particularly if stainable acid mucosubstances form complexes with basic proteins (45). The indisputable electron microscopic demonstration (5,11) that large (~500 nm) peroxidase-positive azurophil granules persist in mature PMNs leaves little doubt that the fairly prominent violet-colored granules visible by light microscopy in mature cells on Wright-stained smears are azurophils whose staining characteristics have altered during maturation. It follows that the most reliable method for visualizing azurophil granules on smears (us-

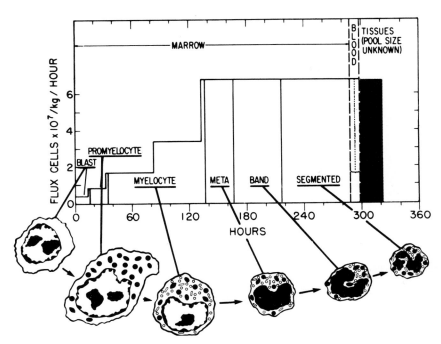

FIG. 1. PMN life span and stages of maturation. See text for discussion. Of every 100 nucleated cells in bone marrow, 2% are myeloblasts, 5% promyelocytes, 12% myelocytes, 22% metamyelocytes and bands, and 20% mature PMNs, yielding a total of ~60% developing PMNs. The times indicated for the various compartments were obtained by isotope labeling techniques (29). The ordinate shows the flux through each compartment, and the abscissa shows the time in each compartment. The stepwise increase in cell numbers through the dividing compartments represents serial divisions. Note that no mitoses occur after the myelocyte stage. (From Bainton, ref. 6.)

ing the light microscope) is to stain the cells for peroxidase. Because most of the specific granules are in a size range (~200 nm; see below) that is at the limit of resolution of the light microscope, they probably cannot be distinguished individually but are responsible for the pink background color of neutrophils during and after the myelocyte stage.

Some mature neutrophils of women have drumstick- or club-shaped nuclear appendages. These appendages are thought to contain an inactivated X chromosome. One study, in which an X chromosome-specific nucleic acid probe was used to detect the position of the X chromosomes in leukocyte nuclei by *in situ* hybridization, provided the first direct evidence of X chromosomal material in the drumstick structures (48).

Stages of Neutrophil Differentiation Observed by Electron Microscopy and Peroxidase Cytochemistry

All of the following observations were derived from specimens of normal human bone marrow and blood tested for peroxidase. The dense enzyme reaction product serves as a marker and stabilizer of azurophil granules (1,11,16,17).

Myeloblast

The earliest cell is a relatively undifferentiated cell with a high nuclear/cytoplasmic ratio and prominent nucleoli. It contains reaction product for peroxidase within the rough-surfaced endoplasmic reticulum (RER) and Golgi

cisternae, and sometimes immature peroxidase-positive azurophil granules.

PMN Promyelocyte

The PMN promyelocyte stage of maturation (Fig. 2) is characterized by the production and accumulation of a large population of peroxidase-positive granules that vary in contour and size; most are spherical (~500 nm), but there are also ellipsoid, crystalline forms, as well as small granules connected by filaments (Fig. 3). Peroxidase is present throughout the secretory apparatus of the promyelocyte, i.e., in cisternae of the RER, in all Golgi cisternae and some vesicles, and in all forming granules. Its presence in these compartments at this stage indicates that it is synthesized and packaged into storage granules by the pathway defined for other secretory proteins (RER → Golgi complex via vesicles → granules).

Hiatal Cell

Peroxidase abruptly disappears from RER and Golgi cisternae at the end of the promyelocyte stage; at this point the production of azurophil granules ceases, and the myelocyte stage and production of the peroxidase-negative specific granules begins. However, cells with the nuclear configuration of the myelocyte, and lacking peroxidase in the RER or Golgi cisternae, often contain mature azurophil but no specific granules; they have large Golgi complexes containing no forming granules of either type.

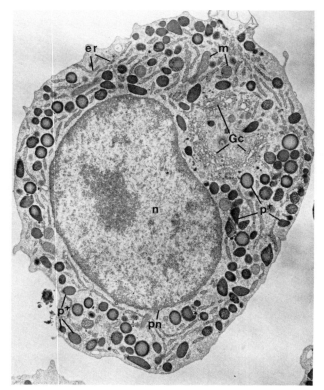

FIG. 2. Electron micrograph of a neutrophilic promyelocyte reacted for peroxidase from normal human bone marrow. This cell is the largest of the neutrophilic series. It has a sizable, slightly indented nucleus (*n*), a prominent Golgi region, and cytoplasm packed with dense peroxidase-positive azurophil granules (*p*⁺) of varying shapes and sizes. Peroxidase reaction product is visible in less concentrated form within all compartments of the secretory apparatus. Endoplasmic reticulum (*er*), perinuclear cisterna (*pn*), and Golgi cisternae (*Gc*). No reaction product is apparent in the cytoplasmic matrix, mitochondria (*m*), or nucleus (*n*). ×9,000. (From Bainton et al., ref. 11.)

Such cells are presumed to exist in a *hiatus* between the two waves of granule formation (5).

PMN Myelocyte

As previously mentioned, the myelocyte stage (Fig. 4) is characterized by the production and accumulation of the peroxidase-negative specific (secondary) granules. The only peroxidase-positive elements present at this stage are the azurophil granules. The specific granules are formed by the Golgi complex (Fig. 5). They vary in size and shape (Figs. 4 and 5) but are typically spherical (~200 nm) or rod-shaped (130 × 1,000 nm). Kinetic studies of human myelocytes (29) indicate that about three divisions occur at this stage of maturation. Mitoses can be observed (Fig.

6), and the two types of granules appear to be distributed to the daughter cells in fairly equal numbers.

Later Stages (Bone Marrow)

The metamyelocyte, band, and mature PMN are nondividing, nonsecretory stages identifiable by their nuclear morphology, mixed granule population, small Golgi regions, and accumulation of glycogen particles (Fig. 1). In the mature PMN the smaller, peroxidase-negative specific granules are twice as abundant as the peroxidase-positive azurophils (Fig. 7). On the average, a cell profile has 200 to 300 granules.

Summary

The data on human PMNs clearly indicate that the peroxidase-positive azurophil and peroxidase-negative specific granules are separate populations of granules that are chemically distinct from the time of their formation and that are both present in the mature PMN. Specific granules become more numerous than azurophils during

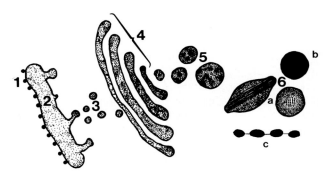

FIG. 3. Hypothetical steps involved in the formation of azurophil granules in normal neutrophilic promyelocytes. Peroxidase reaction product has been observed in increasing concentrations within the RER, Golgi cisternae, and azurophil granules, indicating that in general the pathway of secretion and condensation of this enzyme conforms to that of secretory proteins in the pancreas and in other cell types. These steps include the following: (*1*) synthesis on bound ribosomes, (*2*) segregation within RER cisternae, (*3*) pinching off of vesicles from transitional elements of the RER and their transfer to the Golgi complex via junctional vesicles, (*4*) packing and concentration of the enzyme within the Golgi cisternae and the formation of Golgi-derived vesicles, (*5*) aggregation of smaller vesicles into large, immature azurophil granules, and (*6*) condensation to produce the azurophil granules. Azurophil granules occur in two main forms: Most are spherical (*b*), with dense homogeneous matrices; others are ellipsoid, with crystalline substructures (*a*). Round granule profiles with a central periodicity are presumed to represent ellipsoids cut perpendicular to the crystal axis (*to the right*). A third form (*c*) is distinguished by their small size and the fact that they are interconnected by microtrabeculae (81).

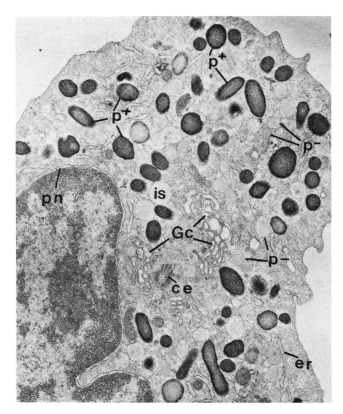

FIG. 4. Neutrophilic myelocyte reacted for peroxidase. At this stage the cell is smaller than the promyelocyte (Fig. 2), the nucleus is more indented, and the cytoplasm contains two types of granule: large, peroxidase-positive azurophils (p^+) and the generally smaller specific granules (p^-), which do not stain for peroxidase. A number of immature specifics (*is*)—larger, less compact, and more irregular in contour than mature granules—appear in the Golgi region. Note that peroxidase reaction product is present only in azurophil granules (p^+) and not in the RER (*er*), perinuclear cisterna (*pn*), or Golgi cisternae (*Gc*). This finding is in keeping with the fact that azurophil granule production has ceased and only peroxidase-negative specifics are produced during the myelocyte stage. *ce* = centriole. ×16,000.

the myelocyte stage because azurophil formation ceases after the promyelocyte stage, the number of azurophils per cell is reduced by mitoses, and specific granules continue to be produced by daughter myelocyte generations. For a more detailed explanation, see Bainton and Farquhar (8). Additional changes that occur during the course of differentiation in regard to surface markers, cytoskeleton elements, and other organelles have been reviewed elsewhere (5).

Contents of Neutrophil Granules

Table 1 lists the components of human neutrophil granules as revealed by both cytochemical and isolation

techniques [see reviews (3,5,53) and references (15a, 47a,71a,84a,104a)]. Because of the marked structural heterogeneity of these granules, investigators have tried several methods for separating their contents into subfractions (22,51,64,74,87,95,100). One ultrastructural and cytochemical study (28) has confirmed previous findings that azurophil granules contain myeloperoxidase and specific granules contain lactoferrin. Other investigators have characterized several bactericidal factors such as defensins (40), ADBF (37a), and BPI (98a), which were previously called phagocytin or cationic proteins (see chapter 24). These factors are found in some azurophil granules. A tertiary granule population containing gelatinase has been tentatively identified (33) but needs further study. Alkaline phosphatase has been localized in the specific granules of the rabbit and several other species (reviewed in references 3,5,53) but appears to be located in a light membrane fraction in human neutrophils. The observations of Garavini et al. (41) are of interest in this regard. They showed that catfish neutrophils are of two types, vacuolated and granulated, and that alkaline phosphatase activity is present only in vacuolated neutrophils, and peroxidase activity only in granulated neutrophils. These findings suggest that the two populations of catfish

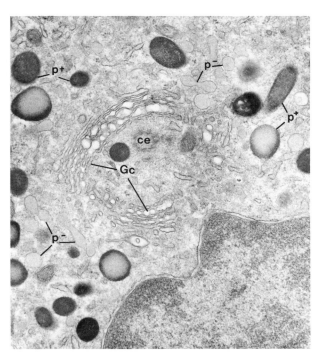

FIG. 5. Golgi region of a neutrophilic myelocyte reacted for peroxidase. As in Fig. 4, peroxidase reaction product is found in azurophils (p^+) but not in specific granules (p^-). The stacked, smooth-surfaced Golgi cisternae (*Gc*) are oriented around the centriole (*ce*). ×23,000.

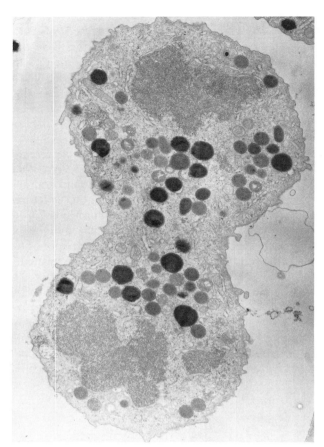

FIG. 6. Myelocyte in the late stage of mitosis from rabbit bone marrow. This myelocyte is in telophase. Note that the granules are being relatively equally distributed to the daughter cells. ×17,000.

neutrophils may have fused later in evolution, and that important steps in neutrophil evolution occurred in fish.

Granule Abnormalities

Some well-documented examples of pathological PMN granulations have been reported, and each can now be classified as a selective abnormality of one granule type or the other. In an attempt to unify the results of studies on the pathology of PMN granules in hereditary or acquired (usually leukemic) disease states, we have proposed the classification shown in Table 2. Additional abnormalities of neutrophils are described elsewhere (see Chapter 26 and refs. 53,106).

Abnormalities of Azurophilic Granules

Quantitative abnormalities

The circulating PMN sometimes contains either a smaller or larger than normal number of azurophils, or

this entire granule population may be missing. Some mature PMNs lack azurophil granules in certain leukemic states, acute myelogenous leukemia (AML) (4,10), and the blastic crisis of chronic myelogenous leukemia (CML) (96). A study (72) of the neutrophilic cells of six children with severe congenital neutropenia and repeated life-threatening infections described several abnormalities, including: (a) the defective synthesis or degeneration of azurophilic (primary) granules, (b) an absence or marked deficiency of specific (secondary) granules, and (c) autophagia. This disease has been called congenital dysgranulopoietic neutropenia.

Qualitative abnormalities

1. *Contents of granules are incomplete.* In some instances azurophil granules may be formed but lack one or more enzymes or other substances. In hereditary myeloperoxidase deficiency, the azurophil granules of neutrophils and monocytes (19,57), but not eosinophils or

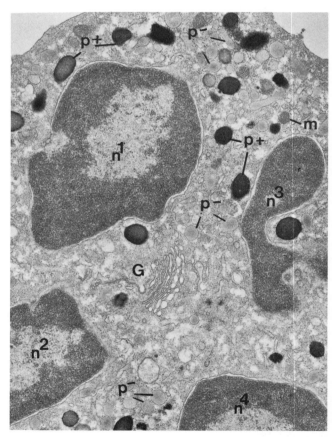

FIG. 7. Mature PMN from normal human bone marrow, reacted for peroxidase. The cytoplasm is filled with granules of the two basic types: the small, pale, peroxidase-negative granules (p^-) and the large, dense, peroxidase-positive granules (p^+). The nucleus is condensed and lobulated (n^1–n^4), the Golgi region (G) is small and without any forming granules, the RER is scant, and mitochondria (m) are few. ×21,000.

TABLE 1. *Constituents of azurophil and specific granules from human neutrophils*

Azurophil granules	Specific granules
Microbicidal enzymes	
Myeloperoxidase	Lysozyme
Lysozyme	
Neutral proteinase	
Elastase	
Cathepsin G	
Proteinase 3	
Acid hydrolases	
β-Glycerophosphatase	Collagenase
β-Glucuronidase	
N-Acetyl-β-	
glucosaminidase	
α-Mannosidase	
Cathepsin B	
Cathepsin D	
Other	
Cationic proteins	Lactoferrin
Defensins	Vitamin B_{12}-binding proteins
Bactericidal permeability	Plasminogen activator
increasing protein (BPI)	Histaminase
Azurophil-derived	Receptors
bactericidal factors	fmet-leu-phe
(ADBF)	CR3 (C3bi)
	Laminin
	Cytochrome b

Subpopulations may exist without these two basic granule types.
Modified from Baggiolini (3).

TABLE 2. *Proposed classification of neutrophil granule abnormalities*

I. Abnormalities of azurophil granules
  A. Quantitative
    1. None
    2. Fewer than normal
    3. More than normal
  B. Qualitative
    1. Contents of granule incomplete
      Example: hereditary peroxidase deficiency (Fig. 8)
    2. Abnormal variants
      Examples: Auer bodies (Fig. 9)
            Chediak-Higashi syndrome (Fig. 10)
II. Abnormalities of specific granules
  A. Quantitative
    1. None
    2. Fewer than normal
    3. More than normal
  B. Qualitative
    1. Contents of granule incomplete
    2. Abnormal variants

Modified from Bainton (7).

basophils, lack peroxidase (Fig. 8). This deficiency occurs in 1/2,000 to 1/5,000 persons (52,76) and is not usually associated with clinical abnormalities. It has been shown (86) that, although not detectable enzymatically, peroxidase can be demonstrated by immunological methods in the neutrophils of individuals with the deficiency. Peroxidase deficiency has also been observed in refractory anemia (58), preleukemia (20), and the blastic crisis of CML (96). In each of these examples of peroxidase deficiency, both types of granules are present and apparently normal, and only the enzyme peroxidase is absent. However, in the hereditary deficiency all of the neutrophils are peroxidase-negative, whereas in the refractory anemias and leukemias (25) the percentage of peroxidase-negative PMNs varies. PMNs lacking peroxidase were observed in

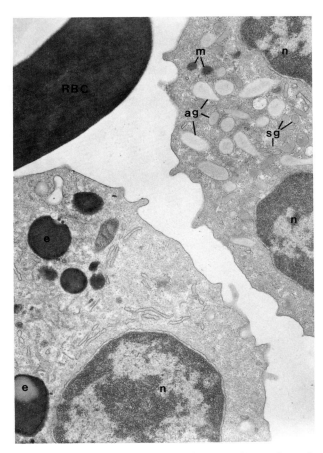

FIG. 8. Neutrophilic PMN, reacted for peroxidase, from the blood of a patient with hereditary peroxidase deficiency. Note that both types of granule are present: the large azurophils (*ag*), pale because of the absence of peroxidase, and the small specific granules (*sg*). Neutrophils and monocytes are devoid of the enzyme, whereas eosinophil and basophil granules are positive. Observe the peroxidase in an eosinophil granule (*e*), as well as the density of the adjacent red blood cell. *m* = mitochondria. *n* = nucleus. ×14,000.

AML (15,25) and in cases of "blast cell transformation" of CML (96). This abnormality, when present, affected 8 to 70% of the circulating PMNs. It has been hypothesized that the deficient PMN may originate from the leukemic precursors (15).

2. *Abnormal variants.* Auer bodies, found in the immature cells of some patients with AML, are abnormally large, elongated, azurophil granules containing peroxidase, lysosomal enzymes, and large crystalline inclusions (reviewed in 10,14,18,94). Although similar to normal azurophil granules in content and staining properties, Auer bodies are "abnormal" because of their gigantic size (Fig. 9). Furthermore, Auer body formation in leukemic blasts and promyelocytes differs markedly from the normal secretory process of azurophil granule formation in that Golgi cisternae contain little peroxidase (10,18).

More Auer bodies can be detected on smears of bone marrow and blood from patients with AML when special stains—peroxidase, chloroacetate esterase, acid phosphatase, or Sudan black—are applied than when Romanovsky stain alone is used. Not all Auer bodies exhibit all these staining characteristics at the same time (7). Hanker et al. (44) modified the Graham and Karnovsky stain for peroxidase (3,3'-diaminobenzidine and H_2O_2 at pH 7.3–

7.6) by poststaining with $Cu(NO_3)_2$. Not surprisingly, this stain reveals additional reactive organelles, "Phi bodies," on smears from patients with AML. The term Phi body was originally introduced to describe the shape of catalase-positive rods in the excretory ducts of mouse salivary glands. Because Auer originally described variably shaped abnormal organelles in leukemia, many hematologists believe that the peroxidase-positive organelles seen in AML leukocytes should be referred to as variants of Auer bodies and not as Phi bodies (7). Finally, it has been suggested that Auer rod formation is an occasional but normal phenomenon in fetal hematopoiesis (66). This observation should be confirmed in other laboratories.

The Chediak-Higashi anomaly or syndrome, a rare autosomal recessive disease, is characterized by oculocutaneous albinism, increased susceptibility to infection, and the presence of abnormally large, lysosome-like organelles in most granule-containing cells. The large inclusions in the PMNs of individuals with Chediak-Higashi syndrome have proved to be enormous abnormal azurophil granules (32,70,82). Normal azurophil granules form early in PMN maturation, but they then fuse to form megagranules; later, during the myelocyte stage, normal specific granules form. The mature circulating PMN contains both the abnormal azurophil and normal specific granules (Fig. 10). The contents of specific granules are present in the megagranules. Giant peroxidase-positive granules have been observed in the PMN of a patient with neutrophil dysfunction (67). These granules were structurally similar to those seen in Chediak-Higashi syndrome, but the PMNs were biochemically different in that there was defective activation of the respiratory burst.

In 1974 giant round granules in leukemic cells were observed on Wright-stained smears from two patients with acute myelomonocytic leukemia (97). Because this acquired morphologic abnormality closely mimicked the giant round granules seen in the Chediak-Higashi anomaly, it was termed the pseudo-Chediak-Higashi anomaly of acute leukemia (35,43). In bone marrow from three patients with AML, we have observed enormous, round, pink inclusions resembling ingested erythrocytes in blasts and promyelocytes. Analysis by electron microscopy and peroxidase cytochemistry showed that these inclusions were large, membrane-bound, peroxidase-positive granules with homogeneous content. We believe that they correspond to the abnormal granules of pseudo-Chediak-Higashi anomaly. Like the Auer rods also seen in AML, these granules appear to be an abnormal variant of peroxidase-positive azurophil granules. Their lack of azurophilia is due to the absence of sulfated glycosaminoglycans (34).

In certain inflammatory disorders, morphological changes may occur in peripheral blood neutrophils. The best-known alteration is the "shift to the left," which de-

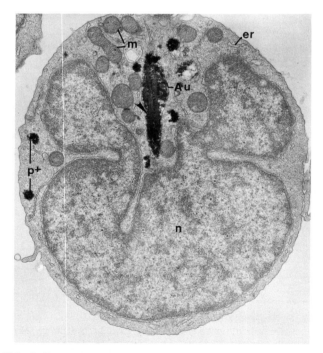

FIG. 9. Peroxidase localization in an abnormal immature cell from a patient with acute myelogenous leukemia. Note the Auer body (*Au*) with its crystalline inclusion (*arrow*) and a matrix containing peroxidase. A few small reactive granules (*p⁺*) are also present. *n* = nucleus. *m* = mitochondria. *er* = RER. ×10,000.

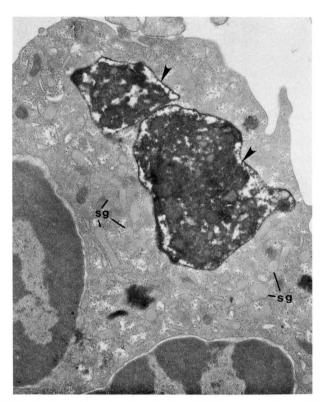

FIG. 10. Peroxidase localization in a PMN from a patient with Chediak-Higashi syndrome. Note that the large megagranules are peroxidase-positive (*arrows*), whereas the specific granules (*sg*) appear normal. ×17,500.

notes the presence of bands, metamyelocytes, and sometimes myelocytes in the circulating blood. The mature PMN may also show certain cytoplasmic modifications including: (a) "toxic" granules, which stain more prominently than those of normal neutrophils; (b) light blue, amorphous inclusion bodies called Dohle bodies; and (c) vacuoles. Toxic granules are azurophils that stain abnormally by light microscopy (62) but which are indistinguishable from normal azurophils by electron microscopy. Dohle bodies are not granules; rather, they have been defined as several rows of RER. They stain as blue bodies in the cytoplasm because of the ribosomes bound to the membrane of the RER (Fig. 11). Functional studies of toxic neutrophils have revealed decreases in chemotaxis and in phagocytic and intracellular bactericidal activities (60,61).

Abnormalities of Specific Granules

Quantitative abnormalities

The three quantitative abnormalities of azurophil granules described above apply to specific granules as well:

circulating PMNs may have smaller or larger than normal quantities of these granules, or may lack them entirely.

The absence of specific granules was first observed in 1974 (91) in a 14-year-old boy with no leukocyte alkaline phosphatase and with recurrent infection. More cases have since been reported (21,39,55). As mentioned above, in congenital dysgranulocytic neutropenia, specific granules may be absent or markedly decreased in number.

The absence or paucity of specific granules in the more mature segmented neutrophils of certain leukemic patients warrants comment. It appears that cytoplasmic development in these cells has ceased after the promyelocytic stage, whereas nuclear maturation has progressed in a fairly normal fashion. The absence of certain normal organelles from mature neutrophils of patients with acute leukemia has been documented by electron microscopy and cytochemistry. For example, we have demonstrated the absence of specific granules in neutrophils from patients with AML (10). We have also observed these abnormal neutrophils quite frequently in acute myeloid leukemia with maturation (i.e., the M_2 variety) as well as in certain cases of hematopoietic dysplasia. Finally, Repine et al. (83) have reported a case of leukemia in which PMNs were deficient in all granules.

Qualitative abnormalities

1. *Contents of granule are incomplete.* The specific granules are present in fairly normal numbers in all PMNs of patients with CML, despite the absence of alkaline phosphatase in most of these PMNs. Thus the low leukocyte alkaline phosphatase score typical of CML seems attributable either to a low activity or to an absence of

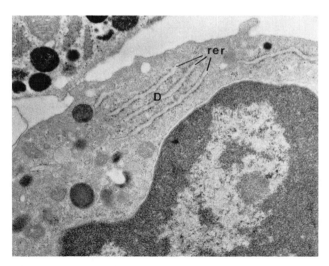

FIG. 11. A portion of a PMN depicts a Dohle body (*D*). It consists of three stacks of RER (*rer*). It stains blue by light microscopy because of the concentration of ribosomes. ×20,000.

the enzyme rather than to a lack of specific granules (96). In addition, studies (68) have shown that the neutrophils of patients with AML lack or are markedly deficient in lactoferrin, a substance found exclusively in the specific granule. Parmely et al. (75) have described a patient with a defect in complex carbohydrate staining that involves both primary and secondary granules.

2. *Abnormal variants.* To our knowledge, no reports of abnormal variants of specific granules have been published.

In Vitro Experiments on Neutrophil Maturation

Cell Lines

Several human acute myeloid leukemia cell lines have become available, as reviewed by Koeffler (54). A cell line developed from a human promyelocyte leukemic cell line in the laboratory of Gallo, and generously distributed to others, has proved to be particularly useful. This cell line, HL-60, was established from the peripheral blood of a patient with acute promyelocytic leukemia (38). It has maintained continuous growth for years in suspension culture without added conditioned medium or colony-stimulating factor, and it is tumorigenic in athymic nude mice. Most HL-60 cells have promyelocytic morphological and histochemical characteristics, but 4 to 15% of them show morphological characteristics of the more mature myeloid cells: myelocytes, metamyelocytes, band forms, and PMNs. Many investigators are now using the HL-60 cell line to analyze the detailed events of early myeloid differentiation, particularly in studies with inducers of differentiation (54).

Enucleated Degranulated PMNs

Roos et al. (85) described the preparation of cytoplasts—vesicles of neutrophil cytoplasm surrounded by plasma membrane and devoid of granules and nucleus. These cytoplasts ingested and killed *Staphylococcus aureus,* proving that neither nucleus nor granules are essential for the killing of these bacteria. Work by Petrequin et al. (78), however, demonstrating some fusion of granule membranes with the plasma membrane of cytoplasts, suggests that degranulation occurs during cytoplast preparation.

Distribution of the Mature Cell in Blood and Tissues

Approximately 100 billion neutrophils enter and leave the circulation daily in normal adults (31,98). The normal sites of destruction of neutrophils have yet to be defined. Many observations suggest that there may be a random loss of granulocytes into the tissues. However, in a study of Jamuar and Cronkite (50), neutrophils were not found in transit through vascular endothelium or in extravascular spaces. Granulocytes did concentrate in the spleen and presumably are destroyed there.

EOSINOPHILS

Light Microscopy of Eosinophils in Bone Marrow and Blood Smears

The earliest identifiable form of the eosinophilic leukocyte is a late myeloblast or early promyelocyte. This cell is about 15 μm in diameter and has a large nucleus, containing nucleoli, and a few granules in intensely basophilic cytoplasm. The later eosinophilic promyelocyte is similar but has less prominent nucleoli and more granules (15–20). Although a few of these granules may stain blue or azure, most are acidophilic. The myelocyte, 18 to 20 μm in diameter, is the largest cell of the development series. It has many more specific (eosinophilic) granules than the promyelocyte, and its nucleoli are difficult to discern. The metamyelocyte is somewhat smaller than the myelocyte and has an indented nucleus. The cytoplasm is tightly packed with eosinophilic granules, but they are somewhat less numerous than in the myelocyte. The band form resembles the metamyelocyte, except that the nucleus has further matured and is shaped like a slightly bent rod. The fully mature eosinophilic leukocyte has a lobed nucleus, and its cytoplasm is filled with larger eosinophilic granules whose rims stain for peroxidase and Sudan black. The nucleus is almost always bilobed, although trilobed forms are sometimes seen. Multilobed nuclei, comparable to those of adult neutrophils, are exceedingly rare (2). Eosinophils are susceptible to mechanical damage during the preparation of blood smears (2). It has been suggested that eosinophilic precursors may degranulate during maturation (24).

Electron Microscopy and Cytochemistry

Early Stages (Promyelocyte and Myelocyte)

When eosinophils of the promyelocyte (Fig. 12) and myelocyte (Fig. 13) stages are stained for peroxidase, reaction product is seen within (a) all cisternae of the RER, including transitional elements, and the perinuclear cisterna; (b) clusters of smooth vesicles at the periphery of the Golgi complex; (c) all cisternae of the Golgi complex; and (d) all immature and mature specific granules (9). The mature granules are completely filled with reaction product except in areas occupied by crystals.

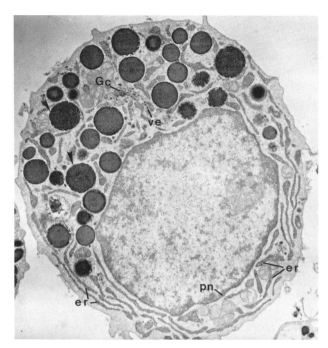

FIG. 12. Human eosinophilic promyelocyte from a preparation incubated for peroxidase. Reaction product appears as a dark flocculent precipitate that fills the entire RER (*er*) including the perinuclear cisterna (*pn*), clusters of smooth vesicles (*ve*) at the periphery of the Golgi complex, all of the cisternae of the Golgi complex (*Gc*), and all the immature granules in the Golgi region and the peripheral cytoplasm. The immature granules (*arrows*) are large and lack the distinctive crystalline bar of mature eosinophils granules. ×10,000.

Later Stages (Metamyelocyte, Band, and Mature Cell)

At the later stages of development, after granule formation has ceased, the eosinophil contains few of the organelles associated with the synthesis and packaging of secretory proteins: RER is sparse or virtually nonexistent, and the Golgi complex is small and inconspicuous. The cytoplasm of the mature eosinophil (Fig. 14) contains primarily granules and glycogen. Most of the granules are specific granules with crystals, which are usually centrally located.

After the myelocyte stage, peroxidase is not detectable in the ER or Golgi elements of the eosinophil by any of the enzyme procedures. It is demonstrable only in the matrix of granules.

Granule Contents

Eosinophil granules contain abundant peroxidase and lysosomal enzymes (9). Eosinophil peroxidase is genetically and biochemically distinct from neutrophil peroxidase, and it appears to play no role in the bactericidal activity of eosinophils (23). Indeed, eosinophils have much less bactericidal activity than neutrophils (102). Immunocytochemical evidence indicates that the specific granules of eosinophils are true peroxisomes in that they also contain catalase (49), two enzymes of peroxisomal lipid β-oxidation [enoyl-CoA hydratase and ketoacyl-CoA thiolase (103)], and a flavoprotein [acyl-CoA oxidase (104)]. All of these substances have been found in the matrix and not the crystalloid of the granule. The eosinophil granule is also known to contain several basic proteins: a major basic protein, eosinophil cationic protein, and eosinophil-derived neurotoxin (77). More than half of the granule protein is the major basic protein, which constitutes the crystalline core of the granule (Fig. 15). It is cytotoxic to parasites as well as normal mammalian cells and induces histamine release from basophils and mast cells. The other two cationic proteins are found in the matrix of the granule (77). One study (105) has shown that eosinophil cationic protein can cause the formation

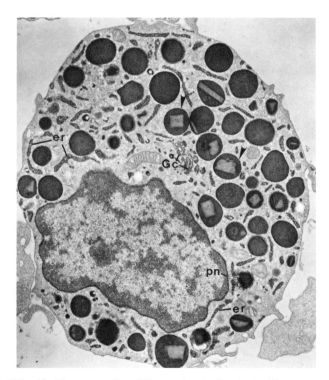

FIG. 13. Human eosinophilic myelocyte incubated for peroxidase. Because peroxidase is still being synthesized, reaction product is present in the ER (*er*), the perinuclear cisterna (*pn*), Golgi elements (*Gc*), and granules. Note that many of the granules now contain a cystalline bar (*arrows*). In mature granules reaction product is not present in the area occupied by the crystalline bar, which stands out sharply against the dark background provided by the remainder of the reactive granule. ×10,000.

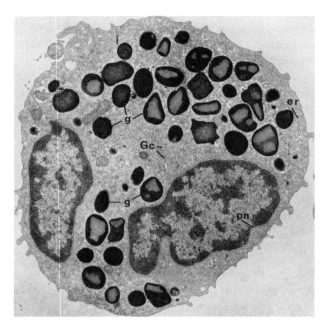

FIG. 14. Human mature eosinophil incubated for peroxidase. Reaction product is present only in granules (*g*). The RER (*er*), including the perinuclear cisterna (*pn*) and the Golgi cisternae (*Gc*), does not contain reaction product. Most of the granules contain the distinctive crystalline bar. ×8,000.

of transmembrane pores and may thereby cause membrane damage. The amino acid sequences of eosinophil cationic protein are remarkably homologous with those of eosinophil-derived neurotoxin, and both sequences show striking homology with those of ribonuclease (42).

The synthesis and secretion of other eosinophil granule substances were reviewed by Spry (90). One long-standing question has been resolved by Weller et al. (99), who showed that Charcot-Leyden crystals, dipyramidal crystals observed in fluids in association with eosinophilic inflammatory reactions, are made of lysophospholipase derived from the plasma membrane of eosinophils. It had previously been assumed that these crystals originated from eosinophil granules.

Granule Abnormalities

Inherited Abnormalities of Eosinophils

Although rare, there are four known inherited abnormalities of eosinophils:

1. The absence of peroxidase and phospholipids in eosinophils is an autosomal-recessive defect that produces no signs of disease (80).

2. In Chediak-Higashi syndrome (32), almost all granulated cells, including eosinophils, contain large abnormal granules.

3. A family was found to have gray inclusions in eosinophils and basophils; the abnormality showed autosomal dominance and had no clinical effects. Electron microscopy revealed cytoplasmic crystals and curved lamella bodies in the cells (93).

Acquired Abnormalities of Eosinophils

Several gross morphologic or cytochemical abnormalities of eosinophils have been observed in leukemias and dysplasias, or in association with benign eosinophilias.

Cytochemistry of abnormal eosinophils in leukemias

In a cytochemical study of eosinophils in acute leukemia (59), the cells were considered normal when they did not show toluidine blue metachromasia or positivity for alkaline phosphatase, chloroacetate esterase, Astra blue, or periodic acid-Schiff (PAS) but did show positivity for peroxidase and Sudan black, and moderate reactivity for naphthol-AS or alpha-naphthyl esterase. The observation of chloroacetate esterase activity in some abnormal eosinophils is of particular interest in view of the subsequent finding that abnormal marrow eosinophils in acute myelomonocytic leukemia (AMML) are associated with the inversion of chromosome 16 (56). Most of the patients studied had a higher than normal percentage of immature

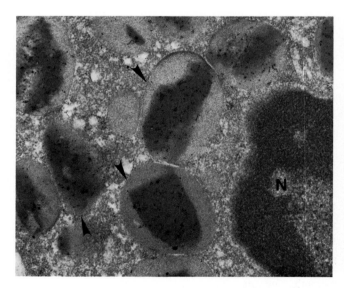

FIG. 15. Localization of major basic protein (MBP) to the core of the eosinophil granule. Sections stained with affinity-purified rabbit anti-human MBP and GCP-goat anti-rabbit IgG show localization of gold particles over the cores of many eosinophil granules (*arrows*). (From Peters et al., ref. 77.)

eosinophils containing a mixture of eosinophilic and basophilic granules. The eosinophilic granules showed abnormal reactivity for chloroacetate esterase and PAS. Electron microscopy revealed that none of the granules had well-formed central crystalloids.

A fairly common abnormality seen in patients with CML is the presence of basophilic and eosinophilic granules in eosinophilic myelocytes and occasionally mature eosinophils (65). Because under normal circumstances eosinophilic and basophilic granules can be viewed as mutually exclusive markers of the respective granulocytic lineages, the presence of both markers in CML cells has been considered a sign of lineage infidelity. This concept deserves further study and confirmation.

Degranulated and light-density eosinophils associated with eosinophilia

The idiopathic hypereosinophilic syndrome (HES) is an interesting disorder defined as follows (46): persistent eosinophilia of 1,500 eosinophils/mm³ for at least 6 months or death before 6 months with signs and symptoms of HES; lack of evidence for parasitic, allergic, or other recognized causes of eosinophilia despite careful evaluation; and signs and symptoms of organ system involvement or dysfunction either directly related to eosinophilia or unexplained in the given clinical setting. Eosinophils with fewer granules than normal can be detected in the blood of patients with a wide variety of eosinophilic disorders and have been reviewed by Spry (90); these cells appear to have undergone degranulation. Metabolic abnormalities of eosinophils (79), and heterogeneity of granule shape and content, as well as lipid inclusions, have also been observed (106).

Intranuclear crystalloids associated with abnormal granules in eosinophilic leukocytes

Eosinophils with abnormal granules and intranuclear crystalloids were observed in a 2-year-old girl with chronic benign neutropenia (73). The father had the same morphologic abnormality but was asymptomatic and had normal leukocyte counts.

Acquired eosinophil nuclear anomaly of pseudo-Pelger-Huet

Incomplete segmentation of the nucleus of mature eosinophils is seen in AML (26) and myelodysplasia (37).

In Vitro Experiments on Eosinophilic Differentiation

The HL-60 leukemic cell line can be induced with specific chemical agents to produce mature cells of the neutrophilic or macrophage lineage. These cells can also dif-

ferentiate to eosinophils and eosinophilic precursors when cultured under mildly alkaline conditions (pH 7.6–7.8) for 7 days without refeeding (36). New cytoplasmic granules are blue in the least mature of these cells and red in the most mature cells when stained with Wright–Giemsa. Most of the cells contain the eosinophil major basic protein, the Charcot-Leyden crystal protein (lysophospholipase), and eosinophil peroxidase. Examination of finely banded chromosomes from these cells has revealed translocation break points at q22 on one chromosome 16 and q23 on the other homolog; abnormalities in this region of the long arm of 16 are a characteristic finding in AMML with abnormal bone marrow eosinophils. Like the bone marrow eosinophils in patients with this disease, the HL-60 eosinophil granules contain material reactive for chloroacetate esterase and PAS, and rarely have crystalloid inclusions. Therefore the HL-60 cell line appears to be suitable for investigating eosinophilopoiesis *in vitro* and may be especially useful for study of the abnormal eosinophils seen in certain malignant conditions (36).

Distribution of the Mature Eosinophil in Blood and Tissues

The turnover time of circulating eosinophils in the rat, as determined by use of tritiated thymidine, is 4.5 days (27). The tissue life span of eosinophils was estimated to be 2 to 4 days in this study and 8 to 12 days in another (71). When blood eosinophils are cultured in the presence of T-cell-conditioned medium, they can survive for 3 weeks or more (90). In a kinetic study of radiolabeled eosinophils in patients with eosinophilia, the mean blood half-life of the cells was 44 hr (30).

Eosinophils are found throughout body tissues and cavities but are most prominent in the gastrointestinal tract. The content of eosinophils in the bowel wall varies; it is usually greatest in the colon. Almost all eosinophils of the alimentary canal are found in the lamina propria and submucosa (2).

It is well recognized that blood and tissue eosinophilia are characteristic of certain types of allergic and parasitic conditions. It is less well recognized that peripheral blood eosinophilia accompanies a wide variety of carcinomas arising from mucin-secreting epithelium (bronchus, gut, pancreas, and uterus) as well as Hodgkin's disease. In this regard, it is of interest that a tumor-derived eosinophilopoietic factor has been extracted from a metastatic pulmonary carcinoma of a patient with an eosinophilic leukemoid reaction (88).

Eosinopenia occurs with acute stress or inflammation. Certain chemotactic substances, e.g., fMLP, have been shown to produce an eosinopenic response in experiments (12,13), but the relevance of this eosinopenic response to acute inflammation is unknown.

REFERENCES

1. Ackerman, G. A., and Clark, M. A. (1971): Ultrastructural localization of peroxidase activity in normal human bone marrow cells. *Z. Zellforsch.,* 117:463–475.
2. Archer, R. K. (1963): *The Eosinophil Leucocytes.* Blackwell Scientific Publications, Oxford.
3. Baggiolini, M. (1980): The neutrophil. In: *The Cell Biology of Inflammation,* edited by G. Weissman, pp. 163–187. Elsevier/North Holland, New York.
4. Bainton, D. F. (1975): Abnormal neutrophils in acute myelogeneous leukemia: identification of subpopulations based on analysis of azurophil and specific granules. *Blood Cells,* 1:191–199.
5. Bainton, D. F. (1977): Differentiation of human neutrophilic granulocytes: normal and abnormal. In: *The Granulocyte: Function and Clinical Utilization,* edited by T. J. Greenwalt and G. A. Jamieson, pp. 1–27. Alan R. Liss, New York.
6. Bainton, D. F. (1980): The cells of inflammation: a general view. In: *The Cell Biology of Inflammation,* Vol. 2, edited by G. Weissman, pp. 1–25. Elsevier/North Holland, New York.
7. Bainton, D. F. (1981): Selective abnormalities of azurophil and specific granules of human neutrophilic leukocytes. *Fed. Proc.,* 40:1443–1450.
8. Bainton, D. F., and Farquhar, M. G. (1966): Origin of granules in polymorphonuclear leukocytes: two types derived from opposite faces of the Golgi complex in developing granulocytes. *J. Cell Biol.,* 28:277–301.
9. Bainton, D. F., and Farquhar, M. G. (1970): Segregation and packaging of granule enzymes in eosinophilic leukocytes. *J. Cell Biol.,* 45:54–73.
10. Bainton, D. F., Friedlander, L. M., and Shohet, S. B. (1977): Abnormalities in granule formation in acute myelogenous leukemia. *Blood,* 49:693–704.
11. Bainton, D. F., Ullyot, J. L., and Farquhar, M. G. (1971): The development of neutrophilic polymorphonuclear leukocytes in human bone marrow: origin and content of azurophil and specific granules. *J. Exp. Med.,* 134:907–934.
12. Bass, D. A. (1975): Behavior of eosinophil leukocytes in acute inflammation. II. Eosinophil dynamics during acute inflammation. *J. Clin. Invest.,* 56:870–879.
13. Bass, D. A., Gonwa, T. A., Szejda, P., Cousart, M. S., De Chatelet, L. R., and McCall, C. E. (1980): Eosinopenia of acute infection: production of eosinopenia by chemotactic factors of acute inflammation. *J. Clin. Invest.,* 65:1265–1271.
14. Beckstead, J. H., Halverson, P. S., Ries, C. A., and Bainton, D. F. (1981): Enzyme histochemistry and immunohistochemistry on biopsy specimens of pathologic human bone marrow. *Blood,* 57:1088–1098.
15. Bendix-Hansen, K., and Nielsen, H. K. (1985): Myeloperoxidase-deficient polymorphonuclear leucocytes (IV): relation to FAB-classification in acute myeloid leukaemia. *Scand J. Haematol.,* 35:174–177.
15a.Borregaard, N., Heiple, J. M., Simons, E. R., and Clark, R. A. (1983): Subcellular localization of the b-cytochrome component of the human neutrophil microbicidal oxidase: translocation during activation. *J. Cell Biol.,* 97:52–61.
16. Brederoo, P., van der Meulen, J., and Daems, W. Th. (1986): Ultrastructural localization of peroxidase activity in developing neutrophil granulocytes from human bone marrow. *Histochemistry,* 84:445–453.
17. Breton-Gorius, J., and Guichard, J. (1969): Etude au microscope electronique de la localisation des peroxydases dane les cellules de la moelle osseuse humaines. *Nouv. Rev. Fr. Hematol.,* 9:678–687.
18. Breton-Gorius, J., and Houssay, D. (1973): Auer bodies in acute promyelocytic leukemia: demonstration of their fine structure and peroxidase localization. *Lab. Invest.,* 28:135–141.
19. Breton-Gorius, J., Coquin, M. Y., and Guichard, J. (1975): Activities peroxydasiques de certaines granulations des neutrophils dans deux cas de déficit congenital en myeloperoxidase. *C. R. Acad. Sci. [D] (Paris),* 280:1753–1756.
20. Breton-Gorius, J., Houssay, D., and Dryfux, B. (1975): Partial myeloperoxidase deficiency in a case of preleukemia. *Br. J. Haematol.,* 30:273–278.
21. Breton-Gorius, J., Mason, D. Y., Buriot, D., Vilde, J. L., and Griscelli, C. (1980): Lactoferrin deficiency as a consequence of a lack of specific granules in neutrophils from a patient with recurrent infections: detection by immunoperoxidase staining for lactoferrin and cytochemical electron microscopy. *Am. J. Pathol.,* 99:413–428.
22. Bretz, U., and Baggiolini, M. (1974): Biochemical and morphological characterization of azurophil and specific granules of human neutrophilic polymorphonuclear leukocytes. *J. Cell Biol.,* 63:251–269.
23. Bujak, J. S., and Root, R. K. (1974): The role of peroxidase in the bactericidal activity of human blood eosinophils. *Blood,* 43:727–736.
24. Butterfield, J. H., Ackerman, S. J., Scott, R. E., Pierre, R. V., and Gleich, G. J. (1984): Evidence for secretion of human eosinophil granule major basic protein and Charcot-Leyden crystal protein during eosinophil maturation. *Exp. Hematol.,* 12:163–170.
25. Catovsky, D., Galton, D. A. G., and Robinson, J. (1972): Myeloperoxidase-deficient neutrophils in acute myeloid leukaemia. *Scand. J. Haematol.,* 9:142–148.
26. Chilosi, M., Fossaluzza, V., and Tosato, F. (1979): Eosinophilic acquired Pelger-Huet anomaly in acute myeloblastic leukemia. *Acta Haematol. (Basel),* 61:198–202.
27. Cohen, N. S., LoBue, J., and Gordon, A. S. (1967): Mechanisms of leukocyte production and release. VIII. Eosinophil and neutrophil kinetics in rats. *Scand. J. Haematol.,* 4:339–350.
28. Cramer, E., Pryzwansky, K. B., Villeval, J-L., Testa, U., and Breton-Gorius, J. (1985): Ultrastructural localization of lactoferrin and myeloperoxidase in human neutrophils by immunogold. *Blood,* 65:423–432.
29. Cronkite, E. P., and Vincent, P. C. (1969): Granulocytopoiesis. *Ser. Haematol.,* 2:3–43.
30. Dale, D. C., Hubert, R. T., and Fauci, A. (1976): Eosinophil kinetics in the hypereosinophilic syndrome. *J. Lab. Clin. Med.,* 3:487–495.
31. Dancey, J. T., Deubelbeiss, K. A., Harker, L. A., and Finch, C. A. (1976): Neutrophil kinetics in man. *J. Clin. Invest.,* 58:705–715.
32. Davis, W. C., and Douglas, S. D. (1972): Defective granule formation and function in the Chediak-Higashi syndrome in man and animals. *Semin. Hematol.,* 9:431–450.
33. Dewald, B., Bretz, U., and Baggiolini, M. (1982): Release of gelatinase from a novel secretory compartment of human neutrophils. *J. Clin. Invest.,* 70:518–525.
34. Dittman, W. A., Kramer, R. J., and Bainton, D. F. (1980): Electron microscopic and peroxidase cytochemical analysis of pink pseudo-Chediak-Higashi granules in acute myelogenous leukemia. *Cancer Res.,* 40:4473–4481.
35. Efrati, P., Nir, E., Kaplan, H., and Dvilanski, A. (1979): Pseudo-Chediak-Higashi anomaly in acute myeloid leukaemia: an electron microscopical study. *Acta Haematol. (Basel),* 61:264–271.
36. Fischkoff, S. A., Pollak, A., Gleich, G. J., Testa, J. R., Misawa, S., and Reber, T. J. (1984): Eosinophilic differentiation of the human promyelocytic leukemia cell line, HL-60. *J. Exp. Med.,* 160:179–196.
37. Fossaluzza, V., and Tosato, F. (1980): Acquired Pelger-Huet anomaly limited to eosinophils. *Acta Haematol. (Basel),* 63:295.
37a.Gabay, J. E., Heiple, J. M., Cohn, Z. A., and Nathan, C. F. (1986): Subcellular location and properties of bactericidal factors from human neutrophils. *J. Exp. Med.,* 164:1407–1421.
38. Gallagher, R., Collins, S., Trujillo, J., McCredie, K., Ahearn, M., Tsai, S., Metzgar, R., Aulakh, G., Ting, R., Ruscetti, F., and Gallo, R. (1979): Characterization of the continuous, differentiating myeloid cell line (HL-60) from a patient with acute promyelocytic leukemia. *Blood,* 54:713–733.
39. Gallin, J. I. (1985): Neutrophil specific granule deficiency. *Ann. Rev. Med.,* 36:263–274.
40. Ganz, T., Selsted, M. E., Szklarek, D., Harwig, S. S. L., Daher, K., Bainton, D. F., and Lehrer, R. I. (1985): Defensins: natural peptide antibiotics of human neutrophils. *J. Clin. Invest.,* 76:1427–1435.
41. Garavini, C., Martelli, P., and Borelli, B. (1981): Alkaline phos-

phatase and peroxidase in neutrophils of the catfish Ictalurus melas (Rafinesque) (Siluriformes ictaluridae). *Histochemistry,* 72:75–81.

42. Gleich, G. J., Loegering, D. A., Bell, M. P., Checkel, J. L., Ackerman, S. J., and McKean, D. J. (1986): Biochemical and functional similarities between human eosinophil-derived neurotoxin and eosinophil cationic protein: homology with ribonuclease. *Proc. Natl. Acad. Sci. USA,* 83:3146–3150.

43. Gorman, A. M., and O'Connell, L. G. (1976): Pseudo-Chediak-Higashi anomaly in acute leukemia. *Am. J. Clin. Pathol.,* 65:1030–1031.

44. Hanker, J. S., Laszlo, J., and Moore, J. O. (1978): The light microscopic demonstration of hydroperoxidase-positive Phi bodies and rods in leukocytes in acute myeloid leukemia. *Histochemistry,* 58:241–252.

45. Hardin, J. H., and Spicer, S. S. (1971): Ultrastructural localization of dialyzed iron-reactive mucosubstance in rabbit heterophils, basophils, and eosinophils. *J. Cell Biol.,* 48:368–386.

46. Harley, J. B. (1982): Clinical manifestations of patients with hypereosinophilic syndrome, pp. 82–84. In: Fauci, A. S., moderator: The idiopathic hypereosinophilic syndrome: clinical pathophysiologic, and therapeutic considerations. *Ann Intern. Med.,* 97:78–92.

47. Hartsock, R. J., Smith, E. B., and Petty, C. S. (1965): Normal variations with aging of the amount of hematopoietic tissue in bone marrow from the anterior iliac crest: a study made from 177 cases of sudden death examined by necropsy. *Am. J. Clin. Pathol.,* 43:326–334.

47a. Heiple, J. M., and Ossowski, L. (1986): Human neutrophil plasminogen activator is localized in specific granules and is translocated to the cell surface by exocytosis. *J. Exp. Med.,* 164:826–840.

48. Hochstenbach, P. F. R., Scheres, J. M. J. C., Hustinx, T. W. J., and Wieringa, B. (1986): Demonstration of X chromatin in drumstick-like nuclear appendages of leukocytes by in situ hybridization on blood smears. *Histochemistry,* 84:383–386.

49. Iozzo, R. V., MacDonald, G. H., and Wight, T. N. (1982): Immunoelectron microscopic localization of catalase in human eosinophilic leukocytes. *J. Histochem. Cytochem.,* 30:697–701.

50. Jamuar, M. P., and Cronkite, E. P. (1980): The fate of granulocytes. *Exp. Hematol.,* 8:884–894.

51. Kane, S. P., and Peters, T. J. (1975): Analytical subcellular fractionation of human granulocytes with reference to the localization of vitamin B_{12}-binding proteins. *Clin. Sci. Mol. Med.,* 49:171–182.

52. Kitahara, M., Eyre, H. J., Simonian, Y., Atkin, C. L., and Hasstedt, S. J. (1981): Hereditary myeloperoxidase deficiency. *Blood,* 57:888–893.

53. Klebanoff, S. J., and Clark, R. A., editors (1978): *The Neutrophil: Function and Clinical Disorders,* pp. 556–557. North Holland, New York.

54. Koeffler, H. P. (1983): Review: induction of differentiation of human acute myelogenous leukemia cells: therapeutic implications. *Blood,* 62:709–721.

55. Komiyama, A., Morosawa, H., Nakahata, T., Miyagawa, Y., and Akabene, T. (1979): Abnormal neutrophil maturation in a neutrophil defect with morphologic abnormality and impaired function. *J. Pediatr.,* 94:19–25.

56. LeBeau, M. M., Larson, R. A., Bitter, M. A., Vardiman, J. W., Golomb, H. M., and Rowley, J. D. (1983): Association of an inversion of chromosome 16 with abnormal marrow eosinophils in acute myelomonocytic leukemia. *N. Engl. J. Med.,* 309:630–636.

57. Lehrer, R. I., and Cline, M. J. (1969): Leukocyte myeloperoxidase deficiency and disseminated candidiasis: the role of myeloperoxidase in resistance to Candida infection. *J. Clin. Invest.,* 48:1478–1488.

58. Lehrer, R. I., Goldberg, L. S., Apple, M. A., Rosenthal, N. P. (1972): Refractory megaloblastic anemia with myeloperoxidase deficient neutrophils. *Ann. Intern. Med.,* 76:447–453.

59. Liso, V., Troccoli, G., Specchia, G., and Magno, M. (1977): Cytochemical "normal" and "abnormal" eosinophils in acute leukemias. *Am. J. Hematol.,* 2:123–131.

60. McCall, C. E., Caves, J., Cooper, R., and DeChatelet, L. (1971): Functional characteristics of human toxic neutrophils. *J. Infect. Dis.,* 124:68–75.

61. McCall, C. E., DeChatelet, L. R., Cooper, M. R., and Shannon, C. (1973): Human toxic neutrophils. III. Metabolic characteristics. *J. Infect. Dis.,* 127:26–33.

62. McCall, C. E., Katayama, I., Cotran, R. S., and Finland, M. (1969): Lysosomal ultrastructural changes in human "toxic" neutrophils during bacterial infection. *J. Exp. Med.,* 129:267–293.

63. Metcalf, D. (1985): The granulocyte-macrophage colony stimulating factors. *Cell,* 43:5–6.

64. Mintz, U., Djaldetti, M., Rozenszajn, L., Pinkhas, J., and de Vries, A. (1973): Giant lysosome-like structures in promyelocytic leukemia: ultrastructural and cytochemical observations. *Biomedicine,* 19:426–430.

65. Mlynek, M-L., and Leder, L-D. (1986): Lineage infidelity in chronic myeloid leukemia: demonstration and significance of hybridoid leukocytes. *Virchows Arch.,* 51:107–114.

66. Newburger, P. E., Novak, T. J., and McCaffrey, R. P. (1983): Eosinophilic cytoplasmic inclusions in fetal leukocytes: are Auer bodies a recapitulation of fetal morphology? *Blood,* 61:593–595.

67. Newburger, P. E., Robinson, J. M., Pryzwansky, K. B., Rosoff, P. M., Greenberger, J. S., and Tauber, A. I. (1983): Human neutrophil dysfunction with giant granules and defective activation of the respiratory burst. *Blood,* 61:1247–1257.

68. Odeberg, H., Olofsson, T., and Olsson, I. (1976): Primary and secondary granule contents and bactericidal capability of neutrophils in acute leukaemia. *Blood Cells,* 2:543–551.

69. Ogawa, M., Porter, P. N., and Nakahata, T. (1983): Renewal and commitment to differentiation of hemopoietic stem cells (an interpretive review). *Blood,* 61:823–829.

70. Oliver, C., and Essner, E. (1975): Formation of anomalous lysosomes in monocytes, neutrophils, and eosinophils from bone marrow of mice with Chediak-Higashi syndrome. *J. Lab. Invest.,* 32:17–27.

71. Osgood, E. E. (1937): Culture of human marrow; length of life of the neutrophils, eosinophils and basophils of normal blood as determined by comparative cultures and sternal marrow from healthy persons. *JAMA,* 109:933–936.

71a. O'Shea, J. J., Brown, E. J., Seligmann, E., Metcalf, J. A., Frank, M. M., and Gallin, J. I. (1985): Evidence for distinct intracellular pools of receptors for C3b and C3bi in human neutrophils. *J. Immunol.,* 134:2580–2587.

72. Parmley, R. T., Crist, W. M., Ragab, A. H., Boxer, L. A., Malluh, A., Lui, V. K., and Darby, C. P. (1980): Congenital dysgranulopoietic neutropenia. *Blood,* 56:465–475.

73. Parmley, R. T., Crist, W. M., Roper, M., Takagi, M., and Austin, R. L. (1981): Intranuclear crystalloids associated with abnormal granules in eosinophilic leukocytes. *Blood,* 58:1134–1140.

74. Parmley, R. T., Dahl, G. V., Austin, R. L., Gauthier, P. A., and Denys, F. R. (1979): Ultrastructure and cytokinetics of leukemic myeloblasts containing giant granules. *Cancer Res.,* 39:3834–3844.

75. Parmley, R. T., Tzeng, D. Y., Baehner, R. L., and Boxer, L. A. (1983): Abnormal distribution of complex carbohydrates in neutrophils of a patient with lactoferrin deficiency. *Blood,* 62:538–548.

76. Parry, M. F., Root, R. K., Metcalf, J. A., Delaney, K. K., Kaplow, L. S., and Richard, W. J. (1981): Myeloperoxidase deficiency. *Ann. Intern. Med.,* 95:293–301.

77. Peters, M. S., Rodriguez, M., and Gleich, G. J. (1986): Localization of human eosinophil granule major basic protein, eosinophil cationic protein, and eosinophil-derived neurotoxin by immunoelectron microscopy. *Lab. Invest.,* 54:656–662.

78. Petrequin, P. R., Todd, R. F., III, Smolen, J. E., and Boxer, L. A. (1986): Expression of specific granule markers on the cell surface of neutrophil cytoplasts. *Blood,* 67:1119–1125.

79. Pincus, S. H., Schooley, W. R., DiNapoli, A. M., and Broder, S. (1981): Metabolic heterogeneity of eosinophils from normal and hypereosinophilic patients. *Blood,* 58:1175–1181.

80. Presentey, B. (1984): Ultrastructure of human eosinophils genetically lacking peroxidase. *Acta Haematol. (Basel),* 71:334–340.

81. Pryzwansky, K. B., and Breton-Gorius, J. (1985): Identification of a subpopulation of primary granules in human neutrophils based upon maturation and distribution: study by transmission electron microscopy cytochemistry and high voltage electron microscopy of whole cell preparations. *Lab. Invest.,* 53:664–671.

82. Rausch, P. G., Pryzwansky, K. B., and Spitznagel, J. K. (1978):

Immunocytochemical identification of azurophilic and specific granule markers in the giant granules of Chediak-Higashi neutrophils. *N. Engl. J. Med.,* 298:694–698.

83. Repine, J. E., Clawson, C. C., and Brunning, R. D. (1976): Abnormal pattern of bactericidal activity of neutrophils deficient in granules, myeloperoxidase, and alkaline phosphatase. *J. Lab. Clin. Med.,* 88:788–795.

84. Rice, W. G., Kinkade, J. M., and Parmley, R. T. (1986): High resolution of heterogeneity among human neutrophil granules: physical, biochemical, and ultrastructural properties of isolated fractions. *Blood,* 68:541–555.

84a. Ringel, E. W., Soter, N. A., and Austen, K. F. (1984): Localization of histaminase to the specific granule of the human neutrophil. *Immunology,* 52:649–658.

85. Roos, D., Voetman, A. A., and Meerhof, L. J. (1983): Functional activity of enucleated human polymorphonuclear leukocytes. *J. Cell Biol.,* 97:368–377.

86. Ross, D. W., and Kaplow, L. S. (1985): Myeloperoxidase deficiency: increased sensitivity for immunocytochemical compared to cytochemical detection of enzyme. *Arch. Pathol. Lab. Med.,* 109:1005–1006.

87. Schrader, J. W., Ziltener, H. J., and Leslie, K. B. (1986): Structural homologies among the hemopoietins *Proc. Natl. Acad. Sci. USA,* 83:2458–2462.

88. Slungaard, A., Ascensao, J., Zanjani, E., and Jacob, H. S. (1983): Pulmonary carcinoma with eosinophilia: demonstration of a tumor-derived eosinophilopoietic factor. *N. Engl. J. Med.,* 309:778–781.

89. Spitznagel, J. K., Dalldorf, F. G., Leffell, M. S., Folds, J. D., Welsh, I. R. H., Cooney, B. S., and Martin, L. E. (1974): Character of azurophil and specific granules purified from human polymorphonuclear leukocytes. *Lab. Invest.,* 30:774–785.

90. Spry, C. J. F. (1985): Synthesis and secretion of eosinophil granule substances. *Immunol. Today,* 6:332–335.

91. Strauss, R. G., Bove, K. E., Jones, J. F., Mauer, A. M., and Filginiti, V. A. (1974): An anomaly of neutrophil morphology with impaired function. *N. Engl. J. Med.,* 290:478–484.

92. Till, J. E., and McCulloch, E. A. (1961): A direct measurement of the radiation sensitivity of normal bone marrow cells. *Radiat. Res.,* 14:213–222.

93. Tracey, R., and Smith, H. (1978): An inherited anomaly of human eosinophils and basophils. *Blood Cells,* 4:291–298.

94. Tulliez, M., and Breton-Gorius, J. (1979): Three types of Auer bodies in acute leukemia. *Lab. Invest.,* 41:419–426.

95. Tulliez, M., Vernant, J. P., Breton-Gorius, J., Imbert, M., and Sul-

tan, C. (1979): Pseudo-Chediak-Higashi anomaly in a case of acute myeloid leukemia: electron microscopic studies. *Blood,* 54:863–871.

96. Ullyot, J. L., and Bainton, D. F. (1974): Azurophil and specific granules of blood neutrophils in chronic myelogeneous leukemia; an ultrastructural and cytochemical analysis. *Blood,* 44:469–482.

97. Van Slyck, E. J., and Rebuck, J. W. (1974): Pseudo-Chediak-Higashi anomaly in acute leukemia: a significant morphologic corollary? *Am. J. Clin. Pathol.,* 62:673–678.

98. Walker, R. I., and Willemze, R. (1980): Neutrophil kinetics and the regulation of granulopoiesis. *Rev. Infect. Dis.,* 2:282–292.

98a. Weiss, J., and Olsson, I. (1987): Cellular and subcellular localization of the bactericidal/permeability-increasing protein of neutrophils. *Blood,* 69:652–659.

99. Weller, P. F., Bach, D. S., and Austen, K. F. (1984): Biochemical characterization of human eosinophil Charcot-Leyden crystal protein (lysophospholipase). *J. Biol. Chem.,* 259:15100–15105.

100. West, B. C., Rosenthal, A. S., Gelb, N. A., and Kimball, H. R. (1974): Separation and characterization of human neutrophil granules. *Am. J. Pathol.,* 77:41–61.

101. Wulffraat, N. M., de Waal, F. C., Stamhuis, I. H., Broekema, G. J., and Loonen, A. H. (1985): Bone marrow mitotic index: a methodological study. *Acta Haematol. (Basel),* 73:89–92.

102. Yazdanbakhsh, M., Eckmann, C. M., Bot, A. A., and Roos, D. (1986): Bactericidal action of eosinophils from normal human blood. *Infect. Immun.,* 53:192–198.

103. Yokota, S., Deimann, W., Hashimoto, T., and Fahimi, H. D. (1983): Immunocytochemical localization of two peroxisomal enzymes of lipid β-oxidation in specific granules of rat eosinophils. *Histochemistry,* 78:425–433.

104. Yokota, S., Deimann, W., Hashimoto, T., and Fahimi, H. D. (1984): Specific granules of rat eosinophils contain peroxisomal acyl-CoA oxidase: possible involvement in production of H_2O_2. *Histochem. J.,* 16:573–577.

104a. Yoon, P. S., Boxer, L. A., Mayo, L. A., Yang, A. Y., and Wicha, M. S. (1987): Human neutrophil laminin receptors: activation-dependent receptor expression. *J. Immunol.,* 138:259–265.

105. Young, J. D-E., Peterson, C. G. B., Venge, P., and Cohn, Z. A. (1986): Mechanism of membrane damage mediated by human eosinophil cationic protein. *Nature,* 321:613–616.

106. Zucker-Franklin, D., Greaves, M. F., Grossi, C. E., and Marmont, A. M. (1981): *Atlas of Blood Cells: Function and Pathology,* pp. 276–284. Lea & Febiger, Philadelphia.

Inflammation: Basic Principles and Clinical Correlates.
Edited by J. I. Gallin, I. M. Goldstein, and R. Snyderman.
Raven Press, Ltd., New York © 1988.

CHAPTER 17

Phagocytic Cells: Development and Distribution of Mononuclear Phagocytes in Normal Steady State and Inflammation

Ralph van Furth

The origin and kinetics of macrophages and monocytes have been studied in great detail, and this research can now be seen to have followed a distinct line. First, studies with chimeras provided information on the bone marrow origin of macrophages (114). Next, studies with labeled cells showed that peritoneal macrophages in an inflammatory exudate derive from circulating blood monocytes (79,81,101,122,126,127). It was then found that in the normal steady-state peritoneal macrophages also arise from blood monocytes; later, the same was found for Kupffer cells (22), pulmonary macrophages (6,7), and spleen macrophages (103).

Before that, however, the precursor cells of the monocytes in the bone marrow were characterized. In 1970 the promonocyte was identified as the direct precursor of the monocyte (102,111), and in 1975 the monoblast was de-

scribed (40,41,104). The precursor of the monoblast is the multipotent stem cell, which is thought to give rise to a bipotent stem cell, the progenitor of the granulocyte and of the mononuclear phagocyte cell lines (5,31,52,53). It is not clear whether this bipotent stem cell leads to other committed stem cells giving rise to a single cell line or directly to myeloblasts and monoblasts.

The present chapter concerns aspects of the origin and kinetics of monocytes and macrophages. It deals mainly with *in vivo* studies done in mice.

CHARACTERIZATION OF MONONUCLEAR PHAGOCYTES

The investigation of mononuclear phagocytes requires adequate characterization of the cells under study. For

TABLE 1. *Characteristic constituents and functions of murine monocytes and macrophages*

Constituents and functions	Promonocytes[a] (%)	Blood monocytes[b] (%)	Resident peritoneal macrophages[b] (%)	Alveolar macrophages[b] (%)	Kupffer cells[b] (%)
Esterase	30	95	99	100	99
Peroxidase	96	60	0	1	0
Lysozyme	100	97	100	c	c
Fcγ receptors	56	99	100	72	84
C3 receptors	32	96	100	2	38
Phagocytosis of ElgG	39	99	91	62	57
Phagocytosis of ElgMC	10	17	13	2	3
Phagocytosis of opsonized bacteria	69	90	98	94	82
Pinocytosis	79	98	99	90	90

[a] Determined in 6-hr cultured cells.
[b] Determined in 24-hr cultured cells.
[c] Not done.

this purpose, use is made of numerous methods that have been published in detail (26). The findings in promonocytes, monocytes, peritoneal macrophages, alveolar macrophages, and Kupffer cells are summarized in Table 1.

Until recently, positive staining of mononuclear phagocytes for nonspecific esterase (with α-naphthyl butyrate or acetate as substrate) was the only characteristic that could reliably differentiate between these cells and other mononuclear cells, e.g., lymphocytes, at sites of inflammation. The availability of monoclonal antibodies specific for mononuclear phagocytes (e.g., monoclonal antibodies for F4/80 antigen on mouse cells and for Mo-2 antigen on human cells) has greatly facilitated the characterization of these cells (3,91,92). Some examples of the binding of a number of monoclonal antibodies to mouse monocytes and peritoneal and alveolar macrophages are given in Table 2. Blood monocytes differ from resident peritoneal macrophages in that they express less F4/80 and M1/70 antigen, and the percentage of monocytes that bind the other monoclonal antibodies studied is considerably smaller. Comparison of blood monocytes with alveolar macrophages revealed another difference in pattern: The C3bi receptor is expressed weakly and the Mac-2 antigen strongly on alveolar macrophages, whereas the reverse is the case for blood monocytes. Resident peritoneal and alveolar macrophages differ in the expression of antigens detected by the monoclonal antibodies F4/80, M1/70, and M3/38. Activated macrophages collected 21 days after infection with BCG express more Ia antigen and less F4/80 antigen and Fc receptor II than do resident macrophages. Compared with corresponding nonactivated cells, activated peritoneal macrophages express more Mac-2 antigen and activated alveolar macrophages more C3bi receptor. Differentiation of the promonocyte to the monocyte is accompanied by an increase in the expression of various surface antigens but not Ia antigens (56); differentiation of monocytes into tissue macrophages does not follow a district pattern (57). The differences in antigen expression by macrophages in different tissues is probably due to differences in local stimuli.

TABLE 2. *Binding of monoclonal antibodies to mouse blood monocytes and peritoneal and alveolar macrophages[a]*

Monoclonal antibody	Antigen	Blood monocytes %	Blood monocytes Intensity	Peritoneal macrophages Resident %	Peritoneal macrophages Resident Intensity	Peritoneal macrophages Activated[b] %	Peritoneal macrophages Activated[b] Intensity	Alveolar macrophages Resident %	Alveolar macrophages Resident Intensity	Alveolar macrophages Activated[b] %	Alveolar macrophages Activated[b] Intensity
F4/80	Macrophage-specific	92	++	100	+++	79	++	94	++	30	+
M1/70	Receptor for C3bi	85	++	99	+++	96	+++	86	+	35	+++
2.4G2	Fc receptor for IgG1/2b	10	+	90	+	21	+	97	+	20	+
M5/114	Ia antigen	16	+	57	+	90	+++	33	+	53	+++
M3/38	Mac-2	48	+	60	+	99	++	100	+++	90	+++

[a] The presence of antigens on the cell surface of freshly isolated murine blood monocytes and macrophages was detected with rat monoclonal antibodies and the biotin-avidin amplification of the immunoperoxidase method (55). The amount of the peroxidase reaction product on cells, which is proportional to the amount of antigen expressed by the cells (57), is graded from 0 (no expression of antigen) and + (weak expression of antigen) to +++ (intense expression of antigen). The percentages refer to cells expressing the antigen.
[b] Activated macrophages were collected 21 days after injection (intravenous) of 10^7 viable BCG.

The presence of peroxidase-positive granules can be used to distinguish between exudate macrophages, which are monocytes recently migrated from the circulation to the site of inflammation and which have not lost their peroxidase activity by degranulation (111), and resident macrophages (Fig. 1). With electron microscopy, peroxidatic activity can be detected in the endoplasmic reticulum, nuclear envelope, Golgi apparatus, and granules of monoblasts and promonocytes. Monocytes and exudate macrophages have only peroxidase-positive granules, and in exudate resident and resident macrophages peroxidatic activity reappears in the rough endoplasmic reticulum and nuclear envelope (Fig. 1).

Receptors for C3bi and the Fc part of IgG occur on the cell surface of mononuclear phagocytes (Table 1). Fc receptors for immunoglobulin G (IgG) mediate the ingestion of opsonized bacteria and IgG-coated red blood cells (immune phagocytosis) (Table 1). Opsonized bacteria are readily ingested by monocytes and macrophages (Table 1). Ingestion of complement-coated red blood cells (EIgMC), which is mediated by C3b receptors, does not occur unless mononuclear phagocytes have been activated by lymphokines or surface-bound fibronectin (132). All mononuclear phagocytes pinocytose avidly (Table 1), but so do other cells (e.g., fibroblasts), albeit to a much smaller degree.

Use of these characteristics makes it possible to define the requirements to be satisfied before a cell can be called a mononuclear phagocyte (100). These requirements are morphological characteristics but include staining obtained with monoclonal antibodies specific for mononuclear phagocytes and the presence of certain enzymes in the cytoplasm. Among the latter are nonspecific esterase, lysozyme, and peroxidatic activity in granules and the rough endoplasmic reticulum, nuclear envelope, and Golgi region (94). Further requirements include the presence of the Fc receptor for IgG as well as C receptors in the cell membrane, and such functional features as phagocytosis of IgG-coated red blood cells or opsonized bacteria and avid pinocytosis. As a rule, not all of the cells are positive for all of these criteria, but it is generally ac-

cepted that a cell must satisfy at least three of them before it can be considered to be a mononuclear phagocyte.

MONONUCLEAR PHAGOCYTES OF THE BONE MARROW

The bone marrow contains various types of mononuclear phagocytes, i.e., monocytes, promonocytes, and monoblasts as well as resident macrophages (Fig. 2). The bone marrow origin of the monocytes has been firmly established. The direct precursor of the monocyte is the promonocyte, a cell that has many characteristics in common with the monocyte. Promonocytes not only stain for nonspecific esterase and lysozyme but also contain peroxidase-positive granules. Furthermore, almost all promonocytes have Fc receptors for IgG and C3b receptors, ingest IgG-coated red blood cells and opsonized bacteria but relatively few C3b-coated red blood cells, and pinocytose avidly (102,104,109).

The monoblast is a less mature cell. It too is positive for esterase and has lysozyme, although only in small amounts. All monoblasts have receptors for IgG and phagocytose IgG-coated red blood cells; opsonized bacteria are ingested much less avidly. C3b receptors occur on only a small percentage of the monoblasts. These cells do not ingest C3b-coated red blood cells and show little ingestion of opsonized bacteria or pinocytosis (41,95, 97,109). These patterns indicate that monoblasts are less mature than promonocytes, and this immaturity is also reflected by the ultrastructure of the cells (94,96,104).

Monocyte Production Under Normal Steady-State Conditions

Adult mice have half as many monoblasts as promonocytes (Table 3). The cell cycle time of the monoblast is shorter than that of promonocytes (40,108) (Table 3). However, the former has been determined only *in vitro* (in cultures with CSF1) and might be shorter than the actual value *in vivo* because the cell cycle time found for promonocytes *in vitro* (40) is also shorter than that de-

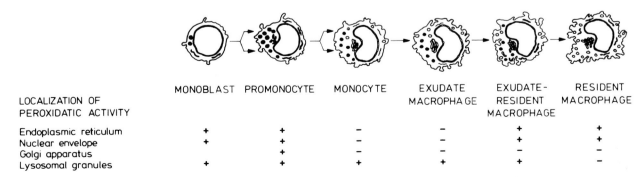

LOCALIZATION OF PEROXIDATIC ACTIVITY	MONOBLAST	PROMONOCYTE	MONOCYTE	EXUDATE MACROPHAGE	EXUDATE- RESIDENT MACROPHAGE	RESIDENT MACROPHAGE
Endoplasmic reticulum	+	+	−	−	+	+
Nuclear envelope	+	+	−	−	+	+
Golgi apparatus		+	+	−	−	+	−
Lysosomal granules	+	+	+	+	+	−

FIG. 1. Peroxidase activity patterns and sequence of development of monocytes and macrophages.

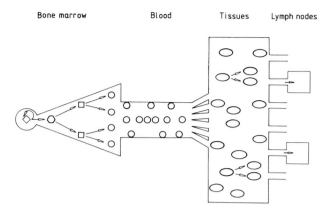

FIG. 2. Current view of the origin and kinetics of mononuclear phagocytes. A stem cell (◇) gives rise to a monoblast (○), which divides once and gives rise to two promonocytes (□). Division of each promonocyte gives rise to two monocytes (○). The monocytes migrate from the bone marrow to the circulation and are distributed over a circulating and a marginating pool. Peripheral blood monocytes migrate to the tissues and body cavities where they differentiate into macrophages. A proportion of the macrophages derive from locally dividing mononuclear phagocytes. The ultimate fate of the macrophages is uncertain: They may die in the tissues and body cavities, migrate to local lymph nodes and die there, or travel to the other sites, e.g., the airspace in the lungs.

termined *in vivo* (108). Although the monoblast could be expected to have stem cell characteristics, i.e., the ability to renew itself after division, which occurs *in vitro* in the presence of CSF1 (115), no indications have been obtained that it is the case *in vivo*.

From the pool sizes and cell cycle times of monoblasts and promonocytes (Table 3) it can be concluded that *in vivo* one dividing monoblast forms two promonocytes and each dividing promonocyte forms two monocytes (Fig. 2). Thus division of these monocyte precursors leads to an amplification from one to four cells. Newly formed monocytes remain in the bone marrow for only a short time (<24 hr) and then migrate to the peripheral blood, which means that they do not pass through a maturation stage in the bone marrow as do the polymorphonuclear leukocytes. The number of monocytes in the bone marrow at any given time is rather small (Table 3).

Bone marrow contains an appreciable number of resident macrophages with a distinctive morphology. These cells are nonspecific esterase-positive and peroxidase-negative, express the F4/80 and Ia antigens, are stained by monoclonal antibody for the Fc IgG1/2b receptor but not by monoclonal antibody for the C3bi receptor, and ingest EIgG (21). Resident bone marrow macrophages are found in close association with dividing hematopoietic cells, which suggests that they play a role in the control of proliferation of these cells (21).

Monocyte Production During Inflammation

During inflammation the number of blood monocytes increases according to the kind of stimulus. Maintenance of an adequate supply of circulating monocytes for more than 24 hr demands increased production of monocyte in the bone marrow because the pool of bone marrow monocytes (Table 3) is not sufficiently large to supply the numbers needed. During an inflammatory response the cell cycle time of the promonocytes is initially shorter (10.8 hr instead of 16.2 hr in the normal steady state) owing to a shorter DNA synthesis time, but it returns to normal after 24 hr when the number of promonocytes is increased for several days (108). Both changes result in substantially increased monocyte production sufficient to maintain larger numbers in the bloodstream. As is discussed in another section, this increased monocyte production is induced by a humoral factor present in the blood and is called factor increasing monocytopoiesis.

Monocyte Production During Treatment with Glucocorticosteroids or Azathioprine

Glucocorticosteroids have an anti-inflammatory effect that is reflected in a decrease of the number of macrophages in the inflammatory exudate, which is accompanied by monocytopenia (see below). Glucocorticosteroids also have an effect on the promonocytes in the bone marrow. After administration of hydrocortisone acetate, which forms a depot, the number of promonocytes drops by roughly one-third, whereas the cell cycle time of these cells is shortened by a few hours (89). Calculation shows that monocyte production is then about 20% lower than that in normal mice. Glucocorticosteroids also inhibit the release of monocytes from bone marrow.

TABLE 3. *Quantitative data on murine mononuclear phagocytes under normal steady-state conditions*[a]

Site	Pool size	Cell cycle (hr)
Bone marrow		
Monoblasts	0.25×10^6	11.9
Promonocytes	0.50×10^6	16.2
Monocytes	2.60×10^6	
Peripheral blood monocytes[b]		
Circulating	0.62×10^6	
Marginating	0.92×10^6	
Tissue macrophages[c]		
Liver	9.0×10^6	
Spleen	4.0×10^6	
Lung	2.0×10^6	
Peritoneal cavity	2.4×10^6	

[a] Average values for adult Swiss mice (~25 g).
[b] Half-time = 17.4 hr.
[c] Mean turnover time: see Table 4.

Hydrocortisone affects monocytopoiesis during an inflammatory response too: The cell cycle time of the promonocytes decreases but does not become shorter than that in normal mice given hydrocortisone, although a shorter cycle would be required for an adequate response to the inflammatory stimulus; the number of promonocytes increases by only 20%. This finding means that monocyte production is increased by 20% in mice given hydrocortisone alone, but the level is still much lower than in normal animals with an acute inflammation (89).

Azathioprine (Imuran) is an antimetabolite that interferes with nucleic acid synthesis, thereby inhibiting cell division. The effect of azathioprine on the promonocytes is expressed in a prolongation of the cell cycle time caused by an effect that occurs late in the DNA synthesis phase of the cell cycle (99,110). This decreased mitotic activity of the promonocytes leads in turn to a decrease in monocyte production, the extent of which depends on the dose and duration of administration of the drug and which induces monocytopenia (see following).

Azathioprine also suppresses the increase in monocyte production normally seen during an inflammatory reaction. This phenomenon is explained by the marked prolongation of the cell cycle time of the promonocytes, which is almost as great as in mice given only azathioprine; under these conditions the number of promonocytes not only does not increase but was even slightly lower than that in mice in the normal steady state (110).

KINETICS OF PERIPHERAL BLOOD MONOCYTES

Normal Steady State

Labeling studies have shown that monocytes enter the circulation within 24 hr after they are produced by division of promonocytes. Until recently it was assumed that blood monocytes occur only in a circulating pool (101). However, a study of the blood volume of the Swiss mice usually used in our kinetic studies showed that in this strain the blood volume is much smaller (7.17 ml for female and 7.14 ml for male Swiss mice per 100 g body weight) (77) than had been assumed from work done by others in Akm mice (49). This finding led to reconsideration of the total number and the localization of monocytes in the peripheral blood. Calculation showed that the total number of monocytes amounts to 1.54×10^6 cells (Table 3) and that monocytes entering the circulation are distributed over a circulating pool containing about 40% of the total pool of blood monocytes, the rest being accounted for by a marginating pool of blood monocytes (106) (Fig. 2). It is conceivable that marginating monocytes, which occur in a layer close to the endothelium to which they are loosely attached, are about to migrate to the tissues and body cavities. In man a marginating pool of monocytes (54) and granulocytes (16) accounting for 75% and 55% of the total pool of cells, respectively, has been reported.

Cells can leave the circulation by a pipeline process, older cells leaving first and younger ones later, or randomly. Studies done in monocytes labeled with [³H]thymidine in vivo, taking into account the disappearance time of the cohort of most heavily labeled monocytes, have shown that the half-time of monocytes in the circulation is 17.4 hr under normal steady-state conditions (108) (Table 3). The average transit time of monocytes in the circulation is 25 hr. A longer monocyte half-time has been reported for normal rats (123,125) and man (129,130).

Labeling studies performed during the normal steady state provide quantitative information about the efflux of monocytes from the blood to various tissues and body cavities. The results summarized in Table 4 show that the proportion of monocytes migrating to various organs corresponds roughly with the size of the organ.

Inflammation

Kinetic studies on monocytes have also been performed during inflammation. During acute or chronic inflammation the number of monocytes in the circulation may increase, the degree depending on the kind of inflam-

TABLE 4. Kinetic parameters of macrophages at various sites

Site	Monocytes leaving the circulation (%)	Rate of monocyte influx[a] ($\times 10^3$/hr)	Rate of local production[a] ($\times 10^3$/hr)	Mean turnover time of macrophages (days)
Liver	71.8	93.3 (92%)	7.7 (8%)	3.8
Spleen	24.7	15.2 (55%)	12.2 (45%)	6.0
Lung	14.7	9.1 (67%)	4.4 (33%)	6.0
Peritoneal cavity	6.7	4.2 (61%)	2.7 (39%)	14.9

[a] The percentages between parentheses give the relative contribution made by influx and local production to the composition of the respective macrophage populations.

matory stimulus. In general, the number of circulating monocytes increases temporarily by a factor of two to three relative to the number under normal steady-state conditions (74,108,117,120). These cells are on their way from the bone marrow to the site of inflammation.

During the first few days of an acute inflammation the number of monocytes entering and the number leaving the circulation of mice are doubled (108). Similar findings concerning the kinetics of monocytes have been reported for rats during a *Salmonella* infection (125). Labeling studies similar to those done in mice under normal steady-state conditions have shown that during the initial phase of an inflammation the total production of monocytes increases by more than 60% and the half-time of circulating monocytes becomes much shorter, i.e., 10 hr, after which there is a return to values found in normal mice (108). These studies have also shown that at least 70% of the increment of monocytes leaving the circulation migrate to the site of inflammation, which leads to a roughly tenfold increase of the number of macrophages in the inflammatory exudate.

HUMORAL REGULATION OF MONOCYTOPOIESIS

Serum and plasma collected during the onset of an inflammatory reaction contain a factor that stimulates monocytopoiesis in the bone marrow of mice and rabbits (73,117,120). This factor, called factor increasing monocytopoiesis (FIM), causes a reduction of the cell cycle time of the promonocytes, an increased rate of division of the monoblasts, and an increase in the number of promonocytes (120), changes similar to those seen in the monocyte precursors during an acute inflammation (108). Labeling studies with [³H]thymidine have shown that FIM causes an increase in the number of labeled monocytes in the circulation compared with that in normal mice, which proves that FIM stimulates monocyte production in the bone marrow. Other investigators have confirmed the presence of a factor that stimulates monocytopoiesis during inflammation (70).

The FIM in mouse and rabbit serum is rather well characterized (Table 5) (73,118). This factor does not have any effect on the production of granulocytes or lymphocytes and can thus be considered cell-line-specific (73,117,120). However, FIM is not species-specific because mouse serum containing it stimulates monocyte production in rabbits and vice versa (73). A concentration–effect relation has been established. FIM is a 18- to 25-kD protein with no carbohydrate moieties essential for its function. FIM has no chemotactic activity and neither stimulates nor enhances the division of monoblasts or promonocytes *in vitro*. It is neither CSF-1, a glycopro-

TABLE 5. *Characteristics of FIM in serum and macrophages*

Characteristics	Serum FIM	Macrophage FIM
In vivo stimulation of		
Monocyte production	Yes	Yes
Granulocyte production	No	No
Lymphocyte production	No	No
Species specificity	No	Not done
Concentration–effect relation	Yes	Yes
Chemical nature	Protein	Protein
Molecular mass (kD)	18–25	10–25
CSF-1 activity	No	No
IL-1 activity	No	No
Chemotactic activity	No	No

Data from refs. 73,76,118.

tein with a molecular mass of 70 kD (82), nor interleukin-1 (76).

Two strains of genetically defined mice, C57BL/10 and CBA, which differ in their ability to react to an inflammatory stimulus by an increase in the number of circulating monocytes and exudate macrophages, exhibit equivalent increases of FIM levels in their serum during inflammation (74). However, only C57BL/10 mice, which develop monocytosis and show increased numbers of macrophages in the inflammatory exudate, react by increasing monocyte production in the bone marrow when stimulated with FIM from either C57BL/10 or CBA mice. CBA mice, which are low responders to an inflammatory stimulus, do not react after injection of FIM, indicating that the ability of monocyte precursors to respond to FIM by intensified division is genetically controlled (74). Because resistance to many kinds of infection is determined by the ability to increase the production of monocytes and migration of these cells to the site of infection, genetically controlled sensitivity to FIM might be a characteristic that plays an important role in the control of such infections.

FIM is present in macrophages and is secreted by them during phagocytosis. Shortly after ingestion of a particle, preformed FIM is secreted and then synthesized and secreted (76). Granulocytes and lymphocytes do not contain or secrete FIM. The characteristics of FIM isolated from macrophages and serum are in all respects similar (Table 4).

The finding that FIM is synthesized and secreted by macrophages at the site of inflammation shows that macrophages themselves regulate the supply of monocytes by inducing increased production of these cells in the bone marrow, leading to an increased number of monocytes in the circulation and consequently at the site of inflammation to act on the inflammatory stimulus. This process represents a form of autoregulation within the mononuclear phagocyte cell line. Autoregulation via FIM does not seem to be restricted to normal mononuclear phagocytes. Findings point to the existence of some form of autoregulation for macrophage cell lines as well. It has been found that cells of two macrophage cell lines, PU5-1.8 and J774.1, contain and secrete FIM, that their proliferation is augmented on exposure to it, and that the rate of proliferation of these cells is inhibited by rabbit anti-mouse FIM IgG (105).

Whether FIM also regulates the production of monocytes under normal steady-state conditions is not known, because it cannot be detected in the serum of mice and rabbits with the methods now available (73,75,120). This factor can be demonstrated in the serum only after the induction of an inflammatory reaction, i.e., when a particle that can be phagocytosed is present at the site of inflammation and the number of macrophages in the exudate is increased. It was found that alveolar macrophages release FIM *in vitro* in the absence of an introduced phagocytosable particle and that resident peritoneal macrophages secrete the factor after phagocytosis of surfactant (78). This finding suggests that *in vivo* alveolar macrophages that have ingested surfactant release FIM into the alveolar space in the absence of an inflammatory stimulus. It is conceivable that the FIM released into the alveolar space is absorbed and transported via the circulation to the bone marrow to maintain the normal production of monocytes. However, the total number of alveolar macrophages is much lower than the number of exudate macrophages, implying that the total amount of FIM secreted by alveolar macrophages under normal conditions is small.

During the latter phase of an inflammatory response the serum contains a factor that inhibits monocytopoiesis (119). This factor, called the monocyte production inhibitor (MPI), has a molecular weight of 50 kD or more but has not yet been further characterized.

ORIGIN AND KINETICS OF MACROPHAGES

Normal Steady State

It is now known with certainty that macrophages in tissues and organ cavities do not derive from lymphocytes or originate from mesenchymal cells, but arise from precursors in the bone marrow. The first evidence indicating the bone marrow origin was obtained in chimera and parabiosis studies (2,4,15,29,33,36,37,42,44,48,61–64,69,87,121,128). Definite proof of the origin of macrophages was provided by cell kinetic studies performed with a stable marker, e.g., [3H]thymidine, which makes it possible to follow the pathway of labeled cells—in this case monocytes—from bone marrow to blood and then

to tissues. Particularly studies in irradiated mice with partial bone marrow shielding gave definite proof of the bone marrow origin of macrophages (6,22,101). The general conclusion drawn from these studies is that under normal steady-state conditions monocytes migrate to tissues and body cavities where they differentiate into macrophages (Fig. 2). A few investigators are of the opinion that macrophages renew only by division in the tissues (11–14,18–20,66–68,85,86,124,126). However, the experimental conditions these investigators applied are open to many objections, either because the animals were not in the steady state or because of the incompleteness of the results; e.g., data on monocyte kinetics are lacking, which partially invalidates the conclusions.

Although we were formerly of the opinion that all macrophages derive from monocytes, we modified this view somewhat a few years ago when we realized that in all of our earlier calculations the small proportion (<5%) of DNA-synthesizing macrophages had not been taken into account. Although the percentage of these cells is low, their total number in tissues and body cavities is considerable. Experiments with double labeling, i.e., [3H]thymidine given *in vivo* and 5-bromodeoxyuridine used as label *in vitro*, showed that these locally dividing cells do not belong to the resident population of macrophages but have recently arrived (about 24 hr before being harvested) in the tissues and body cavities from the bone marrow (*unpublished data*). Furthermore, there is evidence indicating that these cells divide only once outside the bone marrow (109).

These findings led to the development of a new mathematical approach to the origin and kinetics of the macrophage based on the view that renewal of the population of macrophages occurs by the influx of monocytes that differentiate into macrophages and by the production of macrophages by locally dividing cells (7) (Fig. 2). Under normal steady-state conditions the population of macrophages is constant, which means that the rate of monocyte influx plus the rate of local macrophage production equals the rate of disappearance of macrophages. Quantitative data obtained in earlier studies were used to calculate the relevant kinetic parameters summarized in Table 4. These calculations show that the main contribution to the renewal of the macrophage population is made by the influx of monocytes, but the rate of local production is nevertheless appreciable. Table 4 also shows the percentage of monocytes that leave the circulation; it is evident from these data that under normal steady-state conditions the macrophage populations of the liver, spleen, lung, and peritoneal cavity are maintained mainly by the influx of monocytes, although the rate of local production is considerable. The calculations also provided the percentage of monocytes that leave the circulation and migrate to the various sites, as shown in Table 4. In this table the sum is more than 100%, which must be ascribed to the fact that the data originate from experiments done with labeled cells over a period of 20 years during which the condition of the mice was of course not always identical. This statement is true particularly for the period in which experiments with Kupffer cells (22) were performed, for which retrospective analysis showed that the observed numbers of circulating monocytes lay above the usual average value (75,116). Consequently, the previously reported percentage of monocytes migrating to the liver is in all probability too high.

In sum, the calculations provided proof that under normal steady-state conditions the macrophage population is mainly renewed by monocyte influx and that local production takes place as well.

Acute Inflammation

The course of the increase in macrophage numbers during acute and chronic inflammations has been studied with the same approaches as those used for the normal steady state. The use of [³H]thymidine as marker showed that macrophages in the inflammatory exudate derive from blood monocytes (8,9,27,101,113). These cells are called exudate macrophages. *In vitro* labeling with [³H]thymidine showed that the number of DNA-synthesizing cells undergoes a transient rise under inflammatory conditions (8,9,27,101,113) (Table 6), which means that the local production of macrophages also increases temporarily.

In a slightly modified version, the mathematical approach referred to above was also applied to analyze the data obtained during the initial phase of an acute inflammation (Table 6); this approach proved not to be appli-

cable to the further course of the inflammatory response. The results show that during an inflammatory reaction in the peritoneal cavity the increase in the number of macrophages is due mainly to the influx of monocytes; local production does not increase until the second day. In the lung the increasing number of macrophages in the inflammatory exudate during the first 24 hr is determined by a monocyte influx and only after that by an increase of local production as well. With inflammation in the skin, all macrophages are monocyte-derived, and local production of these cells is negligible (Table 6). Kinetic studies done in other animal species also showed that circulating monocytes give rise to exudate macrophages (47,58,59,71,79,81,122,126,127). In sum, proof was obtained that, except for the relatively small share taken by local production during acute inflammation, most of the increase in the number of macrophages in the inflammatory exudate is brought about by an influx of monocytes.

Chronic Inflammation

Chronic inflammatory reactions can be divided into two groups, one without and the other with the formation of granulomas, depending on the agent responsible for the inflammation. In simple chronic inflammation the macrophages at the site of the lesion are bone marrow-derived monocytes, the mechanism underlying cell recruitment being similar to that prevailing during an acute inflammatory reaction. Irritants that cannot be easily disposed of by the macrophages because the material is indigestible usually induce granuloma formation (10,17,24,25,35,51,60,65,84). Granulomas are composed mainly of cells recently recruited from the circulation and

TABLE 6. *Kinetics of macrophages during acute inflammation*

Macrophages	Inflammatory stimulus	Interval after stimulus (hr)	Total monocyte influx (×10⁶)	Total local macrophage production (×10⁶)
Peritoneum	NBCS[a]	6–12	0.17	0.0100
		12–24	1.17	0.0500
		24–48	0.50	0.1900
		NSS[d]	0.10	0.0600
Lung	BCG[b]	2–12	1.96	0.1200
		12–24	0.59	0.1000
		24–48	0.24	0.3200
		NSS	0.22	0.1000
Skin	Glass[c]	0–24	0.10	0.0001

[a] Newborn calf serum 1 ml given intraperitoneally.
[b] Heat-killed BCG 0.25 mg given intravenously.
[c] Coverslip 1.8 cm² inserted subcutanously.
[d] NSS = normal steady state throughout 24-hr interval.

locally dividing mononuclear phagocytes. The share taken by local proliferation is relatively small (25).

Epithelioid cells found in granulomatous lesions are transformed monocytes or macrophages but show much less phagocytic activity than the macrophages. The life span of epithelioid cells is relatively short (on average 1 week; at most 4 weeks) (80). A striking feature of granulomas is the presence of multinucleate giant cells formed by the fusion of mononuclear phagocytes—mainly due to the conjunction of young, newly arrived monocytes with aging macrophages (17,51,80)—rather than by nuclear division of macrophages.

FATE OF MACROPHAGES

When the production of monocytes in the bone marrow is constant and all of these cells migrate to the blood and then to the tissues and body cavities, we must consider their ultimate fate to explain why there is no steady accumulation of macrophages at these sites (109). Little is known about the ultimate fate of macrophages. There are no indications of ineffective monocytopoiesis in the bone marrow, and it is improbable that monocytes die there or in the circulating blood. The only remaining possibilities are that macrophages die in the tissues or body cavities or migrate to still other sites before they die. Firm information concerning recirculation of macrophages via the peripheral blood is lacking. Lung macrophages leave the body through the air space, but the number of cells departing via that route is too small to account for the total efflux of macrophages from the body. It has been shown that macrophages from the liver, lung, and gut migrate to nearby lymph nodes. Because the lymph efferent from lymph nodes does not contain monocytes or macrophages, it is highly probable that macrophages die in lymph nodes. It is also conceivable that cell death occurs in tissues and body cavities. The number of macrophages that die per unit of time must be appreciable in view of the magnitude of the total monocyte production in the normal mouse, which amounts to about 1.5×10^6 cells per 24 hr (99), all of which leave the bone marrow and ultimately become macrophages.

EFFECT OF ANTI-INFLAMMATORY DRUGS AND IRRADIATION ON THE KINETICS OF MONOCYTES AND MACROPHAGES

Treatment with glucocorticosteroids, various cytostatic drugs, and irradiation has an effect on the number of leukocytes in the circulation and the inflammatory exudate. In this section, however, the discussion is limited to the effect on blood monocytes and macrophages as found in experiments with mice.

Glucocorticosteroids

The administration of glucocorticosteroids leads to a rapid decrease (within 3–6 hr) of the number of circulating monocytes, the duration of the effect depending on the nature and dose of the compound used (23,30,72,88,93). Water-soluble dexamethasone is only briefly active (<12 hr), and hydrocortisone acetate, which forms a depot, reduces the number of monocytes for about 2 weeks (Fig. 3), after which monocytes reappear in the blood.

The rapid disappearance of circulating monocytes is attributed to sequestration of these cells in a compartment of unknown localization. The persistent monocytopenia is caused by diminished release of monocytes from the bone marrow in combination with a decrease in the number of promonocytes in bone marrow (89). The mitotic activity of monoblasts (98) and promonocytes (89) diminishes only slightly under glucocorticosteroid treatment.

The number of resident macrophages in normal animals is affected little by glucocorticosteroids, except that the arrested influx of monocytes from the circulation results in a gradual decrease corresponding with the normal turnover of macrophages (88).

Treatment with glucocorticosteroids suppresses the inflammatory response; the substantial increase of the numbers of both blood monocytes and exudate macrophages usually seen after stimulation does not occur (88). There is only a small elevation of monocyte production in the bone marrow; the number of circulating monocytes remains low, and little influx of monocytes to the site of inflammation is observed (88).

Azathioprine

The action of azathioprine gradually decreases the number of circulating monocytes, the extent and duration depending on the dose and duration of administration of the drug (34), as it affects the formation of monocytes in the bone marrow by inhibiting the mitotic activity of the promonocytes (110). A high dose of azathioprine administered daily for 9 days reduces the number of blood monocytes to almost nil (Fig. 3). This effect is known to be reversible; 1 to 2 days after treatment is stopped the number of circulating monocytes starts to increase.

The number of resident macrophages decreases only after prolonged administration of high doses of azathioprine because such treatment leads to prolonged severe monocytopenia, which prevents the normal turnover of macrophages sustained by the influx of blood monocytes (34).

Azathioprine reduces the migration of monocytes to a site of inflammation. Under the influence of the drug the

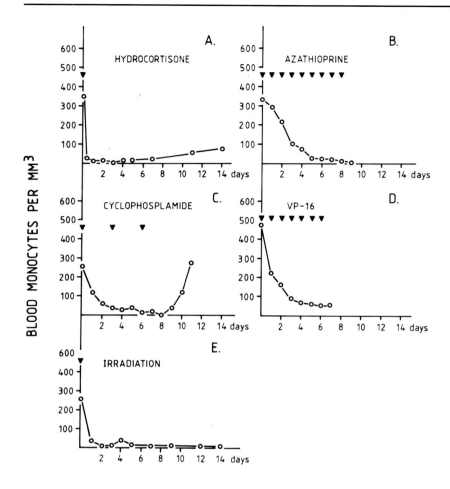

FIG. 3. Course of monocytes during treatment with an anti-inflammatory drug or after irradiation. The interventions are indicated by arrowheads (▼). Swiss mice weighing 25 g received (all subcutaneously): one injection of 15 mg hydrocortisone acetate (**A**); daily injections of 5 mg azathioprine (**B**); one injection of 3.75 mg cyclophosphamide on day 0 and 2.5 mg cyclophosphamide on days 3 and 6 (**C**); or daily injection of 0.3 mg VP-16 (**D**). All mice were irradiated with 8GY on day 0 (**E**). (Data from refs. 34,88,131.)

number of circulating monocytes does not increase during an inflammatory response but, instead, decreases, the degree of the decrease depending on the dose and the duration of administration (110).

Cyclophosphamide

Cyclophosphamide, an alkylating agent that arrests cell division in the post-DNA-synthesis (G2) phase, inhibits the production of monocytes in bone marrow. Intraperitoneal and subcutaneous administration of this agent leads to a gradual decrease of the number of circulating monocytes, which reaches a minimum after 3 days and persists about 3 days (Fig. 3). After that, the number of monocytes starts to increase. Induction of prolonged monocytopenia requires administration of cyclophosphamide at 3-day intervals (131); in mice the subcutaneous route is tolerated better than intraperitoneal administration. The number of resident macrophages decreases slightly and gradually during cyclophosphamide treatment because the drug reduces the normal turnover maintained by the influx of circulating monocytes.

An inflammatory response is severely impaired by prolonged cyclophosphamide treatment because there is no increase of circulating monocytes and exudate macrophages (131).

Etoposide (VP-16)

The administration of VP-16, a derivate of podophyllotoxin, causes monocytopenia (90,131) because it affects the formation of monocytes in the bone marrow by inhibiting DNA synthesis of precursor cells. Daily administration of this drug leads gradually to monocytopenia (Fig. 3) (131). After withdrawal of the drug, the number of blood monocytes returns to normal levels within 2 days. In normal animals the number of macrophages does not change under VP-16 treatment, probably because the drop in the number of circulating monocytes is limited and slow. During an inflammatory response in VP-16-treated mice, the number of monocytes and exudate macrophages does not increase as in untreated mice (131).

Irradiation

Ionizing radiation causes inhibition of mitosis in monocyte precursors. The effect of irradiation on the number of blood monocytes depends on the dose applied. The rate of disappearance of monocytes from the circulation after a sublethal dose of irradiation (Fig. 3) (101,131) corresponds with the average transit time of monocytes in the circulation (108) during total arrest of monocyte production in the bone marrow. The number of resident macrophages decreases slowly after irradiation because due to the monocytopenia there are no cells to migrate to the tissues and body cavities. When an inflammatory stimulus is administered after sublethal irradiation, circulating monocytes remain virtually absent and the number of macrophages at the site of infection does not increase (131).

MONONUCLEAR PHAGOCYTE SYSTEM

The accumulation of information about the origin and kinetics as well as the similarities between the morphological, (immuno)cytochemical, immunological, and functional characteristics of mononuclear phagocytes led to the concept of the mononuclear phagocyte system (107). Before that, monocytes and macrophages were assigned to the reticuloendothelial system by Aschoff in 1924 (1). According to Aschoff, a system is formed by cells sharing a common morphology, origin, and functions as well as other properties, but we now know that the cells of the reticuloendothelial system (reticular cells, endothelial cells, fibrocytes, histiocytes, and monocytes) do not fulfill his criteria. However, the mononuclear phagocytes (monoblasts, promonocytes, monocytes, and macrophages) do satisfy the criteria for a system.

After the mononuclear phagocyte system was first put forward (107) in 1969, more cells were assigned to this system on the basis of new information about the monocyte precursors in bone marrow (112) and about the monocyte-derived macrophages in various localizations under normal and pathological conditions (100). All of these additions to the mononuclear phagocyte system were made mainly on the basis of evidence from studies on cell kinetics. The use of monoclonal antibodies specific for mononuclear phagocytes, especially the monoclonal antibody to the F4/80 antigen in the mouse, has yielded new information about the distribution of macrophages (38,43,45,46). The cells we can now assign to the mononuclear phagocyte system are shown in Table 7. This list includes the precursor cells in the bone marrow, circulating cells, and cells present in the tissues and body cavities under normal conditions as well as during inflammation.

Cells of a number of types cannot yet be assigned to the mononuclear phagocyte system with certainty. They are the Langerhans cells in the skin and the interdigitating cells in the paracortex of lymph nodes. The Langerhans

TABLE 7. *Cells belonging to the mononuclear phagocyte system*

Bone marrow
  Monoblasts
  Promonocytes
  Monocytes

Blood
  Monocytes

Tissues (macrophages occur in the following)
  Connective tissue (histiocytes)
  Skin (histiocytes, Langerhans cells?)
  Liver (Kupffer cells)
  Spleen (red pulp macrophages)
  Lymph nodes (free and fixed macrophages, interdigitating cells?)
  Thymus
  Bone marrow (resident macrophages)
  Bone (osteoclasts)
  Synovia (type A cell)
  Lung (alveolar and tissue macrophages)
  Mucosa-associated lymphoid tissues
  Gastrointestinal tract
  Genitourinary tract
  Endocrine organs
  Central nervous system [macrophages, (reactive) microglia, cerebrospinal fluid macrophages]

Body cavities
  Pleural macrophages
  Peritoneal macrophages

Inflammation
  Exudate macrophages
  Epithelioid cells
  Multinucleated giant cells

cells express several macrophage markers. Freshly isolated Langerhans cells are positive for nonspecific esterase, stain with monoclonal antibodies F4/80 and Mac-1, have Fc receptors, and express Ia antigen. However, these cells do not phagocytose, and after several days of culture they lose all of these characteristics except the expression of Ia antigen (39,83). Langerhans cells probably derive from a precursor cell in the bone marrow (32,50), but it is unlikely that monocytes are the precursor of Langerhans cells. Thus it is impossible to consider Langerhans cells as macrophages and assign them to the mononuclear phagocyte system. Because veiled cells in the lymph, Langerhans cells in the epidermis, and interdigitating cells in lymph nodes share many characteristics, they are probably closely related. Although cell-kinetic studies are not available, a development can be postulated in a sequence from the Langerhans cell in the epidermis to the veiled cell in efferent lymph from the skin to the interdigitating cell in lymph nodes (28,100). Dendritic cells are not assigned to the mononuclear phagocyte system either. These cells, whose precursor resides in the bone marrow, soon become nonadherent in culture, lack Fc receptors, are nonphagocytic, and are negative for F4/80 antigen; however, they do express Ia antigen (83).

TERMINOLOGY FOR MONONUCLEAR PHAGOCYTES PARTICIPATING IN AN INFLAMMATORY REACTION

The mononuclear phagocytes participating in an inflammatory reaction (whether spontaneous or induced) are often carelessly defined. The characteristics of these cells in an exudate depend on the inducing agent, the method of isolation, the developmental stage, and the functional state of the cells. Thus the cells in an inflammatory exudate can be rather heterogeneous and should therefore be characterized cautiously.

The terminology applied to the cells in an inflammatory exudate is generally confusing. For example, terms such as stimulated, activated, elicited, and induced are used interchangeably. Often, too, no distinction is made between the developmental stage of the mononuclear phagocyte and the functional state. To deal with these problems, the following definitions have been proposed (100):

Resident macrophages: macrophages occurring at any given site in the absence of an exogenous or endogenous inflammatory stimulus. These cells are sometimes called normal macrophages; they can also occur in an inflammatory exudate as a small subpopulation present before the stimulus was applied.

Exudate macrophages: macrophages occurring in an exudate and identified by specific markers (e.g., peroxidatic activity and staining with monoclonal antibodies) and by cell-kinetic analysis. Exudate macrophages derive from monocytes and have almost the same characteristics as the latter. The term exudate macrophage should be reserved for this developmental stage of the macrophage.

Exudate-resident macrophages: a transitional form between the resident and the exudate macrophage. These cells can be characterized only electron microscopically after staining for peroxidatic activity.

Activated macrophages: macrophages with increased functional activity induced by a given stimulus. Activation thus implies an increase in one or more functional activities of a cell or a new functional activity. Before activation the cells may have been resident or exudate macrophages. The term can be applied to mononuclear phagocytes stimulated *in vivo* and *in vitro,* but explicit mention should be made of how this activation was accomplished as well as how it was measured.

Elicited macrophages: macrophages attracted to a given site by a given substance. This term refers only to mononuclear phagocytes accumulating at a particular site and

does not indicate the developmental stage or functional state of the cells. An elicited population of cells is usually heterogeneous in both respects. Because elicited and evoked have the same meaning, use of the latter is of course acceptable.

Stimulated macrophages: an imprecise term because stimulation means the application of a stimulus that may result in elicitation of cells, activation of cells, or both. The word stimulus can be used as a noun, as in inflammatory stimulus, but in this context not as an adjective, as in stimulated macrophages. The latter term should not be used.

Induced macrophages: also an inexact term, as it can imply either elicited or activated and therefore should not be used.

Mononuclear cells: a term that should be discarded because it covers cells belonging to different cell lines, i.e., mononuclear phagocytes (monocytes and macrophages) and T- and B-lymphocytes with entirely different functions.

Accumulation, proliferation: terms that are often used erroneously. Proliferation should be reserved for cases in which the increase in the number of cells is known to be due to division of cells already present at or recruited to a site. The term accumulation should be used for the increase in the number of cells caused by migration of (nondividing) cells from other sites.

REFERENCES

1. Aschoff, L. (1924): Das reticulo-endotheliale System. *Ergebn. Inn. Med. Kinderheilk.,* 26:1–118.
2. Ash, P., Loutit, J. F., and Townsend, K. M. S. (1980): Giant lysosomes, a cytoplasmic marker in osteoclasts of beige mice. *J. Pathol.,* 130:237–245.
3. Austyn, J. M., and Gordon, S. (1981): F4/80: a monoclonal antibody directed specifically against the mouse macrophage. *Eur. J. Immunol.,* 11:805–815.
4. Balner, H. (1963): Identification of peritoneal macrophages in mouse radiation chimeras. *Transplantation,* 1:217–223.
5. Bender, J. G., Van Epps, D. E., and Stewart, C. C. (1986): A model for the regulation of myelopoiesis by specific factors. *J. Leukocyte Biol.,* 39:101–111.
6. Blussé van Oud Alblas, A., and Van Furth, R. (1979): The origin, kinetics and characteristics of pulmonary macrophages in the normal steady state. *J. Exp. Med.,* 149:1504–1518.
7. Blussé van Oud Alblas, A., Mattie, H., and Van Furth, R. (1983): A quantitative evaluation of pulmonary macrophage kinetics. *Cell Tissue Kinet.,* 16:211–219.
8. Blussé van Oud Alblas, A., Van der Linden-Schrever, B., and Van Furth, R. (1981): Origin and kinetics of pulmonary macrophages during an inflammatory reaction induced by intravenous administration of heat-killed BCG. *J. Exp. Med.,* 154:235–252.
9. Blussé van Oud Alblas, A., Van der Linden-Schrever, B., and Van Furth, R. (1983): Origin and kinetics of pulmonary macrophages during an inflammatory reaction induced by intra-alveolar administration of aerosolized heat-killed BCG. *Am. Rev. Respir. Dis.,* 128:276–281.
10. Boros, D. L. (1978): Granulomatous inflammations. *Prog. Allergy,* 24:183–267.
11. Bouwens, L., and Wisse, E. (1985): Proliferation, kinetics, and fate

of monocytes in rat liver during a zymosan-induced inflammation. *J. Leukocyte Biol.*, 37:531–543.

12. Bouwens, L., Baekeland, M., and Wisse, E. (1984): Importance of local proliferation in the expanding Kupffer cell population of rat liver after zymosan stimulation and partial hepatectomy. *Hepatology*, 4:213–219.

13. Bouwens, L., Baekeland, M., and Wisse, E. (1986): Cytokinetic analysis of the expanding Kupffer-cell population in rat liver. *Cell Tissue Kinet.*, 19:217–226.

14. Bouwens, L., Knook, D. L., and Wisse, E. (1986): Local proliferation and extrahepatic recruitment of liver macrophages (Kupffer cells) in partial-body irradiated rats. *J. Leukocyte Biol.*, 39:687–697.

15. Brunstetter, M. A., Hardie, J. A., Schiff, R., Lewis, J. P., and Cross, C. E. (1971): The origin of pulmonary alveolar macrophages. *Arch. Intern. Med.*, 127:1064–1068.

16. Cartwright, G. E., Athens, J. W., and Wintrobe, M. M. (1954): The kinetics of granulopoiesis in normal man. *Blood*, 24:780–803.

17. Chambers, T. J. (1978): Multinucleated giant cells. *J. Pathol.*, 126:125–148.

18. Coggle, J. E., and Tarling, J. D. (1982): Cell kinetics of pulmonary alveolar macrophages in the mouse. *Cell Tissue Kinet.*, 15:139–143.

19. Coggle, J. E., and Tarling, J. D. (1984): The proliferation kinetics of pulmonary alveolar macrophages. *J. Leukocyte Biol.*, 35:317–327.

20. Collins, F. M., and Auclair, L. K. (1980): Mononuclear phagocytes within the lungs of unstimulated parabiotic rats. *J. Reticuloendothel. Soc.*, 27:429–441.

21. Crocker, P. R., and Gordon, S. (1985): Isolation and characterization of resident stromal macrophages and hematopoietic cell clusters from mouse bone marrow. *J. Exp. Med.*, 162:993–1014.

22. Crofton, R. W., Diesselhoff-den Dulk, M. M. C., and Van Furth, R. (1978): The origin, kinetics, and characteristics of the Kupffer cells in the normal steady state. *J. Exp. Med.*, 148:1–17.

23. Dale, D. C., Fauci, A. S., and Wolff, S. M. (1974): Alternate day prednisone: leukocyte kinetics and susceptibility to infections. *N. Engl. J. Med.*, 291:1154–1158.

24. Dannenberg, A. M. (1980): Pathogenesis of tuberculosis. In: *Pulmonary Disease and Disorders*, edited by A. P. Fishmann, pp. 1264–1281. McGraw-Hill, New York.

25. Dannenberg, A. M., Ando, M., Shima, K., and Tsuda, T. (1975): Macrophage turnover and activation in tuberculous granulomata. In: *Mononuclear Phagocytes in Immunity, Infection and Pathology*, edited by R. van Furth, pp. 959–980. Blackwell Scientific Publications, Oxford.

26. Diesselhoff-den Dulk, M. M. C., and Van Furth, R. (1981): Characteristics of mononuclear phagocytes from different tissues. In: *Methods for Studying Mononuclear Phagocytes*, edited by D. O. Adams, P. J. Edelson, and H. Koren, pp. 253–282. Academic Press, New York.

27. Diesselhoff-den Dulk, M. M. C., Crofton, R. W., and Van Furth, R. (1979): Origin and kinetics of Kupffer cells during an acute inflammatory response. *Immunology*, 37:7–14.

28. Drexhage, H. A., Lens, L. W., Cvetanov, J., Kamperdijk, E. W. A., Mullink, R., and Balfour, B. M. (1980): Veiled cells resembling Langerhans cells. In: *Mononuclear Phagocytes. Functional Aspects*, edited by R. Van Furth, pp. 235–272. Martinus Nijhoff, Boston.

29. Edwards, J. C. W. (1982): The origin of type A synovial lining cells. *Immunobiology*, 161:227–231.

30. Fauci, A. S., and Dale, D. C. (1974): The effect of in vivo hydrocortisone on subpopulations of human lymphocytes. *J. Clin. Invest.*, 53:240–246.

31. Francis, G. E., and Leaning, M. S. (1985): Stochastic model of human granulocyte-macrophage progenitor cell proliferation and differentiation. I. Setting up the model. *Exp. Hematol.*, 13:92–98.

32. Frelinger, J. G., Hood, L., Hill, S., and Frelinger, J. A. (1979): Mouse epidermal Ia molecules have a bone marrow origin. *Nature*, 282:321–323.

33. Gale, R. P., Sparkes, R. S., and Gode, D. W. (1978): Bone marrow origin of hepatic macrophages (Kupffer cells) in humans. *Science*, 201:937–938.

34. Gassmann, A. E., and Van Furth, R. (1975): The effect of azathioprine (Imuran®) on the kinetics of monocytes and macrophages during the normal steady state and an acute inflammatory reaction. *Blood*, 46:51–64.

35. Ginsburg, I., Mitrani, S., Ne'eman, N., and Lahav, M. (1975): Granulomata in streptococcal inflammation: mechanisms of localization transport and degradation of streptococci in inflammatory sites. In: *Mononuclear Phagocytes in Immunity, Infection and Pathology*, edited by R. Van Furth, pp. 981–1014. Blackwell Scientific Publications, Oxford.

36. Godleski, J. G., and Brain, J. D. (1972): The origin of alveolar macrophages in mouse radiation chimeras. *J. Exp. Med.*, 136:630–643.

37. Goodman, J. W. (1964): The origin of peritoneal fluid cells. *Blood*, 23:18–26.

38. Gordon, S. (1986): Biology of the macrophage. *J. Cell Sci.*, 4(Suppl.):267–286.

39. Gordon, S., Crocker, P. R., Lee, S. H., Morris, L., and Raboniwitz, S. (1986): Trophic and defense functions of murine macrophages. In: *Mechanisms of Host Resistance to Infectious Agents, Tumors, and Allografts*, edited by R. M. Steinman and R. J. North, pp. 121–137. Rockefeller University Press, New York.

40. Goud, Th. J. L. M., and Van Furth, R. (1975): Proliferative characteristics of monoblasts grown in vitro. *J. Exp. Med.*, 142:1200–1217.

41. Goud, Th. J. L. M., Schotte, C., and Van Furth, R. (1975): Identification and characterization of the monoblast in mononuclear phagocyte colonies grown in vitro. *J. Exp. Med.*, 142:1180–1199.

42. Haller, O., Arnheiter, H., and Lindemann, J. (1979): Natural, genetically determined resistance toward influenza virus in hemopoietic mouse chimeras: role of mononuclear phagocytes. *J. Exp. Med.*, 150:117–126.

43. Hirsch, S., and Gordon, S. (1983): Surface antigens as markers of mouse macrophage differentiation. *Int. Rev. Exp. Pathol.*, 25:51–75.

44. Howard, J. G. (1970): The origin and immunological significance of Kupffer cells. In: *Mononuclear Phagocytes*, edited by R. Van Furth, pp. 178–199. Blackwell Scientific Publications, Oxford.

45. Hume, D. A., and Gordon, S. (1983): The mononuclear phagocyte system of the mouse defined by immunohistochemical localisation of antigen F4/80: identification of resident macrophages in renal medullary and cortical interstitium and the juxtaglomerular complex. *J. Exp. Med.*, 157:1704–1709.

46. Hume, D. A. and Gordon, S. (1985): The mononuclear phagocyte system of the mouse defined by immunohistochemical localisation of antigen F4/80. In: *Mononuclear Phagocytes. Characteristics, Physiology and Function*, edited by R. Van Furth, pp. 9–17. Martinus Nijhoff, Boston.

47. Issekutz, T. B., Issekutz, A. C., and Movat, H. Z. (1981): The in vivo quantitation and kinetics of monocyte migration into acute inflammatory tissue. *Am. J. Pathol.*, 103:47–55.

48. Johnson, K. J., Ward, P. A., Stiker, G., and Kunkel, R. (1980): A study of the origin of pulmonary macrophages using the Chédiak-Higashi marker. *Am. J. Pathol.*, 101:365–374.

49. Kaliss, N., and Pressman, D. (1950): Plasma and blood volumes of mouse organs as determined with radioactive iodoproteins. *Proc. Soc. Exp. Biol. Med.*, 75:16–20.

50. Katz, S. I., Tamaki, K., and Sach, D. H. (1979): Epidermal Langerhans cells are derived from cells originating in bone marrow. *Nature*, 282:324–326.

51. Kraus, B. (1981): Mehrkernige Riesenzellen in Granulomen: Multinucleate giant cells in granulomas. In: *Granulome und Granulomatosen*, edited by H. Cain and G. Dhom, pp. 103–125. Gustav Fisher Verlag, Stuttgart.

52. Leaning, M. S., and Francis, G. E. (1985): Stochastic model of human granulocytes-macrophage progenitor cell proliferation and differentiation. II. Validation of the model. *Exp. Hematol.*, 13:99–103.

53. Metcalf, D., and Burgess, A. W. (1982): Clonal analysis of progenitor

cells commitment of granulocyte or macrophage production. *J. Cell. Physiol.*, 111:275–283.

54. Meuret, G., and Hoffmann, G. (1973): Monocyte kinetic studies in normal and disease states. *Br. J. Haematol.*, 24:275–285.

55. Nibbering, P. H., Leijh, P. C. J., and Van Furth, R. (1985): A cytochemical method to quantitate the binding of monoclonal antibodies to individual cells. *J. Histochem. Cytochem.*, 33:453–459.

56. Nibbering, P. H., Leijh, P. C. J., and Van Furth, R. (1987): Quantitative immunocytochemical characterization of mononuclear phagocytes. I. Monoblasts, promonocytes, monocytes, peritoneal and alveolar macrophages. *Cell. Immunol.*, 105:374–385.

57. Nibbering, P. H., Leijh, P. C. J., and Van Furth, R. (1987): Quantitative immunocytochemical characterization of mononuclear phagocytes. II. Monocytes and tissue macrophages. *Immunology*, 62:171–176.

58. Normann, S. J., and Noga, S. J. (1986): Population kinetic study of guinea pig monocytes and their subsets during acute inflammation. *Cell. Immunol.*, 101:534–547.

59. Normann, S. J., and Noga, S. J. (1986): Population kinetic study on the origin of guinea pig monocyte heterogeneity. *Cell. Immunol.*, 99:375–384.

60. Papadimitriou, J. M., and Walters, M. N. (1979): Macrophage polykarya. *C.R.C. Crit. Rev. Toxicol.*, 6:211–255.

61. Parwaresch, M. R., and Wacker, H. H. (1984): Origin and kinetics of resident tissue macrophages: parabiosis studies with radiolabelled leucocytes. *Cell Tissue Kinet.*, 17:25–39.

62. Pinkett, M. O., Cowdrey, C. M., and Nowell, P. C. (1966): Mixed hematopoietic and pulmonary origin of "alveolar macrophages" as demonstrated by chromosome markers. *Am. J. Pathol.*, 48:859–867.

63. Porter, K. A. (1969): Origin of Kupffer cells and endothelial cells in long-surviving human hepatic homografts. In: *Experience in Hepatic Transplantation*, edited by T. E. Starzl, pp. 464–465. Saunders, Philadelphia.

64. Portmann, B., Schindler, A. M., Murray-Lyon, I. M., and Williams, R. (1976): Histological sexing of a reticulum cell sarcoma arising after liver transplantation. *Gastroenterology*, 70:82–84.

65. Ryan, G. B., and Spector, W. G. (1970): Macrophage turnover in inflamed connective tissues. *Proc. R. Soc. [Biol.]*, 175:269–292.

66. Sawyer, R. T. (1986): The cytokinetic behavior of pulmonary alveolar macrophages in monocytic mice. *J. Leukocyte Biol.*, 39:89–99.

67. Sawyer, R. T. (1986): The significance of local resident pulmonary alveolar macrophage proliferation to population renewal. *J. Leukocyte Biol.*, 39:77–87.

68. Sawyer, R. T., Straubauch, P. H., and Volkman, A. (1982): Resident macrophage proliferation in mice depleted of blood monocytes by strontium-89. *Lab. Invest.*, 46:165–170.

69. Shand, F. L., and Bell, E. B. (1972): Studies on the distribution of macrophages derived from rat bone marrow cells in exenogeic radiation chimeras. *Immunology*, 22:549–556.

70. Shum, D. T., and Galsworthy, S. B. (1982): Stimulation of monocyte production by an endogenous mediator induced by a component from Listeria monocytogenes. *Immunology*, 46:343–351.

71. Slonecker, Ch. E. (1971): The cellular composition of an acute inflammatory exudate in rats. *J. Reticuloendothel. Soc.*, 10:269–282.

72. Slonecker, Ch. E., and Lim, W. Ch. (1972): Effects of hydrocortisone on the cells in an acute inflammatory exudate. *Lab. Invest.*, 27:123–128.

73. Sluiter, W., Elzenga-Claasen, I., Hulsing-Hesselink, E., and Van Furth, R. (1983): Presence of the factor increasing monocytopoiesis (FIM) in rabbit peripheral blood during an acute inflammation. *J. Reticuloendothel. Soc.*, 34:235–252.

74. Sluiter, W., Elzenga-Claasen, I., Van der Voort van der Kley-van Andel, A., and Van Furth, R. (1984): Differences in the response of inbred mouse strains to the factor increasing monocytopoiesis. *J. Exp. Med.*, 159:524–536.

75. Sluiter, W., Hulsing-Hesselink, E., Elzenga-Claasen, I., and Van Furth, R. (1985): Method to select mice in the steady state for biological studies. *J. Immunol. Methods*, 760:135–143.

76. Sluiter, W., Hulsing-Hesselink, E., Elzenga-Claasen, I., Van Hems-bergen-Oomens, L. W. M., Van der Voort van der Kley-van Andel, A., and Van Furth, R. (1987): Macrophages as origin of factor increasing monocytopoiesis. *J. Exp. Med.*, 167:909–922.

77. Sluiter, W., Oomens, L. W. M., Brand, A., and Van Furth, R. (1984): Determination of blood volume in the mouse with ^{51}chromium-labelled erythrocytes. *J. Immunol. Methods*, 73:221–225.

78. Sluiter, W., Van Hemsbergen-Oomens, L. W. M., Elzenga-Claasen, I., and Van Furth, R. (1987): Effect of lungsurfactant on the release of factor increasing monocytopoiesis by macrophages. *Exp. Haematol.*, 46:93–97.

79. Spector, W. G., and Coote, E. (1965): Differentially labelled blood cells in the reaction to paraffin oil. *J. Pathol. Bacteriol.*, 90:589–598.

80. Spector, W. G., and Mariano, M. (1975): Macrophage behaviour in experimental granulomas. In: *Mononuclear Phagocytes in Immunity, Infection and Pathology*, edited by R. Van Furth, pp. 927–942. Blackwell Scientific Publications, Oxford.

81. Spector, W. G., Walters, M. N. I., and Willoughby, D. A. (1965): The origin of the mononuclear cells in inflammatory exudates induced by fibrinogen. *J. Pathol. Bacteriol.*, 90:181–192.

82. Stanley, E. R. (1979): Colony-stimulating factor (CSF) radioimmunoassay: detection of a CSF subclass stimulating macrophage production. *Proc. Natl. Acad. Sci. USA*, 76:2969–2973.

83. Steinman, R. M., Inaba, K., Schuler, G., and Witmer, M. (1986): Stimulation of the immune response: contributions of dendritic cells. In: *Mechanisms of Host Resistance to Infectious Agents, Tumors, and Allografts*, edited by R. M. Steinman and R. J. North, pp. 71–97. Rockefeller University Press, New York.

84. Sutton, J. S., and Weiss, L. (1966): Transformation of monocytes in tissue culture into macrophages, epithelioid cells and multinucleate giant cells. *J. Cell Biol.*, 28:303–332.

85. Tarling, J. D., and Coggle, J. E. (1982): Evidence for the pulmonary origin of alveolar macrophages. *Cell Tissue Kinet.*, 15:577–584.

86. Tarling, J. D., and Coggle, J. E. (1982): The absence of effect on pulmonary alveolar macrophage numbers during prolonged periods of monocytopenia. *J. Reticuloendothel. Soc.*, 31:221–224.

87. Thomas, E. D., Ramberg, R. E., and Sale, G. E. (1976): Direct evidence for a bone marrow origin of the alveolar macrophage in man. *Science*, 192:1016–1017.

88. Thompson, J., and Van Furth, R. (1970): The effect of glucocorticosteroids on the kinetics of mononuclear phagocytes. *J. Exp. Med.*, 131:429–449.

89. Thompson, J., and Van Furth, R. (1973): The effect of glucocorticosteroids on the proliferation and kinetics of promonocytes in the bone marrow. *J. Exp. Med.*, 137:10–21.

90. Thörig, L., Thompson, J., Eulderink, F., Emeis, J. J., and Van Furth, R. (1980): Effects of monocytopenia and anticoagulation in experimental Streptococcus sanguis endocarditis. *Br. J. Exp. Pathol.*, 61:108–116.

91. Todd, R. F., and Schlossman, S. F. (1984): Utilization of monoclonal antibodies in the characterization of monocyte-macrophage differentiation antigens. In: *Immunology of the Reticuloendothelial System*, edited by J. A. Bellanti and H. B. Herscowitz, Vol. 6, pp. 87–112. Plenum, New York.

92. Todd, R. F., Biondi, A., and Roach, J. A. (1985): Human macrophage antigens. In: *Mononuclear Phagocytes. Characteristics, Physiology and Function*, edited by R. Van Furth, pp. 31–39. Martinus Nijhoff, Boston.

93. Tompkins, E. H. (1952): The response of monocytes to adrenal cortical extracts. *J. Lab. Clin. Med.*, 39:365–371.

94. Van der Meer, J. W. M., Beelen, R. H. J., Fluitsma, D. M., and Van Furth, R. (1979): Ultrastructure of mononuclear phagocytes developing in liquid bone marrow cultures: a study on peroxidatic activity. *J. Exp. Med.*, 149:17–26.

95. Van der Meer, J. W. M., Van de Gevel, J. S., Diesselhoff-den Dulk, M. M. C., Beelen, R. H. J., and Van Furth, R. (1980): Long-term cultures of murine bone marrow mononuclear phagocytes. In: *Mononuclear Phagocytes. Functional Aspects*, pp. 343–361. Martinus Nijhoff, Boston.

96. Van der Meer, J. W. M., Van de Gevel, J. S., Beelen, R. H. J., Fluitsma, D. M., and Van Furth, R. (1982): Culture of human

bone marrow in the Teflon culture bag: identification of the human monoblast. *J. Reticuloendothel. Soc.,* 34:355–369.

97. Van der Meer, J. W. M., Van de Gevel, J. S., and Van Furth, R. (1983): Characteristics of long-term cultures of proliferating mononuclear phagocytes from bone marrow. *J. Reticuloendothel. Soc.,* 34:203–225.

98. Van der Meer, J. W. M., Van de Gevel, J. S., Westgeest, A. A., and Van Furth, R. (1986): The effect of glucocorticosteroids on bone marrow mononuclear phagocytes in culture. *Immunobiology,* 172:143–150.

99. Van Furth, R. (1975): Modulation of monocyte production. In: *Mononuclear Phagocytes in Immunity, Infection, and Pathology,* edited by R. Van Furth, pp. 161–172. Blackwell Scientific Publications, Oxford.

100. Van Furth, R. (1980): Cells of the mononuclear phagocyte system: nomenclature in terms of sites and conditions. In: *Mononuclear Phagocytes. Functional Aspects,* edited by R. Van Furth, pp. 1–30. Martinus Nijhoff, Boston.

101. Van Furth, R., and Cohn, Z. A. (1968): The origin and kinetics of mononuclear phagocytes. *J. Exp. Med.,* 128:415–435.

102. Van Furth, R., and Diesselhoff-den Dulk, M. M. C. (1970): The kinetics of promonocytes and monocytes in the bone marrow. *J. Exp. Med.,* 132:813–828.

103. Van Furth, R., and Diesselhoff-den Dulk, M. M. C. (1984): Dual origin of mouse spleen macrophages. *J. Exp. Med.,* 160:1273–1283.

104. Van Furth, R., and Fedorko, M. E. (1976): Ultrastructure of mouse mononuclear phagocytes in bone marrow colonies grown in vitro. *Lab. Invest.,* 34:440–450.

105. Van Furth, R., and Sluiter, W. (1985): Macrophages as autoregulators of mononuclear phagocyte proliferation. In: *Macrophage Biology,* Vol. 4, edited by S. Reichard and M. Kojima, pp. 111–123. Alan R. Liss, New York.

106. Van Furth, R., and Sluiter, W. (1986): Distribution of blood monocytes between a marginating and a circulating pool. *J. Exp. Med.,* 163:474–479.

107. Van Furth, R., Cohn, Z. A., Hirsch, J. G., Humphry, J. H., Spector, W. G., and Langevoort, H. L. (1972): The mononuclear phagocyte system: a new classification of macrophages, monocytes and their precursor. *Bull. WHO,* 46:845–852.

108. Van Furth, R., Diesselhoff-den Dulk, M. M. C., and Mattie, H. (1973): Quantitative study on the production and kinetics of mononuclear phagocytes during an acute inflammatory reaction. *J. Exp. Med.,* 138:1314–1330.

109. Van Furth, R., Diesselhoff-den Dulk, M. M. C., Raeburn, J. A., Van Zwet, Th. L., Crofton, R., and Blussé van Oud Alblas, A. (1980): Characteristics, origin and kinetics of human and murine mononuclear phagocytes. In: *Mononuclear Phagocytes. Functional Aspects,* edited by R. Van Furth, pp. 279–298. Martinus Nijhoff, Boston.

110. Van Furth, R., Gassmann, A. E., and Diesselhoff-den Dulk, M. M. C. (1975): The effect of azathioprine (Imuran®) on the cell cycle of promonocytes and the production of monocytes in the bone marrow. *J. Exp. Med.,* 141:531–546.

111. Van Furth, R., Hirsch, J. G., and Fedorko, M. E. (1970): Morphology and peroxidase cytochemistry of mouse promonocytes, monocytes and macrophages. *J. Exp. Med.,* 132:794–812.

112. Van Furth, R., Langevoort, H. L., and Schaberg, A. (1975): Mononuclear phagocytes in human pathology—proposal for an approach to improve classification. In: *Mononuclear Phagocytes in Immunity, Infection, and Pathology,* edited by R. Van Furth, pp. 1–15. Blackwell Scientific Publications, Oxford.

113. Van Furth, R., Nibbering, P. H., Van Dissel, J. T., and Diesselhoff-den Dulk, M. M. C. (1985): The characterization, origin, and ki-

netics of skin macrophages during inflammation. *J. Invest. Dermatol.,* 85:398–402.

114. Van Furth, R., Van der Meer, J. W. M., Blussé van Oud Alblas, A., and Sluiter, W. (1982): Development of mononuclear phagocytes. In: *Self-Defense Mechanisms. Role of Macrophages,* edited by D. Mizuno, Z. A. Cohn, K. Takeya, and N. Ishida, pp. 25–41. Elsevier, New York.

115. Van Furth, R., Van der Meer, J. W. M., Toivonen, H., and Rytömaa, T. (1983): Kinetic analysis of the growth of bone marrow mononuclear phagocytes in long-term cultures. *J. Reticuloendothel. Soc.,* 34:227–234.

116. Van Waarde, D., Bakker, S., Van Vliet, J., Angulo, A. F., and Van Furth, R. (1978): The number of monocytes in mice as a reflection of their contribution and capacity to react to an inflammatory stimulus. *J. Reticuloendothel. Soc.,* 24:197–204.

117. Van Waarde, D., Hulsing-Hesselink, E., and Van Furth, R. (1976): A serum factor inducing monocytosis during an acute inflammatory reaction caused by newborn calf serum. *Cell Tissue Kinet.,* 9:51–63.

118. Van Waarde, D., Hulsing-Hesselink, E., and Van Furth, R. (1977): Properties of a factor increasing monocytopoiesis (FIM) occurring in serum during the early phase of an inflammatory reaction. *Blood,* 50:727–741.

119. Van Waarde, D., Hulsing-Hesselink, E., and Van Furth, R. (1978): Humoral control of monocytopoiesis by an activator and an inhibitor. *Agents Actions,* 8:423–437.

120. Van Waarde, D., Hulsing-Hesselink, E., Sandkuyl, L. A., and Van Furth, R. (1977): Humoral regulation of monocytopoiesis during the early phase of an inflammatory reaction caused by particulate substances. *Blood,* 50:141–153.

121. Virolainen, M. (1968): Hematopoietic origin of macrophages as studied by chromosome markers in mice. *J. Exp. Med.,* 127:943–951.

122. Volkman, A. (1966): The origin and turnover of mononuclear cells in peritoneal exudates in rats. *J. Exp. Med.,* 124:241–254.

123. Volkman, A. (1970): The origin and fate of the monocyte. *Ser. Haematol.,* 2:62–92.

124. Volkman, A. (1976): Disparity in the origin of mononuclear phagocyte populations. *J. Reticuloendothel. Soc.,* 19:249–268.

125. Volkman, A., and Collins, F. M. (1974): The cytokinetics of monocytosis in acute salmonella infection in rat. *J. Exp. Med.,* 139:264–277.

126. Volkman, A., and Gowans, J. L. (1965): The origin of macrophages from bone marrow in the rat. *Br. J. Exp. Pathol.,* 46:62–70.

127. Volkman, A., and Gowans, J. L. (1965): The production of macrophages in the rat. *Br. J. Exp. Pathol.,* 46:50–61.

128. Weiden, P. L., Storb, R., and Tsoi, M. S. (1975): Marrow origin of canine alveolar macrophages. *J. Reticuloendothel. Soc.,* 17:432–345.

129. Whitelaw, D. M. (1966): The intravascular lifespan of monocytes. *Blood,* 28:445–464.

130. Whitelaw, D. M. (1972): Observations on human monocyte kinetics after pulse labeling. *Cell Tissue Kinet.,* 5:311–317.

131. Van't Wout, J. W., Linde, I., Leijh, P. C. J., and Van Furth, R. (1989): Effect of irradiation, cyclophosphamide, and etoposide (VP-16) on number of peripheral blood and peritoneal leukocytes in mice under normal conditions and during acute inflammatory reaction. *Inflammation,* 13:1–14.

132. Wright, S. D., and Silverstein, S. C. (1986): Overview: the function of receptors in phagocytosis. In: *Handbook of Experimental Immunology, Vol. II: Cellular Immunology,* edited by D. M. Weir, L. A. Herzenberg, C. Blackwell, and L. A. Herzenberg, pp. 41.1–41.14. Blackwell Scientific Publications, Oxford.

Inflammation: Basic Principles and Clinical Correlates.
Edited by J. I. Gallin, I. M. Goldstein, and R. Snyderman.
Raven Press, Ltd., New York © 1988.

CHAPTER 18

Phagocytic Cells: Egress from Marrow and Diapedesis

Harry L. Malech

Egress from the Bone Marrow Pool
  Bone Marrow Architecture: Mechanical Factors • Neutrophil Maturational Factors • Humoral Factors in Marrow Egress

Diapedesis
  Blood Flow Characteristics: Mechanical Factors • Cellular Factors • Humoral Factors
References

The kinetics of human neutrophil egress from bone marrow to the circulation is determined by the rate of production of committed neutrophil precursors from stem cells in the marrow, the rate of proliferation of committed neutrophil precursors, the length of time required for each maturational stage, and the maturational stage of neutrophils released into the circulation. In Chapter 16 factors influencing the proliferation of neutrophil precursors, a description of the morphology and biochemistry of cells at each maturational stage, and the time required for each maturational stage are considered. Infection, other types of inflammation, and stress increase the rate of production of neutrophils from precursors, shorten the time usually required for each stage of neutrophil maturation, decrease the time mature neutrophils reside in the marrow, and result in the release of immature neutrophil precursors into the circulation.

In a normal uninfected adult, more than 100 billion neutrophils are in transit from the bone marrow daily. This number may increase to almost a trillion neutrophils daily in the setting of serious infection (25,28,32,73,92). With a circulating blood volume of approximately 5 liters, this daily flux of neutrophils is about 20,000 cells/μl of peripheral blood in the uninfected host and as many as 200,000 cells/μl with severe infection. Because the actual measured peripheral blood neutrophil count is normally only about 3,000 to 5,000 cells/μl and even in severe infection is rarely above 30,000 cells/μl, these rough calculations alone indicate that the circulating blood pool of neutrophils must be in rapid transit from the bone marrow to the postcapillary venule sites of egress into tissues. These observations are consistent with *in vivo* studies of labeled neutrophils which indicate that the normal half-time of the neutrophil in the circulation is about 6 to 10 hr (25,28,32,73,92). This half-time is further shortened in the setting of infection (37). Once in the tissues, neutrophils are capable of surviving several days.

The final tissue destination of most neutrophils in the normal host has not been resolved. Some loss of neutrophils must occur to sites of inapparent infection that develop as a result of minor breaches of the integument. Egress of neutrophils into gingival crevasses around the teeth occurs even with healthy oral tissues and is probably an important mechanism of host defense at this site (27,91). Earlier studies suggested that the gastrointestinal tract is the site of most of the neutrophil egress in normal individuals (73) and is an important mechanism for protecting the host from the heavy burden of microorganisms at this site. More recent studies have called into question these assumptions, as the numbers of neutrophils seen in histological specimens in various tissue sites do not support the concept of neutrophil egress into tissues, including the gut, in the absence of infection or another inflammatory process (52). The spleen and other reticuloendothelial tissues may play some role in the removal of senescent neutrophils, but it is of note that splenectomized individuals do not have major changes in the number of circulating neutrophils.

Neutrophils produced in the bone marrow must cross two endothelial cell barriers in order to arrive at sites of infection or inflammation in the tissues. The interaction between neutrophils in the bone marrow and the endothelial cells of the marrow sinuses may be important in the control of egress from the marrow. The importance of an interaction between neutrophils in the circulation and the endothelial cells of small blood vessels of target tissues has been clearly established and is discussed below. Factors that alter the steady-state flux of neutrophils across these barriers have profound effects on the kinetics of neutrophil egress from the marrow to sites of infection.

EGRESS FROM THE BONE MARROW POOL

Bone Marrow Architecture: Mechanical Factors

Most nonerythroid cellular elements in the bone marrow are neutrophils and neutrophil precursors. Neutrophil precursors are not arranged at random. Early neutrophil precursors are arranged in a reticular pattern as cords of immature cells located away from the marrow sinuses. More mature cells are found at the periphery of these cords of immature cells, where they may be more likely to approach the endothelial cells of the marrow blood vessels (60,73,94). It has been suggested that this architecture makes it more likely for mature neutrophils, rather than precursors, to enter the circulation. However, the location of neutrophils at the periphery of the reticular cords of proliferating myeloid precursors may itself be a consequence of the increasing motile capacity of maturing neutrophils. With *in vitro* cultures of bone marrow, the maturation of granulocyte colonies is associated with movement of mature neutrophils outward at the periphery of the colony (70).

By electron microscopy, the endothelial cells of marrow sinuses appear flattened with tight junctions between cells (60,73,94). Generally there are few or no gaps in the endothelial cell layer except where a blood cell is in transit into the circulation. Neutrophils appear to squeeze between endothelial cells of the sinuses during egress, creating in the process an intercellular space of about 1 μm. The basement membrane of marrow sinus endothelium is patchy and incomplete, which may also facilitate egress of cells from the bone marrow. Ultrastructural studies suggest that infection or endotoxin challenge is associated with a decrease in the adventitial cell cover of the endothelium, as well as with the induction of gaps between endothelial cells of the marrow sinuses, which may allow easier access of neutrophils and neutrophil precursors to the circulation (60,94).

Neutrophil Maturational Factors

In the absence of infection, egress of neutrophils appears to be limited to morphologically mature cells with com-

pletely segmented nuclei. Functional studies of neutrophil precursors have demonstrated the sequential acquisition of increasing motile capacity and increasing chemotactic responsiveness (1,19,58,59). Even band forms have been shown to have motile responses that are inferior to those of morphologically mature neutrophils. A number of studies using precision tapered capillary tubes to measure the viscoelastic properties of individual neutrophil precursors have demonstrated that maturation is associated with increasing cellular deformability (58). Both the marrow bands and morphologically mature neutrophils in the marrow show decreased phagocytic capacity and respiratory burst compared to peripheral blood neutrophils (1,12,98).

Neutrophil maturation is also associated with marked changes in the carbohydrate structure of surface glycoproteins. Such changes appear to consist of an increase in branching and presumably sialic acid content from early precursors to the promyelocyte stage and then a slight decrease with further maturation (40). In the later stages of maturation there is a decrease in negative surface charge, which in part may reflect a decrease in cell surface sialic acid (59). An increase in alkaline phosphatase activity also has been clearly associated with maturation, and a decrease in alkaline phosphatase activity of circulating neutrophils has been used as a marker of enhanced egress of neutrophils from the bone marrow pool (12,36,81). Some of these maturational changes, particularly the acquisition of motile activity and increasing deformability, may be linked to the process that determines egress of neutrophils from the marrow.

Bone marrow neutrophils that have completed the maturational sequence and are morphologically indistinguishable from those in the peripheral blood do not immediately exit to the circulation. This marrow reserve pool of mature neutrophils is estimated to be about 20 times as many cells as is present in the peripheral circulation. These mature neutrophils remain in the bone marrow for about 2 days before entering the circulation (25,28,32,73,92). It is not clear what factors, if any, determine which morphologically mature neutrophils enter the circulation. At this stage the process may be entirely random, but additional maturational processes may occur that continue to increase the tendency of a neutrophil to exit from the marrow. There is some evidence from radioisotope studies that neutrophils exit the marrow pool in the same chronological order in which they were produced from precursor cells (28,65). This finding is in contrast to neutrophils in the peripheral blood pool (discussed below), which appear to exit from the circulation at random (28,38).

It is sometimes assumed that an increase in the number of nuclear lobes relates to the maturational age of a neutrophil and that such changes may be accompanied by other maturational changes. It is of note, however, that no functional or biochemical differences between post-band stage neutrophils with different numbers of nuclear lobes has been demonstrated. It is possible, however, that some of the known differences that exist between band stage and mature neutrophils, relating to functions and to cell surface adhesion molecules or receptors, may be used to distinguish among morphologically mature neutrophils of different ages in the marrow pool.

Studies by Ross and others have indicated that CR2, the receptor for C3d, is normally present on immature neutrophils and is lost only during the most terminal stages of differentiation (78,79). The immature CR2-bearing neutrophils have been reported to be less dense than the more mature neutrophils. More recent studies have demonstrated that peripheral blood neutrophils in patients with localized juvenile periodontitis express CR2 on the cell surface, whereas neutrophils from normal controls do not (46). This phenomenon is not associated with any increase in band forms in the peripheral blood of these patients. A number of studies have indicated that neutrophils from patients with localized juvenile periodontitis have defects in chemotaxis (see Chapter 26). It has been suggested that neutrophils in these patients may be arrested late in differentiation, leading both to retention of CR2 in the neutrophils released from their marrow and to the functional defects observed (46).

We have developed a murine immunoglobulin G_1 (IgG_1) monoclonal antibody, 31D8, that binds heterogeneously to peripheral blood neutrophils (44,56,85). Some observations described below indicate that there are differences in the kinetics of marrow egress of morphologically mature neutrophils expressing different amounts of the antigen detected by this antibody. Using fluorescein-labeled antibodies and fluorescence-activated cell sorting (FACS), it was noted that in most adults more than 90% of circulating neutrophils bind 31D8 strongly, resulting in a single peak of bright fluorescence and either a skew toward the dull region of this peak or a small shoulder indicating that some cells show more dull fluorescence (Fig. 1A). The 31D8 bright cells are functionally more responsive than the 31D8 dull neutrophils in terms of chemotaxis and respiratory burst activity when activated with the bacterial chemoattractant f-met-leu-phe (85). Initial studies of binding to bone marrow cells suggested that the 31D8 antigen can be detected in some neutrophil precursors as early as the late myelocyte stage and that heterogeneity of binding of 31D8 antibody can be seen among all later stages of neutrophil maturation (85). However, a maturation-related increase in expression of this antigen could not be ruled out.

In subsequent studies neonates were shown to have a significant increase in circulating 31D8 dull cells compared to that in adults. In some neonates distinct and only partially overlapping populations of 31D8 bright and dull neutrophils were seen by FACS, whereas this degree

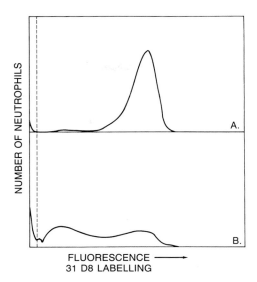

FIG. 1. Fluorescence-activated cell analysis of human neutrophils labeled with murine monoclonal antibody, 31D8. The abscissa shows relative fluorescence intensity on a logarithmic scale (full scale is three $\log_{10}$ cycles). The dashed line parallel to the ordinate represents the upper limit of nonspecific fluorescence. Side scatter and forward scatter characteristics were used to gate on neutrophils in a mixed leukocyte preparation from peripheral blood. All of the nonneutrophils not gated out of the analysis are found by sorting to be to the left of the nonspecific fluorescence cutoff. **A:** Typical analysis of normal adult neutrophils. The single brightly fluorescent curve is skewed to the left, representing some neutrophils that label much less brightly with this antibody. Sorted cells from this area of the curve are all neutrophils. **B:** Representative analysis of neutrophils from an adult admitted for severe trauma. Two populations of fluorescent neutrophils are seen, which by sorting consist of neutrophils or neutrophil band forms. Band forms are enriched in the dull peak, but neither the dull nor the bright peak consist exclusively of bands or mature neutrophils.

of separation was seldom seen in adults (56). Because neonates also have an increase in circulating bands and other neutrophil precursors, FACS separation of the two populations of 31D8-labeled neonate neutrophils was performed in order to determine the number of mature neutrophils and precursors. Although there was a moderate enrichment of band forms in the 31D8 dull population, there were significant numbers of bands in the 31D8 bright population and a significant number of mature neutrophils in the 31D8 dull population (56). These studies suggested that 31D8 antigen expression by neutrophils was only moderately correlated with the maturational level of the neutrophil as indicated by nuclear morphology. Heterogeneity of expression of this antigen was clearly observable in post-band form neutrophils.

In preliminary studies adult patients admitted with severe trauma were found to have a marked increase in 31D8 dull neutrophils leading to FACS patterns similar to that noted in neonates (Fig. 1B) (55). The pattern became more like the normal adult neutrophil pattern seen in Fig. 1A several days after acute trauma. FACS sorting again demonstrated enrichment of band forms in the 31D8 dull peak, but this peak also contained many mature neutrophils.

Human volunteers given endotoxin (4 ng/kg) intravenously develop a drop in the peripheral blood neutrophil count that reached a minimum at 1 hr followed by a progressive rise in peripheral blood neutrophils to levels that were three times the baseline at 8 hr (Fig. 2) (22). The early drop has been attributed to adherence of neutrophils to the endothelium of postcapillary venules (margination). The subsequent increase has been shown to be a result of enhanced egress of neutrophils from the marrow pool (31,95). We have examined 31D8 binding to peripheral blood neutrophils during the response to endotoxin administration (22). There was a profound increase in 31D8 dull cells that slightly preceded the appearance of band forms and thereafter paralleled the increase and eventual decrease in band forms. At 4 hr two distinct, equal-sized 31D8 dull and bright populations of neutrophils were seen by FACS analysis. FACS separation of these neutrophils showed that the 31D8 dull peak was enriched for band forms but contained more than 5% mature forms. Conversely, the 31D8 bright peak contained 5 to 10% band forms. These results further support the notion that the marrow pool of neutrophils contains significant numbers of 31D8 dull, post-band form neutrophils that are mobilized into the peripheral blood with endotoxin administration. One interpretation of these results is that 31D8

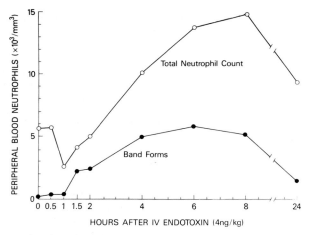

FIG. 2. Analysis of peripheral blood total neutrophil count (bands and mature neutrophils) and neutrophil band count after intravenous administration of endotoxin to human volunteers. The nadir at 1 hr is due to margination of circulating neutrophils. It is followed by a rise in total neutrophils accompanied by a rise in band forms—a result of enhanced marrow egress of both mature neutrophils and band forms from the bone marrow pool. The curves represent the average from six individuals. (Modified from ref. 22.)

antigen expression increases with maturity but does not directly parallel nuclear maturation. These findings raise the possibility that this antigen may provide a marker independent of nuclear morphology that correlates with the maturational and functional state of the neutrophil.

Further studies of the correlation of 31D8 binding, CR2 expression, alkaline phosphatase, or other markers with marrow egress of neutrophils may provide insights into the factors regulating the egress of mature neutrophils from the marrow pool into the circulation in normal versus infected or otherwise stressed individuals.

Humoral Factors in Marrow Egress

A number of humoral factors have been shown to augment the egress of bone marrow pool neutrophils into the circulation. Several studies have demonstrated that bacterial endotoxin greatly increases the rate of egress of bone marrow pool neutrophils into the circulation (31,35,95). A typical time course for this mobilization of bone marrow neutrophils into the circulation is shown in Fig. 2 and was discussed in the previous section.

Intravenous administration of bacterial endotoxin results in a broad array of pathophysiological events, including fever, neutrophilia, and other acute-phase reactions (31,35,95). In animal studies, higher levels of endotoxin administration are associated with shock (18), hemorrhagic damage to a number of organ systems (72), and death of the animal. Whereas endotoxin itself may directly alter cellular functions of a number of cells including macrophages and endothelial cells, it has been shown that two monokines produced by endotoxin-treated macrophages—interleukin 1 (IL-1) (33) and tumor necrosis factor (TNF) (13)—are responsible for many of the most dramatic pathophysiological effects previously attributed to endotoxin.

IL-1 is the primary endogenous pyrogen responsible for mediating the febrile response (see Chapter 12). It is also capable of directly mediating a number of other acute-phase responses, including the neutrophilia usually associated with infection or inflammation (33). Thus IL-1 is an important endogenous factor capable of enhancing marrow egress of neutrophils. The mechanism by which this mediator induces marrow egress of neutrophils is not certain, but it may involve the induction or augmentation of production of yet other mediators, e.g., colony-stimulating factors (see below), by monocytes or other cells (69). It has been reported that IL-1 is capable of activating blood neutrophils in vitro (33). It is possible that it enhances motile activity of marrow neutrophils or primes marrow neutrophils in a way that increases responsiveness to other mediators.

TNF, which is identical to cachexin, has been shown to be one mediator of endotoxin shock and the hemorrhagic tissue damage associated with endotoxin administration (13) (see Chapter 12). TNF is capable of inducing production of IL-1 by macrophages (34) and endothelial cells (57), providing an indirect mechanism by which TNF could enhance marrow egress of neutrophils. TNF also stimulates human endothelial cells to produce granulocyte/monocyte colony-stimulating factor (21). Also of interest is that TNF has direct endogenous pyrogen activity (34). It is not clear from the literature, but it is likely that TNF may have direct effects on marrow egress of neutrophils as well.

Endotoxin is capable of activating the complement system *in vivo,* resulting in margination of neutrophils, particularly in pulmonary small vessels. Of particular importance is the production of C5a, which is a potent chemoattractant and chemokinetic substance (88). It is possible that C5a-induced increased motility of marrow pool mature neutrophils could result in some increased egress of neutrophils from the bone marrow into the circulation.

Patients who are given therapeutic doses of glucocorticoids develop a mild to moderate neutrophilia. Studies by Dale et al. (31) have demonstrated that acute administration of a single oral or intravenous dose of glucocorticoid results in an increase in the peripheral blood neutrophil count first detectable at 2 hr and reaching a maximum at 4 hr. They noted that band forms did not increase and that the neutrophilia consisted of mature neutrophils only. It was suggested that these steroids selectively mobilize the mature neutrophils of the bone marrow pool. It is of note that we do not see an increase in 31D8 dull neutrophils in association with the neutrophilia of glucocorticoid administration (22). (See discussion above regarding results using this antibody after endotoxin administration.) Enhanced bone marrow egress alone cannot explain the chronic neutrophilia associated with chronic administration of glucocorticoids because enhanced egress from the marrow would eventually deplete the marrow pool. There must also be delayed egress into tissues, release of a marginated pool, or enhanced production of neutrophils for a steady-state increase in circulating neutrophils to occur. Steroids do decrease neutrophil adhesion (62,63). Also of note is that glucocorticoids have been reported to enhance proliferation of granulocyte colony-forming units *in vitro* while at the same time depressing growth of eosinophil colonies (16).

It is not known if IL-1, TNF, or corticosteroids play a role in the egress of marrow neutrophils in healthy, uninfected, unstressed individuals. In studies done more than 25 years ago (reviewed in ref. 2) it was shown that rats acutely depleted of neutrophils by repeated peritoneal lavage produced a factor in their serum that induced neutrophilia in rats infused with such sera or made parabiotic with the lavaged rats. Similar studies were done in dogs

by directly removing peripheral blood neutrophils using centrifugation. Such studies have been cited as evidence for humoral factors that regulate marrow egress of neutrophils in the uninfected animal but do not control for the presence of endotoxin, complement activation, and stress to the animals. Subsequent studies using myelosuppressive therapy in dogs (controlled for the presence of endotoxin and stress) indicated the presence of a marrow neutrophil-releasing factor (17). Despite substantial progress in understanding the biochemistry and activity of myeloproliferative factors controlling production and differentiation of neutrophils, there has not been further clarification of the humoral factors involved in regulating marrow egress of neutrophils in the healthy host.

There are other endogenous humoral mediators that could play a role in marrow egress. The availability of recombinant colony-simulating factors (G-CSF and GM-CSF) has resulted in studies demonstrating that these factors have functional effects on mature neutrophils (5,61,74,93) as well as the expected proliferative effects on precursor cells (see Chapter 15). Changes in surface chemotactic receptors have been noted, and an augmentation of activation in response to chemotactic factors was seen after an hour of exposure of mature circulating human neutrophils to GM-CSF. Although the focus of these studies was a demonstration of an effect on peripheral blood neutrophils, it is possible that these factors also affect the marrow pool of mature neutrophils.

DIAPEDESIS

In a normal individual the measured peripheral blood neutrophil count underestimates the number of neutrophils in the circulation, as one-half to two-thirds of peripheral blood neutrophils are in a marginated pool of cells that are sequestered in postcapillary venules (20,54). There may be considerable variability in the size of this marginated pool of neutrophils in different individuals. Some patients with apparent neutropenia may have a normal total number of neutrophils in the peripheral blood pool but have a large fraction of such cells in the marginated pool.

Blood Flow Characteristics: Mechanical Factors

Much of the information about dynamic features of blood flow in small vessels has been obtained from direct microscopic observation in live animals. A number of methods have been developed to analyze the microcirculation *in vivo.* Long-term placement of ear chambers in rabbits, the hamster cheek pouch, and animal mesenteric preparations are some well-studied examples (6,9,10,24). In many studies the microcirculation may have been altered by the process of preparing the tissues for observation. Descriptions of the circulation supposedly in the absence of inflammation must be interpreted with this caveat.

In the precapillary arterioles, blood flow is rapid; there is little evidence of differential spatial arrangement of specific blood cells; and there is little evidence for interaction of leukocytes with the vessel walls. Blood flow is slow in the capillaries, and erythrocytes and leukocytes move through in single file. Neutrophils may occupy the full diameter of a capillary, are often deformed during passage, and occasionally even block blood flow through a capillary for some period. However, neutrophils do not appear to pass into the tissues from capillaries, even in the presence of an inflammatory stimulus. Mechanical factors have been evoked to explain this finding. It has been suggested, based on *in vitro* studies using glass capillary tubes, that the stretched and deformed neutrophil in the blood capillary is prevented mechanically from initiating pseudopod formation and migrating between capillary endothelial cells into the tissues (41). However, neutrophils have been shown to be capable of extreme degrees of deformation *in vitro* during movement into nitrocellulose micropore filters. The limiting pore size restricting movement of the whole neutrophil into the filter is about 0.45 μm (64).

There is often a relative retardation of speed of exit from capillaries into venules by the larger leukocytes relative to erythrocytes. Passive fluid forces result in lateral displacement of such leukocytes entering the postcapillary venules. In the postcapillary venules blood flow is slower than on the arteriole side of the capillary bed, and the diameter is wide enough to allow some differential arrangement of blood cells. In these vessels there is a tendency for leukocytes to segregate toward the lateral, more slowly flowing portion of the moving column of plasma. In this location neutrophils closely approach and transiently adhere to the endothelial cells lining the blood vessel. *In vitro* studies of blood flow in thin-walled glass capillary tubes indicate that in tubes with diameters similar to postcapillary venules and at flow rates found in these vessels, there is rouleau formation by erythrocytes. These stacks of erythrocytes tend to occupy the central, more rapidly moving portion of the moving fluid column. The leukocytes are thus passively displaced toward the periphery of the flow stream (48). Frictional forces with nonmoving surfaces are responsible for slower fluid movement at the periphery of the flow stream. In the absence of erythrocytes there is no peripheral sequestration of leukocytes. Also, larger-diameter vessels and increased rates of flow impede erythrocyte rouleau formation and eliminate the lateral displacement of leukocytes. Thus fluid dynamics of whole blood in postcapillary venules appears to play an important role in bringing the neutrophil into physical contact with endothelial cells. These passive fluid flow factors may be less important during inflammation, where both the neutrophil and endothelial cell become more adhesive (see discussion below).

Cellular Factors

In postcapillary venules *in vivo,* there is some adherence of neutrophils to endothelial cells even in the absence of any inflammatory stimulus. In the absence of inflammation this association between neutrophils and endothelial cells *in vivo* appears to be reversible (6,9,10), influenced by fluid flow (67,83,84) and humoral factors such as epinephrine (20) (see next section). The *in vivo* adherence of neutrophils to endothelium is greatly augmented by tissue damage and other inflammatory stimuli. In the presence of inflammation the adherent neutrophils subsequently migrate between endothelial cells into tissues and do not return to the circulation. With a more intense inflammatory process there is adhesion of circulating neutrophils to other neutrophils that have adhered to, but not migrated through, the endothelial cell layer. This process may result in occlusion of the blood vessel (2,6,9,10).

Adhesion of neutrophils to endothelial cells *in vitro* has been demonstrated in a large number of published studies. Activation of neutrophils by chemotactic factors (C5a, C5a des arg, f-met-leu-phe, leukotriene B$_4$) as well as by nonphysiological stimuli (e.g., phorbol myristate acetate) result in a dramatic increase in the number of neutrophils that adhere to a layer of endothelial cells in culture (47,50,87,89,90). The adherence-promoting activity of chemotactic factors occurs at higher concentrations than is required to stimulate neutrophil chemotaxis (26). Endotoxin, phorbol myristate acetate, and endogenous humoral factors such as IL-1, TNF, and leukotrienes C$_4$ and D$_4$ also have been shown to increase the adherence of neutrophils to endothelial cells by acting on the endothelial cells (15,45,68,77,82).

The identification of patients whose leukocytes lack a family of adherence-related proteins (CR3-deficient patients; see Chapter 21) has indicated that these cell membrane receptors are important for neutrophil adherence to endothelial cells (4,23,49,77). Related studies using antibodies to these receptors indicate that the number of iC3b receptors (CR3) increases severalfold at the neutrophil cell surface upon activation of the neutrophil (11,39,42,75) and that this increase plays an important role in increasing the adherence of neutrophils to other cells and surfaces (42,49,77). It is of note that CR3-deficient patients have a marked leukocytosis, even in the absence of major infection (3,42). It has been suggested that this leukocytosis may be partly a consequence of poor adherence of neutrophils to endothelial cells and thus a shift of neutrophils from the marginated pool to the circulating pool (3,42). The extremely poor delivery of neutrophils to sites of inflammation in these patients would also support this hypothesis and indicate a defect in diapedesis.

As indicated above, endothelial cells are altered by products of infection and inflammation (see Chapter 29). For example, endotoxin acts directly on endothelial cells to increase adherence of neutrophils to the treated cells (15,77,82). This effect is independent of any activation of neutrophils and in most studies is not evident until 1 hr or more after exposure of the endothelial cell to endotoxin. The response requires new protein synthesis by the endothelial cells, which occurs over several hours following exposure to endotoxin (15,45,77,82) and is associated with the appearance of new surface antigens on the endothelial cells (14,76). Figure 3 shows how endotoxin treatment of endothelial cells alters the binding of neutrophils that have not been activated by any stimulus other than exposure to the washed endothelial cell layer.

Endothelial cells may produce factors that activate neutrophils. During the response of endothelial cells to the inflammatory mediators, leukotriene C_4 and D_4, endothelial cells produce platelet-activating factor, which remains at the endothelial cell surface. The platelet-activating factor at the endothelial cell surface is capable of activating neutrophils that come into contact with these cells, further augmenting the adherence process (68).

Studies in our laboratory indicate that endothelial cells readily bind and internalize large amounts of f-met-leu-phe, and that much of the internalized formyl peptide is slowly released intact, without degradation (80). It appears that the endothelial cell can both produce neutrophil activators and take up mediators of neutrophil activation from the extracellular milieu. Endothelial cells may then serve to buffer such inflammatory mediators and present them to the neutrophil at the time of physical contact of the neutrophil with the endothelial cells.

Thus both the endothelial cell and the neutrophil surface membranes may be altered in response to inflammatory stimuli, resulting in increased adherence of neutrophils to endothelial cells and an augmentation of diapedesis into tissues. The marked decrease in peripheral blood circulating neutrophil count at 1 hr after experimental intravenous challenge with endotoxin is a result of increased margination of circulating neutrophils (Fig. 2) and is a consequence of the direct and indirect endotoxin-mediated effects on both neutrophils and endothelial cells indicated in the discussions above.

In the setting of an inflammatory process, adherence of neutrophils to endothelial cells is rapidly followed by the passage of neutrophils between endothelial cells. The process is similar to that described above in the process of egress from the marrow. The neutrophil undergoes considerable deformation during passage between endo-

thelial cells with close approximation of the neutrophil and endothelial cell membranes (51,66). The overall integrity of the vascular endothelial cell layer appears to remain intact during passage of neutrophils (51).

With some sites, e.g., the bladder or peritoneal cavity, neutrophils must also cross an epithelial or mesothelial cell barrier in order to arrive at the site of inflammation. Studies by Cramer and others have shown that at the ultrastructural level this process is similar to that described for passage across endothelium (30,71). Neutrophils may pass between epithelial cells in response to a gradient of chemoattractant without markedly altering the integrity of the epithelial cell layer.

Neutrophils have been shown to secrete granule contents during migration (96). Studies of the movement of neutrophils into experimentally produced skin blisters in human volunteers *in vivo* indicate that the neutrophils in blister fluid are deficient in specific granules and that granule components are present in the blister fluid (101). Secretion of azurophilic granule components such as elastase may also be important during diapedesis for neutrophil penetration of tissues, and such secretion may also damage tissues (53).

Neutrophils respond to a gradient of chemoattractant by orienting toward the source of the gradient (99,100). It is normally associated with movement toward the source. At the endothelial cell layer, movement is impeded by the requirement that the neutrophil insert a leading lamella between endothelial cells and squeeze through this constriction. An *in vitro* model of this barrier can be simulated by placing neutrophils in the upper compartment of a chemotaxis chamber, separated from a lower compartment containing chemoattractant by a nitrocellulose filter. If the pore size is less than 0.6 μm, the neutrophils cannot migrate completely into the filter (64). Despite this impediment, the neutrophils orient at the filter surface in response to the gradient of chemoattractant and remain there for several hours, maintaining a highly specific arrangement of internal organelles in relation to the vector of the gradient, as shown in Fig. 4. This orientation is dynamic and is not a passive effect of an initial, but frustrated, response to the gradient of chemoattractant. If the direction of the chemoattractant gradient is altered, the neutrophils rapidly reorient in the new direction (64). Even if the chemoattractant is merely replaced by buffer in the lower chamber, the orientation rapidly decays. Similar results have been obtained using human monocytes (97). These studies indicate that phagocytic cell movement is not required for sensing the chemoattractant gradient and that neutrophils or monocytes adherent to endothelial cells *in vivo* may be capable of sensing the source of infection or inflammation in the tissues at the time of initial adherence. This observation is further supported by studies showing that the initial direction of neu-

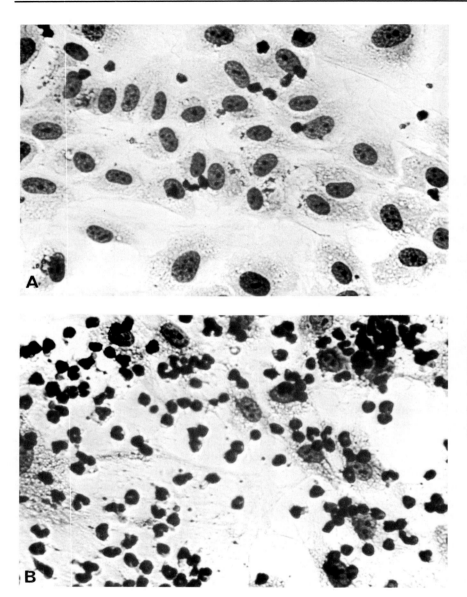

FIG. 3. Human neutrophils were added to 3-day-old primary cultures of human umbilical vein endothelial cells, incubated for 10 min, and then gently rinsed. Plates were stained with hematoxylin. Neutrophils appear as small dark round cells adherent to the much larger flat endothelial cells. **A:** Endothelial cells were not pretreated with endotoxin, and there are few adherent neutrophils. **B:** Endothelial cells had been exposed to endotoxin 100 ng/ml for 6 hr. The endotoxin was washed out of the culture before addition of neutrophils. In other cultures (not shown) endotoxin added to endothelial cells for less than an hour had little effect on neutrophil adherence and the results resembled those in **A.** This finding indicates that residual endotoxin present at the time of addition of neutrophils was not responsible for the effect seen in **B.** (Modified from ref. 22.)

trophil pseudopod formation most often occurs toward the source of the chemoattractant (99,100).

With the *in vitro* micropore filter model, this specific orientation of the neutrophil in response to chemoattractant involves extension of pseudopodia into the filter (Fig. 4). Pyroantimonate staining (not shown) used to localize increased concentrations of cations has shown that in a gradient of chemoattractant there is preferential deposition of submembranous antimonate deposits at the leading edge of the neutrophil pseudopods (29,43).

Other aspects of the neutrophil orientation are that the bulk of the cytoplasmic granules are toward the front of the cell just behind the hyaline, microfilament-filled pseudopods (64). This location may facilitate secretion of

granule contents toward the front portion of the cell during migration.

Near the middle of the oriented neutrophil on the side of the nucleus toward the chemoattractant source are the centrioles with associated microtubule organizing centers and the Golgi apparatus (64). Intact microtubules appear to be essential to the maintenance of this highly specific internal arrangement of cellular organelles in response to the chemotactic vector (64,97). Phagocytic cell chemotactic migration is not ablated by inhibition of microtubule assembly, but the response is blunted. Studies by Singer and Kupfer (86) have emphasized the role of microtubules in the location of the Golgi apparatus to the side of the nucleus in the direction of the vector of movement by

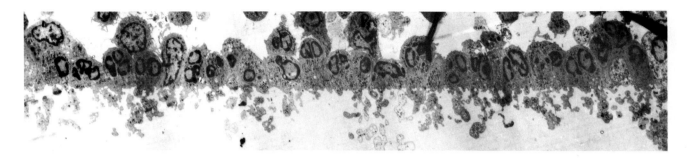

FIG. 4. Human neutrophils incubated for 45 min at 37°C at the surface of a 0.45-μm pore size nitrocellulose filter. The cells are responding to a chemotactic stimulus below the filter (10% human serum activated with zymosan). Note the relative uniformity of the specific orientation of neutrophils in relation to the vector of chemoattractant gradient. Leading pseudopods are inserted deep into the filter pores despite the inability of the entire cell to penetrate the filter.

motile cells in general. Their studies indicate that this orientation of the Golgi may be a general feature of the motility of many cell types and may involve the Golgi as a source of new membrane that preferentially is inserted at the leading portion of the migrating cell, a process that may also be facilitated by microtubules.

Humoral Factors

The role of circulating bacterial products such as endotoxin and f-met-leu-phe in diapedesis was discussed above in the context of cellular factors. There are several endogenous humoral factors that may affect diapedesis. The monokines, IL-1, and TNF act on endothelial cells to enhance the adherence of neutrophils (15,45,77,82).

Another endogenous mediator that appears to markedly influence margination of neutrophils is epinephrine. In the uninfected host the marginated pool of neutrophils can be induced to return to the circulating pool by moderate exercise or the administration of epinephrine. Acute administration of 0.1 to 0.4 mg of epinephrine has been used as a provocative test to determine the size of the marginated pool of neutrophils (7,8,20,54). Studies by Boxer et al. (20) have shown that epinephrine decreases the adherence of neutrophils to endothelial cells in culture. It appears to be an indirect effect. Epinephrine induces the production of cyclic AMP by endothelial or other cells. Increased blood levels of cyclic AMP *in vivo* may act on neutrophils to decrease adhesion to endothelial cells.

A subset of individuals with apparent neutropenia actually have a larger than normal pool of marginated neutrophils (54). The normal rate of exchange between the circulating and marginated pools of neutrophils is not known. Because neutrophils are not seen in significant numbers in most tissues in the absence of infection (52), it is likely that margination in the blood vessels of most uninfected tissues is a temporary and reversible phenomenon.

A number of commonly used drugs, e.g., aspirin, caffeine, and steroids, decrease neutrophil adherence and may influence the size of the marginated pool of neutrophils (63). The physiological consequence of such drug-induced changes in the marginated pool is unknown.

REFERENCES

1. Altman, A. J., and Stossel, T. P. (1974): Functional immaturity of bone marrow bands and polymorphonuclear leucocytes. *Br. J. Haematol.,* 27:241–245.
2. Amundson, B., Jennische, E., and Haljamäe, H. (1980): Correlative analysis of microcirculatory and cellular metabolic events in skeletal muscle during hemorrhagic shock. *Acta Physiol. Scand.,* 108:147–158.
3. Anderson, D. C., Schmalstieg, F. C., Finegold, M. J., Hughes, B. J., Rothlein, R., Miller, L. J., Kohl, S., Tosi, M. F., Jacobs, R. L., Waldrop, T. C., Goldman, A. S., Shearer, W. T., and Springer, T. A. (1985): The severe and moderate phenotypes of heritable Mac-1, LFA-1, p150,95 deficiency: their qualitative definition and relation to leukocyte dysfunction and clinical features. *J. Infect. Dis.,* 152:668–689.
4. Anderson, D. C., Schmalstieg, F. C., Kohl, M. A., Tosi, M. F., Dana, N., Buffone, G. J., Hughes, B. J., Brinkley, B. R., Dickey, W. D., Abramson, J. S., Springer, T., Boxer, L. A., Hollers, J. M., and Smith, C. W. (1984): Abnormalities of polymorphonuclear leukocyte function associated with a heritable deficiency of a high molecular weight surface glycoprotein (GP138): common relationship to diminished cell adherence. *J. Clin. Invest.,* 74:536–551.
5. Arnaout, M. A., Wang, E. A., Clark, S. C., and Sieff, C. A. (1986): Human recombinant granulocyte-macrophage colony-stimulating factor increases cell-to-cell adhesion and surface expression of adhesion-promoting surface glycoproteins on mature granulocytes. *J. Clin. Invest.,* 78:597–601.
6. Asano, M., and Ohkubo, C. (1983): Physiological and pathophysiological events of cutaneous microcirculation observed in the rabbit ear chamber. In: *Intravital Observation of Organ Microcirculation,* edited by M. Tsuchiya, H. Wayland, M. Oda, and I. Okazaki, pp. 31–48. Exerpta Medica, Amsterdam.
7. Athens, J. W. (1972): Granulocyte kinetics in health and disease. *Natl. Cancer Inst. Monogr.,* 30:135–156.
8. Athens, J. W., Haab, O. P., Raab, S. O., Mauer, A. M., Ashenbrucker, H., Cartwright, G. E., and Wintrobe, M. M. (1961): Leukokinetic studies. IV. The total blood, circulatory and marginal pools and the granulocyte turnover rate in normal subjects. *J. Clin. Invest.,* 40:989–995.
9. Atherton, A., and Born, G. V. R. (1972): Quantitative investigations

of the adhesiveness of circulating polymorphonuclear leucocytes to blood vessel walls. *J. Physiol. (Lond.)*, 222:447–474.

10. Atherton, A., and Born, G. V. R. (1973): Relationship between the velocity of rolling granulocytes and that of the blood flow in venules. *J. Physiol. (Lond.)*, 233:157–165.

11. Bainton, D. F., Miller, L. J., Kishimoto, T. K., and Springer, T. A. (1987): Leukocyte adhesion proteins are located in peroxidase-negative granules of human PMN and monocytes: an immunocytochemical study. *Fed. Proc.*, 46:405 (abstract).

12. Berkow, R. L., and Dodson, R. W. (1986): Purification and functional evaluation of mature neutrophils from bone marrow. *Blood*, 68:853–860.

13. Beutler, B., and Cerami, A. (1987): Cachectin: more than a tumor necrosis factor. *N. Engl. J. Med.*, 316:379–385.

14. Bevilacqua, M. P., Pober, J. S., Medrick, D. L., Cotran, R. S., and Gimbrone, M. A., Jr. (1987): Identification of an inducible endothelial-leukocyte adhesion molecule (E-LAM 1) using monoclonal antibodies. *Fed. Proc.*, 46:405 (abstract).

15. Bevilacqua, M. P., Pober, J. S., Wheeler, M. E., Cotran, R. S., and Gimbrone, M. A., Jr. (1985): Interleukin 1 acts on cultured human vascular endothelium to increase the adhesion of polymorphonuclear leukocytes, monocytes, and related leukocyte cell lines. *J. Clin. Invest.*, 76:2003–2011.

16. Bjornson, B. H., Harvey, J. M., and Rose, L. (1985): Differential effect of hydrocortisone on eosinophil and neutrophil proliferation. *J. Clin. Invest.*, 76:924–929.

17. Boggs, D. R., Cartwright, G. E., and Wintrobe, M. M. (1966): Neutrophilia-inducing activity in plasma of dogs recovering from drug-induced myelotoxicity. *Am. J. Physiol.*, 211:51–60.

18. Bond, R. F. (1985): Peripheral circulatory responses to endotoxin. In: *Handbook of Endotoxin, Vol. 2: Pathophysiology of Endotoxin*, edited by L. B. Hinshaw, pp. 36–75. Elsevier, New York.

19. Boner, A., Zeligs, B. J., and Bellanti, J. A. (1982): Chemotactic responses of various differential stages of neutrophils from human cord and adult blood. *Infect. Immun.*, 35:921–928.

20. Boxer, L. A., Allen, J. M., and Baehner, R. L. (1980): Diminished polymorphonuclear leukocyte adherence: function dependent on release of cyclic AMP by endothelial cells after stimulation of β-receptors by epinephrine. *J. Clin. Invest.*, 66:268–274.

21. Broudy, V. C., Kaushansky, K., Segal, G. M., Harlan, J. M., and Adamson, J. W. (1986): Tumor necrosis factor type α stimulates human endothelial cells to produce granulocyte/macrophage colony-stimulating factor. *Proc. Natl. Acad. Sci. USA*, 83:7467–7471.

22. Brown, C. C., Malech, H. L., and Gallin, J. I. (1987): Kinetics of 31D8 defined human neutrophil subpopulations following intravenous endotoxin. *Fed. Proc.*, 46:986 (abstract).

23. Buchanan, M. R., Crowley, C. A., Rosin, R. E., Gimbrone, M. A., Jr., and Babior, B. M. (1982): Studies on the interaction between GP-180-deficient neutrophils and vascular endothelium. *Blood*, 60:160–165.

24. Buckley, I. K. (1963): Delayed secondary damage and leucocyte chemotaxis following focal aseptic heat injury in vivo. *Exp. Mol. Pathol.*, 2:402–417.

25. Cartwright, G. E., Athens, J. W., and Wintrobe, M. M. (1964): The kinetics of neutrophilic cells. *Blood*, 24:780–798.

26. Charo, I. F., Yuen, C., Perez, H. D., and Goldstein, I. M. (1986): Chemotactic peptides modulate adherence of human polymorphonuclear leukocytes to monolayers of cultured endothelial cells. *J. Immunol.*, 136:3412–3419.

27. Charon, J. A., Mergenhagen, S. E., and Gallin, J. I. (1985): Gingivitis and oral ulceration in patients with neutrophil dysfunction. *J. Oral Pathol.*, 14:150–155.

28. Cline, M. J. (1975): *The White Cell*. Harvard University Press, Cambridge.

29. Cramer, E. B., and Gallin, J. I. (1979): Localization of submembranous cations to the leading end of human neutrophils during chemotaxis. *J. Cell Biol.*, 82:369–379.

30. Cramer, E. B., Milks, L. C., and Ojakian, G. K. (1980): Transepithelial migration of human neutrophils: an in vitro model system. *Proc. Natl. Acad. Sci. USA*, 77:4069–4073.

31. Dale, D. C., Fauci, A. S., Guerry, D-P., and Wolff, S. M. (1975): Comparison of agents producing a neutrophilic leukocytosis in man. *J. Clin. Invest.*, 56:808–813.

32. Dancey, J. T., Deubelbeiss, K. A., Harker, L. A., and Finch, C. A. (1976): Neutrophil kinetics in man. *J. Clin. Invest.*, 58:705–715.

33. Dinarello, C. A. (1984): Interleukin-1 and the pathogenesis of the acute-phase response. *N. Engl. J. Med.*, 311:1413–1418.

34. Dinarello, C. A., Cannon, J. G., Wolff, S. M., Bernheim, H., Buetler, B., Cerami, A., Figari, I. S., Palladino, M. A., and O'Conner, J. V. (1986): Tumor necrosis factor (cachectin) is an endogenous pyrogen and induces production of interleukin 1. *J. Exp. Med.*, 163:1433–1450.

35. Elin, R. J., Wolff, S. M., McAdam, K. P. W. J., Chedid, L., Audibert, F., Bernard, C., and Oberling, F. (1981): Properties of reference Escherichia coli endotoxin and its phthalylated derivative in humans. *J. Infect. Dis.*, 144:329–336.

36. Fehr, J., and Grossmann, H. C. (1979): Disparity between circulating and marginated neutrophils: evidence from studies on the granulocyte alkaline phosphatase, a marker of cell maturity. *Am. J. Hematol.*, 7:369–379.

37. Fliedner, T. M., Cronkite, E. P., and Robertson, J. S. (1964): Granulocytopoiesis. I. Senescence and random loss of neutrophilic granulocytes in human beings. *Blood*, 24:402–414.

38. Fliedner, T. M., Cronkite, E. P., Killmann, S. A., and Bond, V. P. (1964): Emergence and pattern of labeling neutrophilic granulocytes in humans. *Blood*, 24:683–700.

39. Friedman, M. M., Falloon, J., Malech, H. L., and Gallin, J. I. (1986): Plasma membrane receptors for iC3b (CR3) increase in density with activation of human neutrophils: analysis by immunoelectron microscopy. *J. Cell Biol.*, 103:211a (abstract).

40. Fukuda, M., Koeffler, H. P., and Minowada, J. (1981): Membrane differentiation in human myeloid cells: expression of unique profiles of cell surface glycoproteins in myeloid leukemic cell lines blocked at different stages of differentiation and maturation. *Proc. Natl. Acad. Sci. USA*, 78:6299–6303.

41. Gaehtgens, P. (1984): Deformation and activation of leukocytes—two contradictory phenomena. In: *White Cell Mechanics: Basic Science and Clinical Aspects*, edited by H. J. Meiselman, M. A. Lichtman, and P. L. LaCelle, pp. 159–165. Alan R. Liss, New York.

42. Gallin, J. I. (1985): Leukocyte adherence-related glycoproteins LFA-1, Mol, and p150,95: a new group of monoclonal antibodies, a new disease, and a possible opportunity to understand the molecular basis of leukocyte adherence. *J. Infect. Dis.*, 152:661–664.

43. Gallin, J. I., Gallin, E. K., Malech, H. L., and Cramer, E. B. (1978): Structural and ionic events during leukocyte chemotaxis. In: *Leukocyte Chemotaxis: Methods, Physiology, and Clinical Implications*, edited by J. I. Gallin and P. G. Quie, pp. 123–141. Raven Press, New York.

44. Gallin, J. I., Jacobson, R. J., Seligmann, B. E., Metcalf, J. A., McKay, J. H., Sacher, R. A., and Malech, H. L. (1986): A neutrophil membrane marker reveals two groups of chronic myelogenous leukemia and its absence may be a marker of disease progression. *Blood*, 68:343–346.

45. Gamble, J. R., Harlan, J. M., Klebanoff, S. J., and Vadas, M. A. (1985): Stimulation of the adherence of neutrophils to umbilical vein endothelium by human recombinant tumor necrosis factor. *Proc. Natl. Acad. Sci. USA*, 82:8667–8671.

46. Genco, R. J., Van Dyke, T. E., Levine, M. J., Nelson, R. D., and Wilson, M. E. (1986): Molecular factors influencing neutrophil defects in periodontal disease. *J. Dent. Res.*, 64:1377–1391.

47. Gimbrone, M. A., Jr., Brock, A. F., and Schafer, A. I. (1984): Leukotriene B₄ stimulates polymorphonuclear leukocyte adhesion to cultured vascular endothelial cells. *J. Clin. Invest.*, 74:1552–1555.

48. Goldsmith, H. L., and Spain, S. (1984): Radial distribution of white cells in tube flow. In: *White Cell Mechanics: Basic Science and Clinical Aspects*, edited by H. J. Meiselman, M. A. Lichtman, and P. L. LaCelle, pp. 131–146. Alan R. Liss, New York.

49. Harlan, J. M., Killen, P. D., Senecal, F. M., Schwartz, B. R., Yee, E. K., Taylor, R. F., Beatty, P. G., Price, T., and Ochs, H. D. (1985): The role of neutrophil membrane glycoprotein GP-150 in neutrophil adherence to endothelium in vitro. *Blood*, 66:167–178.

50. Hoover, R. L., Briggs, R. T., and Karnovsky, M. J. (1978): The adhesive interaction between polymorphonuclear leukocytes and endothelial cells in vitro. *Cell,* 14:423–428.

51. Hurley, J. V. (1963): An electron microscopic study of leucoytic emigration and vascular permeability in rat skin. *Aust. J. Exp. Biol. Med. Sci.,* 41:171–186.

52. Jamuar, M. P., and Cronkite, E. P. (1980): The fate of granulocytes. *Exp. Hematol.,* 8:884–894.

53. Janoff, A. (1985): Elastase in tissue injury. *Annu. Rev. Med.,* 36: 207–216.

54. Joyce, R. A., Boggs, D. R., Hasiba, U., and Srodes, C. H. (1976): Marginal neutrophil pool size in normal subjects and neutropenic patients as measured by epinephrine infusion. *J. Lab. Clin. Med.,* 88:614–620.

55. Krause, P., Maderazo, E. G., Bannon, P., Kosciol, K., and Malech, H. L. (1987): Neutrophil heterogeneity in patients with blunt trauma. *Clin. Res.,* 35:480A (abstract).

56. Krause, P. J., Malech, H. L., Kristie, J., Kosciol, C. M., Herson, V. C., Eisenfeld, L., Pastuszak, W. T., Kraus, A., and Seligmann, B. (1986): Polymorphonuclear leukocyte heterogeneity in neonates and adults. *Blood,* 68:200–204.

57. Libby, P., Ordovas, J. M., Auger, K. R., Robbins, A. H., Birinyi, L. K., and Dinarello, C. A. (1986): Endotoxin and tumor necrosis factor induce interleukin-1 gene expression in adult human vascular endothelial cells. *Am. J. Pathol.,* 124:179–185.

58. Lichtman, M. A. (1970): Cellular deformation during maturation of the myeloblasts—possible role in marrow egress. *N. Engl. J. Med.,* 283:943–948.

59. Lichtman, M. A., and Weed, R. I. (1972): Alteration of the cell periphery during maturation: relationship to cell function. *Blood,* 23:301–316.

60. Lichtman, M. A., Chamberlain, J. K., Weed, R. I., Pincus, A., and Santillo, P. A. (1977): The regulation of the release of granulocytes from normal marrow. *Prog. Clin. Biol. Res.,* 13:53–75.

61. Lopez, A. F., Williamson, D. J., Gamble, J. R., Begley, C. G., Harlan, J. M., Klebanoff, S. J., Waltersdorph, A., Wong, G., Clark, S. C., and Vadas, M. (1986): Recombinant human granulocyte-macrophage colony-stimulating factor stimulates in vitro mature human neutrophil and eosinophil function, surface receptor expression, and survival. *J. Clin. Invest.,* 78:1220–1228.

62. MacGregor, R. R. (1977): Granulocyte adherence changes induced by hemodialysis, endotoxin, epinephrine, and glucocorticoids. *Ann. Intern. Med.,* 86:35–39.

63. MacGregor, R. R., Spagnuolo, B. E., and Lentnek, A. L. (1974): Inhibition of granulocyte adherence by ethanol, prednisone, and aspirin. *N. Engl. J. Med.,* 291:642–645.

64. Malech, H. L., Root, R. K., and Gallin, J. I. (1977): Structural analysis of human neutrophil migration: centriole, microtubule and microfilament orientation and function during chemotaxis. *J. Cell Biol.,* 75:666–693.

65. Maloney, M. A., and Patt, H. M. (1968): Granulocyte transit from bone marrow to blood. *Blood,* 31:195–201.

66. Marchesi, V. T., and Florey, H. W. (1960): Electron micrographic observations on the emigration of leucocytes. *Q. J. Exp. Physiol.,* 45:343–348.

67. McIntire, L. V., and Eskin, S. G. (1984): Mechanical and biochemical aspects of leukocyte interactions with model vessel walls. In: *White Cell Mechanics: Basic Science and Clinical Aspects,* edited by H. J. Meiselman, M. A. Lichtman, and P. L. LaCelle, pp. 209–219. Alan R. Liss, New York.

68. McIntyre, T. M., Zimmerman, G. A., and Prescott, S. M. (1986): Leukotrienes C$_4$ and D$_4$ stimulate human endothelial cells to synthesize platelet-activating factor and bind neutrophils. *Proc. Natl. Acad. Sci. USA,* 83:2204–2208.

69. Metcalf, D. (1982): Sources and biology of regulatory factors active on mouse myeloid leukemic cells. *J. Cell. Physiol. [Suppl. 1],* 23: 175–183.

70. Metcalf, D., Bradley, T. R., and Robinson, W. (1967): Analysis of colonies developing in vitro from mouse bone marrow cells stimulated by kidney feeder layers or leukemic serum. *J. Cell. Physiol.,* 69:93–108.

71. Milks, L. C., Conyers, G. P., and Cramer, E. B. (1986): The effect of neutrophil migration on epithelial permeability. *J. Cell Biol.,* 103:2729–2738.

72. Movat, H. Z., and Burrowes, C. E. (1985): The local Shwartzman reaction: endotoxin-mediated inflammatory and thrombo-hemorrhagic lesions. In: *Handbook of Endotoxin, Vol. 3: Cellular Biology of Endotoxin,* edited by L. J. Berry, pp. 260–302. Elsevier, New York.

73. Murphy, P. (1976): *The Neutrophil,* Plenum, New York.

74. Nicola, N. A. (1987): Granulocyte colony-stimulating factor and differentiation-induction in myeloid leukemic cells. *Int. J. Cell Cloning,* 5:1–15.

75. O'Shea, J. J., Brown, E. J., Seligmann, B. E., Metcalf, J. A., Frank, M. M., and Gallin, J. I. (1985): Evidence for distinct intracellular pools of receptors for C3b and C3bi in human neutrophils. *J. Immunol.,* 134:2580–2587.

76. Pober, J. S., Bevilacqua, M. P., Medrick, D. L., Lapierre, L. A., Fiers, W., and Gimbrone, M. A., Jr. (1986): Two distinct monokines, interleukin 1 and tumor necrosis factor, each independently induce biosynthesis and transient expression of the same antigen on the surface of cultured human vascular endothelial cells. *J. Immunol.,* 136:1680–1687.

77. Pohlman, T. H., Stanness, K. A., Beatty, P. G., Ochs, H. D., and Harlan, J. M. (1986): An endothelial cell surface factor(s) induced in vitro by lipopolysaccharide, interleukin 1, and tumor necrosis factor-α increases neutrophil adherence by a CDw18-dependent mechanism. *J. Immunol.,* 136:4548–4553.

78. Ross, G. D. (1982): Structure and function of membrane complement receptors. *Fed. Proc.,* 41:3089–3093.

79. Ross, G. D., Jarowsky, C. I., Rabellino, E. M., and Winchester, R. J. (1978): The sequential appearance of Ia-like antigens and two different complement receptors during the maturation of human neutrophils. *J. Exp. Med.,* 147:730–744.

80. Rotrosen, D., Malech, H. L., and Gallin, J. I. (1987): Formyl peptide chemoattractant processing by cultured human umbilical vein endothelial cells. *Fed. Proc.,* 46:758 (abstract).

81. Sato, N., Asano, S., Urabe, A., Ohsawa, N., and Takaku, F. (1985): Induction of alkaline phosphatase in neutrophilic granulocytes, a marker of cell maturity, from bone marrow of normal individuals by retinoic acid. *Biochem. Biophys. Res. Commun.,* 131:1181–1186.

82. Schleimer, R. P., and Rutledge, B. K. (1986): Cultured human vascular endothelial cells acquire adhesiveness for neutrophils after stimulation with interleukin 1, endotoxin, and tumor-promoting phorbol diesters. *J. Immunol.,* 136:649–654.

83. Schmid-Schoenbein, G. W., Fung, Y. C., and Zwefach, B. W. (1975): Vascular endothelial-leukocyte interaction. *Circ. Res.,* 36: 173–184.

84. Schmid-Schoenbein, G. W., Usami, S., Skalak, R., and Chien, S. (1980): The interaction of leukocytes and erythrocytes in capillary and postcapillary vessels. *Microvasc. Res.,* 19:45–70.

85. Seligmann, B., Malech, H. L., Melnick, D. A., and Gallin, J. I. (1985): An antibody binding to human neutrophils demonstrates antigenic heterogeneity detected early in myeloid maturation which correlates with functional heterogeneity of mature neutrophils. *J. Immunol.,* 135:2647–2653.

86. Singer, S. J., and Kupfer, A. (1986): The directed migration of eukaryotic cells. *Annu. Rev. Cell Biol. (in press).*

87. Smith, R. P. C., Lackie, J. M., and Wilkinson, P. C. (1979): The effects of chemotactic factors on the adhesiveness of rabbit neutrophil granulocytes. *Exp. Cell Res.,* 122:169–177.

88. Snyderman, R., Gewurz, H., and Mergenhagen, S. E. (1968): Interactions of the complement system with endotoxic lipopolysaccharide: generation of a factor chemotactic for polymorphonuclear leukocytes. *J. Exp. Med.,* 128:259–275.

89. Tonnesen, M. G., Smedly, L. A., and Henson, P. M. (1984): Neutrophil-endothelial cell interactions: modulation of neutrophil adhesiveness induced by complement fragments C5a and C5a des Arg and formyl-methionyl-leucyl-phenylalanine. *J. Clin. Invest.,* 74:1581–1592.

90. Tonneson, M. G., Smedly, L., Goins, A., and Henson, P. M. (1982):

Interaction between neutrophils and vascular endothelial cells. *Agents Actions [Suppl.]*, 11:25–38.

91. Van Dyke, T. E., Levine, M. J., and Genco, R. J. (1985): Neutrophil function and oral disease. *J. Oral Pathol.*, 14:95–120.

92. Walker, R. I., and Willemze, R. (1980): Neutrophil kinetics and the regulation of granulopoiesis. *Rev. Infect. Dis.*, 2:282–292.

93. Weisbart, R. H., Golde, D. W., and Gasson, J. C. (1986): Biosynthetic human GM-CSF modulates the number and affinity of neutrophil f-met-leu-phe receptors. *J. Immunol.*, 137:3584–3587.

94. Weiss, L. (1970): Transmural cellular passage in vascular sinuses of rat bone marrow. *Blood*, 36:189–208.

95. Wolff, S. M., Rubenstein, M., Mulholland, J. H., and Alling, D. W. (1965): Comparison of hematologic and febrile response to endotoxin in man. *Blood*, 26:190–201.

96. Wright, D. G., and Gallin, J. I. (1979): Secretory responses of human neutrophils: exocytosis of specific (secondary) granules by human neutrophils during adherence in vitro and during exudation in vivo. *J. Immunol.*, 123:285–294.

97. Zakhireh, B., and Malech, H. L. (1980): The effect of colchicine and vinblastine on the chemotactic response of human monocytes. *J. Immunol.*, 125:2143–2153.

98. Zakhireh, B., and Root, R. K. (1979): Development of oxidase activity by human bone marrow granulocytes. *Blood*, 54:429–439.

99. Zigmond, S. H. (1977): Ability of polymorphonuclear leukocytes to orient in gradients of chemotactic factors. *J. Cell Biol.*, 75:606–616.

100. Zigmond, S. H., Levitsky, H. I., and Kreel, B. J. (1981): Cell polarity: an examination of its behavioral expression and its consequences for polymorphonuclear leukocyte chemotaxis. *J. Cell Biol.*, 89:585–592.

101. Zimmerli, W., Seligmann, B., and Gallin, J. I. (1986): Exudation primes human and guinea pig neutrophils for subsequent responsiveness to the chemotactic peptide N-formylmethionylleucylphenylalanine and increases complement component C3bi receptor expression. *J. Clin. Invest.*, 77:925–933.

Inflammation: Basic Principles and Clinical Correlates.
Edited by J. I. Gallin, I. M. Goldstein, and R. Snyderman.
Raven Press, Ltd., New York © 1988.

CHAPTER 19

Phagocytic Cells: Stimulus–Response Coupling Mechanisms

Ralph Snyderman and Ronald J. Uhing

<table>
<tr><td>

Nature of Chemoattractant Receptors
Leukocyte Activation via a Receptor/GTP-Binding Protein/Phospholipase C Pathway
Nature of the GTP-Binding Protein Involved in Leukocyte Activation
Calcium Function and Inositide Metabolism in Leukocytes

</td><td>

Diacylglycerol and Protein Kinase C Involvement in Leukocyte Function
Other Mechanisms That May Regulate Leukocyte Function
Termination of Chemoattractant Responses
Summary
References

</td></tr>
</table>

The ability of phagocytes to migrate to sites of inflammation was recognized more than a century ago, and it was speculated that they did so in response to chemical mediators. Studies of leukocyte chemotaxis initially identified a number of factors that led to the accumulation of inflammatory cells. Subsequent investigations have shown that chemotactic factors, at high concentrations, stimulate potentially cytotoxic or microbicidal responses by leukocytes through degranulation of storage vesicles and by the production of toxic oxygen products (see Chapters 22 and 23). Leukocyte responses to chemotactic and other phlogistic stimuli are vital for host defense, and thus substantial interest has been focused on defining the mechanisms of signal transduction in these cells.

Chemoattractants initiate leukocyte activities subsequent to binding to specific receptors on the cell surface (see following). Temporal studies show rapid (≤ 5 sec) increases in phosphoinositide metabolism and cytosolic calcium levels followed by changes in physiological function, e.g., shape change, superoxide production, or degranulation. The ability of pharmacological agents (e.g., calcium ionophores or phorbol esters) to elicit similar functions suggests the central role of calcium, phosphoinositide metabolism, and protein kinase C in leukocyte activation. Although specific receptors are present for the various chemoattractants, they appear to utilize a common mechanism for stimulating phosphoinositide hydrolysis (see following).

In addition to the central role of calcium-mediated activation pathways, the ability of leukocytes to participate in the inflammatory response is regulated by another second messenger system involving cyclic AMP. Prostaglandins (PG) E_1 and E_2 and histamine elevate cyclic AMP concentrations in leukocytes through receptor-mediated activation of adenylate cyclase. The increased cyclic AMP levels attenuate chemoattractant-induced leukocyte activation. Chemoattractants also increase cellular cyclic AMP levels, in this case by a calcium-mediated inhibition of cyclic AMP degradation. This action may serve an autoregulatory role in chemoattractant-induced leukocyte activation.

NATURE OF CHEMOATTRACTANT RECEPTORS

The ability of the various chemoattractant molecules to activate leukocyte responses is mediated via cell surface receptors (Fig. 1). Specific receptors have been characterized for a number of chemoattractants including *N*-for-

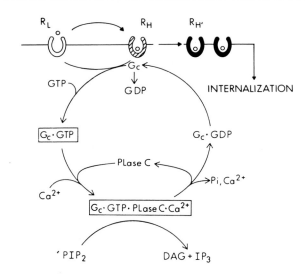

FIG. 1. Model for receptor-mediated stimulation of phospholipase C. The interaction of the chemoattractant receptor with a G-protein (G_c) results in high affinity for chemoattractants (R_H). Chemoattractant binding to the receptor stimulates GTP binding to G_c. The activated $G_c \cdot$ GTP stimulates polyphosphoinositide-specific phospholipase C, enabling it to express activity at physiological Ca^{2+} concentrations. By analogy to other G-proteins, binding of GTP probably promotes dissociation of the heterotrimeric protein. Hydrolysis of GTP terminates the signal by producing the inactive $G_c \cdot$ GDP, which can reform the heterotrimeric structure. Binding of chemoattractants can also result in a slowly dissociating form of the receptor ($R_{H'}$), which is associated with the cytoskeleton and subsequently internalized. (Adapted from refs. 125 and 130.)

mylated peptides, C5a, and leukotriene B_4 (LTB$_4$). Although all appear to utilize a common transduction pathway for cell activation (see below), different receptors are utilized by each. The most extensively studied chemoattractant receptor is that for N-formylated methionyl peptides (123,129,130). Early structure/function studies with polymorphonuclear leukocytes (PMNs) showed that formylation of the aminomethionyl-terminus was essential for the biological activity of formylpeptide chemoattractants (121). The presence of alternative N-terminal modifications (e.g., t-butyloxy) can give rise to potent antagonists. Other studies have suggested that the hydrophobic nature of the peptide is important for binding to leukocyte receptors. Binding of the most active tripeptide fMet-Leu-Phe is further increased by the presence of additional hydrophobic residues (100). Temporal studies of binding versus cellular response show that maximal superoxide production occurs along with maximal receptor occupancy, whereas shape change and maximal stimulation of cyclic AMP accumulation can occur with only about 10% receptor occupancy (123). How receptor occupancy affects directed cellular motility is more complex

to analyze, as the response occurs over a prolonged time and requires the presence of a stimulus gradient to elicit the response.

Direct binding studies with intact human PMNs using fMet-Leu-[^{3}H]Phe (69,151) demonstrated the presence of approximately 50,000 receptor sites per cell. The binding data could be fit to a single class of sites with a Kd of $\sim$20 nM. The ability of various N-formylated peptides to inhibit fMet-Leu-[^{3}H]Phe binding paralleled that seen for eliciting biological responses, indicating that a common receptor is utilized. In contrast, other types of chemoattractant, e.g., C5a or LTB$_4$, do not compete for fMet-Leu-[^{3}H]Phe binding. Binding studies with [^{3}H]LTB$_4$ were best fit to two classes of binding site with Kd values of 0.4 nM ($\sim$4,000 sites/cell) and 61 nM ($\sim$270,000 sites/cell) (51,73). Binding of ^{125}I-labeled C5a to human PMNs exhibits a single class of binding site with a Kd of about 1 nM with about 10,000 sites per cell (61,117).

Various covalent cross-linking techniques have been utilized to identify the receptors involved in chemoattractant responses. Using radiolabeled N-formylated peptides, a cross-linked protein of 60,000 to 70,000 daltons has been identified (35,50,66,98,107,116). The protein is heavily glycosylated with removal of carbohydrate leaving a 32,000-dalton peptide that still exhibits agonist binding (83). Similarly, cross-linking of a 3-aminopropylamide derivative of LTB$_4$, which binds to the high-affinity site, labels a protein of $\sim$60,000 daltons on leukocytes (54). Partial purification of the N-formylated peptide receptor has been reported, although the binding activity of the purified preparations is poor (50,59,60).

Chemoattractant receptors are not static on the cell surface. Cycling of the N-formylated peptide receptor was originally suggested from studies indicating time- and temperature-dependent endocytosis of the peptide (99,136). Subsequent studies have shown that the receptor is internalized following chemoattractant binding (44,123). The internalized peptide–receptor complex appears to be localized in the Golgi fraction. Subsequent to addition of agonist, the number of cell surface receptors initially decreases and then up-regulates, suggesting recycling. In the presence of high concentrations of N-formylated peptide or secretagogues, the number of cell surface receptors can exceed that observed for unstimulated cells, indicating a reserve population of receptors. Fletcher and Gallin (42) and Jesaitis et al. (65) have localized an intracellular population of receptors that co-migrates with the specific granule fraction. Gardner et al. (46) have presented evidence that the specific granule receptor is expressed on the cell surface after exposure to secretagogues and is the same molecular weight as the native surface receptor. Interestingly, receptors for LTB$_4$ appear to be localized exclusively on the plasma membrane (53).

In contrast to intact cells, binding of *N*-formylated peptides to membrane preparations from leukocytes is best fit to two classes of binding site (69,81,131). Chemical and isotopic dilution studies exhibited identical dissociation rates, suggesting two populations of receptor rather than negative cooperativity (69). The Kd values for the sites on human PMN membranes are approximately 0.5 and 20.0 nM, with the high-affinity state representing approximately 25% of the total in a crude membrane preparation (69) or approximately 50% of the total in a plasma membrane preparation (R. Uhing, *unpublished observations*). In other receptor systems multiple binding sites have been shown to be due to aggregation, phosphorylation, or association with a GTP-binding protein. That high- and low-affinity binding sites were detectable in membranes but only a single low-affinity site was found on intact PMNs suggested that the sites might be rapidly interconvertible in whole cells, allowing detection of only a single class using steady-state binding techniques (70). Based on this observation, it was originally suspected that chemoattractant receptors might be coupled to a GTP-binding protein. Guanine nucleotide regulatory proteins (G-proteins) are a group of plasma membrane components that serve a transducing function between a variety of receptors and their effector systems (49). Addition of GDP, GTP, or their nonhydrolyzable analogs (e.g., GppNHp or GTPγS), but not the corresponding adenosine compounds, cause the reversible conversion of high-affinity to low-affinity binding sites for formylpeptides on PMN membranes (70,131). It is presumed that the high-affinity site is represented by the formylpeptide receptor coupled to the G-protein free of either GTP or GDP. A model for the interconvertibility of the affinity of the receptor in intact cells is demonstrated in Fig. 1. The absence of detectable high-affinity binding sites on intact cells using equilibrium binding is presumably due to the high levels of intracellular GTP and GDP, which allow detection of only the low-affinity state (131). Using rapid (<1 min) analysis of peptide–receptor interactions, Sklar et al. (124) have presented evidence for two dissociation rates on intact PMNs, the rapid rate (t ~10 sec) presumably being due to the receptor uncoupled from G-protein or coupled to G-protein bound to GTP or GDP. Using permeabilized cells, GTPγS was shown to increase the rate of dissociation of the entire population of receptor-bound *N*-formylated peptide (124). Association of *N*-formylated peptide receptors with a G-protein is further suggested by the observation that chemoattractant binding to the solubilized receptor is modulated by guanine nucleotides (112). Interestingly, binding to the specific granule fraction of chemoattractant receptors is not modulated by guanine nucleotides (Uhing et al., *manuscript in preparation*). This fact is apparently due to the absence of a G-protein in this fraction. The binding of LTB$_4$ and platelet-activating factor (PAF) to leukocyte membranes is also regulated by guanine nucleotides, suggesting that these receptors are also coupled to G-proteins (53,97).

In addition to guanine nucleotide-interconvertible forms of the receptors, addition of *N*-formylated peptides to PMNs results in the formation of a slowly dissociating state of the receptor (123,156). This form of the receptor remains after detergent lysis of the cells, but its formation is prevented by microtubule disruption. It has been suggested that this slowly dissociating state of the receptor is associated with the cytoskeleton and thus may represent an intermediate in the receptor internalization process (Fig. 1).

LEUKOCYTE ACTIVATION VIA A RECEPTOR/ GTP-BINDING PROTEIN/PHOSPHOLIPASE C PATHWAY

Modulation of receptor binding affinity by guanosine di- and triphosphate suggests the importance of a guanine nucleotide-binding protein (G-protein) in mediating leukocyte responses (70,131). In a variety of cell types hormonal mobilization of intracellular calcium is mediated by stimulated inositol 1,4,5-triphosphate (IP$_3$) formation (10,79,82; see also below). The IP$_3$ is formed from a phospholipase C-mediated phosphodiesteric cleavage of phosphatidylinositol 4,5-bisphosphate (PIP$_2$), a membrane phospholipid (Fig. 2). Inositol-containing phospholipids are minor membrane constituents, although calcium-mobilizing hormones cause rapid metabolism of these substances by activating phospholipase C (10,82; see also following). Addition of chemoattractants to leukocytes results in the rapid formation of inositol phosphates and diacylglycerol and calcium release from intracellular stores (see following), suggesting that chemoattractant receptors activate a phospholipase C (Fig. 2). Analysis of the inositol phosphates produced demonstrate initial formation of IP$_3$ coincident with loss of PIP$_2$ with later formation of IP and loss of phosphotidylinositol (PI) (3,14,15,17,33, 37,76,125), which suggests action of a phospholipase C with preference for polyphosphoinositides (i.e., PIP$_2$). Activation of this phospholipase C appears to be a common mechanism for various chemoattractant receptors including those for *N*-formyl peptides, C5a, LTB$_4$, and PAF (145). Replenishment of PIP$_2$ occurs rapidly via the concerted action of PI and PIP kinases, leading to a decrease in the level of PI. Calcium activation of phospholipase C activities may also be involved in PI reduction (see following). Addition of [γ-^{32}P]ATP to leukocyte plasma membranes results in formation of labeled PIP, PIP$_2$, and phosphatidic acid (23,126). Formation of PIP and PIP$_2$

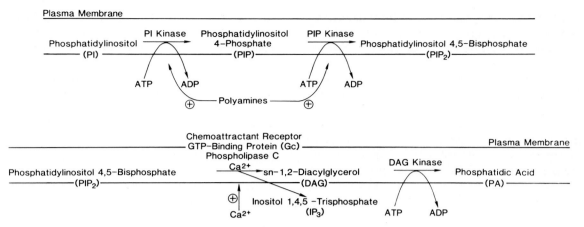

FIG. 2. Plasma membrane components involved in phosphatidylinositol metabolism. The enzymes and metabolites depicted are those that have been shown to be present in plasma membrane preparations from polymorphonuclear leukocytes (see text for details). Stimulatory effects of cytosolic components are depicted by plus.

is accelerated by polyamines at physiological magnesium concentrations, suggesting that cellular polyamine levels may be important in maintaining the rapid flux observed in intact leukocytes (127). In addition to the kinase activities, leukocyte plasma membranes also contain G-proteins and a phospholipase C activity with apparent specificity for the polyphosphoinositides (21,23,125,126). Thus leukocyte plasma membranes contain various components necessary for chemoattractant stimulation of IP_3 formation and replenishment of PIP_2 levels (Fig. 2).

As noted above, the involvement of a G-protein in chemoattractant responses is suggested by the ability of guanine nucleotides to modulate receptor affinity as well as by the ability of *Bordetella pertussis* toxin (which inactivates certain G-proteins) to attenuate phosphoinositide metabolism and leukocyte function (see following). Direct evidence for the involvement of a G-protein in phospholipase C activation was presented by Smith et al. (126), who showed that fMet-Leu-Phe stimulated PIP_2 breakdown in leukocyte plasma membranes only when GTP was present. This action is mediated by a polyphosphoinositide-specific phosphodiesterase (phospholipase C) rather than a phosphomonoesterase, as IP_2 and IP_3 accumulate concomitantly with polyphosphoinositide breakdown (125), and the diacylglycerol formed exhibits a fatty acid composition identical to the PIP_2 (23). Guanine nucleotide activation of phospholipase C exhibits certain properties similar to those that had previously been extensively studied for the activation and inhibition of adenylate cyclase (49). Nonhydrolyzable analogs of GTP activate phospholipase C activity, whereas adenine nucleotides, GDP, and GMP are ineffective (125). Activation by guanine nucleotides is inhibited by GDPβS (21). Chemoattractant stimulation of phospholipase C in leukocyte

plasma membranes is also inhibited by pertussis toxin, indicating that the G-protein involved is a substrate for ADP-ribosylation by this toxin (126).

Little information is available on the nature of the polyphosphoinositide phosphodiesterase involved in leukocyte activation. Stimulation by guanine nucleotides or the synergistic stimulation by chemoattractants plus GTP require the presence of at least low concentrations of calcium, similar to resting cytosolic levels (21,125,126). Stimulation of this enzyme by chemoattractants is primarily due to a reduction in the calcium requirement for maximal activation to ~100 nM, i.e., ambient intracellular levels (125). In the absence of chemoattractants or GTP, supraphysiological concentrations of calcium (≥100 μM) are needed to cause breakdown of polyphosphoinositides in PMN membranes (23,125,126). Specificity for polyphosphoinositides is suggested, as initially only IP_2 and IP_3 accumulate subsequent to stimulation of leukocyte plasma membranes (125), although breakdown of PI at later times has not been excluded.

Most studies on the characteristics of phosphoinositide-specific phospholipase C(s) have been performed using enzyme prepared from cytosolic extracts (82). This enzyme, prepared from a variety of cell types, hydrolyzes PI as well as the polyphosphoinositides. The relative rates of hydrolysis depend on the relative concentrations of phosphoinositides and the calcium concentration, PI being preferred at high calcium concentrations. Whether this enzyme activity represents a component involved in leukocyte activation remains to be established. Deckmyn et al. (28) reported that guanine nucleotide stimulated phospholipase C activity in a 100,000 × g platelet supernatant. It needs to be clarified whether this represents actual soluble cytosolic activity or membrane fragments.

Clearly, more work is necessary to determine subcellular localization as well as substrate specificity of the phospholipase C activity involved in leukocyte activation.

NATURE OF THE GTP-BINDING PROTEIN INVOLVED IN LEUKOCYTE ACTIVATION

A class of G-proteins has been identified as plasma membrane components that couple a variety of receptors to their effector enzymes (11,49,133). The definitively characterized members of this class are G_s and G_i, which couple adenylate cyclase to stimulatory and inhibitory receptors, respectively, and transducin, a G-protein that couples a cyclic GMP-phosphodiesterase to rhodopsin (Table 1). Common characteristics of these proteins are the ability to bind guanine nucleotides, an inherent GTPase activity and a heterotrimeric $\alpha\beta\gamma$ structure. The α subunit confers the specificity for receptor–effector system involvement, is the guanine nucleotide-binding component, and is the potential substrate for bacterial toxin-catalyzed ADP-ribosylation. Bacterial toxins have been useful tools for the investigation of G-protein roles in signal transduction (11,49,133). Cholera toxin catalyzes the ADP-ribosylation of G_s, reducing the GTPase activity (18) and thereby causing persistent activation of adenylate cyclase. Pertussis toxin catalyzes the ADP-ribosylation of G_i and transducin, causing uncoupling with the receptor and thus terminating the hormone signal.

G_o, an abundant G-protein from brain, has the same heterotrimeric structure as G_s and G_i, and the 39,000-dalton α subunit can be ribosylated by pertussis toxin (89,96,135). G_p, a heterotrimeric G-protein with a 21,000-dalton α subunit has been purified from placenta (38). Effector systems involving these latter two G-proteins have yet to be clearly delineated. Other proteins with homology to the above α subunits include eukaryotic elongation factor 2 (ADP-ribosylated by diphtheria toxin) and *ras* gene products.

As described in the previous section, evidence has been obtained in leukocytes demonstrating involvement of a G-protein in chemoattractant activation of phospholipase C. This G-protein shares characteristics of the G-proteins summarized above. fMet-Leu-Phe stimulates both GTPγS binding (128) and GTPase activity (40,106). As suggested from immunochemical evidence for the vasopressin–G-protein complex from liver (41), G-proteins involved in calcium mobilization probably have a heterotrimeric structure. Various lines of evidence suggest that the G-protein involved in chemoattractant responses is a substrate for pertussis toxin-catalyzed ADP-ribosylation. They include attenuation by the toxin of chemoattractant-induced PIP_2-mediated responses (7,13,16,52,64,75,92,104,105,143,146,148), reduction of high-affinity fMet-Leu-Phe binding (74,105,147) and inhibition of fMet-Leu-Phe-receptor/G-protein-mediated events in membrane preparations (106,125, 126,128).

ADP-ribosylation of leukocyte membranes in the presence of pertussis toxin shows a predominance of an ~40-kD substrate. Because of the similarity in molecular weight for the pertussis toxin substrate, it has been investigated whether the G-protein involved in leukocyte activation has identity with G_i. Functional G_i has been demonstrated in intact PMNs by the ability of α_2-agonists to inhibit PGE_1-stimulated cyclic AMP accumulation (142) and in membrane preparations by the ability of α_2-agonists to inhibit cyclic AMP production stimulated by either PGE or β-agonists (12,142). The latter report presented only marginal inhibition by α_2-agonists presumably due to excess $\beta\gamma$ in PMN membranes. The reason for the discrepancy in the degree of inhibition by α_2-agonists is unclear, although different assay conditions were employed in the two reports. Neither report obtained any fMet-Leu-Phe-induced inhibition of agonist-stimulated cyclic AMP formation in PMN membranes (12,142) under conditions similar to those described above (125,126) for hormone-stimulated phospholipase C activity. These results imply that chemoattractant receptors do not couple to adenylate cyclase through G_i. Further evidence against a role for G_i in chemoattractant function is the observation that α_2-agonists that utilize G_i do not cause calcium mobilization in leukocytes (M. Verghese, *unpublished observations*).

An immunological approach has been utilized by Spiegel and co-workers to identify the G-protein coupled to

TABLE 1. *Guanine nucleotide regulatory proteins*

Characteristic	G_s	G_i	G_o	Transducin	G_p	G_c
Receptor coupling	β-Adren., PGE	α_2-Adren.	Musc-cholin.	Rhodopsin	?	CTX
Subunit composition	$\alpha_s\beta\gamma$	$\alpha_i\beta\gamma$	$\alpha_o\beta\gamma$	$\alpha_t\beta\gamma$	$\alpha_p\beta\gamma$	$\alpha_c\beta\gamma$
MW of α subunit (kD)	43–50	41	39	39	21	~40
Ribosylated by	CT	PT	PT	CT/PT	—	CT/PT
Effector	AC^+	AC^-	?	cGMP-PDE	?	PLC

AC = adenylate cyclase. CT = cholera toxin. CTX = chemoattractant. PDE = phosphodiesterase. PLC = phospholipase C. PT = pertussis toxin. Adren. = adrenergic. Musc-cholin. = muscarinic-cholinergic.

chemoattractant receptors. Using antibodies prepared against available G-proteins, these authors have obtained immunochemical evidence that G_i is not present in sufficient quantities in human PMNs to account for the pertussis toxin-catalyzed ADP-ribosylation of ~40-kD protein(s) (48). This lack of antibody reactivity cannot be due to species differences, as the G_i sequence deduced from a human monocyte-like cell line exhibits extensive homology to the G_i sequences previously deduced from other species and tissues (31). Immunochemical evidence also suggests that other previously described pertussis toxin substrates, G_o and transducin, are low or absent in PMNs (48). The G-protein utilized in leukocyte activation is nonetheless probably similar to those previously described, as antibodies to conserved regions of G-proteins exhibit strong reactivity with leukocyte membranes (39).

Other evidence suggestive of a unique G-protein in PMNs comes from studies utilizing cholera toxin. This toxin ADP-ribosylates an ~40-kD protein in phagocytes (1,147) and myeloid cell lines (HL-60, U937) (147) under conditions where little cholera toxin-induced ADP-ribosylation of ~40-kD proteins is evidenced in erythrocytes, liver, or brain (147; *unpublished observations*). Cholera toxin treatment resulted in decreased chemotaxis (1), which could not be accounted for by changes in cyclic AMP concentration. Furthermore, both pertussis and cholera toxins inhibited high-affinity fMet-Leu-Phe binding, suggesting that the same G-protein may be a substrate for both (147).

The above data suggest that leukocytes contain a unique, pertussis/cholera toxin-sensitive G-protein that mediates chemoattractant-induced cell activation (147). However, Kikuchi et al. (67) have reported that either G_i or G_o are capable of reconstituting fMet-Leu-Phe-stimulated phospholipase C activity with similar potencies in plasma membranes prepared from pertussis toxin-treated HL60 cells. It should be noted, however, that brain G_i–G_o preparations have been reported to contain an additional uncharacterized ~40-kD protein (96). The above authors did not comment on the possible presence of this protein in their preparations. Further work is necessary to resolve the specificities of G-proteins involved in phospholipase C coupling.

The most direct approach to identification of the G-protein involved in leukocyte activation is to purify and reconstitute the bacterial toxin substrates present in these cells. Leukocytes contain substantial amounts of high-affinity GTPγS binding (~100 pmol/mg of membrane protein) (128). Furthermore, quantification of pertussis toxin labeling of PMNs suggests amounts of ~40-kD substrates similar to the large amounts found in brain (48). When the G-proteins from HL60 membranes are solubilized, the major GTPγS binding activity and ~40-kD pertussis toxin substrate(s) co-chromatograph during purification (R. J. Uhing et al., *in preparation*). The purified preparation exhibits closely spaced doublets at both ~40 kD and ~35 kD on sodium dodecyl sulfate-polyacrylamide gel electrophoresis (SDS-PAGE) (Fig. 3). Both ~40-kD proteins are ADP-ribosylated by pertussis toxin. The upper protein co-migrates on SDS-PAGE with brain G_i, whereas the lower one migrates more slowly than G_o, suggesting that it may represent a previously undescribed pertussis toxin substrate. Whether this protein couples to chemoattractant receptors remains to be ascertained.

Using a cDNA library prepared from dibutyryl cyclic AMP-differentiated HL60 cells, a cDNA clone that encodes for a unique G-protein has been identified (31). The long open reading frame encodes for a potential pertussis toxin substrate that is highly homologous yet clearly distinct from reported sequences for $G_i\alpha$ subunits. Moreover, both the 5' and 3' noncoding regions of the novel $G\alpha$ are clearly distinct from all reported $G\alpha$ subunit cDNAs.

CALCIUM FUNCTION AND INOSITIDE METABOLISM IN LEUKOCYTES

The role of calcium mobilization in cellular responses to chemoattractants has been extensively studied in leukocytes and appears to be a primary mechanism for receptor-mediated activation. The involvement of calcium in leukocyte activation has been examined using a variety of approaches. Addition of calcium ionophores in the presence of extracellular calcium increases cytosolic calcium levels in leukocytes and stimulates superoxide pro-

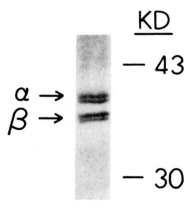

FIG. 3. Pertussis toxin substrates from HL60 cells. GTP-binding proteins were purified from HL60 cells using chromatography on Ultrogel AcA34, heptylamine-Sepharose, and DEAE-Fractogel. Presented is a Coomassie blue stain of a SDS-PAGE gel of the pooled pertussis toxin substrates. Both components of the ~40-kD doublet are ADP-ribosylated by pertussis toxin (not shown).

duction, degranulation, and aggregation (29,77,111,143). Addition of chemoattractants leads to a rapid increase in the cytosolic calcium concentration, which temporally precedes the cellular responses (72,78). The increase in cytosolic calcium and stimulation of response are only partially reduced by chelation of extracellular calcium (78). Depletion of intracellular calcium stores by prior treatment of cells with EGTA in the presence of calcium ionophores attenuates subsequent responses invoked by chemoattractants (77,78). Lew et al. (77,78) have used the fluorescent calcium indicator Quin 2 in the presence of a calcium ionophore and various extracellular calcium concentrations to examine the calcium dependency of various secretory responses. Elevation of cytosolic calcium increased degranulation from secretory vesicles and specific and azurophil granules, with the EC_{50} for the various processes being reduced approximately tenfold by fMet-Leu-Phe. Because fMet-Leu-Phe does not further increase cytosolic calcium under these conditions, the reduction in the calcium dependency probably represents an interaction of the second messengers (i.e., inositol 1,4,5-triphosphate or metabolites thereof and sn-1,2-diacylglycerol) of the phosphoinositide pathway on expression of leukocyte function (see following).

Since the original suggestion that phosphoinositide turnover may trigger calcium mobilization owing to hormone–receptor interaction (88), numerous studies have led to the realization of the involvement of inositol 1,4,5-triphosphate and diacylglycerol as messenger molecules for a diverse group of cellular functions (10,79,82,102). In leukocytes these second messengers are generated in response to chemoattractant receptor-mediated activation of a phospholipase C (see above). Addition of chemoattractants to leukocytes results in the rapid and transient formation of inositol triphosphate (IP_3) (3,14,15,17,33,37,76). Stimulated production of IP_3 occurs even when intracellular calcium stores are depleted, suggesting its importance as a primary event (33,34,104). The initial IP_3 formed, inositol 1,4,5-triphosphate, has been shown to cause the release of calcium from intracellular stores in leukocytes (15,113). Measurement of the intracellular concentration of inositol 1,4,5-triphosphate produced in response to fMet-Leu-Phe [$\sim 1 \ \mu M$ at $10^{-8} \ M$ (15)] suggests sufficient quantities to maximally release calcium from the IP_3-sensitive nonmitochondrial pools (15,113). Subsequent to the initial formation of inositol 1,4,5-triphosphate, a kinase and several phosphatases cause its conversion to a variety of inositol phosphate isomers resulting in the eventual formation of inositol (33) (Fig. 4). Flux through inositol 1,3,4,5-tetrakisphosphate (IP_4) and subsequently inositol 1,3,5-triphosphate appear to be regulated by intracellular calcium (33,76). Functional roles for the various inositol phosphates have not been described in leukocytes, although studies in sea

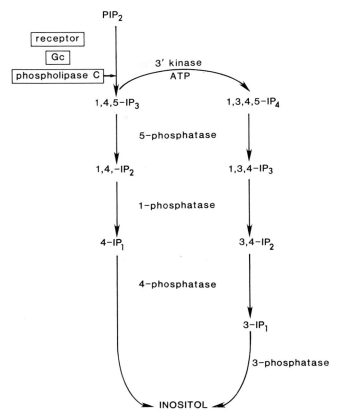

FIG. 4. Pathways of 1,4,5-IP_3 metabolism in PMNs. A PIP_2-specific phospholipase C can be activated via a G-protein (G_c) coupled to chemoattractant receptors. The initial products formed are 1,4,5-IP_3 and 1,2-diacylglycerol. 1,4,5-IP_3 is metabolized via the indicated pathways to free inositol. (Adapted from ref. 33.)

urchin eggs suggest that IP_4 may stimulate calcium influx when cytosolic calcium is also elevated (63).

Measurement of cytosolic calcium with fluorescent indicators reveals that chemoattractants cause a biphasic increase (2,33,77,78). Removal of extracellular calcium eliminates the slower phase, suggesting that it is due to a stimulated influx across the plasma membrane. Chemoattractants stimulate influx of $^{45}Ca^{2+}$, a response that is slower than the initial increase in IP_3 and intracellular calcium (71,72). A role for calcium influx in leukocyte activation is suggested by the fact that chelation of extracellular calcium attenuates fMet-Leu-Phe-stimulated responses in PMNs (72). Interestingly, leukotriene B_4, which is less potent than fMet-Leu-Phe in stimulating superoxide production (108), degranulation (119), or protein kinase C translocation (101), also does not exhibit the slow rise in cytosolic calcium attributable to calcium influx even though initial IP_3 levels are similar to (albeit more transient than) those produced by fMet-Leu-Phe (33). These and other results suggest a role for calcium influx in leukocyte activation and its subsequent role for increased diacylglycerol production independent of PIP$_2$ hydrolysis (see following).

DIACYLGLYCEROL AND PROTEIN KINASE C INVOLVEMENT IN LEUKOCYTE FUNCTION

The diacylglycerol limb of the bifurcating phosphoinositide pathway appears to be of major importance in stimulating leukocyte activation and in feedback regulation. Early studies with the tumor-promoting phorbol esters led to identification of the cellular receptor as protein kinase C (4,19). It is presumed that 1,2-diacylglycerol is the natural product that binds to the same site as do the active phorbols and thus activates protein kinase C. Subsequent studies have utilized phorbol esters to study protein kinase C involvement in many cell types (4,102).

Addition of active phorbol esters to PMNs or monocytes results in the redistribution of protein kinase C from the cytosol to the cells' particulate fraction (47,94,152). The relative potencies of various phorbol esters to cause translocation are similar to their stimulatory effects on superoxide production (94). The NADPH oxidase activity involved appears to be plasma membrane-bound and consists of multiple components (see Chapter 18) (5,85). ATP-dependent protein kinase C-mediated activation of NADPH oxidase activity has been demonstrated in plasma membrane preparations (27,87), suggesting that the determining step in this process is translocation and activation of protein kinase C. Approximately 90% of the protein kinase C activity is cytosolic in unstimulated PMNs (152). In the presence of cytochalasin B, fMet-Leu-Phe increases membrane-associated protein kinase C threefold at doses that stimulate a respiratory burst (86,109). Pharmacological agents that inhibit chemoattractant activation of the respiratory burst specifically inhibit chemoattractant-stimulated translocation of protein kinase C (109). These results further suggest that translocation of protein kinase C to the plasma membrane is required for activation of the respiratory burst by chemoattractants.

As noted in the previous section, calcium ionophores are also capable of stimulating the respiratory burst in leukocytes. Whether the action of Ca^{2+} is also mediated by protein kinase C remains to be resolved. Low concentrations of phorbol esters and calcium ionophores produce a synergistic activation of the respiratory burst (150). It has been shown that elevation of cytosolic calcium increases phorbol ester binding affinity in intact phagocytes (36). Calcium ionophores also increase endogenous diacylglycerol levels (see following).

Other chemoattractant-stimulated leukocyte functions have been suggested to be due to protein kinase C acti-

vation using similar criteria. For example, addition of phorbol myristate acetate (PMA) or chemoattractants in the presence of cytochalasin B stimulates degranulation, primarily of specific granules (6,55). The biochemical events involved in this process are not understood. Data also suggest that differentiation of monocytes to macrophages may be mediated by protein kinase C (57,90,93). In contrast to some of the above-mentioned events, activation of c-fos gene expression in monocytes is not effected by calcium ionophores but is rapidly ($\leq$15 min) stimulated by chemoattractants or PMA (57).

Further evidence that phorbol ester activation mimics changes in cellular diacylglycerol content have been obtained using cell-permeable diacylglycerols (26,30,43,57,103). These analogs also cause superoxide production, degranulation, and enhancement of c-fos gene expression, further supporting a role for protein kinase C. Interestingly, sn-1,2-didecanoylglycerol (diC$_{10}$) stimulated degranulation without increasing superoxide production by PMNs (26). Furthermore, this analog inhibited only a maximum of ~50% of [^{3}H]PDBu binding to protein kinase C in intact PMNs. In contrast, sn-1,2-dioctanoylglycerol (diC8), which stimulated both the respiratory burst and degranulation, completely blocked [^{3}H]PDBu binding in PMNs. These results indicate that secretion and the respiratory burst are regulated differently in PMNs, and that either protein kinase C may be compartmentalized or that different isozymes may exist in PMNs. Studies have demonstrated multiple protein kinase C isozymes based on cDNA sequences (25,62,68).

The above studies support a role for protein kinase C in a variety of leukocyte responses. Changes in diacylglycerol levels have been mainly inferred from the changes in phosphoinositide levels and corresponding manifestations of a leukocyte response with phorbol esters or synthetic diacylglycerols. The development of a sensitive diacylglycerol assay utilizing diacylglycerol kinase has been reported by Preiss et al. (112) and should provide rapid advances in the understanding of the role of diacylglycerol in leukocyte function. Honeycutt and Niedel (58) have utilized this assay to examine formylpeptide enhancement of diacylglycerol levels in PMNs. Although fMet-Leu-Phe alone causes an increase in diacylglycerol, this response is potentiated six- to sevenfold by inclusion of cytochalasin B. These results suggest that the potentiating effect of cytochalasin B on hormone-induced functions may be due to its ability to increase levels of diacylglycerol in cells exposed to chemoattractants. Temporal studies show that cytochalasin B-stimulated diacylglycerol production is slower than that of calcium or IP$_3$ (33,58,71,72,141), suggesting that its formation may be secondary to inositide metabolism. Previous studies have shown that chemoattractant-induced changes in phosphoinositide metabolism exhibit only a slight enhancement by cytochalasin B

(8,14,118), suggesting that most of the diacylglycerol is derived from other sources. It is also suggested by the demonstration that the fatty acid composition of the diacylglycerol produced differs from that observed for PI in neutrophils (22). The source of the diacylglycerol is unknown, although other agents, e.g., PMA and calcium ionophores, similarly increase diacylglycerol, which is apparently not derived from phosphoinositide metabolism (141). Because the same agents that enhance diacylglycerol production also invoke a variety of leukocyte responses, it is important to determine the intracellular source of the phospholipase as well as the mediating signal(s) involved and to determine whether the responses are causative or the result of increased diacylglycerol production. Evidence from this laboratory suggests that diacylglycerol production stimulated by chemoattractants occurs in two phases. The first is due to PIP_2 hydrolysis, and the second requires Ca^{2+} influx from extracellular stores (141). Preliminary data suggest that phosphatidylcholine may provide the source for the second phase of diacylglycerol in PMNs (A. P. Truett et al., *unpublished data*).

OTHER MECHANISMS THAT MAY REGULATE LEUKOCYTE FUNCTION

Addition of chemoattractants to PMNs results in rapid cytosolic acidification with a nadir at approximately 1 min and subsequent alkalinization by 5 min (149,153). Mechanisms involved in the initial acidification have not been clearly characterized, although accelerated metabolism has been suggested as a possible cause (56). Cytosolic acidification has been suggested to be involved in the chemotactic response (153) based on the observation that addition of sodium propionate to PMNs causes rapid acidification as well as a concomitant perpendicular light-scattering response characteristic of that induced by chemoattractants. Previous results have shown that the rapid light-scattering response is indicative of microfilament rearrangement. Pharmacological manipulation of the rapid light-scattering response correlates with effects on the chemotactic response, suggesting that it reflects an initial required cellular response to chemoattractants (154). The alkalinization phase is due to the increased activity of a Na^+/H^+ antiport, as elevation of pH is inhibited by amiloride (149). Activation of the antiport may be mediated by protein kinase C, as addition of PMA also causes alkalinization (149). A role for alkalinization in leukocyte activation is suggested by the observation that amiloride attenuates fMet-Leu-Phe-stimulated superoxide production (149). Sweatt et al. (137,138) have presented evidence that α_2-agonists stimulate Na^+/H^+ exchange in platelets whereupon the resulting alkalinization along with calcium synergistically activates phospholipase A_2. Cy-

clooxygenase products of the liberated arachidonate subsequently activate phospholipase C in platelets (137). A similar system may operate in leukocytes for α_2-agonists. Chemoattractants induce shape changes (morphological polarization) in monocytes due to cytoskeletal rearrangement (20). Morphological polarization of monocytes is also induced by α_2-agonists under conditions where changes in cyclic AMP concentrations are unlikely (134). The polarization induced by α_2-agonist or low concentrations of fMet-Leu-Phe are synergistic when the two are combined, suggesting activation of a common pathway. Muscarinic agonists have also been shown to cause polarization in monocytes (134).

Chemoattractant addition to leukocytes results in a variety of ion fluxes (44; see also above). Evidence in a number of cell types suggests that G-proteins may directly regulate ion channels (11). Patch clamp techniques have suggested the importance of a G-protein in mediating cardiac muscarinic receptor-stimulated K^+ influx. The stimulation can be mimicked by introduction of G_i (11), the active component being the $\beta\gamma$ subunit complex (80). Similarly, G_o has been suggested to mediate voltage-activated Ca^{2+} channels based on patch clamp techniques (11). Whether similar mechanisms are operable in leukocytes remains to be established.

Receptors for various peptide growth factors (e.g., insulin) have been identified on leukocytes, although effects on leukocyte activation have not been established. Studies on their mechanisms of action suggest that circulating concentrations of these agents may serve a modulatory role on leukocyte activation. Using a variety of cell types, various peptide growth factors have been shown to activate a Na^+/H^+ antiport, phosphoinositide metabolism, phospholipase A_2, and protein kinase C (140). In addition, insulin has been shown to activate a novel phospholipase C-type activity (115).

TERMINATION OF CHEMOATTRACTANT RESPONSES

Activation of leukocytes by a single dose of chemoattractant is a transient phenomenon. Superoxide production and degranulation are initiated rapidly but do not persist beyond 2 to 5 min. Similarly, chemoattractant-stimulated increases in IP_3, calcium, and cyclic AMP reach a maximum within 30 sec and return to basal levels by 5 min. These results suggest that mechanisms exist for termination of the chemoattractant signal. Termination of the signal could result from degradation of the chemoattractant, regulation of receptor, or at other steps in the transduction sequence. Studies suggest that multiple controls exist for termination of chemoattractant signaling. Internalization of the receptor can lead to hydrolysis of the peptide after transfer to a lysosomal fraction prior to recycling of the receptor to the cell surface (123). Uptake of N-formylated peptide can far exceed the number of cell surface receptors. It has been shown that the rate of hydrolysis of fMet-Leu-Phe far exceeds that due to cell-mediated uptake (155), indicating that surface-mediated hydrolysis is important for removal of the chemoattractant. Degradation of formylpeptide chemoattractants by intact PMNs or by PMN membranes is rapid and extensive. An enzyme involved in the hydrolysis of fMet-Leu-Phe is a membrane-associated metalloproteinase (155) likely to be an enkephalinase (84).

Addition of chemoattractants to leukocytes causes increases in intracellular cyclic AMP concentrations through a calcium-dependent mechanism (142). The elevated cyclic AMP levels may provide an autoregulatory termination mechanism as suggested from studies using cell-permeable cAMP analogs or cyclic AMP-elevating agents (43,45,114,122,134,144). Elevation of intracellular cyclic AMP concentrations inhibits chemoattractant-induced superoxide production and degranulation but does not inhibit stimulation of the same functions by PMA, indicating regulation of a step proximal to protein kinase C. Binding of fMet-Leu-Phe is not altered by elevated cyclic AMP (132). Superoxide production induced by concanavilin A (which does not utilize a pertussis toxin-sensitive G-protein) is also inhibited by cyclic AMP elevation (144). These results suggest that the inhibitory action of cyclic AMP is not due to effects on the receptor or its associated G-protein. Elevation of cyclic AMP by PGE_2 inhibits the slow phase of the cytosolic calcium increase (139), which has been attributed to calcium influx (see above). In the absence of extracellular calcium, no effects of PGE_2 on cytosolic calcium is witnessed (139). Furthermore, diacylglycerol (A. P. Truett et al., *unpublished observations*) and phosphatidic acid (139) production are inhibited by elevation of cyclic AMP. These results suggest that the inhibitory action of cyclic AMP may be due to effects on hormone-stimulated calcium influx or on the consequences thereof.

Although activation of protein kinase C by PMA stimulates leukocyte function (see above), high concentrations of PMA (≥ 10 ng/ml) inhibit fMet-Leu-Phe and LTB_4-stimulated degranulation and calcium mobilization (95), indicating that increased diacylglycerol production may serve an autoregulatory role. Protein kinase C phosphorylation and activation of an IP_3 5'-phosphomonoesterase have been reported in platelets (24,91). It does not appear to be the primary mechanism for desensitization in leukocytes, as stimulated IP_3 production by concanavilin A is enhanced by PMA (128). The enhancement is due to increased levels of PIP and PIP_2 in PMA-treated cells. Prior treatment of PMNs with PMA inhibits PIP_2 hydrolysis induced by fMet-Leu-Phe, LTB_4, and platelet-acti-

vating factor (128). Inhibition of PIP_2 hydrolysis is mediated differently for PMA versus pertussis toxin. Pertussis toxin inhibits receptor–protein-G coupling as evidenced by reductions in high-affinity binding and hormone-stimulated GTPγS binding. Stimulation of phospholipase C by fMet-Leu-Phe plus GTP is also inhibited by pertussis toxin. Phospholipase C activity stimulated by GTPγS or calcium is not affected by pertussis toxin, indicating that this agent does not prevent effective coupling of the active G protein with phospholipase C (128). In contrast, inhibition by PMA affects G-protein–phospholipase C coupling. Stimulation of phospholipase C by GTPγS but not by a high calcium concentration is disrupted by PMA. Receptor–protein-G interactions, as evidenced by high-affinity fMet-Leu-Phe binding and hormone-stimulated GTPγS binding, are not affected (128). Thus diacylglycerol produced by receptor-mediated cellular activation could feed back to inhibit this transduction pathway by blocking the coupling of the activated G-protein to phospholipase C.

The inhibition of leukocyte activation by cyclic AMP, PMA, and pertussis toxin are examples of heterologous desensitization, i.e., disruption of activation for all agonists using a common transduction mechanism. Homologous desensitization (i.e., receptor-specific) is also suggested based on the observation that exposure of leukocytes to either fMet-Leu-Phe, LTB_4, or platelet-activating factor desensitizes to subsequent exposure with the same agonist (M. Verghese et al., *unpublished observations*). The mechanisms involved for homologous desensitization of chemoattractant receptors in leukocytes have not been ascertained, although homologous desensitization of adrenergic receptors and rhodopsin are due to a kinase that is specific for the agonist-occupied receptor (9,120).

SUMMARY

The data discussed here are consistent with the model for chemoattractant-induced leukocyte activation presented in Fig. 5. As noted above, the biochemical events involved in several of the observed physiological phenomena have not been completely delineated. However, a large body of evidence has accumulated indicating the central role of phosphoinositide metabolism and protein kinase C activation in mediating chemoattractant-stimulated function. Occupancy of chemoattractant receptors activates phospholipase C to produce IP_3 and diacylglycerol. Activation of phospholipase C is mediated by a unique pertussis–cholera toxin-sensitive G-protein termed G_c. Sustained PIP_2 hydrolysis leads to enhanced membrane calcium permeability and a secondary burst of diacylglycerol formation from a precursor other than the phosphoinositides. The latter phenomenon is well cor-

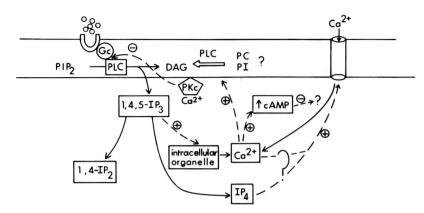

FIG. 5. Model for the regulation of leukocyte responses to chemoattractants. Metabolic pathways are represented by solid arrows and regulatory steps by broken arrows. Positive and negative regulation are represented by plus and minus, respectively. Areas that have not been definitely established include a question mark. Abbreviations used are as described in the text. PKC = protein kinase C. PLC = phospholipase C.

related with activation of the respiratory burst. Attenuation of chemoattractant-induced cellular activation occurs by several mechanisms. The agonist can be hydrolyzed externally or internalized and degraded within leukocytes. Protein kinase C activation and translocation disrupts G-protein–phospholipase C coupling. Elevation of cAMP levels by either the calcium-dependent mechanism involved in chemoattractant-elicited responses or by hormones that act through adenylate cyclase also attenuate the chemoattractant-induced activation of leukocytes, perhaps through inhibition of calcium influx or subsequent responses. Mechanisms for homologous desensitization have not yet been elucidated, but it could be due to receptor sequestration, covalent modification, or both.

ACKNOWLEDGMENTS

This work was supported in part by grant DE03738 from the National Institute of Dental Research and grant CA29589 from the National Cancer Institute.

REFERENCES

1. Aksamit, R. R., Backlund, P. S., Jr., and Cantoni, G. L. (1985): Cholera toxin inhibits chemotaxis by a cAMP-independent mechanism. *Proc. Natl. Acad. Sci. USA,* 82:7475–7479.
2. Andersson, T., Dahlgren, C., Pozzan, T., Stendahl, O., and Lew, D. P. (1986): Characterization of fMet-Leu-Phe receptor-mediated Ca^{2+} influx across the plasma membrane of human neutrophils. *Mol. Pharm.,* 30:437–443.
3. Andersson, T., Schlegel, W., Monod, A., Krause, K-H., Stendahl, O., and Lew, D. P. (1986): Leukotriene B_4 stimulation of phagocytes results in the formation of inositol 1,4,5-triphosphate. *Biochem. J.,* 240:333–340.
4. Ashendel, C. L. (1985): The phorbol ester receptor: a phospholipid-regulated protein kinase. *Biochim. Biophys. Acta,* 822:219–242.
5. Babior, B. M. (1984): The respiratory burst of phagocytes. *J. Clin. Invest.,* 73:599–601.
6. Baggiolini, M., and Dewald, B. (1984): Exocytosis by neutrophils. *Contemp. Top. Immunobiol.,* 14:221–246.
7. Becker, E. L., Kermode, J. C., Naccache, P. H., Yassin, R., Marsh, M. L., Munoz, J. J., and Sha'afi, R. I. (1985): The inhibition of neutrophil granule enzyme secretion and chemotaxis by pertussis toxin. *J. Cell Biol.,* 100:1641–1646.
8. Bennett, J. P., Cockcroft, S., and Gomperts, B. D. (1980): Use of cytochalasin B to distinguish between early and late events in neutrophil activation. *Biochim. Biophys. Acta,* 601:584–591.
9. Benovic, J. C., Strasser, R. H., Caron, M. G., and Lefkowitz, R. J. (1986): β-Adrenergic receptor kinase: identification of a novel protein kinase that phosphorylates the agonist-occupied form of the receptor. *Proc. Natl. Acad. Sci. USA,* 83:2797–2081.
10. Berridge, M. J., and Irvine, R. F. (1984): Inositol triphosphate, a novel second messenger in cellular signal transduction. *Nature,* 312:315–321.
11. Birnbaumer, L., Codina, J., Mattera, R., Yatani, A., Scherer, N., Toro, M-J., and Brown, A. M. (1987): Signal transduction by G proteins. In: *Molecular Biology and the Kidney,* edited by R. Robinson and D. K. Granner (in press).
12. Bokoch, G. M. (1987): The presence of free G protein β/γ subunits in human neutrophils results in suppression of adenylate cyclase activity. *J. Biol. Chem.,* 262:589–594.
13. Bokoch, G. M., and Gilman, A. G. (1984): Inhibition of receptor-mediated release of arachidonic acid by pertussis toxin. *Cell,* 39: 301–308.
14. Bradford, P. G., and Rubin, R. P. (1985): Characterization of formylmethionyl-leucyl-phenylalanine stimulation of inositol triphosphate accumulation in rabbit neutrophils. *Mol. Pharmacol.,* 27:74–78.
15. Bradford, P. G., and Rubin, R. P. (1986): Quantitative changes in inositol 1,4,5-triphosphate in chemoattractant-stimulated neutrophils. *J. Biol. Chem.,* 261:15644–15647.
16. Brandt, S. J., Dougherty, R. W., Lapetina, E. G., and Niedel, J. E. (1985): Pertussis toxin inhibits chemotactic peptide-stimulated generation of inositol phosphates and lysosomal enzyme secretion in human leukemic (HL-60) cells. *Proc. Natl. Acad. Sci. USA,* 82: 3277–3280.
17. Burgess, G. M., McKinney, J. S., Irvine, R. F., and Putney, J. W., Jr. (1985): Inositol 1,4,5-triphosphate and inositol 1,3,4-triphosphate formation in Ca^{2+}-mobilizing-hormone-activated cells. *Biochem. J.,* 232:237–243.
18. Cassel, D., and Selinger, Z. (1977): Mechanism of adenylate cyclase activation by cholera toxin: inhibition of GTP hydrolysis at the regulatory site. *Proc. Natl. Acad. Sci. USA,* 74:3307–3311.
19. Castagna, M., Yoshima, T., Kaibachi, S., Kikkawa, U., and Nishizuka, Y. (1982): Direct activation of calcium-activated, phospholipid-dependent protein kinase by tumour-promoting phorbol esters. *J. Biol. Chem.,* 257:7847–7851.
20. Cianciolo, G. J., and Snyderman, R. (1981): Monocyte responsiveness to chemotactic stimuli is a property of a subpopulation of cells which can respond to multiple chemoattractants. *J. Clin. Invest.,* 67:60–68.
21. Cockcroft, S. (1986): The dependence on Ca^{2+} of the guanine-nucleotide-activated polyphosphoinositide phosphodiesterase in neutrophil plasma membranes. *Biochem. J.,* 240:503–507.
22. Cockcroft, S., and Allan, D. (1984): The fatty acid composition of

phosphatidylinositol, phosphatidate and 1,2-diacylglycerol in stimulated human neutrophils. *Biochem. J., 222*:557–559.

23. Cockcroft, S., Baldwin, J. M., and Allan, D. (1984): The Ca^{2+}-activated polyphosphoinositide phosphodiesterase of human and rabbit neutrophil membranes. *Biochem. J., 221*:477–482.

24. Connolly, T. M., Lawing, W. J., Jr., and Majerus, P. W. (1986): Protein kinase C phosphorylates human platelet inositol triphosphate 5'-phosphomonoesterase increasing the phosphatase activity. *Cell, 46*:951–958.

25. Coussens, L, Parker, P. J., Rhee, L., Yang-Feng, T. L., Chen, E., Waterfield, M. D., Franke, U., and Ullrich, A. (1986): Multiple distinct forms of bovine and human protein kinase C suggest diversity in cellular signaling pathways. *Science, 233*:859–866.

26. Cox, C. C., Dougherty, R. W., Ganong, B. R., Bell, R. M., Niedel, J. E., and Snyderman, R. (1986): Differential stimulation of the respiratory burst and lysosomal enzyme secretion in human polymorphonuclear leukocytes by synthetic diacylglycerols. *J. Immunol., 136*:4611–4616.

27. Cox, J. A., Jeng, A. Y., Sharkey, N. A., Blumberg, P. M., and Tauber, A. I. (1985): Activation of the human neutrophil nicotinamide adenine dinucleotide phosphate (NADPH)-oxidase by protein kinase C. *J. Clin. Invest., 76*:1932–1938.

28. Deckmyn, H., Tu, S-M., and Majerus, P. W. (1986): Guanine nucleotides stimulate phosphoinositide-specific phospholipase C in the absence of membranes. *J. Biol. Chem., 261*:16553–16558.

29. Dewald, B., Bretz, U., and Baggiolini, M. (1982): Release of gelatinase from a novel secretory compartment of human neutrophils. *J. Clin. Invest., 70*:518–525.

30. Dewald, B., Payne, T. G., and Baggiolini, M. (1984): Activation of NADPH oxidase of human neutrophils: potentiation of chemotactic peptide by a diacylglycerol. *Biochem. Biophys. Res. Commun., 125*:367–373.

31. Didsbury, J. R., and Snyderman, R. (1987): Molecular cloning of a novel human GTP-binding protein and its potential role in chemoattractant stimulus-response coupling. *Clin. Res.* (abstract) (*in press*).

32. Didsbury, J. R., Ho, Y-S., and Snyderman, R. (1987): Human G_i protein α-subunit deduction of amino acid structure from a cloned cDNA. *FEBS Lett., 211*:160–164.

33. Dillon, S. B., Murray, J. J., Verghese, M. W., and Snyderman, R. (1987): Regulation of inositol phosphate metabolism in chemoattractant-stimulated human polymorphonuclear leukocytes: definition of distinct dephosphorylation pathways for IP_3 isomers. Submitted for publication.

34. DiVirgilio, F., Vicentini, L. M., Treves, S., Riz, G., and Pozzan, T. (1985): Inositol phosphate formation in fMet-Leu-Phe-stimulated human neutrophils does not require an increase in the cytosolic free Ca^{2+} concentration. *Biochem. J., 229*:361–367.

35. Dolmatch, B., and Niedel, J. (1983): Formyl peptide chemotactic receptor: evidence for an active proteolytic fragment. *J. Biol. Chem., 258*:7570–7577.

36. Dougherty, R. W., and Niedel, J. E. (1986): Cytosolic calcium regulates phorbol diester binding affinity in intact phagocytes. *J. Biol. Chem., 261*:4097–4100.

37. Dougherty, R. W., Godfrey, P. P., Hoyle, P. C., Putney, J. W., Jr., and Freer, R. J. (1984): Secretagogue-induced phosphoinositide metabolism in human leucocytes. *Biochem. J., 222*:307–314.

38. Evans, T., Brown, M. L., Fraser, E. D., and Northup, J. K. (1986): Purification of the major GTP-binding proteins from human placental membranes. *J. Biol. Chem., 261*:7052–7059.

39. Falloon, J., Malech, H., Milligan, G., Unson, C., Kahn, R., Goldsmith, P., and Spiegel, A. (1986): Detection of the major toxin substrate of human leukocytes with antisera raised against synthetic peptides. *FEBS Lett., 209*:352–356.

40. Feltner, D. E., Smith, R. H., and Marasco, W. A. (1986): Characterization of the plasma membrane GTPase from rabbit neutrophils. I. Evidence for an N_i-like protein coupled to the formyl peptide, C5a, and leukotriene B_4 chemotaxis receptors. *J. Immunol., 137*:1961–1970.

41. Fitzgerald, T. J., Uhing, R. J., and Exton, J. H. (1986): Solubilization of the vasopressin receptor from rat liver plasma membranes: evidence for a receptor-GTP-binding protein complex. *J. Biol. Chem., 261*:16871–16877.

42. Fletcher, M. P., and Gallin, J. I. (1982): Human neutrophils contain an intracellular pool of putative receptors for the chemoattractant N-formyl methionylleucylphenylalanine with a density of specific granules. *J. Cell. Biol., 95*:444a.

43. Fujita, I., Irita, K., Takeshige, K., and Minakami, S. (1984): Diacylglycerol, 1-oleoyl-2-acetylglycerol, stimulates superoxide-generation from human neutrophils. *Biochem. Biophys. Res. Commun., 120*:318–324.

44. Gallin, J. I., and Seligmann, B. E. (1984): Neutrophil chemoattractant fMet-Leu-Phe receptor expression and ionic events following activation. *Contemp. Top. Immunobiol., 14*:83–108.

45. Gallin, J. I., Sandler, J. A., Clyman, R. I., Manganiello, V. C., and Vaughan, M. (1978): Agents that increase cyclic AMP inhibit accumulation of cGMP and depress human monocyte locomotion. *J. Immunol., 120*:492–496.

46. Gardner, J. P., Melnick, D. A., and Malech, H. L. (1986): Characterization of the formyl peptide chemotactic receptor appearing at the phagocytic cell surface after exposure to phorbol myristate acetate. *J. Immunol., 136*:1400–1405.

47. Gennaro, R., Florio, C., and Romeo, D. (1986): Coactivation of protein kinase C and NADPH oxidase in the plasma membrane of neutrophil cytoplasts. *Biochem. Biophys. Res. Commun., 134*:305–312.

48. Giershik, P., Falloon, J., Milligan, G., Pines, M., Gallin, J. I., and Spiegel, A. (1986): Immunochemical evidence for a novel pertussis toxin substrate in human neutrophils. *J. Biol. Chem., 261*:8058–8062.

49. Gilman, A. G. (1984): G proteins and dual control of adenylate cyclase. *Cell, 36*:577–579.

50. Goetzl, E. J., Foster, D. W., and Goldman, D. W. (1981): Isolation and partial characterization of membrane protein constituents of human neutrophil receptors for chemotactic formylmethionyl peptides. *Biochemistry, 20*:5717–5722.

51. Goldman, D. W., and Goetzl, E. J. (1984): Heterogeneity of human polymorphonuclear leukocyte receptors for leukotriene B_4. *J. Exp. Med., 159*:1027–1041.

52. Goldman, D. W., Chang, F. H., Gifford, L. A., Goetzl, E. J., and Bourne, H. R. (1985): Pertussis toxin inhibition of chemotactic factor-induced calcium mobilization and function in human polymorphonuclear leukocytes. *J. Exp. Med., 162*:145–156.

53. Goldman, D. W., Gifford, L. A., Marotti, T., Koo, C. H., and Goetzl, E. J. (1987): Molecular and cellular properties of human polymorphonuclear leukocyte receptors for leukotriene B_4. *Fed. Proc., 46*:200–203.

54. Goldman, D. W., Gifford, L. A., Young, R. N., and Goetzl, E. J. (1985): Affinity labeling of human neutrophil receptors for leukotriene B_4. *Fed. Proc., 44*:781 (abstract).

55. Goldstein, I. M. (1984): Neutrophil degranulation. *Contemp. Top. Immunobiol., 14*:189–220.

56. Grinstein, S., and Furuya, W. (1986): Cytoplasmic pH regulation in phorbol ester-activated human neutrophils. *Am. J. Physiol. 251*:C55–C65.

57. Ho, Y-S., Lee, W. M. F., and Snyderman, R. (1987): Chemoattractant-induced activation of c-fos gene expression. *J. Exp. Med.* (*in press*).

58. Honeycutt, P. J., and Niedel, J. E. (1986): Cytochalasin B enhancement of the diacylglycerol response in formyl-stimulated neutrophils. *J. Biol. Chem., 261*:15900–15905.

59. Hoyle, P. C., and Freer, R. J. (1984): Isolation and reconstitution of the N-formylpeptide receptor from HL-60 derived neutrophils. *FEBS Lett., 167*:277–280.

60. Huang, C-K. (1987): Partial purification and characterization of formylpeptide receptor from rabbit peritoneal neutrophils. *J. Leuk. Biol., 41*:63–69.

61. Hugli, T. E. (1984): Structure and function of anaphylatoxins. *Springer Semin. Immunopathol., 7*:193–219.

62. Inagaki, M., Yokukura, H., Sakoh, T., and Hidaka, H. (1987): Tissue specific expression of three distinct types of rabbit protein kinase C. *Nature, 325*:161–166.

63. Irvine, R. F., and Moor, R. M. (1986): Micro-injection of inositol 1,3,4,5-tetrakisphosphate activates sea urchin eggs by a mechanism dependent on external Ca^{2+}. *Biochem. J.*, 240:917–920.

64. Jackowski, S., and Sha'afi, R. I. (1979): Response of adenosine cyclic 3',5'-monophosphate level in rabbit neutrophils to the chemotactic peptide formyl-methionyl-leucyl-phenylalanine. *Mol. Pharmacol.*, 16:473–481.

65. Jesaitis, A. J., Naemura, J. R., Painter, R. G., Sklar, L. A., and Cochrane, C. G. (1982): Intracellular localization of N-formyl chemotactic receptor and Mg^{2+} dependent ATPase in human granulocytes. *Biophys. Biochim. Acta*, 719:556–568.

66. Kay, G. E., Lane, B. C., and Snyderman, R. (1983): Induction of selective biological responses to chemoattractants in a human monocyte-like cell line. *Infect. Immun.*, 41:1166–1174.

67. Kikuchi, A., Kozawa, O., Kaibuchi, K., Katada, T., Ui, M., and Takai, Y. (1986): Direct evidence for involvement of a guanine nucleotide-binding protein in chemotactic peptide-stimulated formation of inositol biphosphate and triphosphate in differentiated leukemic (HL-60) cells: reconstitution with G_i or G_o of the plasma membranes ADP-ribosylated by pertussis toxin. *J. Biol. Chem.*, 257:11558–11562.

68. Knopf, J. L., Lee, M-H., Sultzman, L. A., Kriz, R. W., Loomis, C. R., Hewick, R. M., and Bell, R. M. (1986): Cloning and expression of multiple protein kinase C cDNAs. *Cell*, 46:491–502.

69. Koo, C., Lefkowitz, R. J., and Snyderman, R. (1982): The oligopeptide chemotactic factor receptor on human polymorphonuclear leukocyte membranes exists in two affinity states. *Biochem. Biophys. Res. Commun.*, 106:442–449.

70. Koo, C., Lefkowitz, R. J., and Snyderman, R. (1983): Guanine nucleotides modulate the binding affinity of the oligopeptide chemoattractant receptor on human polymorphonuclear leukocytes. *J. Clin. Invest.*, 72:748–753.

71. Korchak, H. M., Rutherford, L. E., and Weissmann, G. (1984): Stimulus response coupling in the human neutrophil. I. Kinetic analysis of changes in calcium permeability. *J. Biol. Chem.*, 259:4070–4075.

72. Korchak, H. M., Vienne, K., Rutherford, L. E., Wilkenfeld, C., Finkelstein, M. C., and Weissmann, G. (1984): Stimulus response coupling in the human neutrophil. II. Temporal analysis of changes in cytosolic calcium and calcium efflux. *J. Biol. Chem.*, 259:4076–4082.

73. Kreisle, R. A., and Parker, D. W. (1983): Specific binding of leukotriene B_4 to a receptor on human polymorphonuclear leukocytes. *J. Exp. Med.*, 157:628–634.

74. Lad, P. M., Olson, C. V., and Smiley, P. A. (1985): Association of the N-formyl-Met-Leu-Phe receptor in human neutrophils with a GTP-binding protein sensitive to pertussis toxin. *Proc. Natl. Acad. Sci. USA*, 82:869–873.

75. Lad, P. M., Olson, C. V., Grewal, I. S., and Scott, S. J. (1985): A pertussis toxin-sensitive GTP-binding protein in the human neutrophil regulates multiple receptors, calcium mobilization, and lectin-induced capping. *Proc. Natl. Acad. Sci. USA*, 82:8643–8647.

76. Lew, P. D., Monod, A., Krause, K-H., Waldvogel, F. A., Biden, T. J., and Schlegel, W. (1986): The role of cytosolic calcium in the generation of inositol 1,4,5-triphosphate and inositol 1,3,4-triphosphate in HL-60 cells: differential effects of chemotactic peptide receptor stimulation at distinct Ca^{2+} levels. *J. Biol. Chem.*, 261:13121–13127.

77. Lew, P. D., Monod, A., Waldvogel, F. A., Dewald, B., Baggiolini, M., and Pozzan, T. (1986): Quantitative analysis of the cytosolic free calcium dependency of exocytosis from three subcellular compartments in intact neutrophils. *J. Cell Biol.*, 102:2197–2204.

78. Lew, P. D., Wollheim, C. B., Waldvogel, F. A., and Pozzan, T. (1984): Modulation of cytosolic-free calcium transients by changes in intracellular calcium-buffering capacity: correlation with exocytosis and O_2^- production in human neutrophils. *J. Cell Biol.*, 99:1212–1220.

79. Litosch, I., and Fain, J. N. (1986): Regulation of phosphoinositide breakdown by guanine nucleotides. *Life Sci.*, 39:187–194.

80. Logothetis, D. E., Kurachi, Y., Galper, J., Neer, E. J., and Clapham, D. E. (1987): The $\beta\gamma$ subunits of GTP-binding proteins activate the muscarinic K^+ channel in heart. *Nature*, 324:321–326.

81. Mackin, W. M., Huang, C. K., and Becker, E. L. (1982): The formyl peptide chemotactic receptor on rabbit peritoneal neutrophils. *J. Immunol.*, 129:1608–1611.

82. Majerus, P. W., Connolly, T. M., Deckmyn, H., Ross, T. S., Bross, T. E., Ishii, H., Bansal, V. S., and Wilson, D. B. (1986): The metabolism of phosphoinositide-derived messenger molecules. *Science*, 234:1519–1526.

83. Malech, H. L., Gardner, J. P., Heiman, D. F., and Rosenzweig, S. A. (1985): Asparagine-linked oligosaccharides on formyl peptide chemotactic receptors of human phagocytic cells. *J. Biol. Chem.*, 260:2509–2514.

84. Malfroy, B. and Schwartz, J.-C. (1984): Enkephalinase from rat kidney: Purification, characterization, and study of substrate specificity. *J. Biol. Chem.*, 259(23): 14365–14370.

85. McPhail, L. C., and Snyderman, R. (1984): Mechanisms of regulating the respiratory burst in leukocytes. *Contemp. Top. Immunobiol.*, 14:247–281.

86. McPhail, L. C., Wolfson, M., Clayton, C., and Snyderman, R. (1984): Protein kinase C and neutrophil (PMN) activation: differential effects of chemoattractants and phorbol myristate acetate (PMA). *Fed. Proc.*, 43:1661 (abstract).

87. Melloni, E., Pontremoli, S., Salamino, F., Sparatore, B., Michetti, M., Sacco, O., and Horeker, B. L. (1986): ATP induces the release of a neutral serine proteinase and enhances the production of superoxide anion in membranes from phorbol ester-activated neutrophils. *J. Biol. Chem.*, 261:11437–11439.

88. Michell, R. H. (1975): Inositol phospholipids and cell surface receptor function. *Biochim. Biophys. Acta*, 415:81–147.

89. Milligan, G., and Klee, W. A. (1985): The inhibitory guanine nucleotide-binding protein (N_i) purified from bovine brain is a high affinity GTPase. *J. Biol. Chem.*, 260:2057–2063.

90. Mitchell, R. L., Zokas, L., Schreiber, R. D., and Yema, I. M. (1985): Rapid induction of the expression of proto-oncogene fos during human monocytic differentiation. *Cell*, 40:209–217.

91. Molina, Y., Vedia, L., and Lapetina, E. G. (1986): Phorbol 12,13-dibutyrate and 1-oleyl-2-acetyldiacylglycerol stimulate inositol triphosphate dephosphorylation in human platelets. *J. Biol. Chem.*, 261:10493–10495.

92. Molski, T. F. P., Naccache, P. H., Marsah, M. L., Kermode, J., Becker, E. L., and Sha'afi, R. I. (1984): Pertussis toxin inhibits the rise in the intracellular concentration of free calcium that is induced by chemotactic factors in rabbit neutrophils: possible role of the "G proteins" in calcium mobilization. *Biochem. Biophys. Res. Commun.*, 124:644–650.

93. Muller, R., Muller, D., and Guilbert, L. (1984): Differential expression of c-fos in hematopoietic cells: correlation with differentiation of monomyelocytic cells in vitro. *EMBO J.*, 3:1887–1890.

94. Myers, M. A., McPhail, L. C., and Snyderman, R. (1985): Redistribution of protein kinase C activity in human monocytes: correlation with activation of the respiratory burst. *J. Immunol.*, 135:3411–3416.

95. Naccache, P. H., Molski, T. F. P., Borgeat, P., White, J. R., and Sha'afi, R. I. (1985): Phorbol esters inhibit the fMet-Leu-Phe- and leukotriene B_4-stimulated calcium mobilization and enzyme secretion in rabbit neutrophils. *J. Biol. Chem.*, 260:2125–2131.

96. Neer, E. J., Lok, J. M., and Wolf, L. G. (1984): Purification and properties of the inhibitory guanine nucleotide regulatory unit of brain adenylate cyclase. *J. Biol. Chem.*, 259:14222–14229.

97. Ng, D. S., and Wong, K. (1986): GTP regulation of platelet-activating factor binding to human neutrophil membranes. *Biochem. Biophys. Res. Commun.*, 141:353–359.

98. Niedel, J., David, J., and Cuatrecasas, P. (1980): Covalent affinity labeling of the formyl peptide chemotactic receptor. *J. Biol. Chem.*, 255:7063–7066.

99. Niedel, J., Kahane, I., and Cuatrecasas, P. (1979): Receptor-mediated internalization of fluorescent chemotactic peptide by human neutrophils. *Science*, 205:1412–1414.

100. Niedel, J., Wilkinson, S., and Cuatrecasas, P. (1979): Receptor-

mediated uptake and degradation of ^{125}I-chemotactic peptide by human neutrophils. *J. Biol. Chem.*, 254:10700–10706.

101. Nishihira, J., McPhail, L. C., and O'Flaherty, J. T. (1986): Stimulus-dependent mobilization of protein kinase C. *Biochem. Biophys. Res. Commun.*, 134:587–594.

102. Nishizuka, Y. (1986): Studies and perspectives of protein kinase C. *Science*, 233:305–312.

103. O'Flaherty, J. T., Schmitt, J. D., McCall, C. E., and Wykle, R. L. (1984): Diacylglycerols enhance human neutrophil degranulation responses: relevancy to a multiple mediator hypothesis of cell function. *Biochem. Biophys. Res. Commun.*, 123:64–70.

104. Ohta, H., Okajima, F., and Ui, M. (1985): Inhibition by islet-activating protein of a chemotactic peptide-induced early breakdown of inositol phospholipids and Ca^{2+} mobilization in guinea pig neutrophils. *J. Biol. Chem.*, 260:15771–15780.

105. Okajima, F., and Ui, M. (1984): ADP-ribosylation of the specific membrane protein by islet-activating protein, pertussis toxin, associated with inhibition of a chemotactic peptide-induced arachidonate release in neutrophils. *J. Biol. Chem.*, 259:13863–13871.

106. Okajima, F., Katada, T., and Ui, M. (1985): Coupling of the guanine nucleotide regulatory protein to chemotactic peptide receptors in neutrophil membranes and its uncoupling by islet-activating protein, pertussis toxin: a possible role of the toxin substrate in Ca^{2+}-mobilizing receptor-mediated signal transduction. *J. Biol. Chem.*, 260:6761–6768.

107. Painter, R. G., Schmitt, M., Jesaitis, A. J., Sklar, L. A., Aissnar, K., and Cochrane, C. G. (1982): Photoaffinity labeling of the N-formyl peptide receptor on human polymorphonuclear leukocytes. *J. Cell. Biochem.*, 20:203–214.

108. Palmblad, J., Gyllenhammar, H., Lindgren, J. A., and Malmsten, C. L. (1984): Effects of leukotrienes and f-Met-Leu-Phe on oxidative metabolism of neutrophils and eosinophils. *J. Immunol.*, 132:3041–3045.

109. Pike, M. C., Jakoi, L., McPhail, L. C., and Snyderman, R. (1986): Chemoattractant-mediated stimulation of the respiratory burst in human polymorphonuclear leukocytes may require appearance of protein kinase activity in the cells' particulate fraction. *Blood*, 67:909–913.

110. Polakis, P., and Snyderman, R. (1987): G-protein-chemoattractant receptor interaction: co-purification of the formylpeptide receptor with a guanine nucleotide binding protein. *Clin. Res.* (abstract) (in press).

111. Pozzan, T., Lew, D. P., Wollheim, C. B., and Tsien, R. Y. (1983): Is cytosolic ionized calcium regulating neutrophil activation? *Science*, 221:1413–1415.

112. Preiss, J., Loomis, C. R., Bishop, W. R., Stein, R., Niedel, J. E., and Bell, R. M. (1986): Quantitative measurement of sn-1,2-diacylglycerols present in platelets, hepatocytes and ras- and sis-transformed normal rat kidney cells. *J. Biol. Chem.*, 261:8597–8600.

113. Prentki, M., Wollheim, C. G., and Lew, P. D. (1984): Ca^{2+} homeostasis in permeabilized human neutrophils: characterization of Ca^{2+}-sequestering pools and the action of inositol 1,4,5-triphosphate. *J. Biol. Chem.*, 259:13777–13782.

114. Rivkin, I., Rosenblatt, J., and Becker, E. L. (1975): The role of cyclic AMP in the chemotactic responsiveness and spontaneous motility of rabbit peritoneal neutrophils. *J. Immunol.*, 115:1126–1134.

115. Saltiel, A. R., and Cuatrecasas, P. (1986): Insulin stimulates the generation from hepatic plasma membranes of modulators derived from an inositol glycolipid. *Proc. Natl. Acad. Sci. USA*, 83:5793–5797.

116. Schmitt, M., Painter, R. G., Jesaitis, A. J., Preissner, K., Sklar, L. A., and Cochrane, C. G. (1983): Photoaffinity labeling of the N-formyl peptide receptor binding site of intact human polymorphonuclear leukocytes. *J. Biol. Chem.*, 258:649–654.

117. Schreiber, R. D. (1984): The chemistry and biology of complement receptors. *Springer Semin. Immunopathol.*, 7:221–249.

118. Serhan, C. N., Broekman, M. J., Korchak, H. M., Smolen, J. E., Marcus, A. J., and Weissmann, G. (1983): Changes in phosphatidylinositol and phosphatidic acid in stimulated human neutrophils:

119. Serhan, C. N., Radin, A., Smolen, J. E., Korchak, H., Samuelsson, B., and Weissman, G. (1982): Leukotriene B$_4$ is a complete secretagogue in human neutrophils: a kinetic analysis. *Biochem. Biophys. Res. Commun.*, 107:1006–1012.

120. Shichi, H., and Somers, R. L. (1978): Light-dependent phosphorylation of rhodopsin: purification and properties of rhodopsin kinase. *J. Biol. Chem.*, 253:7040–7046.

121. Showell, H. J., Freer, R. J., Zigmond, S. H., Schiffmann, E., Aswanikumar, S., Corcoran, B., and Becker, E. L. (1976): The structure-activity relations of synthetic peptides as chemotactic factors and inducers of lysozymal enzyme secretion for neutrophils. *J. Exp. Med.*, 143:1154–1169.

122. Simchowitz, L., Fischbein, L. C., Spilberg, I., and Atkinson, J. P. (1980): Induction of a transient elevation in intracellular levels of adenosine-3′,5′-cyclic monophosphate by chemotactic factors: an early event in human neutrophil activation. *J. Immunol.*, 124:1482–1491.

123. Sklar, A., Jesaitis, A. J., and Painter, R. G. (1984): The neutrophil N-formyl peptide receptor: dynamics of ligand-receptor interactions and their relationship to cellular responses. *Contemp. Top. Immunobiol.*, 14:29–82.

124. Sklar, L. A., Bokoch, G. M., Button, D., and Smolen, J. E. (1987): Regulation of ligand-receptor dynamics by guanine nucleotides: real-time analysis of interconverting states for the neutrophil formylpeptide receptor. *J. Biol. Chem.*, 262:135–139.

125. Smith, C. D., Cox, C. C., and Snyderman, R. (1986): Receptor-coupled activation of phosphoinositide-specific phospholipase C by an N protein. *Science*, 232:97–100.

126. Smith, C. D., Lane, B. C., Kusaka, I., Verghese, M. W., and Snyderman, R. (1985): Chemoattractant-receptor induced hydrolysis of phosphatidylinositol 4,5-biphosphate in human polymorphonuclear leukocyte membranes: requirement of a guanine nucleotide regulatory protein. *J. Biol. Chem.*, 260:5875–5878.

127. Smith, C. D., Sharp, J. J., and Snyderman, R. (1987): Modulation of inositol phospholipid metabolism by polyamines. Submitted for publication.

128. Smith, C. D., Uhing, R. J., and Snyderman, R. (1987): Nucleotide regulatory protein-mediated activation of phospholipase C in human polymorphonuclear leukocytes is disrupted by phorbol esters. *J. Biol. Chem.* (in press).

129. Snyderman, R., and Pike, M. C. (1984): Chemoattractant receptors on phagocytic cells. *Annu. Rev. Immunol.*, 2:257–281.

130. Snyderman, R., and Pike, M. C. (1984): Regulation of leukocyte function. *Contemp. Top. Immunobiol.*, 14:1–28.

131. Snyderman, R., Pike, M. C., Edge, S., and Lane, B. (1984): A chemoattractant receptor on macrophages exists in two affinity states regulated by guanine nucleotides. *J. Cell Biol.*, 98:444–448.

132. Snyderman, R., Smith, C. D., and Verghese, M. W. (1986): Model for leukocyte regulation by chemoattractant receptors: roles of a guanine nucleotide regulatory protein and polyphosphoinositide metabolism. *J. Leuk. Biol.*, 40:785–800.

133. Spiegel, A. M. (1987): Signal transduction by guanine nucleotide binding proteins. *Mol. Cell. Endocrinol.*, 49:1–16.

134. Stephens, C. G., and Snyderman, R. (1982): Cyclic nucleotides regulate the morphologic alterations required for chemotaxis in monocytes. *J. Immunol.*, 128:1192–1197.

135. Sternweis, P. C., and Robishaw, J. D. (1984): Isolation of two proteins with high affinity for guanine nucleotides from membranes of bovine brain. *J. Biol. Chem.*, 259:13806–13813.

136. Sullivan, S., and Zigmond, S. (1980): Chemotactic peptide receptor modulation in polymorphonuclear leukocytes. *J. Cell Biol.*, 85:703–711.

137. Sweatt, J. D., Blair, I. A., Cragoe, E. J., and Limbird, L. E. (1986): Inhibitors of Na$^+$/H$^+$ exchange block epinephrine- and ADP-induced stimulation of human platelet phospholipase C by blockade of arachidonic acid release at a prior step. *J. Biol. Chem.*, 261:8660–8666.

138. Sweatt, J. D., Connolly, T. M., Cragoe, E. J., and Limbird, L. E. (1986): Evidence that Na$^+$/H$^+$ exchange regulates receptor-mediated

phospholipase A_2 activation in human platelets. *J. Biol. Chem.*, 261:8667–8673.

139. Takenawa, T., Ishitoya, J., and Nagai, Y. (1986): Inhibitory effect of prostaglandin E_2, forskolin, and dibutyryl cAMP on arachidonic acid release and inositol phospholipid metabolism in guinea pig neutrophils. *J. Biol. Chem.*, 261:1092–1098.

140. Taylor, C. W. (1986): Growth factors control a network of interacting messengers. *Trends Pharmacol. Sci.*, 7:467–471.

141. Truett, A. P., III, Verghese, M. W., Dillon, S. B., and Snyderman, R. (1987): Leukocyte (PMN) activation by chemoattractants (CTX): a two phase sequential pathway mediates the respiratory burst. *Clin. Res.* (abstract) (*in press*).

142. Verghese, M. W., Fox, K., McPhail, L. C., and Snyderman, R. (1985): Chemoattractant-elicited alterations of cAMP levels in human polymorphonuclear leukocytes require a Ca^{++}-dependent mechanism which is independent of transmembrane activation of adenylate cyclase. *J. Biol. Chem.*, 260:6769–6775.

143. Verghese, M. W., Smith, C. D., and Snyderman, R. (1985): Potential role for a guanine nucleotide regulatory protein in chemoattractant receptor mediated polyphosphoinositide metabolism, Ca^{++} mobilization and cellular responses by leukocytes. *Biochem. Biophys. Res. Commun.*, 127:450–457.

144. Verghese, M. W., Smith, C. D., and Snyderman, R. (1985): Role for a guanine nucleotide regulatory (N) protein in chemoattractant mediated Ca^{2+} mobilization and cAMP formation in human neutrophils (PMNs). *Clin. Res.*, 33:566A.

145. Verghese, M. W., Smith, C. D., Charles, L. A., and Snyderman, R. (1986): A common transduction pathway for leukocyte chemoattractant receptors: phospholipase C activation by a guanine nucleotide regulatory protein. *Clin. Res.*, 34:679A.

146. Verghese, M. W., Smith, C. D., Charles, L. A., Jakoi, L., and Snyderman, R. (1986): A guanine nucleotide regulatory protein controls polyphosphoinositide metabolism, Ca^{2+} mobilization and cellular responses to chemoattractants in human monocytes. *J. Immunol.*, 137:271–275.

147. Verghese, M. W., Uhing, R. J., and Snyderman, R. (1986): A pertussis/cholera toxin-sensitive N protein may mediate chemoat-tractant receptor signal transduction. *Biochem. Biophys. Res. Commun.*, 138:887–894.

148. Volpi, M., Nacchache, P. H., Molski, T. F. P., Shefcyk, J., Huang, C. K., Marsh, M. L., Munoz, J., Becker, E. L., and Sha'afi, R. I. (1985): Pertussis toxin inhibits fMet-Leu-Phe- but not phorbol ester-stimulated changes in rabbit neutrophils: role of G proteins in excitation response coupling. *Proc. Natl. Acad. Sci. USA*, 82:2708–2712.

149. Weisman, S. J., Punzo, A., Ford, C., and Sha'afi, R. I. (1987): Intracellular pH changes during neutrophil activation: Na^+/H^+ antiport. *J. Leuk. Biol.*, 41:25–32.

150. White, J. R., Huang, C-K., Hill, J. M., Jr., Naccache, P. H., Becker, E. L., and Sha'afi, R. I. (1984): Effect of phorbol 12-myristate 13-acetate and its analogue 4α-phorbol 12,13-didecanoate on protein phosphorylation and lysosomal enzyme release in rabbit neutrophils. *J. Biol. Chem.*, 259:8605–8611.

151. Williams, L. T., Snyderman, R., Pike, M. C., and Lefkowitz, R. J. (1977): Specific receptor sites for chemotactic peptides on human polymorphonuclear leukocytes. *Proc. Natl. Acad. Sci. USA*, 74:1204–1208.

152. Wolfson, M., McPhail, L. C., Nasrallah, V. N., and Snyderman, R. (1985): Phorbol myristate acetate mediates redistribution of protein kinase C in human neutrophils: potential role in the activation of the respiratory burst enzyme. *J. Immunol.*, 135:2057–2062.

153. Yuli, I., and Oplatka, A. (1987): Cytosolic acidification as an early transductory signal of human neutrophil chemotaxis. *Science*, 235:340–342.

154. Yuli, I., and Snyderman, R. (1984): Light scattering by polymorphonuclear leukocytes stimulated to aggregate under various pharmacologic conditions. *Blood*, 64:649–655.

155. Yuli, I., and Snyderman, R. (1986): Extensive hydrolysis of N-formyl-L-methionyl-L-leucyl-L-[^{3}H]phenylalanine by human polymorphonuclear leukocytes: a potential mechanism for modulation of the chemoattractant signal. *J. Biol. Chem.*, 261:4902–4908.

156. Zigmond, S. H., and Tranquillo, A. W. (1986): Chemotactic peptide binding by rabbit polymorphonuclear leukocytes: presence of two compartments having similar affinities but different kinetics. *J. Biol. Chem.*, 261:5283–5288.

Inflammation: Basic Principles and Clinical Correlates.
Edited by J. I. Gallin, I. M. Goldstein, and R. Snyderman.
Raven Press, Ltd., New York © 1988.

CHAPTER 20

The Mechanical Responses of White Blood Cells

Thomas P. Stossel

Locomotion, pinocytosis (endocytosis), phagocytosis, and exocytosis are mechanical responses of leukocytes because they involve movements of the plasma membrane and the cytoplasm. Information concerning these mechanical responses, reviewed in this chapter, is only part of the more general subject of eukaryotic cell motility, and attention is called to reviews of this topic (111,128).

Phagocytosis, locomotion, and granule movements were the first activities of leukocytes to be recognized. The descriptions of these events made with the light microscope still form an important basis for attempting to understand the mechanism of these aspects of leukocyte behavior.

LEUKOCYTE MECHANICAL RESPONSE: IMPORTANCE OF PERIPHERAL CYTOPLASM

Locomotion

The earliest descriptions of leukocyte movements reveal an appreciation that the leukocyte crawls rather than swims, that it acquires an asymmetrical shape, and that from its periphery extend organelle-excluding hyaline pseudopodia (often called lamellipodia) in the direction of locomotion (Fig. 1). The lamellipodia become briefly adherent to the substrate to provide the frictional force for movement, whereas the cell body from which the pseudopod extends appears to be pulled passively forward by the advancement of the lamellipodia. Sometimes the rear of the cell, which can acquire a knob-like protuberance called the uropod or simply the tail, adheres to the surface. This tail is the site where molecules on the cell membrane that have become cross-linked by various ligands migrate (cap) and are subsequently shed or internalized.

Occasionally, as the cell moves forward, the attached tail stretches to form one or more thin strings; either motion is totally retarded by the tethered tail or else the strings (sometimes called retraction fibers) break. Most large organelles within the moving cell, e.g., the nucleus and hydrolase-containing granules, are relatively immobile, although they sometimes move anteriorly in concert with

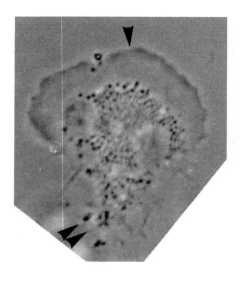

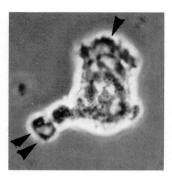

FIG. 1. Appearance of two crawling neutrophils photographed with the phase-contrast microscope showing the anterior lamellipod (*single arrow*) and the tail (uropod) at the rear (*double arrows*). ×1,200.

streaming of the internal cytoplasm from the rear to the front of the cell. On the other hand, relatively rapid granule movements take place just proximal to the lamellipodia (103,137).

With better optics it became apparent that the moving leukocyte's anterior pseudopodia are comprised of a relatively broad and somewhat flattened region from which extend blebs and little spikes at the leading edge. Two separate lamellipodia can transiently be splayed into different directions separated by as much as 180 degrees, as if they were in competition for pulling the cell; this situation does not persist, however, and one lamellipod or group of lamellipodia takes precedence. At this point the "losing" lamellipodia retract back to the cell body. Frequent reference has been made to a contractile ring immediately behind the lamellipodia that forms from time to time and persists as cytoplasm moves forward through it (27,37,56,71,93). The effects of molecules that induce chemotaxis of leukocytes in orienting the direction of leukocyte movement and the interaction of these molecules with receptors on phagocyte membranes are discussed elsewhere in this text.

Because of their propensity to polarize and move rapidly, the morphological properties summarized above have been most frequently described in neutrophils. Mononuclear phagocytes, especially macrophages, have a tendency to spread a completely circumferential hyaline lamella that folds upward at the edge, a process called ruffling (Fig. 2). Macrophages also form pleats on and extend spikes from the nonadherent surface of the cell; these phenomena are best appreciated with the scanning electron microscope (9,55,84).

The dominance of the peripheral cytoplasm in light microscopic descriptions of leukocyte movement implies but does not prove that this region is of primary importance to the mechanism of motility. A critical observation

made by Keller and Bessis (56) and confirmed by Malawista and Boisfleury Chevance (73) is that neutrophils heated to 40°C release lamellipodia from their cell bodies, and that these "cytokinetoplasts" persist in a rudimentary form of movement and even exhibit chemotaxis. This discovery comes close to proving that the "motor" of leukocytes resides in the cell periphery and that events at the front of the cell, rather than a squeezing at the rear, for example, are adequate for locomotion, at least under these experimental conditions.

Phagocytosis and Pinocytosis

The peripheral cytoplasm is also of great importance in phagocytosis. This fact is particularly clear when the observer watches polymorphonuclear leukocytes migrate on a glass slide in the presence of objects they ingest, e.g., bacteria or yeast particles. The leukocytes move toward the target particles guided by a gradient of chemotactic molecules emanating from them. The act of engulfment appears to be a variant of locomotion. The organelle-excluding leading lamellipod surrounds an appropriately opsonized object and fuses at its distal end (47). For leukocytes in suspension or macrophages spread on a surface, the phagocytic act is more difficult to visualize by light microscopy because it is not limited to any one focal plane. However, scanning electron microscope images of leukocytes suspended with ingestible particles or adherent macrophages ingesting particles on their free surfaces reveal the extension of a thin lamella around the object (55,84).

Further evidence that the protrusive pseudopodial movements underlying phagocytosis represent, like locomotion, events within a localized region of membrane and peripheral cytoplasm comes from experiments of Silverstein and co-workers (40,41). They showed that a mac-

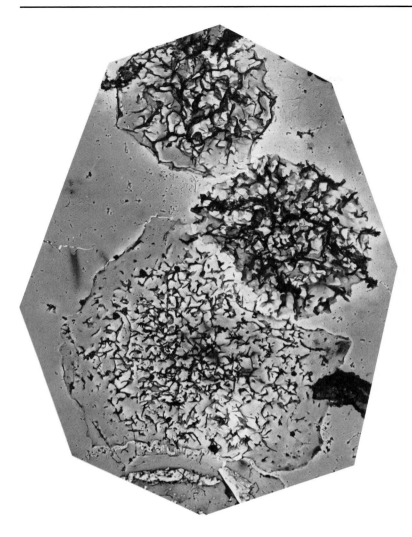

FIG. 2. Appearance of three spread macrophages that were rapidly frozen, rotary-shadowed with carbon–platinum, and photographed in the electron microscope, showing the peripheral spread lamellae and projecting veils on the dorsal surface of the cell. ×3,500.

rophage advances pseudopodia only over the regions of a target particle that express recognition molecules (opsonins). Conversely, the phagocyte membrane must express receptors for the opsonin in order for the pseudopod advancement to propagate. These observations explain how a polymorphonuclear leukocyte can "pit" the nucleus out of a damaged lymphocyte in serum containing antinuclear antibodies without ingesting the remainder of the cell—an event known to earlier clinicians as the LE cell phenomenon and which was used as a diagnostic test for systemic lupus erythematosus.

In the region of the ruffled membrane of macrophages is the point of origin of pinocytic vesicles visible with the light microscope, and these vesicles move centripetally to the perinuclear region.

Exocytosis

In polymorphonuclear leukocytes, granule movements become prominent at the base of the forming phagocytic vacuole, and the disappearance (degranulation) of the granules corresponds to a secretory act in which there is exocytosis of granule contents into the phagosomal vacuole (47). Because leukocytes release granule-associated enzymes into the medium during locomotion (7) it is possible that the movement of granules behind the advancing lamella during locomotion also represents an exocytic event.

Agonal Events

After leukocytes have exhibited the morphology described above for a time under observation with the light microscope, they may begin to display extensive blebbing of the surface. The blebs are initially spherical and about 1 μm in diameter. Later they can become confluent and extend like sausages for impressive distances from the cell body, from which they are easily separated by minimal mechanical agitation. For the most part, the blebs continue to exclude granules, but when a granule enters the bleb it may demonstrate extensive movement that may be either saltatory or apparently brownian in form. In such cells, which are evidently dying, internal granules may become much more mobile than in more viable leukocytes. Eventually all movements cease (9).

CONSISTENCY OF PERIPHERAL CYTOPLASM

The organelle exclusion that usually characterizes peripheral cytoplasm led early investigators to infer that it was in some kind of gelled state (27,72). To obtain detailed information about the mechanical properties of a delicate rim of such small cells has been a formidable assignment attacked by such ingenious methods as the determination of the centrifugal force needed for ingested oil droplets to float a bit of peripheral cytoplasm into a protrusion facing the opposite direction of the sedimenting cell (107). Aspiration of a piece of membrane with underlying cytoplasm with micropipettes has indicated that the peripheral cytoplasm of a resting polymorphonuclear leukocyte resists initial deformation in a manner expected for an elastic or gel-like material, but on prolonged aspiration it flows. This kind of mechanical behavior is called viscoelastic behavior. Because the plasma membrane of the leukocyte in isotonic medium has numerous folds and is widely believed to be a relatively delicate and fluid lipid bilayer, it is presumed to be passively deformed in such experiments and does not contribute to the measurement. Similar determinations on pseudopodia extended from a leukocyte show them to resist deformation in a manner characteristic of a solid or a gel; but unlike the case of the resting cell, they do not flow in response to relatively prolonged stress, suggesting that the pseudopod is more gelled than the peripheral cytoplasm of the resting cell. Similarly, the overall deformability of lymphocytes diminishes, i.e., they become more rigid, when the cells are activated by mitogens (87).

MOLECULAR COMPONENTS OF PERIPHERAL CYTOPLASM: IMPORTANCE OF ACTIN

For the past 15 years considerable evidence has accumulated that actin filaments are principal structures of leukocyte peripheral cytoplasm and therefore probably responsible for its mechanical properties (described above). The initial information was that transmission electron micrographs of thin sections of leukocytes revealed 4 to 6 nm diameter filaments as the dominant element in peripheral cytoplasm (59). Reaction of permeabilized cells with myosin fragments, heavy meromyosin, or myosin subfragment I caused the filaments to appear thickened in thin-section electron micrographs, and favorable images revealed an arrowhead configuration on the filaments characteristic for actomyosin complexes (4). Subsequently, staining of leukocytes by immunoflu-

orescence, immunoperoxidase, and immunogold techniques with antibodies specific for actin and for actin-associated proteins indicated that these proteins are localized and probably concentrated in the peripheral cytoplasm and are present in pseudopodia (83,86, 105,119,120,134,142). These conclusions were supported by biochemical analyses of blebs released from the peripheral cytoplasm of leukocytes showing that the total actin concentration in these structures was as high as 20 mg/ml (26). Finally, the cytochalasins, fungal metabolites now known to react with actin filaments and to inhibit their assembly from monomeric subunits (see following), powerfully inhibit leukocyte locomotion and phagocytosis, enhance exocytosis, and cause retraction of the leukocyte cortical cytoplasm (4,6,39,43,86). In addition, the cytochalasins decrease the "stiffness" of leukocytes, as assessed by a variety of rheological techniques, reflecting a reduction in the consistency of the actin-rich peripheral cytoplasm (76,87,114,133). One exception is the report of Miller (78), which states that cytochalasin increased the resistance of neutrophils to deformation by a micropipette.

In contrast to the prominence of actin and actin-associated proteins in the leukocyte peripheral cytoplasm, immunofluorescence microscopy suggests that the other known cytoskeletal protein systems, the tubulin polymers (microtubules), and the intermediate filaments, assemblies of the protein called vimentin in leukocytes, are relatively few in number and are restricted to the cell body, although they penetrate the actin-rich peripheral cytoplasm to some extent (5,20,74,91,100). Chemicals that affect tubulin assembly, i.e., colchicine, podophyllotoxin, and vinca alkaloids, inhibit the polymerization and cause net depolymerization of microtubules in leukocytes but do not have the profound inhibitory effects on leukocyte mechanical functions caused by the cytochalasins (57). On the other hand, it has been shown that the centriole of leukocytes tends to orient itself on the side of the nucleus in the direction of cell migration (74), and it has been argued that a centriolar–Golgi apparatus complex may be important for recycling of plasma membrane in a way that helps to maintain the polarity of the cell (111).

The isolation and characterization of leukocyte actin and actin-associated proteins (summarized in Table 1) have also been useful steps in furthering understanding of leukocyte mechanics, beginning with the pioneering studies of Senda and co-workers more than 15 years ago (110). Investigations of mechanical phenomena occurring in cytoplasmic extracts of leukocytes and of proteins purified from these extracts later suggested that actin might be essential for the properties of peripheral cytoplasm. Appropriately prepared, initially liquid leukocyte extract gel and actin filaments are the major components of these solidified extracts. Two proteins, *actin-binding protein* and

TABLE 1. *Actin-modulating proteins of leukocytes*

Protein	Function *in vitro*	Native M_r (kD)	Number of subunits and M_r of each subunit (kD)	Regulated by
Actin-binding protein (ABP)	Isotropic (orthogonal) gelation of actin filaments	540	2×270	?
α-Actinin	Anisotropic (bundling) gelation of actin filaments	220	2×105	Calcium
Profilin	Actin monomer sequestration	15	1×15	PIP$_2$
42K	Blockade of the "fast" ends of actin filaments	42	1×42	Calcium
Gelsolin	Severing of actin filaments Nucleation of actin filament growth	84	1×84	Calcium, PIP$_2$
Acumentin	?	64	1×64	?
Tropomyosin	Stabilization of actin filaments	70	2×35	
Myosin	Contraction	460	2×200, 20 and 15	Calcium (myosin light-chain kinase + calmodulin)

α-*actinin,* which were found capable of gelling actin *in vitro,* were purified from leukocytes. Another protein, *spectrin* (also called *fodrin*), which is known to produce actin gels *in vitro,* has been identified by immunofluorescence in lymphocytes (67). A different mechanical event documentable in leukocyte extracts was contraction of the actin gel in the presence of ATP. The contracted gels concentrated *myosin* molecules, and purified leukocyte myosin was capable of contracting actin gels *in vitro,* suggesting that myosin was responsible for the contractile activity (12,122).

Gelation and contractile phenomena can be complex and may be caused by a number of very different molecular interactions. Furthermore, there is no assurance that the events taking place in disrupted systems such as cytoplasmic extracts bear more than a chance relation to gelation and contraction in peripheral cytoplasm. Therefore it is reasonable to look to the structure of actin filaments in peripheral cytoplasm as a clue as to the molecular interactions that might underlie gelatin and contraction in the cell.

ARCHITECTURE OF ACTIN FILAMENTS IN PERIPHERAL CYTOPLASM: PSEUDOPODIAL ACTIN NETWORK

New ultrastructural techniques have permitted investigators to obtain a clearer picture of cortical cytoplasm than was possible with earlier thin-sectioning methods (Fig. 3). Using mechanical shear to remove the tops of leukocytes adherent to glass slides or ingesting zymosan particles, Boyles and Bainton (13,14) were able to obtain scanning electron micrographs of the attached surface of the plasma membrane. These images revealed a network

of filaments, many of which converged onto foci. More recent pictures utilizing this technique also have shown that clathrin-encased coated vesicles are abundant at these attachment sites as well and represent either pinocytic or exocytic vesicles (2,3,125). Pyrzwanski and co-workers (91) and Ryder et al. (95) utilized critical point drying to preserve the three-dimensionality of fixed and detergent-permeabilized leukocytes and examined the structure of cortical filaments. These studies documented that the peripheral filaments were actin by their ability to bind heavy meromyosin molecules; they also showed that some of the actin filaments tended to branch at right angles.

Hartwig and Shevlin (42) have examined the architecture of the cortical cytoplasm of macrophages fixed and detergent-extracted while spreading on a surface. These investigators employed both rapid freezing and critical point drying to prepare the specimens for electron microscopy in order to provide better reassurance that the three-dimensional structure observed was not affected by shrinkage artifacts. They confirmed with immunohistochemical techniques that most of the filaments in the cell cortex are actin. Using a computer-assisted morphometric technique to analyze stereo pair electron micrographs, they determined that the actin filament concentration in the macrophage periphery was about 15 mg/ml ($\sim$200 μM), that the average spacing between filament overlaps was about 120 nm with a narrow distribution, and that the branch angle at filament overlaps was strongly biased toward the perpendicular. Relatively few free filament ends could be seen in these images; most were observed either attaching to the adherent surface of the lamellipod or extending upward from the free surface.

The ultrastructural examinations of the peripheral cytoplasm of leukocytes provide plausible explanations for the apparent rigidity and the organelle exclusion of the

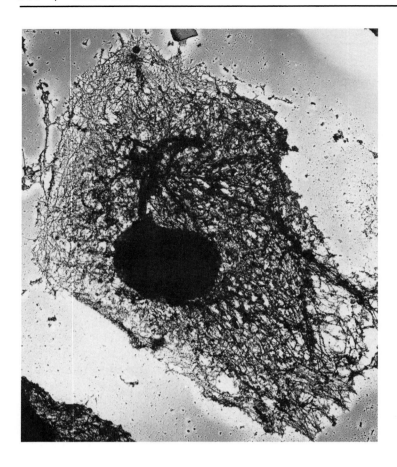

FIG. 3. Ultrastructural appearance of a macrophage lamellar cytoskeleton. A spread cell was permeabilized with the nonionic detergent Triton X-100, rapidly frozen, rotary-shadowed with platinum–carbon, and photographed in the electron microscope. ×3,500.

lamellipod. An orthogonal network of actin filaments with the dimensions observed could provide maximal extension of the lamellipod with an economy of mass, permitting solutes, water, and small vesicles to percolate through the network. On the other hand, the pore size of the network is sufficiently small to produce the organelle exclusion observed for so many years. Although the study of Hartwig and Shevlin (42) indicated that an orthogonal actin network comprises the bulk of the pseudopodial network, they also observed some filaments that align side by side and then diverge.

Molecular Basis of the Architecture of the Pseudopodial Actin Network

The ultrastructural images of cortical cytoplasm can be combined with studies of purified proteins *in vitro* to begin to formulate conclusions as to how these structures arise *in vivo.*

Purified monomeric (G) actin forms double helical filaments (F-actin), which morphologically appear as relatively straight rods that align at random with a bias toward parallel arrays (80). These pictures fit with the structural

models inferred from the most recent physical studies of actin. These studies have concluded that actin monomers (G-actin) and dilute actin filaments (F-actin) short enough not to overlap in solution exhibit ideal behavior; that is, they have a newtonian viscosity and diffusional properties expected for spheres (G-actin) or rods (F-actin) (53,79,149). Actin filaments sufficiently long or concentrated to overlap hinder one anothers' rotational movements exhibit nonnewtonian viscoelastic behavior known as "semidilute" in the parlance of contemporary polymer chemistry (30). Semidilute rods such as actin filaments, however, retain translational and limited rotational motions that permit them to line up and flow under stress (147,149). This view of pure F-actin as a system of constrained interpenetrating rods contrasts with earlier ones ascribing the rheological behavior of actin to the unspecified bonding of actin filaments to one another, although some persist in this interpretation (98).

It is obvious that the cross-linking of actin filaments, especially if it promotes high-angle branching, should markedly inhibit the mobility of actin filaments and lead to the formation of a gel or near-gel. Thus far the only agent shown *in vitro* to be capable of producing the perpendicular branching of actin documented in leukocyte cortical cytoplasm is actin-binding protein (45,80) (Fig. 4). The ability of this protein to affect the right-angle branching of actin is based on its large size and filamentous shape and explains its efficiency in causing a sol-to-gel transition of actin filaments of a given length. High-angle junctions minimize the opportunity for redundant cross-links to accumulate between adjacent filaments (15,45, 121). The actin gel composed of actin and actin-binding protein could be rigid at the concentrations of these re-agents estimated to exist in cortical cytoplasm, and ex-perimental results support this prediction (147).

The other principal actin cross-linking agent identified in leukocytes, α-actinin, binds to F-actin with an affinity of about 10^7 M^{-1} and joins the actin filaments side-to-side as bundles. α-Actinin is a short (100 nm) rod that, based on electron micrograph findings, binds end onto the sides of adjacent actin filaments to cross-link them. α-Actinin is inefficient in producing a sol-to-gel transformation of actin filaments *in vitro* compared with actin-binding pro-tein at 37°C, as would be expected for low-angle cross-linking (8). At lower temperatures this difference is less striking because the ability of α-actinin to cause actin to gel becomes much stronger as the temperature falls toward 0°C. With respect to this property, leukocyte α-actinin resembles skeletal muscle α-actinin (75). This finding may be a consequence of actin filaments becoming longer at the lower temperatures because the amount of a polymer cross-linking agent required for gelation of linear polymers is inversely proportional to the end-to-end distance of the polymer chains. There is as much α-actinin as actin-bind-ing protein in the leukocyte (about 1% of the total cell protein), and it is reasonable to conclude that α-actinin may stabilize points where actin filaments are observed to align in parallel in the cortical cytoplasm. An interesting feature of leukocyte and other nonmuscle cell α-actinins is that micromolar calcium concentrations decrease their ability to bind F-actin by about two orders of magnitude (8). Although the function of α-actinin may be to stabilize side-by-side alignments of actin filaments, this role must be considered much more tentative than the function proposed for actin-binding protein (ABP).

MECHANISM OF CONTRACTION OF THE PSEUDOPODIAL NETWORK

Leukocyte Myosins

The evidence that myosin powers the contraction of leukocyte peripheral cytoplasm are the observations that myosin collects in aggregates formed by the contraction of leukocyte extract gels *in vitro*, that addition of myosin

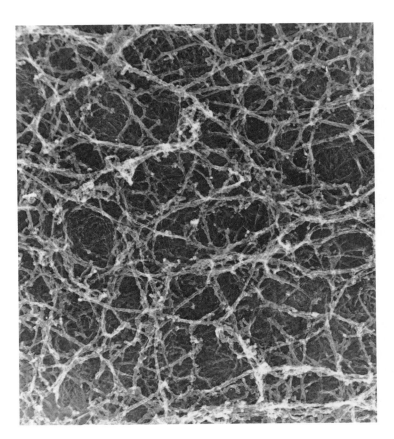

FIG. 4. Ultrastructural appearance of purified actin as-sembled with actin-binding protein and prepared for electron microscopy as in Fig. 3. ×44,800.

and suitable myosin-activating factors to actin gels leads to their contraction in the presence of ATP *in vitro,* and that anti-myosin antibodies inhibit the contraction of leukocyte cytoplasmic extracts (12,119,120,122).

Myosin has been purified from a variety of leukocyte types, including neutrophils, macrophages, and lymphocytes (33,43,101,110,123). The initial characterizations of leukocyte myosins showed that the myosin molecules resemble muscle and most other nonmuscle myosins in having two sets of heavy chains (M_r 200,000) and two sets of light chains ($M_r \sim$ 20,000 and 15,000). Under appropriate conditions these molecules form short (300 nm) bipolar filaments in which rod-like tails form the backbone of the filament and globular heads project from the shafts of the filament at each end. These heads interact with F-actin to form characteristic arrowhead configurations. Tight binding of the myosins to actin takes place in the absence but not the presence of millimolar ATP concentrations.

Regulation of Contractility

Purified leukocyte myosins, like muscle and other nonmuscle myosins, have low magnesium-dependent ATPase activity. Purified striated muscle myosin shows a marked increase in this activity in the presence of actin, and the actin-activated Mg^{2+}-ATPase activity of the myosin is an integral feature of the cyclic myosin head–actin monomer interaction that generates the contraction of muscle. The Mg^{2+}-ATPase activity of leukocyte myosins, unlike that of striated muscle myosin, is not increased directly by addition of F-actin. Because this ATPase activity is associated with contractile activity of actinomyosin, it is not surprising that mixtures of purified leukocyte myosin and actin do not contract readily. However, in the presence of crude fractions from leukocyte extracts, activation of the myosin Mg^{2+}-ATPase activity and contraction occurred (122). The work of Trotter and Adelstein (130) indicated that the actin-activated Mg^{2+}-ATPase activity of macrophage myosin correlated with the extent to which the 15-kD light chains of the myosin were phosphorylated. Phosphorylation of the myosin heavy chains has also been documented in leukocytes (132).

These results suggest that the mechanism of regulation of leukocyte myosin is similar to what is thought to obtain in platelets and smooth muscle where a calcium–*calmodulin* complex activates a *myosin light chain kinase,* which in turn phosphorylates the 15-kD myosin light chain. The purification of a myosin light-chain kinase from neutrophils has been reported (138) as well as of calmodulins from neutrophils and macrophages (69,145). Presumably a *phosphatase* in the cell reverses this activation (Fig. 5). In support of this idea, stimulation of neutrophils with chemotactic peptides and induction of capping in lymphocytes, stimuli that can increase intracellular calcium,

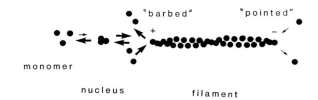

FIG. 5. Scheme for the assembly of purified actin. Actin monomers may form nuclei, although this reaction is thermodynamically unfavorable. Formed nuclei, however, elongate by monomer addition. Exchange of monomers with filaments is much more rapid at the (+; "barbed") than at the (−; "pointed") end of the filament. A critical monomer concentration is in equilibrium with filaments at steady state.

result in the phosphorylation of a 15-kD polypeptide in the cell (10) as well as a redistribution of myosin and of calmodulin and myosin light-chain kinase into the cap (10,97,102).

Scholey et al. (101) observed that the ability of thymocyte myosin to form bipolar filaments was influenced positively by the extent of phosphorylation of the molecule. Therefore the available information concerning regulation of the oligomeric state of myosin and its interactive properties with actin suggests that the cytosolic calcium concentration can control filament formation and the interaction of myosin with actin. However, there is another dimension of "regulation" in leukocytes. In muscle the contractile apparatus is fixed so that the regulatory problem can be a relatively straightforward "switch on/switch off" mechanism. In leukocytes and many nonmuscle cells, the pseudopodial network on which myosin acts to produce a contraction may be built and destroyed at different times and in different places. A "contraction" in the sense of something being pulled or aggregated depends on that something having sufficient structure for the contraction to propagate across the entire scaffolding.

ASSEMBLY OF THE PSEUDOPODIAL ACTIN NETWORK

Assembly of Actin

To discuss the assembly of actin it is first necessary to summarize briefly some information concerning its polymerization. Actin is a highly conserved molecule. Although vertebrates possess several genes encoding actin, the proteins produced differ only slightly in primary structure and functional properties, at least as currently understood (135). Leukocytes contain two of these gene products, typical for nonmuscle cells, which are designated beta and gamma based on their isoelectric points and are present in cytoplasm respectively in molar ratios of about 5:1.

Pure monomeric actin is a slightly asymmetrical globular protein of M_r 42,500, which in the presence of neutral salts spontaneously assembles to form the double helical actin filament (Fig. 5). A rate-limiting step in this assembly is the formation of a nucleus composed of two or three monomers. Therefore the presence of preexisting actin nuclei, filaments, or other agents that substitute as nuclei can have an important effect on the kinetics of actin assembly. At the completion of polymerization from monomers, the monomers continue to exchange with the ends of filaments that have a large and exponential length distribution, varying from a few that are more than 10 μm in length to many that are a few monomers in composition.

The concentration of actin monomers is one important determinant of the assembly process. As in any bimolecular reaction, the rate of assembly is influenced by the concentration of the reactants and by the association and dissociation rate constants. In the case of actin, these constants are different for the opposite ends of actin nuclei or filaments. This difference in rate constants is one of several examples of the polarity of the actin filament, which was first recognized by the fact that proteolytically derived actin-binding fragments of myosin such as heavy meromyosin bind to actin filaments at an angle that produces arrowheads that are visible in the electron microscope. In the case of actin assembly, it is the barbed filament end with respect to the heavy meromyosin arrowheads that has association and dissociation rate constants that are about 30 times faster than at the pointed ends. Therefore under steady-state conditions actin monomers exchange with the opposite ends of filaments at different rates. In addition, the concentration of G-actin in dynamic equilibrium with actin filaments is different at the opposite filament ends. This concentration, known as the critical monomer concentration, is also about 15 times lower for the barbed as contrasted with the pointed filament end. Because exchange is so much faster at the barbed than at the pointed end, the critical concentration of pure actin is essentially that of the barbed end. Under ionic conditions believed to be reasonably physiological, this concentration is about 0.1 μM. In this circumstance the rate of addition of actin monomers to the barbed filament end is ~20 monomers/μM actin monomer concentration per second, and the off-rate is ~2/sec.

The absolute values for these rate constants and critical concentrations vary depending on the temperature, the salt conditions, and on other ambient metabolites. For example, monomeric actin binds one ATP molecule (G-ATP actin), which becomes hydrolyzed to ADP during assembly (F-ADP actin). When a monomer dissociates from F-actin, it exchanges its ADP for ATP, provided ATP is present in the medium. Depending on the rates of assembly and depolymerization, ATP hydrolysis and ATP–ADP exchange may or not be kinetically coupled to the assembly. Therefore G-ATP actin may coexist with F-ATP actin or with F-ADP actin, depending on the conditions. The affinity of G-ATP actin for F-ATP actin is lower than that of G-ATP actin for F-ADP actin and much lower than that of G-ADP actin for F-ADP actin. It is therefore apparent that adenine nucleotides can play an important role in regulating the polarity of assembly of actin. Readers interested in more information about this fascinating and complex problem should consult the reviews by Frieden (36) and Pollard and Cooper (152). Because ATP levels tend to remain fairly constant (in the millimolar range) in living cells, a regulatory role of adenine nucleotides seems unlikely, but ATP depletion could possibly affect the function of actin in cells with impaired energy metabolism.

Assembly of Actin in Leukocytes

In the resting leukocyte, about half of the total actin is in the form of filaments that remain in a cellular "cytoskeleton" of leukocytes subjected to detergent solubilization of their membranes. The rest is in a form that is extracted along with other "soluble" proteins by detergent treatment. When leukocytes are stimulated by addition of the chemotaxis-inducing oligopeptide fMet-Leu-Phe, by tumor-promoting phorbol esters, by a calcium ionophore in the presence of extracellular calcium, and by a number of other agonists, the fraction of detergent-insoluble actin transiently rises (34,48–50,54,113,136,139).

Because the total actin concentration in the peripheral cytoplasm is on the order of 400 μm, all but a tiny fraction (0.1 μM) ought to be polymerized based on the critical concentration of pure actin under ionic, thermal, and metabolic conditions thought to exist in the cytoplasm of a resting leukocyte. Furthermore, the length distribution of actin filaments in the cytoplasm is not the broad exponential characteristic of actin filaments assembled from pure monomers. Therefore the assembly of actin in the leukocyte must be regulated to keep so much of the actin unpolymerized in resting cells and to allow for rapid polymerization and depolymerization of actin in response to stimulation. There are two theoretical approaches to this regulation. In one, a molecule sequesters actin monomers with sufficient affinity to prevent their nucleation or exchange onto filaments. In a second, molecules bind the ends of filaments to prevent monomer addition or loss. Both mechanisms seem to be active in leukocytes (Fig. 6).

Regulatory Actin-Binding Proteins of Leukocytes

Monomer Sequestration

A basic protein (M_r 20,000) originally isolated from spleen by Lindberg and colleagues in Sweden and named profilin sequesters actin monomers (18). Profilins have subsequently been purified from many cell types including

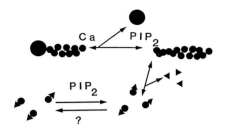

FIG. 6. Scheme for the coordinate regulation of actin (•) assembly in leukocytes by profilin (▲), gelsolin (●), calcium, and PIP₂. When profilin is in a high-affinity complex with actin and gelsolin blocks the (+) ends of actin filaments, there is minimal exchange of actin monomers with filaments. PIP₂ promotes actin assembly by reducing the affinity of profilin for actin monomers and removing the gelsolin block at the (+) filament ends, which compete successfully with low-affinity profilin for actin monomers. Calcium promotes the blocking of (+) filament ends by gelsolin; the signal for restoration of high-affinity profilin binding to actin is unknown. Conversion of profilin from low- to high-affinity binding to actin when gelsolin is not on the (+) filament ends would promote rapid depolymerization.

leukocytes (29). Profilin has been isolated in either of two states: a high-affinity state that complexes actin monomers so tightly that only denaturing conditions can separate this association *in vitro*. On the other hand, free profilin can be isolated from cells, but this form has a relatively low affinity ($\sim 10^7 M^{-1}$) for actin and therefore competes poorly with actin filament ends, especially the fast-exchanging ends, for monomers. If profilin has any regulatory role in leukocytes, there must be some control that governs a shift of profilin between its high- and low-affinity states for binding to actin (Fig. 5). Preliminary evidence suggests that lipids of the inositol cycle, especially phosphatidylinositol-4,5-biphosphate (PIP₂), may play a role in this regulation by lowering the affinity of profilin for actin (66) (Fig. 6). Interconversion between high and low affinity states of profilin has recently been documented in platelet extracts (153).

The ability of profilin to keep actin unpolymerized has several important implications, especially if its actin-sequestering function can be regulated. First, the profilin–actin complex can diffuse throughout the peripheral cytoplasm to serve as a source of monomers for assembly on demand. Second, profilin can keep unpolymerized actin so far above the critical concentration that upon dissociation of the profilin–actin complex assembly could be rapid. However, this characteristic has the possible disadvantage that nucleation of actin would occur randomly in space. One way to gain spatial control is to couple changes in the affinity of profilin for actin with regulation at the rapidly growing, barbed end of actin filaments.

Actin Filament End-Blockade

The first cytoplasmic molecule recognized to confer this kind of regulation and the prototype of the most powerful type of actin filament length-controlling factor recognized is a protein (M_r 84,000) purified from leukocytes and named *gelsolin*. This protein binds the fast growing ends of actin filaments and prevents exchange of monomers with that end. In addition to blocking the ends of actin filaments, gelsolin severs actin–actin bonds in filaments, thereby rupturing the filaments. It is obvious how such an action could dissolve an actin network gel such as was described above, explaining why the protein is named gelsolin (52,140,141,144) (Fig. 6). Because gelsolin binds to the barbed end of actin filaments, only the pointed filament ends exchange monomers. Therefore the critical concentration of gelsolin-blocked actin filaments rises to that of the pointed end, and it follows that gelsolin produces partial depolymerization as well as fragmentation of F-actin. The cytochalasins resemble gelsolin in that these molecules inhibit the exchange of actin monomers with the fast-growing ends of actin filaments and thereby shorten the average actin filament length.

The severing and blocking action of gelsolin is activated by micromolar calcium concentrations. In the presence of calcium, gelsolin first binds one actin molecule. This binding, which has an affinity constant of more than 10^8 M^{-1}, exposes a cryptic actin binding site that binds a second actin with even higher affinity ($>10^{10} M^{-1}$) (53). This binding of a second actin is required for gelsolin to sever an actin filament. The molecular structure of gelsolin has been analyzed by proteolytic mapping and partial amino acid sequencing, and its primary structure has been deduced by the sequencing of a full-length cDNA clone. Such analyses have shown that the severing site is at the amino-terminus of the molecule, whereas the calcium-sensitive binding site resides in the carboxy-terminal half of gelsolin (16,21,63–65,143).

Once gelsolin has interacted with actin in the presence of calcium, only the first actin bound can be removed by chelation of calcium with EGTA, whereas the actin bound to the severing site is EGTA-resistant (52). The EGTA-resistant gelsolin–actin complex can block the fast ends of actin filaments, but it neither severs actin filaments nor nucleates actin monomer assembly. In the presence of calcium, nucleating activity but not severing activity is regained. The EGTA-resistant actin monomer can, however, be dissociated from gelsolin by PIP₂, the phospholipid previously shown to dissociate profilin–actin complexes. PIP₂ also inhibits the severing of actin filaments by gelsolin, even in the presence of micromolar calcium (53a). The observation that gelsolin binds to PIP₂ suggests that gelsolin, like protein kinase C, may operate in both cytosolic and membrane domains of the cell. Hence gelsolin is under dual regulation: Calcium promotes its binding to actin, its severing of actin filaments, and its blocking of monomer addition at the fast-growing filament end—all effects leading to actin depolymerization and to the solation of a cross-linked actin gel. Therefore it follows that the reversal of gelsolin's tight binding to actin must be essential for assembly of the pseudopodial network. PIP_2 could be responsible for this reversal, with the implication that gelsolin, in being regulated by the two known intracellular messengers—calcium and an intermediate of the phosphoinositide cycle—is positioned centrally in the transduction of surface stimulation into mechanical events in the cell. This reversal process may be sufficiently effective to keep gelsolin from forming tight complexes with actin even in the presence of micromolar calcium concentrations. The balance of these mechanisms presumably regulates actin assembly in the cell (Figs. 6 and 7).

Immunoprecipitation experiments utilizing high-affinity monoclonal anti-gelsolin antibodies conjugated to Sepharose beads to quantitatively recover gelsolin from cell extracts have shown that the EGTA-resistant complex can form in the cell and that the cell can reverse this complex, presumably by its interaction with PIP_2. The cells are extracted in EGTA (low calcium) to prevent further complex formation between gelsolin and actin. The anti-gelsolin beads are incubated with the extract, and gelsolin, with or without actin bound to it, binds to the antibody. The beads are centrifuged and washed with EGTA-containing solutions and the proteins associated with the beads analyzed electrophoretically (23). Freshly harvested leukocytes have most of their gelsolin in a free state, uncomplexed to actin. However, when the cells are suspended at 37°C, the fraction of gelsolin in an EGTA irreversible 1:1 complex with actin increases. As expected, addition of a calcium ionophore plus calcium to the cells rapidly increases the amount of this complex. In contrast,

a chemotactic peptide, fMet-Leu-Phe, decreases the amount of complex (23), even though this peptide is known to increase the resting intracellular calcium concentration from nanomolar to submicromolar levels (46,90). Plating the cells onto plastic, which causes spreading of the cell and concomitant formation of the pseudopodial actin network in the spread lamellae, rapidly dissociates all actin–gelsolin complexes present, despite the observation that induction of spreading causes a transient rise in the cytosolic calcium concentration of macrophages (61). Furthermore, the addition of a calcium ionophore plus calcium does not produce complexes in the plated cells, even though it increases the cytosolic calcium levels.

The discovery that PIP_2 can promote actin assembly by "unblocking" the fast ends of actin filaments and by dissociating actin–profilin complexes is consistent with much data documenting that surface stimuli that promote cellular actin stimuli either increase PIP_2 (phorbol esters) or cause it to be resynthesized after it is initially hydrolyzed (chemotactic peptides). It seems reasonable to speculate that the mechanism(s) reversing the tight binding of gelsolin to actin and of profilin to actin are coupled. If profilin and gelsolin simultaneously have a lowering of their respective binding affinities for actin, the actin monomers liberated from profilin can add rapidly onto the ends of actin filaments unblocked by the release of gelsolin.

Other Actin-Modulating Proteins of Leukocytes

At least two other proteins have been isolated from leukocytes that affect actin assembly. One is *acumentin,* an M_r 65,000 protein, which in the purified state binds the actin filaments with relatively low affinity (115–117). An M_r 42,000 calcium-binding protein binds to the barbed end of actin filaments in the presence but not the absence of calcium. This protein binds to actin with much lower affinity than gelsolin and, unlike gelsolin, does not sever actin filaments. It is difficult to imagine a role for these proteins at the present time.

ACTIN ASSEMBLY; EXTENSION OF AND CONTRACTION WITHIN PSEUDOPODIA ASSOCIATED WITH CELL SPREADING, LOCOMOTION, AND PHAGOCYTOSIS

Although it is intuitively simple to understand that assembly from subunits might be necessary to produce the pseudopodial actin network, it is not so easy to picture how this assembly could induce protrusion of a pseudopod. The major problem is that whenever microscopists have visualized how the ends of actin filaments interact with the cytoplasmic face of the plasma membrane, it is invariably the barbed end that hitherto has been captured

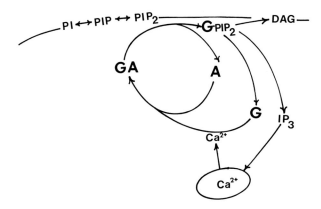

FIG. 7. Scheme for the regulation of gelsolin (G) function during leukocyte activation. Stimulation by agonists coupled to PIP_2 hydrolysis results in accumulation of inositol triphosphate (IP_3) and diacylglycerol (DAG). The former releases calcium from internal stores. Gelsolin in the presence of calcium forms a tight complex with actin (A), possibly resulting in actin filament severing, (+) end blockade, and nucleation. PIP_2 resynthesis and reuptake and the extrusion of calcium reverse the interaction of gelsolin with actin.

abutting that membrane in electron micrographs (4,91). Because it is believed that rapid assembly takes place at the barbed filament end, a problem arises as to how actin monomers are to attach to that end if it is pushed up against a planar surface.

An attractive theoretical solution to this dilemma has been offered by Oster (85). He proposed that the driving force for protrusion is osmotic rather than mechanical. According to his view, osmotic swelling of an actin gel takes place when it is dissolved by an actin-severing protein such as gelsolin. Polymer gels have a swelling pressure that is balanced by mechanical restraints imposed by the cross-links between filaments in the gel, and the release of these restraints allows the gel to swell further. Osmotic swelling would cause the plasma membrane to bleb away from the underlying actin matrix and permit monomers to add on to barbed ends of actin filaments.

A modified version of this basic idea that incorporates the biochemical information available concerning leukocyte actin assembly can be offered in speculation as to how actin assembly might be associated with propulsive pseudopodial movement (Fig. 8). In response to the rise in intracellular free calcium from nanomolar to submicromolar concentrations following binding of chemotactic peptides to their receptors (46,90), the action of gelsolin in fragmenting and depolymerizing actin would be expected to effect a rise in the osmotic pressure, causing the membrane to lift away from the underlying network. For these events to take place, in the resting cell the barbed ends of actin filaments would need to be blocked with gelsolin to prevent spontaneous elongation or shortening,

and spontaneous nucleation and polymerization of monomeric actin would also have to be inhibited, presumably by its being bound tightly to the high-affinity actin-binding form of profilin. An initial solation of the pseudopodial actin network by an increase in calcium and severing of F-actin by gelsolin might also be predicted to facilitate the ability of vesicles containing chemotactic factor receptors to diffuse toward and ultimately fuse with the plasma membrane, thereby allowing the expression or "up-regulation" of receptors, which has been documented to occur when chemotactic peptides bind to their receptors on leukocytes (35).

After the initial rise in calcium and solation of the pseudopodial network, activation of the mechanism for reversing gelsolin's binding to filament ends, possibly the interaction between gelsolin and PIP_2, would expose many barbed actin filament ends, and conversion of profilin to a low-affinity state would facilitate rapid actin polymerization onto those ends. As actin polymerizes, the reduction in the number of osmotically active particles might actually induce a compressive effect. In effect, the actin would initially perform propulsive work osmotically and then stabilize its accomplishment mechanically. Although there is little experimental evidence to support this hypothesis, it has been shown that addition of chemotactic peptides to leukocytes in suspension produced a generalized swelling, at least as defined by changes in cell volume measured with an electronic cell counter (82).

This hypothetical mechanism solves a conceptual problem posed by the evidence that a rise in cytosolic calcium activates the contraction of the actin network by

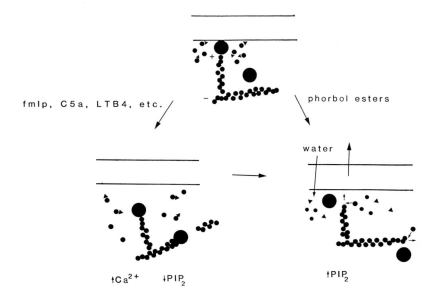

FIG. 8. Possible mechanisms of membrane propulsion coupled to actin (●) assembly following stimulation of leukocytes. In the resting cell, (+) filament ends are blocked by gelsolin (●); therefore profilin (▲) can be in its low-affinity binding state for actin monomers and still prevent spontaneous nucleation. In response to stimulation with phorbol ester, PIP_2 hypothetically increases and interacts with gelsolin, reversing the blockade of actin filaments. Profilin is in the low-affinity state and gives monomers up to the filament ends. The transient dissociation reactions increase osmotic pressure, cause swelling, and propel the membrane, behind which advances the polymerizing actin. Following stimulation with agonists such as chemotactic peptides a rise in cytosolic calcium promotes the severing of actin filaments by free gelsolin molecules which then block monomer exchange with the (+) ends of the severed actin filaments. An initial PIP_2 hydrolysis is followed by resynthesis, which reverses the gelsolin blockade of the (+) filament ends and dissociates high-affinity actin–profilin complexes. Actin filament assembly is more rapid than in the case of phorbol stimulation because of the greater quantity of filament ends created by gelsolin's severing action.

myosin. The problem is that if calcium were causing gelsolin to shred the pseudopodial network at the same time that it was activating myosin for contraction, no useful contractile work could be done (119,120), although Taylor and colleagues (127) have argued that a loosening of an actin network is required for contraction in amebas. On the other hand, if restoration of the PIP₂ level following its initial hydrolysis after cell activation by chemotactic peptides prevents gelsolin from severing actin filaments, the assembling pseudopodial network is protected even in the presence of calcium, and the myosin in that network can get a grip on an intact meshwork to produce contraction. If the advancing pseudopod is adherent to the substrate, this contraction pulls the cell body forward, or if the pseudopod is free it retracts that pseudopod back to the cell body.

The exact manner in which the propulsive and contractile activity would propagate itself is difficult to imagine without more information as to how the calcium-dependent regulation of gelsolin balances with the PIP₂-dependent reversal mechanism at the biochemical level and as to how the high-affinity binding of profilin to actin is restored. Once cytosolic calcium increases, the calcium is rapidly pumped back out into the extracellular medium or is sequestered by intracellular vesicles (69,70,81,94). For this reason there may be calcium transients, gradients, or waves moving through the pseudopod that might regulate the propulsive activity of the pseudopod. However, there is evidence that an increase in the average cytosolic calcium concentration may not be necessary or sufficient for leukocyte actin assembly (106,139). Furthermore, particles opsonized with iC3b (70), and in some experiments with IgG (77), reportedly elicit pseudopod extension (phagocytosis), and certain phorbol esters cause exocytosis of granules (146) without a detectable rise in the average cytosolic calcium to levels associated with activation of calcium-regulated biochemical effects. In addition, evidence is accumulating that certain agonists can induce actin polymerization in leukocytes irrespective of whether the cytosolic calcium concentration rises (106,139). In such cases it is conceivable that the PIP₂-mediated release of actin from profilin and from gelsolin alone is responsible. Because the dissociation of the profilin–actin complex doubles the number of osmotically active particles, this action might provide the osmotic force for pseudopod propulsion. It seems that this mechanism would be less efficient and slower than the one involving an initial severing of actin filaments by calcium activation of gelsolin.

Whatever the regulation, the advancement of the network at the leading edge requires an adequate supply of component subunits. If the mechanisms for dissociation of gelsolin–actin and profilin–actin complexes are at the leading edge of the cell, the concentrations of free profilin and free gelsolin would become higher at this front than elsewhere. This concentration differential would create a bidirectional gradient in which free profilin and gelsolin diffuse toward the rear of the pseudopodial network and profilin–actin diffuses forward. These gradients would provide a continuous source of monomers for actin assembly at the front of the network as well as a supply of free profilin to complex actin depolymerizing from the rear of the network.

INTERACTION BETWEEN PSEUDOPODIAL ACTIN NETWORK AND PLASMA MEMBRANE

If one accepts that the pseudopod advances under an osmotic drive that produces a submembrane cushion of fluid behind which grows the pseudopodial network, how can the network establish a foothold by which either to drag the cell body toward the advancing pseudopod or retract a pseudopod toward the cell body? It seems that there is no alternative but that some part of the network be attached to the cell membrane, which in turn must attach to the substrate on which the cell moves when the cell is advancing; failing such an attachment to the substrate, the pseudopod will retract.

One logical place for actin filament membrane attachment is the surface of the pseudopod that lies on the substrate. Another is where the actin filament assembly catches up to the leading edge when the stimulus for advancement ceases. Once the barbed ends of actin filaments reach the membrane, they are in a position to bind molecules diffusing in the plane of the membrane. These molecules would provide maximal stability to the actin–membrane attachment if they are transmembrane proteins. In contrast to the extensive fund of knowledge concerning the association between the red cell cytoskeleton and the plasma membrane, there is relatively little information on the molecular basis of leukocyte actin–membrane interaction. Associations of leukocyte actin with various membrane receptors, including cell surface immunoglobulin, histocompatibility antigens, and the vitamin D-binding protein have been described, but the specificity or importance of these associations are unknown (38,60,88,89). The electron microscopy studies of the cell edge of phagocytes described above have not revealed any structure resembling the two-dimensional spectrin–actin shell that laminates the cytoplasmic surface of the red cell membrane, although fodrin, a spectrin-like protein, has been localized to the periphery of lymphocytes by immunofluorescence (67). The ultrastructure of the cytoplasmic aspect of the lymphocyte periphery has not yet been carefully analyzed.

Because either or both actin–membrane and membrane–substrate attachments must be transient for translocation to occur, and because pseudopodia can alternate between states of advancement and retraction, these attachments must be reversible. The attachment at the interface between the plasma membrane and the substrate could be broken by a hydrolytic event or endocytosis. Except for the possible scission of actin filaments near the membrane by gelsolin, we have no information as to possible molecular mechanisms for how such associations might be reversed on the cytoplasmic side.

Another unresolved question concerns the response of the membrane bilayer to changes in cell shape. A resting cell is relatively spherical, although adorned with surface ruffles and pleats. Whether these protuberances provide sufficient redundancy to account for passive accommodation to localized extensions of pseudopodia in activated cells is unclear. Because membrane turnover can be extensive in leukocytes (118) a more complex mechanism wherein membrane insertion and retrieval takes place as pseudopodia are extended and retracted, respectively, is also possible.

PSEUDOPODIAL ACTIN NETWORK AND SECRETION

For exocytosis to take place at the base of a forming phagocytic vacuole, attenuation of the pseudopodial actin network is evidently required to permit granule movements and granule fusion with the plasmalemma. From the biochemical data presented, one mechanism to account for these findings would be for the calcium concentration to be sufficiently high at that region to keep gelsolin active and the network dissolved. One study attempting to establish the localized free calcium concentration in locomoting and phagocytosing neutrophils reported that the highest calcium concentrations existed at the pit of newly forming phagocytic vacuoles (99). The cycle of network components proposed to be associated with advancement of pseudopodia could also account for the network attenuation at the base of a phagocytic vacuole. The network decomposes at the base of the advancing pseudopod, whether during phagocytosis or locomotion, and this decomposition facilitates the fusion of granules with the plasma membrane at that location.

The phenomenon of leukocytes' exocytosis of granule-associated enzymes when stimulated by various agonists in suspension is more difficult to explain because there is insufficient anatomical information to define the secretory pathway. Some have proposed, however, that cell-to-cell aggregation is a prerequisite for such secretion (25), which means that the mechanism would be similar to that in spreading, locomoting, or phagocytosing cells.

One repeated observation has been that cytochalasins enhance exocytosis by agonist-stimulated phagocytes, provided the cytochalasin is present before stimulation.

Cytochalasins alone do not directly elicit secretion nor enhance it if added after a secretory stimulus (45a). This phenomenon has been taken as evidence that cortical actin filaments keep cytoplasmic granules away from the plasma membrane, as cytochalasins can disrupt actin networks by blocking actin filaments at their fast-growing ends (44). These findings are consistent with the model for agonist-activated actin assembly described here, because actin assembly following unblocking of fast-growing ends by signals resulting from stimulation would be blocked by cytochalasins, and the peripheral actin gel would not assemble and granule access to the plasmalemma would not be impaired. Once actin assembly was well established, however, its blockade by cytochalasins would not be expected to impair network formation, and despite the activation of processes that permit granule fusion with the plasma membrane, granules would be separated from that site by the growing actin network.

PSEUDOPODIAL ACTIN NETWORK AND AGONAL EVENTS

The increase in peripheral granule movements and the generalized blebbing of the cell that occurs in leukocytes after prolonged incubation, exposure to sonication, or various toxic substances (9,26,104) could result from a pathological disruption of the peripheral actin network. Because the plasma membrane is mechanically weak, even partial destruction of the underlying actin matrix might predispose the membrane to rupture, and it is common for membrane blebs to break away from the cell. Sonic waves close to the dimensions of the network can be predicted to disrupt it mechanically. Metabolic toxicity to the cell might cause the intracellular calcium concentration to increase, thereby activating gelsolin and resulting in widespread severing of the actin network. This simple idea is complicated by the discovery that the cell can reverse gelsolin's binding to actin (22). A study of oxidant injury to macrophages showed an increase in the amount of polymerized actin.

The metabolic functions of the cell may be optimal when energy-producing enzyme cascades are organized in association with the cortical actin network. For example, there is evidence that the activity of glycolytic enzymes is influenced by association with actin filaments (28,62). Therefore better understanding of the changes in actin and actin-associated proteins accompanying cell injury and metabolic deprivation may be useful in devising strategies for protecting cells against irreversible damage.

CONCLUDING COMMENTS

The complexity of the mechanical responses of leukocytes is of an order associated with those of whole organisms. Particularly in the case of directional locomotion, an orchestration of several systems must be understood. First, extracellular gradients of chemotactically active agonists guide the direction of cell polarization, which establishes directionality of movement. Second is the expression, binding activity, mobility, and disposition of chemotactic factor receptors, with and without bound ligands, and their possible cycling from the front to the rear and back to the leading edge of the cell. Third, the binding of the agonists to the receptors generates messages that activate the cytoplasm for protrusive and retractive movements. One strongly implicated message is calcium; and phosphoinositides such as PIP_2, shown to interact with actin-binding proteins, may be equally or even more important. A major aspect of the cytoplasmic response that has been emphasized in this chapter is the assembly and contraction of the pseudopodial actin network. Its contribution to directional movement may be both osmotic and mechanical. In addition, the polarity it establishes in the cell, in terms of cell shape and whatever effects it has on the traffic of receptors and of intracellular gradients of network components, may also be important for maintaining a degree of persistence in motility that has been documented in behavioral studies of leukocytes subjected to changes in the direction of chemotactic factor gradients (58,150,151).

The ongoing discovery of molecules involved in the mechanical responses of leukocytes has facilitated presentation of the increasingly explicit hypotheses in an attempt to provide general explanations for these responses. Although the theories are contaminated with large lacunae of speculation, the rate of accumulation of useful facts that have made these notions possible is encouraging and implies that more plausible and testable ideas will be forthcoming.

ACKNOWLEDGMENTS

This work was supported by USPHS grant HL19429 and grants from the Council for Tobacco Research, the Edwin S. Webster Foundation, The Richard Saltonstall Trust, and Edwin W. Hiam.

REFERENCES

1. Adelstein, R. S. (1983): Regulation of contractile proteins by phosphorylation. *J. Clin. Invest.,* 72:1863–1865.
2. Aggeler, J., and Werb, Z. (1982): Initial events during phagocytosis by macrophages viewed from outside and inside the cell membrane-particle interactions and clathrin. *J. Cell Biol.,* 94:613–623.
3. Aggeler, J. R., Takemura, R., and Werb, Z. (1983): High-resolution three dimensional views of membrane-associated clathrin and cytoskeleton in critical-point-dried macrophages. *J. Cell Biol.,* 97:1542–1548.
4. Allison, A. C., Davies, P., and DePetris, S. (1971): Subplasmalemmal microfilaments in macrophage movement and endocytosis. *Nature,* 232:153–155.
5. Anderson, D. C., Wible, L. J., Hughes, B. J., Smith, C. W., and Brinkley, B. R. (1982): Cytoplasmic microtubules in polymorphonuclear leukocytes: effects of chemotactic stimulation and colchicine. *Cell,* 31:719–729.
6. Axline, S. G., and Reaven, E. P. (1974): Inhibition of phagocytosis and plasma membrane mobility of the cultivated macrophage by cytochalasin B. Role of subplasmalemmal microfilaments. *J. Cell Biol.,* 62:647–659.
7. Becker, E. L., Showell, H. J., Henson, P. M., and Hsu, L. S. (1974): The ability of chemotactic factors to induce lysosomal enzyme release. I. The characteristics of the release, the importance of surfaces and the relation of enzyme release to chemotactic responsiveness. *J. Immunol.,* 112:2047–2054.
8. Bennett, J. P., Zaner, K. S., and Stossel, T. P. (1984): Isolation and some properties of macrophage α-actinin: evidence that it is not an actin gelling protein. *Biochemistry,* 23:5081–5086.
9. Bessis, M. (1971): *Living Blood Cells and Their Ultrastructure.* Heidelberg, Springer-Verlag.
10. Bourguignon, L. Y. W., Nagpal, M. L., and Shing, Y-C. (1981): Phosphorylation of myosin light chain during capping of mouse T-lymphoma cells. *J. Cell Biol.,* 91:889–894.
11. Bourguignon, L. Y. W., Walker, G., Suchard, S. J., and Balazovich, K. (1986): A lymphoma plasma membrane-associated protein with ankyrin-like properties. *J. Cell Biol.,* 102:2115–2124.
12. Boxer, L. A., and Stossel, T. P. (1976): Isolation and properties of actin, myosin, and a new actin-binding protein of chronic myelogenous leukemia leukocytes. *J. Clin. Invest.,* 57:5696–5705.
13. Boyles, J., and Bainton, D. F. (1979): Changing patterns of plasma membrane-associated filaments during the initial phases of polymorphonuclear leukocyte adherence. *J. Cell Biol.,* 82:347–368.
14. Boyles, J., and Bainton, D. F. (1981): Changes in plasma-membrane-associated filaments during endocytosis and exocytosis in polymorphonuclear leukocytes. *Cell,* 24:905–914.
15. Brotschi, E. A., Hartwig, J. H., and Stossel, T. P. (1978): The gelation of actin by actin-binding protein. *J. Cell Biol.,* 253:8988–8993.
16. Bryan, J., and Hwo, S. (1986): Definition of an N-terminal actin-binding domain and a C-terminal Ca^{2+} regulatory domain in human brevin. *J. Cell Biol.,* 102:1439–1446.
17. Bryan, J., and Kurth, M. (1984): Actin-gelsolin interactions: evidence for two actin-binding sites. *J. Cell Biol.,* 259:7480–7487.
18. Carlsson, L., Nystrom, L. E., Sundkvist, I., Markey, F., and Lindberg, U. (1976): Profilin, a low molecular weight protein controlling actin polymerisability. In: *Contractile Systems in Non-muscle Tissues,* edited by S. V. Perry, A. Margreth, and R. S. Adelstein, pp. 39–48. Elsevier/North Holland, Amsterdam.
19. Carson, M., Weber, A., and Zigmond, S. H. (1986): An actin-nucleating activity in polymorphonuclear leukocytes is modulated by chemotactic peptides. *J. Cell Biol.,* 103:2707–2714.
20. Cassimeris, L. U., Wadsworth, P., and Salmon, E. D. (1986): Dynamics of microtubule depolymerization in monocytes. *J. Cell Biol.,* 102:2023–2032.
21. Chaponnier, C., Janmey, P. A., and Yin, H. L. (1986): The actin filament-severing domain of plasma gelsolin. *J. Cell Biol.,* 103:1473–1481.
22. Chaponnier, C., Janmey, P. A., Yin, H. L., and Stossel, T. P. (1985): Reversal of gelsolin:actin complexes by macrophages in vivo. *J. Cell Biol.,* 102:650a.
23. Chaponnier, C., Yin, H. L., and Stossel, T. P. (1987): Reversibility of gelsolin/actin interaction in macrophages: evidence of Ca^{2+}-dependent and Ca^{2+}-independent pathways. *J. Exp. Med.,* 165:97–106.
24. Chien, S., Schmid-Schonbein, G. W., Sung, K-L. P., Schmalzer, E. A., and Skalak, R. (1984): Viscoelastic properties of leukocytes. In: *White Cell Mechanics: Basic Science and Clinical Aspects,* edited by P. LaCelle and M. A. Lichtman, pp. 19–51. Alan R. Liss, New York.
25. Dahinden, C. A., Fehr, J., and Hugli, T. E. (1983): Role of cell surface contact in the kinetics of superoxide production by granulocytes. *J. Clin. Invest.,* 72:113–121.
26. Davies, W. A., and Stossel, T. P. (1977): Peripheral hyaline blebs (podosomes) of macrophages. *J. Cell Biol.,* 75:941–955.
27. DeBruyn, P. P. H. (1946): The amoeboid movement of the mammalian leucocyte in tissue culture. *Anat. Rec.,* 95:117–191.

28. Dedman, J. R., Payne, D. M., and Harris, B. G. (1975): Increased proteolytic susceptibility of aldolase induced by actin binding. *Biochem. Biophys. Res. Commun.*, 65:1170–1176.

29. DiNubile, M. J., and Southwick, F. S. (1985): Effects of macrophage profilin on actin in the presence and absence of acumentin and gelsolin. *J. Biol. Chem.*, 260:7402–7409.

30. Doi, M., and Edwards, S. F. (1986): *The Theory of Polymer Dynamics.* Clarendon Press, Oxford.

31. Dyett, D. E., Malawista, S. E., Naccache, P. H., and Sha'afi, R. I. (1986): Stimulated cytokineplasts from human polymorphonuclear leukocytes mobilize calcium and polymerize actin: cytoplasts made in cytochalasin B retain a defect in actin polymerization. *J. Clin. Invest.*, 77:34–37.

32. Euteneuer, U., and Schliwa, M. (1985): Evidence for an involvement of actin in the positioning and motility of centrosomes. *J. Cell Biol.*, 101:96–103.

33. Fechheimer, M., and Cebra, J. J. (1982): Phosphorylation of lymphocyte myosin catalyzed in vitro and in intact cells. *J. Cell Biol.*, 93:261–268.

34. Fechheimer, M., and Zigmond, S. H. (1983): Changes in cytoskeletal proteins of polymorphonuclear leukocytes induced by chemotactic peptides. *Cell Motil.*, 3:349–361.

35. Fletcher, M. P., and Gallin, J. I. (1980): Degranulating stimuli increase the availability of receptors on human neutrophils for the chemoattractant f-Met-Leu-Phe. *J. Immunol.*, 124:1585–1588.

36. Frieden, C. (1985): Actin and tubulin polymerization: the use of kinetic methods to determine mechanism. *Annu. Rev. Biophys. Chem.*, 14:189–210.

37. Fukushima, K., Senda, N., Miura, S., Ishagami, S., and Murakami, Y. (1954): Dynamic pattern in the movement of leukocyte I and II. *Med. J. Osaka Univ.*, 5:1–56.

38. Gabbiani, G., Chaponnier, C., Zumbe, A., and Vassalli, P. (1977): Actin and tubulin co-cap with surface immunoglobulins in mouse B-lymphocytes. *Nature*, 269:697–698.

39. Goldstein, I., Hoffstein, S., Gallin, J., and Weissman, G. (1973): Mechanisms of lysosomal enzyme release from human leukocytes: microtubule assembly and membrane fusion induced by a component of complement. *Proc. Natl. Acad. Sci. USA*, 70:2916–2920.

40. Griffin, F. M., Griffin, J. A., and Silverstein, S. C. (1976): Studies on the mechanism of phagocytosis. II. The interaction of macrophages with anti-immunoglobulin IgG-coated bone marrow derived lymphocytes. *J. Exp. Med.*, 144:788–809.

41. Griffin, F. M. Jr., Griffin, J. A., Leider, J. E., and Silverstein, S. C. (1975): Studies on the mechanism of phagocytosis. I. Requirements for circumfirential attachment of particle-bound ligands to specific receptors on the macrophage plasma membrane. *J. Exp. Med.*, 142:1263–1282.

42. Hartwig, J. H., and Shevlin, P. A. (1986): The architecture of actin filaments and the ultrastructural location of actin-binding protein in the periphery of lung macrophages. *J. Cell Biol.*, 103:1007–1020.

43. Hartwig, J. H., and Stossel, T. P. (1975): Isolation and properties of actin, myosin, and a new actin-binding protein in rabbit alveolar macrophages. *J. Biol. Chem.*, 250:5696–5705.

44. Hartwig, J. H., and Stossel, T. P. (1979): Cytochalasin B and the structure of actin gels. *J. Mol. Biol.*, 134:539–554.

45. Hartwig, J. H., and Stossel, T. P. (1981): The structure of actin-binding protein molecules in solution and interacting with actin filaments. *J. Mol. Biol.*, 145:563–581.

45a. Henson, P. M., Zanolari, B., Schwartzman, N. A., and Hong, S. R. (1978): Intracellular control of human neutrophil secretion. I. C5a-induced stimulus-specific desensitization and the effects of cytochalasin B. *J. Immunol.*, 121:851–855.

46. Hirata, M., Hamachi, T., Suematsu, E., and Koga, T. (1983): Stimulation of Ca^{2+}-efflux by N-formyl chemotactic peptides in guinea-pig peritoneal macrophages. *Biochim. Biophys. Acta*, 763:339–345.

47. Hirsch, J. G. (1962): Cinemicrophotographic observations on granule lysis in polymorphonuclear leucocytes during phagocytosis. *J. Exp. Med.*, 116:827–833.

48. Howard, T. H., and Meyer, W. (1984): Chemotactic peptide modulation of actin assembly and locomotion in neutrophils. *J. Cell Biol.*, 98:1265–1271.

49. Howard, T. H., and Oresajo, C. O. (1985): A method for quantifying F-actin in chemotactic peptide activated neutrophils: study of the effect of tBOC peptide. *Cell Motil.*, 5:545–557.

50. Howard, T. H., and Oresajo, C. O. (1985): The kinetics of chemotactic peptide-induced change in F-actin content, F-actin distribution, and the shape of neutrophils. *J. Cell Biol.*, 101:1078–1085.

51. Hwo, S., and Bryan, J. (1985): Immuno-identification of Ca^{2+}-induced conformational changes in human gelsolin and brevin. *J. Cell Biol.*, 102:227–236.

52. Janmey, P. A., Chaponnier, C., Lind, S. E., Zaner, K. S., Stossel, T. P., and Yin, H. L. (1985): Interactions of gelsolin and gelsolin actin complexes with actin: effects of calcium on actin nucleation, filament severing and end blocking. *Biochemistry*, 24:3714–3723.

53. Janmey, P. A., Peetermans, J., Zaner, K. S., Stossel, T. P., and Tanaka, T. (1986): Structure and mobility of actin as measured by quasielastic light scattering, viscometry and electron microscopy. *J. Biol. Chem. (in press)*.

53a. Janmey, P. A., and Stossel, T. P. (1987): Modulation of gelsolin function by phosphatidylinositol-4,5-bis phosphate. *Nature*, 325:362–364.

54. Jesaitis, A. J., Naemura, J. R., Cochrane, C. G., and Painter, R. G. (1984): Rapid modulation of N-formyl chemotactic peptide receptors on the surface of human granulocytes: formation of high-affinity ligand-receptor complexes in transient association with the cytoskeleton. *J. Cell Biol.*, 98:1378–1387.

55. Kaplan, G. (1977): Differences in the mode of phagocytosis with Fc and C3 receptors in macrophages. *J. Immunol.*, 6:797–807.

56. Keller, H. U., and Bessis, M. (1975): Migration and chemotaxis of a nucleate cytoplasmic fragment. *Nature*, 258:723–724.

57. Keller, H. U., Naef, A., and Zimmerman, A. (1984): Effects of colchicine, vinblastine and nocodazole on polarity, motility, chemotaxis and cAMP levels of human polymorphonuclear leukocytes. *Exp. Cell. Res.*, 153:173–185.

58. Keller, H. U., Zimmermann, A., and Cottier, H. (1983): Crawling-like movements, adhesion to solid substrata and chemokinesis of neutrophil granulocytes. *J. Cell Sci.*, 64:89–106.

59. Keyserlingk, D. G. (1968): Elektronenmikroskopische untersuchung uber die Differenzierungsvorgange in Cytoplasma von segmentierten neutrophilen Leukozyten wahrend der Zellbewegung. *Exp. Cell Res.*, 51:79–91.

60. Koch, G. L. E., and Smith, M. J. (1978): An association between actin and the major histocompatibility antigen H-2. *Nature*, 273:274–278.

61. Kruskal, B. A., Shak, S., and Maxfield, F. R. (1986): Spreading of human neutrophils is immediately preceded by a large increase in cytoplasmic free calcium. *Proc. Natl. Acad. Sci. USA*, 83:2919–2923.

62. Kuo, H-J., Malencik, D. A., Liou, R-S., and Anderson, S. R. (1986): Factors affecting the activation of rabbit muscle phosphofructokinase by actin. *Biochemistry*, 25:1278–1286.

63. Kwiatkowski, D. J., Stossel, T. P., Colten, H. R., Mole, J. E., Orkin, S. H., and Yin, H. L. (1986): *Nature*, 323:455–458.

64. Kwiatkowski, D. J., Janmey, P. A., Mole, J. E., and Yin, H. L. (1985): Isolation and properties of two actin-binding domains in gelsolin. *J. Biol. Chem.*, 260:15232–15238.

65. Kwiatkowski, D. J., Mehl, R., and Yin, H. L. (1987): Genomic organization and biosynthesis of gelsolin. Submitted for publication.

66. Lassing, I., and Lindberg, U. (1985): Specific interaction between phosphatidylinositol 4,5-biphosphate and profilactin. *Nature*, 314:472–473.

67. Levine, J., and Willard, M. (1983): Redistribution of fodrin (a component of the cortical cytoplasm) accompanying capping of cell surface surface molecules. *proc. Natl. Acad. Sci. USA*, 80:191–195.

68. Lew, P. D., and Stossel, T. P. (1980): Calcium transport by macrophage plasma membranes. *J. Biol. Chem.*, 255:5841–5846.

69. Lew, P. D., and Stossel, T. P. (1981): Effect of calcium on superoxide production by phagocytic vesicles from rabbit alveolar macrophages. *J. Clin. Invest.*, 67:1–9.

70. Lew, P. D., Andersson, T., Hed, J., Di Virgilio, F., Pozzan, T., and

Stendahl, O. (1985): Ca²⁺-dependent and Ca²⁺-independent phagocytosis in human neutrophils. *Nature,* 315:509–511.

71. Lewis, W. H. (1934): On the locomotion of the polymorphonuclear neutrophils of the rat in autoplasma cultures. *Bull. Johns Hopkins Hosp.,* 55:273–279.

72. Lewis, W. H. (1939): The role of a superficial plasmagel layer in changes of form, locomotion and division of cells in tissue cultures. *Arch. Exp. Zellforsch.,* 23:7–13.

73. Malawista, S. E., and Boisfleury Chevance, A. (1982): The cytokineplast: purified, stable, and functional motile machinery from human blood polymorphonuclear leukocytes: possible formative role of heat-induced centrosomal dysfunction. *J. Cell Biol.,* 95: 960–973.

74. Malech, H. L., Root, R. K., and Gallin, J. I. (1977): Structural analysis of human neutrophil migration: centriole, microtubule, and microfilament orientation and function during chemotaxis. *J. Cell Biol.,* 75:666–693.

75. Maruyama, K., and Ebashi, S. (1964): Alpha actinin, a new structural protein from striated muscle. II. Action on actin. *J. Biochem.,* 58:13–19.

76. Mazur, M. T., and Williamson, J. R. (1977): Macrophage deformability and phagocytosis. *J. Cell Biol.,* 75:185–198.

77. McNeil, P. L., Swanson, J. A., Wright, S. D., Silverstein, S. C., and Taylor, D. L. (1986): Fc-receptor-mediated phagocytosis occurs in macrophages without an increase in average [Ca⁺⁺]i. *J. Cell Biol.,* 102:1586–1592.

78. Miller, M. E. (1979): Cell elastimetry in the study of normal and abnormal movement of human neutrophils. *Clin. Immunol. Immunopathol.,* 14:302–310.

79. Mozo-Villarias, A., and Ware, B. R. (1985): Actin oligomers below the critical concentration detected by fluorescence photobleaching recovery. *Biochemistry,* 24:1544–1548.

80. Niederman, R., Amrein, P., and Hartwig, J. H. (1983): The three dimensional structure of actin filaments in solution and an actin gel made with actin-binding protein. *J. Cell Biol.,* 96:1400–1413.

81. Ochs, D. L., and Reed, P. W. (1984): Ca²⁺-stimulated, Mg²⁺-dependent ATPase activity in neutrophil plasma membrane vesicles: coupling to Ca²⁺ transport. *J. Biol. Chem.,* 259:102–106.

82. O'Flaherty, J. T., Kreutzer, D. L., and Ward, P. A. (1977): Neutrophil aggregation and swelling induced by chemotactic agents. *J. Immunol.,* 119:232–239.

83. Oliver, J. M., Lalchandani, R., and Becker, E. L. (1977): Actin redistribution during concanavalin A cap formation in rabbit neutrophils. *J. Reticuloendothelial. Soc.,* 21:359–364.

84. Orenstein, J. M., and Shelton, E. (1977): Membrane phenomena accompanying erythrophagocytosis: a scanning electron microscope study. *Lab. Invest.,* 36:363–374.

85. Oster, G. F. (1984): On the crawling of cells. *J. Embryol. Exp. Morphol.,* 83(Suppl.):329–364.

86. Painter, R. G., Whisenand, J., and McIntosh, A. T. (1981): Effects of cytochalasin B on actin and myosin association with particle binding sites in mouse macrophages: implications with regard to the mechanism of action of the cytochalasins. *J. Cell Biol.,* 91:373–384.

87. Pasternak, C., and Elson, E. (1985): Lymphocyte mechanical response triggered by cross-linking surface receptors. *J. Cell Biol.,* 100:860–872.

88. Petrini, M., Emerson, D. L., and Galbraith, R. M. (1983): Linkage between surface immunoglobulin and cytoskeleton of B lymphocytes may involve Gc protein. *Nature,* 306:73–74.

89. Pober, J. S., Guild, B. C., Strominger, J. L., and Veatch, W. R. (1981): Purification of HLA-A2 antigen, fluorescent labeling of its intracellular region, and demonstration of an interaction between fluorescently labeled HLA-A2 antigen and lymphoblastoid cell cytoskeleton proteins. *Biochemistry,* 20:5625–5633.

90. Pozzan, T., Lew, P. D., Wollheim, C. B., and Tsien, R. Y. (1983): Is cytosolic ionized calcium regulating neutrophil activation? *Science,* 221:1413–1415.

91. Pryzwansky, K. B., Schliwa, M., and Porter, K. R. (1983): Comparison of the three-dimensional organization of unextracted and triton-extracted human neutrophilic polymorphonuclear leukocytes. *Eur. J. Cell Biol.,* 30:112–125.

92. Rikihisa, Y., and Mizuno, D. (1977): Demonstration of myosin on the cytoplasmic side of plasma membranes of guinea pig polymorphonuclear leukocytes with immunoferritin. *Exp. Cell Res.,* 110:87–92.

93. Robineaux, R. (1954): Mouvements cellulaires et fonction phagocytaire des granulocytes neutrophiles. *Rev. Hematol.,* 9:364–402.

94. Romeo, D. (1982): Transmembrane signalling and modulation of neutrophil behaviour. *Trends Biochem. Sci.,* 7:408–411.

95. Ryder, M. I., Weinreb, R. N., and Niederman, R. (1984): The organization of actin filaments in human polymorphonuclear leukocytes. *Anat. Rec.,* 209:7–20.

96. Sagara, J., Nagata, K., and Ichikawa, Y. (1982): A cofactor protein required for actin activation of myosin Mg²⁺ATPase activity in leukemic myeloblasts. *J. Biochem.,* 92:1845–1851.

97. Salisbury, J. L., Condeelis, J. S., Maihle, N. J., and Satir, P. (1981): Calmodulin localization during capping and receptor-mediated endocytosis. *Nature,* 294:163–166.

98. Sato, M., Leimbach, G., Schwarz, W. H., and Pollard, T. D. (1985): Mechanical properties of actin. *J. Biol. Chem.,* 260:8585–8592.

99. Sawyer, D. W., Sullivan, J. A., and Mandell, G. L. (1985): Intracellular free calcium localization in neutrophils during phagocytosis. *Science,* 230:663–666.

100. Schliwa, M., Pryzwansky, K. B., and Euteneuer, U. (1982): Centrosome splitting in neutrophils: an unusual phenomenon related to cell activation and motility. *Cell,* 31:705–717.

101. Scholey, J. M., Smith, R. C., Drenckhahn, D., Groschel-Stewart, U., and Kendrick-Jones, J. (1982): Thymus myosin: isolation and characterization of myosin from calf thymus and thymic lymphocytes, and studies on the effect of phosphorylation of its Mᵣ = 20,000 light chain. *J. Biol. Chem.,* 257:7737–7745.

102. Schreiner, G. F., Fujiwara, K., Pollard, T. D., and Unanue, E. R. (1977): Redistribution of myosin accompanying capping of surface Ig. *J. Exp. Med.,* 145:1393–1398.

103. Schultze, M. (1865): Ein Heizbarer objekttisch und seine Verwendung bei Untersuchung des Blutes. *Arch. Mikrosk. Anat.,* 1:1–42.

104. Scott, R. E., and Maercklein, P. B. (1977): Plasma membrane vesiculation: correlation between macrophage spreading and the shedding of cell surface vesicles. *Lab. Invest.,* 37:430–436.

105. Senda, N., Tamura, H., Shibata, N., Yoshitake, J., Kondo, K., and Tanaka, K. (1975): The mechanism of the movement of leucocytes. *Exp. Cell Res.,* 70:55–94.

106. Sha'afi, R. I., Naccache, P. H., Alobaidi, T., Molski, T. F. P., and Volpi, M. (1981): Effect of arachidonic acid and the chemotactic factor f-Met-Leu-Phe on cation transport in rabbit neutrophils. *J. Cell. Physiol.,* 106:215–223.

107. Shapiro, H., and Harvey, E. N. (1936): The tension at the surface of macrophages. *J. Cell. Comp. Physiol.,* 8:21–30.

108. Sheterline, P., Rickard, J. E., and Richards, R. C. (1984): Fc-receptor-directed phagocytic stimuli induce transient actin assembly at an early stage of phagocytosis in neutrophil leukocytes. *Eur. J. Cell Biol.,* 34:80–87.

109. Sheterline, P., Rickard, J. E., Boothroyd, B., and Richards, R. C. (1986): Phorbol ester induces rapid actin assembly in neutrophil leucocytes independently of changes in [Ca²⁺]i and pHi. *J. Muscle Res. Cell Motil.,* 7:405–412.

110. Shibata, N., Tatsumi, N., Tanaka, K., Okamura, Y., and Senda, N. (1972): A contractile protein possessing Ca²⁺ sensitivity (natural actomyosin) from leucocytes: its extraction and some of its properties. *Biochim. Biophys. Acta,* 256:565–576.

111. Singer, S. J., and Kupfer, A. (1986): The directed migration of eukaryotic cells. *Annu. Rev. Cell Biol.,* 2:337–365.

112. Skalak, R., Chien, S., and Schmid-Schonbein, G. W. (1984): Viscoelastic deformation of white cells: theory and analysis. In: *White Cell Mechanics: Basic Science and Clinical Aspects,* edited by P. LaCelle and M. A. Lichtman, pp. 3–18. Alan R. Liss, New York.

113. Sklar, L. A., Hyslop, P. A., Oades, Z. G., Omann, G. M., Jesaitis, A. J., Painter, R. J., and Cochrane, C. G. (1985): Signal transduction and ligand-receptor dynamics in the human neutrophil: transient responses and occupancy response relations at the formyl peptide receptor. *J. Biol. Chem.,* 260:11461–11467.

114. Smith, C. M., Tukey, D. P., Mundshenk, D., Krivit, W., White,

J. G., Repine, J. E., and Hoidal, J. R. (1982): Filtration deformability of rabbit pulmonary macrophage. *J. Lab. Clin. Med.,* 99:568–579.

115. Southwick, F. S., and Hartwig, J. H. (1982): Acumentin, a protein of macrophages which caps the "pointed" end of actin filaments. *Nature,* 297:303–307.

116. Southwick, F. S., and Stossel, T. P. (1981): Isolation of an inhibitor of actin polymerization from human polymorphonuclear leukocytes. *J. Biol. Chem.,* 256:3030–3036.

117. Southwick, F. S., Tatsumi, N., and Stossel, T. P. (1982): Acumentin, an actin-modulating protein of rabbit pulmonary macrophages. *Biochemistry,* 21:6321–6326.

118. Steinman, R. M., Mellman, I. S., Muller, W. A., and Cohn, Z. A. (1983): Endocytosis and the recycling of plasma membrane. *J. Cell Biol.,* 96:1–27.

119. Stendahl, O. I., and Stossel, T. P. (1980): Actin-binding protein amplifies actomyosin contraction and gelsolin confers calcium controls in the direction of contraction. *Biochem. Biophys. Res. Commun.,* 92:675–681.

120. Stendahl, O. I., Hartwig, J. H., Brotschi, E. A., and Stossel, T. P. (1980): Distribution of actin-binding protein and myosin in macrophages during spreading and phagocytosis. *J. Cell Biol.,* 84:215–224.

121. Stossel, T. P. (1984): Contribution of actin to the structure of the cytoplasmic matrix. *J. Cell Biol.,* 99:15s–21s.

122. Stossel, T. P., and Hartwig, J. H. (1976): Interaction of actin, myosin, and a new actin-binding protein of rabbit pulmonary macrophages. II. Role in cytoplasmic movement and phagocytosis. *J. Cell Biol.,* 68:602–614.

123. Stossel, T. P., and Pollard, T. D. (1973): Myosin in polymorphonuclear leukocytes. *J. Biol. Chem.,* 248:8288–8294.

124. Stossel, T. P., Chaponnier, C., Ezzell, R. M., Hartwig, J. H., Janmey, P. A., Kwiatkowski, D. J., Lind, S. E., et al. (1985): Nonmuscle actin-binding proteins. *Annu. Rev. Cell Biol.,* 1:353–402.

125. Takemura, R., Stenberg, P. E., Bainton, D. F., and Werb, Z. (1986): Rapid distribution of clathrin onto macrophage plasma membranes in response to Fc receptor-ligand interaction during frustrated phagocytosis. *J. Cell Biol.,* 102:55–69.

126. Takeuchi, K. (1985): Properties of porcine myosin. I. Similarity between vertebrate smooth muscle and nonmuscle myosins in their binding properties with F-actin. *J. Biochem.,* 97:295–305.

127. Taylor, D. L., and Fechheimer, M. (1982): Cytoplasmic structure and contractility: the solation–contraction coupling hypothesis. *Philos. Trans. R. Soc. Lond.* [*Biol.*], 299:185–197.

128. Trinkaus, J. P. (1984): *Cells into Organs: The Forces that Shape the Embryo.* Prentice-Hall, Englewood Cliffs, New Jersey.

129. Trotter, J. A. (1982): Living macrophages phosphorylate the 20,000 dalton light chains and heavy chains of myosin. *Biochem. Biophys. Res. Commun.,* 106:1071–1077.

130. Trotter, J. A., and Adelstein, R. S. (1979): Macrophage myosin: regulation of actin-activated ATPase activity by phosphorylation of the 20,000-dalton light chain. *J. Biol. Chem.,* 254:8781–8785.

131. Trotter, J. A., Nixon, C. S., and Johnson, M. A. (1985): The heavy chain of macrophage myosin is phosphorylated at the tip of the tail. *J. Biol. Chem.,* 260:14374–14378.

132. Trotter, J. A., Scordilis, S. P., and Margossian, S. S. (1983): Macrophages contain at least two myosins. *FEBS Lett.,* 156:135–140.

133. Valberg, P. A., and Albertini, D. F. (1985): Cytoplasmic motions, rheology, and structure probed by a novel magnetic particle method. *J. Cell Biol.,* 101:130–140.

134. Valerius, N. H., Stendahl, O., Hartwig, J. H., and Stossel, T. P. (1981): Distribution of actin-binding protein and myosin in polymorphonuclear leukocytes during locomotion and phagocytosis. *Cell,* 24:195–202.

135. Vanderkerckhove, J., and Weber, K. (1978): At least six different actins are expressed in a higher mammal: an analysis based on the amino acid sequence of the amino-terminal peptide. *J. Mol. Biol.,* 126:783–802.

136. Wallace, P. J., Wersto, R. P., Packman, C. H., and Lichtman, M. A. (1984): Chemotactic peptide-induced changes in neutrophil actin conformation. *J. Cell Biol.,* 99:1060–1065.

137. Wharton Jones, T. (1846): The blood-corpuscle considered in its different phases of development in the animal series. *Philos. Trans. R. Soc. Lond.,* 63–87.

138. Yang, H. H., and Boxer, L. A. (1981): Purification of myosin light chain kinase from rabbit polymorphonuclear leukocytes. *Pediatr. Res.,* 15:229–234.

139. Yassin, R., Shefcyk, J., White, J. R., Tao, W., Volpi, M., Molski, T. F. P., Naccache, P. H., and Sha'afi, R. I. (1985): Effects of chemotactic factors and other agents on the amounts of actin and a 65,000-mol-wt protein associated with the cytoskeleton of rabbit and human neutrophils. *J. Cell Biol.,* 101:182–188.

140. Yin, H. L., and Stossel, T. P. (1979): Control of cytoplasmic actin gel-sol transformation by gelsolin, a calcium-dependent regulatory protein. *Nature,* 281:583–586.

141. Yin, H. L., and Stossel, T. P. (1980): Purification and structural properties of gelsolin, a Ca^{2+}-activated regulatory protein of macrophages. *J. Biol. Chem.,* 255:9490–9493.

142. Yin, H. L., Albrecht, J., and Fattoum, A. (1981): Identification of gelsolin, a Ca^{2+}-dependent regulatory protein of actin gel-sol transformation: its intracellular distribution in a variety of cells and tissues. *J. Cell Biol.,* 91:901–906.

143. Yin, H. L., Kwiatkowski, D. J., Mole, J. E., and Cole, F. S. (1984): Structure and biosynthesis of cytoplasmic and secreted variants of gelsolin. *J. Biol. Chem.,* 259:5271–5276.

144. Yin, H. L., Zaner, K. S., and Stossel, T. P. (1980): Ca^+ control of actin gelation. *J. Biol. Chem.,* 255:9494–9500.

145. Young, N., Gergely, P., and Crawford, N. (1981): Platelet and leukocyte calmodulins: isolation and characterisation. *Eur. J. Biochem.,* 120:303–308.

146. Yuli, I., and Snyderman, R. (1984): Rapid changes in light scattering from human polymorphonuclear leukocytes exposed to chemoattractants: discrete responses correlated with chemotactic and secretory functions. *J. Clin. Invest.,* 73:1408–1417.

147. Zaner, K. S. (1986): The effect of the 540 kilodalton actin cross-linking protein, actin-binding protein (ABP) on the mechanical properties of F-actin. *J. Biol. Chem.,* 261:7615–7620.

148. Zaner, K. S., and Stossel, T. P. (1982): Some perspectives on the viscosity of actin filaments. *J. Cell Biol.,* 93:987–991.

149. Zaner, K. S., and Stossel, T. P. (1983): Physical basis of the rheologic properties of F-actin. *J. Biol. Chem.,* 258:11004–11009.

150. Zigmond, S. H. (1974): Mechanisms of sensing chemical gradients by polymorphonuclear leucocytes. *Nature,* 249:450–452.

151. Zigmond, S. H., and Sullivan, S. J. (1979): Sensory adaptation of leukocytes to chemotactic peptides. *J. Cell Biol.,* 82:517–527.

152. Pollard, T. D. and Cooper, J. A. (1986): Actin and actin-binding proteins: A critical evaluation of mechanisms and functions. *Annu. Rev. Biochem.,* 55:987–1035.

153. Lind, S. E., Janmey, P. A., Chaponnier, C., Hersert, T. J., and Stossel, T. P. (1987): Reversible binding of actin to gelsolin and profilin in human platelet extracts. *J. Cell Biol.,* 105:833–842.

Inflammation: Basic Principles and Clinical Correlates.
Edited by J. I. Gallin, I. M. Goldstein, and R. Snyderman.
Raven Press, Ltd., New York © 1988.

CHAPTER 21

Phagocytic Cells: Fc$_\gamma$ and Complement Receptors

Jay C. Unkeless and Samuel D. Wright

The basic mechanisms by which phagocytes recognize foreign organisms have been known for more than 80 years. In 1903 Wright and Douglas (192) showed that human serum contains heat-stable and heat-labile factors that dramatically enhance the ability of blood phagocytes to ingest staphylococci. These factors, now known to include immunoglobulin G (IgG) and C3, were shown to act by binding to the bacteria. The phagocytes then recognized the coated bacteria via specific receptors for IgG and C3. The structure and function of IgG and C3 are addressed in greater detail elsewhere in this text. Here we primarily discuss the receptors for these ligands.

Fc$_\gamma$ RECEPTORS

The existence of Fc receptors for IgG (Fc$_\gamma$R) has been appreciated since the early studies of Berken and Benacerraf (17). The rapid progress in this field is due largely to the isolation of monoclonal antibodies (MAbs) specific for different receptors. The Fc$_\gamma$R family probably evolved in parallel with the immunoglobulins; indeed, cloning studies of Ravetch et al. (150), Lewis et al. (109), and Hogarth et al. (73) showed that Fc$_\gamma$Rs form a subgroup of the immunoglobulin supergene family. The Fc$_\gamma$Rs provide a crucial link between the phagocytic effector cells and the lymphocytes that secrete Ig, as the macrophage/monocyte, polymorphonuclear leukocyte, and NK cell Fc$_\gamma$Rs confer the element of specific recognition on the effector cells. Phagocytic cells thus have several mechanisms whereby friend can be distinguished from foe, in-

cluding Fc$_\gamma$Rs, complement receptors, and receptors for oligosaccharides discussed here and elsewhere in this volume (see Chapter 17). Because complement and Fc$_\gamma$Rs have been the subject of several reviews (38,180,193) we concentrate here primarily on recent data.

Human Receptors for IgG

Human leukocytes have three distinguishable receptors for IgG. The first, Fc$_\gamma$R, characterized by Huber and Fudenberg (76) and Huber et al (77), is a receptor found on monocytes and macrophages that binds monomeric IgG with high avidity with the rank order IgG1 > IgG3 > IgG4 $\gg$ IgG2. The Ka is $\sim 1 \times 10^8$ to 3×10^8. Competitive binding studies performed by Anderson and Abraham (5) of different subclasses of IgG to the U937 cell line have failed to reveal heterogeneity in the high-avidity binding sites. The protein responsible for the high-avidity binding has now been identified as a 72-kilodalton (kD) peptide first by affinity chromatography (4) and then later by immunoprecipitation with a goat antiserum obtained following immunization with affinity-purified Fc-binding protein (8). Most recently, Anderson et al. (6) have isolated a monoclonal antibody (MAb) that immunoprecipitates the 72-kD protein from U937 cells. This MAb immunoprecipitates but does not inhibit receptor activity of Fc$_\gamma$R$_{p72}$, indicating that MAb 32 is directed against an epitope distinct from the binding site. Similarly, immune complex-triggered superoxide production was not blocked by MAb 32 but was strongly inhibited by IgG.

The valence of the $Fc_\gamma R_{p72}$ molecule is thought to be 1, based on mixing experiments by O'Grady et al. (134). They saturated U937 cells with mixtures of labeled and unlabeled IgG1 kappa and lambda, lysed the cells, and adsorbed the lysates on an anti-kappa immunoadsorbent. If the $Fc_\gamma R_{p72}$ was a multimer, some labeled lambda IgG1 would be precipitated by the anti-kappa adsorbent, but essentially no labeled IgG1 lambda was found. However, in the presence of MAb 32, which would render the receptor bivalent, labeled IgG1 lambda binding to the anti-kappa immunoadsorbent was observed.

The CH2 domain of IgG is generally thought to interact with $Fc_\gamma R_{p72}$, and it seems likely that carbohydrate plays an important role in maintenance of the proper conformation for binding to $Fc_\gamma R$. Nose and Wigzell (133) reported that aglycosylated IgG2a, isolated by growing myeloma cells in the presence of tunicamycin, was unable to fix complement or to bind to macrophage $Fc_\gamma R$. Leatherbarrow et al. (108) also found that oligosaccharides play a role in maintenance of the conformation required for binding, as aglycosylated IgG2a bound with a 50-fold lower affinity to human monocytes. However, the capacity of the aglycosylated IgG2a to activate C1 was approximately the same as the native protein.

In general it appears that γ-interferon, among its many other effects, primes monocytes and macrophages for enhanced cellular defenses (165). $Fc_\gamma R_{p72}$ is likely to be centrally involved in antibody-dependent cellular cytotoxicity (ADCC) mechanisms. Guyre et al. (63) have shown that $Fc_\gamma R_{p72}$ is induced in monocytes and the U937 cell line eight- to tenfold by γ-interferon, with a time course of 12 to 18 hr. This striking result suggests that $Fc_\gamma R_{p72}$ may play a role in the enhanced effector function often associated with γ-interferon stimulation. Akiyama et al. (2) demonstrated that γ-interferon induction of U937 cells induces mouse IgG2a- and IgG3-dependent ADCC.

Additional compelling evidence for this role of the $Fc_\gamma R_{p72}$ was provided by Shen et al. (167). They reported that covalent heteroconjugates formed with intact 32.2 MAb or its Fab fragment, and antibody directed against chicken erythrocytes mediates efficient ADCC by monocytes and U937 cells. This ADCC was not due simply to formation of cell–cell conjugates, as heteroconjugates formed from anti-HLA and anti-chicken erythrocyte IgG had no effect. The extent of the ADCC was enhanced by pretreatment of the cells with γ-interferon. The most significant aspect of the study was the observation that the ADCC mediated by the heteroantibody was not inhibited by IgG at 2 mg/ml, in striking contrast to the inhibition of anti-erythrocyte antibody ADCC by IgG1 at 40 μg/ml. Similar results were reported by Graziano and Fanger (56), who found that monocyte ADCC against hybridoma cells bearing MAb 32.2 on their surface was stimulated by γ-interferon, but that no ADCC was seen against hybrido-

mas bearing MAbs directed against other antigens such as the iC3b receptor or class I histocompatibility antigens. The results provide a possible rationale for specific anti-tumor/anti-$Fc_\gamma R_{p72}$ heteroconjugates in therapy of malignancy, assuming that appropriate antibodies directed against tumor antigens are selected.

The second $Fc_\gamma R$ identified on human leukocytes is a low-avidity $Fc_\gamma R$ with broad electrophoretic mobility (M_r 50,000–70,000) in sodium dodecyl sulfate (SDS)-acrylamide gels ($Fc_\gamma R_{p50-70}$). This antigen, assigned the name CD16, is present on a variety of cell types, including neutrophils, NK cells, and tissue macrophages (50,138–140). The receptor appears to be a late differentiation antigen in both the myeloid and monocytic differentiation pathways. Fleit et al. (51) found that $Fc_\gamma R_{p50-70}$ was present in bone marrow at the metamyelocyte stage but was not present in promyelocytes. In agreement with this result, $Fc_\gamma R_{p50-70}$ was not detectable on uninduced HL-60 cells, which are arrested at the promyelocyte stage, but it was induced by retinoic acid and dimethylsulfoxide, both of which induce differentiation of HL-60 toward a more mature neutrophil morphology. Similarly, monocytes do not express $Fc_\gamma R_{p50-70}$, but the antigen is expressed at high levels on tissue macrophages present in liver, spleen, and lung. Culture of blood monocytes in vitro for 1 week, which results in cells that have many macrophage-like characteristics, results in induction of the antigen. No agents were found that induce $Fc_\gamma R_{p50-70}$ on U937 or HL-60 cells.

There are several MAbs that are directed against the CD16, or $Fc_\gamma R_{p50-70}$ molecule, including 3G8, B73.1, Leu-11a,b, and VEP-13 (141). These MAbs are directed against different epitopes on the receptor and thus differ in the efficacy with which they block binding of IgG complexes. MAb 3G8 is the most efficient inhibitor of antibody binding but is unsuitable for ablation of populations of cells by complement cytotoxicity, as it is a mouse IgG1 and fixes complement poorly. Leu-11a, a mouse IgM, is preferable in this regard. B73.1 was initially isolated as a reagent specific for NK cells and was reported to bind to neutrophils of 50% of the population, suggesting that it binds to an alloantigen. However, B73.1 reacts with all NK cells regardless of reactivity of the antibody with neutrophils of the individual. Werner et al. (185) have found that NA1 and NA2 antigens, reported to be neutrophil-specific, are $Fc_\gamma R_{p50-70}$ alloantigens. A good correlation has been found between autoimmune neutropenia and NA1/NA2-specific antibody in patients' sera (99,114). There is, however, no information on the presence of NA1 and NA2 determinants on tissue macrophages, nor is the distribution of these antigens on NK cells understood.

$Fc_\gamma R_{p50-70}$ is a receptor of low avidity that preferentially binds immune complexes. Kurlander and Batker (94) found that neutrophils, which do not express the high-avidity $Fc_\gamma R_{p72}$, bind IgG1 dimers with an avidity 100 to 1,000 times lower than do monocytes. These results were confirmed by Fleit et al. (50) who found negligible binding of monomeric IgG1 to neutrophils, although these cells obviously bear $Fc_\gamma R$ and saturate with MAb 3G8 at more than 1×10^5 sites per cell. Kurlander et al. (98) have shown by Scatchard analysis of the binding of IgG1 dimers to monocytes and peritoneal macrophages that macrophages acquire a new low-avidity IgG binding site not present on blood monocytes. Peritoneal macrophages exhibit biphasic Scatchard plots of binding of IgG1 dimers, with a low-avidity site ($1.1 \times 10^7 M^{-1}$) and a high-avidity site with a Ka 200-fold higher. The number of low-avidity sites on peritoneal macrophages was more than 2×10^5 sites/cell, some fivefold higher than the number of high-avidity sites present on the same cells. Clarkson et al. (28) found strong reactivity with MAb 3G8 in sites where there are high concentrations of tissue macrophages—in the red pulp of the spleen and in the liver on Kupffer cells.

The phagocytic potential of $Fc_\gamma R_{p50-70}$ on neutrophils can be modulated by a small ($M_r < 10,000$) cytokine first analyzed with respect to its stimulation of the C3b receptor that results in phagocytosis. This lymphokine, which is released from T-cells in response to monocytes incubated with immune complexes and from a human T-cell line MO(t) (59,62), rapidly stimulates phagocytosis but not binding of IgG-sensitized erythrocytes by polymorphonuclear neutrophils (PMNs) (58). The binding of the anti-$Fc_\gamma R_{p50-70}$ MAb 3G8 was unaffected by the cytokine. A MAb against neutrophils has been described that inhibits only the portion of the phagocytic index *stimulated* by the cytokine (58). This result suggests that although virtually all the binding and phagocytosis was inhibited by MAb 3G8 there are nonetheless functionally different classes of $Fc_\gamma R_{p50-70}$ on the surface of the PMN. Along these lines, Jack and Fearon (82) found that 50% of PMN $Fc_\gamma R_{p50-70}$ co-caps with the C3b receptor, implying that $Fc_\gamma R$ may exist in different states depending on whether it is associated with the cell cytoskeleton. There is no evidence for phosphorylation of $Fc_\gamma Rs$, although if it is a transitory event it might have been missed.

The receptor on human leukocytes most recently described is $Fc_\gamma R_{p40}$, which was initially observed following affinity chromatography of U937 lysates on IgG-Sepharose (4) and then immunoprecipitated with a goat-anti-$Fc_\gamma R$ antibody elicited by immunization with affinity-purified protein (8). Rosenfeld et al. (152) then made an MAb, IV.3, directed against this antigen. The protein immunoprecipitated by this antibody has a mass of 40 kD and is distributed on a wide variety of cell types, including monocytes, platelets, neutrophils, possibly B-cells, and the K562 cell line. $Fc_\gamma R_{p40}$ is the only receptor detected on K562 cells and on platelets. The IV.3 MAb (and the Fab fragment) blocks aggregation of platelets triggered by IgG aggregates but has no effect on aggregation triggered by other agents such as thrombin or collagen. Neutrophils also have two distinguishable receptors, $Fc_\gamma R_{p50-70}$ and $Fc_\gamma R_{p40}$, whereas tissue macrophages have $Fc_\gamma R_{p72}$ in addition to these two. Kulczycki (92) found that neutrophils and eosinophils have different $Fc_\gamma Rs$ and reported that the M_r of the eosinophil $Fc_\gamma R$ is 43,000. It seems likely that the eosinophil $Fc_\gamma R$ may be $Fc_\gamma R_{p40}$, and Looney et al. (111) reported that $Fc_\gamma R_{p40}$ is present on eosinophils.

The $Fc_\gamma R_{p40}$ is of low avidity and is the human receptor responsible for the binding of murine IgG2b aggregates. Jones et al. (85) reported that binding of this ligand to U937 cells was greatly enhanced by lowering the ionic strength of the medium. In contrast, the binding of murine IgG2a to macrophages was unaffected by changes in ionic strength. The binding of IgG2b aggregates was poorly inhibited by murine IgG2a and vice versa. All of these properties serve to distinguish the low-avidity $Fc_\gamma R_{p40}$ from the high-avidity $Fc_\gamma R_{p72}$, although both receptors are present on U937 cells. McCool et al. (118) examined binding of IgG to K562 and U937 cells and found that K562 had too low an affinity for IgG to measure monomer binding accurately. High-avidity binding of murine IgG2a, but not IgG2b, to U937 cells was found. Studies with switch mutants demonstrated that binding of IgG2a to human $Fc_\gamma R$ required, in addition to the C_H3 domain, amino-terminal domains.

Given the complexity of the $Fc_\gamma R$ system, with multiple receptors on the same cells, it is difficult to sort out the role of each $Fc_\gamma R$. There are, however, some intriguing clues. As discussed above, the $Fc_\gamma R_{p72}$ is induced eight-to tenfold by γ-interferon, which primes macrophages and monocytes for cytotoxicity against tumor cells (165). It is likely that $Fc_\gamma R_{p72}$ plays a role in ADCC, which is elevated following γ-interferon treatment of monocytes.

The role of $Fc_\gamma R_{p40}$, which is found on an extraordinary variety of cells, is not well understood, but some experiments of Anderson et al. (7) suggested that it is involved in T-cell proliferative responses driven by murine IgG1 anti-Leu-4 (T3) MAbs. Tax et al. (171) reported that in 30% of otherwise normal individuals there was no T-cell mitogenic response in the presence of monocytes to IgG1 anti-T3 MAbs, although these antibodies would drive a mitogenic response when coupled to Sepharose. Monocytes from nonresponding individuals did not rosette with IgG1-coated erythrocytes (170). Similar results suggesting the presence of multiple receptors on monocytes were published by Clement et al. (29), who found that the lack of response to IgG1 anti-T3 antibodies was not absolute but could be driven with high concentrations of antibody. The monocyte-driven response is thought to be Fc-dependent and probably occurs through cross-linking of the antigen on the T-cell surface. The IgG1 anti-T3 polymorphism in stimulation of the T-cell mitogenic response is likely to be mediated by the $Fc_\gamma R_{p40}$, as this response is blocked by an anti-$Fc_\gamma R_{p40}$ MAb (110), providing strong evidence that the $Fc_\gamma R_{p40}$ is involved in this response. Anderson et al. (7) observed an isoelectric point polymorphism in $Fc_\gamma R_{p40}$ that correlates well with the observed gene frequencies in the population. A different type of polymorphism was reported by Rosenfeld et al. (153), who found that there are reproducible differences (which correlate with the sensitivity of platelet aggregation by IgG aggregates) in the amount of $Fc_\gamma R_{p40}$ on platelets from different individuals.

Another possible polymorphism in human $Fc_\gamma Rs$ may be associated with HLA-DR2 and HLA-DR3 allotypes. Salmon et al. (161) reported statistically significant decreased $Fc_\gamma R$-mediated phagocytosis by monocytes from normal individuals bearing DR2 and DR3 antigens. Salmon and Kimberly (160) also found that these individuals have decreased ability to phagocytize concanavalin A-coated rabbit erythrocytes. They believed that the membrane binding protein for concanavalin A and the monocyte $Fc_\gamma R$ are related because a dramatic inhibition in phagocytosis of both IgG- and concanavalin A-sensitized erythrocytes is seen following adherence of monocytes on aggregated IgG-coated coverslips. Under these conditions there was no inhibition of phagocytosis of erythrocytes treated with tannic acid or wheat germ lectin, nor was phagocytosis of zymosan affected.

$Fc_\gamma R_{p40}$ may act as a target for NK cell activity, an interesting observation in light of the widespread distribution of this antigen. Perl et al. (137) reported a correlation of $Fc_\gamma R_{p40}$ density, determined by binding of anti-$Fc_\gamma R$, and NK susceptibility. More direct evidence for $Fc_\gamma R_{p40}$ acting as a NK target is the observation that intact IV.3 MAb and its Fab fragment partially block NK activity directed against K562 and U937 cells. The transferrin receptor is also proposed to be a recognition site for NK cytolysis (3,183). Perl et al. (137) found that a combination of anti-transferrin receptor MAb and anti-$Fc_\gamma R_{p40}$ MAb can totally block NK cytolysis of K562 cells. The anti-$Fc_\gamma R_{p40}$ MAb has no effect on cells not bearing the epitope, as would be predicted. Single cell binding and cytolysis experiments suggested that the transferrin receptor and $Fc_\gamma R_{p40}$ serve as recognition elements and do not play a role in subsequent events.

One function in which $Fc_\gamma R$ clearly must play a role is the clearance of immune complexes. One approach to dissection of the role of the various human $Fc_\gamma R$ species is to study the effect on immune complex clearance of *in vivo* administration of MAbs that inhibit $Fc_\gamma R$ function. This approach has been used by Clarkson et al. (28) to study the role of $Fc_\gamma R_{p50-70}$ *in vivo*. The epitope recognized by MAb 3G8 is present only on human and chimpanzee leukocytes, necessitating the use of chimpanzees for the *in vivo* experiments. The clearance of $[^{51}Cr]O_4$-labeled autologous erythrocytes sensitized with chimpanzee anti-$a^cb^cd^c$ serum was measured in lightly anesthetized animals following methodology developed by Frank et al. (52) for performing clearance studies in humans. Infusion of MAb 3G8 at doses as low as 0.25 mg/kg body weight resulted in a dramatic (20-fold) increase in clearance time of the sensitized erythrocytes compared to the preinfusion clearance $T_\frac{1}{2}$ of 1 hr. Infusion of 3G8 IgG resulted in a transient (4 days) neutropenia, which may be due to the opsonization of the neutrophils with intact 3G8 IgG. The Fab fragment of 3G8 also blocked clearance, but there were no peripheral leukocyte changes associated with infusion, although the density of 3G8 Fab on peripheral neutrophils was similar to that found with the intact antibody. These experiments demonstrated that the $Fc_\gamma R$ *primarily* responsible for clearance of the IgG-sensitized erythrocyte is $Fc_\gamma R_{p50-70}$, although they do not rule out a lesser role for other $Fc_\gamma R$ and complement receptors.

The ability of the anti-$Fc_\gamma R_{p50-70}$ MAb 3G8 to block immune complex clearance in the chimpanzee led Clarkson et al. (27) to test the therapeutic usefulness of the MAb for patients with immune thrombocytopenic purpura (ITP). In the one reported case, infusion of 3G8 at 1 mg/kg in a patient with refractory ITP led to a dramatic increase to normal levels in circulating platelets, which subsided in about 2 weeks. A second infusion of MAb 3G8 led to a smaller, but still clinically significant, increase in platelet number. In this patient there was also prolongation of the clearance $T_\frac{1}{2}$. Although the dramatic increases in platelet number were limited in time, the patient stabilized at a somewhat higher platelet number and once again became responsive to intravenous γ-globulin. However, it remains to be determined if it is a practical therapy in the more general sense.

The analysis of all the factors that modulate or enhance phagocytosis mediated by IgG or other ligands clearly will keep immunologists and cell biologists occupied for some time to come. Ehlenberger and Nussenzweig (45) demonstrated a synergistic effect of complement and IgG on phagocytosis by macrophages. Loos (112) and Heinz et al. (66) have reported that C1q on macrophages functions as an $Fc_\gamma R$, based on inhibition of the binding of erythrocytes coated with IgG by polyvalent and monoclonal anti-C1q antibodies and F(ab')$_2$ fragments thereof. These results are echoed in the work of Bobak et al. (21), who found that C1q-coated surfaces markedly enhance the phagocytosis of IgG-opsonized targets by monocytes. The stimulation is blocked by anti-C1q F(ab')$_2$ and is not seen for PMNs. That these interactions are significant is suggested by the results of Hamada and Greene (64), who found that C1q enhances IgG-dependent killing of *Schistosoma mansoni*. The collagenous domain of C1q is thought to be responsible for the enhanced killing and phagocytosis seen in the two systems.

Murine Receptors for IgG

The mouse, like man, has a wealth of complexity in FcγRs, with many unanswered questions remaining. Previous work, reviewed by Dickler (38) and Unkeless et al. (180), led to the identification of three receptors on mouse leukocytes. There is a high-avidity FcγR specific for murine IgG2a (Fcγ2aR) that is found only on macrophages (179). The Fcγ2aR is somewhat trypsin-sensitive (177). Diamond and Scharff (34) and Unkeless (178) demonstrated a second FcγR specific for IgG2b and IgG1 (Fcγ2b/γ1R), and Diamond and Yelton (35) characterized an FcγR specific for IgG3 (Fcγ3R). The identification of these receptors was accomplished by competition experiments, in which the binding of ligands (usually erythrocytes coated with monoclonal anti-erythrocyte antibody) was inhibited by addition of aggregated Ig of different subclasses and by inhibition studies using proteolytic enzymes or an anti-FcγR MAb 2.4G2 (178).

The assignment of specificity for the FcγR recognized by 2.4G2 as IgG2b/IgG1 may be too narrow. It is clear from several reports that MAb 2.4G2 recognizes, in addition to a low-affinity receptor on macrophages, an analogous receptor on lymphocytes (14,101,144,172). In these studies, however, the receptor reactive with MAb 2.4G2 bound IgG1, IgG2b, *and* IgG2a, in contrast to the reports on mouse macrophages, where the FcγR reactive with MAb 2.4G2 was found not to bind mouse IgG2a. The lymphocyte/macrophage FcγR has now been cloned (see below) and expressed in non-FcγR-bearing cells. The results unequivocally demonstrate (R. Weinshank, J. V. Ravetch, and J. C. Unkeless, *unpublished results*) that the receptor binds, with low avidity, IgG2b, IgG1, and IgG2a. The IgG2a-specific high-avidity trypsin-sensitive FcγR on macrophages probably masked the weaker IgG2a binding activity detected with the transfected receptor and on lymphocytes, which lack the high-avidity FcγR.

The evidence from cloning studies to date suggests that macrophage and lymphocyte receptors reactive with MAb 2.4G2 are, in their extracellular domains, identical in protein sequence. However, studies by Kulczycki et al. (93), suggested that the FcγR on mouse suppressor T-cell hybridomas, which react with the anti-FcγR MAb 2.4G2, differ in specificity from those on B-cells, as the receptor from the T-cell hybridomas does not bind either IgG3 or IgG2a. The size of the T-cell receptor from ^{125}I-labeled cells was M_r 56,000 to 61,000, which is consistent with previous reports of the size of the FcγR isolated from the S49.1 T-cell line by Mellman and Unkeless (123). The biochemical bases for these differences in specificity are unclear but are likely to be due to differences in posttranslational modification rather than different genes.

One of the more intriguing results is the demonstration by two independent groups (70,74) that the Ly-17 locus

defines a polymorphism of the FcγR recognized by MAb 2.4G2. Ly-17 antisera block FcγR activity and were used, in combination with MAb 2.4G2, in preclearing experiments that show that both sera recognize different determinants on the same molecules. It is of interest because Ly-17 [called Ly-m20.2 earlier by Mark et al. (115)] is tightly linked to Mls. Disparities at Mls trigger strong mixed lymphocyte reaction mitogenic responses but do not generate cytotoxic T-cells. Ly-17 maps to the distal arm of chromosome 1, as does the gene for cloned murine FcγR (150). These results seem to be contradictory to the results of Baum et al. (14), who found that a polymorphism of murine B-cell FcγR that results in an altered affinity for rat IgG mapped to chromosome 12 distal to the Igh locus. Perhaps secondary binding sites, such as the C1q interaction discussed earlier, account for these results.

Progress on the characterization of the Fcγ2aR and Fcγ3R has been slow. Lane and Cooper (100) isolated, by affinity chromatography, Fcγ binding proteins from IgG2a, IgG1, and IgG2b immunoadsorbents and found the IgG2a-binding proteins were somewhat more acidic and slightly different in size from the proteins that bound to IgG2b and IgG1. There is nothing reported on the characterization of the proteins responsible for IgG3 binding.

In addition to the studies of Nose and Wigzell (133) and Leatherbarrow et al. (108) indicating that oligosaccharide is important in the maintenance of the conformation required for interaction with FcγR, Diamond et al. (36) have used a series of switch variants to examine the domains that interact with the various FcγR on mouse macrophages. They concluded that IgG2b binds via the C_H2 domain, as a mutant IgG2b with a deleted C_H3 still bound to the Fcγ2b/γ1R. Another mutant with an IgG2b-like C_H2 domain and an IgG2a-like C_H3 domain bound to both Fcγ2aR and Fcγ2b/γ1R. Clearly the situation is complex, however, because in a later paper (19) they described a mutant with an IgG2b-like CH1 and hinge region and an IgG2a-like C_H2 and C_H3 region, which does not bind to Fcγ2aR, although the Fc fragment of the mutant IgG did. The level of discrimination of the Fcγ2aR and the Fcγ2b/γ1R is remarkable. Diamond et al. (37) looked at the inhibition of rosetting of EIgG2a and EIgG2b to macrophages by cyanogen bromide (CNBr) fragments of IgG2a and IgG2b. Specific inhibition was found for IgG2a and IgG2b by homologous CNBr fragments from the C_H2 domain of the respective antibodies. The inhibitory CNBr peptides from IgG2a and IgG2b differed by only four residues in 62 amino acids. Only one peptide from IgG2b was inhibitory, but two IgG2a peptides, one from the C_H2 domain and one from the C_H3 domain, were inhibitory for EIgG2a binding. These results suggest that there may be two domains that are involved in separate binding sites for the $Fc_{\gamma 2a}R$. Binding of both IgG2a CNBr peptides was sensitive to trypsin, as would have been predicted from previous studies.

Function of Murine $Fc_\gamma R$

In contrast to some other receptor–ligand systems, e.g., the transferrin receptor and the asialoglycoprotein receptor, following internalization of immune aggregates the murine $Fc_\gamma R$ reactive with MAb 2.4G2 apparently does not recycle. Mellman et al. (124) found that as much as 50% of macrophage $Fc_\gamma R$ could be driven inside the cell by presentation of IgG-sensitized erythrocyte ghosts, and the amount of $Fc_\gamma R$ on the cell surface remained depressed for many hours, whereas a series of other plasma membrane antigens was unaffected. Furthermore, the $T_{\frac{1}{2}}$ of the ^{125}I-labeled $Fc_\gamma R$ internalized along with immune complexes was 2 hr compared to a $T_{\frac{1}{2}}$ of 10 hr in the absence of ligand.

Evidence from several groups has suggested that $Fc_\gamma Rs$ bound with monomeric ligand (i.e., IgG) do not deliver ligand to the endosomal compartment but, rather, recycle with bound antibody (86,95). The determining factor in whether bound ligand is cleared to the lysosomes seems to be the valence of the complex. Monomers and dimers were poorly internalized, whereas larger complexes were efficiently catabolized. Ukkonen et al. (176), Mellman et al. (123), and Mellman and Plutner (121) demonstrated that monomeric 2.4G2 Fab fragment is not taken into lysosomes and degraded, but it cycles with the receptor through the endocytic compartment and is found in low-density endosomes. Pointing out once again the importance of valence, when the 2.4G2 Fab was rendered multivalent by adsorption to colloidal gold it again was transferred to the lysosomal compartment.

The $Fc_\gamma R$ recognized by MAb 2.4G2, like the human $Fc_\gamma R_{p50-70}$ described previously, is a low-avidity receptor that binds monomeric IgG poorly. Studies by Kurlander et al. (97) and Kurlander and Hall (96) have established that this $Fc_\gamma R$ is involved in the clearance of immune complexes, as infusion of MAb 2.4G2 in mice was a potent inhibitor of this $Fc_\gamma R$ function. It is, however, difficult to assign functions to the different receptors, as all of them often coexist on the same macrophage and as the isotype specificity discussed previously is relative, not absolute. Ralph et al. (201) found that all classes of murine IgG mediate phagocytosis and lysis of erythrocytes, but to extrapolate from that experimental result to the conclusion that all $Fc_\gamma Rs$ mediate phagocytosis may not be warranted.

One system in which there does exist some evidence for activity attributable to specific subclass is in antibody-dependent cytotoxicity mediated by thioglycollate-elicited macrophages. Results of Matthews et al. (117) and Herlyn and Koprowski (68) implicate IgG2a as the subclass of IgG that mediates macrophage cytotoxicity. In these studies both groups used either an *in vivo* nude mouse model or a homologous animal tumor model to demonstrate protection, which gives these results validity greater than might be obtained with *in vitro* experiments. Langlois et al. (102) have also developed an *in vitro* model that mimics the *in vivo* results on the efficacy of IgG2a antibody. Nathan et al. (130), however, found that MAb 2.4G2 inhibits ADCC mediated by BCG-stimulated macrophages 70%, which implicates the low-avidity macrophage $Fc_\gamma R$ as well as the high-avidity $Fc_{\gamma 2a}R$ implicated by the results discussed above by Matthews et al. (117) and Herlyn and Koprowski (68).

The function of $Fc_\gamma R$ on B-cells is still not clear. The studies of Phillips and Parker (142–144) seem to suggest that immune complexes *in vivo* would be inhibitory for B-cell differentiation and that anti-idiotypic antibodies reactive with surface Ig, if they bind to $Fc_\gamma R$, would also be inhibitory. They observed, as had others, that rabbit anti-μ IgG would not trigger a mitogenic B-cell response, although the $F(ab')_2$ fragment was stimulatory. However, if the $Fc_\gamma R$ was occupied by MAb 2.4G2, the intact rabbit anti-μ antibody was stimulatory. Thus they concluded that for anti-μ antibody to effectively inhibit a mitogenic B-cell response it must form a ternary complex with the surface Ig and $Fc_\gamma R$. How the formation of this ternary complex differs from binding of the anti-$Fc_\gamma R$ MAb with respect to $Fc_\gamma R$ signaling is unclear.

The mechanism for transduction of the signal by ligation of the $Fc_\gamma R$ is suggested to involve depolarization. Young et al. (206) used tetraphenyl phosphonium ion to measure depolarization of macrophages in response to immune complexes and found that there was a progressive depolarization in response to the increased size of the complexes. Similar results were found with membrane vesicles, and the depolarization was assigned to an inward Na^+ flow (207). However, Wilson et al. (186) did not find any depolarization of B-cells by $Fc_\gamma R$ cross-linking but reported a lower Ca^{2+} and inositol triphosphate elevation in response to anti-Ig. Nelson et al. (131), studying human alveolar macrophages by patch clamping techniques, reported large ion channels induced by aggregated immunoglobulin. The channels were cation-specific, without selectivity for Na^+ relative to K^+, similar to the studies of Young et al. (208), in which purified $Fc_\gamma R$ was incorporated into planar lipid bilayers and current measured in a voltage clamp apparatus in response to ligand. In view of the complexity revealed in the cloning studies (see below), further study of the contributions of each individual receptor are clearly warranted.

Cloning Studies

Murine $Fc_\gamma Rs$ have now been cloned by three groups, which should lead to rapid progress in elucidation of the relation between structure and function for these important molecules. The results from the various laboratories are in substantial agreement (71,73,109,150). Fc$_\gamma$R is another member of the immunoglobulin gene superfamily, with closest homology to class II histocompatibility antigens. Following a leader sequence there is an extracellular portion that consists of two repeated immunoglobulin-like domains. Each domain, of approximately 85 amino acids, has two sites for *N*-linked oligosaccharide, and two cysteine residues, which are separated by 42 and 45 amino acids. This finding is in good agreement with the experimental evidence of Green et al. (57) demonstrating four *N*-linked glycosylation sites. The external repeated domains show homology to immunoglobulins, MHC class I and II products, β_2-microglobulin, and other members of the immunoglobulin supergene family. The most striking homology, however, is to the β_2 domain of the Eβ class II gene, with 32% homology over 91 amino acid stretch. The Fc$_\gamma$R has a single transmembrane hydrophobic domain, and a cytoplasmic domain.

The method used by Ravetch et al. (150) to clone the Fc$_\gamma$R was to construct an oligonucleotide probe based on *N*-terminal sequence of protein purified by affinity chromatography on MAb 2.4G2-Sepharose. This method resulted in the isolation of two Fc$_\gamma$R genes, termed α and β. These two genes show a 95% homology when the extracellular immunoglobulin-like region is examined, but there is a complete lack of homology in the leader sequences, the transmembrane and cytoplasmic domains, and in the 3' and 5' noncoding region of the complementary DNA (cDNA). The α gene transcript is found only in macrophage cell lines and was not detected in any Fc$_\gamma$R-positive B-cell or T-cell line examined, whereas the β gene is found in all Fc$_\gamma$R-positive lines examined to date. It is clear from transfection experiments that the β gene encodes the 2.4G2 MAb determinant, as cloning of the β cDNA into the pcEXV-3 eukaryotic expression vector followed by transfection into a mouse melanoma cell resulted in expression of Fc$_\gamma$R inhibited by MAb 2.4G2. Also, Lewis et al. (109) found that a B-cell mutant lacking Fc$_\gamma$R lacks the β gene transcript. The function of the α gene is under study. The element of macrophage specificity makes the identification of the α gene product as high-avidity Fc$_{\gamma 2a}$R an attractive hypothesis.

In addition to the presence of two different genes, Ravetch et al. (150) also found evidence for differential messenger RNA (mRNA) processing. Two β gene (β_1 and β_2) transcripts were found, identical save for a 138-nucleotide insertion in the cytoplasmic domain. The 138-nucleotide insertion would code for an additional 46 amino acids, and tryptic fragments with sequence in this area were in fact found, ruling out a cloning artifact. In addition, ribonuclease protection experiments demonstrated the presence of both transcripts in all Fc$_\gamma$R-positive B- and T-cell lines but only the smaller of the two β transcripts

(β_2) in macrophages. The functions of the transmembrane and cytoplasmic domains of the α and β receptors are not understood, but it seems likely that, given the striking differences, there are also differences in the types of signal transmitted to the cell. The significance of the insertion of 46 amino acids in the β_1 compared to the β_2 transcripts likewise is not understood. However, one may expect rapid progress in all these areas with the availability of the cloned genes and the ability to transfect them or mutations thereof into various cell types. Detailed study of the interaction of Fc$_\gamma$R, a member of the immunoglobulin gene superfamily, with IgG may provide a fascinating glimpse into the parallel evolution of ligand–receptor systems.

RECEPTORS FOR COMPLEMENT

Ligands of Complement Receptors

Activation of the complement cascade with resultant proteolytic cleavages liberates several potential ligands for receptors on leukocytes (Table 1). These ligands may be divided into two categories: (a) soluble ligands, which cause chemotactic movement of leukocytes to sites of complement activation; and (b) surface-bound ligands, which function as opsonins. Receptors for the soluble fragments C3a and C5a are described elsewhere in this text and are not addressed here. Essentially all of the opsonic activity of complement resides in the surface-bound fragments of C3 and receptors for these fragments (Table 2) are the principal focus of this section.

C3 is the most abundant complement protein in serum (1.3 mg/ml), and it can be deposited on target particles by either of two pathways: (a) the classic pathway, which is activated by prior binding of immune IgG or IgM to the target; or (b) the alternative pathway, which is antibody-independent. Both pathways initiate a remarkable reaction that causes C3 to bind covalently to the target (103). Upon proteolytic activation, an internal thioester bond in C3 is rearranged to yield a free sulfhydryl group on C3 (83) and an ester link between C3 and a hydroxyl group on the target (105) (Fig. 1). The resulting covalently bound molecule is termed C3b and is recognized by a receptor termed CR1 (complement receptor type 1). After C3b is deposited on the surface of particles that activate the classic pathway, its lifetime is short (132). The α chain of C3b is cleaved in minutes by the combined action of the binding protein, factor H, and the enzyme, factor I (C3b inactivator) (104) to yield iC3b, a form that is stable in serum for several hours. However, if C3b is deposited on the surface of an alternative pathway-activating particle, a fraction of the C3b resists the action of factor I and may survive in serum for more than an hour (132). Thus the dominant fragment of C3 displayed depends on the nature of the particle to which it is attached.

TABLE 1. *Complement proteins recognized by receptors on leukocytes*

Protein	Receptor	Cell type	Function	Comments
C3a	C3a receptor	MC, PMN	Secretion	Ligand is soluble
C5a	C5a receptor	MC, PMN	Chemotaxis/secretion	Ligand is soluble
C1q	C1q receptor	MC	?	[a]
C3b/C4b	CR1	MC, MO, PMN	Phagocytosis	Enhances cleavage of C3b by factor I
C3bi	CR3	MC, MO, PMN	Phagocytosis	Also recognizes LPS
C3dg	CR2	B-lymphocytes	?	EBV receptor
C3dg	CR4	PMNs, platelets	?	

[a] C1qrs is deposited; then C1r and C1s are removed by the action of the C1 inhibitor to yield exposed C1q (173). MC = monocyte. MO = macrophage. PMN = polymorphonuclear leukocyte.

If particles coated with C3b, iC3b, or both are not removed by phagocytes, the C3 is converted to C3dg by the further action of factor I. Although phagocytes have been reported to express receptors for C3dg (termed CR4) (181,182), these receptors have not been shown to mediate phagocytosis or clearance. C3dg is also recognized by a receptor on B-lymphocytes termed CR2 (44,81,156,184). This receptor serves as the site of attachment of Epstein-Barr virus (EBV) to B-cells (49) and may function together with receptors for cytokines to control the proliferation of B-cells (120).

Complement protein C4 is structurally homologous to C3 and binds to surfaces in a similar covalent fashion (106). C4b is recognized by CR1 (30), but it is not degraded further to biologically active fragments.

Structure and Cellular Distribution of Complement Receptors

CR1

CR1 binds dimeric C3b with an affinity of $\sim 5 \times 10^7$ M^{-1} (13). Native, uncleaved C3 is not recognized (15), nor is C3dg. C3bi is recognized by CR1 (119), but this binding is weak and may not be of physiological importance. Although the binding affinity of CR1 appears to be low in comparison with receptors for hormones, phagocytes normally encounter particles coated with hundreds or thousands of C3b molecules, and effective binding is ensured by the ensuing multivalent interaction.

CR1 is a glycosylated protein with a molecular weight between 160 and 250 kD. In the human population, four allelic forms of CR1 have been described with molecular weights of 160, 190, 220, and 250 kD (41–43,190). These alleles are expressed in a co-dominant fashion, and thus individuals may be either homozygous and express CR1 of a single molecular weight or heterozygous and express CR1 of two distinct molecular weights. The large heterogeneity in molecular weight is not the result of variant patterns of glycosylation (113,190) but derives from alternative polypeptide structures (see below). The expression of any one allele has yet to be linked with functional abnormalities or enhanced susceptibility to disease.

The gene for CR1 has been cloned and partially sequenced by Fearon and co-workers (90,188,189). The protein is predicted to have a single membrane-spanning domain of 25 amino acids and a short cytoplasmic C-terminal domain of 43 amino acids. The large extracellular domain is comprised of at least 30 repeated units arranged in tandem. Each of these small consensus repeats (SCRs) encompasses 60 to 70 amino acids. Variation is observed in the length and sequence among the 30 SCRs, but 29 of the 60 to 70 amino acids are highly conserved, and the location of four half-cysteines is invariant. The cysteines within an SCR are thought to be joined to one another and not to cysteines in neighboring SCRs, thereby causing each SCR to be a rigid, cross-linked unit.

The consensus sequence observed in SCRs is found in additional proteins beyond CR1. For example, factor H contains 20 copies of this repeated domain, C4 binding protein has eight copies, CR2 has four copies, factor B and C2 each have three copies, clotting factor XIIIb has 10 copies, and the interleukin-2 (IL-2) receptor has two copies. (See ref. 151 for a review of these findings.) Al-

TABLE 2. *Receptors for bound fragments of C3*

Receptor	Ligands	Cellular distribution	Ion requirements
CR1	C3b, C4b	PMNs, monocytes, macrophages, glomerular podocytes, lymphocytes	None
CR3	C3bi, LPS	PMNs, monocytes, macrophages	Ca^{2+} and Mg^{2+}
CR2	C3bi, C3dg	B-lymphocytes	None
CR4	C3bi, C3dg	PMNs, B-lymphocytes, platelets	None

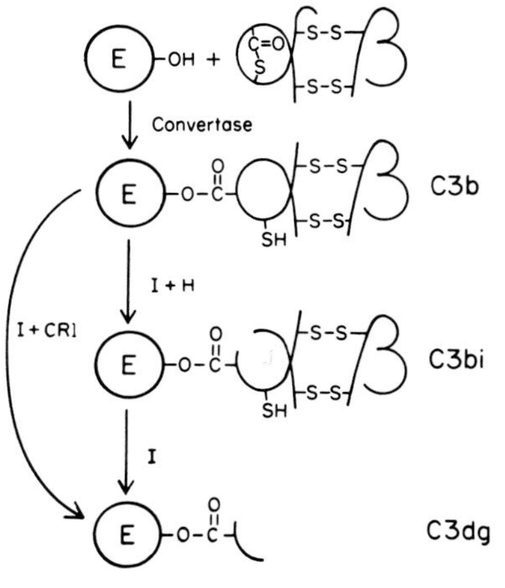

FIG. 1. Active fragments of bound C3. The α and β chains of C3 are represented by the corresponding characters. Upon proteolytic activation, C3 binds to hydroxyl groups on the surface of an erythrocyte (E) or other particulate substance. The resulting surface-bound C3b is subsequently degraded to C3bi and C3dg.

though several of these proteins share the capacity to bind C3b or C4b, others do not, and the functional significance of the SCRs remains unclear.

An additional, larger, repeat pattern is also observed in the extracellular domain of CR1 (90). At least four tandem repeats of 450 amino acids are visible, each in turn composed of seven SCRs. These "long homologous repeats" (LHRs) are similar in sequence to one another (70–99% identical) and may form the basis for the different allelic forms of CR1: It is hypothesized that the 160-kD receptor contains four LHRs, the 190 kD contains five LHRs, etc. The LHRs might also represent individual binding domains for C3b, but to date there is no information regarding the functional significance of LHRs.

CR1 functions as an opsonin receptor, and it is therefore not surprising that it is found on all phagocytic leukocytes (monocytes, PMNs, macrophages) (47). In addition, CR1 is expressed on erythrocytes, a subpopulation of lymphocytes (187), and glomerular podocytes (88). The function of the receptor in the latter cells is uncertain but may be related to the observation that CR1 functions as a cofactor in the breakdown of its ligand, C3b (80). As mentioned above, factor I cleaves C3b to C3bi, and this cleavage is accelerated when C3b is complexed with the serum factor H. Upon binding to C3b, CR1 also accelerates the cleavage by factor I. Because the cleaved C3b cannot participate in the amplification of the alternative pathway, this cleavage serves to dampen alternative pathway activity and may act to prevent gratuitous complement deposition on host cells. It should also be noted that the cleavage of C3b promoted by CR1 is not to C3bi but to C3dg (119) (Fig. 1). Thus CR1 may function to prevent the generation of C3bi.

CR3

CR3 recognizes C3bi but does not recognize either the precursor, C3b, or the product of further cleavage, C3dg (24,154,197). Binding of monomeric or dimeric C3bi to CR3 has not been reported, presumably because of a low binding affinity, and the above statements on the specificity of the receptor rest primarily on studies of the binding of particles coated with defined complement fragments to CR3-bearing cells. These particles, usually sheep erythrocytes, bear 10^4 to 10^5 C3bi per erythrocyte, and the resulting multivalent interaction with phagocytes is avid.

In contrast with other opsonin receptors (CR1, FcR), CR3 requires relatively high concentrations of divalent cations (about 0.5 mM Ca and Mg) in order to interact effectively with ligand (197). In addition, the binding capacity of CR3 is temperature-dependent and is absent in cells held at 5°C (194).

The region of the C3bi molecule that is recognized by CR3 has been defined by the use of synthetic peptides (204). CR3 binds particles coated with a 21-amino-acid peptide that spans residues 1383 to 1403 of C3. This peptide contains the triplet Arg-Gly-Asp (RGD) in its midsection. As discussed below, the RGD triplet serves as a recognition structure for many receptors involved in cell adhesion events, and CR3 thus appears to be a member of a larger family of adhesion-promoting receptors.

CR3 is composed of two polypeptides, an α of 185 kD and a β of 95 kD, noncovalently linked as $α_1β_1$ dimers (163,164,203). Both chains are exposed at the cell surface. Two lines of evidence suggest that the binding site for C3bi is located, at least in part, on the α polypeptide. First, monoclonal antibodies directed against the α polypeptide have been raised, and a subset of these antibodies block the binding of C3bi, whereas antibodies against the β chain do not (203). Further evidence for the role of the α chain in the binding of C3bi comes from observations of the β chain in dimeric association with alternative α chains. Antibodies against the β chain immunoprecipitate three distinct $α_1β_1$ dimers from macrophages. One is CR3, a second is a molecule termed LFA-1, and the third is termed p150,95 (Fig. 2). The β chains in LFA-1 and p150,95 are identical with those in CR3, but the α chains are structurally and antigenically distinct (163). Neither

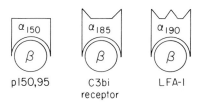

FIG. 2. LFA-1, CR3, p150,95 family of leukocyte antigens. Each protein is a dimer composed of a unique α chain in association with a β chain that is identical in all three proteins.

LFA-1 nor p150,95 recognizes C3bi (194), and because both of these receptors express β chain it is unlikely that the β chain binds C3bi.

CR3: Relation to the Leukocyte Antigens LFA-1 and p150,95

CR3, LFA-1, and p150,95 comprise a family of leukocyte proteins, the properties of which are described in Table 3. Several observations suggest that the CR3/LFA family functions in cell–cell and cell–substrate adhesion. CR3 mediates the adhesion of C3bi-coated particles to phagocytes. LFA-1 appears to mediate the adhesion between cytolytic T-cells (91,162), NK cells (126), and tumorilytic macrophages (168) and their respective targets. Monoclonal antibodies against LFA-1 block each of these cytotoxicity phenomena by interfering with the binding of killer to target (116). The LFA-1-mediated binding of cytolytic lymphocytes to targets is similar to the binding of CR3 to C3bi in that divalent cations and warm temperatures are required (166). A unique function for p150,95 has not yet been described.

Additional evidence for the function of CR3, LFA-1, and p150,95 in adhesion phenomena comes from observations on more than 20 patients that exhibit a genetic deficiency in the CR3/LFA family (11,12). These patients present with recurrent life-threatening infections. Phagocytes from these patients fail to bind C3bi-coated particles (9) and show defective cytocidal activity in vitro (125). All of the patients exhibit neutrophilia but fail to form pus at sites of infection (10), and PMNs from these patients fail to adhere to protein-coated glass surfaces and to endothelial cells in vitro (65). Thus CR3, LFA-1, and p150,95 appear essential for defense against infectious agents and for emigration of leukocytes from the vasculature.

CR3, LFA-1, and p150,95: Relation to Adhesion-Promoting Receptors on Other Cells

Work from several laboratories indicates that there exists a large family of structurally homologous proteins that promote cell adhesion (78,159). This family includes the fibronectin receptor (147), vitronectin receptor (146), platelet glycoproteins IIb and IIIa (54,148), and the VLA antigen series (67). All of these receptors mediate cell adhesion, all share the capacity to recognize protein ligands that contain the sequence Arg-Gly-Asp (RGD), and all require divalent cations. CR3 also shares these properties, as it promotes the attachment of cells to surface-bound ligands by recognizing an RGD-containing region of C3bi (204), and this recognition requires divalent cations (197). CR3 also appears to be structurally related to the other RGD-recognizing proteins, as all of these proteins consist of a noncovalently linked dimer of glycoproteins having molecular masses in the range of 95 to 190 kD. Finally, evidence (89,107) indicates substantial sequence homology between the β chain of the CR3/LFA-1 family and one of the chains of a fibronectin receptor (169). Because LFA-1 and p150,95 have β chains that are identical to that of CR3 and function in cell adhesion, they are also likely to be members of the family of RGD-recognizing cell adhesion molecules.

CR3: Recognition of Ligands Other than C3bi

Several workers have discovered that antibodies against CR3 not only inhibited the binding of C3bi-coated particles but also partially inhibited binding of particles such as zymosan (46,155), Leishmania (20,129), and Staphylococcus (157). Because these binding experiments were performed in the absence of a source of complement, it was proposed that CR3 interacts not with C3bi but with the particles directly. Further support for this idea came from the observation that patients who are deficient in CR3, LFA-1, and p150,95 exhibited defective recognition of zymosan (157) and Escherichia coli (S. D. Wright, unpublished observations), again in the absence of serum opsonins.

More detailed experiments have indicated that CR3, LFA-1, and p150,95 each share the capacity to directly bind the microbes Histoplasma capsulatum (23) and E. coli (194). In these experiments individual receptors were

TABLE 3. Adhesion-promoting receptors of leukocytes

Receptor	mAbs against α chain	Cellular distribution	Function
CR3	OKM1, OKM10, 44a	Monocytes, macrophages	C3bi receptor
		PMNs	LPS receptor
LFA-1	TA-1, TS1/22	Monocytes, macrophages	NK target binding
		PMNs, T- and B-cells	T-cell target binding
			MO tumor binding
			LPS receptor
p150,95	LeuM5, 3.9	Monocytes, macrophages	?
		PMNs	LPS receptor

removed from the macrophage membrane by allowing the cells to spread on surfaces derivatized with specific anti-receptor monoclonal antibodies. The receptors diffuse in the plane of the membrane and are trapped by antibody at the basal surface of the macrophage, leaving the apical surface devoid of a particular receptor. By this means it was shown that removal of all three receptors—CR3, LFA-1, and p150,95—caused inhibition of the binding of microbes, but binding is still observed if any one of these receptors is present. Thus each of these homologous receptors is individually capable of binding to *H. capsulatum* and *E. coli*. The observation that CR3, LFA-1, and p150,95 may bind directly to microbes without the intervention of antibody or complement suggests a novel mechanism by which macrophages may recognize potential pathogens before the onset of adaptive immunity.

CR3, LFA-1, and p150,95 Recognition of Bacterial Lipopolysaccharide

The binding of *E. coli* by CR3, LFA-1, and p150,95 exhibits the same dependence on divalent cations and warm temperatures as does the binding of C3bi-coated particles by CR3 (194). However, the chemical nature of the ligands on *E. coli* are different from the protein C3bi. Macrophages bind *E. coli* by recognizing the most prevalent molecule on the surface of the bacterium, lipopolysaccharide (LPS) (194). The portion of the LPS molecule that is recognized is the lipid A region, which consists of a fatty-acylated diglucosamine biphosphate. Because the fatty acids of lipid A are buried in the outer membrane of the bacterium, it is likely that the diglucosamine phosphate provides the recognition structure bound by CR3, LFA-1, and p150,95. It is also likely that sugar phosphates on the surface of *H. capsulatum,* zymosan, and *Leishmania* account for their recognition by these receptors.

Bacterial LPS (endotoxin) causes profound physiological effects in man and animals, including fever, shock, and induction of the acute-phase response (128). The cell type primarily responsible for these effects is the macrophage that synthesizes large amounts of interleukin-1 and tumor necrosis factor (TNF) cachectin in response to LPS (18,40). The experiments described above indicate that CR3, LFA-1, and p150,95 can bind LPS, but whether these receptors directly mediate the many biological effects of LPS is not yet certain.

Cellular Distribution of CR3

CR3 is expressed on all phagocytic leukocytes. Monocytes express high levels of CR3, which increase further during maturation of monocytes to macrophages, and CR3 has been detected on all mature macrophage pop-

ulations (peritoneal macrophages, splenic macrophages, Kuppfer cells) so far examined (S. D. Wright, *unpublished observations*). Resting PMNs express relatively little CR3 per cell, but these phagocytes possess a large intracellular pool of receptors that can be rapidly externalized upon stimulation with chemotactic agents, phorbol esters, or isolation procedures (see following).

Unlike CR1, CR3 is not found on lymphocytes or erythrocytes. It is also noteworthy that CR3 does not act as a cofactor to hasten the cleavage of C3bi by factor I; thus unlike CR1, CR3 is not capable of protecting cells from the action of the alternative pathway.

Function of Complement Receptors

The principal role for CR3 is to mediate the uptake of infectious microorganisms. This conclusion derives from observations of patients who are genetically deficient in C3 (32) or CR3 (11,12). Both types of patient suffer recurrent, life-threatening infections caused by a variety of organisms. CR1 is also likely to have an important function in the clearance of pathogens, but to date no CR1 deficiencies have been recognized.

Regulation of the Function of Complement Receptors

In order for a receptor to successfully mediate phagocytosis, it must perform two tasks. The first is to bind the ligand and thereby attach a ligand-coated particle to the phagocyte. This function is subserved by the extracellular domain of a transmembrane receptor protein. The second task is to signal the cell to elaborate pseudopods that engulf the attached particle. This function is presumably mediated by the cytoplasmic domain of an opsonic receptor. Experiments indicate that both the binding and the signaling functions of C3 receptors are regulated in phagocytic leukocytes.

Binding step

One of the principal cytokines that influence macrophage function is γ-interferon, and studies show that γ-interferon regulates complement receptors on mononuclear phagocytes in an unexpected fashion (201). CR1 and CR3 on resting human monocytes and macrophages avidly mediate binding of the corresponding ligand-coated erythrocyte. Half-maximal binding occurs with about 15,000 C3b per erythrocyte and about 5,000 C3bi per erythrocyte (197). Culture of the phagocytes for 48 hr with γ-interferon (but not α-interferon) causes a striking decrease in the binding capacity of C3 receptors: Half-maximal binding of erythrocytes is not obtained even with 120,000 C3b or C3bi per erythrocyte (201). This result contrasts with the behavior of Fc receptors in that γ-interferon causes dramatically enhanced expression of $Fc_\gamma R_{p72}$ (63) and enhanced binding of IgG-coated erythrocytes (201).

The reduced binding activity of CR1 and CR3 in γ-interferon-treated cells is not associated with changes in the number of cell surface receptor molecules, nor is it associated with proteolytic inactivation of the receptors (201). Rather, depression of binding activity of CR1 and CR3 by γ-interferon appears to be caused by reversible changes in the conformation of existing receptors. This point is emphasized by the observation that the binding capacity of C3 receptors can be fully restored within minutes by allowing the phagocytes to interact with surfaces coated with the extracellular matrix protein fibronectin (see following).

The physiological significance of this "deactivation" of C3 receptors by γ-interferon is not currently clear, but γ-interferon can be expected to shut off complement receptor activity on all macrophages except those in contact with the appropriate extracellular matrix components. Because γ-interferon-treated macrophages possess extremely potent cytolytic activity, such a shutoff may prevent unwanted cytolysis. The observation that receptors may exist in a form that cannot bind ligand suggests that assays of ligand binding are poor indicators of the absence of receptors from a particular cell.

The binding activity of CR1 and CR3 on granulocytes is also regulated but in a manner different from that seen in mononuclear cells. Resting PMNs have low capacity to bind C3-coated particles. This binding activity is rapidly up-regulated by several agents including phorbol myristate acetate (PMA) and C5a. Though PMA is not a physiological stimulus, its activities are the best characterized and are described in detail below.

Stimulation of PMNs with PMA produces a biphasic response (196). During the first 10 min the capacity of CR1 and CR3 to bind (and phagocytose) C3b- and C3bi-coated erythrocytes is dramatically enhanced. During the following 30 min, the capacity to bind and phagocytose is depressed to levels below those shown by resting cells. The "activation" step that occurs during the first 10 min appears to be a process separable from the "deactivation" that occurs thereafter, and therefore the processes of activation and deactivation are described separately.

Activation. Treatment of PMNs with PMA or chemotactic factors causes a rapid rise in the expression of both CR1 and CR3 on the cell surface (16,48,87,135,175,196). Fusion of specific granules with the plasma membrane provides the newly expressed CR3 (135,175), but the source of the CR1 is not yet certain. The magnitude of the increase in surface CR1 and CR3 reported by different authors varies from two- to tenfold. A likely explanation for this apparent discrepancy is that the procedures used

for purifying PMNs are themselves capable of causing increases in receptor expression (48), and spreading of PMNs on culture dishes causes further increases. Thus purified, adherent PMNs show relatively small changes in surface expression of CR1 and CR3 after stimulation.

Though increased expression of CR1 and CR3 is temporally associated with the enhanced capacity to bind and ingest C3-coated particles caused by PMA, an increased number of receptors is unlikely to be responsible for either the increased binding or the phagocytosis. During activation of adherent PMNs by PMA, the attachment of C3bi-coated erythrocytes increases eight- to tenfold, and phagocytosis increases 30- to 40-fold, whereas the number of CR3 per cell increases only threefold (196). Because other studies have shown that the attachment of ligand-coated erythrocytes increases linearly with increases in the number of cell-surface receptors (127), these results suggest that the receptors on the resting PMNs bind C3bi inefficiently with respect to CR3 on stimulated cells. The inefficient binding activity of CR3 on resting cells cannot be overcome by increasing the concentration of ligand on the C3bi-coated erythrocyte (196). Thus it appears that CR3 on resting cells is functionally inactive, and that PMA enhances binding and phagocytosis of C3bi-coated particles by a combination of two effects: an increase in the number of cell surface CR3 and a change in the nature of the CR3 that allows it to efficiently bind surface-bound ligands and to promote phagocytosis.

PMA causes a 30-fold increase in the capacity of CR1 to promote phagocytosis. Because PMA increases surface CR1 only twofold, it causes a qualitative change in the behavior of CR1. The capacity of CR1 to bind ligand, however, does not appear to change in PMA-stimulated cells as the number of C3b/E required for half-maximal binding remains constant (196).

Deactivation. Incubation of activated PMNs with PMA for 65 min causes a six- to eightfold decrease in the capacity of CR1 to bind EC3b and a 12- to 20-fold decrease in the capacity of CR3 to bind EC3bi (196). Similarly, the capacity of both CR1 and CR3 to promote phagocytosis is eliminated during this time. Because the expression of cell surface CR3 does not change and the expression of CR1 decreases only twofold during this time, the loss of receptor activity appears not to be caused by decreased expression of receptor protein. Rather, PMA appears to cause a qualitative change in CR1 and CR3 that renders them incapable of either binding surface-bound C3 or promoting phagocytosis.

The physiological significance of this type of deactivation is not clear but may reflect the need of cells to detach from a ligand-coated surface. PMNs attach firmly to complement-coated epithelial cells, but the PMNs detach and migrate through the epithelium upon stimulation with the formylpeptide chemoattractant fMet-Leu-Phe

(31). Deactivation of adhesion-promoting receptors may permit locomotion by allowing successive rounds of adhesion to and detachment from the substrate. Deactivation may also prevent unwanted cytolytic interactions with host tissues unless an ancillary signal is received.

Engulfment step

The capacity of CR1 and CR3 to initiate the movement of pseudopods around a particle is also subject to physiological regulation. This regulation is most clearly shown in the human macrophage (197). CR1 and CR3 avidly mediate the attachment of C3-coated particles to these cells, but neither receptor is capable of promoting phagocytosis. However, the human macrophage can be stimulated in such a way that CR1 and CR3 are independently capable of efficiently promoting phagocytosis. Within minutes of being exposed to the tumor-promoting phorbol ester PMA, macrophages become capable of ingesting large numbers of C3b- and C3bi-coated erythrocytes (197). PMA affects only the ability of CR1 and CR3 to signal phagocytosis, not their ability to bind ligand. Furthermore, it affects the phagocytosis-promoting activities only of CR1 and CR3, not of Fc receptors.

Several naturally occurring substances are capable of activating the signaling capacity of CR1 and CR3. We consider first the insoluble stimuli and later the soluble stimuli.

Activation of C3 Receptors by Components of the Extracellular Matrix. Macrophages that are spread on human serum albumin or collagen exhibit low resting levels of C3b and C3bi receptor-mediated phagocytosis. However, when they spread on surfaces coated with fibronectin (145,200), serum amyloid P component (200), or laminin (22), their receptors are activated and they promote phagocytosis. Several aspects of this type of activation of C3 receptors are worthy of note. First, fibronectin and serum amyloid P that are covalently bound to the substrate can activate the phagocytosis-promoting capacity of C3 receptors that are located on the apical portion of the phagocyte (200). Thus it is clear that fibronectin and serum amyloid P are not acting as opsonins. Rather, these proteins act to regulate the activity of receptors for opsonins. Second, in order for fibronectin to activate C3 receptors, it *must* be bound to a substrate: Soluble fibronectin is not capable of activating C3 receptors (195,200).

Fibronectin, serum amyloid P, and laminin share the capacity to bind tightly to a variety of components of the extracellular matrix. Fibronectin is the best studied of these three molecules and has the most complicated spectrum of binding capabilities. It is an elongated molecule that possesses separate binding sites for collagen, heparin, fibrin, and bacteria (79). SAP is a disc-shaped decamer that binds to amyloid (136), to a 4,6-pyruvate acetal of galactose (a carbohydrate structure prevalent in some yeasts and bacterial cell walls) (72), and to components of the basement membrane (136). Laminin is a large (10^6 daltons) T-shaped molecule (174) that binds to type IV collagen (191), the collagen of basement membranes. Fibronectin, serum amyloid P, and laminin each function as components of the extracellular matrix at specialized locations in tissues. All three proteins are found in basal lamina and are attached to elastin fibers in loose connective tissue. Thus we may expect that macrophages in contact with basal lamina will have active C3 receptors. Of greater interest, however, is that fibronectin is present in high concentrations as a soluble molecule in plasma. This soluble fibronectin can rapidly bind to thrombi, bacteria, and denatured collagen. The binding capabilities of fibronectin allow it to target the phagocytic capacities of macrophages to select regions of the body where extra phagocytic potential may be required.

Fibronectin, laminin, and serum amyloid P presumably exert their effects by interacting with receptors on macrophages. As mentioned above, the fibronectin receptor of fibroblasts recognizes a region of fibronectin that contains the amino acid sequence Arg-Gly-Asp. Although the studies of Hosein and Bianco (75) suggested that the fibronectin receptor of macrophages is immunologically distinct from that on fibroblasts, the fibronectin receptor of macrophages does recognize Arg-Gly-Asp (195). Surface-bound synthetic peptides with this sequence readily activate CR1 and CR3 on macrophages. Furthermore, soluble, monomeric peptides competitively inhibit activation by surface-bound fibronectin. These experiments indicate that the activating effect of fibronectin is mediated by a receptor that recognizes the sequence Arg-Gly-Asp, and that fibronectin receptors must be cross-linked or immobilized in order to activate CR1 and CR3.

Soluble Activators of Complement Receptors. Complement receptors on macrophages may also be activated by soluble factors that are generated by stimulated T-lymphocytes. Griffin and colleagues have described a lymphokine of approximately 10 kD that activates the phagocytosis-promoting capacity of C3 receptors on murine peritoneal macrophages (59,62). A unique sequence of cellular interactions initiates release of this lymphokine. Upon ingestion of IgG-coated particles, macrophages elaborate a factor that in turn causes T-lymphocytes to secrete the lymphokine. The lymphokine appears to be different from other lymphokines, e.g., γ-interferon and interleukin-2, and cannot be elicited by classic mechanisms of lymphokine productions such as antigenic stimulation of appropriate T-cell clones (62). The lymphokine acts by binding to a fucosidase-sensitive receptor on macrophages (60).

The lymphokine studied by Griffin appears to function *in vivo* just as it does *in vitro* (61). Injection of immune complexes into the peritoneal cavity of mice activates the

C3 receptors of peritoneal macrophages. As is the case *in vitro*, T-lymphocytes are required for receptor activation as athymic mice did not exhibit this response. This means of activating C3 receptors may have special importance in situations in which Fc receptors are blockaded or overwhelmed by an excess of immune complexes.

Mechanisms by Which C3 Receptors Are Activated

The activation of C3 receptors on phagocytes poses an intriguing question in cell biology. How does ligation of one type of receptor (the receptor for lymphokine, fibronectin, or PMA) alter the behavior of a second type of receptor (CR1 or CR3)? The answer to this question is not in hand, but several solutions have been suggested.

Activation of C3 receptors for phagocytosis does not require protein synthesis, as activation by either lymphokine or PMA occurs in the presence of inhibitors of protein synthesis (62,197). Thus the manufacture of new receptors does not explain activation. Activation is not accompanied by changes in the number of cell surface receptors, as neither PMA nor fibronectin caused changes in the number of cell surface CR1s or CR3s (202). This observation suggested that activation is caused by a change in the nature of existing C3 receptors. Activation of C3 receptors is reversible. Observations with lymphokine, PMA, and fibronectin show that receptors can be switched from inactive to active and back in the course of an hour (62,202). Thus activation is not the result of irreversible modifications such as proteolysis.

What biochemical events could explain activation? Several observations suggest that phosphorylation may provide an answer. The time course, reversibility, and independence from protein synthesis of C3 receptor activation are consistent with the hypothesis that phosphorylation controls receptor activity. Furthermore, PMA is a potent activator of a Ca^{2+}-activated, phospholipid-dependent protein kinase (25). Finally, loading PMNs (196) or macrophages (S. D. Wright, *unpublished observations*) with inorganic thiophosphate (thioP) allows irreversible activation of C3 receptors. ThioP resembles phosphate and is incorporated into nucleotides and phosphoproteins, but the resulting thiophosphoproteins are resistant to phosphatases. One would thus expect that in a cell loaded with thioP, phosphorylation caused by stimulation of a kinase would result in a pool of thiophosphorylated proteins that are resistant to dephosphorylation. It is thus likely that the irreversible activation of receptors observed in loaded cells is a consequence of irreversible thiophosphorylation.

Changelian and Fearon (26) have shown that PMA does cause phosphorylation of CR1 in PMNs. The phosphorylation is transient and follows a time course similar to that observed for activation and deactivation. Phosphorylation of CR3, however, has not yet been documented.

How could phosphorylation of C3 receptors alter their capacity to bind ligand and promote phagocytosis? Work by Detmers (33) suggested a novel mechanism for this type of regulation. Treatment of PMNs with PMA caused CR3 to move from a random, monomeric, distribution on the cell surface into clusters of six to ten receptors. The time course of aggregation corresponded precisely with the time course of activation, and further incubation with PMA caused disaggregation of CR3 with a time course that matched deactivation of the receptors. Phosphorylation may thus allow C3 receptors to move into an active, clustered configuration.

A possible mechanism by which clustering of receptors may endow them with enhanced binding activity is suggested by studies on the spatial distribution of the ligand, C3b or C3bi, on the surface of ligand-coated particles (69). When C3 was deposited as random monomers, the resulting C3b- or C3bi-coated erythrocytes were not bound by macrophages. However, if an equivalent number of C3 molecules were deposited in clusters, binding to macrophages was avid. Thus it appears that for successful interaction between CR3 and C3bi both receptor and ligand need to be in clusters. The multivalent interactions of adjacent clusters of ligand and receptor may provide the stabilization needed for effective binding.

Significance of C3 Receptor Regulation in Host Defense

The exact physiological importance of the regulated behavior of complement receptors is not certain, and readers are referred to ref. 193 for a detailed treatment of this topic. We assume that because regulated behavior is observed in both man and mouse, however, it must be a conserved trait that confers reproductive advantage. Regulated behavior may be a general property of adhesion-promoting receptors that allows these receptors to perform their unique functions in the cells' economy. Cells may synthesize and express large amounts of a receptor in inactive form so that it can be deployed rapidly when needed. For example, members of the CR3/LFA family are thought to mediate binding and migration of blood cells through endothelia, and maintenance of these receptors in an inactive state could serve to keep leukocytes in circulation and may further serve to allow detachment of leukocytes from the endothelial cells following diapedesis. C3 receptor may be kept in an inactive state in tissue macrophages to prevent the phagocytes from damaging host cells inadvertently coated with complement.

Responses of Cells to Ligation of Adhesion-Promoting Receptors

During Fc receptor-mediated phagocytosis, macrophages press the leading edge of their advancing pseudopod against the ligand-coated target. So tight is the contact between pseudopod and target that soluble protein molecules in the medium are excluded from the zone of contact between phagocyte and target (199). This observation suggests a mechanism by which macrophages kill targets that are too large to eat: Toxic molecules secreted into the protected compartment between phagocyte and target act preferentially and swiftly on the target and leave bystanders unharmed. The C3 receptors of resting phagocytes do not initiate movement of pseudopods and, not surprisingly, do not promote formation of a protein-tight seal (199). Active C3 receptors, on the other hand, do initiate movement of pseudopods and do promote formation of a protein-tight seal. Thus we can expect that Fc and C3 receptors function in a similar fashion to engulf small particles and to digest particles too large to eat.

The behavior of C3 receptors differs from that of Fc receptors in two other respects. During Fc receptor-mediated phagocytosis, phagocytes release large amounts of oxygen metabolites (superoxide and hydrogen peroxide) and arachidonic acid metabolites (prostaglandins and leukotrienes). Secretion of these substances does not require engulfment and closure of the phagosome, as IgG-coated beads or substrates that are too large to be ingested readily promote release of both peroxide (84) and arachidonate (158). In contrast, neither active nor inactive C3 receptors trigger release of either hydrogen peroxide (198,205) or arachidonic acid metabolites (1). The observation that C3 receptors do not promote secretion of these inflammatory compounds suggests that C3 receptor-mediated phagocytosis may provide a means of clearing opsonized particles without initiating or perpetuating an inflammatory response.

We must point out that studies on the effects of ligation of CR3 have thus far employed only the protein ligand C3bi. Because CR3 also recognizes LPS and components on other microbes, it is possible that binding of these ligands may induce a different spectrum of responses, a possibility first suggested by Ross and colleagues (155). Several observations make this suggestion likely. For example, binding of the yeast *Histoplasma capsulatum* to human macrophages is absolutely dependent on CR3, LFA-1, and p150,95, but unexpectedly this binding event initiates a strong oxidative burst (23). Ligation of CR3 may also cause long-term effects. Ding et al. (39) have shown that ligation of murine CR3 with a monoclonal antibody causes the slow (2 days) differentiative changes normally observed in response to γ-interferon. Finally, LPS is known to induce dramatic changes in the patterns of protein synthesis of macrophages (18,40), and other work suggests that CR3, along with LFA-1 and p150,95, may mediate these changes (S. D. Wright, *unpublished observations*). Future studies may thus uncover additional roles for complement receptors in inflammation and host responsiveness to pathogens.

ACKNOWLEDGMENTS

We thank Drs. Patricia A. Detmers, Eileen Scigliano, and Victoria Freedman for critical reading of the manuscript. The work reported herein was supported by USPHS grants AI-22003 (S.D.W.) and AI-24322 (J.C.U.), and by JRFA103 from the American Cancer Society (S.D.W.).

REFERENCES

1. Aderem, A. A., Wright, S. D., Silverstein, S. C., and Cohn, Z. A. (1985): Ligated complement receptors do not activate the arachidonic acid cascade in resident peritoneal macrophages. *J. Exp. Med.*, 161:617–622.
2. Akiyama, Y., Lubeck, M. D., Steplewkski, Z., and Koprowski, H. (1984): Induction of mouse IgG2a- and IgG3-dependent cellular cytotoxicity in human monocytic cells (U937) by immune interferon. *Cancer Res.*, 44:5127–5131.
3. Alarcon, B., and Fresno, M. (1985): Specific effect of anti-transferrin antibodies on natural killer cells directed against tumor cells: evidence for the transferrin receptor being one of the target structures recognized by NK cells. *J. Immunol.*, 134:1286–1291.
4. Anderson, C. L. (1982): Isolation of the receptor for IgG from a human monocyte cell line (U937) and from human peripheral blood monocytes. *J. Exp. Med.*, 156:1794–1806.
5. Anderson, C. L., and Abraham, G. N. (1980): Characterization of the Fc receptor for IgG on a human macrophage cell line, U937. *J. Immunol.*, 125:2735–2741.
6. Anderson, C. L., Guyre, P. M., Whitin, J. C., Ryan, D. H., Looney, R. J., and Fanger, M. W. (1986): Monoclonal antibodies to Fc receptors for IgG on human mononuclear phagocytes: antibody characterization and induction of superoxide production in a monocyte cell line. *J. Biol. Chem.*, 261:12856–12864.
7. Anderson, C. L., Ryan, D. H., Looney, R. J., and Leary, P. C. (1987): Structural polymorphism of the human monocyte 40 kilodalton Fc receptor for IgG. *J. Immunol. (in press)*.
8. Anderson, C. L., Spence, J. M., Edwards, T. S., and Nusbacher, J. (1985): Characterization of a polyvalent antibody directed against the IgG Fc receptor of human mononuclear phagocytes. *J. Immunol.*, 134:465–470.
9. Anderson, D. C., Schmalstieg, F. C., Arnaout, M. A., Kohl, S., Tosi, M. F., Dana, N., Buffone, G. J., Hughes, B. J., Brinkley, B. R., Dickey, W. D., Abramson, J. S., Springer, T. A., Boxer, L. A., Hollers, J. M., and Smith, C. W. (1984): Abnormalities of polymorphonuclear leukocyte function associated with a heritable deficiency of high molecular weight surface glyco-proteins (GP138): common relationship to diminished cell adherence. *J. Clin. Invest.*, 74:536–551.
10. Anderson, D. C., Schmalstein, F. C., Finegold, M. J., Hughes, B. J., Rothlein, R., Miller, L. J., Kohl, S., Tosi, M. F., Jacobs, R. L., Waldrop, T. C., Goldman, A. S., Shearer, W. T., and Springer, T. A. (1985): The severe and moderate phenotypes of heritable Mac-1, LFA-1 deficiency: their quantitative definition and relation to leukocyte dysfunction and clinical features. *J. Infect. Dis.*, 4:668–689.
11. Anderson, D. C., Schmalstieg, F. C., Shearer, W., Becker-Freeman, K., Kohl, S., Smith, C. W., Tosi, M. F., and Springer, T. (1985): Leukocyte LFA-1, OKM1, p150,95 deficiency syndrome: functional

and biosynthetic studies of three kindreds. *Fed. Proc.*, 44:2671–2677.

12. Arnaout, M. A., Dana, N., Pitt, J., and Todd, R. F., III (1985): Deficiency of two human leukocyte surface membrane glycoproteins (Mol and LFA-1). *Fed Proc.*, 44:2664.

13. Arnaout, M. A., Melamed, J., Tack, B., and Colten, H. R. (1981): Characterization of the human complement (C3b) receptor with a fluid phase C3b dimer. *J. Immunol.*, 127:1348–1354.

14. Baum, C. M., McKearn, J. P., Riblet, R., and Davie, J. M. (1985): Polymorphism of Fc receptor on murine B cells is Igh-linked. *J. Exp. Med.*, 162:282–296.

15. Berger, M., Gaither, T. A., Hammer, C. H., and Frank, M. M. (1981): Lack of binding of human C3, in its native state, to C3b receptors. *J. Immunol.*, 127:1329–1334.

16. Berger, M., O'Shea, J., Cross, A. S., Folks, T. M., Chused, T. M., Brown, E. J., and Frank, M. M. (1984): Human neutrophils increase expression of C3bi as well as C3b receptors upon activation. *J. Clin. Invest.*, 74:1566.

17. Berken, A., and Benacerraf, B. (1966): Properties of antibodies cytophilic for macrophages. *J. Exp. Med.*, 123:119–144.

18. Beutler, B., Mahoney, J., LeTrang, N., Pekala, P., and Cerami, A. (1985): Purification of cachectin, a lipoprotein lipase-supressing hormone secreted by endotoxin-treated RAW 264.7 cells. *J. Exp. Med.*, 161:984–995.

19. Birshtein, B. K., Campbell, R., and Diamond, B. (1982): Effects of immunoglobulin (structure) on (Fc receptor) binding: a mouse myeloma variant immunoglobulin with a gamma 2b-gamma 2a hybrid heavy chain having a complete gamma 2a (Fc) region fails to bind to gamma 2a (Fc) receptors on mouse macrophages. *J. Immunol.*, 129:610–614.

20. Blackwell, J. M., Ezekowitz, R. A. B., Roberts, M. B., Channon, J. Y., Sim, R. B., and Gordon, S. (1985): Macrophage complement and lectin-like receptors bind Leishmania in the absence of serum. *J. Exp. Med.*, 162:324–331.

21. Bobak, D. A., Gaither, T. A., Frank, M. M., and Tenner, A. J. (1987): Modulation of FcR function by complement: subcomponent C1q enhances the phagocytosis of IgG-opsonized targets by human monocytes and culture-derived macrophages. *J. Immunol.*, 138:1150–1156.

22. Bohnsack, J. F., Kleinman, H. K., Takahashi, T., O'Shea, J. J., and Brown, E. J. (1985): Connective tissue proteins and phagocytic cell function: laminin enhances complement and Fc-mediated phagocytosis by cultured human phagocytes. *J. Exp. Med.*, 161:912–923.

23. Bullock, W. E., and Wright, S. D. (1987): The role of adherence-promoting receptors, CR3, LFA-1, and p150,95 in binding of Histoplasma capsulatum by human macrophages. *J. Exp. Med.*, 165:195–210.

24. Carlo, J. R., Ruddy, S., and Studer, E. J. (1979): Complement receptor binding of C3b-coated cells treated with C3b inactivator, betalH globulin and trypsin. *J. Immunol.*, 123:523.

25. Castagna, M., Takai, Y., Kaibuchi, K., Sano, K., Kikkawa, U., and Nishizuka, Y. (1982): Direct activation of calcium-activated, phospholipid-dependent protein kinase by tumor-promoting phorbol esters. *J. Biol. Chem.*, 257:7847–7851.

26. Changelian, P. S., and Fearon, D. T. (1986): The tissue-specific phosphorylation of complement receptors CR1 and CR2. *J. Exp. Med.*, 163:101–115.

27. Clarkson, S. B., Bussel, J. B., Kimberly, R. P., Valinsky, J. E., Nachman, R. L., and Unkeless, J. C. (1986): Treatment of refractory immune thrombocytopenic purpura with an anti-Fc gamma-receptor antibody. *N. Engl. J. Med.*, 314:1236–1239.

28. Clarkson, S. B., Kimberly, R. P., Valinsky, J. E., Witmer, M. D., Bussel, J. B., Nachman, R. L., and Unkeless, J. C. (1986): Blockade of clearance of immune complexes by an anti-Fc gamma receptor monoclonal antibody. *J. Exp. Med.*, 164:474–489.

29. Clement, L. T., Tilden, A. B., and Dunlap, N. E. (1985): Analysis of the monocyte Fc receptors and antibody-mediated cellular interactions required for the induction of T cell proliferation by anti-T3 antibodies. *J. Immunol.*, 135:165–171.

30. Cooper, N. R. (1969): Immune adherence by the fourth component of complement. *Science*, 165:396–398.

31. Cramer, E. B., Milks, L. C., Brontoli, M. J., Ojakian, G. K., Wright, S. D., and Showell, H. (1986): Effect of human serum and some of its components on neutrophil adherence and migration across an epithelium. *J. Cell Biol.*, 102:1868–1877.

32. Day, N. K., and Good, R. A. (1975): Deficiencies of the complement system in man. *Birth Defects*, 11:306–311.

33. Detmers, P. A., Wright, S. D., Olsen, E., Kimball, B., and Cohn, Z. A. (1987): Aggregation of complement receptors on human neutrophils in the absence of ligand. *J. Cell Biol.*, 105:(in press).

34. Diamond, B., and Scharff, M. D. (1980): IgG1 and IgG2b share the Fc receptor on mouse macrophages. *J. Immunol.*, 125:631–633.

35. Diamond, B., and Yelton, D. E. (1981): A new Fc receptor on mouse macrophages binding IgG3. *J. Exp. Med.*, 153:514–519.

36. Diamond, B., Birshtein, B. K., and Scharff, D. M. (1979): Site of binding of mouse IgG2b to the Fc receptor on mouse macrophages. *J. Exp. Med.*, 150:721–726.

37. Diamond, B., Boccumini, L., and Birshtein, B. K. (1985): Site of binding of IgG2b and IgG2a by mouse macrophage Fc receptors by using cyanogen bromide fragments. *J. Immunol.*, 134:1080–1083.

38. Dickler, H. B. (1976): Lymphocyte receptors for immunoglobulin. *Adv. Immunol.*, 24:167–214.

39. Ding, A., Wright, S. D., and Nathan, C. F. (1987): Activation of mouse peritoneal macrophages by monoclonal antibodies to Mac-1 (complement receptor type 3). *J. Exp. Med.*, 165:733–749.

40. Durum, S. K., Schmidt, J. A., and Oppenheim, J. J. (1985): Interleukin-1: an immunological perspective. *Annu. Rev. Immunol.*, 3:263–287.

41. Dykman, T. R., Cole, J. L., Iida, K., and Atkinson, J. P. (1983): Polymorphism of human erythrocyte C3b/C4b receptor. *J. Immunol.*, 80:1698–1702.

42. Dykman, T. R., Hatch, J. A., and Atkinson, J. P. (1984): Polymorphism of the human C3b/C4b receptor: identification of a third allele and analysis of receptor phenotypes in families and patients with systemic lupus erythematosus. *J. Exp. Med.*, 159:691–703.

43. Dykman, T. R., Hatch, J. A., Aqua, M. S., and Atkinson, J. P. (1985): Polymorphism of the C3b/C4b receptor (CR1): characterization of a fourth allele. *J. Immunol.*, 134:1787–1789.

44. Eden, A., Miller, G. W., and Nussenzweig, V. (1973): Human lymphocytes bear membrane receptors for C3b and C3d. *J. Clin. Invest.*, 52:3239.

45. Ehlenberger, A. G., and Nussenzweig, V. (1977): The role of membrane receptors for C3b and C3d in phagocytosis. *J. Exp. Med.*, 145:357–371.

46. Ezekowitz, R. A. B., Sim, R. B., Hill, M., and Gordon, S. (1984): Local opsonization by secreted macrophage complement components: role of receptors for complement in uptake of zymosan. *J. Exp. Med.*, 159:244–260.

47. Fearon, D. T. (1980): Identification of the membrane glycoprotein that is the C3b receptor of the human erythrocyte, polymorphonuclear leukocyte, β lymphocyte, and monocyte. *J. Exp. Med.*, 152:20–30.

48. Fearon, D. T., and Collins, L. A. (1983): Increased expression of C3b receptors on polymorphonuclear leukocytes induced by chemotactic factors and by purification procedures. *J. Immunol.*, 130:370.

49. Fingeroth, J. D., Wells, J. J., Tedder, T. F., Strominger, J. L., Bird, P. A., and Fearon, D. T. (1984): Epstein-Barr virus receptor of human B lymphocytes is the C3d receptor CR2. *Proc. Natl. Acad. Sci. USA*, 81:4510–4516.

50. Fleit, H. B., Wright, S. D., and Unkeless, J. C. (1982): Human neutrophil Fcγ receptor distribution and structure. *Proc. Natl. Acad. Sci. USA*, 79:3275–3279.

51. Fleit, H. B., Wright, S. D., Durie, C. J., Valinsky, J. E., and Unkeless, J. C. (1984): Ontogeny of Fc receptors and complement receptor (CR3) during human myeloid differentiation. *J. Clin. Invest.*, 73:516–525.

52. Frank, M. M., Hamburger, M. I., Lawley, T. J., Kimberly, R. P., and Plotz, P. H. (1979): Defective reticuloendothelial system Fc receptor function in systemic lupus erythematosus. *N. Engl. J. Med.*, 300:518–520.

53. Frey, J., Janes, M., Engelhardt, W., Afting, E. G., Geerds, C., and Moller, B. (1986): Fc gamma-receptor-mediated changes in the plasma membrane potential induce prostaglandin release from human fibroblasts. *Eur. J. Biochem.,* 158:85–89.

54. Gardner, J. M., and Hynes, R. O. (1985): Interaction of fibronectin with its receptor on platelets. *Cell,* 42:439–448.

56. Graziano, R. F., and Fanger, M. W. (1987): Human monocyte-mediated cytotoxicity: the use of Ig-bearing hybridomas as target cells to detect trigger molecules on the monocyte cell surface. *J. Immunol.,* 138:945–950.

57. Green, S. A., Plutner, H., and Mellman, I. (1985): Biosynthesis and intracellular transport of the mouse macrophage Fc receptor. *J. Biol. Chem.,* 260:9867–9874.

58. Gresham, H. D., Clement, L. T., Lehmeyer, J. E., Griffin, F. M., Jr., and Volonakis, J. E. (1986): Stimulation of human neutrophil Fc receptor-mediated phagocytosis by a low molecular weight cytokine. *J. Immunol.,* 137:868–875.

59. Griffin, F. M., Jr., and Griffin, J. A. (1980): Augmentation of macrophage complement receptor function in vitro. II. Characterization of the effects of a unique lymphokine upon the phagocytic capabilities of macrophages. *J. Immunol.,* 125:844–849.

60. Griffin, F. M., Jr., and Mullinax, P. J. (1984): Augmentation of macrophage complement receptor function in vitro. IV. The lymphokine that activates macrophage C3 receptors for phagocytosis binds to a fucose-bearing glycoprotein on the macrophage plasma membrane. *J. Exp. Med.,* 160:1206.

61. Griffin, F. M., Jr., and Mullinax, P. J. (1985): In vivo activation of macrophage C3 receptors for phagocytosis. *J. Exp. Med.,* 162: 352–357.

62. Griffin, J. A., and Griffin, F. M., Jr. (1979): Augmentation of macrophage complement receptor function in vitro. I. Characterization of the cellular interactions required for the generation of a T-lymphocyte product that enhances macrophage complement receptor function. *J. Exp. Med.,* 150:653–675.

63. Guyre, P. M., Morganelli, P. M., and Miller, R. (1983): Recombinant immune interferon increases immunoglobulin G Fc receptors on cultured human mononuclear phagocytes. *J. Clin. Invest.,* 72:393–397.

64. Hamada, A., and Greene, B. M. (1987): C1q enhancement of IgG-dependent eosinophil-mediated killing of schistosomula in vitro. *J. Immunol.,* 138:1240–1245.

65. Harlan, J. M., Killen, P. D., Senecal, F. M., Schwartz, B. R., Yee, E. K., Taylor, F. R., Beatty, P. G., Price, T. H., and Ochs, H. (1985): The role of neutrophil membrane protein GP-150 in neutrophil adhesion to endothelia in vitro. *Blood,* 66:167–178.

66. Heinz, H. P., Dlugonska, H., Rude, E., and Loos, M. (1984): Monoclonal anti-mouse macrophage antibodies recognize the globular portions of C1q, a subcomponent of the first component of complement. *J. Immunol.,* 133:400–404.

67. Hemler, M. E., Huang, C., and Schwarz, L. (1987): The VLA protein family: characterization of five distinct cell surface heterodimers each with a common 130,000 M_r beta subunit. *J. Biol. Chem.,* 262:3300–3308.

68. Herlyn, D., and Koprowski, H. (1982): IgG2a monoclonal antibodies inhibit human tumor growth through interaction with effector cells. *Proc. Natl. Acad. Sci. USA,* 79:4761–4765.

69. Hermanowski-Vosatka, A., Detmers, P. A., Goetze, O., Silverstein, S. C., and Wright, S. D. (1987): Clustered, surface-bound ligand, but not monomeric ligand, is recognized by complement receptors on human macrophages. Submitted for publication.

70. Hibbs, M. L., Hogarth, P. M., and McKenzie, I. F. (1985): The mouse Ly-17 locus identifies a polymorphism of the Fc receptor. *Immunogenetics,* 22:335–348.

71. Hibbs, M. L., Walker, I. D., Kirszbaum, L., Pietersz, G. A., Deacon, N. J., Chambers, G. W., McKenzie, I. F., and Hogarth, P. M. (1986): The murine Fc receptor for immunoglobulin: purification, partial amino acid sequence, and isolation of cDNA clones. *Proc. Natl. Acad. Sci. USA,* 83:6980–6984.

72. Hind, C. R. K., Collins, P. M., Rinn, D., Cook, R. B., Caspi, D., Baltz, M. L., and Pepys, M. B. (1984): Binding specificity of serum amyloid P component for the pyruvate acetal of galactose. *J. Exp. Med.,* 159:1058–1069.

73. Hogarth, P. M., Hibbs, M. L., Bonadonna, L., Scott, B. M., Witort, E., Pietersz, G. A., and FcKenzie, I. F. C. (1987): The murine Fc receptor for IgG (Ly-17): molecular cloning and specificity. *Immunogenetics (in press).*

74. Holmes, K. L., Palfree, R. G., Hammerling, U., and Morse, H. C., III (1985): Alleles of the Ly-17 alloantigen define polymorphisms of the murine IgG Fc receptor. *Proc. Natl. Acad. Sci. USA,* 82: 7706–7710.

75. Hosein, B., and Bianco, C. (1985): Monocyte receptors for fibronectin characterized by a monoclonal antibody that interferes with receptor activity. *J. Exp. Med.,* 162:157–170.

76. Huber, H., and Fudenberg, H. H. (1970): The interaction of monocytes and macrophages with immunoglobulins and complement. *Ser. Haematol.,* 3:160–175.

77. Huber, H., Douglas, S. D., Nusbacher, J., Kochwa, S., and Rosenfield, R. E. (1971): IgG subclass specificity of human monocyte receptor sites. *Nature,* 229:419–420.

78. Hynes, R. O. (1987): Integrins: a family of cell surface receptors. *Cell,* 48:549–554.

79. Hynes, R. O., and Yamada, K. M. (1982): Fibronectins: multifunctional modular glycoproteins. *J. Cell Biol.,* 95:369.

80. Iida, K., and Nussenzweig, V. (1981): Complement receptor is an inhibitor of the complement cascade. *J. Exp. Med.,* 153:1138–1150.

81. Iida, K., Nadler, L., and Nussenzweig, V. (1983): Identification of the membrane receptor for the complement fragment C3d by means of a monoclonal antibody. *J. Exp. Med.,* 158:1021–1033.

82. Jack, R. M., and Fearon, D. T. (1984): Altered surface distribution of both C3b receptors and Fc receptors on neutrophils induced by anti-C3b receptor or aggregated IgG. *J. Immunol.,* 132:3028–3033.

83. Janatova, J., Lorenz, P. E., Schechter, A. N., Prahl, J. W., and Tack, B. F. (1980): The third component of human complement: appearance of a sulfhydryl group following chemical or enzymatic inactivation. *Biochemistry,* 19:4471–4478.

84. Johnston, R. B., Jr., Lehmeyer, J. E., and Guthrie, L. A. (1976): Generation of superoxide anion and chemiluminescence by human monocytes during phagocytosis and on contact with surface-bound immunoglobulin G. *J. Exp. Med.,* 143:1551–1556.

85. Jones, D. H., Looney, R. J., and Anderson, C. L. (1985): Two distinct classes of IgG Fc receptors on a human monocyte line (U937) defined by differences in binding of murine IgG subclasses at low ionic strength. *J. Immunol.,* 135:3348–3353.

86. Jones, D. H., Nusbacher, J., and Anderson, C. L. (1985): Fc receptor-mediated binding and endocytosis by human mononuclear phagocytes: monomeric IgG is not endocytosed by U937 cells and monocytes. *J. Cell Biol.,* 100:558–564.

87. Kay, A. B., Glass, J., and Salter, D. M. (1979): Leucoattractants enhance complement receptors on human phagocytic cells. *Clin. Exp. Immunol.,* 38:294–299.

88. Kazatchkine, M. D., Fearon, D. T., Appay, M. D., Mandet, C., and Bariety, J. (1982): Immunohistochemical study of the human glomerular C3b receptor in normal kidney and in seventy-five cases of renal disease. *J. Clin. Invest.,* 69:900–912.

89. Kishimoto, T. K., O'Connor, K., Lee, A., Roberts, T. M., and Springer, T. A. (1987): Cloning of the beta subunit of the leukocyte adhesion proteins: homology to an extracellular matrix receptor defines a novel supergene family. *Cell,* 48:681–690.

90. Klickstein, L. B., Wong, W. W., Smith, J. A., Weis, H. J., Wilson, J. G., and Fearon, D. T. (1987): Human C3b/C4b receptor (CR1): demonstration of long homologous repeating domains that are composed of the short consensus repeats characteristic of C3/C4 binding proteins. *J. Exp. Med.,* 165:1095–1112.

91. Krensky, A. M., Sanchez-Madrid, F., Robbins, E., Nagy, J. A., Springer, T. A., and Burakoff, S. J. (1983): The functional significance, distribution, and structure of LFA-1, LFA-2, and LFA-3: cell surface antigens associated with CTL-target interaction. *J. Immunol.,* 131:611.

92. Kulczycki, A., Jr. (1984): Human neutrophils and eosinophils have structurally distinct Fc gamma receptors. *J. Immunol.,* 133:849–854.

93. Kulczycki, A., Jr., Trial, J., Connolly, J. M., Sharp, S., and Kapp,

J. A. (1986): Structure and expression of Fc gamma receptors on mouse suppressor T cell hybridomas. *J. Immunol.,* 137:2325–2330.

94. Kurlander, R. J., and Batker, J. (1982): The binding of human immunoglobulin G1 monomer and small, covalently cross-linked polymers of immunoglobulin G1 to human peripheral blood monocytes and polymorphonuclear leukocytes. *J. Clin. Invest.,* 69: 1–8.

95. Kurlander, R. J., and Gartrell, J. E. (1983): The binding and processing of monoclonal human IgG1 by cells of a human macrophage-like cell line (U937). *Blood,* 62:652–662.

96. Kurlander, R. J., and Hall, J. (1986): Comparison of intravenous gamma globulin and a monoclonal anti-Fc receptor antibody as inhibitors of immune clearance in vivo in mice. *J. Clin. Invest.,* 77:2010–2018.

97. Kurlander, R. J., Ellison, D. M., and Hall, J. (1984): The blockade of Fc receptor-mediated clearance of immune complexes in vivo by a monoclonal antibody (2.4G2) directed against Fc receptors on murine leukocytes. *J. Immunol.,* 133:855–862.

98. Kurlander, R. J., Haney, A. F., and Gartrell, J. (1984): Human peritoneal macrophages possess two populations of IgG Fc receptors. *Cell Immunol.,* 86:479–490.

99. Lalezari, P., Khorshidi, M., and Petrosova, M. (1986): Autoimmune neutropenia of infancy. *J. Pediatr.,* 109:764–769.

100. Lane, B. C., and Cooper, S. M. (1982): Fc receptors of mouse cell lines. I. Distinct proteins mediate the IgG subclass-specific Fc binding activities of macrophages. *J. Immunol.,* 128:1819–1824.

101. Lane, B. C., Bricker, M. D., and Cooper, S. M. (1982): Fc receptors of mouse cell lines. II. IgG binding specificity and identification of the Fc receptor on a lymphoid leukemia. *J. Immunol.,* 128:1825–1831.

102. Langlois, A. J., Matthews, T. J., Weinhild, K. J., and Bolognesi, D. P. (1985): Immunologic control of a retrovirus associated murine adenocarcinoma. VII. Tumor cell destruction by macrophages and IgG2a. *J. Natl. Cancer Inst.* 75:709–715.

103. Law, S. K., and Levine, R. P. (1977): Interaction between the third complement protein and cell surface macromolecules. *Proc. Natl. Acad. Sci. USA,* 74:2701–2705.

104. Law, S. K., Fearon, D. T., and Levine, R. P. (1979): Action of the C3b-inactivator on cell-bound C3b. *J. Immunol.,* 122:759–765.

105. Law, S. K., Lichtenberg, N. A., and Levine, R. P. (1979): Evidence for an ester linkage between the labile binding site of C3b and receptive surfaces. *J. Immunol.,* 123:1388–1394.

106. Law, S. K., Lichtenberg, N. A., and Levine, R. P. (1980): Covalent binding and hemolytic activity of complement proteins. *Proc. Natl. Acad. Sci. USA,* 77:7194–7198.

107. Law, S. K. A., Gagnon, J., Hildreth, J. E., Wells, C. E., Willis, A. C., and Wong, A. J. (1987): The primary structure of the beta-subunit of the cell surface adhesion glycoproteins LFA-1, CR3 and p150,95 and its relationship to the fibronectin receptor. *EMBO J.,* 6:915–919.

108. Leatherbarrow, R. J., Rademacher, T. W., Dwek, R. A., Woof, J. M., Clark, A., Burton, D. R., Richardson, N., and Feinstein, A. (1985): Effector functions of a monoclonal aglycosylated mouse IgG2a: binding and activation of complement component C1 and interaction with human monocyte Fc receptor. *Mol. Immunol.,* 22:407–415.

109. Lewis, V. A., Koch, T., Plutner, H., and Mellman, I. (1986): A complementary DNA clone for a macrophage-lymphocyte Fc receptor. *Nature,* 324:372–375.

110. Looney, R. J., Abraham, G. N., and Anderson, C. L. (1986): Human monocytes and U937 cells bear two distinct Fc receptors for IgG. *J. Immunol.,* 136:1641–1647.

111. Looney, R. J., Ryan, D. H., Takahashi, K., Fleit, H. B., Cohen, H. J., Abraham, G. N., and Anderson, C. L. (1986): Identification of a second class of IgG Fc receptors on human neutrophils: a 40 kilodalton molecule also found on eosinophils. *J. Exp. Med.,* 163: 826–836.

112. Loos, M. (1982): The functions of endogenous C1q, a subcomponent of the first component of complement, as a receptor on the membrane of macrophages. *Mol. Immunol.,* 19:1229–1238.

113. Lublin, D. M., Griffith, R. C., and Atkinson, J. P. (1986): Influence of glycosylation on allelic and cell specific M_r variation, receptor

114. Madyastha, P. R., Fudenberg, H. H., Glassman, A. B., Madyastha, K. R., and Smith, C. L. (1982): Autoimmune neutropenia in early infancy: a review. *Ann. Clin. Lab. Sci.,* 12:356–367.

115. Mark, W. H., Kimura, S., and Hammerling, U. (1985): Biochemical characterization of murine lymphoid alloantigen Ly-m20.2, a cell surface marker controlled by a gene linked to the (Mls locus.). *J. Immunol.,* 135:2635–2641.

116. Martz, E. (1986): LFA-1 and other accessory molecules functioning in adhesions of T and B lymphocytes. *Hum. Immunol.,* 18:3–37.

117. Matthews, T. J., Collins, J. J., Roloson, G. J., Thiel, H. J., and Bolognesi, D. P. (1981): Immunologic control of the ascites form of murine adenocarcinoma 755. IV. Characterization of the protective antibody in hyperimmune serum. *J. Immunol.,* 126:2332–2336.

118. McCool, D., Birchstein, B. K., and Painter, R. H. (1985): Structural requirements of immunoglobulin G for binding to the fc receptor of human tumor cell lines U937, HL-60, ML-1, and K562. *J. Immunol.,* 135:1975–1980.

119. Medof, M. E., Iida, K., Mold, C., and Nussenzweig, V. (1982): Unique role of the complement receptor CR1 in the degradation of C3b associated with immune complexes. *J. Exp. Med.,* 156: 1739–1754.

120. Melchers, F., Erdei, A., Schulz, T., and Dierich, M. P. (1985): Growth control of activated, synchronized murine B cells by the C3d fragment of human complement. *Nature,* 317:264–267.

121. Mellman, I., and Plutner, H. (1984): Internalization and degradation of macrophage Fc receptors bound to polyvalent immune complexes. *J. Cell Biol.,* 98:1170–1177.

122. Mellman, I., Plutner, H., and Ukkonen, P. (1984): Internalization and rapid recycling of macrophage Fc receptors tagged with monovalent antireceptor antibody: possible role of a prelysosomal compartment. *J. Cell Biol.,* 98:1163–1169.

123. Mellman, I. S., and Unkeless, J. C. (1980): Purification of a functional mouse Fc receptor through the use of a monoclonal antibody. *J. Exp. Med.,* 152:1048–1069.

124. Mellman, I. S., Plutner, H., Steinman, R. M., Unkeless, J. C., and Cohn, Z. A. (1983): Internalization and degradation of macrophage Fc receptors during receptor-mediated phagocytosis. *J. Cell Biol.,* 96:887–895.

125. Mentzer, S. J., Bierer, B. E., Anderson, D. C., Springer, T. A., and Burakoff, S. J. (1986): Abnormal cytolytic activity of lymphocyte function-associated antigen-1-deficient cytolytic T lymphocyte clones. *J. Clin. Invest.,* 78:1387–1391.

126. Mentzer, S. J., Krensky, A. M., and Burakoff, S. J. (1986): Mapping functional epitopes of the LFA-1 glycoprotein: monoclonal antibody inhibition of NK and CTL effectors. *Hum. Immunol.,* 17:288–296.

127. Michl, J., Unkeless, J. C., Pieczonka, M. M., and Silverstein, S. C. (1983): Modulation of Fc receptors of mononuclear phagocytes by immobilized antigen-antibody complexes: quantitative analysis of the relationship between ligand concentration and Fc receptor response. *J. Exp. Med.,* 157:1746.

128. Morrison, D. C., and Ulevitch, R. J. (1978): The effects of bacterial endotoxins on host mediating systems. *Am. J. Pathol.,* 93:527–617.

129. Mosser, D. M., and Edelson, P. J. (1985): The mouse macrophage receptor for C3bi (CR3) is a major mechanism in the phagocytosis of Leishmania promastigotes. *J. Exp. Med.,* 135:2785.

130. Nathan, C., Brukner, L., Kaplan, G., Unkeless, J., and Cohn, Z. (1980): Role of activated macrophages in antibody-dependent lysis of tumor cells. *J. Exp. Med.,* 152:183–197.

131. Nelson, D. J., Jacobs, E. R., Tang, J. M., Zeller, J. M., and Bone, R. C. (1985): Immunoglobulin G-induced single ionic channels in human alveolar macrophage membranes. *J. Clin. Invest.,* 76:500–507.

132. Newman, S. L., and Mikus, L. K. (1985): Deposition of C3b and iC3b onto particulate activators of the human complement system: quantitation with monoclonal antibodies to human C3. *J. Exp. Med.,* 161:1414–1431.

133. Nose, M., and Wigzell, H. (1983): Biological significance of car-

bohydrate chains on monoclonal antibodies. *Proc. Natl. Acad. Sci. USA*, 80:6632–6636.

134. O'Grady, J. H., Looney, R. J., and Anderson, C. L. (1986): The valence for ligand of the human mononuclear phagocyte 72 kD high-affinity IgG Fc receptor is one. *J. Immunol.*, 137:2307–2310.

135. O'Shea, J., Brown, E. J., Seligmann, B. E., Metcalf, J. A., Frank, M. M., and Gallin, J. I. (1985): Evidence for distinct intracellular pools of receptors for C3b and C3bi in human neutrophils. *J. Immunol.*, 134:2580.

136. Pepys, M. B., Baltz, M. L., deBeer, F. C., Dyck, R. F., Holford, S., Breathnach, S. M., Black, M. M., Tribe, C. R., Evans, D. J., and Feinstein, A. (1982): Biology of serum amyloid P component. *Ann. N.Y. Acad. Sci.*, 389:286–297.

137. Perl, A., Looney, R. J., Ryan, D. H., and Abraham, G. N. (1986): The low affinity 40,000 Fc gamma receptor and the transferrin receptor can be alternative or simultaneous target structures on cells sensitive for natural killing. *J. Immunol.*, 136:4714–4720.

138. Perussia, B., Acuto, O., Terhorst, C., Faust, J., Lazarus, R., Fanning, V., and Trinchieri, G. (1983): Human natural killer cells analyzed by B73.1, a monoclonal antibody blocking Fc receptor functions. II. Studies of B73.1 antibody-antigen interaction on the lymphocyte membrane. *J. Immunol.*, 130:2142–2148.

139. Perussia, B., and Trinchieri, G. (1984): Antibody 3G8, specific for the human neutrophil Fc receptor, reacts with natural killer cells. *J. Immunol.*, 132:1410–1415.

140. Perussia, B., Starr, S., Abraham, S., Fanning, V., and Trinchieri, G. (1983): Human natural killer cells analyzed by B73.1, a monoclonal antibody blocking Fc receptor functions. I. Characterization of the lymphocyte subset reactive with B73.1. *J. Immunol.*, 130: 2133–2141.

141. Perussia, B., Trinchieri, G., Jackson, A., Warner, N. L., Faust, J., Rumpold, H., Kraft, D., and Lanier, L. L. (1984): The Fc receptor for IgG on human natural killer cells: phenotypic, functional, and comparative studies with monoclonal antibodies. *J. Immunol.*, 133: 180–189.

142. Phillips, N. E., and Parker, D. C. (1983): Fc-dependent inhibition of mouse B cell activation by whole anti-mu antibodies. *J. Immunol.*, 130:602–606.

143. Phillips, N. E., and Parker, D. C. (1984): Cross-linking of B (lymphocyte) Fc gamma receptors and membrane immunoglobulin inhibits anti-immunoglobulin-induced blastogenesis. *J. Immunol.*, 132:627–632.

144. Phillips, N. E., and Parker, D. C. (1985): Subclass specificity of Fc gamma receptor-mediated inhibition of mouse B cell activation. *J. Immunol.*, 134:2835–2838.

145. Pommier, C. G., Inada, S., Fries, L. F., Takahashi, T., Frank, M. M., and Brown, E. J. (1983): Plasma fibronectin enhances phagocytosis of opsonized particles by human peripheral blood monocytes. *J. Exp. Med.*, 157:1844.

146. Pytela, R., Pierschbacher, M. D., and Ruoslahti, E. (1985): A 125/ 115-kDa cell surface receptor specific for vitronectin interacts with the arginine-glycine-aspartic acid adhesion sequence derived from fibronectin. *Proc. Natl. Acad. Sci. USA*, 82:5766–5770.

147. Pytela, R., Pierschbacher, M. D., and Ruoslahti, E. (1985): Identification and isolation of a 140 Kd cell surface glycoprotein with properties expected of a fibronectin receptor. *Cell*, 40:191.

148. Pytela, R., Peirschbacher, M. D., Ginsberg, M. H., Plow, E. F., and Ruoslahti, E. (1986): Platelet membrane glycoprotein IIb/IIIa: member of a family of Arg-Gly-Asp-specific adhesion receptors. *Science*, 231:1559–1562.

149. Ralph, P., Nakoinz, I., Diamond, B., and Yelton, D. (1980): All classes of murine (IgG) antibody mediate macrophage phagocytosis and lysis of erythrocytes. *J. Immunol.*, 125:1885–1888.

150. Ravetch, J. V., Luster, A. D., Weinshank, R., Kochan, J., Pavlovec, A., Portnoy, D. A., Hulmes, J., Pan, Y. C., and Unkeless, J. C. (1986): Structural heterogeneity and functional domains of murine immunoglobulin G Fc receptors. *Science*, 234:718–725.

151. Reid, K. B. M., Bentley, D. R., Campbell, R. D., Chung, L. P., Sim, R. B., Kristensen, T., and Tack, B. F. (1986): Complement system proteins which interact with C3b or C4b: a superfamily of structurally related proteins. *Immunol. Today*, 7:230–234.

152. Rosenfeld, S. I., Looney, R. J., Leddy, J. P., Phipps, D. C., Abraham, G. N., and Anderson, C. L. (1985): Human platelet Fc receptor for immunoglobulin G: identification as a 40,000-molecular-weight membrane protein shared by monocytes. *J. Clin. Invest.*, 76:2317–2322.

153. Rosenfeld, S. I., Ryan, D. H., Looney, R. J., Anderson, C. L., Abraham, G. N., and Leddy, J. P. (1987): Human Fc gamma receptors: stable inter-donor variation in quantitative expression on platelets correlates with functional responses. *J. Immunol. (in press)*.

154. Ross, G. D., and Lambris, J. D. (1982): Identification of a C3bi-specific membrane complement receptor that is expressed on lymphocytes, monocytes, neutrophils, and erythrocytes. *J. Exp. Med.*, 155:96–110.

155. Ross, G. D., Cain, J. A., and Lachman, P. J. (1985): Membrane complement receptor type three (CR3) has lectin-like properties analogous to bovine conglutinin and functions as a receptor for zymosan and rabbit erythrocytes as well as a receptor for iC3b. *J. Immunol.*, 134:3307–3315.

156. Ross, G. D., Polley, M. J., Rabellino, E. M., and Grey, H. M. (1973): Two different complement receptors on human lymphocytes: one specific for C3b and one specific for C3b inactivator-cleaved C3b. *J. Exp. Med.*, 138:798.

157. Ross, G. D., Thompson, R. A., Walport, M. J., Springer, T. A., Watson, J. V., Ward, R. H. R., Lida, J., and Newman, S. L. (1985): Characterization of patients with an increased susceptibility to bacterial infections and a genetic deficiency of leukocyte membrane complement receptor type 3 and the related membrane antigen LFA-1. *Blood*, 66:882–890.

158. Rouzer, C. A., Scott, W. A., Kempe, J., and Cohn, Z. A. (1980): Prostaglandin synthesis by macrophages requires a specific receptor-ligand interaction. *Proc. Natl. Acad. Sci. USA*, 77:4279–4282.

159. Ruoslahti, E., and Pierschbacher, M. D. (1986): Arg-Gly-Asp: a versatile cell recognition signal. *Cell*, 44:517–518.

160. Salmon, J. E., and Kimberly, R. P. (1986): Phagocytosis of concanavalin A-treated erythrocytes is mediated by the Fc gamma receptor. *J. Immunol.*, 137:456–462.

161. Salmon, J. E., Kimberly, R. P., Gibofsky, A., and Fotino, M. (1986): Altered phagocytosis by monocytes from HLA-DR2 and DR3-positive healthy adults is Fc gamma receptor specific. *J. Immunol.*, 136:3625–3630.

162. Sanchez-Madrid, F., Krensky, A. M., Ware, C. F., Robbins, E., Strominger, J. L., Burakoff, S. J., and Springer, T. A. (1982): Three distinct antigens associated with human T-lymphocyte-mediated cytolysis: LFA-1, LFA-2, and LFA-3. *Proc. Natl. Acad. Sci. USA*, 79:7489–7493.

163. Sanchez-Madrid, F., Nagy, J. A., Robbins, E., Simon, P., and Springer, T. A. (1983): Characterization of a human leukocyte differentiation antigen family with distinct α subunits and a common β subunit: the lymphocyte-function associated antigen (LFA-1), the C3bi complement receptor (OKM1/Mac1), and the p150,95 molecule. *J. Exp. Med.*, 158:1785–1803.

164. Sanchez-Madrid, F., Simon, P., Thompson, S., and Springer, T. A. (1983): Mapping of antigenic and functional epitopes on the α- and β-subunits of two related mouse glycoproteins involved in cell interactions, LFA-1 and Mac1. *J. Exp. Med.*, 158:586–602.

165. Schreiber, R. D. (1984): Identification of gamma-interferon as a murine macrophage-activating factor for tumor cytotoxicity. *Contemp. Top. Immunobiol.*, 13:171–198.

166. Shaw, S., Luce, G. E. G., Quinones, R., Gress, R. E., Springer, T. A., and Sanders, M. E. (1986): Two antigen-independent adhesion pathways used by human cytotoxic T cell clones. *Nature*, 323: 262–264.

167. Shen, L., Guyre, P. M., Anderson, C. L., and Fanger, M. W. (1986): Heteroantibody-mediated cytotoxicity: antibody to the high affinity Fc receptor for IgG mediates cytotoxicity by human monocytes that is enhanced by interferon-gamma and is not blocked by human IgG. *J. Immunol.*, 137:3378–3382.

168. Strassman, G., Springer, T. A., Somers, S. D., and Adams, D. O. (1986): Mechanisms of tumor cell capture by activated macrophages: evidence for involvement of lymphocyte function-associated (LFA)-1 antigen. *J. Immunol.*, 136:4329–4333.

169. Tamkun, J. W., DeSimone, D. W., Fonda, D., Patel, R. S., Buck, C., Horwitz, A. F., and Hynes, R. O. (1986): Structure of integrin,

a glycoprotein involved in the transmembrane linkage between fibronectin and actin. *Cell,* 46:271–282.

170. Tax, W. J., Hermes, F. F., Willems, R. W., Capel, P. J., and Koene, R. A. (1984): Fc receptors for mouse IgG1 on human monocytes: polymorphism and role in antibody-induced T cell proliferation. *J. Immunol.,* 133:1185–1189.

171. Tax, W. J., Willems, H. W., Reekers, P. P., Capel, P. J., and Koene, R. A. (1983): Polymorphism in mitogenic effect of IgG1 monoclonal antibodies against T3 antigen on human T cells. *Nature,* 304:445–447.

172. Teillaud, J. L., Diamond, B., Pollock, R. R., Fajtova, V., and Scharff, M. D. (1985): Fc receptors on cultured myeloma and hybridoma cells. *J. Immunol.,* 134:1774–1779.

173. Tenner, A. J., and Cooper, N. R. (1980): Analysis of receptor-mediated C1q binding to human peripheral blood mononuclear cells. *J. Immunol.,* 125:1658.

174. Timpl, R., Rohde, M., Robey, P. G., Rennard, S. I., Foidart, J. M., and Martin, G. M. (1979): Laminin—a glycoprotein from basement membranes. *J. Biol. Chem.,* 254:9933.

175. Todd, R. F., III, Arnaout, M. A., Rosin, R. E., Crowley, C. A., Peters, W. A., and Babior, B. M. (1984): Subcellular localization of the large subunit of Mol (Mol: formerly gp 110), a surface glycoprotein associated with neutrophil adhesion. *J. Clin. Invest.,* 74:1280.

176. Ukkonen, P., Lewis, V., Marsh, M., Helenius, A., and Mellman, I. (1986): Transport of macrophage Fc receptors and Fc receptor-bound ligands to lysosomes. *J. Exp. Med.,* 163:952–971.

177. Unkeless, J. C. (1977): The presence of two Fc receptors on mouse macrophages: evidence from a variant cell line and differential trypsin sensitivity. *J. Exp. Med.,* 145:931–945.

178. Unkeless, J. C. (1979): Characterization of a monoclonal antibody directed against mouse macrophage and lymphocyte Fc receptors. *J. Exp. Med.,* 150:580–596.

179. Unkeless, J. C., and Eisen, H. N. (1975): Binding of monomeric immunoglobulins to Fc receptors of mouse macrophages. *J. Exp. Med.,* 142:1520–1533.

180. Unkeless, J. C., Fleit, H., and Mellman, I. S. (1981): Structural aspects and heterogeneity of immunoglobulin Fc receptors. *Adv. Immunol.,* 31:247–270.

181. Vik, D. P., and Fearon, D. T. (1985): Neutrophils express a receptor for iC3b, C3dg, and C3d that is distinct from CR1, CR2, and CR3. *J. Immunol.,* 134:2571–2579.

182. Vik, D. P., and Fearon, D. T. (1987): Cellular distribution of complement receptor type 4 (CR4): expression on human platelets. *J. Immunol.,* 138:254–258.

183. Vodinelich, L., Sutherland, R., Schneider, C., Newman, R., and Greaves, M. (1983): Receptor for transferrin may be a "target" structure for natural killer cells. *Proc. Natl. Acad. Sci. USA,* 80:835–839.

184. Weis, J. J., Tedder, T. F., and Fearon, D. T. (1984): Identification of a 145,000 M_r membrane protein as the C3d receptor (CR2) of human B lymphocytes. *Proc. Natl. Acad. Sci. USA,* 81:881–885.

185. Werner, G., von dem Borne, A. E. G. Kr., Bos, M. J. E., Tromp, J. F., van der Plas-van Dalen, C. M., Visser, F. J., Engelfriet, C. P., and Tetteroo, P. A. T. (1986): Localization of the human NA1 alloantigen on neutrophil Fc-γ receptors. In: *Leukocyte Typing II V. 3 Human Myeloid and Hematopoietic Cells,* edited by E. L. Reinherz, B. F. Haynes, L. M. Nadler, and I. D. Bernstein, pp. 109–121. Springer-Verlag, New York.

186. Wilson, H. A., Greenblatt, D., Taylor, C. W., Putney, J. W., Tsien, R. Y., Finkelman, F. D., and Chused, T. M. (1987): The B lymphocyte calcium response to anti-Ig is diminished by membrane immunoglobulin cross-linkage to the Fc gamma receptor. *J. Immunol.,* 138:1712–1718.

187. Wilson, J. G., Tedder, T. F., and Fearon, D. T. (1983): Characterization of human T lymphocytes that express the C3b receptor. *J. Immunol.,* 131:684–689.

188. Wong, W. W., Kennedy, C. A., Bonaccio, E. T., Wilson, J. G., Klickstein, L. B., Weis, J. H., and Fearon, D. T. (1986): Analysis of multiple restriction fragment length polymorphisms of the gene for the human complement receptor type I: duplication of genomic

sequences occurs in association with a high molecular mass receptor allotype. *J. Exp. Med.,* 164:1531–1546.

189. Wong, W. W., Klickstein, L. B., Smith, J. A., Weis, J. H., and Fearon, D. T. (1985): Identification of a partial cDNA clone for the human receptor for complement fragments C3b/C4b. *Proc. Natl. Acad. Sci. USA,* 82:7711–7715.

190. Wong, W. W., Wilson, J. G., and Fearon, D. T. (1983): Genetic regulation of a structural polymorphism of human C3b receptor. *J. Clin. Invest.,* 72:685–693.

191. Woodley, D. T., Rao, C. N., Hassell, J. R., Liotta, L., Martin, G. R., and Kleinman, H. F. (1983): Interaction of basement membrane components. *Biochim. Biophys. Acta,* 761:278.

192. Wright, A. E., and Douglas, S. R. (1903): An experimental investigation of the role of the body fluids in connection with phagocytosis. *Proc. R. Soc. Lond.,* 72:357–370.

193. Wright, S. D., and Griffin, F. M., Jr. (1985): Activation of phagocytic cells' C3 receptors for phagocytosis. *J. Leuk. Biol.,* 38:327–339.

194. Wright, S. D., and Jong, M. T. C. (1986): Adhesion-promoting receptors on human macrophages recognize E. coli by binding to lipopolysaccharide. *J. Exp. Med.,* 164:1876–1888.

195. Wright, S. D., and Meyer, B. C. (1985): The fibronectin receptor of human macrophages recognizes the amino acid sequence, Arg-Gly-Asp-Ser. *J. Exp. Med.,* 162:762.

196. Wright, S. D., and Meyer, B. C. (1986): Phorbol esters cause sequential activation and deactivation of complement receptors on polymorphonuclear leukocytes. *J. Immunol.,* 136:1759–1764.

197. Wright, S. D., and Silverstein, S. C. (1982): Tumor-promoting phorbol esters stimulate C3b and C3b' receptor-mediated phagocytosis in cultured human monocytes. *J. Exp. Med.,* 156:1149–1164.

198. Wright, S. D., and Silverstein, S. C. (1983): Receptors for C3b and C3bi promote phagocytosis but not the release of toxic oxygen from human phagocytes. *J. Exp. Med.,* 158:2016–2023.

199. Wright, S. D., and Silverstein, S. C. (1984): Phagocytosing macrophages exclude proteins from the zones of contact with opsonized targets. *Nature,* 309:359–361.

200. Wright, S. D., Craigmyle, L. S., and Silverstein, S. C. (1983): Fibronectin and serum amyloid P component stimulate C3b- and C3bi-mediated phagocytosis in cultured human monocytes. *J. Exp. Med.,* 158:1338–1343.

201. Wright, S. D., Detmers, P. A., Jong, M. T. C., and Meyer, B. C. (1986): Interferon-gamma depresses binding of ligand by C3b and C3bi receptors on cultured human monocytes, an effect reversed by fibronectin. *J. Exp. Med.,* 163:1245–1259.

202. Wright, S. D., Licht, M. R., Craigmyle, L. S., and Silverstein, S. C. (1984): Communication between receptors for different ligands on a single cell: ligation of fibronectin receptors induces a reversible alteration in the function of C3 receptors in cultured human monocytes. *J. Cell Biol.,* 99:336–339.

203. Wright, S. D., Rao, P. E., Van Voorhis, W. C., Craigmyle, L. S., Iida, K., Talle, M. A., Goldstein, G., and Silverstein, S. C. (1983): Identification of the C3bi receptor on human monocytes and macrophages by using monoclonal antibodies. *Proc. Natl. Acad. Sci. USA,* 80:5699–5703.

204. Wright, S. D., Reddy, P. A., Jong, M. T. C., and Erickson, B. W. (1987): The C3bi receptor (CR3) recognizes a region of complement protein C3 containing the sequence Arg-Gly-Asp. *Proc. Natl. Acad. Sci. USA,* 84:1965–1968.

205. Yamamoto, K., and Johnston, R. B., Jr. (1984): Dissociation of phagocytosis from stimulation of the oxidative metabolic burst in macrophages. *J. Exp. Med.,* 159:405–416.

206. Young, J. D., Unkeless, J. C., Kaback, H. R., and Cohn, Z. A. (1983): Macrophage membrane potential changes associated with γ2b/γ1 Fc receptor-ligand binding. *Proc. Natl. Acad. Sci. USA,* 80:1357–1361.

207. Young, J. D., Unkeless, J. C., Young, T. M., Mauro, A., and Cohn, Z. A. (1983): Mouse macrophage Fc receptor for IgGγ2b/γ1 in artificial and plasma membrane vesicles functions as a ligand-dependent ionophore. *Proc. Natl. Acad. Sci. USA,* 80:1636–1640.

208. Young, J. D., Unkeless, J. C., Young, T. M., Mauro, A., and Cohn, Z. A. (1983): Role for mouse macrophage IgG Fc receptor as ligand-dependent ion channel. *Nature,* 306:186–189.

Inflammation: Basic Principles and Clinical Correlates.
Edited by J. I. Gallin, I. M. Goldstein, and R. Snyderman.
Raven Press, Ltd., New York © 1988.

CHAPTER 22

Phagocytic Cells: Degranulation and Secretion

Peter M. Henson, Janet E. Henson, Claus Fittschen,
Gachuhi Kimani, Donna L. Bratton,
and David W. H. Riches

The emigration of inflammatory cells from the blood into the tissues represents one of the most important components of the inflammatory response. However, it is not the actual accumulation of these cells that is so critical but, rather, what they do in the tissue upon their arrival. Central to these activities are endocytosis and exocytosis (secretion). The phagocytic process is discussed in Chapter 21. Here the mechanisms, products, and consequences of secretion by phagocytic inflammatory cells are considered. The emphasis on phagocytic cells (i.e., cells that have been termed "professional phagocytes" to distinguish them from the wide variety of tissue cells that *can* undertake the phagocytic process under specific conditions) raises an important additional consideration. Thus we must consider not only the release of constituents of these cells to the external milieu but also the discharge of these materials into the phagocytic vacuole, the phagosome. That these two processes are likely to be related seems sound and at this point is supported, but by no means proved, by experimental observations.

The category of phagocytic inflammatory cells includes neutrophils, eosinophils, and the mononuclear phagocytic series. Here we distinguish between monocytes and macrophages but assume for the purposes of this discussion that the wide variety of macrophage phenotypes use the same mechanisms for secretion, even if the major products they secrete are different. Monocytes, on the other hand, seem in their secretory capacity to more closely resemble neutrophils and eosinophils and are considered in that context. Arguments for the latter designation include the following: (a) These three cell types are highly motile and respond readily to chemoattractants *in vitro* and *in vivo*. (b) They have performed their major synthetic processes in the bone marrow and circulate in the blood in a relatively quiescent state. (c) They contain preformed granules, the contents of which can be discharged into phagosomes or, under the appropriate circumstances, to the outside of the cell. (d) There seems to be a remarkable similarity in the stimuli to which these three cell types respond. In fact, a major difference between monocytes and the granulocyte series (apart from obvious differences in granule content, which are not considered here as a functional distinction) is the ability of the former to mature (differentiate, adapt) into the wide variety of cells that make up the mononuclear phagocyte series (see Chapters 17 and 25).

Degranulation and secretion in granulocytes is usually considered in the context of discharge of proteinaceous, occasionally proteoglycan, materials found in the lysosomes or other granular structures. Macrophages are now recognized as cells that synthesize new proteins destined for passage to the extracellular environment, but again the emphasis in terms of mechanisms of secretion is predominantly on proteins. In addition, it seems appropriate therefore to devote some attention to what is (or is not) known about secretion of lipids from these cell types. Because lipid molecules are gaining prominence as key mediators and modulators of physiological, allergic, inflammatory, and even immunological reactions, the mechanisms by which they gain access to the blood or tissue space seems to represent an important area for investigation. A similar question can be raised for oxygen metabolites. Here, however, evidence is accumulating that the reduction of molecular oxygen that occurs as part of the respiratory burst of inflammatory cells takes place in or on the plasma membrane so that active secretory processes do not necessarily need to be invoked (see Chapter 23). If, as may be argued, the release of constituents from inflammatory cells is a central process in both the protective and detrimental aspects of inflammation, is involved in the initial accumulation of the cells themselves, and determines the final outcome of the response, how this process occurs deserves major attention.

Much of the work on secretion from inflammatory cells has focused on the discharge of lysosomal hydrolases, often those with pH optima significantly in the acidic range (e.g., pH 4.5). The reason for this emphasis has been experimental ease and custom, certainly not proved biological relevance. In fact, the importance of release of acid hydrolases into well-buffered tissue spaces has frequently been challenged, it being argued that such enzymes are appropriately liberated into phagosomes where the pH is low but would be inactive in the extracellular milieu *in vivo*. Even now this issue is unresolved. Those of us who have worked with acid hydrolase release have invoked a number of possibilities to validate the studies, all of them yet unproved. (a) The local pH at sites of leukocyte secretion and cell contact *in vivo* is not known, although work with osteoclasts, macrophages, and chondrocytes indicates that the pH at the attachment site is approximately 5.0 (26,55,62,63). If the overall inflammatory exudate (i.e., an average) is slightly acidic, as it usually is, local pH values would be expected to be much lower and, moreover, may be influenced significantly by surface

charges (184,287). (b) Inflammatory cells produce (and may release) hydrogen ions during stimulation (145,316). (c) Most of the enzymes are in fact weakly active at pH values around those found in samples of inflammatory fluid; it is just that they are much less effective than at pH levels nearer their optima. (d) Environments with conditions that are not optimal for enzyme activity provide closer control of such activities. (e) Because secretion of these enzymes clearly occurs, it must have some importance, even if we do not yet perceive what that might be.

Irrespective of these somewhat teleological concepts, we suggest that to investigate the *mechanisms* of secretion from such cells is intrinsically important. In fact, as investigators turn their attention to proteins of different activity and environmental limitations (e.g., neutral proteases, cytokines), the secretory processes previously found for acid phosphatase or β-glucuronidase seem to be applicable here also.

SECRETION AND CELL LYSIS

It has long been known that inflammatory exudate fluid contains constituents that were derived from the incoming inflammatory cells (98,153,162,313). Early concepts as to the source of these materials focused on *in situ* lysis of the inflammatory cells with concurrent discharge of their contents. Products of bacteria with cytocidal properties (128) as well as endogenous lytic events mediated by intracellular disruption (188) were the types of mechanism suggested as causes. The development of the lysosome concept, and the demonstration of granule discharge into the phagosomes in neutrophils (121) did nothing to dispel this prevailing viewpoint. It was not until the early 1970s that the mounting evidence that neutrophils and macrophages could *secrete* constituents without lysis became generally accepted (110,290,314,331). Now, by contrast, secretion is seen as a major function of macrophages (37) and is recognized as a key process in granulocytes.

It seems important in this discussion, therefore, to try and present a balanced viewpoint on the issue of lysis versus secretion. Numerous studies have shown inflammatory cells to secrete constituents *in vitro* without loss of membrane integrity or discharge of cytoplasmic constituents. Given the fact that many of these materials are toxic for other cells, some intrinsic resistance of the inflammatory cell to these agents seems likely and deserving of further study. Additionally, or alternatively, the conditions of the *in vitro* assays may minimize autotoxicity and underrepresent this process.

In vivo study of inflammatory exudates (or ultrastructural examination of inflammatory reactions) (Fig. 1) usually reveals intact inflammatory cells. In fact, exudate

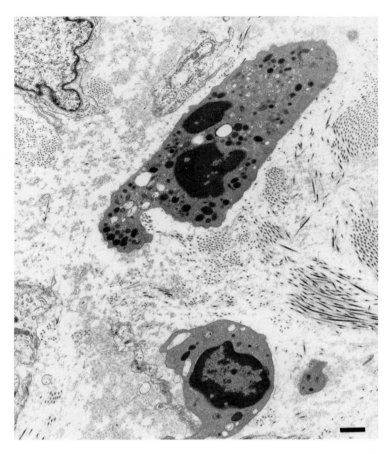

FIG. 1. Intact neutrophils in an inflammatory lesion. Section is from the pulmonary interstitium of a patient with eosinophilic granuloma. The cells are in contact with collagen bundles and surrounded by flocculent material, perhaps protein derived from the extensive edema, perhaps immature collagen. Bar = 1 μm.

cells are still perfectly capable of normal (even heightened) functional responses (201,330). However, the focus in more recent studies has indeed been on intact cells, and those that are inactive or disrupted have tended to be ignored. Few investigators have considered the life span and fate of granulocytes or mononuclear phagocytes in inflammatory lesions, partly because of the difficulties of quantitative investigation of these phenomena *in vivo.* Neutrophils (and by inference eosinophils) do undergo an aging process that results in surface changes associated with recognition and removal by macrophages (118,319). During the aging process *in vitro,* neutrophils undergo morphological changes characteristic of the apoptotic process (102,196), which appears to be closely, possibly critically, linked to recognition by macrophages (239). Apoptosis in other cells, e.g., thymocytes, is a "programmed" form of cell senescence that causes shut-down of the cell (but organelles and membrane function remain intact initially) and surface changes, leading to recognition and phagocytosis by macrophages (319).

However, what is unknown is the proportion of inflammatory cells that is removed in this way in any given type of inflammatory lesion. If sought for, it is just as easy to find morphologically disrupted neutrophils in old inflammatory lesions (Fig. 2). How important this fact is to the overall process must vary with the type of inflammatory response but certainly should not be ignored. What are the mechanisms? Taking a teleological perspective, does this lysis usually occur only at times in the life history of the inflammation when appropriate inhibitors are present to minimize the potential injury (i.e., what is the temporal relation of neutrophil lysis to the exudative process?). Do cytoplasmic inhibitors of proteases (45,135), for example, significantly reduce the impact of granular constituents released during lysis? Answers to these questions and the quantitative issues raised above will help balance our view of the sources of critical molecules in the inflammatory response.

Lysis of granulocytes and release of their contents *in vivo* may be particularly associated with bacterial infections. As an example of a bacterial product that can induce release of neutrophil constituents, the molecule leucocidin might be cited. Much work was carried out with leucocidin by Woodin and associates (308; see also 22), demonstrating that neutrophil cytolysis induced by this material was preceded or accompanied by more active secretory processes. Studies in this area have not continued but could shed insight on secretory mechanisms as well as on cy-

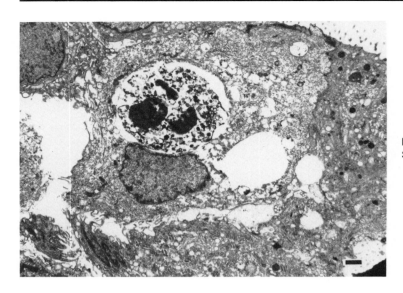

FIG. 2. Degenerate neutrophil in an inflammatory lesion. Section is from human nasal epithelium.

totoxic events in inflammation. Among a group of endogenous lytic agents worth considering might be included lysophospholipids, particularly those derived from alkyl acyl compounds, which because of the ether linkage are resistant to the action of lysophospholipases.

Finally, however, it is important to emphasize that in most inflammatory reactions (possibly excluding those involving certain bacteria) the *early* response involves emigration of granulocytes and monocytes and release of cell constituents without overt cell lysis. At these time points, then, an active secretory process can be inferred as the major source of mediators, modulators, enzymes, and other inflammatory molecules.

MOBILIZATION OF PREFORMED GRANULE CONSTITUENTS FROM NEUTROPHILS, EOSINOPHILS, AND MONOCYTES: DEGRANULATION AND SECRETION

Neutrophils, eosinophils, and monocytes emerge from the bone marrow with a complement of morphologically distinct granules (see Chapters 16, 17, and 25) containing proteins and glycosaminoglycans that are presumably destined for discharge into either endocytic vesicles and vacuoles or the external environment. In the literature the term "degranulation" has been used loosely in this context, sometimes referring to discharge into phagosomes, sometimes more broadly to release to the outside of the cell as well. Strictly "degranulation" could be used exclusively for morphological loss of granules (i.e., liberation of contents to any structure). However, this definition suffers from problems related to the type of microscopic observation employed and the distinction of primary from secondary lysosomes in macrophages, the latter resulting from lysosome fusion events. The process

of discharge of granules into phagosomes can legitimately be termed phagosome–lysosome fusion when the structure involved is a lysosome. However, the cells in question contain nonlysosomal granules as well (e.g., the specific granules of the neutrophil), which may lead to confusion. Accordingly, *degranulation* in this chapter is used to indicate discharge of neutrophil, eosinophil, or monocyte preformed granules into phagosomes (or other endocytic structures), and the term *secretion* (exocytosis) applies to release of granule contents to the outside of the cell. Secretion also encompasses active, nonlytic release of proteins, carbohydrates, and lipids from inflammatory cells, even if these molecules were not originally packaged into granules.

Degranulation

Engulfment of particles is accompanied by the assembly of contractile elements around the developing phagosome (see Chapter 20). These elements are then removed, probably sequentially, starting at the apex of the phagosome as it moves toward the center of the cell (Figs. 3 and 4). Granules (lysosomes) may be seen at this site fusing with the phagosome and discharging their contents into this structure (290,331). It has been presumed (largely on intuitive grounds backed by morphological observations) that the granules cannot penetrate the matrix of contractile protein and that fusion can occur only after it has been removed (113,205,218,262,317; see also 106).

During phagocytosis, most granule fusion occurs with the phagosomal membrane, not the plasma membrane (see below). Accordingly, it may reasonably be argued that local changes in the invaginating plasma membrane permit first recognition of the cytoplasmic surface of the granules and then the complicated and poorly understood processes that encompass membrane fusion (see below).

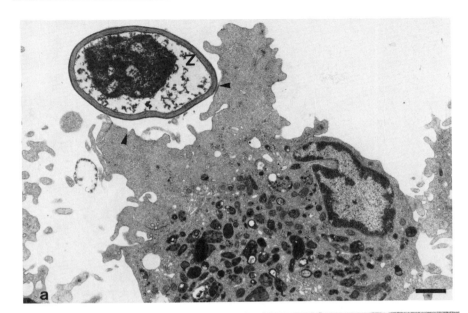

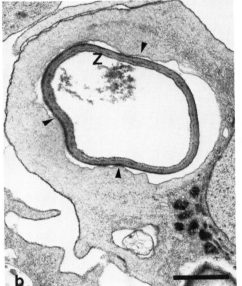

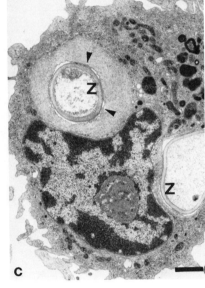

FIG. 3. Early morphological changes in phagocytosing and secreting rabbit alveolar macrophages. These electron micrographs depict organelle clearance (*arrows*) due to contractile protein assembly and rearrangement around the zymosan (Z) particles as they are engulfed. **b:** The cells were exposed to cationized ferritin after fixation, which binds the membranes to which it has access; it can be seen as the dark deposit on the macrophage surface but not in the phagosome, showing the latter to be sealed off from the extracellular environment. Bars = 1 μm.

In this context there is no reason to suppose that this type of event is any different mechanistically from phagolysosome fusion and secretory processes in other cells (18,113,248,305). However, the neutrophil contains at least three morphologically distinct populations of granules (storage organelles), and evidence has been obtained to indicate that secretion from them may be under separate control (51,168,315). Specific granules interact with the phagosome earlier than do the azurophil granules (15,23,111). Because there are more specific granules in the cell, the explanation for this observation could simply be their numerical difference. However, an argument is presented below that degranulation and secretion of specific granules indeed precede and can be separated from

that of azurophil granules. If accepted, it implies that there are separate and sequential recognition processes between the granule types and the phagosome. It has been suggested that such a sequence would allow the action of molecules from the specific granules with functional pH optima near neutrality to act on the phagosomal contents before the pH drops (123) and the azurophil granule enzymes (including the lysosomal acid hydrolases) gain their maximal effectiveness (15). This teleological concept may indeed have validity, but it is complicated by the knowledge that a variety of enzymes that are now thought to reside (in part) in the azurophil granule are optimally active at neutral pH (e.g., elastase, myeloperoxidase, lysozyme). Perhaps it is more reasonable to suggest that the overall ac-

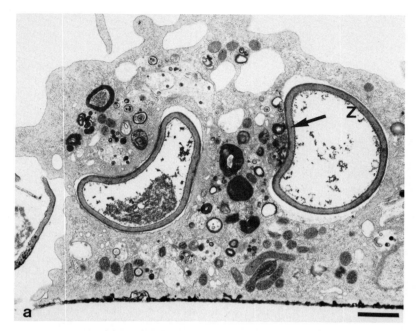

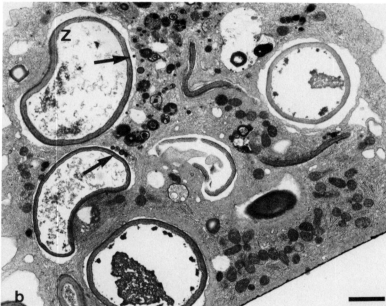

FIG. 4. Later morphological changes in phagocytosing and secreting macrophages (30 min after addition of zymosan). Most of the areas of organelle clearance around the phagosomes have disappeared, and multiple examples of lysosome–phagosome fusion (*arrows*) may be seen. Bars = 1 μm.

tivity of the granule phagosome contents is continuously modified by the pH (which is probably seldom at optimal levels for any of the enzymes, thereby ensuring greater control) and that granule contents that reach the external, and better-buffered, milieu may exhibit different types of dominant activity compared with those seen in the phagosomes.

Secretion of Granule Contents

Phagocytosis of particles by neutrophils, eosinophils, or monocytes results in release of preformed granule (or lysosomal) contents to the outside of the cell without concomitant liberation of cytoplasmic materials (22,104,111,116,152,167). These steps are characteristic of secretory events and are now considered to represent active secretion from these cell types. At issue, however, is exactly how such secretion occurs. As indicated above, for the purposes of this discussion it is argued that the mechanisms are similar, if not identical, for neutrophils, eosinophils, and monocytes. Therefore the three cells are considered together, although the neutrophil receives major emphasis because it has undergone by far the most investigation.

The earliest observations that neutrophils actively secreted some of their constituents (111,181,190) were soon followed by attempts to determine mechanisms for the process. The problem was compounded by *in vivo* observations of neutrophils interacting with glomerular basement membranes during inflammatory reactions in which a clear area of organelle exclusion was observed under the adherent cytoplasmic membrane, even though neutrophil granule enzymes and digested products of the basement membrane were found in the urine (106).

There is still no final explanation of this observation except to argue that sampling error minimized the opportunity to observe granule fusion events or to argue for a completely different secretory process (see below). Studies of neutrophils phagocytosing bacteria, opsonized yeast cell walls (zymosan particles), or immune complexes suggested that the degranulation process and extracellular secretion might be one and the same (112,219,290). Discharge of granules into developing phagosomes that were not yet closed off from the external environment would result in release of contents to the outside, i.e., secretion. Various circumstances were suggested under which the phagosomes might retain, or gain, access to the outside (112), and the process was colloquially termed "regurgitation while feeding" (290).

In an attempt to mimic the interaction of neutrophils with surfaces in the body (e.g., the glomerular basement membrane mentioned above), secretory events were studied also when such cells interacted with collagen, filters, or culture dishes coated with neutrophil stimuli (103,111,119). Secretion of granule constituents was readily observed, and the process was considered to be akin to granule fusion with the phagosome; but given the physical constraints of the system, internalization of the altered plasma membrane could not occur, so the discharge was directly to the outside. We used the term "frustrated phagocytosis" to describe this phenomenon and to suggest its mechanism.

The observation of surface stimulation of secretion has been extended to eosinophils (85,203) and monocytes (59,139,152), and its potential importance in inflammatory processes is mentioned below. However, both "frustrated phagocytosis" and "regurgitation while feeding" encompass underlying implications about secretory mechanisms that may be significantly incomplete or even wrong. Thus both concepts suggest an inefficiency of what is essentially a "normal" process, i.e., discharge of granules into phagosomes.

Little is known of the actual molecular events that occur during fusion of secretory vesicles or granules with the plasma membrane in neutrophils undergoing exocytosis. Much of our understanding of this process has stemmed from the study of permeabilized cells and cell-free systems derived from a variety of tissues with active exocytosis,

as well as model membrane systems. For clarity, the process of exocytosis can be broken down into the following events: (a) An intracellular signal (triggering event) causes the translocation of secretory vesicles to the inner surface of the plasma membrane; (b) repulsive forces are overcome enabling contact of the two opposing membranes; (c) the membrane bilayers undergo a focal destabilization; and (d) fusion of the secretory vesicle membrane and the plasma membrane occurs with reestablishment of the membrane bilayer structure, thereby maintaining the integrity of the cell while expelling vesicle contents to the external milieu.

Many data support a central role for an increase in intracellular ionized calcium as the triggering event in neutrophils to a variety of stimuli on which subsequent exocytosis depends. An increase in intracellular calcium concentration to 200 to 300 nM (as determined by the fluorescent calcium indicator quin 2) has been determined as the threshold for exocytosis in ionomycin-treated neutrophils (168). As such, the use of neutrophils treated with calcium ionophores resembles studies with permeabilized adrenal medullary cells and platelets, which have greatly enhanced our understanding of exocytosis (31,155). After permeabilization by electroporation, detergents (saponin or digitonin), ATP, or Sendai virus, the intracellular calcium concentration of these cells may be manipulated via the external milieu (31,48,155). In these "leaky" cell preparations micromolar calcium (1–100 μM) serves as the trigger for granule translocation and secretion (31,48,100,155) with further enhancement of calcium sensitivity possible with addition of GTP analogs (91,100). Further dissection of the exocytotic process has been possible with calcium-dependent fusion of purified adrenal chromaffin granules to adrenal medullary cell plasma membranes in cell-free preparations (31,156). Thus these models appear to mimic the triggering events in the neutrophil as we know them. The translocation of secretory granules in response to triggering has led investigators to search for interactions of secretory granules with cytosolic or cytoskeletal proteins. The use of affinity absorption columns has allowed the isolation of various proteins, from several cell sources, that adhere in a calcium-dependent manner to immobilized purified membranes (granule or plasma membranes) (31). Using these techniques, calmodulin, synexin, protein kinase C, and other possible granule–plasma membrane recognition proteins have been identified as proteins that may play a role in either translocation or adherence (recognition) of secretory vesicles to the plasma membrane (42,48). Furthermore, the sequence homology of a variety of proteins (calelectrin, endonexin, and protein pII) identified in this manner from various cell sources suggests a common role in exocytosis (80,159). The role of calmodulin in the final adherence process along the plasma membrane has also been suggested by experiments using calmodulin inhibitors (48) and specific calmodulin antibodies (259,271). Phosphorylation of several chromaffin granule membrane proteins either by calmodulin or protein kinase C appears to occur following activation with calcium (79,265).

Contact of opposing membranes—that of secretory vesicle and the plasma membrane—in addition to overcoming the repulsive forces of the net negative charges present on both membrane surfaces (53) must overcome hydration forces of the "hydration shell" overlying each bilayer (220). In model systems using vesicles of anionic phospholipids the affinity of opposed bilayers for calcium is sufficient to dehydrate the polar heads and result in vesicle–vesicle fusion at millimolar concentrations of calcium (122,208,307). The addition of synexin to this model system markedly lowers the calcium required for fusion to the micromolar range (126). Model vesicle–vesicle fusion appears to be highly dependent on negatively charged phospholipids (with even small amounts of neutral lipids decreasing fusion efficiency) (208), fluidity of the lipid bilayers (307), and polar head hydration (122). Model systems employing vesicle–bilayer fusion are more dependent on physical stresses within the vesicle and are sensitive to increases in osmotic pressure (67), the role of which may be important in exocytosis in some cellular systems (215,216).

Following contact of the secretory vesicle and plasma membranes, a nonbilayer focal destabilization occurs that, based on the rarity with which it is found in morphological studies of cells undergoing exocytosis, must be extremely short-lived (48). Lipidic particles have been identified in interacting model lipid bilayer systems and are thought perhaps to represent inverted micelles (220,278). These nonbilayer perturbations have been identified for cardiolipin, phosphatidylethanolamines, and diacylglycerols, lipids known to exhibit hexagonal phases that may represent the destabilized fusion intermediate of exocytosis (220,278). In any event, restabilization of the membrane bilayer occurs rapidly, fully integrating the secretory vesicle membrane into the plasma membrane. Data suggest that extensive phospholipid recycling follows to conserve cell surface area and maintain function (260).

Alternative Mechanisms for Inflammatory Cell Secretion

On the basis of little *direct* evidence, but as an explanation of a number of problems with the above-mentioned concepts of granule discharge, we raise the possibility that there are multiple pathways for secretion in these cell types, even of preformed proteinaceous materials (let alone for lipid molecules).

One of these pathways certainly would be fusion of granules–lysosomes with developing phagosomal membranes as indicated above and would perhaps be exaggerated in conditions of surface stimulation (frustrated phagocytosis).

A second process might explain the selective secretory involvement of the neutrophil specific granules. The contents of these granules are discharged (a) earlier (15,111, but see also 219), (b) with different stimuli (313,315), (c) to a greater extent, and (d) under different physical and environmental circumstances (89,252) than are materials in azurophil granules. This finding has led some authors to suggest that specific granules represent the true secretory granules of the neutrophil (70,76). The implication here is that direct fusion of the membrane of this granule with the plasma membrane results in an exocytosis that can be unrelated to endocytic events and the membrane invagination that accompanies it. That specific granule secretion can be initiated by calcium ionophores (315), alterations in extracellular calcium concentration (89), and a variety of soluble stimuli (313,315) supports this contention, even though direct ultrastructural evidence of fusion events has been difficult to demonstrate. A concern here is that although the stimuli and conditions mentioned certainly produce a selective secretion of specific granule contents, maximal stimulation under these conditions still results only in discharge of less than half of the contained specific granule materials. Moreover, small amounts of azurophil materials are usually discharged as well, especially at higher stimulus concentrations. Does this argue against a unique mechanism for specific granule secretion? No. It does, however, raise further questions about the relation of secretory processes involving the two granule types. Furthermore, the role and secretory pattern of additional, less characterized granule types must be considered in this context (51,81,191,302).

Third, one of us has suggested that vesicle transport (shuttling) may contribute to secretion from preformed stores within neutrophils and mononuclear phagocytes (113). At present, this idea is based on flimsy evidence indeed, but it would be consistent with vesicle shuttling in other cell types (127,260) and would explain a number of currently inexplicable problems. For example, secretion occurs in neutrophils, monocytes, and macrophages within the first few minutes of exposure to phagocytosable particles, at a time when only the earliest contact of particle and phagocyte membrane can be observed (113) and when large contractile protein barriers of "organelle exclusion" exist between the adherent particle and the "granules" from which the secreted products are presumed to be coming (Figs. 3 and 4). The lack of direct evidence of granule fusion with membrane sites distant from the area of membrane associated with the phagocytic events led to the concept of fusion events with smaller vesicles, which would not be apparent by simple ultrastructural observation. This hypothesis was deduced from morphological changes that have been observed by us (113) and others (24,38) in granules of secreting neutrophils, even when those granules were apparently located at some distance from the plasma membrane (Fig. 5). The changes are characterized by apparent dissolution of contents and occur within stimulated neutrophils *in vivo* as well as in the test tube. Similar changes have been seen in basophils (where they were ascribed to a process of "piecemeal"

degranulation and where more direct evidence of vesicle transport was actually provided (76)), eosinophils (107), and, although with less frequency because of interpretational difficulties, in mononuclear phagocytes.

Clearly, these arguments (113) are circumstantial and could be countered with legitimate alternative explanations. For example, the granule changes may be due to altered granule membrane permeability, influx of fluid, and increases in volume and thus could be unrelated to

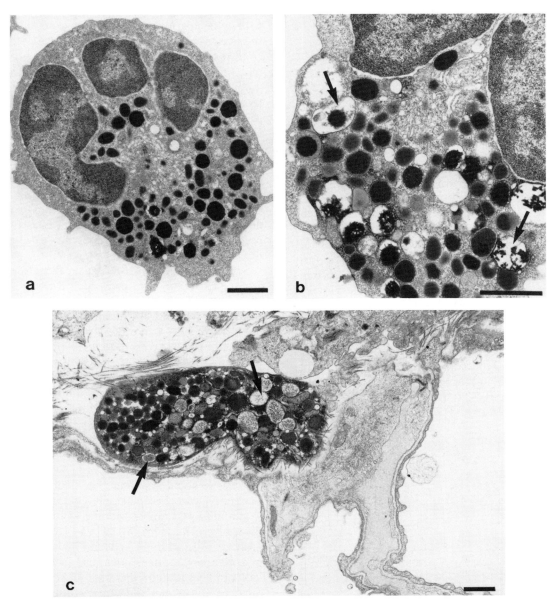

FIG. 5. Alterations in granule structure in neutrophils accompanying stimulation and secretion. **a:** Normal unstimulated rabbit neutrophil. **b:** Rabbit neutrophil stimulated with C5a and showing *in situ* dissolution of granule material. **c:** Rabbit neutrophil in the pulmonary interstitium showing similar changes in granule structure. Bars = 1 μm.

secretory events. Nevertheless, we put forward the possibility of additional secretory pathways as legitimate areas for further investigation.

Why might the physical mechanisms of secretion be important? Selective therapeutic inhibition of the putative secretory pathways labeled 2 and 3 in Fig. 6 might limit the degree of tissue injury in inflammation while preserving the discharge of granule contents into phagosomes, thereby sparing the protective functions of the phagocytic inflammatory cells. By contrast, suppression of the first mechanism could conceivably lead to the enhanced susceptibility to infections already known to result from impairment of inflammatory cell function.

Effects of Cytochalasins

Cytochalasins enhance the secretion of preformed constituents from inflammatory cells (105,114,332). In addition, they convert stimuli that are inactive or poorly active secretagogues into agents that are highly effective in this regard. As such, they have been used extensively in the study of inflammatory cell secretion (especially with neutrophils), even to the point that it is frequently necessary to delve carefully into the methods section of a manuscript to determine if cytochalasin was added to the reaction. The problem here is that we still do not know how the enhancement is brought about, and it probably does not reflect events and circumstances that are operative *in vivo*. Thus the usefulness of cytochalasins as tools for dissection of mechanisms may need a reevaluation that would lead to their more judicious use or at least interpretation.

Cytochalasins inhibit the uptake of particles during phagocytosis presumably because of their well-known effects on actin, and morphological evidence of granule discharge at membrane sites associated with particle contact can be readily observed (332). However, the interpretation

that now the phagosomes cannot be sealed off, i.e., that this situation may resemble the aforementioned frustrated phagocytosis, may be far too simplistic, even though we and others have earlier made such suggestions (117,123).

It is perhaps appropriate at this point to raise again a hypothesis developed by Poste and Allison (218). A submembranous marginal "bundle" of filamentous elements could limit access of vesicles–granules to the cytoplasmic face of the plasma membrane. Removal of this "barrier" naturally during cell stimulation (particularly as a consequence of general clearance of contractile elements following phagocytosis, as mentioned above) or artificially with cytochalasins could enhance secretion by rendering the necessary contacts easier to achieve. Although these concepts do not seem to have much following at the current time, they have not been disproved, and some element of such control processes may in fact contribute to secretory events. Cytochalasin produces profound morphological alterations in the whole cell following stimulation (113,123) with deep invaginations of plasma membrane. It has been suggested that these invaginations actually result from directed granule fusion (34), accompanied also by a nondirected vesicle and granule fusion that can be separated from the former process depending on the source of calcium. However, these concepts were derived from freeze-fracture pictures that could be interpreted also in relation to proposed opposing contractile forces in the cell (123).

Soluble, chemotactic stimuli can induce extensive granule secretion from cytochalasin-treated cells. Cytochalasins enhance not only secretion but most of the stimulated responses of the neutrophil including oxygen metabolism (90), leukotriene production, and adhesion (41). Thus it seems reasonable to emphasize the likelihood that cytochalasins also (or even rather) enhance the stimulus–response coupling process in general. Reports that their presence is associated with increased production of diacylglycerol (125) may relate to such a process.

Priming and Enhanced Cell Reactivity

It has become apparent that neutrophils and mononuclear phagocytes can exhibit different states of reactivity to stimulation. Emphasized first with bacterial endotoxin (lipopolysaccharide, LPS) (97,204) but now extended to a variety of stimuli, the cells can apparently be "primed" in a manner that does not cause the response in and of itself but does result in the subsequent response to another (or even sometimes the same) stimulus being of much greater magnitude. Originally, the priming phenomenon was studied largely in the context of oxygen metabolite production, but it is now clear that it extends to secretion of a wide variety of materials including lysosomal con-

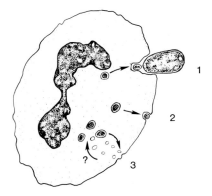

FIG. 6. Three possible mechanisms of secretion of granule contents in neutrophils.

stituents (68), to the production and release of lipid mediators (312), and to a number of other cellular responses. Interestingly, a similar or identical phenomenon has been observed *in vivo* in that neutrophils derived from inflammatory exudates in rabbits (P. M. Henson and E. L. Becker *unpublished observations*) or man (330) exhibited enhanced responsiveness to stimulation.

"Priming" of macrophages for enhanced production of oxygen metabolites (204) may or may not represent the same process as is observed with neutrophils. So many agents (including such diverse materials as LPS, muramyl dipeptide, interferons, polynucleotides, lymphokines, and prostanoids) alter macrophage phenotypic characters and their subsequent responsiveness to additional stimuli that the processes in mononuclear phagocytes may be much more varied and more complex than those seen in neutrophils. This complexity should not, however, diminish the potential importance of combinations of stimuli for induction of macrophage responses; in fact, it focuses on the need for further study in this area.

The mechanisms involved in priming of neutrophils are not understood, although a great deal of effort is being extended in this area. We have suggested (97) that the priming process does not lie at the level of receptor number or affinity, and the observation that cells can be primed to the subsequent action of phorbol myristate acetate would imply (though not emphatically) that the priming process preceded, in the stimulus-secretion coupling pathway, the involvement of protein kinase C.

The observation that cells can be primed by a variety of materials including LPS (97,204) have a number of important implications for inflammatory reactions.

1. Circulating cells in "normal" animals or individuals are in even more of a resting state than was often thought. It is difficult to rid isolated cell preparations of the LPS (1–10 ng/ml) that is required for priming, and it must be concluded that for years most of us were studying cells that were already raised to this intermediate state of stimulation.

2. A class of stimuli can be defined that encompass agents that predominantly induce the priming phenomenon and that are weak direct cell stimulants or secretagogues (e.g., LPS). Other stimuli (e.g., immune complexes) can induce both priming and further cell responses such as secretion. However, for neutrophils natural stimuli that directly induce azurophil granule or a major degree of specific granule secretion are usually particulate or surface-bound unless cytochalasin is used. Does it mean that the intracellular events that are induced during the priming phenomenon are related to the effect of surfaces (see above) of particle uptake and even perhaps of cytochalasin? Do neutrophils have to proceed through a "primed" step in any activation sequence, this requirement having been missed in many circumstances previously studied because the stages were not temporarily separable?

3. Because bacterial endotoxin is such a potent priming agent, its effect on neutrophils *in vivo* may lead to greater degrees of tissue injury. In this context, LPS and chemotactic factors together have been shown to enhance neutrophil-dependent pulmonary vascular injury *in vivo* (310) and neutrophil-mediated damage to endothelial monolayers *in vitro* (250). The recent demonstration of a high correlation between the presence of both LPS and C5 fragments in the blood of patients at risk for adult respiratory distress syndrome (ARDS) with those who actually develop the syndrome (211) lends support to the suspicion that priming processes may contribute to inflammatory injury and disease.

4. Increasingly, phenomena such as those described above emphasize the likelihood that *in vivo* complex combinations of cellular stimuli interact to produce the overall observed effect, or cellular response. A mediator network (193) seems to be a useful way of conceptualizing this idea, and its therapeutic implications are significant.

SECRETION OF NEWLY SYNTHESIZED PROTEINS BY MACROPHAGES

Stimulation of macrophages, e.g., by the act of phagocytosis, initiates secretion of a wide variety of proteinaceous materials. These secretory processes can be readily separated into the discharge of preformed constituents (see above) and the secretion of newly synthesized materials by use of protein-synthesis inhibitors (183,240). Figure 7 depicts the secretion of hexosaminidase from macrophages and distinguishes the early, protein synthesis-independent process from the release of this enzyme over days, which is prevented by cycloheximide. A further group of proteins are, however, synthesized and secreted constitutively, i.e., independent of added macrophage stimuli. This discharge also is prevented by inhibitors of protein synthesis.

Constitutive Secretion

The constant release of lysozyme by macrophages in culture is often used as the typical example of constitutive secretion. A few other materials that behave in this way (e.g., apolipoprotein E) are indicated in Table 1, and the spontaneous discharge of many proteins is clearly seen in the electrophoresis gel depicted in Fig. 8.

The clear implication from the term "constitutive," from the literature and from the above remarks, is that the macrophage synthesizes a group of such proteins at a relatively constant rate and that they are then packaged directly for export to the exterior. For cells in culture *in*

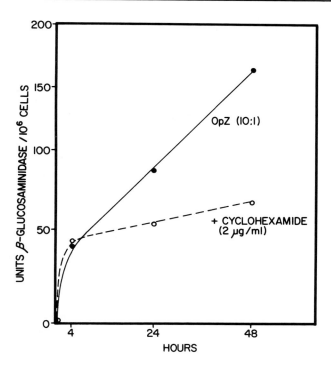

FIG. 7. Synthesis-dependent and synthesis-independent secretion from rabbit alveolar macrophages. Cells were stimulated with serum-opsonized zymosan (OpZ) at the indicated ratios. Enzymes released to the exterior were measured, and here the glucosaminidase is depicted. Cycloheximide, which inhibited protein synthesis in these cells by more than 80%, prevented the prolonged secretion of enzymes but not the discharge seen over the first 4 hr. The cytoplasmic enzyme lactic dehydrogenase was not liberated, indicating that lysosomal enzymes were actively secreted and not released subsequent to cell lysis. (From ref. 102.)

vitro, this situation certainly appears to be the case. Nevertheless, it seems appropriate to question the validity of this concept of nonstimulated secretion for cells *in vivo.* The acts of isolation and culture for cells that are as responsive to their environments as mononuclear phagocytes could conceivably provide stimulus enough to initiate the synthesis of secretory proteins such as lysozyme. For example, the synthetic, secretory, and functional properties of macrophages differ appreciably when they are in contact with different types of surface (147,263). Certainly, it might be argued that because lysozyme (for example) can be found in fluids lavaged from body spaces inhabited by macrophages that constitutive secretion of this protein occurs *in vivo.* Here again, however, the stimuli impinging on the macrophage are not completely known, and the situation might be complicated by the presence of alternative cellular sources of lysozyme (neutrophils, for example, where the protein is stored in the granules and released only upon stimulation). In the case of apolipoprotein E, Werb and Chin (298) have suggested that constitutive secretion of this protein by macrophages is important in the physiological transport of lipids. This conclusion was based in part on the observation that the synthesis and secretion of apolipoprotein E by macrophages is strongly inhibited by exposure to lipopolysaccharide. It was speculated that this down-regulation of apolipoprotein E synthesis may contribute to the triglyceridemia associated with infections with gram-negative organisms. With the increasing availability of complimentary DNA probes specific for macrophage secretory proteins, it should soon prove possible using the techniques of *in situ* hybridization to conclusively identify

TABLE 1. *Secretory products of macrophages*

Constitutive	Preformed	Induced
Proteins		
Apolipoprotein E (21,298)	Acid hydrolases (183,224,242)	Acid hydrolases (182,183,240)
α_2-Macroglobulin (129)		Angiogenesis factor(s) (217)
C1q, C2, C4 (303)		Arginase (4)
Factor H, factor I (303)		β-Interferon (69)
Fibronectin (2,137)		Cachectin/tumor necrosis factor (25)
Lipoprotein lipase (178)		Collagenase (280,300)
Lysozyme (93)		Colony-stimulating factor (189)
		Elastase (299)
		Factor B, C3 (225,264)
		Interleukin-1 (82)
		Macrophage-derived growth factors (165)
		Plasminogen activator (275)
Lipids		Leukotriene C_4 (234)
		Platelet-activating factor (187)
		Prostaglandin E_2 (132)
		Prostaglandin F_2 (132)
		6-Keto-prostaglandin $F_{1\alpha}$ (132)
Others		
Thymidine (255,256)	Protons (by implication)	Hydrogen peroxide (194)
		Superoxide anion (138)

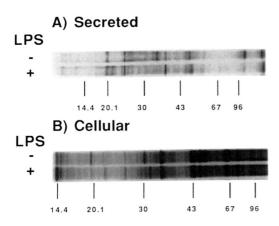

FIG. 8. Changes in the total protein biosynthetic phenotype after incubation of resident peritoneal macrophages in the presence or absence of bacterial lipopolysaccharide (LPS; 1 µg/ml) for 24 hr. The cells were then biosynthetically labeled with 200 µCi of L-[^{35}S]methionine dissolved in methionine-free DMEM for 1 hr. They were then either chased in nonradioactive methionine (1 mM) for 18 hr for measurement of the secreted products (**A**) or were harvested immediately for measurement of the cellular products (**B**). Cells were lysed in a detergent–enzyme inhibitor mixture as described (204), and samples were electrophoresed through 5 to 15% SDS–polyacrylamide gels under reducing conditions. Radioactive bands were visualized by fluorography as described (223).

those macrophages that have the *potential* to secrete "constitutive" proteins *in vivo* in fixed sections of normal and pathological tissue.

Induced (Synthesis-Dependent) Secretion

As indicated above, induced secretion may in fact encompass the entire array of secretory processes that involve newly synthesized proteins (i.e., that process which has been called constitutive as well). Remarkably little is known about the secretory processes in this complicated cell type; the status of investigation lies mostly at the level of what is secreted and to a limited extent to how it is controlled, e.g., by icosanoids or by different groups of impinging stimuli and inhibitors. Nevertheless, a few generalizations can be made and some questions raised.

It seems reasonable to assume that there is nothing unique about macrophage secretion and that it follows pathways similar to those in other cell types (e.g., hepatocytes). Current dogma therefore would imply synthesis on the rough endoplasmic reticulum, co-translational glycosylation and translocation into the lumen of the endoplasmic reticulum, transport to the Golgi, and vesicle transport to the plasma membrane (27). In this scenario, stimulation might occur at two levels: (a) At the level of transcription or translation. In its simplest form, this situation would imply that any newly synthesized protein bearing a suitable signal peptide would be secreted. (b) At

the level of packaging, processing, transport, or membrane fusion. In this case, the macrophage is viewed as continually synthesizing specific secretory proteins, but unless the cells are stimulated the secretory proteins are degraded intracellularly so as to prevent buildup of the material within the cell. For example, deprivation of fibroblasts of ascorbic acid does not change the rate of collagen synthesis, but the collagen so produced is recognized as being abnormal and is rapidly degraded before reaching the secretory pathway (261).

Probably different proteins are controlled by one or both of these broad mechanisms, and each may have to be studied in detail to sort out its point(s) of control. Because of the importance of the macrophage and its secreted products (proteolysis, control of lymphocyte activity, wound healing) this area seems to be a fruitful one for investigation.

Some of the proteins that are secreted in a fashion that requires protein synthesis following stimulation are also proteins that reside in the lysosomes and can be discharged in synthesis-independent processes (182,183,240) (Fig. 7). This point raises an important question. Are the actual mechanisms identical? The pathways of lysosomal enzyme synthesis, intracellular transport, and targeting to the lysosome have been largely elucidated (Fig. 9) using as examples β-glucuronidase, hexosaminidase, and cathepsin D. Unlike most proteins destined for intracellular distribution (e.g., mitochondrial proteins), lysosomal enzymes are synthesized along with secretory proteins on the rough endoplasmic reticulum (233). During translocation to the lumen of the endoplasmic reticulum, an *N*-terminal signal peptide is cleaved from the lengthening nascent chain. Dolichol phosphate-dependent core glycosylation, with a high mannose-type oligosaccharide chain, also takes place co-translationally.

The mechanism of transport to the Golgi apparatus has not been determined, although on the basis of inhibition of this process by 1-deoxynojirimycin, a glucose analog known to inhibit trimming glucosidases (166), it has been speculated that the deglucosylation of the oligosaccharide side chain may in some undefined manner promote the transport of lysosomal enzymes to the region of the cis-Golgi (166). Because lysosomal enzymes are initially cosegregated into the lumen of the endoplasmic reticulum along with other secretory proteins, a sorting mechanism must exist to prevent their constitutive secretion to the extracellular milieu and promote their targeting to the lysosomes. The passage through the Golgi apparatus is crucial to this sorting process. During this period the high mannose oligosaccharide is phosphorylated in the 6-position in a complex conversion process (158). The unique mannose-6-phosphate residue engages with specific mannose-6-phosphate receptors that cycle between the Golgi and the lysosomes (and, to a limited though nevertheless potentially important extent, to the plasma membrane as

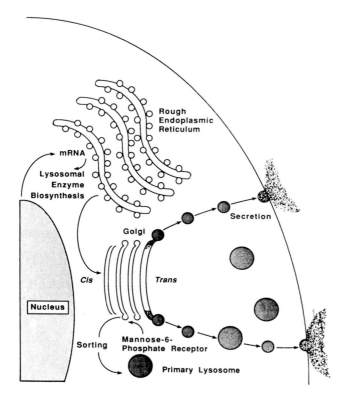

FIG. 9. Possible pathways of lysosomal enzyme biosynthesis and secretion in macrophages. Transcription of the genes for lysosomal enzymes yields mRNA, which is translated in the rough endoplasmic reticulum. A signal peptide directs the vectoral translocation of the lengthening polypeptide chain into the lumen of the rough endoplasmic reticulum. Dolichol phosphate-dependent asparagine-linked core glycosylation of the lysosomal enzymes takes place co-translationally. After removal of the signal peptide by signal peptidase, the lysosomal enzymes are transported to the Golgi apparatus, during which some trimming of the oligosaccharide side chain occurs. Passage through the Golgi apparatus results in phosphorylation of mannose residues at the 6-position to produce a ligand that is recognized by a specific receptor (mannose-6-phosphate receptor). Mannose-6-phosphate receptors remove phosphorylated lysosomal enzymes from other bulk secreted proteins and transport the former to the lysosomes (here defined as primary lysosomes). Stimulus-dependent secretion of performed lysosomal enzymes probably takes place from primary lysosomes. The mechanism of synthesis-dependent lysosomal enzyme secretion is unknown but potentially could occur owing to: (a) an absence of lysosomal enzyme phosphorylation; (b) down-regulation of the mannose-6-phosphate receptor system; or (c) alteration of the secretion-recapture mechanism.

well). Two types of mannose-6-phosphate receptors have been identified. The major form utilized by most cell types so far studied has a molecular weight of 215 kD (30,83,236), whereas a smaller receptor (46 kD) has been found to be involved in lysosomal enzyme sorting and targeting in certain cell lines deficient in the 215-kD receptor (124). Upon forming primary lysosomes, the acidic

intralysosomal pH promotes dissociation of the lysosomal enzymes from the mannose-6-phosphate receptors, and the receptors are free to recycle to the Golgi apparatus to begin another cycle of transport (92). Studies conducted with fibroblasts derived from individuals with lysosomal storage diseases have indicated the importance of the mannose-6-phosphate residues of lysosomal enzymes in directing their transport to the lysosomes, because in their absence these lysosomal enzymes are directly secreted to the exterior of the cells (222).

On the basis of these data, several intriguing possibilities can be raised concerning the synthesis-dependent secretion of lysosomal enzymes from stimulated macrophages.

1. Do secreted enzymes lack mannose-6-phosphate residues? If so, it suggests that after macrophage stimulation the increased level of lysosomal enzyme synthesis may overload the capacity of the cells to efficiently phosphorylate all lysosomal enzymes, or the activity of the phosphorylating enzymes may have been actively down-regulated.

2. To what extent are secreted enzymes reinternalized by plasma membrane mannose and mannose-6-phosphate receptors? Measurements of total cellular and secreted enzyme activities clearly do not address this possibility. As alluded to earlier, mannose-6-phosphate residues are also expressed at the plasma membrane, as are mannose receptors. Lysosomal enzyme secretion and recapture has been reported to occur in fibroblasts and macrophages (54). It is thus conceivable that after stimulation the recapture mechanism becomes inactivated (perhaps as a consequence of plasma membrane internalization during endocytic stimulation) or down-regulated. Interestingly, treatment of macrophages with dexamethasone increases the expression of surface mannose receptors, leading to an apparent decrease in spontaneous lysosomal secretion, which in fact is due to an increase in the reuptake of secreted lysosomal enzymes (246). Clearly the answer to some of these questions could be determined by examining the mannose-6-phosphate receptor status of stimulated cells.

3. Most lysosomal enzymes so far investigated have been shown to undergo limited proteolytic cleavage in the lysosomal compartment (249). In the case of β-glucuronidase, this situation reduces the molecular weight of the molecule by 2 to 3 kD. This fact may provide a useful "handle" with which to determine if the secreted molecule has passed through the lysosomal system. One might predict that in protein synthesis-dependent secretion of lysosomal enzymes by macrophages the secreted enzymes have not undergone proteolytic cleavage.

In addition to stimulating lysosomal enzyme biosynthesis, stimulation of macrophages in vitro also induces changes in the synthesis of a variety of other proteins, some of which are retained intracellularly, others of which are secreted. Some of the changes in the synthesis of certain proteins appear to correlate with changes in the functional phenotype of the cell (177). The identification of these proteins is clearly of value in determining the biochemical and signal transduction mechanisms that are involved in macrophage phenotypic differentiation, studies of which are currently in their infancy.

A fascinating series of investigations during the 1960s by Cohn and collaborators showed that enzyme induction (later associated with secretion) depended on the ingestion of digestible particles. Equal uptake of nondigestible material, e.g., particles composed of D-amino acids (8), were inactive. The mechanisms underlying the ability of the macrophage to discriminate between such materials remain enigmatic, though intriguing. The importance of these observations to inflammatory processes may be in discrimination (crude recognition) by macrophages exposed to environmental particulates in vivo. For example, inhalation of bacteria (digestible) or coal dust (nondigestible) produce quite different types of pulmonary response; and if the alveolar macrophages really orchestrate the initial pulmonary inflammatory reactions (as is often suggested), the secretory response to their ingestion of digestible particles may be a critical factor.

Macrophages, like any cell, have limited synthetic resources. Interestingly, then, stimulation of such cells induces on the one hand new protein synthesis and, on the other, suppression of synthesis of another group of proteins (Fig. 8). Oldstone and Buchmeier (202) suggested, in the context of viral infection, that cells shut down their synthesis of nonessential "housekeeping" proteins to direct the machinery and intracellular resources to production of the stimulated (viral) proteins. Such a concept seems logical for the macrophage and seems particularly applicable to secreted proteins. Early studies of the control of this process are suggestive of an extremely complex series of controlling factors and mechanisms that lead to the precise array of secreted materials seen under each environmental and stimulating circumstance. As examples may be cited the suppression of apolipoprotein E (298) and β-glucuronidase (223) synthesis and secretion by lipopolysaccharide at the same time the synthesis and secretion of C3 and factor B are initiated (240). By complete contrast, exposure to dextran sulfate enhanced the production of acid hydrolases but did not initiate synthesis of C3. At this point, with a few proteins studied (e.g., apolipoprotein E, β-glucuronidase, C3, factor B), control appears to occur largely at the level of transcription (225,264). However, it may not be the case for all the proteins whose synthesis and secretion is altered by each new stimulus or group of stimuli (Fig. 8).

In summary, we reemphasize that the macrophage is a pluripotential cell. Endocytosis and secretion then encompass two of its major functions, the latter being of critical importance in the initiation, progression, and especially the resolution of the inflammatory process. Because of the extremely wide array of materials that this cell type can secrete, it becomes of critical importance to determine how the patterns of secretion are controlled. Understanding the differential control of such secretory events represents an exciting and significant line of endeavor if we see release of proteases to be destructive, discharge of fibroblast growth factors to be useful in the skin but perhaps disastrous in the lung, or secretion of parenchymal cell replication factors to promote healing and a return to normal function.

SECRETION OF NONPROTEINACEOUS, NONGRANULE MATERIALS FROM INFLAMMATORY CELLS

Most of the emphasis on cellular secretory processes has been placed on discharge of proteins. However, inflammatory cells release critically important molecules that are neither proteinaceous nor derived from granules or lysosomes. Here, we consider briefly the "secretion" of lipid "mediators" and oxygen metabolites. Surprisingly little is known about the mechanisms by which such molecules are released, so the discussion is of necessity speculative and we hope stimulatory.

Lipids

When secretion of lipids is considered, attention is usually drawn to hepatocytes (65) or "professional" lipid secretors, e.g., the type II alveolar epithelial cells that synthesize and secrete pulmonary surfactant (179,229). In the latter circumstance, the phospholipids destined for extracellular transport are packaged in special, membrane-bound organelles (the lamellar bodies) in association with what is turning out to be an array of apoproteins (179,229). Upon appropriate stimulation of the cells, these lamellar bodies are then discharged directly to the exterior (272,273).

Inflammatory cells synthesize and release platelet-activating factor (PAF), which is a phospholipid, and a wide variety of arachidonate metabolites (see below). Critical to tracing the pathways and mechanisms of secretion of such molecules is an understanding of the geography of the system, i.e., where in the cell the molecules are synthesized. Increasingly, a body of indirect evidence (195,251) is pointing toward the nuclear envelope as a major site for liberation of arachidonate from phospholipid precursors and thus for the production of the substrates for icosanoid and PAF synthesis. If the synthetic processes also occur deep within the cell, we need to account for transport across the cytoplasm as well as through the plasma membrane.

A number of possibilities exist, with but meager evidence in support of any of them.

1. Packaging in vesicles with transport to the extracellular environment in a manner similar to any other group of secreted products. Intuitively, this mechanism is attractive, being somewhat conservative in concept and having precedence in some sense in the type II epithelial cell. Additionally, it would fit with one hypothesis for the intracellular transport and insertion of membrane phospholipids (148,149,279). Nevertheless, there is no direct evidence for such a process and no details of any mechanisms whereby such packaging might occur.

2. Carrier proteins. Some interest is now being generated in phospholipid transport proteins (148,329) for movement of phospholipids within cells. These proteins could carry such molecules across the cytoplasm and conceivably aid their passage through the membrane. Additionally, the presence of a proposed carrier protein for PAF has been reported in plasma (172) that might serve to "extract" PAF from a membrane-associated site. However, specific proteins have been difficult to identify; their role in secretion is completely unknown, and none has yet been identified that interacts with arachidonate metabolites (perhaps they have not yet been looked for). Interestingly, however, most experiments on icosanoid release from inflammatory cells employ extracellular albumin to "trap" the released icosanoid. Does albumin play such a role *in vivo,* and is it the carrier protein that "extracts" such molecules from the cell? Critically lacking in these concepts is knowledge of the physical forces involved in association of given icosanoids with the membrane, the aqueous environment, and albumin, respectively.

3. Diffusion. The molecules in question all have, to a greater or lesser extent, hydrophilic properties in comparison with most membrane phospholipids. Accordingly, it is conceivable that they pass to the outside of the cell along diffusion gradients, perhaps aided by their hydrophilicity and aforementioned carrier proteins. However, in a study of removal of lysophosphatides from membranes, those with acyl chains of 16 or more carbon atoms (which would include molecules such as PAF) appeared to be tightly bound (297).

As outlined above, such concepts are clearly unsophisticated in the extreme. Nevertheless, they do raise some experimentally approachable questions. For example, if diffusional mechanisms were operative, by manipulating the external environment it should be possible to create circumstances wherein the intracellular levels of the lipids in question remained high. In fact, high intracellular levels for PAF are usually seen (173), although it is not the case

for icosanoids, which generally seem to be released soon after synthesis (251). By contrast, intracellular buildup of these molecules following interference with known vesicular secretory pathways might point toward these types of processes as likely candidates. Because of the importance of secretion of lipid mediators to the overall outcome of the inflammatory response, pursuit of these mechanisms may be important, with the possible ultimate objective of being able to provide external control over them.

Oxygen Metabolites

Phagocytic responses to appropriate particulate or soluble stimuli include the generation and release of a variety of reactive oxygen species (64,230). The presumed parent compound of these oxidants, superoxide anion (O_2^-) is formed at the plasma and phagosomal membrane by transfer onto oxygen of an electron from an electron transport chain driven by the plasma membrane-associated NADPH oxidase (9,50,186). Although the precise location of this enzyme is unknown, restriction of its substrate, NADPH, to the cytoplasm suggests an association with the inner leaflet of the plasma membrane. How, then is O_2^- transported across the plasma membrane without prior inactivation by cytoplasmic superoxide dismutase (SOD)? Does the electron transport chain perhaps span the inner leaflet of the lipid bilayer, receiving electrons on the plasma side but forming the oxidants in between both lipid leaflets of the plasma membrane? Such a location might protect O_2^- from the action of SOD. Moreover, because the chemical composition of lipid membranes influences their permeability to O_2^- (96,235), the cell could ensure unidirectional flow of the oxidant by differential structuring of inner and outer leaflets of the membrane bilayer. Whether O_2^- generated by phagocytes indiscriminately diffuses across lipid membranes or utilizes specialized transmembrane pathways is unclear. In liposomes (96) and erythrocytes (175,176) the transmembrane diffusion of O_2^- was markedly accelerated by the presence of anion channels. Although it is entirely possible that phagocyte plasma membranes contain specialized regions where the O_2^--forming apparatus is associated with such channels, clear evidence is lacking.

RELATION OF SECRETION TO OTHER CELL FUNCTIONS

In some respects this section is a compendium of the information provided in most of the chapters of this section. Nevertheless, a few key points are made herein for the purpose of putting the secretory processes of inflammatory cells into perspective.

Cell functions such as phagocytosis, the oxidative burst,

cellular polarization (orientation, shape change), adhesion, movement, and chemotaxis can in many circumstances be induced by the same stimuli as are effective in the initiation of secretion (e.g., immunoglobulin Fc fragments, complement fragments). On the other hand, it has been possible to create experimental conditions that allow the dissociation of nearly every one of the above-mentioned cellular processes from any other (40,115,253,281). However, because some of these conditions are highly artificial, it is worth noting that secretory processes and the oxidative burst have frequently been found separable from chemotaxis, adhesion, and shape change (and may in fact involve different pools of protein kinase C) (40), and that phagocytosis is often seen in a different category again.

Nevertheless, for the purposes of this discussion we argue that these actions are integrated responses of the cell and that in inflammation *they occur together*. In fact, we suggest that these various responses may be required for the complete cellular response in inflammation. A few examples are given for the neutrophil and should be considered in the context of the discussion below.

It has been suggested that normal secretion of specific granules is required for a maximal chemotactic response (see Chapters 18 and 26). The concept is that new receptors for the chemoattractant are translocated to the plasma membrane by this process. In this context, then, it is interesting that a monoclonal antibody (directed to a human neutrophil surface protein) that inhibited secretion also blocked chemotactic responsiveness (39).

Chemotaxis and cell movement are surface phenomena: The inflammatory cells crawl, they do not swim. Thus adhesion is a critical part of the migratory process. This point is best exemplified by the inability of neutrophils that lack the adhesive CDw18 surface glycoprotein complex (or have had it deliberately blocked) to migrate *in vitro* or *in vivo* (4). Another intriguing possibility is that phagocytosis and these adherence and migratory responses share common features. Griffin et al. (95) have suggested that the "zipper" hypothesis for phagocytosis might also account for directed cell movement over surface-bound gradients of chemotactic factors (52,285). Although most investigators of chemotaxis consider that the cell is able to recognize a fluid phase gradient of chemoattractant, the surface concept and its similarity to phagocytosis remain as possibilities to fit into the puzzle.

Finally, movement of cells *in vivo* is clearly much more complex than that seen in chemotaxis chambers *in vitro*, and as is mentioned briefly it seems increasingly likely that secretory events and even release of oxygen metabolites may be involved in the maximal emigratory response in tissues, even if arguably required *in vitro* (but see above).

We have considered broad categories of cellular response. Clearly they must ultimately be translated to specific intracellular stimulus–response transduction pathways (see Chapter 19). However, it seems clear already that, despite the likely presence of more than one receptor type (or affinity state) for many of these cell stimuli, the disparate and complex interacting cellular responses to such stimuli cannot all be accounted for at the receptor level and must result from as yet poorly understood diverging intracellular response pathways.

PRODUCTS OF PHAGOCYTIC INFLAMMATORY CELL SECRETION

The recognition of phagocytic inflammatory cells as having major secretory functions has led to the demonstration of an enormously wide variety of secreted products, especially in the case of mononuclear phagocytes. A detailed discussion of these materials is far beyond the scope of this chapter. Rather, we have included Tables 1 through 4, which list *some* of the materials that have been reported to be secreted from neutrophils, eosinophils, and macrophages. Macrophages here are defined as cells of the mononuclear phagocyte lineage that are found within tissues (or induced by culture), rather than in the circulation, that exhibit secondary lysosomes. Criteria that are more quantitative in nature might include such elements as significant prestimulation vacuolation, large cytoplasm/nuclear ratios, multiple Golgi apparati, and extensive rough endoplasmic reticulum.

Various types, sources, and states of activation of macrophages have not been distinguished in these tables. Instead, a *potential* list of secreted materials is indicated. In fact, for all three cell types different stimuli and circumstances may induce proportionally more or less secretion of different groups of products.

Finally, these lists are not, and could not be, exhaustive. Emphasis has arbitrarily been placed on materials of particular interest and abundance. The authors' bias is clearly apparent. Furthermore, the references in this section are likewise intended to provide access to, rather than coverage of, the literature to given secretory products, as the bibliography is in some cases extensive. Accordingly, apologies are offered up front for any oversight of a favorite secretory product or reference.

EFFECTS OF SECRETION FROM INFLAMMATORY CELLS

Given the plethora of materials that are secreted from these cell types, and their potential spectrum of biological activities, the subject of effects is clearly large and in fact encompasses much of what this whole book and the subject of inflammation in general is about. Therefore only

TABLE 2. *Possible secretory products of neutrophils: enzymes, proteins, and glycosaminoglycans*

Azurophil granules	Specific granules	Other granule types	Membranes
Peroxidase ($R_{13,14,16}$; $H_{11,57,146}$)		Acid phosphatase ($R_{11,13,14,302}$; H_{11})	Acid phosphatase (R_{11}, H_{11})
Acid phosphatase ($R_{11,13,14,16,302}$; $H_{11,146,254}$)		Heparitinase (H_{180})	5'-Nucleotidase (H_{146})
β-Glucosaminidase ($R_{11,13,14}$; H_{254})	Alkaline phosphatase ($R_{11,13,14,302}$)	β-Glucosaminidase (R_{11}; $H_{11,146}$)	Alkaline phosphatase (H_{146})
5'-Nucleotidase (R_{16}; H_{17})	Histaminase (H_{227})	α-Mannosidase (R_{11}; H_{11})	Neutral α-glucosidase (H_{146})
α-Mannosidase ($R_{11,13,14}$; $H_{11,146}$)		Acid proteinase (H_{146})	Deoxyribonuclease ? (H_{61})
Arylsulfatase (R_{16}; H_{17})			Ribonuclease ? (H_{221})
α-Fucosidase (H_7)			Leucyl-β-naphthylaminidase (H_{146})
Neuraminidase ? (H_{320})			
Esterase (H_{213})			
Cathepsin A ? (R_{282})			
Cathepsin D ? (R_{258}; H_{134})			
Cathepsin E ? (R_{258})			
Cathepsin F ? ($O_{157,161}$)			
Cathepsin G ? (acid) ($O_{157,161}$)			
Collagenolytic cathepsin (R_{84}; O_3)		Collagenolytic cathepsin ? (R_{84})	Elastase (*de novo* synthesis) (H_{35})
Elastase ($H_{35,200}$)		Elastase ? (H_{35})	
Cathepsin G (neutral) ($H_{146,200}$)	Collagenase (R_{228}; H_{192})	Gelatinase (H_{51})	Plasminogen activator ? (*de novo* synthesis) (H_{94})
Histonase (H_{45})			
Lysozyme ($R_{11,13,14}$; $H_{11,146}$)	Lysozyme ($R_{11,13,14}$; $H_{11,146,164}$)		
	Vitamin B_{12} binding protein (H_{146})		
Phospholipase A ($R_{72,160}$)			
Cationic proteins (R_{328}; H_{198})	Laminin receptor (H_{324})	Laminin receptor (H_{324})	Phospholipase (H_{73})
Bactericidal/permeability-inducing protein ($R_{60,327}$; H_{286})	C3bi receptor ($H_{6,237,318}$)		
Defensins (R_{243}; H_{78})	fMet-Leu-Phe receptor (H_{70})		
Glycosaminoglycans ($R_{99,191}$; H_{210})	Lactoferrin (R_{12}; H_{164})	Glycosaminoglycans ($R_{99,191}$; H_{210})	
Chondroitin sulfate (H_{210})	Cytochrome b_{245} (H_{29})		
Heparin sulfate (H_{210})	Flavoproteins (H_{28})		

R = rabbit. H = human. O = other species.   Subscript numbers are the reference numbers.

a few points are made here, mostly for the purpose of integrating the secretory processes themselves with the rest of the inflammatory responses.

TABLE 3. *Other neutrophil secretory products*

Lipids	Reductants and oxidants
Platelet-activating factor (PAF) (171,174)	Hydrogen ion (H^+) (136,145)
Arachidonic acid (296)	Superoxide anion (O_2^-) (10,56)
Thromboxane B_2 (TxB_2)[a] (207)	Hydroxyl radical ($OH\cdot$) (268,289)
Leukotriene B_4 (LTB_4) (207,306)	Singlet oxygen ($^1O_2$) (212,232)
5-Hydroxyeicosatetraenoic acid (5-HETE) (306)	Hydrogen peroxide (H_2O_2) (46,231)
	N-Chloramines (288)
	Hypochlorous acid (HOCl) (36)

[a] Stable breakdown product of thromboxane A_2.

Effects on the Cells Themselves

It is now commonplace to conceptualize secretion from inflammatory cells as resulting in toxic consequences to the surrounding tissue. Although we argue below that this concept may be somewhat overplayed, it has an interesting sidelight in that the sources of these "toxic" materials seem themselves to be remarkably resistant to such effects. Close examination of inflammatory lesions usually reveals a remarkably large percentage of intact inflammatory cells (see above) presumably bathed in a figurative cesspool of toxic cellular wastes. *In vitro* we go even further, stimulating populations of inflammatory cells that are a monoculture (almost never seen *in vivo*) in concentrations up to 10^8 per milliliter (also seldom seen). Amazingly, our criteria for observing a secretory event (release of materials without cell lysis or disruption) clearly indicate that over a period of hours even supposedly fragile cells such as neutrophils survive this onslaught with impunity, and macrophages in this context seem indestructable.

TABLE 4. *Possible secretory products of eosinophils*

Products	Intracellular source	Refs.
Proteins, peptides, enzymes		
Major basic protein	Granules	32,33,66,75,86,154,199,284
Eosinophil cationic protein	Granules	1,44,74,185,277
Eosinophil-derived neurotoxins	Granules	58,74
Eosinophil peroxidases	Granules	49,87,108,109,140–143,170,197,266
Phospholipases	"Membranes"	151,276
Lysophospholipases	"Membranes"	291–293
Histaminase	Lysosomes	325,326
Lysosomal hydrolases	Lysosomes/granules	5,323
Arylsulfatase		5,209,283,294
β-Glucuronidase		5,323
Acid phosphatase		19
Alkaline phosphatase	Granules + plasma membrane	5,304
β-Glycerophosphatase		301
Ribonuclease		5
Peroxisomes	Granules	5,323
Catalase		5,133,323
Acyl-CoA oxidase		323
Enoyl-CoA hydratase		322
3-Ketoacyl CoA thiolase		322
NaDPH oxidase		47
Serine pyruvate aminotransferase		321
Proteinases		
Collagenase	?	20,120
Cathepsin	Granules	5,323
Lipids		
LTC$_4$, LTD$_4$		144,206,245,267,295
HETE		88,274
PAF		163
Prostanoids		71,130,131
Others		
Oxygen metabolites		214,247,269

Are inflammatory cells really resistant to the toxic effects attributed to them in relation to tissue cells? Probably to some degree they are, e.g., by virtue of higher intracellular oxygen metabolite inactivating mechanisms. However, we also suggest that the inflammatory sea of toxic agents has been overemphasized. In fact, it is extremely difficult to induce inflammatory cells to kill target cells *in vitro* and then usually only when close cell contact is achieved. The surrounding milieu in fact usually comprises more of an inhibitory environment. Nevertheless, it is still true that with opposing adherent membranes the inflammatory cell often seems to escape injury whereas the tissue cell, e.g., endothelial cell (88) (Fig. 10b), is susceptible.

Another important area in which inflammatory cell secretion affects the cells doing the secreting lies in the potentially autocrine nature of many of the mediators secreted. *In vitro* it is easy to show that secretion of prostanoids by macrophages, for example, serves to diminish some other cellular response by demonstrating an enhancing action of cyclooxygenase inhibitors (241). However, once again these cultures are pure, and it seems reasonable to suggest that the time has come to demonstrate that the levels of such molecules in inflammatory environments reach those that are required to modulate cell functions. Conceptually, the secretory activities of a variety of inflammatory cells provide a network (101) of both positive and negative stimuli, for the cells of origin themselves, their inflammatory cell neighbors (whether of like or unlike type), and the tissue cells in the environment. Surely the outcome at any one point in time is the consequence of the precise mix of mediators at that time—the whole process being highly dynamic.

Effects on Tissues

The points made above apply equally to tissue cells and structures. Here we make two points.

1. Accumulation of inflammatory cells in tissues may require secretory processes; and

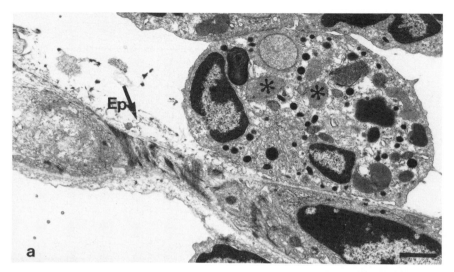

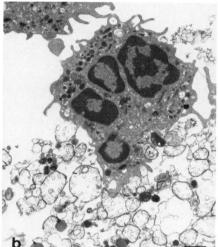

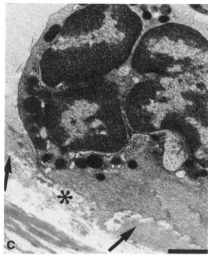

FIG. 10. Examples of morphological alterations to tissue cells presumably produced by inflammatory cell (neutrophil) secretion. **a:** Destruction of alveolar epithelium (*Ep, arrow*) beneath an adherent neutrophil in the lung of a rabbit with immune complex-induced alveolitis (137). The neutrophil itself shows phagosomes containing material that is probably ingested immune complexes (*asterisks*) **b:** Neutrophil amid the debris of the endothelial cells it has destroyed. The neutrophils (human) were stimulated with a combination of bacterial endotoxin and chemotactic factors and were added to monolayers of cultured human microvascular endothelial cells. **c:** Rabbit neutrophil in contact with, and presumably digesting, the internal elastic lamina of the carotid artery. Chemotactic factors were placed on the adventitial surface of the exposed artery 4 hr previously and resulted in massive penetration of the vessel wall by neutrophils. The granular debris immediately beneath the neutrophil (*asterisk*) is reminiscent of digested elastin and spans the space between the two ends of the intact internal elastic lamina (*arrows*). Bars = 1 μm.

2. Despite this fact and the potential toxicity of such secretion, tissue injury is not the inevitable consequence of such migration.

As indicated above and in Chapters 18 and 26, secretion of neutrophil secondary granules has been suggested to be required for chemotactic responsiveness *in vitro* and *in vivo*. Additionally, there is a great deal of current interest being directed toward the likelihood that neutrophil secretion of proteases is required for emigration through connective tissue barriers such as the basement membrane (169,238,270). Although not yet proved and the precise proteases not yet identified, it nevertheless seems to us that this suggestion most effectively encompasses the available information on inflammatory cell (particularly neutrophil) emigration. If valid, it provides an additional *requirement* for secretion in the generation, as well as the outcome, of the inflammatory reaction.

Nevertheless, on many occasions examination of inflammatory lesions morphologically reveals no evidence

of injury to the cells or structures past which the inflammatory cells are presumably migrating (244,311). Measurements of altered vascular permeability (which certainly results from endothelial injury although probably occurring by physiological processes as well) also have demonstrated occasions of neutrophil emigration without concurrent (detectable) alterations in permeability (257,309). Presumably, if secretion of potentially toxic agents is occurring, the agents are either severely limited in action or so localized in effect that no generalized changes occur. In either event, knowledge of the mechanisms involved would have extreme value as we attempt to preserve the beneficial, protective aspects of inflammatory cell accumulation while seeking to limit the injurious effects that are their common accompaniment.

ACKNOWLEDGMENTS

This work was supported by NIH grant GM24834. The work was performed in the F. L. Bryant Jr. Research Laboratory for the Mechanisms of Lung Disease, Department of Pediatrics.

REFERENCES

1. Ackerman, S. J., Gleich, G. J., Loegering, D. A., Richardson, B. A., and Butterworth, A. E. (1985): Comparative toxicity of purified human eosinophil granule cationic proteins for schistosomula of Schistosoma mansoni. *Am. J. Trop. Med. Hyg.*, 34:735–745.

2. Alitale, K., Hovi, T., and Vahen, A. (1980): Fibronectin is produced by human macrophages. *J. Exp. Med.*, 151:602–613.

3. Anderson, A. J. (1971): Enzyme system in rat leukocyte granules which degrades insoluble collagen. *Ann. Rheumatol. Dis.*, 30:299–302.

4. Anderson, D. C., and Springer, T. A. (1987): Leukocyte adhesion deficiency: an inherited defect in the Mac-1, LFA-1, and p150,95 glycoproteins. *Annu. Rev. Med. (in press).*

5. Archer, G. T., and Hirsch, J. G. (1963): Isolation of granules from eosinophil leucocytes and study of their enzyme content. *J. Exp. Med.*, 118:277–285.

6. Arnaout, M. A., Spits, H., Terhorst, C., Pitt, J., and Todd, R. F., III. (1984): Deficiency of a leukocyte surface glycoprotein (LFA-1) in two patients with Mo 1 deficiency: effects of cell activation on Mo 1/LFA-1 surface expression in normal and deficient leukocytes. *J. Clin. Invest.*, 74:1291–1300.

7. Avila, J. L., and Convit, J. (1974): Studies on human polymorphonuclear enzymes. IV. Intracellular distribution and properties of alpha-L-glucosidase. *Biochim. Biophys. Acta*, 358:308–318.

8. Axline, S. G., and Cohn, Z. A. (1970): In vitro induction of lysosomal enzymes by phagocytosis. *J. Exp. Med.*, 131:1239–1260.

9. Babior, B. M. (1982): The enzymatic basis of O_2^- production by human neutrophils. *Can. J. Physiol. Pharmacol.*, 60:1353–1358.

10. Babior, B. R., Kipnes, R., and Curnutte, J. (1973): Biological defense mechanism: the production by leukocytes of superoxide, a potential bactericidal agent. *J. Clin. Invest.*, 52:741–744.

11. Baggiolini, M., Bretz, U., and Gusus, B. (1974): Biochemical characterization of azurophil and specific granules from human and rabbit polymorphonuclear leukocytes. *Schweiz. Med. Wochenschr.*, 104:129–132.

12. Baggiolini, M., deDuve, C., Masson, P. L., and Heremans, J. F. (1970): Association of lactoferrin with specific granules in rabbit heterophil leukocytes. *J. Exp. Med.*, 131:559–570.

13. Baggiolini, M., Hirsch, J. G., and deDuve, C. (1969): Resolution of granules from rabbit heterophil leukocytes into distinct populations by zonal centrifugation. *J. Cell Biol.*, 40:529–541.

14. Baggiolini, M., Hirsch, J. G., and deDuve, C. (1970): Further biochemical and morphological studies of granule fractions from rabbit heterophil leukocytes. *J. Cell Biol.*, 45:586–597.

15. Bainton, D. F. (1973): Sequential degranulation of the two types of polymorphonuclear leukocyte granules during phagocytosis of microorganisms. *J. Cell Biol.*, 58:249–264.

16. Bainton, D. F., and Farquhar, M. G. (1968): Differences in granule content of azurophil and specific granules of polymorphonuclear leukocytes. II. Cytochemistry and electron microscopy of bone marrow cells. *J. Cell Biol.*, 39:299–317.

17. Bainton, D. F., Ullyot, J. L., and Farquhar, M. G. (1971): The development of neutrophilic leukocytes in human bone marrow: origin and content of azurophil and specific granules. *J. Exp. Med.*, 134:907–934.

18. Baker, P. F., and Knight, D. E. (1986): Exocytosis: control by calcium and other factors. *Br. Med. Bull.*, 42:399–404.

19. Bass, D. A., Lewis, J. C., Szejda, P., Cowley, L., and McCall, E. (1981): Activation of lysosomal acid phosphatase of eosinophil leukocytes. *Lab. Invest.*, 44:403–409.

20. Bassett, E. G., Baker, J. R., Baker, P. A., and Myers, D. B. (1976): Comparison of collagenase activity in eosinophil and neutrophil fractions from rat peritoneal exudates. *A.J.E.B.A.K.*, 54:459–465.

21. Basu, S. K., Brown, M. S., Ho, T. K., Havel, R. J., and Goldstein, J. L. (1981): Mouse macrophages synthesize and secrete a protein resembling apopolyprotein E. *Proc. Natl. Acad. Sci. USA*, 78:7545–7549.

22. Becker, E. L., and Henson, P. M. (1973): In vitro studies of immunologically induced secretion of mediators from cells and related phenomena. *Adv. Immunol.*, 17:93–193.

23. Bentwood, B. J., and Henson, P. M. (1980): The sequential release of granule constituents from human neutrophils. *J. Immunol.*, 124:855–862.

24. Bertram, T. A., and Coignoul, F. L. (1982): Morphometry of equine neutrophils isolated at different temperatures. *Vet. Pathol.*, 19:534–543.

25. Beutler, B., Greenwald, D., Hulmes, J. D., Chang, M., Pan, Y. C., Mathison, J., Ulevitch, R., and Cerami, A. (1985): Identity of tumour necrosis factor and the macrophage-secreted factor cachectin. *Nature*, 316:552–554.

26. Blair, H. C., Kahn, A. J., Crouch, E. C., Jeffrey, J. J., and Teitelbaum, S. L. (1986): Isolated osteoclasts resorb the organic and inorganic components of bone. *J. Cell Biol.*, 102:1164–1172.

27. Blobel, G. (1983): Control of intracellular protein traffic. *Methods Enzymol.*, 96:663–682.

28. Borregaard, N. (1985): The respiratory burst of phagocytosis: biochemistry and subcellular localization. *Immunol. Lett.*, 11:165–171.

29. Borregaard, N., Heiple, J. M., Simons, E. R., and Clark, R. A. (1983): Subcellular localization of the b-cytochrome component of the human neutrophil microbicidal oxidase: translocation during activation. *J. Cell Biol.*, 97:52–61.

30. Brown, W. J., and Farquhar, M. G. (1984): The mannose-6-phosphate receptor for lysosomal enzymes is concentrated in cis Golgi cisternae. *Cell*, 36:295–307.

31. Burgoyne, R. D. (1984): Mechanisms of secretion from adrenal chromaffin cells. *Biochim. Biophys. Acta*, 779:201–216.

32. Butterfield, J. H., Kephart, G. M., Banks, P. M., and Gleich, G. J. (1986): Extracellular deposition of eosinophil major basic protein in lymph nodes of patients with Hodgkin's disease. *Blood*, 68:1250–1256.

33. Butterworth, A. E., Wassom, D. L., Gleich, G. J., Loegering, A. A., and David, J. R. (1979): Damage to schistosomula of Schistosoma mansoni induced directly by eosinophil major basic protein. *J. Immunol.*, 122:221–229.

34. Chandler, D. E., and Kazilek, C. J. (1986): Chemotactic peptide-induced exocytosis in neutrophils: granule fusion patterns depend on the source of messenger calcium. *J. Cell Sci.*, 83:293–311.

35. Clark, J. M., Vaughan, D. W., Aiken, B. M., and Kagan, H. M. (1980): Elastase-like enzymes in human neutrophils localized by ultrastructural cytochemistry. *J. Cell Biol.*, 84:102–119.

36. Clark, R. A., and Klebanoff, S. J. (1975): Neutrophil-mediated tumor cell cytotoxicity: role of the peroxidase system. *J. Exp. Med.*, 141:1442–1447.

37. Cohn, Z. A. (1981–1982): The macrophage—versatile element of inflammation. *Harvey Lect.*, 77:63–80.

38. Coignoul, F. L., Bertram, T. A., Roth, J. A., and Cheville, N. F. (1984): Functional and ultrastructural evaluation of neutrophils from foals and lactating and nonlactating mares. *Am. J. Vet. Res.*, 45:898–902.

39. Cotter, T. G., Spears, P., and Henson, P. M. (1981): A monoclonal antibody inhibiting human neutrophil chemotaxis and degranulation. *J. Immunol.*, 127:1355–1360.

40. Cox, C. C., Dougherty, R. W., Ganong, B. R., Bell, R. M., Niedel, J. E., and Snyderman, R. (1986): Differential stimulation of the respiratory burst and lysosomal enzyme secretion in human polymorphonuclear leukocytes by synthetic diacylglycerols. *J. Immunol.*, 136:4611–4616.

41. Craddock, P. R., White, J. G., and Jacob, H. S. (1978): Potentiation of complement (C5a)-induced granulocyte aggregation by cytochalasin B. *J. Lab. Clin. Med.*, 91:490–499.

42. Creutz, C. E., Dowling, L. G., Sando, J. J., Villar-Palasi, C., Whipple, J. H., and Zaks, W. J. (1983): Characterization of the chromobindins. *J. Biol. Chem.*, 258:14664–14674.

43. Currie, G. A. (1978): Activated macrophages kill tumour cells by releasing arginase. *Nature*, 273:758–759.

44. Dahl, R., and Venge, P. (1979): Enhancement of urokinase-induced plasminogen activation by the cationic protein of human eosinophil granulocytes. *Thromb. Res.,* 14:559–608.

45. Davies, P., Rita, G. A., Krakauer, K., and Weissmann, G. (1971): Characterization of a neutral protease from lysosomes of rabbit polymorphonuclear leukocytes. *Biochem. J.,* 123:559–569.

46. DeChatelet, L. R. (1975): Oxidative bactericidal mechanisms of polymorphonuclear leukocytes. *J. Infect. Dis.,* 131:295–303.

47. DeChatelet, L. R., Shirley, P. S., McPhail, L. C., Huntley, C. C., Muss, H. B., and Bass, D. A. (1977): Oxidative metabolism of the human eosinophil. *Blood,* 50:525–535.

48. DeLisle, R. C., and Williams, J. A. (1986): Regulation of membrane fusion in secretory exocytosis. *Annu. Rev. Physiol.,* 48:225–238.

49. DeSimone, C., Ferrari, M., Pugnaloni, L., Ferrarelli, G., Rumi, C., and Sorice, F. (1986): Eosinophil-mediated cellular cytotoxicity induced by zymosan activated serum. *Immunol. Lett.,* 12:37–41.

50. Dewald, B., Baggiolini, M., Curnutte, J. T., and Babior, B. M. (1979): Subcellular localization of the superoxide-forming enzyme in human neutrophils. *J. Clin. Invest.,* 63:21–29.

51. Dewald, B., Bretz, U., and Baggiolini, M. (1982): Release of gelatinase from a novel secretory compartment of human neutrophils. *J. Clin. Invest.,* 70:518–525.

52. Dierich, M. P., Wilhelmi, D., and Till, G. (1977): Essential role of surface-bound chemoattractant in leukocyte migration. *Nature,* 270:351–352.

53. Diliberto, E. J., Jr., Viveros, O. H., and Axelrod, J. (1976): Subcellular distribution of protein carboxymethylase and its endogenous substrates in the adrenal medulla: possible role in excitation-secretion coupling. *Proc. Natl. Acad. Sci. USA,* 73:4050–4054.

54. Diment, S., and Dean, M. F. (1983): Receptor-mediated endocytosis of fibroblast beta-glucuronidase by peritoneal macrophages. *Biochim. Biophys. Acta,* 762:165–174.

55. Dingle, J. T. (1975): The secretion of enzymes into the pericellular environment. *Philos. Trans. R. Soc. Lond. [Biol.],* 27:315–324.

56. Drath, D. B., and Karnovsky, M. L. (1975): Superoxide production by phagocytic leukocytes. *J. Exp. Med.,* 141:257–261.

57. Dunn, W. B., Hardin, J. H., and Spicer, S. S. (1968): Ultrastructural localization of myeloperoxidase in human neutrophil and rabbit heterophil and eosinophil leukocytes. *Blood,* 32:935–944.

58. Durack, D. T., Ackerman, S. J., Loegering, D. A., and Gleich, G. J. (1981): Purification of human eosinophil derived neurotoxin. *Proc. Natl. Acad. Sci. USA,* 78:5165–5169.

59. Eccles, M. H., and Glauert, A. M. (1984): The response of human monocytes to interaction with immobilized immune complexes. *J. Cell Sci.,* 71:141–157.

60. Elsbach, P., Weiss, J., Fransson, R. C., Beckerdite-Quagliata, S., Schneider, A., and Harris, L. (1979): Separation and purification of a potent bactericidal/permeability-increasing protein and a closely associated phospholipase A_2 from rabbit polymorphonuclear leukocytes. *J. Biol. Chem.,* 254:11000–11009.

61. Eschenbach, C. (1970): Zytochemischer Nachweis von saurer Desoxyribonuclease in Zytoplasma von Blutzellen. *Histochemie,* 24:85–98.

62. Etherington, D. J. (1980): Proteinases in connective tissue breakdown. *Ciba Found. Symp.,* 75:57–63.

63. Fallon, M. D. (1984): Bone resorbing fluid from osteoclasts is acidic—an in vitro micropuncture study. In: *Endocrine Control of Bone and Calcium Metabolism,* Vol. 8A, edited by C. V. Cohn, T. Fujita, J. T. Potts, and R. V. Talmadge, pp. 144–146. Elsevier, Amsterdam.

64. Fantone, J. C., and Ward, P. A. (1982): Role of oxygen-derived free radicals and metabolites in leukocyte-dependent inflammatory reactions. *Am. J. Pathol.,* 107:397–418.

65. Fielding, C. J., and Fielding, P. E. (1985): Metabolism of cholesterol and lipoproteins. In: *Biochemistry of Lipids and Membranes,* edited by D. E. Vance and J. E. Vance, pp. 429–433. Benjamin Cummings Publishing, Menlo Park, California.

66. Filley, W. V., Holley, K. E., Kephart, G. M., and Gleich, G. J. (1982): Identification by immunofluorescence of eosinophil major basic protein in lung tissues of patients with bronchial asthma. *Lancet,* 2:11–16.

67. Finkelstein, A., Zimmerberg, J., and Cohen, F. S. (1986): Osmotic swelling of vesicles: its role in the fusion of vesicles with planar phospholipid bilayer membranes and its possible role in exocytosis. *Annu. Rev. Physiol.,* 48:163–174.

68. Fittschen, C., Sandhaus, R. A., Worthen, G. S., and Henson, P. M. (1987): Bacterial lipopolysaccharide enhances chemoattractant-induced elastase secretion by human neutrophils. Submitted for publication.

69. Fleit, H. B., and Rabinovitch, M. (1982): Production of interferon by in vitro derived bone marrow macrophages. *Cell Immunol.,* 57:495–504.

70. Fletcher, M. P., Seligmann, B. E., and Gallin, J. I. (1982): Correlation of human neutrophil secretion, chemoattractant receptor mobilization and enhanced functional capacity. *J. Immunol.,* 128:941–948.

71. Foegh, M. L., Maddox, Y. T., and Ramwell, P. W. (1986): Human peritoneal eosinophils and formation of arachidonate cyclooxygenase products. *Scand. J. Immunol.,* 23:599–603.

72. Franson, R., Patriarchia, P., and Elsbach, P. (1974): Phospholipid metabolism by phagocytic cells: phospholipase A_2 associated with rabbit polymorphonuclear leukocyte granules. *J. Lipid Res.,* 15:380–388.

73. Franson, R., Weiss, J., Martin, L., Spitznagel, J. K., and Elsbach, P. (1977): Phospholipase A activity associated with the membranes of human polymorphonuclear leukocytes. *Biochem. J.,* 167:839–841.

74. Fredens, K., Dahl, R., and Venge, P. (1982): The Gordon phenomena induced by the eosinophil cationic protein and eosinophil protein X. *J. Allergy Clin. Immunol.,* 70:361–366.

75. Frigas, E., Loegering, D. A., and Gleich, G. J. (1980): Cytotoxic effects of the guinea pig eosinophil major basic protein on tracheal epithelium. *Lab. Invest.,* 42:35–43.

76. Galli, S. J., Dvorak, A. M., and Dvorak, H. F. (1984): Basophils and mast cells: morphologic insights into their biology, secretory patterns and function. *Prog. Allergy,* 34:1–141.

77. Gallin, J. I. (1984): Neutrophil specific granules: a fuse that ignites the inflammatory response. *Clin. Res.,* 32:320–328.

78. Ganz, T., Selsted, M. E., Szklatek, D., Harwig, S. S. L., Daher, K., Bainton, D. F., and Lehrer, R. I. (1985): Natural peptide antibiotics of human neutrophils. *J. Clin. Invest.,* 76:1427–1435.

79. Geisow, M. J., Burgoyne, R. D., and Harris, A. (1982): Interaction of calmodulin with adrenal chromaffin granule membranes. *FEBS Lett.,* 143:69–72.

80. Geisow, M. J., Fritsche, U., Hexham, J. M., Dash, B., and Johnston, T. (1986): A consensus amino-acid sequence repeat in Torpedo and mammalian Ca^{2+}-dependent membrane-binding proteins. *Nature,* 320:636–638.

81. Gennaro, R., DeWald, B., Horrisberger, U., Gubler, H. U., and Baggiolini, M. (1983): A novel type of cytoplasmic granule in bovine neutrophils. *J. Cell Biol.,* 96:1651–1661.

82. Gery, I., Davies, P., Derr, J., Krett, N., and Barranger, J. A. (1981): Anti-IgD enhancement of primary antibody responses in rats. *Cell Immunol.,* 64:293–303.

83. Geuze, H. J., Slot, J. W., Strouse, G. J. A. M., Hasilik, A., and von Figura, K. (1984): Ultrastructural localization of the mannose-6-phosphate receptor in rat liver. *J. Cell Biol.,* 98:2047–2054.

84. Gibson, W. T., Milsom, D. W., Stevens, F. S., and Lowe, J. S. (1978): Collagenolytic cathepsin activity in rabbit leukocytes. *Biochem. J.,* 172:83–89.

85. Glauert, A. M., and Butterworth, A. E. (1977): Morphological evidence for the ability of eosinophils to damage antibody-coated schistosomula. *Trans. R. Soc. Trop. Med. Hyg.,* 71:392–395.

86. Gleich, G. J., Frigas, E., Loegering, D. A., Wassom, D. L., and Steinmuller, D. (1979): Cytotoxic properties of the eosinophil major basic protein. *J. Immunol.,* 123:2925–2927.

87. Goetzl, E. J. (1982): The conversion of leukotriene C_4 to isomers of leukotriene B_4 by human eosinophil peroxidase. *Biochem. Biophys. Res. Commun.,* 106:270–275.

88. Goetzl, E. J., Weller, P. F., and Sun, F. F. (1980): The regulation of human eosinophil function by endogenous mono-hydroxy-eicosatetraenoic acids (HETES). *J. Immunol.,* 124:926–933.

89. Goldstein, I. M., Horn, J. K., Kaplan, H. B., and Weissmann, G. (1974): Calcium-induced lysozyme secretion from human polymorphonuclear leukocytes. *Biochem. Biophys. Res. Commun.*, 60: 647–652.

90. Goldstein, I. M., Roos, D., Kaplan, H. B., and Weissmann, G. (1975): Complement and immunoglobulins stimulate superoxide production by human leukocytes independently of phagocytosis. *J. Clin. Invest.*, 56:1155–1163.

91. Gomperts, B. D. (1983): Involvement of guanine nucleotide-binding protein in the gating of Ca^{2+} by receptors. *Nature*, 306:64–66.

92. Gonzales-Noriega, A., Grubb, J. H., Talkod, V., and Sly, W. S. (1980): Chloroquine inhibits lysosomal enzyme pinocytosis and enhances lysosomal enzyme secretion by impairing receptor recycling. *J. Cell Biol.*, 85:839–852.

93. Gordon, S., Todd, J., and Cohn, Z. A. (1974): In vitro synthesis and secretion of lysozyme by mononuclear phagocytes. *J. Exp. Med.*, 139:1228–1248.

94. Granelli-Piperno, A., Vasalli, J-D., and Reich, E. (1977): Secretion of plasminogen activator by human polymorphonuclear leukocytes: modulation by glucocorticoids and other effectors. *J. Exp. Med.*, 146:1693–1706.

95. Griffin, F. M., Jr., Griffin, J. A., and Silverstein, S. C. (1976): Studies on the mechanism of phagocytosis. II. The interaction of macrophages with anti-immunoglobulin IgG-coated bone marrow-derived lymphocytes. *J. Exp. Med.*, 144:788–809.

96. Gus'Kova, R. A., Ivanov, I. I., Koltover, V. K., Akhobadze, V. V., and Rubin, A. B. (1984): Permeability of bilayer lipid membranes for superoxide (O_2^-) radicals. *Biochim. Biophys. Acta*, 778:579–585.

97. Guthrie, L. A., McPhail, L. C., Henson, P. M., and Johnston, R. B., Jr. (1984): Priming of neutrophils for enhanced release of oxygen metabolites by bacterial lipopolysaccharide: evidence for increased activity of the superoxide-producing enzyme. *J. Exp. Med.*, 160:1656–1671.

98. Hallgren, R., Bjelle, A., and Venge, P. (1984): Eosinophil cationic protein in synovial effusions as evidence of eosinophil involvement. *Ann. Rheum. Dis.*, 43:556–562.

99. Hardin, J. H., and Spicer, S. S. (1971): Ultrastructural localization of dialyzed iron-reactive mucosubstance in rabbit heterophils, basophils, and eosinophils. *J. Cell Biol.*, 48:368–386.

100. Haslam, R. J., and Davidson, M. M. L. (1984): Guanine nucleotides decrease the free Ca^{2+} required for secretion of serotonin from permeabilized blood platelets: evidence of a role for a GTP-binding protein in platelet activation. *FEBS Lett.*, 174:90–95.

101. Haslett, C., and Henson, P. M. (1987): Resolution of inflammation (in press).

102. Haslett, C., Lee, A., Wyllie, A. H., and Henson, P. M. (1987): Programmed cell senescence in neutrophils aging in vitro. Manuscript in preparation.

103. Hawkins, D. (1971): Biopolymer membrane: a model system for the study of the neutrophilic leukocyte response to immune complexes. *J. Immunol.*, 107:344–352.

104. Hawkins, D. (1972): Neutrophilic leukocytes in immunologic reactions: evidence for the selective release of lysosomal constituents. *J. Immunol.*, 108:310–317.

105. Hawkins, D. (1973): Neutrophilic leukocytes in immunologic reactions in vitro: effect of cytochalasin B. *J. Immunol.*, 110:294–296.

106. Hawkins, D., and Cochrane, C. G. (1968): Glomerular basement membrane damage in immunological glomerulonephritis. *Immunology*, 14:665–681.

107. Henderson, W. R., and Chi, E. Y. (1985): Ultrastructural characterization and morphometric analysis of human eosinophil degranulation. *J. Cell Sci.*, 73:33–48.

108. Henderson, W. R., Chi, E., and Klebanoff, S. J. (1980): Eosinophil peroxidase-induced mast cell secretion. *J. Exp. Med.*, 152:265–279.

109. Henderson, W. R., Jorg, A., and Klebanoff, S. J. (1982): Eosinophil peroxidase-mediated inactivation of leukotrienes B_4, C_4, and D_4. *J. Immunol.*, 128:2609–2613.

110. Henson, P. M. (1971): Interaction of cells with immune complexes: adherence, release of constituents, and tissue injury. *J. Exp. Med.*, 134:114s–135s.

111. Henson, P. M. (1971): The immunologic release of constituents from neutrophil leukocytes. II. Mechanisms of release during phagocytosis and adherence to nonphagocytosable surfaces. *J. Immunol.*, 107:1547–1557.

112. Henson, P. M. (1973): Mechanisms of release of granule enzymes from human neutrophils phagocytosing aggregated immunoglobulin: an electron microscopic study. *Arthritis Rheum.*, 16:208–216.

113. Henson, P. M. (1980): Mechanisms of exocytosis in phagocytic inflammatory cells. *Am. J. Pathol.*, 101:494–511.

114. Henson, P. M., and Oades, Z. G. (1973): Enhancement of immunologically induced granule exocytosis from neutrophils by cytochalasin B. *J. Immunol.*, 110:290–293.

115. Henson, P. M., and Oades, Z. G. (1975): Stimulation of human neutrophils by soluble and insoluble immunoglobulin aggregates: secretion of granule constituents and increased oxidation of glucose. *J. Clin. Invest.*, 56:1053–1061.

116. Henson, P. M., Ginsberg, M. H., and Morrison, D. C. (1978): Mechanisms of mediator release by inflammatory cells. In: *Membrane Fusion*, edited by G. Poste and G. L. Nicolson, pp. 407–508. Biomedical Press/Elsevier/North Holland, Amsterdam.

117. Henson, P. M., Hollister, J. R., Musson, R. A., Webster, O., Spears, P., Henson, J. E., and McCarthy, K. M. (1979): Inflammation as a surface phenomenon: initiation of inflammatory processes by surface-bound immunologic components. *Adv. Inflamm. Res.*, 1: 341–352.

118. Henson, P. M., Larsen, G. L., Henson, J. E., Newman, S. L., Musson, R. A., and Leslie, C. C. (1984): Resolution of pulmonary inflammation. *Fed. Proc.*, 43:2799–2806.

119. Henson, P. M., Webster, R. O., and Henson, J. E. (1981): Neutrophil and monocyte activation and secretion: role of surfaces in inflammatory reactions and in vitro. In: *Cellular Interactions*, edited by J. C. Dingle and J. L. Gordon, pp. 43–56. Biomedical Press/Elsevier/North Holland, Amsterdam.

120. Hibbs, M., Mainardi, C. L., and Kang, A. H. (1982): Type-specific collagen degradation by eosinophils. *Biochem. J.*, 207:621–624.

121. Hirsch, J. G., and Cohn, Z. A. (1960): Degranulation of polymorphonuclear leukocytes following phagocytosis of microorganisms. *J. Exp. Med.*, 112:1005–1022.

122. Hoekstra, D. (1982): Role of lipid phase separations and membrane hydration in phospholipid vesicle fusion. *Biochemistry*, 21:2833–2840.

123. Hoffstein, S., and Weissmann, G. (1978): Microfilaments and microtubules in calcium ionophore-induced secretion of lysosomal enzymes from polymorphonuclear leukocytes. *J. Cell Biol.*, 78: 769–781.

124. Hoflack, B., and Kornfeld, S. (1985): Purification and characterization of a cation-dependent mannose-6-phosphate receptor from murine P388D, macrophages and bovine liver. *J. Biol. Chem.*, 260: 12008–12014.

125. Honeycutt, P. J., and Niedel, J. E. (1986): Cytochalasin B augments diacylglycerol levels in stimulated neutrophils. *Fed. Proc.*, 45:1135 (abstract).

126. Hong, K., Duzgunes, N., and Papahadjopoulos, D. (1982): Modulation of membrane fusion by calcium-binding proteins. *Biophys. J.*, 37:297–305.

127. Hopkins, C. R. (1983): Intracellular routing of transferrin and transferrin receptor in epidermoid carcinoma A431 cells. *Cell*, 35: 321–330.

128. Horwitz, M. A. (1982): Phagocytosis of microorganisms. *Rev. Infect. Dis.*, 4:104–123.

129. Hovi, T., Mosher, D., and Valeri, A. (1977): Cultured human monocytes synthesize and secrete gamma-2-macroglobulin. *J. Exp. Med.*, 145:1580–1589.

130. Hubscher, T. (1975): Role of the eosinophil in the allergic reaction. I. EDI: an eosinophil-derived inhibitor of histamine release. *J. Immunol.*, 114:1379–1388.

131. Hubscher, T. (1975): Role of eosinophils in the allergic reaction. II. Release of prostaglandins from human eosinophilic leukocytes. *J. Immunol.*, 114:1389–1393.

132. Humes, J. L., Bonney, R. J., Pelus, L., Dahlgren, M. E., Sadowski, S. J., Kuehl, F. A., and Davies, P. (1977): Macrophages synthesize and release prostaglandins in response to inflammatory stimuli. *Nature*, 269:149–151.

133. Iozzo, R. V., MacDonald, G. H., and Wright, T. N. (1982): Immunoelectron microscopic localisation of catalase in human eosinophilic leukocytes. *J. Histochem. Cytochem.*, 300:697–701.

134. Ishikawa, I., and Cimason, G. (1977): Isolation of cathepsin D from human leukocytes. *Biochim. Biophys. Acta*, 480:228–240.

135. Janoff, A., and Blondin, J. (1971): Further studies on an esterase inhibitor in human leukocyte cytosol. *Lab. Invest.*, 25:565–571.

136. Jensen, M. S., and Bainton, D. F. (1973): Temporal changes in pH within the phagocytic vacuole of the polymorphonuclear leukocyte. *J. Cell Biol.*, 56:379–388.

137. Johansson, S., Rubin, K., Hook, M., Ahlgren, T., and Seljelid, R. (1979): In vitro biosynthesis of cold insoluble globulin (fibronectin) by mouse peritoneal macrophages. *FEBS Lett.*, 105:313–316.

138. Johnston, R. B., Jr., Godzik, C. A., and Cohn, Z. A. (1978): Increased superoxide anion production by immunologically activated and chemically elicited macrophages. *J. Exp. Med.*, 148:115–127.

139. Johnston, R. B., Jr., Lehmeyer, J. E., and Guthrie, L. A. (1976): Generation of superoxide anion and chemiluminescence by human monocytes during phagocytosis and on contact with surface-bound immunoglobulin G. *J. Exp. Med.*, 143:1551–1556.

140. Jong, E., and Klebanoff, S. J. (1980): Eosinophil-mediated mammalian tumour cell cytotoxicity: role of the peroxidase system. *J. Immunol.*, 124:1949–1953.

141. Jong, E., Chi, E., and Klebanoff, S. J. (1984): Human neutrophil-mediated killing of schistosomula of Schistosoma mansoni: augmentation by schistosomal binding of eosinophil peroxidase. *Am. J. Trop. Med. Hyg.*, 33:104–115.

142. Jong, E., Henderson, W., and Klebanoff, S. J. (1980): Bactericidal activity of eosinophil peroxidase. *J. Immunol.*, 124:1378–1382.

143. Jong, E., Mahmoud, A. A. F., and Klebanoff, S. J. (1981): Peroxidase mediated toxicity to schistosomula of Schistosoma mansoni. *J. Immunol.*, 126:468–471.

144. Jorg, A., Henderson, W. R., Murphy, R. C., and Klebanoff, S. J. (1982): Leukotriene generation by eosinophils. *J. Exp. Med.*, 155:390–402.

145. Kakinuma, K. (1970): Metabolic control and intracellular pH during phagocytosis by polymorphonuclear leukocytes. *J. Biochem.*, 68:177–185.

146. Kane, S. P., and Peters, T. J. (1975): Analytical subcellular fractionation of human granulocytes with reference to the localization of vit B_{12}-binding proteins. *Clin. Sci. Mol. Med.*, 49:171–182.

147. Kaplan, G. (1983): In vitro differentiation of human monocytes: monocytes cultured on glass are cytotoxic to tumor cells but monocytes cultured on Teflon are not. *J. Exp. Med.*, 157:2061–2072.

148. Kaplan, M. R., and Simoni, R. D. (1985): Transport of cholesterol from the endoplasmic reticulum to the plasma membrane. *J. Cell Biol.*, 101:446–453.

149. Kaplan, M. R., and Simoni, R. O. (1985): Intracellular transport of phosphatidylcholine to the plasma membrane. *J. Cell Biol.*, 101:441–445.

150. Kaplan, R. L., Schocket, A. L., King, T. E., Maulitz, R. M., Good, J. T., Jr., and Sahn, S. A. (1980): A model of immune complex-mediated pleuropulmonary injury: evidence of deposition of circulating immune complexes in the lung. *Am. J. Pathol.*, 100:115–130.

151. Kater, L. A., Goetzl, E. J., and Austen, K. F. (1980): Isolation of human eosinophil phosphalipase D. *J. Clin. Invest.*, 57:1173–1180.

152. Keeling, P. J., and Henson, P. M. (1981): Lysosomal enzyme release from human monocytes in response to particulate stimuli. *J. Immunol.*, 128:563–567.

153. Kerby, G. P., and Taylor, S. M. (1967): Enzymatic activity in human synovial fluid from rheumatoid and non-rheumatoid patients. *Proc. Soc. Exp. Biol. Med.*, 126:865–868.

154. Kierszenbaum, F., Ackerman, S. J., and Gleich, G. J. (1981): Destruction of bloodstream forms of Trypanosoma cruzi by eosinophil granule major basic protein. *Am. J. Trop. Med. Hyg.*, 30:775–779.

155. Knight, D. E., Hallam, T. J., and Scrutton, M. C. (1982): Agonist selectivity and second messenger concentration in Ca^{2+}-mediated secretion. *Nature*, 296:256–257.

156. Konings, F., Majchrowicz, B., and DePotter, W. (1983): Release of chromaffin granular content on interaction with plasma membranes. *Am. J. Physiol.*, 244:C309–C312.

157. Kopitar, M., Kregar, I., and Lebez, D. (1971): Leukocyte proteinases. II. Partial purification of proteinases present in cathepsin D preparations. *Enzymologia*, 41:129–139.

158. Kornfeld, S. (1986): Trafficking of lysosomal enzymes in normal and disease states. *J. Clin. Invest.*, 77:1–6.

159. Kretsinger, R. H., and Creutz, C. E. (1986): Consensus in exocytosis. *Nature*, 320:573.

160. Lanni, C., and Becker, E. L. (1983): Release of phospholipase A_2 activity from rabbit peritoneal neutrophils by f-Met-Leu-Phe. *Am. J. Pathol.*, 113:90–94.

161. Lebez, D., and Kopitar, M. (1970): Leukocyte proteinases. I. Low molecular weight cathepsin of F and G types. *Enzymologia*, 39:271–283.

162. Lee, C. T., Fein, A. M., Lippmann, M., Holtzmann, H., Kimbel, P., and Weinbaum, G. (1981): Electrolytic activity in pulmonary lavage fluid from patients with adult respiratory distress syndrome. *N. Engl. J. Med.*, 304:192–196.

163. Lee, T., Lenihan, D. J., Malone, B., Roddy, L., and Wasserman, S. I. (1984): Increased biosynthesis of platelet-activating factor in activated human eosinophils. *J. Biol. Chem.*, 259:5526–5530.

164. Leffel, M. S., and Spitznagel, J. K. (1972): Association of lactoferrin with lysozyme in granules of human polymorphonuclear leukocytes. *Infect. Immun.*, 6:761–765.

165. Leibovitch, S. J., and Ross, R. (1976): A macrophage-dependent factor that stimulates the proliferation of fibroblasts in vitro. *Am. J. Pathol.*, 84:501–513.

166. Lemansky, P., Gieselmann, V., Hasailik, A., and von Figura, K. (1984): Cathepsin D and beta-hexosaminidase synthesized in the presence of 1-deoxynojirimycin accumulate in the endoplasmic reticulum. *J. Biol. Chem.*, 259:10129–10135.

167. Leoni, P., and Dean, R. T. (1983): Mechanisms of lysosomal enzyme secretion by human monocytes. *Biochim. Biophys. Acta*, 762:378–389.

168. Lew, P. D., Monod, A., Waldvogel, F. A., Dewald, B., and Baggiolini, M. (1986): Quantitative analysis of the cytosolic free calcium dependency of exocytosis from three subcellular compartments in intact human neutrophils. *J. Cell Biol.*, 102:2197–2204.

169. Liotta, L. A., Tryggvason, K., Gambisa, S., Hart, I., Foltz, E. M., and Shafie, S. (1980): Metastatic potential correlates with enzymatic degradation of basement membrane collagen. *Nature*, 284:67–68.

170. Locksley, R. M., Wilson, C. B., and Klebanoff, S. J. (1982): Role of endogenous and acquired peroxidase in the toxoplasmicidal activity of murine and human mononuclear phagocytes. *J. Clin. Invest.*, 69:1099–1111.

171. Lotner, G. Z., Lynch, J. M., Betz, S. J., and Henson, P. M. (1980): Human neutrophil-derived platelet activating factor. *J. Immunol.*, 124:676–684.

172. Lumb, R. H., Pool, G. L., Bubacz, D. G., Blank, M. L., and Snyder, F. (1983): Spontaneous and protein-catalized transfer of 1-alkyl-2-acetyl-sn-glycero-3-phosphocholine (platelet-activity factor) between phospholipid bilayers. *Biochim. Biophys. Acta*, 750:217–222.

173. Lynch, J. M., and Henson, P. M. (1986): The intracellular retention of newly synthesized platelet-activating factor. *J. Immunol.*, 137:2653–2661.

174. Lynch, J. M., Lotner, G. Z., Betz, S. J., and Henson, P. M. (1979): The release of a platelet-activating factor by stimulated rabbit neutrophils. *J. Immunol.*, 123:1219–1226.

175. Lynch, R. E., and Fridovich, I. (1978): Effects of superoxide on the erythrocyte membrane. *J. Biol. Chem.*, 253:1838–1845.

176. Lynch, R. E., and Fridovich, I. (1978): Permeation of the erythrocyte stroma by superoxide radical. *J. Biol. Chem.*, 253:4697–4699.

177. Mackay, R. J., and Russell, S. W. (1986): Protein changes associated with stages of activation of mouse macrophages for tumor cell killing. *J. Immunol.*, 137:1392–1398.

178. Mahoney, E. M., Khoo, J. C., and Steinberg, D. (1982): Lipoprotein

lipase secretion by human monocytes and rabbit alveolar macrophages in culture. *Proc. Natl. Acad. Sci. USA,* 79:1639–1642.

179. Mason, R. J., Cott, G. R., Robinson, P. C., Sugahara, K., Leslie, C. C., and Dobbs, L. G. (1984): Pharmacology of alveolar type II cells. *Prog. Respir. Res.,* 18:279–287.

180. Matzner, Y., Bar-Ner, M., Yahalom, J., Ishai-Michaeli, R., Fuks, Z., and Vlodavsky, I. (1985): Degradation of heparan sulfate in the subendothelial extracellular matrix by a readily released heparanase from human neutrophils: possible role in invasion through basement membranes. *J. Clin. Invest.,* 76:1306–1313.

181. May, C. D., Levine, B. B., and Weissmann, G. (1970): Effects of compounds which inhibit antigenic release of histamine and phagocytic release of lysosomal enzyme on glucose utilization by leukocytes in humans. *Proc. Soc. Exp. Biol. Med.,* 133:758–763.

182. McCarthy, K., and Henson, P. M. (1979): Induction of lysosomal enzyme secretion by alveolar macrophages in response to the purified complement fragments C5a and C5a Des Arg. *J. Immunol.,* 123:2511–2517.

183. McCarthy, K. M., Musson, R. A., and Henson, P. M. (1982): Protein synthesis dependent and protein synthesis independent secretion of lysosomal hydrolases from rabbit and human macrophages. *J. Reticuloendothelial Soc.,* 31:131–144.

184. McLaren, A. D. (1957): Concerning the pH dependence of enzyme reactions on cells, particulates, and in solution. *Science,* 125:692.

185. McLaren, D. J., McKean, J. R., Olsson, I., Venge, P., and Kay, A. B. (1981): Morphological studies of the killing of schistosomula of Schistosoma mansoni by human eosinophil and neutrophil cationic proteins in vitro. *Parasite Immunol.,* 3:359–373.

186. McPhail, L. C., Henson, P. M., and Johnston, R. B., Jr. (1981): Respiratory burst enzyme in human neutrophils: evidence for multiple mechanism of activation. *J. Clin. Invest.,* 67:710–716.

187. Mencia-Huerta, J. M., and Benveniste, J. (1979): Platelet-activating factor and macrophages. I. Evidence for the release from rat and mouse peritoneal macrophages and not from mastocytes. *Eur. J. Immunol.,* 9:409–415.

188. Metchnikov, E. (1905): *Immunity in Infectious Diseases.* 1968 Reprint. Johnson Reprint Co., New York.

189. Moore, R. N., Urbaschek, R., Wahl, L. M., and Mergenhagen, S. E. (1979): Prostaglandin regulation of colony-stimulating factor production by lipopolysaccharide-stimulated murine leukocytes. *Infect. Immun.,* 26:408–414.

190. Movat, H. Z., Uriuhara, T., MacMorine, D. L., and Bunke, J. S. (1964): A permeability factor released from leukocytes after phagocytosis of immune complexes and its possible role in the Arthus reaction. *Life Sci.,* 3:1025–1032.

191. Murata, F., and Spicer, S. S. (1973): Morphologic and cytochemical studies of rabbit heterophilic leukocytes: evidence for tertiary granules. *Lab. Invest.,* 29:65–72.

192. Murphy, G., Reynolds, J. J., Bretz, U., and Baggiolini, M. (1977): Collagenase is a component of the specific granules of human neutrophil leukocytes. *Biochem. J.,* 162:195–197.

193. Murphy, R. C., and Henson, P. M. (1985): Mediator network. *Ann. Inst. Pasteur Immunol.,* 219–221.

194. Nathan, C. F., and Root, R. K. (1977): H_2O_2 release from mouse peritoneal macrophages: dependence on sequential activation and triggering. *J. Exp. Med.,* 146:1648–1662.

195. Neufeld, E. J., Majerus, P. W., Krueger, C. M., and Saffitz, J. E. (1985): Uptake and subcellular distribution of ^3H arachidonic acid in murine fibrosarcoma cells measured by electron microscope autoradiography. *J. Cell Biol.,* 101:573–581.

196. Newman, S. L., Henson, J. E., and Henson, P. M. (1982): Phagocytosis of senescent neutrophils by human monocyte-derived macrophages and rabbit inflammatory macrophages. *J. Exp. Med.,* 156:430–442.

197. Nogueira, N. M., Klebanoff, S. J., and Cohn, Z. (1982): T. cruzi: sensitisation to macrophage killing by eosinophil peroxidase. *J. Immunol.,* 128(4):1705–1708.

198. Odeberg, H., Olsson, I., and Venge, P. (1975): Cationic proteins of human granulocytes. IV. Esterase activity. *Lab. Invest.,* 32:86–90.

199. O'Donnell, M. C., Ackerman, S. J., Gleich, G. J., and Thomas, L. L. (1983): Activation of basophil and mast cell histamine release by eosinophil major basic protein. *J. Exp. Med.,* 157:1981–1991.

200. Ohlsson, K. K., Olsson, I., and Spitznagel, J. K. (1977): Localization of chymotrypsin-like cationic protein, collagenase, and elastase in azurophil granules of human neutrophilic polymorphonuclear leukocytes. *Hoppe Seylers Z. Physiol. Chem.,* 358:361–366.

201. Ohura, K., Katona, I., Chenoweth, D., Wahl, L., and Wahl, S. (1985): Chemoattractant receptors on peripheral blood (PB) monocytes and receptor modulation in inflammation. *Fed. Proc.,* 44:1268 (abstract).

202. Oldstone, M. B. A., and Buchmeier, M. J. (1982): Restricted expression of viral glycoproteins in cells of persistently infected mice. *Nature,* 300:360–362.

203. Oliver, R. C., Glauert, A. M., and Thorne, K. J. I. (1982): Mechanism of Fc mediated interaction of eosinophils with immobilized immune complexes. I. Effects of inhibitors and activators of eosinophil function. *J. Cell Sci.,* 56:337–356.

204. Pabst, M. J., and Johnston, R. B., Jr. (1980): Increased production of superoxide anion by macrophages exposed in vivo to muramyl dipeptide or lipopolysaccharide. *J. Exp. Med.,* 151:101–114.

205. Painter, R. G., and McIntosh, A. J. (1979): The regional association of actin and myosin with sites of particle phagocytosis. *J. Supramol. Struct.,* 12:369–384.

206. Palmblad, J., Gyllenhammar, H., Lindgren, J. A., and Malmsten, C. L. (1984): Effects of leukotrienes and f-Met-Leu-Phe on oxidative metabolism of neutrophils and eosinophils. *J. Immunol.,* 132:3041–3045.

207. Palmer, R. M. J., and Salmon, J. A. (1985): Comparison of the effects of some compounds on human neutrophil degranulation and leukotriene B_4 and thromboxane B_2 synthesis. *Biochem. Pharmacol.,* 34:1485–1490.

208. Papahadjopoulos, D., Poste, G., Schaeffer, B. E., and Vail, W. J. (1974): Membrane fusion and molecular segregation in phospholipid vesicles. *Biochim. Biophys. Acta,* 352:10–28.

209. Parker, C. W., Koch, D. A., Huber, M. M., and Falkenhein, S. F. (1980): Arylsulfatase inactivation of slow reacting substance: evidence for proteolysis as a major mechanism when ordinary commercial preparations of the enzyme are used. *Prostaglandins,* 20:887–908.

210. Parmley, R. T., Hurst, R. E., Takagi, M., Spicer, S. S., and Austin, R. L. (1983): Glycoaminoglycans in human neutrophils and leukemic myeloblasts: ultrastructural, cytochemical, immunological and biochemical characterization. *Blood,* 61:257–266.

211. Parsons, P. E., Tate, R. M., Worthen, G. S., and Henson, P. M. (1986): Endotoxin and complement fragments (C5f) in plasma, but not elevated C5f levels done, correlate with the development of ARDS. *Am. Rev. Respir. Dis.,* 133:A277.

212. Piatt, J. F., and O'Brien, P. J. (1979): Singlet oxygen formation by a peroxidase, H_2O_2, and halide system. *Eur. J. Biochem.,* 93:323–332.

213. Piette, C., and Piette, M. (1976): Localisation par voie cytoenzymologique de l'esterase active sur le chloroacetate de naphthol AS-D dans les granulations primaire des granulocytes neutrophiles du sang humain. *Ann. Pharm. Fr.,* 34:19–24.

214. Pincus, S., DiNapoli, A., and Schooley, W. R. (1982): Superoxide production by eosinophils: activation by histamine. *J. Invest. Dermatol.,* 79:53–57.

215. Pollard, H. B., Pazoles, C. J., Creutz, C. E., Scott, J. H., Zinder, O., and Hotchkiss, A. (1984): An osmotic mechanism for exocytosis from dissociated chromaffin cells. *J. Biol. Chem.,* 259:1114–1121.

216. Pollard, H. B., Tack-Goldman, K., Pazoles, C. J., Creutz, C. E., and Shulman, N. R. (1977): Evidence for control of serotonin secretion from human platelets by hydroxyl ion transport and osmotic lysis. *Proc. Natl. Acad. Sci. USA,* 74:5295–5299.

217. Polverini, P. J., Cotran, R. S., Gimbrone, M. A., and Unanue, E. R. (1977): Activated macrophages induce vascular proliferation. *Nature,* 269:804–806.

218. Poste, G., and Allison, A. C. (1973): Membrane fusion. *Biochim. Biophys. Acta,* 300:421–465.

219. Pryzwansky, K. B., MacRae, E. K., Spitznagel, J. K., and Cooney,

M. H. (1979): Early degranulation of human neutrophils: immunocytochemical studies of surface and intracellular phagocytic events. *Cell,* 18:1025–1033.

220. Rand, R. P., and Parsegian, V. A. (1986): Mimicry and mechanism in phospholipid models of membrane fusion. *Annu. Rev. Physiol.,* 48:201–212.

221. Reddi, K. K. (1976): Human granulocyte ribonuclease. *Biochem. Biophys. Res. Commun.,* 68:1119–1125.

222. Reitman, M. L., Varki, A., and Kornfeld, S. (1981): Fibroblasts from patients with I-cell disease and pseudo-Hurler polydystrophy are deficient in uridine 5^1-diphosphate-N-acetylglucosamine: glycoprotein N-acetylglucosaminylphosphotransferase. *J. Clin. Invest.,* 67:1574–1579.

223. Riches, D. W. H., and Henson, P. M. (1986): Bacterial lipopolysaccharide suppresses the production of catalytically active lysosomal acid hydrolases in human macrophages. *J. Cell Biol.,* 102:1606–1614.

224. Riches, D. W. H., and Stanworth, D. R. (1982): Evidence for a mechanism for the initiation of acid hydrolase secretion by macrophages that is functionally independent of alternative pathway complement activation. *Biochem. J.,* 202:639–645.

225. Riches, D. W. H., Henson, P. M., Caterall, J. F., Remigio, L. K., Wheat, W. H., and Strunk, R. C. (1987): Regulation of the synthesis of factor B, C3 and β-glucuronidase during macrophage activation with a polyribonucleotide: the role of endogenously-derived interferon. In preparation.

226. Rindler-Ludwig, R., and Braunsteiner, H. (1975): Cationic proteins from human neutrophil granulocytes: evidence for their chymotrypsin-like properties. *Biochim. Biophys. Acta,* 379:606–617.

227. Ringel, E. W., Soter, N. A., and Austen, K. F. (1984): Localization of histaminase to the specific granule of the human neutrophil. *Immunology,* 52:649–658.

228. Robertson, P. B., Ryel, R. B., Taylor, R. E., Shyn, K. W., and Fullmer, H. M. (1972): Collagenase: localization in polymorphonuclear leukocyte granules in the rabbit. *Science,* 177:64–65.

229. Rooney, S. A. (1985): The surfactant system and lung phospholipid biochemistry. *Am. Rev. Respir. Dis.,* 131:439–460.

230. Root, R. K., and Cohen, M. S. (1981): The microbicidal mechanisms of human neutrophils and eosinophils. *Rev. Infect. Dis.,* 3:565–598.

231. Root, R. K., Metcalf, J., Oshino, N., and Chance, B. (1975): H_2O_2 release from human granulocytes during phagocytosis. I. Documentation, quantitation, and some regulating factor. *J. Clin. Invest.,* 55:945–955.

232. Rosen, H., and Klebanoff, S. J. (1977): Formation of singlet oxygen by the myeloperoxidase-mediated antimicrobial system. *J. Biol. Biochem.,* 252:4803–4810.

233. Rosenfeld, M. G., Kreibich, G., Popov, D., Kato, K., and Sabatini, D. D. (1982): Biosynthesis of lysosomal hydrolases: their synthesis in bound polysomes and the role of co- and post-translational processing in determining their subcellular distribution. *J. Cell Biol.,* 93:135–143.

234. Rouzer, C. A., Scott, W. A., Cohn, Z. A., Blackburn, P., and Manning, J. M. (1980): Mouse peritoneal macrophages release leukotriene C in response to a phagocytic stimulus. *Proc. Natl. Acad. Sci. USA,* 77:4928–4932.

235. Rumyantseva, G. V., Weiner, L. M., Molin, Y. N., and Budver, V. G. (1979): Permeation of liposome membrane by superoxide radical. *FEBS Lett.,* 108:477–480.

236. Sahagian, G. G., Distler, J., and Jourdian, G. W. (1981): Characterization of a membrane-associated receptor from bovine liver that binds phosphomannosyl residues of bovine testicular betagalactosidase. *Proc. Natl. Acad. Sci. USA,* 78:4289–4293.

237. Sanchez-Madrid, F., Nagy, J. A., Robbins, E., Simon, P., and Springer, T. A. (1983): A human leukocyte differentiation antigen family with distinct alpha-subunits and a common beta-subunit: the lymphocyte function-associated antigen (LFA-1), the C3bi complement receptor (OKM-1/Mac-1), and the p150,95 molecule. *J. Exp. Med.,* 158:1785–1803.

238. Sandhaus, R. A., and Henson, P. M. (1987): Elastin degradation is required for directed migration of neutrophils through an elastin rich barrier in vitro. Submitted for publication.

239. Savill, J., Lee, A., Henson, P. M., and Haslett, C. (1987): Macrophages specifically recognize and engulf apoptotic cells in an aging neutrophil population. Manuscript in preparation.

240. Schnyder, J., and Baggiolini, M. (1978): Secretion of lysosomal hydrolases by stimulated and non-stimulated macrophages. *J. Exp. Med.,* 148:435–450.

241. Schnyder, J., Dewald, B., and Baggiolini, M. (1982): Prostaglandin E$_2$ is a feed-back regulator of macrophage activation. In: *Macrophages and Natural Killer Cells, Regulation and Function,* edited by S. J. Norman and E. Sorkin, pp. 535–540. Plenum Press, New York.

242. Schorlemmer, H. U., Edwards, J. H., Davies, P., and Allison, A. C. (1977): Macrophage responses to mouldy hay dust, Micropolyspora faeni and zymosan, activators of complement by the alternate pathway. *Clin. Exp. Immunol.,* 27:198–207.

243. Selsted, M. E., Szklarek, D., and Lehrer, R. I. (1984): Purification and antibactericidal activity of antimicrobial peptides of rabbit granulocytes. *Infect. Immun.,* 45:150–154.

244. Shaw, J. O. (1980): Leukocytes in chemotactic-fragment-induced lung inflammation: vascular emigration and alveolar surface emigration. *Am. J. Pathol.,* 101:283–302.

245. Shaw, R. J., Walsh, G. M., Cromwell, O., Mogbel, R., Spry, C. J. F., and Kay, A. B. (1985): Activated human eosinophils generate SRS-A leukotrienes following IgG-dependent stimulation. *Nature,* 316:150–152.

246. Shephard, V. L., Konish, M. G., and Stahl, P. (1985): Dexamethasone increases expression of mannose receptors and decreases extracellular lysosomal enzyme accumulation in macrophages. *J. Biol. Chem.,* 260:160–164.

247. Shult, P. A., Graziano, F. M., Wallow, I. H., and Busse, W. W. (1985): Comparison of superoxide generation and luminol dependent chemiluminescence with eosinophils and neutrophils from normal individuals. *J. Lab. Clin. Med.,* 106:638–645.

248. Silverstein, S. C., Steinman, R. M., and Cohn, Z. A. (1977): Endocytosis. *Annu. Rev. Biochem.,* 46:669–722.

249. Skudlarek, M. D., and Swank, R. T. (1981): Turnover of two lysosomal enzymes in macrophages. *J. Biol. Chem.,* 256:10137–10144.

250. Smedley, L. A., Tonnesen, M. G., Sandhaus, R. A., Haslett, C., Guthrie, L. A., Johnston, R. B., Jr., Henson, P. M., and Worthen, G. S. (1986): Neutrophil-mediated injury to endothelial cells: enhancement by endotoxin and essential role of neutrophil elastase. *J. Clin. Invest.,* 77:1233–1243.

251. Smith, W. L., and Borgeat, P. (1985): The eicosanoids: prostaglandins, leukotrienes and hydroxy-eicosaenoic acids. In: *Biochemistry of Lipids and Membranes,* edited by D. E. Vance and J. E. Vance, p. 343. Benjamin Cummings Publishing, Menlo Park, California.

252. Smolen, J. E., Todd, R. F., III, and Boxer, L. A. (1986): Expression of a granule membrane marker on the surface of neutrophils permeabilized with digitonin: correlations with Ca^{2+}-induced degranulation. *Am. J. Pathol.,* 124:281–285.

253. Snyderman, R., and Pike, M. C. (1984): Chemoattractant receptors on phagocytic cells. *Annu. Rev. Immunol.,* 2:257–281.

254. Spitznagel, J. K., Dalldorf, F. G., Leffell, M. S., Folds, J. D., Welsh, I. R. H., Cooney, M. H., and Martin, L. E. (1974): Character of azurophil and specific granules purified from human polymorphonuclear leukocytes. *Lab. Invest.,* 30:774–785.

255. Stadecker, M. J., and Unanue, E. R. (1979): The regulation of thymidine secretion by macrophages. *J. Immunol.,* 123:568–571.

256. Stadecker, M. J., Calderon, J., Karnovsky, M. L., and Unanue, E. R. (1977): Synthesis and release of thymidine by macrophages. *J. Immunol.,* 119:1738–1743.

257. Staub, N. C., Schultz, E. L., Koike, K., and Albertine, K. H. (1983): Effect of neutrophil migration induced by leukotriene B$_4$ on protein permeability in sheep lung. *Fed. Proc.,* 44:30–35.

258. Stefanovic, J., Webb, T., and Lapresle, C. (1962): Etude des cathepsines D et E dans des preparations de polynucleaires, de macrophages et de lymphocytes de lapin. *Ann. Inst. Pasteur,* 103:276–284.

259. Steinhardt, R. A., and Alderton, J. M. (1982): Calmodulin confers calcium sensitivity on secretory exocytosis. *Nature,* 295:154–155.

260. Steinman, R. M., Mellman, J. S., Muller, W. A., and Cohn, Z. A.

(1983): Endocytosis and the recycling of plasma membrane. *J. Cell Biol.*, 96:1–27.

261. Steinmann, B., Rao, V. H., and Gitzelmann, R. (1981): Intracellular degradation of newly synthesized collagen is conformation-dependent studies: studies in human skin fibroblasts. *FEBS Lett.*, 133: 142–144.

262. Stossel, T. P. (1977): Contractile proteins during phagocytosis: an example of cell-to-cytoplasm communication. *Fed. Proc.*, 36:2181–2184.

263. Strunk, R. C., Kunke, K. S., and Musson, R. A. (1980): Lack of requirement for spreading for macrophages to synthesize complement. *J. Reticuloendothel. Soc.*, 28:483–493.

264. Strunk, R. C., Whitehead, A. S., and Cole, F. S. (1985): Pretranslational regulation of the synthesis of the third component in human mononuclear phagocytes by the lipid A portion of lipopolysaccharide. *J. Clin. Invest.*, 76:985–990.

265. Summers, T. A., and Creutz, C. E. (1985): Phosphorylation of a chromaffin granule-binding protein by protein kinase C. *J. Biol. Chem.*, 260:2437–2443.

266. Takenaka, T., Okuda, M., Kawabori, S., and Kubo, K. (1977): Extracellular release of peroxidase from eosinophils by interaction with immune complexes. *Clin. Exp. Immunol.*, 28:56–60.

267. Taniguchi, N., Mita, H., Saito, H., Yui, Y., Kajita, T., and Shida, T. (1985): Increased generation of leukotriene C_4 from eosinophils in asthmatic patients. *Allergy*, 40:571–573.

268. Tauber, A. I., and Babior, B. M. (1977): Evidence for hydroxyl radical production by human neutrophils. *J. Clin. Invest.*, 60:374–379.

269. Tauber, A. I., Goetzl, E. J., and Babior, B. M. (1979): Unique characteristics of superoxide production by human eosinophils in eosinophilic states. *Inflammation*, 3:261–272.

270. Thorgeirsson, U. P., Liotta, L. A., Kalebic, T., Margulies, I. M., Thomas, K., Rios-Candelore, M., and Russo, R. G. (1982): Effect of natural proteinase inhibitors and a chemoattractant on tumor cell invasion in vitro. *J. Natl. Cancer Inst.*, 69:1049–1054.

271. Trifaro, J. M., and Kenigsberg, R. L. (1983): Microinjection of calmodulin antibodies into chromaffin cells provides direct evidence for a role of calmodulin in the secretory process. *Fed. Proc.*, 42: 456.

272. Tsilibary, E. C., and Williams, M. C. (1983): Actin and secretion of surfactant. *J. Histochem. Cytochem.*, 31:1298–1304.

273. Tsilibary, E. C., and Williams, M. C. (1983): Actin in peripheral rat lung: S_1 labeling and structural changes induced by cytochalasin. *J. Histochem. Cytochem.*, 31:1289–1297.

274. Turk, J., Maas, R. L., Brash, A. R., Roberts, L. J., and Oates, J. A. (1982): Arachidonic acid 15-lipoxygenase products from human eosinophils. *J. Biol. Chem.*, 257:7068–7076.

275. Unkeless, J. C., Gordon, S., and Reich, E. (1974): Secretion of plasminogen activator by stimulated macrophages. *J. Exp. Med.*, 139:834–850.

276. Valone, F. H., Whitmer, D., Pickett, W. C., Austen, K. F., and Goetzl, E. J. (1979): The immunological generation of a platelet-activating factor and a platelet-lytic factor in the rat. *Immunology*, 37:841–848.

277. Venge, P., Dahl, R., and Hallgren, R. (1979): Enhancement of factor XII dependent reactions by eosinophil cationic protein. *Thromb. Res.*, 14:641–649.

278. Verkleij, A. J. (1984): Lipidic intramembranous particles. *Biochim. Biophys. Acta*, 779:43–63.

279. Voelker, D. R. (1985): Lipid assembly into cell membranes. In: *Biochemistry of Lipids and Membrane*, edited by D. E. Vance and J. E. Vance, pp. 475–502. Benjamin Cummings Publishing, Menlo Park, California.

280. Wahl, L. M., Wahl, S. M., Mergenhagen, S. E., and Martin, G. R. (1974): Collagenase production by endotoxin activated macrophages. *Proc. Natl. Acad. Sci. USA*, 71:3598–3601.

281. Ward, P. A., Sulavik, M. C., and Johnson, K. J. (1985): Activated rat neutrophils: correlation of arachidonate products with enzyme secretion but not with O_2 generation. *Am. J. Pathol.*, 120:112–120.

282. Wasi, S., Murray, R. K., MacMorine, D. L., and Movat, H. Z. (1966): The role of PMN-leucocyte lysosomes in tissue injury, inflammation and hypersensitivity. II. Studies on the proteolytic activity of PMN-leucocyte lysosomes of the rabbit. *Br. J. Exp. Pathol.*, 47:411–423.

283. Wasserman, S. I., Goetzl, E. J., and Austen, K. F. (1975): Inactivation of slow reacting substances of anaphylaxis by human eosinophil arylsulfatase. *J. Immunol.*, 114:645–649.

284. Wassom, D. L., and Gleich, G. J. (1979): Damage to Trichinella spiralis newborn larvae by eosinophil major basic protein. *Am. J. Trop. Med. Hyg.*, 28:860–863.

285. Webster, R. O., Zanolari, B., and Henson, P. M. (1980): Neutrophil chemotaxis in response to surface-bound C5a. *Exp. Cell Res.*, 129: 55–62.

286. Weiss, J., Elsbach, P., Olsson, I., and Odeberg, H. (1978): Purification and characterization of a potent bactericidal and membrane-active protein from the granules of human polymorphonuclear leukocytes. *J. Biol. Chem.*, 253:2664–2672.

287. Weiss, L. (1963): The pH value at the surface of Bacillus subtilis. *J. Gen. Microbiol.*, 32:331–340.

288. Weiss, S. J., Lampert, M. B., and Test, S. T. (1983): Long lived oxidants generated by human neutrophils: characterization and bioactivity. *Science*, 222:625–628.

289. Weiss, S. S., Rustagi, P. K., and LoBuglio, A. F. (1978): Human granulocyte generation of hydroxyl radical. *J. Exp. Med.*, 147:316–324.

290. Weissmann, G., Zurier, R. B., Spielen, P. J., and Goldstein, I. M. (1971): Mechanisms of lysosomal enzyme release from leukocytes exposed to immune complexes and other particles. *J. Exp. Med.*, 134:149–165s.

291. Weller, P. F., Bach, D., and Austen, K. F. (1981): Expression of lysopholipase activity by intact human eosinophils and their Charcot-Leyden crystals. *Trans. Assoc. Am. Physicians*, 94:165–171.

292. Weller, P. F., Bach, D., and Austen, K. F. (1982): Human eosinophil lysophospholipase: the sole protein constituent of Charcot-Leyden crystals. *J. Immunol.*, 128:1346–1349.

293. Weller, P. F., Bach, D., and Austen, K. F. (1984): Biochemical characterisation of human eosinophil Charcot-Leyden crystal protein (lysophospholipase). *J. Biol. Chem.*, 259:15100–15105.

294. Weller, P. F., Corey, E. J., Austen, K. F., and Lewis, R. A. (1986): Inhibition of homogeneous human eosinophil arylsulfatase by sulfidopeptide leukotrienes. *J. Biol. Chem.*, 261:1737–1744.

295. Weller, P. F., Lee, C. W., Foster, D. W., Corey, E. J., Austen, K. F., and Lewis, R. A. (1983): Generation and metabolism of 5-lipoxygenase pathway leukotrienes by human eosinophils: predominant production of leukotriene C_4. *Proc. Natl. Acad. Sci. USA*, 80:7626–7630.

296. Welsh, C. E., Waite, B. M., Thomas, M. J., and DeChatelet, L. R. (1981): Release and metabolism of arachidonic acid in human neutrophils. *J. Biol. Chem.*, 256:7228–7234.

297. Weltzien, H. U. (1979): Cytolytic and membrane perturbing properties of lysophosphatidylcholine. *Biochim. Biophys. Acta*, 559:259–287.

298. Werb, Z., and Chin, J. R. (1983): Endotoxin suppresses expression of apoprotein E by mouse macrophages in vivo and in culture. *J. Biol. Chem.*, 258:10642–10648.

299. Werb, Z., and Gordon, S. (1974): Elastase secretion by stimulated macrophages. *J. Exp. Med.*, 142:361–377.

300. Werb, Z., and Gordon, S. (1974): Secretion of a specific collagenase by stimulated macrophages. *J. Exp. Med.*, 142:346–360.

301. West, B. C. (1985): Heparin inhibition of human neutrophil and eosinophil-enriched leukocyte acid glycerophosphatase (42020). *Proc. Soc. Exp. Biol. Med.*, 178:373–384.

302. Wetzel, B. K., Spicer, S. S., and Horn, R. G. (1967): Fine structural localization of acid and alkaline phosphatases in cells of rabbit blood and bone marrow. *J. Histochem. Cytochem.*, 15:311–334.

303. Whaley, K. (1980): Biosynthesis of the complement components and the regulatory proteins of the alternative complement pathway by human peripheral blood monocytes. *J. Exp. Med.*, 151:501–516.

304. Williams, D. M., Linder, J. E., Hill, M. W., and Gillett, R. (1978): Ultrastructural localisation of alkaline phosphatases in rat eosinophil leucocytes. *J. Histochem. Cytochem.*, 26:862–864.

305. Williams, J. A. (1984): Regulatory mechanisms in pancreas and salivary acini. *Annu. Rev. Physiol.,* 46:361–375.
306. Williams, J. D., Lee, T. H., Lewis, R. A., and Austen, F. (1985): Intracellular retention of the 5-lipoxygenase pathway product, leukotriene B$_4$, by human neutrophils activated with unopsonized zymosan. *J. Immunol.,* 134:2624–2630.
307. Wilschut, J., Duzgunes, N., Hoekstra, D., and Papahadjopoulos, D. (1985): Modulation of membrane fusion by membrane fluidity: temperature dependence of divalent cation induced fusion of phosphatidylserine vesicles. *Biochemistry,* 24:8–14.
308. Woodin, A. M., and Wieneke, A. A. (1970): Leukocidin, tetraethylammonium ions, and the membrane acyl phosphatases in relation to the leukocyte potassium pump. *J. Gen. Physiol.,* 56:16–32.
309. Worthen, G. S., Gumbay, R. S., Larsen, G. L., and Henson, P. M. (1983): Prostaglandin E$_2$ enhances platelet-activity factor induced lung neutrophil migration but not vascular permeability. *Am. Rev. Respir. Dis.,* 127:57 (abstract).
310. Worthen, G. S., Haslett, C., Rees, A. J., Gumbay, R. S., Henson, J. E., and Henson, P. M. (1987): Neutrophil-mediated pulmonary vascular injury: synergistic effect of trace amounts of LPS and neutrophil stimuli on vascular permeability and neutrophil sequestration in the lung. Submitted for publication.
311. Worthen, G. S., Lien, D. C., Tonnesen, M. G., and Henson, P. M. (1987): Interaction of leukocytes with the pulmonary endothelium. In: *Pulmonary Endothelium,* edited by U. Ryan. Marcel Dekker, New York (in press).
312. Worthen, G. S., Seccombe, J. F., Guthrie, L. A., Clay, K., and Johnston, R. B., Jr. (1987): Priming of neutrophils by lipopolysaccharide for the intracellular production of platelet-activity factor. Submitted for publication.
313. Wright, D. G., and Gallin, J. I. (1979): Secretory responses of human neutrophils: exocytosis of specific (secretory) granules by human neutrophils during adherence in vitro and during exudation in vivo. *J. Immunol.,* 123:285–294.
314. Wright, D. G., and Malawista, S. E. (1972): The mobilization and extracellular release of granule enzymes from human leukocytes during phagocytosis. *J. Cell Biol.,* 53:788–797.
315. Wright, D. G., Bralove, D. A., and Gallin, J. I. (1977): The differential mobilization of human neutrophil granules: effects of phorbol myristate acetate and ionophore A23187. *Am. J. Pathol.,* 87:273–284.
316. Wright, J., Schwartz, J. H., Olson, R., Kosowsky, J. M., and Tauber, A. I. (1986): Proton secretion by the sodium/hydrogen ion antiporter in the human neutrophil. *J. Clin. Invest.,* 77:782–788.
317. Wright, S. D., and Silverstein, S. C. (1984): Phagocytosing macrophages exclude proteins from the zones of contact with opsonized targets. *Nature,* 309:359–361.
318. Wright, S. D., Rao, P. E., van Voorhis, W. C., Craigmyle, L. S., Iida, K., Talle, M. A., Westberg, E. F., Goldstein, G., and Silverstein, S. C. (1983): Identification of the C3bi receptor of human monocytes and macrophages by using monoclonal antibodies. *Proc. Natl. Acad. Sci. USA,* 80:5699–5703.
319. Wyllie, A. H., Kerr, J. F. R., and Currie, A. C. (1982): Cell death: the significance of apoptosis. *Int. Rev. Cytol.,* 68:251–306.
320. Yeh, A. K., Tulsiani, D. R. P., and Carubelli, R. (1971): Neuraminidase activity in human leukocytes. *J. Lab. Clin. Med.,* 78:771–778.
321. Yokota, S., and Oda, T. (1983): Immunoelectron microscopic localisation of serine: pyruvate aminotransferase in rat eosinophil leukocytes. *Histochemistry,* 78:417–424.
322. Yokota, S., Deimann, W., Hashimoto, T., and Fahimi, H. D. (1983): Immunocytochemical localisation of two peroxisomal enzymes of lipid oxidation in specific granules of rat eosinophils. *Histochemistry,* 78:425–433.
323. Yokota, S., Tsuji, H., and Kato, K. (1984): Localisation of lysosomal and peroxisomal enzymes in the specific granules of rat interstitial eosinophil leukocytes revealed by immunoelectron microscopic techniques. *J. Histochem. Cytochem.,* 32:267–273.
324. Yoon, P. S., Boxer, L. A., Mayo, L. A., Yang, A. Y., and Wicha, M. S. (1987): Human neutrophil laminin receptors: activation-dependent receptor expression. *J. Immunol.,* 138:259–265.
325. Zeiger, R. S., and Colten, H. R. (1977): Histaminase release from human eosinophils. *J. Immunol.,* 118:540–543.
326. Zeiger, R. S., Yurdin, D. L., and Colten, H. R. (1976): Histamine metabolism: cellular and subcellular localisation of the catabolic enzymes, histaminase and histamine methyl transferase in human leukocytes. *J. Allergy Clin. Immunol.,* 58:172–179.
327. Zeya, H. I., and Spitznagel, J. K. (1968): Arginine-rich proteins of polymorphonuclear lysosomes: antimicrobial specificity and biochemical heterogeneity. *J. Exp. Med.,* 127:927–941.
328. Zeya, H. I., and Spitznagel, J. K. (1971): Characterization of cationic protein-bearing granules of polymorphonuclear leukocytes. *Lab. Invest.,* 24:229–236.
329. Zilversmith, D. B. (1984): Lipid transfer proteins. *J. Lipid Res.,* 25:1563–1569.
330. Zimmerli, W., Seligmann, B., and Gallin, I. J. (1986): Exudation primes human and guinea pig neutrophils for subsequent responsiveness to the chemotactic peptide N-formylmethionyl leucylphenylamine and increases complement component C3bi receptor expression. *J. Clin. Invest.,* 77:925–933.
331. Zucker-Franklin, D., and Hirsch, J. G. (1964): Electronmicroscopic studies on the degranulation of rabbit peritoneal leucocytes during phagocytosis. *J. Exp. Med.,* 120:569–576.
332. Zurier, R. B., Hoffstein, S., and Weissmann, G. (1973): Cytochalasin B: effect on lysosomal enzyme release from human leukocytes. *Proc. Natl. Acad. Sci. USA,* 70:844–848.

Inflammation: Basic Principles and Clinical Correlates.
Edited by J. I. Gallin, I. M. Goldstein, and R. Snyderman.
Raven Press, Ltd., New York © 1988.

CHAPTER 23

Phagocytic Cells: Products of Oxygen Metabolism

Seymour J. Klebanoff

Neutrophils
   Respiratory Burst • Superoxide Anion • Hydrogen Peroxide • Peroxidase/H_2O_2/Halide System • Hydroxyl Radical • H_2O_2/Fe^{2+}/Iodide Antimicrobial System • Singlet Oxygen

Eosinophils
   Respiratory Burst • Eosinophil Peroxidase
Mononuclear Phagocytes
   Monocytes • Macrophages
References

Professional phagocytes (neutrophils, eosinophils, monocytes/macrophages) have among their functions the phagocytosis and destruction of microorganisms. These cells, when appropriately stimulated, also can release toxic agents to the outside of the cell, with the potential for attack on adjacent normal tissue, malignant cells, invading organisms too large to be ingested, and certain soluble mediators. They perform these functions through a variety of mechanisms (424) that can be conveniently divided into those which are dependent on oxygen and those which are not. This chapter considers the microbicidal and cytotoxic systems that are oxygen-dependent. The oxygen-independent toxic systems are considered in Chapter 24.

Oxygen is a reactive molecule thermodynamically and thus can react with most elements and many organic molecules. However, from a kinetic standpoint, oxygen is rather inert and in most instances requires a catalyst to overcome this kinetic barrier. This property is necessary because without the kinetic barrier the high reactivity of oxygen would result in its depletion from the environment and the loss of aerobic life as we know it. The basis of the kinetic inertness of oxygen is its electronic configuration. In most instances electrons occur in pairs stabilized by spins in the opposite direction. When it is not the case, i.e., an electron is unpaired, the molecule is a highly reactive free radical. Molecular oxygen is a diradical in

which two of its valence electrons, located in different orbitals, are unpaired and have parallel spins (Fig. 1). In oxidation reactions, oxygen accepts electrons from the molecule, which it oxidizes, and in the process is reduced. In reactions with a nonradical, this transfer of electrons occurs from an electron pair with opposite spins, and thus inversion of spin is necessary if both of the vacant spaces in the unfilled orbitals of oxygen are to be filled. This restriction to electron transfer accounts for the sluggishness of oxygen reactivity.

The reactivity of oxygen can be increased by either reduction or excitation. Oxygen is reduced ultimately to water by the acceptance of four electrons; however, partial reduction can occur with the formation of highly reactive intermediates, i.e., the superoxide anion (O_2^-), hydrogen peroxide (H_2O_2), and the hydroxyl radical ($OH\cdot$) (Fig. 1). Excitation occurs when an absorption of energy shifts one of the unpaired electrons of oxygen to an orbital of higher energy with an inversion of spin. The product (singlet oxygen, $^1O_2$) can occur in two forms: delta singlet oxygen ($^1\Delta_g O_2$) in which the newly paired electrons occupy the same orbital (with the other orbital empty) and sigma singlet oxygen ($^1\Sigma_g^+ O_2$) in which the two electrons now with opposite spins occupy different orbitals. The formation of these toxic oxygen products and their involvement in the activity of phagocytes are considered here (39,48,306,418).

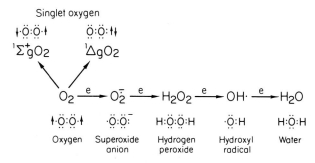

FIG. 1. Reduction and excitation of oxygen.

NEUTROPHILS

Respiratory Burst

A striking feature of neutrophils is their response to stimulation with a marked increase in oxygen consumption. Early findings indicated that the respiratory burst of neutrophils was not needed for the generation of the metabolic energy required for phagocytosis; rather, the respiratory burst appeared to be required for optimum microbicidal activity as indicated by the decrease (but not loss) of microbicidal activity on exposure of neutrophils to hypoxic conditions (480,756) and by the association of a microbicidal defect (601) with the absence of the respiratory burst (342) in the leukocytes of patients with chronic granulomatous disease (CGD). This finding has focused attention on the enzyme systems responsible for the respiratory burst and on the nature of the toxic products formed.

NADPH Oxidase

The most widely held view is that phagocytes respond to stimulation with the activation of a transmembrane electron transport system in which a reduced pyridine nucleotide (predominantly nicotinamide adenine dinucleotide, or NADPH) on the cytoplasmic side of the membrane reduces oxygen in the extracellular fluid, or when the membrane is invaginated in the phagosome, through a series of reactions involving the oxidation and reduction of a flavin, a b-cytochrome, and possibly a quinone (Fig. 2). Each component of this system is considered below.

Electron donor

That NADPH is the primary electron donor for the reduction of oxygen during the respiratory burst is based on the demonstration of an enzyme system in leukocytes which catalyzes the reaction

$$NADPH + O_2 \rightarrow O_2^- + NADP^+ + H^+$$

This NADPH oxidase was first described in 1964 (631), and its preference for NADPH as the electron donor is based on the considerably greater affinity (lower Km) of the enzyme for NADPH than for NADH (45,82,255,766). The NADPH binding site of the oxidase extends into the cytoplasm, with the remainder of the enzyme system embedded into the plasma membrane (46,282,524,818). The NADPH binding component of the NADPH oxidase is reported to be a protein of 66 kilodaltons (kD) (754). A sulfhydryl group essential for enzyme activity has been described in close proximity to the NADPH binding site (257). Although NADPH is believed to be the predominant electron donor for the oxidase, most preparations also react with NADH, although with a lower affinity, raising the possibility that there is some contribution of electrons from NADH as well as NADPH.

Flavoprotein

The early finding that cyanide did not inhibit the respiratory burst of neutrophils distinguished this activity from the mitochondrial respiratory chain. A flavin requirement for the oxidase was supported by reconstitution experiments in which the loss of NADPH oxidase activity on extraction of a human neutrophil preparation with detergent was prevented by the addition of flavin adenine dinucleotide (FAD) (41,255,258,765). Flavin mononucleotide (FMN) was less effective. Furthermore, flavin analogs were found to inhibit O_2^- production by a partially purified oxidase preparation (467).

FAD has been detected in neutrophil membrane fractions with a flavin/b-cytochrome ratio of 1:1 in cell membranes and 2.3:1.0 in phagosome membranes (180). Membranes of resting and phorbol myristate acetate (PMA)-stimulated neutrophil cytoplasts contained equal amounts of noncovalently bound FAD with the flavin/b-cytochrome ratio being 0.5:1.0 (473). FAD also has been detected in specific granules of neutrophils with a flavin/b-cytochrome ratio of 0.5:1.0 (102), in a subcellular particulate fraction of human neutrophils enriched in NADPH oxidase activity (254), and in solubilized NADPH oxidase preparations (42). It has been localized in the major 65-kD protein of a purified NADPH oxidase preparation from human neutrophils (482), which may

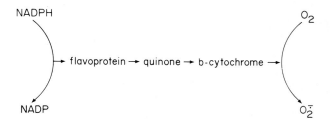

FIG. 2. NADPH oxidase of phagocytes.

be the same protein that binds NADPH (754). The FAD of neutrophil preparations is decreased or absent in some patients with CGD (102,180,256,561).

Flavoprotein dehydrogenases generally accept electrons from reduced pyridine nucleotides and transmit them to an electron acceptor molecule. The FAD of pig neutrophil membranes from either resting or stimulated cells has a midpoint potential of -280 mV at pH 7.0 (379). Addition of NADPH to the plasma membranes of stimulated cells resulted in the formation of a flavin-free radical that was not seen when NADPH was added to membranes of resting cells. The midpoint potential of FAD lies between that of the $NADP^+/NADPH$ couple (-320 mV) and that of the b-cytochrome (-245 mV), suggesting that the flavoprotein may catalyze a two-electron transfer from NADPH and a one-electron transfer to the b-cytochrome. However, the reduced flavoprotein also may be oxidized by oxygen directly.

Flavin-linked dehydrogenases generally can reduce artificial electron receptors such as dichlorophenolindophenol (DCIP), and this NADPH diaphorase activity has been detected in human neutrophil NADPH oxidase preparations in some studies (278–280,283,766) but not in others (40,83). The absence of diaphorase activity indicates either that a flavoprotein dehydrogenase is not a component of the NADPH oxidase or that the active site of the complex is inaccessible to the artificial electron acceptor.

A role for FAD in the NADPH oxidase activity of neutrophils has been questioned based on the low levels of FAD relative to b-cytochrome in partially purified NADPH oxidase of pig neutrophils (84). In this study the cytochrome b/FAD ratio fell from 1.13:1.00 to 18.95:1.00 with purification. These data suggest either that the NADPH oxidase lacks FAD or that each flavoprotein molecule is associated with a large number of b-cytochrome molecules (84). Similarly, FAD could not be detected in a purified preparation of bovine neutrophil NADPH oxidase, although a firmly bound flavin was not excluded (220).

Quinone

Involvement of a quinone in the transfer of electrons from reduced pyridine nucleotides to oxygen remains controversial. A quinone has been detected in neutrophil preparations (175,183,500,687) that was identified as ubiquinone-50 (now termed ubiquinone-10) (176,183). It was not primarily located in the plasma membrane (687) or in specific or azurophil granules (177), but it was enriched in phagolysosomes and in a distinct tertiary granule (501). A membrane-associated NADPH oxidase complex has been described that consists of a flavoprotein, ubiquinone-10, and a b-cytochrome in an approximate molar ratio

of 1.3:1.0:2.0 and a mechanism for the respiratory burst proposed in which electrons flow from NADPH through FAD to ubiquinone-10 in resting cells and continue through the b-cytochrome to oxygen in stimulated cells (257).

Other investigators have been unable to detect a quinone in intact neutrophils (473), neutrophil cytoplasts (473), a plasma membrane fraction (178), or NADPH oxidase preparations (84). Although ubiquinone-10 was detected in a mitochondrial fraction, it was not enriched in phagolysosomes in contrast to O_2^--generating activity and b-cytochrome (181). These conflicting studies leave open the question of the role of ubiquinone-10 in the respiratory burst.

Cytochrome b_{559}

Leukocytes contain a novel low-potential b-cytochrome in high concentration (183,321,562,653,675). The oxidation–reduction midpoint potential ($E_{m\ 7.0}$) was -245 mV (178), which is lower than that reported for any other mammalian b-cytochrome. The b-cytochrome of phagocytes has been designated cytochrome b_{-245} to indicate its uniquely low midpoint potential or cytochrome b_{558} or b_{559} to indicate the wavelength of the α band of the reduced cytochrome. The latter is in line with the nomenclature used for other b-cytochromes.

The molecular weight of the b-cytochrome purified in a number of laboratories (310,311,474,583,673) has varied widely [68–78 kD (310); 235 kD (474); three bands of 14, 12, and 11 kD (583); and 32 kD for a complex containing phospholipid, b-cytochrome, and NADPH oxidase activity (673). It is a glycoprotein with carbohydrate, in one study, accounting for approximately 15% of the molecular weight, with the major sugars being N-acetylglucosamine and galactose (311). A b-cytochrome could not be detected in a purified bovine NADPH oxidase preparation (220).

The involvement of cytochrome b_{559} in the respiratory burst is suggested by a number of findings.

1. The low midpoint potential [-245 mV (178); -225 mV (583); -218 mV and -407 mV for the unpurified and purified cytochrome, respectively (474)] is close to that (-330 mV) reported for the $O_2 \rightleftharpoons O_2^-$ couple (350,808), which is compatible with the b-cytochrome being the terminal component in the NADPH oxidase electron transport chain.

2. The b-cytochrome is reduced when intact neutrophils are stimulated, particularly under anaerobic conditions, and reoxidation occurs on the reintroduction of air (104,654). The b-cytochrome of cell-free preparations also is reduced by NADPH and NADH (81,179,182,259,675), and the reduced cytochrome is rapidly oxidized by oxygen (178,467). In some studies the reduction of the b-cytochrome by NADPH occurred

slowly or not at all (178,179,259,467,504), raising a question about the invariant participation of the b-cytochrome in the transfer of electrons from NADPH to oxygen (40,259,504).

3. The b-cytochrome in its reduced form binds carbon monoxide (CO) (81,259,474,583,653,675), and it is generally believed that a cytochrome that binds CO also can react with oxygen. The significance of the binding of CO as evidence for the participation of the b-cytochrome as the terminal oxidase has been questioned based on the slow kinetics of binding (474) and the absence of inhibition of the respiratory burst of intact neutrophils by CO (504).

4. The b-cytochrome of unstimulated neutrophils has a dual distribution with a portion present in the plasma membrane and the remainder in the membrane of the specific granules (98,102,106,261,338,560,575,655,687). In one study (501) the b-cytochrome was reported to be concentrated in a tertiary granule that was resolved from both specific and azurophil granules. Following stimulation there is a translocation of b-cytochrome from the specific granules to the plasma membrane, findings compatible with the assembly of the components of the oxidase at the membrane surface in response to neutrophil stimulation.

5. HL-60 cells are induced to differentiate into relatively mature granulocytes by treatment with dimethylsulfoxide (DMSO) or certain other reagents (169). Maturation is associated with an increased respiratory burst, increased NADPH oxidase activity, and an increase in b-cytochrome levels (543,611).

6. The b-cytochrome is absent from the leukocytes of most patients with X-linked CGD (561,653,657,660). One patient with X-linked inheritance and the presence of b-cytochrome (99,103) was found to be atypical in that the leukocyte oxidase was not totally defective, and as a result PMA-stimulated nitroblue tetrazolium reduction in a slide test was normal in contrast to other measures of the respiratory burst (105). Another patient with probable X-linked inheritance and normal cytochrome b_{559} levels also has been described (561).

In contrast to X-linked CGD, the neutrophils of CGD patients with autosomal recessive inheritance contained b-cytochrome (99,103) that was normal in its midpoint potential, its ability to bind to CO, and its subcellular distribution (660); however, it was not normally reduced during neutrophil stimulation (656,660). Occasional patients with probable autosomal recessive inheritance (as distinct from extreme lyonization of an X-linked heterozygote) and cytochrome b_{559} deficiency have been described (561,769).

Mechanism of activation

The components of the oxidase described above are those that may be directly involved in the transfer of elec-

trons to oxygen. However, a striking feature of the oxidase is its conversion from an inactive dormant state when the cell is at rest to an activated state when the phagocyte is exposed to a stimulus. A number of factors have been implicated in this activation process.

Transmembrane potential. A change in transmembrane potential is one of the earliest consequences of neutrophil stimulation (see Chapter 21) (164,442,443,466,507, 666,668,788), although the use of different methods of measurement has led to conflicting results as to the direction of the change (668). Thus in early studies in which the resting membrane potential was low, stimulation produced a triphasic response of hyperpolarization, depolarization, and hyperpolarization (442); whereas in other studies in which the resting potential was generally higher, stimulation produced a biphasic response of depolarization followed by hyperpolarization, or only depolarization, depending on the stimulus (164,369,666,788). The membrane depolarization was greatly decreased or absent when CGD neutrophils were used (164,667,788; however, see 465 for normal depolarization in a variant of CGD). The apparent hyperpolarization that followed depolarization was due largely to myeloperoxidase (MPO)-catalyzed oxidation of the probe by H_2O_2 (789). The ability to respond to stimulation with superoxide (O_2^-) production and membrane potential change (depolarization) develop concomitantly as the granulocytes differentiate and mature (407).

The early membrane depolarization on stimulation and its absence in CGD suggests a relation to activation of the neutrophil oxidase. Whether the transmembrane potential change is a required component of the initial triggering of the respiratory burst or is an epiphenomenon (507) is unclear.

Ca^{2+}. The stimulation of neutrophils by a variety of particulate and soluble stimuli is associated with an increase in free cytoplasmic Ca^{2+} (267,444,466,598,786), which occurs within seconds of addition of the stimulus (444,451,786); indeed it was reported to precede membrane depolarization and to be the earliest evidence of stimulation yet described (451).

It has been proposed that intracellular free Ca^{2+} is a requirement for triggering the respiratory burst by a variety of stimuli based on inhibition of the respiratory burst by inhibitors of intracellular calcium mobilization and of calmodulin (225,692,721); the specificity of the inhibitors, however, may not be absolute. Although intracellular free Ca^{2+} may be required, its increased concentration is not by itself sufficient to induce a respiratory burst because an increase in cytosolic Ca^{2+} with little or no respiratory burst activity is observed when stimuli are added to CGD neutrophils (466) or when low levels of the chemotactic peptide formylmethionyl-leucyl-phenylalanine (fMLP) (444), ionomycin (598), or monoclonal antibody PMN7C3 (30) is added to normal neutrophils. Furthermore, the respiratory burst induced by PMA occurs in the absence of an increase in intracellular free Ca^{2+} (217,267,674); indeed there is a net loss of Ca^{2+} presumably due to the activation of a Ca^{2+} efflux pump (507,674).

Protein kinase C. Protein kinase C is a Ca^{2+}-activated, phospholipid-dependent phosphorylating enzyme that plays an important role in signal transduction in a variety of tissues (550). It is present in an inactive form in the cytoplasm and is activated by 1,2-diacylglycerol, with translocation to the plasma membrane. Diacylglycerol is formed by the hydrolysis of membrane (poly)phosphatidylinositol by phospholipase C in response to external signals (see Chapter 20). Activation appears to result from the transient binding of diacylglycerol to protein kinase C, which increases its affinity for Ca^{2+} so that Ca^{2+} is now effective at physiological concentrations. A phospholipid, particularly phosphatidylserine, also is needed for activation. The requirement for diacylglycerol for protein kinase C activation can be bypassed by phorbol esters such as PMA or 12-*o*-tetradecanoyl-phorbol-13-acetate (TPA) or by certain synthetic diacylglycerols, e.g., 1-oleoyl-2-acetylglycerol (OAG), which can intercalate into the membrane. A second product of phosphatidylinositol 4,5-biphosphate (PIP$_2$) hydrolysis, inositol 1,4,5-triphosphate (IP$_3$), has been implicated as a mediator of Ca^{2+} mobilization from endoplasmic reticular stores.

The long-recognized stimulation of the respiratory burst of phagocytes by phorbol esters (613), the synergistic effect of suboptimal concentrations of phorbol esters and agents such as the Ca^{2+} ionophore A23187 or ionomycin, which increase intracellular Ca^{2+} levels (191,217), the stimulation of the respiratory burst by OAG either alone or synergistically with other agents (172,191,205,252,376, 558,585), and the decrease in the respiratory burst induced by inhibitors of protein kinase C (268,597; however, see 810) have suggested that protein kinase C is involved in the activation of leukocytic NADPH oxidase. The rapid decrease in phosphatidylinositol 4,5-biphosphate in neutrophils stimulated by fMLP (219,689,762,824) supports the involvement of this pathway. One mechanism for the rise in intracellular free Ca^{2+} associated with neutrophil stimulation by many but not all agents may be the release of Ca^{2+} from intracellular stores by IP$_3$ (599).

Limited proteolysis of protein kinase C by a Ca^{2+}-requiring proteinase (calpain) in neutrophils converts it to a form that is fully active in the absence of Ca^{2+} and phospholipid (493,494). It has been proposed that stimulation of neutrophils results in the binding of cytosolic protein kinase C and calpain to the plasma membrane, where activation of the proteinase leads to the conversion of protein kinase C to its Ca^{2+}/phospholipid-independent form, which is released from the membrane into the cytosol where it can phosphorylate intracellular proteins. Protein kinase C phosphorylates a variety of proteins (550), and it is therefore assumed that its effect on NADPH

oxidase results from the phosphorylation of a key component of the system. Stimulation of neutrophils is associated with the phosphorylation of multiple proteins and polypeptides (25,26,252,326,339,573,648,662,787); dephosphorylation of one protein band also has been observed (25,26). These proteins have been characterized in regard to their molecular weight, but in most instances their function in the cell is unknown [exceptions are the phosphorylation of lipomodulin (339) and a component of a purified preparation of NADPH oxidase (573)]. A variety of stimuli have been employed, suggesting that phosphorylation is a general response to stimulation, although the degree and rate of phosphorylation varied to some degree with the nature of the stimulus (26,323). Most of the phosphorylated proteins were cytosolic, although some were present in the cytoskeleton, the nuclear pellet, and the plasma membrane (787). In an early study (25), PMA-treated neutrophils from patients with CGD were found to form the same phosphorylated products as did normal neutrophils. However, subsequent studies with neutrophils from four patients with autosomal recessive CGD (662) and four male patients with CGD (323) indicated the absence of phosphorylation of a 44-kD (662) or 48-kD (323) protein. The role of this protein in the respiratory burst is not known.

Cyclic nucleotides. Cyclic adenosine monophosphate (cyclic AMP)-dependent protein kinase (protein kinase A), like protein kinase C, is a phosphorylating enzyme involved in signal transduction in cells. Cyclic AMP levels of neutrophils increase transiently with stimulation (100,335,353,682,690,691), an effect that precedes O_2^- production (691). However, the increase in cyclic AMP levels could be dissociated from the increased respiratory burst by replacement of extracellular Na^+ and K^+ with choline (691), use of a low concentration of stimulator (691), addition of certain agents that increase intracellular cyclic AMP levels (682), addition of an inhibitor of adenylate cyclase (683), or the substitution of CGD for normal neutrophils (335). Furthermore, although protein kinase A has been detected in neutrophils, inhibitor studies suggest that phosphorylation is due predominantly to protein kinase C (326). Indeed agents that raise cyclic AMP levels in leukocytes inhibit the respiratory burst (see Chapter 20). These findings suggest that the transient increase in cyclic AMP is not required for triggering the respiratory burst. No change in cyclic guanosine monophosphate (cyclic GMP) levels was observed on neutrophil stimulation (682,691; however, see 320).

Guanosine triphosphate-binding protein. Guanosine triphosphate (GTP) binding regulatory proteins (designated G- or N-proteins) have been implicated in the coupling of receptor stimulation to the activation of adenylate cyclase in a number of cell types (see Chapter 20). In some instances adenylate cyclase is activated by the GTP-binding protein Ns (or Gs), and in other instances adenylate cyclase is inhibited by the GTP binding protein Ni (or Gi). Cholera toxin induces adenosine diphosphate (ADP)-ribosylation of the α subunit of N_S thereby stabilizing it in an active form with persistent activation of adenylate cyclase, whereas pertussis toxin induces ADP-ribosylation of the α subunit of Ni, thereby perpetuating its inhibitory effect on adenylate cyclase. The GTP-binding proteins have been implicated in signal transduction from chemotactic factor receptors in neutrophils (76,272, 346,440,502,563,693,758,763) and macrophages (694); however, a mechanism other than a direct effect on adenylate cyclase activity appears to be involved (759). It has been proposed that the N-proteins are required for polyphosphoinositide hydrolysis (77,110,273,689) and thus for activation of protein kinase C.

Translocation of components from intracellular stores. The neutrophil oxidase is a multicomponent complex that has been localized in the plasma membrane of stimulated cells (203,819). A high proportion of the b-cytochrome (98,102,106) and the flavin (98,102) of unstimulated neutrophils is present in the specific granules and is transferred to the plasma membrane during stimulation. This fact is compatible with the intracellular storage of important components of the leukocyte oxidase and their assembly at the cell surface or on the phagosome membrane by degranulation during the activation process.

Translocation of b-cytochrome and flavin in this way does not appear to be essential for activation of the leukocyte oxidase, as cells devoid of specific granules such as the HL-60 promyelocyte cell line (611), neutrophils from patients with specific granule deficiency (109,560), and neutrophils depleted of nuclei and granules (cytoplasts) (338,473,560,575) respond to stimulation with a respiratory burst. In some instances the burst is less than that seen with comparably stimulated normal cells, whereas in other cases, e.g., patients who lack specific granules (109), the respiratory burst is greater than that of normal neutrophils. Cytoplasts have been reported to contain higher levels of plasma membrane b-cytochrome than do intact resting neutrophils (338,587; however, see 473), suggesting some fusion of granule and plasma membranes during cytoplast preparation. Although translocation of components from specific granules to the plasma membrane may not be essential for initiation of the respiratory burst, a continued supply of components by translocation from an intracellular pool may be required for maintenance of activity.

Translocation of protein kinase C from the cytosol to the membrane fraction with associated phosphorylation of a number of polypeptides occurred when neutrophil cytoplasts were stimulated with PMA (268,269,805). This translocation preceded activation of NADPH oxidase, and both responses to stimulation occurred at comparable PMA concentrations. Both phosphorylation and O_2^- pro-

duction by PMA-stimulated cytoplasts were inhibited by trifluoperazine, a protein kinase C inhibitor (268) (but see below). These findings suggest that the translocation of protein kinase C from the cytosol to the plasma membrane may be one of the mechanisms by which the respiratory burst is triggered.

Serine proteinase. Certain serine proteinase inhibitors or synthetic substrates decrease O_2^- production by stimulated neutrophils (and monocytes) (404–406,681), raising the possibility that a serine proteinase may be involved in triggering the respiratory burst.

Other requirements. Crude *phospholipids* or pure phosphatidylethanolamine (but not phosphatidylcholine or phosphatidylserine) were found to stimulate O_2^- production by detergent-solubilized NADPH oxidase, and a phospholipid requirement for oxidase activity was therefore proposed (255). Phospholipids have been detected in a partially purified NADPH oxidase from pig neutrophils (84).

The involvement of *calmodulin* in the activation of the oxidase is based on the inhibitory effect of calmodulin inhibitors on the respiratory burst of intact neutrophils (225,721,810), on NADPH oxidase activity of subcellular particles (721), and on a solubilized NADPH oxidase preparation (68,82). The specificity of the inhibitors, however, is not absolute. For example, trifluoperazine inhibits both calmodulin-dependent protein kinase and protein kinase C.

Activation in vitro. Arachidonic acid, as well as other fatty acids stimulate the respiratory burst of intact leukocytes (49,52,165,186,336,377,378). This effect of fatty acids on intact cells led to the important finding that NADPH oxidase can be activated in cell-free preparations by arachidonic acid (116,184,337,491), as well as other unsaturated fatty acids (116), and by anionic detergents such as sodium dodecyl sulfate and sodium dodecyl sulfonate (117). Activation was not associated with enzymatic oxidation of the fatty acid (116). It was proposed that the sodium salts of long-chain unsaturated fatty acids activate the oxidase by functioning as anionic detergents (117). The stimulatory effect of arachidonic acid is prevented by delipidated albumin, as arachidonic acid binds to albumin to form an inactive complex (52,186).

NADPH oxidase preparations activated *in vitro* could be separated by centrifugation into a particulate (membrane) fraction and a soluble (cytosolic) fraction, both of which were required for optimum activity. Stimulation of intact leukocytes with PMA or fMLP decreased the requirement for the cytosolic factor (117,491). The oxidase activity of the cell-free preparation did not require Ca^{2+} (184,337) but was dependent on Mg^{2+} for optimum activity (337). The cytosolic factor is heat-sensitive (117,184). *In vitro* activated cell-free preparations from patients with b-cytochrome-deficient CGD lacked

NADPH oxidase activity (184,337). The defect appeared to reside in the particulate fraction, as arachidonic acid + CGD particulate fraction + normal soluble fraction lacked NADPH oxidase activity, whereas arachidonic acid + normal particulate fraction + CGD soluble fraction was active (184).

The activation of the NADPH oxidase of a neutrophil membrane fraction by PMA, phospholipid (phosphatidylserine, phosphatidylinositol), adenosine triphosphate (ATP), Ca^{2+}, and a cytosolic factor has been reported (171). Purified protein kinase C could substitute for the cytosolic fraction, which together with the other requirements for activation suggested that the cytosolic factor was protein kinase C. This mechanism of activation appears to differ from that of fatty acid-induced activation, suggesting that several mechanisms of activation exist in the intact cell that are dependent in part on the nature of the stimulus.

NADH Oxidase

Although the current emphasis is on the primary role of an NADPH oxidase in the respiratory burst, there may be a contribution by an NADH oxidase in some species. A soluble NADH oxidase from guinea pig neutrophils has been well characterized (47). It contains flavin, generates both O_2^- and H_2O_2, has a Km for NADH of 400 μM, and is present in amounts sufficient to account for the oxygen consumed during the respiratory burst (47). The other electron donors tested including NADPH were ≤15% as effective as NADH. An NADH diaphorase was purified from a human neutrophil membrane fraction but was not believed to be a component of the respiratory burst oxidase (280). An NADH–cytochrome C reductase has been detected in the plasma membrane fraction of human neutrophils (478). Activation of neutrophils resulted in a twofold increase in this enzyme activity in contrast to a 30-fold increase in NADPH oxidase activity. An NADH–cytochrome b_5 reductase is present in the light membrane fraction of human neutrophils (51,726). However, it was not detected in the membrane of the phagocytic vacuole (726), and it reacts poorly with oxygen (51). It is thus unlikely to be a component of the respiratory burst oxidase.

Other Enzyme Systems

A contribution by xanthine oxidase to the killing mechanisms of neutrophils and macrophages was proposed (750,751) based on the increased level of xanthine oxidase in the leukocytes of infected mice and on the inhibitory effect of allopurinol or adenine and the stimulatory effect of xanthine on the microbicidal activity of mouse neutrophils. Further confirmatory studies are needed in this and other species.

An unusual aldehyde oxidase has been detected in the phagosome membrane of guinea pig granulocytes that oxidizes a number of aldehydes with the formation of O_2^- and H_2O_2 (50). The aldehydes may be formed in the phagosome by the MPO-catalyzed oxidative deamination of amino acids. This enzyme is not the primary source of toxic oxygen metabolites, as it is inhibited by cyanide whereas the respiratory burst is not; and it requires a source of aldehydes whose generation by the MPO/H_2O_2/C1 system presupposes a preexisting respiratory burst; it may, however, be an ancillary source of oxidants.

Superoxide Anion

The initial product of the respiratory burst formed when oxygen accepts a single electron is O_2^- (43,68).

$$O_2 + e \rightarrow O_2^-$$

Reports of the redox potential of the O_2/O_2^- couple have ranged from +0.5 to −590 mV; a value of −330 mV has been proposed by several investigators (350,808). O_2^- is in equilibrium with its protonated form, the perhydroxyl radical (HO$_2^-$) with the pKa of the dissociation

$$HO_2^- \rightleftharpoons O_2^- + H^+$$

being 4.88 (78,90). Thus the radical exists almost entirely as O_2^- at neutral or alkaline pH. O_2^- is predominantly a reductant, as for example in the reduction of ferricytochrome C, where it loses an electron and is converted back to oxygen. It can also act as an oxidant, however, as for example in the oxidation of epinephrine, where it gains an electron and is converted to H_2O_2. When two molecules interact, one is oxidized and the other reduced in a dismutation reaction with the formation of oxygen and H_2O_2.

$$O_2^- + O_2^- + 2H^+ \rightarrow O_2 + H_2O_2$$

This reaction can occur spontaneously or be catalyzed by the enzyme superoxide dismutase (SOD). Three distinct SODs exist that vary in their metal component (copper–zinc SOD, manganese SOD, iron SOD) and in their distribution in cells (250).

Spontaneous dismutation occurs optimally at pH 4.8, where O_2^- and HO$_2^-$ are present in equal concentrations. At this pH the rate constant for spontaneous dismutation [$8.5 \times 10^7 M^{-1}s^{-1}$ (78)] approaches that of SOD-catalyzed dismutation [$1.9 \times 19^9 M^{-1}s^{-1}$ (602)]. The rate constant for spontaneous dismutation decreases when the pH is lowered and HO$_2^-$ predominates, and it is particularly low at alkaline pH where O_2^- predominates (78,90). Indeed it is probable that spontaneous dismutation does not occur when O_2^- is the sole species. The rate constant for SOD-catalyzed dismutation is little affected by pH over the range 5.0 to 10.0 (602) and is thus a particularly effective catalyst at neutral or alkaline pH where spontaneous dismutation is low. Although SOD is present in neutrophils (609), its release into the phagosome has not been demonstrated. SOD, however, can be introduced there as a component of the ingested organism. Most studies of the pH within the phagosome have indicated it to be acidic (424,619; however, see 659), i.e., in the region where spontaneous dismutation is rapid.

The direct toxicity of O_2^- has been the subject of some controversy (231,250). O_2^- reacts rather sluggishly with many biologically important compounds, e.g., amino acids (92) and carboxylic acids (91), leading to the suggestion by some (231,647) that O_2^- does not have the necessary reactivity to be directly toxic to cells. A few words of caution are in order, however. The chemical reactivity of O_2^- is considerably increased in a nonpolar environment as may exist in the hydrophobic region of a membrane (610,647) where its reactions are not in competition with the proton-requiring dismutation reaction. Under these conditions O_2^- is a powerful base with considerable nucleophilicity and reducing activity. Furthermore, the protonated form, HO_2, is a considerably stronger oxidant than is O_2^- (93,263), raising the possibility that a local decrease in pH as might occur within a phagosome or at a membrane surface may cause a shift in the $HO_2 \rightleftharpoons O_2^-$ equilibrium toward the more reactive protonated form with local damage to the target cell membrane. Furthermore, the low steady-state concentration of O_2^- would limit its dissipation by spontaneous dismutation (250), and this situation together with its relatively low reactivity may allow it to diffuse over significant distances where it can be toxic through a local decrease in pH or the formation of more reactive oxidants. In this regard, O_2^- can penetrate some cell membranes, including those of granulocytes (266), by passage through anion channels (475,476, 620,772). O_2^- permeated liposome membranes made from dipalmitoylphosphatidylcholine at temperatures above that of the lipid-phase transition (41°C) (636). However, it passed slowly if at all through phospholipid bilayers and chloroplast thyakoids under other conditions (720).

A direct toxic effect of O_2^- is suggested when the toxicity of an O_2^--generating system is inhibited by SOD but not by catalase or by OH· scavengers. O_2^--generating systems are toxic to a variety of cells and compounds, and the inhibitory effect of SOD has implicated O_2^- either as a direct toxin or in the generation of a more distal oxidant (306). In some studies SOD was the only inhibitor tested. In other instances toxicity also was inhibited by catalase and OH· scavengers, implicating OH·. In yet other studies catalase or OH· scavengers were inhibitory, but not both. However, in some cases only SOD was inhibitory [e.g., bleaching of bilirubin and biliverdin (612), oxidation of

tocopherols (549), O_2^--dependent glycolate formation by transketolase (719)], thereby implicating a direct effect of O_2^-. *Streptococcus sanguis* contains an NADH reductase that forms O_2^- and H_2O_2 on the addition of quinones such as plumbagin (216). The addition of plumbagin to the organisms increases oxygen consumption and induces damage that is inhibited by high concentrations of intracellular SOD but not by DMSO, an OH· scavenger that can permeate freely into the organisms. It was concluded that in *S. sanguis* O_2^- can be toxic independent of OH· (216).

Hydrogen Peroxide

H_2O_2 is formed in large amounts by stimulated phagocytes (352). Its formation is predominantly by dismutation of O_2^-, which occurs rapidly and efficiently (768). However, under some conditions H_2O_2 may be formed in part directly from oxygen by divalent reduction without an O_2^- intermediate (185,281).

H_2O_2 is a well known germicidal agent, and its involvement in the microbicidal activity of phagocytes was therefore proposed (352). A number of points should be made regarding the toxicity of H_2O_2.

1. The reactivity of H_2O_2 is relatively low compared to some of the other toxic products of the respiratory burst (e.g., OH·, hypohalous acids). This low reactivity allows H_2O_2 to pass intact through cell membranes (251) and through complex biological fluids, rebounding intact from collisions to be toxic at a distance under conditions in which the more reactive oxygen products are readily scavenged. Thus when toxicity occurs at a distance through a fluid rich in proteins and other scavengers, H_2O_2 may be the chief (perhaps only) product of the respiratory burst that is toxic. However, when there is close apposition between effector and target cell, diffusion distances are short, and proteins and other scavengers may be excluded, thereby favoring the activity of the more reactive products of the respiratory burst.

2. In complex biological fluids, the toxicity of H_2O_2 can be reduced not only by degradation by catalase but also by peroxidase and a halide, presumably due to the utilization of H_2O_2 for the formation of more powerful oxidants, which are scavenged by the components of the reaction mixture prior to their reaching the target cells. Thus neutrophil and eosinophil granule pellets that contained peroxidase inhibited killing of the newborn larvae of *Trichinella spiralis* by an H_2O_2-generating enzyme system in a complex serum-containing tissue culture fluid, an effect that was reversed by the heme enzyme inhibitors azide and cyanide, and by preheating the granule pellets (73). Similarly, lactoperoxidase and iodide inhibited the toxicity of PMA-stimulated peritoneal macrophages to

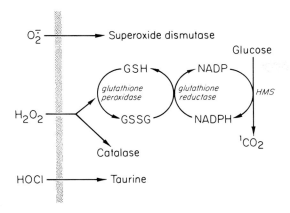

FIG. 3. Scavengers of reactive oxygen species.

tumor cells in tissue culture medium containing serum (536). Although extracellular protein strongly inhibits the toxicity of the peroxidase/H_2O_2/halide system when the peroxidase is in the fluid phase, protein is much less inhibitory when the peroxidase is bound to the surface of the target cell (373,531; see also following).

3. Organisms vary widely in their susceptibility to H_2O_2, and in general this correlates with the level of H_2O_2-scavenging enzymes in the target cell. These enzymes include catalase, which breaks down H_2O_2 to oxygen and water, and the glutathione cycle (Fig. 3). The glutathione cycle is a sequence of reactions by which the degradation of H_2O_2 is coupled to the increased activity of the hexose monophosphate shunt (HMS). The first two enzymes of the HMS, glucose-6-phosphate dehydrogenase and 6-phosphogluconate dehydrogenase, reduce $NADP^+$ to NADPH, and the continued activity of the shunt depends on the reoxidation of NADPH. The latter can be accomplished by the glutathione cycle, which is initiated by the oxidation of reduced glutathione (GSH) by H_2O_2 catalyzed by glutathione peroxidase. The oxidized glutathione (GSSG) formed is reduced by NADPH in the presence of glutathione reductase with the formation of $NADP^+$. The HMS is thus a sink for excess H_2O_2 with the increased oxidation of glucose carbon-1 to CO_2 as evidence of its use.

H_2O_2 released by phagocytes is toxic nonenzymatically to a number of targets *in vitro*. Thus H_2O_2 has been implicated as the toxic species responsible for the killing of the newborn larvae of *Trichinella spiralis* by human neutrophils and eosinophils in the presence of immune serum (72,73). Similarly activated macrophages, when appropriately stimulated (as by PMA), are toxic to tumor cells in a complex tissue culture medium through the formation of H_2O_2 (535,536). Furthermore, H_2O_2 has been implicated in the autotoxicity of stimulated neutrophils (56,741), although in this (744) and other systems H_2O_2

may not act alone but in conjunction with some other component of the reaction mixture or cell. Neutrophils are protected from the toxic effects of exogenous or endogenous H_2O_2 by their content of catalase (618,760) and the components of the glutathione cycle (617,698).

The toxicity of H_2O_2 can be increased considerably by a number of mechanisms, including reactions with ascorbic acid and a trace metal such as Cu^{2+} or Co^{2+} (197,221,229,386,417; see also below) and a synergism between H_2O_2 and proteinases. A neutral serine proteinase is present in the plasma membrane fraction of human neutrophils that is released into the medium on stimulation of the cells with low concentrations of PMA or by treatment of neutrophil membranes with 1 M NaCl (596). The neutral serine proteinase was lytic to erythrocytes only after pretreatment of the target cells with nonlytic concentrations of H_2O_2. Serine proteinase inhibitors decreased erythrocyte lysis by stimulated neutrophils. These findings suggest that sublytic concentrations of H_2O_2 and a neutrophil plasma membrane neutral serine proteinase may act synergistically to lyse the target cell. H_2O_2 also reacts synergistically with a neutral proteinase released from activated macrophages to lyse tumor cells (2). Two other mechanisms by which the toxicity of H_2O_2 can be increased many orders of magnitude—reaction with peroxidase and a halide and reaction with ferrous iron—are considered in detail below.

Peroxidase/H_2O_2/Halide System

A number of distinct peroxidases exist in mammalian tissues that differ in primary structure and in their heme prosthetic group but which have in common the ability to increase the rate of H_2O_2-dependent reactions many orders of magnitude. Peroxidases alone have not been shown to exert an antimicrobial effect, although the strongly basic nature of some peroxidases, e.g., eosinophil peroxidase (EPO) and to a lesser degree MPO, suggests that, like other basic proteins, they may be antimicrobial at high concentrations. However, peroxidase can exert an antimicrobial effect indirectly by catalyzing the conversion of a substance with little or no antimicrobial activity to one that is strongly toxic. The peroxidase/H_2O_2/halide system appears to be operative in phagocytes and is considered in detail here.

Myeloperoxidase

A peroxidase first appears in the developing human granulocyte in the promyelocyte stage, where it is synthesized and packaged into the azurophil (primary) granules (59) (see Chapter 17). This process ceases at the end of the promyelocyte stage, and the peroxidase-positive azurophil granules are distributed to daughter cells and intermingled with the newly formed peroxidase-negative specific (secondary) granules during the myelocyte stage of granulocyte development. Mature neutrophils contain their total complement of MPO in azurophil granules. In human cells these granules are morphologically heterogeneous, varying in shape from spherical to ellipsoid (59), and they can be separated into two peroxidase-positive populations on the basis of density (403,699,781). Following phagocytosis degranulation occurs, with the release of MPO into the phagosome; leakage or secretion of MPO to the outside of the cell can occur either during phagocytosis or after exposure of neutrophils to an antibody-coated surface or a soluble stimulus. In addition, MPO can be released by cell lysis.

MPO is present in human neutrophils in exceptionally high concentrations, with estimates varying from 1 to 2% of the dry weight of the cell (4) to more than 5% (614,650); it is an intense green, and the green color of pus is due to its presence. MPO is a complex protein with a molecular weight that ranges among estimates from 120 to 160 kD (424,649). Its subunit structure has been studied extensively (23,27,62,315,316,485,541). Current evidence suggests that the native enzyme consists of two heavy (α) (55–60 kD) and two light (β) (10.5–15.0 kD) subunits (27,316,566) with both heme and carbohydrate bound to the heavy subunit (36,316,566; see 566 for the association of heme also with the light subunit). It was initially proposed that the subunits were associated in a linear $\alpha\beta\beta\alpha$ structure, with the predominant cross-linking between the two light subunits (316). However, it was subsequently suggested that MPO consisted of two heavy–light protomers linked by a single disulfide bond between the two heavy subunits along their long axis (27). Reduction and alkylation separated the two protomers into hemi-MPO consisting of a heavy and a light subunit, which retained enzymatic and bactericidal activity (27,29). A green heme protein, isolated from bovine spleen, has the same spectroscopic properties as MPO and similar but not identical substrate specificities (38,196). It is a monomer of 57 kD and may be the heavy α subunit of MPO. It has been reported that the two heavy subunits of MPO differ in their chymotryptic digest maps, and that one but not the other has a reducible intrapeptide disulfide bond (540).

MPO has been resolved by ion-exchange chromatography into three distinct forms in the same individual that vary in solubility, enzymatic activity, sensitivity to inhibition by aminotriazole, subunit structure, distribution in azurophil granule subpopulations, and release on neutrophil stimulation (580,581,582), suggesting that heterogeneity of MPO in normal neutrophils may exist. MPO from a patient with chronic myelogenous leukemia was abnormal in that one of the 55-kD α subunits was replaced by a 39-kD peptide, a mixture of smaller peptides, and a heme-containing component (36).

The human promyelocyte cell line HL-60 has been employed to study the biosynthesis of MPO. A small (79 kD) and a large (153 kD) form of MPO was detected in a ratio of 4:1, with 40% in the cytosol and the remainder in the granules (816). The small and large enzymes contained the same two subunits of 59 and 14 kD (817). When HL-60 cells were induced to differentiate to more mature granulocytes by DMSO or retinoic acid, the MPO content of the cells decreased (814,816) owing to decreased synthesis associated with the absence of MPO mRNA (814). Pulse-chase labeling studies of the posttranslational processing of MPO in HL-60 cells have revealed intermediates of approximately 91, 81, and 74 kD (14,319,438,568,813). Human MPO has been cloned using an HL-60 expression cDNA library (364).

MPO contains two iron-containing prosthetic groups per molecule (9) that are covalently linked to the heavy subunits (5,316,544), possibly by an amide bond (812). Magnetic circular dichroism (226) and resonance Raman spectroscopy (38,678) suggested that the prosthetic groups are iron chlorins. There has been some controversy as to whether the two iron centers are identical in structure and function, with some studies indicating equivalence (38,347,678) and others inequivalence (9,315,553). It has been proposed that at low concentrations H_2O_2 reacts with only one of the two iron atoms, whereas at high concentrations H_2O_2 binds to both and is degraded catalatically to O_2 and H_2O with associated inactivation of the enzyme (11). The latter reaction would serve to modulate the activity of the peroxidase system by both the degradation of H_2O_2 and the inactivation of MPO.

H_2O_2

The respiratory burst of phagocytes serves as the primary source of H_2O_2 for MPO-catalyzed reactions. In addition, certain ingested microorganisms can generate H_2O_2 and thus contribute to their own destruction by the peroxidase system. Lactic acid bacteria (e.g., pneumococci, streptococci, lactobacilli) lack heme and as a result do not utilize the cytochrome system (which reduces oxygen to water) for terminal oxidations. Rather, flavoproteins are employed that reduce oxygen to H_2O_2, which in the absence of the heme protein catalase is released into the medium (790). H_2O_2 also is produced by certain mycoplasmal strains (163,168,695,696) and by *Candida albicans* (195).

MPO forms three distinct complexes on reaction with H_2O_2 or certain other oxidants: compounds I, II, and III. H_2O_2 at relatively low (equimolar) concentrations reacts with the iron of MPO to form compound I (554). Compound I also appears to be formed on reaction of MPO with hypochlorous acid (HOCl) (313). It is the primary catalytic peroxide compound of MPO, is highly unstable, and is at an oxidized level two equivalents above that of ferric MPO. Its structure is unknown. Compound II is formed on the addition of an excess of H_2O_2 and is at an oxidized level one equivalent above that of the ferric enzyme (554). It is an inactive form of MPO in respect to the oxidation of chloride (313). Compound III is an oxyperoxidase that, like oxyhemoglobin or oxymyoglobin, has oxygen attached to the heme iron (804,821). It is at the three-equivalent oxidized level above ferric MPO and is formed by reaction of compound II with H_2O_2 (554), by the aerobic oxidation of NADH (554), by the reaction of ferrous MPO with oxygen (554), or by the reaction of ferric MPO with O_2^- (554,555,803).

Although the primary substrate for peroxidase is H_2O_2, peroxidases also can react with molecular oxygen (oxidatic reaction) and with O_2^-. The number of substances that can be oxidized by peroxidase and oxygen in the absence of H_2O_2 are limited. They include NADH and NADPH (13), a reaction that is strongly stimulated by Mn^{2+}, and by certain phenolic compounds such as the thyroid hormones (410) and estrogens (410,791). H_2O_2 is formed in the reaction and utilized either for the oxidation of the reduced pyridine nucleotides or for coupled oxidations of other substances (411). O_2^- is formed when peroxidase acts as an oxidase (822,825) and may serve as an intermediate in H_2O_2 formation or react directly with peroxidase to form compound III (554,555).

Compound III is unstable, decaying to ferric peroxidase with a half-decay time of several minutes at room temperature (588,804). It can react with a number of electron donors (722,804,825,826) and with certain electron acceptors (826), raising the possibility that MPO compound III formed by reaction with O_2^- may be a catalytic form of MPO in neutrophils. In this regard, spectral changes suggestive of MPO compound III formation have been detected in intact stimulated neutrophils or on incubation of purified MPO with either PMA-stimulated neutrophils or the xanthine oxidase system in the presence of chloride (803).

Halides

Iodide, bromide, chloride (412,413), or the pseudohalide thiocyanate (427,433) can serve as the halide component of the MPO-mediated antimicrobial system. Of the halides, iodide is the most effective on a molar basis (413). The concentration of inorganic iodide in serum, however, is low (<1 μg/dl), and its contribution to the peroxidase system may therefore be small. Iodide also can be provided by deiodination of the thyroid hormones (412). Bromide is intermediate in effectiveness between iodide and chloride (413), although its concentration in biological fluids is considerably higher than that of iodide (343), raising the possibility that bromide may serve as a

physiological halide. Thiocyanate is oxidized by intact neutrophils to the antimicrobial agent hypothiocyanite when the concentration of thiocyanate is high relative to that of chloride, as occurs in saliva; but under conditions similar to those in plasma where the thiocyanate concentration is low relative to chloride, chloride is preferentially oxidized (734). The concentration of chloride in biological fluids is considerably greater than that required for the isolated MPO-mediated antimicrobial system, suggesting that it is the primary halide utilized by the MPO system *in situ*.

The halides at high concentration can inhibit the MPO-mediated antimicrobial system. Thus bromide was consistently less effective as the halide component of the MPO system at high than at low concentration (413), and an inhibitory effect of thiocyanate on the MPO/H_2O_2/halide system has been described (412,413,424,734,785). Two distinct binding sites for chloride on MPO have been proposed: (a) the substrate binding site is unaffected by pH and leads to the production of HOCl; and (b) the inhibitor binding site requires prior protonation (acidic pH) and leads to the competitive inhibition of H_2O_2 binding to MPO (28,63,313,837). The substrate binding site for chloride appears to be at or close to the heme (chlorin) iron of MPO (347,349,703,782).

Toxic Products Formed

The halides are oxidized by compound I and possibly also by compound III (803) to form toxic agents that vary with the halide, its concentration, the pH, and other factors; the products include hypohalous acids, halogens, long-lived oxidants such as chloramines or aldehydes, and possibly hydroxyl radicals and singlet oxygen.

Hypohalous acids

Chloride is oxidized to HOCl by MPO and H_2O_2 (10,12,314). Because HOCl has a pKa of 7.53, it exists as a mixture of the undissociated acid and the hypochlorite ion at physiological pH levels. When the pH is lowered, as may occur within the phagosome, HOCl predominates. Hypobromous acid (HOBr) and hypothiocyanous acid (HOSCN) and the corresponding hypohalite ions appear to be the primary products formed by the peroxidase-catalyzed oxidation of bromide and thiocyanate; and although hypoiodous acid (HOI) may be formed by iodide oxidation by peroxidases, it is not clear whether it or iodine is the predominant species formed.

The formation of HOCl by stimulated neutrophils has been demonstrated by its reaction with taurine or other nitrogenous compounds to form stable chloramines (736,777) or by the chlorination of 1,3,5-trimethoxybenzene (247). Using these techniques, a high proportion of the oxygen consumed by stimulated neutrophils could be accounted for by the formation of HOCl. Thus Thomas et al. (736) reported a chloramine yield of 31 to 55% of the oxygen consumed using PMA-stimulated neutrophils and 72% with zymosan-stimulated neutrophils; and Foote et al. (247) could account for at least 28% of the oxygen consumed by neutrophils stimulated with polystyrene beads coated with PMA by the formation of a chlorinating species, presumably HOCl. The latter workers considered this value to be minimum, which did not take into account the competing effects of protein and other scavengers. Weiss et al. (777) concluded that approximately 40% of the H_2O_2 detected was utilized to generate HOCl under their conditions.

Halogens

The halogens chlorine (Cl_2), bromine (Br_2), iodine (I_2), and the pseudohalogen thiocyanogen [$(SCN)_2$] may be formed by halide oxidation, although the predominant species (at least with chloride, bromide, and thiocyanate) appears to be the hypohalous acid. Iodine is a major product of iodide oxidation by peroxidase and H_2O_2. The MPO/H_2O_2/iodide antimicrobial system is effective at an iodide concentration that is considerably lower than that of the reagent iodine needed to produce a comparable antimicrobial effect (412). However, this discrepancy has been explained by the catalytic activity of iodide in which iodide is oxidized by peroxidase and H_2O_2 to iodine, and the iodine is then reduced by reaction with a surface sulfhydryl or other oxidizable group and reutilized by the peroxidase system (731,732) (Fig. 4). Reactions of this sort with other halogens may amplify their contribution to the antimicrobial effect.

Chloramines

HOCl formed by neutrophils can react with nitrogen-containing compounds to form nitrogen–chlorine derivatives with retention of oxidizing activity (Fig. 5) (288,642,727,728,778). Some of these compounds are relatively long-lived, thereby providing a mechanism for prolongation of the oxidant activity of the peroxidase system. The toxicity of the chloramine can occur in a number of ways.

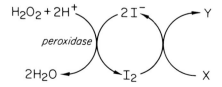

FIG. 4. Amplification of cytotoxicity by the redox activity of iodide.

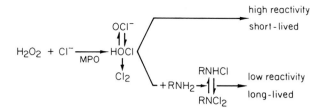

FIG. 5. Products of chloride oxidation by MPO and H_2O_2.

1. The nitrogen–chlorine derivative may be directly toxic. Taurine, which is present in neutrophils in high concentration (697), forms a relatively stable chloramine, and it was proposed that taurine chloramine formed by the MPO/H_2O_2/chloride system may serve a microbicidal function (836). Taurine, however, inhibits the bactericidal activity of the MPO/H_2O_2/chloride system (712,730), suggesting that the formation of taurine chloramine is competitive with, rather than required for, microbicidal activity. *N*-Chlorotaurine, however, can oxidize sulfhydryl or sulfur–ether groups (728) and thus may have sufficient oxidant activity to inactivate soluble mediators dependent on an intact sulfur–ether group such as α_1-proteinase inhibitor or chemotactic peptides (778) but have insufficient activity to induce a microbicidal effect (577). This finding has been attributed to the hydrophilic nature of the organic chloramines. In contrast, reaction of HOCl with ammonium ions forms a lipophilic oxidizing agent monochloramine (NH_2Cl) with considerably increased toxic activity (287,288,730). The relative toxicity of the oxidants varies with the target. Thus in one study (288) NH_2Cl was 50 times as effective as HOCl, taurine chloramine, or H_2O_2 in the oxidation of hemoglobin, whereas HOCl was three times as effective as NH_2Cl, and taurine chloramine and H_2O_2 were ineffective in the lysis of erythrocytes. It has been concluded that taurine and other organic amines protect certain targets including neutrophils by scavenging HOCl in a form that is relatively nontoxic (Fig. 3). The taurine chloramine can pass through the anion channels of the erythrocyte membrane and be reduced intracellularly to taurine, which is trapped, thereby preventing its accumulation in the extracellular fluid (737).

2. Chloramines are generally unstable, hydrolyzing to continuously release their "available chlorine" in an activated form such as HOCl (716) or NH_2Cl (288).

3. Degradation of unstable chloramines may result in the formation of a nonchloride-containing derivative with toxic properties. The formation of toxic aldehydes by the deamination and decarboxylation of amino acids by MPO, H_2O_2, and chloride (835,836) was proposed to be a microbicidal mechanism (712). Although certain aldehydes are toxic to microorganisms in high concentrations, the involvement of free aldehydes in the toxicity of the

peroxidase system *in situ* remains to be established. Chlorination of glycine or glycylpeptides can yield hydrogen cyanide (HCN), which can be chlorinated to cyanogen chloride (ClCN) (702,704,834). It is not known if these agents are produced in sufficient quantities to contribute to the toxic effect.

4. The long lived *N*-chloramines can react with iodide to form a highly toxic species, which may be free iodine or some other oxidized product (577).

5. The organic monochloramine (RNHCl) can undergo dismutation to form the more powerful dichloramine (RNCl$_2$) (737).

6. The amine chlorinated by the MPO/H$_2$O$_2$/chloride system can be covalently bound to protein (735). However, this reaction is slow, is quantitatively minor, and requires a high pH, suggesting that it does not contribute significantly to the antimicrobial activity of the MPO system. Glucosamine is incorporated into protein by stimulated neutrophils by an MPO-dependent process (74); and although the mechanism of incorporation was not established, a chlorinated intermediate may be involved. 3-Amino-1-methyl-5*H*-pyrido[4,3-*b*] indole also is incorporated into protein by the MPO system (815).

Hydroxyl radicals

It has been proposed that OH· may be generated by the MPO/H$_2$O$_2$/Cl$^-$ system (66) as follows

$$H_2O_2 + Cl \underset{MPO}{\rightarrow} HOCl + OH^-$$

$$HOCl + O_2^- \rightarrow Cl^- + O_2 + OH\cdot$$

HOCl can react with O$_2^-$ at an appreciable rate, which varies with the pH; and both OH· and singlet oxygen (^{1}O$_2$) have been proposed as products (472). In contrast, MPO has been reported to be an effective inhibitor of the formation of OH· by the iron-catalyzed Haber-Weiss reaction through reaction with H$_2$O$_2$ (799).

Singlet oxygen

The formation of ^{1}O$_2$ by the MPO system is considered elsewhere (see Peroxide/H$_2$O$_2$/Halide System, below).

Nature of the Destructive Lesion

The products of halide oxidation are powerful oxidants that can attack the target at a variety of chemical sites. The nature of the lesion in the cell that causes death is not known. Perhaps no single lesion will be found. The attack on the microorganism is rapid. In one study (15) HOCl prevented replication of *Escherichia coli,* as measured by colony formation, in milliseconds. The highly reactive nature of the oxidants formed suggests that the attack is at, or close to, the surface of the organism, i.e., at the cell membrane. An early effect of the MPO system and its product HOCl on microorganisms is the loss of membrane transport function with associated leakage of small molecules (17,424,685), an effect that correlated closely to the loss of viability as measured by replication (17,685). The loss of transport function is not due to membrane lysis, as some membrane functions, e.g., transmembrane proton conductance and glycerol permeability, are unaffected by HOCl (17); it may be due to a direct oxidative attack on transport proteins or to the dissipation of adenylate energy reserves (71).

There are two main modes of attack by the peroxidase system: (a) halogenation in which the halide is covalently bound to cellular constituents; and (b) oxidation in which exposed groups are oxidized.

Halogenation

MPO and H$_2$O$_2$ oxidize the halide to a form that binds in covalent linkage to components on the ingested organism. With iodide as the halide, iodination is indicated by the conversion of radioiodide to a trichloroacetic acid (TCA)-precipitable form and by the radioautographic localization of the fixed iodide on the organism (412). Tyrosine residues of protein are readily iodinated to form mono- and diiodotyrosine, and the exposed tyrosine residues of the organism appear to be the primary site of iodination by the peroxidase system (733). In addition, unsaturated fatty acids (752), sulfhydryl groups (733), and a number of other compounds may be iodinated. Bromination of cell surface constituents also occurs. Chlorination of microorganisms by purified MPO, H$_2$O$_2$, and chloride and by granulocytes that have ingested bacteria is indicated by ^{36}Cl incorporation (833). This fact, together with the formation of chlorinated derivatives on the addition of taurine or 1,3,5-trimethoxybenzene to stimulated neutrophils (247,736,777) or monocytes (488), suggests that chlorination of components of the ingested organism occurs. The chlorinated derivatives include monochloramines and dichloramines (see above) and preferentially involve the *N*-terminal amino group of peptides or proteins (704). The glycine residues of bacterial peptidoglycan (702) and reduced pyridine nucleotides (670) also are chlorinated. Chlorinated NAD(P)H is no longer catalytically active. The chlorination of tryptophan residues of protein by the MPO system results in chemiluminescence (838). The substitution of a bulky halide atom for a hydrogen atom at a crucial location on the cell surface or the subsequent degradative changes initiated by the halogenation reaction may contribute to the toxicity.

Oxidation

It is probable that toxicity results primarily from the oxidation of essential cell constituents. HOCl and the other products of halide oxidation are powerful oxidants capable of the oxidation of a number of biologically important substances (16,798) through reaction with a variety of chemical groups, some of which are considered below.

Sulfhydryl groups. A number of enzymes and other biologically important compounds require a free sulfhydryl group for optimum activity, and the oxidation of essential sulfhydryl groups by the peroxidase system may contribute to its toxicity. The sulfhydryl groups of *E. coli* are readily oxidized by peroxidase, H_2O_2, and iodide as well as by one of the products of that system, I_2 (733), and by MPO, H_2O_2, and chloride and its major product HOCl (730). Only a portion of the oxidizing equivalents consumed could be accounted for by sulfhydryl oxidation, although there was a close correlation between the oxidation of bacterial sulfhydryl groups and cell death.

The MPO/H_2O_2/halide system oxidizes GSH to GSSG with the effectiveness of the halides, being of the order I > Br > Cl (753). GSH is also oxidized by stimulated neutrophils through formation of a product of the MPO system (642). It is not known, however, if GSH is oxidized within intact organisms, and if it is, if it contributes to cell death or serves a protective function.

Iron–sulfur centers. The iron–sulfur centers of ferredoxin are rapidly oxidized by the MPO/H_2O_2/chloride system and by its product HOCl (16,629), raising the possibility that proteins with iron–sulfur centers, which are important constituents of the electron transport system of the microbial cytoplasmic membrane, may be a site of attack by the peroxidase system. This idea is supported by the finding that the microbicidal effect of the MPO/H_2O_2/halide system on *E. coli* is associated with the loss of iron into the medium as measured by the release of ^{59}Fe from prelabeled organisms (628). Iron loss, which reached levels in excess of 70% of the total microbial iron, was observed with chloride or bromide but not with iodide as the halide. That a portion of the iron loss was due to the oxidation of *E. coli* iron–sulfur centers by the peroxidase system was suggested by the loss of labile sulfide content (629). In contrast to iron loss, the effectiveness of the halides, on a molar basis, in inducing labile sulfide oxidation was in the order I > Br > Cl. Thus iodide-derived oxidants appeared to oxidize microbial iron–sulfur centers without the release of iron into the medium.

Heme proteins. Porphyrins, hemes, and heme proteins are rapidly oxidized by HOCl and by the peroxidase/H_2O_2/halide system (16,628,798). The oxidation of cytochrome C by the MPO/H_2O_2/halide system was associated with the release of the heme iron; and as with iron

release from the intact organism, chloride or bromide but not iodide could meet the halide requirement (628). MPO, which is a heme protein, is inactivated by H_2O_2 and a halide (525).

Sulfur–ether groups. The MPO/H_2O_2/Cl⁻ system oxidizes the sulfur–ether group of free (743) and peptide-bound methionine and of the sulfidopeptide leukotrienes (see sections under Targets of the MPO System, below) to the corresponding sulfoxide, and thus the oxidation of sulfur–ether groups in the target organism may contribute to cell death.

Oxidative decarboxylation, deamination, and peptide cleavage of proteins. The oxidative decarboxylation and deamination of free and peptide-linked amino acids (3,669,712,835,836) occurs with associated peptide cleavage (669). The amino acids of particulate proteins are decarboxylated in the phagosome by the peroxidase system, whereas free soluble amino acids pass into the cytoplasm where they are decarboxylated predominantly after transamination by the normal, nonperoxidase, cellular amino acid oxidative pathway (3). It is not clear whether peptide cleavage is a direct consequence of the action of the peroxidase system in intact cells or decarboxylation of amino acids or peptides follows cleavage of the protein by proteases released into the phagosome.

Lipid peroxidation. Lipid peroxidation, i.e., the oxidation of polyunsaturated fatty acids, has been implicated in membrane damage. It can be initiated by a variety of oxygen species and is maintained in a chain reaction (propagation) by radical species formed. Lipid peroxidation occurs in phagocytes following particle ingestion (677,711), and its relation to the respiratory burst is indicated by its absence in CGD leukocytes (677,711) unless an H_2O_2-generating organism is ingested (677). The peroxidase/H_2O_2/halide system can initiate lipid peroxidation (380), raising the possibility that this effect may contribute to its toxicity.

Evidence for Involvement in Intact Leukocytes

There are a number of lines of evidence that support involvement of the MPO system in the toxic activity of neutrophils.

1. The components of the MPO system are present in neutrophils, and their formation or release occurs at a time appropriate to the microbicidal act.

2. Cytochemical studies have demonstrated the presence of both MPO (415) and H_2O_2 (113,114) in the phagosome following particle ingestion, and their interaction there with a halide is indicated by the iodination reaction that occurs when neutrophils ingest microorganisms (412). Iodination of the microorganisms by the cell-free MPO/H_2O_2/iodide system is evident autoradio-

graphically (412). In intact leukocytes the fixed iodide can be localized in part in the phagosome by autoradiographic techniques (415) and the analysis of isolated phagosomes (622). Extracellular proteins also are iodinated when intact neutrophils ingest bacteria (425,556); and although autoradiographic studies indicate the presence of silver grains on the organism surface in the phagosome (415), other neutrophil constituents also are iodinated (415,662).

Other evidence for the interaction of MPO, H_2O_2, and a halide either in the phagosome or in the extracellular medium include the decarboxylation of amino acids by intact neutrophils (712), a reaction that requires MPO, H_2O_2, and chloride (835), and the formation of HOCl, the product of chloride oxidation by MPO and H_2O_2, by intact neutrophils (247,736,777).

3. Patients with CGD have severe and repeated infections owing to the inability of their neutrophils to kill certain ingested organisms (601). This microbicidal defect is associated with, and presumably a result of, the absence of a respiratory burst (342), thereby emphasizing the role of the products of the respiratory burst in the killing of some organisms. The importance of H_2O_2 deficiency in the microbicidal defect has been emphasized by its partial reversal by the introduction of H_2O_2 into the cell (366,621). Glucose oxidase, an enzyme that forms H_2O_2 without an apparent O_2^- intermediate, can be employed for this purpose, emphasizing that H_2O_2 is effective even when O_2^- remains deficient in these cells. Some organisms (i.e., lactic acid bacteria such as the streptococci and pneumococci) generate H_2O_2 and are killed well by CGD leukocytes (385,432,481) unless mutant strains are employed, which are relatively deficient in H_2O_2 production (595,677). Thus the susceptibility of H_2O_2-generating organisms to the intracellular microbicidal systems appears to be due to replacement of a defective leukocytic H_2O_2-generating system with H_2O_2 of microbial origin.

4. The neutrophils of patients with hereditary MPO deficiency have a microbicidal defect, although it is not as severe as that seen in patients with CGD. Hereditary MPO deficiency is a genetic disorder in which MPO is absent from neutrophils and monocytes. It was first described in 1963 in healthy siblings (285); however, interest in this condition intensified with the finding of the microbicidal activity of MPO when combined with H_2O_2 and a halide (412,413) and the description of a patient with MPO deficiency and systemic candidiasis in whom a neutrophil microbicidal defect was demonstrated (458). Although initially the few sporadic cases of MPO deficiency described suggested a rare condition, the introduction of an automated flow cytochemical system for routine leukocyte differential counts that utilized cellular peroxidase activity indicated a more frequent occurrence of this condition (174,576), with an incidence of complete deficiency of 1 in 4,000 in one study (576). Individuals

with this condition generally do not have an increased incidence of infection, although some have had major systemic infections, particularly with *Candida albicans* (133,458,576). Partial deficiency of MPO also has been described. Partially MPO-deficient neutrophils contain MPO that is electrophoretically and immunologically normal but present in decreased amounts, whereas completely MPO-deficient neutrophils lack any evidence of MPO protein (541).

The isolated leukocytes of patients with MPO deficiency have decreased microbicidal activity (133,174,408, 416,458,461,576,705), suggesting a requirement for MPO for optimum killing. This defect is particularly apparent with *C. albicans* as the test organism (458,459). The bactericidal defect is characterized by a lag period following which the organisms are killed (461); it is not as severe as in the leukocytes of patients with CGD, and in some patients it has been reported to be mild (576). These findings, although implicating MPO in the microbicidal activity of phagocytes, also indicate the presence of MPO-independent antimicrobial systems in these cells that are adequate to maintain most patients in good health.

Does the microbicidal activity of MPO-deficient neutrophils accurately reflect the relative role of MPO-dependent and MPO-independent antimicrobial systems in normal cells? A number of lines of evidence suggests that it does not.

1. Agents such as azide or cyanide that inhibit peroxidase-catalyzed reactions decrease the bactericidal activity of normal leukocytes to a level below that of similarly treated MPO-deficient leukocytes (416,705), suggesting that the MPO-independent antimicrobial systems are more highly developed in MPO-deficient than normal cells.

2. The respiratory burst, as measured by oxygen consumption, O_2^- production, H_2O_2 production, or hexose monophosphate shunt activity, is considerably greater in MPO-deficient than in normal neutrophils (133,173, 200,408,425,428,541,623,705,707). Those measures of the respiratory burst dependent in part or totally on MPO (e.g., iodination, chemiluminescence), as would be anticipated, are decreased in MPO-deficient neutrophils (200,408,423,623,705,707) unless peroxidase is added (423,471). The increased respiratory burst of MPO-deficient neutrophils is due to at least two mechanisms. First, MPO appears to be required for termination of the respiratory burst through inactivation of the NADPH oxidase (355), and thus its absence would lead to increased oxygen consumption and production of toxic oxygen metabolites. Second, because H_2O_2 is degraded in part by the MPO system, the absence of MPO would be expected to lead to a buildup of H_2O_2 with associated increased production of oxidants (e.g., OH·) dependent on H_2O_2

for their formation. It would be particularly evident in the phagosome or extracellular fluid, as cytosolic H_2O_2-degrading systems, e.g., catalase, glutathione cycle, appear to be normal in MPO deficiency (542).

3. Phagocytosis by MPO-deficient neutrophils of IgG- or C3b-coated yeast particles is enhanced (707) owing to the inhibitory effect of MPO and H_2O_2 on the Fc (707) and C3b (301,707) receptors on the cell surface.

Despite the increased phagocytosis and respiratory burst of MPO-deficient neutrophils, which would favor microbial killing, a microbicidal defect is present. This finding raises the possibility that the toxicity induced by the MPO system in normal neutrophils is replaced in the absence of MPO in part by another toxic mechanism dependent on the products of the heightened respiratory burst.

Studies of the degradation of leukotriene C_4 (LTC_4) (see below) by normal and MPO-deficient neutrophils suggests that an adaptation of this sort occurs (328). LTC_4 was degraded by the MPO/H_2O_2/chloride system, and, as anticipated, this degradation was inhibited by catalase and by the heme protein inhibitor azide at low concentrations (10^{-5} M) but was unaffected by SOD or by the $OH\cdot$ scavengers mannitol or ethanol. LTC_4 also was degraded by the xanthine oxidase system; however, the inhibitor profile was different. Both catalase and SOD were strongly inhibitory, as were mannitol and ethanol. Azide was inhibitory at relatively high concentrations (10^{-3} M) but not at the low concentrations inhibitory to the peroxidase system. This inhibitor profile is that expected for a reaction dependent on $OH\cdot$ generated by the Haber-Weiss reaction (see following). Thus LTC_4 is degraded by the MPO system and by $OH\cdot$.

Intact normal neutrophils stimulated by the Ca^{2+} ionophore A23187 degrade LTC_4, and the inhibitor profile suggested involvement of the MPO system; degradation was inhibited by catalase and azide at concentrations down to 10^{-5} M but was unaffected by SOD, mannitol, or ethanol. MPO-deficient neutrophils stimulated with A23187 were also found to completely degrade LTC_4; however, in this instance degradation was inhibited by catalase, SOD, the $OH\cdot$ scavengers mannitol and ethanol, and azide only at high concentration (10^{-3} M). Thus MPO-deficient neutrophils, like the xanthine oxidase system, degrade LTC_4 by $OH\cdot$ generated by the Haber-Weiss reaction. These findings suggest that the predominant LTC_4-degrading system in normal neutrophils is the MPO/H_2O_2/halide system, but that when MPO is absent there is an increased respiratory burst resulting in the formation of $OH\cdot$ in amounts able to degrade LTC_4.

In summary, the general good health of most persons with MPO deficiency has raised the issue of the importance of MPO in the microbicidal activity of neutrophils (738). The studies described above suggest that neutrophils

which lack MPO adapt to its loss with an increase in respiratory burst activity and an associated increase in the toxicity of oxygen metabolites that do not require MPO for their formation.

Targets of the MPO System

The targets of the MPO system may be intracellular or extracellular. The primary function of neutrophils is the phagocytosis and destruction of microorganisms (424). Organisms ingested by neutrophils initiate a process by which H_2O_2 formed by the respiratory burst reacts in the phagosome with MPO released by degranulation, as well as chloride or possibly other halides, to form a potent oxidant or oxidants that can diffuse from their site of origin to attack the ingested organism (Fig. 6). The components of the MPO system also can be released to the outside of the cell, where they can attack extracellular targets (140) such as normal or malignant cells, connective tissue components, organisms such as fungal forms or helminths that are too large to be ingested, and a number of soluble mediators. Although generally inhibitory in its action, the peroxidase system under certain conditions can stimulate cells to secrete biological mediators or can activate certain enzymes.

The following lines of evidence have been employed in support of a role for the MPO system in the toxic effect of neutrophils on a particular target.

1. Toxicity is produced by a purified preparation of MPO when combined with H_2O_2 (or a H_2O_2-generating enzyme system) and a halide. This toxicity requires each component of the MPO system and is inhibited by peroxidase inhibitors such as azide and cyanide, and by catalase. Protein inhibits the peroxidase/H_2O_2/halide system by scavenging its toxic products; and when maintenance of target cell viability requires the presence of protein in the medium, the toxicity of the peroxidase system may not be demonstrable (373,531). Preincubation of the target cell with the peroxidase for a short period allows the dem-

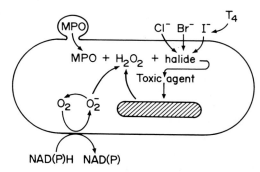

FIG. 6. Myeloperoxidase/H_2O_2/halide antimicrobial system in the phagosome.

onstration of toxicity of the peroxidase system, even in the presence of large amounts of protein. MPO and particularly EPO are strongly basic proteins that bind firmly to anionic surfaces, including those of target cells. Thus after preincubation the toxic products are directed to the target cell surface by the bound peroxidase (373,531) (see Eosinophil Peroxidase, below). The peroxidase system can be targeted to a particular cell type by conjugation of either the H_2O_2-generating enzyme glucose oxidase (436,589,590) or both glucose oxidase and peroxidase (584) to specific antibody.

2. Toxicity produced by intact phagocytes has the following properties.

a. Toxicity is dependent on stimulation of the phagocytes.

b. A halide is required for optimum activity. If possible an incubation medium is employed that lacks chloride, unless it is added as a component of the MPO system, in order to be able to detect a chloride requirement. When intact cells are employed, isotonic solutions in which chloride is replaced by sulfate or nitrate can generally be used, as incubations are usually short (<2 hr). If chloride is an absolute requirement for maintenance of the viability of the cells in the suspension medium, a halide requirement can be inferred from the inhibitory effect of agents, e.g., methionine and taurine, which react with HOCl, although the specificity of this reaction is not absolute. Furthermore, the addition of a second halide, i.e., iodide or bromide, may increase the toxicity of the peroxidase system. Iodination of the target is compatible with halide involvement, as it demonstrates an interaction between a product of halide oxidation by the MPO system and the target. However, it should be emphasized that iodination per se is not the mechanism of toxicity.

c. Toxicity is decreased by peroxidase inhibitors such as azide or cyanide and by catalase. When the target cell is sensitive to both H_2O_2 alone and the peroxidase/H_2O_2/halide system (at lower H_2O_2 concentrations), the addition of a heme–enzyme inhibitor such as azide may not inhibit toxicity and may even increase it. Azide, by inhibiting the degradation of H_2O_2 by the peroxidase (and catalase) of the phagocyte, causes buildup of H_2O_2 to relatively high levels, which can be toxic in the absence of peroxidase. Furthermore, inhibition of the catalase of the target cell by the heme–enzyme inhibitor may increase its sensitivity to H_2O_2 toxicity. This paradoxical effect of heme–enzyme inhibitors has been observed with the release of platelet constituents by neutrophils activated by phagocytosis (149) and the inactivation of granule enzymes by phagocytosing neutrophils (761). An additional problem with the use of inhibitors, particularly those of high molecular weight, is the possible exclusion of the inhibitor from the site of action of the peroxidase (or other) antimicrobial system.

d. Toxicity is decreased when CGD leukocytes are employed, and this decrease in toxicity is reversed by H_2O_2 or an H_2O_2-generating enzyme system. This finding indicates a requirement for H_2O_2 in the toxicity.

e. Toxicity is decreased when MPO-deficient leukocytes are employed, and this decrease in toxicity is reversed by the addition of MPO. As described above, MPO-deficient leukocytes may substitute an MPO-independent system for the normally operative MPO-dependent one, and it is sometimes possible through the use of inhibitors to determine the nature of the toxic system.

The MPO-mediated antimicrobial system has been implicated in the effects of neutrophils on a variety of targets (Table 1) through studies of this kind. The peroxidase system is generally inhibitory in its activity, although in some instances it is stimulatory.

Inhibitory activity

Microorganisms. The MPO/H_2O_2/halide system is toxic to bacteria (412,413,492) [including *Mycoplasma* (354), *Chlamydia* (827), *Mycobacterium leprae* (430), and *Legionella pneumophila* (470)], fungi (207,209–213, 344,416,456,460,464,811), viruses (79), protozoa such as *Trypanosoma dionisii* (739,740) and *Leishmania donovani* (135,579), and multicellular organisms such as the schistosomula of *Schistosoma mansoni* (372,389). In most instances the microorganisms are ingested, and toxicity occurs in the phagosome; however, the toxic effect of the MPO system may be extracellular. For example, neutrophils attach to and damage *Candida albicans* pseudohyphae (211) by oxidative mechanisms (209) and the toxicity of the cell-free MPO/H_2O_2/halide system, inhibitor studies with intact cells, and the decrease or absence of damage when CGD or MPO-deficient leukocytes are employed (209,213,764) suggest that *C. albicans* pseudohyphae are killed in part by the MPO system released by attached

TABLE 1. *Effects of the myeloperoxidase system*

In vitro inhibitory effects
  Microorganisms: bacteria, fungi, viruses, protozoa, helminths
  Mammalian cells: spermatozoa, blood cells (granulocytes, lymphocytes, erythrocytes, platelets), tumor cells
  Soluble agents: chemotactic factors (C5a, fMLP), α_1-proteinase inhibitor, bacterial toxins (diphtheria toxin, pneumolysin, clostridial toxins), neutrophil granule components (lysosomal enzymes, vitamin B_{12} binding protein), arachidonic acid metabolites (prostaglandins, leukotrienes), elastin, fluorescent probes
In vitro stimulatory effects
  Cell secretion (platelets, mast cells), enzyme activation (collagenase, gelatinase)
In vivo effects
  Pulmonary injury, renal injury, tumor cell destruction

neutrophils. MPO binds to the mannan of the *Candida* cell wall (811).

Bacterial toxins. The first demonstration of the inactivation of a biological product by MPO was that of Agner (6–8) who observed that diphtheria toxin was detoxified by MPO, H_2O_2, and a dialyzable cofactor found in casein hydrolysates, urine, and other materials. Although partially purified, the nature of the dialyzable cofactor was not established at that time. More recently detoxification of the cytotoxin of *Clostridium difficile* by MPO, H_2O_2, and a halide has been demonstrated (569). PMA-stimulated normal neutrophils also inactivated this toxin, and this inactivation was decreased by azide, cyanide, or catalase, by the removal of halides from the medium, or by replacement of the normal neutrophils with CGD or MPO-deficient leukocytes. Added H_2O_2 restored the activity of CGD leukocytes and MPO that of the MPO-deficient leukocytes. Similarly, pneumolysin, a thiol-activated, oxygen-labile hemolytic toxin from *Streptococcus pneumoniae,* is inactivated by the isolated MPO/H_2O_2/halide system and by stimulated neutrophils through the release of this system (141). The rapid inactivation of *C. difficile* cytotoxin and *C. perfringens* phospholipase C by whole human neutrophils and cell sonicates also has been demonstrated (450); however, no evidence for the involvement of the MPO/H_2O_2/halide system in the inactivation was found. Rather, inactivating activity was localized in the azurophil granules and was inhibited by protease inhibitors, implicating neutral proteases.

Tumor cells. Tumor cells are readily killed by the cell-free peroxidase/H_2O_2/halide system (152,224,589) and a combination of inhibitor studies with the use of neutrophils from patients with CGD or MPO deficiency suggest that the destruction of tumor cells by intact neutrophils stimulated by phagocytosis (143), concanavalin A (148), or PMA (150,192,370,686,773) occurs via the release of the components of the peroxidase system.

The antibody-dependent tumor cell cytotoxic activity of neutrophils does not appear to depend on MPO. Thus toxicity to a mouse lymphoma line was unaffected by azide or by the substitution of MPO-deficient leukocytes for normal ones, although toxicity was decreased when CGD leukocytes were employed, suggesting a requirement for the respiratory burst for optimum activity (145). Antibody-coated tumor cells were found to trigger a respiratory burst in neutrophils, and the associated toxicity to the tumor cells was inhibited by hypoxia or agents that block the respiratory burst; however, the peroxidase inhibitors azide and cyanide had no effect (300). In both of these studies cytotoxicity was unaffected by catalase and SOD.

Blood cells. 1. *Granulocytes:* The MPO/H_2O_2/halide system is toxic to neutrophils as well as to blood mononuclear cells (144), raising the possibility that this system may be autotoxic to stimulated phagocytes. Self-destruction of neutrophils during stimulation has been reported; and although H_2O_2 has been implicated (56,741,744), involvement of the peroxidase system has not been shown.

An inhibitory effect of the MPO system on phagocytosis by human neutrophils has been described (706). The addition of MPO to normal neutrophils inhibited the ingestion of immunoglobulin G (IgG)-coated, and to a lesser extent C3b-coated, yeast particles without affecting the oxidative response to PMA or the chemotactic response to fMLP. This effect of MPO was inhibited by azide, catalase, and methionine, implicating the reaction of endogenously formed H_2O_2 with the added MPO. Phagocytosis by adherent MPO-deficient neutrophils was greater than that by normal cells, and as with normal cells the addition of MPO to MPO-deficient neutrophils produced a catalase-sensitive inhibition of phagocytosis. Preincubation of the opsonized particles with the MPO/H_2O_2/halide system also inhibited their phagocytic uptake (159), suggesting that the MPO system can affect both the receptors on the cell and the ligands on the particle. The binding of FITC-labeled anti-IgG or anti-C3b to the yeast particles was decreased following exposure of the opsonized particles to the peroxidase system (159), suggesting either the loss of the ligand from the particle surface or its modification to a form unreactive with specific antibody. IgG exposed to MPO, H_2O_2, and catechol forms large amounts of heavy IgG aggregates that behave like immune complexes in that they consume complement, precipitate with monoclonal rheumatoid factor, and are detected by the Raji cell and solid-phase C1q assays (359). This finding indicates that IgG can be modified by MPO; however, the requirement for catechol for cross-linking raises the question of its physiological counterpart *in situ.*

Neutrophils stimulated by phagocytosis of opsonized zymosan or by PMA inactivate their own granule enzymes (lysozyme, β-glucuronidase) (761). Studies with the enzyme α-glucosidase suggested that enzyme inactivation occurred within the phagolysosome rather than in the extracellular fluid. Enzyme inactivation was not observed with CGD leukocytes or under anaerobic conditions, suggesting a requirement for products of the respiratory burst. The absence of granule enzyme inactivation by MPO-deficient leukocytes pointed to the MPO/H_2O_2 system; however, the addition of glucose oxidase as a source of H_2O_2 to CGD neutrophils did not induce inactivation nor did the addition of catalase either alone or in combination with SOD inhibit inactivation by normal neutrophils. Furthermore, enzyme inactivation was increased by the heme protein inhibitor azide. The lack of inhibition by catalase could be due to the inability of the added enzyme to penetrate the phagolysosome. The possibility was raised that inactivation of granule enzymes by normal neutrophils was due to MPO and H_2O_2, whereas when

MPO was inhibited by azide the H_2O_2 concentration was increased to a level where it induced inactivation in the absence of peroxidase.

The inactivation of lysosomal enzymes by neutrophils during phagocytosis was confirmed and evidence presented that this inactivation was due to the $MPO/H_2O_2/$ halide system (437). In this study lysosomal enzyme inactivation did not occur when CGD neutrophils were employed, thereby implicating the respiratory burst. Furthermore, secreted components from PMA-stimulated normal, but not CGD, neutrophils were found to inactivate lysosomal enzymes released from stimulated CGD neutrophils. Catalase, azide, and histidine inhibited lysosomal enzyme inactivation, whereas SOD and mannitol did not. PMA-stimulated neutrophils could be replaced by MPO plus the glucose/glucose oxidase system or by HOCl, thereby implicating the $MPO/H_2O_2/$halide system.

Another granule component inactivated by substances released from stimulated neutrophils is the vitamin B_{12} binding protein (142). This inactivation, which occurred extracellularly, was inhibited by the heme–enzyme inhibitors azide and cyanide, by catalase, or by use of a halide-free medium; and the intact cell system could be replaced by purified MPO, H_2O_2, and a halide, thereby implicating the MPO system.

2. *Lymphocytes:* Natural killer (NK) cell activity, lymphocyte proliferation in response to mitogens, and generation of immunoglobulin-secreting cells were suppressed on exposure of human mononuclear leukocytes to the $MPO/H_2O_2/$halide system (227,228). When the H_2O_2 flux was increased or the number of mononuclear leukocytes decreased, lymphocyte suppression could be mediated by H_2O_2 alone. The various lymphocyte functions tested were affected to a different degree by the MPO system, and removal of the monocytes from the mononuclear cell preparation increased the susceptibility of the lymphocytes to oxidant injury. The toxic nature of the MPO system raises the possibility that the effect on function is secondary to a loss of viability of lymphocytes. Normal trypan blue exclusion, fluorescein diacetate uptake, and target cell binding frequency by the treated mononuclear leukocytes, as well as the reversibility of the lesion, argue against loss of viability as the mechanism for loss of function and thus point to an immunoregulatory role for the MPO system.

3. *Erythrocytes:* Erythrocytes can be lysed by exposure to the $MPO/H_2O_2/$halide system (422) and by reactive oxygen species formed by stimulated neutrophils (101,193,284,388,680,771). The nature of the oxygen species responsible for erythrocyte lysis by intact neutrophils has varied in these studies (140). In general the $MPO/H_2O_2/$halide system was not implicated, although in one study (193) inhibition of the lysis of chicken erythrocytes by azide, catalase, and the substitution of CGD for normal

neutrophils suggested that the MPO system may be involved.

Oxidant injury to erythrocytes that does not progress to lysis also can be induced by stimulated neutrophils. Thus the GSH level of glucose-6-phosphate dehydrogenase-deficient (but not normal) erythrocytes was depressed by phagocytosing neutrophils with associated rapid removal of the cells from the circulation; H_2O_2 was implicated as the toxic species (55). When erythrocytes are exposed to stimulated neutrophils, some hydrophilic products of the peroxidase system, e.g., taurine chloramine, can enter the cell through anion channels and be trapped intracellularly as taurine following reduction by GSH (737), whereas lipophilic oxidants, e.g., NH_2Cl, penetrate the lipid bilayer and produce oxidant damage (288).

4. *Platelets:* The granule marker serotonin and the cytoplasmic marker adenine were released by platelets exposed either to the cell-free $MPO/H_2O_2/$halide system (146) or to intact neutrophils stimulated by phagocytosis (149). The considerably greater serotonin than adenine release by the cell-free system suggested in part a nonlytic secretory process (see below), whereas serotonin and adenine were released by platelets exposed to intact neutrophils in equivalent amounts, suggesting a lytic event (149). In the intact cell system release was prevented by omission of halides, the addition of catalase, the use of MPO-deficient neutrophils unless MPO was added, or the use of CGD neutrophils unless H_2O_2 was added. These data strongly suggest involvement of the peroxidase system. Paradoxically, the heme protein inhibitors azide and cyanide did not inhibit release but, rather, increased it. This effect of heme protein inhibitors also was observed with MPO-deficient neutrophils (but not with CGD neutrophils) or when the neutrophils were replaced by reagent H_2O_2 or a H_2O_2-generating enzyme system. It was concluded that neutrophils activated by phagocytosis induce release of platelet constituents by a lytic process through the action of the peroxidase system. However, when MPO and platelet catalase is inhibited by heme–enzyme inhibitors, H_2O_2 can accumulate to levels that are lytic in the absence of peroxidase.

Spermatozoa. A number of peroxidases, including MPO, when combined with H_2O_2 and a halide (or the pseudohalide thiocyanate) are toxic to spermatozoa (431,688). H_2O_2 is formed by spermatozoa in the presence of phenylalanine or certain other amino acids, and the H_2O_2 so formed is autoinhibitory in the presence of the other components of the peroxidase system (431).

Liposomes. Exposure of liposomes made up of phosphatidylcholine with or without dicetyl phosphate and cholesterol and containing ^{51}Cr as the aqueous space marker to the $MPO/H_2O_2/$halide system resulted in rapid lysis with release of ^{51}Cr (671). Lysis also was observed when the liposomes were exposed to PMA-stimulated neutrophils; the demonstration of a halide requirement and inhibition by azide, cyanide, and catalase suggested involvement of the MPO system (672). It was supported by the absence of lysis when MPO-deficient or CGD leukocytes were employed unless MPO or H_2O_2, respectively, was added. Introduction of tocopherol or β-carotene into the liposome or the use of dipalmitoyl phosphatidylcholine (which contains no double bonds) as the structural lipid led to resistance to lysis induced by the MPO/H_2O_2/chloride system; this protection was decreased or lost when iodide was added. Tocopherol and dipalmitoyl phosphatidylcholine also prevented liposome lysis by PMA-stimulated neutrophils.

Chemotactic factors. The chemotactic factors C5a Des Arg and fMLP were inactivated by the MPO/H_2O_2/halide system (147) with the halides being effective in the order Br > I > Cl. Inactivation was inhibited by both catalase and azide, and correlated with a decrease in binding of the peptide to the leukocyte receptor (153). The biochemical basis for the inactivation of fMLP by the peroxidase system was oxidation of the methionine residue (153). Thus synthetic peptides containing methionine were inactivated, whereas those that lacked methionine were not. Inactivation was inhibited by reducing agents (2-mercaptoethanol, ascorbic acid) and by methionine but not methionine sulfoxide, and the product formed migrated on thin-layer chromatography as did the peptide with chemically oxidized methionine. Free methionine is oxidized by the MPO/H_2O_2/halide system (742).

Intact neutrophils when exposed to a particulate or soluble stimulus also inactivated fMLP (151,449,745), and the MPO/H_2O_2/halide system was implicated by the inhibitory effect of peroxidase inhibitors and catalase and by the absence of inactivation when either CGD or MPO-deficient neutrophils were employed unless H_2O_2 was added to the former or MPO to the latter. As with the cell-free MPO/H_2O_2/halide system, inactivation of fMLP by intact leukocytes resulted in oxidation of the methionine residue and was associated with decreased binding to surface receptors. Among the stimuli that induced neutrophils to inactivate fMLP by the release of the peroxidase system was the chemotactic factor itself (139,707). C5a also was inactivated by the peroxidase system released from stimulated neutrophils (151).

The functional activity of the sulfoxide and sulfone derivatives of fMLP have been investigated (318). Both derivatives were ineffective as chemotactic factors for neutrophils over a 10^{-9} to 10^{-3} M concentration range, whereas monocytes did respond, although a 10- to 100-fold higher concentration of the oxidized peptide was required for chemotaxis equivalent to that produced by the parent compound. The oxidized derivatives also increased superoxide production by neutrophils and monocytes and

bound to these cells; however, again concentrations 10 to 100 times those that were optimal for the parent peptide were required.

Although oxidant damage to chemoattractants by stimulated neutrophils has been clearly demonstrated under some experimental conditions, other mechanisms of chemotactic factor degradation by phagocytes also exist. Thus hydrolysis of chemotactic peptides by neutrophils can occur either by stimulation of proteinase secretion at relatively high chemotactic peptide concentration (35,260) or at the cell surface by a mechanism independent of degranulation (830). The latter occurred at low (0.01–1.00 μM) concentrations of the chemoattractant. Similarly, C5a can be inactivated by neutrophil granule components, presumably by proteolysis (118,757,809).

α_1-Proteinase inhibitor. α_1-Proteinase inhibitor (α_1-antitrypsin) inhibits a number of serine proteinases of biological importance and indeed is the major serine proteinase inhibitor of plasma. It has a molecular weight of approximately 52,000 and is present at a concentration of about 130 mg/dl of plasma. Its importance is emphasized by the increased incidence of emphysema in persons genetically deficient in this inhibitor (505). This finding raises the possibility that in those persons with normal production of α_1-proteinase inhibitor its increased inactivation may contribute to uncontrolled destruction of lung elastin and other proteins by tissue proteinases. The reactive site of α_1-proteinase inhibitor contains a methionine residue (360,361) whose oxidation by N-chlorosuccinimide (which oxidizes methionyl residues to the corresponding sulfoxide) inhibits antiproteinase activity (361).

The MPO/H_2O_2/halide system converts the methionine residue of α_1-proteinase inhibitor to the sulfoxide with a loss of biological activity (129,154,484,486). Intact neutrophils when appropriately stimulated also inactivate α_1-proteinase inhibitor, and this inactivation is inhibited by the peroxidase inhibitors azide and cyanide, by catalase, and by halide depletion (128,129,154); it is not observed when CGD neutrophils are employed (129,154) unless H_2O_2 is added (154) or when MPO-deficient neutrophils are used unless MPO is added (154), thereby implicating the peroxidase system. Both HOCl and long-lived N-chloramines can be utilized by stimulated neutrophils to inactivate α_1-proteinase inhibitor with HOCl being the predominant oxidant over short distances and N-chloramines being effective even when the neutrophils were separated from the α_1-proteinase inhibitor by a dialyzing membrane (570). Among the proteinases inhibited by α_1-proteinase inhibitor is human neutrophil elastase (570,831), and the inactivation of α_1-proteinase inhibitor by the MPO system is associated with its inability to form stable complexes with this elastase (154,361,831). Although recombinant α_1-proteinase inhibitor containing methionine at the active site (position 358) was more sensitive to inactivation by N-chlorosuccinimide, the MPO/H_2O_2/halide system, activated neutrophils, and gas-phase cigarette smoke than was a mutant in which the methionine was replaced by valine, prolonged exposure to the oxidants produced partial inactivation of the mutant inhibitor (357). Thus oxidation of sites other than methionine-358 in the inhibitor may contribute to the inactivation.

Oxidant inactivation of α_1-proteinase inhibitor can be prevented by antioxidants such as ascorbate, cysteine, and dapsone (729) by certain antiarthritic drugs (483) and by methionine or methionine-containing proteins that compete with the methionine residues of α_1-proteinase inhibitor for the oxidant formed by phagocytes (65). An enzyme, methionine sulfoxide-peptide reductase, which can reduce methionine sulfoxide residues in proteins, restores the biological activity of oxidatively inactivated α_1-proteinase inhibitor (1). This enzyme has been detected in human lung homogenates, human neutrophils, and rabbit alveolar type II cells (131).

Although the MPO system appears to be the predominant source of oxidants for the inactivation of α_1-proteinase inhibitor by neutrophils, other oxidants, specifically OH·, also have been implicated (128,129). Inactivation of α_1-proteinase inhibitor by nonoxidative mechanisms, i.e., proteolysis, also may occur, and this mechanism appears to be the major one for its inactivation by rabbit alveolar macrophages (65), which lacks a granule peroxidase. Some proteolysis of the α_1-proteinase inhibitor by stimulated neutrophils has been observed (570).

A number of studies have suggested that oxidative inactivation of α_1-proteinase inhibitor also occurs *in vivo*. Thus α_1-proteinase inhibitor isolated from the synovial fluid of patients with rheumatoid arthritis contained oxidized methionine residues and was unable to form complexes with elastase (806). Functionally inactive α_1-proteinase inhibitor also has been detected in the bronchoalveolar lavage fluid of patients with respiratory distress syndrome (119,160,161,453,495) and of smokers (130), as well as in certain animal models (356,832).

Elastin. The lysine side chains of elastin are oxidized by the cell-free MPO/H_2O_2/halide system and by neutrophils stimulated by PMA (155). Oxidation by the intact cell system was inhibited by azide, cyanide, and catalase and was not observed when MPO-deficient neutrophils were employed unless exogenous MPO was added, thereby implicating the MPO system.

Arachidonic acid metabolites. 1. *Prostaglandins:* Human neutrophils when stimulated by PMA or opsonized zymosan transform 6-keto-PGF$_\alpha$, PGE$_2$, and PGF$_{2\alpha}$ to unidentified products (574). This transformation was inhibited by catalase and azide but not by SOD, suggesting the involvement of the MPO/H_2O_2/halide system. This idea was supported by the transformation of the prostaglandins

to the same products by the cell-free MPO/H_2O_2/chloride system.

2. *Leukotrienes:* LTC$_4$, the slow-reacting substance of anaphylaxis (SRS-A), is a lipoxygenase product of arachidonic acid metabolism that contains glutathione bound covalently to C6 of the arachidonic acid backbone by a sulfur–ether bond. SRS-A, obtained from the peritoneal cavity of rats injected intraperitoneally with rabbit anti-rat IgE, was inactivated by horseradish peroxidase or mast cell peroxidase when combined with H_2O_2 (321). The SRS-A activity of LTC$_4$ and LTD$_4$ and the chemotactic activity of LTB$_4$ also was decreased by EPO, H_2O_2, and either iodide, bromide, or to a lesser degree chloride, and by HPO, H_2O_2, and chloride (332). H_2O_2 alone, at a higher concentration, inactivated LTC$_4$ and LTD$_4$ (but not LTB$_4$). Horse eosinophils, which generated large amounts of LTC$_4$ when stimulated by the Ca^{2+} ionophore A23187 (374), also released both H_2O_2 and EPO when stimulated in this way (332). Azide (which inhibits EPO) and catalase (which degrades H_2O_2) increased the amount of SRS activity detected following A23187 stimulation of intact eosinophils (332), suggesting that eosinophils may modulate the amount of LTC$_4$ at an inflammatory site by both its production and degradation. The two 6-*trans* stereoisomers of LTB$_4$ [5-(S),12-(S)-6-*trans* LTB$_4$ and 5-(S),12-(R)-6-*trans* LTB$_4$] were detected as products of the degradation of LTC$_4$ by PMA-stimulated human eosinophils and by the cell-free EPO/H_2O_2/iodide system (271); a detailed study of the products formed by the degradation of LTC$_4$, LTD$_4$, or LTE$_4$ by PMA-stimulated neutrophils, by the cell free MPO/H_2O_2/chloride system, and by HOCl indicated the formation of the corresponding S-diasterioisomeric sulfoxides in addition to the 5-(S),12(R)- and 5-(S),12(S)-6-*trans* isomers of LTB$_4$ (454,455). The inhibition of degradation by peroxidase inhibitors and by catalase suggested involvement of the peroxidase system in the degradation of LTC$_4$ by PMA-stimulated (454,455) or A23187-stimulated (333) neutrophils and by PMA-stimulated eosinophils (271).

Fluorescent probes. An early consequence of stimulation of neutrophils is a change in transmembrane potential, with membrane depolarization occurring within 6 sec of stimulation (666,788), followed by an apparent hyperpolarization (788). The initial depolarization was not observed when CGD leukocytes were employed (667,788) but was normal with stimulated MPO-deficient neutrophils (789). The subsequent apparent hyperpolarization, which was indicated by a decrease in the fluorescence of the lipophilic probe of membrane potential 3,3-dipropylthiodicarbocyanine, was diminished by anaerobiasis (788) and was not observed in MPO-deficient cells unless purified MPO was added (789). The decrease in fluorescence with normal neutrophils was inhibited by azide, cyanide, and catalase; and the addition of MPO, H_2O_2, and a halide to 3,3-dipropylthiodicarbocyanine in a cell-free system produced a rapid decrease in fluorescence. This finding suggested that the secondary decrease in fluorescence is not a consequence of membrane hyperpolarization but is due to the reaction of the probe with MPO and H_2O_2 released from the stimulated neutrophils.

Fluorescein is a pH-sensitive dye that has been employed to measure intralysosomal pH (559). A fall in pH results in a decrease in fluorescence. HOCl, either added as such or generated by the MPO/H_2O_2/chloride system, rapidly chlorinates fluorescein, and the chlorinated products have altered fluorescence properties (345). The fluorescence intensity of the dianionic form of the dye is decreased, and proton equilibrium constants are shifted to a more acidic pH. As a result, a greater fall in pH would be required before the fluorescence intensity of the dye decreases. The fluorescence changes associated with the uptake of fluorescein-labeled particles by neutrophils were consistent with chlorination of the indicator by the MPO/H_2O_2/chloride system. Thus the use of fluorescein as an indicator of intraphagosomal pH in peroxidase-containing phagocytes (659) should be interpreted with caution (345,619).

Stimulatory activity

The peroxidase system, although predominantly inhibitory in its action, can be stimulatory under some conditions. The latter occurs with intact cells as targets when the concentration of the components of the peroxidase system are relatively low, so that reaction with the cell surface is sufficient to trigger a secretory response without inducing irreversible membrane damage. In addition, certain enzymes are activated by exposure to the products of the MPO system.

Platelet secretion. The MPO/H_2O_2/halide system caused the release of the dense-granule marker serotonin from platelets to a significantly greater degree than the release of the cytoplasmic marker adenine, suggesting in part a nonlytic process analogous to the platelet release reaction (146). Serotonin release was rapid, reaching maximum levels at 2 to 5 min; it was blocked by agents that inhibit the peroxidase system (azide, cyanide, catalase) and by agents that affect platelet metabolism (dinitrophenol, deoxyglucose) or chelate Mg^{2+} (EDTA but not Mg-EGTA). The requirement for divalent cations and intact platelet metabolic activity supported an active nonlytic secretory process. The MPO system released from stimulated neutrophils also caused release of the platelet markers (149); however, in this instance equivalent amounts of serotonin and adenine were released, suggesting a lytic process (see Inhibitory Activity, Blood Cells, above).

Mast cell secretion. EPO or MPO at relatively low concentrations, when combined with H_2O_2 and a halide, induced mast cell secretion, as indicated by the release of the granule component histamine without the concomitant release of the cytoplasmic marker lactate dehydrogenase (LDH) (329) and by ultrastructural changes typical of those seen when mast cells are stimulated to secrete by classic secretagogues (138,329). Each component of the EPO/H_2O_2/iodide system was required, and histamine release was inhibited by the heme–enzyme inhibitors azide, cyanide, and aminotriazole. An increase in EPO to relatively high levels when combined with H_2O_2 and a halide was cytotoxic to mast cells, as indicated by the release of both histamine and LDH and by morphological evidence of cell damage (138,329). Intact neutrophils stimulated by the phagocytosis of zymosan also initiated mast cell degranulation through release of the components of the peroxidase system (158,706), an effect that was inhibited by the sulfones dapsone and sulfapyridine. In contrast, mast cell degranulation induced by PMA-stimulated neutrophils did not require the peroxidase system; histamine release was unaffected by azide and catalase and by the substitution of MPO-deficient neutrophils for normal neutrophils.

Enzyme activation. Neutrophils contain a collagenase that is stored in a latent, inactive form in the specific granules (477,508,746). It is a metalloenzyme that attacks interstitial collagens type I, II, and III. When neutrophils are stimulated, this enzyme is released and simultaneously activated. The activation of latent collagenase was unaffected by SOD but was inhibited by catalase, thereby implicating H_2O_2 (779). The absence of collagenase activation by CGD neutrophils unless H_2O_2 was added further supported H_2O_2 involvement. The activation of latent collagenase by neutrophils also was inhibited by the peroxidase inhibitor azide and by methionine, which can scavenge HOCl. The addition of HOCl activated the latent collagenase. These findings suggest that collagenase activation is a consequence of the formation of HOCl by the peroxidase system.

Gelatinase is a metalloenzyme different from collagenase that is stored in a latent form in a distinct secretory granule (204). This enzyme attacks denatured collagen (gelatin) and solubilizes type IV and V collagens. Like collagenase, this latent gelatinase is activated by stimulated neutrophils in part through the formation of chlorinated oxidants (586). However, activation also occurs in part by an oxygen-independent mechanism, as some activation was observed when CGD neutrophils were employed.

In vivo *effects of administered MPO*

Pulmonary injury. Instillation into rat lung of either a low dose of glucose oxidase as a source of H_2O_2, or peroxidase [lactoperoxidase (LPO), MPO] produced little lung injury; however, when both glucose oxidase and peroxidase were instilled, severe acute lung injury was observed that progressed to interstitial fibrosis (363). The pulmonary injury could be prevented by catalase but not by SOD. Similarly, the neutrophil-mediated pulmonary injury induced by immune complexes was inhibited by catalase but not by SOD, thereby implicating H_2O_2 (362). Intratracheal injection of MPO and H_2O_2 into hamsters produced a partial inactivation of α_1-proteinase inhibitor as measured by decreased binding to elastase (832), suggesting that, in addition to a direct toxic effect of the products of the MPO system, indirect toxicity may occur through the increase in proteinase activity resulting from inhibitor inactivation.

Renal injury. MPO is a highly cationic protein that when administered intravenously to mice binds on the basis of charge and size to anionic sites in the glomerular capillary wall and to mesangial cells (275). Similarly, MPO was detected throughout the glomerular basement membrane following infusion into the renal artery of rats, with concentration in the subepithelial space at the base of the epithelial cell foot processes (365a). MPO administered alone did not produce glomerular injury. However, when the MPO infusion was followed by H_2O_2 at a concentration that was not toxic alone, injury was evidenced by proteinuria and marked endothelial cell swelling and epithelial cell foot process effacement. When radioiodide was added to the last infusion, iodination of glomerular structures was observed, with concentration in the glomerular basement membrane and mesangial cells. Iodination is a consequence of the oxidation of iodide by peroxidase and H_2O_2 and thus indicates the interaction of these components in the glomerular capillary wall. Iodination of glomeruli occurs in the neutrophil-mediated concanavalin A/anticoncanavalin A model of glomerulonephritis, raising the possibility of the involvement of the MPO system.

Antitumor cell activity. Intraperitoneal or subcutaneous injection into mice of glucose oxidase covalently coupled to polystyrene microspheres suppressed the growth of some locally transplanted tumor cells and prolonged survival (530). This protective effect of glucose oxidase was prevented by the co-injection of catalase coupled to latex beads, thus implicating H_2O_2 as the protective agent. The H_2O_2 could theoretically limit tumor cell growth directly or via the formation of a more reactive oxidant such as a product of the MPO system or OH·. MPO injected daily into mammary tumor-bearing mice in conjunction with an antitumor agent thiotepa was shown to significantly decrease the rate of tumor growth (651).

Hydroxyl Radical

Haber-Weiss Reaction

Another mechanism by which the toxicity of H_2O_2 can be increased is by reaction with ferrous iron to form OH·. Fenton (232) described the strong oxidizing activity of a mixture of ferrous sulfate and H_2O_2, and it was subsequently proposed (299) that the powerful oxidant formed by Fenton's reagent was OH·.

$$H_2O_2 + Fe^{2+} \rightarrow Fe^{3+} + OH^- + OH\cdot$$

When the iron concentration is limiting, the reduction of the ferric iron formed by Fenton's reagent is needed for the complete conversion of H_2O_2 to OH·. It can be accomplished by O_2^-.

$$O_2^- + Fe^{3+} \rightarrow Fe^{2+} + O_2$$

with the overall reaction being the iron-catalyzed interaction of H_2O_2 and O_2^- (Haber-Weiss reaction).

$$H_2O_2 + O_2^- \rightarrow O_2 + OH^- + OH\cdot$$

A direct interaction between H_2O_2 and O_2^- (actually its protonated form HO_2^-) to form OH· was originally proposed (299). However, there is abundant evidence that O_2^- does not react directly with H_2O_2 at an appreciable rate compared to competing reactions such as the spontaneous dismutation of O_2^-. Thus a rate constant of 0.50 $M^{-1}s^{-1}$ for $HO_2^- + H_2O_2$ and 0.13 $M^{-1}s^{-1}$ for $O_2^- + H_2O_2$ has been reported (770), which can be compared to a rate constant of $8.5 \times 10^7 M^{-1}s^{-1}$ for spontaneous dismutation at pH 4.8 ($HO_2^- + O_2^-$) (78). Trace metal catalysis is now an accepted requirement for the generation of OH· by the Haber-Weiss reaction (187,295,302,303,489).

Although OH· is generally believed to be the product of the Haber-Weiss reaction, other radicals functionally similar to OH· have been suggested. They include the "crypto-OH radical" of unknown structure that mimics free OH· but is more discriminating in its reactions (828,829), the ferryl radical ($FeOH^{3+}$ or FeO^{2+}) (441,637,638), or the perferryl radical (FeO^+ or Fe^{3+} -O_2^-). The ferryl radical has an appreciably longer lifetime than OH· in aqueous solution when complexed with simple ligands such as hydroxide ions (637) and is more discriminating than OH· in its actions. Its reactivity is greater than that of the perferryl radical. When xanthine oxidase was used as the source of O_2^- and H_2O_2 and Fe^{2+}-ethylenediaminetetraacetic acid (EDTA) was the catalyst, the oxidant formed had the properties of OH·. However, in the absence of EDTA, Fe^{2+} catalyzed the formation of an oxidant that differed from free OH· (801). The iron bound with high affinity to the enzyme, and the possibility of a bound iron–oxygen species was considered.

O_2^- requirement

In the iron-catalyzed Haber-Weiss reaction, the Fe^{3+} formed by Fenton's reagent is reduced by O_2^-. However, under certain conditions, thiols such as GSH or cysteine (632,640,652), the reduced pyridine nucleotides NADH and NADPH (633), paraquat (715,796,800), and ascorbic acid (111,286,634,635,794,795,807) can replace O_2^- as the reductant required for the formation of OH·. Enzymatic reduction of Fe^{3+}-chelates also may occur (793). This pro-oxidant activity of the reducing agents may be offset by antioxidant activity due to the scavenging of O_2^- (304,548), OH· (286), or H_2O_2, particularly when the concentration of the reducing agent is high. Although reductants such as GSH or ascorbic acid are present in neutrophils, their release into the phagosome has not been demonstrated (802), suggesting that they function not as pro-oxidants in the phagosome but in a protective role as scavengers of reactive oxygen species in the cytoplasm (700,701). In this regard, stimulation of neutrophils with opsonized zymosan or PMA oxidized a portion (30–40%) of the cellular ascorbate to dehydroascorbate without affecting total (reduced + oxidized) ascorbate levels (802).

Metal requirement

Iron has been most often implicated as the trace metal catalyst of the Haber-Weiss reaction (302,489,627). However, other metals also may be involved. Co^{2+} reacts with H_2O_2 to form an oxidant that can hydroxylate aromatic compounds and degrade deoxyribose (503). These reactions are stimulated by EDTA and are inhibited by scavengers of OH·, particularly in the presence of EDTA, raising the possibility that the reactive species is OH· formed by a Fenton-type reaction

$$H_2O_2 + Co^{2+} \rightarrow Co^{3+} + OH^- + OH\cdot$$

The addition of an O_2^--generating system did not potentiate the reactivity of H_2O_2 and Co^{2+}, suggesting that cobalt does not catalyze the Haber-Weiss reaction. Cupric ions (Cu^{2+}) appear to catalyze the formation of OH· by a mechanism analogous to the Haber-Weiss reaction (294,635,643,676). Cu^{2+} is reduced by O_2^-

$$Cu^{2+} + O_2^- \rightarrow Cu^+ + O_2$$

and the Cu^+ formed reacts with H_2O_2 to generate OH·

$$Cu^+ + H_2O_2 \rightarrow Cu^{2+} + OH^- + OH\cdot$$

with the overall reaction being a copper-catalyzed Haber-Weiss reaction.

$$O_2^- + H_2O_2 \xrightarrow{Cu} O_2 + OH^- + OH\cdot$$

O_2^- can be replaced by ascorbate (635,644,676) or thiols (708). When the copper is bound to certain amino acids or proteins, the release of free OH· into solution is inhibited; however, site-specific damage to the protein, presumably by localized formation of OH·, occurs (294,643,676). The degradation of DNA and deoxyribose by a copper–phenanthroline complex required a reductant such as NADH, 2-mercaptoethanol, or O_2^- and was inhibited by catalase but not by OH· scavengers (293). SOD was inhibitory when O_2^- was used but not with the other reductants. It was proposed that Cu^{2+}-phenanthroline is reduced to Cu^+-phenanthroline by the reductant, and that Cu^+-phenanthroline reacts with H_2O_2 to form an oxidant that can attack DNA and deoxyribose. This oxidant did not appear to be free OH·, as OH· scavengers were not inhibitory; however, the formation of OH· in close association with the DNA was not excluded.

Chelator requirement

The catalytic effect of iron on the Haber-Weiss reaction is increased considerably under some experimental conditions by the chelator EDTA (120,295,302,303,489,627). Optimum catalysis occurred in the vicinity of iron and EDTA equivalence, with activity decreasing when either iron or EDTA was in great excess (295,627). The nature of the iron chelator complex appears to be critical for catalysis, as other chelators (e.g., diethylenetriaminepentaacetic acid (DTPA), bathophenanthrolinesulfonate, or desferrioxamine) decrease rather than increase the iron-catalyzed Haber-Weiss reaction (120,121,134,295,302,303,627). The inhibition by the latter chelators is generally believed to be due to the chelation of iron in a nonreactive form; however, inhibition by desferrioxamine may be due in part to the scavenging of O_2^- (684) and OH· (340).

Ferric iron is poorly soluble in aqueous solution at physiological pH levels, as hydrated iron complexes are formed that precipitate as polynuclear complexes (238,627). Chelation of iron by EDTA maintains iron in solution in a form that is catalytically active, i.e., can be oxidized and reduced (123,124,489) and thus can catalyze the Haber-Weiss reaction.

$$H_2O_2 + Fe^{2+}\text{–EDTA} \rightarrow Fe^{3+}\text{–EDTA} + OH^- + OH\cdot$$

$$O_2^- + Fe^{3+}\text{–EDTA} \rightarrow Fe^{2+}\text{–EDTA} + O_2$$

$$\overline{H_2O_2 + O_2^- \rightarrow O_2 + OH^- + OH}$$

In contrast, iron chelates of DTPA, bathophenanthroline, and desferrioxamine react much more slowly with O_2^- (124).

It has been proposed that the chemical basis for the reactivity of the Fe–EDTA chelate is the presence of an aquo coordination site that is catalytically active in contrast to other chelates, in which all coordination sites are bound (627). Iron has six coordination sites, and in aqueous solution water is bound to each to form the hexaaquo coordinate written for Fe^{3+} as $[Fe(H_2O)_6]^{3+}$. When iron is chelated, the chelator displaces water and is coordinately bound to the iron. A multidentate chelator such as DTPA or desferrioxamine may bind to all six coordination sites, completely displacing water; and because a free aquo site appears to be required for catalysis, the chelated iron is in a catalytically inactive form. Although EDTA also is multidentate, it is too small to completely encompass the iron atom. As a result, there is the retention of a catalytically active aquo coordination site possibly resulting from distortion of the usual symmetry of coordination with the formation of a seventh coordination site to which water can bind. This hypothesis has been tested (274) using 12 iron chelates; a direct correlation was found between the presence of at least one open coordination site (or one occupied by a readily dissociable ligand such as water) and the ability of the chelated iron to catalyze the formation of OH· by the Haber-Weiss reaction.

Is a chelator required for iron catalysis of the Haber-Weiss reaction *in vivo;* and, if so, what is its nature? The concentration of free iron in biological fluids is low, with the bulk of the iron bound to protein either for storage and transport in a releasable form or as a catalytic center in a more firmly bound form. The ability of a bound form of iron to catalyze the Haber-Weiss reaction in biological fluids would considerably increase the amount of iron available for this reaction.

Most interest has centered around the iron–lactoferrin chelate as the physiological catalyst of the Haber-Weiss reaction. Lactoferrin is present in the specific granules of neutrophils and is released into the phagosome following particle ingestion. It is an iron-binding protein that when fully saturated contains two Fe^{3+} atoms per molecule. Iron-saturated lactoferrin can act as a catalyst of the Haber-Weiss reaction (21), with formation of OH· by intact neutrophils, particulate neutrophil fractions, or the xanthine oxidase system being enhanced by this chelate. The enhanced production of OH· by iron-saturated lactoferrin was confirmed (67); however, lactoferrin saturated with an exact equivalence of iron had little or no stimulatory effect on OH· formation (64,797), and partially iron-saturated lactoferrin was inhibitory (64,297,797). Under physiological conditions, lactoferrin is largely unsaturated, containing 20% or less of its total iron capacity. Under these conditions chelation of iron in a nonreactive form decreases its availability as a catalyst of the Haber-Weiss reaction; whereas when lactoferrin is fully iron-saturated, excess iron bound to the protein at nonspecific sites (or released into the medium) may be catalytically active. This finding was supported by the fact that apolactoferrin protects rats from acute lung injury induced by systemic activation of complement with cobra venom factor, whereas infusion of iron-saturated lactoferrin had no effect, and ionic iron potentiated the tissue injury (767). Leukocytes with less than 8% of normal lactoferrin levels due to specific granule deficiency had more than 80% of normal OH· production when stimulated by opsonized zymosan (109).

Transferrin also catalyzed OH· formation when fully iron-loaded (69,489,506) but not when partially saturated with iron (64,479). When the iron concentration is low, phosphate ions can form a reactive chelate (238); and

OH· formation catalyzed by Fe^{2+} bound to α-picolinic acid [an intermediate in the metabolic degradation of tryptophan (70)], to the di- and triphosphate nucleotides of adenosine, cytidine, thymidine, and guanosine (240,241,839), and to DNA (239) has been reported. However, iron bound to pyrophosphate, DTPA, citrate, ATP, or ADP in phosphate or Tris buffer pH 7.3 was considerably less effective than Fe^{2+}–EDTA as the catalyst of the Haber-Weiss reaction (714). Iron compounds capable of catalyzing the formation of OH· have been detected in biological fluids in some studies (290,296,298) but not in others (795).

When the Fe^{2+} concentration is high, recycling of the iron by reducing the Fe^{3+} formed is not necessary. It has been proposed that hemoglobin (Hb)–Fe^{2+} can react with H_2O_2 to form OH·.

$$Hb\text{–}Fe^{2+} + H_2O_2 \rightarrow Hb\text{–}Fe^{3+} + OH^- + OH\cdot$$

(639), a reaction facilitated by the reduction of the methemoglobin formed by ascorbic acid (85). The H_2O_2 needed for this reaction can be generated by the interaction of ascorbic acid and oxyhemoglobin (85). Although this mechanism may serve to generate OH· in erythrocytes, it cannot do so in leukocytes. An additional source of free or chelated iron is the microorganism. Bacteria grown in a high-iron medium increased their iron content and were more susceptible to destruction by H_2O_2 (606). The inhibition of this H_2O_2-dependent toxicity by OH· scavengers suggested the involvement of OH· formed by the interaction of Fe^{2+} and H_2O_2. However, growth of organisms in a high-iron medium did not increase their susceptibility to killing by neutrophils (608). Iron is released from organisms killed by the MPO system (628) and could theoretically be utilized for destruction of adjacent viable organisms. However, a chelator (EDTA) was needed for passage of the iron of MPO-killed organisms into the medium.

When the pH is lowered, iron-catalysis of OH· formation occurs readily in the absence of a chelator as measured by the OH·-dependent conversion of iodide to organic form (iodination) (419). Iodination was optimal in acetate buffer pH 5.0 to 5.5 and was inhibited by phosphate, lactate, and citrate buffer at this pH, as well as by EDTA. When the pH was increased free iron-dependent OH· formation by the xanthine oxidase system fell sharply, whereas OH· formation in the presence of iron–EDTA increased, so that at pH 7.0 the iron–EDTA chelate was considerably more effective than free iron. Thus a low pH within the phagosome may make a chelator unnecessary or even inhibitory. An acidic pH optimum (4.8) for the Haber-Weiss reaction has been reported (60); however, in this study, in which phosphate was the buffer used, Fe–EDTA was considerably more effective than free iron at this pH. An acidic pH greatly increased the catalysis of OH· formation by a number of iron chelates (61).

Aerobic Oxidation of Fe^{2+}

Hydroxyl radicals can be generated by the aerobic oxidation of Fe^{2+} in the absence of an exogenous source of O_2^- and H_2O_2 (162,289,291,292,305,497,807). The following sequence of reactions was proposed.

$$Fe^{2+} + O_2 \rightarrow [Fe^{3+}-O_2^-] \rightarrow Fe^{3+} + O_2^-$$

$$2O_2^- + 2H^+ \rightarrow O_2 + H_2O_2$$

$$Fe^{2+} + H_2O_2 \rightarrow O_2 + OH^- + OH\cdot$$

This reaction has a requirement for phosphate (289,291,312,497), EDTA (292,312), or certain other iron chelators for optimum activity.

Formation by Leukocytes

The formation of O_2^- and H_2O_2 by stimulated phagocytes suggests that these cells can generate $OH\cdot$ by the Haber-Weiss reaction. Hydroxyl radical formation by phagocytes has been sought using a variety of techniques; and although the totality of the evidence strongly supports the formation of this (or a functionally similar) radical, its formation has not been unequivocably demonstrated.

Ethylene formation from thiol ethers

Ethylene is formed from methional by abstraction of an electron from the sulfur atom to form the radical cation, which is converted under nucleophilic attack by OH^- to form ethylene, methyldisulfide, and formic acid, with the ethylene readily detected by gas chromatography (823). 2-Keto-4-thiomethylbutyric acid (KMB) is similarly degraded, except that the final products are ethylene, methyldisulfide, and carbon dioxide (823). Hydroxyl radicals are powerful one-electron oxidants capable of forming ethylene from methional (75) or KMB (215), a fact that prompted the use of ethylene formation from these thiol ethers by stimulated phagocytes as a measure of $OH\cdot$ formation. Ethylene formation by stimulated neutrophils (222,429,605,724,775), eosinophils (429), and mononuclear phagocytes (222,774) was demonstrated; and the partial inhibition of this reaction by SOD, catalase, and $OH\cdot$ scavengers implicated $OH\cdot$ generated by the Haber-Weiss reaction.

A number of other oxidants can initiate the formation of ethylene from methional or KMB (107,429,600,645). Thus organic free radicals are effective with the relative reactivity being $\cdot OH > RO\cdot > ROO\cdot > RCO\text{-}O\cdot > R\cdot$ (600), and O_2^- reacts sluggishly with methional to form ethylene (107). Ethylene formation by neutrophils is dependent largely on MPO; it is inhibited by the peroxidase inhibitors azide and cyanide and is less than 10% of normal when neutrophils that lack MPO are employed (429).

The addition of MPO to MPO-deficient neutrophils increases ethylene formation from KMB to levels greater than those observed with normal neutrophils (429), which presumably reflects the greater respiratory burst of MPO-deficient neutrophils (see above). These studies suggest that ethylene formation by neutrophils is due predominantly to an MPO-dependent mechanism, and a cell-free MPO-dependent system has been described that can form ethylene from methional or KMB (429). This system required MPO, H_2O_2, EDTA, and either chloride or bromide for optimum activity and was inhibited by catalase, SOD, azide, cyanide, and the divalent cations Mn^{2+}, Zn^{2+}, Co^{2+}, and Cu^{2+} at concentrations higher than that of EDTA, as well as by methanol, ethanol, DABCO, and histidine. The nature of the oxidant(s) which initiates ethylene formation by the cell-free system or by an MPO-dependent reaction in intact neutrophils is unknown.

Methane or formaldehyde formation from DMSO

Hydroxyl radicals react readily with DMSO with the formation of methane, and this reaction was employed as a measure of $OH\cdot$ formation by stimulated neutrophils, monocytes, or alveolar macrophages (605). The inhibition of methane formation by SOD, catalase, and $OH\cdot$ scavengers suggested that it was due in part to $OH\cdot$ formation by the Haber-Weiss reaction. Formaldehyde also is formed by the interaction of DMSO and $OH\cdot$, and its formation is more sensitive than that of methane as a measure of $OH\cdot$ formation (435). It is not known if MPO is required for methane or formaldehyde formation from DMSO by neutrophils as it is for ethylene formation from thiolethers.

CO_2 release from benzoic acid

The release of $^{14}CO_2$ by the decarboxylation of carboxyl-labeled ^{14}C-benzoic acid has been employed as a measure of $OH\cdot$ formation by the xanthine oxidase system and by stimulated neutrophils (641). Decarboxylation of benzoic acid by phagocytes was inhibited by SOD, catalase, azide, and mannitol and was absent when CGD neutrophils were employed. Studies with neutrophils that lack MPO were not performed.

Electron paramagnetic resonance spectrometry

Electron paramagnetic resonance (EPR) spectrometry using a spin trap has been employed in an attempt to detect $OH\cdot$ formation by phagocytes. EPR spectrometry detects free radicals, and when the radical is unstable it is often possible to trap it as a more stable radical adduct using a nitrone or nitroso compound as a spin trap. Hydroxyl radicals form an adduct with the nitrone compound 5,5-dimethylpyrroline-*N*-oxide (DMPO), which is sufficiently long-lived for detection by its characteristic EPR spectrum (309,358).

Neutrophils stimulated in the presence of DMPO form the OH· adduct (277,564,626). The adduct is not formed by CGD neutrophils, and its formation is greater than normal when MPO-deficient leukocytes are employed, an effect that is not observed when MPO is added (626). DMPO-OH· adduct formation also is increased when the peroxidase inhibitors azide and cyanide are added to normal neutrophils stimulated by phagocytosis (277). The increased DMPO-OH· adduct formation is presumably an additional measure of the greater respiratory burst of MPO-deficient leukocytes (see above).

It should be emphasized that detection of the DMPO-OH· adduct does not unequivocably establish the formation of OH· by stimulated leukocytes. DMPO also forms a radical adduct with O_2^- (or HO_2^-), and reduction of the DMPO-OOH· adduct to DMPO-OH· can occur (233–236). It is therefore possible that the DMPO-OOH· adduct is initially formed by stimulated neutrophils and is subsequently reduced to DMPO-OH·, which would account for the observation that DMPO-OH· adduct formation by neutrophils is inhibited by SOD but not by catalase (277,626). However, it would not explain the inhibition of DMPO-OH· adduct formation by the OH· scavenger mannitol (626). The DMPO-OOH· adduct, which has an EPR spectrum distinct from that of the OH· adduct (233,309), was detected along with the DMPO-OH· adduct when neutrophils were stimulated with PMA (115,277,322), whereas only the DMPO-OH· spectrum was detected when neutrophils were stimulated by phagocytosis of latex or zymosan (115,277,322,626). However, when the zymosan concentration was increased to 3 mg/ml, both the DMPO-OOH· and the DMPO-OH· adducts were detected (115). Both adducts also were found when azide and, to a lesser degree, cyanide were added to neutrophils stimulated by ingestion of latex particles (277). In contrast to the studies described above with human neutrophils, when mixed rat leukocytes were incubated with opsonized *E. coli* and either phenyl-ter-butyl nitrone (PBN), 2-methyl-2-nitrosopropane (MNP), or DMPO as a spin trap, an adduct was formed only with MNP, which appeared to be identical to that formed with O_2^- (488).

The presence of both the DMPO-OOH· and the DMPO-OH· adducts could reflect (a) the formation of both O_2^- and OH· by phagocytes; (b) the primary formation of DMPO-OOH· by phagocytes with its bioreduction to DMPO-OH· (115); and (c) the formation of OH· and its reaction with excess H_2O_2 to form HO_2^- (571). In regard to the latter, the incubation of O_2^- with DMPO in acetonitrile resulted in the formation of a compound with an EPR spectrum that was not in agreement with that of either the O_2^- or the HO_2^- adduct of DMPO; it was thought to be that of a reduction product of DMPO of unknown structure. The addition of 1% H_2O_2 to the reaction mixture resulted in the appearance of a spectrum characteristic of the DMPO-OH· adduct. When the H_2O_2 was increased to 5%, a new spectrum appeared that was characteristic of the DMPO-OOH adduct. The following sequence of reactions was suggested.

$$O_2^- + H_2O_2 \rightarrow O_2 + OH· + OH^-$$

$$OH· + H_2O_2 \rightarrow H_2O + HO_2^-$$

$$HO_2^- \rightarrow H^+ + O_2^-$$

This finding is in agreement with another (308,309) that the electrochemical dissociation of H_2O_2 at low concentration in the presence of DMPO resulted in the formation of DMPO-OH·; whereas when high concentrations of H_2O_2 were employed, the DMPO-OOH· radical adduct was formed. The rate constant for the reaction of DMPO with OH· ($3.4 \times 10^9 M^{-1}s^{-1}$) is considerably greater than that for reaction with HO_2^- ($6.6 \times 10^3 M^{-1}s^{-1}$), which is greater than that for the reaction of DMPO with O_2^- ($10 M^{-1}s^{-1}$) (234). The interpretation of the detection of DMPO-OH· adduct formation is further complicated by the possibility that DMPO can form an adduct with $^1O_2$, which on hydration would form the OH· adduct (243).

Role in Leukocytes

The hydroxyl radical is an extremely powerful oxidant (218) and as such is not discriminating in its action, reacting with essentially the first molecule it meets. It therefore can be readily scavenged by compounds in the medium or by nonessential components of the target. However, a variety of studies have implicated OH· as a toxic species in cell-free O_2^- and H_2O_2-generating systems (39,48,306,307), and it is logical to assume therefore that OH· production by intact neutrophils contributes to the toxicity of the cell. In general, the evidence implicating OH· formed by the Haber-Weiss reaction in a toxic reaction consists of the inhibition by catalase, SOD, and OH· scavengers.

The xanthine oxidase system, with either xanthine, hypoxanthine, or acetaldehyde as substrate forms O_2^-, H_2O_2, and OH· (75,249) and thus has been employed as a model of the oxygen-dependent microbicidal mechanisms of phagocytes. In early studies of the bactericidal activity of xanthine oxidase, inhibition by catalase implicated H_2O_2 (276,468). However, the discovery of SOD and its use with catalase and OH· scavengers to detect OH· formation by the Haber-Weiss reaction, has led to the identification of OH· as a microbicidal product of the xanthine oxidase system (513,625,627). In some instances the bactericidal activity of the xanthine oxidase system was inhibited by catalase but not by SOD (44,351), or by catalase and SOD but not by OH· scavengers (44), suggesting that with some targets and under some experimental conditions products of the xanthine oxidase system other than OH· may be the toxic agent.

The participation of OH· in the microbicidal activity of neutrophils has been proposed based on the inhibition of the bactericidal activity of intact leukocytes by SOD and catalase bound to latex beads (367) and by some OH· scavengers (367,607). When DMSO was employed as the scavenger, the OH· product methane was detected (607). The O_2^- and H_2O_2 required for OH· formation are provided by the respiratory burst, and the iron needed for catalysis may come from leukocytic or microbial sources. Chelation of the iron in the phagosome by iron-unsaturated lactoferrin would be expected to inhibit rather than to stimulate the formation of OH· by the Haber-Weiss reaction. However, a chelator may not be required for iron catalysis of the Haber-Weiss reaction at the acidic pH believed to exist in the phagosome (419). Different mechanisms of toxicity may be operative in neutrophils depending on the target, the state of stimulation, and pathological variations. Thus, for example, normal neutrophils degrade LTC_4 by the MPO system; whereas when MPO is absent, as in hereditary MPO deficiency, degradation occurs by an OH·-dependent mechanism (328; see also above).

H_2O_2/Fe^{2+}/Iodide Antimicrobial System

H_2O_2 reacts with ferrous ions and iodide to form an antimicrobial system effective against bacteria (420) and fungi (463,713). The properties of the H_2O_2/Fe^{2+}/iodide system differ from those of the H_2O_2/MPO/halide system in several respects (420). Both systems are inhibited by catalase and are unaffected by SOD. However, the Fe^{2+}/H_2O_2/iodide system is strongly inhibited by the OH· scavengers mannitol and ethanol at concentrations that do not affect the MPO-dependent system. Although both systems are inhibited by azide, a considerably higher concentration is required for inhibition of the Fe^{2+}- than the MPO-dependent system. The pH optimum of the Fe^{2+}-dependent system was 5.5; 0.2 M acetate buffer could be employed at this pH, whereas phosphate and lactate buffers at the same pH and molarity were ineffective and indeed inhibited the bactericidal activity of the system in acetate buffer (or when unbuffered). In contrast, the pH optimum of the MPO/H_2O_2/iodide system was 5.0, and all three buffers could be employed at this pH with comparable results. EDTA inhibited the Fe^{2+}- but not the MPO-dependent system. Whereas the MPO system was effective with iodide, bromide, or chloride as the halide, only iodide was effective when MPO was replaced by iron. Thyroxine could serve as the source of iodide for the

MPO/H_2O_2/iodide system but not for the Fe^{2+}/H_2O_2/iodide system. It was proposed that Fe^{2+} and H_2O_2 (Fenton's reagent) interact to form OH·

$$Fe^{2+} + H_2O_2 \rightarrow Fe^{3+} + OH^- + OH·$$

which reacts with iodide to form a toxic species

$$OH· + I^- \rightarrow OH^- + I*$$

with the overall reaction being

$$Fe^{2+} + H_2O_2 + I \rightarrow Fe^{3+} + 2OH^- + I*$$

Singlet Oxygen

Of the two forms of $^1O_2$, $^1\Sigma_g^+O_2$ has a higher energy above ground state (37.5 kcal) than does $^1\Delta_gO_2$ (22.4 kcal) but a considerably shorter lifetime. In aqueous solution the lifetime of $^1\Sigma_g^+O_2$ does not exceed 10^{-11} sec, whereas that of $^1\Delta_gO_2$ is approximately 2 μsec (390). The lifetime of $^1\Delta_gO_2$ is increased considerably in a number of solvents (up to 1,000 μsec with Freon) and is increased at least tenfold by the substitution of deuterium oxide (D_2O) for water (390). The increase in a chemical reaction by the substitution of D_2O for H_2O has been employed as evidence for $^1O_2$ involvement.

$^1\Delta_gO_2$, the reactive form of $^1O_2$ in solution, is a strong electrophile that reacts with compounds in areas of high electron density to form characteristic, generally oxygenated products. That such reactions can be toxic is indicated by the photodynamic action of dyes. Certain dyes in the presence of light and oxygen are toxic to cells and other targets, and one of the mechanisms proposed is the reaction of the light-sensitized dye with oxygen to form $^1O_2$, which can attack the cell or other target (242). This fact, together with the chemiluminescence observed when neutrophils are stimulated (20), raised the possibility of the formation of $^1O_2$ by phagocytes and its involvement in microbicidal activity. $^1O_2$ can be formed by a variety of reactions; only three of probable pertinence to the neutrophil are considered here.

Spontaneous Dismutation

It has been proposed that the oxygen formed during the spontaneous dismutation of O_2^- is in part in the excited state, i.e., $^1O_2$ (394). Although the evidence was initially indirect and dependent on techniques (chemiluminescence, chemical scavengers) that have been criticized because of their lack of specificity, the development of a sensitive spectrometer capable of the detection of the characteristic emission of $^1\Delta_gO_2$ decay at 1,268 nm (400) has allowed the detection of $^1O_2$ in the reaction of water with potassium superoxide suspended in chloroform (395). Although this evidence supports the generation of $^1O_2$ by the spontaneous dismutation of O_2^- under the experimental conditions employed, unequivocal evidence for its formation by spontaneous dismutation under biological conditions has not been provided. It seems unlikely that $^1O_2$ formed by dismutation could be responsible for the biological toxicity of O_2^-, as in one study $^1O_2$ accounted for less than 0.2% of the oxygen produced in the dismutation reaction (244,245).

Haber-Weiss Reaction

The formation of $^1O_2$ by the Haber-Weiss reaction has been proposed (391,392). However, in subsequent studies from the same laboratory, $^1O_2$ was found to account for no more than 0.1% of the O_2^- formed by the aerobic xanthine oxidase system and was thus, at best, a minor product of the Haber-Weiss reaction (521).

Peroxidase/H_2O_2/Halide System

A well-established mechanism for the formation of $^1O_2$ is by the interaction of hypochlorite and H_2O_2.

$$OCl^- + H_2O_2 \rightarrow Cl^- + H_2O_2 + {}^1O_2$$

This reaction emits a weak red chemiluminescence, and spectroscopic studies have established that the metastable product formed is $^1\Delta_gO_2$ (387,547). The formation of $^1O_2$ by the interaction of HOCl and O_2^- also has been proposed (472). The finding that HOCl is the primary product formed by the oxidation of chloride by MPO and H_2O_2 (10,314) has raised the possibility that its reaction with excess H_2O_2 or O_2^- may result in the formation of $^1O_2$.

$^1O_2$ reacts with a number of compounds to yield characteristic products whose formation have been employed for the detection of $^1O_2$. One such reaction is the conversion of 2,5-diphenylfuran to cis-dibenzoylethylene (402). The MPO/H_2O_2/halide system was found to initiate this reaction, and $^1O_2$ was implicated by the stimulation of conversion by D_2O and by the inhibition of conversion by the $^1O_2$ quenchers β-carotene, bilirubin, histidine, and 1,4-diazabicyclo[2,2,2]octane (DABCO) (624). HOCl also converted diphenylfuran to cis-dibenzoylethylene, and this reaction exhibited properties comparable to those of the enzyme system (624). Diphenylfuran conversion by HOCl at acidic pH was increased by the addition of chloride but not by H_2O_2, suggesting that the classic reaction for the formation of $^1O_2$, the interaction of hypochlorite and H_2O_2, was not operative. The conversion of diphenylisobenzofuran to o-dibenzoylbenzene by the LPO/H_2O_2/bromide system also has been observed and an $^1O_2$-dependent mechanism proposed (591,592). HOCl (317,

325,755) or Cl_2 formed by the interaction of HOCl and chloride at acidic pH (624) may initiate furan conversion directly, i.e., without $^1O_2$ involvement, thus bringing into question the validity of this reaction for the detection of $^1O_2$ formation by the MPO system.

Early studies had indicated that the MPO/H_2O_2/halide system emits light with the effectiveness of the halides decreasing in the order Br > Cl > I (18,19,623). The pH optimum of the chemiluminescence was 4.4 to 5.0 (19), and the light emission was increased by the addition of zymosan or bacteria (623). Presumably, excitation of surface components on the particle was the primary source of the chemiluminescence. The development of instrumentation for detection of the infrared emission band at 1,268 nm characteristic of $^1\Delta_gO_2$ decay to the ground state (381,400,445) has renewed interest in the formation of $^1O_2$ by the peroxidase system. Using this technique, $^1\Delta_gO_2$ has been detected as a product of the interaction of LPO, H_2O_2, and bromide (381,396,398) and of chloroperoxidase, H_2O_2, and chloride or bromide (382,396,398,401). The formation of $^1O_2$ with high efficiency by the MPO/H_2O_2/bromide system also has been observed by this technique (383,399). In contrast, $^1O_2$ formation by the MPO/H_2O_2/chloride system was much less efficient. It was concluded (383) that although the MPO/H_2O_2/bromide system can form $^1O_2$ the conditions required were not physiological. The poor yield of $^1O_2$ by the MPO/H_2O_2/chloride system was associated with MPO inactivation (383). The finding that ascorbic acid in micromolar quantities protected MPO from inactivation (97) prompted a study of the effect of ascorbic acid on the yield of $^1O_2$ from the MPO/H_2O_2/halide system (384). No increased production was found.

Intact Leukocytes

The formation of $^1O_2$ by intact leukocytes was first proposed by Allen et al. (20) based on the chemiluminescence of stimulated neutrophils. Chemiluminescence indicates the formation of electronically excited states but without spectral analysis does not indicate the nature of the excited species. Analysis of the light emitted by stimulated neutrophils revealed broad peak activity with a maximum at about 570 nm, rather than the characteristic spectrum of $^1O_2$ decay (22,137). This finding suggests that the light emitted by phagocytes is not due primarily to $^1O_2$ decay but to secondary excitations that could be induced by reaction of a number of the oxidants formed by stimulated leukocytes with cellular constituents.

Another mechanism for the detection of $^1O_2$ formation by phagocytes is by product analysis. A compound that reacts with $^1O_2$ is added to the leukocytes and the product formed by the reaction of that compound with $^1O_2$ sought.

However the chemical traps for $^1O_2$ are generally nonspecific, leaving open the possibility that the chemical conversion is by another mechanism (see above). Cholesterol is believed to be a specific chemical trap for $^1O_2$ with the product formed, 3 β-hydroxy-5α-cholest-6-ene-5-hydroperoxide, being different from that produced by radical oxidation (447). Cholesterol, however, is an inefficient $^1O_2$ scavenger compared to other less specific traps. Incubation of polystyrene latex microbeads or mineral oil droplets containing ^{14}C-cholesterol with neutrophils or macrophages did not result in the formation of the $^1O_2$ product, leading to the conclusion that $^1O_2$ is at best a minor product of the respiratory burst of phagocytes (245,246). The observation that carotenoid-containing wild-type *Sarcina lutea* are less readily killed by neutrophils than are mutant pigmentless mutants (446) was proposed as evidence of $^1O_2$ involvement, as carotenoid pigments are efficient $^1O_2$ scavengers. However, other interpretations are possible. Thus a role for $^1O_2$ in the microbicidal activity of phagocytes has not been established.

EOSINOPHILS

Eosinophils can ingest and kill microorganisms; however, in general they do this less effectively than do neutrophils (53,122,156,199,498), a fact that in most studies has been related to their decreased phagocytic activity (53,122,157,498). The primary cytotoxic role of this cell thus may be against such extracellular targets as helminths and tumor cells.

Eosinophils have potent cytotoxic constituents in cytoplasmic granules (270) and, like neutrophils, respond to stimulation with degranulation and with a respiratory burst forming O_2^- (198,434,725), H_2O_2 (53,198,389, 434,498), and probably OH· (429). Among the granule components are a group of basic proteins whose properties and function have been extensively studied (270). Their cytotoxic activity is independent of oxygen and thus is not considered here (see Chapter 26).

Respiratory Burst

With most stimuli the respiratory burst of eosinophils is greater than that of equivalent numbers of neutrophils comparably stimulated (53,198,434,452,498,593, 594,820). An NADPH oxidase similar to that present in neutrophils appears to be involved (53,198,725). NADPH oxidase activity was reported to be three to six times greater in eosinophils than in comparable neutrophil preparations (198), and eosinophils have a cytochrome b_{559} concentration that is twice that of neutrophils or monocytes (658). As with neutrophils, oxygen does not appear to be required for phagocytosis by eosinophils (156) but, rather, is utilized for the generation of toxic oxygen metabolites.

Eosinophil Peroxidase

The eosinophil is exceptionally rich in peroxidase. Cytochemical studies have localized the peroxidase in the matrix of the specific granules of the mature eosinophil surrounding the central crystalline core (58). These granules form during the myelocyte stage of eosinophil development, where peroxidase activity can be detected in the cisternae of the rough endoplasmic reticulum and Golgi complex as well as in the developing granules (58). Following phagocytosis peroxidase is detected in the phagosome surrounding the ingested organism (170); eosinophils adherent to a target too large to be ingested release their granule components, including peroxidase, extracellularly, and the peroxidase can be detected on the target cell surface (373,490). The peroxidase also can be released extracellularly by soluble stimuli (333) and peroxidase-containing granules can be released by lysis of eosinophils in tissues (630).

EPO has been purified from rat (31,32), guinea pig (202), horse (375), and human (127,565,784) eosinophils. The human enzyme is a glycoprotein of approximately 77 kD that can be separated into a large (approximately 50 kD) and small (10–15 kD) subunit under reducing conditions (96,127,565,567), with the carbohydrate associated with the large subunit and consisting of mannose and N-acetylglucosamine residues (567). The heme prosthetic group of EPO is a protoporphyrin (96,783) that is similar to that of LPO in optical and EPR spectra (96,783) but which differs to some degree from LPO in its resonance Raman spectrum (679).

EPO, like MPO, has toxic properties when combined with H_2O_2 and a halide. In early studies human eosinophil granules were found to be candidacidal (456) and sonicates bactericidal (499) when combined with H_2O_2 and iodide but not chloride; these findings were supported by the finding that EPO did not catalyze the oxidative deamination and decarboxylation of amino acids when combined with H_2O_2 and chloride under conditions in which MPO was active (499). However, when purified EPO was employed, toxic activity was observed with chloride as well as iodide or bromide as the halide (125,372,373,375), although chloride was less effective relative to iodide or bromide with EPO than with MPO. The effect of chloride was more evident when the pH was lowered (370,371, 372,375). Additional evidence for the utilization of chloride by the EPO system was the chlorination of monochlorodimedon by EPO, H_2O_2, and chloride (784).

The relative ineffectiveness of chloride with EPO compared to MPO raises the question of the physiological halide for an EPO-mediated antimicrobial system (603). Chloride at physiological concentration (0.1 M) has little effect at neutral pH but is effective at this concentration when the pH is lowered to 5.0. Because the pH within the phagosome (or in the space between an adherent eosinophil and a target too large to be ingested) may fall to this level, there may be a contribution by chloride to the effective halide pool in these locations. Iodide is the most effective halide on a molar basis; however, its concentration in biological fluids is low (<1 μg/dl), suggesting that its contribution is small. Bromide is nearly as effective as iodide in the EPO/H_2O_2/halide system and is present in biological fluids in considerably higher concentrations. Thus the level of bromide in blood ranges from 130 to 810 μg/dl and that of urine from 213 to 520 μg/dl (343). In one study (603) bromide was effective as a component of the EPO-mediated antimicrobial system at pH 5.0 at a concentration of 8 μg/dl and at pH 7.0 at 80 μg/dl, raising the possibility that bromide is the physiological halide. In this regard, EPO released from eosinophils by a cationic detergent can catalyze the bromide-dependent decarboxylation of amino acids, whereas no decarboxylation occurs with chloride, fluoride, or iodide as the halide (173). Strong support for bromide involvement in intact cells comes from the finding that intact human eosinophils stimulated by PMA or opsonized zymosan preferentially utilized bromide to generate a halogenating oxidant (presumably hypobromous acid) when both bromide and chloride were present in physiological concentrations (780).

The cell-free EPO/H_2O_2/halide system is toxic to bacteria including *Escherichia coli* (371,375,499) *Staphylococcus aureus* (499,603), *Legionella pneumophila* (470), and *Mycobacterium leprae* (430), as well as to fungi, (456), the schistosomula of *Schistosoma mansoni* (372,373), the newborn larvae of *Trichinella spiralis* (125,126), *Trypanosoma cruzi* trypomastigotes (551), *Toxoplasma gondii* (469), tumor cells (370), and mast cells (329). EPO is a highly basic protein that binds avidly to negatively charged surfaces with retention of peroxidatic activity. Among the surfaces to which it binds is that of the target cell. If H_2O_2 and a halide are added to target cells with surface-bound EPO, the target cells are rapidly killed under conditions in which control cells without bound peroxidase are unaffected. This phenomenon has been observed with *S. aureus* (603), *L. pneumophila* (470), *T. gondii* (469), *T. cruzi* (551), schistosomula of *S. mansoni* (373), and tumor cells (531) as the target. The toxicity of the EPO/H_2O_2/halide system is strongly inhibited by protein when the EPO is free in solution owing to competition with the target cell for the toxic products of the peroxidase system. Protein is much less inhibitory when EPO is bound to the target cell surface (373,531) presumably due to proximity

of toxic oxidant production to critical sites on the membrane. The toxic effect of intact neutrophils (373) or macrophages (see below) is considerably increased when EPO is bound to the target cell surface because of more efficient utilization of the H_2O_2 generated by the phagocyte.

EPO also binds to the negatively charged mast cell granule to form a complex that retains toxic activity when combined with H_2O_2 and a halide (330); indeed the bactericidal (330) and tumoricidal (331) activity of the complex is greater than that of free EPO when standardized to the same guaiacol units of peroxidase activity. The finding that H_2O_2 alone at high concentration and the EPO/H_2O_2/halide system at lower H_2O_2 concentrations can initiate mast cell secretion with the release of mast cell granules (329) (see above) raises the possibility that in an inflammatory lesion mast cell granules released by the EPO system bind EPO with potentiation of its toxic activity. Mast cells contain a small amount of peroxidase in their cytoplasmic granules (327), which may be synthesized by the cell (230) or acquired by endocytosis of exogenous EPO. EPO binds to the surface of guinea pig basophils and cloned mouse mast cells and is internalized by a vesicular transport system and incorporated into cytoplasmic granules (223). Mast cells when incubated with H_2O_2 and a halide were toxic to tumor cells (331) or schistosomula (334); the mechanism proposed was the initiation of mast cell secretion by H_2O_2 and the reaction of the endogenous peroxidase of the mast cell granule with H_2O_2 and a halide to form a toxic system.

When eosinophils adhere to a target, they discharge their granule contents, including EPO (373,393,490) as well as a number of other basic proteins (270). Eosinophils when stimulated generate H_2O_2 in large amounts (53,198,389,434,498), and thus the interaction of EPO and H_2O_2 with a halide at the target cell surface might be anticipated. Support for the involvement of the peroxidase system in the toxicity of eosinophils against tumor cells (370) and the schistosomula of *S. mansoni* (389) has been provided, although other studies have emphasized the involvement of other basic granule proteins (270). Although the basic proteins of eosinophils have well-recognized direct toxic properties, the major basic protein (MBP) of eosinophils also can scavenge the toxic product of the EPO/H_2O_2/halide system and in this way inhibit EPO-mediated killing (126).

MONONUCLEAR PHAGOCYTES

Mononuclear phagocytes are a continuum of changing cells beginning with bone marrow precursors and continuing through the blood monocyte to the fully activated tissue macrophage. The latter vary in their morphological and functional characteristics depending on their location and state of activation.

All mononuclear phagocytes respond to a greater or lesser degree to stimulation with a burst of oxygen consumption. The mechanism of the respiratory burst in mononuclear phagocytes appears to be in part comparable to that of neutrophils. An NADPH oxidase is present in the particulate fraction of stimulated human monocytes and is present in low concentration or absent in unstimulated cells or in stimulated CGD monocytes (136). The monocyte NADPH oxidase does not react with NADH and has a lower affinity for NADPH (Km 83 μM) than does the neutrophil enzyme (Km 31 μM) (136). An NADPH oxidase also is present in the plasma membrane of mature macrophages (80,86,87,248,341,615,646). The low potential (-245 mV) b-cytochrome is present in monocytes (658) and macrophages (132,748) in concentrations comparable to that found in neutrophils. As with neutrophils and eosinophils, the respiratory burst appears to contribute oxidants required for optimum microbicidal activity. The role of toxic oxygen metabolites in the effector function of macrophages has been reviewed (421,527,528,532).

Monocytes

Of the mononuclear phagocytes, the blood monocyte most closely resembles the neutrophil in its antimicrobial systems. Monocytes respond to stimulation with a brisk respiratory burst, although its magnitude is less than that of equivalent numbers of neutrophils comparably stimulated (616). In one study in which paired measurements were made using monocytes and neutrophils from the same blood sample, oxygen consumption and H_2O_2 production by opsonized zymosan-stimulated monocytes were 39% and 19%, respectively, of that of similarly treated neutrophils (604). The blood monocyte contains a peroxidase in cytoplasmic granules that is identical to that of the MPO of neutrophils, as indicated by comparable structural and functional properties (108) and by the absence of a granule peroxidase from both neutrophils and monocytes in hereditary MPO deficiency in which there is a genetic absence of this enzyme (285). However, monocytes contain less MPO than do neutrophils. Thus the average number of peroxidase-positive granules in human monocytes is 34 per thin section (546) compared to 75 per thin section in human neutrophils (59); quantitative analysis revealed approximately three times as much MPO in neutrophils as in monocytes (54,108).

The MPO of monocytes is released into the phagosome following particle ingestion (190), where it can react with H_2O_2 and a halide to form a microbicidal system. Thus iodination, which is a measure of the interaction of MPO, H_2O_2, and iodide, occurs in monocytes, although its level is less than that of comparably stimulated neutrophils

(54,108,457,471). Furthermore, monocytes when stimulated form a chlorinating species, presumably HOCl (448). The involvement of the MPO/H_2O_2/halide system in the killing of C. albicans (208,457) and Aspergillus fumigatus (214) by human monocytes was suggested by the decreased fungicidal activity induced by peroxidase inhibitors or the substitution of MPO-deficient monocytes for normal monocytes. However, MPO-independent and nonoxidative fungicidal mechanisms also were detected in monocytes. Toxoplasma gondii was killed at a slower rate by MPO-deficient monocytes than by normal cells, and this defect was abolished by the introduction of EPO into the phagosome bound to the surface of the organism (469). In contrast, the toxoplasmacidal defect of CGD monocytes was unaffected by surface-bound EPO. As with neutrophils, the respiratory burst of monocytes as measured by O_2^- production or by iodination in the presence of added MPO, was greater in MPO-deficient than in normal monocytes (471).

Monocytes also are toxic to extracellular targets such as erythrocytes or tumor cells. In some instances toxic oxygen species do not appear to be major contributors to the toxicity (237,409,665), whereas a contribution by oxygen metabolites has been proposed in other studies. The toxic oxygen metabolites primarily involved have varied with the experimental conditions; they include products of the MPO/H_2O_2/halide system (773), H_2O_2 operating in the absence of MPO (487), a combination of O_2^- and H_2O_2 (487,776), OH· (101), or an unidentified oxygen product (409,439).

Macrophages

Monocytes that transform into macrophage-like cells in tissue culture develop multiple synthetic and secretory functions (167), but the change is associated with a decrease in microbicidal potency (see Chapters 15 and 18). This decrease results in a marked decrease in antimicrobial activity against a variety of pathogens including Listeria monocytogenes (188), Cryptococcus neoformans (206), Toxoplasma gondii (792), Leishmania donovani (512), and type 1 herpes simplex virus (194). It presents a problem to the host, as these and other organisms may survive and replicate in macrophages, producing disease.

The basis for the decreased potency of macrophages is, in part, a decrease in oxygen-dependent mechanisms of toxicity. Blood monocytes retain their granule peroxidase for a time following passage into the extravascular space (253), and this peroxidase is released into the phagosome following particle ingestion (190). Because many of the macrophages in a granulomatous lesion are relatively recent immigrants (24,552) their granule peroxidase may contribute to their antimicrobial effect. However, as tissue monocytes mature into macrophages *in vivo* (253) or *in vitro* (365,522,664,709) their granule peroxidase is lost.

The magnitude of the respiratory burst also decreases markedly when monocytes mature into macrophages. This situation is indicated by the weak respiratory burst of resident macrophages (368,533) and by the sharp decrease in the respiratory burst when monocytes differentiate into macrophages *in vitro* (512,520,522,572). Some studies have indicated an early decrease in the respiratory burst at about day 1 of culture (522,663) followed by a rise at day 3 (520,522,663) prior to the sharp decrease with continued culture (520,522). The decreased potency is presumably due in part to the decreased respiratory burst and MPO content of the mature resident macrophage.

Activation is a process by which macrophages develop morphological and metabolic changes associated with heightened microbicidal activity following exposure to activating agents for periods generally measured in days (see Chapters 15 and 26). In contrast, stimulation is an acute process, generally measured in minutes, in which phagocytes respond to phagocytosis or a soluble stimulus such as PMA with a respiratory burst and degranulation. The respiratory burst of resident macrophages in response to stimulation is increased severalfold when the macrophages are activated *in vivo* (368,533). Activation of cultured monocyte-derived macrophages also can be induced *in vitro* by the addition of lymphokine, with an associated increase in the respiratory burst (262,512,523). Crude lymphokine preparations, i.e., supernatants from mitogen- or antigen-stimulated human mononuclear cells (262,512,523), or purified recombinant γ-interferon (IFN) (132,518,538) can be used for this purpose whereas a number of other cytokine preparations—native α-IFN, recombinant α-IFN-A, recombinant α-IFN-D, recombinant β-IFN, colony-stimulating factor type 1 (CSF-1), colony-stimulating factor for granulocytes and macrophages (GM-CSF), pluripotent colony stimulating factor, tumor necrosis factor, native interleukin-2, and recombinant interleukin 2—were ineffective (539). A migration inhibitory factor (MIF) preparation increased macrophage respiratory burst activity, although it was not as effective in this regard as γ-IFN (539). The respiratory burst of activated macrophages can be suppressed (deactivation) by exposure of the cells to a factor in the culture medium of a wide variety of malignant and some nonmalignant cells (717,718).

These changes in the respiratory burst as macrophages differentiate and are activated and deactivated appear to result from changes in the kinetics of the NADPH oxidase. Thus when human blood monocytes mature into macrophages in culture, the decrease in the respiratory burst is associated with a decrease in the affinity of NADPH oxidase for its substrate (increase in Km); and when the

monocyte-derived macrophages are activated by γ-IFN, the affinity of the enzyme for NADPH is increased (132). Similarly, the NADPH oxidase of *in vivo*-activated mouse macrophages has a higher affinity for NADPH than does the oxidase of resident (nonactivated) macrophages (88,646,748); and the deactivation of macrophages induced by medium conditioned by a variety of malignant and some nonmalignant cells is associated with a decreased affinity of NADPH oxidase for NADPH (749). In contrast to the Km, there is little or no change in the V_{max} of the NADPH oxidase (88,132,646,748) or the b-cytochrome content of the cell (89,748) with activation. The oxygen-dependent microbicidal activity of mature activated macrophages is presumably due to the formation of toxic oxygen metabolites.

H_2O_2

H_2O_2 has been implicated in the toxic activity of macrophages. Thus *Leishmania* promastigotes are readily killed by resident mouse peritoneal macrophages, and this leishmanicidal activity is inhibited by catalase or glucose deprivation (which decreases H_2O_2 production by the macrophages) but not by SOD or by the OH· scavengers mannitol or benzoate, thus implicating H_2O_2 (509). Similar findings were obtained when the lymphokine-treated macrophage cell line J744G8 was employed (510). Sensitivity to H_2O_2 is related to the level of H_2O_2 scavenging enzymes. Thus *Leishmania* promastigotes, which are considerably more sensitive to H_2O_2 than is *Toxoplasma gondii,* contain lower levels of catalase and glutathione peroxidase (509). Furthermore, *Leishmania donovani* amastigotes are more resistant to H_2O_2 and to the toxic activity of macrophages than are promastigotes and have correspondingly higher levels of catalase (511). The killing of *Leishmania donovani* promastigotes and amastigotes by human monocyte-derived macrophages stimulated with lymphokine (γ-IFN) also correlated with H_2O_2 production by the cells (512,517,518). However, similarly treated cells from patients with CGD retained partial leishmanicidal activity, indicating a contribution by oxygen-independent mechanisms.

Trypanosoma cruzi trypomastigotes survive in normal mouse peritoneal macrophages but are killed by macrophages activated *in vitro* or *in vivo* by lymphokines; this trypanocidal activity correlated well with the amount of H_2O_2 formed on stimulation of the macrophages with PMA (534). A variant macrophage cell line defective in the respiratory burst was unable to kill epimastigotes of *Trypanosoma cruzi* unless glucose oxidase, an enzyme that generates H_2O_2 without an O_2^- intermediate, was introduced into the cell covalently bound to zymosan particles (723).

H₂O₂ also has been identified as the toxic species responsible for the killing of tumor cells by activated macrophages stimulated by PMA (526,535,536). Although an oxidative mechanism appeared to be involved in the lysis of tumor cells by activated macrophages in the presence of anti-tumor cell antibody, H_2O_2 was not definitively established as the product responsible, as catalase was not inhibitory (529). However, the scavenging of H_2O_2 by the glutathione oxidation–reduction cycle in murine tumor cells is important to their susceptibility to lysis by macrophages plus anti-tumor cell antibody, as well as by PMA-triggered macrophages and by H_2O_2 generated by glucose oxidase (33,34,537). Some human tumor cells use the glutathione redox system as the primary defense against H_2O_2, whereas others appeared to utilize catalase (557). H_2O_2 can react synergistically with a cytolytic protease to lyse tumor cells (2). The capacity to secrete H_2O_2 can be dissociated from the tumor cell cytolytic activity of activated macrophages under some conditions (166).

H_2O_2 also has been implicated in the inhibitory effect of *C. parvum* or thioglycollate-induced mouse peritoneal macrophages on lymphocyte transformation (496) and in the cytotoxic activity of human pulmonary macrophages on human skin fibroblasts (462).

Because mature tissue macrophages in general lack a granule peroxidase, they cannot amplify the toxicity of H_2O_2 through the release of this enzyme into the phagosome (or extracellularly) by degranulation. Many resident macrophages contain cytochemically identifiable peroxidase in the perinuclear cisternae, rough endoplasmic reticulum, and in some instances the Golgi lamellae (57,189). Other mononuclear phagocytes that do not contain a peroxidase in the endoplasmic reticulum can develop a peroxidase there transiently when the cells adhere to a surface *in vitro* (57,94,95). The nature of this peroxidase is unknown. It is not MPO, as it appears in the endoplasmic reticulum of adherent monocytes from patients with hereditary MPO deficiency (57,112). The release of prostanoids corresponded to the appearance of the peroxidase, raising the possibility that it is associated with arachidonic acid metabolism (201). The peroxidase of the endoplasmic reticulum is not packaged into granules, nor is it released into the phagosome (190), suggesting that it is not involved in microbicidal activity. Although catalase generally inhibits H_2O_2-dependent microbicidal systems, it can be microbicidal when the pH is low (i.e., 4.5), the H_2O_2 is maintained at low steady-state concentrations, and iodide (or thyroxine) is added as the halide (414,426). Catalase, present in high concentration in rabbit alveolar macrophages (264), is released in part into the phagosome (710); and granule preparations from these cells are bactericidal at acidic pH when combined with iodide and low levels of H_2O_2 (578). This finding raises the possibility that catalase may serve a microbicidal

function in these cells. However, procedures that decreased (265,426) the catalase content of rabbit alveolar macrophages did not decrease their bactericidal activity, suggesting that catalase either is present in considerable excess or is not involved in microbicidal activity.

Mature macrophages can acquire peroxidase by endocytosis, and this exogenous peroxidase could theoretically greatly amplify the toxicity of the small amount of H_2O_2 formed by these cells. Fluid-phase peroxidase can be taken up by pinocytosis, with the peroxidase being transported via coated vesicles and tubules to pinosomes (545). Lysosomal enzymes can be discharged into the pinocytic organelles, which in some instances open to the outside of the cell. Peroxidase released from adjacent neutrophils, eosinophils, or monocytes in particulate form can be taken up by phagocytosis (37,324,630). Phagocytic cell peroxidases, especially EPO, are strongly basic proteins that bind avidly to the surface of microorganisms and mammalian cells (see above). Peroxidase-coated targets are killed much more readily by macrophages than are uncoated targets through an H_2O_2-dependent mechanism, which has been observed with *S. aureus* (603), *T. gondii* (469), *T. cruzi* (551), and tumor cells (531).

OH·

Hydroxyl radicals have been implicated in the toxic activity of macrophages against some targets. Thus *T. gondi* are rich in catalase and glutathione peroxidase and are relatively resistant to destruction by H_2O_2 (516). *T. gondii*, however, are killed by the xanthine/xanthine oxidase system (521), by macrophages from immune mice chronically infected with *T. gondii* or from these mice immune-boosted with *Toxoplasma* (515), and by normal macrophages co-cultivated *in vitro* with lymphokine and heart infusion broth (514). This toxicity is inhibited by catalase, SOD, and the OH· scavengers mannitol and benzoate, thus implicating OH·. Similarly, human normal or lymphokine-activated monocyte-derived macrophages kill *T. gondii* predominantly by an oxygen-dependent mechanism that is inhibited by glucose deprivation or by the addition of catalase, SOD, or mannitol (519). However, studies with CGD monocytes and macrophages indicated the presence in these cells of an oxygen-independent toxoplasmacidal system as well (518,519).

REFERENCES

1. Abrams, W. R., Weinbaum, G., Weissbach, L., Weissbach, H., and Brot, N. (1981): Enzymatic reduction of oxidized α-1-proteinase inhibitor restores biological activity. *Proc. Natl. Acad. Sci. USA,* 78:7483–7486.
2. Adams, D. O., Johnson, W. J., Fiorito, E., and Nathan, C. F. (1981): Hydrogen peroxide and cytolytic factor can interact synergistically

in effecting cytolysis of neoplastic targets. *J. Immunol.*, 127:1973–1977.

3. Adeniyi-Jones, S. K., and Karnovsky, M. L. (1981): Oxidative decarboxylation of free and peptide-linked amino acids in phagocytizing guinea pig granulocytes. *J. Clin. Invest.*, 68:365–373.

4. Agner, K. (1941): Verdoperoxidase: a ferment isolated from leucocytes. *Acta Chem. Scand. [Suppl. 8]*, 2:1–62.

5. Agner, K. (1943): Verdoperoxidase. *Adv. Enzymol.*, 3:137–148.

6. Agner, K. (1947): Detoxicating effect of verdoperoxidase on toxins. *Nature*, 159:271–272.

7. Agner, K. (1950): Studies on peroxidative detoxification of purified diphtheria toxin. *J. Exp. Med.*, 92:337–347.

8. Agner, K. (1955): Peroxidative detoxification of diphtheria toxin studied by using I^{131}. *Rec. Trav. Chim.*, 74:373–376.

9. Agner, K. (1958): Crystalline myeloperoxidase. *Acta Chem. Scand.*, 12:89–94.

10. Agner, K. (1958): Peroxidative oxidation of chloride ions. *Proc. Int. Congr. Biochem. 4th Vienna*, 15:64.

11. Agner, K. (1963): Studies on myeloperoxidase activity. 1. Spectrophotometry of the MPO-H$_2$O$_2$ compound. *Acta Chem. Scand.*, 17:332–338.

12. Agner, K. (1972): Biological effects of hypochlorous acid formed by "MPO"-peroxidation in the presence of chloride ions. In: *Structure and Function of Oxidation-Reduction Enzymes, Vol. 18*, edited by A. Akeson and A. Ehrenberg, pp. 329–335. Pergamon Press, New York.

13. Akazawa, T., and Conn, E. E. (1958): The oxidation of reduced pyridine nucleotides by peroxidase. *J. Biol. Chem.*, 232:403–415.

14. Akin, D. T., and Kinkade, J. M., Jr. (1986): Processing of a newly identified intermediate of human myeloperoxidase in isolated granules occurs at neutral pH. *J. Biol. Chem.*, 261:8370–8375.

15. Albrich, J. M., and Hurst, J. K. (1982): Oxidative inactivation of *Escherichia coli* by hypochlorous acid: rates and differentiation of respiratory from other reaction sites. *FEBS Lett.*, 144:157–161.

16. Albrich, J. M., McCarthy, C. A., and Hurst, J. K. (1981): Biological reactivity of hypochlorous acid: implications for microbicidal mechanisms of leukocyte myeloperoxidase. *Proc. Natl. Acad. Sci. USA*, 78:210–214.

17. Albrich, J. M., Gilbaugh, J. H., III, Callahan, K. B., and Hurst, J. K. (1986): Effects of the putative neutrophil-generating toxin, hypochlorous acid, on membrane permeability and transport systems of *Escherichia coli. J. Clin. Invest.*, 78:177–184.

18. Allen, R. C. (1975): Halide dependence of the myeloperoxidase-mediated antimicrobial system of the polymorphonuclear leukocyte in the phenomenon of electronic excitation. *Biochem. Biophys. Res. Commun.*, 63:675–683.

19. Allen, R. C. (1975): The role of pH in the chemiluminescent response of the myeloperoxidase-halide-HOOH antimicrobial system. *Biochem. Biophys. Res. Commun.*, 63:684–691.

20. Allen, R. C., Stjernholm, R. L., and Steele, R. H. (1972): Evidence for the generation of an electronic excitation state(s) in human polymorphonuclear leukocytes and its participation in bactericidal activity. *Biochem. Biophys. Res. Commun.*, 47:679–684.

21. Ambruso, D. R., and Johnston R. B. (1981): Lactoferrin enhances hydroxyl radical production by human neutrophils, neutrophil particulate fractions and an enzymatic generating system. *J. Clin. Invest.*, 67:352–360.

22. Andersen, B. R., Brendzel, A. M., and Lint, T. F. (1977): Chemiluminescence spectra of human myeloperoxidase and polymorphonuclear leukocytes. *Infect. Immun.*, 17:62–66.

23. Andersen, M. R., Atkins, C. L., and Eyre, H. J. (1982): Intact form of myeloperoxidase from normal human neutrophils. *Arch. Biochem. Biophys.*, 214:273–283.

24. Ando, M., Dannenberg, A. M., Jr., and Shima, K. (1972): Macrophage accumulation, division, maturation and digestion and microbicidal capacities in tuberculous lesions. II. Rate at which mononuclear cells enter and divide in primary BCG lesions and those of reinfection. *J. Immunol.*, 109:8–19.

25. Andrews, P. C., and Babior, B. M. (1983): Endogenous protein phosphorylation by resting and activated human neutrophils. *Blood*, 61:333–340.

26. Andrews, P. C., and Babior, B. M. (1984): Phosphorylation of cytosolic proteins by resting and activated human neutrophils. *Blood*, 64:883–890.

27. Andrews, P. C., and Krinsky, N. I. (1981): The reductive cleavage of myeloperoxidase in half, producing enzymatically active hemi-myeloperoxidase. *J. Biol. Chem.*, 256:4211–4218.

28. Andrews, P. C., and Krinsky, N. I. (1982): A kinetic analysis of the interaction of human myeloperoxidase with hydrogen peroxide, chloride ions, and protons. *J. Biol. Chem.*, 247:13240–13245.

29. Andrews, P. C., Parnes, C., and Krinsky, N. I. (1984): Comparison of myeloperoxidase and hemi-myeloperoxidase with respect to catalysis, regulation, and bactericidal activity. *Arch. Biochem. Biophys.*, 228:439–442.

30. Apfeldorf, W. J., Melnick, D. A., Meshulam, T., Rasmussen, H., and Malech, H. L. (1985): A transient rise in intracellular free calcium is not a sufficient stimulus for respiratory burst activation in human polymorphonuclear leukocytes. *Biochem. Biophys. Res. Commun.*, 132:674–680.

31. Archer, G. T., and Jackas, M. (1965): Disruption of mast cells by a component of eosinophil granules. *Nature*, 205:599–600.

32. Archer, G. T., Air, G., Jackas, M., and Morell, D. B. (1965): Studies on rat eosinophil peroxidase. *Biochim. Biophys. Acta*, 99:96–101.

33. Arrick, B. A., Nathan, C. F., Griffith, O. W., and Cohn, Z. A. (1982): Glutathione depletion sensitizes tumor cells to oxidative cytolysis. *J. Biol. Chem.*, 257:1231–1237.

34. Arrick, B. A., Nathan, C. F., and Cohn, Z. A. (1983): Inhibition of glutathione synthesis augments lysis of murine tumor cells by sulfhydryl-reactive antineoplastics. *J. Clin. Invest.*, 71:258–267.

35. Aswanikumar, S., Schiffmann, E., Corcoran, B. A., and Whal, S. M. (1976): Role of a peptidase in phagocyte chemotaxis. *Proc. Natl. Acad. Sci. USA*, 73:2439–2442.

36. Atkin, C. L., Andersen, M. R., and Eyre, H. J. (1982): Abnormal neutrophil myeloperoxidase from a patient with chronic myelocytic leukemia. *Arch. Biochem. Biophys.*, 214:284–292.

37. Atwal, O. S. (1971): Cytoenzymological behavior in peritoneal exudate cells of rat *in vivo*. 1. Histochemical study of enzymatic function of peroxidase. *J. Reticuloendothel. Soc.*, 10:163–172.

38. Babcock, G. T., Ingle, R. T., Oertling, W. A., Davis, J. C., Averill, B. A., Hulse, C. L., Stufkens, D. J., Bolscher, B. G. J. M., and Wever, R. (1985): Raman characterization of human leukocyte myeloperoxidase and bovine spleen green haemoprotein: insight into chromophore structure and evidence that the chromophores of myeloperoxidase are equivalent. *Biochim. Biophys. Acta*, 828:58–66.

39. Babior, B. M. (1978): Oxygen-dependent microbial killing by phagocytes. *N. Engl. J. Med.*, 298:659–668, 721–725.

40. Babior, B. M. (1983): The nature of the NADPH oxidase. *Adv. Host Def. Mech.*, 3:91–119.

41. Babior, B. M., and Kipnes, R. S. (1977): Superoxide-forming enzyme from human neutrophils: evidence for a flavin requirement. *Blood*, 50:517–524.

42. Babior, B. M., and Peters, W. A. (1981): The O$_2^-$-producing enzyme of human neutrophils: further properties. *J. Biol. Chem.*, 256:2321–2323.

43. Babior, B. M., Kipnes, R. S., and Curnutte, J. T. (1973): Biological defense mechanisms: the production by leukocytes of superoxide, a potential bactericidal agent. *J. Clin. Invest.*, 52:741–744.

44. Babior, B. M., Curnutte, J. T., and Kipnes, R. S. (1975): Biological defense mechanisms: evidence for the participation of superoxide in bacterial killing by xanthine oxidase. *J. Lab. Clin. Med.*, 85:235–244.

45. Babior, B. M., Curnutte, J. T., and Kipnes, R. S. (1975): Pyridine nucleotide-dependent superoxide production by a cell-free system from human granulocytes. *J. Clin. Invest.*, 56:1035–1042.

46. Babior, G. L., Rosin, R. E., McMurrich, B. J., Peters, W. A., and Babior, B. M. (1981): Arrangement of the respiratory burst oxidase in the plasma membrane of the neutrophil. *J. Clin. Invest.*, 67:1724–1728.

47. Badwey, J. A., and Karnovsky, M. L. (1979): Production of superoxide and hydrogen peroxide by an NADH-oxidase in guinea

pig polymorphonuclear leukocytes: modulation by nucleotides and divalent cations. *J. Biol. Chem.*, 254:11530–11537.

48. Badwey, J. A., and Karnovsky, M. J. (1980): Active oxygen species and the functions of phagocytic leukocytes. *Annu. Rev. Biochem.*, 49:695–726.

49. Badwey, J. A., Curnutte, J. T., and Karnovsky, M. L. (1981): Cis-polyunsaturated fatty acids induce high levels of superoxide production by human neutrophils. *J. Biol. Chem.*, 256:12640–12643.

50. Badwey, J. A., Robinson, J. M., Karnovsky, M. J., and Karnovsky, M. L. (1981): Superoxide production by an unusual aldehyde oxidase in guinea pig granulocytes: characterization and cytochemical localization. *J. Biol. Chem.*, 246:3479–3486.

51. Badwey, J. A., and Karnovsky, M. L. (1983): Properties of NADH-cytochrome-b_5 reductase from human neutrophils. *Blood*, 62:152–157.

52. Badwey, J. A., Curnutte, J. T., Robinson, J. M., Berde, C. B., Karnovsky, M. J., and Karnovsky, M. L. (1984): Effects of free fatty acids on release of superoxide and on change of shape by human neutrophils: reversibility by albumin. *J. Biol. Chem.*, 259:7870–7877.

53. Baehner, R. L., and Johnston, R. B., Jr. (1971): Metabolic and bactericidal activities of human eosinophils. *Br. J. Haematol.*, 20:277–285.

54. Baehner, R. L., and Johnston, R. B. Jr. (1972): Monocyte function in children with neutropenia and chronic infections. *Blood*, 40:31–41.

55. Baehner, R. L., Nathan, D. G., and Castle, W. B. (1971): Oxidant injury of Caucasian glucose-6-phosphate dehydrogenase-deficient red blood cells by phagocytosing leukocytes during infection. *J. Clin. Invest.*, 50:2466–2473.

56. Baehner, R. L., Boxer, L. A., Allen, J. M., and Davis, J. (1977): Auto-oxidation as a basis for altered function by polymorphonuclear leukocytes. *Blood*, 50:327–335.

57. Bainton, D. F. (1980): Changes in peroxidase distribution within organelles of blood monocytes and peritoneal macrophages after surface adherence *in vitro* and *in vivo*. In: *Mononuclear Phagocytes Functional Aspects*, edited by R. van Furth, pp. 61–86. Martinus Nijhoff, The Hague.

58. Bainton, D. F., and Farquhar, M. G. (1970): Segregation and packaging of granule enzymes in eosinophilic leukocytes. *J. Cell Biol.*, 45:54–73.

59. Bainton, D. F., Ullyot, J. L., and Farquhar, M. G. (1971): The development of neutrophilic polymorphonuclear leukocytes in human bone marrow: origin and content of azurophil and specific granules. *J. Exp. Med.*, 134:907–934.

60. Baker, M. S., and Gebicki, J. M. (1984): The effect of pH on the conversion of superoxide to hydroxyl free radicals. *Arch. Biochem. Biophys.*, 234:258–264.

61. Baker, M. S., and Gebicki, J. M. (1986): The effect of pH on yields of hydroxyl radicals produced from superoxide by potential biological iron chelators. *Arch. Biochem. Biophys.*, 246:581–588.

62. Bakkenist, A. R. J., Wever, R., Vulsma, T., Plat, H., and Van Gelder, B. F. (1978): Isolation procedure and some properties of myeloperoxidase from human leukocytes. *Biochim. Biophys. Acta*, 524:45–54.

63. Bakkenist, A. R. J., DeBoer, J. E. G., Plat, H., and Wever, R. (1980): The halide complexes of myeloperoxidase and the mechanism of the halogenation reactions. *Biochim. Biophys. Acta*, 613:337–348.

64. Baldwin, D. A., Jenny, E. R., and Aisen, P. (1984): The effect of human serum transferrin and milk lactoferrin on hydroxyl radical formation from superoxide and hydrogen peroxide. *J. Biol. Chem.*, 259:13391–13394.

65. Banda, M. J., Clark, E. J., and Werb, Z. (1985): Regulation of alpha$_1$ proteinase inhibitor function by rabbit alveolar macrophages: evidence for proteolytic rather than oxidative inactivation. *J. Clin. Invest.*, 75:1758–1762.

66. Bannister, J. V., Bannister, W. H., Hill, H. A. O., and Thornalley, P. J. (1982): Some current aspects of oxygen radicals in biological systems. *Life Chem. Rep.*, 1:49–53.

67. Bannister, J. V., Bannister, W. H., Hill, H. A. O., and Thornalley, P. J. (1982): Enhanced production of hydroxyl radicals by the xan-thine-xanthine oxidase reaction in the presence of lactoferrin. *Biochim. Biophys. Acta*, 715:116–120.

68. Bannister, J. V., Ballavite, P., Serra, M. C., Thornalley, P. J., and Rossi, F. (1982): An EPR study of the production of superoxide radicals by neutrophil NADPH oxidase. *FEBS Lett.*, 145:323–326.

69. Bannister, J. V., Bellavite, P., Davoli, A., Thornalley, P. J., and Rossi, F. (1982): The generation of hydroxyl radicals following superoxide production by neutrophil NADPH oxidase. *FEBS Lett.*, 150:300–302.

70. Bannister, W. H., Bannister, J. V., Searle, A. J. F., and Thornalley, P. J. (1983): The reaction of superoxide radicals with metal picolinate complexes. *Inorg. Chim. Acta*, 78:139–142.

71. Barrette, W. C., Jr., Albrich, J. M., and Hurst, J. K. Hypochlorous acid-promoted loss of metabolic energy in *Escherichia coli*: *Inf. Immun*. (in press).

72. Bass, D. A., and Szejda, P. (1979): Eosinophils versus neutrophils in host defense: killing of newborn larvae of *Trichinella spiralis* by human granulocytes *in vitro. J. Clin. Invest.*, 64:1415–1422.

73. Bass, D. A., and Szejda, P. (1979): Mechanism of killing of newborn larvae of *Trichinella spiralis* by neutrophils and eosinophils: killing by generators of hydrogen peroxide *in vitro. J. Clin. Invest.*, 64:1558–1564.

74. Bearman, S. I., Schwarting, G. A., Kolodny, E. H., and Babior, B. M. (1980): Incorporation of glucosamine by activated human neutrophils: a myeloperoxidase-mediated process. *J. Lab. Clin. Med.*, 96:893–902.

75. Beauchamp, C., and Fridovich, I. (1970): A mechanism for the production of ethylene from methional: the generation of hydroxyl radical by xanthine oxidase. *J. Biol. Chem.*, 245:4641–4646.

76. Becker, E. L. (1986): Leukocyte stimulation: receptor, membrane, and metabolic events. *Fed. Proc.*, 45:2148–2150.

77. Becker, E. L., Kermode, J. C., Naccache, P. H., Yassin, R., Munoz, J. J., Marsh, M. L., Huang, C-K., and Sha'afi, R. I. (1986): Pertussis toxin as a probe of neutrophil activation. *Fed. Proc.*, 45:2151–2155.

78. Behar, D., Czapski, G., Rabani, J., Dorfman, L. M., and Schwarz, H. A. (1970): The acid dissociation constant and decay kinetics of the perhydroxyl radical. *J. Phys. Chem.*, 74:3209–3213.

79. Belding, M. E., Klebanoff, S. J., and Ray, C. G. (1970): Peroxidase-mediated virucidal systems. *Science*, 167:195–196.

80. Bellavite, P., Berton, G., Dri, P., and Soranzo, M. R. (1981): Enzymatic basis of the respiratory burst of guinea pig resident peritoneal macrophages. *J. Reticuloendothel. Soc.*, 29:47–60.

81. Bellavite, P., Cross, A. R., Serra, M. C., Davioli, A., Jones, O. T. G., and Rossi, F. (1983): The cytochrome b and flavin content and properties of the O$_2^-$-forming NADPH oxidase solubilized from activated neutrophils. *Biochim. Biophys. Acta*, 746:40–47.

82. Bellavite, P., Serra, M. C., Davoli, A., Bannister, J. V., and Rossi, F. (1983): The NADPH oxidase of guinea pig polymorphonuclear leucocytes: properties of the deoxycholate extracted enzyme. *Mol. Cell. Biochem.*, 52:17–25.

83. Bellavite, P., Bianca, V. D., Serra, C., Papini, E., and Rossi, F. (1984): NADPH oxidase of neutrophils forms superoxide anion but does not reduce cytochrome C and dichlorophenolindophenol. *FEBS Lett.*, 170:157–161.

84. Bellavite, P., Jones, O. T. G., Cross, A. R., Papini, E., and Rossi, F. (1984): Composition of partially purified NADPH oxidase from pig neutrophils. *Biochem. J.*, 223:639–648.

85. Benatti, U., Morelli, A., Guida, L., and De Flora, A. (1983): The production of activated oxygen species by an interaction of methemoglobin with ascorbate. *Biochem. Biophys. Res. Commun.*, 111:980–987.

86. Berton, G., Bellavite, P., De Nicola, G., Dri, P., and Rossi, F. (1982): Plasma membrane and phagosome localization of the activated NADPH oxidase in elicited peritoneal macrophages of the guinea pig. *J. Pathol.*, 136:241–252.

87. Berton, G., Bellavite, P., Dri, P., De Togni, P., and Rossi, F. (1982): The enzyme responsible for the respiratory burst in elicited guinea pig peritoneal macrophages. *J. Pathol.*, 136:273–290.

88. Berton, G., Cassatella, M., Cabrini, G., and Rossi, F. (1985): Activation of mouse macrophages causes no change in expression and function of phorbol diesters' receptors, but is accompanied by al-

terations in the activity and kinetic parameters of NADPH oxidase. *Immunology*, 54:371–379.

89. Berton, G., Cassatella, M. A., Bellavite, P., and Rossi, F. (1986): Molecular basis of macrophage activation: expression of the low potential cytochrome b and its reduction upon cell stimulation in activated macrophages. *J. Immunol.*, 136:1393–1399.

90. Bielski, B. H. J., and Allen, A. O. (1977): Mechanism of the disproportionation of superoxide radicals. *J. Phys. Chem.*, 81:1048–1050.

91. Bielski, B. H. J., and Richter, H. W. (1977): A study of the superoxide radical chemistry by stopped-flow radiolysis and radiation induced oxygen consumption. *J. Am. Chem. Soc.*, 99:3019–3023.

92. Bielski, B. H. J., and Shiue, G. G. (1979): Reaction rates of superoxide radicals with the essential amino acids. In: *Oxygen Free Radicals and Tissue Damage, Ciba Foundation Symposium 65*, pp. 43–48. Excerpta Medica, Amsterdam.

93. Bielski, B. H. J., Arudi, R. L., and Sutherland, M. W. (1983): A study of the reactivity of HO_2/O_2^- with unsaturated fatty acids. *J. Biol. Chem.*, 258:4759–4761.

94. Bodel, P. T., Nichols, B. A., and Bainton, D. F. (1977): Appearance of peroxidase activity within the rough endoplasmic reticulum of blood monocytes after surface adherence. *J. Exp. Med.*, 145:264–274.

95. Bodel, P. T., Nichols, B. A., and Bainton, D. F. (1978): Difference in peroxidase localization of rabbit peritoneal macrophages after surface adherence. *Am. J. Pathol.*, 91:107–117.

96. Bolscher, B. G. J. M., Plat, H., and Wever, R. (1984): Some properties of human eosinophil peroxidase, a comparison with other peroxidases. *Biochim. Biophys. Acta*, 784:177–186.

97. Bolscher, B. G. J. M., Zoutberg, G. R., Cuperus, R. A., and Wever, R. (1984): Vitamin C stimulates the chlorinating activity of human myeloperoxidase. *Biochim. Biophys. Acta*, 784:189–191.

98. Borregaard, N. (1985): The respiratory burst of phagocytosis: biochemistry and subcellular localization. *Immunol. Lett.*, 11:165–171.

99. Borregaard, N., and Johansen, K. S. (1979): Cytochrome and chronic granulomatous disease. *Lancet*, 1:1397–1398.

100. Borregaard, N., and Juhl, H. (1981): Activation of the glycogenolytic cascade in human polymorphonuclear leucocytes by different phagocytic stimuli. *Eur. J. Clin. Invest.*, 11:257–263.

101. Borregaard, N., and Kragbelle, K. (1980): Role of oxygen in antibody-dependent cytotoxicity mediated by monocytes and neutrophils. *J. Clin. Invest*, 66:676–683.

102. Borregaard, N., and Tauber, A. I. (1984): Subcellular localization of the human neutrophil NADPH oxidase: b-cytochrome and associated flavoprotein. *J. Biol. Chem.*, 259:47–52.

103. Borregaard, N., Johansen, K. S., Taudorff, E., and Wandall, J. H. (1979): Cytochrome b is present in neutrophils from patients with chronic granulomatous disease. *Lancet*, 1:949–951.

104. Borregaard, N., Simons, E. R., and Clark, R. A. (1982): Involvement of cytochrome b-245 in the respiratory burst of human neutrophils. *Infect. Immun.*, 38:1301–1303.

105. Borregaard, N., Cross, A. R., Herlin, T., Jones, O. T. G., Segal, A. W., and Valerius, N. H. (1983): A variant form of X-linked chronic granulomatous disease with normal nitroblue tetrazolium slide test and cytochrome b. *Eur. J. Clin. Invest.*, 13:243–247.

106. Borregaard, N., Heiple, J. M., Simons, E. R., and Clark, R. A. (1983): Subcellular localization of the b-cytochrome component of the human neutrophil microbicidal oxidase—translocation during activation. *J. Cell Biol.*, 97:52–61.

107. Bors, W., Lengfelder, E., Saran, M., Fuchs, C., and Michel, C. (1976): Reactions of oxygen radical species with methional: a pulse radiolysis study. *Biochem. Biophys. Res. Commun.*, 70:81–87.

108. Bos, A., Wever, R., and Roos, D. (1978): Characterization and quantification of the peroxidase in human monocytes. *Biochim. Biophys. Acta*, 525:37–44.

109. Boxer, L. A., Coats, T. D., Haak, R. A., Wolach, J. B., Hoffstein, S., and Baehner, R. L. (1982): Lactoferrin deficiency associated with altered granulocyte function. *N. Engl. J. Med.*, 307:404–410.

110. Brandt, S. J., Dougherty, R. W., Lapetina, E. G., and Niedel, J. E. (1985): Pertussis toxin inhibits chemotactic peptide-stimulated generation of inositol phosphates and lysosomal enzyme secretion

in human leukemic (HL-60) cells. *Proc. Natl. Acad. Sci. USA*, 82:3277–3280.

111. Breslow, R., and Lukens, L. N. (1960): On the mechanism of action of an ascorbic acid-dependent nonenzymatic hydroxylating system. *J. Biol. Chem.*, 235:292–296.

112. Breton-Gorius, J., Guichard, J., Vainchenker, W., and Vilde, J. L. (1980): Ultrastructural and cytochemical changes induced by short and prolonged culture of human monocytes. *J. Reticuloendothel. Soc.*, 27:289–301.

113. Briggs, R. T., Karnovsky, M. L., and Karnovsky, M. J. (1975): Cytochemical demonstration of hydrogen peroxide in the polymorphonuclear leukocyte phagosomes. *J. Cell Biol.*, 64:254–260.

114. Briggs, R. T., Drath, D. B., Karnovsky, M. L., and Karnovsky, M. J. (1975): Localization of NADH oxidase on the surface of human polymorphonuclear leukocytes by a new cytochemical method. *J. Cell Biol.*, 67:566–586.

115. Britigan, B. E., Rosen, G. M., Chai, Y., and Cohen, M. S. (1986): Do human neutrophils make hydroxyl radical? Determination of free radicals generated by human neutrophils activated with a soluble or particulate stimulus using electron paramagnetic resonance spectrometry. *J. Biol. Chem.*, 261:4426–4431.

116. Bromberg, Y., and Pick, E. (1984): Unsaturated fatty acids stimulate NADPH-dependent superoxide production by cell-free system derived from macrophages. *Cell. Immunol.*, 88:213–221.

117. Bromberg, Y., and Pick, E. (1985): Activation of NADPH-dependent superoxide production in a cell-free system by sodium dodecyl sulfate. *J. Biol. Chem.*, 260:13539–13545.

118. Brozna, J. P., Senior, R. M., Kreutzer, D. L., and Ward, P. A. (1977): Chemotactic factor inactivators of human granulocytes. *J. Clin. Invest.*, 60:1280–1288.

119. Bruce, M., Boat, T., Martin, R. J., Dearborn, D., and Fanaroff, A. (1982): Proteinase inhibitors and inhibitor inactivation of neonatal airways secretions. *Chest*, 81(Suppl.):44S–45S.

120. Buettner, G. R., Oberley, L. W., and Chan Leuthauser, S. W. H. (1978): The effect of iron on the distribution of superoxide and hydroxyl radicals as seen by spin trapping and on the superoxide dismutase assay. *Photochem. Photobiol.*, 28:693–695.

121. Buettner, G. R., Doherty, T. P., and Patterson, L. K. (1983): The kinetics of the reaction of superoxide radical with Fe(III) complexes of EDTA, DETAPAC and HEDTA. *FEBS Lett.*, 158:143–146.

122. Bujak, J. S., and Root, R. K. (1974): The role of peroxidase in the bactericidal activity of human blood eosinophils. *Blood*, 43:727–736.

123. Bull, C., McClune, J., and Fee, J. A. (1983): The mechanisms of Fe-EDTA catalyzed dismutation. *J. Am. Chem. Soc.*, 105:5290–5300.

124. Butler, J., and Halliwell, B. (1982): Reaction of iron-EDTA chelates with the superoxide radical. *Arch. Biochem. Biophys.*, 218:174–178.

125. Buys, J., Wever, R., van Stigt, R., and Ruitenberg, E. J. (1981): The killing of newborn larvae of *Trichinella spiralis* by eosinophil peroxidase *in vitro*. *Eur. J. Immunol.*, 11:843–845.

126. Buys, J., Wever, R., and Ruitenberg, E. J. (1984): Myeloperoxidase is more efficient than eosinophil peroxidase in the *in vitro* killing of newborn larvae of *Trichinella spiralis*. *Immunology*, 51:601–607.

127. Carlson, M. G. Ch., Peterson, C. G. B., and Venge, P. (1985): Human eosinophil peroxidase: purification and characterization. *J. Immunol.*, 134:1875–1879.

128. Carp, H., and Janoff, A. (1979): *In vitro* suppression of serum elastase-inhibitory capacity by reactive oxygen species generated by phagocytosing polymorphonuclear leukocytes. *J. Clin. Invest.*, 63:793–797.

129. Carp, H., and Janoff, A. (1980): Potential mediator of inflammation: phagocyte-derived oxidants suppress the elastase-inhibitory capacity of alpha₁-proteinase inhibitor *in vitro*. *J. Clin. Invest.*, 66:987–995.

130. Carp, H., Miller, F., Hoidal, J. R., and Janoff, A. (1982): Potential mechanism of emphysema: α_1-proteinase inhibitor recovered from lungs of cigarette smokers contains oxidized methionine and has decreased elastase inhibitory activity. *Proc. Natl. Acad. Sci. USA*, 79:2041–2045.

131. Carp, H., Janoff, A., Abrams, W., Weinbaum, G., Drew, R. T.,

Weissbach, H., and Brot, N. (1983): Human methionine sulfoxide-peptide reductase, an enzyme capable of reactivating oxidized alpha-1-proteinase inhibitor *in vitro. Am. Rev. Respir. Dis.,* 127:301–305.

132. Cassetella, M. A., Della Bianca, V., Berton, G., and Rossi, F. (1985): Activation by gamma interferon of human macrophage capability to produce toxic oxygen molecules is accompanied by decreased Km of the superoxide-generating NADPH oxidase. *Biochem. Biophys. Res. Commun.,* 132:908–914.

133. Cech, P., Papathanassiou, A., Boreux, G., Roth, P., and Miescher, P. A. (1979): Hereditary myeloperoxidase deficiency. *Blood,* 53:403–411.

134. Cederbaum, A. I., and Dicker, E. (1983): Inhibition of microsomal oxidation of alcohols and of hydroxyl-radical-scavenging agents by the iron-chelating agent desferrioxamine. *Biochem. J.,* 210:107–113.

135. Chang, K.-P. (1981): Leishmanicidal mechanisms of human polymorphonuclear phagocytes. *Am. J. Trop. Med. Hyg.,* 30:322–333.

136. Chaudhry, A. N., Santinga, J. T., and Gabig, T. G. (1982): The subcellular particulate NADPH-dependent O_2^--generating oxidase from human blood monocytes: comparison to the neutrophil system. *Blood,* 60:979–983.

137. Cheson, B. D., Christensen, R. L., Sperling, R., Kohler, B. E., and Babior, B. M. (1976): The origin of the chemiluminescence of phagocytosing granulocytes. *J. Clin. Invest.,* 58:789–796.

138. Chi, E. Y., and Henderson, W. R. (1984): Ultrastructure of mast cell degranulation induced by eosinophil peroxidase: use of diaminobenzidine cytochemistry by scanning electron microscopy. *J. Histochem. Cytochem.,* 32:332–341.

139. Clark, R. A. (1982): Chemotactic factors trigger their own oxidative inactivation by human neutrophils. *J. Immunol.,* 129:2725–2728.

140. Clark, R. A. (1983): Extracellular effects of the myeloperoxidase-hydrogen peroxide-halide system. In: *Advances in Inflammation Research, Vol. 5,* edited by G. Weissmann, pp. 107–146. Raven Press, New York.

141. Clark, R. A. (1986): Oxidative inactivation of pneumolysin by the myeloperoxidase system and stimulated human neutrophils. *J. Immunol.,* 136:4617–4622.

142. Clark, R. A., and Borregaard, N. (1985): Neutrophils autoinactivate secretory products by myeloperoxidase-catalyzed oxidation. *Blood,* 65:375–381.

143. Clark, R. A., and Klebanoff, S. J. (1975): Neutrophil mediated tumor cell cytotoxicity: role of the peroxidase system. *J. Exp. Med.,* 141:1442–1447.

144. Clark, R. A., and Klebanoff, S. J. (1977): Myeloperoxidase-H_2O_2-halide system: cytotoxic effect on human blood leukocytes. *Blood,* 50:65–70.

145. Clark, R. A., and Klebanoff, S. J. (1977): Studies on the mechanism of antibody-dependent polymorphonuclear leukocyte-mediated cytotoxicity. *J. Immunol.,* 119:1413–1418.

146. Clark, R. A., and Klebanoff, S. J. (1979): Myeloperoxidase-mediated platelet release reaction. *J. Clin. Invest.,* 63:177–183.

147. Clark, R. A., and Klebanoff, S. J. (1979): Chemotactic factor inactivation by the myeloperoxidase-hydrogen peroxide-halide system: an inflammatory control mechanism. *J. Clin. Invest.,* 64:913–920.

148. Clark, R. A., and Klebanoff, S. J. (1979): Role of the myeloperoxidase-H_2O_2-halide system in concanavalin A-induced tumor cell killing by human neutrophils. *J. Immunol.,* 122:2605–2610.

149. Clark, R. A., and Klebanoff, S. J. (1980): Neutrophil-platelet interaction mediated by myeloperoxidase and hydrogen peroxide. *J. Immunol.,* 124:399–405.

150. Clark, R. A., and Szot, S. (1981): The myeloperoxidase-hydrogen peroxide-halide system as effector of neutrophil-mediated tumor cell cytotoxicity. *J. Immunol.,* 126:1295–1301.

151. Clark, R. A., and Szot, S. (1982): Chemotactic factor inactivation by stimulated human neutrophils mediated by myeloperoxidase-catalyzed methionine oxidation. *J. Immunol.,* 128:1507–1513.

152. Clark, R. A., Klebanoff, S. J., Einstein, A. B., and Fefer, A. (1975): Peroxidase-H_2O_2-halide system: cytotoxic effect on mammalian tumor cells. *Blood,* 45:161–170.

153. Clark, R. A., Szot, S., Venkatasubramanian, K., and Schiffmann,

E. (1980): Chemotactic factor inactivation by myeloperoxidase-mediated oxidation of methionine. *J. Immunol.,* 124:2020–2026.

154. Clark, R. A., Stone, P. J., El Hag, A., Calore, J. D., and Franzblau, C. (1981): Myeloperoxidase-catalyzed inactivation of α_1-protease inhibitor by human neutrophils. *J. Biol. Chem.,* 256:3348–3353.

155. Clark, R. A., Szot, S., Williams, M. A., and Kagan, H. M. (1986): Oxidation of lysine side-chains of elastin by the myeloperoxidase system and by stimulated human neutrophils. *Biochem. Biophys. Res. Commun.,* 135:451–457.

156. Cline, M. J. (1972): Microbicidal activity of human eosinphils. *J. Reticuloendothel. Soc.,* 12:332–339.

157. Cline, M. J., Hanifin, J., and Lehrer, R. I. (1968): Phagocytosis by human eosinophils. *Blood,* 32:922–934.

158. Coble, B-I., Lindroth, M., Molin, L., and Stendahl, O. (1984): Histamine release from mast cells during phagocytosis and interaction with activated neutrophils. *Int. Arch. Allergy Appl. Immunol.,* 75:32–37.

159. Coble, B-I., Dahlgren, C., Hed, J., and Stendahl, O. (1984): Myeloperoxidase reduces the opsonizing activity of immunoglobulin G and complement component C3b. *Biochim. Biophys. Acta,* 802:501–505.

160. Cochrane, C. G., Spragg, R. G., and Revak, S. D. (1983): Studies on the pathogenesis of the adult respiratory distress syndrome: evidence of oxidant activity in bronchoalveolar lavage fluid. *J. Clin. Invest.,* 71:754–761.

161. Cochrane, C. G., Spragg, R. G., Revak, S. D., Cohen, A. B., and McGuire, W. W. (1983): The presence of neutrophil elastase and evidence of oxidant activity of bronchoalveolar lavage fluid of patients with adult respiratory distress syndrome. *Am. Rev. Respir. Dis.,* 127:S25–S27.

162. Cohen, G., and Sinet, P. M. (1980): Fenton's reagent-once more revisited. *Dev. Biochem.,* 11A:27–37.

163. Cohen, G., and Somerson, N. L. (1969): Glucose-dependent secretion and destruction of hydrogen peroxide by *Mycoplasma pneumoniae. J. Bacteriol.,* 98:547–551.

164. Cohen, H. J., Newburger, P. E., Chovaniec, M. E., Whitin, J. C., and Simons, E. R. (1981): Opsonized zymosan-stimulated granulocytes—activation and activity of the superoxide generating system and membrane potential changes. *Blood,* 58:975–982.

165. Cohen, H. J., Chovaniec, M. E., Takahashi, K., and Whitin, J. C. (1986): Activation of human granulocytes by arachidonic acid: its use and limitations for investigating granulocyte functions. *Blood,* 67:1103–1109.

166. Cohen, M. S., Taffet, S. M., and Adams, D. O. (1982): The relationship between competence for secretion of H_2O_2 and completion of tumor cytotoxicity by BCG-elicited murine macrophages. *J. Immunol.,* 128:1781–1785.

167. Cohn, Z. A. (1983): The macrophage—versatile element of inflammation. *Harvey Lect.,* 77:63–80.

168. Cole, B. C., Ward, J. R., and Martin, C. H. (1968): Hemolysin and peroxide activity of Mycoplasma species. *J. Bacteriol.,* 95:2022–2030.

169. Collins, S. J., Ruscetti, F. W., Gallagher, R. E., and Gallo, R. C. (1978): Terminal differentiation of human promyelocytic leukemia cells induced by dimethyl sulfoxide and other polar compounds. *Proc. Natl. Acad. Sci. USA,* 75:2458–2462.

170. Cotran, R. S., and Litt, M. (1969): The entry of granule-associated peroxidase into the phagocytic vacuole of eosinophils. *J. Exp. Med.,* 129:1291–1306.

171. Cox, J. A., Jeng, A. Y., Sharkey, N. A., Blumberg, P. M., and Tauber, A. I. (1985): Activation of the human neutrophil nicotinamide adenine dinucleotide phosphate (NADPH)-oxidase by protein kinase C. *J. Clin. Invest.,* 76:1932–1938.

172. Cox, C. C., Dougherty, R. W., Ganong, B. R., Bell, R. M., Niedel, J. E., and Snyderman, R. (1986): Differential stimulation of the respiratory burst and lysosomal enzyme secretion in human polymorphonuclear leukocytes by synthetic diacylglycerols. *J. Immunol.,* 136:4611–4616.

173. Cramer, R., Soranzo, M. R., and Patriarca, P. (1981): Evidence that eosinophils catalyze the bromide-dependent decarboxylation of amino acids. *Blood,* 58:1112–1118.

174. Cramer, R., Soranzo, M. R., Dri, P., Rottini, G. D., Bramezza,

M., Cirielli, S., and Patriarca, P. (1982): Incidence of myeloperoxidase deficiency in an area of northern Italy: histochemical, biochemical and functional studies. *Br. J. Haematol.*, 51:81–87.

175. Crawford, D. R., and Schneider, D. L. (1981): Evidence that a quinone may be required for the production of superoxide and hydrogen peroxide in neutrophils. *Biochem. Biophys. Res. Commun.*, 99:1277–1286.

176. Crawford, D. R., and Schneider, D. L. (1982): Identification of ubiquinone-50 in human neutrophils and its role in microbicidal events. *J. Biol. Chem.*, 257:6662–6668.

177. Crawford, D. R., and Schneider, D. L. (1983): Ubiquinone content and respiratory burst activity of latex-filled phagolysosomes isolated from human neutrophils and evidence for the probable involvement of a third granule. *J. Biol. Chem.*, 258:5363–5367.

178. Cross, A. R., Jones, O. T. G., Harper, A. M., and Segal, A. W. (1981): Oxidation-reduction properties of the cytochrome b found in the plasma-membrane fraction of human neutrophils: a possible oxidase in the respiratory burst. *Biochem. J.*, 194:599–606.

179. Cross, A. R., Higson, F. K., Jones, O. T. G., Harper, A. M., and Segal, A. W. (1982): The enzymic reduction and kinetics of oxidation of cytochrome b$_{-245}$ of neutrophils. *Biochem. J.*, 204:479–485.

180. Cross, A. R., Jones, O. T. G., Garcia, R., and Segal, A. W. (1982): The association of FAD with the cytochrome b$_{-245}$ of human neutrophils. *Biochem. J.*, 208:759–763.

181. Cross, A. R., Jones, O. T. G., Garcia, R., and Segal, A. W. (1983): The subcellular localization of ubiquinone in human neutrophils. *Biochem. J.*, 216:765–768.

182. Cross, A. R., Parkinson, J. F., and Jones, O. T. G. (1984): The superoxide-generating oxidase of leucocytes: NADPH-dependent reduction of flavin and cytochrome b in solubilized preparations. *Biochem. J.*, 223:337–344.

183. Cunningham, C. C., DeChatelet, L. R., Spach, P. I., Parce, J. W., Thomas, M. J., Lees, C. J., and Shirley, P. S. (1982): Identification and quantitation of electron-transport components in human polymorphonuclear neutrophils. *Biochim. Biophys. Acta*, 682:430–435.

184. Curnutte, J. T. (1985): Activation of human neutrophil nicotinamide adenine dinucleotide phosphate, reduced (triphosphopyridine nucleotide, reduced) oxidase by arachidonic acid in a cell-free system. *J. Clin. Invest.*, 75:1740–1743.

185. Curnutte, J. T., and Tauber, A. I. (1983): Failure to detect superoxide in human neutrophils stimulated with latex particles. *Pediatr. Res.*, 17:281–284.

186. Curnutte, J. T., Badway, J. A., Robinson, J. M., Karnovsky, M. J., and Karnovsky, M. L. (1984): Studies on the mechanism of superoxide release from human neutrophils stimulated with arachidonate. *J. Biol. Chem.*, 259:11851–11857.

187. Czapski, G., and Ilan, Y. A. (1978): On the generation of the hydroxylation agent from the superoxide radical: can the Haber-Weiss reaction be the source of ·OH radicals? *Photochem. Photobiol.*, 28:651–653.

188. Czuprynski, C. J., Campbell, P. A., and Henson, P. M. (1983): Killing of *Listeria monocytogenes* by human neutrophils and monocytes, but not by monocyte-derived macrophages. *J. Reticuloendothel. Soc.*, 34:29–44.

189. Daems, W. Th., and van der Rhee, H. J. (1980): Peroxidase and catalase in monocytes, macrophages, epithelioid cells and giant cells of the rat. In: *Mononuclear Phagocytes. Functional Aspects*, edited by R. van Furth, pp. 43–60. Martinus Nijhoff, The Hague.

190. Daems, W. T., Poelmann, R. E., and Brederoo, P. (1973): Peroxidatic activity in resident peritoneal macrophages and exudate monocytes of the guinea pig after ingestion of latex particles. *J. Histochem. Cytochem.*, 21:93–95.

191. Dale, M. M., and Penfield, A. (1984): Synergism between phorbol ester and A23187 in superoxide production by neutrophils. *FEBS Lett.*, 175:170–172.

192. Dallegri, F., Frumento, G., and Patrone, F. (1983): Mechanisms of tumour cell destruction by PMA-activated human neutrophils. *Immunology*, 48:273–279.

193. Dallegri, F., Patrone, F., Frumento, G., Banchi, L., and Succhetti, C. (1984): Phagocytosis-dependent neutrophil-mediated extracellular cytotoxicity against different target cells. *Acta Haematol. (Basel)*, 71:371–375.

194. Daniels, C. A., Kleinerman, E. S., and Snyderman, R. (1978): Abortive and productive infections of human mononuclear phagocytes by type I herpes simplex virus. *Am. J. Pathol.*, 91:119–130.

195. Danley, D. L., Hilger, A. E., and Winkel, C. A. (1983): Generation of hydrogen peroxide by *Candida albicans* and influence on murine polymorphonuclear leukocyte activity. *Infect. Immun.*, 40:97–102.

196. Davis, J. C., and Averill, B. A. (1981): Isolation from bovine spleen of a green heme protein with properties of myeloperoxidase. *J. Biol. Chem.*, 256:5992–5996.

197. DeChatelet, L. R., Cooper, M. R., and McCall, C. E. (1972): Stimulation of the hexosemonophosphate shunt in human neutrophils by ascorbic acid: mechanism of action. *Antimicrob. Agents Chemother.*, 1:12–16.

198. DeChatelet, L. R., Shirley, P. S., McPhail, L. C., Huntley, C. C., Muss, H. B., and Bass, D. A. (1977): Oxidative metabolism of the human eosinophil. *Blood*, 50:525–535.

199. DeChatelet, L. R., Migler, R. A., Shirley, P. S., Muss, H. B., Szejda, P., and Bass, D. A. (1978): Comparison of intracellular bactericidal activities of human neutrophils and eosinophils. *Blood*, 52:609–617.

200. DeChatelet, L. R., Long, G. D., Shirley, P. S., Bass, D. A., Thomas, M. J., Henderson, F. W., and Cohen, M. S. (1982): Mechanism of the luminol-dependent chemiluminescence of human neutrophils. *J. Immunol.*, 129:1589–1593.

201. Deimann, W., Seitz, M., Gemsa, D., and Fahimi, H. D. (1984): Endogenous peroxidase in the nuclear envelope and endoplasmic reticulum of human monocytes *in vitro*: association with arachidonic acid metabolism. *Blood*, 64:491–498.

202. Desser, R. K., Himmelhoch, S. R., Evans, W. H., Januska, M., Mage, M., and Shelton, E. (1972): Guinea pig heterophil and eosinophil peroxidase. *Arch. Biochem. Biophys.*, 148:452–465.

203. Dewald, B., Baggiolini, M., Curnutte, J. T., and Babior, B. M. (1979): Subcellular localization of the superoxide-forming enzyme in human neutrophils. *J. Clin. Invest.*, 63:21–29.

204. Dewald, B., Bretz, U., and Baggiolini, M. (1982): Release of gelatinase from a novel secretory compartment of human neutrophils. *J. Clin. Invest.*, 70:518–525.

205. Dewald, B., Payne, T. G., and Baggiolini, M. (1984): Activation of NADPH oxidase of human neutrophils: potentiation of chemotactic peptide by a diacylglycerol. *Biochem. Biophys. Res. Commun.*, 125:367–373.

206. Diamond, R. D., and Bennett, J. E. (1973): Growth of *Cryptococcus neoformans* within human macrophages *in vitro*. *Infect. Immun.*, 7:231–236.

207. Diamond, R. D., and Clark, R. A. (1982): Damage to *Aspergillus fumigatus* and *Rizopus oryzae hyphae* by oxidative and non oxidative microbicidal products of human neutrophils *in vitro*. *Infect. Immun.*, 38:487–495.

208. Diamond, R. D., and Haudenschild, C. C. (1981): Monocyte-mediated serum-independent damage to hyphal and pseudohyphal forms of *Candida albicans in vitro*. *J. Clin. Invest.*, 67:173–182.

209. Diamond, R. D., and Krzesicki, R. (1978): Mechanisms of attachment of neutrophils to *Candida albicans* pseudohyphae in the absence of serum, and of subsequent damage to pseudohyphae by microbicidal processes of neutrophils *in vitro*. *J. Clin. Invest.*, 61:360–369.

210. Diamond, R. D., Root, R. K., and Bennett, J. E. (1972): Factors influencing killing of *Cryptococcus neoformans* by human leukocytes *in vitro*. *J. Infect. Dis.*, 125:367–376.

211. Diamond, R. D., Krzesicki, R., and Jao, W. (1978): Damage to pseudohyphyl forms of *Candida albicans* by neutrophils in the absence of serum *in vitro*. *J. Clin. Invest.*, 61:349–359.

212. Diamond, R. D., Krzesicki, R., Epstein, B., and Jao, W. (1978): Damage to hyphal forms of fungi by human leukocytes *in vitro*: a possible host defense mechanism in aspergillosis and mucormycosis. *Am. J. Pathol.*, 91:313–328.

213. Diamond, R. D., Clark, R. A., and Haudenschild, C. C. (1980): Damage to *Candida albicans* hyphae and pseudohyphae by the myeloperoxidase system and oxidative products of neutrophil metabolism *in vitro*. *J. Clin. Invest.*, 66:908–917.

214. Diamond, R. D., Huber, E., and Haudenschild, C. C. (1983): Mechanisms of destruction of *Aspergillus fumigatus* hypae mediated by human monocytes. *J. Infect. Dis.,* 147:474–483.

215. Diguiseppi, J., and Fridovich, I. (1980): Ethylene from 2-keto-4-thiomethyl butyric acid: the Haber-Weiss reaction. *Arch. Biochem. Biophys.,* 205:323–329.

216. DiGuiseppi, J., and Fridovich, I. (1982): Oxygen toxicity in *Streptococcus sanguis:* the relative importance of superoxide and hydroxyl radicals. *J. Biol. Chem.,* 257:4046–4051.

217. DiVirgilio, F., Lew, D. P., and Pozzan, T. (1984): Protein kinase C activation of physiological processes in human neutrophils at vanishingly small cytosolic Ca^{2+} levels. *Nature,* 310:691–693.

218. Dorfman, L. M., and Adams, G. E. (1973): Reactivity of the hydroxyl radical in aqueous solutions. In: *National Standard Reference Data System, National Bureau of Standards,* No. 46, pp. 1–59.

219. Dougherty, R. W., Godfrey, P. P., Hoyle, P. C., Putney, J. M., Jr., and Freer, R. J. (1984): Secretagogue-induced phosphoinositide metabolism in human leukocytes. *Biochem. J.,* 222:307–314.

220. Doussiere, J., and Vignais, P. V. (1985): Purification and properties of an O$_2^-$-generating oxidase from bovine polymorphonuclear neutrophils. *Biochemistry,* 24:7231–7239.

221. Drath, D. V., and Karnovsky, M. L. (1974): Bactericidal activity of metal-mediated peroxide-ascorbate systems. *Infect. Immun.,* 10:1077–1083.

222. Drath, D. B., Karnovsky, M. L., and Huber, G. L. (1979): Hydroxyl radical formation in phagocytic cells of the rat. *J. Appl. Physiol.,* 46:136–140.

223. Dvorak, A. M., Klebanoff, S. J., Henderson, W. R., Monahan, R. A., Pyne, K., and Galli, S. J. (1985): Vesicular uptake of eosinophil peroxidase by guinea pig basophils and by cloned mouse mast cells and granule-containing lymphoid cells. *Am. J. Pathol.,* 118:425–438.

224. Edelson, P. J., and Cohn, Z. A. (1973): Peroxidase-mediated mammalian cell cytotoxicity. *J. Exp. Med.,* 138:318–323.

225. Edwards, D. L., and Unger, B. W. (1980): Inhibition of the respiratory burst of human polymorphonuclear leukocytes by phenothiazine drugs. *Biochem. Int.,* 1:364–370.

226. Eglinton, D. G., Barber, D., Thomson, A. J., Greenwood, C., and Segal, A. W. (1982): Studies of cyanide binding to myeloperoxidase by electron paramagnetic resonance and magnetic circular dichroism spectroscopies. *Biochim. Biophys. Acta,* 703:187–195.

227. El-Hag, A., and Clark, R. A. (1984): Down-regulation of human natural killer activity against tumors by the neutrophil myeloperoxidase system and hydrogen peroxide. *J. Immunol.,* 133:3291–3297.

228. El-Hag, A., Lipsky, P. E., Bennett, M., and Clark, R. A. (1986): Immunomodulation by neutrophil myeloperoxidase and hydrogen peroxide: differential susceptibility of human lymphocyte functions. *J. Immunol.,* 136:3420–3426.

229. Ericsson, Y., and Lundbeck, H. (1955): Antimicrobial effect *in vitro* of the ascorbic acid oxidation. I. Effect on bacteria, fungi and viruses in pure culture. *Acta Pathol. Microbiol. Scand.,* 37:493–506.

230. Escribano, L. M., Gabriel, L. C., Sainz, T., Rocamora, A., Arrazola, J. M., and Navarro, J. L. (1984): Peroxidase activity in human cutaneous mast cells: an ultrastructural demonstration. *J. Histochem. Cytochem.,* 32:573–578.

231. Fee, J. A. (1980): Is superoxide toxic? *Dev. Biochem.,* 11B:41–48.

232. Fenton, H. J. H. (1894): Oxidation of tartaric acid in the presence of iron. *J. Chem. Soc.,* 65:899–910.

233. Finkelstein, E., Rosen, G. M., Rauckman, E. J., and Paxton, J. (1979): Spin trapping of superoxide. *Mol. Pharmacol.,* 16:676–685.

234. Finkelstein, E., Rosen, G. M., and Rauckman, E. J. (1980): Spin trapping: kinetics of the reaction of superoxide and hydroxyl radicals with nitrones. *J. Am. Chem. Soc.,* 102:4994–4999.

235. Finkelstein, E., Rosen, G. M., and Rauckman, E. J. (1980): Spin trapping of superoxide and hydroxyl radical: practical aspects. *Arch. Biochem. Biophys.,* 200:1–16.

236. Finkelstein, E., Rosen, G. M., and Rauckman, E. J. (1982): Production of hydroxyl radical by decomposition of superoxide spin-trapped adducts. *Mol. Pharmacol.,* 21:262–265.

237. Fleer, A., Roos, D., von dem Borne, A. E. G. Kr., and Engelfriet, C. P. (1979): Cytotoxic activity of human monocytes toward sensitized red cells is not dependent on the generation of reactive oxygen species. *Blood,* 54:407–411.

238. Flitter, W. A., Rowley, D., and Halliwell, B. (1983): Superoxide-dependent formation of hydroxyl radicals in the presence of iron salts: what is the physiological iron chelator? *FEBS Lett.,* 158:310–312.

239. Floyd, R. A. (1981): DNA-ferrous iron catalyzed hydroxyl free radical formation from hydrogen peroxide. *Biochem. Biophys. Res. Commun.,* 99:1209–1215.

240. Floyd, R. A. (1983): Direct demonstration that ferrous ion complexes of di- and triphosphate nucleotides catalyse hydroxyl free radical formation from hydrogen peroxide. *Arch. Biochem. Biophys.,* 225:263–270.

241. Floyd, R. A., and Lewis, C. A. (1983): Hydroxyl free radical formation from hydrogen peroxide by ferrous iron-nucleotide complexes. *Biochemistry,* 22:2645–2649.

242. Foote, C. S. (1976): Photosensitized oxidation and singlet oxygen: consequences in biological systems. In: *Free Radicals in Biology, Vol. 2,* edited by W. A. Pryor, pp. 85–133. Academic Press, New York.

243. Foote, C. S. (1979): Detection of singlet oxygen in complex systems: a critique. In: *Biochemical and Clinical Aspects of Oxygen,* edited by W. S. Caughey, pp. 603–625. Academic Press, New York.

244. Foote, C. S., Shook, F. C., and Abakerli, R. B. (1980): Chemistry of superoxide ion. 4. Singlet oxygen is not a major product of dismutation. *J. Am. Chem. Soc.,* 102:2503–2504.

245. Foote, C. S., Abakerli, R. B., Clough, R. L., and Shook, F. C. (1980): On the question of singlet oxygen production in leukocytes, macrophages and the dismutation of superoxide anion. *Dev. Biochem.,* 11B:222–230.

246. Foote, C. S., Abakerli, R. B., Clough, R. L., and Lehrer, R. I. (1980): On the question of singlet oxygen production in polymorphonuclear leucocytes. In: *Bioluminescence and Chemiluminescence,* edited by M. A. DeLuca and W. D. McElroy, pp. 81–88. Academic Press, New York.

247. Foote, C. S., Goyne, T. E., and Lehrer, R. I. (1983): Assessment of chlorination by human neutrophils. *Nature,* 301:715–716.

248. Forman, H. J., Nelson, J., and Fisher, A. B. (1980): Rat alveolar macrophages require NADPH for superoxide production in the respiratory burst: effect of NADPH depletion by paraquat. *J. Biol. Chem.,* 255:9879–9883.

249. Fridovich, I. (1970): Quantitative aspects of the production of superoxide anion radical by milk xanthine oxidase. *J. Biol. Chem.,* 245:4053–4057.

250. Fridovich, I. (1983): Superoxide radical: an endogenous toxicant. *Annu. Rev. Pharmacol. Toxicol.,* 23:239–257.

251. Frimer, A. A., Forman, A., and Borg, D. C. (1983): H$_2$O$_2$-diffusion through lysosomes. *Isr. J. Chem.,* 23:442–445.

252. Fujita, I., Irita, K., Takeshige, K., and Minakami, S. (1984): Diacylglycerol, 1-oleoyl-2-acetyl-glycerol, stimulates superoxide-generation from human neutrophils. *Biochem. Biophys. Res. Commun.,* 120:318–324.

253. Furth, R., van, Hirsch, J. G., and Fedorko, M. E. (1970): Morphology and peroxidase cytochemistry of mouse promonocytes, monocytes and macrophages. *J. Exp. Med.,* 132:794–812.

254. Gabig, T. G. (1983): The NADPH-dependent O$_2^-$-generating oxidase from human neutrophils: identification of a flavoprotein component that is deficient in a patient with chronic granulomatous disease. *J. Biol. Chem.,* 258:6352–6356.

255. Gabig, T. G., and Babior, B. M. (1979): The O$_2^-$ forming oxidase responsible for the respiratory burst in human neutrophils: properties of the solubilized enzyme. *J. Biol. Chem.,* 254:9070–9074.

256. Gabig, T. G., and Lefker, B. A. (1984): Deficient flavoprotein component of the NADPH-dependent O$_2^-$ generating oxidase in the neutrophils from three male patients with chronic granulomatous disease. *J. Clin. Invest.,* 73:701–705.

257. Gabig, T. G., and Lefker, B. A. (1985): Activation of the human neutrophil NADPH oxidase results in coupling of electron carrier function between ubiquinone and cytochrome b$_{559}$. *J. Biol. Chem.,* 260:3991–3995.

258. Gabig, T. G., Kipnes, R. S., and Babior, B. M. (1978): Solubilization

of the O_2^--forming activity responsible for the respiratory burst in human neutrophils. *J. Biol. Chem.*, 253:6663–6665.

259. Gabig, T. G., Schervish, E. W., and Santinga, J. T. (1982): Functional relationship of the cytochrome b to the superoxide-generating oxidase of human neutrophils. *J. Biol. Chem.*, 257:4114–4119.

260. Gallin, J. I., Wright, D. G., and Schiffmann, E. (1978): Role of secretory events in modulating human neutrophil chemotaxis. *J. Clin. Invest.*, 62:1364–1374.

261. Garcia, R. C., and Segal, A. W. (1984): Changes in the subcellular distribution of the cytochrome b_{-245} on stimulation of human neutrophils. *Biochem. J.*, 219:233–242.

262. Gately, C. L., Wahl, S. M., and Oppenheim, J. J. (1983): Characterization of hydrogen peroxide-potentiating factor: a lymphokine that increases the capacity of human monocytes and monocyte-like cell lines to produce hydrogen peroxide. *J. Immunol.*, 131: 2853–2858.

263. Gebicki, J. M., and Bielski, B. H. J. (1981): Comparison of the capacities of the perhydroxyl and the superoxide radicals to initiate chain oxidation of linoleic acid. *J. Am. Chem. Soc.*, 103:7020–7022.

264. Gee, J. B. L., Vassallo, C. L., Bell, P., Kaskin, J., Basford, R. E., and Field, J. B. (1970): Catalase-dependent peroxidative metabolism in the alveolar macrophage during phagocytosis. *J. Clin. Invest.*, 49:1280–1287.

265. Gee, J. B. L., Kaskin, J., Duncombe, M. P., and Vassallo, C. L. (1974): The effect of ethanol on some metabolic features of phagocytosis in the alveolar macrophage. *J. Reticuloendothel. Soc.*, 15: 61–68.

266. Gennaro, R., and Romeo, D. (1979): The release of superoxide anion from granulocytes: effect of inhibitors of anion permeability. *Biochem. Biophys. Res. Commun.*, 88:44–49.

267. Gennaro, R., Possan, T., and Romeo, D. (1984): Monitoring of cytosolic free Ca^{2+} in C5a-stimulated neutrophils: loss of receptor-modulated Ca^{2+} stores and Ca^{2+} uptake in granule-free cytoplasts. *Proc. Natl. Acad. Sci. USA*, 81:1416–1420.

268. Gennaro, R., Florio, C., and Romeo, D. (1985): Activation of protein kinase C in neutrophil cytoplasts: localization of protein substrates and possible relationship with stimulus-response coupling. *FEBS Lett.*, 180:185–190.

269. Gennaro, R., Florio, C., and Romeo, D. (1986): Coactivation of protein kinase C and NADPH oxidase in the plasma membrane of neutrophil cytoplasts. *Biochem. Biophys. Res. Commun.*, 134: 305–312.

270. Gleich, G. J., and Adolphson, C. R. (1986): The eosinophilic leukocyte: structure and function. *Adv. Immunol.*, 39:177–253.

271. Geotzl, E. J. (1982): The conversion of leukotriene C_4 to isomers of leukotriene B_4 by human eosinophil peroxidase. *Biochem. Biophys. Res. Commun.*, 106:270–275.

272. Goldman, D. W., Chang, F. H., Gifford, L. A., Goetzl, E. J., and Bourne, H. R. (1985): Pertussis toxin inhibition of chemotactic factor-induced calcium mobilization and function in human polymorphonuclear leukocytes. *J. Exp. Med.*, 162:145–156.

273. Gomperts, B. D., Barrowman, M. M., and Cockcroft, S. (1986): Dual role for guanine nucleotides in stimulus-secretion coupling. *Fed. Proc.*, 45:2156–2161.

274. Graf, E., Mahoney, J. R., Bryant, R. G., and Eaton, J. W. (1984): Iron catalyzed hydroxyl radical formation: stringent requirement for free iron coordination site. *J. Biol. Chem.*, 25:3620–3624.

275. Graham, R. C., and Karnovsky, M. J. (1966): Glomerular permeability: ultrastructural cytochemical studies using peroxidases as protein tracers. *J. Exp. Med.*, 124:1123–1134.

276. Green, D. E., and Pauli, R. (1943): The anti-bacterial action of the xanthine oxidase system. *Proc. Soc. Exp. Biol. Med.*, 54:148–150.

277. Green, M. R., Hill, H. A. O., Okolow-Zubkowska, M. J., and Segal, A. W. (1979): The production of hydroxyl and superoxide radicals by stimulated human neutrophils: measurements by EPR spectroscopy. *FEBS Lett.*, 100:23–26.

278. Green, T. R., and Schaefer, R. E. (1981): Intrinsic dichlorophenolindophenol reductase activity associated with the superoxide-generating oxidoreductase of human granulocytes. *Biochemistry*, 20:7483–7487.

279. Green, T. R., and Wu, D. E. (1985): Detection of NADPH diaph-

orase activity associated with human neutrophil NADPH-O_2 oxidoreductase activity. *FEBS Lett.*, 179:82–86.

280. Green, T. R., and Wu, D. E. (1985): Purification and resolution of NADH diaphorase activity from NADPH diaphorase-linked: O_2 oxidoreductase activity of human neutrophils. *Biochim. Biophys. Acta*, 831:74–81.

281. Green, T. R., and Wu, D. E. (1986): The NADPH:O_2 oxidoreductase of human neutrophils: stoichiometry of univalent and divalent reduction of O_2. *J. Biol. Chem.*, 261:6010–6015.

282. Green, T. R., Shaefer, R. E., and Makler, M. T. (1980): Orientation of the NADPH dependent superoxide generating oxidoreductase of the outer membrane of human PMNs. *Biochem. Biophys. Res. Commun.*, 94:262–269.

283. Green, T. R., Wirtz, M. K., and Wu, D. E. (1983): Delineation of the catalytic components of the NADPH-dependent O_2^- generating oxidoreductase of human neutrophils. *Biochem. Biophys. Res. Commun.*, 110:873–879.

284. Greene, W. H., Colclough, L., Anton, A., and Root, R. K. (1980): Lectin-dependent neutrophil-mediated cytotoxicity against chicken erythrocytes: a model of non-myeloperoxidase-mediated oxygen-dependent killing by human neutrophils. *J. Immunol.*, 125:2727–2734.

285. Grignaschi, V. I., Sperperato, A. M., Etcheverry, M. J., and Macario, A. J. L. (1963): Un nuevo cuadro citoquimico: negatividad espontanea de las reacciones de peroxidasas, oxidasas y lipido en la progenie neutrofila y en los monocitos de dos hermanos. *Rev. Assoc. Med. Argent.*, 77:218–221.

286. Grinstead, R. R. (1960): The oxidation of ascorbic acid by hydrogen peroxide: catalysis by ethylenediaminetetraacetato-iron (III). *J. Am. Chem. Soc.*, 82:3464–3471.

287. Grisham, M. B., Jefferson, M. M., and Thomas, E. L. (1984): Role of monochloramine in the oxidation of erythrocyte hemoglobin by stimulated neutrophils. *J. Biol. Chem.*, 259:6757–6765.

288. Grisham, M. B., Jefferson, M. M., Melton, D. F., and Thomas, E. L. (1984): Chlorination of endogenous amines by isolated neutrophils: ammonia-dependent bactericidal, cytotoxic and cytolytic activities of the chloramines. *J. Biol. Chem.*, 259:10404–10413.

289. Gutteridge, J. M. C. (1981): Thiobarbituric acid-reactivity following iron-dependent free-radical damage to amino acids and carbohydrates. *FEBS Lett.*, 128:343–346.

290. Gutteridge, J. M. C. (1982): Fate of oxygen free radicals in extracellular fluids. *Biochem. Soc. Trans.*, 10:72–73.

291. Gutteridge, J. M. C. (1984): Ferrous ion-EDTA-stimulated phospholipid peroxidation—a reaction changing from alkoxyl-radical-dependent to hydroxyl-radical-dependent initiation. *Biochem. J.*, 224:697–701.

292. Gutteridge, J. M. C. (1984): Reactivity of hydroxyl and hydroxyl-like radicals discriminated by release of thiobarbituric acid-reactive material from deoxy sugars, nucleosides and benzoate. *Biochem. J.*, 224:761–767.

293. Gutteridge, J. M. C., and Halliwell, B. (1982): The role of superoxide and hydroxyl radicals in the degradation of DNA and deoxyribose induced by a copper-phenanthroline complex. *Biochem. Pharmacol.*, 31:2801–2805.

294. Gutteridge, J. M. C., and Wilkins, S. (1983): Copper salt-dependent hydroxyl radical formation: damage to proteins acting as antioxidants. *Biochim. Biophys. Acta*, 759:38–41.

295. Gutteridge, J. M. C., Richmond, R., and Halliwell, B. (1979): Inhibition of the iron-catalyzed formation of hydroxyl radicals from superoxide and of lipid peroxidation by desferrioxamine. *Biochem. J.*, 184:469–472.

296. Gutteridge, J. M. C., Rowley, D. A., and Halliwell, B. (1981): Superoxide-dependent formation of hydroxyl radicals in the presence of iron salts: detection of "free" iron in biological systems by using bleomycin-dependent degradation of DNA. *Biochem. J.*, 199:263–265.

297. Gutteridge, J. M. C., Paterson, S. K., Segal, A. W., and Halliwell, B. (1981): Inhibition of lipid peroxidation by the iron-binding protein lactoferrin. *Biochem. J.*, 199:259–261.

298. Gutteridge, J. M. C., Rowley, D. A., and Halliwell, B. (1982): Superoxide-dependent formation of hydroxyl radicals and lipid peroxidation in the presence of iron salts: detection of "catalytic" iron

and anti-oxidant activity in extracellular fluids. *Biochem. J.,* 206: 605–609.

299. Haber, F., and Weiss, J. (1934): The catalytic decomposition of hydrogen peroxide by iron salts. *Proc. R. Soc. Lond.* [*A*], 147:332–351.

300. Hafeman, D. G., and Lucas, Z. J. (1979): Polymorphonuclear leukocyte-mediated, antibody-dependent, cellular cytotoxicity against tumor cells: dependence on oxygen and the respiratory burst. *J. Immunol.,* 123:55–62.

301. Håkansson, L., and Venge, P. (1982): Kinetic studies of neutrophil phagocytosis. V. Studies on the co-operation between the Fc and C3b receptors. *Immunology,* 47:687–694.

302. Halliwell, B. (1978): Superoxide-dependent formation of hydroxyl radicals in the presence of iron chelates: is it a mechanism for hydroxyl radical production in biochemical systems? *FEBS Lett.,* 92:321–326.

303. Halliwell, B. (1978): Superoxide-dependent formation of hydroxyl radicals in the presence of iron salts: its role in degradation of hyaluronic acid by a superoxide-generating system. *FEBS Lett.,* 96: 238–242.

304. Halliwell, B., and Foyer, C. H. (1976): Ascorbic acid, metal ions and the superoxide radical. *Biochem. J.,* 155:697–700.

305. Halliwell, B., and Gutteridge, J. M. C. (1981): Formation of a thiobarbituric-acid-reactive substance from deoxyribose in the presence of iron salts: the role of superoxide and hydroxyl radicals. *FEBS Lett.,* 128:347–352.

306. Halliwell, B., and Gutteridge, J. M. C. (1985): The role of transition metals in superoxide-mediated toxicity. In: *Superoxide Dismutase, Vol. III,* edited by L. W. Oberley, pp. 45–82. CRC Press, Boca Raton, Florida.

307. Halliwell, B., and Gutteridge, J. M. C. (1986): Oxygen free radicals and iron in relation to biology and medicine: some problems and concepts. *Arch. Biochem. Biophys.,* 246:501–513.

308. Harbour, J. R., and Bolton, J. R. (1975): Superoxide formation in spinach chloroplasts: electron spin resonance detection by spin trapping. *Biochem. Biophys. Res. Commun.,* 64:803–807.

309. Harbour, J. R., Chow, V., and Bolton, J. R. (1974): An electron spin resonance study of the spin adducts of OH and HO_2 radicals with nitrones in the ultraviolet photolysis of aqueous hydrogen peroxide solutions. *Can. J. Chem.,* 52:3549–3553.

310. Harper, A. M., Dunne, M. J., and Segal, A. W. (1984): Purification of cytochrome b_{-245} from human neutrophils. *Biochem. J.,* 219: 519–527.

311. Harper, A. M., Chaplin, M. F., and Segal, A. W. (1985): Cytochrome b_{-245} from human neutrophils is a glycoprotein. *Biochem. J.,* 227: 783–788.

312. Harris, D. C., and Aisen, P. (1973): Facilitation of Fe(II) autoxidation by Fe(III) complexing agents. *Biochim. Biophys. Acta,* 329: 156–158.

313. Harrison, J. E. (1976): The functional mechanism of myeloperoxidase. In: *Cancer Enzymology,* edited by J. Schultz and F. Ahmad, pp. 305–317. Academic Press, New York.

314. Harrison, J. E., and Schultz, J. (1976): Studies on the chlorinating activity of myeloperoxidase. *J. Biol. Chem.,* 251:1371–1374.

315. Harrison, J. E., and Schultz, J. (1978): Myeloperoxidase: confirmation and nature of heme-binding inequivalence. *Biochim. Biophys. Acta,* 536:341–349.

316. Harrison, J. E., Pabalan, S., and Schultz, J. (1977): The subunit structure of crystalline canine myeloperoxidase. *Biochim. Biophys. Acta,* 493:247–259.

317. Harrison, J. E., Watson, B. D., and Schultz, J. (1978): Myeloperoxidase and singlet oxygen: a reappraisal. *FEBS Lett.,* 92:327–332.

318. Harvath, L., and Aksamit, R. R. (1984): Oxidized N-formylmethionyl-leucyl-phenylalanine: effect on the activation of human monocyte and neutrophil chemotaxis and superoxide production. *J. Immunol.,* 133:1471–1476.

319. Hasilik, A., Pohlmann, R., Olsen, R. L., and von Figura, K. (1984): Myeloperoxidase is synthesized as larger phosphorylated precursor. *EMBO J.,* 3:2671–2676.

320. Hatch, G. E., Nichols, W. K., and Hill, H. R. (1977): Cyclic nucleotide changes in human neutrophils induced by chemoattractants and chemotactic modulators. *J. Immunol.,* 119:450–456.

321. Hattori, H. (1961): Studies on the labile, stable NADI oxidase and peroxidase staining reactions in the isolated particles of horse granulocytes. *Nagoya J. Med. Sci.,* 23:362–378.

322. Hawley, D. A., Kleinhans, F. W., and Biesecker, J. L. (1983): Determination of alternate pathway complement kinetics by electron spin resonance spectroscopy. *Am. J. Clin. Pathol.,* 79:673–677.

323. Hayakawa, T., Suzuki, K., Suzuki, S., Andrews, P. C., and Babior, B. M. (1986): A possible role for protein phosphorylation in the activation of the respiratory burst in human neutrophils: evidence from studies with cells from patients with chronic granulomatous disease. *J. Biol. Chem.,* 261:9109–9115.

324. Heifets, L., Imai, K., and Goren, M. B. (1980): Expression of peroxidase-dependent iodination by macrophages ingesting neutrophil debris. *J. Reticuloendothel. Soc.,* 28:391–404.

325. Held, A. M., and Hurst, J. K. (1978): Ambiguity associated with use of singlet oxygen trapping agents in myeloperoxidase-catalyzed oxidations. *Biochem. Biophys. Res. Commun.,* 81:878–885.

326. Helfman, D. M., Appelbaum, B. D., Vogler, N. R., and Kuo, J. F. (1983): Phospholipid-sensitive Ca^{2+} dependent protein kinase and its substrates in human neutrophils. *Biochem. Biophys. Res. Commun.,* 111:847–853.

327. Henderson, W. R., and Kaliner, M. (1979): Mast cell granule peroxidase: location, secretion and SRS-A inactivation. *J. Immunol.,* 122:1322–1328.

328. Henderson, W. R., and Klebanoff, S. J. (1983): Leukotriene production and inactivation by normal, chronic granulomatous disease and myeloperoxidase-deficient neutrophils. *J. Biol. Chem.,* 258: 13522–13527.

329. Henderson, W. R., Chi, E. Y., and Klebanoff, S. J. (1980): Eosinophil peroxidase-induced mast cell secretion. *J. Exp. Med.,* 152: 265–279.

330. Henderson, W. R., Jong, E. C., and Klebanoff, S. J. (1980): Binding of eosinophil peroxidase to mast cell granules with retention of peroxidatic activity. *J. Immunol.,* 124:1383–1388.

331. Henderson, W. R., Chi, E. Y., Jong, E. C., and Klebanoff, S. J. (1981): Mast cell-mediated tumor-cell cytotoxicity: role of the peroxidase system. *J. Exp. Med.,* 153:520–533.

332. Henderson, W. R., Jörg, A., and Klebanoff, S. J. (1982): Eosinophil peroxidase-mediated inactivation of leukotrienes B_4, C_4 and D_4. *J. Immunol.,* 128:2609–2613.

333. Henderson, W. R., Chi, E. Y., Jörg, A., and Klebanoff, S. J. (1983): Horse eosinophil degranulation induced by the ionophore A23187: ultrastructure and role of phospholipase A_2. *Am. J. Pathol.,* 111: 341–349.

334. Henderson, W. R., Chi, E. Y., Jong, E. C., and Klebanoff, S. J. (1986): Mast cell-mediated toxicity to schistosomula of *Schistosoma mansoni*: potentiation by exogenous peroxidase. *J. Immunol.,* 137: 2695–2699.

335. Herlin, T., and Borregaard, N. (1983): Early changes in cyclic AMP and calcium efflux during phagocytosis by neutrophils from normals and patients with chronic granulomatous disease. *Immunology,* 48:17–26.

336. Heyneman, R. A. (1983): Subcellular localization and properties of the NAD(P)H oxidase from equine polymorphonuclear leukocytes. *Enzyme,* 29:198–207.

337. Heyneman, R. A., and Vercauteren, R. E. (1984): Activation of a NADPH oxidase from horse polymorphonuclear leukocytes in a cell-free system. *J. Leukocyte Biol.,* 36:751–759.

338. Higson, F. K., Durbin, L., Pavlotsky, N., and Tauber, A. I. (1985): Studies of cytochrome B_{-245} translocation in the PMA stimulation of the human neutrophil NADPH-oxidase. *J. Immunol.,* 135:519–524.

339. Hirata, F. (1981): The regulation of lipomodulin, a phospholipase inhibitory protein, in rabbit neutrophils by phosphorylation. *J. Biol. Chem.,* 256:7730–7733.

340. Hoe, S., Rowley, D. A., and Halliwell, B. (1981): Reactions of ferrioxamine and desferrioxamine with the hydroxyl radical. *Chem. Biol. Interact.,* 41:75–81.

341. Hoffman, M., and Autor, A. P. (1980): Production of superoxide anion by an NADPH-oxidase from rat pulmonary macrophages. *FEBS Lett.,* 121:352–354.

342. Holmes, B., Page, A. R., and Good, R. A. (1967): Studies of the

metabolic activity of leukocytes from patients with a genetic abnormality of phagocytic function. *J. Clin. Invest.*, 46:1422–1432.

343. Holzbecher, J., and Ryan, D. E. (1980): The rapid determination of total bromine and iodine in biological fluids by neutron activation. *Clin. Biochem.*, 13:277–278.

344. Howard, D. H. (1973): Fate of *Histoplasma capsulatum* in guinea pig polymorphonuclear leukocytes. *Infect. Immun.*, 8:412–419.

345. Hurst, J. K., Albrich, J. M., Green, T. R., Rosen, H., and Klebanoff, S. J. (1984): Myeloperoxidase-dependent fluorescein chlorination by stimulated neutrophils. *J. Biol. Chem.*, 259:4812–4821.

346. Hyslop, P. A., Oades, Z. G., Jesaitis, A. J., Painter, R. G., Cochrane, C. G., and Sklar, L. A. (1984): Evidence for N-formyl chemotactic peptide-stimulated GTPase activity in human neutrophil homogenates. *FEBS Lett.*, 166:165–169.

347. Ikeda-Saito, M., and Prince, R. C. (1985): The effect of chloride on the redox and EPR properties of myeloperoxidase. *J. Biol. Chem.*, 260:8301–8305.

349. Ikeda-Saito, M., Argade, P. V., and Rousseau, D. L. (1985): Resonance raman evidence of chloride binding to the heme iron in myeloperoxidase. *FEBS Lett.*, 184:52–55.

350. Ilan, Y. A., Czapski, G., and Meisel, D. (1976): The one-electron transfer redox potentials of free radicals. 1. The oxygen/superoxide system. *Biochim. Biophys. Acta*, 430:209–224.

351. Ismail, G., Sawyer, W. D., and Wegener, W. S. (1977): Effect of hydrogen peroxide and superoxide radical on viability of *Neisseria gonorrhoeae* and related bacteria. *Proc. Soc. Exp. Biol. Med.*, 155: 264–269.

352. Iyer, G. Y. N., Islam, D. M. F., and Quastel, J. H. (1961): Biochemical aspects of phagocytosis. *Nature*, 192:535–541.

353. Jackowski, S., and Sha'afi, R. I. (1979): Response of adenosine cyclic 3′,5′-monophosphate level in rabbit neutrophils to the chemotactic peptide formyl-methionyl-leucyl-phenylalanine. *Mol. Pharmacol.*, 16:473–481.

354. Jacobs, A. A., Low, I. E., Paul, B. B., Strauss, R. R., and Sbarra, A. J. (1972): Mycoplasmacidal activity of peroxidase-H$_2$O$_2$-halide systems. *Infect. Immun.*, 5:127–131.

355. Jandl, R. C., André-Schwartz, J., Borges-Dubois, L., Kipnes, R. S., McMurrich, B. J., and Babior, B. M. (1978): Termination of the respiratory burst in human neutrophils. *J. Clin. Invest.*, 61:1176–1177.

356. Janoff, A., Carp, H., Lee, D. K., and Drew, R. T. (1979): Cigarette smoke inhalation decreases α_1-antitrypsin activity in rat lung. *Science*, 206:1313–1314.

357. Janoff, A., George-Nascimento, C., and Rosenberg, S. (1986): A genetically engineered, mutant human alpha-1-proteinase inhibitor is more resistant than the normal inhibitor to oxidative inactivation by chemicals, enzymes, cells, and cigarette smoke. *Am. Rev. Respir. Dis.*, 133:353–356.

358. Janzen, E. G., Nutter, D. E., Jr., Davis, E. R., Blackburn, B. J., Poyer, J. L., and McCay, P. B. (1978): On spin trapping hydroxyl and hydroperoxyl radicals. *Can. J. Chem.*, 56:2237–2242.

359. Jasin, H. E. (1983): Generation of IgG aggregates by the myeloperoxidase-hydrogen peroxide system. *J. Immunol.*, 130:1918–1923.

360. Johnson, D., and Travis, J. (1978): Structural evidence for methionine at the reactive site of human α-1-proteinase inhibitor. *J. Biol. Chem.*, 253:7142–7144.

361. Johnson, D., and Travis, J. (1979): The oxidative inactivation of human α-1-proteinase inhibitor: further evidence for methionine at the reactive center. *J. Biol. Chem.*, 254:4022–4026.

362. Johnson, K. J., and Ward, P. A. (1981): Role of oxygen metabolites in immune complex injury of lung. *J. Immunol.*, 126:2365–2369.

363. Johnson, K. J., Fantone, J. C., III, Kaplan, J., and Ward, P. A. (1981): In vivo damage of rat lungs by oxygen metabolites. *J. Clin. Invest.*, 67:983–993.

364. Johnson, K., Nauseef, W. M., Wheelock, M., Caré, A., and Rovera, G. (1986): Molecular cloning of human myeloperoxidase using an HL-60 expression cDNA library. *Clin. Res.*, 34:521A.

365. Johnson, W. D., Jr., Mei, B., and Cohn, Z. A. (1977): The separation, long-term cultivation and maturation of the human monocyte. *J. Exp. Med.*, 146:1613–1626.

365a. Johnson, R. J., Couser, W. G., Chi, E. Y., Adler, S., and Klebanoff, S. J. (1987): A new mechanism for glomerular injury: the myelo-

peroxidase-hydrogen peroxide-halide system. *J. Clin. Invest.*, 79: 1379–1387.

366. Johnston, R. B., Jr., and Baehner, R. L. (1970): Improvement of leukocyte bactericidal activity in chronic granulomatous disease. *Blood*, 35:350–355.

367. Johnston, R. B., Jr., Keele, B. B., Jr., Misra, H. P., Lehmeyer, J. E., Webb, L. S., Baehner, R. L., and Rajagopalan, K. V. (1975): The role of superoxide anion generation in phagocytic bactericidal activity: studies with normal and chronic granulomatous disease leukocytes. *J. Clin. Invest.*, 55:1357–1372.

368. Johnston, R. B., Jr., Godzik, C. A., and Cohn, Z. A. (1978): Increased superoxide anion production by immunologically activated and chemically elicited macrophages. *J. Exp. Med.*, 148:115–127.

369. Jones, G. S., Van Dyke, K., and Castranova, V. (1981): Transmembrane potential changes associated with superoxide release from human granulocytes. *J. Cell. Physiol.*, 106:75–83.

370. Jong, E. C., and Klebanoff, S. J. (1980): Eosinophil-mediated mammalian tumor cell cytotoxicity: role of the peroxidase system. *J. Immunol.*, 124:1949–1953.

371. Jong, E. C., Henderson, W. R., and Klebanoff, S. J. (1980): Bactericidal activity of eosinophil peroxidase. *J. Immunol.*, 124:1378–1382.

372. Jong, E. C., Mahmoud, A. A. F., and Klebanoff, S. J. (1981): Peroxidase-mediated toxicity to schistosomula of *Schistosoma mansoni*. *J. Immunol.*, 126:468–471.

373. Jong, E. C., Chi, E. Y., and Klebanoff, S. J. (1984): Human neutrophil-mediated killing of schistosomula of *Schistosoma mansoni*: augmentation by schistosomal binding of eosinophil peroxidase. *Am. J. Trop. Med. Hyg.*, 33:104–115.

374. Jörg, A., Henderson, W. R., Murphy, R. C., and Klebanoff, S. J. (1982): Leukotriene generation by eosinophils. *J. Exp. Med.*, 155: 390–402.

375. Jörg, A., Pasquier, J-M., and Klebanoff, S. J. (1982): Purification of horse eosinophil peroxidase. *Biochim. Biophys. Acta*, 701:185–191.

376. Kajikawa, N., Kaibuchi, K., Matsubara, T., Kikkawa, U., Takai, Y., Nishizuka, Y., Ito, K., and Tomioka, C. (1983): A possible role of protein kinase C in signal-induced lysosomal enzyme release. *Biochem. Biophys. Res. Commun.*, 116:743–750.

377. Kakinuma, K. (1974): Effects of fatty acids on the oxidative metabolism of leukocytes. *Biochim. Biophys. Acta*, 348:76–85.

378. Kakinuma, K., and Minakami, S. (1978): Effects of fatty acids on superoxide radical generation in leukocytes. *Biochim. Biophys. Acta*, 538:50–59.

379. Kakinuma, K., Kaneda, M., Chiba, T., and Ohnishi, T. (1986): Electron spin resonance studies on a flavoprotein in neutrophil plasma membranes: redox potentials of the flavin and its participation in NADPH oxidase. *J. Biol. Chem.*, 261:9426–9432.

380. Kanner, J., and Kinsella, J. E. (1983): Initiation of lipid peroxidation by a peroxidase/hydrogen peroxide/halide system. *Lipids*, 18:204–210.

381. Kanofsky, J. R. (1983): Singlet oxygen production by lactoperoxidase: evidence from 1270 nm chemiluminescence. *J. Biol. Chem.*, 258:5991–5993.

382. Kanofsky, J. R. (1984): Singlet oxygen production by chloroperoxidase-hydrogen peroxide-halide systems. *J. Biol. Chem.*, 259: 5596–5600.

383. Kanofsky, J. R., Wright, J., Miles-Richardson, G. E., and Tauber, A. I. (1984): Biochemical requirement for singlet oxygen production by purified human myeloperoxidase. *J. Clin. Invest.*, 74:1489–1495.

384. Kanofsky, J. R., Wright, J., and Tauber, A. J. (1985): Effect of ascorbic acid on the production of singlet oxygen by purified human myeloperoxidase. *FEBS Lett.*, 187:299–301.

385. Kaplan, E. L., Laxdal, T., and Quie, P. G. (1968): Studies of polymorphonuclear leukocytes from patients with chronic granulomatous disease of childhood: bactericidal capacity for streptococci. *Pediatrics*, 41:591–599.

386. Karnovsky, M. L. (1975): Biochemical aspects of the functions of polymorphonuclear and mononuclear leukocytes. In: *The Phagocytic Cell in Host Resistance*, edited by J. A. Bellanti and D. H. Dayton, pp. 25–43. Raven Press, New York.

387. Kasha, M., and Khan, A. U. (1970): The physics, chemistry and

biology of singlet molecular oxygen. *Ann. N.Y. Acad. Sci.,* 171:5–23.

388. Katz, P., Simone, C. B., Henkart, P. A., and Fauci, A. S. (1980): Mechanisms of antibody-dependent cellular cytotoxicity: use of effector cells from chronic granulomatous disease patients as investigative probes. *J. Clin. Invest.,* 65:55–63.

389. Kazura, J. W., Fanning, M. M., Blumer, J. L., and Mahmoud, A. A. F. (1981): Role of cell-generated hydrogen peroxide in granulocyte-mediated killing of schistosomula of *Schistosoma mansoni in vitro. J. Clin. Invest.,* 67:93–102.

390. Kearns, D. R. (1979): Solvent and solvent isotope effects on the lifetime of singlet oxygen. In: *Singlet Oxygen,* edited by H. H. Wasserman and R. W. Murray, pp. 115–137. Academic Press, New York.

391. Kellogg, E. W., III, and Fridovich, I. (1975): Superoxide, hydrogen peroxide, and singlet oxygen in lipid peroxidation by a xanthine oxidase system. *J. Biol. Chem.,* 250:8812–8817.

392. Kellogg, E. W., III, and Fridovich, I. (1977): Liposome oxidation and erythrocyte lysis by enzymically generated superoxide and hydrogen peroxide. *J. Biol. Chem.,* 252:6721–6728.

393. Khalife, J., Capron, M., Grzych, J-M., Bazin, H., and Capron, A. (1985): Extracellular release of rat eosinophil peroxidase (EPO). I. Role of anaphylactic immunoglobulin. *J. Immunol.,* 134:1968–1974.

394. Khan, A. U. (1978): Activated oxygen: singlet molecular oxygen and superoxide anion. *Photochem. Photobiol.,* 28:615–627.

395. Khan, A. U. (1981): Direct spectral evidence of the generation of singlet molecular oxygen ($^1\Delta$g) in the reaction of potassium superoxide with water. *J. Am. Chem. Soc.,* 103:6516–6517.

396. Khan, A. U. (1983): Enzyme system generation of singlet ($^1\Delta$g) molecular oxygen observed directly by 1.0–1.8 μm luminescence spectroscopy. *J. Am. Chem. Soc.,* 105:7195–7197.

398. Khan, A. U. (1984): Discovery of enzyme generation of $^1\Delta$g molecular oxygen: spectra of (0,0) $^1\Delta$g → $^3\Sigma$g$^-$ IR emission. *J. Photochem.,* 25:327–333.

399. Khan, A. U. (1984): Myeloperoxidase singlet molecular oxygen generation detected by direct infrared electronic emission. *Biochem. Biophys. Res. Commun.,* 122:668–675.

400. Khan, A. U., and Kasha, M. (1979): Direct spectroscopic observation of singlet oxygen emission at 1268 nm excited by sensitizing dyes of biological interest in liquid solution. *Proc. Natl. Acad. Sci. USA,* 76:6047–6049.

401. Khan, A. U., Bebauer, P., and Hager, L. P. (1983): Chloroperoxidase generation of singlet Δ molecular oxygen observed directly by spectroscopy in the 1- to 1.6-μm region. *Proc. Natl. Acad. Sci. USA,* 80:5195–5197.

402. King, M. M., Lai, E. K., and McCay, P. B. (1975): Singlet oxygen production associated with enzyme-catalyzed lipid peroxidation in liver microsomes. *J. Biol. Chem.,* 250:6496–6502.

403. Kinkade, J. M., Jr., Pember, S. O., Barnes, K. C., Shapira, R., Spitznagel, J. K., and Martin, L. E. (1983): Differential distribution of distinct forms of myeloperoxidase in different azurophilic granule subpopulations from human neutrophils. *Biochem. Biophys. Res. Commun.,* 114:296–303.

404. Kitagawa, S., Takaku, F., and Sakamoto, S. (1979): Possible involvement of proteases in superoxide production by human polymorphonuclear leukocytes. *FEBS Lett.,* 99:275–278.

405. Kitagawa, S., Takaku, F., and Sakamoto, S. (1979): Serine protease inhibitors inhibit superoxide production by human polymorphonuclear leukocytes and monocytes stimulated by various surface active agents. *FEBS Lett.,* 107:331–334.

406. Kitagawa, S., Takaku, F., and Sakamoto, S. (1980): Evidence that proteases are involved in superoxide production by human polymorphonuclear leukocytes and monocytes. *J. Clin. Invest.,* 65:74–81.

407. Kitagawa, S., Ohta, M., Nojiri, H., Kakinuma, K., Saito, M., Takaku, F., and Miura, Y. (1984): Functional maturation of membrane potential changes and superoxide-producing capacity during differentiation of human granulocytes. *J. Clin. Invest.,* 73:1062–1071.

408. Kitahara, M., Eyre, H. J., Simonian, Y., Atkin, C. L., and Hasstedt, S. J. (1981): Hereditary myeloperoxidase deficiency. *Blood,* 57:888–893.

409. Klassen, D. K., and Sagone, A. L., Jr. (1980): Evidence for both oxygen and non-oxygen dependent mechanisms of antibody sensitized target cell lysis by human monocytes. *Blood,* 56:985–992.

410. Klebanoff, S. J. (1959): An effect of thyroxine on the oxidation of reduced pyridine nucleotides by the peroxidase system. *J. Biol. Chem.,* 234:2480–2485.

411. Klebanoff, S. J. (1960): Reduced pyridine nucleotides as activators of certain reactions catalyzed by peroxidase. *Biochim. Biophys. Acta,* 44:501–509.

412. Klebanoff, S. J. (1967): Iodination of bacteria: a bactericidal mechanism. *J. Exp. Med.,* 126:1063–1078.

413. Klebanoff, S. J. (1968): Myeloperoxidase-halide-hydrogen peroxide antimicrobial system. *J. Bacteriol.,* 95:2131–2138.

414. Klebanoff, S. J. (1969): Antimicrobial activity of catalase at acid pH. *Proc. Soc. Exp. Biol. Med.,* 132:571–574.

415. Klebanoff, S. J. (1970): Myeloperoxidase-mediated antimicrobial systems and their role in leukocyte function. In: *Biochemistry of the Phagocytic Process,* edited by J. Schultz, pp. 89–110. North Holland, Amsterdam.

416. Klebanoff, S. J. (1970): Myeloperoxidase: contribution to the microbicidal activity of intact leukocytes. *Science,* 169:1095–1097.

417. Klebanoff, S. J. (1975): Antimicrobial systems of the polymorphonuclear leukocyte. In: *The Phagocytic Cell in Host Resistance,* edited by J. A. Bellanti and D. H. Dayton, pp. 45–59. Raven Press, New York.

418. Klebanoff, S. J. (1982): Oxygen-dependent cytotoxic mechanisms of phagocytes. *Adv. Host. Def. Mech.,* 1:111–162.

419. Klebanoff, S. J. (1982): Iodination catalyzed by the xanthine oxidase system: role of hydroxyl radicals. *Biochemistry,* 21:4110–4116.

420. Klebanoff, S. J. (1982): The iron-H_2O_2-iodide cytotoxic system. *J. Exp. Med.,* 156:1262–1267.

421. Klebanoff, S. J. (1985): Oxygen-dependent antimicrobial systems in mononuclear phagocytes. In: *Progress in Leukocyte Biology, Vol. 4: Macrophage Biology,* edited by S. Reichard and M. Kojima, pp. 487–503. Alan R. Liss, New York.

422. Klebanoff, S. J., and Clark, R. A. (1975): Hemolysis and iodination of erythrocyte components by a myeloperoxidase mediated system. *Blood,* 45:699–707.

423. Klebanoff, S. J., and Clark, R. A. (1977): Iodination by human polymorphonuclear leukocytes: a re-evaluation. *J. Lab. Clin. Med.,* 89:675–686.

424. Klebanoff, S. J., and Clark, R. A. (1978): *The Neutrophil: Function and Clinical Disorders.* North Holland, Amsterdam.

425. Klebanoff, S. J., and Hamon, C. B. (1972): Role of myeloperoxidase-mediated antimicrobial systems in intact leukocytes. *J. Reticuloendothel. Soc.,* 12:170–196.

426. Klebanoff, S. J., and Hamon, C. B. (1975): Antimicrobial systems of mononuclear phagocytes. In: *Mononuclear Phagocytes in Immunity Infection and Pathology,* pp. 507–531. Blackwell, Oxford.

427. Klebanoff, S. J., and Luebke, R. G. (1965): The antilactobacillus system of saliva: role of salivary peroxidase. *Proc. Soc. Exp. Biol. Med.,* 118:483–486.

428. Klebanoff, S. J., and Pincus, S. H. (1971): Hydrogen peroxide utilization in myeloperoxidase-deficient leukocytes: a possible microbicidal control mechanism. *J. Clin. Invest.,* 50:2226–2229.

429. Klebanoff, S. J., and Rosen, H. (1978): Ethylene formation by polymorphonuclear leukocytes: role of myeloperoxidase. *J. Exp. Med.,* 148:490–506.

430. Klebanoff, S. J., and Shepard, C. C. (1984): Toxic effect of the peroxidase-hydrogen peroxide-halide antimicrobial system on *Mycobacterium leprae. Infect. Immun.,* 44:534–536.

431. Klebanoff, S. J., and Smith, D. C. (1970): The source of H_2O_2 for the uterine fluid-mediated sperm-inhibitory system. *Biol. Reprod.,* 3:236–242.

432. Klebanoff, S. J., and White, L. R. (1969): Iodination defect in the leukocytes of a patient with chronic granulomatous disease of childhood. *N. Engl. J. Med.,* 280:460–466.

433. Klebanoff, S. J., Clem, W. H., and Luebke, R. G. (1966): The peroxidase-thiocyanate-hydrogen peroxide antimicrobial system. *Biochim. Biophys. Acta,* 117:63–72.

434. Klebanoff, S. J., Durack, D. T., Rosen, H., and Clark, R. A. (1977):

Functional studies on human peritoneal eosinophils. *Infect. Immun.,* 17:167–173.

435. Klein, S. M., Cohen, G., and Cederbaum, A. I. (1980): The interaction of hydroxyl radicals with dimethylsulfoxide produces formaldehyde. *FEBS Lett.,* 116:220–222.

436. Knowles, D. M., II, Sullivan, T. J., III, Parker, C. W., and Williams, R. C., Jr. (1973): *In vitro* antibody-enzyme conjugates with specific bactericidal activity. *J. Clin. Invest.,* 52:1443–1452.

437. Kobayashi, M., Tanaka, T., and Usui, T. (1982): Inactivation of lysosomal enzymes by the respiratory burst of polymorphonuclear leukocytes: possible involvement of myeloperoxidase-H_2O_2-halide system. *J. Lab. Clin. Med.,* 100:896–907.

438. Koeffler, H. P., Ranyard, J., and Pertcheck, M. (1985): Myeloperoxidase: its structure and expression during myeloid differentiation. *Blood,* 65:484–491.

439. Koller, C. A., and LoBuglio, A. F. (1981): Monocyte-mediated antibody-dependent cell-mediated cytotoxicity: the role of the metabolic burst. *Blood,* 58:293–299.

440. Koo, C., Lefkowitz, R. J., and Snyderman, R. (1983): Guanine nucleotides modulate the binding affinity of the oligopeptide chemoattractant receptor on human polymorphonuclear leukocytes. *J. Clin. Invest.,* 72:748–753.

441. Koppenol, W. H., and Liebman, J. F. (1984): The oxidizing nature of the hydroxyl radical: a comparison with the ferryl ion (FeO^{2+}). *J. Phys. Chem.,* 88:99–101.

442. Korchak, H. M., and Weissmann, G. (1978): Changes in membrane potential of human granulocytes antecede the metabolic responses to surface stimulation. *Proc. Natl. Acad. Sci. USA,* 75:3818–3822.

443. Korchak, H. M., and Weissmann, G. (1980): Stimulus-response coupling in the human neutrophil: transmembrane potential and the role of extracellular Na^+. *Biochim. Biophys. Acta,* 601:180–194.

444. Korchak, H. M., Vienne, K., Rutherford, L. E., Winkenfeld, C., Finkelstein, M. C., and Weissmann, G. (1984): Stimulus response coupling in the human neutrophil. II. Temporal analysis of changes in cytosolic calcium and calcium efflux. *J. Biol. Chem.,* 259:4076–4082.

445. Krasnovsky, A. A., Jr. (1976): Photoluminescence of singlet oxygen in pigment solutions. *Photochem. Photobiol.,* 29:29–36.

446. Krinsky, N. I. (1974): Singlet excited oxygen as a mediator of the antibacterial action of leukocytes. *Science,* 186:363–365.

447. Kulig, M. J., and Smith, L. L. (1973): Sterol metabolism. XXV. Cholesterol oxidation by singlet molecular oxygen. *J. Org. Chem.,* 38:3639–3642.

448. Lampert, M. B., and Weiss, S. J. (1983): The chlorinating potential of the human monocyte. *Blood,* 62:645–651.

449. Lane, T. A., and Lamkin, G. E. (1983): Myeloperoxidase-mediated modulation of chemotactic peptide binding to human neutrophils. *Blood,* 61:1203–1207.

450. Larson, H. E., Smith, G. P., and Shah, L. (1985): Antitoxin activity of human polymorphonuclear leucocytes. *Br. J. Exp. Pathol.,* 66:243–249.

451. Lazzari, K. G., Proto, P. J., and Simons, E. R. (1986): Simultaneous measurement of stimulus-induced changes in cytoplasmic Ca^{2+} and in membrane potential of human neutrophils. *J. Biol. Chem.,* 261:9710–9713.

452. Learn, D. B., and Brestel, E. P. (1982): A comparison of superoxide production by human eosinophils and neutrophils. *Agents Actions,* 12:485–488.

453. Lee, C. T., Fein, A. M., Lippmann, M., Holtzman, H., Kimbel, P., and Weinbaum, G. (1981): Elastolytic activity in pulmonary lavage fluid from patients with adult respiratory distress syndrome. *N. Engl. J. Med.,* 304:192–196.

454. Lee, C. W., Lewis, R. A., Corey, E. J., Barton, A., Oh, H., Tauber, A. I., and Austen, K. F. (1982): Oxidative inactivation of leukotriene C_4 by stimulated human polymorphonuclear leukocytes. *Proc. Natl. Acad. Sci. USA,* 79:4166–4170.

455. Lee, C. W., Lewis, R. A., Tauber, A. I., Mehrotra, M., Corey, E. J., and Austen, K. F. (1983): The myeloperoxidase-dependent metabolism of leukotriene C_4, D_4 and E_4 to 6-trans-leukotriene B_4 diastereoisomers and the subclass specific S-diastereoisomeric sulfoxides. *J. Biol. Chem.,* 258:15004–15010.

456. Lehrer, R. I. (1969): Antifungal effects of peroxidase systems. *J. Bacteriol.,* 99:361–365.

457. Lehrer, R. I. (1975): The fungicidal mechanisms of human monocyte. I. Evidence for myeloperoxidase-linked and myeloperoxidase-independent candidacidal mechanisms. *J. Clin. Invest.,* 55:338–346.

458. Lehrer, R. I., and Cline, M. J. (1969): Leukocyte myeloperoxidase deficiency and disseminated candidiasis: the role of myeloperoxidase in resistance to *Candida* infection. *J. Clin. Invest.,* 48:1478–1488.

459. Lehrer, R. I., and Cline, M. J. (1969): Interaction of *Candida albicans* with human leukocytes and serum. *J. Bacteriol.,* 98:996–1004.

460. Lehrer, R. I., and Jan, R. G. (1970): Interaction of *Aspergillus fumigatus* spores with human leukocytes and serum. *Infect. Immun.,* 1:345–350.

461. Lehrer, R. I., Hanifin, J., and Cline, M. J. (1969): Defective bactericidal activity in myeloperoxidase-deficient human neutrophils. *Nature,* 223:78–79.

462. Lemarbre, P., Hoidal, J., Vesella, R., and Rinehart, J. (1980): Human pulmonary macrophage tumor cell cytotoxicity. *Blood,* 55:612–617.

463. Levitz, S. M., and Diamond, R. D. (1984): Killing of *Aspergillus fumigatus* spores and *Candida albicans* yeast phase by the iron-hydrogen peroxide-iodide cytotoxic system: comparison with the myeloperoxidase-hydrogen peroxide-halide system. *Infect. Immun.,* 43:1100–1102.

464. Levitz, S. M., and Diamond, R. D. (1985): Mechanisms of resistance of *Aspergillus fumigatus* conidia to killing by neutrophils *in vitro*. *J. Infect. Dis.,* 152:33–42.

465. Lew, P. D., Southwick, F. S., Stossel, T. P., Whitin, J. C., Simons, E., and Cohen, H. J. (1981): A variant of chronic granulomatous disease: deficient oxidative metabolism due to a low affinity NADPH oxidase. *N. Engl. J. Med.,* 305:1329–1333.

466. Lew, P. D., Wolheim, C., Seger, R. A., and Pozzan, T. (1984): Cytosolic free calcium changes induced by chemotactic peptide in neutrophils from patients with chronic granulomatous disease. *Blood,* 63:231–233.

467. Light, D. R., Walsh, C., O'Callaghan, A. M., Goetzl, E. J., and Tauber, A. I. (1981): Characteristics of the cofactor requirements for the superoxide-generating NADPH oxidase of human polymorphonuclear leukocytes. *Biochemistry,* 20:1468–1476.

468. Lipmann, F., and Owen, C. R. (1943): The antibacterial effect of enzymatic xanthine oxidation. *Science,* 98:246–248.

469. Locksley, R. M., Wilson, C. B., and Klebanoff, S. J. (1982): Role for endogenous and acquired peroxidase in the toxoplasmacidal activity of murine and human mononuclear phagocytes. *J. Clin. Invest.,* 69:1099–1111.

470. Locksley, R. M., Jacobs, R. F., Wilson, C. B., Weaver, W. M., and Klebanoff, S. J. (1982): Susceptibility of *Legionella pneumophila* to oxygen-dependent microbicidal systems. *J. Immunol.,* 129:2192–2197.

471. Locksley, R. M., Wilson, C. B., and Klebanoff, S. J. (1983): Increased respiratory burst in myeloperoxidase-deficient monocytes. *Blood,* 62:902–909.

472. Long, C. A., and Bielski, B. H. J. (1980): Rate of reaction of superoxide radical with chloride-containing species. *J. Phys. Chem.,* 84:555–557.

473. Lutter, R., van Zwieten, R., Weening, R. S., Hamer, M. N., and Roos, D. (1984): Cytochrome b, flavins and ubiquinone-50 in enucleated human neutrophils (polymorphonuclear leukocyte cytoplasts). *J. Biol. Chem.,* 259:9603–9606.

474. Lutter, R., van Schaik, M. J. L., van Zwieten, R., Wever, R., Roos, D., and Hamers, M. N. J. (1985): Purification and partial characterization of the b-type cytochrome from human polymorphonuclear leukocytes. *J. Biol. Chem.,* 260:2237–2244.

475. Lynch, R. E., and Fridovich, I. (1978): Effects of superoxide on the erythrocyte membrane. *J. Biol. Chem.,* 253:1838–1845.

476. Lynch, R. E., and Fridovich, I. (1978): Permeation of the erythrocyte stroma by superoxide radical. *J. Biol. Chem.,* 253:4697–4699.

477. Macartney, H., and Tschesche, H. (1983): Latent and active human polymorphonuclear leukocyte collagenases: isolation, purification and characterization. *Eur. J. Biochem.,* 130:71–78.

478. Mackler, B., Person, R., Davis, K. A., and Ochs, H. (1985): Studies of pyridine nucleotide oxidizing enzymes from human neutrophils. *Biochem. Int.*, 11:319–325.

479. Maguire, J. J., Kellogg, E. W., III, and Packer, L. (1982): Protection against free radical formation by protein bound iron. *Toxicol. Lett.*, 14:27–34.

480. Mandell, G. L. (1974): Bactericidal activity of aerobic and anaerobic polymorphonuclear neutrophils. *Infect. Immun.*, 9:337–341.

481. Mandell, G. L., and Hook, E. W. (1969): Leukocyte bactericidal activity in chronic granulomatous disease: correlation of bacterial hydrogen peroxide production and susceptibility to intracellular killing. *J. Bacteriol.*, 100:531–532.

482. Markert, M., Glass, G. A., and Babior, B. M. (1985): Respiratory burst oxidase from human neutrophils: purification and some properties. *Proc. Natl. Acad. Sci. USA*, 82:3144–3148.

483. Matheson, N. R. (1982): The effect of antiarthritic drugs and related compounds on the human neutrophil myeloperoxidase system. *Biochem. Biophys. Res. Commun.*, 108:259–265.

484. Matheson, N. R., Wong, P. S., and Travis, J. (1979): Enzymatic inactivation of human alpha-1-proteinase inhibitor by neutrophil myeloperoxidase. *Biochem. Biophys. Res. Commun.*, 88:402–409.

485. Matheson, N. R., Wong, P. S., and Travis, J. (1981): Isolation and properties of human neutrophil myeloperoxidase. *Biochemistry*, 20:325–330.

486. Matheson, N. R., Wong, P. S., Schuyler, M., and Travis, J. (1981): Interaction of human α-1-proteinase inhibitor with neutrophil myeloperoxidase. *Biochemistry*, 20:331–336.

487. Mavier, P., and Edgington, T. S. (1984): Human monocyte-mediated tumor cytotoxicity. *J. Immunol.*, 132:1980–1986.

488. McCay, P. B., Noguchi, T., Fong, K-L., Lai, E. K., and Poyer, J. L. (1980): Production of radicals from enzyme systems and the use of spin traps. In: *Free Radicals in Biology*, Vol. 4, edited by W. A. Pryor, pp. 155–186. Academic Press, New York.

489. McCord, J. M., and Day, E. D., Jr. (1978): Superoxide-dependent production of hydroxyl radical catalyzed by iron-EDTA complex. *FEBS Lett.*, 86:139–142.

490. McLaren, D. J., Mackenzie, C. D., and Ramalho-Pinto, F. J. (1977): Ultrastructural observations on the *in vitro* interaction between rat eosinophils and some parasitic helminths (*Schistosoma mansoni, Trichinella spiralis* and *Nippostrongylus brasiliensis*). *Clin. Exp. Immunol.*, 30:105–118.

491. McPhail, L. C., Shirley, P. S., Clayton, C. C., and Snyderman, R. (1985): Activation of the respiratory burst enzyme from human neutrophils in a cell-free system: evidence for a soluble cofactor. *J. Clin. Invest.*, 75:1735–1739.

492. McRipley, R. J., and Sbarra, A. J. (1967): Role of the phagocyte in host-parasite interactions. XII. Hydrogen peroxide-myeloperoxidase bactericidal system in the phagocyte. *J. Bacteriol.*, 94:1425–1430.

493. Melloni, E., Pontremoli, S., Michetti, M., Sacco, O., Sparatore, B., Salamino, F., and Horecker, B. L. (1985): Binding of protein kinase C to neutrophil membranes in the presence of Ca²⁺-requiring proteinase. *Proc. Natl. Acad. Sci USA*, 82:6435–6439.

494. Melloni, E., Pontremoli, S., Michetti, M., Sacco, O., Sparatore, B., and Horecker, B. L. (1986): The involvement of calpain in the activation of protein kinase C in neutrophils stimulated by phorbol myristic acid. *J. Biol. Chem.*, 261:4101–4105.

495. Merritt, T. A., Cochrane, C., Holcomb, K., Bohl, B., Hallman, M., Strayer, D., Edwards, D. K., and Gluck, L. (1983): Elastase and α₁ proteinase inhibitor activity in tracheal aspirates during respiratory distress syndrome: role of inflammation in the pathogenesis of bronchopulmonary dysplasia. *J. Clin. Invest.*, 72:656–666.

496. Metzger, Z., Hoffeld, J. T., and Oppenheim, J. J. (1980): Macrophage-mediated suppression. I. Evidence for participation of both hydrogen peroxide and prostaglandins in suppression of murine lymphocyte proliferation. *J. Immunol.*, 124:983–988.

497. Michelson, A. M. (1973): Studies in bioluminescence. X. Chemical models of enzymic oxidations. *Biochimie*, 55:465–479.

498. Mickenberg, I. D., Root, R. K., and Wolff, S. M. (1972): Bactericidal and metabolic properties of human eosinophils. *Blood*, 39:67–80.

499. Migler, R., DeChatelet, L. R., and Bass, D. A. (1978): Human

500. Millard, J. A., Gerard, K. W., and Schneider, D. L. (1979): The isolation from rat peritoneal leukocytes of plasma membrane enriched in alkaline phosphatase and a B-type cytochrome. *Biochem. Biophys. Res. Commun.*, 90:312–319.

501. Mollinedo, F., and Schneider, D. L. (1984): Subcellular localization of cytochrome b and ubiquinone in a tertiary granule of resting human neutrophils and evidence for a proton pump ATPase. *J. Biol. Chem.*, 259:7143–7150.

502. Molski, T. F. P., Naccache, P. H., Marsh, M. L., Kermode, J., Becker, E. L., and Sha'afi, R. I. (1984): Pertussis toxin inhibits the rise in the intracellular concentration of free calcium that is induced by chemotactic factors in rabbit neutrophils: possible role of the "G proteins" in calcium mobilization. *Biochem. Biophys. Res. Commun.*, 124:644–650.

503. Moorhouse, C. P., Halliwell, B., Grootveld, M., and Gutteridge, J. M. C. (1985): Cobalt (II) ion is a promoter of hydroxyl radical and possible "crypto-hydroxyl" radical formation under physiological conditions: differential effects of hydroxyl radical scavengers. *Biochim. Biophys. Acta*, 843:261–268.

504. Morel, F., and Vignais, P. V. (1984): Examination of the oxidase function of the b-type cytochrome in human polymorphonuclear leucocytes. *Biochim. Biophys. Acta*, 764:213–225.

505. Morse, J. O. (1978): Alpha₁-antitrypsin deficiency. *N. Engl. J. Med.*, 299:1045–1048, 1099–1105.

506. Motohashi, N., and Mori, I. (1983): Superoxide-dependent formation of hydroxyl radical catalyzed by transferrin. *FEBS Lett.*, 157:197–199.

507. Mottola, C., and Romeo, D. (1982): Calcium movement and membrane potential changes in the early phase of neutrophil activation by phorbol myristate acetate: a study with ion-selective electrodes. *J. Cell Biol.*, 93:129–134.

508. Murphy, G., Reynolds, J., Bretz, U., and Baggiolini, M. (1982): Partial purification of collagenase and gelatinase from human polymorphonuclear leukocytes. *Biochem. J.*, 203:209–221.

509. Murray, H. W. (1981): Susceptibility of *Leishmania* to oxygen intermediates and killing by normal macrophages. *J. Exp. Med.*, 153:1302–1315.

510. Murray, H. W. (1981): Interaction of *Leishmania* with a macrophage cell line: correlation between intracellular killing and the generation of oxygen intermediates. *J. Exp. Med.*, 153:1690–1695.

511. Murray, H. W. (1982): Cell-mediated immune response in experimental visceral leishmaniasis. II. Oxygen-dependent killing of intracellular *Leishmania donovani* amastigotes. *J. Immunol.*, 129:351–357.

512. Murray, H. W., and Cartelli, D. M. (1983): Killing of intracellular *Leishmania donovani* by human mononuclear phagocytes: evidence for oxygen-dependent and -independent leishmanicidal activity. *J. Clin. Invest.*, 72:32–44.

513. Murray, H. W., and Cohn, Z. A. (1979): Macrophage oxygen-dependent antimicrobial activity. I. Susceptibility of *Toxoplasma gondii* to oxygen intermediates. *J. Exp. Med.*, 150:938–949.

514. Murray, H. W., and Cohn, Z. A. (1980): Macrophages oxygen-dependent antimicrobial activity. III. Enhanced oxidative metabolism as an expression of macrophage activation. *J. Exp. Med.*, 152:1596–1609.

515. Murray, H. W., Juangbhanich, C. W., Nathan, C. F., and Cohn, Z. A. (1979): Macrophage oxygen-dependent antimicrobial activity. II. The role of oxygen intermediates. *J. Exp. Med.*, 150:950–964.

516. Murray, H. W., Nathan, C. F., and Cohn, Z. A. (1980): Macrophage oxygen-dependent antimicrobial activity. IV. Role of endogenous scavengers of oxygen intermediates. *J. Exp. Med.*, 152:1610–1624.

517. Murray, H. W., Byrne, G. I., Rothermel, C. D., and Cartelli, D. M. (1983): Lymphokine enhances oxygen-independent activity against intracellular pathogens. *J. Exp. Med.*, 158:234–239.

518. Murray, H. W., Rubin, B. Y., and Rothermel, C. D. (1983): Killing of intracellular *Leishmania donovani* by lymphokine-stimulated human mononuclear phagocytes: evidence that interferon-γ is the activating lymphokine. *J. Clin. Invest.*, 72:1506–1510.

519. Murray, H. W., Rubin, B. Y., Carriero, S. M., Harris, A. M., and Jaffee, E. A. (1985): Human mononuclear phagocyte antiprotozoal

mechanisms: oxygen-dependent vs. oxygen-independent activity against intracellular *Toxoplasma gondii. J. Immunol.,* 134:1982–1988.

520. Musson, R. A., McPhail, L. C., Shafran, H., and Johnston, R. B., Jr. (1982): Differences in the ability of human peripheral blood monocytes and *in vitro* monocyte-derived macrophages to produce superoxide anion: studies with cells from normals and patients with chronic granulomatous disease. *J. Reticuloendothel. Soc.,* 31:261–266.

521. Nagano, T., and Fridovich, I. (1985): Does the aerobic xanthine oxidase reaction generate singlet oxygen? *Photochem. Photobiol.,* 41:33–37.

522. Nakagawara, A., Nathan, C. F., and Cohn, Z. A. (1981): Hydrogen peroxide metabolism in human monocytes during differentiation *in vitro. J. Clin. Invest.,* 68:1243–1252.

523. Nakagawara, A., DeSantis, N. M., Nogueira, N., and Nathan, C. F. (1982): Lymphokines enhance the capacity of human monocytes to secrete reactive oxygen intermediates. *J. Clin. Invest.,* 70:1042–1048.

524. Nakamura, M., Baxter, C. R., and Masters, B. S. S. (1981): Simultaneous demonstration of phagocytosis-connected oxygen consumption and corresponding NAD(P)H oxidase activity: direct evidence for NADPH as the predominant electron donor to oxygen in phagocytizing human neutrophils. *Biochem. Biophys. Res. Commun.,* 98:743–751.

525. Naskalski, J. W. (1977): Myeloperoxidase inactivation in the course of catalysis of chlorination of taurine. *Biochim. Biophys. Acta,* 485:291–300.

526. Nathan, C. F. (1980): The release of hydrogen peroxide from mononuclear phagocytes and its role in extracellular cytolysis. In: *Mononuclear Phagocytes—Functional Aspects,* edited by R. van Furth, pp. 1105–1137. Martinus Nijhoff, The Hague.

527. Nathan, C. F. (1982): Secretion of oxygen intermediates: role in effector functions of activated macrophages. *Fed. Proc.,* 41:2206–2211.

528. Nathan, C. F. (1983): Mechanisms of macrophage antimicrobial activity. *Trans. R. Soc. Trop. Med. Hyg.,* 77:620–630.

529. Nathan, C., and Cohn, Z. (1980): Role of oxygen-dependent mechanisms in antibody-induced lysis of tumor cells by activated macrophages. *J. Exp. Med.,* 152:198–208.

530. Nathan, C. F., and Cohn, Z. A. (1981): Antitumor effects of hydrogen peroxide *in vivo. J. Exp. Med.,* 154:1539–1553.

531. Nathan, C. F., and Klebanoff, S. J. (1982): Augmentation of spontaneous macrophage-mediated cytolysis of eosinophil peroxidase. *J. Exp. Med.,* 155:1291–1308.

532. Nathan, C. F., and Nakagawara, A. (1982): Role of reactive oxygen intermediates in macrophage killing of intracellular pathogens: a review. In: *Self-Defense Mechanisms. Role of Macrophages,* edited by D. Mizuno, Z. A. Cohn, K. Takeya, and N. Ishida, pp. 279–294. University of Tokyo Press, Tokyo.

533. Nathan, C. F., and Root, R. K. (1977): Hydrogen peroxide release from mouse peritoneal macrophages: dependence on sequential activation and triggering. *J. Exp. Med.,* 146:1648–1662.

534. Nathan, C., Nogueira, N., Juangbhanich, C., Ellis, J., and Cohn, Z. (1979): Activation of macrophages *in vivo* and *in vitro:* correlation between hydrogen peroxide release and killing of *Trypanosoma cruzi. J. Exp. Med.,* 149:1056–1068.

535. Nathan, C. F., Brukner, L. H., Silverstein, S. C., and Cohn, Z. A. (1979): Extracellular cytolysis by activated macrophages and granulocytes. 1. Pharmacologic triggering of effector cells and the release of hydrogen peroxide. *J. Exp. Med.,* 149:84–99.

536. Nathan, C. F., Silverstein, S. C., Brukner, L. H., and Cohn, Z. A. (1979): Extracellular cytolysis by activated macrophages and granulocytes. II. Hydrogen peroxide as a mediator of cytotoxicity. *J. Exp. Med.,* 149:100–113.

537. Nathan, C. F., Arrick, B. A., Murray, H. W., DeSantis, N. M., and Cohn, Z. A. (1981): Tumor cell anti-oxidant defenses: inhibition of the glutathione redox cycle enhances macrophage-mediated cytolysis. *J. Exp. Med.,* 153:766–782.

538. Nathan, C. F., Murray, H. W., Wiebe, M. E., and Rubin, B. Y. (1983): Identification of interferon-γ as the lymphokine that activates human macrophage oxidative metabolism and antimicrobial activity. *J. Exp. Med.,* 158:670–689.

539. Nathan, C. F., Prendergast, T. J., Wiebe, M. E., Stanley, E. R., Platzer, E., Remold, H. G., Welte, K., Rubin, B. Y., and Murray, H. W. (1984): Activation of human macrophages: comparison of other cytokines with interferon-γ. *J. Exp. Med.,* 160:600–605.

540. Nauseef, W. M., and Malech, H. L. (1986): Analysis of the peptide subunits of human neutrophil myeloperoxidase. *Blood,* 67:1504–1507.

541. Nauseef, W. M., Root, R. K., and Malech, H. L. (1983): Biochemical and immunologic analysis of hereditary myeloperoxidase deficiency. *J. Clin. Invest.,* 71:1297–1307.

542. Nauseef, W. M., Metcalf, J. A., and Root, R. K. (1983): Role of myeloperoxidase in the respiratory burst of human neutrophils. *Blood,* 61:483–492.

543. Newburger, P. E., Speier, C., Borregaard, N., Walsh, C. E., Whitin, J. C., and Simons, E. R. (1984): Development of the superoxide-generating system during differentiation of the HL-60 human promyelocytic leukemia cell line. *J. Biol. Chem.,* 259:3771–3776.

544. Newton, N., Morell, D. B., Clarke, L., and Clezy, P. S. (1965): The haem prosthetic groups of some animal peroxidases. II. Myeloperoxidase. *Biochim. Biophys. Acta,* 96:476–486.

545. Nichols, B. A. (1982): Uptake and digestion of horseradish peroxidase in rabbit alveolar macrophages: formation of a pathway connecting lysosomes to the cell surface. *Lab. Invest.,* 47:235–246.

546. Nichols, B. A., and Bainton, D. F. (1973): Differentiation of human monocytes in bone marrow and blood: sequential formation of two granule populations. *Lab. Invest.,* 29:27–40.

547. Nilsson, R., and Kearns, D. R. (1974): Role of singlet oxygen in some chemiluminescence and enzyme oxidation reactions. *J. Phys. Chem.,* 78:1681–1683.

548. Nishikimi, M. (1975): Oxidation of ascorbic acid with superoxide generated by the xanthine-xanthine oxidase system. *Biochem. Biophys. Res. Commun.,* 63:463–468.

549. Nishikimi, M., Yamada, H., and Yagi, K. (1980): Oxidation by superoxide of tocopherols dispersed in aqueous media with deoxycholate. *Biochim. Biophys. Acta,* 627:101–108.

550. Nishizuka, Y. (1986): Studies and perspectives of protein kinase C. *Science,* 233:305–312.

551. Nogueira, N. M., Klebanoff, S. J., and Cohn, Z. A. (1982): T. cruzi: sensitization to macrophage killing by eosinophil peroxidase. *J. Immunol.,* 128:1705–1708.

552. North, R. J. (1970): The relative importance of blood monocytes and fixed macrophages to the expression of cell-mediated immunity to infection. *J. Exp. Med.,* 132:521–534.

553. Odajima, T. (1980): Myeloperoxidase of the leukocyte of normal blood: nature of the prosthetic group of myeloperoxidase. *J. Biochem.,* 87:379–391.

554. Odajima, T., and Yamazaki, I. (1970): Myeloperoxidase of the leukocyte of normal blood. I. Reaction of myeloperoxidase with hydrogen peroxide. *Biochim. Biophys. Acta,* 206:71–77.

555. Odajima, T., and Yamazaki, I. (1972): Myeloperoxidase of the leukocyte of normal blood. III. The reaction of ferric myeloperoxidase with superoxide anion. *Biochim. Biophys. Acta,* 284:355–359.

556. Odeberg, H., Olofsson, T., and Olsson, I. (1974): Myeloperoxidase-mediated extracellular iodination during phagocytosis in granulocytes. *Scand. J. Haematol.,* 12:155–160.

557. O'Donnell-Tormey, J., DeBoer, C. J., and Nathan, C. F. (1985): Resistance of human tumor cells *in vitro* to oxidative cytolysis. *J. Clin. Invest.,* 76:80–86.

558. O'Flaherty, J. T., Schmitt, J. D., and Wykle, R. L. (1985): Interactions of arachidonate metabolism and protein kinase C in mediating neutrophil function. *Biochem. Biophys. Res. Commun.,* 127:916–923.

559. Ohkuma, S., and Poole, B. (1978): Fluorescence probe measurement of the intralysosomal pH in living cells and the perturbation of pH by various agents. *Proc. Natl. Acad. Sci. USA,* 75:3327–3331.

560. Ohno, Y., Seligmann, B. E., and Gallin, J. I. (1985): Cytochrome b translocation to human neutrophil plasma membranes and superoxide release: differential effects of N-formylmethionylleucyl-

phenylalanine, phorbol myristate acetate and A23187. *J. Biol. Chem.,* 260:2409–2415.

561. Ohno, Y., Buescher, E. S., Roberts, R., Metcalf, J. A., and Gallin, J. (1986): Reevaluation of cytochrome b and flavin adenine dinucleotide in neutrophils from patients with chronic granulomatous disease and description of a family with probable autosomal recessive inheritance of cytochrome b deficiency. *Blood,* 67:1132–1138.

562. Ohta, H., Takahashi, H., Hattori, H., Yamada, H., and Takikawa, K. (1966): Some oxidative enzymes and cytochrome in the specific granules of neutrophil leukocytes. *Acta Haematol. Jpn.,* 29:799–808.

563. Okajima, F., Katada, T., and Ui, M. (1985): Coupling of the guanine nucleotide regulatory protein to chemotactic peptide receptors in neutrophil membranes and its uncoupling by islet-activating protein, pertussis toxin: a possible role of the toxin substrate in Ca^{2+}-mobilizing receptor-mediator signal transduction. *J. Biol. Chem.,* 260:6761–6768.

564. Okolow-Zubkowska, M. J., and Hill, H. A. O. (1980): Spin trapping of superoxide and hydroxyl radicals produced by stimulated human neutrophils. *Dev. Biochem.,* 11B:201–210.

565. Olsen, R. L., and Little, C. (1983): Purification and some properties of myeloperoxidase and eosinophil peroxidase from human blood. *Biochem. J.,* 209:781–787.

566. Olsen, R. L., and Little, C. (1984): Studies on the subunits of human myeloperoxidase. *Biochem. J.,* 222:701–709.

567. Olsen, R. L., Syse, K., Little, C., and Christensen, T. B. (1985): Further characterization of human eosinophil peroxidase. *Biochem. J.,* 229:779–784.

568. Olsson, I., Persson, A., and Strömberg, K. (1984): Biosynthesis, transport and processing of myeloperoxidase in the human leukaemic promyelocytic cell line HL-60 and normal marrow cells. *Biochem. J.,* 223:911–919.

569. Ooi, W., Levine, H. G., LaMont, J. T., and Clark, R. A. (1984): Inactivation of *Clostridium difficile* cytotoxin by the neutrophil myeloperoxidase system. *J. Infect. Dis.,* 149:215–219.

570. Ossanna, P. J., Test, S. T., Matheson, N. R., Regiani, S., and Weiss, S. J. (1986): Oxidative regulation of neutrophil elastase-alpha-1-proteinase inhibitor interactions. *J. Clin. Invest.,* 77:1939–1951.

571. Ozawa, T., and Hanaki, A. (1978): Hydroxyl radical produced by the reaction of superoxide ion with hydrogen peroxide: electron spin resonance detection by spin trapping. *Chem. Pharm. Bull.,* 26:2572–2575.

572. Pabst, M. J., Hedegaard, H. B., and Johnston, R. B., Jr. (1982): Cultured human monocytes require exposure to bacterial products to maintain an optimal oxygen radical response. *J. Immunol.,* 128:123–128.

573. Papini, E., Grzeskowiak, M., Bellavite, P., and Rossi, F. (1985): Protein kinase C phosphorylates a component of NADPH oxidase of neutrophils. *FEBS Lett.,* 190:204–208.

574. Paredes, J. M., and Weiss, S. J. (1982): Human neutrophils transform prostaglandins by a myeloperoxidase-dependent mechanism. *J. Biol. Chem.,* 257:2738–2740.

575. Parkos, C. A., Cochrane, C. G., Schmitt, M., and Jesaitis, A. J. (1985): Regulation of the oxidative response of human granulocytes to chemoattractants: no evidence for stimulated traffic of redox enzymes between endo and plasma membranes. *J. Biol. Chem.,* 260:6541–6547.

576. Parry, M. F., Root, R. K., Metcalf, J. A., Delaney, K. K., Kaplow, L. S., and Richar, W. J. (1981): Myeloperoxidase deficiency: prevalence and clinical significance. *Ann. Intern. Med.,* 95:293–301.

577. Passo, S. A., and Weiss, S. J. (1984): Oxidative mechanisms utilized by human neutrophils to destroy *Escherichia coli. Blood,* 63:1361–1368.

578. Paul, B. B., Strauss, R. R., Selvaraj, R. J., and Sbarra, A. J. (1973): Peroxidase mediated antimicrobial activities of alveolar macrophage granules. *Science,* 181:849–850.

579. Pearson, R. D., and Steigbigel, R. T. (1981): Phagocytosis and killing of the protozoan *Leishmania donovani* by human polymorphonuclear leukocytes. *J. Immunol.,* 127:1438–1443.

580. Pember, S. O., and Kinkade, J. M., Jr. (1983): Differences in myeloperoxidase activity from neutrophilic polymorphonuclear leukocytes of differing density: relationship to selective exocytosis of distinct forms of the enzyme. *Blood,* 61:1116–1124.

581. Pember, S. O., Fuhrer-Krusi, S. M., Barnes, K. C., and Kinkade, J. M., Jr. (1982): Isolation of three native forms of myeloperoxidase from human polymorphonuclear leukocytes. *FEBS Lett.,* 140:103–108.

582. Pember, S. O., Shapira, R., and Kinkade, J. M., Jr. (1983): Multiple forms of myeloperoxidase from human neutrophilic granulocytes; evidence for differences in compartmentalization, enzymic activity, and subunit structure. *Arch. Biochem. Biophys.,* 221:391–403.

583. Pember, S. O., Heyl, B. L., Kinkade, J. M., Jr., and Lambeth, J. D. (1984): Cytochrome b_{558} from (bovine) granulocytes: partial purification from Triton X-114 extracts and properties of the isolated cytochrome. *J. Biol. Chem.,* 259:10590–10595.

584. Pene, J., Rousseau, V., and Stanislawski, M. (1986): *In-vitro* cytolysis of myeloma tumor cells with glucose oxidase and lactoperoxidase antibody conjugates. *Biochem. Int.,* 13:233–243.

585. Penfield, A., and Dale, M. M. (1984): Synergism between A23187 and 1-oleoyl-2-acetyl-glycerol in superoxide production by human neutrophils. *Biochem. Biophys. Res. Commun.,* 125:332–336.

586. Peppin, G. J., and Weiss, S. J. (1986): Activation of the endogenous metalloproteinase, gelatinase, by triggered human neutrophils. *Proc. Natl. Acad. Sci. USA,* 83:4322–4326.

587. Petrequin, P. R., Todd, R. F., III, Smolen, J. E., and Boxer, L. A. (1986): Expression of specific granule markers on the cell surface of neutrophil cytoplasts. *Blood,* 67:1119–1125.

588. Phelps, C. F., Antonini, E., Giacometti, G., and Brunori, M. (1974): The kinetics of oxidation of ferroperoxidase by molecular oxygen. *Biochem. J.,* 141:265–272.

589. Philpott, G. W., Bower, R. J., and Parker, C. W. (1973): Selective iodination and cytotoxicity of tumor cells with an antibody-enzyme conjugate. *Surgery,* 74:51–58.

590. Philpott, G. W., Shearer, W. T., Bower, R. J., and Parker, C. W. (1973): Selective cytotoxicity of hapten-substituted cells with an antibody-enzyme conjugate. *J. Immunol.,* 111:921–929.

591. Piatt, J., and O'Brien, P. J. (1979): Singlet oxygen formation by a peroxidase, H_2O_2 and halide system. *Eur. J. Biochem.,* 93:323–332.

592. Piatt, J. F., Cheema, A. S., and O'Brien, P. J. (1977): Peroxidase catalyzed singlet oxygen formation from hydrogen peroxide. *FEBS Lett.,* 74:251–254.

593. Pincus, S. H. (1980): Peroxidase-mediated iodination by guinea pig peritoneal exudate eosinophils. *Inflammation,* 4:89–106.

594. Pincus, S. H. (1980): Comparative metabolism of guinea pig peritoneal exudate neutrophils and eosinophils. *Proc. Soc. Exp. Biol. Med.,* 163:482–489.

595. Pitt, J., and Bernheimer, H. P. (1974): Role of peroxide in phagocytic killing of pneumococci. *Infect. Immun.,* 9:48–52.

596. Pontremoli, S., Melloni, E., Michetti, M., Sacco, O., Sparatore, B., Salamino, F., Damiano, G., and Horecker, B. L. (1986): Cytolytic effects of neutrophils: role for a membrane-bound neutral proteinase. *Proc. Natl. Acad. Sci. USA,* 83:1685–1689.

597. Pontremoli, S., Melloni, E., Michetti, M., Sacco, O., Salamino, F., Sparatore, B., and Horecker, B. L. (1986): Biochemical responses in activated human neutrophils mediated by protein kinase C and a Ca^{2+}-requiring proteinase. *J. Biol. Chem.,* 261:8309–8313.

598. Pozzan, T., Lew, D. P., Wollheim, C. B., and Tsien, R. Y. (1983): Is cytosolic ionized calcium regulating neutrophil activation? *Science,* 221:1413–1415.

599. Prentki, M., Wollheim, C. B., and Lew, P. D. (1984): Ca^{2+} homeostasis in permeabilized human neutrophils: characterization of Ca^{2+}-sequestering pools and the action of inositol 1,4,5-triphosphate. *J. Biol. Chem.,* 259:13777–13782.

600. Pryor, W. A., and Tang, R. H. (1978): Ethylene formation from methional. *Biochem. Biophys. Res. Commun.,* 81:498–503.

601. Quie, P. G., White, J. G., Holmes, B., and Good, R. A. (1967): *In vitro* bactericidal capacity of human polymorphonuclear leukocytes: diminished activity in chronic granulomatous disease in childhood. *J. Clin. Invest.,* 46:668–679.

602. Rabani, J., Klug, D., and Fridovich, I. (1972): Decay of the HO_2 and O_2^- radicals catalyzed by superoxide dismutase: a pulse radiolytic investigation. *Isr. J. Chem.,* 10:1095–1106.

603. Ramsey, P. G., Martin, T., Chi, E., and Klebanoff, S. J. (1982): Arming of mononuclear phagocytes by eosinophil peroxidase bound to Staphylococcus aureus. J. Immunol., 128:415–420.

604. Reiss, M., and Roos, D. (1978): Differences in oxygen metabolism of phagocytosing monocytes and neutrophils. J. Clin. Invest., 61:480–488.

605. Repine, J. E., Eaton, J. W., Anders, M. W., Hoidal, J. R., and Fox, R. B. (1979): Generation of hydroxyl radical by enzymes, chemicals, and human phagocytes in vitro: detection with the anti-inflammatory agent, dimethyl sulfoxide. J. Clin. Invest., 64:1642–1651.

606. Repine, J. E., Fox, R. B., and Berger, E. M. (1981): Hydrogen peroxide kills Staphylococcus aureus by reacting with staphylococcal iron to form hydroxyl radical. J. Biol. Chem., 256:7094–7096.

607. Repine, J. E., Fox, R. B., and Berger, E. M. (1981): Dimethyl sulfoxide inhibits killing of Staphylococcus aureus by polymorphonuclear leukocytes. Infect. Immun., 31:510–513.

608. Repine, J. E., Fox, R. B., Berger, E. M., and Harada, R. N. (1981): Effect of staphylococcal iron content on the killing of Staphylococcus aureus by polymorphonuclear leukocytes. Infect. Immun., 32:407–410.

609. Rest, R. F., and Spitznagel, J. K. (1977): Subcellular distribution of superoxide dismutases in human neutrophils: influence of myeloperoxidase on the measurement of superoxide dismutase activity. Biochem. J., 166:145–153.

610. Roberts, J. L., Jr., and Sawyer, D. T. (1983): Activation of superoxide ion by reactions with protons, electrophiles, secondary amines, radicals and reduced metal ions. Isr. J. Chem., 23:430–438.

611. Roberts, P. J., Cross, A. R., Jones, O. T. G., and Segal, A. W. (1982): Development of cytochrome b and an active oxidase system in association with maturation of a human promyelocytic (HL-60) cell line. J. Cell. Biol., 95:720–726.

612. Robertson, P., Jr., and Fridovich, I. (1982): A reaction of the superoxide radical with tetrapyrroles. Arch. Biochem. Biophys., 213:353–357.

613. Robinson, J. M., Badwey, J. A., Karnovsky, M. L., and Karnovsky, M. J. (1985): Release of superoxide and change in morphology by neutrophils in response to phorbol esters: antagonism by inhibitors of calcium-binding proteins. J. Cell Biol., 101:1052–1058.

614. Rohrer, G. F., von Wartburg, J. P., and Aebi, H. (1966): Myeloperoxidase aus menschlichen Leukocyten. I. Isolierung und Charakterisierung des Enzymes. Biochem. Z., 344:478–491.

615. Romeo, D., Zabucchi, G., Soranzo, M. R., and Rossi, F. (1971): Macrophage metabolism: activation of NADPH oxidation by phagocytosis. Biochem. Biophys. Res. Commun., 45:1056–1062.

616. Roos, D., and Balm, A. J. M. (1980): The oxidative metabolism of monocytes. In: The Reticuloendothelial System. A Comprehensive Treatise. 2. Biochemistry and Metabolism, edited by A. J. Sbarra and R. R. Strauss, pp. 189–229. Plenum Press, New York.

617. Roos, D., Weening, R. S., Voetman, A. A., Vanschaik, M. L. J., Bot, A. A. M., Meerhof, L. J., and Loos, J. A. (1979): Protection of phagocytic leukocytes by endogenous glutathione: studies in a family with glutathione reductase deficiency. Blood, 53:851–866.

618. Roos, D., Weening, R. S., Wyss, S. R., and Aebi, H. E. (1980): Protection of human neutrophils by endogenous catalase: studies with cells from catalase-deficient individuals. J. Clin. Invest., 65:1515–1522.

619. Roos, D., Hamers, M. N., van Zwieten, R., and Weening, R. S. (1983): Acidification of the phagocytic vacuole: a possible defect in chronic granulomatous disease? Adv. Host. Def. Mech., 3:145–193.

620. Roos, D., Eckmann, C. M., Yazdanbakhsh, M., Hamers, M. N., and deBoer, M. (1984): Excretion of superoxide by phagocytes measured with cytochrome c entrapped in resealed erythrocyte ghosts. J. Biol. Chem., 259:1770–1775.

621. Root, R. K. (1974): Correction of the function of chronic granulomatous disease (CGD) granulocytes (PMN) with extracellular H_2O_2. Clin. Res., 22:452.

622. Root, R. K., and Stossel, T. P. (1974): Myeloperoxidase-mediated iodination by granulocytes: intracellular site of operation and some regulating factors. J. Clin. Invest., 53:1207–1215.

623. Rosen, H., and Klebanoff, S. J. (1976): Chemiluminescence and superoxide production by myeloperoxidase-deficient leukocytes. J. Clin. Invest., 58:50–60.

624. Rosen, H., and Klebanoff, S. J. (1977): Formation of singlet oxygen by the myeloperoxidase-mediated antimicrobial system. J. Biol. Chem., 252:4803–4810.

625. Rosen, H., and Klebanoff, S. J. (1979): Bactericidal activity of a superoxide anion generating system: a model for the polymorphonuclear leukocyte. J. Exp. Med., 149:27–39.

626. Rosen, H., and Klebanoff, S. J. (1979): Hydroxyl radical generation by polymorphonuclear leukocytes measured by electron spin resonance spectroscopy. J. Clin. Invest., 64:1725–1729.

627. Rosen, H., and Klebanoff, S. J. (1981): Role of iron and ethylenediaminetetraacetic acid in the bactericidal activity of a superoxide anion-generating system. Arch. Biochem. Biophys., 208:512–519.

628. Rosen, H., and Klebanoff, S. J. (1982): Oxidation of Escherichia coli iron centers by the myeloperoxidase-mediated microbicidal system. J. Biol. Chem., 257:13731–13735.

629. Rosen, H., and Klebanoff, S. J. (1985): Oxidation of microbial iron-sulfur centers by the myeloperoxidase-H_2O_2-halide antimicrobial system. Infect. Immun., 47:613–618.

630. Ross, R., and Klebanoff, S. J. (1966): The eosinophilic leukocyte: fine structure of changes in the uterus during the estrous cycle. J. Exp. Med., 124:653–660.

631. Rossi, F., and Zatti, M. (1964): Biochemical aspects of phagocytosis in polymorphonuclear leucocytes: NADH and NADPH oxidation by the granules of resting and phagocytizing cells. Experientia, 20:21–23.

632. Rowley, D. A., and Halliwell, B. (1982): Superoxide-dependent formation of hydroxyl radicals in the presence of thiol compounds. FEBS Lett., 138:33–36.

633. Rowley, D. A., and Halliwell, B. (1982): Superoxide-dependent formation of hydroxyl radicals from NADH and NADPH in the presence of iron salts. FEBS Lett., 142:39–41.

634. Rowley, D. A., and Halliwell, B. (1983): Formation of hydroxyl radicals from hydrogen peroxide and iron salts by superoxide- and ascorbate-dependent mechanisms: relevance to the pathology of rheumatoid disease. Clin. Sci., 64:649–653.

635. Rowley, D. A., and Halliwell, B. (1983): Superoxide-dependent and ascorbate-dependent formation of hydroxyl radicals in the presence of copper salts: a physiologically significant reaction? Arch. Biochem. Biophys., 225:279–284.

636. Rumyantseva, G. V., Weiner, L. M., Molin, Yu. N., and Budker, V. G. (1979): Permeation of liposome membrane by superoxide radical. FEBS Lett., 108:477–480.

637. Rush, J. D., and Bielski, B. H. J. (1986): Pulse radiolysis studies of alkaline Fe (III) and Fe (VI) solutions: observation of transient iron complexes with intermediate oxidation states. J. Am. Chem. Soc., 108:523–525.

638. Rush, J. D., and Koppenol, W. H. (1986): Oxidizing intermediates in the reaction of ferrous EDTA with hydrogen peroxide: reactions with organic molecules and ferrocytochrome C. J. Biol. Chem., 261:6730–6733.

639. Sadrzadeh, S. M. H., Graf, E., Panter, S. S., Hallaway, P. E., and Eaton, J. W. (1984): Hemoglobin: a biologic Fenton reagent. J. Biol. Chem., 259:14354–14356.

640. Saez, G., Thornalley, P. J., Hill, H. A. O., Hems, R., and Bannister, J. V. (1982): The production of free radicals during the autoxidation of cysteine and their effect on isolated rat hepatocytes. Biochim. Biophys. Acta, 719:24–31.

641. Sagone, A. L., Jr., Decker, M. A., Wells, R. M., and DeMocko, C. (1980): A new method for the detection of hydroxyl radical production by phagocytic cells. Biochim. Biophys. Acta, 628:90–97.

642. Sagone, A. L., Jr., Husney, R. M., O'Dorisio, M. S., and Metz, E. N. (1984): Mechanisms for the oxidation of reduced glutathione by stimulated granulocytes. Blood, 63:96–104.

643. Samuni, A., Chevion, M., and Czapski, G. (1981): Unusual copper-induced sensitization of the biological damage due to superoxide radicals. J. Biol. Chem., 256:12632–12635.

644. Samuni, A., Aronovitch, J., Godinger, D., Chevion, M., and Czapski, G. (1983): On the cytotoxicity of vitamin C and metal ions: a site-specific Fenton mechanism. Eur. J. Biochem., 137:119–124.

645. Saran, M., Bors, W., Michel, C., and Elstner, E. F. (1980): Formation

of ethylene from methionine: reactivity of radiolytically produced oxygen radicals and effect of substrate activation. *Int. J. Radiat. Biol.*, 37:521–527.

646. Sasada, M., Pabst, M. J., and Johnston, R. B., Jr. (1983): Activation of mouse peritoneal macrophages by lipopolysaccharide alters the kinetic parameters of the superoxide-producing NADPH oxidase. *J. Biol. Chem.*, 258:9631–9635.

647. Sawyer, D. T., and Valentine, J. S. (1981): How super is superoxide. *Acc. Chem. Res.*, 14:393–400.

648. Schneider, C., Zanetti, M., and Romeo, D. (1981): Surface-reactive stimuli selectively increase protein phosphorylation in human neutrophils. *FEBS Lett.*, 127:4–8.

649. Schultz, J. (1980): Myeloperoxidase. In: *The Reticuloendothelial System. A Comprehensive Treatise. 2. Biochemistry and Metabolism,* edited by A. J. Sbarra and R. R. Strauss, pp. 231–254. Plenum Press, New York.

650. Schultz, J., and Kaminker, K. (1962): Myeloperoxidase of the leucocyte of normal human blood. I. Content and localization. *Arch. Biochem. Biophys.*, 96:465–467.

651. Schultz, J., Baker, A., and Tucker, B. (1976): Myeloperoxidase-enzyme therapy on rat mammary tumors. In: *Cancer Enzymology,* edited by J. Schultz and F. Ahmad, pp. 319–333. Academic Press, New York.

652. Searle, A. J. F., and Tomasi, A. (1982): Hydroxyl free radical production in iron-cysteine solutions and protection by zinc. *J. Inorg. Biochem.*, 17:161–166.

653. Segal, A. W., and Jones, O. T. G. (1978): Novel cytochrome b system in phagocytic vacuoles of human granulocytes. *Nature,* 276:515–517.

654. Segal, A. W., and Jones, O. T. G. (1979): Reduction and subsequent oxidation of a cytochrome b of human neutrophils after stimulation with phorbol myristate acetate. *Biochem. Biophys. Res. Commun.,* 88:130–134.

655. Segal, A. W., and Jones, O. T. G. (1979): The subcellular distribution and some properties of the cytochrome b component of the microbicidal oxidase system of human neutrophils. *Biochem. J.,* 182:181–188.

656. Segal, A. W., and Jones, O. T. G. (1980): Absence of cytochrome b reduction in stimulated neutrophils from both female and male patients with chronic granulomatous disease. *FEBS Lett.,* 110:111–114.

657. Segal, A. W., Jones, O. T. G., Webster, D., and Allison, A. C. (1978): Absence of a newly described cytochrome b from neutrophils of patients with chronic granulomatous disease. *Lancet,* 2:446–449.

658. Segal, A. W., Garcia, R., Goldstone, A. H., Cross, A. R., and Jones, O. T. G. (1981): Cytochrome b$_{-245}$ of neutrophils is also present in human monocytes, macrophages and eosinophils. *Biochem. J.,* 196:363–367.

659. Segal, A. W., Geisow, M., Garcia, R., Harper, A., and Miller, R. (1981): The respiratory burst of phagocytic cells is associated with a rise in vacuolar pH. *Nature,* 290:406–409.

660. Segal, A. W., Cross, A. R., Garcia, R. C., Borregaard, N., Valerius, N. H., Soothill, J. F., and Jones, O. T. G. (1983): Absence of cytochrome b$_{-245}$ in chronic granulomatous disease: a multicenter European evaluation of its incidence and relevance. *N. Engl. J. Med.,* 308:245–251.

661. Segal, A. W., Garcia, R. D., and Harper, A. M. (1983): Iodination by stimulated human neutrophils: studies on its stoichiometry, subcellular localization and relevance to microbial killing. *Biochem. J.,* 210:215–225.

662. Segal, A. W., Heyworth, P. G., Cockcroft, S., and Barrowman, M. M. (1985): Stimulated neutrophils from patients with autosomal recessive chronic granulomatous disease fail to phosphorylate a M$_r$-44,000 protein. *Nature,* 316:547–549.

663. Seim, S. (1982): Production of reactive oxygen species and chemiluminescence by human monocytes during differentiation and lymphokine activation *in vitro. Acta Pathol. Microbiol. Immunol. Scand. [C],* 90:179–185.

664. Seim, S. (1983): Role of myeloperoxidase in the luminol-dependent chemiluminescence response of phagocytosing human monocytes. *Acta Pathol. Microbiol. Immunol. Scand. [C],* 91:123–128.

665. Seim, S., and Espevik, T. (1983): Toxic oxygen species in monocyte-mediated antibody-dependent cytotoxicity. *J. Reticuloendothel. Soc.,* 33:417–428.

666. Seligmann, B., and Gallin, J. I. (1980): Secretagogue modulation of the response of human neutrophils to chemoattractants: studies with a membrane potential sensitive cyanine dye. *Mol. Immunol.,* 17:191–200.

667. Seligmann, B. E., and Gallin, J. I. (1980): Use of lipophilic probes of membrane potential to assess human neutrophil activation—abnormality in chronic granulomatous disease. *J. Clin. Invest.,* 66:493–503.

668. Seligmann, B., and Gallin, J. I. (1983): Abnormalities in elicited membrane potential changes in neutrophils from patients with chronic granulomatous disease. *Adv. Host Def. Mech.,* 3:195–226.

669. Selvaraj, R. J., Paul, B. B., Strauss, R. R., Jacobs, A. A., and Sbarra, A. J. (1974): Oxidative peptide cleavage and decarboxylation by the MPO-H$_2$O$_2$-Cl$^-$ antimicrobial system. *Infect. Immun.,* 9:255–260.

670. Selvaraj, R. J., Zgliczynski, J. M., Paul, B. B., and Sbarra, A. J. (1980): Chlorination of reduced nicotinamide adenine dinucleotides by myeloperoxidase: a novel bactericidal mechanism. *J. Reticuloendothel. Soc.,* 27:31–38.

671. Sepe, S. M., and Clark, R. A. (1985): Oxidant membrane injury by the neutrophil myeloperoxidase system. I. Characterization of a liposome model and injury by myeloperoxidase, hydrogen peroxide, and halides. *J. Immunol.,* 134:1888–1895.

672. Sepe, S. M., and Clark, R. A. (1985): Oxidant membrane injury by the neutrophil myeloperoxidase system. II. Injury by stimulated neutrophils and protection by lipid-soluble antioxidants. *J. Immunol.,* 134:1896–1901.

673. Serra, M. C., Bellavite, P., Davoli, A., Bannister, J. V., and Rossi, F. (1984): Isolation from neutrophil membranes of a complex containing active NADPH oxidase and cytochrome b$_{-245}$. *Biochim. Biophys. Acta,* 788:138–146.

674. Sha'afi, R. I., White, J. R., Molski, T. F. R., Shefcyk, J., Volpi, M., Naccache, P. N., and Feinstein, N. B. (1983): Phorbol 12-myristate 13-acetate activates rabbit neutrophils without an apparent rise in the level of intracellular free calcium. *Biochem. Biophys. Res. Commun.,* 114:638–645.

675. Shinagawa, Y., Shinagawa, Y., Tanaka, C., and Teraoka, A. (1966): Electron microscopic and biochemical study of the neutrophilic granules from leucocytes. *J. Electron Microsc.,* 15:81–85.

676. Shinar, E., Navok, T., and Chevion, M. (1983): The analogous mechanisms of enzymatic inactivation induced by ascorbate and superoxide in the presence of copper. *J. Biol. Chem.,* 258:14778–14783.

677. Shohet, S. B., Pitt, J., Baehner, R. L., and Poplack, D. G. (1974): Lipid peroxidation in the killing of phagocytized pneumococci. *Infect. Immun.,* 10:1321–1328.

678. Sibbett, S. S., and Hurst, J. K. (1984): Structural analysis of myeloperoxidase by resonance Raman spectroscopy. *Biochemistry,* 23:3007–3013.

679. Sibbett, S. S., Klebanoff, S. J., and Hurst, J. K. (1985): Resonance Raman characterization of the heme prosthetic group in eosinophil peroxidase. *FEBS Lett.,* 189:271–275.

680. Simchowitz, L., and Spilberg, I. (1979): Evidence for the role of superoxide radicals in neutrophil-mediated cytotoxicity. *Immunology,* 37:301–309.

681. Simchowitz, L., Mehta, J., and Spilberg, I. (1979): Chemotactic factor-induced superoxide radical generation by human neutrophils: requirement for proteinase (esterase) activity. *J. Lab. Clin. Med.,* 94:403–413.

682. Simchowitz, L., Fischbein, L. C., Spilberg, I., and Atkinson, J. P. (1980): Induction of a transient elevation in intracellular levels of adenosine-3′,5′-cyclic monophosphate by chemotactic factors: an early event in human neutrophil activation. *J. Immunol.,* 124:1482–1491.

683. Simchowitz, L., Spilberg, I., and Atkinson, J. P. (1983): Evidence that the functional responses of human neutrophils occur independently of transient elevations in cyclic AMP levels. *J. Cyclic Nucleotide Protein Phosphor. Res.,* 9:35–47.

684. Sinaceur, J., Ribière, C., Nordmann, J., and Nordmann, R. (1984):

Desferrioxamine: a scavenger of superoxide radicals? *Biochem. Pharmacol.,* 33:1693–1694.

685. Sips, H. J., and Hamers, M. N. (1981): Mechanism of the bactericidal action of myeloperoxidase: increased permeability of the *Escherichia coli* cell envelope. *Infect. Immun.,* 31:11–16.

686. Slivka, A., LoBuglio, A. F., and Weiss, S. J. (1980): A potential role of hypochlorous acid in granulocyte-mediated tumor cell cytotoxicity. *Blood,* 55:347–350.

687. Sloan, E. P., Crawford, D. R., and Schneider, D. L. (1981): Isolation of plasma membrane from human neutrophils and determination of cytochrome b and quinone content. *J. Exp. Med.,* 153:1316–1328.

688. Smith, D. C., and Klebanoff, S. J. (1970): A uterine fluid-mediated sperm-inhibitory system. *Biol. Reprod.,* 3:229–235.

689. Smith, C. D., Lane, B. C., Kusaka, I., Verghese, M. W., and Snyderman, R. (1985): Chemoattractant-receptor induced hydrolysis of phosphatidylinositol 4,5-biphosphate in human polymorphonuclear leukocyte membranes: requirement for a guanine nucleotide regulatory protein. *J. Biol. Chem.,* 260:5875–5878.

690. Smolen, J. E., and Weissmann, G. (1981): Stimuli which provoke secretion of azurophil enzymes from human neutrophils induce increments in adenosine cyclic 3'-5'-monophosphate. *Biochim. Biophys. Acta,* 672:197–206.

691. Smolen, J. E., Korchak, H. M., and Weissmann, G. (1980): Increased levels of cyclic adenosine-3',5'-monophosphate in human polymorphonuclear leukocytes after surface stimulation. *J. Clin. Invest.,* 65:1077–1085.

692. Smolen, J. E., Korchak, H. M., and Weissmann, G. (1981): The roles of extracellular and intracellular calcium in lysosomal enzyme release and superoxide anion generation by human neutrophils. *Biochim. Biophys. Acta,* 677:512–520.

693. Snyderman, R., and Pike, M. C. (1984): Chemoattractant receptors on phagocytic cells. *Annu. Rev. Immunol.,* 2:257–281.

694. Snyderman, R., Pike, M. C., Edge, S., and Lane, B. (1984): A chemoattractant receptor on macrophages exists in two affinity states regulated by guanine nucleotides. *J. Cell Biol.,* 98:444–448.

695. Sobeslavsky, O., and Chanock, R. M. (1968): Peroxide formation by mycoplasmas which infect man. *Proc. Soc. Exp. Biol. Med.,* 129:531–535.

696. Somerson, N. L., Walls, B. E., and Chanock, R. M. (1965): Hemolysin of *Mycoplasma pneumoniae:* tentative identification as a peroxide. *Science,* 150:226–228.

697. Soupart, P. (1962): Free amino acids in blood and urine in the human. In: *Amino Acid Pools,* edited by J. T. Holden, pp. 220–262. Elsevier, Amsterdam.

698. Spielberg, S. P., Boxer, L. A., Oliver, J. M., Allen, J. M., and Schulman, J. D. (1979): Oxidative damage to neutrophils in glutathione synthetase deficiency. *Br. J. Haematol.,* 42:215–223.

699. Spitznagel, J. K., Dalldorf, F. G., Leffell, M. S., Folds, J. D., Welsh, I. R. H., Cooney, M. H., and Martin, L. E. (1974): Character of azurophil and specific granules purified from human polymorphonuclear leukocytes. *Lab. Invest.,* 30:774–785.

700. Stankova, L., Rigas, D. A., Keown, P., and Bigley, R. (1977): Leukocyte ascorbate and glutathione: potential capacity for inactivating oxidants and free radicals. *J. Reticuloendothel. Soc.,* 21:97–102.

701. Stankova, L., Bigley, R., Wyss, S. R., and Aebi, H. (1979): Catalase and dehydroascorbate reductase in human polymorphonuclear leukocytes (PMN): possible functional relationship. *Experientia,* 35:852–853.

702. Stelmaszyńska, T. (1985): Formation of HCN by human phagocytosing neutrophils. 1. Chlorination of *Staphylococcus epidermidis* as a source of HCN. *Int. J. Biochem.,* 17:373–379.

703. Stelmaszyńska, T., and Zgliczynski, J. M. (1974): Myeloperoxidase of human neutrophilic granulocytes as chlorinating enzyme. *Eur. J. Biochem.,* 45:305–312.

704. Stelmaszyńska, T., and Zgliczynski, J. M. (1978): N-(2-Oxoacyl) amino acids and nitriles as final products of dipeptide chlorination mediated by the myeloperoxidase/H_2O_2/Cl^- system. *Eur. J. Biochem.,* 92:301–308.

705. Stendahl, O., and Lindgren, S. (1976): Function of granulocytes with deficient myeloperoxidase-mediated iodination in a patient with generalized pustular psoriasis. *Scand. J. Haematol.,* 16:144–153.

706. Stendahl, O., Molin, L., and Lindroth, M. (1983): Granulocyte-mediated release of histamine from mast cells: effect of myeloperoxidase and its inhibition by antiinflammatory sulfone compounds. *Int. Arch. Allergy Appl. Immunol.,* 70:277–284.

707. Stendahl, O., Coble, B-I., Dahlgren, C., Hed, J., and Molin, L. (1984): Myeloperoxidase modulates the phagocytic activity of polymorphonuclear neutrophil leukocytes: studies with cells from a myeloperoxidase-deficient patient. *J. Clin. Invest.,* 73:366–373.

708. Steveninick, J., van, van der Zee, J., and Dubbelman, T. M. A. R. (1985): Site-specific and bulk-phase generation of hydroxyl radicals in the presence of cupric ions and thiol compounds. *Biochem. J.,* 232:309–311.

709. Stevenson, H. C., Katz, P., Wright, D. G., Contreras, T. J., Jemionek, J. F., Hartwig, V. M., Flor, W. J., and Fauci, A. S. (1981): Human blood monocytes: characterization of negatively selected human monocytes and their suspension cell culture derivatives. *Scand. J. Immunol.,* 14:243–256.

710. Stossel, T. P., Mason, R. J., Pollard, T. D., and Vaughan, M. (1972): Isolation and properties of phagocytic vesicles. II. Alveolar macrophages. *J. Clin. Invest.,* 51:604–614.

711. Stossel, T. P., Mason, R. J., and Smith, A. L. (1974): Lipid peroxidation by human blood phagocytes. *J. Clin. Invest.,* 54:638–645.

712. Strauss, R. R., Paul, B. B., Jacobs, A. A., and Sbarra, A. J. (1971): Role of the phagocyte in host parasite interactions. XXVII. Myeloperoxidase-H_2O_2-Cl^--mediated aldehyde formation and its relationship to antimicrobial activity. *Infect. Immun.,* 3:595–602.

713. Sugar, A. M., Chahal, R. S., Brummer, E., and Stevens, D. A. (1984): The iron-hydrogen peroxide-iodide system is fungicidal: activity against the yeast phase of *Blastomyces dermatitidis. J. Leuk. Biol.,* 36:545–548.

714. Sutton, H. C. (1985): Efficiency of chelated iron compounds as catalysts for the Haber-Weiss reaction. *J. Free Rad. Biol. Med.,* 1:195–202.

715. Sutton, H. C., and Winterbourn, C. C. (1984): Chelated iron-catalyzed OH· formation from paraquat radicals and H_2O_2: mechanism of formate oxidation. *Arch. Biochem. Biophys.,* 235:106–115.

716. Sykes, G. (1965): The halogens. In: *Disinfection and Sterilization,* 2nd ed., pp. 381–410. Lippincott, Philadelphia.

717. Szuro-Sudol, A., and Nathan, C. F. (1982): Suppression of macrophage oxidative metabolism by products of malignant and nonmalignant cells. *J. Exp. Med.,* 156:945–961.

718. Szuro-Sudol, A., Murray, H. W., and Nathan, C. F. (1983): Suppression of macrophage antimicrobial activity by a tumor cell product. *J. Immunol.,* 131:384–387.

719. Takabe, T., Asami, S., and Akazawa, T. (1980): Glycolate formation catalyzed by spinach leaf transketolase utilizing the superoxide radical. *Biochemistry,* 19:3985–3989.

720. Takahashi, M. A., and Asada, K. (1983): Superoxide anion permeability of phospholipid membranes and chloroplast thylakoids. *Arch. Biochem. Biophys.,* 226:558–566.

721. Takeshige, K., and Minakami, S. (1981): Involvement of calmodulin in phagocytotic respiratory burst of leukocytes. *Biochem. Biophys. Res. Commun.,* 99:484–490.

722. Tamura, M., and Yamazaki, I. (1972): Reactions of the oxyform of horseradish peroxidase. *J. Biochem.,* 71:311–319.

723. Tanaka, Y., Kiyotaki, C., Tanowitz, H., and Bloom, B. R. (1982): Reconstitution of a variant macrophage cell line defective in oxygen metabolism with a H_2O_2-generating system. *Proc. Natl. Acad. Sci. USA,* 79:2584–2588.

724. Tauber, A. I., and Babior, B. M. (1977): Evidence for hydroxyl radical production by human neutrophils. *J. Clin. Invest.,* 60:374–379.

725. Tauber, A. I., Goetzl, E. J., and Babior, B. M. (1979): Unique characteristics of superoxide production by human eosinophils in eosinophilic states. *Inflammation,* 3:261–272.

726. Tauber, A. I., Wright, J., Higson, F. K., Edelman, S. A., and Waxman, D. J. (1985): Purification and characterization of the human neutrophil NADH-cytochrome b_5 reductase. *Blood,* 66:673–678.

727. Test, S. T., and Weiss, S. J. (1986): The generation and utilization

of chlorinated oxidants by human neutrophils. *Adv. Free Rad. Biol. Med.,* 2:91–116.

728. Test, S. T., Lampert, M. B., Ossanna, P. J., Thoene, J. G., and Weiss, S. J. (1984): Generation of nitrogen-chlorine oxidants by human phagocytes. *J. Clin. Invest.,* 74:1341–1349.

729. Theron, A., and Anderson, R. (1985): Investigation of the protective effects of the antioxidants ascorbate, cysteine, and dapsone on the phagocyte-mediated oxidative inactivation of human alpha-1-protease inhibitor *in vitro. Am. Rev. Respir. Dis.,* 132:1049–1054.

730. Thomas, E. L. (1979): Myeloperoxidase-hydrogen peroxide-chloride antimicrobial system: effect of exogenous amines on antibacterial action against *Escherichia coli. Infect. Immun.,* 25:110–116.

731. Thomas, E. L., and Aune, T. M. (1977): Peroxidase-catalyzed oxidation of protein sulfhydryls mediated by iodine. *Biochemistry,* 16:3581–3586.

732. Thomas, E. L., and Aune, T. M. (1978): Cofactor role of iodide in peroxidase antimicrobial action against *Escherichia coli. Antimicrob. Agents Chemother.,* 13:1000–1005.

733. Thomas, E. L., and Aune, T. M. (1978): Oxidation of *Escherichia coli* sulfhydryl components by the peroxidase-hydrogen peroxide-iodide antimicrobial system. *Antimicrob. Agents Chemother.,* 13: 1006–1010.

734. Thomas, E. L., and Fishman, M. (1986): Oxidation of chloride and thiocyanate by isolated leukocytes. *J. Biol. Chem.,* 261:9694–9702.

735. Thomas, E. L., Jefferson, M. M., and Grisham, M. B. (1982): Myeloperoxidase-catalyzed incorporation of amines into proteins: role of hypochlorous acid and dichloramines. *Biochemistry,* 21:6299–6308.

736. Thomas, E. L., Grisham, M. B., and Jefferson, M. M. (1983): Myeloperoxidase-dependent effect of amines on functions of isolated neutrophils. *J. Clin. Invest.,* 72:441–454.

737. Thomas, E. L., Grisham, M. B., Melton, D. F., and Jefferson, M. M. (1985): Evidence for a role of taurine in the *in vitro* oxidative toxicity of neutrophils toward erythrocytes. *J. Biol. Chem.,* 260:3321–3329.

738. Thong, Y. H. (1982): How important is the myeloperoxidase microbicidal system of phagocytic cells? *Med. Hypoth.,* 8:249–254.

739. Thorne, K. J. I., Svvennsen, R. J., and Franks, D. (1978): Role of hydrogen peroxide and peroxidase in the cytotoxicity of *Trypanosoma dionisii* by human granulocytes. *Infect. Immun.,* 21:798–805.

740. Thorne, K. J. I., Glauert, A. M., Svvennsen, R. J., Thomas, H., Morris, J., and Franks, D. (1981): Evasion of the oxidative microbicidal activity of human monocytes by trypomastigotes of *Trypanosoma dionisii. Parasitology,* 83:115–123.

741. Tsan, M-F. (1980): Phorbol myristate acetate-induced neutrophil autotoxicity. *J. Cell. Physiol.,* 105:327–334.

742. Tsan, M-F. (1982): Myeloperoxidase-mediated oxidation of methionine. *J. Cell. Physiol.,* 111:49–54.

743. Tsan, M.-F., and Chen, J. W. (1980): Oxidation of methionine by human polymorphonuclear leukocytes. *J. Clin. Invest.,* 65:1041–1050.

744. Tsan, M-F., and Denison, R. C. (1980): Phorbol myristate acetate-induced neutrophil autotoxicity: a comparison with H_2O_2 toxicity. *Inflammation,* 4:371–380.

745. Tsan, M-F., and Denison, R. C. (1981): Oxidation of n-formyl methionyl chemotactic peptide by human neutrophils. *J. Immunol.,* 126:1387–1389.

746. Tschesche, H., and Macartney, H. (1981): A new principle of regulation of enzymic activity: activation and regulation of human polymorphonuclear leukocyte collagenase via disulfide-thiol exchange as catalyzed by the glutathione cycle in a peroxidase coupled reaction to glucose metabolism. *Eur. J. Biochem.,* 120:183–190.

748. Tsunawaki, S., and Nathan, C. F. (1984): Enzymatic basis of macrophage activation: kinetic analysis of superoxide production in lysates of resident and activated mouse peritoneal macrophages and granulocytes. *J. Biol. Chem.,* 259:4305–4312.

749. Tsunawaki, S., and Nathan, C. F. (1986): Macrophage deactivation: altered kinetic properties of the superoxide-producing enzyme after exposure to tumor cell-conditioned medium. *J. Exp. Med.,* 164:1319–1331.

750. Tubaro, E., Lotti, B., Santiangeli, C., and Cavallo, G. (1980): Xanthine oxidase increase in polymorphonuclear leucocytes and mac-

rophages in mice in three pathological situations. *Biochem. Pharmacol.,* 29:1945–1948.

751. Tubaro, E., Lotti, B., Santiangeli, C., and Cavallo, G. (1980): Xanthine oxidase: an enzyme playing a role in the killing mechanism of polymorphonuclear leucocytes. *Biochem. Pharmacol.,* 29:3018–3019.

752. Turk, J., Henderson, W. R., Klebanoff, S. J., and Hubbard, W. C. (1983): Iodination of arachidonic acid mediated by eosinophil peroxidase, myeloperoxidase and lactoperoxidase: identification and comparison of products. *Biochim. Biophys. Acta,* 751:189–200.

753. Turkall, R. M., and Tsan, M. F. (1982): Oxidation of glutathione by the myeloperoxidase system. *J. Reticuloendothel. Soc.,* 31:353–360.

754. Umei, T., Takeshige, K., and Minakami, S. (1986): NADPH binding component of neutrophil superoxide-generating oxidase. *J. Biol. Chem.,* 261:5229–5232.

755. Ushijima, Y., and Nakano, M. (1980): No or little production of singlet molecular oxygen in HOCl or $HOCl/H_2O_2$: a model system for myeloperoxidase/H_2O_2/Cl. *Biochem. Biophys. Res. Commun.,* 93:1232–1237.

756. Vel, W. A. C., Namavar, F., Verweij, A., Marian, J. J., Pubben, A. N. B., and MacLaren, D. M. (1984): Killing capacity of human polymorphonuclear leukocytes in aerobic and anaerobic conditions. *J. Med. Microbiol.,* 18:173–180.

757. Venge, P., and Olsson, I. (1975): Cationic proteins of human granulocytes. VI. Effects on the complement system and mediation of chemotactic activity. *J. Immunol.,* 115:1505–1508.

758. Verghese, M. W., Smith, C. D., and Snyderman, R. (1985): Involvement of a guanine nucleotide regulatory protein in chemoattractant receptor mediated polyphosphoinositide metabolism, Ca^{++} mobilization and cellular responses by leukocytes. *Biochem. Biophys. Res. Commun.,* 127:450–457.

759. Verghese, M. W., Fox, K., McPhail, L. C., and Snyderman, R. (1985): Chemoattractant-elicited alterations of cAMP levels in human polymorphonuclear leukocytes require a Ca^{2+}-dependent mechanism which is independent of transmembrane activation of adenylate cyclase. *J. Biol. Chem.,* 260:6769–6775.

760. Voetman, A. A., and Roos, D. (1980): Endogenous catalase protects human blood phagocytes against oxidative damage by extracellularly generated hydrogen peroxide. *Blood,* 56:846–852.

761. Voetman, A. A., Weening, R. S., Hamers, M. W., Meerhof, L. J., Bot, A. A. A. M., and Roos, D. (1981): Phagocytosing human neutrophils inactivate their own granular enzymes. *J. Clin. Invest.,* 67:1541–1549.

762. Volpi, M., Yassin, R., Naccache, P. H., and Sha'afi, R. I. (1983): Chemotactic factor causes rapid decreases in phosphatidylinositol 4,5-biphosphate and phosphatidylinositol 4-monophosphate in rabbit neutrophils. *Biochem. Biophys. Res. Commun.,* 112:957–964.

763. Volpi, M., Naccache, P. H., Molski, T. F. P., Shefcyk, J., Huang, C-K., Marsh, M. L., Munoz, J., Becker, E. L., and Sha'afi, R. I. (1985): Pertussis toxin inhibits fMet-Leu-Phe but not phorbol ester-stimulated changes in rabbit neutrophils: role of G proteins in excitation response coupling. *Proc. Natl. Acad. Sci. USA,* 82:2708–2712.

764. Wagner, D. K., Collins-Lech, C., and Sohnol, P. G. (1986): Inhibition of neutrophil killing of *Candida albicans* pseudohyphae by substances which quench hypochlorous acid and chloramines. *Infect. Immun.,* 51:731–735.

765. Wakeyama, H., Takeshige, K., Takayanagi, R., and Minakami, S. (1982): Superoxide-forming NADPH oxidase preparation of pig polymorphonuclear leucocytes. *Biochem. J.,* 205:593–601.

766. Wakeyama, H., Takeshige, K., and Minakami, S. (1983): NADPH-dependent reduction of 2,6-dichlorophenol-indophenol by the phagocytic vesicles of pig polymorphonuclear leucocytes. *Biochem. J.,* 210:577–581.

767. Ward, P. A., Till, G. O., Kunkel, R., and Beauchamp, C. (1983): Evidence for the role of hydroxyl radical in complement and neutrophil-dependent tissue injury. *J. Clin. Invest.,* 72:789–801.

768. Weening, R. S., Wever, R., and Roos, D. (1975): Quantitative aspects of the production of superoxide radicals by phagocytizing human granulocytes. *J. Lab. Clin. Med.,* 85:245–252.

769. Weening, R. S., Corbeel, L., de Boer, M., Lutter, R., van Zwieten, R., Hamers, M. N., and Roos, D. (1985): Cytochrome b deficiency in an autosomal form of chronic granulomatous disease: a third form of chronic granulomatous disease recognized by monocyte hybridization. *J. Clin. Invest.,* 75:915–920.

770. Weinstein, J., and Bielski, B. H. J. (1979): Kinetics of the interaction of HO_2 and O_2^- radicals with hydrogen peroxide: the Haber-Weiss reaction. *J. Am. Chem. Soc.,* 101:58–62.

771. Weiss, S. J. (1980): The role of superoxide in the destruction of erythrocyte targets by human neutrophils. *J. Biol. Chem.,* 255:9912–9917.

772. Weiss, S. J. (1982): Neutrophil-mediated methemoglobin formation in the erythrocyte: the role of superoxide and hydrogen peroxide. *J. Biol. Chem.,* 257:2947–2953.

773. Weiss, S. J., and Slivka, A. (1982): Monocyte and granulocyte-mediated tumor cell destruction: a role for the hydrogen peroxide-myeloperoxidase-chloride system. *J. Clin. Invest.,* 69:255–262.

774. Weiss, S. J., King, G. W., and LoBuglio, A. F. (1977): Evidence for hydroxyl radical generation by human monocytes. *J. Clin. Invest.,* 60:370–373.

775. Weiss, S. J., Rustagi, P. K., and LoBuglio, A. F. (1978): Human granulocyte generation of hydroxyl radical. *J. Exp. Med.,* 147:316–323.

776. Weiss, S. J., LoBuglio, A. F., and Kessler, H. B. (1980): Oxidative mechanisms of monocyte-mediated cytotoxicity. *Proc. Natl. Acad. Sci. USA,* 77:584–587.

777. Weiss, S. J., Klein, R., Slivka, A., and Wei, M. (1982): Chlorination of taurine by human neutrophils: evidence for hypochlorous acid generation. *J. Clin. Invest.,* 70:598–607.

778. Weiss, S. J., Lampert, M. B., and Test, S. T. (1983): Long lived oxidants generated by human neutrophils: characterization and bioactivity. *Science,* 222:625–628.

779. Weiss, S. J., Peppin, G., Ortiz, X., Ragsdale, C., and Test, S. T. (1985): Oxidative autoactivation of latent collagenase by human neutrophils. *Science,* 227:747–749.

780. Weiss, S. J., Test, S. T., Eckmann, C. M., Roos, D., and Regiani, S. (1986): Brominating oxidants generated by human eosinophils. *Science,* 234:200–203.

781. West, B. C., Rosenthal, A. S., Gelb, N. A., and Kimball, H. R. (1974): Separation and characterization of human neutrophil granules. *Am. J. Pathol.,* 77:41–62.

782. Wever, R., and Bakkenist, A. R. J. (1980): The interaction of myeloperoxidase with ligands as studied by EPR. *Biochim. Biophys. Acta,* 612:178–184.

783. Wever, R., Hamers, M. N., Weening, R. S., and Roos, D. (1980): Characterization of the peroxidase in human eosinophils. *Eur. J. Biochem.,* 108:491–495.

784. Wever, R., Plat, H., and Hamers, M. N. (1981): Human eosinophil peroxidase: a novel isolation procedure, spectral properties and chlorinating activity. *FEBS Lett.,* 123:327–331.

785. Wever, R., Kast, W. M., Kasinoedin, J., and Boelens, R. (1982): The peroxidation of thiocyanate catalyzed by myeloperoxidase and lactoperoxidase. *Biochim. Biophys. Acta,* 709:212–219.

786. White, J. R., Naccache, P. H., Molski, T. F. P., Borgeat, P., and Sha'afi, R. I. (1983): Direct demonstration of increased intracellular concentration of free calcium in rabbit and human neutrophils following stimulation by chemotactic factor. *Biochem. Biophys. Res. Commun.,* 113:44–50.

787. White, J. R., Huang, C. K., Hill, J. M., Naccache, P. H., Becker, E. L., and Sha'afi, R. I. (1984): Effect of phorbol 12-myristate 13-acetate and its analogue 4 phorbol 12,13-didecanoate on protein phosphorylation and lysosomal enzyme release in rabbit neutrophils. *J. Biol. Chem.,* 259:8605–8611.

788. Whitin, J. C., Chapman, C. E., Simons, E. R., Chovaniec, M. E., and Cohen, H. J. (1980): Correlation between membrane potential changes and superoxide production in human granulocytes stimulated by phorbol myristate acetate: evidence for defective activation in chronic granulomatous disease. *J. Biol. Chem.,* 255:1874–1878.

789. Whitin, J. C., Clark, R. A., Simons, E. R., and Cohen, H. J. (1981): Effects of the myeloperoxidase system on fluorescent probes of granulocyte membrane potential. *J. Biol. Chem.,* 256:8904–8906.

790. Whittenbury, R. (1964): Hydrogen peroxide formation and catalase activity in the lactic acid bacteria. *J. Gen. Microbiol.,* 35:13–26.

791. Williams-Ashman, H. G., Cassman, M., and Klavins, M. (1959): Two enzymic mechanisms for hydrogen transport by phenolic oestrogens. *Nature,* 184:427–429.

792. Wilson, C. B., Tsai, V., and Remington, J. S. (1980): Failure to trigger the oxidative metabolic burst by normal macrophages: possible mechanism for survival of intracellular pathogens. *J. Exp. Med.,* 151:328–346.

793. Winston, G. W., Feierman, D. E., and Cederbaum, A. I. (1984): The role of iron chelates in hydroxyl radical production by rat liver microsomes, NADPH-cytochrome P-450 reductase and xanthine oxidase. *Arch. Biochem. Biophys.,* 232:378–390.

794. Winterbourn, C. C. (1979): Comparison of superoxide and other reducing agents in the biological production of hydroxyl radicals. *Biochem. J.,* 182:625–628.

795. Winterbourn, C. C. (1981): Hydroxyl radical production in body fluids: role of metal ions, ascorbate and superoxide. *Biochem. J.,* 198:125–131.

796. Winterbourn, C. C. (1981): Production of hydroxyl radicals from paraquat radicals and H_2O_2. *FEBS Lett.,* 128:339–342.

797. Winterbourn, C. C. (1983): Lactoferrin-catalyzed hydroxyl radical production: additional requirement for a chelating agent. *Biochem. J.,* 210:15–19.

798. Winterbourn, C. C. (1985): Comparative reactivities of various biological compounds with myeloperoxidase-hydrogen peroxide-chloride, and similarity of the oxidant to hypochlorite. *Biochim. Biophys. Acta,* 840:204–210.

799. Winterbourn, C. C. (1986): Myeloperoxidase as an effective inhibitor of hydroxyl radical production: implications for the oxidative reactions of neutrophils. *J. Clin. Invest.,* 78:545–550.

800. Winterbourn, C. C., and Sutton, H. C. (1984): Hydroxyl radical production from hydrogen peroxide and enzymatically generated paraquat radicals: catalytic requirements and oxygen dependence. *Arch. Biochem. Biophys.,* 235:116–126.

801. Winterbourn, C. C., and Sutton, H. C. (1986): Iron and xanthine oxidase catalyze formation of an oxidant species distinguishable from OH·: comparison with the Haber-Weiss reaction. *Arch. Biochem. Biophys.,* 244:27–34.

802. Winterbourn, C. C., and Vissers, M. C. M. (1983): Changes in ascorbate levels on stimulation of human neutrophils. *Biochim. Biophys. Acta,* 763:175–179.

803. Winterbourn, C. C., Garcia, R. C., and Segal, A. W. (1985): Production of the superoxide adduct of myeloperoxidase (compound III) by stimulated human neutrophils and its reactivity with hydrogen peroxide and chloride. *Biochem. J.,* 228:583–592.

804. Wittenberg, J. B., Noble, R. W., Wittenberg, B. A., Antonini, E., Brunori, M., and Wyman, J. (1967): Studies on the equilibria and kinetics of the reactions of peroxidase with ligands. II. The reaction of ferroperoxidase with oxygen. *J. Biol. Chem.,* 242:626–634.

805. Wolfson, M., McPhail, L. C., Nasrallah, V. N., and Snyderman, R. (1985): Phorbol myristate acetate mediates redistribution of protein kinase C in human neutrophils: potential role in the activation of the respiratory burst enzyme. *J. Immunol.,* 135:2057–2062.

806. Wong, P. S., and Travis, J. (1980): Isolation and properties of oxidized alpha-1-proteinase inhibitor from human rheumatoid synovial fluid. *Biochem. Biophys. Res. Commun.,* 96:1449–1454.

807. Wong, S. F., Halliwell, B., Richmond, R., and Skowroneck, W. R. (1981): The role of superoxide and hydroxyl radicals in the degradation of hyaluronic acid induced by metal ions and by ascorbic acid. *J. Inorg. Biochem.,* 14:127–134.

808. Wood, P. M. (1974): The redox potential of the system oxygen-superoxide. *FEBS Lett.,* 44:22–24.

809. Wright, D. G., and Gallin, J. I. (1977): A functional differentiation of human neutrophil granules: generation of C5a by a specific (secondary) granule product and inactivation of C5a by azurophil (primary) granule products. *J. Immunol.,* 119:1068–1076.

810. Wright, C. D., and Hoffman, M. D. (1986): The protein kinase C inhibitors H-7 and H-9 fail to inhibit human neutrophil activation. *Biochem. Biophys. Res. Commun.,* 135:749–755.

811. Wright, C. D., Bowie, J. U., Gray, G. R., and Nelson, R. D. (1983):

Candidacidal activity of myeloperoxidase: mechanisms of inhibitory influence of soluble cell wall mannan. *Infect. Immun.,* 42:76–80.

812. Wu, N. C., and Schultz, J. (1975): The prosthetic group of myeloperoxidase. *FEBS Lett.,* 60:141–144.

813. Yamada, M. (1982): Myeloperoxidase precursors in human myeloid leukemia HL-60 cells. *J. Biol. Chem.,* 257:5980–5982.

814. Yamada, M., and Kurahashi, K. (1984): Regulation of myeloperoxidase gene expression during differentiation of human myeloid leukemia HL-60 cells. *J. Biol. Chem.,* 259:3021–3025.

815. Yamada, M., Mori, M., and Sugimura, T. (1980): Myeloperoxidase-catalyzed binding of 3-amino-1-methyl-5H-pyrido [4,3-β] indole, a tryptophan pyrolysis product, to protein. *Chem. Biol. Interact.,* 33:19–33.

816. Yamada, M., Mori, M., and Sugimura, T. (1981): Myeloperoxidase in cultured human promyelocytic leukemia cell line HL-60. *Biochem. Biophys. Res. Commun.,* 98:219–226.

817. Yamada, M., Mori, M., and Sugimura, T. (1981): Purification and characterization of small molecular weight myeloperoxidase from human promyelocytic leukemia HL-60 cells. *Biochemistry,* 20:766–771.

818. Yamaguchi, T., and Kakinuma, K. (1982): Inhibitory effect of Cibacron blue F3GA on the O_2^- generating enzyme of guinea pig polymorphonuclear leukocytes. *Biochem. Biophys. Res. Commun.,* 104:200–206.

819. Yamaguchi, T., Sato, K., Shimada, K., and Kakinuma, K. (1982): Subcellular localization of O_2^- generating enzyme in guinea pig polymorphonuclear leukocytes; fractionation of subcellular particles by using a Percoll density gradient. *J. Biochem.,* 91:31–40.

820. Yamashita, T., Someya, A., and Hara, E. (1985): Response of superoxide anion production by guinea pig eosinophils to various soluble stimuli: comparison to neutrophils. *Arch. Biochem. Biophys.,* 241:447–452.

821. Yamazaki, I., and Yokota, K. N. (1973): Oxidation states of peroxidase. *Mol. Cell. Biochem.,* 2:39–52.

822. Yamazaki, I., Yokota, K., and Nakajima, R. (1965): A mechanism and model of peroxidase-oxidase reaction. In: *Oxidases and Related Redox Systems, Vol. I,* edited by T. E. King, H. C. Mason, and M. Morrison, pp. 485–513. Wiley, New York.

823. Yang, S. F. (1969): Further studies on ethylene formation from ketomethylthiobutyric acid or β-methylthiopropionaldehyde by peroxidase in the presence of sulfite and oxygen. *J. Biol. Chem.,* 244:4360–4365.

824. Yano, K., Nakashima, S., and Nozawa, Y. (1983): Coupling of polyphosphoinositide breakdown with calcium efflux in formyl-methionyl-leucyl-phenylalanine-stimulated rabbit neutrophils. *FEBS Lett.,* 161:296–300.

825. Yokota, K., and Yamazaki, I. (1965): Reaction of peroxidase with reduced nicotinamide-adenine dinucleotide and reduced nicotinamide-adenine dinucleotide phosphate. *Biochim. Biophys. Acta,* 105:301–312.

826. Yokota, K., and Yamazaki, I. (1965): The activity of the horseradish peroxidase compound III. *Biochem. Biophys. Res. Commun.,* 18:48–53.

827. Yong, E. C., Klebanoff, S. J., and Kuo, C-C. (1982): Toxic effect of human polymorphonuclear leukocytes on *Chlamydia trachomatis. Infect. Immun.,* 37:422–426.

828. Youngman, R. J. (1984): Oxygen activation—is the hydroxyl radical always biologically relevant. *Trends Biochem. Sci.,* 9:280–283.

829. Youngman, R. J., and Elstner, E. F. (1981): Oxygen species in paraquat toxicity: the crypto-OH radical. *FEBS Lett.,* 129:265–268.

830. Yuli, I., and Snyderman, R. (1986): Extensive hydrolysis of N-formyl-L-methionyl-L-leucyl-L-[^{3}H] phenylalanine by human polymorphonuclear leukocytes: a potential mechanism for modulation of the chemoattractant signal. *J. Biol. Chem.,* 261:4902–4908.

831. Zaslow, M. C., Clark, R. A., Stone, P. J., Calore, J. D., Snider, G. L., and Franzblau, C. (1983): Human neutrophil elastase does not bind to alpha 1-protease inhibitor that has been exposed to activated human neutrophils. *Am. Rev. Respir. Dis.,* 128:434–439.

832. Zaslow, M. C., Clark, R. A., Stone, P. J., Calore, J., Snider, G. L., and Franzblau, C. (1985): Myeloperoxidase-induced inactivation of α_1-antiprotease in hamsters. *J. Lab. Clin. Med.,* 105:178–184.

833. Zgliczyński, J. M., and Stelmaszyńska, T. (1975): Chlorinating ability of human phagocytosing leucocytes. *Eur. J. Biochem.,* 56:157–162.

834. Zgliczyński, J. M., and Stelmaszyńska, T. (1979): Hydrogen cyanide and cyanogen chloride formation by the myeloperoxidase-H_2O_2-Cl^- system. *Biochim. Biophys. Acta,* 567:309–314.

835. Zgliczyński, J. M., Stelmaszyńska, T., Ostrowski, W., Naskalski, J., and Sznajd, J. (1968): Myeloperoxidase of human leukemic leucocytes: oxidation of amino acids in the presence of hydrogen peroxide. *Eur. J. Biochem.,* 4:540–547.

836. Zgliczyński, J. M., Stelmaszyńska, T., Domański, J., and Ostrowski, W. (1971): Chloramines as intermediates of oxidative reaction of amino acids by myeloperoxidase. *Biochim. Biophys. Acta,* 235:419–424.

837. Zgliczyński, J. M., Selvaraj, R. J., Paul, B. B., Stelmaszyńska, T., Poskitt, P. K. F., and Sbarra, A. J. (1977): Chorination by the myeloperoxidase-H_2O_2-Cl^- antimicrobial system at acid and neutral pH. *Proc. Soc. Exp. Biol. Med.,* 154:418–422.

838. Zgliczyński, J. M., Olszowska, E., Olszowski, S., Stelmaszyńska, T., and Kwasnowska, E. (1985): A possible origin of chemiluminescence in phagocytosing neutrophils: myeloperoxidase-mediated chlorination of proteins and tryptophan. *Int. J. Biochem.,* 17:393–397.

839. Zs-Nagy, I., and Floyd, R. A. (1984): Hydroxyl free radical reactions with amino acids and proteins studied by electron spin resonance spectroscopy and spin trapping. *Biochim. Biophys. Acta,* 790:238–250.

Inflammation: Basic Principles and Clinical Correlates.
Edited by J. I. Gallin, I. M. Goldstein, and R. Snyderman.
Raven Press, Ltd., New York © 1988.

CHAPTER 24

Phagocytic Cells: Oxygen-Independent Antimicrobial Systems

Peter Elsbach and Jerrold Weiss

Evolution of Evidence for O_2-Independent Antimicrobial
  Action of Phagocytes
Antimicrobial Proteins of Phagocytes
Properties of Purified Proteins with Well-Established O_2-
  Independent Antimicrobial Activity
  Bactericidal/Permeability-Increasing Protein • Defen-
  sins • Cathepsin G • Lactoferrin • Lysozyme • Major
  Basic Protein of Eosinophils • Eosinophil Cationic Pro-
  tein

Role of Degradative Enzymes in (O_2-Independent) Anti-
  microbial Activity
  Proteases • Lipid Hydrolases • Nucleases
Role of O_2-Independent Agents in the Bactericidal Activity
  of Intact Phagocytes
Future
References

EVOLUTION OF EVIDENCE FOR O_2-INDEPENDENT ANTIMICROBIAL ACTION OF PHAGOCYTES

In addition to the O_2-dependent cytotoxic systems discussed in Chapter 23 (*this volume*), phagocytes are
equipped with O_2-independent means of killing microorganisms. In fact, the earliest attempts at identifying specific agents that might be involved in the antimicrobial
activity of phagocytes preceded recognition of the respiratory burst as a source of antibacterial activity and were
made in broken-cell preparations that did not generate
toxic O_2 derivatives (1,2). These initial studies were conducted with polymorphonuclear leukocytes (PMN), not
only because of their central role in host defense against
most bacterial infections, but also because PMN were
more readily available than other inflammatory cells, such
as mononuclear phagocytes or eosinophils, for which sat-
isfactory isolation procedures had not yet been developed.
Particularly useful were the large homogeneous (>90%)
populations of PMN obtainable from sterile inflammatory
exudates elicited in the peritoneal cavities of experimental
animals such as rabbits and guinea pigs (1,2). Crude (rabbit) PMN fractions were shown to be capable of killing a

range of both gram-positive and gram-negative bacterial
species (1,2). Hirsch was the first to show that a protein-
rich fraction from acid-extracted PMN, named *phagocytin,* had potent bactericidal activity (1). Further focus
on antibacterial proteins followed from the discovery, by
Robineaux (3) and Hirsch and Cohn (4–6), of the degranulation phenomenon that accompanies phagocytosis.
Owing to the development of the lysosome concept and
a simple cell-fractionation technique for the isolation of
a granule-rich fraction from rabbit PMN, Cohn and
Hirsch could show that in these cells the characteristic
lysosomal hydrolases (capable of degrading bacterial
macromolecules) and bactericidal phagocytin were also
packaged in discrete cytoplasmic granules (4,6). During
degranulation the granules fuse with newly formed
phagocytic vacuoles, thus exposing ingested material (e.g.,
bacteria) to the action of these granule proteins.

Certain other isolated cellular constituents that are not
granule-associated, such as the highly positively charged
histones and polyamines in very high concentrations, can
also be bactericidal (2,7). In the intact phagocyte, however,
no mechanism is evident by which these agents can gain
access to sequestered microorganisms. It is the compartmentalization of antibacterial substances in the granules

that provides the phagocyte with a highly selective delivery system during degranulation.

After the description of the properties of phagocytin, it seemed that more precise definition of the components of this still-crude protein fraction should soon follow. However, in the subsequent few years the further dissection of PMN granule constituents with bactericidal activity was almost entirely limited to the work of Zeya and Spitznagel (8–13), leading to a partial resolution of a phagocytin-like fraction into a series of apparently low M_r (4,000–8,000) proteins with overlapping bactericidal activity toward a spectrum of both gram-positive and gram-negative bacterial species. When it became established at the same time that products of the respiratory burst provide the PMN with a cytotoxic system that is capable of killing most microbes, and even viruses and eukaryotic cells, interest in the possible contribution of O_2-independent bactericidal mechanisms to the overall antimicrobial activity of PMN waned. The fatal infections in patients with classical chronic granulomatous disease (CGD), whose phagocytes cannot generate toxic O_2 derivatives, lent credence to the view that O_2-independent bactericidal mechanisms are an inadequate back-up system (14). However, as more observations on patients with CGD were being gathered, it became evident that the clinical course is highly variable, ranging from inevitably fatal to a near normal incidence of infections. In different patients with CGD, different biochemical defects (see Chapter 23, *this volume*) can account for a similar inability to mount the respiratory burst, further implying a heterogeneous disease with a complex genetic origin. Why this should result in a variable clinical course is not clear (15,16). Although there is no evidence that in the more serious cases of CGD other antimicrobial deficiencies (O_2-independent?) may coexist, such a possibility has not yet been excluded. That bactericidal mechanisms not dependent on O_2 are protective in CGD is evident from the fact that even patients who die of their infections can deal effectively with many potentially pathogenic microbial species. While some of these are H_2O_2 producers and thus contribute a missing component of the defective O_2-requiring bactericidal systems, other species are also well killed by CGD PMN *in vitro* without "correcting" the respiratory defect. Studies on normal human and rabbit PMN strengthen the evidence that generation of toxic oxygen derivatives is not essential for effective killing of a number of common pathogens (17–19). Specifically, several species of Gram-negative bacteria such as *Escherichia coli* and *Salmonella typhimurium* are killed after ingestion just as well when O_2 is depleted in the ambient air (virtually eliminating O_2 metabolism) as when O_2 is present and during an active respiratory burst (18,19). Moreover, the rate and extent of killing of these bacterial species by disrupted PMN that do not produce O_2-derivatives are equal to the bactericidal activity of an equivalent number of intact PMN (20–22).

In the early 1970s a renewed attempt to define the bactericidal agents capable of acting without apparent need of O_2 was triggered by the finding that prompt killing (i.e., loss of ability to multiply) of *E. coli* by either intact or disrupted PMN was accompanied by surprisingly little structural and functional disorganization of the organism (20–26). On the whole, students of the interaction of phagocytes and microorganisms had restricted their assessment of the fate of the target cells by assaying for a reduction in colony formation. Because it takes about 20 divisions (usually 20–30 min per generation) to yield a visible colony, it is obvious that the events leading to loss of viability may stretch over many hours. To examine in greater detail the consequences of the actions of PMN on target bacteria, we have measured bacterial metabolism under conditions of >90% loss of colony-forming ability. Whereas all biosynthetic activity of nonpathogenic gram-positive bacteria such as *Micrococcus lysodeikticus* and *Bacillus megaterium* exposed to PMN *in vitro* stops almost immediately, gram-negative *E. coli,* under our experimental conditions, retained the ability to incorporate radiolabeled precursors into macromolecular constituents, including nucleic acids, proteins, lipids, peptidoglycans, and lipopolysaccharides (LPS) for at least 1 hr (20). The continued operation of its biochemical machinery enables the *E. coli,* although no longer viable, to respond (for periods of up to 1 hr) to environmental changes with adjustments in its biochemical activity (20,21,23). A remarkable example of this preservation of integrated biochemical functioning by *E. coli,* well beyond the time it takes for the antimicrobial arsenal of either intact or disrupted PMN to initiate lethal events, is the response of nonviable *E. coli* to an appropriate inducer with the synthesis of an inducible enzyme (20,24). The biochemical apparatus of gram-negative bacteria is largely associated with the cytoplasmic (or "inner") membrane. The very slow deterioration of biochemical functions implies therefore that this layer of the *E. coli* envelope (Fig. 1) at least initially escapes major damage during killing by PMN. This conclusion is supported by fine-structural studies (25) and by studies on K^+ transport (21), showing continued K^+ influx at control rates for at least 30 min, even in the face of increased efflux (leakage). However, subtle envelope alterations, involving the outer membrane, are in fact a very early (<1 min) event in the interaction between disrupted PMN and *E. coli* (21,22). These changes are detected as an increased permeability of the outer membrane (OM) to normally impermeant substances, such as the antibiotics actinomycin D and rifampin (21,22). Quantitative measurement of this envelope effect is possible because passage of these transcription-inhibiting agents through the outer membrane

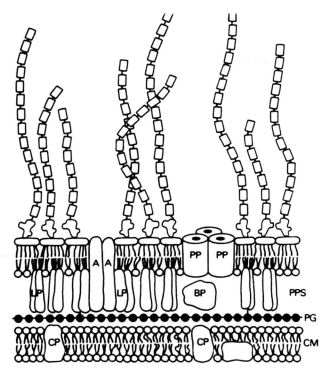

FIG. 1. Molecular organization of the outer membrane of *Enterobacteriaceae.* The most likely positions of outer-membrane constituents are schematically indicated. LPS and phospholipid molecules are the major constituents of an asymmetric bilayer. Divalent cations (not indicated) are supposed to play important roles in interactions of LPS. Only three types of proteins have been drawn, namely pore proteins including LamB protein (PP), OmpA protein (A), and lipoprotein (LP). Pore proteins have been drawn without interactions with peptidoglycan and lipoprotein, although such interactions cannot be excluded. Several *O*-antigen chains are much longer than visualized. Enterobacterial common antigen has not been drawn for reasons of simplicity. Other aspects of the cell envelope, such as the periplasmic space with a nutrient-binding protein (BP), the peptidoglycan layer (PG), and the cytoplasmic or inner membrane (CM) with a carrier protein (CP) involved in transport, have also been drawn. (PPS) Periplasmic space. For further explanation, see text. (From ref. 50).

ANTIMICROBIAL PROTEINS OF PHAGOCYTES

Table 1 lists the numerous granule-associated proteins with antimicrobial activity that have been identified to date in PMN, eosinophils, and mononuclear phagocytes. Many of these proteins exhibit catalytic activity [e.g., the typical lysosomal hydrolases capable of degrading (microbial) macromolecules, including nucleic acids, proteins, polysaccharides, peptidoglycans, and lipids]. Also listed are proteins and peptides without known catalytic activity, as well as the enzyme (myelo)peroxidase, an important granule-associated element in the O_2-dependent cytotoxic systems of all phagocytes.

The following general statements should be made at the outset: (a) As isolated proteins the hydrolases of macromolecules (e.g., lysozyme) exhibit little or no microbicidal activity against most microorganisms. However, the extent to which these enzymes may contribute to the overall antimicrobial potency of the intact phagocyte has not been clearly established. In contrast, some of the apparently noncatalytic proteins by themselves are potent cytotoxins. (b) Each of the three main cell-types involved in antimicrobial activity contain a different mix of antimicrobial proteins, reflecting their specialized roles in the defense against the enormous diversity of microbial predators to which the host is exposed. (c) Although this review

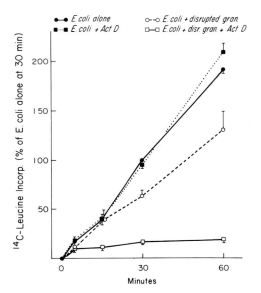

FIG. 2. Effect of disrupted granulocytes on sensitivity of *E. coli* to actinomycin D. *E. coli* W (2.5×10^8 organisms) were incubated with 1.25×10^7 disrupted rabbit granulocytes in a total volume of 0.25 ml of sterile saline supplemented with 40 mM Tris-maleate buffer (pH 7.4), 10% Hanks' balanced salt solution, 20 μg casamino acid mixture and, where added, 12.5 μg of actinomycin D. (From ref. 21.)

barrier promptly blocks incorporation of radiolabeled precursors into bacterial macromolecules that otherwise continues despite the bactericidal effects of the disrupted PMN (Fig. 2; 20–25).

These observations set in motion a renewed search for substance(s) in the PMN, apparently acting without need for O_2 and capable of inflicting a highly discrete lethal lesion. The granule-associated PMN proteins appeared to be the most likely source of such agent(s) because the granules had already been recognized as a repository of antimicrobial proteins and also as a vehicle for their delivery to ingested microbes through fusion with the phagocytic vacuole.

TABLE 1. *Granule-associated proteins with (possible) antimicrobial properties[a]*

Proteins	PMN Primary granules	PMN Secondary granules	Mononuclear phagocytes	Eosinophils
Catalytically active:				
Elastase	+	−	+	?
Collagenases	+	+	+	?
Chymotrypsin-like protease (cathepsin G)	+	−	?	?
Lipases (triacylglycerol hydrolases)*	+		+	?
Phospholipase A2	+		+	?
Phospholipase A1*	?		?	?
Phospholipase C*	?		?	?
Phospholipase D*	?		?	+
Lysophospholipases*	+		+	+
(Deoxy)ribonucleases	+		+	+
Polysaccharidases*	+		+	?
Sulfatases*	+		+	+
(Myelo)peroxidase	+	−	+	+
Cytochrome b-245	−	+	?	?
Phosphatases*	+		+	?
No known catalytic activity				
BPI	+	−	−	−
Defensins	+	−	+	−
Lactoferrin	−	+	−	−
B$_{12}$-binding protein*	−	+	?	?
Major basic protein	−		−	+
Eosinophil cationic protein	−		−	+
Eosinophil-derived neurotoxin	−		−	+

[a] Proteins or catalytic activities that have not been purified or for which no information is available concerning any role in antimicrobial activity of phagocytes are denoted with an asterisk and are not discussed in the text.

of O$_2$-independent microbicidal mechanisms concerns mainly the roles of constituents of phagocytes, it must be recognized that the effectiveness of host-defense against infection depends also on participation of the complement system (see Chapter 4, *this volume*), specific antibody-producing cells (see Chapter 31, *this volume*), and quite possibly killer T-cells in at least some instances.

The biosynthesis and processing of proteins destined for assembly into the cytoplasmic granules of PMN, eosinophils, and mononuclear phagocytes have not yet been studied as extensively as in tissues such as liver (27). However, recent studies of phagocytic cells suggest that the translocation of newly synthesized proteins from endoplasmic reticulum, via the Golgi cisternae into the granules (lysosomes), requires similar posttranslational modifications of sequential glycosylations, phosphorylation, and proteolytic cleavage. References to specific information will be provided in the discussion of individual granule proteins.

The mononuclear phagocyte actively synthesizes protein, including granule-associated proteins (28) during its long life-span. In fact, under certain conditions *in vitro,*

these cells secrete large quantities of proteases and other degradative enzymes (28). Thus, its sustained biosynthetic capabilities provide the mononuclear phagocyte with the means of replenishing antibacterial proteins and of assembling new granules, permitting repeated phagocytic events (29,30). In contrast, the short-lived PMN synthesizes its granule proteins and assembles its granules only during the promyelocyte/myelocyte stages of maturation. Beyond that level of differentiation the PMN exhibits little biosynthetic activity. The biosynthesis of individual antimicrobial proteins and their insertion during myeloid differentiation into primary and/or secondary granules occur therefore in a relatively narrow time frame, suitable for analysis. Because adequate numbers of reasonably homogeneous populations of cells in the bone marrow at a particular stage of differentiation cannot readily be obtained, investigators have turned, for their study of granule protein synthesis and processing, to stable cell lines such as the promyelocytic human leukemic HL-60 cell. This cell can be directed with various agents to differentiate into either granulocyte- or monocyte-like cells (31–35). Although stable leukemic cell lines differ both morphologically and functionally from normal cells, they do serve as a useful model for the study of production of granule-associated proteins.

We will now review salient features of each of the proteins or category of proteins listed in Table 1. The order of presentation is based on the apparent potency and the extent of characterization of the antimicrobial action of the various proteins.

PROPERTIES OF PURIFIED PROTEINS WITH WELL-ESTABLISHED O₂-INDEPENDENT ANTIMICROBIAL ACTIVITY

Bactericidal/Permeability-Increasing Protein

The search for an agent acting in O₂-independent fashion and capable of killing *E. coli* with minimal apparent initial damage to bacterial structure and function led to the isolation of a single protein from human as well as rabbit PMN (36,37). This protein, for its biological effects, was called *bactericidal/permeability increasing protein* (BPI). Our view that BPI may indeed be primarily responsible for the killing of *E. coli* and other BPI-sensitive microorganisms by intact PMN is supported by the following findings: (a) Nearly all activity in crude PMN fractions toward BPI-sensitive bacteria can be accounted for by their BPI content; (b) The discrete envelope alterations produced by intact PMN and by crude PMN fractions on the target bacteria are also elicited by pure BPI; (c) IgG fractions from goats immunized with BPI abolish all effects of whole PMN homogenates with regard to viability and permeability of target bacteria. Moreover, intact human and rabbit PMN kill BPI-sensitive bacteria (but *not* BPI-insensitive bacteria) as effectively after O₂-depletion as in the presence of O₂ (18,19).

Human and rabbit BPI are similar molecules with respect to M_r (approximately 60,000 and 50,000, respectively), high net positive charge (pI > 9.6), amino acid composition, NH₂-terminal amino acid sequence showing 80% homology among the first 17 residues (Table 2), and as judged by immunological cross-reactivity (38).

The two proteins are also similar in their biological effects and show identical target specificity. BPI is potently bactericidal toward a broad range of enteric gram-negative bacterial species and strains; however, at concentrations of up to 100-fold higher, it is nontoxic to all of the Gram-positive bacteria and eukaryotic cells tested so far (Table 3). For the same bactericidal effect on some BPI-sensitive

strains, up to fivefold higher molar concentrations are required of human BPI than of rabbit BPI (39).

By sensitive immunological assays, BPI can only be detected in cells of the myeloid series (40). Thus, this bactericidal protein exhibits two levels of specificity, namely, (i) with respect to its cytotoxicity, and (ii) in its occurrence in PMN only, i.e., in those phagocytes that are the principal defenders against BPI-sensitive bacterial species.

BPI produced by PMN obtained from patients with chronic myelocytic leukemia cannot be distinguished from BPI isolated from normal human PMN. Immunofluorescent staining of human bone marrow preparations, utilizing rabbit anti-human BPI IgG, shows that BPI first appears in cells of the myeloid series at the promyelocyte stage of differentiation. In line with the immunological assay of whole cells, neutralized acid extracts of peripheral white blood cells from patients with promyelocytic leukemia contain BPI, whereas those of cells from a patient with myeloblastic leukemia (blast crisis) do not, as determined by immunological (ELISA) or biological assays. Double staining of bone marrow preparations for BPI and lactoferrin reveals that BPI appears before lactoferrin during myeloid differentiation (40). Consistent with this observation, cell fractionation studies show that BPI is located in the primary granules (40). Treatment of isolated granules with salt or weak acid solubilizes nearly all myeloperoxidase, lactoferrin, and elastase (another primary granule protein), but little BPI (40), indicating that BPI is more tightly associated with the granules than are other granule proteins. That BPI is held more tightly within the granule structure is further suggested by the finding that treatment of intact PMN with cytochalasin *b* and *f*-Met-Leu-Phe results in the extracellular appearance of much less BPI than of myeloperoxidase, lactoferrin, and elastase (40). This property of BPI should be viewed in the context of evidence indicating that the bactericidal effect of BPI appears to be restricted to the intracellular environment and that upon incubation of *E. coli* with intact PMN, only intracellular and not uningested bacteria show subsequent fluorescent staining for BPI (19). How BPI is transferred from the granule to the bacterium within the phagosome is not yet known.

Effects of BPI on Target Bacteria

Four elements have been identified in the interaction of BPI with susceptible bacteria: (i) insertion into the outer

TABLE 2. NH₂-terminal sequences of human and rabbit BPI[a]

	1	2	3	4	5	6	7	8	9	10	11	12	13	14	15	16	17
Human BPI:	V	N	P	G	V	V	V	R	I	S	Q	K	G	L	D	Y	A	S	Q	Q
Rabbit BPI:	T	N	P	G	F	T	T	R	I	S	Q	K	G	L	(D)	Y	(A)	(S)	(Q)	(Q)

[a] The single letter code is used to designate amino acids. Letters within parentheses represent tentative amino acid assignments. Identical amino acids (including those tentatively identified) in human BPI and rabbit BPI are underlined.

TABLE 3. *Antimicrobial spectrum of BPI*[a]

Target cell	Rabbit	Human
Gram-negative bacteria		
Escherichia coli		
Short-chain LPS (± capsule)	+++	+++
Long-chain LPS (± capsule)	++	+
Salmonella typhimurium		
Short-chain LPS	+++	+++
Long-chain LPS	++	+
Salmonella typhi	++/+++	++/+++
Shigella boydii	++/+++	++/+++
Pseudomonas aeruginosa		
(mucoid or nonmucoid)	++/+++	++/+++
Neisseria gonorrhoeae	++	++
Klebsiella pneumoniae		
(encapsulated)	+	+
Enterobacter aerogenes	+/++	+/++
Serratia marcescens	−	−
Gram-positive bacteria		
Staphylococcus aureus	−	−
Staphylococcus epidermidis	−	−
Streptococcus faecalis	−	−
Bacillus megaterium	−	−
Micrococcus lysodeikticus	−	−
Listeria monocytogenes	−	−
Fungi		
Candida albicans	−	−
Candida parapsilosis	−	−
Red blood cells (human, rabbit, sheep)	−	−

[a] +++, >90% killing of 10^7 microorganisms/ml by 0.5–2.5-μg BPI/ml; ++, >90% killing of 10^7 microorganisms/ml by 2.5–20-μg BPI/ml; +, >90% killing of 10^7 microorganisms/ml by 20–100-μg BPI/mg; −, Little or no killing by 100–200-μg BPI/ml.

membrane of the Gram-negative bacterial envelope through electrostatic and hydrophobic forces (41); (ii) irreversible loss of colony-forming ability within 30 sec after exposure to BPI at 37°C (41); (iii) a reversible increase in the permeability of the outer membrane for normally impermeant hydrophobic substances (42,43); and (iv) a reversible and highly selective activation of enzymes degrading bacterial phospholipids and peptidoglycans (42,44–48).

The remarkable specificity of BPI for gram-negative bacteria and the highly discrete envelope alterations that are associated with its actions appear to be explained by the unique composition and organization of the gram-negative bacterial outer membrane (see Fig. 1). With the exception of the phospholipids of the outer membrane, which are similar to those in the inner membrane, the lipopolysaccharides (LPS) or endotoxins, outer membrane lipoproteins, and the major outer membrane proteins are

all unique to the outer membrane (49–51). None of the outer-membrane macromolecular constituents, except the phospholipids, are readily detected in purified inner-membrane preparations. This is remarkable because the biosynthesis of all outer membrane constituents takes place in association with the inner membrane and, to a lesser extent, in the cytoplasm (49–51). The outer membrane is almost completely devoid of biosynthetic capabilities. This implies that translocation of newly synthesized products destined for assembly of the outer membrane must be unidirectional and extraordinarily efficient. By what route the individual outer membrane components reach the final assembly site is not entirely clear. Most likely the limited number (a few hundred per bacterium) of so-called adhesion zones (52,53) between inner and outer membrane serve as pathways for transport. The highly unusual functional properties of the outer membrane, as studied mainly in *E. coli* and *S. typhimurium,* reflect its chemical anatomy. The outer membrane provides gram-negative bacteria with a barrier against hydrophobic substances such as the antibiotics actinomycin and rifampicin and certain detergents (49–51). This barrier function has been explained by the uniquely asymmetric arrangement of the hydrophobic bilayer in this membrane (Fig. 1; 49,50), in which most of the phospholipids occupy only the inner leaflet, whereas the outer leaflet is made up of the lipid portion of the LPS. The outwardly directed polysaccharide chains create a hydrophilic shield against hydrophobic substances. In *E. coli* and *S. typhimurium,* and presumably other gram-negative bacteria, the barrier and the outer membrane as a whole are stabilized by the divalent cations Mg^{2+} and Ca^{2+}, which cross-link the LPS molecules into a cohesive layer through charge interactions with clusters of anionic sites at the base of the polysaccharide chains (50). Thus, chelation of the cross-linking ions destabilizes the outer membrane and breaks down the barrier against hydrophobic substances (54).

The outer membrane also acts as a molecular sieve for hydrophilic substances, permitting only molecules of M_r < 600 to reach the periplasmic space through aqueous pores of limited size that are formed by oligomers of the major outer membrane proteins or porins (51).

It is in this structural and functional framework of the outer membrane that the scheme depicting the effects of BPI is presented (Fig. 3). It must be emphasized that several aspects of the properties of the gram-negative bacterial envelope as discussed here, as well as the proposed interaction with BPI, are still hypothetical.

The antimicrobial specificity of BPI for gram-negative bacteria is explained by the dependence of the expression of all biological effects on binding of the protein to the target cell. Homing-in of the highly basic BPI involves an initial electrostatic interaction with negatively charged surface sites (15,41,55). Presumably these sites are pro-

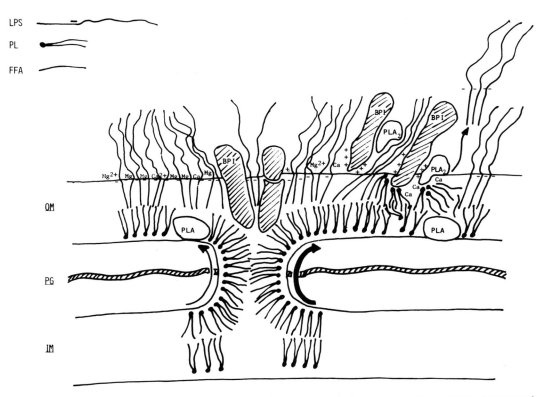

FIG. 3. Hypothetical scheme of BPI action on susceptible gram-negative bacteria. Sequential electrostatic and hydrophobic interactions of BPI with the outer membrane (OM) cause displacement of cross-linking divalent cations and LPS, thereby exposing hydrophobic permeation channels that are normally inaccessible to lipophilic substances. These membrane perturbations also result in hydrolysis of OM phospholipids by bacterial and PMN phospholipases. Net hydrolysis of phospholipids in the OM may stimulate phospholipid biosynthesis by pathways associated with the inner membrane (IM) and hence stimulate phospholipid migration through adhesion zones toward the OM. High concentrations of Mg^{2+} (or Ca^{2+}) release BPI from exposed sites, abruptly stopping degradation of phospholipids and initiating the repair of the OM. Viability is not regained, however, possibly because BPI reaches specialized regions, such as the fusion zones between inner and outer membranes, where irreversible lethal effects are initiated. (PLA) Phospholipase A; (PG) peptidoglycan; (PL) phospholipid; (FFA) free fatty acid; and (LPS) lipopolysaccharide. (From ref. 15.)

vided [particularly by the cluster of negatively charged sugars (2-keto-3-deoxyoctonate, KDO) and phosphate groups at the junction between the lipid A moiety and the polysaccharide chain of LPS] that are also the anchoring points for the cross-linking divalent cations (43,46,50,54,57,58). BPI binds by competing for these sites and thus displaces Mg^{2+} and Ca^{2+}, thereby destabilizing the LPS layer and the surrounding structures (15,16). Supraphysiological concentrations of these ions prevent binding and hence all biological effects of BPI (22). Once BPI is bound, addition of high concentrations of Mg^{2+} (or Ca^{2+}) to the bacterial suspension reverses the competitive advantage of BPI, and more than 80% of the bound BPI is displaced from the bacterial surface (41). That the greater portion of bound BPI is located at or near the surface is further indicated by the finding that trypsin treatment of BPI-coated *E. coli* results in the freeing of nearly the same number of binding sites as ini-

tially occupied (55). At saturation binding, roughly one BPI molecule is bound for every five LPS molecules, i.e., approximately 5×10^5 BPI molecules/*E. coli* (55). The amount of BPI bound at maximally bactericidal concentrations is closely similar for strains of *E. coli* or *S. typhimurium* with LPS of widely differing polysaccharide chain length. However, the ambient concentration of BPI required to kill >90% of the bacterial population increases with increasing polysaccharide chain length, indicating that the sites of attachment become less accessible, thus reducing the affinity for BPI and explaining why smooth strains show greater resistance to BPI (55). Rough strains at concentrations of 10^7/ml are killed by approximately 1 to 5×10^{-8} *M* BPI. Smooth strains may require up to 20-fold higher concentrations (39,55). Encapsulated (or mucoid) and nonencapsulated strains, by contrast, are equally sensitive to BPI (58).

Binding is necessary for the effects of BPI on bacterial

multiplication and envelope but is not sufficient. Post-binding steps, apparently involving hydrophobic interactions, must follow (41). At 37°C these physical interactions are fast, resulting in irreversible loss of colony-forming ability and the various envelope alterations after exposure of the bacteria to BPI for only a fraction of a minute. The dependence of the bactericidal effect of BPI on postbinding steps can be demonstrated by creating conditions that impede hydrophobic interactions without preventing binding. Under such conditions the bacteria can be rescued from the bactericidal effect (41).

The breakdown of the permeability barrier, as measured by the sensitivity of previously insensitive *E. coli* to actinomycin D, can be explained by the destabilizing effect of the insertion of BPI into the LPS layer. As a consequence the asymmetric position of the phospholipids in the bilayer may also be disturbed, causing formation of phospholipid bilayer regions and externally exposed hydrophobic channels that render the outer membrane permeable to actinomycin D.

The lethal action of BPI on *E. coli* is also accompanied by the immediate onset of net hydrolysis of bacterial phospholipids by bacterial phospholipases A and by certain exogenous phospholipases A2 (42,44–48). The action of added phospholipases can be demonstrated by using *E. coli* mutants lacking phospholipase A (44–48). Activation of hydrolysis of bacterial phospholipids, which, under physiological conditions, exhibit almost no turnover, is a complex phenomenon in which the displacement of Ca^{2+} and Mg^{2+} by cationic bactericidal peptides or proteins (such as polymixin B and BPI) appears to be an important element (65). First, the resulting rearrangement of phospholipids, as proposed above, facilitates enzyme-substrate interaction. Second, the release of Ca^{2+} from sites in close proximity to the hydrophobic bilayer apparently supplies the Ca^{2+} needed for catalytic activity of strictly Ca^{2+}-dependent phospholipases A (45,65). Evidence supporting these contentions has been obtained in experiments with polymixin B, a highly basic peptide antibiotic with effects on the outer membrane that resemble those of BPI (65). However, in contrast to polymixin B, which, at bactericidal concentrations, triggers the action of any added phospholipase A2, BPI only activates a few of many phospholipases A2 (45–48). Among the BPI-responsive enzymes are the phospholipase A2 purified from PMN (37), a phospholipase A2 present in cell-free supernatant of inflammatory exudates produced in rabbits (59), and two snake-venom phospholipases A2 (47,59).

Phospholipases A2 are highly conserved proteins in which common structural and functional properties have been identified (47,48,59). Among these is a functionally important NH_2-terminal region that has an alpha-helical conformation (47,48). Chemical modification of one BPI-responsive phospholipase A2 (46,47) and comparison of

the structures of multiple phospholipases A2 suggest that the BPI-responsive phospholipases A2 share an unusual composition and sequence of the polar face of this NH_2-terminal alpha-helix (47,48). How this structural variability affects the BPI-mediated functions of these phospholipases A2 is not known.

Lethal concentrations of BPI also trigger in *E. coli* degradation of peptidoglycans by endogenous degradative enzymes (*unpublished observations*) but not by added lysozyme, further indicating that the envelope alterations produced by BPI are too discrete to render bacterial macromolecules generally accessible to degradative enzymes. That the effect of BPI on digestion of killed *E. coli* is selective is also shown by the finding that bacterial proteins and nucleic acids do not undergo detectable autolysis.

There is no evidence that the BPI-mediated degradation of envelope phospholipids and peptidoglycans plays a role in the killing of *E. coli* by BPI. In fact, the bactericidal action of BPI is the same on three strains of *E. coli*, differing only in their phospholipase A content, namely: (i) a typical wild-type phospholipase A content (BPI-mediated hydrolysis 15–20%); (ii) a mutant lacking phospholipase A (no hydrolysis); (iii) this mutant into which a plasmid had been introduced containing the *E. coli* phospholipase A gene (Pld A) in high copy number (hydrolysis up to 70%) (60,61).

It remains to be determined to what extent envelope phospholipid hydrolysis is a variable in the overall digestive process that accompanies phagocytosis.

Reversibility of Envelope Effects of BPI

The extraordinarily discrete lethal lesion that BPI produces in the target bacteria is evident from the preservation of K^+ gradients (21) and the ability to carry out macromolecular biosynthesis for at least 1 hr (22,36,37), indicating that the inner-membrane-associated biochemical machinery escapes major damage during this period. In fact, not only is biosynthesis of bacterial protein and RNA not markedly impaired after addition of saturating amounts of BPI, but incorporation of radioactive precursors into LPS and phospholipids is actually stimulated (43,62). Moreover, removal of previously bound BPI from bacterial surface sites, by raising the ambient concentrations of Mg^{2+} or Ca^{2+} (to 40 mM) or by adding trypsin, further increases new LPS synthesis and initiates repair of the permeability barrier (42–44). This time- and temperature-dependent repair process is linked to biosynthesis of LPS, as demonstrated by the fact that repair is blocked by an inhibitor specific for LPS synthesis or by incubation of a temperature-sensitive *S. typhimurium* mutant defective in LPS synthesis at the nonpermissive temperature (43). Inhibitors of protein synthesis do not interfere with repair (43).

Another reversal of an effect of BPI on the *E. coli* envelope, when high concentrations of Mg^{2+} or /Ca^{2+} are added, is an immediate cessation of net degradation of phospholipids and peptidoglycans (42,44; *unpublished observations*), accompanied by a gradual reincorporation of the products of phospholipid hydrolysis (namely, free fatty acids and lysocompounds) into diacylphosphatides (42,44). Although the breakdown of the envelope phospholipids and the permeability barrier for hydrophobic substances (as well as their repair when BPI is removed) coincide, the two phenomena are not causally connected, because BPI produces the same permeability alterations when no phospholipid hydrolysis occurs (using a phospholipase-A-less *E. coli* mutant).

Nature of Bactericidal Effect of BPI

What the primary irreversible event is that leads to bacterial death is unknown. The fact that BPI produces reversible envelope alterations as well as an almost immediately irreversible effect on bacterial viability may mean that BPI has different actions depending on where it interacts with the bacterial envelope. Thus, the lethal action of BPI might be confined to a small subpopulation of bound protein that reaches specialized envelope sites from where it cannot be removed by divalent cations or proteases (15,41). The adhesion zones between inner and outer membranes represent examples of such microanatomically and chemically distinct sites (49–53). In order for the BPI molecules to find the limited number of such sites (approximately 100 per bacterium in the case of adhesion zones), saturation binding may be necessary; however, once the critical sites are occupied, removal of the other bound BPI molecules would not rescue the bacteria. Alternatively, randomly bound BPI may promptly produce a discrete and as yet unidentified lesion that leads irreversibly to bacterial death, even after release or digestion of nearly all bound protein.

Whereas BPI under our usual experimental conditions kills susceptible bacteria with minimal structural and functional alterations, there are conditions under which BPI treatment causes rapid and profound inhibition of amino acid incorporation into bacterial protein. This has also been observed by Hovde and Gray, who have reported the purification of a potent 55,000-M_r bactericidal protein from the granules of human PMN (63). They found that the immediate inhibition of amino acid uptake and incorporation into protein of *P. aeruginosa* and *E. coli* correlated with an equally prompt reduction in bacterial O_2 consumption and motility (63). It is conceivable that these different biological effects are caused by different granule proteins. However, despite small differences in M_r as measured by sodium dodecylsulfate polyacrylamide gel electrophoresis (SDS-PAGE), the conditions used for purification of this protein and of a 57,000-M_r protein with an amino acid composition nearly identical to that of BPI, isolated by Shafer et al. (64), suggest that all three proteins are similar or closely related.

We have attempted to relate different effects of BPI on bacterial metabolism to the timing of bacterial growth arrest. Enumeration of BPI-treated *E. coli* in a bacterial counting chamber under the light microscope has revealed that BPI promptly arrests normal bacterial growth and division, evident either as abrupt cessation of growth or as limited growth for up to three generations without septation and/or daughter cell separation, resulting in chain formation. Even when growth is immediately blocked, macromolecular biosynthesis may continue for at least 1 hr, indicating that disruption of the biosynthetic apparatus or other related energy-dependent processes such as transport are not primary events in the bactericidal action of BPI.

BPI does produce one dramatic and irreversible effect on bacterial macromolecular synthesis, namely an immediate arrest of the synthesis of one of the OM pore proteins [Omp F (outer-membrane protein F)] and a concomitant increase in the synthesis of another porin, Omp C (Fig. 4). These two proteins serve closely similar pore functions in *E. coli*. Their biosynthesis is reciprocally controlled by a complex gene system that is responsive to environmental conditions (50,51,66). Radioautography of the detergent-extracted proteins of ^{14}C-amino-acid-labeled control and BPI-killed *E. coli* confirms that except for the respective inhibition and stimulation of OmpF and OmpC, biosynthesis of the other proteins is comparable in the control and BPI-treated bacterial populations. It appears unlikely that this effect of BPI (which is not reversed by removal of bound BPI) is directly linked to its bactericidal action, because: (a) OmpC substitutes effectively for loss of OmpF (31), and neither OmpF$^-$ nor OmpC$^-$ mutants exhibit functional or growth disturbances; and (b) OmpF$^-$ or OmpC$^-$ mutants are as BPI-sensitive as are wild-type *E. coli*.

Defensins

Another set of well-defined cytotoxic proteins has been isolated recently from alveolar macrophages and peritoneal granulocytes of rabbits and from human peripheral blood neutrophils by Lehrer and co-workers (67–71). These small proteins of $M_r < 4000$ appear to be the pure components of an arginine- and cystine-rich cationic protein fraction first described by Zeya and Spitznagel (10,12). Acid extraction (0.1 M citrate or 10% acetic acid) of granule-rich cell fractions solubilizes large quantities of these cationic peptides that can be resolved by preparative elec-

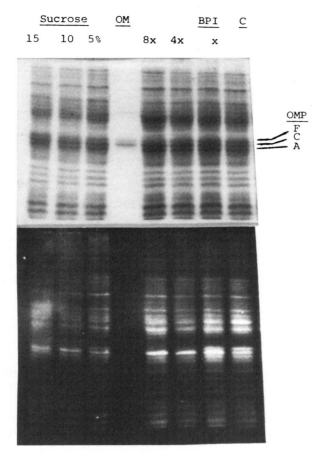

FIG. 4. Effect of BPI on porin synthesis by *E. coli* PL2. Detergent-extracted proteins of *E. coli* PL2 incubated alone (control, C) or with increasing concentrations of BPI or sucrose, in the presence of [¹⁴C]amino acids, were submitted to SDS-PAGE and Coomassie Blue staining (**top**) and subsequent radioautography (**bottom**). [Increasing medium osmolality is known to inhibit expression of OMP F and to stimulate synthesis of OMP C (50,51,66).] An extract of outer membranes isolated from *E. coli* PL2 was run in the lane marked OM to identify OM proteins OMP F, C, and A.

2), six from rabbit peritoneal granulocytes (NP 1, NP 2, NP 3a, NP 3b, NP 4, and NP 5) (68,69), and three from human neutrophils (HNP 1, HNP 2, and HNP 3) (70,71). These peptides, for their antimicrobial activity, have been named *defensins*. The primary structure of all 11 defensins has been determined (67,69,71), and the rabbit granulocyte peptide NP 2 has been crystallized (72). Peptides MCP 1 and 2 are identical to peptides NP 1 and 2, respectively (69), and the other sequenced peptides exhibit a high degree of homology (Fig. 5). All 11 peptides contain between 32 and 34 amino acid residues and share at least 11 residues, including six cystines without apparent free SH groups. If these peptides indeed contain three S-S bridges they would be exceedingly compact molecules, which apparently contributes to their biological properties (71). All defensins carry a net positive charge, attributable to the arginine content, which ranges between 4 and 10 residues.

Despite their common structural features, the biological potency of individual peptides varies considerably. The more basic peptides, NP 1 (MCP 1) and NP 2 (MCP 2), with the highest arginine content, exhibit the greatest potency and the broadest cytotoxicity. These two peptides and HNP 1-3 combined kill both gram-positive (*Staphylococcus epidermidis,* several strains of *Staphylococcus aureus,* and *Streptococcus* and *Listeria monocytogenes*) and, less effectively, gram-negative (*E. coli, Pseudomonas aeruginosa, Klebsiella pneumoniae*) bacterial species (68,73,74), as well as various fungi (75–77) and viruses (78). Some of the peptides lack virucidal activity and are less active or more limited in their bactericidal activity (68,78). Expression of bactericidal activity requires approximately neutral pH, as well as a hypotonic medium that contains certain nutrients (70). Addition of physiological concentrations of NaCl or other salts competitively inhibits bactericidal and fungicidal activity (68). The apparent need of some nutrient source for the antibacterial action of the defensins is different for different microorganisms (70), but no activity is evident in nutrient-free medium. In contrast, *Cryptococcus neoformans* is effectively killed in such a medium (70). The fungicidal activity of the various defensins against *Candida albicans* correlates with their relative binding affinity for surface sites

trophoresis and reverse-phase high-performance liquid chromatography (HPLC) into several closely homologous single peptides. Two have been purified to homogeneity from rabbit alveolar macrophages (67) (MCP 1 and MCP

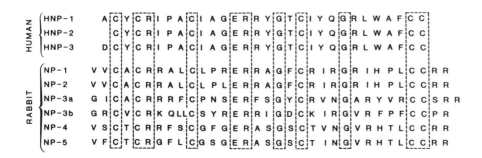

FIG. 5. Sequence comparison of human and rabbit defensins. Each sequence is represented by the single-letter amino acid symbol. The sequences were maximally aligned to show the structural homology conferred by the 11 residues common to both the human and rabbit peptides (enclosed in boxes). (From ref. 71.)

on the organism. As has been observed with BPI (41), initial binding of the agents is temperature-independent, reversible, and insufficient for microbicidal activity. Postbinding events are temperature-dependent and are linked to the candidacidal activity (79). The secondary phase of interaction of the defensins with the *Candida* envelope is inhibitable by millimolar calcium but not by magnesium (79).

On a molar basis the defensins are much less potent than BPI. Nearly complete killing of 10^6 bacteria per milliliter requires a defensin concentration of 10^{-5} *M*. (For comparison: More than 90% of 10^7 *E. coli* or *S. typhimurium* are killed by BPI concentrations of $\geq 10^{-8}$ *M*.) However, the defensins are so abundant in the granules [as determined in granulocytes (75)] that it may be expected that sufficient amounts are available in the intact cell for antimicrobial activity if other intracellular conditions, such as ionic strength and composition, are permissive. The defensins are constituents of the primary (azurophilic) granules of (human) PMN (70) and, upon degranulation, they appear in the extracellular medium (80). As isolated agents *in vitro* they can express cytotoxicity toward both transformed and normal mammalian cells (81). Especially because serum inhibits cytotoxicity it remains to be determined whether, under physiological conditions, release of defensins from intact cells may reach cytotoxic levels, as has been proposed (81).

How the defensins exert their cytotoxic effect on target cells is apparently unknown. Experiments with *Candida albicans* have shown that bactericidal concentrations of MCP-1 and MCP-2 (5 μg/ml) cause rapid suppression of O_2 consumption and loss of intracellular $^{86}Rb^+$ (77), possibly signifying envelope damage.

Cathepsin G

This chymotrypsin-like protease is one of the neutral proteases present in the primary granules of human PMN (82). This enzyme or group of enzymes has been isolated in several laboratories, yielding proteins with different apparent M_r and similar, but not identical, amino acid composition (83–86), raising questions about the degree of purity of the various isolates. Olsson and Venge (83) have obtained four immunologically indistinguishable isozymic forms with virtually identical amino acid composition and identical catalytic properties, but ranging in M_r from 25,000 to 29,000. The authors suggest that the M_r differences may be attributable to differences in carbohydrate content or extent of amidation of carboxylic residues. The high net positive charge of the enzyme(s) cannot be accounted for by the content of basic amino acids and suggests therefore that acidic residues are in the amide form (83).

Several groups have reported that cathepsin G has antimicrobial properties. Odeberg et al. (87) were the first to show that their chymotrypsin-like proteins at 10^{-6} *M* kill >90% of 2×10^6 *S. aureus* and other gram-positive bacterial species. Gram-negative *E. coli* and *P. aeruginosa* were also killed, but at protein concentrations 2.5 times higher (87). The four isozymes are also similar in their bactericidal activity. Table 4 shows some of the characteristics of the antimicrobial activity of cathepsin G, as determined by Odeberg and co-workers (86,87). The bactericidal activity seems unrelated to the enzymatic action of the purified protein because heating to 90°C or 100°C destroys the catalytic, but not the bactericidal, activity (87). Thorne et al. (88) confirmed these findings, showing that purified cathepsin G killed *Acinetobacter* 199A independent of catalytic activity, and Lehrer et al. (89) showed heat-stable fungicidal activity (against *Candida parapsilosis*) in protein fractions from human PMN granules that were electrophoretically comparable to the proteins of Odeberg and co-workers (86,87).

The possibility always remains that the microbicidal activity preserved after heating is actually a property of a protein contaminating the protease. This seems unlikely because of the similar specific bactericidal activity of the four isozymic proteins isolated by Olsson and co-workers (83,86,87).

The bactericidal action of cathepsin G on *S. aureus* or *E. coli* requires neutral pH and an environment of physiological or lower ionic strength. The inhibitory effect of 5 to 10 m*M* Mg^{2+} and NaCl concentrations >0.1 *M* suggests that these highly cationic proteins also bind to their targets by charge interactions (86,87). The loss of colony-forming ability coincides with early effects on bacterial O_2 consumption, presumably the basis for the inhibition of $^{86}Rb^+$ uptake and incorporation of specific radioactive precursors in the synthesis of bacterial protein, RNA, and DNA (90). This effect of cathepsin G on bacterial metabolism may be mediated by a rather discrete one on the cytoplasmic membrane because $^{86}Rb^+$ efflux from *S. aureus* preloaded with Rb is affected little in the first 20 min.

TABLE 4. *Microbicidal activity of chymotrypsin-like proteins*[a]

Neutral pH-optimum
Heat stable (resists boiling)
Low optimal ionic strength
Inhibited by 5–10 m*M* Mg^{2+}
Inhibited by serum protease inhibitors
Inhibits bacterial:
Oxygen consumption
Protein synthesis
DNA synthesis
RNA synthesis
$^{86}Rb^+$ influx

[a] From Odeberg et al. (86).

Very recently Shafer et al. (91) have purified a protein fraction from the granules of human PMN consisting of two recognizable components with M_r 24,000 and 25,500 as well as carrying both cathepsin G and bactericidal activity against *Neisseria gonorrhoeae* (91). Again, the esterase activity was heat-labile and inhibited by diisopropyl fluorophosphate (DFP), whereas the bactericidal activity was not. However, the heat-treated protein fraction was tested for its effect on the gonococcal viability at a concentration 100 times higher than the untreated fraction. It has not been reported which of the two protein components has the bactericidal activity. The bactericidal potency of the protein fraction was much greater (66-fold) toward a gonococcal mutant with an apparently very low LPS content, characterized by short polysaccharide chains as judged by their electrophoretic mobility in SDS-PAGE (91). Surprising is the finding of Shafer et al. (64) that the parent strain (with a more typical LPS content and composition) and the mutant gonococcus showed equal sensitivity to a 57,000-M_r bactericidal protein purified from human PMN by Shafer et al. (64) by a procedure similar to that used by Weiss et al. (36) for the purification of BPI; the two proteins also exhibit a nearly identical amino acid composition. All evidence presented by Weiss et al. (39,55) indicates that the relative sensitivities of different strains of *E. coli* and *S. typhimurium* to BPI is determined by the length of the polysaccharide chains of the LPS of these bacterial species. These observations may mean that the surface properties that render the gonococcus sensitive to BPI (R. Rest, J. Weiss, and P. Elsbach, *unpublished observations*) or to a similar cationic protein (91) are very different from those that determine the sensitivity of other gram-negative bacterial species.

Shafer et al. (64,91) also have isolated a 37,000-M_r protein that at high protein concentrations can kill *E. coli* and *S. typhimurium* as well as *N. gonorrhoeae*.

Lactoferrin

Lactoferrin is an ~80,000-M_r iron-binding glycoprotein (92) that, in phagocytic cells, is only found in the specific granules of PMN (93–95) but that occurs also in most secretory fluids (for a recent comprehensive review, see ref. 13). At present, few details are known about the molecular properties of lactoferrin. Such information should be forthcoming soon, however, because progress has been reported in the isolation of mRNA of this protein (96,97). The role of lactoferrin as an isolated antimicrobial agent, at concentrations in the micromolar range, appears to be related, in part, to its iron-binding [two ferric ions per molecule (98)] and, hence, its ability to compete with iron-requiring bacteria for an essential growth factor. This property of lactoferrin explains its growth-inhibitory effect (reversible) on a range of microbial species, including

gram-positive as well as gram-negative bacteria (13,99). However, iron-depleted lactoferrin also exhibits bactericidal activity against *Streptococcus mutans* (100,101) and *Legionella pneumophila* (102) which is not mimicked by iron depletion. Because iron saturated lactoferrin is entirely nontoxic, it appears that iron removal from the microbial environment is necessary but is not sufficient for the bactericidal effect of lactoferrin. The antimicrobial activity of lactoferrin against *Legionella pneumophila* is blocked by 8 mM $MgCl_2$, but 100 mM $MgCl_2$ has no effect on killing of *S. mutans* by iron-depleted lactoferrin (102).

It has been proposed that iron-saturated lactoferrin at low concentrations (10 nM) may also contribute to antimicrobial activity within the PMN environment by stimulating production of hydroxyl radical as an effective donor of iron (103). This function of lactoferrin has been questioned, however (104). Other very recent evidence, using spin-trapping of hydroxyl radical, suggests that lactoferrin may either enhance or prevent hydroxyl radical formation, depending on its level of iron saturation and the availability of exogenous iron salts (105,106).

Individuals whose PMN lack lactoferrin or specific granules may be prone to bacterial infections (13,107–109). Experimental *in-vitro* depletion of PMN of specific granules and lactoferrin results in diminished bactericidal activity at high bacteria-to-PMN ratios (110). Theoretically, lactoferrin deficiency could impair host defense against infection, not only because the protein can act as an antimicrobial agent, but also because lactoferrin may be a determinant of the adhesive properties of neutrophils (111), thereby influencing neutrophil function during phagocytosis (111–114). In addition, lactoferrin appears to be a modulator of granulopoiesis (98,99,115–117). To our knowledge, it has not yet been determined to what extent extracellular lactoferrin from other cellular sources is also lacking in this congenital condition or may be capable of fulfilling some of these latter functions. It is also unknown what the consequences are for PMN function of the absence or deficiency of other constituents of the specific granules (see Chapter 34).

Lysozyme

This small (M_r ~ 14,500), very cationic (pI > 10) enzyme is widely distributed in tissues and body fluids and occurs also in the granules of mononuclear and polymorphonuclear phagocytes. In PMN it is a constituent of both primary and secondary granules. Few enzymes have been characterized as well as lysozyme, whose three-dimensional structure is precisely defined (118). Nevertheless, the role, in nature, of this very abundant enzyme is still not very clear. Because lysozyme is potently bactericidal for some microorganisms, whose cell-wall peptidoglycans are exquisitely susceptible to the highly specific cleavage of the beta(1-4)glycosidic link between *N*-acetylglucosamine and *N*-acetylmuramic acid, resulting in prompt bacterial lysis, the protein usually is listed prominently among bactericidal agents of phagocytes. Actually, only a few nonpathogenic gram-positive bacteria are lysed by lysozyme. Resistance to its action is the rule among gram-negative bacteria and is common among gram-positive species (13). The inability of lysozyme to hydrolyze the peptidoglycans of most microorganisms is attributable to at least two factors (119): First, the overall complexity of the peptidoglycan matrix, the extent of cross-linking, and the length of the cross-bridges determine if lysozyme can penetrate the peptidoglycan mesh to reach the glycosidic bonds; second, the degree of *O*-acetylation of the peptidoglycans is an important variable in the susceptibility to hydrolysis by lysozyme. The outer membrane of gram-negative bacteria provides an additional barrier to the action of lysozyme on its substrate. It is also uncertain if lysozyme is an essential element in the disassembly of microorganisms during phagocytosis by the complete degradative apparatus of the phagocyte. For example, bactericidal concentrations of BPI initiate prompt and extensive net degradation of the peptidoglycans of *E. coli* by bacterial degradative enzymes (*unpublished observations*) but do not facilitate the action of added lysozyme, indicating that cell-wall digestion may be effectively carried out by autolytic enzymes, without participation of the host's lysozyme. Further, several animals, including the cow (13,120), lack lysozyme in their PMN as well as in some of their secretions (120) but exhibit no diminished defense against infection.

The biological usefulness of the secretion by mononuclear phagocytes of large quantities of lysozyme (121) is also unclear. Naturally occurring substrates for lysozyme, other than bacterial cell-wall polysaccharides, have not been recognized.

Major Basic Protein of Eosinophils

The major basic protein (MBP) of eosinophils is a small-M_r (9,000–11,000), highly basic (pI > 10) polypeptide that has been isolated from the large specific granules of guinea-pig, human, and rat eosinophils by Gleich and co-workers (122–124). Immunoelectron microscopy and subcellular fractionation have shown that MBP is localized in the crystalloid core of these granules (122,125). So named for its abundance, MBP accounts for up to 50% of the eosinophil's granule protein content (126). The histamine- and heparin-containing granules of basophils contain a protein immunochemically indistinguishable from MBP, albeit in much smaller quantity (127). Human placenta also appears to produce a molecule immunochemically similar to eosinophil MBP but of greater apparent molecular size (128).

MBP contains nearly 13 mol % arginine (which largely accounts for its basicity) and six half-cystine residues, two of which exist as free sulfhydryls in the isolated protein (129). At high protein concentrations, these sulfhydryls readily oxidize to form reversible aggregates of disulfide-linked polymers with reduced biological activity (130). Reduced and alkylated (and hence monomeric) MBP is biologically active (131), suggesting that the monomeric form, but not free sulfhydryls, is needed for bioactivity.

Isolated MBP exhibits minimal antibacterial activity (129) but is cytotoxic toward a range of parasites, including larval forms of *Schistosoma mansoni* and *Trichinella spiralis* and bloodstream and amastigote forms of *Trypanosoma cruzi* (132–135), consistent with accumulating evidence of a role for the eosinophil and its granule contents in host defense against helminth infections (130). Although relatively high concentrations (10^{-4}–10^{-6} *M*) of MBP are required to produce parasite damage, these concentrations may be achieved during eosinophil-parasite interaction by virtue of the high concentration of MBP in eosinophil granules and the localized delivery of these granule contents to intracellular or adherent extracellular targets during degranulation (132,135). At similar concentrations, MBP can also damage many types of mammalian cells *in vitro* (130,136). While dilutional effects may normally protect "innocent bystander" host cells from secreted MBP, sufficient extracellular MBP accumulates in certain inflammatory diseases associated with eosinophilia to contribute possibly to tissue damage and organ dysfunction (130,136–138).

How MBP damages cells is unknown. Manifestations of parasite damage include loss of motility, dye uptake, [^{51}Cr]- and [^{3}H]uridine release from prelabeled cells, and "ballooning" of the surface (tegumental) membrane following exposure to MBP for periods ranging from several hours up to 1 to 2 days (132,135). Clearly, these studies lack the molecular and temporal resolution needed to identify the primary loci of MBP action. Considering the highly cationic properties of MBP and the relatively low potency and selectivity of its action, cell damage may reflect essentially nonspecific membrane alterations resulting from surface charge interactions between MBP and negatively charged cell membranes. The ability of polyanions, such as heparin, to block MBP binding and cytotoxicity is consistent with this view. However, the inability of many polycations to mimic MBP action (132,136) may mean that other physical-chemical determinants, besides overall basicity, are important for cytotoxicity.

Eosinophil Cationic Protein

Another extremely basic (pI > 11) protein of the large specific granules of eosinophils is the eosinophil cationic protein (ECP). Olsson and Venge (83) originally isolated ECP from acid extracts of leukocytes obtained from patients with eosinophilia. The origin of ECP in eosinophils was subsequently confirmed by localization of ECP in the matrix of the unique crystalloid-containing large eosinophil granule by subcellular fractionation (139) and immunoelectron microscopy (140).

ECP appears to represent a family of arginine-rich glycoproteins. Preparative electrophoresis (83) or cation-exchange chromatography (141,142) can resolve ECP into at least four subspecies. These subspecies appear to be immunochemically identical (83,141), with virtually the same amino acid composition (141) and NH₂-terminal amino acid sequence (142), but they can be separated by SDS-PAGE (apparent M_r 17,000–21,000) (141,142). Treatment with endoglycosidase F (but not endoglycosidase H) reduces the electrophoretic heterogeneity, suggesting that at least some of the ECP species differ in complex N-linked oligosaccharide content (142). ECP biosynthesis can be studied *in vitro* with marrow cells from patients with eosinophilia (141), which may help elucidate further the biochemical origin of the multiple ECP species. The biological significance, if any, of this microheterogeneity is unknown.

Like the eosinophil's major basic protein, cytotoxic effects of ECP have been detected toward parasites (131,143) and cultured mammalian cells (144) but not against bacteria (139). ECP damages schistosomula at approximately one-tenth the molar concentration required for MBP-mediated toxicity (131), but eosinophils contain up to 10-fold more MBP (126). The MBP and ECP content of eosinophils can vary considerably, however, possibly because of secretion of these proteins during (hyper)eosinophilia (126,127,130).

The action of ECP against schistosomula differs from that of MBP not only in potency, but also in its effects on cell architecture. At minimum cytotoxic doses of ECP ($\sim 10^{-6}\ M$), effects on parasite motility, dye uptake, and internal granulation are seen within 1 hr without gross membrane disorganization (131), suggesting early and relatively discrete effects on membrane structure and function, possibly depleting energy stores needed for motility. At later times and at higher doses of ECP, formation of surface blebs, membrane detachment, and extrusion of internal contents are seen, followed eventually by gross fragmentation of the tegumental membrane (131,143).

ECP shares with another cationic eosinophil granule protein, the eosinophil-derived neurotoxin (EDN), the ability to produce a neurological syndrome characterized by stiffness and ataxia, as well as muscle weakness and wasting (Gordon phenomenon), following intrathecal injection (142,145). A monoclonal antibody has been isolated that recognizes the secreted (but not the storage) form of both proteins (146), indicating the presence of a common epitope in ECP and EDN. Whether this corresponds to common structural determinants involved in interaction with components of the granule matrix (e.g., proteoglycans) or in neurotoxic activity is not known. Further evidence of structural homology between ECP and EDN has been obtained by NH₂-terminal amino acid sequence analysis, which revealed identity at 37 of 55 residues, including all four cysteines in this region (142). Even more remarkable, ECP and EDN show significant homology with ribonucleases of various animal species, including all four cysteines in perfect alignment (142) and also highly conserved amino acids involved in substrate-binding and catalysis. The significance of these observations has been confirmed by the demonstration that ECP and EDN possess RNase activity (I. Olsson and G. J. Gleich, *unpublished communications*). It remains to be shown whether or not RNase activity contributes to the cytotoxic activity of these two eosinophil proteins. Because EDN exhibits little or no helminthotoxic activity (131), it seems likely that other properties of ECP are required for parasite killing, such as the channel-forming activity of ECP recently described by Young et al. (147). At cytotoxic concentrations ($10^{-6}\ M$), ECP, but not MBP or eosinophil protein-X [probably EDN (130)], causes lipid vesicles to become leaky to ions, sucrose, and small fluorescent molecules and also induces current steps in voltage-clamped phospholipid planar bilayers. Channel formation by ECP shows no specific lipid requirements but is markedly enhanced at higher temperatures. Insertion of ECP into the phospholipid bilayer therefore probably depends on membrane fluidity and possibly on temperature-induced changes in protein conformation (148–150). ECP channels exhibit little ion selectivity or voltage sensitivity, suggesting that ECP forms large and stable aqueous pores. ECP also causes rapid and sustained membrane depolarization in nucleated cells and hemolysis of erythrocytes, indicating channel formation in biological as well as model membranes.

Because of the growing evidence of pore formation by many cytotoxic proteins produced throughout evolution [e.g., membrane-attack complex (or isolated C9) of complement (148,149); perforins of cytotoxic T and NK cells (149,151); and cytotoxins from protozoa (152), yeast (153), and bacteria (154)], it is tempting to speculate that ECP belongs to a family of conserved proteins capable of killing cells by producing holes in their membranes (147,149,155). Indeed, ECP channels functionally resemble channels formed by poly-C9 and by perforin-1 (147,149), two proteins that show immunological cross-reactivity and, hence, may be of common ancestral origin (149). However, it must be recognized that similar membrane damage can be produced by a wide variety of cytotoxic agents of diverse structure (156), possibly involving different molecular mechanisms of membrane alteration.

Moreover, in virtually all instances, the precise relation of channel formation to cell death remains uncertain, partly because the characteristics of the channel vary with the dose of cytotoxin added (148,149,156) and partly because the effects of membrane damage on cell integrity vary with the repair capabilities of the target cell (156,157). In the case of ECP, this relation is further complicated by the apparent multifunctional properties of this protein (i.e., channel-forming and nuclease activities). Do ECP channels promote internalization of ECP or of an enzymatically active fragment [as in other multifunctional cytotoxins (158)] that digests cellular RNA? If so, is RNA degradation necessary for cell killing, or does it merely amplify cell destruction after lethal injury by pore formation? Monoclonal antibodies and/or limited proteolysis may facilitate dissection of the multiple activities of ECP and help define the steps required for cytotoxicity.

ROLE OF DEGRADATIVE ENZYMES IN (O₂-INDEPENDENT) ANTIMICROBIAL ACTIVITY

Theoretically, any one of the lysosomal hydrolases that abound in the granules of phagocytes may contribute to the demise of the target cells in one of several ways: (i) by a direct lethal effect through its catalytic activity; (ii) by a mechanism independent of enzymatic action; (iii) in conjunction with other antimicrobial agents; or (iv) by aiding in the digestion of a cell already killed by another agent (or agents).

Except for lysozyme (see above), which, by its catalytic action, lyses and kills a few harmless saprophytes such as gram-positive *Micrococcus lysodeikticus* and *Bacillus megaterium,* convincing evidence is lacking that the enzymatic action of any of the phagocyte's other hydrolases alone can be effectively microbicidal for pathogenic microorganisms. In fact, as has been pointed out in a recent review (159), even the role of the phagocyte's hydrolases (as opposed to autolysis by the target cell's own degradative enzymes) in the digestion of killed microorganisms is not well-defined. However, several reports suggest that certain combinations of hydrolytic enzymes have synergistic antimicrobial effects, but not necessarily by virtue of their catalytic activity (86,87,91,160,161).

Proteases

The granules of PMN and other phagocytes of all animal species studied contain many proteases (82). Some of these have acid pH optima (predominantly the proteases of rodent PMN) (82,88); others, the so-called neutral proteases, which are prevalent in human PMN, are most active at physiological pH (82,86,88).

So far, the only apparently pure protease that is micro-

bicidal by itself, although independently of its enzymatic action, is cathepsin G (discussed earlier). Other purified and presumably well-characterized proteases such as elastase and collagenase have no clear-cut independent antibacterial activity. Purified elastase can digest some of the outer-membrane proteins of the intact gonococcus (162), but without lethal consequences for the organism. However, whereas lysosomal proteases or lysozyme as single agents do little damage to *Acinetobacter* 199A, the addition of purified elastase or one of several cathepsins, followed by lysozyme, causes lysis of the bacterium, perhaps because the proteolytic attack on the outer membrane of this organism paves the way for peptidoglycan degradation by lysozyme (88). Odeberg, Olsson, and co-workers (86,161) have shown that purified elastase also potentiates the bactericidal activity of the myeloperoxidase-H₂O₂ (glucose-oxidase) system and of cathepsin G toward *E. coli* as well as *S. aureus,* mainly by increasing the initial rate of killing. Potentiation of killing of *S. aureus* was evident only at pH 5.5, and that of *E. coli* was evident at pH 7.4, in accord with the finding that at pH 7.4 elastase binds to *E. coli,* but not to *S. aureus.* The potentiating effect of elastase on MPO-mediated bacterial killing in this instance is again unaffected by heating (i.e., unrelated to the proteolytic activity of elastase).

Unpublished observations in Olsson's laboratory have shown that the action of BPI can also be potentiated as much as 10-fold by either heated or unheated cathepsin G or elastase (mentioned in ref. 86). These findings need to be reconciled with those of Weiss and co-workers (36,37), which indicated that the bactericidal activity of crude extracts of PMN (which are rich in proteases) against *E. coli* can be accounted for by the BPI content (confirmed by RIA) of these extracts, calculating their activity on the basis of the organism's sensitivity to pure BPI (36,37).

Appraisal of the antimicrobial role of proteases, particularly in the intact cell, is complicated by the fact that the activity of enzymes such as elastase and collagenase is regulated by ubiquitous protein inhibitors (163). The interaction of the enzyme and its inhibitor(s) is apparently controlled by the cell's respiration (164–169). Thus the respiratory burst may release inhibition of proteases by their protein inhibitors (166–169).

Lipid Hydrolases

Of the neutral lipid and phospholipid-degrading enzymatic activities that have been recognized in PMN and macrophages (170), several take place in the granules and hence might play a role in the fate of ingested bacteria. Since most pathogenic bacteria are essentially devoid of neutral lipids, only phospholipid-degrading enzymes may be expected to contribute to destruction of ingested bacteria. It has been shown that phospholipases of the PMN indeed participate in the degradation of the phospholipids of *E. coli* killed by the PMN (37,45,171). However, there is no evidence that phospholipases of phagocytes, or any other source, can act as independent antibacterial agents (45). In fact, normally the phospholipids of intact bacteria (*E. coli*) are not degraded by either bacterial or exogenous phospholipases, except when the latter are added at enormously high concentrations (37,45,48,172). For net phospholipid hydrolysis to occur, the bacterial envelope must be perturbed, usually by conditions that are incompatible with survival [e.g., phage infection or exposure to bactericidal agents such as polymixin B and BPI or the activated complement system (42,44,45,48,173–176)]. The exploration of phospholipid degradation as a variable in the interaction between bacteria and phagocytes or their products has been limited largely to studies on *E. coli*, because: (a) *E. coli* has been one of the favored test organisms for assessment of bactericidal activities; (b) much is known about the phospholipases of *E. coli* (48,177); and (c) mutants are available that lack phospholipases A (60,61). Experiments with *E. coli* provide no evidence that bacterial phospholipid degradation enhances the microbicidal efficiency of isolated microbicidal agents such as BPI or other cytotoxins (44,48,176). For example, the bactericidal potency of BPI, which appears to be the principal activator in PMN of both bacterial and PMN phospholipases A (48), is the same for (a) wild-type *E. coli* (endowed with the typical *E. coli* phospholipid-degrading equipment), (b) an *E. coli* mutant devoid of detectable phospholipase A, and (c) this mutant into which a plasmid carrying the *E. coli* phospholipase A gene is introduced (60), raising the phospholipase A content to 20-fold higher levels than in the parent strain (60; this laboratory, *unpublished observations*), even though net phospholipid degradation ranged from <5% to 70% in the three strains. Whether killing by phagocytes of other microorganisms may be more efficient when bacterial and/or the phagocyte's phospholipases are activated is not known.

How important degradation of bacterial phospholipids is for the rate and extent of overall digestion and killed bacteria has also not been clearly established.

Nucleases

Nucleases with acid pH are present in the granules of both PMN and mononuclear phagocytes (28,178). Lysates of human peripheral blood mononuclear phagocytes contain, per cell equivalent, 15- to 20-fold more DNase activity with a pH optimum of ~5.0 than do lysates of PMN from the same donor, as measured against chromosomal DNA isolated from *E. coli* (179). *E. coli* ingested and killed by PMN exhibit almost no degradation of either

chromosomal (20,179,180) or plasmid DNA (179). In contrast, mononuclear phagocytes degrade, into small fragments, 50% to 60% of the [^{3}H]thymidine-labeled DNA of unencapsulated phagocytosed *E. coli* but do not degrade DNA of encapsulated *E. coli* (179,180). Unlike chromosomal DNA of unencapsulated *E. coli* engulfed and killed by mononuclear phagocytes, plasmid DNA is refractory to degradation and retains its transforming capabilities (179). One of the limiting factors in the degradation of chromosomal DNA of *E. coli* is the level of DNase in the phagocyte because addition of exogenous (pancreas or spleen) DNase to lysates of PMN, prepared after ingestion of *E. coli*, resulted in extensive degradation of bacterial DNA (179). To our knowledge, the antibacterial activity of DNases or RNases isolated from the granules of PMN or macrophages and purified to the point that these proteins can be tested as independent agents has not been examined. However, the intriguing demonstration of significant primary structure homology between the eosinophil cationic protein, the eosinophil-derived neurotoxin, and a highly conserved region of pancreatic RNase encompassing the catalytic site (142), plus the independent and unpublished observations in the laboratories of Olsson and Gleich indicating that these eosinophil cytotoxins possess the ability to degrade RNA, raise anew the question of the role of nuclease activity in cytotoxicity.

ROLE OF O$_2$-INDEPENDENT AGENTS IN THE BACTERICIDAL ACTIVITY OF INTACT PHAGOCYTES

The demonstration that a given agent, isolated from a phagocyte, is potently bactericidal under certain conditions *in vitro* does not permit the conclusion that this agent also serves a significant function within the intact cell. In fact, it must be recognized that convincing evidence is not easily obtained that any one of the numerous products and components of the phagocyte's antimicrobial systems is primarily responsible for the killing of a particular microorganism *in vivo*. Conditions in the intact cell may either amplify or diminish the antimicrobial potency of a given substance. For example, delivery of the agent to intravacuolar bacteria, competition for the same target among substances with similar properties, or the composition of the intracellular environment may be either more or less favorable for activity. Furthermore, the speed of action of two or more antimicrobial agents may be so different that only the most rapidly acting one is likely to play an active role. To complicate matters further, in assigning relative importance, any order in the kinetics of action of several agents may differ for different microbial species. The most compelling arguments for the importance of a defined antimicrobial system in the intact phagocyte stem, of course, from clinical observations on the consequences of the inborn absence or deficiency of that system for the antimicrobial activity of the host cells. However, such conditions are rare. So far the study of only one disease, chronic granulomatous disease (CGD) of childhood, has provided apparently unequivocal evidence that one cytotoxic system (O_2-dependent) is essential for the killing of a number of bacterial species. But even in this case the highly variable clinical course of patients with this disease indicates that a defective respiratory burst does not necessarily have predictable consequences for the ability of the phagocyte to deal with certain microbial predators, suggesting that additional variables contribute to its antimicrobial effectiveness. These considerations should be kept in mind when attempts are made to assign a role to isolated factors or systems in host defense against infection.

Reports showing that O_2-deprived PMN, as well as PMN from patients with CGD, effectively kill a range of microbial species lend credence to the claim that O_2-independent microbicidal systems are adequate for host defense against such organisms (13,15,17–19). Since it is notoriously difficult to remove O_2 completely from incubation vessels, it has been questioned whether residual killing activity of O_2-depleted PMN is actually O_2-independent. However, in at least some of the reported experiments, the juxtaposition of results for bacteria that are killed and for those that are not killed, both under O_2-depleted conditions (18), gives confidence that the bactericidal activity was indeed O_2-independent, particularly when the killed bacteria produce both superoxide dismutase and catalase (18).

An example of such an experiment is shown in Table 5. Rabbit PMN were incubated either with a rough strain of S. typhimurium (BPI-sensitive) or with Staphylococcus epidermidis (BPI-insensitive) in room air (permitting full respiratory burst activation) or after O_2-depletion by N_2-flushing (virtually abolishing respiratory burst activity). Whereas killing of ingested S. typhimurium was equally prompt and nearly complete in room air and under N_2, minimal killing of S. epidermidis occurred after O_2 depletion. When S. typhimurium and S. epidermidis were presented simultaneously, both were ingested, but only S. typhimurium was killed effectively. The bactericidal capacity of aerobically and anaerobically incubated PMN toward rough as well as smooth S. typhimurium was the same over a wide range of presented and ingested bacteria (Fig. 6), indicating that O_2-independent bactericidal mechanisms are sufficient to deal with maximal numbers of ingested bacteria (18).

Similar experiments have been carried out with human PMN (19,181), showing that ingested E. coli and S. typhimurium are killed as effectively under N_2 as in room air. Further support for the effectiveness of O_2 depletion in these experiments and the adequacy of O_2-independent bactericidal mechanisms for killing of these species of gram-negative bacteria comes from observations on PMN from patients with CGD showing that these cells and normal O_2-depleted PMN killed ingested E. coli and S. typhimurium equally well (18,19). The fact that, among the

TABLE 5. N_2 flushing of rabbit PMN: Effect on bactericidal and respiratory burst activity[a]

Incubation conditions		Bacterial survival		$[1\text{-}^{14}C]Glucose \rightarrow {}^{14}CO_2$	O_2^- formed
Bacteria	N_2	−Sonic.[b]	+Sonic.	(% Stimulation)	(nmole)
S. typhimurium MR10	−	4.9 ± 1.9	3.4 ± 1.6	1410 ± 240	3.9
(20/1)	+	6.4 ± 4.1	6.2 ± 4.3	49 ± 24	0.2
Staph. epidermidis (10/1)	−	17.8 ± 4.3	23.6 ± 3.3	480	
	+	18.8 ± 5.0	70.8 ± 8.2	10	
S. typhimurium MR10	−	3.7 ± 2.0	3.6 ± 1.8		
(20/1)	+	0.3 ± 0.2	0.4 ± 0.1		
Staph. epidermidis (10/1)	−	13.2 ± 1.1	29.2 ± 9.5		
	+	19.3 ± 6.8	85.7 ± 6.7		

[a] After preincubation of 10^7 rabbit PMN in room air or under a nitrogen atmosphere, S. typhimurium MR10 and/or Staph. epidermidis (160K), were added. The numbers in parentheses indicate the bacteria/PMN ratio. Following incubation at 37°C for 30 min, bacterial survival, hexose monophosphate shunt activity, or superoxide (O_2^-) production by PMN was measured. Bacterial survival is expressed as percent of viability of bacteria incubated alone. Oxidation of $[1\text{-}^{14}C]glucose \rightarrow {}^{14}CO_2$ by PMN incubated with bacteria is expressed as the percent stimulation over the amount of glucose oxidized by PMN incubated alone. Superoxide (O_2^-) production, measured as superoxide dismutase-inhibitable cytochrome C reduction, is shown as the increase in O_2^- formation (nmole) by 10^7 phagocytosing (vs. resting) PMN in 30 min. These values represent the mean of two experiments. All other results shown represent the mean and, where indicated, standard error of the mean of three or more experiments. (From ref. 18.)

[b] Sonic., sonication.

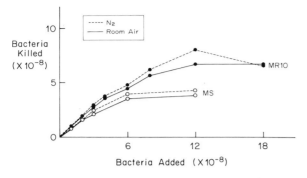

FIG. 6. O_2-independent bactericidal capacity of rabbit PMN toward *S. typhimurium* 395 MR10 and MS. After pretreatment of 10^7 PMN in room air (—) or nitrogen (---), various amounts of either MR-10 (●) or opsonized MS (○) were added. After incubation at 37°C for 30 min, bacterial killing was measured. The loss of bacterial viability measured before and after sonication of cell suspensions was the same; for purposes of clarity, only the values obtained after sonication are shown. The values shown represent the mean of the results of two or more experiments. (From ref. 18.)

various agents of the PMN capable of O_2-independent killing, BPI plays the major role is most strongly suggested by the finding that, in whole homogenates or sonicates, anti-BPI IgG, but not nonimmune IgG, nearly abolishes killing of BPI-sensitive bacteria. Moreover, intracellular (but not extracellular) *E. coli* incubated with intact PMN for 15 min stain brightly with fluorescent anti-BPI IgG, indicating that BPI is efficiently transferred to ingested bacteria (19).

How does the presence of multiple cationic granule proteins affect the binding of any one protein to available binding sites on ingested bacteria?

The very different target specificity of different cationic proteins indicates that electrostatic interactions are not sufficient to define the attraction of a bactericidal protein for a particular microorganism. Hence, other physical-chemical properties of both the bactericidal agent and the microbial envelope must determine the ability of a given cationic protein to find attachment sites.

In the case of BPI, the interaction with susceptible gram-negative bacteria is not noticeably affected by the presence of other highly cationic proteins. Neither lysozyme (pI > 10), MPO (pI > 10), nor the other very basic proteins present in crude extracts diminish the BPI binding to *E. coli,* as judged by immunofluorescence and radioimmune assays of the treated bacteria. Further, the bactericidal potency of whole homogenates or sonicates of PMN, crude extracts, or purified BPI corresponds to the amount of BPI present (36,37). It is conceivable that the concentration of positive charge in a particular domain of the protein (rather than overall net charge) and/or the ability of the protein to engage in hydrophobic interactions deter-

mines the effectiveness of competition for sites and bactericidal action. As structural information on molecules such as BPI is gathered, such speculations can be further explored.

FUTURE

Where should future efforts in the further analysis of O_2-independent microbicidal systems be directed?

The isolation, from phagocytes, of specific molecules with cytotoxic properties and a more precise determination, in some instances, of the nature of their effects on the target microorganism (20–22,26,36,63) have lifted the study of O_2-independent microbicidal mechanisms above the level of mere phenomenology. Thus far, however, the exploration of O_2-independent cytocidal substances has been largely limited to the neutrophil and eosinophil. Further progress in the identification of antimicrobial substances is likely to come from mononuclear phagocytes, particularly activated macrophages, where the existence of nonoxidative antimicrobial systems has become increasingly apparent (182–184), although the molecules involved in this cytotoxicity have remained largely unknown.

Beyond the possible isolation of as yet unrecognized cytotoxic proteins, many questions concerning the function and elaboration of the phagocytes' antimicrobial proteins remain unanswered. For example: (a) What is the molecular basis of their cytotoxicity? (b) What are the determinants of their production and assembly into storage granules during differentiation of the phagocyte, and of their transfer from the granule to the target?; (c) Can insight into the structure of these naturally occurring mammalian antimicrobial agents be used to design new classes of antibiotics?

Our knowledge of the relationship between structure and function of the cytotoxins of phagocytes still lags far behind what is known about the molecular and functional properties of cytotoxins from other sources, such as bacterial toxins acting on eukaryotic cells [e.g., diphtheria (158) and cholera (185) toxins] or on other bacteria [the bacteriocins (186,187)]. The structures and some related functions of numerous cytotoxic proteins produced by plants or secreted in the venoms of insects and snakes have also been defined (188,189). Considerable progress has been made recently in the analysis of the structure and apparent mode of action of mammalian cytotoxins that are pore-forming proteins. This progress involves: (a) the membrane-attack complex (MAC) formed in the complement cascade and specifically the properties of the 9th complement component that polymerizes, when properly triggered, into a transmembrane aqueous pore in the target cell (148,149); (b) the lymphocyte granule cytolysins, the so-called *perforins,* that are constituents of the granules of cytotoxic T and killer lymphocytes (149,151).

Although these different cytotoxins may kill by very different mechanisms such as formation of large holes (pores) or more discrete ion-channels in membranes, thereby causing lysis or energy depletion (148,149,186), or by catalytic action on nucleic acids (186) or other intracellular substrates (158,185,188), their interaction with the target cells also exhibits similar principles. Among events that appear to be common to most, if not all, cytotoxins are the homing-in of the molecules onto the target envelope and insertion into, and partial or complete penetration of, the surface membrane, resulting in disturbances of membrane structure and function. These effects are produced by agents as diverse as detergents, by low-M_r cationic peptides such as the antibiotic polymyxin B (51,190), melittin (191) and the defensins (70), and by numerous cytotoxic proteins ranging in M_r from approximately 20,000 to $>10^6$. How can such very different molecules cause apparently similar disturbances of biological and artificial membranes. Beyond the fact that many of the cytotoxins carry net positive charge and are capable of hydrophobic interactions, can any of their effects on the target cell be traced more specifically to shared structural characteristics? The rapidly growing ability to determine the primary structure and, in some cases, the three-dimensional structure of these molecules has led to many attempts to find "domains" in the larger proteins involved in binding, penetration, and channel (pore) formation, as well as other defined effects on the target cell. It is particularly the dissection of the bacterial toxins (such as the bacteriocins and diphtheria toxin) into fragments by limited proteolysis (158,186,192) that has led to the recognition of well-defined domains involved in different actions and interactions of individual cytotoxic proteins (158).

Monospecific polyclonal and monoclonal antibodies are being used to detect common antigenic determinants as markers of relatedness among cytotoxins. Thus, structural homology has been found by these immunological criteria between the pore-formers, MAC and the lymphocytic perforin (149,193), in support of the possibility that different proteins may be capable of similar functions because of shared structures. Note, however, that homology has also been found between C_9 and the low-density lipoprotein receptor (193) so that the common regions may only reflect the structural requirements of proteins whose function is membrane-related. The extrapolation of primary structural information to function is further complicated by the growing evidence that insertion of (cytotoxic) proteins into membranes may be accompanied by profound conformational changes (148–151,194,195) causing the formation of structural domains not evident

from knowledge of the primary structure alone. It is conceivable, therefore, that induced conformational transitions bring about similar functional capabilities, even in proteins that lack extensive primary structural homology.

It follows that in order to establish convincing structure-function relationships in any newly isolated cytotoxin, multiple approaches must be coordinated. These should include, on the molecular level: (a) primary structural analysis; (b) where possible, evaluation of three-dimensional structure [as has already been done for the defensins (72)]; (c) fragmentation of larger molecules by limited proteolysis, which may reveal preferred cleavage sites that separate functionally distinct fragments (158). For further functional studies, the fragments can be tested for biological activity, can be examined in competition experiments, and can be used to generate (neutralizing?) antibodies as another means of localizing regions involved in such functions as binding, envelope alterations, and cytocidal activity (158). Whenever expression of the pertinent DNA in a suitable vector is possible, manipulation of the nucleotide sequence will permit more stringent verification of the structural determinants of functionally essential regions. For smaller polypeptides, like the defensins, similar analyses may be possible by solid-phase synthesis of peptide analogs (196).

It should be emphasized that elucidation of the molecular basis of cytotoxicity also requires a molecular description of the cellular alterations that accompany injury and death. Too often, cytotoxicity against microorganisms or eukaryotic cells has been measured only as loss of colony-forming ability or lysis, respectively. A better definition of the lethal action of the agent may be obtained by timing its effects on multiple cellular functions. Such studies have been carried out extensively with BPI and BPI-like molecules (41,43,48,55,63).

The production of cytotoxins by the various types of phagocytes appears to be a highly regulated process. Thus, because several of the cytotoxins are cell-specific, their biosynthesis must be integrated into the differentiation program of these cytotoxic cells. Further, the biosynthesis of the granules of neutrophils and eosinophils occurs at distinct stages in the maturation of these cells, and formation of primary and secondary granules in the neutrophil is temporally separated (197), implying therefore that the synthesis of the various proteins is precisely coordinated with the assembly of a particular granule population.

With the availability of purified proteins and monospecific antibodies and, soon to be expected, of cDNA probes, these regulatory processes can now be further monitored.

The incorporation of radiolabeled precursors into individual cytotoxins during the course of differentiation into immunoprecipitable products should serve to detect peak biosynthetic activity, as does determination of levels and stability of specific mRNA. For such studies it will be necessary to isolate the various precursor cell populations from the mixed bone marrow cells.

Monoclonal antibodies to surface antigens, transiently present during differentiation, are now becoming available (198,199) and should provide the means to mark and sequester such (sub)populations. Alternatively, one can use stable cell lines derived from immature leukemic cells (such as the human leukemia, promyelocytic HL-60 cells) that can be induced to take on the characteristics of neutrophil-, eosinophil-, or monocyte-like cells (31–34,200). The HL-60 cell has provided a useful model for the study of at least one primary granule protein of the neutrophil, myeloperoxidase (201,202), and several eosinophilic granule proteins, including MBP (200,203). However, because production of other granule proteins, including BPI, ECP, and lactoferrin, by currently available cell lines is either subnormal or absent (31,33,35,40,96), it should be recognized that the fidelity of the differentiation program in such abnormal cell lines may be incomplete. The search for other cell populations should therefore continue.

A particularly profitable approach will be *in-situ* hybridization with cDNA probes generated after cloning of individual cytotoxins, permitting the identification in mixed cell preparations of individual cells actively engaged in expression of specific cytotoxins and of environmental factors that promote growth and differentiation and, hence, modulate expression. Cloning of genes may also help identify regulatory DNA sequences involved in control of granule biogenesis.

The longer-lived mononuclear phagocyte, in contrast to the neutrophil, is capable of vigorous protein biosynthesis during its life-span outside of the bone marrow. Production of any cytotoxin by this cell can therefore be studied during further differentiation (as resident or activated tissue macrophages) or after destruction of target cells to replenish consumed cytotoxic components. For example, *in vitro* conditions known to activate nonoxidative macrophage cytotoxicity (182,184) can be tested for effects on production, accumulation, or perhaps conversion from inactive to active form of either known macrophage-associated cytotoxins [e.g., defensins (73)] or of other cytotoxic proteins not present in mononuclear phagocytes prior to activation [e.g., BPI (40)]. Examination of the defensins may be particularly interesting, since only two (NP1 and 2) of the six rabbit granulocyte species are present in alveolar macrophages (67,69) and these two species are absent in peritoneal macrophages and present at fourfold higher levels in alveolar macrophages from BCG-treated animals (73,74,77), suggesting differential regulation of the various defensin species.

The molecular basis of the passage of the phagocyte's antimicrobial proteins into or out of the structure of the cytoplasmic granules can also be explored by following granule biogenesis *in vitro*. Studies in other cells and tissues (e.g., liver) have shown that the sequential movement of proteins from the site of biosynthesis in the rough endoplasmic reticulum to their final location in lysosomes or in secretory granules is directed by several recognition markers on the protein that may be provided by peptide extensions (signal peptides) to be removed later, by post-translational carbohydrate additions or modifications, or perhaps by the primary or secondary structure of a protein domain that may be unique to proteins that are directed to a particular organelle (27). These insights can now guide studies on phagocytes actively synthesizing granule proteins using pulse-chase labeling of newly synthesized proteins and subcellular fractionation to follow the molecular processing and intracellular sorting that directs these proteins to the various types of storage granules. Recent studies with normal human bone marrow cells and the leukemic HL-60 cells have shown that myeloperoxidase acquires the classical lysosomal recognition marker, high mannose-phosphate, en route to the primary granules (204,205). A comparison of the processing of proteins such as MPO [a primary granule (lysosome-like) constituent] and lactoferrin [a secondary granule (secretory granule-like) protein] may reveal distinct mechanisms of intracellular sorting.

The importance of degranulation in the delivery of the phagocyte's antimicrobial proteins to target cells is well-appreciated (5,6,13–15), but the physical-chemical properties of the granules and their constituents that determine release remain largely obscure. The possible role of interactions, depending on varying affinity between the strongly acidic mucopolysaccharides of the granule matrix and the granule's basic proteins, was suggested more than a decade ago (206). Recently, this concept has been revived as a possible basis for the anchoring and regulation of the activity of the granule cytolysins of cytotoxic lymphocytes and, hence, as a mechanism of self-protection (207,208). If charge interactions are important in protein-proteoglycan associations, then changes in the pH and ion composition in the environment of the granule proteins that accompany degranulation (209), as well as changes in the charge (and hydrophobic?) properties of the target cell envelope, may determine protein release and transfer to the target cell. These hypotheses can be put to the test as more of the participants in such putative interactions become available as reasonably well-defined molecules.

The isolation of native proteins with potent activity raises the obvious question of their usefulness as therapeutic agents. For agents like the defensins and the eosinophil's cytolysins, which manifest broad cytotoxicity, with the potential of damaging the host's own cells (81,136,144), such use may only be possible if delivery systems can be devised that permit specific targeting [e.g., by conjugation to antibodies (158) or by incorporation into liposomes (210)]. In the case of the defensins, their use may be limited also by the fact that the electrolyte composition of the extracellular fluid is inhibitory to their activity (see pertinent earlier section). In contrast, BPI is only toxic for gram-negative bacteria and is therefore worthy of consideration. Unfortunately BPI, although unaffected by physiological ion concentrations, is inactive in serum, probably because of complexing by serum (lipo)proteins (*unpublished observations*). Moreover, the tight association of BPI with the granule structure may mean that this protein is destined for intracellular action and is not suitable for parenteral administration. However, by linking identification of structural determinants of antimicrobial activity of BPI with recombinant DNA technology, it may be possible to construct (smaller) modified molecules that are still bactericidal and retain their target cell specificity but that are no longer inactivated by serum. Hopefully, such modified molecules do not elicit an immune response in the host from which the native BPI was obtained. Because pure rabbit BPI is in hand and closely homologous with human BPI (38), these approaches and their usefulness can be tested in a suitable animal model.

ACKNOWLEDGMENTS

The work in our laboratory reviewed in this chapter was supported by USPHS Grants AM 05472 and AI 18571.

The superb assistance of Ruth Hecht in the preparation of the manuscript is gratefully acknowledged.

REFERENCES

1. Hirsch, J. G. (1956): Phagocytin: A bactericidal substance from polymorphonuclear leukocytes. *J. Exp. Med.,* 103:589.
2. Hirsch, J. G. (1960): Antimicrobial factors in tissues and phagocytic cells. *Bacteriol. Rev.,* 21:133.
3. Robineaux, J., and Frederic, J. (1955): Contribution à l'étude des granulations neutrophiles des polynucléaires par la microcinématographie en contraste de phase. *C. R. Soc. Biol. (Paris),* 149:486.
4. Cohn, Z. A., and Hirsch, J. G. (1960): The isolation and properties of the specific cytoplasmic granules of rabbit polymorphonuclear leukocytes. *J. Exp. Med.,* 112:983.
5. Hirsch, J. G., and Cohn, Z. A. (1960): Degranulation of polymorphonuclear leukocytes following phagocytosis of microorganisms. *J. Exp. Med.,* 112:1005.
6. Cohn, Z. A., and Hirsch, J. G. (1960): The influence of phagocytosis on the intracellular distribution of granule-associated components of polymorphonuclear leukocytes. *J. Exp. Med.,* 112:1015.
7. Hirsch, J. G. (1958): Bactericidal action of histone. *J. Exp. Med.,* 108:925.
8. Zeya, H. I., and Spitznagel, J. K. (1963): Antibacterial and enzymatic basic proteins from leukocyte lysosomes: Separation and identification. *Science,* 142:1085.
9. Zeya, H. I., and Spitznagel, J. K. (1966): Cationic proteins of polymorphonuclear leukocytes. I. Resolution of antibacterial and enzymatic activities. *J. Bacteriol.,* 91:750.
10. Zeya, H. I., and Spitznagel, J. K. (1966): Cationic proteins of polymorphonuclear leukocytes. II. Composition, properties and mechanisms of antibacterial action. *J. Bacteriol.,* 91:755.
11. Zeya, H. I., and Spitznagel, J. K. (1966): Antimicrobial specificity of leukocyte lysosomal cationic proteins. *Science,* 154:1059.
12. Zeya, H. I., and Spitznagel, J. K. (1968): Arginine-rich proteins of polymorphonuclear leukocyte lysosomes. Antimicrobial specificity and biochemical heterogeneity. *J. Exp. Med.,* 127:927.
13. Spitznagel, J. K. (1984): Non-oxidative antimicrobial reactions of leukocytes. In: *Contemporary Topics in Immunobiology, Vol. 14: Regulation of Leukocyte Function,* edited by R. Snyderman, Chapter 10, p. 283. Plenum Press, New York.
14. Klebanoff, S. J. (1975): Antimicrobial mechanisms in neutrophilic polymorphonuclear leukocytes. *Semin. Hematol.,* 12:116.
15. Elsbach, P., and Weiss, J. (1983): A reevaluation of the roles of the O_2-dependent and O_2-independent microbicidal systems of phagocytes. *Rev. Infect. Dis.,* 5:843.
16. Elsbach, P., and Weiss, J. (1985): Oxygen-dependent and oxygen-independent mechanisms of microbicidal activity of neutrophils. *Immunol. Lett.,* 11:159.
17. Mandell, G. L. (1974): Bactericidal activity of aerobic and anaerobic polymorphonuclear neutrophils. *Infect. Immun.,* 9:337.
18. Weiss, J., Victor, M., Stendahl, O., and Elsbach, P. (1982): Killing of gram-negative bacteria by polymorphonuclear leukocytes. Role of an O_2-independent bactericidal system. *J. Clin. Invest.,* 69:959.
19. Weiss, J., Kao, L., Victor, M., and Elsbach, P. (1985): Oxygen-independent intracellular and oxygen-dependent extracellular killing of *Escherichia coli* S15 by human polymorphonuclear leukocytes. *J. Clin. Invest.,* 76:206.
20. Elsbach, P., Pettis, P., Beckerdite, S., and Franson, R. (1973): The effect of phagocytosis by rabbit granulocytes on macromolecular synthesis and degradation in different species of bacteria. *J. Bacteriol.,* 115:490.
21. Beckerdite, S., Mooney, C., Weiss, J., Franson, R., and Elsbach, P. (1974): Early and discrete changes in permeability of E. coli and certain other gram negative bacteria during killing by granulocytes. *J. Exp. Med.,* 140:396.
22. Weiss, J., Franson, R. C., Beckerdite, S., Schmeidler, K., and Elsbach, P. (1975): Partial characterization and purification of a rabbit granulocyte factor that increases permeability of *E. coli. J. Clin. Invest.,* 55:33.
23. Elsbach, P., Beckerdite, S., Pettis, P., and Franson, R. (1974): Persistence of regulation of macromolecular synthesis by Escherichia coli during killing by disrupted granulocytes. *Infect. Immun.,* 9: 663.
24. Elsbach, P. (1973): On the interaction between phagocytes and microorganisms. *N. Engl. J. Med.,* 289:846.
25. Zucker-Franklin, D., Elsbach, P., and Simon, E. J. (1971): The effect of levorphanol, a morphine analog on phagocytizing leukocytes—An electron microscope study. *Lab. Invest.,* 25:415.
26. Elsbach, P. (1977): Cell surface changes in phagocytosis. In: *Cell Surface Reviews, Vol. IV,* edited by G. L. Nicolson and G. Poste, p. 363. North-Holland, Amsterdam.
27. Kornfeld, S. (1986): Trafficking of lysosomal enzymes in normal and disease states. *J. Clin. Invest.,* 77:1.
28. Nathan, C. F., Murray, H. W., and Cohn, Z. A. (1980): The macrophage as an effector cell. *N. Engl. J. Med.,* 303:662.
29. Werb, Z., and Cohn, Z. A. (1972): Plasma membrane synthesis in the macrophage following phagocytosis of polystyrene latex particles. *J. Biol. Chem.,* 247:2439.
30. Cohn, Z. A. (1982): The macrophage—Versatile element of inflammation. *Harvey Lect.,* 77:63.
31. Newburger, P. E., Chovaniec, M. E., Greenberger, J. S., and Cohen, H. J. (1979): Functional changes in human leukemic cell line HL-60. A model for myeloid differentiation. *J. Cell Biol.,* 82:315.
32. Breitman, T. R., Selarick, S. E., and Collins, S. J. (1980): Induction of differentiation in the human promyelocytic leukemic cell line (HL-60) by retinoic acid. *Proc. Natl. Acad. Sci. USA,* 77:2936.
33. Koeffler, H. P., and Golde, D. W. (1980): Human myeloid leukemic cell-lines: A review. *Blood,* 56:344.
34. Rovera, G., Santoli, D., and Damsky, C. (1979): Human granulocytic leukemia cells in culture differentiate into macrophage-like cells when treated with phorbol diester. *Proc. Natl. Acad. Sci. USA,* 76:2779.
35. Olsson, I., and Olofsson, T. (1981): Induction of differentiation in a human promyelocytic leukemic cell line (HL-60). Production of granule proteins. *Exp. Cell Res.,* 131:225.

36. Weiss, J., Elsbach, P., Olsson, I., and Odeberg, H. (1978): Purification and characterization of a potent bactericidal and membrane-active protein from the granules of human polymorphonuclear leukocytes. *J. Biol. Chem.*, 235:2664.

37. Elsbach, P., Weiss, J., Franson, R. C., Beckerdite-Quagliata, S., Schneider, A., and Harris, L. (1979): Separation and purification of a potent bactericidal/permeability increasing protein and a closely associated phospholipase A2 from rabbit polymorphonuclear leukocytes. Observations on their relationship. *J. Biol. Chem.*, 254: 11000.

38. Weiss, J., Ooi, C. E., and Elsbach, P. (1986): Structural and immunological dissection of highly conserved neutrophil bactericidal/permeability-increasing proteins. *Clin. Res.*, 34:537A.

39. Weiss, J., Hutzler, M., and Kao, L. (1986): Environmental modulation of lipopolysaccharide chain length alters the sensitivity of *Escherichia coli* to the neutrophil bactericidal/permeability-increasing protein. *Infect. Immun.*, 51:594.

40. Weiss, J., and Olsson, I. (1987): Cellular and subcellular localization of the bactericidal/permeability-increasing protein of neutrophils. *Blood*, 69:652.

41. Weiss, J., Victor, M., and Elsbach, P. (1983): The role of charge and hydrophobic interactions in the action of the bactericidal/permeability increasing protein of neutrophils on Gram-negative bacteria. *J. Clin. Invest.*, 71:540.

42. Weiss, J., Schmeidler, K., Beckerdite-Quagliata, S., Franson, R. C., and Elsbach, P. (1976): Reversible envelope effects during and after killing of *Escherichia coli* by a highly-purified rabbit polymorphonuclear leukocyte fraction. *Biochim. Biophys. Acta*, 436: 154.

43. Weiss, J., Muello, K., Victor, M., and Elsbach, P. (1984): The role of lipopolysaccharides in the action of the bactericidal/permeability increasing protein on the bacterial envelope. *J. Immunol.*, 132: 3109.

44. Weiss, J., and Elsbach, P. (1977): The use of a phospholipase A-less *Escherichia coli* mutant to establish the action of granulocyte phospholipase A on bacterial phospholipids during killing by a highly purified granulocyte fraction. *Biochim. Biophys. Acta (Biomembranes)*, 466:23.

45. Weiss, J., Beckerdite-Quagliata, S., and Elsbach, P. (1979): Determinants of the action of phospholipases A on the envelope phospholipids of *Escherichia coli*. *J. Biol. Chem.*, 254:11010.

46. Forst, S., Weiss, J., and Elsbach, P. (1982): The role of phospholipase A2 lysines in phospholipolysis of *Escherichia coli* killed by a membrane-active neutrophil protein. *J. Biol. Chem.*, 257:14055.

47. Forst, S., Weiss, J., Blackburn, P., Frangione, B., Goni, F., and Elsbach, P. (1986): Amino acid sequence of a basic *Agkistrodon halys blomhoffii* phospholipase A2. Possible role of NH$_2$-terminal lysines in action on phospholipids of *Escherichia coli*. *Biochemistry*, 25:4309.

48. Elsbach, P., Weiss, J., and Forst, S. (1986): Determinants of the action of phospholipases on the phospholipids of gram-negative bacteria (*E. coli*) In: *Lipids and Biomembranes: Past, Present and Future*, edited by J. A. F. Op den Kamp, B. Roelofsen, and K. W. A. Wirtz, p. 259. Elsevier, Amsterdam.

49. Osborn, M. J. (1983): Biogenesis of the outer membrane of Salmonella. *Harvey Lect.*, 78:87.

50. Lugtenberg, B., and van Alphen, M. (1985): Molecular architecture and functioning of the outer membrane of *Escherichia coli* and other gram-negative bacteria. *Biochim. Biophys. Acta*, 737:51.

51. Nikaido, H., and Vaara, M. (1975): Molecular basis of bacterial outer membrane permeability. *Microbiol Rev.*, 49:1.

52. Bayer, M. E. (1979): The fusion sites between outer membrane and cytoplasmic membrane of bacteria: their role in membrane assembly and virus infection. In: *Bacterial Outer Membranes*, edited by M. Inouye, p. 167. John Wiley & Sons, New York.

53. Ishidate, K., Creeger, E. S., Zrike, J., Deb, S., Glauner, B., MacAlister, T. J., and Rothfield, L. I. (1986): Isolation of differentiated membrane domains from *Escherichia coli* and *Salmonella typhimurium*, including a fraction containing attachment sites between the inner and outer membranes and the murein skeleton of the cell envelope. *J. Biol. Chem.*, 261:428.

54. Leive, L. (1974): The barrier function of the gram-negative envelope. *Ann. NY Acad. Sci.*, 235:109.

55. Weiss, J., Beckerdite-Quagliata, S., and Elsbach, P. (1980): Resistance of gram-negative bacteria to purified bactericidal leukocyte proteins. Relation to binding and bacterial lipopolysaccharide structure. *J. Clin. Invest.*, 65:619.

56. Coughlin, R. T., Tonsager, S., and McGroarty, E. J. (1983): Quantitation of metal cations bound to membranes and extracted lipopolysaccharides of *Escherichia coli*. *Biochemistry*, 22:2002.

57. Schindler, M., and Osborn, M. J. (1979): Interaction of divalent cations and polymyxin B with lipopolysaccharide. *Biochemistry*, 18:4425.

58. Weiss, J., Victor, M., Cross, A. S., and Elsbach, P. (1982): Sensitivity of K1-encapsulated *Escherichia coli* to killing by the bactericidal/permeability-increasing protein of rabbit and human neutrophils. *Infect. Immun.*, 38:1149.

59. Forst, S., Weiss, J., Elsbach, P., Maraganore, J. M., Reardon, I., and Heinrikson, R. L. (1986): Structural and functional properties of a phospholipase A2 purified from an inflammatory exudate. *Biochemistry*, 25:8381.

60. de Geus, P., van Die, I., Bergmans, H., Tommassen, J., and de Haas, G. (1983): Molecular cloning of pld A, the structural gene for outer membrane phospholipase of *E. coli* K12. *Mol. Gen. Genet.*, 190:150.

61. Homma, H., Kobayashi, T., Chiba, N., Karasawa, K., Mizushima, H., Kudo, I., Inoue, K., Ikeda, H., Sekiguchi, M., and Nojima, S. (1984): The DNA sequence encoding pld A gene, the structural gene for detergent-resistant phospholipase A of *E. coli*. *J. Biochem.*, 96:1655.

62. Mooney, C., and Elsbach, P. (1975): Altered phospholipid metabolism in *Escherichia coli* accompanying killing by disrupted granulocytes. *Infect. Immun.*, 11:1269.

63. Hovde, C. J., and Gray, B. H. (1986): Physiological effects of a bactericidal protein from human polymorphonuclear leukocytes on *Pseudomonas aeruginosa*. *Infect. Immun.*, 52:90.

64. Shafer, W. M., Martin, L. E., and Spitznagel, J. K. (1984): Cationic antimicrobial proteins isolated from human neutrophil granulocytes in the presence of diisopropyl fluorophosphate. *Infect. Immun.*, 45: 29.

65. Elsbach, P., Weiss, J., and Kao, L. (1985): The role of intramembrane Ca^{2+} in the hydrolysis of the phospholipids of *Escherichia coli* by Ca^{2+}-dependent phospholipases. *J. Biol. Chem.*, 260:1618.

66. Hall, M. N., and Silhavy, T. J. (1981): Genetic analysis of the major outer membrane proteins of *Escherichia coli*. *Annu. Rev. Genet.*, 15:91.

67. Selsted, M. E., Brown, D. M., DeLange, R. J., and Lehrer, R. I. (1983): Primary structures of MCP-1 and MCP-2, natural peptide antibiotics of rabbit lung macrophages. *J. Biol. Chem.*, 258:14485.

68. Selsted, M. E., Szklarek, D., and Lehrer, R. I. (1984): Purification and antibacterial activity of antimicrobial peptides of rabbit granulocytes. *Infect. Immun.*, 45:150.

69. Selsted, M. E., Brown, D. M., DeLange, R. J., Harwig, S. S. L., and Lehrer, R. I. (1985): Primary structures of six antimicrobial peptides of rabbit peritoneal neutrophils. *J. Biol. Chem.*, 260:4579.

70. Ganz, T., Selsted, M. E., Szklarek, D., Harwig, S. S. L., Daher, K., Bainton, D. F., and Lehrer, R. I. (1985): Natural peptide antibiotics of human neutrophils. *J. Clin. Invest.*, 76:1427.

71. Selsted, M. E., Harwig, S. S. L., Ganz, T., Schilling, J. W., and Lehrer, R. I. (1985): Primary structures of three human neutrophil defensins. *J. Clin. Invest.*, 76:1436.

72. Westbrook, E. M., Lehrer, R. I., and Selsted, M. E. (1984): Characterization of two crystal forms of neutrophil cationic protein NP2, a naturally occurring broad-spectrum antimicrobial agent from leukocytes. *J. Mol. Biol.*, 178:783.

73. Patterson-Delafield, J., Martinez, R. J., and Lehrer, R. I. (1980): Microbicidal cationic proteins in rabbit alveolar macrophages: A potential host defense mechanism. *Infect. Immun.*, 30:180.

74. Lehrer, R. I., Selsted, M. E., Szklarek, D., and Fleischmann, J. (1983): Antibacterial activity of microbicidal cationic proteins 1 and 2, natural peptide antibiotics of rabbit lung macrophages. *Infect. Immun.*, 42:10.

75. Selsted, M. E., Szklarek, D., Ganz, T., and Lehrer, R. I. (1985):

Activity of rabbit leukocyte peptides against *Candida albicans. Infect. Immun.,* 49:202.

76. Segal, G. P., Lehrer, R. I., and Selsted, M. E. (1985): *In vitro* effect of phagocyte cationic peptides on *Coccidioides immitis. J. Infect. Dis.,* 151:890.

77. Paterson-Delafield, J., Szklarek, D., Martinez, R. J., and Lehrer, R. I. (1981): Microbicidal cationic proteins of rabbit alveolar macrophages: Amino acid composition and functional attributes. *Infect. Immun.,* 31:725.

78. Lehrer, R. I., Daher, K., Ganz, T., and Selsted, M. E. (1985): Direct inactivation of viruses by MCP-1 and MCP-2, natural peptide antibiotics from rabbit leukocytes. *J. Virol.,* 54:467.

79. Lehrer, R. I., Szklarek, D., Ganz, T., and Selsted, M. E. (1985): Correlation of binding of rabbit granulocyte peptides to *Candida albicans* with candidacidal activity. *Inf. Immun.,* 49:207.

80. Ganz, T., Cardaci, C., Selsted, M. E., and Lehrer, R. I. (1986): Secretion of antimicrobial defensins by human neutrophils. *Clin. Res.,* 34:458A.

81. Lichtenstein, A., Ganz, T., Selsted, M. E., and Lehrer, R. I. (1986): Cytocidal effects of human defensins, cationic peptides of neutralized primary granules. *Clin. Res.,* 34:462A.

82. Baggiolini, M., Bretz, U., and Dewald, B. (1978): Subcellular localization of granulocyte enzymes. In: *Neutral Proteases of Human Polymorphonuclear Leukocytes,* edited by K. Havemann and A. Janoff, p. 3. Urban & Schwartzenberg, Baltimore.

83. Olsson, I., and Venge, P. (1974): Cationic proteins of human granulocytes. II. Separation of the cationic proteins of the granules of leukemic myeloid cells. *Blood,* 44:235.

84. Feinstein, G., and Janoff, A. (1975): A rapid method for purification of human granulocyte cationic neutral proteases: Purification and characterization of human granulocyte chymotrypsin-like enzyme. *Biochim. Biophys. Acta,* 403:477.

85. Rindler-Ludwig, R., and Braunsteiner, H. (1975): Cationic proteins from human neutrophil granulocytes. Evidence for their chymotrypsin-like properties. *Biochim. Biophys. Acta,* 379:606.

86. Olsson, I., Odeberg, H., Weiss, J., and Elsbach, P. (1980): Bactericidal cationic proteins of human granulocytes. In: *Neutral Proteases of Human Polymorphonuclear Leukocytes,* edited by K. Havemann and A. Janoff, p. 18. Urban & Schwartzenberg, Baltimore.

87. Odeberg, H., Olsson, I., and Venge, P. (1975): Antibacterial cationic proteins of human granulocytes. *J. Clin. Invest.,* 56:1118.

88. Thorne, K. J. I., Oliver, R. C., and Barrett, A. J. (1976): Lysis and killing of bacteria by lysosomal proteinases. *Infect. Immun.,* 14:555.

89. Lehrer, R. I., Ladra, K. M., and Hake, R. B. (1975): Nonoxidative fungicidal mechanisms of mammalian granulocytes: Demonstration of components with candidacidal activity in human, rabbit and guinea pig leukocytes. *Infect. Immun.,* 11:1226.

90. Odeberg, H., and Olsson, I. (1976): Mechanisms for the microbicidal activity of cationic proteins of human granulocytes. *Infect. Immun.,* 14:1269.

91. Shafer, W. M., Onunka, V., and Hitchock, P. J. (1986): A spontaneous mutant of Neisseria gonorrhoeae with decreased resistance to neutrophil granule proteins. *J. Infect. Dis.,* 153:910.

92. Masson, P. L., Heremans, J. F., and Schonne, E. (1969): Lactoferrin, an iron-binding protein in neutrophilic leukocytes. *J. Exp. Med.,* 130:643.

93. Bennett, R. M., and Kokocinsky, T. (1978): Lactoferrin content of peripheral blood cells. *Br. J. Haematol.,* 39:509.

94. Baggiolini, M., de Duve, C., Masson, P. L., and Heremans, J. F. (1970): Association of lactoferrin with specific granules in rabbit heterophil leukocytes. *J. Exp. Med.,* 131:559.

95. Spitznagel, J. K., Dalldorf, F. G., Lefell, M. S., Folds, J. D., Welsh, I. R. H., Cooney, M. H., and Martin, L. E. (1974): Character of azurophil and specific granules purified from human polymorphonuclear leukocytes. *Lab. Invest.,* 30:774.

96. Rado, T. A., Bollekens, J., St. Laurent, G., Parker, L., and Benz, E. J., Jr. (1984): Lactoferrin biosynthesis during granulocytopoiesis. *Blood,* 64:1103.

97. Lomax, K., Rado, T., and Benz, E. J., Jr. (1986): Lactoferrin mRNA accumulation in granulocyte precursors and leukemia cell lines. *Clin. Res.,* 34:660A (abstract).

98. Masson, P. L., and Heremans, J. F. (1968): Metal combining properties of human lactoferrin (red milk protein). 1. The involvement of bicarbonate in the reaction. *Eur. J. Biochem.,* 6:579.

99. Bullen, J. J., Rogers, H. J., and Griffiths, E. (1978): Role of iron in bacterial infection. *Curr. Top. Microbiol. Immunol.,* 35:792.

100. Arnold, R. R., Brewer, M., and Gauthier, J. J. (1980): Bactericidal activity of human lactoferrin: sensitivity of a variety of microorganisms. *Infect. Immun.,* 28:893.

101. Arnold, R. R., Russell, J. E., Champion, W. J., Brewer, M., and Gauthier, J. J. (1982): Bactericidal activity of human lactoferrin. Differentiation from the stasis of iron deprivation. *Infect. Immun.,* 35:792.

102. Bortner, C. A., Miller, R. D., and Arnold, R. R. (1986): Bactericidal effect of lactoferrin on *Legionella pneumophila. Infect. Immun.,* 51:373.

103. Ambruso, D. R., and Johnson, R. B., Jr. (1981): Lactoferrin enhances hydroxyl radical production by human neutrophils, neutrophil particulate fractions, and an enzymatic generating system. *J. Clin. Invest.,* 67:352.

104. Winterbourn, C. C. (1986): Myeloperoxidase as an effective inhibitor of hydroxyl radical production. Implications for the oxidative reactions of neutrophils. *J. Clin. Invest.,* 78:545.

105. Britigan, B. E., Rosen, G. M., Chai, Y., and Cohen, M. S. (1986): Do human neutrophils make hydroxyl radical? Determination of free radicals generated by human neutrophils activated by soluble or particulate stimulus using electron paramagnetic resonance spectrometry. *J. Biol. Chem.,* 261:4426.

106. Britigan, B. E., Rosen, G. M., Thompson, B. Y., Chai, Y., and Cohen, M. S. (1986): Stimulated human neutrophils limit iron-catalyzed hydroxyl radical formation as detected by spin trapping techniques. *J. Biol. Chem. (in press).*

107. Spitznagel, J. K., Cooper, M. R., McCall, A. E., De Chatelet, L. R., and Welsh, I. R. H. (1972): Selective deficiency of granules associated with lysozyme and lactoferrin in human polymorphs with reduced microbicidal activity. *J. Clin. Invest.,* 51:93a.

108. Strauss, R. G., Bove, K. E., Jones, J. F., Mauer, A. M., and Fulginiti, V. A. (1974): An anomaly of neutrophil morphology with impaired function. *N. Engl. J. Med.,* 290:478.

109. Breton-Gorius, J., Mason, D. Y., Buriot, D., Vilde, J. L., and Griscelli, C. (1980): Lactoferrin deficiency as a consequence of a lack of specific granules in neutrophils from a patient with recurrent infections. *Am. J. Pathol.,* 99:413.

110. Wang-Iverson, P., Pryzwansky, K. B., Spitznagel, J. K., and Cooney, M. H. (1978): Bactericidal capacity of phorbol myristate acetate-treated human polymorphonuclear leukocytes. *Infect. Immun.,* 22:945.

111. Oseas, R., Yang, H-H., Baehner, R. L., and Boxer, L. A. (1981): Lactoferrin: A promoter of polymorphonuclear leukocyte adhesiveness. *Blood,* 57:939.

112. Boxer, L. A., Hack, R. A., Yang, H-H., Wallace, J. B., Whitcomb, J. A., Butterick, C. J., and Baehner, R. L. (1982): Membrane-bound lactoferrin alters the surface properties of polymorphonuclear leukocytes. *J. Clin. Invest.,* 79:1049.

113. Boxer, L. A., Coates, T. D., Haak, R. A., Wolach, J. B., Hoffstein, S., and Baehner, R. L. (1982): Lactoferrin deficiency associated with altered granulocyte function. *N. Engl. J. Med.,* 307:404.

114. Gallin, J. I., Fletcher, M. P., Seligman, B. E., Hoffstein, S., Cehrs, K., and Mounessa, N. (1982): Human neutrophil-specific granule deficiency: A model to assess the role of neutrophil-specific granules in the evolution of the inflammatory response. *Blood,* 59:1317.

115. Broxmeyer, H. E., De Sousa, M., Smithyman, A., Ralph, P., Kurland, J. L., and Bogmacki, J. (1980): Specificity and modulation of lactoferrin, a negative feedback regulator of myelopoiesis. *Blood,* 55:324.

116. Bagley, G. C., Jr., McCall, E., and Layman, D. L. (1983): Regulation of colony stimulating activity production. *J. Clin. Invest.,* 71:340.

117. Gentile, P., and Broxmeyer, H. E. (1983): Suppression of mouse myelopoiesis by administration of human lactoferrin *in vivo* and the comparative action of human lactoferrin. *Blood,* 61:982.

118. Stryer, L. (1981): *Biochemistry,* 2nd edition, p. 135. W. H. Freeman, San Francisco.
119. Johnson, K. G., and Campbell, J. N. (1972): Effect of growth conditions on peptidoglycan structure and susceptibility to lytic enzymes in cell walls of *Micrococcus sodonensis. Biochemistry,* 11: 277.
120. Padgett, G. A., and Hirsch, J. G. (1967): Lysozyme: Its absence in tears and leukocytes of cattle. *Aust. J. Exp. Biol. Med. Sci.,* 45: 569.
121. Gordon, S., Todd, J., and Cohn, Z. A. (1974): *In vitro* synthesis and secretion of lysozyme by mononuclear phagocytes. *J. Exp. Med.,* 139:1228.
122. Gleich, G. J., Loegering, D. A., and Maldonado, J. E. (1973): Identification of a major basic protein in guinea pig eosinophil granules. *J. Exp. Med.,* 137:1459.
123. Gleich, G. J., Loegering, D. A., Mann, K. G., and Maldonado, J. E. (1976): Comparative properties of the Charcot-Leyden crystal protein and the major basic protein from human eosinophils. *J. Clin. Invest.,* 57:633.
124. Lewis, D. M., Loegering, D. A., and Gleich, G. J. (1976): Isolation and partial characterization of a major basic protein from rat eosinophil granules. *Proc. Soc. Exp. Biol. Med.,* 152:512.
125. Lewis, D. M., Lewis, J. C., Loegering, D. A., and Gleich, G. J. (1978): Localization of the guinea pig eosinophil major basic protein to the core of the granules. *J. Cell Biol.,* 77:702.
126. Ackerman, S. J., Loegering, D. A., Venge, P., Olsson, I., Harley, J. B., Fauci, A. S., and Gleich, G. J. (1983): Distinctive cationic proteins of the human eosinophil granule: Major basic protein, eosinophil cationic protein and eosinophil-derived neurotoxin. *J. Immunol.,* 131:297.
127. Ackerman, S. J., Kephart, G. M., Haberman, T. M., Gripp, P. R., and Gleich, G. J. (1983): Localization of eosinophil major basic protein in human basophils. *J. Exp. Med.,* 158:946.
128. Maddox, D. E., Kephart, G. M., Coulam, C. B., Butterfield, J. H., Benitschke, K., and Gleich, G. J. (1984): Localization of a molecule immunochemically similar to eosinophil major basic protein in human placenta. *J. Exp. Med.,* 160:29.
129. Gleich, G. J., Loegering, D. A., Kueppers, F., Bajaj, S. P., and Mann, K. D. (1974): Physicochemical and biological properties of the major basic protein from guinea pig eosinophil granules. *J. Exp. Med.,* 140:313.
130. Gleich, G. J., and Loegering, D. A. (1984): Immunobiology of eosinophils. *Annu. Rev. Immunol.,* 2:429.
131. Ackerman, S. J., Gleich, G. J., Loegering, D. A., Richardson, B. A., and Butterworth, A. E. (1985): Comparative toxicity of purified human eosinophil granule cationic proteins for schistosomula of *Schistosoma mansoni. Am. J. Trop. Med. Hyg.,* 34:735.
132. Butterworth, A. E., Wassom, D. L., Gleich, G. J., Loegering, D. A., and David, J. R. (1979): Damage of schistosomula of *Schistosoma mansoni* induced directly by eosinophil major basic protein. *J. Immunol.,* 122:221.
133. Wassom, D. L., and Gleich, G. J. (1979): Damage of *Trichinella spiralis* newborn larvae by eosinophil major basic protein. *Am. J. Trop. Med. Hyg.,* 28:860.
134. Kierszenbaum, F., Ackerman, S. J., and Gleich, G. J. (1981): Destruction of bloodstream forms of *Trypanosomal cruzi* by eosinophil granule major basic protein. *Am. J. Trop. Med. Hyg.,* 30:775.
135. Villalta, F., and Kierszenbaum, F. (1984): Role of inflammatory cells in Chagas' disease. I. Uptake and mechanisms of destruction of intracellular (amastigote) forms of *Trypanosoma cruzi* by human eosinophils. *J. Immunol.,* 312:1053.
136. Gleich, G. J., Frigas, E., Loegering, D. A., Wassom, D. L., and Steinmuller, D. (1979): Cytotoxic properties of the eosinophil major basic protein. *J. Immunol.,* 123:2925.
137. Wassom, D. L., Loegering, D. A., Solley, G. O., Moore, S. B., Schooley, R. T., Fanci, A. S., and Gleich, G. J. (1981): Elevated serum levels of the eosinophil granule major basic protein in patients with eosinophilia. *J. Clin. Invest.,* 67:651.
138. Filley, W. V., Holley, K. E., Kephart, G. J., and Gleich, G. J. (1981): Identification by immunofluorescence of eosinophil granule major basic protein in lung tissues of patients with bronchial asthma. *Lancet,* 2:11.
139. Olsson, I., Venge, P., Spitznagel, J. K., and Lehrer, R. I. (1977): Arginine-rich cationic proteins of human eosinophil granules. Comparison of the constituents of eosinophilic and neutrophilic leukocytes. *Lab. Invest.,* 36:493.
140. Peters, M. S., Rodriguez, M., and Gleich, G. J. (1986): Localization of human eosinophil granule major basic protein, eosinophil cationic protein, and eosinophil-derived neurotoxin by immunoelectron microscopy. *Lab. Invest.,* 54:656.
141. Olsson, I., Persson, A.-M., and Winquist, I. (1986): Biochemical properties of the eosinophil cationic protein and demonstration of its biosynthesis *in vitro* in marrow cells from patients with an eosinophilia. *Blood,* 67:498.
142. Gleich, G. J., Loegering, D. A., Bell, M. P., Checkel, J. L., Ackerman, S. J., and McKean, D. J. (1986): Biochemical and functional similarities between human eosinophil-derived neurotoxin and eosinophil cationic protein: Homology and ribonuclease. *Proc. Natl. Acad. Sci. USA,* 83:3146.
143. McLaren, D. J., McKean, J. R., Olsson, I., Venge, P., and Kay, A. B. (1981): Morphological studies on the killing of schistosomula of *Schistosoma mansoni* by human eosinophil and neutrophil cationic proteins *in vitro. Parasite Immunol.,* 3:359.
144. Tai, P. C., Hayes, D. J., Clark, J. B., and Spry, C. J. F. (1982): Toxic effects of eosinophil secretion products on isolated rat heart cells *in vitro. Biochem. J.,* 204:75.
145. Durack, D. T., Ackerman, S. J., Loegering, D. A., and Gleich, G. J. (1981): Purification of human eosinophil-derived neurotoxin. *Proc. Natl. Acad. Sci. USA,* 78:5165.
146. Tai, P. C., Spry, C. J. F., Peterson, C., Venge, P., and Olsson, I. (1984): Monoclonal antibodies distinguish between storage and secreted forms of eosinophil cationic protein. *Nature,* 309:182.
147. Young, J. D.-E., Peterson, C. G. B., Venge, P., and Cohn, Z. A. (1986): Mechanism of membrane damage mediated by human eosinophil cationic protein. *Nature,* 321:613.
148. Müller-Eberhard, H. J. (1986): The membrane attack complex of complement. *Annu. Rev. Immunol.,* 4:503.
149. Young, J. D.-E., Cohn, Z. A., and Podack, E. R. (1986): The ninth component of complement and the pore-forming protein (perforin 1) from cytotoxic T cells: Structural, immunological, and functional similarities. *Science,* 233:184.
150. Zhao, J.-M., and London, E. (1986): Similarity of the conformation of diphtheria toxin at high temperature to that in the membrane-penetrating low-pH state. *Proc. Natl. Acad. Sci. USA,* 83:2002.
151. Masson, D., and Tschopp, J. (1985): Isolation of a lytic, pore-forming protein (perforin) from cytolytic T lymphocytes. *J. Biol. Chem.,* 260:9069.
152. Young, J. D.-E., Young, T. M., Lu, L. P., Unkeless, J. C., and Cohn, Z. A. (1982): Characterization of a membrane pore-forming protein from *Entamoeba histolytica. J. Exp. Med.,* 156:1677.
153. Kagan, B. L. (1983): Mode of action of yeast killer toxins: Channel formation in lipid bilayer membranes. *Nature,* 320:709.
154. Fussle, R., Bhakdi, S., Sziegoleit, A., Tranum-Jensen, J., Kranz, T., and Wellensink, J. (1981): On the mechanism of membrane damage by *S. aureus* alpha toxin. *J. Cell Biol.,* 81:83.
155. Lachmann, P. J. (1986): A common form of killing. *Nature,* 321: 560.
156. Bashford, C. L., Alder, G. M., Menestrina, G., Micklem, K. J., Murphy, J. J., and Pasternak, C. A. (1986): Membrane damage by hemolytic viruses, toxins, complement, and other cytotoxic agents. A common mechanism blocked by divalent cations. *J. Biol. Chem.,* 261:9300.
157. Wiedner, T., and Sims, P. J. (1985): Effect of complement proteins C58-9 on blood platelets. Evidence for reversible depolarization of membrane potential. *J. Biol. Chem.,* 260:8014.
158. Collier, R. J., and Kaplan, D. A. (1984): Immunotoxins. *Sci. Am.,* 254:56.
159. Elsbach, P. (1980): Degradation of microorganisms by phagocytic cells. *Rev. Infect. Dis.,* 2:106.
160. Ginsburg, I., and Sela, M. N. (1976): The role of leukocytes and

their hydrolases in the persistence of degradation and transport of bacterial constituents in tissues: Relation to chronic inflammatory processes in staphylococcal, streptococcal and mycobacterial infections and in chronic periodontal disease. *Crit. Rev. Microbiol.,* 4:249.

161. Odeberg, H., and Olsson, I. (1976): Microbicidal mechanisms of human granulocytes: Synergistic effects of granulocyte elastase and myeloperoxidase or chymotrypsin-like cationic protein. *Infect. Immun.,* 14:1276.

162. Rest, R. F., and Pretzer, E. (1981): Degradation of gonococcal outer membrane proteins by human neutrophil lysosomal proteases. *Infect. Immun.,* 34:62.

163. Ohlsson, K. (1978): Interaction of granulocyte neutral proteases with alpha$_1$-antitrypsin, alpha$_2$-macroglobulin and alpha$_1$-antichymotrypsin. In: *Neutral Proteases of Human Polymorphonuclear Leukocytes,* edited by K. Havemann and A. Janoff, p. 167. Urban & Schwartzenberg, Baltimore.

164. Johnson, D., and Travis, J. (1979): The oxidative inactivation of human alpha$_1$-proteinase inhibitor. *J. Biol. Chem.,* 254:4022.

165. Matheson, N. R., Wong, P. S., and Travis, J. (1979): Enzymatic inactivation of alpha-1-proteinase inhibitor by neutrophil myeloperoxidase. *Biochem. Biophys. Res. Commun.,* 88:402.

166. Carp, H., and Janoff, A. (1979): *In vitro* suppression of serum elastase-inhibiting capacity by reactive oxygen species generated by phagocytosing polymorphonuclear leukocytes. *J. Clin. Invest.,* 63:793.

167. Weiss, S. J., Peppin, G., Ortiz, X., Ragsdale, C., and Tost, S. T. (1985): Oxidative autoactivation of latent collagenase by human neutrophils. *Science,* 227:747.

168. Tschesche, H., and Macartney, H. W. (1981): A new principle of regulation of enzymatic activity. Activation and regulation of human polymorphonuclear leucocyte collagenase via disulfide-thiol exchange as catalyzed by the glutathione cycle in a peroxidase-coupled reaction to glucose metabolism. *Eur. J. Biochem.,* 120:183.

169. Peppin, G. J., and Weiss, S. J. (1986): Activation of the endogenous metalloproteinase, gelatinase, by triggered human neutrophils. *Proc. Natl. Acad. Sci. USA,* 83:4322.

170. Elsbach, P., and Weiss, J. (1980): Lipid metabolism by phagocytic cells. In: *The Reticoloendothelial System: A Comprehensive Treatise. Vol. II. Biochemistry of the RES,* edited by R. Strauss and A. Sbarra, (M. Escobar, H. Friedman, and S. Reichard, series editors), p. 91. Plenum Press, New York.

171. Patriarca, P., Beckerdite, S., Pettis, P., and Elsbach, P. (1972): Phospholipid metabolism by phagocytic cells. VII. The degradation and utilization of phospholipids of various microbial species by rabbit granulocytes. *Biochim. Biophys. Acta,* 280:45.

172. Duckworth, D. H., Bevers, E. K., Verkleij, A. J., Op den Kamp, J. A. F., and van Deenen, L. L. M. (1974): Action of phospholipase A2 and phospholipase C on *Escherichia coli. Arch. Biochem. Biophys.,* 165:379.

173. Wurster, N., Elsbach, P., Rand, J., and Simon, E. J. (1971): Effects of levorphanol on phospholipid metabolism and composition in *E. coli. Biochim. Biophys. Acta,* 248:282.

174. Patriarca, P., Beckerdite, S., and Elsbach, P. (1972): Phospholipases and phospholipid turnover in *Escherichia coli* spheroplasts. *Biochim. Biophys. Acta,* 260:593.

175. Vos, M., Op den Kamp, J., Beckerdite-Quagliata, S., and Elsbach, P. (1978): Acylation of monoacylglycerophosphoethanolamine in the inner and outer membranes of the envelope of an *Escherichia coli* K12 strain and its phospholipase-A deficient mutant. *Biochim. Biophys. Acta (Biomembranes),* 508:165.

176. Beckerdite-Quagliata, S., Simberkoff, M., and Elsbach, P. (1975): Effects of human and rabbit serum on viability, permeability, and envelope lipids of *Serratia marcescens. Inf. Immun.,* 11:758.

177. Raetz, C. R. H. (1978): Enzymology, genetics, and regulation of membrane phospholipid synthesis in *Escherichia coli. Microbiol. Rev.,* 42:614.

178. Hirschhorn, R. (1974): Lysosomal mechanisms in the inflammatory process. In: *The Inflammatory Process,* edited by B. W. Zweifach,

L. Grant, and R. T. McCluskey, p. 259. Academic Press, New York.

179. Rozenberg-Arska, M., van Strijp, J. A. G., Hoekstra, W. P. M., and Verhoef, J. (1984): Effect of human polymorphonuclear and mononuclear leukocytes on chromosomal and plasmid DNA of *Escherichia coli.* Role of acid DNase. *J. Clin. Invest.,* 73:1254.

180. Hamers, M. C., De Groot, E. R., and Roos, D. (1981): Phagocytosis and degradation of DNA-anti-DNA complexes by human phagocytes. I. Assay conditions, quantitative aspects and differences between human blood monocytes and neutrophils. *Eur. J. Immunol.,* 11:757.

181. Okamura, N., and Spitznagel, J. (1982): Outer membrane mutants of *Salmonella typhimurium* LT2 have lipopolysaccharide-dependent resistance to the bactericidal activity of anaerobic human neutrophils. *Infect. Immun.,* 36:1086.

182. Murray, H. W., Byrne, G. I., Rothermel, C. D., and Cartelli, D. M. (1983): Lymphokine enhances oxygen-independent activity against intracellular pathogens. *J. Exp. Med.,* 158:234.

183. Scott, P., James, S., and Sher, A. (1985): The respiratory burst is not required for killing of intracellular and extracellular parasites by a lymphokine-activated macrophage cell line. *Eur. J. Immunol.,* 15:553.

184. Catterall, J. R., Sharma, S. D., and Remington, J. S. (1986): Oxygen-independent killing by alveolar macrophages. *J. Exp. Med.,* 163:1113.

185. Ludwig, D. S., Holmes, R. K., and Schoolnik, G. K. (1985): Chemical and immunochemical studies on the receptor binding domain of cholera toxin B subunit. *J. Biol. Chem.,* 260:12528.

186. Konisky, J. (1982): Colicin and other bacteriocins with established modes of action. *Annu. Rev. Microbiol.,* 36:125.

187. Jakes, K. S. (1982): In: *Molecular Action of Toxins and Viruses,* edited by P. Cohen and S. van Heyningen, p. 131. Elsevier, Amsterdam.

188. Ready, M., Wilson, K., Piatak, M., and Robertus, J. D. (1984): Ricin-like plant toxins are evolutionarily related to single-chain ribosome-inhibiting proteins from phytolacca. *J. Biol. Chem.,* 259:15252.

189. Gariepy, J., O'Hanley, P., Waldman, S. A., Murad, F., and Schoolnik, G. K. (1984): A common antigenic determinant found in two functionally unrelated toxins. *J. Exp. Med.,* 160:1253.

190. Storm, D. R., Rosenthal, K. S., and Swanson, P. E. (1977): Polymixin and related peptide antibiotics. *Annu. Rev. Biochem.,* 46:723.

191. Esser, A. F. (1986): In: *Membrane-Mediated Cytotoxicity,* UCLA Symposia New Series 56 (*in press*).

192. Mekalanos, J. J., Collier, R. J., and Romig, W. R. (1979): Enzyme activity of cholera toxin. II. Relationships to proteolytic processing, disulfide bond reduction, and subunit composition. *J. Biol. Chem.,* 254:5855.

193. Tschopp, J., Masson, D., and Stanley, K. K. (1986): Structural/functional similarity between proteins involved in complement- and cytotoxic T-lymphocyte-mediated cytolysis. *Nature,* 322:831.

194. Escuyer, V., Boquet, P., Perrin, D., Montecucco, C., and Mock, M. (1986): A pH-induced increase in hydrophobicity as a possible step in the penetration of colicin E3 through bacterial membranes. *J. Biol. Chem.,* 261:10891.

195. Briggs, M. S., Cornell, D. G., Dluhy, R. A., and Gierasch, L. M. (1986): Conformations of signal peptides induced by lipids suggest initial steps in protein export. *Science,* 233:206.

196. Heath, W. F., and Merrifield, R. B. (1986): A synthetic approach to structure-function relationships in the murine epidermal growth factor molecule. *Proc. Natl. Acad. Sci. USA,* 83:6367.

197. Bainton, D. F., and Farquhar, K. (1966): Origin of the granules in polymorphonuclear leukocytes: Two types derived from opposite faces of the Golgi complex in developing granulocytes. *J. Cell Biol.,* 28:277.

198. Foon, K. A., and Todd, R. F., III (1986): Immunologic classification of leukemia and lymphoma. *Blood,* 68:1.

199. Todd, M. B., and Malech, H. L. (1986): Identification of a differ-

entiation-specific cell surface antigen on HL60 cells that is associated with proliferation. *Cancer Res.,* 46:113.

200. Fischkoff, S. A., Pollak, A., Gleich, G. J., Testa, J. R., Misawa, S., and Reber, T. J. (1984): Eosinophilic differentiation of the human promyelocytic cell line, HL60. *J. Exp. Med.,* 160:179.

201. Yamada, M., Kurahashi, K. (1984): Regulation of myeloperoxidase gene expression during differentiation of human myeloid leukemia HL-60 cells. *J. Biol. Chem.,* 259:3021.

202. Koeffler, H. P., Ranyard, J., Pertchek, K. (1985): Myeloperoxidase: Its structure and expression during myeloid differentiation. *Blood,* 65:494.

203. Fischkoff, S. A., Brown, G. E., and Pollak, A. (1986): Synthesis of eosinophil-associated enzymes in HL-60 promyelocytic leukemia cells. *Blood,* 68:185.

204. Olsson, I., Persson, A. M., Stroemberg, K. (1984): Biosynthesis, transport and processing of myeloperoxidase in the human leukemic promyelocytic cell line HL-60 and normal marrow cells. *Biochem. J.,* 223:911.

205. Nauseef, W. M. (1986): Glycosylation of human myeloperoxidase during biosynthesis. *Clin. Res.,* 34:527A.

206. Avila, J. L., and Convit, J. (1976): Physicochemical characteristics of the glycosaminoglycan-lysosomal enzyme interactions *in vitro. Biochem. J.,* 160:129.

207. Tschopp, J., and Conzelmann, A. (1986): Proteoglycans in secretory granules of NK cells. *Immunol. Today,* 7:135.

208. MacDermott, R. P., Schmidt, R. E., Canfield, J. P., Hein, A., Bartley, G. T., Ritz, J., Schlossman, S. F., Austen, K. F., and Stevens, R. L. (1985): Proteoglycans in cell-mediated cytotoxicity. Identification, localization and exocytosis of a chondroitin sulfate proteoglycan from human coned natural killer cells during target cell lysis. *J. Exp. Med.,* 162:1771.

209. Segal, A. W. (1981): The respiratory burst of phagocytic cells is associated with a rise in vacuolar pH. *Nature,* 290:407.

210. Smirnov, V. N., Domagatsky, S. P., Dolgov, V. V., Hvatov, V. B., Klibanov, A. L., Koteliansky, V. E., Muzykantov, V. R., Repin, V. S., Samokhin, G. P., Shekhonin, B. V., Smirnov, M. D., Sviridov, D. D., Torchilin, V. P., and Chazov, E. I. (1986): Carrier-directed targeting of liposomes and erythrocytes to denuded areas of vessel wall. *Proc. Natl. Acad. Sci. USA,* 83:6603.

Inflammation: Basic Principles and Clinical Correlates.
Edited by J. I. Gallin, I. M. Goldstein, and R. Snyderman.
Raven Press, Ltd., New York © 1988.

CHAPTER 25

Phagocytic Cells: Cytotoxic Activities of Macrophages

Dolph O. Adams and T. A. Hamilton

Mononuclear phagocytes effect and regulate many aspects of acute and chronic inflammation (1–11). Since their discovery over a century ago by Elia Metchnikoff (12), macrophages have become well established as a major protective element in host defenses against microbes and, over the past $2\frac{1}{2}$ decades, against neoplastic cells as well. Integral to macrophage protection against replicating cells of either microbial or neoplastic origin is the basic physiology and biochemistry of these cells, which permits them to change functional potential in response to stimuli in their environment and thus gain the ability to effect such destruction (1). The molecular mechanisms, which regulate the potent injurious forces of macrophages, are particularly worth considering, because the host must balance delicately the protective role of macrophages against their potential to cause injury and destruction of host tissues (1,2).

Macrophages play several other major parts in the inflammatory response (see Fig. 1) (1,2). First, macrophages and their secretory products make essential contributions to controlling acute inflammation, by their secretion and regulation of elements of the complement cascade, by their secretion of cytokines such as interleukin-1, and by their

secretion of metabolites of arachidonic acid. Second, macrophages govern any ongoing inflammatory response by regulating both T- and B-lymphocytes, growth and replication of other cells such as fibroblasts, hemostasis, fibrinolysis, and by secretion of both proteases and antiproteases. Finally, macrophages serve as scavengers that not only remove cellular and molecular debris but also detoxify and/or sequester toxic materials.

This chapter reviews the general biology of macrophages, macrophages as protective cells, the regulation of macrophage functions, and the destructive effects of macrophages *in vivo*. The data, unless otherwise stated, were obtained in experiments employing macrophages from small rodents, such as mice. It is worth emphasizing, however, that the majority of these conclusions do pertain to human mononuclear phagocytes as well.

GENERAL BIOLOGY OF MACROPHAGES

Life History

Macrophages represent one element of a host-wide collection of cells, which comprise the *mononuclear phago-*

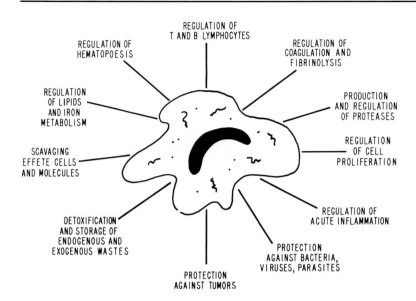

FIG. 1. General functions of the macrophage in the host. Depicted are multiple functions of macrophages. These include, beginning at the 12 o'clock position: homeostatic regulation of cellular and molecular host systems; protection against rapidly replicating cells; and detoxification/scavenging.

cyte system (MPS) (7,11) (see chapter by van Furth for details). Central to any understanding of mononuclear phagocytes is the fact that these are not end cells—in either sense of that term. Macrophages in the tissues, after having left the bone marrow, are capable of both further replication and further maturation. Both of these potentials are essential to ability of the MPS to protect the host against replicating invaders. The development or the appearance of new mononuclear phagocytes in sites of inflammation represents a combination of immigration of young monocytes into such sites and local proliferation (13).

The general development of mononuclear phagocytes begins in the marrow (see Fig. 2) with the development of colony-forming-unit granulocytes and monocytes (CFU-GM) into monoblasts, promonocytes, and ultimately into monocytes (11). In the steady state, monocytes immigrate into the tissues at a reasonably constant rate and form the various pools of local tissue macrophages. The functional potential of such local tissue phagocytes has been down-regulated, by comparison with monocytes, in terms of many physiologic properties (1). In sites of acute inflammation, relatively large numbers of monocytes enter the tissues and accumulate. When these young monocytes confront a variety of acute inflammatory mediators, they mature and develop into large macrophages that have potent secretory and endocytic capacities (1). These so-called *inflammatory macrophages,* when driven by products from specifically sensitized T-lymphocytes or from replicating invaders such as microorganisms, undergo further development and gain powerful destructive properties. This process has been termed *activation* (1,14,15).

The concept of macrophage activation dates back to Elia Metchnikoff, who noted in 1905 that macrophages

could perfect their powers of chemotaxis and microbicidal destruction (12). Since that time, the precise definition of *macrophage activation* has been a subject of controversy (1,2,14,15). Macrophages can be activated to destroy not only microbes but tumor cells as well. Some workers restrict the definition of activation to enhanced ability to kill microbes and tumor cells or even to kill microbes alone. Macrophages recently immigrated into sites of inflammation have a large and diverse potential for further development (Fig. 3). Mononuclear phagocytes, acting under the regulatory influence of a variety of stimuli, can develop in many potential directions, some of which are mutually exclusive (1). Most of these developmental paths lead to an enhanced ability to carry out a complex function, such as destruction of tumor cells or orchestration of the acute inflammatory response (1,16). Alternatively then, *macrophage activation* represents development of enhanced potential for completion of any complex function; activation for the destruction of tumor cells, for example, would represent just one example of activation. In support of this general concept, macrophages can be activated for four distinct modes of tumor cell destruction, each requiring a different form of cellular development (see below). Whether one uses a narrow or a broad definition of activation, the key concept is that mononuclear phagocytes are multipotential cells, whose subsequent development can be both induced and suppressed by a complex network of regulatory molecules (1).

The developmental potential of macrophages is currently believed to be both large and diverse (1) (see Fig. 3). Appropriately *responsive macrophages* are multipotential cells, which can develop in a variety of ways depending on the signals they receive. In a hypothetical model of development (Fig. 3), such responsive macrophages can be activated for a certain function (e.g., func-

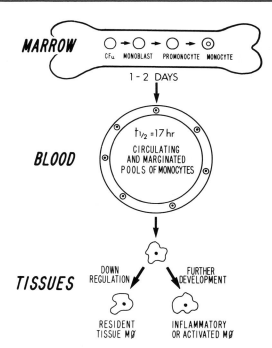

FIG. 2. The life history of mononuclear phagocytes. Mononuclear phagocytes arise in the marrow from colony-forming units (CFU) and mature into monocytes. Monocytes then leave the marrow and circulate in the blood for brief periods of time, after which they enter the tissues to become macrophages. In general, the recently immigrated cells are down-regulated in the unperturbed host to become resident tissue macrophages. They can, however, undergo further development and maturation/modulation in sites of inflammatory stimulation. The resident and inflammatory macrophages are maintained by both local division and immigration from the blood. (Mφ) Macrophage.

tion W) by receiving one of two signals (e.g., signal 8 or signal 9), while only another signal (e.g., signal 10) induces activation for a distinct function (e.g., function Q). Two signals (S6 *plus* S7) may be required for inducing activation for other functions (e.g., function Z). By contrast, activation for some functions (e.g., X and Y) is complex and may require two signals in sequence (S1/S2 or S3/S4) but can be achieved by one signal alone (S5). Many of these developmental paths can be blocked by various suppressive signals (e.g., the effects of inhibitor IN_a on activation for function Q). In sum, the developmental potential of mononuclear phagocytes is large. When these cells commit to one line of development they frequently lose the potential to develop in other ways—at least temporarily.

Morphology and Physiology

The fine morphology of mononuclear phagocytes, which are medium-to-large irregularly shaped cells with one single-lobed nucleus, is elegantly revealed when these cells are allowed to spread in culture (see Figs. 4–6) (3,17). The abundant cytoplasm, which surrounds a central or slightly eccentric reniform nucleus, contains large numbers of rod-like mitochondria, phase-lucent pinosomes, and phase-dense lysosomes (Fig. 4). The cytoplasm, particularly at the periphery, is marked by numerous flanges, ruffles, and pseudopodia (Fig. 5), which undulate slowly in a wave-like action toward the nucleus. Ultrastructurally, the cytoplasm contains a well-developed Golgi zone in the "hof" of the nucleus (i.e., the space formed by the U-shaped nucleus) as well as containing a complex and well-organized cytoskeleton of both actin filaments and microtubules. Of note, complexity of the cytoplasm and of its organelles increases markedly with the maturation and activation of these cells.

The macrophage, even when in an apparent resting state, is extremely active metabolically (1,2). At the surface, macrophages form pinosomes rapidly, such that macrophages are estimated to turn over the equivalent of their entire plasma membrane every 30 min (18). The pinosomes flow through the cytoplasm in a well-regulated characteristic pattern toward the Golgi apparatus, where many are filled with acid hydrolases to become primary lysosomes. As in other endocytic cells, there are multiple, complex recycling pathways for endocytosed proteins, which may be degraded within the lysosome, passed into

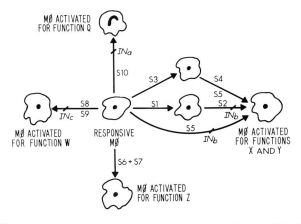

FIG. 3. A general model of macrophage development in the tissues. Macrophages can be activated in a variety of ways, which include enhanced competence for complex functions *Q, W, X, Y,* and *Z*. Competence for functions *X* and *Y* are acquired jointly but independently of functions *Z, Q,* or *W*. Such development begins when newly immigrated or responsive macrophages are subjected to one or more stimulatory signals (S1-S11). In some cases, only one signal is required (application of S10 to induce function *Q*); in other cases, however, multiple signals are required (application of S6 and S7 to activate the macrophages for function *Z*). There may be multiple routes of activation for a given function (activation for functions *X* and *Y*). Many of these paths are specifically blocked by inhibitors (In_a, In_b, or In_c). The sum of these inductive and suppressive interactions can result in multiple and mutually exclusive paths of activation.

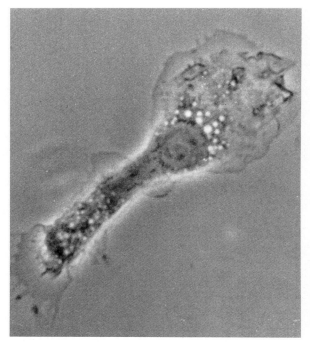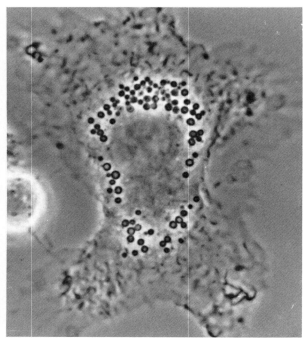

a,b

FIG. 4. Phase micrographs of macrophages. **(a)** In this low-powered micrograph, the body of the macrophage is seen (*upper right*), and a trailing pseudopod is also seen (*lower left*). The macrophage has moved most of its body ahead of the nucleus (*upper right*), and the cytoplasm there has numerous ruffles and flanges. ×595. **(b)** In this high-powered figure, the phase dark nucleus is surrounded by phase-lucent pinosomes. Below the nucleus with chromatin fragments is an amorphous granular region, which, when examined ultrastructurally, is the Golgi apparatus. Surrounding the nucleus and Golgi zone are phase dark lysosomes. At the periphery are dark rod-like mitochondria. ×1,445. Phase micrographs of BCG-activated murine macrophages fixed in glutaraldehyde.

the cytosol itself, or recycled to the surface. With respect to protein synthesis, macrophages are highly active (1,2). These basal metabolic activities are supported by both glycolysis and oxidative phosphorylation, though the predominant source of energy depends on the origin of the macrophage (19).

The surface of macrophages is generously endowed with a variety of proteins (1,2,11). For example, important immunogenic proteins, such as class I and class II products of the major histocompatibility complex and adsorbed proteins typified by molecules that regulate the coagulation response, are present at the surface. The variety and number of specific receptors on macrophages which can be classified into several broad categories is almost staggering (over 50) (Table 1). First, receptors important for endocytosis include those recognizing various isotypes of immunoglobulin, various components of the complement cascade, specific carbohydrates, modified and unmodified lipoproteins, and proteins such as transferrin and lactoferrin. Second, a wide variety of receptors for regulatory molecules such as colony-stimulating factor-1 (CSF-1), interferons, neuropeptides, adrenergic agents, cholinergic

agents, and histamine exist, although the functional role of all has yet to be defined.

The cytoskeleton of macrophages is complexly organized (20,21) (Fig. 6). Beneath the plasma membrane and the hyaline ectoplasm lies a complex meshwork of actin microfilaments, which appear to be responsible for localized movements such as ruffling, pseudopod formation, and locomotion. The microtubular network serves to order pinocytosis and establish the polarity of migration in response to chemotactic stimuli.

Macrophages are powerful secretory cells and are currently known to produce at least 80 defined molecular products (1,2,22) (see Table 2). In broad terms, macrophages can secrete at least 10 components of the complement cascade, six coagulation factors, a wide variety of neutral proteases and acid hydrolases, several antiproteases, a variety of metabolites of arachidonic acid, and various factors both defined and undefined, which regulate the proliferation and function of other cells [e.g., interleukin-1, interferon-γ (IFNγ), IFNα, and IFNβ]. Regulation of secretion, which differs markedly from molecule to molecule, is complex. Some products, such as lysozyme,

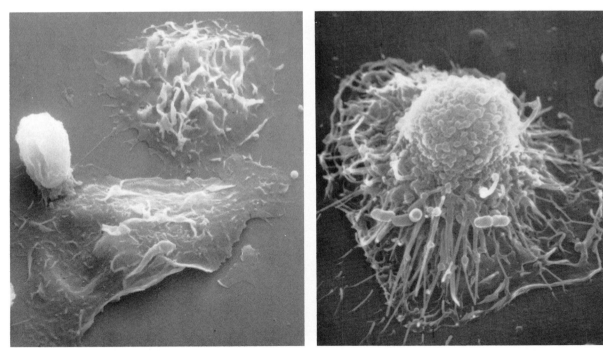

a,b

FIG. 5. Scanning electron micrographs of macrophages. **(a)** Scanning micrograph of two BCG-activated macrophages, showing the complex surface structure with ruffles, ridges, flanges, and various pseudopods in both the flattened, elongated, triangular macrophage at the bottom and the rounded macrophage above ×3,485. **(b)** Closer magnification of a macrophage showing the complex surface morphology in more detail and several adherent bacteria. ∼×5,950. (Courtesy of Lennart Nilsson/Boehringer Ingelheim GmbH.)

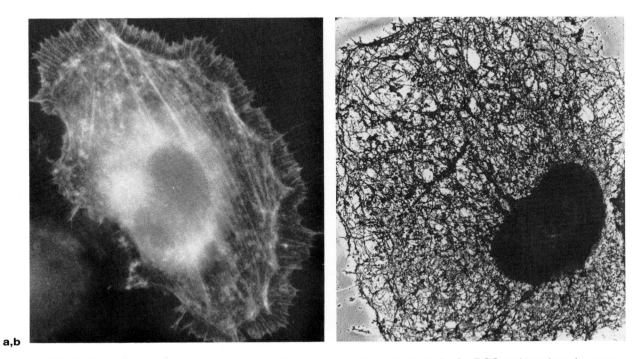

a,b

FIG. 6. The cytoskeleton of macrophages. **(a)** Fluorescent photomicrograph of a BCG-activated murine macrophage stained with an antibody against actin, showing the diffuse arrangement of actin filaments throughout the cytoplasm. ×1,445. **(b)** Electron micrograph showing the cytoskeleton of the entire macrophage. ×3,655. (Electron micrograph courtesy of Dr. John Hartwig.)

TABLE 1. *Some ligands binding to defined receptors of macrophages from various species[a]*

Regulatory proteins
  IFN α and IFN β
  IFNγ
  CSF-1
  TNF
  α-2 Macroglobulin–protease complexes
  Insulin
  Glucocorticosteroids
  Platelet-activating factor
  MIF
  GM-CSF
  IL-2
  IL-3
Immunoglobulins
  IgG_{2a}
  IgG_{2b}/IgG_1
  IgG_3
  IgE
  IgA
Complement components
  $C1_q$
  C3b
  C3bi
  C3d
  C5a
Additional proteins
  Transferrin
  Lactoferrin
  Fibrin
  Fibronectin
  Fibrinogen products
  Coagulation factor VII
  Coagulation factor VIIa
  Maleylated proteins
  α_1-Antithrombin
  Laminin
  Substance P
  Angiotensin
Glycoproteins and carbohydrates
  Mannose/fucose terminal glycoproteins
  Mannose-6-phosphate terminal glycoproteins
  Galactose terminal glycoproteins
  Heparin
Peptides and small molecules
  Enkephalins/endorphins
  Arg-vasopressin
  Histamine (H_1 and H_2 receptors)
  N-formylated peptides
  1,2,5-Dihydroxy vitamin D_3
  Serotonin
Lipids and lipoproteins
  LDL
  β VLDL
  Modified LDL (e.g., acetylated-LDL)
  Leukotriene C
  Leukotriene D_4
  Leukotriene B_4
  Prostaglandin E_2
Other molecules
  Cholinergic agonists
  α Adrenergic agonists
  β Adrenergic agonists

[a] Adapted from refs. 1 and 2.

are apparently secreted constitutively, but most are released following occupancy of a specific receptor or receptors. In many cases, secretion is regulated by two signals: (i) A priming signal prepares the macrophages, and (ii) a triggering signal stimulates actual release. Secreted products may be released via several routes, including fusion of vesicles or lysosomes with the membrane or by opening of a phagolysome to the surface.

The basal metabolism of macrophages can be profoundly altered by receptor-ligand interactions (1,2). Many of these trigger a respiratory burst similar to that observed in neutrophils. One consequence of the respiratory burst, apparently mediated in part through protein kinase C (see following), is altered activity of the membrane-bound oxidase complex to generate reactive oxygen compounds, such as superoxide anion (O_2^-) and subsequently H_2O_2 and hydroxyl radical (OH·). A second consequence of receptor-ligand interaction is the phospholipase-A_2-mediated release of arachidonic acid from cellular stores of phospholipids and its subsequent conversion via either lipooxygenases or cyclooxygenases to a series of leukotrienes or prostaglandins, respectively.

Almost all of the foregoing events can be altered by the development or activation of macrophages (1). Macrophages, which have undergone activation, have profound differences in the number and display of membrane proteins, in the arrangement of the cytoskeleton, in the regulation of protein translation and transcription, and in the synthesis, expression, location, and covalent modifications of both cell-bound and secreted proteins. The precise pattern of alteration in each category is stringently regulated, such that characteristic and requisite changes in cellular physiology are observed for the various forms of macrophage activation. Most forms of activation include precise deemphasis or down-regulation of certain physiologic characteristics as well as emphasis or up-regulation of others. Regulatory control mechanisms, including modulation of signal transduction, are also strikingly altered in activated cells. Thus, occupancy of a given receptor may have profoundly different consequences in activated as opposed to unactivated macrophages.

These various physiologic properties and their alterations during activation can be effectively integrated into striking alterations of function (1). In so doing, it is useful to distinguish between capacities and functions (for reviews, see refs. 1 and 16). A *capacity* is a defined physiologic or biochemical property, which can be quantified biochemically; examples would be the number/affinity of a given receptor, the number of molecules of a given membranous protein, the number of molecules/functional activity of a given enzyme, or the number of molecules of a given secreted protein. By contrast, a *function* is the completion of a complex task, which is quantified by determining the rate or extent of completion of the action

TABLE 2. *Secretory products of macrophages*[a]

Enzymes	Factor D
Lysozyme	Properdin
Plasminogen activator	C3b inactivator
Collagenase	βIH
Elastase	Additional proteins
Angiotensin convertase	Transferrin
Acid proteases	Transcobalomin II
Acid lipases	Fibronectin
Acid nucleases	Apolipoprotein E
Acid phosphatases	Tumor necrosis factor
Acid glycosidases	Interleukin 1
Acid sulfatases	Colony-stimulating factor(s)
Arginase	Erythropoietin
Lipoprotein lipase	Thymosin B_4
Phospholipase A_2	Serum amyloid A
Cytolytic proteinase	Serum amyloid P
Inhibitors of enzymes	Haptoglobin
α-2 Macroglobulin	Interferons α/β
α-1 Antiprotease	Platelet-derived growth factor
Lipocortin	TGF-β
α-1 Antichymotrypsin	Reactive oxygen intermediates
Coagulation factors	O_2^-
Factor X	H_2O_2
Factor IX	OH$\cdot$
Factor VII	Hypohalous acids
Factor V	Lipids
Protein kinase	PGE_2
Thromboplastin	$PGF_2\alpha$
Prothrombin	Prostacylin
Thrombospondin	Thromboxane A_2
Fibrinolysis inhibitor	Leukotrienes B, C, D, and E
Components of complement cascade	Mono-HETES
C_1	Di-HETES
C_4	Platelet-activating factor
C_2	Small molecules
C_3	Purines
C_5	Pyrimidines
Factor B	Glutathione

[a] Adapted from refs. 1 and 2.

in a physiologic assay. Capacities thus generally represent the expression of separate and independently regulated gene products, whereas functions generally represent operative interactions between these gene products. For example, endocytosis requires coordinated interaction between surface receptors and cytoskeletal elements and can be significantly and selectively altered during macrophage development (see chapter by Wright and Unkeless). Likewise, occupancy of the receptor for chemotactic peptides initiates a complex signal transduction cascade, leading to an intricate pattern of change in membrane, cytoskeletal, and cytosolic proteins that are ultimately responsible for change in directed motility and execution of the respiratory burst (see chapter by Snyderman). The ability of macrophages to present antigen effectively to T-lymphocytes is an acquired property, which requires the following: competence to endocytose and degrade proteins;

transport of the modified proteins to the surface; surface expression of immune-associated (Ia) or class II histocompatibility antigens; and the appearance of IL-1 on the plasma membrane of the macrophages (see Fig. 7) (23). The first two of these physiologic capacities are apparently constitutive in most populations of macrophages, whereas the other two must be induced. These latter two capacities are induced by interferon-γ and lipopolysaccharide in macrophages, and their appearance leads to macrophage functional competence for antigen presentation (i.e., activation for antigen presentation) (see ref. 23 for review). The physiologic properties required for the destruction of various microbes and tumor cells are discussed extensively below. In brief, activation for the direct kill of tumor cells mandates that the macrophages must acquire the capacity to bind tumor cells strongly and the capacity to secrete effector molecules, such as cytolytic protease (CP) and

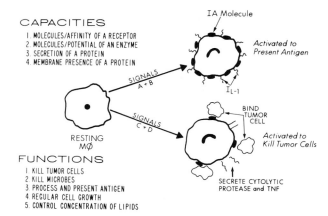

CAPACITIES
1. MOLECULES/AFFINITY OF A RECEPTOR
2. MOLECULES/POTENTIAL OF AN ENZYME
3. SECRETION OF A PROTEIN
4. MEMBRANE PRESENCE OF A PROTEIN

IA Molecule

SIGNALS A + B

Activated to Present Antigen

IL-1

RESTING MØ

SIGNALS C + D

BIND TUMOR CELL

Activated to Kill Tumor Cells

SECRETE CYTOLYTIC PROTEASE and TNF

FUNCTIONS
1. KILL TUMOR CELLS
2. KILL MICROBES
3. PROCESS AND PRESENT ANTIGEN
4. REGULAR CELL GROWTH
5. CONTROL CONCENTRATION OF LIPIDS

FIG. 7. Schematic of activation of macrophages for two discrete functions. At the left are shown some general examples of capacities and functions. Macrophages in the basal state receive one or more signals and then express two capacities [a Class II histocompatibility molecule (e.g., I-A) and interleukin-1 (IL-1)] on the surface; these macrophages have thus become activated to present antigen to T-cells. Application of other activating signals induces the capacity to bind tumor cells and the capacity to secrete lytic mediators such as cytolytic protease and tumor necrosis factor; these macrophages are activated to kill tumor cells.

tumor necrosis factor (TNF) (see Fig. 7). Although the molecular and biochemical requirements for many macrophage functions are yet to be defined, it is useful to think of *activation for a given function* as induction of those physiologic properties and biochemical characteristics that are necessary for execution of that function (1,16). Less information is currently available about the functional roles served by down-regulation of other physiologic properties, but this may represent, in part, a mechanism for conserving scarce cellular resources.

MACROPHAGES AS PROTECTIVE CELLS

General Rules of Destruction

Macrophages can destroy a wide range of prokaryotic and eukaryotic microorganisms, and a variety of isogeneic and allogeneic cells, including erythrocytes, normal tissue cells, and tumor cells (24–26). Although the basic mechanisms employed vary considerably, some general principles of killing may be formulated, since destruction in most cases involves three basic steps. First, the replicating intruder must be recognized as foreign, if destruction is to proceed efficiently. Recognition via cell-cell contact is often, but not always, mediated by receptor-ligand interactions. Second, some decision must be made as to disposition of the microorganism or noxious cell. Macrophages retain many replicating cells (tumor cells are an excellent example) at the surface. Alternatively, macro-

phages may actively endocytose microorganisms by pinocytosis in the case of viruses or by phagocytosis in the case of bacteria. Once endocytosed, the intruder may remain in the lysosomal system or pass into the cytosol from the lysosomal compartment. Other microorganisms (e.g., trypanosomes) invade the cytosol directly from the exterior surface of the cell. Very little is presently known about the molecular determinants that control and affect this decision-making process. Third, the replicating organism may be killed by the secretion of lytic effector substances from the macrophages. Such secretion is often triggered by stimulation of the receptor(s) involved in recognition and may involve secretion or release into the lysosomal compartment or secretion into the extracellular space, particularly into the space between macrophages and foreign organisms they have captured. The precise mechanisms of recognition and killing, which ultimately result in the destruction of a given invader, depend on many variables, including the specific invader, state of the macrophages, other host inflammatory systems which have been put into play (e.g., the presence of complement components or antibodies on the surface of the parasite), and the stage of development of the intruder. Failure to kill can result from passive failure at the stages of recognition, disposition, or killing or from active subversion of the destructive process by the microorganism or by host cells themselves. Macrophages in culture can also injure targets that are not in contact, particularly by release of noxious substances; cytostasis of tumor cells or of fungi, in some experimental settings, represent excellent examples of this. Imperfections in this process, by inappropriate recognition or inadequately controlled secretion, can also injure normal cells.

Destruction of Microorganisms

Macrophages represent a major defense against invasion of the host by a wide variety of microorganisms, including viruses, bacteria, fungi, and protozoa. The mechanisms for destruction of these organisms have been studied in a number of experimental settings, and detailed discussions of them are provided (see chapters by Klebanoff and by Elsbach). This brief section will focus on those elements of antimicrobial action particularly important to macrophages.

The initial requirement for antimicrobial activity involves recognition (see Fig. 8) (24–26). Macrophages may recognize the foreign invader primarily via the action of opsonins, which are molecules that bind to specific sites on both the invader and the macrophage (26). Opsonins may be of several categories, the most well documented being immunoglobulin G and fragments of the third component of complement. Macrophages bear receptors,

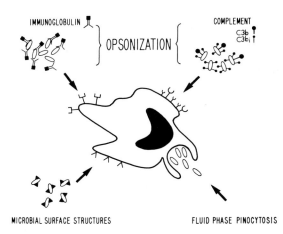

FIG. 8. Recognition of microorganisms by macrophages. In most cases, foreign microbes are recognized by immunoglobulins and/or complement components and are thus opsonized. In some cases, microbial surface structures are directly recognized by receptors on the macrophages (e.g., the mannose receptor) and are endocytosed, whereas in other cases the organisms are ingested during fluid phase pinocytosis.

which specifically bind several isotypes of IgG and which specifically bind several distinct fragments of complement (see Table 1). Circulating immunoglobulins frequently recognize and bind common bacterial cell-wall components, and large quantities of specific antibody against less common determinants can be generated through the specific immune response. Many microbes are also capable of activating the complement cascade, thus generating complement fragments that coat the organism and thus opsonize it. The macrophage itself is an important source of complement components and, indeed, macrophage-derived complement factors can opsonize microbial organisms for subsequent destruction in the absence of other sources (27). Adsorption and/or internalization of microbes may occur without opsonization per se, i.e. if the microbe expresses molecular determinants on its surface which the macrophage recognizes directly. These include carbohydrate residues (28), which can interact with the mannose-fucose receptor or proteins capable of recognition by scavenger receptors of various types (see Table 1). Finally, limited microbial destruction may occur without specific recognition, because macrophages may internalize some microbes during pinocytosis or phagocytosis of other materials or may destroy organisms in the surrounding microenvironment by the secretion of toxic materials. Opsonic phagocytosis is, however, the principal route to macrophage-mediated destruction of microbes.

A major antimicrobial mechanism of macrophages is the production and intracellular release of reactive oxygen intermediate species (ROI), including O_2^-, H_2O_2, and OH· (see chapter by Klebanoff). For example, destruction of

numerous pathogens, including leishmania, toxoplasma, trypanosome, mycobacteria, and candida, can be correlated with the ability of appropriately stimulated macrophages to secrete H_2O_2 (25). The exact mechanisms involved in microbial kill remain unresolved, but generation of OH· by either the Haber-Weiss reaction or by interaction with Fenton's reagent (iron) are likely candidates. Although the importance of the peroxidase-H_2O_2-halide antimicrobial system has been clearly demonstrated in neutrophils, macrophages do not express substantial levels of myeloperoxidase, and thus the contribution of this system to microbial killing by macrophages is questionable. Macrophages also possess potent nonoxidative mechanisms of killing (see chapter by Elsbach).

Destruction of Tumor Cells

The destruction of tumor cells by macrophages occurs in at least four distinct circumstances, which exhibit substantial differences in requirements, selectivity, state of macrophage activation, and mechanisms. Within each major circumstance, multiple effector mechanisms may operate.

Inhibition of Proliferation

Macrophage-mediated cytostasis can be defined strictly as the inhibition of target cell division and, experimentally, can be readily distinguished from cell destruction or cytolysis (29–31) (see Table 3). Inhibition of proliferation is observed in two circumstances. The first, termed *suppression*, refers to the ability of macrophages in certain stages of activation to block proliferation of lymphocytes in response to either specific antigens or polyclonal mitogens. Suppression, which requires relatively few macrophages (as few as 1% of the total cell population), probably acts by preventing the initial mitogenic response; it may well be mediated by the secretion of metabolites of arachidonic acid, such as prostaglandin E_2.

The second circumstance, termed *cytostasis*, affects a very broad spectrum of target cells (including tumor cells), requires a substantially larger number of macrophages (60% or more of the total cell population), and may be important beyond immunoregulatory function. Cytostasis is not selective for neoplastic or malignant cells, since both normal and transformed target cell types are equally susceptible. It is also effective across histocompatibility barriers, since targets from allogeneic or xenogenic sources are sensitive. Because there is little specificity in the recognition process and little evidence for contact, the actual cytostatic effect is likely carried out by soluble mediators that act upon all proliferating cells present in the local microenvironment. Candidate molecules for such media-

TABLE 3. *Four basic modes of injury to tumor cells[a]*

Characteristic	Cytostasis	MTC	Rapid ADCC	Slow ADCC
Stages of target injury	No current evidence for discrete stages	Binding and lysis	Binding and lysis	Binding and lysis
Contact-dependent	No?	Yes	Yes	Yes
Activation of macrophage necessary	Yes	Yes	Yes	Yes
Stage of effector activation where macrophage is most effective	Fully activated	Fully activated	Fully activated	Responsive or primed (selected populations)
Target selectivity	Any proliferating cell	Cells neoplastically transformed	Antibody-dependent	Antibody-dependent
Mediator(s)	Unknown	CP TNF	H_2O_2 Other?	H_2O_2 Other?
Recognition system	None?	Binding site for tumor cells	FcR's	FcR's
Time for completion	<2 hr	24–48 hr	4–6 hr	24–48 hr

[a] Adapted from ref. 31.

tors include prostaglandins, thymidine, and arginase Il-1 and TNF, but unequivocal evidence supporting even the concept of soluble antiproliferative activity has not yet been forthcoming. The inhibitory effects, which occur rapidly, can also be partially reversed quite rapidly. The primary effect on targets appears to be at the level of DNA synthesis, since activated macrophages block the movement of target cells through the cell cycle, principally by preventing entry into S phase, replication of DNA, or both. In contrast to suppression, cytostatic macrophages block proliferative responses even after they have been initiated in the targets.

Antibody-Independent Tumor Cytolysis

Macrophage-mediated tumor cytolysis (MTC), which occurs in the absence of specific anti-target-cell antibody, was first described in 1971–1972 (32,33). MTC, which occurs over 1–3 days, is contact dependent, nonphagocytic, selective for neoplastic cells (as opposed to their non-neoplastic and nontumorigenic counterparts), and requires the macrophages to be activated in a specific fashion (1,16).

A remarkable feature of MTC is its selectivity for targets (16). Activated macrophages kill a wide variety of malignant cells of syngeneic, allogeneic, and xenogeneic origin without the destruction of tissue-matched nonmalignant cells. The cytolytic process is dependent on cell-cell contact. By cinemicroscopy, one can observe the macrophages to cluster selectively around malignant versus normal cells and, in fact, to bind such targets avidly (see Fig. 9). The selectivity of such binding reflects the selectivity of cytolytic activity, implying this form of recognition is a major determinant of target cell destruction.

Destruction of tumor cells in MTC can be divided into two clearly separable events, which must occur in a precise sequence (1,34). First, macrophages selectively capture tumor cells and bind them to their surface (Fig. 9). Second, macrophages secrete toxic substances, which result in the eventual lysis of the bound target cells. Substantial evidence indicates that these lytic effector molecules may be secreted into a diffusion-limited space, formed between the junction of macrophage and tumor cell (see Fig. 10).

The binding and capture of target cells by macrophages is a complex process (35). Analysis of binding has been greatly aided by a novel technique that permits precise

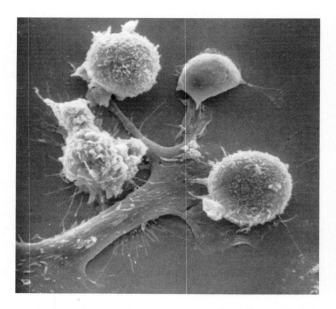

FIG. 9. Scanning electron micrograph of an activated macrophage binding tumor cells. A BCG-activated murine macrophage has captured four tumor cells by strong binding. ×2,320. (From ref. 87.)

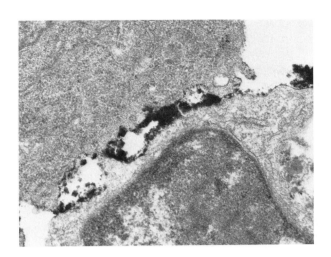

FIG. 10. Electron micrograph of the diffusion-limited space in binding. This electron micrograph is a cross section through a BCG-activated murine macrophage (below) and a bound P815 tumor cell (above). Between the two cells is a small cleft, the edges of which are extremely narrowed. The cells, before binding, were stained with ruthenium red, which has been mostly eluted from the sections by acetone rinses. The buildup of the ruthenium red in the cleft between the macrophages and targets suggests that this space may not be readily permeable. ×18,200.

quantification of the actual strength of cell-cell adhesion between various cell pairs. The antibody-independent binding of various cellular targets by macrophages begins initially as a very weak interaction which can be readily disrupted, which has no metabolic requirements for its establishment, and which may be mediated by physical forces such as van der Waals interactions. In the case where the macrophages are primed or activated and the target is a neoplastic cell, the weak binding is converted to stronger binding that requires at least 20 times more force to disrupt. This strong binding, which has precise metabolic requirements for its establishment, including a need for an hour's interaction at 37°C and intact microtubular and microfilamentous systems, is a multistep process and may require modification and/or reorganization of surface proteins on the macrophages. The precise molecular basis for the interaction between activated macrophages and neoplastic cells remains undefined, although several lines of evidence raise the possibility that this process is mediated by specific cell surface receptor(s) on the macrophages. For example, recognition structures on tumor cells can be demonstrated in the plasma membranes from disparate tumor cell populations, and these heterologously compete for the binding of intact tumor cells; these structures can be adsorbed onto activated macrophages. Tumor cell binding is abrogated when macrophage surfaces are digested with proteases, indicating the

putative receptor activity is at least partially composed of, or dependent upon, protein(s). Finally, the binding of tumor cells to the macrophage surface does initiate secretion of cytolytic protease and may initiate the subsequent performance of cytolytic function. To date, no specific molecular structures have been isolated from, or identified in, the macrophage plasma membrane which might be responsible for selective recognition and binding.

Macrophages secrete a large variety of toxic or lytic products (36). Although the precise role of all these products in MTC is not known, multiple lines of evidence support the participation of a novel serine protease and of TNF. The CP is a neutral serine protease of approximately 40 kilodaltons and is secreted only by fully activated macrophages. The activity of CP is highly sensitive to the antiproteases of serum, so its measurement must be done under serum-free conditions. Multiple lines of evidence indicate a major role for CP in lysis, but it remains to be established whether it is directly toxic to targets or in some way initiates or potentiates injury by other molecules. The secretory protein, TNF, has also received considerable attention as a cytolytic mediator (37). Antibodies specific for TNF can abrogate MTC in some experimental systems, and the production of TNF by macrophages correlates closely with expression of cytolytic function. The relative significance of TNF in MTC must, however, be assessed in light of the limited range of targets that are apparently sensitive to its destructive effect *in vivo* and *in vitro*. Of course, other secretory products may also participate in MTC. For example, ROI, though not the principal mediators of MTC, can potentiate the activity of the cytolytic protease when present in nontoxic quantities. While the precise mechanistic details of MTC remain obscure, the picture emerging of this phenomenon is one of a complex process involving multiple toxic mediators, which may not only interact but may also vary from target to target.

Antibody-Dependent Cellular Cytotoxicity (ADCC)

The ability of leukocytes, including macrophages, to destroy various target cells in the presence of specific antibodies has been well studied (1,35,38). Because the selectivity is based principally, if not entirely, upon the antibody, ADCC reactions are not restricted to tumor cells but may be used to destroy normal cells as well. Nevertheless, the importance of macrophage-mediated ADCC in antitumor function is underscored by recent experimental observations documenting the therapeutic efficacy of certain monoclonal antibodies directed against tumor cells. Such therapy is dependent on both the number of macrophages in the tumor bed and their relative state of function with respect to ADCC (39).

TABLE 4. *Suppressive substances acting on macrophage*

Agent	Effect
Lipopolysaccharide (endotoxin)	↓ Expression of Ia ↓ Fc receptor function
Immune complexes	↓ Antitumor function and expression of Ia
Corticosteroids	↓ Expression of Ia and activity of phospholipase A$_2$
α-2 Macroglobulin	↓ Secretion of H$_2$O$_2$, proteases, tumor cytolysis, and Ia
Prostaglandin (E series)	↓ Expression of Ia and tumor cytolysis

^{a} Adapted from refs. 1 and 45–49.

The primary determinant of recognition is the interaction between Fab portions of immunoglobulins to surface antigens on the target cells and the Fc portions of the immunoglobulin to surface receptors on the macrophage, which specifically bind the Fc fragment of such antibodies. Macrophages possess at least four classes of Fc receptors corresponding to several isotypes of immunoglobulin G (i.e.: IgG; Ig$_1$/IgG$_{2b}$; IgG$_{2a}$; IgG$_3$; and IgE) (see chapter by Wright and Unkeless). At least the first three of these receptors on macrophages can mediate ADCC (35,38). The binding of antibody-coated targets to macrophages resembles that seen in the absence of antibody with respect to morphology, but avidity of the resultant interaction is stronger. Fc-receptor-mediated binding of target cells occurs readily at 4°C (or higher) and is complete within 5 min. As in MTC, the binding of antibody-coated target cells is necessary but is not sufficient for completion of ADCC (35).

The second step in ADCC is lytic attack (35,38). Secretion of mediators occurs upon occupancy and cross-linking of the Fc receptor, at least in part. Evidence of multiple sorts indicates a major role for ROI (in particular H$_2$O$_2$) in completion of cytolysis (40). For example, anaerobiasis or glucose deprivation limits secretion of ROI and ADCC at the stage of lytic attack. Furthermore, immune complexes are well known triggers of the respiratory burst. The participation of other toxic mediators remains unclear (36).

Macrophages perform the lysis of antibody-coated targets under two quite distinct circumstances. These have been termed *rapid ADCC* and *slow ADCC,* although the two forms of kill are distinct in several ways other than time required for completion (see Table 3). In rapid ADCC, fully activated macrophages can lyse some targets, principally targets that are quite sensitive to relatively low amounts of ROI, over 5 to 6 hr (39,40). Macrophages competent for ADCC in this circumstance are all capable of mounting a rapid and extensive respiratory burst in response to pharmacologic triggering by phorbol myristate acetate (PMA). In slow ADCC, selected populations of

macrophages from the responsive and primed states of development can lyse antibody-coated targets over 24 to 48 hr (see refs. 41 and 42). Of interest, conversion of these macrophages to the fully activated state by addition of the appropriate inductive signals suppresses competence for this latter form of ADCC. A broad range of targets are lysed in this fashion, including lymphomas, carcinomas, melanomas, and sarcomas. In both cases, considerable evidence indicates that a major lytic mediator is an ROI, although the potential role of other substances remains undefined. Both reactions are similar in that they depend upon antibody coating the targets, upon an initial antibody-dependent capture of the targets, and apparently upon subsequent release of reactive oxygen intermediates. The two differ, however, in the targets that are lysed and in the types of macrophages that are able to lyse the various targets. At present, evidence suggests that these two forms of killing are variants of the same fundamental form of lysis and that the difference between the two may reside in whether the targets can be killed rapidly by relatively low amounts of hydrogen peroxide or whether the targets require prolonged incubation with H$_2$O$_2$ and perhaps with other mediators for target injury (41).

The ADCC reaction by macrophages, whether of the rapid or slow variant, is dependent upon the isotype of antibody coating the targets. Although antibodies of the IgG$_1$, IgG$_{2a}$, IgG$_{2b}$, and IgG$_3$ isotypes can all mediate such lysis, antibodies of the IgG$_{2a}$ isotype may be as much as twofold more efficient (43); the reasons for this difference remain to be defined.

REGULATION OF MACROPHAGE FUNCTION

Induction of Functional Competence

One of the cardinal features of the mononuclear phagocyte system is its great plasticity (see Fig. 3). Although neutrophils perform many similar (though not identical) functions, their potential for development after maturation in the marrow is restricted. By contrast, most functions of tissue macrophages are not constitutively expressed and require further development of these cells (1). This process, when applied to the acquisition of nonspecific immunity to invading microbes and subsequently to the destruction of tumor cells, has been termed *macrophage activation*. The term has now been extended to encompass the development of competence to perform any complex function.

Macrophages acquire competence for antitumor function in discrete steps, based upon sensitivity of the cells to various activating signals (see Fig. 11) (44–46). Two major signals are lymphokines and bacterial products. *Resting tissue macrophages* are relatively insensitive to activating stimuli. Young macrophages (*responsive macrophages*) from sites of inflammation remain relatively insensitive to bacterial lipopolysaccharide (LPS) but are

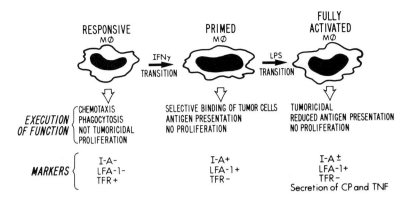

FIG. 11. The two-signal model of macrophage tumoricidal activation. Responsive tissue macrophages acquire tumoricidal function in two stages, following exposure to IFNγ and a second signal such as LPS. The different stages of activation (responsive, primed, and fully activated) can be distinguished from one another on the basis of their expression of objective markers or capacities. These capacities reflect the ability of macrophages in any given stage to execute particular functions. Following treatment with an activating stimulus, the macrophage undergoes transition to the next stage and thereby acquires the capacities requisite for further functional competence.

responsive to macrophage-activating factors (MAF), the most well-characterized of which is IFNγ (47). Macrophages primed by interaction with MAF (*primed macrophages*) now become sensitive to a second signal, the prototype of which is LPS. Upon such exposure, they acquire full competence for MTC (*fully activated macrophages*). Although synergy or cooperativity does exist between first and second signals, these agents alone are able to activate macrophages fully in most cases if provided in high concentration. Thus, first signals generally increase macrophage sensitivity to second signals and become more active themselves when used in concert with a second signal.

Although this model has been developed primarily with respect to the acquisition of tumoricidal function, many other functional responses are modulated by these classes of activating signals (1). Responsive macrophages, which are fully competent for chemotaxis and phagocytosis, must acquire competence for antigen presentation to T-lymphocytes and competence for kill of tumor cells; they concomitantly lose competence for multiplication (see Fig. 11). Such changes in function are paralleled by changes in various physiologic capacities. As representative examples, changes in the surface expression of Ia molecules (for example, I-A), leukocyte function antigen 1 (LFA-1), and the receptor for transferrin (TFR) or change in secretion of CP and TNF are observed during these developmental stages (Fig. 11). These two signals may also act independently, in parallel, cooperatively, and even antagonistically (41).

The two signals requisite for induction of MTC relate directly to the acquisition of the physiologic capacities needed to complete MTC (1). Responsive macrophages, upon treatment with MAF or IFNγ, acquire the capacity to capture tumor cells selectively. Secretion of lytic mediators, such as the cytolytic protease or TNF, is regulated by both signals. The lymphokine prepares or primes the cell for secretion, but the second signal triggers actual synthesis and release. Of note, binding of tumor cells to fully activated macrophages stimulates more rapid and more extensive secretion of cytolytic activity. Thus, the re-

quirement for two signals (e.g., IFNγ and LPS) given in a defined order is, at least partially, explained by how these signals regulate the physiologic capacities necessary for completion of MTC.

Other cytotoxic mechanisms of macrophages (i.e., cytostasis and ADCC) are also acquired functions (31). For example, macrophages exhibit cytostatic function following exposure to both IFNγ and LPS. The events regulating competence for ADCC remain poorly defined. Competence for ADCC can be induced by lymphokines or LPS *in vitro* (48). When manipulated *in vivo,* macrophages having high competence for release of hydrogen peroxide in response to PMA are the most competent for mediating the rapid form of ADCC (40); such macrophages, while frequently also activated for MTC, can be obtained in ways such that they do not have competence for MTC (e.g., intraperitoneal injection of the sterile irritant casein) (39). Thus, activation for MTC and for rapid ADCC are closely related but distinct. Some macrophages in the responsive and primed stages of activation (i.e., elicited by some agents but not others) have competence for the slow form of ADCC, while fully activated macrophages have reduced competence (42). The regulation of competence for ADCC in response to specific stimulating signals is less well understood. Macrophage-activating factors such as IFNγ can induce heightened capacity to release ROI and for rapid ADCC over several days (49). Whereas IFNγ plus LPS suppress competence for slow ADCC when added to responsive macrophages, this effect is induced in primed macrophages by LPS alone (42). In considering this problem, the complexities of regulating the respiratory burst and the many effects on various Fc receptors induced by both IFNγ and LPS must obviously be kept in mind (see Chapter by Nathan) (1,2).

Mechanisms of Signal Transduction

How signals generated by external stimuli are transduced into altered cellular behavior is a major problem in modern cell biology. Although currently understood in rudimentary terms, the general cascade of events probably includes the following: ligand-receptor interactions; generation of immediate second messengers; modulation of existing proteins (e.g., by phosphorylation or myristilation); modulation of gene expression; synthesis of new proteins; altered disposition of the modulated and new proteins; and alteration in other cellular elements, such as glycolipids. Although the central themes are doubtless played out in many different cells and responses, the specific ways in which each system utilizes these common elements doubtless determines the specificity of the response that ultimately ensues (see Fig. 12). The regulation of macrophage activation has recently been reviewed (50,51).

Responses to IFNγ

A specific surface receptor for IFNγ exists on macrophages (52). Although immediate second messengers have not been identified, alteration in intracellular metabolism of Ca^{2+} are induced by IFNγ in macrophages (for reviews, see refs. 50 and 51). Since all of the IFNγ-induced changes in macrophage physiology cannot be accounted for by changes in levels of Ca^{2+}, other mechanisms of signal transduction may operate. IFNγ is also established to raise the *potential* function of protein kinase C in macrophages (though not to initiate phosphorylation via this enzyme)— a change symbolized by the conversion of PK_c to PK_c^* (see Fig. 12). Interferons of all three classes induce the expression of novel polypeptides in various cells. For example, IFNγ induces expression of class II histocompatibility antigens on macrophages; this cell-surface protein complex is necessary in order for macrophages to present antigen to thymus-derived lymphocytes (23). Most of the documented changes in functional activity induced by IFNγ do not require protein synthesis during the early times following stimulation.

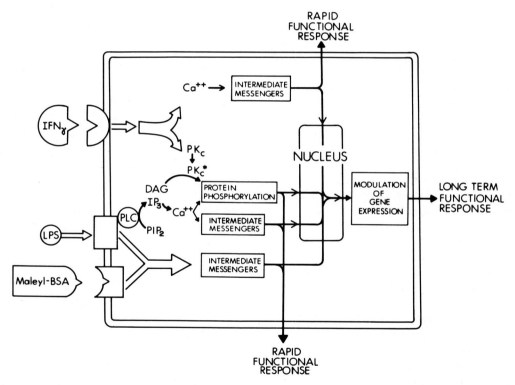

FIG. 12. Schematic model of signal transduction mechanisms induced in macrophages by IFNγ and LPS. IFNγ, acting via its receptor, may initiate early messengers, which are as-yet unidentified. These putative early second messengers lead to slow fluxes of calcium and alterations in the *potential* activity of protein kinase C (PK$_c$). LPS may act via at least two pathways. The first is the hydrolysis, mediated by a phospholipase C (PLC), of phosphatidylinositol-4,5-bisphosphate (PIP$_2$) into inositol triphosphate (IP$_3$) and diacylglycerol (DAG). These two molecules, in turn and respectively, initiate rapid elevation of cytosolic Ca^{2+} and protein phosphorylation via protein kinase C. LPS, acting through as-yet undefined early messengers, induces expression of early "competence" genes. These rapid and intermediate responses, such as fluxes of Ca^{2+} and protein phosphorylation, can lead to immediate rapid functional responses such as the respiratory burst and secretion of arachidonic acid metabolites. In conjunction with the protein products of the competence genes, they may also regulate expression of genes whose products are requisite to the activated function (e.g., Ia or TNF molecules). (For reviews, see refs. 50 and 51.)

Responses to LPS

Lipopolysaccharide is a potent modifier of immune function, but little is known of how the cell perceives this signal (53). Recent evidence has indicated a role for the breakdown products of phosphatidylinositol metabolism as immediate second messengers generated in macrophages by LPS (50,51). These include the generation of various isomers of inositol trisphosphate (IP_3) and diacylglycerol (DAG). Rapid spikes in intracellular Ca^{2+} levels and changes in endogenous patterns of protein phosphorylation, similar to those induced in response to specific stimuli of protein kinase C, are induced by LPS and/or its active lipid-A moiety. Other early effects of LPS are apparently independent of polyphosphoinositol hydrolysis and lead to the synthesis of new proteins. A number of early gene products induced by LPS in macrophages have been studied and share at least some similarities with the early responses of fibroblasts to platelet-derived growth factor (54). Such early gene products may, in some way, endow cells with competence for a particular function, whether it be cell division in the case of the fibroblasts or development toward tumoricidal function in the case of the macrophage, possibly by regulating the transcription and/or translation of genes whose products are more specific for the function in question. Alternative second signals, produced by defined molecules such as maleylated bovine serum albumin (mal-BSA), can mimic, to some extent, the functional and biochemical effects of LPS (51).

The cooperation between IFNγ and LPS in induction of macrophage development is mirrored in the biochemical events the signals induce (50,51). The phosphorylation induced by LPS via protein kinase C can be enhanced by previous modulation of protein kinase C with IFNγ. A reduction in protein phosphorylation, mediated via the cyclic adenosine monophosphate(cAMP)-dependent protein kinase A, can also be a cooperative effect between IFNγ and LPS (55). These events can lead to rapid functional responses (for review, see ref. 50). Cooperation between changes in intracellular levels of Ca^{2+} and the stimulation of protein kinase C can, for example, initiate chemotaxis, release of metabolites of arachidonic acid, and the secretion of ROI. Such, cooperation between early transductional signals also regulates expression of many genes, although such expression may be either enhanced, diminished, or dependent upon the presence of both signals. Current evidence indicates (at least for the limited number of gene products studied to date) that activating signals regulate the long-term expression of surface or secreted proteins by regulating the relevant genes (50,51). That is to say, changes in surface or secreted proteins during activation appear to involve initiating or shutting off transcription or altering stability of mRNA for the genes under study. Macrophage activation, which is es-

tablished to occur over 1 to 2 days, at present thus appears to be, at least in good part, a problem in regulation and control of genes encoding the proteins necessary for completion of the complex function under study. Further elucidation of these intricate genomic mechanisms will be necessary before pharmacologic intervention in the regulation of macrophage function can be further developed.

Suppression of Functional Competence

The broad range of macrophage functions and the potential injurious consequences of these to the host would both predict, *a priori,* the existence of mechanisms to diminish or suppress macrophage functions. A variety of agents, frequently encountered by macrophages in inflammatory sites, suppress various functions of macrophages (1,56–60) (Table 4, page 482). Analysis of suppression is, however, complex because some signals enhance or suppress, depending on the physiologic capacity being measured, as well as because the effect of a particular signal may depend on the state of development of the macrophages. For example, LPS and other second signals derived from invading microbes activate antimicrobial and antitumor mechanisms and also suppress the IFNγ-mediated induction of Ia or DR antigens (1,56). Exposure of other populations of macrophages to LPS for long time periods leads to a selective loss in the ability of Fc receptors to stimulate the respiratory burst (1,60). Immune complexes, in turn, suppress the development of antitumor function and of the ability of macrophages to present antigen (57,58). At least a portion of the anti-inflammatory activity of corticosteroids is mediated at the level of the mononuclear phagocyte system (59). Steroids, for example, indirectly inhibit phospholipase-A_2 activity, thereby suppressing arachidonic acid metabolism, and also inhibit the expression of Ia antigens.

Two kinds of potent suppressive agents derive from macrophages themselves. First, the antiprotease alpha-2-macroglobulin (α_2M) of serum is secreted by macrophages (1). When α_2M interacts with proteases in the inflammatory environment, it undergoes a conformational change to expose a binding site recognized by a specific receptor expressed on a number of cells, including macrophages (61). Exposure of activated macrophages to such α_2M-protease complexes, in turn, suppresses (a) secretion of neutral and cytolytic proteases, (b) MTC, (c) respiratory burst, and (d) induction of Ia antigen by macrophages (1,61). Second, prostaglandins are secreted by macrophages (and other cell types as well) (1,2). Following stimulation with various inflammatory agents, prostaglandin E_2 (PGE$_2$), which may be recognized by receptors on macrophages which are coupled to adenylate cyclase, can increase intracellular concentration of cAMP in macrophages (62). PGE$_2$ suppresses the antitumor function and the ability to present antigen. The latter effect reflects suppressed expression of Ia or DR antigens, which are normally induced or maintained by IFNγ.

With the exception of modulating cAMP levels by PGE$_2$, little information is currently available about the molecular mechanisms of suppressing macrophage function. Such mechanisms likely involve suppressive effects upon the generation of immediate second messengers as well as upon the systems that lead to the modification of existing proteins or to expression of genes for other proteins.

Regulation of Execution

The functions that macrophages perform after they have been activated are large and diverse, so the mechanisms that regulate such functions are likely to be equally large and diverse. Detailed examples of functions other than destruction are covered in several other chapters (see chapters by Snyderman; Unkeless; Stossel; Klebanoff; Elsbach; Henson; and Rosenthal). In general, macrophages must first become activated (1). Once activated, they are triggered in one form or another by another signal to execute that function. *A priori,* the execution of further responses by macrophages involves at least three broad categories of events: (i) ligand-receptor interactions; (ii) stimulus-response coupling; and (iii) stimulation of the output system itself.

Exogenous stimuli are most frequently perceived by the macrophage via a receptor-ligand interaction. The number of receptors for a particular ligand and the function of these will thus be important determinants of the overall response. Alteration in the number of receptors for a particular ligand has been demonstrated in macrophages and may be responsible for certain examples of altered function (1). For example, the number of Fc$_{\gamma2b}$R is significantly decreased upon activation with IFNγ and LPS (see chapter by Wright and Unkeless). In other cases, the function of the receptor is altered by activation. For example, the lateral mobility of receptors for fragments of C3 is modulated by signals, which macrophages may well encounter in inflammatory responses.

Following occupancy of a receptor, second messengers or signals must be generated that are ultimately transduced or coupled to output systems for the function in question (for review, see ref. 50). Perhaps the most thoroughly studied example is the receptor for chemotactic peptides, which is coupled to chemotaxis as well as to secretory responses (see chapter by Snyderman). This system involves the receptor-stimulated breakdown of polyphosphoinositides via a nucleotide regulatory protein coupled to phospholipase C. These metabolic products (e.g., inositol trisphosphate or IP$_3$ and diacylglycerol or DAG), in turn, independently modulate internal levels of Ca^{2+} and stimulate the phospholipid-Ca^{2+}-dependent protein kinase C. Of note, changes in Ca^{2+} and in endogenous protein phosphorylation have both been implicated in the activation of the NADP(H)-oxidase complex that generates O$_2^-$ (63). Other signal transduction mechanisms undoubtedly also participate in this, although details of such have yet to be described. Finally, the ligation of Fc receptors has been reported to initiate the influx of monovalent cations into macrophages, to perturb intracellular levels of Ca^{2+}, and to activate phospholipases as well (64,65; for review, see ref. 50). Thus, stimulus-response coupling is an important locus through which the magnitude and/or character of inflammatory responses can be controlled.

The third and last component necessary for execution of a given response is the actual output system itself. In the case of respiratory burst/secretory responses, this includes (a) the vesicles from which acidic hydrolases may be secreted, (b) enzymes of the hexose monophosphate shunt, and (c) the NADP(H)-oxidase referred to above (1,2). Although the actual amount of a given enzyme present in the cell will doubtless be an important determinant of such a response, modification of existing enzyme molecules may also endow them with greater activity. For example, the NADP(H)-oxidase of macrophage shows a decreased K_m for NADP(H) as the cells acquire the ability to generate O$_2^-$ (66–68). Thus, such cells exhibit higher production of O$_2^-$ at equivalent concentrations of NADP(H). Activation of the oxidase itself appears to involve stimulation of protein kinase C, and components of the oxidase or other associated molecules may be substrates for phosphorylation by this enzyme (63).

DESTRUCTIVE EFFECTS OF MACROPHAGES IN VIVO

Cellular Resistance to Microbial Infection

Host resistance to facultative and obligate intracellular bacteria and parasites, such as *Mycobacterium tuberculosis, Listeria monocytogenes, Schistosoma mansoni,* or *Trypanosoma cruzi,* is effected by cooperation between specifically sensitized T-lymphocytes and mononuclear phagocytes; antibodies apparently play little role in such immunity (69,70). Typically, the number of viable organisms after infection rises dramatically until the development of specifically sensitized cells, at which time there is a precipitous fall in their number (see Fig. 13). This entire process is accelerated in animals previously sensitized to the organism. The specifically sensitized T-cells

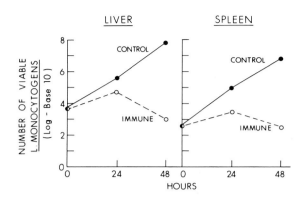

FIG. 13. Growth of *L. monocytogenese* in mice that have acquired cellular resistance to this organism. Immune and control mice have received *L. monocytogenese*. The number of microorganisms in liver or spleen rises dramatically for 1 day and then falls in the immune mice but continues to rise in the unprotected animals. Data replotted from ref. 86.

are essential for this process but do not carry out the microbicidal destruction. Rather, destruction occurs within macrophages, and the accelerated destruction of the replicating parasite, which is essential for host survival, depends on two changes in the mononuclear phagocytes of the affected organ or organs. First, a profound increase in the number of mononuclear phagocytes, which stems from enhanced inward migration of young monocytes plus extensive proliferation of macrophages in the tissues, is observed. Second, the macrophages have become activated, as defined by a wide variety of criteria (including enhanced competence), to destroy the organism in question. To date, the enhanced ability to secrete ROI such as H_2O_2 correlates best with the expression of enhanced microbicidal destruction either by the macrophages or in the tissues (25).

Host Resistance to Tumors

Host resistance to neoplasia, when it is observed, is obviously a complex phenomenon, which may depend on nonspecific host factors as well as various elements of the immune system, including T-lymphocytes, B-lymphocytes, antibodies, natural killer (NK) cells, and macrophages (71). The precise circumstances that determine whether host resistance to a given neoplasm will develop, whether it will involve elements of the immune system, and, if so, what elements will participate, is poorly understood. Current evidence suggests that, at minimum, the presence or absence of T-suppressor cells, the location and size of the neoplastic lesion, the overall burden of tumor, and the previous history of nonspecific or specific stimulation or suppression of the overall immune system are all important.

Macrophages, nevertheless, can be implicated in the destruction of neoplasms under some circumstances (24). First, the hypothesis that macrophages participate in immune surveillance against nascent neoplasms remains intriguing but neither proven nor disproven (72). Second, the degree of protection offered by macrophages to established tumors in unperturbed hosts is also unsettled (71). Although there is not a clear correlation between the number of macrophages in various tumors (which can be considerable) and their behavior (71), recent studies in one experimental system have shown that progressive variants of ultraviolet-induced sarcomas, which are usually rejected, have become resistant to lysis by activated macrophages and by tumor-specific T-cells (73). Of interest, cooperation between specifically sensitized T-cells and host macrophages has been implicated in the destruction of transplanted syngeneic tumors. Third, macrophages appear to participate in some examples of tumor rejection by induced immunotherapy (74). A wide variety of nonspecific immunomodulators such as bacillus Calmette Guerin (BCG) or muramyl-dipeptide (MDP) activate macrophages for MTC. Tumors undergoing such immune-mediated attack may contain increased numbers of macrophages. Recently in one experimental system, macrophages activated for MTC have been isolated from such regressing tumors (75). Tumors whose rejection is induced by antibodies may also depend on participation of host-derived macrophages (41). Recent studies on two disparate experimental models of antibody-induced rejection have documented that the rejection is accompanied by two cardinal changes in the population of intratumoral macrophages. First, the number of macrophages within the tumors is increased two- to threefold and, second, the macrophages have become activated for the slow form of ADCC. In all of these settings, the data do not preclude the participation of other effector leukocytes in destruction of the tumors (71). More critical studies of this important problem are needed in order to determine whether these isolated instances, in which macrophages appear to lead the attack upon tumors, represent a phenomenon of any widespread applicability.

Tissue Injury by Macrophages

Sites of inflammation, containing mononuclear phagocytes, frequently exhibit extensive damage to normal cells, which may be manifested by subtle evidence of cell injury, extensive fibrosis, overgrowth of normal tissues, or even massive destruction and necrosis (76–79). Such injury is not surprising when one considers the large number of destructive products secreted by macrophages (see Fig. 14). Hydrolytic enzymes (which are effective optimally at

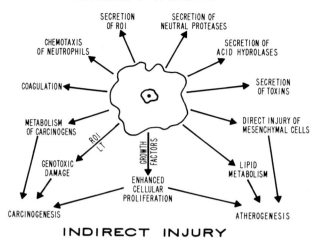

FIG. 14. Tissue injury by macrophages. Macrophages, as shown in the upper half of the figure, can *directly* injure tissues by their secretion of noxious substances as well as by calling forth other leukocytes or changing the vascular flow in a tissue. Macrophages can also cause more subtle and long-lasting forms of *indirect* injury, such as atherogenesis and formation of tumors by modulating the growth of cells, regulating extracellular lipids, causing genotoxic damage, metabolizing carcinogens to their ultimate forms, and directly injuring target cells.

acidic pH), proteases such as elastases and collagenase (which are effective optimally at neutral pH), and ROI such as O_2^-, H_2O_2, and O_2 are all capable of producing injury to cells and interstitium of various tissues. In addition, the mechanisms by which macrophages injure and destroy invading cells can also be turned against host cells, particularly if recognition molecules such as antibodies directed against host cells are present. Regulation of these destructive products is controlled at a minimum of four levels: (i) *when* secretion occurs, since release of these toxic products must be triggered by specific signals and is also controlled by preparatory signals; (ii) *where* secretion occurs, which is regulated, in part, by the formation of phagosomes (e.g., passive leaking of destructive elements during the phagocytic process); (iii) the presence or absence of a variety of suppressive factors, which can dampen both preparation and triggering of secretion; and (iv) the presence or absence of native inhibitors of the toxic products in the tissues (1). Obviously, ultimate regulation at these disparate levels is complex and remains to be understood fully in sites of inflammation. Nevertheless, it is interesting to note that for all of the classes of destructive elements (i.e., acid hydrolyses, neutral proteases, and ROI), lymphokines enhance the content and potential for secretion, whereas the uptake of foreign particles such as bacteria can trigger release. An additional

postulated mechanism of tissue injury is death of macrophages resulting from ingestion of toxic materials and subsequent spilling of enzymes into the environment.

Macrophages can also induce damage to normal host tissues indirectly. Considerable evidence now implies that macrophages may potentiate the development of carcinogenesis. Macrophages, as potent scavenger cells, ultimately collect and contain xenobiotics of a wide assortment, including chemical carcinogens (79). Mononuclear phagocytes can metabolize ingested carcinogens to their proximate forms, which may inflict genomic damage upon bystander cells (80). In the development of tumors in the liver by carcinogens, macrophages have actually been shown to play such a role (81). Macrophages can also cause genomic injury in bystander cells via the secretion of ROI and metabolites of arachidonic acid, which have the potential for enhancing mutagenesis (82; for review of oxidative DNA damage, see ref. 83). By these two routes, macrophages can thus potentially enhance both the initiation and promotion phases of carcinogenesis. Since both of these activities of macrophages may depend on the state of development of the macrophages and since other xenobiotics, which are themselves not directly carcinogenetic, can influence macrophage development, this process may be accelerated by environmental pollutants (79). Although the long-term biological relevance of these observations remains to be established, macrophages may thus be important in secondary or indirect injury as well as primary or direct damage.

Granulomatous Inflammation

The granuloma represents a useful model for analyzing some of the roles of macrophages in inflammation (84,85). Granulomas, which may be usefully defined as focal collections of macrophages, consist of two basic types. Foreign body granulomas, which are generally induced by a high local concentration of a wide variety of inert materials, constitute collections of incompletely developed macrophages. Epithelioid granulomas, which are usually induced by microorganisms capable of inducing specifically sensitized T-cells, constitute collections of activated macrophages. Thus, these two types of granulomas mirror the basic observation that sterile irritants induce the inflammatory macrophages, while the presence of lymphokines is required to induce fully activated macrophages (see Fig. 15). Necrosis frequently accompanies the epithelioid granuloma and is usually observed when the delayed hypersensitivity reaction, mediated by specifically mediated T-cells, is at its height. Yet, host protection against the invading organisms is strongly correlated with activation of the macrophages in the granulomas and the

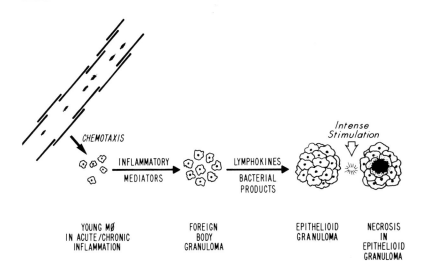

FIG. 15. Schematic of granulomatous inflammation. Granulomatous inflammation begins when mononuclear phagocytes are chemotactically attracted into an area of inflammation. In response to local inflammatory mediators such as products of the complement cascade, these macrophages become partially developed (i.e., become inflammatory macrophages) and loosely aggregated into foreign body granulomas. If the inciting agent is a bacterium that has stimulatory lipids such as the tubercle bacillus or incites a vigorous delayed hypersensitivity response resulting in the generation of local lymphokines, these macrophages become activated *in situ*, enlarge, and form epithelioid granulomas. In some cases, stimulation of the macrophages is particularly intense, leading to central necrosis in the granulomas, presumably as a result of secretion of noxious substances from the macrophages such as ROI or proteases.

development of specifically sensitized T-cells; failure of either lowers resistance. Thus, delayed hypersensitivity promotes both host protection and destruction of normal tissues.

CONCLUSIONS

Macrophages constitute a host-wide system of multifaceted and highly versatile regulatory cells. First discovered to be important in host protection against microbes, macrophages are admirably equipped to recognize and destroy, both intracellularly and extracellularly, a wide variety of rapidly replicating invaders, whether these be of prokaryotic or eukaryotic origin. Macrophages also serve as important scavengers for effector cells and molecules of host origin and for exogenous compounds (e.g., drugs or pollutants) that macrophages take up, detoxify, and degrade fully or contain. Over the past decade, it has become clear that macrophages fulfill many other important roles in the host. Although beyond the scope of this chapter, macrophages are known to regulate a large number of bodily functions and systems. By virtue of their many receptors and large endocytic capacity for fluids as well as particles, they are critical to the regulation of lipid and iron metabolism and general homeostasis. By virtue of their enormous array of secretory products, they also regulate the proliferation and function of other cells such as fibroblasts or development of myeloid elements in the marrow.

The regulation of these diverse functions by macrophages is tightly controlled. Macrophages resident in the tissues are generally cells that have been extensively down-regulated. These tissue macrophages, as well as young

monocytes recently immigrated into the tissues, can have their functions profoundly and dramatically up-regulated after the macrophages have received a wide variety of extracellular stimuli. This stimulation or up-regulation has been termed *activation,* in terms of the macrophage's capacity to destroy microbes and/or tumor cells. Over the past 5 years, it has become apparent that the other functions of macrophages become up-regulated as well and that the up-regulation of macrophage function is extremely diverse. Thus, macrophages can develop in many different ways, and development of one function is almost surely accompanied by loss of other functions. From such considerations, we have begun to appreciate that the macrophage is a multipotential cell that can develop in a wide variety of ways, depending on the precise signals that it has received. For these reasons, the control of macrophage function in molecular terms has become a topic of considerable interest. Although we have just begun to understand the complexities of such regulation, an eventual understanding of the precise molecular mechanisms that distinguish one form of macrophage development and activation from another may provide cardinal points for pharmacologic intervention into the mononuclear phagocyte system.

Certainly, the appropriate maintenance of this delicate and tightly regulated system in both the unperturbed host and in areas of inflammation and injury is essential to the well-being of the entire body. On the one hand, inability to activate the mononuclear phagocyte system (by virtue for example of insufficient amounts of stimulatory factors) can lead to inability to destroy microbes and may have profound deleterious consequences for the host (e.g., lepromatous leprosy). On the other hand, inappropriate regulation of activation, by virtue of excess stimulation or insufficient suppression, can lead to extensive tissue injury and damage. The potent destructive forces of mononuclear phagocytes are obviously difficult to control, so it is not surprising that areas of intense macrophage destructive effort (e.g., the center of a tuberculous granuloma) is often accompanied by focal necrosis. Of more consequence to the host are chronic or long-lasting and widespread failures in such control, which can lead to, or contribute to, chronic destructive diseases such as multiple sclerosis or rheumatoid arthritis. Over the past few years, an increased understanding that macrophages may participate in a more indirect fashion in diseases such as development of atherosclerosis or neoplasia has emerged. In these diseases, the regulatory destructive and homeostatic mechanisms of macrophages are apparently impaired individually or collectively, so that macrophages contribute to the pathogenesis of these diseases; such impairments or derangements may, of course, be inherent in the mononuclear phagocyte system (MPS), the regulatory signals (both inductive and suppressive) they receive, or both. These observations put further emphasis on the need to understand, in fine detail, the exquisite mechanisms that control macrophage development and execution of function.

Mononuclear phagocytes, in sum, represent a major body of host defense and regulatory system, which may well be essential not only for the integrity of the host but for life itself. Derangements in the regulation of this system, whether they be overexuberant responses to challenge or ineffective responses to challenge, have serious, and often lethal, consequences to the host.

REFERENCES

General References for Further Reading

1. Adams, D. O., and Hamilton, T. A. (1984): The cell biology of macrophage activation. *Annu. Rev. Immunol.,* 2:283–318.
2. Nathan, C. F., and Cohn, Z. A. (1980): Cellular components of inflammation: Monocytes and macrophages. In: *Textbook of Rheumatology,* edited by W. Kelley, E. Harris, S. Ruddey, and R. Hedge, p. 186. W. B. Saunders, New York.
3. Steinman, R. M., and Cohn, Z. A. (1974): The metabolism and physiology of mononuclear phagocytes. In: *The Inflammatory Process,* 2nd edition, edited by B. W. Zweifach et al., pp. 450–510. Academic Press, New York.
4. Cohn, Z. A. (1983): The macrophage-versatile element of inflammation. *Harvey Lect.,* 77:63–80.
5. Snyderman, R. (1985): Structure and function of monocytes and macrophages. In: *Arthritis and Allied Conditions,* edited by D. McCarty, pp. 287–305. Lea and Febiger, Philadelphia.
6. Cohn, Z. A. (1968): The structure and function of monocytes and macrophages. *Adv. Immunol.,* 8:163–215.
7. Van Furth, R. (1978): Mononuclear phagocytes and inflammation. In: *Inflammation,* edited by J. R. Vane and S. H. Ferreira, pp. 68–108. Springer-Verlag, Berlin.
8. Nelson, D. S., editor (1976): *Immunobiology of the Macrophages.* Academic Press, New York.
9. Reichard, S., and Kojima, M., editors (1985): *Macrophage Biology.* Alan R. Liss, New York.
10. Van Furth, R., editor (1985): *Mononuclear Phagocytes: Characteristics, Physiology and Function.* Martinus Nijhoff, Amsterdam.
11. Gordon, S. (1986): Biology of the macrophage. *J. Cell. Sci. (Suppl.),* 4:267–286.
12. Metchnikoff, E. (1905): *Immunity to Infectious Diseases.* Cambridge University Press, London.

Specific References

13. Spector, W. G., and Mariano, M. (1975): Macrophage behaviour in experimental granulomas, In: *Mononuclear Phagocytes in Immunity Infection and Pathology,* edited by R. van Furth, pp. 927–942. Blackwell Scientific Publishers, Oxford.
14. Cohn, Z. A. (1978): The activation of mononuclear phagocytes: Fact, fancy, and future. *J. Immunol.,* 121:813–816.
15. North, R. J. (1978): The concept of the activated macrophage. *J. Immunol.,* 121:806–809.
16. Adams, D. O., and Marino, P. (1984): Activation of mononuclear phagocytes for destruction of tumor cells as a model for study of macrophage development. In: *Contemporary Topics in Hematology-Oncology, Vol. III,* edited by A. S. Gordon, R. Silver, and J. LoBue, pp. 69–1361. Plenum Press, N.Y.
17. Fedorko, M. E., and Hirsch, J. G. (1970): Structure of monocytes and macrophages. *Semin. Hematol.,* 7:109–124.
18. Steinman, R. M., Mellman, I. S., Muller, W. A., and Cohn, Z. A. (1983): Endocytosis and the recycling of plasma membrane. *J. Cell. Biol.,* 96:1–27.
19. Axline, S. (1970): Functional biochemistry of the macrophages. *Semin. Hematol.,* 7:142.
20. Stossell, T. P. (1981): Actin filaments and secretion. The macrophage model. *Methods Cell Biol.,* 23:215–230.
21. Cain, H., Krauspe, R., and Kraus, B. (1982): The cytoskeleton in activated and functionally disordered cells of the macrophage system. *Pathol. Res. Pract.,* 175:162–179.
22. Unanue, E. R. (1986): Secretory function of mononuclear phagocytes. *Am. J. Pathol.,* 83:396–417.
23. Unanue, E. R. (1984): Mechanisms of action of antigen presenting cells. *Annu. Rev. Immunol.,* 2:395–428.
24. Nelson, D. S. (1972): Macrophages as effectors of cell-mediated immunity, In: *Macrophages and Cellular Immunity,* edited by A. I. Laskin and H. LeChevalier, pp. 45–76. CRC Press, Cleveland.
25. Nathan, C. F. (1986): Mechanisms of macrophage antimicrobial activity. *Trans. R. Soc. Trop. Med. Hyg.,* 77:620–630.
26. Edelson, P. J. (1982): Intracellular parasites and phagocytic cells: Cell biology and pathophysiology. *Rev. Infect. Dis.,* 4:124.
27. Ezehowitz, R. A. B., Sim, R. B., Hill, M., and Gordon, S. (1983): Local opsonization by secreted macrophage complement components: Role of receptors for complement in uptake of zymosan. *J. Exp. Med.,* 159:244–260.
28. Sung, S. S., Nelson, R. S., and Silverstein, S. C. (1983): Yeast mannans inhibit binding and phagocytosis of zymosan by mouse peritoneal macrophages. *J. Cell Biol.,* 96:160–166.
29. Gynongyossy, M. C., Liabeu, F. A., and Goldstein, P. (1979): Cell-mediated cytostasis: A critical analysis of methodological problems. *Cell. Immunol.,* 45:1.
30. Allison, A. C. (1978): Mechanisms by which activated macrophages inhibit lymphocyte responses. *Immunol. Rev.,* 40:3–27.
31. Hamilton, T. A., and Adams, D. O. (1987): Mechanisms of macrophage mediated tumor injury. In: *Tumor Immunology: Mechanisms, Diagnosis, Therapy,* edited by W. den Otter and E. J. Rutenberg. Elsevier, Amsterdam (*in press*).
32. Alexander, P., and Evans, R. (1971): Endotoxin and double stranded RNA render macrophages cytotoxic. *Nature New Biol.,* 232:76–79.
33. Hibbs, J. B., Lambert, L. H., and Remington, J. S. (1972): *In vitro* nonimmunologic destruction of cells with abnormal characteristics by adjuvant activated macrophages. *Proc. Soc. Exp. Biol. Med.,* 139:1049.

34. Adams, D. O., Johnson, W. J., and Marino, P. A. (1982): Mechanisms of target recognition and destruction in macrophage mediated tumor cytotoxicity. *Fed. Proc.,* 41:134.

35. Somers, S. D., Johnson, W. J., and Adams, D. O. (1986): Destruction of tumor cells by macrophages: Mechanisms of recognition and lysis and their regulation. In: *Basic and Clinical Tumor Immunology,* edited by R. Herberman, p. 69.

36. Adams, D. O., and Nathan, C. F. (1983): Molecular mechanisms in tumor-cell killing by activated macrophages. *Immunol. Today,* 4:166–170.

37. Beutler, B., and Cerami, A. (1986): Cachetin and tumor necrosis factor as two sides of the same biological coin. *Nature,* 320:584.

38. Adams, D. O., Cohen, M. S., and Koren, H. S. (1983): Activation of mononuclear phagocytes for cytolysis: Parallels and contrasts between activation for tumor cytotoxicity and for ADCC. In: *Macrophage Mediated Antibody-Dependent Cellular Cytotoxicity,* edited by H. S. Koren, pp. 43–52. Marcel Dekker, New York.

39. Adams, D. O., Hall, T., Steplewski, Z., and Koprowski, H. (1984): Tumor undergoing rejection induced by monoclonal antibodies of the IgG$_{2a}$ isotype contain increased numbers of macrophages activated for a distinctive form of antibody-dependent cytolysis. *Proc. Natl. Acad. Sci. USA,* 81:3506–3510.

40. Nathan, C. F. (1982): Reactive oxygen intermediates in lysis of antibody-coated tumor cells. In: *Macrophage-mediated antibody-dependent cellular cytotoxicity,* edited by H. S. Koren. Plenum Press, New York.

41. Adams, D. O., and Hamilton, T. A. (1986): *Destruction of Tumor Cells by Mononuclear Phagocyte Models for Analyzing Effector Mechanisms and Regulation of Macrophage Activation in Mechanisms of Host Resistance to Infectious Agents, Tumors, and Allografts,* edited by R. Steinman and R. J. North, pp. 185–204. Rockefeller University Press, New York.

42. Johnson, W. J., Steplewski, Z., Matthews, T. J., Koprowski, H., and Adams, D. O. (1986): Characterization of lytic conditions and requirements for effector activation. *J. Immunol.,* 136:4704–4713.

43. Kipps, B. J., Parham, P., Punt, J., and Herzenberg, A. L. (1985): Importance of immunoglobulin isotype in human antibody-dependent cell-mediated cytotoxicity directed by murine monoclonal antibodies. *J. Exp. Med.,* 161:1–17.

44. Hibbs, J. B., Taintor, R. R., Chapman, H. A., and Weinberg, J. B. (1977): Macrophage tumor killing: Influence of the local environment. *Science,* 197:279–282.

45. Meltzer, M. S., Ruco, L. P., Boraschi, D., and Nacy, C. A. (1979): Macrophage activation for tumor cytotoxicity: Analysis of intermediary reactions. *J. Reticuloendothel. Soc.,* 26:403–416.

46. Russell, S. W., Doe, W. F., and McIntosh, A. J. (1977): Functional characterization of a stable, noncytolytic stage of macrophage activation in tumors. *J. Exp. Med.,* 146:1511–1520.

47. Schreiber, R. (1984): Identification of γ-interferon as murine macrophage activating factor for tumor cytotoxicity. *Contemp. Top. Immunobiol.,* 13:174.

48. Ralph, P., Williams, N., Nakoinz, I., Jackson, H., and Watson, J. D. (1982): Distinct signals for antibody-dependent and nonspecific killing of tumor targets mediated by macrophages. *J. Immunol.,* 129:427.

49. Nathan, C. F., Murry, H. W., Weibe, M. E., and Rubin, B. Y. (1983): Identification of IFNγ as the lymphokine that activates human macrophage oxidative metabolism and antimicrobial activity. *J. Exp. Med.,* 1158:670–689.

50. Hamilton, T. A., and Adams, D. O. (1987): Molecular mechanisms of signal transduction in macrophage activation. *Immunol. Today,* 8:151–158.

51. Adams, D. O., and Hamilton, T. A. (1987): Molecular bases of signal transduction in macrophage activation induced by IFNγ and by second signals. *Immunol. Rev.,* 97:1–27.

52. Celada, A., Gray, P. W., Rinderknecht, E., and Schreiber, R. D. (1984): Evidence for a γ-interferon receptor that regulates macrophage tumoricidal activity. *J. Exp. Med.,* 160:55.

53. Morrison, D. C., and Rudback, J. A. (1981): Endotoxin-cell membrane interactions leading to transmembrane signalling. *Contemp. Top. Mol. Immunol.,* 8:187–218.

54. Stiles, C. D. (1983): The molecular biology of platelet derived growth factor. *Cancer Res.,* 33:653.

55. Justement, L. B., Aldrich, W. A., Wenger, G. D., O'dorisio, M. S., and Zwilling, B. S. (1986): Modulation of cyclic AMP dependent protein kinase isozyme expression associated with activation of a macrophage cell line. *J. Immunol.,* 136:270–277.

56. Steeg, P. S., Johnson, H. M., and Oppenheim, J. J. (1982): Regulation of murine macrophage I-A antigen expression by an immune interferon-like lymphokine: Inhibitory effect of endotoxins. *J. Immunol.,* 129:2402.

57. Esparza, I., Green, R., and Schreiber, R. D. (1983): Inhibition of macrophage tumoricidal activity by immune complexes and altered erythrocytes. *J. Immunol.,* 131:2117.

58. Virgin, H. W., Henberg, G. F. W., and Unanue, E. R. (1985): Immune complex effects on murine macrophages. Immune complexes suppress interferon-gamma induction of I-A expression. *J. Immunol.,* 135:3735.

59. Warren, M. K., and Vogel, S. N. (1985): Opposing effects of glucocorticoids on IFNγ-induced murine macrophage Fc receptor and I-A antigen expression. *J. Immunol.,* 134:2462–2469.

60. Johnston, P. A., Adams, D. O., and Hamilton, T. A. (1985): Regulation of Fc receptor mediated respiratory burst: Treatment of primed murine peritoneal macrophages with lipopolysaccharide selectively inhibits H$_2$O$_2$ secretion stimulated by immune complexes. *J. Immunol.,* 135:513–518.

61. Feldman, S. R., Gonias, S. L., and Pizzo, S. V. (1985): A model of α_2-macroglobulin structure and function. *Proc. Natl. Acad. Sci. USA,* 82:5700–5704.

62. Gemsa, D. (1981): *Stimulation of Prostaglandin E Release from Macrophages and Possible Role in the Immune Response in Lymphokines, Vol. IV,* edited by E. Pick, p. 335. Academic Press, New York.

63. Babior, B. M. (1984): Oxidants from phagocytes: Agents of defenses and destruction. *Blood,* 64:959.

64. Young, J. D.-E., Unkeless, J. C., Kaback, H. R., and Cohn, Z. A. (1983): Mouse macrophage Fc receptor for IgG$_{2b/A1}$ and artifical and plasma membrane vesicles functions as a ligand-dependent ionophore. *Proc. Natl. Acad. Sci. USA,* 80:1636–1640.

65. Nitta, T., and Suzuki, T. (1982): Biochemical signals transmitted by Fc$_\gamma$ receptors: Triggering synthesis of the increased synthesis of adenosine 3'5'-cyclic monophosphate mediated by Fc$_{\gamma 2a}$ and Fc$_{\gamma 2b}$-receptors on a murine macrophage like cell line (P388D$_1$). *J. Immunol.,* 129:2708.

66. Sasada, M., Pabst, M. J., and Johnston, R. B., Jr. (1983): Activation of mouse peritoneal macrophages alters the kinetic parameters of the superoxide-producing NADPH oxidase. *J. Biol. Chem.,* 258:9631.

67. Tsunawaki, S., and Nathan, C. F. (1984): Enzymatic basis of macrophage activation. *J. Biol. Chem.,* 259:4305–4312.

68. Browning, Y., and Pick, E. (1985): Activation of NADPH-dependent superoxide production in a cell-free system by sodium dodecyl sulfate. *J. Biol. Chem.,* 260:13539–13545.

69. Mackaness, G. B. (1972): The mechanism of macrophage activation. In: *Infectious Agents and Host Reactions,* edited by S. Mudd, p. 61. W. B. Saunders, Philadelphia.

70. North, R. J. (1974): Cell-mediated immunity and the response to infection. In: *Mechanisms of Cell-Mediated Immunity,* edited by R. T. McClosky and S. Cohen, pp. 185–220. John Wiley & Sons, New York.

71. Evans, R. (1986): The immunological network at the site of tumor rejection. *Biochim. Biophys. Acta,* 865:1–11.

72. Adams, D. O., and Snyderman, R. (1979): Do macrophages destroy nascent tumors? *J. Natl. Cancer Inst.,* 16:1341–1345.

73. Urban, J., and Schreiber, H. (1984): The surveillance role of various leukocytes in preventing the outgrowth of potential and malignant cells. *Contemp. Top. Immunobiol.,* 13:225–242.

74. Hibbs, J. B., Remington, J. S., and Stewart, C. C. (1980): Modulation of immunity and host resistance by micro-organisms. *Pharmacol. Ther.,* 8:37–69.

75. Key, M. E., et al. (1982): Isolation of tumoricidal macrophages from lung melanoma metastases of mice treated systemically with lipo-

somes containing a lipophylic derivative of murimyldipeptide. *J. Natl. Cancer Inst.,* 69:1189–1198.

76. Fantone, J. C., and Ward, P. A. (1984): Mechanisms of lung parenchymal injury. *Am. Rev. Resp. Dis.,* 130:484–491.

77. Tracey, D. E. (1982): Macrophage-mediated injury. In: *The RES: A Comprehensive Treatise, Vol. 4, Immunopathology,* edited by N. R. Rose and B. V. Siegel, pp. 77–101. Plenum Press, New York.

78. Weiss, S. J. (1983): Oxygen as a weapon in the phagocyte armamentarium. In: *Handbook of Inflammation, Vol. 4, Immunology of Inflammation,* edited by P. A. Ward, pp. 37–87. Elsevier, Amsterdam.

79. Adams, D. O., Lewis, J. G., and Dean, J. H. (1986): Activation of mononuclear phagocytes by xenobiotics of environmental concern: Analysis and host effects. In: *Target Organ Toxicity: Lung,* edited by J. D. Crapo, D. E. Gardner, and E. J. Masara. Raven Press, New York *(in press).*

80. Harris, C. C., Hsu, I. C., Stoner, G. D., Trump, B. F., and Selkirk, J. K. (1978): Human pulmonary alveolar macrophages metabolize benzo[*A*]pyrene to proximate and ultimate mutagens. *Nature,* 272: 633–634.

81. Lewis, J. G., and Swenberg, J. A. (1983): The kinetics of DNA alkylation, repair, and replication in hepatocytes, Kupffer cells, and sinusoidal endothelial cells during continuous exposure to 1,2 dimethylhydrazine. *Carcinogenesis,* 4:529–536.

82. Lewis, J. G., and Adams, D. O. (1985): Induction of 5,6-saturated thymine bases in NIH3T3 cells by phorbol ester-stimulated macrophages: Role of reactive oxygen intermediates. *Cancer Res.,* 45: 1270.

83. Cerutti, P. A. (1985): Prooxidant states and tumor promotion. *Science,* 227:375–381.

84. Adams, D. O. (1983): The biology of the granuloma. In: *Pathology of Granulomas,* edited by H. L. Ioachim, pp. 1–20. Raven Press, New York.

85. Adams, D. O. (1976): The granulomatous inflammatory response: A review. *Am. J. Pathol.,* 84:164–191.

86. Mackaness, G. B. (1970): The monocyte in cellular immunity. *Semin. Hematol.,* 7:172–184.

87. Marino, P. A., and Adams, D. O. (1980): Interaction of BCG activated Mϕ and neoplastic cells *in vitro.* I. Conditions of binding and its selectivity. *Cell Immunol.,* 54:11.

Inflammation: Basic Principles and Clinical Correlates.
Edited by J. I. Gallin, I. M. Goldstein, and R. Snyderman.
Raven Press, Ltd., New York © 1988.

CHAPTER 26

Phagocytic Cells: Disorders of Function

John I. Gallin

Ehrlich (49) and Metchnikoff (108) predicted that abnormal function of any element of the defense system would lead to disease. Perhaps no deficiency of the host defenses dramatizes this point better than patients with absent or severely impaired inflammation due to dysfunction of the phagocytic cells. Absent inflammation causes a compromised host (64), and inadequate turnoff of inflammation contributes to diseases such as rheumatoid arthritis, vasculitis, lupus, and the adult respiratory distress syndrome (see Chapters 38, 41, and 46, *this volume*). The purpose of this chapter is to illustrate how disease models demonstrate salient features of the role of phagocytes in inflammation. Neutropenia and monocytopenia are obvious extreme examples of absent function and demonstrate the critical importance of phagocytes in inflammation. However, they offer few insights into specific functions of the cells and therefore will not be reviewed here (reviews of these subjects can be found in refs. 36, 95, and 99. The molecular basis for the pathologic defects listed in Table 1 have only been defined in a few congenital disorders of phagocyte function. An understanding of several of these diseases has provided understanding phagocytic cell function in inflammation, including cell adherence, function of neutrophil granules, and the respiratory burst (hydrogen peroxide formation). This chapter will focus on the congenital phagocyte defects that serve as models of the physiological processes (Table 2).

LEUKOCYTE ADHESION DEFICIENCY[1]

The ability of phagocytes to form aggregates in the circulation and to adhere to endothelial cells is critical for margination, diapedesis (migration out of the circulation) (see Chapter 18, *this volume*), and phagocytosis. These events require cell-cell adhesion. Without cell adhesion, an inflammatory process cannot be established. The mechanism of phagocyte adhesion is unknown. However, the discovery of monoclonal antibodies that bind to adhesion sites has provided a breakthrough in understanding these processes and understanding the abnormality of a group of patients with abnormal phagocyte adherence and depressed inflammation (4,63,151,159).

In 1979 Springer et al. (150) and subsequently other colleagues developed a series of monoclonal antibodies specific for leukocyte antigens (4,147,148,159). Some of these monoclonal antibodies were shown to bind to a common antigen on neutrophils and monocytes (called Mo1 antigen and also known as Mac-1), whereas other antibodies bound to a different antigen, called *lymphocyte function-associated antigen* (LFA-1) found on lymphocytes [T cells and natural killer (NK) cells], B cells, mono-

---

[1] Other terminology includes CR3 (iC3B receptor) deficiency or LFA-1, Mac-1, p150,95 antigen deficiency, or CD11/CD18 leukocyte glycoprotein deficiency.

TABLE 1. *Types of neutrophil dysfunction*

Function	Acquired disease	Congenital disorder
Adherence-aggregation	Neonates; hemodialysis	iC3b-receptor (CR3) deficiency
Deformability	Leukemia; neonates; diabetes mellitus; immature neutrophils	
Chemokinesis-chemotaxis	Thermal injury; malignancy; malnutrition; periodontal disease; neonates; systemic lupus erythematosus; rheumatoid arthritis; diabetes mellitus; sepsis; influenza virus infection; herpes simplex virus infection; acrodermatitis enteropathica; Down's syndrome; α-mannosidase deficiency; severe combined immunodeficiency; Wiskott-Aldrich syndrome	Hyper-IgE-recurrent infection (Job's) syndrome; Chédiak-Higashi syndrome; specific-granule deficiency
Microbicidal activity	Leukemia; aplastic anemia; certain neutropenias; thermal injury; sepsis; neonates; diabetes mellitus; malnutrition	Chédiak-Higashi syndrome; neutrophil specific-granule deficiency; chronic granulomatous diseases

cytes, and neutrophils (Table 3). A third glycoprotein called p150,95 was found on granulocytes and mononuclear phagocytes (100,104). It became clear that the Mo1 and LFA-1 antigens contained an alpha chain of 150 to 177 kilodaltons (kD) and a beta chain of 95 kD, held together in a noncovalent linkage. There are no intersubunit disulfide bonds. The beta chain is identical among the three different antigens; however, there are different alpha chains, called alpha M, alpha L, and alpha X, which define Mac-1, LFA-1, and p150,95, respectively. The glycoproteins LFA-1, Mac-1, and p150,95 are also referred to by the cluster designation of the alpha and beta subunits as CD11$_{a-c}$/CD18, respectively (159) (Table 3).

The distinction among the three alpha subunits and the identity of the beta subunits was confirmed by peptide mapping, amino acid sequencing, and physiochemical characteristics. The amino acid sequences of the alpha M, alpha L, and alpha X subunits show 33% to 55% identity, and therefore the subunits are considered a protein family (4). Mac-1 corresponds to the iC3b receptor [complement receptor 3 (CR3) on granulocytes and macrophages (10)] and is important for cell adherence and phagocytosis and production of hydrogen peroxide upon contact with IgG-coated particles (7). LFA-1 participates in lymphocyte and monocyte adherence to cells (149) and is required for (a) T-lymphocyte antigen-dependent adhesion and killing of some target cells (133), (b) natural killing and antibody-dependent killing by killer lymphocytes and granulocytes, and (c) T-lymphocyte–helper-cell interactions (97). LFA-1 is also important for B-lymphocyte aggregation (25,106) and proper antibody production (109). Although p150,95 has been shown to bind iC3b and is important in cell adherence to surfaces (7), less is known about its functional significance. The clinical importance of these proteins became apparent with the de-

scription of patients lacking these proteins (reviewed in ref. 4).

Clinical Presentation

In the 1970s there were reports of patients with recurrent bacterial infections, defective neutrophil mobility, and delayed separation of the umbilical cord (12,38,51,81). Other patients with recurrent infections who had abnormal initiation of the respiratory burst to particulate, but not soluble, stimuli were also recognized (79). A patient was reported to have actin dysfunction (18), but later evaluation suggested the patient had adhesion protein deficiency (145).

Crowley et al. (35) were the first to propose that a phagocyte defect was related to defective phagocyte adherence. Their patient's neutrophils had defective spreading on a surface. In addition, Crowley et al. described a glycoprotein deficiency in the patient's neutrophils. Subsequently Arnaout et al. (5,6), Bowens et al. (15), and others (3,37,148,151) reported that, in patients with a similar abnormality, neutrophil aggregation was defective (Fig. 1) and the cells lacked glycoproteins of 150,000 to 180,000 daltons. Buescher et al. (25) confirmed these findings in another patient and showed that the abnormality of the neutrophil extended to similar defects of mononuclear phagocytes as well as Epstein-Barr (EB)-virus-transformed B cells. Subsequently these patients' leukocytes were shown to lack, or have markedly reduced amounts of, CR3, LFA-1, and p150,95.

Aside from recurrent severe infections, these patients have a persistent leukocytosis, with a neutrophilia of about twice that in normal patients (Table 2). There is a severe deficiency in mobilizing an inflammatory response, which

TABLE 2. *Distinguishing features of congenital phagocyte dysfunction syndromes*

Disease	Inheritance	Defect	Clinical manifestations
Leukocyte adhesion protein deficiency [iC3b-receptor (CR3) deficiency (abnormal β-chain synthesis)]	Autosomal recessive; localized to chromosome 21	Adherence; aggregation; spreading chemotaxis; neutrophilia gingivitis; periodontal diseases	Delayed separation of umbilical stump; depressed inflammation; bacterial infections
Hyper-IgE-recurrent infection (Job's) syndrome	Usually non-X-linked	Variable chemotactic defects, very high IgE with anti-*S. aureus* IgE; low anti-*S. aureus* IgA in serum and saliva	"Coarse" facies in most patients; "cold" cutaneous abscesses; recurrent pulmonary, bone, upper-airway infections with *S. aureus* or *Haemophilius influenzae*; mild eosinophilia; mucocutaneous candidiasis
Myeloperoxidase deficiency	Autosomal recessive; localized to chromosome 17	Absent myeloperoxidase	Minimal unless another defect, then *Candida albicans* or other fungal infections
Chédiak-Higashi syndrome	Autosomal recessive	Giant lysosomal granules; neutropenia; decreased chemotaxis, degranulation, and microbicidal activity; excess O_2 consumption and H_2O_2 production; deficient neutrophil cathepsin G and elastase	Recurrent pyogenic infections, especially with *S. aureus*; periodontal disease; partial oculocutaneous albinism; nystagmus; progressive peripheral neuropathy; many patients develop lymphomatous-like illness during adolescence
Neutrophil specific-granule deficiency	Possibly autosomal recessive	Absent neutrophil-specific granules; decreased chemotaxis; decreased O_2 production; decreased bactericidal activity; absent neutrophil gelatinase and defensins	Recurrent cutaneous, ear, and sinopulmonary bacterial infections; diminished inflammation
Chronic granulomatous diseases	X-linked (Xp21.3); autosomal recessive, autosomal dominant	H_2O_2 production absent in neutrophils and monocytes; defective "turn-off" of inflammation	Severe infections of skin, ears, lungs, liver, and bone with catalase (+) microorganisms such as *S. aureus, Pseudomonas cepacia, Aspergillus* sp, and *Chromobacterium violaceum*; often hard to culture organism; excessive inflammation with granulomas and frequent lymph-node suppuration; granulomas can obstruct vital structures such as gastrointestinal or genitourinary tracts; gingivitis, aphthous ulcers

most likely relates to impaired leukocyte adhesiveness. Patients also have severe gingivitis and periodontitis. To date, over 30 patients have been described (reviewed in ref. 4). Since the primary defect appears to relate to impaired myeloid cell adhesiveness, "leukocyte adhesion deficiency" is a reasonable name for the disease (4).

Two forms of leukocyte adhesion deficiency exist, one with severe and the other with moderate clinical manifestations (3). Patients with severe deficiency have no detectable expression of the three alpha and beta chain complexes described above, whereas patients with moderate deficiency express 2.5% to 6% of the three complexes.

TABLE 3. *Leukocyte adhesion proteins*

Glycoprotein designation	Cells	Polypeptide subunit designation (molecular weight, kD)	Antigenic epitope cluster designation (CD)	Representative monoclonal antibodies
LFA-1	Neutrophils, monocytes, lymphocytes, large granular lymphocytes	α L (170–185) β (94–105)[a]	CD11a CD18	TS1/22, L1, TA-1 1B4, 60.3, TS1/18
Mac-1, Mo.1, OKM1	Neutrophils, monocytes, macrophages, large granular lymphocytes	α M (155–165) β (94–105)	CD11b CD18	Anti-Mo.1, OKM1, Mac-1, Leu-15
p150,95	Neutrophils, monocytes, macrophages	α X (130–153) β (94–105)	CD11c CD18	Anti-Leu-M5, Ki-M1

[a] β chain is identical for each glycoprotein.

In most families there is a history of consanguinity; in all the parents, neutrophils express about 50% of the gene product. The disease is thought to be inherited as an autosomal recessive inheritance.

Biosynthesis of the glycoproteins listed in Table 3 has been studied both in mouse and human cells (88,151), and translation and glycosylation of the proteins has been studied in mouse cells (134,135). Using cloned probes, the murine Mac-1 subunit messenger RNA (mRNA) of 6 kilobases (134) and the human beta subunit mRNA of 3.2 kilobases (135) have been defined. Utilizing this information, Anderson and Springer developed a model of biosynthesis of the subunits (4). Each of the three alpha subunits and the common beta subunit is encoded by a separate mRNA. The subunits are synthesized as precursors which are cotranslationally glycosylated with N-linked high-mannose carbohydrate groups. After alpha and beta subunit association, which occurs 1 to 2 hr after synthesis, most of the high-mannose groups are converted to complex-type carbohydrates in the Golgi apparatus, and the subunits increase slightly in molecular weight. The mature glycoproteins are then transported to the cell surface or to storage sites in intracellular secretory vesicles.

In the normal neutrophil the storage pool for Mac-1 antigen or CR3 has been localized to the specific granules (119). The expression of the CR3 receptor is increased with specific granule discharge, and the concept has emerged that up-regulation of these epitopes in neutrophils occurs through specific granule mobilization (see below). The probable importance of CR3 mobilization in phagocyte margination *in vivo* is demonstrated by studies in normal volunteers in whom there is up-regulation of neutrophil CR3 following intravenous endotoxin or following exudation into an experimental inflammatory le-

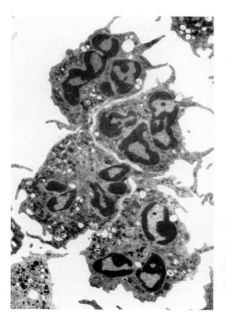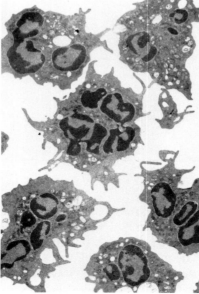

FIG. 1. Formyl-peptide-stimulated shape change and aggregation in normal (**left**) and iC3b-receptor-deficient (**right**) neutrophils (×500). Note failure to aggregate despite shape change in iC3b-receptor-deficient cells. (From ref. 129.)

sion (see Fig. 2). Patients with leukocyte adhesion deficiency have no intracellular pool of neutrophil CR3 and have a poor inflammatory response (119).

The Genetic Lesion

The molecular basis of leukocyte adhesion deficiency has been studied by biosynthesis studies and studies of human × mouse hybrids (reviewed in ref. 4). Biosynthesis experiments have utilized (EB)-virus-transformed B cells and mitogen-stimulated T-lymphocyte cell lines, which, from normal cells, express alpha L and common beta subunit on their surface. Initial studies showed that the patient cell lines synthesized normal LFA-1 alpha-subunit precursor. However, the alpha L precursor failed to undergo carbohydrate processing and did not form an alpha-beta complex, and neither subunit was expressed on the cell surface.

In human × mouse lymphocyte hybrids, normal human LFA-1 alpha and beta subunits associated with mouse LFA-1 subunits to form interspecies hybrid alpha-beta complexes (105). In hybrids of patient and mouse cells, instead of only seeing incompletely developed alpha units, interspecies complexes appeared. These experiments indicate that incompletely developed alpha-subunit expression can occur in patient cells and that the genetic lesion involves the beta subunit. The alpha subunits re-

quire normal beta subunits for complete maturation and expression on the cell surface. In the absence of beta subunits the alpha subunits are degraded.

Recently Springer's group developed a rabbit anti-human beta-subunit serum (4). This enabled immunoprecipitation and sodium dodecylsulfate polyacrylamide gel electrophoresis (SDS-PAGE) studies of the immunoprecipitates in normal and patient cells. Beta-subunit precursors were present in some, but not all, patients. Within family groups with beta-subunit precursors, the immunoprecipitates were the same molecular weight. But there was variability among families. Therefore, it is likely that distinct mutations in the beta-subunit gene exist. The ability of the beta-subunit precursors to complex to alpha-chain subunits in some patients may explain moderate clinical expression of the disease. In mouse × human hybrids, the beta subunit, and hence the genetic lesion, has been mapped to chromosome 21, which is in agreement with autosomal inheritance (105).

The identification of the genetic lesion to the common beta subunit found on chromosome 21 indicates that introduction of a normal beta-subunit gene into hematopoietic cells could cure the disease. The feasibility of doing this is suggested by experiments in which mouse beta subunits are complexed with human alpha L subunits of LFA-1 in mouse × patient human hybrids (105). Springer's laboratory has recently obtained a cDNA clone for the beta subunit, and efforts are underway to introduce the

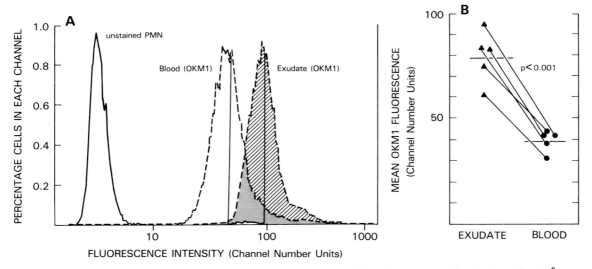

FIG. 2. The iC3b-receptor expression of human exudate (▲) and blood (●) neutrophils. Neutrophils (10⁶) were incubated with 5 µg of OKM1 for 30 min on ice and subsequently with 25 µl of fluoresceinated F(ab)₂ fragments of goat anti-mouse IgG for an additional 30 min. Green fluorescence is measured on paraformaldehyde-fixed cells on a cell sorter and is reported as mean fluorescence of the >95% cells that were OKM1-positive. **(A)** Plot of data from individual experiment, showing autofluorescence of exudate PMN, OKM1 fluorescence of blood, and exudate PMN. The vertical lines give the mean fluorescence. **(B)** Mean OKM1 fluorescence on paired exudate and blood samples. The significance of the difference between the arithmetic means was determined by the two-tailed Student's t test. (From ref. 174.)

missing gene into patient bone marrow cells using retroviral vectors (4). If this works, correction of the disease by gene therapy may be possible in the foreseeable future.

ABNORMAL NEUTROPHIL GRANULE FORMATION AND FUNCTION

Striking morphologic derangements of neutrophils are seen in patients with abnormal granules. The morphologic abnormalities of toxic neutrophil granulations seen with acute infection of normal subjects, Auer bodies seen in acute myelogenous leukemia, giant granules of Chédiak-Higashi syndrome and leukemia, specific granule deficiency, and deficiency of all granules in a patient with leukemia have been described in depth in Chapter 16 (this volume).

Neutrophil granule contents have potentially important roles in modulating inflammation (60). Specific (secondary) granule contents can amplify the function of the neutrophil and recruit inflammatory mediators. For example, the specific granules contain receptors for the chemoattractant f-Met-Leu-Phe (52,75,90), iC3b (119,138,158), and laminin (172), as well as a complement activator (170), a monocyte chemoattractant (171), and cytochrome b (14,84,136,171). The presence of several receptors within the specific granule compartment has resulted in the hypothesis that the specific granules function as an important reservoir of certain plasma membrane receptors that are used during chemotaxis and phagocytosis (see Fig. 3). Another specific granule product, lactoferrin, may have a role in regulating neutrophil adhesiveness (16,17,118) as well as a role in myelopoiesis (22) and iron homeostasis (94). The anemia of chronic inflammation may relate to chelation of iron by lactoferrin as well as to its subsequent irreversible sequestration by the mononuclear phagocyte system (94). Gelatinase (83) and histaminase (129), which is important in modulating the effects of histamine on

inflammation [see Chapter 11 (this volume) and ref. 141] have also been localized to neutrophil specific granules. Azurophil (primary) granules contain elastase and myeloperoxidase (see Chapters 23, 30, and 45, this volume), which are potentially important modulators of inflammation. Several patient models, in which neutrophil granules are abnormal, emphasize the importance of neutrophil granules in the regulation of inflammation.

Neutrophil Specific-Granule Deficiency

The neutrophil specific granules are the most prevalent granules within the cell, and their contents are released into the circulation in response to inflammatory stimuli [see Chapter 16 (this volume) and ref. 174]. In certain leukemic patients, absence or deficiency of neutrophil specific granules has been described as a congenital deficiency in neutrophils from neonates and in neutrophils from thermally injured patients (reviewed in refs. 50 and 62; also see refs. 16,21,69,98,146, and 154).

The depressed inflammatory response in patients congenitally deficient in neutrophil specific granules is a dramatic demonstration of the importance of these granules (reviewed in refs. 60 and 62). General comments can be made about the patients (Table 2). Most patients are products of nonconsanguineous marriages, although the parents of one patient are first cousins once removed. Both sexes are affected about equally. There are no documented examples of siblings with the disease, but the sister of the patient whose parents were related died of infection at 1 year of age. Therefore, if the disease is inherited it probably follows an autosomal recessive pattern of inheritance.

All patients have recurrent infections with bacteria without increased susceptibility to a particular pathogen. The peripheral white blood count is usually normal, but on Wright's stain, which stains specific granules, the neu-

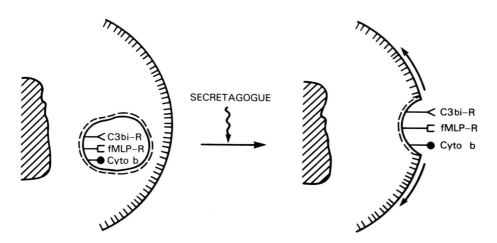

FIG. 3. Diagram illustrating how neutrophil granule-membrane-bound components could get translocated from granule membranes to the cell surface with secretion.

trophils appear to lack granules. Azurophil granules, however, are evident on peroxidase stain. Nuclei are bilobed, and the nuclear membrane may be distorted by blebs, clefts, and pockets. Normal specific granule contents such as lactoferrin, vitamin B_{12}-binding protein, and cytochrome *b* are either absent or markedly reduced, and cells are deficient in the plasma membrane marker alkaline phosphatase. Parmley et al. (121) studied neutrophils and bone marrow of a specific-granule-deficient patient using a periodic-acid–thiocarbohydrazide staining method to identify vicinal glycol-containing complex carbohydrates. It was inferred that the patient's cells contained "empty" specific granules, since small, abnormal, elongated organelles appeared late in neutrophil maturation and were "secreted" in response to phorbol myristate acetate. However, the underlying defect in granule genesis probably differs among patients, since ultrastructural studies have not demonstrated "empty" granules in all patients studied (129).

Other neutrophil granule markers are also absent in specific granule deficiency. For example, gelatinase, which has recently been shown to be in a specific granule location (83), was absent from one patient with specific granule deficiency (Gallin, Dewald, and Baggiolini, *unpublished observations*). Defensins, normally localized to the azurophil granules, were recently found to be absent from neutrophils of a patient with specific granule deficiency (74). Neutrophil azurophil granules from patients with specific granule deficiency sediment with a decreased density as compared to normal azurophil granules. The abnormalities of azurophil granules in specific granule deficiency indicate that the fundamental defect is not restricted to a regulatory system controlling specific granule formation but, rather, represents an abnormal gene(s) that regulates the packaging of a group of proteins present in both the specific and azurophil granules.

The accumulation of neutrophils and monocytes *in vivo* into Rebuck skin windows and skin blister devices, as well as *in-vitro* chemotaxis of neutrophils, is impaired in neutrophil specific-granule deficiency (62). In one patient, monocyte chemotaxis *in vitro* was normal (69), suggesting that the impaired monocyte recruitment seen *in vivo* reflects deficient release of monocyte chemoattractants or of factors capable of generating chemoattractants. In support of this, secretory products from the patient's neutrophils exposed to specific-granule secretagogues failed to generate C5a upon activation with endotoxin (69). Neutrophils from patients with congenital deficiency of specific granules also exhibit impaired up-regulation of formyl peptide receptors and CR3, impaired respiratory burst to certain stimuli, and deficient bacterial killing (62). Whether or not the latter finding is a consequence of absent specific granules or absence of another important neutrophil component, such as defensins, is not known.

Thus, patients with neutrophil specific-granule deficiency constitute an important model illustrating the critical role that granules normally play in modulating inflammation.

Acquired forms of neutrophil specific-granule deficiency further emphasize these points. For example, neutrophils from patients with thermal injury are deficient in specific granules (39,164,168) but appear "activated" with increased surface area and iC3b-receptor expression (48,110). This may represent premature granule discharge. The granule defect is temporally associated with the appearance of a chemotactic defect, defective oxidative metabolism, and elevation of serum lysozyme and lactoferrin (39,110,168). The increased neutrophil surface marker expression and decreased specific-granule content correlate with the degree of neutrophil functional impairment, suggesting that the acquired deficiency of specific granules in thermal injury plays a role in the increased susceptibility of burn patients to infection.

Other models of neutrophil specific-granule deficiency include neonatal cells, normal cells (2,5,4) experimentally depleted of organelles (cytoplasts) (72), and HL-60 promyelocytic leukemia cells induced *in vitro* toward a neutrophil-like phenotype (for review see ref. 62). *In-vitro* studies of these cells also support an important role for specific granules in amplification of early phases of inflammation (60).

Chédiak-Higashi Syndrome

The Chédiak-Higashi syndrome is a rare inherited disease (autosomal recessive) characterized clinically by partial oculocutaneous albinism, photophobia, nystagmus, progressive peripheral neuropathy, neutropenia, gingivitis, periodontal disease, and recurrent pyogenic infections (13,169). In many cells, giant lysosomal granules are seen (see Chapter 16, *this volume*). These giant granules result from fusion of predominately azurophil, but also secondary granules, with each other (167). A similar disease has been described in Aleutian mink, partial albino Hereford cattle, albino whales, and beige mice. The increased susceptibility to infection is related to a depressed inflammatory response. This cannot be explained by the degree of neutropenia. During infection the patients can mount a leukocytosis, although it is somewhat less than normal. Impaired neutrophil and monocyte migration (31,71) and defective degranulation (127) are thought to be the basis for the delayed inflammatory response and increased susceptibility to infection (169). In addition, neutrophils from beige mice and humans with Chédiak-Higashi syndrome are deficient in cathepsin G and elastase (74,156).

Factors underlying the abnormal phagocyte function in Chédiak-Higashi syndrome include abnormal cyclic nucleotide metabolism, disorders of microtubule assembly, and markedly increased tyrosinolyation of the alpha chain of tubulin (111; for review see ref. 129). The abnormalities of microtubules may relate to a profound abnormality of orientation of intracellular elements of neutrophils in a gradient of chemoattractant (Fig. 4). Oxygen consumption and hydrogen peroxide production is greatly exaggerated for unknown reasons and probably compensates, at least in part, for the compromised defenses in this disease. Abnormal phagocyte plasma membrane fluidity has been reported (77). It is not known how any of these defects relate to the pathogenesis of the disease.

Boxer et al. (19) noted markedly elevated levels of cAMP in an 11-month-old girl who was in the accelerated (lymphoma-like) stage of Chédiak-Higashi syndrome. The patient responded clinically to ascorbate. It has been suggested that the improvement in neutrophil function in response to ascorbate results from enhanced microtubule assembly and correction of the abnormal cyclic nucleotide metabolism. However, in a study using two adult brothers with Chédiak-Higashi syndrome, who were not in the accelerated phase of the disease, benefit from ascorbate was not confirmed (67). However, in the latter study, neutrophil function in beige mice was improved by ascorbate.

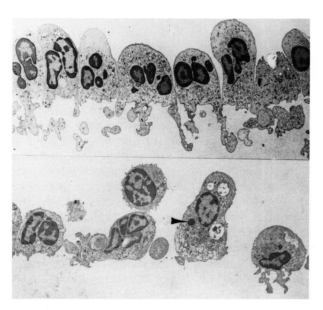

FIG. 4. Abnormal orientation of Chédiak-Higashi neutrophils in a gradient of *E. coli* endotoxin-activated serum (5% vol/vol). Normal neutrophils (**upper panel**) or neutrophils from a patient with Chédiak-Higashi syndrome (**lower panel**) were oriented for 45 min at 37°C on 0.45-μm cellulose nitrate filters. Arrowhead points to giant granule in Chédiak-Higashi cell. Note the characteristic orientation of normal neutrophils with nuclei toward the rear; also note the long pseudopods projecting into the filter. The Chédiak-Higashi cells send pseudopods out poorly, and in some cells the nucleus is in the wrong position, toward the bottom (leading edge) of the cell. ×2,400.

The different results with ascorbate are not understood, but it is possible that in Chédiak-Higashi syndrome the stage of the underlying disease determines responsiveness.

DISORDERS OF OXYGEN-DEPENDENT ANTIMICROBIAL SYSTEMS

Chronic Granulomatous Diseases (CGD) of Childhood

Since the initial descriptions of CGD in the mid-1950s, over 300 cases have been reported (reviewed in detail in refs. 66 and 157) and have been presented in a monograph (68). The disease represents a group of disorders of phagocyte oxidative metabolism with a common phenotype. Neutrophils, mononuclear phagocytes, and eosinophils are abnormal. In addition, abnormal oxidative metabolism has been reported in EB virus-transformed B cells (163). The disease is inherited as X-linked, autosomal recessive, and autosomal dominant patterns (66). The patients have recurrent infections and, in response to inflammation, they develop severe chronic inflammation leading to granuloma formation. Thus, there are two clinical features to the disease: recurrent life-threatening infection and excessive inflammation with granuloma formation.

The phenotypic expression of CGD is rare, affecting only about one in 1,000,000 persons; nonetheless, the disease has engendered tremendous interest as a prototype for abnormalities of phagocyte oxidative metabolism. Elucidation of the underlying defects has been critical to developing an understanding of the structure, activation, and function of the reduced nicotinamide adenine dinucleotide (NADPH) oxidase [see Chapter 23 (*this volume*) and Fig. 5].

Nearly all males with X-linked CGD have absent or grossly abnormal cytochrome b_{558}, an essential component of the electron transport chain coupled to NADPH oxidase (136). In female carriers the concentration of cytochrome b_{558} in the neutrophil population as a whole correlates directly with the population of cells demonstrating inactivation of the abnormal X-chromosome. Ohno et al. (115) described a male patient with normal levels of cytochrome b_{558} in association with apparent X-linked transmission; these facts suggest the X-chromosome may code for additional factors important in the function of the oxidase. In about 15% of reported cases of CGD, an autosomal recessive pattern of transmission seems most likely; the vast majority of such patients have normal levels of the cytochrome, although two patients with apparent autosomal recessive transmission and cytochrome deficiency have been reported (115,166). We speculated that a structural gene for the cytochrome might be found on an autosomal chromosome, whereas the X-

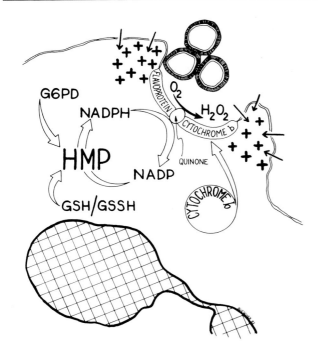

FIG. 5. Scheme of events leading to hydrogen peroxide formation that may be abnormal in some patients with chronic granulomatous disease. Soluble or particulate stimuli (depicted in upper right) bind to the cell and trigger a membrane depolarization (+'s) which may or may not trigger the hexose monophosphate shunt (HMP) that utilizes NADPH oxidase and an associated membrane-bound electron transport system containing flavoprotein, possibly quinone, and cytochrome *b*. Full activation results in conversion of oxygen to hydrogen peroxide. Cytochrome *b* may be added to the membrane from an intracellular pool present in specific granules. A lesion anywhere in the scheme may lead to CGD.

chromosome may encode a putative *b*-cytochrome gene activator (an "enhancer element" required for appropriate transcription) or a protein (possibly a component of the oxidase) necessary for normal insertion of the cytochrome in the oxidase chain (115).

In some patients with X-linked *b*-cytochrome-deficient CGD there is coexistence of other diseases. A patient with retinitis pigmentosa and Duchenne's muscular dystrophy and CGD has been particularly helpful in localizing the genetic defect in CGD (8). The chromosomal lesion in the patient has been localized near the locus for Duchenne's muscular dystrophy on the short arm of the X-chromosome at position Xp 21.3.

Orkin and co-workers (130) used clones of the involved region and cDNAs from induced HL-60 cells to do subtraction studies with cDNAs from CGD EB-virus-transformed B cells. With this approach a particularly interesting gene that probably is responsible for the X-linked *b*-cytochrome deficient form of CGD was cloned; the transcript of the gene was expressed in phagocytic myeloid

cells but was absent or structurally abnormal in four patients with X-linked CGD. The nucleotide sequence of complementary DNA clones predicts a polypeptide of at least 468 amino acids. Recent studies indicate the protein is a 91-kD subunit of the *b*-cytochrome that interacts with a 22-kD subunit to form the functional *b*-cytochrome. The 91-kD subunit that is absent in CGD is an integral membrane protein that may be critical to anchor the rest of the *b*-cytochrome to the plasma membrane (41).

Diminished flavin adenine dinucleotide (FAD) has been reported in some CGD patient's neutrophils (55,115,157). In general, the results support a close relationship between cytochrome b_{558} deficiency and reduced FAD content. To demonstrate FAD deficiency, assays must be done with partially purified particulate neutrophil material. While FAD deficiency probably occurs only in a setting of *b*-cytochrome deficiency, a normal content of FAD in the setting of *b*-cytochrome deficiency is probably at least as common (115). The significance of FAD deficiency is not settled. It also is still unclear whether the reported deficiency of another possible component of the electron transport chain, membrane quinone (66,157), is a cause of CGD.

Patients with an autosomal recessive pattern of inheritance of CGD have a less frequent incidence of infection than do patients with the X-linked form of the disease (165). Neutrophils from some of our patients with the autosomal recessive CGD produce superoxide in response to phorbol myristate acetate if the cells are previously exposed to gamma interferon (Sechler and Gallin, *unpublished observations*). Therefore, unlike patients with X-linked CGD, patients with autosomal recessive form of CGD have the biochemical machinery but lack proper regulation of phagocyte oxidative metabolism.

A defect in phosphorylation of a 44-kD protein in stimulated neutrophils from patients with autosomal (but not X-linked) CGD has been reported in several laboratories (137). This is consistent with the concept that the 44-kD protein is an important link in activation of the oxidase or that it may serve as an electron transporting molecule in the oxidase chain. In this regard, Rossi et al. (128) have presented data suggesting that the *b*-cytochrome is, itself, phosphorylated in stimulated guinea-pig neutrophils.

Other examples of the heterogeneity of the defect in CGD have been described. For example, patients have been reported with defects in hydrogen peroxide generation in response to particulate, but not soluble, stimuli or by soluble, but not particulate, stimuli (79). Whether or not these observations relate to a slow rate of phagocytosis and abnormal C3b receptor (CR1) expression in CGD neutrophils is not known (57,58,153).

Several patients with CGD have been reported with a greatly diminished, but not absent, respiratory burst (102,114,139,155). In these patients the defect has been attributed to abnormal NADPH oxidase arising from a decreased affinity of the oxidase for its substrate, NADPH. These patients, who have X-linked or autosomal recessive inheritance, have deficient b-cytochrome and normal or sluggish neutrophil transmembrane depolarization in response to formyl peptides or phorbol myristate acetate. The essentially normal elicited depolarization of membrane potential is in contrast to all other patients with CGD who have an abnormality in membrane depolarization in response to the chemoattractant f-Met-Leu-Phe or to phorbol myristate acetate (66). In this regard, the nature of the relationship between abnormal elicited changes in neutrophil membrane potential and defective hydrogen peroxide generation in CGD remains obscure, since depolarization of CGD cells by calcium ionophores or extracellular potassium does not correct the defect. It has been suggested that the abnormality of neutrophil depolarization in CGD may relate to abnormal acidification of the phagosome (126).

Severe deficiency of the enzyme glucose-6-phosphate dehydrogenase (G6PD) may result in the CGD phenotype (157). NADPH oxidase activity is normal in neutrophil G6PD deficiency. A laboratory distinction between G6PD deficiency and abnormal NADPH oxidase can be made by addition of methylene blue, which serves as an electron donor and will drive the hexose monophosphate shunt in cells with abnormal NADPH oxidase but not in neutrophils deficient in G6PD (66).

The multiple abnormalities that can lead to CGD demonstrate that numerous biochemical lesions can result in the same phenotype. The variability of CGD is characterized by experiments demonstrating that monocyte hybrids from patients with genetically distinct forms of CGD are complementary, with a resulting product capable of reducing nitroblue tetrazolium (NBT) (78). Ultimately, in all patients with CGD the clinical features can be accounted for solely on the basis of impaired activity of the hexose monophosphate shunt, which furnishes reducing equivalents (NADPH) for superoxide production.

Clinical Manifestations of CGD (Table 2)

Patients with CGD develop serious infections early in life, usually in the first year. Common infectious syndromes include pneumonia and lung abscesses, skin and soft tissue infections, lymphadenopathy, suppurative lymphadenitis, osteomyelitis (usually involving the small bones of the hands and feet), and hepatic abscesses. Septicemia, meningitis, brain abscesses, and infection of the gastrointestinal and genitourinary tracts are not common. Though severe, infection in CGD may follow a rather indolent course characterized initially only by malaise, low-grade fever, and a mild leukocytosis or elevation of the erythrocyte sedimentation rate (66). The diagnosis of CGD is readily established by an inability of neutrophils to reduce the dye nitroblue tetrazolium or by other tests of phagocyte oxidative metabolism. Diagnosis is often delayed, with potentially catastrophic consequences.

Staphylococcus aureus and gram-negative bacilli account for the majority of serious infections, but infections with *Aspergillus sp.* and other fungi are also observed (66). Organisms that produce hydrogen peroxide but that are catalase negative (e.g., streptococci, pneumococci, and lactobacilli) are not major pathogens. It has been suggested that the production of hydrogen peroxide within the phagosome by catalase negative microorganisms (no microbial catalase to break down the hydrogen peroxide), in concert with host cell myeloperoxidase, results in efficient bactericidal activity against these organisms (see Chapter 23, *this volume*). Alternatively, oxygen-independent microbicidal mechanisms (see Chapter 24, *this volume*) may be sufficient to kill certain pathogens by CGD phagocytes.

The granulomas characteristic of CGD can obstruct vital structures such as the gastrointestinal and genitourinary tracts. The mechanism for the granulomatous process in CGD is unknown but may be represented by the scheme outlined in Fig. 6. Normal neutrophils inactivate chemoattractants and other mediators via the myeloperoxidase–hydrogen-peroxide–halide (MPO–H_2O_2–Cl$^-$) system (ref. 29; see also Chapter 23, *this volume*), and failure to do so may account for prolonged leukocyte recruitment (65). In addition, inefficient degradation of antigen by the MPO–H_2O_2–Cl$^-$ system could result in chronic release of mediators, such as gamma interferon, which may play an important role in monocyte recruitment (Sechler and Gallin, *unpublished observations*) and polykaryon (giant cell) formation (see Chapter 14, *this volume*). Clearly, abnormal turn-off of inflammation is a major problem in CGD. It is of interest that obstruction from granulomas in CGD can be dramatically reversed by hydrocortisone (29), presumably by "turning off" the granulomatous process.

Myeloperoxidase Deficiency

The development in the early 1980s of an automated flow cytochemical system for performing leukocyte differential counts enabled screening of large populations for neutrophil myeloperoxidase deficiency. It is now apparent that myeloperoxidase deficiency is a relatively common disorder, occurring in approximately 1 in 2,000 individuals (see also Chapter 23, *this volume*) (113,122). Most patients with phagocyte myeloperoxidase deficiency are not at increased risk of serious infection. Disseminated infection with *Candida albicans* has been noted infre-

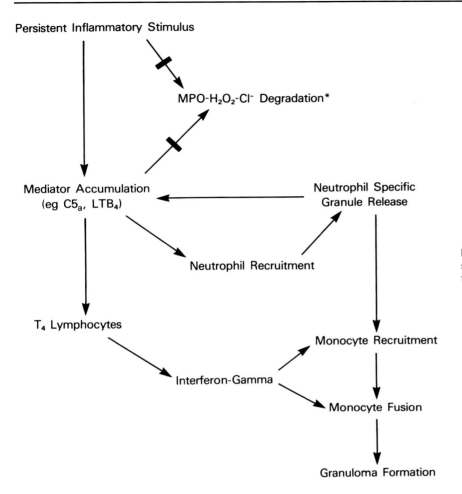

Persistent Inflammatory Stimulus

MPO-H$_2$O$_2$-Cl$^-$ Degradation*

Mediator Accumulation
(eg C5$_a$, LTB$_4$)

Neutrophil Specific
Granule Release

Neutrophil Recruitment

T$_4$ Lymphocytes

Interferon-Gamma

Monocyte Recruitment

Monocyte Fusion

Granuloma Formation

FIG. 6. Hypothetical sequence of events resulting in unusual propensity to granuloma formation in CGD.

*Absent in CGD

quently; in these patients, underlying immunosuppressive conditions, such as poorly controlled diabetes mellitus, probably contributes to the risk of infection.

Phagocytosis in myeloperoxidase deficiency is normal or increased, probably as a result of a failure to down-regulate receptor-mediated recognition mechanisms (152). Deactivation of the respiratory burst is likewise delayed, and hydrogen peroxide generation is markedly exaggerated. Bactericidal activity is usually normal, whereas candidacidal activity may be moderately-to-severely impaired (122). Unlike patients with CGD, patients with myeloperoxidase deficiency do not get granulomas as a complication of their disease. Presumably this is because, as a result of excessive hydrogen peroxide generation, patients with myeloperoxidase deficiency do not have difficulty metabolizing chemoattractants and other mediators of inflammation (82).

Approximately 50% of patients with myeloperoxidase deficiency are totally deficient in myeloperoxidase; the other patients have a partial deficiency associated with decreased amounts of structurally and functionally normal myeloperoxidase (113,122). Native myeloperoxidase consists of two heavy-light chain dimers, each with a heavy chain of approximately 59 kD and a light chain of about 14 kD. The interrelationships between the subunits and the location of heme groups have not been fully established (96,112). Recent studies indicate that myeloperoxidase synthesis ceases with neutrophil maturation and that myeloperoxidase deficiency is not due to absence of the gene encoding for myeloperoxidase but, instead, is due to a defect in cotranslational or posttranslational processing of a myeloperoxidase precursor that results in a failure to package the enzyme correctly into the azurophil granule (96). While current concepts of the defect would not exclude a single gene mutation, transmission patterns in myeloperoxidase deficiency are not consistent with simple autosomal recessive inheritance (122). Recently the genetic lesion in myeloperoxidase deficiency has been localized to chromosome 17 (Nauseef, *personal communication*).

HYPERIMMUNOGLOBULIN E-RECURRENT INFECTION (JOB'S) SYNDROME

In 1966, Davis et al. (40) described two girls with persistent weeping eczematoid lesions and large subcutaneous staphylococcal abscesses that were termed "cold" because they lacked typical signs of inflammation. Otitis, sinusitis, staphylococcal pneumonia, furunculosis, and cellulitis were prominent features. The severe problem with furunculosis resulted in the eponym "Job's syndrome." Patients described in subsequent reports have had similar clinical features in addition to characteristic coarse facies with hypertelorism, prominent jaw, cranial synostosis, and osteoporosis (for reviews see refs. 24,44,85, and 87). Recurrent cutaneous and sinopulmonary infection with *Staphylococcus aureus* is the major problem clinically, but infection with *Hemophilus influenzae* is also common. Following pneumonia, these patients have difficulty healing and often develop pneumatoceles and cavitary lung lesions that may get infected with *Aspergillus* sp. In addition, approximately 50% of the patients have mucocutaneous candidiasis. Characteristically the patients have extreme elevation of serum IgE, particularly against *S. aureus* and *Candida albicans* (11). The IgE is usually higher than in patients with eczema and recurrent cutaneous *S. aureus* infection and has been shown to be related to increased IgE synthesis and decreased catabolism (46). In addition, there is low or absent serum and salivary anti-*S. aureus* IgA, slight elevation of IgM, and normal IgD (45). The low anti-*S. aureus* IgA correlates with sinopulmonary infections (45). There is a low-grade eosinophilia and prominent eosinophil enrichment at infected foci (24).

Patients with this syndrome have striking depression of acute inflammation, as evidenced by the "cold" abscesses despite overwhelming local infection. The basis for the depressed inflammation and recurrent infections is unknown. Abnormal neutrophil and monocyte chemotaxis has also been documented, and it has been argued that too few phagocytes arrive too late (32,42). A chemotactic inhibitory factor produced *in vitro* by mononuclear cells from Job's patients has been described (42,43). The material was partially purified and was shown to be heterogeneous, with molecular weights of approximately 61,000 and 30,000 to 45,000; it was also shown to be sensitive to proteolytic digestion and stable at 56°C. Although the abnormality of phagocyte chemotaxis may contribute to the recurrent infections, the chemotactic defect is variable and unlikely fully explains the depressed inflammation (42).

Other factors may contribute to the compromised host defenses in this syndrome. Hill (85,86) suggested that elevated histamine, which is known to inhibit neutrophil function (141), would be released locally as organisms interacted with organism-specific IgE. There have been reports of the efficacy of antihistamines (H2 blockers) in association with improved *in-vitro* leukocyte chemotaxis (86). However, elevation of urinary histamine has been seen in only some patients, and the increased urinary histamine appears to be related to eczematoid dermatitis and not to infection (47). The latter observations, together with our impression that antihistamines have not helped our patients (Gallin, *unpublished observations*), raises some question of the clinical importance of histamine in these patients' compromised defenses.

Lymphocyte function in the hyper-IgE-recurrent infection syndrome is also abnormal (76). Delayed hypersensitivity responses to a variety of skin-test antigens are impaired in some, but not all, patients (73). Mitogen-induced and antigen-induced lymphocyte transformation is also impaired, especially with regard to candida antigen and tetanus toxoid, and is perhaps related to the mucocutaneous candidiasis in many patients. The patients have deficient suppressor T-cell numbers, which may account for increased IgE. There has been no evidence of increased percentages of IgE-bearing B cells. All the patients have low or absent salivary and plasma antistaphylococcal IgA despite recurrent infection with *S. aureus* (45). This latter finding likely contributes to the propensity to mucosal infections.

Thus, although there is little question that patients with hyper-IgE-recurrent infection syndrome comprise a separate clinical entity, the specific abnormality is not known. It is clear that there is a profound abnormality of inflammation, with defects of phagocytes, lymphocytes, and immunoglobulins. In addition there are abnormalities of bone with hypertelorism, protruding jaw, and cranial synostosis. The broad spectrum of abnormalities suggests a regulatory defect that has yet to be defined.

Several patients with the hyper-IgE-recurrent infection syndrome also have osteogenesis imperfecta (20), a genetic disease with an abnormality localized to chromosome 7. Other patients who do not have Job's syndrome have been reported with defective chemotaxis where the only other abnormality is a deletion on chromosome 7 (92,131). Speculation has risen concerning the possible existence of a "neutrophil migration factor" in the region of chromosome 7q22 to 7qter (56,120). A gene for the alpha-II chain of Type-1 collagen is located at 7q21-7q22 (125). Although the karyotypes we have examined in patients with hyper-IgE-recurrent infection syndrome have so far been normal, it is possible that a small defect in the 7q21 to 7qter region may lead to manifestations of the hyper-IgE-recurrent infection syndrome, disordered chemotaxis as well as to connective tissue abnormalities manifested clinically as coarse facies and scoliosis. We are currently investigating this possibility using chromosome-7-specific

DNA probes in our patients with the hyper-IgE-recurrent infection syndrome.

LOCALIZED JUVENILE PERIODONTITIS

In patients with neutropenia or functional phagocyte impairment, mucosal ulcerations, gingivitis, and periodontitis occur frequently and are often severe. In most cases, intraoral infection is associated with recurrent infection at other sites. In contrast, localized juvenile periodontitis is an adolescent disease of the supporting structures of the permanent dentition, characterized by severe alveolar bone loss limited primarily to the first molars and incisors. Patients are not predisposed to extraoral infection (160–162).

Genco and co-workers (161,162) have demonstrated in patients with localized juvenile periodontitis a moderate, but reproducible, impairment of chemotaxis to formyl peptides and C5a; neutrophil adherence is normal. Defective chemotaxis persists following aggressive local therapy and has been demonstrated in siblings prior to the development of the clinical syndrome. Limited data suggest that formyl peptide receptor numbers and affinities are normal; however, receptor up-regulation or internalization is impaired (161). It remains unclear whether the suspected abnormalities in receptor processing in localized juvenile periodontitis are causally related or are only secondary. If confirmed, studies indicating that neutrophils from patients with localized juvenile periodontitis are deficient in a 108-kD surface protein would suggest a role for the latter in the organizing and processing of chemotactic receptors (160).

NEUTROPHIL HETEROGENEITY AS A POSSIBLE EXPLANATION FOR CERTAIN ACQUIRED CHEMOTACTIC DEFECTS

Neutrophil heterogeneity was first suggested by Florence Sabin in 1923 (132). She observed that myelocytes had poor locomotory capacity and speculated that the poor movement of immature myeloid cells kept them in the marrow. The wide range of individual rates of neutrophil locomotion was described in the same year (103). Based on clot preparation studies, Howard (89) subsequently divided neutrophils into fast-moving (>7 μm/min) and slow-moving (<7 μm/min) populations. Harvath and Leonard (80) described two neutrophil populations separable on the basis of their chemotactic responsiveness. Using a fluorescence-activated cell sorter, Seligmann et al. (140) demonstrated a heterogeneous response of neutrophil binding of the chemotactic peptide f-Met-Leu-Phe.

Monoclonal antibodies that bind to neutrophils in a heterogeneous fashion have been described. Ball et al. (9) reported a monoclonal antibody (AML-2-23) made against acute myelogenous leukemia myeloblasts that labeled from 85% to 90% of normal neutrophils. The fluorescence staining pattern of each individual studied showed a single peak, and nonstaining cells were defined as those cells on the peak that overlapped in the negative control range. Clement et al. (34) described two anti-neutrophil monoclonal antibodies (1B5 and 4D1) that recognized a mean of 57% and 51% of neutrophils, respectively. The fluorescence staining pattern was that of two distinct peaks, with the more negative peak overlapping the negative control peak. A mouse IgG1 monoclonal antibody (31D8) that binds heterogeneously to neutrophils, exhibiting a bright and dull staining pattern, has been described (142). When neutrophils are stained with fluorochrome-labeled 31D8, the vast majority stain in a bright pattern. The dull staining cells tend to be less capable of chemotaxis, NBT reduction, and membrane depolarization. Band forms are 31D8-dull, but clearly many 31D8-dull-staining neutrophils appear morphologically mature (Brown, Gallin, and Malech, *unpublished observations*). It is not clear at this point how 31D8 relates to neutrophil maturity. Of interest, however, is the demonstration that 31D8 expression becomes undetectable in a select group of chronic myelogenous leukemia patients who, within a year, develop blast crisis (70).

A new anti-neutrophil IgG monoclonal antibody, C10, clearly binds neutrophils heterogeneously, with distinct positive and negative peaks (23). Whereas variation between individuals in percent positive staining of neutrophils is great, the variation in the same individual over time is small. Furthermore, while the negative population number and staining pattern remains constant, the positive population increases its expression of C10 with activation *in vitro* or in the circulation after endotoxin injection or following exudation *in vivo* (23).

Although work is ongoing, neutrophil heterogeneity has not yet been proven to be important in normal or pathologic phagocyte function. However, the possibility that shifts in the distribution of populations of neutrophils may lead to phagocyte defects, as reported following acute infection or other examples of inflammation (61), emphasizes the potential importance of neutrophil heterogeneity in the pathogenesis of certain acquired phagocyte disorders.

DISORDERS OF THE MONONUCLEAR PHAGOCYTE SYSTEM

Many disorders of the neutrophils extend to the mononuclear phagocyte system. Thus patients with CR3 deficiency, hyper IgE-recurrent infection (Job's) syndrome, Chédiak-Higashi syndrome, and chronic granulomatous diseases of childhood all have abnormalities of their mononuclear phagocytes.

Certain viral infections impair mononuclear phagocyte function. For example, influenza and herpes simplex virus infection are associated with abnormal monocyte chemotaxis (93,101,144). Abnormal monocyte chemotaxis and clearance of IgG-coated erythrocytes (discussed below) is also seen in the acquired immunodeficiency syndrome (AIDS), which is caused by a human retrovirus (143). It is likely that the defects of the monocyte-macrophage system in AIDS contribute to the increased susceptibility to opportunistic infection due to intracellular microorganisms such as *Pneumocystis carinii* and *Mycobacterium avium-intracellulare*. T lymphocytes produce a factor, possibly deficient in AIDS, that induces Fc-receptor expression and phagocytosis by mononuclear phagocytes. In other diseases, such as T-cell lymphomas, excessive release of such a T-cell factor is thought to cause erythrophagocytosis by splenic macrophages (64).

Specific defects of the mononuclear phagocytes have been described in neoplasms (see Chapter 49, *this volume*) and in certain autoimmune diseases. Removal of IgG-coated radiolabeled autologous erythrocytes, presumably via the Fc receptor of splenic macrophages, is profoundly abnormal in patients with active systemic lupus erythematosus (53). Patients with other autoimmune diseases characterized by tissue deposition of immune complexes, as seen in Sjogren's syndrome, mixed cryoglobulinemia, dermatitis herpetiformis, and chronic progressive multiple sclerosis, also have defects in Fc-receptor function, as judged by clearance of IgG-coated erythrocytes. The basis for the abnormality in Fc-receptor clearance is not known. It is of interest that clinically normal subjects with genetic haplotypes commonly associated with autoimmune disease (e.g., HLA-B8/DRw3) also have an increased incidence of defective Fc-receptor-specific functional activity, suggesting that individuals with this defect and this genetic profile are predisposed to immune complex disease.

DIAGNOSIS AND MANAGEMENT OF PHAGOCYTE DYSFUNCTION

Most patients with disorders of phagocyte function present with clinical evidence for impaired inflammation (64). Patients often have aphthous ulcers of the mucous membranes (gray ulcers without pus). Gingivitis is common and periodontal disease is frequent in some patient groups (28). Characteristically, patients with phagocyte defects have recurrent, and often severe, bacterial or fungal infections that often present as difficult management problems. Patients with congenital defects can have infections within the first few days of life. In some disorders, the frequency of infection is variable, and patients can go months or even years without major infection. Adults over 30 years of age with congenital defects are rare, suggesting that patients with such defects die at an early age.

However, in recent years with aggressive management, adults with these diseases are being seen with increasing frequency. Skin, ear, upper and lower respiratory tract, and bone infections are common. For unexplained reasons, meningitis and sepsis are rare in this group of patients.

Initial studies of white-blood-cell count and differential (and often bone marrow) examinations are followed by assessment of bone marrow reserves (steroid challenge test), marginated circulating pool (epinephrine challenge test), and marginating ability (endotoxin challenge test) (see Chapter 18, *this volume*). *In vivo* assessment of inflammation is possible with a Rebuck skin window test, in which the ability of leukocytes to accumulate at a superficial abrasion and adhere to a glass coverslip is tested. Quantitation of neutrophil and monocyte responses, as well as of mediator production *in vivo*, is readily accomplished with a blister apparatus in which phagocyte accumulation into blisters created by suction over forearm skin is monitored over time (173). *In vivo* clearance of IgG-coated erythrocytes provides a useful way to monitor the mononuclear-phagocyte system (53). *In vitro* tests of phagocyte aggregation, adherence, chemotaxis, phagocytosis, degranulation, and microbicidal activity (for *Staphylococcus aureus*) help pinpoint cellular or humoral defects which can then be further characterized at the molecular level. Deficiencies of oxidative metabolism are screened with the nitroblue tetrazolium dye (NBT) test, which is based on the ability of products of oxidative metabolism to reduce yellow, soluble NBT to blue-black formazan, an insoluble material that precipitates intracellularly and can be seen microscopically. Further aspects of neutrophil oxidative metabolism are defined by studies of superoxide and hydrogen peroxide production. (Details of phagocyte function assays can be obtained in ref. 107.)

The most important aspect of patient management is to appreciate that patients often have delayed inflammatory responses. Therefore, clinical manifestations may be minimal despite overwhelming infection, and unusual infections must always be suspected in some patients. The aggressive management of early infection is essential and described elsewhere (27). White-blood-cell transfusions appear to be an important adjunct to therapy in patients with CGD (26,123). In CGD patients it has been shown that transfused phagocytes arrive at inflammatory foci functionally intact (26). Hydrogen peroxide from the normal cells will diffuse into the CGD cells (116), and it is suspected that a few normal cells have the capacity to reconstitute the function of multiple CGD cells; this may explain why some CGD heterozygotes, who only have 15% normal phagocytes, live normal lives. In patients with CGD, prophylactic antibiotics (trimethoprim-sulfamethoxazole) diminishes the frequency of life-threatening infections (66). In CGD, when excessive granulomas lead to obstruction of vital structures such as the esophagus or ureter, steroids can bring prompt relief (29). Cure of some congenital phagocyte defects has been reported by bone marrow transplantation (3,51,91). However, complications of bone marrow transplantation are still great, and, with rigorous medical care, many patients with disorders of phagocyte function can go for years without a life-threatening infection. Therefore, bone marrow transplantation is not currently used as a form of therapy for most patients. Ultimately, gene therapy is the goal for curing the phagocyte defects. Development of gene therapy for certain phagocyte defects is being aggressively pursued in several laboratories.

REFERENCES

1. Abramson, J. S., Mills, E. L., Sawyer, M. K., Regelmann, W. R., Nelson, J. D., and Quie, P. G. (1981): Recurrent infections and delayed separation of the umbilical cord in an infant with abnormal phagocytic cell locomotion and oxidative response during particle phagocytosis. *J. Pediatr.,* 99:887–894.
2. Ambruso, D. R., Sasada, M., Nishiyama, H., Kubo, A., Koiyama, A., and Allen, R. H. (1984): Defective bacterial activity and absence of specific granules in neutrophils from a patient with recurrent bacterial infections. *J. Clin. Immunol.,* 4:23–30.
3. Anderson, D. C., Schmalstieg, F. C., Arnaout, M. A., Kohl, S., Tosi, M. F., Dana, N., Buffone, G. J., Hughes, B. J., Brinkley, B. R., Dickey, W. D., Abramson, J. S., Springer, T., Boxer, L. A., Hollers, J. M., and Smith, C. W. (1984): Abnormalities of polymorphonuclear leukocyte function associated with a heritable deficiency of high molecular weight surface glycoproteins (gp138): Common relationship to diminished cell adherence. *J. Clin. Invest.,* 74:536–551.
4. Anderson, D. C., and Springer, T. A. (1987): Leukocyte adhesion deficiency: An inherited defect in the Mac-1, LFA-1, and p150,95 glycoproteins. *Am. Rev. Med.,* 38:175–194.
5. Arnaout, M. A., Pitt, J., Cohen, H. J., Melamed, J., Rosen, F. S., and Cohen, H. R. (1982): Deficiency of a granulocyte membrane glycoprotein (gp150) in a boy with recurrent bacterial infections. *N. Engl. J. Med.,* 306:693–699.
6. Arnaout, M. A., Spits, H., Terhorst, C., Pitt, J., and Todel, R. F. (1984): Deficiency of a leukocyte surface glycoprotein (LFA-1) in two patients with MO1 deficiency: Effects of cell activation on MO1/LFA-1 surface expression on normal and deficient leukocytes. *J. Clin. Invest.,* 74:1291–1300.
7. Arnaout, M. A., Todd, R. F., Dana, N., Melamed, J., Schlossman, S. F., and Colten, H. R. (1983): Inhibition of phagocytosis of complement C3- or immunoglobulin G-coated particles and C3bi binding by monoclonal antibodies to a monocyte-granulocyte membrane glycoprotein (Mol). *J. Clin. Invest.,* 72:171–179.
8. Baehner, R. L., Kunkel, L. M., Monaco, A. P., Haines, J. L., Conneally, P. M., Palmer, C., Heerema, N., and Orkin, S. H. (1986): DNA linkage analysis of X-chromosome-linked chronic granulomatous disease. *Proc. Natl. Acad. Sci. USA,* 83:3398–3401.
9. Ball, E. D., Graziano, R. F., Shen, L., and Fanger, M. W. (1982): Monoclonal antibodies to novel myeloid antigens reveal human neutrophil heterogeneity. *Proc. Natl. Acad. Sci. USA,* 79:5374–5378.
10. Beller, D. I., Springer, T. A., and Scheiber, R. D. (1982): Anti-Mac-1 selectively inhibits the mouse and human type three complement receptor. *J. Exp. Med.,* 56:1000–1009.
11. Berger, M., Kirkpatrick, C. H., Goldsmith, P. K., and Gallin, J. I. (1980): IgE antibodies to *Staphylococcus aureus* and *Candida albicans* in patients with the syndrome of hyperimmunoglobulin E and recurrent infections. *J. Immunol.,* 125:2437–2443.
12. Bissenden, J. G., Haeney, M. R., Tarlow, M. J., and Thompson,

13. R. (1981): Delayed separation of the umbilical cord, severe widespread infections, and immunodeficiency. *Arch. Dis. Child.,* 56: 397–399.
14. Blume, R. S., and Wolff, S. M. (1972): The Chédiak-Higashi syndrome: Studies in four patients and a review of the literature. *Medicine,* 51:247–280.
15. Borregaard, N., Heiple, J. M., Simons, E. R., and Clark, R. A. (1983): Subcellular localization of the *b*-cytochrome component of the human neutrophil microbicidal oxidase. *J. Cell Biol.,* 97: 25–61.
16. Bowens, T. S., Ochs, H. D., Altman, L. C., Perksin, W. D., Babior, B. M., Klebanoff, S. J., and Wedgwood, R. J. (1982): Severe recurrent bacterial infectious associated with defective adherrence and chemotaxis in two patients with neutrophils deficient in cell-associated glycoproteins. *J. Pediatr.,* 101:932–940.
17. Boxer, L. A., Coates, T. D., Haak, R. A., Wolach, J. B., Hoffstein, S., and Baehner, R. L. (1982): Lactoferrin deficiency associated with altered granulocyte function. *N. Engl. J. Med.,* 307:404–409.
18. Boxer, L. A., Haak, R. A., Yang, H-H., et al. (1982): Membrane-bound lactoferrin alters the surface properties of polymorphonuclear leukocytes. *J. Clin. Invest.,* 70:1049–1057.
19. Boxer, L. A., Hedley-Whyte, E. T., and Stossel, T. P. (1974): Neutrophil actin dysfunction and abnormal neutrophil behavior. *N. Engl. J. Med.,* 291:1093–1099.
20. Boxer, L. A., Watanabe, A. M., Rister, M., Besch, H. R., Jr., Allen, J., and Baehner, R. L. (1976): Correction of leukocyte function in Chédiak-Higashi syndrome by ascorbate. *N. Engl. J. Med.,* 295: 1041–1045.
21. Brestel, E. P., Klingberg, W. G., Veltri, R. W., and Donn, J. S. (1982): Osteogenesis imperfecta tarda in a child with hyper-IgE syndrome. *Am. J. Dis. Child.,* 136:774–776.
22. Brenton-Gorius, J., Mason, D. Y., Bruiot, D., Vilde, J. L., and Griscelli, C. (1980): Lactoferrin deficiency as a consequence of a lack of specific granule in neutrophils from a patient with recurrent infection. *Am. J. Pathol.,* 99:413–419.
23. Broxmeyer, H. E., DeSousa, M., Smithyman, A., et al. (1980): Specificity and modulation of the action of lactoferrin, a negative feedback regulator of myelopoiesis. *Blood,* 55:324–333.
24. Brown, C. C., Malech, H. L., Shrimpton, C. F., Beverly, P. C., Segal, T., and Gallin, J. I. (1987): Unique human neutrophil populations defined by monoclonal antibody ED12F8C10. *Clin. Res.,* 35:421a.
25. Buckley, R. H., and Sampson, H. A. (1981): The hyperimmunoglobulinema E Syndrome. In: *Clinical Immunology Update,* edited by E. C. Franklin, pp. 148–167. Elsevier/North-Holland, Amsterdam.
26. Buescher, E. S., Gaither, T., Nath, J., and Gallin, J. I. (1985): Abnormal adherence-related functions of neutrophils, monocytes, and Epstein-Barr virus-transformed B cells in a patient with C3bi receptor deficiency. *Blood,* 65:1382–1390.
27. Buescher, E. S., and Gallin, J. I. (1982): Leukocyte transfusions in chronic granulomatous disease. *N. Engl. J. Med.,* 307:800–803.
28. Buescher, E. S., and Gallin, J. I. (1983): Disorders of phagocyte function, In: *Current Therapy in Allergy and Immunology,* edited by A. S. Fauci, pp. 287–293. Decker, Philadelphia.
29. Charon, J. A., Mergenhagen, S. E., and Gallin, J. I. (1985): Gingivitis and oral ulceration in patients with neutrophil dysfunction. *J. Oral Pathol.,* 14:150–155.
30. Chin, T. W., Stiehin, E. R., Falloon, J., and Gallin, J. I. (1987): Corticosteroids in the treatment of obstructive lesions of chronic granulomatous disease. *J. Pediatr.,* accepted for publication.
31. Clark, R. A. (1983): Extracellular effects of the myeloperoxidase-hydrogen peroxide-halide system. In: Weissmann, G., ed. *Advances in Inflammation Research, Vol. 5,* p. 107. Raven Press, New York.
32. Clark, R. A., and Kimball, H. R. (1971): Defective granulocyte chemotaxis in the Chédiak-Higashi syndrome. *J. Clin. Invest.,* 50: 2645–2652.
33. Clark, R. A., Root, R. K., Kimball, H. R., and Kirkpatrick, C. H. (1973): Defective neutrophil chemotaxis and cellular immunity in a child with recurrent infections. *Ann. Intern. Med.,* 78:515–519.
34. Clawson, C. C., Repine, J. E., and White, J. G. (1979): The Chédiak-

Higashi syndrome: Quantitation of a deficiency in maximal bactericidal capacity. *Am. J. Pathol.,* 94:539–551.

34. Clement, L. T., Lehmeryer, J. E., and Gartland, G. L. (1983): Identification of neutrophil subpopulations with monoclonal antibodies. *Blood,* 61:326–332.

35. Crowley, C. A., Curnutte, J. T., Rosin, R. E., Andre-Schwartz, J., Gallin, J. I., Klempner, M., Snyderman, R., Southwick, F. S., Stossel, T. P., and Babior, B. M. (1980): An inherited abnormality of neutrophil adhesion. Its genetic transmission and its association with a missing protein. *N. Engl. J. Med.,* 302:1163–1168.

36. Dale, D. C., Guerry, DuPont, Wewerka, J. R., Bull, J. M., and Chusid, M. J. (1979): Chronic neutropenia. *Medicine,* 58:128–144.

37. Dana, N., Todd, R. F., Pitt, J., Springer, T. A., and Arnaout, M. A. (1984): Deficiency of a surface membrane glycoprotein (Mol) in man. *J. Clin. Invest.,* 73:153–159.

38. Davies, E. G., Isaacs, D., and Levinsky, R. J. (1982): Defective immune interferon production and natural killer activity associated with poor neutrophil mobility and delayed umbilical cord separation. *Clin. Exp. Immunol.,* 50:454–660.

39. Davis, J. M., Dineen, P., and Gallin, J. I. (1980): Neutrophil degranulation and abnormal chemotaxis after thermal injury. *J. Immunol.,* 124:1467–1471.

40. Davis, S. D., Schaller, J., and Wedgwood, R. J. (1966): Job's syndrome: Recurrent "cold" staphyloccal abscesses. *Lancet,* 1:1013–1015.

41. Dinauer, M., Parkos, C. A., Jesaitis, A. J., and Orkin, S. H. (1987): Identification of the in vivo protein encoded by the gene mutated in X-linked chronic granulomatous disease. *Clin. Res.,* 35:598A.

42. Donabedian, H., and Gallin, J. I. (1982): Mononuclear cells from patients with the hyperimmunoglobulin E-recurrent infection syndrome produce an inhibitor of leukocyte chemotaxis. *J. Clin. Invest.,* 69:1155–1163.

43. Donabedian, H., and Gallin, J. I. (1983): Two inhibitors of neutrophil chemotaxis are produced by hyperimmunoglobulin E recurrent infection syndrome mononuclear cells exposed to heat-killed staphlococci. *Infect. Immun.,* 40:1030–1037.

44. Donabedian, H., and Gallin, J. I. (1983): The hyperimmunoglobulin E recurrent infection (Job's) syndrome. *Medicine,* 62:195–208.

45. Dreskin, S. C., Goldsmith, P. K., and Gallin, J. I. (1985): Immunoglobulins in the hyperimmunoglobulin E and recurrent infection (Job's) syndrome. *J. Clin. Invest.,* 75:26–34.

46. Dreskin, S. C., Goldsmith, P. K., Strober, W., Zech, L. A., and Gallin, J. I. (1987): The metabolism of IgE in patients with markedly elevated serum IgE levels. *J. Clin. Invest.* (in press).

47. Dreskin, S. C., Kaliner, M. A., and Gallin, J. I. (1987): Elevated urinary histamine in the hyperimmunoglobulin-E and recurrent infection (Job's) syndrome: Association with eczematoid dermatits and not with infection. *J. Allergy Clin. Immunol.* (in press).

48. Duque, R. E., Phan, S. H., Hudson, J. L., Till, G. O., and Ward, P. A. (1985): Functional defects in phagocytic cells following thermal injury: Application of flow cytometric analysis. *Am. J. Pathol.,* 118:116–121.

49. Ehrlich, P. (1900): Leukocytose. In: *13th Congress of Internal Medicine,* Paris.

50. Falloon, J., and Gallin, J. I. (1986): Neutrophil granules in health and disease. *J. Allergy Clin. Immunol.,* 77:653–662.

51. Fisher, A., Trung, P. H., Descamps-Latsdra, B., Lisowska-Grospierre, B., Gerota, I., Perez, N., Scheinmetzler, C., Durandy, A., Virelizier, J. L., and Griscelli, C. (1983): Bone marrow-transplantation for inborn error of phagocytic cells associated with defective adherence, chemotaxis, and oxidative response during opsonized particle phagocytosis. *Lancet,* 2:473–476.

52. Fletcher, M., and Gallin, J. I. (1983): Human neutrophils contain an intracellular pool of putative receptors for the chemoattractant *N*-formymethionyl leucylphenylalanine. *Blood,* 62:792–799.

53. Frank, M. M., Lawley, T. J., Hamberger, M. I., and Brown, E. J. (1983): Immunoglobulin G Fc receptor-mediated clearance in autoimmune diseases. *Ann. Intern. Med.,* 98:206–218.

54. Freeman, K. B., Huges, B. J., Buffone, G., and Anderson, D. C. (1984): Abnormal motility of neonatal PMNs: Relationships to impaired "upregulation" of chemotactic factor receptors and lactoferrin secretion. *Proc. Infect. Immunocomp. Host,* III:27 (abstract).

55. Gabig, T. G., and Lefker, B. A. (1984): Deficient flavoprotein component of the NADPH-dependent O_2 generating oxidase in the neutrophils from three male patients with chronic granulomatous disease. *J. Clin. Invest.,* 73:701–705.

56. Gahmberg, C. G., Anderson, L. C., Ruutu, P., et al. (1979): Decrease of the major high molecular weight surface glycoprotein of human granulocytes in monosomy-7 associated with defective chemotaxis. *Blood,* 54:401–406.

57. Gaither, T. A., Gallin, J. I., Iida, K., Nussenzweig, V., and Frank, M. M. (1984): Deficiency in C3b receptors on neutrophils of patients with chronic granulomatous disease and hyperimmunoglobulin-E recurrent infection (Job's) syndrome. *Inflammation,* 82:429–444.

58. Gaither, T. A., Medley, S. R., Gallin, J. I., and Frank, M. M. (1987): Studies of phagocytosis in chronic granulomatous disease. *Inflammation,* 11:211–227.

59. Gallin, J. I. (1981): Abnormal phagocyte chemotaxis: Pathophysiology, clinical manifestations, and management of patients. *Rev. Infect. Dis.,* 3:1196–1220.

60. Gallin, J. I. (1984): Neutrophil specific granules: A fuse that ignites the inflammatory response. *Clin. Res.,* 32:320–328.

61. Gallin, J. I. (1984): Human neutrophil heterogeneity exists but is it meaningful? *Blood,* 63:977–983.

62. Gallin, J. I. (1985): Neutrophil specific granule deficiency. *Annu. Rev. Med.,* 36:263–274.

63. Gallin, J. I. (1985): Leukocyte adherence-related glycoproteins LFA-1, Mol, and p150,95: A new group of monoclonal antibodies, a new disease, and a possible opportunity to understand the molecular basis of leukocyte adherence. *J. Infect. Dis.,* 152:661–664.

64. Gallin, J. I. (1987): Disorders of phagocytic cells. In: *Harrison's Principles of Internal Medicine,* 11th edition, edited by E. Braunwald, K. J. Isselbacher, R. G. Petersdorf, J. D. Wilson, J. B. Martin, and A. S. Fauci, pp. 278–283, McGraw-Hill, New York.

65. Gallin, J. I., and Buescher, E. S. (1983): Abnormal regulation of inflammatory skin responded in male patients with chronic granulomatous diseases. *Inflammation,* 7:227–232.

66. Gallin, J. I., Buescher, E. S., Seligmann, B. E., Nath, J., Gaither, T. E., and Katz, P. (1983): Recent advances in chronic granulomatous disease. *Ann. Intern. Med.,* 99:657–674.

67. Gallin, J. I., Elin, R. J., Hubert, R. T., Fauci, A. S., Kaliner, M. A., and Wolff, S. M. (1979): Efficacy of ascorbic acid in Chédiak-Higashi Syndrome (CHS): Studies in humans and mice. *Blood,* 226–234.

68. Gallin, J. I., and Fauci, A. S., editors (1982): *Advances in Host Defense Mechanisms, Vol. 3, Chronic Granulomatous Disease.* Raven Press, New York.

69. Gallin, J. I., Fletcher, M. P., Seligmann, B. E., Hoffstein, S., Cehrs, K., and Mounessa, N. (1982): Human neutrophil-specific granule deficiency: A model to assess the role of neutrophil-specific granules in the evolution of the inflammatory response. *Blood,* 59:1317–1329.

70. Gallin, J. I., Jacobson, R. J., Seligmann, B. E., Metcalf, J. A., McKay, J. H., Sacher, R. A., and Malech, H. L. (1986): A neutrophil membrane marker reveals two groups of chronic myelogenous leukemia and its absence may be a marker of disease progression. *Blood,* 68:343–346.

71. Gallin, J. I., Klimerman, J. A., Padgett, G. A., and Wolff, S. M. (1975): Defective mononuclear leukocyte chemotaxis in the Chédiak-Higashi syndrome of humans, mink, and cattle. *Blood,* 45:863–870.

72. Gallin, J. I., Metcalf, J. A., Roos, D., Seligmann, B. E., and Friedman, M. M. (1984): Organelle-depleted human neutrophil cytoplasts used to study fmet-leu-phe receptor modulation and cell functions. *J. Immunol.,* 133:415–421.

73. Gallin, J. I., Wright, D. G., Malech, H. L., Davis, J. M., Klempner, M. S., Kirkpatrick, C. H. (1980): Disorders of phagocyte chemotaxis. *Ann. Intern. Med.,* 92:520–538.

74. Ganz, T., Metcalf, J. A., Gallin, J. I., and Lehrer, R. I. (1987): Two genetic disorders that affect human neutrophils are associated with deficiencies of microbicidal and cytotoxic granule proteins. *Clin. Res.,* 35:424A.

75. Gardner, J. P., Melnick, D. A., and Malech, H. L. (1986): Characterization of the formyl peptide chemotactic receptor appearing

at the phagocyte cell surface after exposure to phorbol myristate acetate. *J. Immunol.,* 136:1400–1405.

76. Geha, R. S., Reinherz, E., Lung, D., McKee, K. T., Schlossman, S., and Rosen, F. S. (1981): Deficiency of Suppressor T cells in the hyperimmunoglobulin E syndrome. *J. Clin. Invest.,* 68:783–791.

77. Haak, R. A., Ingraham, L. M., Baehner, R. L., and Boxer, L. A. (1979): Membrane fluidity in human and mouse Chédiak-Higashi leukocytes. *J. Clin. Invest.,* 64:138–144.

78. Hamers, M. N., de Boer, M., Meerhof, L. J., Weening, R. S., Roos, D. (1984): Complementation in monocyte hybrids revealing genetic heterogeneity in chronic granulomatous disease. *Nature,* 307:553–555.

79. Harvath, L., and Andersen, B. R. (1979): Defective initiation of oxidative metabolism in polymorphonuclear leukocytes. *N. Engl. J. Med.,* 300:1130–1135.

80. Harvath, L., and Leonard, E. J. (1982): Two neutrophil populations in human blood with different chemotactic activities: Separation and chemoattractant binding. *Infect. Immun.,* 36:443–451.

81. Hayward, A. R., Leonard, J., Wood, C. B. S., Harvey, B. A. M., Greenwood, M. C., and Soothill, J. F. (1979): Delayed separation of the umbilical cord, widespread infections and defective neutrophil mobility. *Lancet,* 1:1099–1101 (letter).

82. Henderson, W. R., and Klebanoff, S. J. (1983): Leukotriene production and inactivation by normal, chronic granulomatous disease and myeloperoxidase-deficient neutrophils. *J. Biol. Chem.,* 258:13522–13527.

83. Hibbs, M. S., Kang, A. H., and Bainton, D. F. (1986): Ultrastructural localization of gelatinase. *Clin. Res.,* 34:459A (abstract).

84. Higson, F. K., Durbin, L., Pavlotsky, N., and Tauber, A. I. (1985): Studies of cytochrome b_{245} translocation in the PMA stimulation of the human neutrophil NADPH-oxidase. *J. Immunol.,* 135:519–524.

85. Hill, H. R. (1982): The syndrome of hyperimmunoglobulin E and recurrent infections. *Am. J. Dis. Child.,* 136:767–771.

86. Hill, H. R. (1984): Clinical disorders of leukocyte function. In: *Contemporary Topics in Immunobiology, Vol. 14,* edited by R. Snydermann, pp. 345–393. Plenum, New York.

87. Hill, H. R. (1982): The syndrome of hyperimmunoglobulinemia E and recurrent infections. *Am. J. Dis. Child.,* 136:767–771.

88. Ho, M. K., and Springer, T. A. (1983): Biosynthesis and assembly of the alpha and beta subunits of Mac-1, a macrophage glycoprotein associated with complement receptor function. *J. Biol. Chem.,* 258:2766–2769.

89. Howard, T. H. (1982): Quantitation of the locomotive behavior of polymorphonuclear leukocytes in clot preparations. *Blood,* 59:946–951.

90. Jesaitis, A. J., Naemura, J. R., Painter, R. G., Sklar, L. A., and Cochrane, C. G. (1982): Intracellular localization of *N*-formyl chemotactic receptor and Mg^{++} dependent ATPase in human granulocytes. *Biophys. Biochem. Acta,* 719:556–568.

91. Kamani, N., August, C. S., Douglas, S. D., Burkey, E., Etzioni, A., and Lischner, H. W. (1984): Bone marrow transplantation in chronic granulomatous disease. *J. Pediatr.,* 105:42–46.

92. Kere, J., Rwutu, T., and de la Chapelle, A. (1986): Monosomy 7 in granulocytes and monocytes in myelodysplastic syndrome. *N. Engl. J. Med.,* 316:499–503.

93. Kleinerman, E. S., Snyderman, R., and Daniels, C. A. (1974): Depression of human monocyte chemotaxis by herpes simplex and influenza viruses. *J. Immunol.,* 113:1562–1567.

94. Klempner, M. S., Dinarello, C. A., and Gallin, J. I. (1978): Human leukocyte pyrogen induces release of specific granule contents from human neutrophils. *J. Clin. Invest.,* 61:1330–1336.

95. Klempner, M. S., and Wolff, S. M. (1980): The neutrophil in host defense: Congenital, acquired and drug-induced abnormalities. In: *Infections in Abnormal Host,* edited by Michael Grieco, pp. 11–37. Yorke Medical Books.

96. Koeffler, H. P., Ranyard, J., and Pertcheck, M. (1985): Myeloperoxidase. Its structure and expression during myeloid differentiation. *Blood,* 65:484–491.

97. Kohl, S., Springer, T. A., Shmalsteig, F. C., Loo, L. S., and Anderson, D. C. (1984): Defective natural killer cytotoxicity and polymorphonuclear leukocyte antibody-dependent cellular cytoxicity

in patients with LFA-1/OKM-1 deficiency. *J. Immunol.,* 133:2972–2978.

98. Komiyama, A., Morosawa, H., Nakahata, T., Miyagawa, Y., and Akabane, T. (1979): Abnormal neutrophil maturation in a neutrophil defect with morphologic abnormality and impaired function. *J. Pediatr.,* 94:19–25.

99. Kyle, R. A. (1980): Natural history of chronic neutropenia. *N. Engl. J. Med.,* 302:908–909.

100. Lanier, L. L., Arnaout, M. A., Schwarting, R., Warner, N. L., and Ross, G. D. (1985): p150/95 a third member of the LFA-1/CR3 polypeptide family identified by anti Leu M5 monoclonal antibody. *Eur. J. Immunol.,* 15:713–718.

101. Larson, H. E., and Blades, R. (1976): Impairment of human polymorphonuclear leukocyte function by influenza virus. *Lancet,* 1:283–284.

102. Lew, D. P., Southwick, F. S., Stossel, T. P., Whitin, J. C., Simons, E., and Cohen, H. J. (1981): A variant of chronic granulomatous disease: Deficient oxidative metabolism due to a low-affinity NADPH oxidase. *N. Engl. J. Med.,* 305:1329–1333.

103. McCutcheon, M. (1923): Studies on the locomotion of leukocytes. I. The normal rate of locomotion of human neutrophilic leukocytes *in vitro. Am. J. Physiol.,* 66:180–195.

104. McDonald, S. M., Pulford, K., Falini, B., Micklem, K., and Mason, D. Y. (1986): A monoclonal antibody recognizing the p150/95 leukocyte differentiation antigen. *Immunology,* 59:427–431.

105. Marlin, S. D., Mortin, C. C., Anderson, D. C., and Springer, T. A. (1986): LFA-1 immunodeficiency disease: Definition of the genetic defect and chromosomal mapping of alpha and beta subunits by complementation in hybrid cells. *J. Exp. Med.,* 164:855–867.

106. Mentzer, S. J., Gromkowski, S. H., Krensky, A. M., Burakoff, S. J., and Marz, E. (1985): LFA-1 membrane molecule in the regulation of homotypic adhesions of human B lymphocytes. *J. Immunol.,* 135:9–11.

107. Metcalf, J. A., Gallin, J. I., Nauseef, W. M., and Root, R. K. (1986): *Laboratory Manual of Neutrophil Function.* Raven Press, New York.

108. Metchnikoff, E. (1905): *Immunity in Infective Diseases.* Cambridge University Press, Cambridge, England.

109. Miedema, F., Tetteroo, P. A. T., Tepstra, F. G., Keizer, G., Roos, M., Weening, R. S., Weemaes, C. M. R., Roos, D., and Melief, C. J. M. (1985): Immunologic studies with LFA-1 and Mol-deficient lymphocytes from a patient with recurrent bacterial infections. *J. Immunol.,* 134:3075–3081.

110. Moore, F. D., Davis, C., Rodrick, M., Mannick, J. A., and Fearon, D. T. (1986): Neutrophil activation in thermal injury as assessed by increased expression of complement receptors. *N. Engl. J. Med.,* 948–953.

111. Nath, J., Flavin, M., and Gallin, J. I. (1982): Tubulin tyrosinolation in human polymorphonuclear leukocytes: Studies in normal subjects and in patients with the Chédiak-Higashi syndrome. *J. Cell Biol.,* 95:519–526.

112. Nauseef, W. M. (1986): Myeloperoxidase biosynthesis by a human promyelocytic leukemia cell line: Insight into myeloperoxidase deficiency. *Blood,* 67:965–972.

113. Nauseef, W. M., Root, R. K., and Malech, H. L. (1983): Biochemical and immunologic analysis of hereditary myeloperoxidase deficiency. *J. Clin. Invest.,* 71:1297–1307.

114. Newburger, P. E., Luscinskas, F. W., Ryan, T., Beard, C. J., Wright, J., Platt, O. S., Simons, E. R., and Tauber, A. I. (1986): Variant chronic granulomatous disease: Modulation of the neutrophil defect by severe infection. *Blood,* 68:914–919.

115. Ohno, Y., Buescher, E. S., Roberts, R., Metcalf, J. A., and Gallin, J. I. (1986): Reevaluation of cytochrome *b* and flavin adenine dinucleotide in neutrophils from patients with chronic granulomatous disease and description of a family with probably autosomal recessive inheritance of cytochrome *b* deficiency. *Blood,* 67:1132–1138.

116. Ohno, Y., and Gallin, J. I. (1985): Diffusion of extracellular hydrogen peroxide into intracellular compartments of human neutrophils. *J. Biol. Chem.,* 260:8438–8446.

117. Ohno, Y., Seligmann, B. E., and Gallin, J. I. (1985): Cytochrome

b translocation to human neutrophil plasma membranes and superoxide release. *J. Biol. Chem.*, 260:2409–2414.

118. Oseas, R., Yang, H-H, Baehner, R. L., and Boxer, L. A. (1981): Lactoferrin: A promoter of polymorphonuclear leukocyte adhesiveness. *Blood*, 57:939–948.

119. O'Shea, J. J., Brown, E. J., Seligmann, B. E., Metcalf, J. A., Frank, M. M., and Gallin, J. I. (1985): Evidence for distinct intracellular pools of receptors for C3b and C3bi in human neutrophils. *J. Immunol.*, 134:2580–2587.

120. Pedersen-Bjergaard, J., Vindelov, L., Phillip, P., et al. (1982): Varying involvement of peripheral granulocytes in the clonal abnormality-7 in bone marrow cells in preleukemia secondary to treatment of other malignant tumors: Cytogenetic results compared with cytometric DNA analysis and neutrophil chemotaxis. *Blood*, 60:172–179.

121. Parmley, R. T., Tzeng, D. Y., Baehner, R. L., and Boxer, L. A. (1983): Abnormal distribution of complex carbohydrates in neutrophils of a patient with lactoferrin deficiency. *Blood*, 62:538–548.

122. Parry, M. F., Root, R. K., Metcalf, J. A., Delaney, K. K., Kaplow, L. S., and Richar, W. J. (1981): Myeloperoxidase deficiency: Prevalence and clinical significance. *Ann. Intern. Med.*, 95:293–301.

123. Quie, P. G. (1987): The white cells: Use of granulocyte transfusions. *Rev. Infect Dis.*, 9:189–193.

124. Ringel, E. W., Soter, N. A., and Austen, K. F. (1984): Localization of histaminase to the specific granule of the human neutrophil. *Immunology*, 52:649–653.

125. Robson, E. G., and Meera, K. P. (1982): Report of the committee on the genetic constitution of chromosomes 7,8, and 9. *Cytogenet. Cell Genet.*, 32:144–152.

126. Roos, D., Hammers, M. N., Van Zwietey, R., and Weening, R. S. (1983): Acidification of the phagocytic vacuole: A possible defect in chronic granulomatous disease. In: *Advances in Host Defense Mechanisms, Vol. 3, Chronic Granulomatous Diseases*, edited by J. I. Gallin and A. S. Fauci, pp. 145–194. Raven Press, New York.

127. Root, R. K., Rosenthal, A. S., and Balestra, D. J. (1972): Abnormal bactericidal, metabolic, and lysosomal functions of Chédiak-Higashi syndrome leukocytes. *J. Clin. Invest.*, 51:649–665.

128. Rossi, F., Bellavite, P., and Papini, E. (1986): Respiratory response of phagocytes: Terminal NADPH oxidase and the mechanisms of its activation. In: *Biochemistry of Macrophages, Vol. 118*, pp. 172–195. Pittman, London.

129. Rotrosen, D., and Gallin, J. I. (1987): Disorders of phagocyte function. *Annu. Rev. Immunol.*, 5:127–150.

130. Royer-Pokora, B., Kunkel, L. M., Monaco, A. P., Goff, S. C., Newburger, P. E., Baehner, R. L., Cole, F. S., Curnutte, J. T., and Orkin, S. H. (1986): Cloning the gene for an inherited human disorder-chronic granulomatous disease-on the basis of its chromosomal location. *Nature*, 322:32–38.

131. Ruutu, P., Ruutu, T. P., Kosunen, T. U., and de la Chapell, A. (1977): Defective chemotaxis in monosomy-7. *Nature*, 265:146–147.

132. Sabin, F. B. (1923): Studies of living human blood cells. *Bull. Johns Hopkins Hosp.*, 34:277–288.

133. Sanchez-Madrid, F. A., Krensky, A. M., Ware, C. F., Robbins, E., Strominger, J. L., Burakoff, S. J., and Springer, T. A. (1982): Three distinct antigens associated with human T lymphocyte-mediated cytolysis: LFA-1, LFA, and LFA-3. *Proc. Natl. Acad. Sci. USA*, 79:7489–7493.

134. Sastre, L., Kishimoto, T. K., Gee, C., Roberts, T., and Springer, T. A. (1986): The mouse leukocyte adhesion proteins Mac-1 and LFA-1. Studies on mRNA translation and protein glycosylation with emphasis on Mdc-1. *J. Immunol.*, 137:1060–1065.

135. Sastre, L., Roman, J., Teplow, D., Dreyer, W., Gee, C., Larson, R., Roberts, T., and Springer, T. A. (1986): A partial genomic DNA clone for the alpha subunit of the mouse complement receptor type 3 and cellular adhesion molecule Mac-1. *Proc. Natl. Acad. Sci. USA*, 83:5644–5648.

136. Segal, A. W., Cross, A. R., Garcia, R. C., Borregaard, N., Valerius, N. H., Soothill, J. F., and Jones, O. T. G. (1983): Absence of cytochrome B-245 in chronic granulomatous diseases: A multicenter

European evaluation of its incidence and relevance. *N. Engl. J. Med.*, 308:245–251.

137. Segal, A. W., Heyworth, P. G., Cockcroft, S., and Barrowman, M. M. (1985): Stimulated neutrophils from patients with autosomal recessive chronic granulomatous disease fail to phosphorylate a M_r-44,000 protein. *Nature*, 316:547–549.

138. Segal, A. W., and Jones, O. T. G. (1979): The subcellular distribution and some properties of the cytochrome *b* component of the microbicidal oxidase system of human neutrophils. *Biochem. J.*, 182:181–188.

139. Seger, R. A., Tiefenauer, L., Matsunaga, T., Wildfever, A., and Newbuger, P. E. (1983): Chronic ganulomatous disease due to granulocytes with abnormal NADPH oxidase activity and deficient cytochrome-b. *Blood*, 61:228–243.

140. Seligmann, B., Chused, T. M., and Gallin, J. I. (1984): Differential binding of chemoattractant peptide to subpopulations of human neutrophils. *J. Immunol.*, 133:2641–2646.

141. Seligmann, B. E., Fletcher, M. P., and Gallin, J. I. (1983): Histamine modulation of human neutrophil oxidative metabolism, locomotion, degranulation and membrane potential changes. *J. Immunol.*, 130:1902–1909.

142. Seligmann, B., Malech, H. L., Melnick, D. A., and Gallin, J. I. (1985): An antibody binding to human neutrophils demonstrates antigenic heterogeneity detected early in myeloid maturation which correlates with functional heterogeneity of mature neutrophils. *J. Immunol.*, 135:2647–2653.

143. Smith, P. D., Ohura, K., Masur, H., Lane, H. C., Fauci, A. S., and Wahl, S. M. (1984): Munocyte function in the acquired immune deficiency syndrome. Defective chemotaxis. *J. Clin. Invest.*, 74:2121–2128.

144. Snyderman, R., and Pike, M. C. (1978): Pathophysiologic aspects of leukocyte chemotaxis: Identification of a specific chemotactic factor binding site on human granulocytes and defects of macrophage function associated with neoplasia. In: *Leukocyte Chemotaxis: Methods, Physiology and Clinical Implications*, edited by J. I. Gallin and P. G. Quie, pp. 357–378. Raven Press, New York.

145. Southwick, F. S., Holbrook, T., Howard, T., Springer, T., Stossel, T. P., Arnaout, M. A. (1986): Neutrophil actin dysfunction is associated with a deficiency of Mol. *Clin. Res.*, 34:533A (abstract).

146. Spitznagle, J. K., Cooper, M. R., McCall, A. E., DeChatelet, L. R., and Welsh, I. R. H. (1972): Selective deficiency of granules associated with lysozyme and lactoferrin in human polymorphs with reduced microbicidal capacity. *J. Clin. Invest.*, 51:93a.

147. Springer, J. A. (1985): The LFA-1, Mac 1 glycoprotein family and its deficiency in an inherited disease. *Fed. Proc.*, 44:2660–2663.

148. Springer, T. A., and Anderson, D. C. (1986): The importance of the Mac-1, LFA-1 glycoprotein family in monocyte and granulocyte adherence, chemotaxis, and migration into inflammatory sites: Insights from an experiment of nature. In: *Biochemistry of Macrophages, Ciba Foundation Symposium 118*, edited by D. Evered, J. Nugent, and M. O'Connor, pp. 102–126. Pittman, London.

149. Springer, T. A., Dustin, M. L., Kishimoto, T. K., and Marlin, S. (1987): The Lymphocyte function associated (LFA) molecules: Cell adhesion receptors of the immune system. *Annu. Rev. Immunol.*, 5:223–252.

150. Springer, T., Galfre, G., Secher, D. S., and Milstein, C. (1979): Mac-1: A macrophage differentiation antigen identified by monoclonal antibody. *Eur. J. Immunol.*, 9:301–306.

151. Springer, T. A., Thomspon, W. S., Miller, J., Schmalstieg, F. C., and Anderson, D. C. (1984): Inherited deficiency of the Mac-1, LFA-1, P150,95 glycoprotein family and its molecular basis. *J. Exp. Med.*, 160:1901–1918.

152. Stendahl, O., Coble, B. I., Dahlgre, C., Hed, J., and Molin, L. (1984): Myeloperoxidase modulates the phagocytic activity of polymorphonuclear neutrophil leukocytes. Studies with cells from a myeloperoxidase-deficient patient. *J. Clin. Invest.*, 73:366–373.

153. Stossel, T. P. (1973): Evaluation of opsonic and leukocyte function with a spectrophotometric test in patients with infection and with phagocytic disorders. *Blood*, 42:121–130.

154. Strauss, R. G., Bove, K. E., Jones, J. R., Mauer, A. M., and Fulginiti,

V. A. (1974): An anomaly of neutrophil morphology with impaired function. *N. Engl. J. Med.,* 290:478–484.

155. Styrt, B., and Klempner, M. S. (1984): Late-presenting variant to chronic granulomatous disease. *Pediatr. Infect. Dis.,* 3:456–459.

156. Takeughi, K., Wood, H., and Swank, R. T. (1986): Lysosomal elastase and cathepsin G in beige mice. *J. Exp. Med.,* 163:665–677.

157. Tauber, A. I., Borregaard, N., Simons, E., and Wright, J. (1983): Chronic granulomatous disease: A syndrome of phagocyte oxidase deficiencies. *Medicine,* 62:286–309.

158. Todd, T. F., III, Arnaout, M. A., Rosin, R. E., Crowley, C. A., Peters, W. A., and Babior, B. M. (1984): Subcellular localization of the large subunit of Mol (Molα; formerly, gp100), surface glycoprotein associated with neutrophil adhesion. *J. Clin. Invest.,* 74:1280–1290.

159. Todd, R. F., and Freyer, D. O. (1987): The CD11/CD18 leukocyte glycoprotein deficiency. *Hemotol. Oncol. Clin. (in press).*

160. Van Dyke, T. E. (1985): Role of the neutrophil in oral disease: Receptor deficiency in leukocytes from patients with juvenile periodontitis. *Rev. Infect. Dis.,* 7:419–425.

161. Van Dyke, T. E., Levine, M. J., Tabak, L. A., and Genco, R. J. (1981): Reduced chemotactic peptide binding in juvenile periodontitis: A model for neutrophil function. *Biochem. Biophys. Res. Commun.,* 100:1278–1284.

162. Van Dyke, T. E., Levine, M. J., and Genco, R. J. (1985): Neutrophil function and oral disease. *J. Oral Pathol.,* 14:95–120.

163. Volkman, D. J., Buescher, E. S., Gallin, J. I., and Fauci, A. S. (1984): B cell lines as models for inherited phagocytic diseases: Abnormal superoxide generation in chronic granulomatous disease and giant granules in Chédiak-Higashi syndrome. *J. Immunol.,* 133:3006–3009.

164. Warden, G. D., Mason, A. D., and Pruitt, B. A. (1974): Evaluation of leukocyte chemotaxis *in vitro* in thermally injured patients. *J. Clin. Invest.,* 54:1001–1003.

165. Weening, R. S., Adriaansz, L. H., Weemaes, C. M. R., Lutter, R., and Roos, D. (1985): Clinical differences in chronic granulomatous disease in patients with cytochrome b-negative or cytochrome b-positive neutrophils. *J. Pediatr.,* 107:102–104.

166. Weening, R. S., Corbeel, L., de Boer, M., Lutter, R., van Zwieten, R., Hamers, M. N., and Roos, D. (1985): Cytochrome *b* deficiency in an autosomal form of chronic granulomatous disease. *J. Clin. Invest.,* 75:915–920.

167. White, J. G., and Clawson, C. C. (1980): The Chédiak-Higashi syndrome: The nature of the giant neutrophil granules and their interactions with cytoplasm and foreign particulates. *Am. J. Pathol.,* 98:151–167.

168. Wolach, B., Coates, T. D., Hugli, T. E., Baehner, R. L., and Boxer, L. A. (1984): Plasma lactoferrin reflects granulocyte activation via complement in burn patients. *J. Lab. Clin. Med.,* 103:284–293.

169. Wolff, S. M., Dale, D. C., Clark, R. A., Root, R. K., and Kimball, H. R. (1972): The Chédiak-Higashi syndrome: Studies of host defenses. *Ann. Intern. Med.,* 76:293–306.

170. Wright, D. G., and Gallin, J. I. (1977): A functional differentiation of human neutrophil granules: Generation of C5a by a specific (secondary) granule product and inactivation of C5a by azurophil (primary) granule products. *J. Immunol.,* 199:1068–1076.

171. Wright, D. G., and Greenwald, D. (1979): Increased motility and maturation of human blood monocytes stimulated by products released from neutrophil secondary granules. *Blood,* 54(Suppl. 1):95A.

172. Yoon, P. S., Boxer, L. A., Mayo, L. A., Yang, A. Y., and Wicha, M. S. (1987): Human neutrophil laminin receptors: activation-dependent receptor expression. *J. Immunol.,* 138:259–265.

173. Zimmerli, W., and Gallin, J. I. (1987): Monocytes accumulate on Rebuck skin window converships but not in skin chamber fluid: A comparative evaluation of two *in vivo* migration methods. *J. Immunol. Methods,* 96:11–17.

174. Zimmerli, W., Seligmann, B., and Gallin, J. I. (1986): Exudation primes human and guinea pig neutrophils for subsequent responsiveness to the chemotactic peptide N-formylmethionylleucylphenylalanine and increases complement component C3bi receptor expression. *J. Clin. Invest.,* 77:925–933.

Inflammation: Basic Principles and Clinical Correlates.
Edited by J. I. Gallin, I. M. Goldstein, and R. Snyderman.
Raven Press, Ltd., New York © 1988.

CHAPTER 27

Mast Cells and Basophils

Reuben P. Siraganian

Mast cells and basophils were first described by Paul
Ehrlich, more than 100 years ago, as being cells that have
prominent cytoplasmic granules and that stain with basic
dyes. The basophils are present in the blood, whereas mast
cells are found in connective tissues. However, it was many
years before it was recognized that mast cells and basophils
play a critical role in immediate hypersensitivity reactions
and that they contain histamine and other inflammatory
mediators.

The stimulation of basophils or mast cells is initiated
by the interaction of a number of secretagogues with cell-
surface receptors. This results in a series of biochemical
events that eventually culminate in the release of biologically active mediators. This chapter reviews our current
knowledge of the cell biology of basophils and mast cells,
including their structure, their origin, the mediators present in the cells, and the biochemical mechanisms involved
in the release reaction. Some of the older literature
has been summarized in a number of reviews
(121,133,189,242–244).

Recent progress in the understanding of the biology of
basophils and mast cells has been largely due to the development of techniques to obtain large number of these
cells. Basophils and mast cells are sparsely distributed in
the blood or tissues. Therefore, the earliest experiments
with human materials utilized peripheral blood leukocytes
or organ fragments in which only a small fraction of the
cells were basophils or mast cells. More recently, methods
have been described to obtain purified basophils or mast
cells from either peripheral blood or lung fragments.
However, even with these techniques, the number of cells
obtained are small, and few biochemical studies can be
performed (163,235). In contrast, rat peritoneal mast cells
can be purified easily and, in general, yield about 1×10^6
cells per rat. This low number also limits the biochemical
studies that can be accomplished; a further complication
is that conclusions drawn from experiments with rat mast
cells might not be applicable to human basophils or mast
cells. The development of cultured cell lines has had an
important influence on recent mast-cell–basophil studies

(7,8). Rat basophilic leukemia cell lines have been characterized that can be activated for histamine release (7). Variants of these cells have also been isolated which are incapable of release and can be used in the characterization of the biochemical events in the release process (182,250). Unlike these cell lines, which were developed from tumors, the use of growth factors has allowed the isolation of untransformed cell lines (196,233). The culture of mouse bone marrow or spleen cells with IL-3, a growth factor from T-lymphocytes, stimulates pluripotential stem cells to grow and differentiate into mast cells (233). The cells require the continued presence of growth factors. Using growth factors, cells similar to human mast cells or basophils have been grown from cord blood or bone marrow (114,205,270). However, unlike the murine system, the human model has not been well standardized. In studies with cultured cell lines, distinctions between different phenotypes are not as clear-cut because the characteristics of the cell depend on the culture conditions.

CHARACTERISTICS OF MAST CELLS AND BASOPHILS

Mast cells and basophils have several features in common. Both have prominent cytoplasmic granules containing histamine and other chemical mediators. Both cell types have surface receptors ($Fc_\epsilon R$) that bind the Fc portion of IgE with high affinity. The exposure of basophils or mast cells that have IgE on their surface receptors to multivalent antigen stimulates the cells to secrete mediators. Mast cells and basophils both develop from a common bone-marrow-derived hematopoietic precursor cell.

There are a number of differences between basophils and mast cells. Basophils differentiate and mature in the bone marrow, then enter the circulation and rarely migrate into tissues. They are short-lived (<2 weeks) and are probably end-cells. There is no evidence that basophils enter tissue and transform into mast cells. In contrast, the mast cells are distributed in connective tissues and the skin, and they are often adjacent to blood vessels and beneath epithelial surfaces such as the gastrointestinal and respiratory tracts. Mast cells normally do not circulate, are long-lived, and appear to retain the capacity to proliferate. Studies in several mammalian species suggest an inverse quantitative relationship between basophils and mast cells; e.g., species that have abundant mast cells have few basophils. Humans, however, have a large number of both mast cells and basophils.

Basophil and Mast-Cell Ultrastructure

Human basophils have a nucleus that appears lobular, bilobed, or multilobed (71,81). The cytoplasm contains granules that have bilayer membranes as well as membrane aggregates or whorls. Some cells have smaller granules that contain a homogeneous dense material. There are frequently cytoplasmic vesicles containing glycogen. There are also mitochondria, but the Golgi apparatus and endoplasmic reticulum are not prominent. There appears to be some heterogeneity among human basophils because of the variation in their granule content. Some of the cells observed by electron microscopy have granules filled uniformly with electron-dense material, whereas other cells also have granules that lack some of the dense materials.

Human mast cells have a different ultrastructural appearance (71). The cell surface has many long thin projections that appear as villi by scanning electron microscopy. The nucleus is generally round and can be aggregated, although it is not as densely clumped as that in basophils. There are some mitochondria, but the endoplasmic reticulum and the Golgi apparatus is not prominent. Mast cells also contain intermediate filaments that can be quite abundant. These cells contain lipid bodies that are not membrane-bound and can be radiolabeled with arachidonic acid. The exact functional significance of these lipid bodies is not clear. The mast-cell granules are more heterogeneous in substructural pattern than are the basophil granules. Occasional granular matrices have a scroll-like appearance, whereas others have an amorphous electron-dense matrix. Some of this variation in the granular appearance depends on the tissue from which the mast cells are isolated.

Mast-Cell Heterogeneity

The concept of heterogeneity in the population of mast cells is based principally on studies in rodents (14,54,132). Histological studies dating back to Maximow in 1905 described "typical" staining mast cells in the rat intestinal mucosa. These staining differences can now be explained on the basis of the different proteoglycans present in the granules of these cells.

There appear to be two major populations of mast cells in rats and mice. The differences between the two cell types are summarized in Table 1. Although different authors have used different terms, these atypical appearing mast cells are frequently called the "mucosal" mast cells in contrast to those that are predominantly in the "connective" tissues, e.g., in the peritoneal cavity. There are a number of differences seen in the staining characteristics; berberine binds well to heparin and therefore stains well the connective type of mast cells. With Alcian blue-safranin the mucosal mast cells stain blue, whereas the connective tissue type has a red-blue color. The mucosal mast cells, as the name implies, are found predominantly in the intestinal wall. The mucosal mast cell is about half

TABLE 1. *Properties of the different types of mast cells*[a]

Property	Connective-tissue-type mast cells	Mucosal-type mast cells
Staining (Alcian blue/safranin)	Red-blue	Blue
Size	9–20 μm	Smaller
Granules	Large, many, uniform size	Smaller, variable size
T-cell-dependent proliferation	−	+
Migratory	Non-migratory	Migratory
Life-span	Long	Short
Half-life	>6 months	<40 days
Proteoglycan	Heparin	Chondroitin sulfates
Histamine	10–30 pg/cell	<2 pg/cell
Protease type	RMCP-I (chymase, carboxypeptidase)	RMCP-II
Secretagogues		
IgE	+	+
Ca^{2+} ionophore	+	+
Compound 48/80	+	−
Bradykinin	+	−
Somatostatin	+	−
Opiate drugs	+	−
Arachidonic acid metabolite	PGD$_2$	LTC$_4 \gg$ PGD$_2$

[a] RMCP, rat mast-cell protease; +, positive response; −, absent or failed to respond.

the size of the connective tissue cell and contains only about 1.3 μg of histamine per 10^6 cells. In contrast, the connective-tissue-type cells contain about 10-fold more histamine. The number of mucosal mast cells increases dramatically in parasitized rats and mice because of a T-cell-derived factor, interleukin-3. Similarly, *in vitro* culture of bone-marrow or spleen cells with this factor results in the development of these mucosal-type mast cells.

There is a significant difference in the proteoglycan content of the two mast-cell populations. The connective tissue mast cells contain heparin with a molecular weight of 750,000, whereas the mucosal-type mast cells have chondroitin sulfate di-B with a molecular weight of about 200,000 (215,261). Similarly, there are differences in the content of the serine protease enzyme present in the different mast cells: The connective-tissue-type cells contain the rat mast-cell protease I, which is also called *chymase,* whereas the mucosal cells have rat mast cell protease II. Interestingly, the rat basophilic leukemia cells contain a chondroitin sulfate and rat mast-cell protease II, suggesting that they have homology with mucosal mast cells (139,238). The use of secretagogues can demonstrate differences between mucosal and connective-tissue-type mast cells. Both types of cells respond to IgE-receptor or ionophore stimulation with the release of mediators. Compound 48/80 or a bee-venom peptide causes histamine release from the connective tissue mast cell but not from the mucosal-type cell. Similarly, a number of other compounds cause secretion from the connective-tissue-type mast cells only; these include bradykinin, vasoactive polypeptide, somatostatin, endorphins, and opiate-type

drugs. Phosphatidylserine enhances the release from the connective-type mast cells but has no effect on the secretion from mucosal cells. Heterogeneity in the response to different secretagogues has also been described when mast cells are isolated from different tissue in the body.

There are also differences in the mediators released from the different cell types. Both cell types release histamine and in rodents they contain and release serotonin. The main arachidonic acid metabolite synthesized and released by the connective tissue type cells is prostaglandin D_2, whereas the mucosal-type cells form more LTC$_4$ (216,217).

At present there is some histological evidence for the presence of more than one type of mast cells in human tissues. However, the isolation of mast cells from different tissue sites in humans has not demonstrated any functional heterogeneity. The observations described above indicate that there are clearly differences in mast cells isolated from different tissues in rodents. These results should be interpreted in light of two important experimental results. First, as will be discussed in the next section, the two types of mast cells can change their phenotype from one to the other. Secondly, mast cells at different points in their cell cycle or maturation can respond differently to various secretagogues (191,234).

Origin and Differentiation of Basophils and Mast Cells

The present knowledge on the origin and differentiation of mast cells is based on a series of studies by Kitamura and associates that have utilized transplantation studies in several mouse strains (142,200). There are two congenitally mast-cell-deficient mouse strains called W/W^v and Sl/Sl^d, and the beige (bg/bg) mouse has characteristically large granules that can be easily recognized. By transplantation studies with cells from congenic mice, the precursors of the mast cells and their differentiation have been determined.

Mast cell precursors first appear during embryogenesis in the yolk sac, then decrease rapidly, followed by the appearance of precursors in the fetal liver. The appearance of precursors in other tissues, e.g., the skin, occurred later; these precursors seemed to originate in the liver. These mast cells produced during embryo development probably survive through adult life as a result of the long life-span of tissue-localized mast cells. In adult animals, the bone marrow is the main source of the mast-cell precursors. In contrast to the other hematopoietic cells that differentiate fully in the bone marrow (e.g., the erythrocytes or the granulocytes), the mast-cell precursors leave the bone marrow and differentiate to their final stage in tissues. Although no mast cells are detectable in the blood of these mice, transplantation experiments demonstrate the presence of mast-cell precursors in the circulation and also in the spleen. However, they occur with the highest frequency in the bone marrow. The precursor cells appear to proliferate in tissues before differentiating into mast cells. Therefore, the bone marrow is the important source of the precursors of mast cells.

Recent interest has centered on the heterogeneity of mast cells. Both the connective tissue and mucosal mast cells have a common precursor. The type of cell that a precursor forms depends on the microenvironment. Even after morphological differentiation, mast cells retain their capacity to proliferate, as demonstrated by transplantation experiments. The cells also can transdifferentiate into the different types. When peritoneal mast cells formed in culture were injected into the skin, they had the characteristics of the connective tissue type; however, when they were injected into the wall of the stomach, they differentiated into the mucosal type (143,255). The transplantation of a single peritoneal connective-tissue-type mast cell into the stomach wall results in the development of mucosal-type cells (254). Similarly, mucosal-type mast cells developed in culture containing the growth factor (interleukin-3), when injected into the peritoneal cavity of mice, gave rise to connective type of mast cells (200). When bone-marrow or spleen cells are cultured *in vitro* with interleukin-3, there is the development of mucosal-type mast cells. In contrast, when the culture is on fibroblast layers, the result is the formation of both the mucosal- and the connective-tissue-type mast cell (25,75). Peritoneal mast cells also retain their connective-tissue-type characteristics when cultured on fibroblast mono-layers (149). Similarly, when mucosal-type mast cells developed by growth in interleukin-3 are transferred to fibroblast monolayers, they develop the characteristics of the connective-type mast cell (150). These results indicate that two types of mast cells can change their phenotype, depending on the microenvironment.

Mice of the mutant genotypes W/W^v and Sl/Sl^d lack both mucosal and connective-tissue-type mast cells. The genetic defects in the two mouse strains appear to be different. In the W/W^v the precursor cells are defective in their capacity to invade and differentiate in the tissues. In contrast, the tissue of the Sl/Sl^d mice do not support the invasion and proliferation of the mast-cell precursors.

These results have provided a great deal of knowledge on the lineage of mast cells in rodents. In contrast, there is little information on basophils, except for the fact that they develop in the bone marrow. In studies with human tissues, there have been reports on the growth of metachromatically staining cells that contain histamine and have high-affinity IgE receptors (114,205,270). However, in most of these cases it is not clear whether the cultured cells were basophils or some type of mast cell. Further development of tissue culture techniques and growth factors will help to shed more light on human mast cells and basophils.

Growth Factors (Interleukin-3)

Interleukin-3 (IL-3) is a T-cell lymphokine that stimulates the growth of permanent lines of myeloid cells or mast cells. Hemopoietic progenitor cells respond to IL-3 to generate neutrophils, macrophages, megakaryocytes, and mast cells (102,233). Therefore, this lymphokine stimulates the progenitors of multiple lineages of hemopoietic cells and thus has colony-stimulating-factor activity. The culture of murine bone marrow or spleens with IL-3 generates cell lines that have the characteristics of mucosal mast cells.

Purified IL-3 is a glycoprotein with an apparent molecular weight of 28,000. Through the use of recombinant DNA technology, murine and human IL-3 cDNA have been isolated (102,291). For murine IL-3 the nucleotide sequence predicts a polypeptide of 166 amino acids, which is cleaved to 140- and 134-amino-acid polypeptides. The predicted molecular weight of this material would be 15,000, indicating that the IL-3 is heavily glycosylated. The nucleotide sequence of the human IL-3 predicts a 152-amino-acid polypeptide (291). The first 19 amino acids are very hydrophobic and are probably cleaved in the secreted molecule, which would consist of 133 amino acids. Interestingly, although the gene has been cloned, the human material has not yet been isolated.

IL-3 is released *in vivo* when T-cells are activated by

antigen stimulation, and, when released, its effects are local. However, during parasitic infestations, when there is a more potent immunological challenge, the IL-3 appears in the serum and is also secreted in the urine. The half-life of the material in the serum is very short. The action of IL-3 depends on the presence of cell-surface receptors. IL-3-dependent cell lines have specific receptors (estimates are between 1,500 and 5,000 per cell), with a K_d of about 1 to 5 $\times$ 10^{-11} M (173).

Mediators from Basophils and Mast Cells

Basophils and mast cells secrete substances that mediate allergic reactions. These mediators released from basophils and mast cells are either preformed and stored in secretory granules or are newly generated (Table 2).

Preformed Mediators

Biogenic amines

The biogenic amines such as histamine and serotonin are the major components of the secretory granules on a molar basis. Human basophils and mast cells contain only histamine; however, serotonin is present in the mast cells of some species, e.g., rodents.

Histamine. Histamine is produced from the amino acid L-histidine by histidine decarboxylase. This enzyme is located in the cytoplasm of the basophils and mast cells, but the histamine is concentrated and stored in secretory granules. In the granule, histamine is associated with the

TABLE 2. *Mediators from mast cells and basophils*

A. Preformed mediators
  1. Biogenic amines
    Histamine
    Serotonin
  2. Neutral protease
    Rat mast-cell protease I and II
  3. Proteoglycans
    Heparin
    Chondroitin sulfate
  4. Acid hydrolase
    β-Hexosaminidase
    β-Glucuronidase
    β-D-Galactosidase
    Arylsulfatase
  5. Chemotactic factors
    Eosinophil chemotactic factors
    High-MW neutrophil chemotactic factor
B. Newly generated mediators
  1. Arachidonic acid products
    Cyclooxygenase products: PGD$_2$
    Leukotriene products: LTC$_4$, LTD$_4$, LTE$_4$
  2. Platelet-activating factor

carboxyl groups of proteoglycans and/or proteins by ionic binding (20,282). During secretion, the interior of the granule is exposed to the extracellular ions, and histamine is released by a cation exchange mechanism from the binding sites. The amount of histamine in mast cells is clearly greater than that in basophils; human basophils contain approximately 1 to 3 μg of histamine per 10^6 cells, whereas human mast cells appear to have 5- to 10-fold higher concentrations.

The biological effects due to histamine are the result of its binding and activating either H$_1$ or H$_2$ cell-surface receptors. The H$_1$ receptors are blocked by the classical antihistamines such as mepyramine and are involved in the histamine-induced contraction of bronchial and gastrointestinal smooth muscle. However, part of the bronchial effects *in vivo* are due to histamine reacting with irritant receptors and by reflex vagal action. The H$_2$ receptors are involved prominently in gastric acid secretion by parietal cells and are present on a number of other cell types. These H$_2$ receptors are blocked by cimetidine. These receptors function in the down-regulation of a number of different cell systems; histamine activating the H$_2$ receptors on lymphocytes inhibits proliferation, cell-mediated cytotoxicity, and decreases lymphokine production. Histamine acting through H$_2$ receptors on basophils has a negative feedback effect on secretion (154). Histamine enhances vascular permeability by acting on the endothelial cells in the postcapillary venules. This effect is to allow transudation into tissue spaces of plasma proteins and possible deposition of immune complexes from the serum.

Histamine is rapidly inactivated *in vivo* by two mechanisms; in one pathway it is sequentially metabolized by histamine-N-methyltransferase to methylhistamine and to methylimidazole acetic acid by monamine oxidase. In the second pathway, it is metabolized to imidazole acetic acid by diamine oxidase (histaminase), and is then conjugated to form ribosyl imidazole acetic acid.

Serotonin. The addition of a hydroxyl group to the tryptophan molecule followed by decarboxylation results in the formation of 5-hydroxytryptamine, commonly called *serotonin*. It is present primarily in (a) enterochromaffin cells in the gastrointestinal tract, (b) platelets, and (c) the central nervous system. In some species, e.g., rodents, it is also present in mast cells. Serotonin in rat mast-cell granules is bound to the enzymatic site of the chymase enzyme. Other serotonin binding proteins have been described in the cytoplasm of the rat basophilic leukemia cells. There is some suggestive evidence that cells might be capable of releasing serotonin in the absence of the release of histamine.

There is considerable species variation in the physiological response to serotonin. In rats and mice it causes edema and plays an important role in anaphylactic reactions. Human bronchial tissue is not constricted by serotonin. Antagonists of serotonin include methysergide, LSD, and cyproheptadine. Serotonin is catabolized by monoamine oxidase, which is present in a number of tissues such as monocytes and pulmonary endothelial cells.

Neutral proteases

The neutral proteases are a major component of the secretory granules of mast cells and basophils. These proteolytic enzymes are present in the granules of mast cells and, following IgE receptor activation, are released bound to proteoglycans. The amounts and the types of these enzymes appear to vary within different cell populations. The rat connective-tissue mast cells contain both chymase [molecular weight (MW) 26,000–29,000] and carboxypeptidase A (MW 35,000–40,000); the chymase has also been called *rat mast-cell protease I*. In contrast, the rat mucosal mast cells contain a different protease, which is called *rat mast-cell protease II*. Human mast cells contain a tryptase with an MW of 144,000. Pulmonary mast cells appear to contain and release other proteolytic enzymes that activate prekallikrein or have kallikrein-like properties and generate kinin from low-molecular-weight kininogen. Other chymotrypsin-like proteinases have been postulated to be present in skin mast cells. Human basophils release a kallikrein-like endopeptidase (MW 1,200,000) that generates bradykinin from plasma kininogen (202,203).

Proteoglycans

The characteristic metachromatic staining of basophils and mast cells is due to the presence of proteoglycans in their granules. There are differences in the proteoglycans present in different cell types: The connective-tissue mast cell contains predominantly heparin, the mucosal-type mast cells have chondroitin sulfate E, and basophils contain chondroitin monosulfate proteoglycans.

Heparin. In this molecule, glycosaminoglycan chains are attached by O-linkage to a small protein core composed predominantly of glycine and serine residues. Heparin from rat mast cells has an MW of 750,000, whereas that isolated from human lung tissues (mast cells?) is much smaller.

Heparin is a negatively charged molecule that has anticoagulant activities. In the mast cell, it forms the matrix of the secretory granule to which many preformed basically charged mediators are bound by ionic linkage. The proteases in the mast-cell granules are also tightly bound to heparin.

Heparin has effects on a number of enzymatic reactions. Besides its well-recognized anticoagulant property, it also inhibits the activity of a number of lysosomal enzymes. A number of other activities involve the attachment of fibronectin to fibroblasts and the stimulation of capillary endothelial cell migration.

Chondroitin sulfate. These glycosaminoglycans have a different carbohydrate linkage than does heparin. The chondroitin sulfates are the predominant proteoglycans in basophils and in the mucosal-type mast cells. Chondroitin monosulfates are the major proteoglycan of basophils, whereas the mucosal mast cells grown in culture contain the disulfate, chondroitin sulfate E, but not heparin.

A number of acid hydrolases are present in the mast-cell secretory granules and, by analogy, are probably also present in basophils. Several of these enzymes have been shown to be released in parallel to histamine during cell secretion from mast cells. These include β-hexosaminidase and β-glucuronidase, which are both acid exoglycosidases; β-D-galactosidase and arylsulfatase. A number of other typical lysosomal enzymes (e.g., acid phosphatase) are also present in mast cells but not in secretory granules.

Other enzymes

The mast-cell granule material has superoxide dismutase activity and peroxidase. Both of these enzymes appear to be bound to the granular proteoglycan.

Chemotactic factors

A number of chemotactic molecules are generated during secretion from mast cells or basophils. A number of these are preformed mediators and include histamine, which is chemotactic for eosinophils. The tetrapeptides Val-Gly-Ser-Glu and Ala-Gly-Ser-Glu are chemotactic for eosinophils. A 1,400-MW peptide that induces an inflammatory response in the skin has been purified from mast cells. There is also a high-MW (over 750,000) neutrophil chemotactic factor present in mast cells. A number of other chemotactic factors are newly generated and are described in the next section.

Newly Generated Mediators

These mediators are generated from the cells after an appropriate stimulus. They are not present preformed in the cell and therefore cannot be released by breaking up the cells by physical means.

Arachidonic acid metabolites

The metabolism of the arachidonic acid along either the cyclooxygenase or lipoxygenase pathways results in the generation of a number of potent inflammatory mediators. During the release process, arachidonic acid is released from cellular phospholipids as a result of the activation of phospholipase enzymes (see section on biochemical mechanisms of the release reaction). The metabolism of this arachidonic acid can then proceed along different pathways depending on the enzymes present. If it is metabolized along the cyclooxygenase pathway, it results in the formation of the prostaglandins, whereas the lipoxygenase pathway leads to the formation of the leukotrienes. These pathways and the resulting mediators are discussed in detail in some of the other chapters of this volume.

There are differences in these mediators generated by different cell types. The rat serosal mast cell predominantly forms PGD_2, whereas the mucosal mast cells generate more lipoxygenase products. Human mast cells make PGD_2 but also produce LTC_4 and other leukotrienes. In contrast, human basophils do not generate PGD_2 and only produce small amounts of the leukotrienes.

Platelet-activating factor

Platelet-activating factor (PAF) is a low-MW phospholipid first recognized as a mediator released from rabbit basophils following IgE-mediated reactions. The structure of this molecule has been determined and shown to be 1-*O*-alkyl-2-acetyl-*sn*-glyceryl-3-phosphorylcholine. This is generated from alkyl phospholipids in the cell by the sequential reaction of a phospholipase A2 and an acetyltransferase. This material has a number of potent biological activities.

THE HIGH-AFFINITY RECEPTOR FOR IgE

A variety of cells have membrane receptors that bind the Fc portion of immunoglobulin molecules. In the case of the IgE molecule, there are receptors on a number of different cell types that can be divided into two distinct groups. The first group of receptors consists of those that are on mast cells or basophils and that are characterized by having a very high affinity for monomeric IgE; these are called the *high-affinity Fc$_ε$ receptors* (Fc$_ε$R). In contrast, other cells such as lymphocytes, eosinophils, and macrophages have receptors that bind IgE with much lower affinity, and accordingly are called the *low-affinity IgE receptor*. This low-affinity IgE receptor has been isolated from human B-lymphocytes, and its structure has been determined (141,256). Structurally, it appears to be related to the IgE-binding factors that are released in cultures of some B-lymphocytes.

The study of the IgE receptor has been greatly facilitated by several factors. A first step was the isolation and characterization of IgE, followed by the availability of IgE myeloma or hybridomas from several species (e.g., human, rat, and mouse). The availability of cell lines that have IgE receptors has further aided these studies. The most extensive studies have been with the rat basophilic leu-

kemia cell line; however, more recent work has been with several other cell lines, e.g., human and mouse cultured lines that have IgE receptors. Some short-term cultured cell lines have been obtained with the use of IL-3 and other growth factors and probably will prove more useful in the future. Mast cells or basophils can also be purified from blood or tissues, but their use has been more problematic because of the difficulty of recovering adequate numbers of cells.

IgE-Receptor Interactions

Reaction Mechanism and Kinetics

The binding of IgE to its receptor on mast cells follows the kinetics of a simple reversible bimolecular reaction:

$$IgE + R \rightleftharpoons R - IgE$$

In such reactions the molar concentration of the IgE, R, and R-IgE determines the equilibrium constants. The forward rate constant, k_1, is 10^5 M^{-1} sec^{-1}. The rate is 30-fold greater for solubilized receptors. The reaction has a very small first-order reverse rate constant, k_{-1}, of 10^{-5} sec^{-1}. Therefore, the affinity (K_a) of the receptor for IgE is high and has been estimated as being 10^{10} M^{-1} (65,144,283). The dissociation rate of IgE from cells is therefore very slow, with variable estimates on the half-life for cell-bound IgE of 20 to over 100 hr (106,221). However, in a biological setting the effective half-life of IgE is probably even longer because the IgE that dissociates from cells is functionally normal and can rebind to the same or other cells. By using the Prausnitz-Kustner reaction, it has been estimated that the half-life of IgE in the skin is 13 days (2).

Specificity

The reaction of IgE with its high-affinity receptor on mast cells is not effectively inhibited by immunoglobulins of other classes. The only exception is the inhibition, by very high concentrations of IgG$_a$, of IgE binding to purified receptors.

There is also species specificity of IgE binding to receptors. In general, IgE from one species binds only to the receptors on the cells from the same or closely related species; e.g., human IgE binds to human and monkey basophils or mast cells but not to mouse or rat mast cells. Exceptions to this have recently been demonstrated where monoclonal mouse hybridomas were shown to bind to human basophils (34) and where human IgE were shown to bind to mouse mast cells (260). However, human IgE does not bind to the rat basophilic leukemia cell line used extensively in experimental studies (108,145,185).

Binding Sites on IgE

The IgE binds to its receptor through the Fc portion of the molecule, as demonstrated in studies with the digestion of IgE myelomas, to obtain the whole Fc portion of the molecule. The 95-kilodalton Fc fragment obtained by papain digestion, containing the $C_\epsilon2$, $C_\epsilon3$, and $C_\epsilon4$ portions of the molecule, is biologically active and presumably binds to the receptor; in contrast, the F(ab')$_2$ fragment obtained by pepsin digestion is inactive (16,257,258). Some smaller fragments obtained by the further digestion of the Fc portion of the molecule, although quite large, have no biological activity; an example of this is the 38-kilodalton Fc$_\epsilon''$ (110).

The reduction of disulfide bonds in the IgE molecule will also abolish its capacity to bind to the receptor on mast cells (272). Some studies on the denaturation of IgE conclude that the $C_\epsilon3$ and $C_\epsilon4$ domains are involved in the binding to the receptor, although studies on renaturation do not support that conclusion (49). Studies comparing the digestion of IgE bound to the receptor with that of IgE in solution have suggested that a region close to the $C_\epsilon2$:$C_\epsilon3$ juncture might interact with the receptor (209).

Recent experiments have utilized human IgE cloned in bacteria to produce smaller portions of the IgE molecule. Two laboratories have produced molecules that contain most of the Fc portion of IgE. These molecules produced by bacteria are unglycosylated but retain their capacity to bind, with high affinity, to human basophils (116,138,157). Therefore, the carbohydrate on the IgE is not critical for binding to its receptor. These Fc fragments encode portions of the second, third, and fourth domains of the constant region of the ϵ-chain of the IgE molecule. One of these fragments is missing a portion of the NH$_2$-terminal third of the $C_\epsilon2$ region. Therefore, this portion of the molecule is not critical for binding to basophils. Additional studies with different fragments that lack different portions of the constant region will probably better define the sites that are critical for binding to cells.

Another approach to define regions on the IgE molecule that are critical for binding to receptors is by the use of monoclonal antibodies (mAb). An mAb that is reacting with IgE in solution, but not when it is in its receptor, would indicate that the epitope is unavailable when the IgE is on the cell surface. These epitopes could be either a result of sites that are actually hidden in the receptor or a result of allosteric conformational changes when IgE binds to the receptor. In the analysis of a series of monoclonal antibodies to human IgE, it has been found that several have these characteristics (94). By analysis of reactivity with IgE fragments, it was also shown that these react with the $C_\epsilon1$, $C_\epsilon2$ and $C_\epsilon3$-4 regions. Therefore, sites in several domains are in contact with the receptor. How-

ever, other antibodies to other sites in both $C_\epsilon1$ and $C_\epsilon3$-4 regions were still capable of binding to IgE in its receptor. The other type of experiment tests whether the monoclonal antibodies are capable of inhibiting the binding of IgE to its receptor. By this analysis, other sites were also defined which are more distant than the previous sites; this inhibition could be due to stearic factors. In studies with seven monoclonal antibodies to mouse IgE, some inhibited partially the binding of IgE to cells (4). However, all these mAb were capable of releasing histamine and therefore could bind to epitopes on the IgE molecule sitting on the basophil surface. Binding studies demonstrated less binding of the mAb to IgE on the cell surface than in solution. The results suggest a heterogeneity, either of epitopes on the IgE or of IgE receptors (5).

Studies have also utilized energy transfer measurements to define the interaction of IgE with its receptor (3,91,93). The $C_\epsilon4$ portion of the IgE is not hidden in the receptor and is available for binding by antibodies (93). The data are also interpreted to indicate that the IgE binds to the receptor via only one face of the Fc region, although this conflicts with the results with the monoclonal antibodies to IgE (94). There is also some suggestion that the Fc region bends at the $C_\epsilon2$:$C_\epsilon3$ interface when the IgE is in the receptor. However, there appear to be no significant changes in the flexibility of IgE following its binding to the receptor (252).

In summary, it appears that the binding of the IgE to its receptor is due to contact between several domains of the molecule and the receptor. Studies with fragments of IgE have not demonstrated any that would bind to the receptor with affinities that are significantly different than the parent molecule. There are conflicting reports in the literature on the capacity of high concentrations of IgE-inhibiting allergic reactions. Clearly this would depend on a number of factors, including the concentration of IgE, the ratio of specific to nonspecific IgE, and the length of time allowed for the nonspecific IgE to reach equilibrium with the cell-surface IgE. The definition of the binding sites on the IgE molecule could eventually lead to the design of better drugs that could interfere with the IgE-receptor interaction.

Distribution of Fc$_\epsilon$R

The Fc$_\epsilon$R are distributed diffusely over the surface of the cell (264). There is no significant pool of receptors in the cytoplasm (105,221). The monomeric-IgE–receptor complex is freely mobile in the plane of the membrane, as determined by a number of different techniques (181,293). By use of photobleaching techniques, the diffusion coefficient of the IgE receptor was determined to be similar to other membrane proteins. The IgE receptors appear to be univalent (i.e., one IgE per receptor) and are independently mobile by these techniques (184), although co-internalization studies (see below) suggest that there is some interaction between different IgE receptors (70,119).

The presence of monomeric IgE bound to the $Fc_\epsilon R$ decreases the rate of receptor turnover (69). The half-life of receptors on the rat basophilic leukemia cells is 8 to 13 hr (69,214). If occupied by IgE, the half-life is much longer, with estimates of greater than 32 hr (69). Therefore, the binding of IgE to its receptor has an effect on the rate at which it turns over. However, the results do not distinguish between the possibility that there are changes in the lability of the receptor or that the IgE protects the $Fc_\epsilon R$ from digestion when the complex is exposed to lysosomal enzymes following internalization (190).

The estimate of the number of $Fc_\epsilon R$ has varied between 10^3 and 10^6 per cell on different cell preparations (34,105,167,262). Basophils from individuals with high levels of serum IgE have increased numbers of $Fc_\epsilon R$ receptors (35,170). Similarly, in culture, the presence of IgE in the medium increased the number of IgE receptors on the rat basophilic leukemia cells (69,214). This up-regulation of the $Fc_\epsilon R$ receptor number by the presence of IgE is different than the observation with a number of other receptor systems where increased concentration of the ligand causes a down-regulation in the receptor number.

Internalization and Recycling of the $Fc_\epsilon R$

The addition of antigen or anti-IgE to basophils or mast cells results in the bridging of the IgE molecules, with the formation of aggregates and patches, finally resulting in the capping of these to one pole of the cell and eventual internalization and degradation of these complexes (13,148). This type of phenomenon has been observed in numerous cell types following the cross-linking of their surface receptors. The binding of multivalent antigen to the IgE on the cell surface results in the immobilization of the receptor, as measured by photobleaching techniques (187,188). This immobilization does not require Ca^{2+} in the medium. There is some evidence that this immobilization is due to the interaction of the receptors with cytoskeletal elements in the cell (187).

The internalization and recycling of the IgE receptors on rat basophilic leukemia cells has been studied in detail (66–68,70,106,107,218). The aggregation of the IgE with multivalent antigen results in rapid internalization of the complexes; the $t_{1/2}$ for this reaction is 3 to 5 min and is similar for rat basophilic leukemia and rat mast cells, which have very different rates of histamine release. This internalization appears to be through the coated pits, as has been described for other ligand systems. The internalized IgE and receptor do not reappear on the cell surface and are probably degraded. Even when the internalization reaction has gone to completion, a significant portion of the IgE is left on the cell surface. The internalization does not require external Ca^{2+}, conditions that completely inhibit the release process. Even simple IgE dimers can initiate the internalization process, although they are less efficient than larger oligomers. Internalization requires the continued antigen-induced aggregation of the IgE molecules. During the endocytosis of IgE-antigen aggregates, there is co-internalization of receptors that have monomeric IgE. This is not due to random co-internalization of membrane proteins. Therefore, the cross-linking of the IgE receptors results in the internalization of these aggregates. The observation that this occurs in the absence of Ca^{2+} in the medium suggests that this is an event that precedes, and is independent of, a number of biochemical changes that accompany secretion (e.g., the influx of Ca^{2+} into the cell and the hydrolysis of phosphatidylinositol). However, it is not clear whether this internalization process plays any role in cross-membrane signaling.

Structure of $Fc_\epsilon R$

The purification of these receptors has been undertaken by a number of different laboratories (65,190). These purifications have utilized the capacity of the receptors to bind IgE with either high-affinity antibodies or monoclonal antibodies against the receptor (9). Most studies have used the rat basophilic leukemia cells because of the ready access to a large number of cells; however, some studies have been undertaken with other cells, which indicate that this is a good model for structural study of the receptor. Metzger et al. (190) have presented a model of the receptor containing four polypeptide chains (Table 3). The α-chain is 45 to 60 kilodaltons, contains carbohydrate, and is exposed on the outer surface of the cell.

TABLE 3. *Properties of the high-affinity $Fc_\epsilon R$ components[a]*

Property	Subunits		
	Alpha	Beta	Gamma
Molecular weight	45,000–60,000	33,000	9,000
Molecules per receptor	1	1	2
Glycosylation	+	−	−
Surface labeled	+	−	−
Intrinsic labeling			
Leucine, lysine	+	+	+
Methionine	+	+	−
Fatty acids	+	+	+
Phosphorus	?	+	+

[a] +, positive response; −, absent or failed to respond; ?, undetermined.

It is composed of two domains that are about equal in size. This component is the one to which the IgE molecule binds. The other receptor components do not contain carbohydrate and cannot be surface-labeled. The β-component is 33 kilodaltons and is an intramembranous protein exposed on the inner surface of the plasma membrane. The γ-component is also an intramembranous protein present as two disulfide-linked chains; each is 9 kilodaltons. It is also an intramembranous protein. The β- and γ-receptor components are not exposed on the cell surface but are exposed to the cytoplasmic side. The different receptor components dissociate, depending on the detergent concentrations. The β- and γ-dimer dissociate in unison from these complexes, suggesting that these two components might not interact independently with the α-chain. All receptor components have some covalently linked lipids, and there is evidence for some tightly bound lipids that might be important in the association of the different components. In intrinsic labeling studies, it has been observed that the γ-component does not label with [^{14}C]methionine, whereas the β-component labels well.

Full knowledge of the structure of the receptor will depend on the cloning of the genes of the receptor components. The injection of mRNA from the rat basophilic leukemia cell line into oocytes induced IgE-binding capacity in those cells (159,213). The cDNA from such mRNA was cloned, and positive clones were selected with antireceptor antibodies (158). The material that was originally seen in the injected oocytes was 31 kilodaltons, and the cloned sequence appears to be of similar size. The molecule has no glycosylation sites and has a large number of proline residues. Structurally, it does not appear to be related to the above components of the receptor but might correspond to a similar-sized molecule described in some experiments (92).

STIMULI FOR MAST CELL OR BASOPHIL SECRETION

A large number of different stimuli can stimulate basophils and mast cells to secrete a variety of mediators that have been discussed in other chapters. Both basophils and mast cells respond to the physiologically relevant stimulation through the IgE receptor. However, there appear to be numerous other differences in their response to other secretagogues; for example, compound 48/80 causes histamine release from rat mast cells and human cutaneous mast cells but not from human-lung mast cells or basophils (167). There are also differences in the response of mast cells or basophils from different species to the same stimulus. It seems very likely that some of the different secretagogues activate different biochemical pathways in the release process.

IgE-Receptor-Mediated System

As already discussed in previous sections, a characteristic of mast cells and basophils is the presence of the high-affinity IgE receptors on their cell surface. The IgE binds through the Fc portion of the molecule while the Fab portions are available for interacting with antigen. Activation of the cell is then due to bridging of the IgE molecules by antigen (249). Antibodies to the IgE receptor can activate cells in the absence of IgE (9,109,120). This indicates that the function of IgE is to confer antigenic specificity to the Fc$_\epsilon$R.

Basophils and mast cells can also be activated to release with heterologous antisera that react with the IgE on the cell surface (e.g., antibody that recognizes the immunoglobulin light or heavy chain). Similar reactions could occur in vivo with autoimmune rheumatoid-type antibodies that react with IgE on cells. Mitogens such as concanavalin A or phytohemagglutinin (PHA) can cross-link cell-surface IgE by binding to the carbohydrates on the IgE molecules (241,251). Protein A from *Staphylococcus aureus* can also react with IgE and release histamine (55). Recently there have also been reports of a cytokine that reacts with IgE on the basophil surface and releases histamine.

IgG-Receptor-Mediated System

Basophils and mast cells have an Fc$_\gamma$R that binds IG and is different from the Fc$_\epsilon$R (111,123,236). The binding of IgG is of much lower affinity than the binding of IgE to the Fc$_\epsilon$R. The IgG bound to the receptor easily dissociates from the cell surface unless it is in the form of antigen-IgG aggregates (39,40,64,236). Basophils or mast cells, especially from rodents, can be activated through this receptor to release histamine. However, this appears to be a less efficient system and requires much more antibody than does the IgE receptor.

Alloantisera directed toward the major histocompatibility complex can trigger mast cells. In mouse cells it has been shown that these IgG alloantisera bind to the mast cell surface by the antibody-binding sites and trigger the cell through the Fc portion of the molecule binding to the Fc$_\gamma$ receptors. The digestion of the allo-antibodies to remove the Fc portion abolished the reaction (39).

Complement Receptors

The two major complement-derived anaphylatoxins, C5a and C3a, can release mediators from mast cells and basophils (96,98,99). The cells have distinct receptors for both C5a and C3a which are separate from the immunoglobulin receptors (99). Another anaphylatoxin, C4a, is of low activity and appears to interact with the C3a receptor. On a molar basis, C5a is much more potent than C3a in stimulating cells for histamine release. Both mast cells and basophils have C3b receptors; however, they do not cause the activation of cells to release. With human basophils the activation of the C3b receptor results in enhancement of IgE-mediated histamine release (276,277).

Cytokines

There are lymphocyte- and/or macrophage-derived mediators that induce histamine release from human basophils (278,279). At the present time it is not clear whether there are different factors or if the difference is in the methods of generating and testing. Some of these factors might, in fact, release histamine by reacting with IgE on the cell surface (160,284). Other lymphokines, namely the interferons, enhance the IgE-mediated histamine release from human basophils (100,101). These effects are due to the induction of new RNA synthesis in the cells (85). Such modulation of mediator release may explain the exacerbations of asthma which are observed during viral infections.

Formyl Methionine Peptides

Formyl-methionine-containing tripeptides are chemotactic for a number of cell types and have similarities to chemotactic factors produced by bacteria. They bind to specific receptors and induce histamine release from human basophils but not from rat mast cells (95,247).

Eosinophilic-Granule-Derived Proteins

Approximately half the eosinophil granule protein consists of the arginine-rich major basic protein. This protein has been shown to damage a number of different cells, and it activates basophils and mast cells for histamine release (292).

Other Compounds

A large number of compounds have been described that activate mast cells or basophils for histamine release. Ionophores are lipophilic compounds that insert themselves into cell membranes and transport ions across the membrane. The calcium ionophore A23187 triggers mediator release from basophils and mast cells in the presence of calcium in the medium. Other compounds that are of experimental interest are tumor promoters (e.g., phorbol myristic acid), which release histamine from human ba-

sophils without a requirement for extracellular calcium (229,230). The recent interest in the mechanism of this release is a result of the finding that this compound binds and activates protein kinase C (see discussion below on the role of the phosphatidylinositol in the release pathway). Other secretagogues include polycationic compounds such as polymyxin B, compound 48/80, polylysine, and poly-arginine. Other compounds that cause mediator release are neuropeptides such as substance P, luteinizing-hormone-releasing hormone, morphine, tubocurarine, adenosine triphosphate, dextran, mellitin, chymotrypsin, and proteins released from neutrophils (76).

BIOCHEMICAL MECHANISMS OF THE RELEASE REACTION

The initial event in the stimulation of basophils and mast cells to secrete mediators is the interaction of antigen with IgE on the cell surface. The antigen then bridges two IgE molecules to initiate a series of biochemical events that eventually result in the secretion of mediators from the cells (Table 4). The release of histamine and other mediators from the cells is a rapid process that is complete in less than 30 min. Mediator release is a secretory (exocytotic) event that is noncytotoxic and occurs in the ab-

TABLE 4. *Biochemical events during basophil–mast-cell secretion*

Calcium-independent events
  1. IgE reacting with receptors on the cell surface
  2. IgE bridging by antigen
  3. Morphological changes
  4. Immobilization of receptors
  5. Internalization of receptors
  6. Changes in membrane potential
  7. Role for cGMP-binding proteins?
  8. Activation of protease enzymes
  9. Drop of internal $[Ca^{2+}]_i$ due to Ca^{2+} extrusion
  10. Rise in cAMP
  11. Protein phosphorylation
  12. Hydrolysis of phosphatidyl-inositides?
Calcium-dependent events
  13. Activation of methyl transferase
  14. Hydrolysis of phosphatidyl inosities
  15. Opening of Ca^{2+} channels and rise of $[Ca^{2+}]_i$
  16. Phosphorylation of proteins
  17. Release of arachidonic acid due to phospholipase-A2 and phospholipase-C activation
  18. Phosphorylation of several proteins, including a 92-kilodalton polypeptide
  19. Changes in the cytoskeleton, with movement of the granules
  20. Fusion of the granular membrane to the plasma membrane
  21. Opening of the granule to the extracellular space, with the release of granular contents

sence of serum. However, there is an absolute requirement for the presence of calcium in the medium for the IgE-receptor-mediated release reactions. The release reaction is temperature-dependent, with optimal release at 37°C. The reaction depends on the presence of IgE on the basophil–mast-cell surface. The concentration of antigen-specific IgE antibody on the membrane and its antigen-binding affinity are important parameters for the triggering of cells (30,43–45). Therefore, the optimal conditions for the release of histamine depends on the concentration of IgE, the concentration of the antigen, and the affinity of the IgE for the antigen. *In vitro* it has been shown that as little as 1 ng of ragweed antigen E (2.5×10^{-11} M) can trigger basophils from ragweed-allergic individuals.

The following sections will describe the biochemical events that have been described during basophil–mast-cell activation (Table 4). The recognition of these biochemical events has been either by direct measurement or by studying the action of inhibitors on the release process. Examples of direct measurement would be the changes in intracellular Ca^{2+} following cell stimulation. In contrast, the evidence for the activation of protease enzymes is deduced from the inhibition of secretion by inhibitors of proteolytic enzymes. The measurement of a biochemical change is the most unequivocal result, especially because of the notorious nonspecific activity of most inhibitors. It should also be noted that not all of these biochemical steps have been observed in all cell types and that there is controversy concerning some of these observations. These discrepancies will be pointed out in the following sections. It should also be pointed out that some of these biochemical events are bypassed when cells are activated by different secretagogues or by nonphysiological means; e.g., the calcium ionophore, by directly transporting calcium into the cell, bypasses some of the early steps in the activation of the cell.

The studies of the different biochemical changes do not unequivocally lead to a hypothesis of the sequence of events that occur in the cell. However, the changes in the absence of extracellular Ca^{2+} are early events. In the following sections, these steps in the release process are described in more detail.

Receptor Bridging and Aggregation

Studies with defined-length bivalent haptens have shown that bridging of two IgE molecules initiates the cell-triggering signal (249). Bivalent haptens with a different antigenic site at each end will activate cells, indicating that the bridging is between adjacent IgE molecules on the cell surface (249). Preformed, chemically cross-linked IgE dimers were active in triggering both rodent mast cells and human basophils (129,237). In contrast,

studies with the rat basophilic leukemia cell line have shown that IgE dimers were much less effective than trimers in releasing histamine (59). With human basophils, studies suggest that the dimeric triggering signal could be qualitatively different from trimer or oligomer stimulation (166). More recent studies by MacGlashan et al. (165) have found that the basophils from some donors respond to dimers as well as larger oligomers, whereas those from others require at least trimers to release mediators. This difference in response correlates with the capacity of the cells to release histamine, a parameter that has been called *releasability* (see discussion below on releasability). These studies suggest that although dimers can form the unit signal for activating cells, there could be variation in mast cell types or in cells from different donors. Furthermore, biochemical changes in the cell could change the sensitivity of a cell to an external signal. It is also possible that dimers, once they are bound to the cell surface, coalesce to form larger aggregates because of intrinsic changes in the receptor, or because of the interaction of the IgE-receptor complex with the cytoskeleton (186).

Number of Aggregates for Cell Activation

Activation of basophils or mast cells requires the bridging of a very few IgE molecules on the cell surface. Most studies suggest that bridging of 100 or less IgE molecules will fully activate the cell for histamine release. With the knowledge that mast cells and basophils appear to have 10^5 receptors per cell, it is obvious that bridging of less than 1% of the total IgE molecules on the cell surface activates biochemical events in the cell and also activates the release of histamine (44,59,161). In studies with rat mast cells, the addition of secretagogues immobilized on beads induces localized degranulation; therefore, full secretion from the cell would require the bridging of IgE molecules on different sectors of the cell surface (147).

The aggregation of the receptors results in a number of biochemical events in the basophils and mast cells (Table 4). There are two ways that these events could be activated by the aggregation of receptors. The aggregation of the receptors could result in a number of intrinsic activities; for example, other cell receptors form ion channels on aggregation or have enzymatic activity. So far, no intrinsic function for the $Fc_\epsilon R$ has been reported. An alternative mechanism for the activation of cellular biochemical events is the interaction of the aggregated receptors with other components. No direct interaction of other cellular components with the receptor have been described. As indicated in Table 4, a number of these biochemical events occur in the absence of any added Ca^{2+} in the medium. Some of these Ca^{2+}-independent reactions might be the initial trigger that transmits a signal across the membrane to activate the cell for secretion.

Morphological Study of Degranulation

Microscopic studies have detected a number of changes that occur in mast cells and basophils during mediator release (71,146). Under phase-contrast microscopy, when antigen is added to basophils *in vitro* the cells lose their oriented motility and spread out on the slide, extending pseudopodia in several directions (80). Some cells that exhibit this change do not go on to degranulate. The degranulating basophils develop small "vesicles" in their cytoplasm which rapidly increase in size and coalesce. The increase in the vesicles is accompanied by a decrease in the number of specific granules. The basophils remain sticky but regain their motility. By electron microscopic studies, the surface of the rat basophilic leukemia cells shows numerous microvilli (212). Within 30 sec of the addition of antigen, the microvillous surface transforms to a plicated appearance; the cells spread with increased adhesion to the substrate (212). There is also increased fluid pinocytosis. These changes occur in the absence of added Ca^{2+} and in cells during mitosis when secretion does not occur (206), although there is an increase in the $[Ca^{2+}]_i$ following receptor activation (86).

A number of transmission microscopic studies have described the changes that occur in basophils or mast cells of different species during secretion (for a review see ref. 71).

The stimulation of human basophils with antigen to release histamine results in a series of characteristic morphological changes (51,52,71). The granular membranes fuse with the plasma membrane around the circumference of the cell, resulting in the extrusion of the granular material to the outside. The diameter of the openings to the exterior are variable. There are occasional interconnected chains of granules opened to the exterior at a single point on the cell surface. The granule matrix is released as a whole to the outside, but the granule membrane is left behind. Frequently, membrane-free granular contents are seen attached to the cell exterior. In a fully degranulated basophil there is a complete loss of recognizable cytoplasmic granules. In contrast, a different morphological picture of degranulation is seen in basophils infiltrating sites of delayed hypersensitivity reactions. The process has been termed "piecemeal" degranulation; the granules never fuse with the cell membrane, and they lose their matrix in a "piecemeal" manner over a period of days. This type of degranulation probably does not occur in the type of reaction under discussion here.

The degranulation of human mast cells following IgE-receptor activation has similar morphological characteristics (29,53). There is swelling of the individual granules, with a change in the electron-dense granular contents. The individual granular contents fuse with each other to form an interconnected chain filled with altered granule matrix. These channels then open to the exterior by fusion with the plasma membrane. During the release process, there are prominent cytoplasmic filaments observed close to the granules. In very rapid freeze-fracture studies of rat mast cells, Chandler and Heuser (31) demonstrated that the earliest event in degranulation was the formation of single narrow-necked pores joining the membranes of the granules with the plasma membrane.

Changes in Receptor Mobility

The IgE receptors are diffusely distributed on the cell surface (13). The interaction of the IgE with multivalent antigen results in the interaction of the receptors with the cytoskeleton (188,219). There is the formation of clusters, aggregates, and patches, finally leading to capping of these into one pole of the cell (see section on receptors for full description).

Requirement for Metabolic Energy

The secretion of mediators from mast cells or basophils depends on energy generated from metabolic pathways. Energy is required for maintaining general cell functions. A number of inhibitors have been used to block energy utilization; these include anoxia in the absence of glucose as well as cyanide, 2-deoxyglucose, or antimycin A. The results from these experiments suggest that energy for histamine release may be obtained from either aerobic or anaerobic glycolysis. Direct experiments have also demonstrated energy use during mediator release with a number of isolated cell systems in which oxidative phosphorylation (aerobic glycolysis) plays the dominant role (127,128).

Changes in Transmembrane Potential

In many cells there are changes in the transmembrane potential as an early step in stimulus-response coupling. Transmembrane potentials can be measured by microelectrodes or by the use of fluorescence or isotopic techniques. The cell membrane potential depends on the ionic gradient of K^+ maintained across the plasma membrane. Changing the K^+ in the medium has no effect on the release of histamine from human basophils, although it is known that it should result in membrane potential changes in cells. Similarly, there is no other monovalent cation or anion requirement for histamine release from human basophils as long as Ca^{2+} is available in the medium (97). Membrane potential changes have been observed in rat mast cells and rat basophilic leukemia cells following cell stimulation for histamine release (130,211,224,226). In the rat mast-cell experiments, the membrane potential changes could have been secondary to the release of mediators. The changes in the rat basophilic leukemia cells have been interpreted as either being due to true membrane potential change or as being secondary to Ca^{2+} uptake by the mitochondria. There is also disagreement on whether the membrane potential changes are dependent on extracellular Ca^{2+}. In a further study, Kanner and Metzger (131) reported the uptake of $^{22}Na^+$ following IgE receptor aggregation in the absence of Ca^{2+}. These authors suggested that the plasma membrane channels are specific for Ca^{2+} only at millimolar concentrations of this cation. The question of whether the membrane potential changes are independent of the changes in intracellular Ca^{2+} requires further study.

Activation of Proteases

Inhibitors and substrates of proteolytic enzymes block secretion from mast cells and basophils (121). These inhibitors have included diisopropyl fluorophosphate, its analogs, and a number of trypsin and chymotrypsin substrates and inhibitors. Diisopropyl fluorophosphate phosphorylates serine residues in proteins and inactivates enzymes that contain serine in their active sites; i.e., the enzyme is a serine protease. Therefore, the proteolytic enzyme might be a serine esterase. These inhibitors block phospholipid methylation, the rise in $[Ca^{2+}]_i$, the cAMP increase, and cell secretion (121). In some experimental systems, the inhibitors are only effective during actual cell stimulation; if the cells are incubated with the inhibitor and washed prior to the addition of the secretagogue, there is normal release. This implies that the proteolytic enzyme is activated only after the start of the secretory process. The activation of this protease appears to be Ca^{2+}-independent. There is also evidence that a second protease enzyme is activated which is involved in cell desensitization (see section below on desensitization). The activation of this protease occurs in the absence of Ca^{2+} and is sensitive to lower concentrations of the protease inhibitors (122,134). In studies with rat mast-cell-membrane fragments, proteolytic inhibitors blocked the IgE-receptor-mediated increase in phospholipid methylation and adenylate cyclase activation (118). Therefore, a membrane-associated proteolytic enzyme might be an early step that activates the subsequent biochemical reactions.

Activation of Methyltransferases

Methylation reactions regulate a number of biochemical reactions in cells, including chemotaxis and gene expression (281). These reactions depend on different methyltransferase enzymes that transfer a methyl group from *S*-adenosylmethionine, a high-energy methyl donor, to lipids, proteins, or nucleic acids. Inhibitors of methylation reactions block IgE-mediated secretion from a variety of mast cells and basophils (37,38,113,117). There is also inhibition of the increase in the $[Ca^{2+}]_i$ as well as abrogation of the early rise in cAMP levels and of the release of arachidonic acid (37,38,118,183). This inhibition is limited to the IgE-receptor-mediated cell activation but not to stimulation with either compound 48/80, the calcium ionophore A23187, formyl methionine peptides, or C5a (88,193,194). Therefore, only the IgE-receptor-mediated activation requires this methyltransferase enzyme.

A critical role for signal transduction across the plasma membrane has been suggested for the phospholipid methyl transferase enzymes present in membranes (87). In the hypothesis suggested by Hirata and Axelrod (87), the phospholipid methyltransferase I enzyme faces the cytoplasmic surface and transfers one methyl group from *S*-adenosylmethionine, a high-energy methyl donor, to phosphatidylethanolamine. This results in the formation of monomethylethanolamine. The second enzyme, phospholipid methyltransferase II, then adds two more methyl groups, resulting in the formation of phosphatidylcholine. Most of the cellular phosphatidylcholine is synthesized through the UDP-choline pathway; however, the suggestion is that the small fraction formed by this methylation pathway is crucial for signaling across the plasma membrane.

A number of studies have demonstrated an early transient increase in phospholipid methylation following IgE-receptor activation of mast cells or basophils (38,117,121). This transient increase temporally preceded the $[Ca^{2+}]_i$ increase and histamine secretion (38). In some of these studies, no changes in methylation of proteins was observed (37). In membrane preparations from rat mast cells, there is activation of methyltransferase enzymes following IgE-receptor cross-linking (118). In studies with rat basophilic leukemia cells, variants were identified which were defective in either one of the two phospholipid methyltransferase enzymes (182). These two lines failed to demonstrate increased phospholipid methylation, Ca^{2+} influx, or histamine release after IgE-mediated cell stimulation. Fusion of these lines reconstituted the phospholipid methyltransferase I and II enzyme activities and, on IgE-receptor activation, resulted in Ca^{2+} influx and histamine release.

Recently, a number of questions have been raised with regard to the role of the phospholipid methyltransferase enzymes in secretion. First, there are questions as to whether two different phospholipid methyltransferase enzymes in fact exist. This can only be answered when the enzymes have been fully purified. Second, the experiments described above were performed by measuring the total incorporation of radioactive counts into a lipid soluble fraction. The amount of counts actually in this fraction is a very small fraction of the total added and incorporated into the cell. In experiments where the different phospholipids were fractionated, the predicted changes in the phospholipids were not observed (18,192). Third, the effect of the methyltransferase inhibitors could be at multiple sites in the cell (195). Therefore, although inhibitors of methylation reaction block histamine release, the mechanism of their reaction is not completely clear.

Hydrolysis of Phosphatidyl Inositides

There has been much recent interest on (a) the receptor-activated breakdown of myoinositol-containing phospholipids on cell activation and (b) the possible role of some of the products generated as intracellular second messengers (21,22,169,204). There are three myoinositol-containing phosphatides: phosphatidylinositol (PI), phosphatidylinositol-4-phosphate (PIP or diphosphoinositide), and phosphoinositol-4,5-bisphosphate (PIP_2 or triphosphoinositide). They account for less than 10% of the total phospholipids of the cell, with PI accounting for over 90% of the inositides. Receptor stimulation in a number of systems (hormones) results in the hydrolysis of the inositides with the release of water-soluble inositol phosphates and 1,2-diacylglycerol. These two are important second messengers within the cell; the 1,2-diacylglycerol activates protein kinase C, whereas the inositol phosphates release Ca^{2+} from the endoplasmic reticulum (23,24,28).

Receptor-mediated hydrolysis of membrane inositol phospholipids requires the activation of phospholipase C. There probably is a requirement for the interaction of receptors with GTP-regulatory proteins. The hydrolysis of phosphatidylinositol-4,5-bisphosphate results in the formation of 1,4,5-triphosphate and 1,2-diacylglycerol. The 1,4,5-triphosphate can release Ca^{2+} ions from ATP-dependent Ca^{2+} stores in the endoplasmic reticulum of several cell systems, whereas the 1,2-diacylglycerol activated protein kinase C (140). These then provide synergistic stimulatory signals for cells. Cells also contain phosphatidylinositol and inositides. Hydrolysis of this also occurs and might be secondary to the rise in the intracellular Ca^{2+}. There are other enzymatic pathways in the cell which result in the rapid conversion of inositol-1,4,5-triphosphate to inositol-1,3,4,5-tetrakisphosphate and subsequently to inositol-1,3,4-triphosphate. Several of these molecules appear to have the capacity to release Ca^{2+} from intracellular stores (104).

In rat mast cells there is increased turnover in phosphatidylinositol, phosphatidylcholine, and phosphatidic acid (32,103,124–126,136,227). The changes in phosphatidic acid occur prior to the onset of mediator release. The phosphatidic acid was probably formed from the 1,2-diacylglycerol generated by the action of the phospholipase C on the phosphatidyl inositides. In rat mast cells there is an increase in 1,2-diacylglycerol following cell activation; however, this appears to be slower than the time course of histamine release (137). Parallel inhibition of mediator release and phospholipid turnover was observed with a number of pharmacological agents. The changes in the phospholipids were blocked by drugs that increase intracellular cAMP levels (135). The generation of the 1,2-diacylglycerol activates protein kinase C, with resulting phosphorylation of proteins. Protein kinase C can also be directly activated by the binding of phorbol esters. This could be the mechanism by which phorbol ester stimulates secretion from basophils and mast cells (222,225,230). In the activated state there is more membrane association of the protein kinase C (286).

The IgE-receptor stimulation of rat basophilic leukemia cells results in a rapid breakdown of the phosphatidylinositides (11,168). The hydrolysis of the phosphatidyl inositides was originally thought to be absolutely dependent on Ca^{2+} in the medium; however, in more recent experiments there is evidence for some hydrolysis on cell stimulation independent of Ca^{2+}. By the use of La^{3+} it has been shown that the hydrolysis of inositides does not require an increase in $[Ca^{2+}]_i$. There is no significant hydrolysis of phosphatidyl inositides following stimulation with the calcium ionophore A23187 (11,19). The experiments, however, have not clearly defined a water-soluble inositol phosphate that could be important in releasing intracellular pools of Ca^{2+}.

There is indirect evidence for the involvement of the GTP-regulatory proteins in the activation of phospholipase C in cells. This could be distinct from the well-characterized molecules known as G_s, G_i, and transducin.

Role of G(GTP)-Binding Proteins

The G proteins are a family of molecules that form an important link between membrane receptors and intracellular effectors (263). A number of these proteins have been described in different tissues; several of these are well characterized and include G_s, G_i, G_o, and transducin. Whereas G_s and G_i appear to be present in most cells, G_o was described in the brain and transducin was described in the retina. These proteins are heterotrimers consisting of three polypeptides: the 39- to 52-kilodalton α chain, which has guanyl-nucleotide-binding activity; the 35- to 36-kilodalton β chain, and the 8-kilodalton γ chain. The three components associate (forming the GDP$\alpha\beta\gamma$ complex) when GDP is bound to the α chain. This complex is inactive and membrane-bound. A conformational change in the cell-surface receptor triggers G-protein activation, and this catalyzes the activation of the G protein by exchanging of GTP for the bound GDP. This results in the dissociation of the α chain from the other two components, leaving the G$\beta\gamma$ complex. Although the α components from the different proteins demonstrate a number of differences, the β chains are nearly identical. The β chain of the G, G_s, and G_i proteins can be specifically ADP-ribosylated, respectively, by bacterial toxins, cholera toxin, and pertussis.

There is some evidence for a role of these proteins in histamine release from cells. The release of histamine and other mediators from cells is altered by the addition of either cholera toxin or pertussis toxin (197). With human basophils, cholera toxin inhibits the IgE-mediated release reaction, whereas pertussis has no effect (26,27). With rat mast cells, pertussis inhibits the compound-48/80-induced histamine release and, to some extent, the release by IgE-mediated reactions (198). This inhibition has been suggested to occur at an early step in the release process because $^{45}Ca^{2+}$ uptake and arachidonic acid release were also inhibited (199). However, with rat basophilic leukemia cells there was no inhibition of IgE-mediated histamine release, although there was ADP ribosylation of a cellular protein.

There is indirect evidence for the involvement of the GTP-regulatory proteins in the activation of phospholipase C in cells (33,42). This could be distinct from the well-characterized molecules known as G_s, G_i, and transducin. In permeabilized rat mast cells, nonhydrolyzable GTP analogs stimulate secretion of histamine (77). This is not inhibited by neomycin, which prevents hydrolysis of phosphatidylinositol-4,5-bisphosphate. Similarly, pertussis toxin inhibits the hydrolysis of inositol phospholipids, and compound 48/80 stimulates secretion in rat mast cells and is shown to inhibit G_i through ADP ribosylation.

When GTP is introduced into mast cells through patch pipettes, it can induce Ca^{2+}-independent exocytosis (57). This suggests that GTP can act at least at two distinct sites: One site is critical for the activation of the phospholipase C, whereas the other site is at a later stage in the release process (6).

Activation of Adenylate Cyclase

Adenylate cyclase is a membrane-associated enzyme that is activated by binding of ligands to specific cell-surface receptors. The cyclic 3′,5′-adenosine monophosphate (cAMP) that is formed then acts as an intracellular second messenger in a number of cells. In most of these systems, increased levels of cAMP provide the signal for cell activation. The activation of mast cells by an IgE-mediated mechanism results in the increase of intracellular cAMP levels which is very rapid and parallels the rise and fall in phospholipid methylation (112,113,266). The rise in cAMP can be blocked by both methylation and protease

inhibitors. It occurs in the absence of extracellular Ca^{2+} prior to the increase in $[Ca^{2+}]_i$ (121,122). A late rise in cAMP has also been observed; this is a secondary effect resulting from the released PGD_2 (152). In rat basophilic leukemia cells, the IgE-receptor activation is not accompanied by an increase in the intracellular cAMP level (194). Other investigators have noted either a drop or no change in intracellular cAMP levels during secretion from human or rat mast cells and basophils (155,167,265). Therefore, a rise in cAMP is not critical for secretion but might be related to the modulation of other intracellular reactions.

The adenylate cyclase system includes a catalytic subunit that converts ATP to cAMP; it also includes several GTP-binding proteins that form the link between the membrane receptors and the catalytic unit (see section above on G-binding proteins). Adenosine can bind to several sites, one of which is on the external surface (R site) and increases adenylate cyclase activity; in contrast, adenosine also acts on an intracellular site (P site) and inhibits adenylate cyclase. Analogs of adenosine, which have only one or the other activity, either enhance or inhibit mediator release from mast cells. The addition of R-site agonists results in enhanced IgE-induced mediator release from rat mast cells and an increase in the peak-stimulated cAMP levels. However, the addition of such an agonist alone will result in an increased intracellular cAMP level without release of histamine. The addition of the P-site agonists blocks IgE-receptor-mediated cAMP rise and mediator release (90).

The intracellular effects of cAMP are mediated by the cAMP-dependent protein kinases. The increased intracellular cAMP levels can activate the cAMP-dependent protein kinase, which then phosphorylates its respective protein substrate. In rat mast cells, both type-I and type-II cAMP-dependent protein kinase activity is present in the cytoplasm and is activated after IgE-mediated cell triggering (287–289). The phosphorylation of the cell proteins could then play a modulating role in the release process. However, the increased intracellular cAMP level following the addition of PGD_2 or theophylline does not activate the protein kinase enzymes (289). There are conflicting reports in the literature with regard to the importance of cAMP in the release of histamine from cells (1,48,268,269).

Cyclic nucleotides appear to modulate the secretion of mediators from mast cells and basophils (267,288). A number of compounds can change the intracellular cAMP levels by interacting with specific cell-surface receptors which then activate the adenylate cyclase. These compounds include the β-adrenergic agents, prostaglandins, histamine (acting through the H_2 receptors), and cholera toxin. The intracellular levels of cAMP can also be raised by the addition of exogenous cAMP or its analog and by the addition of inhibitors of the phosphodiesterase enzyme involved in the breakdown of cAMP. All of these agents have been reported to inhibit mediator release in a variety of systems, including human basophils and mast cells. The compounds that raise intracellular cAMP levels inhibit phospholipid methylation and Ca^{2+} influx. Therefore, the increased cAMP levels could be a turn-off signal for secretion in some of these cell systems.

Changes in Intracellular Calcium

A requirement for calcium has long been recognized as essential for secretion from mast cells and basophils (207). There is extensive evidence for the essential role of calcium in the release process. First, Ca^{2+} chelators inhibit the release process. Second, the Ca^{2+} ionophore A23187 transports Ca^{2+} into the cell and initiates the secretory event (61). Third, the introduction of Ca^{2+} into the cytoplasm by microinjection, by fusion with Ca^{2+}-containing vesicles, or by permeabilization of the cell membrane activates the cell for secretion (15,274). Fourth, measurements with isotope-labeled Ca^{2+} demonstrate the uptake of this cation into the cell before the release of mediators (38,60,115). Fifth, measurement of the intracellular Ca^{2+} (abbreviated $[Ca^{2+}]_i$) with fluorescent dyes demonstrates an increase in the $[Ca^{2+}]_i$ when the cells are stimulated (12,285). The $[Ca^{2+}]_i$ concentration of ~105 nM in the cytoplasm is low compared to the 2 mM level in the extracellular space and is maintained by an energy-dependent pump that moves Ca^{2+} out of the cell. Following IgE-receptor cell stimulation there is a 100-fold increase in $[Ca^{2+}]_i$ in rat basophilic leukemia cells (8). This rise in $[Ca^{2+}]_i$ depends on the presence of Ca^{2+} in the medium. A mutant cell line has been isolated that can be stimulated to release mediators without a measurable increase in the $[Ca^{2+}]_i$ levels (290). Even in this cell line the release process is dependent on the presence of extracellular calcium. Therefore, a rise in $[Ca^{2+}]_i$ is not essential for the release process.

Accurate time-course measurements have demonstrated the uptake of isotopically labeled Ca^{2+} by basophils or mast cells early after IgE-receptor activation. The movement of Ca^{2+} into the cell occurs prior to the release of mediators. The increase in the $[Ca^{2+}]_i$ concentration can be due to several different mechanisms: first, mobilization of Ca^{2+} from intracellular or membrane stores; second, increased influx of extracellular Ca^{2+} by either increased permeability of the plasma membrane to Ca^{2+} or the opening of specific channels; third, a decrease in the efflux of intracellular Ca^{2+}. Direct isotopic measurements have shown that the stimulation of the rat basophilic leukemia cell for release results in a net increase in $[Ca^{2+}]_i$ to above the control levels (271). There appears to be little mobilization of Ca^{2+} from internal stores in most cells, with the possible exception of rat mast cells. The rise in $[Ca^{2+}]_i$ is too rapid to be explained on the basis of a decrease in the rate of pumping Ca^{2+} out of the cell.

The IgE-receptor activation of rat basophilic leukemia cells also results in the stimulation of Ca^{2+} efflux from the cell (271). This is independent of the increase in $[Ca^{2+}]_i$ and is an early event during cell stimulation. When there is an increase in $[Ca^{2+}]_i$, this reaction would function to return the cytoplasmic Ca^{2+} levels to normal.

A number of inhibitors block the IgE-receptor-mediated increase in $[Ca^{2+}]_i$. These include (a) compounds that raise intracellular cAMP levels, (b) metabolic inhibitors, and (c) inhibitors of transmethylation (280). By the use of two-dimensional gel analysis of the total cellular proteins, a number of polypeptides were found to be phosphorylated in the absence of extracellular Ca^{2+} and in the absence of a rise in $[Ca^{2+}]_i$. Therefore, there are a number of enzymatic steps that precede the increase of the $[Ca^{2+}]_i$.

A series of investigations by Marurek, Pecht, and co-workers (174–180) suggest that there is a specific Ca^{2+}-channel-forming protein in rat basophilic leukemia cells. These investigations are based on the observation that the drug cromolyn inhibits mediator release from mast cells as a result of inhibition of Ca^{2+} channels. Rat mast cells and leukemic basophils bind to cromolyn immobilized on beads (177). By the use of immobilized cromolyn, a protein was isolated from the rat basophilic leukemia cells and used for producing monoclonal antibodies (175). They have also isolated variant rat basophilic cell lines that do not bind cromolyn and that do not secrete (176). The addition of the purified cromolyn-binding protein in vesicles restored the secretory capacity of the cells (174). Conductance changes were measured when the monoclonal antibody was added to the purified protein reconstituted into planar bilayers (180). In other experiments, when both purified IgE receptors and this protein were reconstituted into the planar membranes, there were conductance changes when the IgE receptors were aggregated (36,178). Although these observations are very intriguing, a number of questions have been raised (190). Other investigators, utilizing patch-clamp techniques in whole rat basophilic leukemia cells have not been able to demonstrate the presence of a Ca^{2+} channel (156). The observation that a number of inhibitors block the rise in $[Ca^{2+}]_i$ are also in conflict with the idea that the aggregation of IgE receptors directly interacts with, as well as opens, Ca^{2+} channels.

The intracellular regulatory functions of Ca^{2+} are primarily due to its binding to ubiquitous Ca^{2+}-binding protein, calmodulin. This protein has a molecular weight of 17,000 and contains four Ca^{2+}-binding sites. The binding of Ca^{2+} to any of the four binding sites results in a conformational change that brings about the association of the complex with enzymes. The Ca^{2+}-calmodulin complex regulates a large number of enzyme systems, including phospholipase A$_2$ and microtubule assembly. A number of inhibitors (e.g., trifluoperazine) bind to calmodulin and inhibit its action in isolated systems; however, when these inhibitors are added to cells they probably affect a number of other systems.

Phosphorylation of Cellular Proteins

In a number of biological systems, extracellular signals activate cell-surface receptors and generate intracellular signals, which consequently activate protein kinase enzymes. The protein kinase results in the phosphorylation of cellular proteins. Many intracellular processes are regulated by the phosphorylation-dephosphorylation of proteins. A number of such protein kinases have been described, including: (a) cAMP-dependent protein kinase; (b) cGMP-dependent protein kinase; and (c) calcium-dependent protein kinases, which are of two types—a calmodulin-dependent and a phospholipid-dependent protein kinase. The Ca^{2+}- and phospholipid-dependent enzyme is called *protein kinase C* and, as discussed in the previous sections, might be activated by the 1,2-diacylglycerol generated by the breakdown of phophatidyl inositides. The proteins phosphorylated by these kinases are then dephosphorylated by phosphatases that limit the effect of the phosphorylated proteins.

A number of cell-surface receptors have kinase activity. For example, insulin and epidermal growth factor receptors have kinase activity and are also substrates for this activity. The α chain of the Fc$_\epsilon$R on rat mast cells was normally phosphorylated, and there was a further increase during mast-cell activation (83,84). However, these changes in the α component have not been observed with the rat basophilic leukemia cells (58,208). The changes with mast cells have also been observed following ionophore A23187 stimulation, suggesting that they could be secondary. The β and γ components of the Fc$_\epsilon$R are normally phosphorylated (58,208). Following receptor activation there is approximately a 45% increase in the phosphorylation of the β subunit, whereas there was a 35% decrease in the phosphorylation of the γ component (208). However, only a small fraction of the receptors incorporate labeled phosphate. The evidence from these experiments is inconclusive as to whether phosphorylation plays an essential role in signal transduction across the membrane.

The stimulation of rat mast cells for secretion results in the rapid phosphorylation of proteins with molecular weights of 78,000, 68,000, 59,000, and 42,000 (239). The phosphorylation of the three lower-MW proteins is rapid and parallels the rate of histamine release. In contrast, the phosphorylation of the 78,000-MW protein is slower than histamine secretion. Several inhibitors of mast-cell secretion, including cromolyn, transiently increase the phosphorylation of a 78,000-MW protein, which might be identical to that phosphorylated during cell stimulation (240,275). Interestingly, the inhibitory effect of cromolyn on mast-cell secretion is also transient. Therefore, the phosphorylation of this 78,000-MW protein might play a role in the turn-off signals for histamine secretion.

In rat basophilic leukemia cells, IgE- or ionophore-mediated histamine release is accompanied by the rapid phosphorylation of a 92,000-MW protein (82). This phosphorylation required the presence of extracellular Ca^{2+} in the medium, although this was not due to the rise in the [Ca^{2+}]$_i$. The number of changes in phosphorylated proteins that could be identified was much greater when the cells were analyzed by two-dimensional gel electrophoresis (56). Several polypeptides were phosphorylated in the absence of extracellular Ca^{2+} and therefore might function in steps leading to an increase in the [Ca^{2+}]$_i$. Other proteins have been described that are phosphorylated in the rat basophilic leukemia cell during cell secretion (223,273). The role of these phosphorylations in cell secretion needs further study.

Release of Arachidonic Acid

The activation of basophils or mast cells results in the release of arachidonic acid (an unsaturated fatty acid) from the cellular phospholipids (37,183). Arachidonic acid is commonly present in the *sn*-2 position of the glycerol backbone of phospholipids. The major membrane phospholipid is phosphatidylcholine, with lower amounts of phosphatidylethanolamine, phosphatidylserine, and phosphatidylinositides. There are different cellular pools of phospholipids, and the source from which the arachidonic acid is released depends on the stimulus.

There are several possible pathways for the release of arachidonic acid during cell stimulation. Activation of the cell results in the stimulation of phospholipase-C and phospholipase-A$_2$ enzymes. In one pathway, the action of phospholipase C on phosphatidyl inositides results in the formation of 1,2-diacylglycerol (DAG). This diacylglycerol can then be hydrolyzed by DAG lipase to release arachidonic acid. In the second pathway, arachidonic acid is released by phospholipase A2 from a number of different phospholipids, including phosphatidylcholine, phosphatidylethanolamine, and phosphatidylinositol. There is evidence for the presence of both pathways in rat mast cells and rat basophilic leukemia cells (72,137).

In rat basophilic leukemia cells the time course of the release of arachidonic acid parallels the release of histamine and appears to be slower than the increase in [Ca^{2+}]$_i$ (37,183). The release is observed only in the presence of extracellular Ca^{2+}. Phospholipase-A2 activation was present in cell homogenates following cell activation (73). Although arachidonic acid is released by both IgE and Ca^{2+}-ionophore stimulation of cells, there are a number of differences in the release induced by these two secretagogues. With the Ca^{2+} ionophore, more of the total arachidonic acid of the cell is released, and it is derived predominantly from the cellular phosphatidylethanolamine (72). In contrast, with IgE-mediated release the major source of the arachidonic acid was phosphatidylinositol/phosphatidylserine. This suggests that different phospholipase enzymes are activated by the two stimulants or that there are different pools of phospholipids that are accessible to the activated enzymes.

Glucocorticoids inhibit mediator release in a number of *in vitro* models of allergic reactions. The exposure of human basophils to steroids causes an inhibition of IgE-mediated histamine release (41,220,231,232). This inhibition is limited to the IgE-receptor-mediated system, whereas release due to stimulation with either Ca^{2+}-ionophore A23184, f-Met-Leu-Phe, or the phorbol ester is not blocked. With human mast cells there is no inhibition of the IgE-mediated release of histamine or prostaglandin D_2, although there are decreases in the release of some cyclooxygenase products (228). In mouse mast cells and rat basophilic leukemia cells, dexamethasone inhibited the release of histamine and arachidonic acid as well as increasing the uptake of Ca^{2+} from the extracellular fluid (19,41,220). In these systems the release process is slow and requires the culture of cells with the steroid for several hours, suggesting the requirement for the synthesis of a protein or molecule for this effect. In a number of systems it has been suggested that the action of the steroids is due to their induction of the synthesis of a phospholipase-A_2 inhibitory protein (89). Although such molecules can explain the inhibition of the release of the arachidonic acid following cell stimulation, they do not explain the inhibition of the $^{45}Ca^{2+}$ entry into the cells. Furthermore, the experiments with the rat basophilic leukemia cells have demonstrated that culture of the cells with steroids also results in the inhibition of the IgE-receptor-mediated phosphoinositide breakdown. Therefore, steroids should also have an effect on the phosphoinositol pathway of the generation of arachidonic acid in cells. A possible site for the action of steroids could be at an early step in the release process. Guanosine-5′-triphosphate-binding proteins have been proposed to play a role in the receptor-mediated stimulation of phospholipase C. Therefore, the action of steroids could occur at some of these early stages in cell activation.

The arachidonic acid released can be metabolized by either the cyclooxygenase or the lipoxygenase pathways (79,151). The products of the lipoxygenase pathway are the leukotrienes (see the detailed discussion elsewhere in this volume). There is some suggestive evidence for a role of an unknown product from this lipoxygenase pathway in cell secretion. Inhibitors of arachidonic acid metabolism block histamine release, whereas the selective inhibition of the cyclooxygenase pathway (with indomethacin or aspirin), by diverting the arachidonic acid to the lipoxygenase pathway, enhances histamine release (78,171,201,210,259). In contrast, lipoxygenase inhibition blocks some release reactions (201). Among the lipoxygenase products, several compounds (e.g., 5-HPETE, 5-HETE, and 12-HETE) enhance IgE-mediated release; also, 5-HPETE can release histamine in the presence of cytochalasin B, an agent that disrupts microfilaments (210). However, with rat basophilic leukemia cells, the inhibition of the lipoxygenase pathway with indomethacin has no effect on the histamine release (183). Therefore, the role of the lipoxygenase product in the release process is not clearly established.

The arachidonic acid released from the mast cells and basophils can also be metabolized by the cyclooxygenase pathway. This pathway leads predominantly to the formation of prostaglandin D_2 in these cells (153,183). There is also the formation of some thromboxane A_2 and prostacyclin. The addition of prostaglandin D_2 to basophils or mast cells has variable effects; in some systems it has been reported to inhibit histamine release.

The Cytoskeleton

The cytoskeletal structures of eukaryotic cells determine the characteristic shape of the cell and the cytoplasm. The cytoskeletal structures consist of the microtubules, actin microfilaments, and intermediate filaments. These are not static structures; instead, they undergo rapid changes responsible for cell motility and for movement in the cytoplasm. The cytoskeletal components are thought to insert, either directly or through other proteins, into the cell membrane and might also bind to granules. Receptors on the cell surface may exist in two interconvertible states, either (i) free where they can diffuse in the cell membrane or (ii) bound in some way to the microtubular or microfilament structures in the cell. Therefore, the distribution of cell-surface receptors is influenced by their interaction with the cytoskeleton; conversely, the binding of ligands to cell-surface receptors influences the organization of the cytoskeleton. The cytoskeletal elements are involved in the aggregation of receptors into patches, leading to their eventual coalescence into caps at one end of the cell. Therefore, skeletal components could play an important role in histamine release.

Microtubules are present in mast cells and basophils. They have a characteristic tubular structure consisting of heterodimers formed from α- and β-tubulin polypeptides.

The microtubules are filamentous protein polymers (which are labile structures) and are in a state of constant dynamic equilibrium with a pool of tubulin subunits. The assembly of the tubules is controlled by the level of Ca^{2+} as well as by the oxidation state of tubulin sulfhydryl groups and of cyclic nucleotides. There are a number of microtubule-associated proteins that may play a role in regulating the polymerization of tubulin. Microtubules are inserted into both the cell membrane and granules and could be either passive direction markers for the secretion of granules or actively involved in the movement of the granule. Colchicine and vinblastine bind to tubulin dimers and prevent their polymerization into microtubules. Colchicine also binds to cell-surface proteins and inhibits nucleoside transport into the cell. Colchicine and vinblastine inhibit histamine release from both basophils and mast cells. Conversely, deuterium oxide (heavy water) stabilizes microtubules and enhances IgE-mediated histamine release (74). However, heavy water also enhances phosphoinositide hydrolysis, indicating that it could also have effects at early steps of the release process (168). Inhibitors of microtubular function blocked the release of arachidonic acid without affecting the increase in $[Ca^{2+}]_i$ (280). Therefore, the coupling of the IgE receptor and Ca^{2+} influx to phospholipase activation requires the microtubular system.

Microfilaments are filamentous structures observed in many cells and are usually distributed close to the cell surface. They are thought to be actin-like polymers, and there is some evidence that they interact with the cell membrane. The cytochalasins are fungal products that inhibit cellular movements. Although they were originally thought to act directly on microfilaments, more recent studies suggest that they have a number of effects, including inhibition of membrane transport systems. Cytochalasin B inhibits the lateral diffusion of IgE molecules in the membrane of cells. These agents also enhance IgE-receptor-mediated histamine release from mast cells or basophils but inhibit leukotriene formation. From these inhibitor data it appears that microtubules and microfilaments probably are involved in the secretory function of basophils and mast cells.

RELEASABILITY

There is variation in the extent of histamine release from the cells of different donors; this has been termed the *releasability* of the cells (248). The extent of histamine release from the cells of any one individual can vary from as low as being no different than the spontaneous release to values as high as 90% to 100%. Similarly, the releasability of the cells can be different with different secretagogues; i.e., the cells of a donor could release well with

an IgE stimulus but poorly with another secretagogue, e.g., f-Met-Leu-Phe or C5a and vice versa (95,246,247). The release by IgE-receptor-mediated activation of the cells has drawn the most interest because it may relate to clinical allergy. In a number of studies, no correlation has been found between the number of IgE molecules present on the cell surface of cells from donors that respond well and donors that do not release histamine. Variations have also been observed over time as to the releasability of the cells of the same donor. In studies comparing mono- and dizygotic twins, there was good correlation in IgE-induced histamine release only among the monozygotic twins (172).

Recent evidence suggests that the difference in the releasability of different donors could be due to the sensitivity of their basophils to different stimuli. As the density of IgE molecules on the cell surface appears to be the same on the cells of different donors with marked variation in cell sensitivity, the difference is probably at the cellular level. The sensitivity of cells to different stimuli can be modified by a number of factors, e.g., variation in lymphokine factors, steroids, or dietary lipids that can incorporate into the membranes. The cells of donors who are high responders release histamine with chemically cross-linked IgE dimers, whereas the cells of the low responders release with chemically cross-linked trimers but release very poorly with dimers (165).

DESENSITIZATION FOR THE RELEASE REACTION

The cross-linking of the IgE receptors on the basophil or mast cell results in the activation of a number of biochemical reactions, leading to the secretion of mediators. Some of these biochemical reactions also function either directly or indirectly to regulate the extent of the release reaction. This process is called *desensitization;* similar phenomena have been observed in a number of biological systems. Under experimental conditions the desensitization process is initiated by the addition of the secretagogue under nonpermissive conditions. That is, the cells are first exposed to these secretagogues under conditions that do not result in secretion (e.g., the addition of an antigen in the absence of Ca^{2+} in the medium); then, after a defined incubation period, the permissive conditions are restored (e.g., by the addition of Ca^{2+} in this case). Desensitization has been observed (a) when the secretagogue has been added in the absence of either Ca^{2+} or another essential ingredient of the reaction mixture (e.g., phosphatidylserine for rat mast-cell antigen release), (b) when the concentration of the antigen has been supraoptimal, or (c) when the reaction temperature has been nonoptimal (45–47,50,64,245). When different secretagogues are used with human basophils, the desensitization is specific for the stimulus; e.g., desensitization for IgE-mediated release does not inactivate the cells for release with C5a or with the formyl-methionine peptides (246,247). The IgE-receptor-mediated desensitization requires receptor aggregation and can be initiated by dimers, although larger oligomers are more effective. In experiments with IgE-mediated release reactions, the desensitization can either be specific (i.e., specific to the antigen that was used for the desensitization process) or it could be nonspecific (i.e., the cells would not respond to challenge with any antigen) (253). Depending on the density of the IgE on the cell surface, specific or nonspecific desensitization can be obtained. At low IgE densities there is specific desensitization, whereas at high IgE levels there is nonspecific desensitization (164). The fact that it occurs in the absence of added Ca^{2+} suggests that it involves a step prior to the rise in the intracellular Ca^{2+} concentration. Further evidence is the lack of an enhanced $^{45}Ca^{2+}$ in desensitized cells following receptor cross-linking (122). Desensitization is an active process with similarities to the events that result in cell secretion; e.g., desensitization is not observed at low temperatures. The desensitization reaction can be blocked by the addition of some inhibitors; e.g., with human basophils the serine esterase inhibitor diisopropylfluorophosphate (DFP), when added at a narrow concentration range, decreased desensitization and enhanced release (134). With mouse mast cells, both DFP (a serine esterase inhibitor) and inhibitors of methyltransferases blocked desensitization (122). It has been suggested that the extent of desensitization directly regulates the extent of the release process (10). In rat mast cells, manipulations that influence the desensitization reaction had parallel effects on the extent of histamine release. With human basophils, DFP can inhibit desensitization and enhance basophil histamine release; again there was correlation between the amount of inhibition of desensitization by DFP and the subsequent enhancement of histamine release.

The biochemical basis of the desensitization phenomena is not understood. Desensitization is not due to the cell-surface loss of antigen-specific IgE caused by endocytosis or shedding of IgE-antigen complexes (161,162). There is a rapid endocytosis of IgE-antigen complexes from the cell surface; however, even under these conditions there are enough IgE-receptor complexes remaining on the cell surface to stimulate release. Alternatively, there could be the decay of an unstable intermediate formed by the cross-linked receptors interacting with a secondary component (46,47). With human basophils the data suggest that the endocytosis of the antigen-receptor complexes from the cell surface does not occur in the absence of Ca^{2+}; however, this is not true for the rat basophilic leukemia cell line. There is also continued capacity of antigen

binding to the IgE on the cell surface (162). Similarly, nonspecific desensitization does not appear to be due to the co-internalization of all cell-surface IgE when the specific IgE is cross-linked. Evidence with human basophils suggests that specific desensitization is due to alterations in some very early biochemical event, whereas the nonspecific desensitization results from changes in biochemical events in more distal reactions.

Secretion from cells results from a balance between activation and deactivation signals (10). It is possible that signals are generated early in the secretory event, resulting in cell secretion; these signals decay as a result of degradative enzymatic pathways. If the signals cannot be processed because of the unfavorable experimental conditions (e.g., in the absence of calcium in the medium), there is decay in the signal.

COMPARISON OF MAST-CELL AND BASOPHIL RELEASE REACTIONS

A crucial question exists with regard to whether or not the mechanism for mediator release is similar among the various cell systems studied (e.g., human mast cells or basophils versus rat mast cells). There are differences in the response of various cells to diverse nonphysiologic stimuli; e.g., the rat mast cell releases very well to compound 48/80, whereas human basophils do not respond. However, all systems respond to the physiologically relevant system of IgE-antigen. The rate of release with human basophils and mast cells is slower than with rat mast cells; e.g., histamine release with human cells requires 15 to 40 min, as opposed to 1 to 2 min with rat mast cells. The rate with human mast cells is faster than with human basophils. The use of inhibitors suggests that there are similarities in the release mechanism of basophils and mast cells. However, there are differences between human basophils and mast cells (Table 5).

Basophils are smaller cells that enter the circulation and have a short half-life in comparison to the mast cells located in the tissues. As discussed above, there are morphological differences in degranulation, as observed by electron microscopy: that of the basophils is of the "compound" type, with granules fusing with each other, whereas the mast cell granules fuse directly with the plasma membrane. Both cell types respond to IgE-receptor activation with the release of mediators. However, mast cells require higher concentrations of anti-IgE for activation. When tested with different secretagogues, a number of differences have been observed between mast cells and basophils, as observed in Table 5. In contrast, the isolated mast cells do not respond to the complement factors C5a and C3a, nor do they respond to formyl peptides. Basophils also release when activated with the phor-

TABLE 5. *Comparison of basophils and mast cells*[a]

Property	Basophil	Mast cell
Size (microns)	7–10	14–20
Nucleus	Multilobed	Single-lobed
Histamine content	1 pg/cell	3 pg/cell
Life-span	Short (hours)	Long (months)
Degranulation morphology	Compound fusion	Single-granule fusion
Arachidonic acid metabolites		
Leukotriene	LTC_4	LTC_4
Cyclooxygenase	−	PGD_2, thromboxanes
Platelet-activating factor	−	+ (synthesized)
Secretagogues		
IgE	+	+
Ca^{2+} ionophore	+	+
Polyarginine	+	+
Hyperosmolarity	+	+
C5a	+	−
C3a	+	−
F-Met-Leu-Phe	+	−
TPA	+	−
5HPETE (+ cytochalasin)	+	−
Morphine	−	+/−
Compound 48/80	−	+/−
Pharmacological modulation		
β-adrenergic	+/−	+
Theophylline	+	+
H_2 agonist	+	−
Adenosine	+	−
Prostaglandins	+	+
Steroids	+	−
Indomethacin	Enhances	−

[a] +, responds to secretagogue, or the pharmacological agent will inhibit the release process; −, does not respond to the secretagogue, or pharmacological agent has no effect.

bol ester TPA, whereas this has no effect on the mast cells. Similarly, the lipoxygenase product, 5HPETE, releases histamine only from basophils but not from mast cells. Most of these studies were with mast cells isolated from lung tissues by techniques that require treatment with protease enzymes. It is therefore not completely clear whether these differences are partly due to the fact that this treatment removes a number of cell-surface receptors. A number of other studies have isolated mast cells either from skin tissues or from intestinal sites; the few reports with these cells show little differences from the cells isolated from the lungs (17,62,63).

There are also differences in the response of basophils and mast cells to different pharmacological agents. Inhibitors of the cyclooxygenase pathway enhance release from basophils but not from mast cells. The H_2 agonists inhibit release from basophils but have no effect on mast cells, and PGD_2 enhances the release from human basophils but is without effect on mast cells (167). Other differences include the effect of dexamethasone, which inhibits mediator release from human basophils but not from human mast cells. Adenosine inhibits the basophil's release but slightly enhances the release from mast cells. Some of

these differences in the effects of pharmacological agents could be due to the presence or absence of agonist-specific receptors on these cells.

A number of differences have been observed in the mediators released by mast cells as compared to those released by basophils. In contrast to mast cells, human basophils release very little, if any, of the cyclooxygenase-derived products of arachidonic acid such as PGD_2. However, both mast cells and basophils release the leukotriene LTC_4. These are secondary mediators generated by enzymes acting on released arachidonic acid. The difference seen here between the basophils and mast cells could be due to the presence or absence of the enzymes involved in the production of these metabolites. Although there are clear differences between the basophil and mast cell, there is little evidence to suggest that the secretory process is fundamentally different in the two cell types.

CONCLUDING REMARKS

A better understanding of the mast cell and the basophil is crucial for advancing our knowledge of immediate hypersensitivity reactions. As discussed in this chapter, there have been major advances made in understanding the origin and development of these cells in animal models. However, adequate human basophil or mast-cell lines for these studies are still lacking. It is hoped that the next major advance will be the development of such tools to further our understanding and allow the control of allergic reactions. The understanding of the mechanisms involved in the secretion of mediators from mast cells and basophils could allow the better utilization of tools to abrogate this secretory event.

ACKNOWLEDGMENTS

I would like to acknowledge the excellent secretarial help of Ms. Peggy Swift as well as to thank William Hook and Elsa Berenstein for reviewing the manuscript.

REFERENCES

1. Alm, E., and Bloom, G. D. (1982): Cyclic nucleotide involvement in histamine release from mast cells—A reevaluation. *Life Sci.,* 30:213–218.
2. Augustin, R. (1967): Demonstration of reagin in the serum of allergic subjects. In: *Handbook of Experimental Immunology,* edited by D. M. Weir, pp. 1076–1151. Blackwell Scientific Publications, Oxford.
3. Baird, B., and Holowka, D. (1985): Structural mapping of Fc receptor bound immunoglobulin E: Proximity to the membrane surface of the antibody combining site and another site in the Fab segments. *Biochemistry,* 24:6252–6259.
4. Baniyash, M., and Eshhar, Z. (1984): Inhibition of IgE binding to mast cells and basophils by monoclonal antibodies to murine IgE. *Eur. J. Immunol.,* 14:799–807.
5. Baniyash, M., Eshhar, Z., and Rivnay, B. (1986): Relationships between epitopes on IgE recognized by defined monoclonal antibodies and by the FC epsilon receptor on basophils. *J. Immunol.,* 136:588–593.
6. Barrowman, M. M., Cockcroft, S., and Gomperts, B. D. (1986): Two roles for guanine nucleotides in the stimulus-secretion sequence of neutrophils. *Nature,* 319:504–507.
7. Barsumian, E. L., Isersky, C., Petrino, M. G., and Siraganian, R. P. (1981): IgE-induced histamine release from rat basophilic leukemia cell lines: Isolation of releasing and nonreleasing clones. *Eur. J. Immunol.,* 11:317–323.
8. Barsumian, E. L., McGivney, A., Basciano, L. K., and Siraganian, R. P. (1985): Establishment of four mouse mastocytoma cell lines. *Cell Immunol.,* 90:131–141.
9. Basciano, L. K., Berenstein, E. H., Kmak, L., and Siraganian, R. P. (1986): Monoclonal antibodies that inhibit IgE binding. *J. Biol. Chem.,* 261:11823–11831.
10. Baxter, J. H., and Adamik, R. (1975): Control of histamine release: Effects of various conditions on rate of release and rate of cell desensitization. *J. Immunol.,* 114:1034–1041.
11. Beaven, M. A., Moore, J. P., Smith, G. A., Hesketh, T. R., and Metcalfe, J. C. (1984): The calcium signal and phosphatidylinositol breakdown in 2H3 cells. *J. Biol. Chem.,* 259:7137–7142.
12. Beaven, M. A., Rogers, J., Moore, J. P., Hesketh, T. R., Smith, G. A., and Metcalfe, J. C. (1984): The mechanism of the calcium signal and correlation with histamine release in 2H3 cells. *J. Biol. Chem.,* 259:7129–7136.
13. Becker, K. E., Ishizaka, T., Metzger, H., Ishizaka, K., and Grimley, P. M. (1973): Surface IgE on human basophils during histamine release. *J. Exp. Med.,* 138:394–409.
14. Befus, A. D., Bienenstock, J. and Denburg, J. A., editors (1986):

Mast Cell Differentiation and Heterogeneity, pp. 1–426. Raven Press, New York.
15. Bennett, J. P., Cockcroft, S., and Gomperts, B. D. (1981): Rat mast cells permeabilized with ATP secrete histamine in response to calcium ions buffered in the micromolar range. *J. Physiol. (Lond.),* 317:335–345.
16. Bennich, H., and Johansson, S. G. (1971): Structure and function of human immunoglobulin E. *Adv. Immunol.,* 13:1–55.
17. Benyon, R. C., Church, M. K., Clegg, L. S., and Holgate, S. T. (1986): Dispersion and characterisation of mast cells from human skin. *Int. Arch. Allergy Appl. Immunol.,* 79:332–334.
18. Benyon, R. C., Church, M. K., and Holgate, S. T. (1986): IgE-dependent activation of mast cells is not associated with enhanced phospholipid methylation. *Biochem. Pharmacol.,* 35:2535–2544.
19. Berenstein, E. H., Garcia-Gil, M., and Siraganian, R. P. (1987): Dexamethasone inhibits receptor-activated phosphoinositide breakdown in rat basophilic leukemia (RBL-2H3) cells. *J. Immunology,* 138:1914–1918.
20. Bergendorff, A., and Uvnäs, B. (1972): Storage of 5-hydroxytryptamine in rat mast cells. Evidence for an ionic binding to carboxyl groups in a granule heparin-protein complex. *Acta Physiol. Scand.,* 84:320–331.
21. Berridge, M. J. (1984): Inositol trisphosphate and diacylglycerol as second messengers. *Biochem. J.,* 220:345–360.
22. Berridge, M. J. (1986): Regulation of ion channels by inositol trisphosphate and diacylglycerol. *J. Exp. Biol.,* 124:323–335.
23. Berridge, M. J., and Irvine, R. F. (1984): Inositol trisphosphate, a novel second messenger in cellular signal transduction. *Nature,* 312:315–321.
24. Biden, T. J., Prentki, M., Irvine, R. F., Berridge, M. J., and Wollheim, C. B. (1984): Inositol 1,4,5-trisphosphate mobilizes intracellular Ca^{2+} from permeabilized insulin-secreting cells. *Biochem. J.,* 223:467–473.
25. Bland, C. E., Ginsburg, H., Silbert, J. E., and Metcalfe, D. D. (1982): Mouse heparin proteoglycan. Synthesis by mast cell-fibroblast monolayers during lymphocyte-dependent mast cell proliferation. *J. Biol. Chem.,* 257:8661–8666.
26. Bourne, H. R., Lehrer, R. I., Lichtenstein, L. M., Weissmann, G., and Zurier, R. (1973): Effects of cholera enterotoxin on adenosine 3',5'-monophosphate and neutrophil function. Comparison with other compounds which stimulate leukocyte adenyl cyclase. *J. Clin. Invest.,* 52:698–708.
27. Bourne, H. R., Lichtenstein, L. M., Melmon, K. L., Henney, C. S., Weinstein, Y., and Shearer, G. M. (1974): Modulation of inflammation and immunity by cyclic AMP. *Science,* 184:19–28.
28. Burgess, G. M., Godfrey, P. P., McKinney, J. S., Berridge, M. J., Irvine, R. F., and Putney, J. W., Jr. (1984): The second messenger linking receptor activation to internal Ca release in liver. *Nature,* 309:63–66.
29. Caulfield, J. P., Lewis, R. A., Hein, A., and Austen, K. F. (1980): Secretion in dissociated human pulmonary mast cells. Evidence for solubilization of granule contents before discharge. *J. Cell Biol.,* 85:299–312.
30. Chabay, R., DeLisi, C., Hook, W. A., and Siraganian, R. P. (1980): Receptor cross-linking and histamine release in basophils. *J. Biol. Chem.,* 255:4628–4635.
31. Chandler, D. E., and Heuser, J. E. (1980): Arrest of membrane fusion events in mast cells by quick-freezing. *J. Cell Biol.,* 86:666–674.
32. Cockcroft, S. (1982): Phosphatidylinositol metabolism in mast cells and neutrophils. *Cell Calcium,* 3:337–349.
33. Cockcroft, S., and Gomperts, B. D. (1985): Role of guanine nucleotide binding protein in the activation of polyphosphoinositide phosphodiesterase. *Nature,* 314:534–536.
34. Conrad, D. H., Wingard, J. R., and Ishizaka, T. (1983): The interaction of human and rodent IgE with the human basophil IgE receptor. *J. Immunol.,* 130:327–333.
35. Conroy, M. C., Adkinson, N. F., Jr., and Lichtenstein, L. M. (1977): Measurement of IgE on human basophils: relation to serum IgE and anti-IgE-induced histamine release. *J. Immunol.,* 118:1317–1321.
36. Corcia, A., Schweitzer-Stenner, R., Pecht, I., and Rivnay, B. (1986):

Characterization of the ion channel activity in planar bilayers containing IgE-Fc epsilon receptor and the cromolyn-binding protein. *EMBO J.,* 5:849–854.

37. Crews, F. T., Morita, Y., Hirata, F., Axelrod, J., and Siraganian, R. P. (1980): Phospholipid methylation affects immunoglobulin E-mediated histamine and arachidonic acid release in rat leukemia basophils. *Biochem. Biophys. Res. Commun.,* 93:42–49.

38. Crews, F. T., Morita, Y., McGivney, A., Hirata, F., Siraganian, R. P., and Axelrod, J. (1981): IgE-mediated histamine release in rat basophilic leukemia cells: Receptor activation, phospholipid methylation, Ca^{2+} flux, and release of arachidonic acid. *Arch. Biochem. Biophys.,* 212:561–571.

39. Daëron, M., Couderc, J., Ventura, M., Liacopoulos, P., and Voisin, G. A. (1982): Anaphylactic properties of mouse monoclonal IgG2a antibodies. *Cell Immunol.,* 70:27–40.

40. Daëron, M., Prouvost-Danon, A., and Voisin, G. A. (1980): Mast cell membrane antigens and Fc receptors in anaphylaxis. II. Functionally distinct receptors for IgG and for IgE on mouse mast cells. *Cell Immunol.,* 49:178–189.

41. Daëron, M., Sterk, A. R., Hirata, F., and Ishizaka, T. (1982): Biochemical analysis of glucocorticoid-induced inhibition of IgE-mediated histamine release from mouse mast cells. *J. Immunol.,* 129:1212–1218.

42. Deckmyn, H., Tu, S. M., and Majerus, P. W. (1986): Guanine nucleotides stimulate soluble phosphoinositide-specific phospholipase C in the absence of membranes. *J. Biol. Chem.,* 261:16553–16558.

43. DeLisi, C., and Siraganian, R. P. (1979): Receptor cross-linking and histamine release. II. Interpretation and analysis of anomalous dose response patterns. *J. Immunol.,* 122:2293–2299.

44. DeLisi, C., and Siraganian, R. P. (1979): Receptor cross-linking and histamine release. I. The quantitative dependence of basophil degranulation on the number of receptor doublets. *J. Immunol.,* 122:2286–2292.

45. Dembo, M., and Goldstein, B. (1980): A model of cell activation and desensitization by surface immunoglobin: The case of histamine release from human basophils. *Cell,* 22:59–67.

46. Dembo, M., Goldstein, B., Sobotka, A. K., and Lichtenstein, L. M. (1979): Histamine release due to bivalent penicilloyl haptens the relation of activation and desensitization of basophils to dynamic aspects of ligand binding to cell surface antibody. *J. Immunol.,* 122:518–528.

47. Dembo, M., Goldstein, B., Sobotka, A. K., and Lichtenstein, L. M. (1979): Degranulation of human basophils: Quantitative analysis of histamine release and desensitization, due to a bivalent penicilloyl hapten. *J. Immunol.,* 123:1864–1872.

48. Diamant, B., Kazimierczak, W., and Patkar, S. A. (1978): Does cyclic AMP play any role in histamine release from rat mast cells. *Allergy,* 33:50–51.

49. Dorrington, K. J., and Bennich, H. H. (1978): Structure-function relationships in human immunoglobulin E. *Immunol. Rev.,* 41:3–25.

50. Drobis, J. D., and Siraganian, R. P. (1976): Histamine release from cultured human basophils: Lack of histamine resynthesis after antigenic release. *J. Immunol.,* 117:1049–1053.

51. Dvorak, A. M., Ishizaka, T., and Galli, S. J. (1985): Ultrastructure of human basophils developing *in vitro.* Evidence for the acquisition of peroxidase by basophils and for different effects of human and murine growth factors on human basophil and eosinophil maturation. *Lab Invest.,* 53:57–71.

52. Dvorak, A. M., Lett-Brown, M. A., Thueson, D. O., Pyne, K., Raghuprasad, P. K., Galli, S. J., and Grant, J. A. (1984): Histamine-releasing activity (HRA). III. HRA induces human basophil histamine release by provoking noncytotoxic granule exocytosis. *Clin. Immunol. Immunopathol.,* 32:142–150.

53. Dvorak, A. M., Schulman, E. S., Peters, S. P., MacGlashan, D. W., Jr., Newball, H. H., Schleimer, R. P., and Lichtenstein, L. M. (1985): Immunoglobulin E-mediated degranulation of isolated human lung mast cells. *Lab Invest.,* 53:45–56.

54. Ennis, M., and Pearce, F. L. (1980): Differential reactivity of isolated mast cells from the rat and guinea pig. *Eur. J. Pharmacol.,* 66:339–345.

55. Espersen, F., Jarlv, J. O., Jensen, C., Skov, P. S., and Norn, S. (1984): Staphylococcus aureus peptidoglycan induces histamine release from basophil human leukocytes *in vitro. Infect. Immun.,* 46:710–714.

56. Essani, N., Essani, K., and Siraganian, R. P. (1986): Protein phosphorylation in rat basophilic leukemia cells following stimulation for histamine release. *Fed. Proc.,* 45:243.

57. Fernandez, J. M., Neher, E., and Gomperts, B. D. (1984): Capacitance measurements reveal stepwise fusion events in degranulating mast cells. *Nature,* 312:453–455.

58. Fewtrell, C., Davis, C. L., and Metzger, H. (1982): Phosphorylation of the receptor of immunoglobulin E. *Biochemistry,* 21:2004–2010.

59. Fewtrell, C., and Metzger, H. (1980): Larger oligomers of IgE are more effective than dimers in stimulating rat basophilic leukemia cells. *J. Immunol.,* 125:701–710.

60. Foreman, J. C., Hallett, M. B., and Mongar, J. L. (1977): The relationship between histamine secretion and ^{45}calcium uptake by mast cells. *J. Physiol. (Lond.),* 271:193–214.

61. Foreman, J. C., Mongar, J. L., and Gomperts, B. D. (1973): Calcium ionophores and movement of calcium ions following the physiological stimulus to a secretory process. *Nature,* 245:249–251.

62. Fox, C. C., Dvorak, A. M., MacGlashan, D. W., Jr., and Lichtenstein, L. M. (1984): Histamine-containing cells in human peritoneal fluid. *J. Immunol.,* 132:2177–2179.

63. Fox, C. C., Dvorak, A. M., Peters, S. P., Kagey-Sobotka, A., and Lichtenstein, L. M. (1985): Isolation and characterization of human intestinal mucosal mast cells. *J. Immunol.,* 135:483–491.

64. Fox, P. C., Basciano, L. K., and Siraganian, R. P. (1982): Mouse mast cell activation and desensitization for immune aggregate-induced histamine release. *J. Immunol.,* 129:314–319.

65. Froese, A. (1984): Receptors for IgE on mast cells and basophils. *Prog. Allergy,* 34:142–187.

66. Furuichi, K., Ra, C., Isersky, C., and Rivera, J. (1986): Comparative evaluation of the effect of pharmacological agents on endocytosis and coendocytosis of IgE by rat basophilic leukaemia cells. *Immunology,* 58:105–110.

67. Furuichi, K., Rivera, J., Buonocore, L. M., and Isersky, C. (1986): Recycling of receptor-bound IgE by rat basophilic leukemia cells. *J. Immunol.,* 136:1015–1022.

68. Furuichi, K., Rivera, J., and Isersky, C. (1984): The fate of IgE bound to rat basophilic leukemia cells. III. Relationship between antigen-induced endocytosis and serotonin release. *J. Immunol.,* 133:1513–1520.

69. Furuichi, K., Rivera, J., and Isersky, C. (1985): The receptor for immunoglobulin E on rat basophilic leukemia cells: Effect of ligand binding on receptor expression. *Proc. Natl. Acad. Sci. USA,* 82:1522–1525.

70. Furuichi, K., Rivera, J., Triche, T., and Isersky, C. (1985): The fate of IgE bound to rat basophilic leukemia cells. IV. Functional association between the receptors for IgE. *J. Immunol.,* 134:1766–1773.

71. Galli, S. J., Dvorak, A. M., and Dvorak, H. F. (1984): Basophils and mast cells: Morphologic insights into their biology, secretory patterns, and function. *Prog. Allergy,* 34:1–141.

72. Garcia-Gil, M., and Siraganian, R. P. (1986): Source of the arachidonic acid released on stimulation of rat basophilic leukemia cells. *J. Immunol.,* 136:3825–3828.

73. Garcia-Gil, M., and Siraganian, R. P. (1986): Phospholipase A2 stimulation during cell secretion in rat basophilic leukemia cells. *J. Immunol.,* 136:259–263.

74. Gillespie, E., and Lichtenstein, L. M. (1972): Histamine release from human leukocytes: Studies with deuterium oxide, colchicine, and cytochalasin B. *J. Clin. Invest.,* 51:2941–2947.

75. Ginsburg, H., Ben-Shahar, D., and Ben-David, E. (1982): Mast cell growth on fibroblast monolayers: two-cell entities. *Immunology,* 45:371–380.

76. Goetzl, E. J., Chernov, T., Renold, F., and Payan, D. G. (1985): Neuropeptide regulation of the expression of immediate hypersensitivity. *J. Immunol.,* 135:802s–805s.

77. Gomperts, B. D. (1983): Involvement of guanine nucleotide-binding protein in the gating of Ca^{2+} by receptors. *Nature,* 306:64–66.

78. Hamasaki, Y., and Tai, H. H. (1984): Calcium stimulation of a

novel 12-lipoxygenase from rat basophilic leukemia (RBL-1) cells. *Biochim. Biophys. Acta,* 793:393–398.

79. Hammarström, S. (1983): Leukotrienes. *Annu. Rev. Biochem.,* 52: 355–377.

80. Hastie, R. (1971): The antigen-induced degranulation of basophil leucocytes from atopic subjects, studied by phase-contrast microscopy. *Clin. Exp. Immunol.,* 8:45–61.

81. Hastie, R. (1974): A study of the ultrastructure of human basophil leukocytes. *Lab Invest.,* 31:223–231.

82. Hattori, Y., and Siraganian, R. P. (1987): Rapid phosphorylation of a 92,000 MW protein on activation of rat basophilic leukemia cells for histamine release. *Immunology,* 60 (*in press*).

83. Hempstead, B. L., Kulczycki, A., Jr., and Parker, C. W. (1981): Phosphorylation of the IgE receptor from ionophore A23187 stimulated intact rat mast cells. *Biochem. Biophys. Res. Commun.,* 98: 815–822.

84. Hempstead, B. L., Parker, C. W., and Kulczycki A., Jr. (1983): Selective phosphorylation of the IgE receptor in antigen-stimulated rat mast cells. *Proc. Natl. Acad. Sci. USA,* 80:3050–3053.

85. Hernandez-Asensio, M., Hooks, J. J., Ida, S., Siraganian, R. P., and Notkins, A. L. (1979): Interferon-induced enhancement of IgE-mediated histamine release from human basophils requires RNA synthesis. *J. Immunol.,* 122:1601–1603.

86. Hesketh, T. R., Beaven, M. A., Rogers, J., Burke, B., and Warren, G. B. (1984): Stimulated release of histamine by a rat mast cell line is inhibited during mitosis. *J. Cell Biol.,* 98:2250–2254.

87. Hirata, F., and Axelrod, J. (1980): Phospholipid methylation and biological signal transmission. *Science,* 209:1082–1090.

88. Hirata, F., Axelrod, J., and Crews, F. T. (1979): Concanavalin A stimulates phospholipid methylation and phosphatidylserine decarboxylation in rat mast cells. *Proc. Natl. Acad. Sci. USA,* 76: 4813–4816.

89. Hirata, F., Schiffmann, E., Venkatasubramanian, K., Salomon, D., and Axelrod, J. (1980): A phospholipase A_2 inhibitory protein in rabbit neutrophils induced by glucocorticoids. *Proc. Natl. Acad. Sci. USA,* 77:2533–2536.

90. Holgate, S. T., Lewis, R. A., and Austen, K. F. (1980): Role of adenylate cyclase in immunologic release of mediators from rat mast cells: Agonist and antagonist effects of purine- and ribose-modified adenosine analogs. *Proc. Natl. Acad. Sci. USA,* 77:6800–6804.

91. Holowka, D., and Baird, B. (1983): Structural studies on the membrane-bound immunoglobulin E-receptor complex. 1. Characterization of large plasma membrane vesicles from rat basophilic leukemia cells and insertion of amphipathic fluorescent probes. *Biochemistry,* 22:3466–3474.

92. Holowka, D., and Baird, B. (1984): Lactoperoxidase-catalyzed iodination of the receptor for immunoglobulin E at the cytoplasmic side of the plasma membrane. *J. Biol. Chem.,* 259:3720–3728.

93. Holowka, D., Conrad, D. H., and Baird, B. (1985): Structural mapping of membrane-bound immunoglobulin E-receptor complexes: Use of monoclonal anti-IgE antibodies to probe the conformation of receptor-bound IgE. *Biochemistry,* 24:6260–6267.

94. Hook, W. A., Berenstein, E. H., Wahl, L. M., and Siraganian, R. P. (1985): Differential binding by monoclonal antibodies to fluid phase vs. basophil-bound IgE. *Clin. Res.,* 33:515A.

95. Hook, W. A., Schiffmann, E., Aswanikumar, S., and Siraganian, R. P. (1976): Histamine release by chemotactic, formyl methionine-containing peptides. *J. Immunol.,* 117:594–596.

96. Hook, W. A., and Siraganian, R. P. (1977): Complement-induced histamine release from human basophils. III. Effect of pharmacologic agents. *J. Immunol.,* 118:679–684.

97. Hook, W. A., and Siraganian, R. P. (1981): Influence of anions, cations and osmolarity on IgE-mediated histamine release from human basophils. *Immunology.,* 43:723–731.

98. Hook, W. A., Siraganian, R. P., and Wahl, S. M. (1975): Complement-induced histamine release from human basophils. I. Generation of activity in human serum. *J. Immunol.,* 114:1185–1190.

99. Hugli, T. E., and Müller-Eberhard, H. J. (1978): Anaphylatoxins: C3a and C5a. *Adv. Immunol.,* 26:1–53.

100. Ida, S., Hooks, J. J., Siraganian, R. P., and Notkins, A. L. (1977): Enhancement of IgE-mediated histamine release from human basophils by viruses: Role of interferon. *J. Exp. Med.,* 145:892–906.

101. Ida, S., Hooks, J. J., Siraganian, R. P., and Notkins, A. L. (1980): Enhancement of IgE-mediated histamine release from human basophils by immune-specific lymphokines. *Clin. Exp. Immunol.,* 41:380–387.

102. Ihle, J. N., and Weinstein, Y. (1986): Immunological regulation of hematopoietic/lymphoid stem cell differentiation by interleukin 3. *Adv. Immunol.,* 39:1–50.

103. Imai, A., Ishizuka, Y., Nakashima, S., and Nozawa, Y. (1984): Differential activation of membrane phospholipid turnover by compound 48/80 and ionophore A23187 in rat mast cells. *Arch. Biochem. Biophys.,* 232:259–268.

104. Irvine, R. F., Letcher, A. J., Heslop, J. P., and Berridge, M. J. (1986): The inositol tris/tetrakisphosphate pathway—Demonstration of Ins(1,4,5)P3 3-kinase activity in animal tissues. *Nature,* 320: 631–634.

105. Isersky, C., Metzger, H., and Buell, D. N. (1975): Cell cycle-associated changes in receptors for IgE during growth and differentiation of a rat basophilic leukemia cell line. *J. Exp. Med.,* 141:1147–1162.

106. Isersky, C., Rivera, J., Mims, S., and Triche, T. J. (1979): The fate of IgE bound to rat basophilic leukemia cells. *J. Immunol.,* 122: 1926–1936.

107. Isersky, C., Rivera, J., Segal, D. M., and Triche, T. (1983): The fate of IgE bound to rat basophilic leukemia cells. II. Endocytosis of IgE oligomers and effect on receptor turnover. *J. Immunol.,* 131: 388–396.

108. Isersky, C., Rivera, J., Triche, T. J., and Metzger, H. (1982): Characterization of the receptors for IgE on membranes isolated from rats basophilic leukemia cells. *Mol. Immunol.,* 19:925–941.

109. Isersky, C., Taurog, J. D., Poy, G., and Metzger, H. (1978): Triggering of cultured neoplastic mast cells by antibodies to the receptor for IgE. *J. Immunol.,* 121:549–558.

110. Ishizaka, K., Ishizaka, T., and Lee, E. H. (1970): Biologic function of the Fc fragments of E myeloma protein. *Immunochemistry,* 7: 687–702.

111. Ishizaka, K., Tomioka, H., and Ishizaka, T. (1970): Mechanisms of passive sensitization. I. Presence of IgE and IgG molecules on human leukocytes. *J. Immunol.,* 105:1459–1467.

112. Ishizaka, T. (1982): Biochemical analysis of triggering signals induced by bridging of IgE receptors. *Fed. Proc.,* 41:17–21.

113. Ishizaka, T., Conrad, D. H., Schulman, E. S., Sterk, A. R., and Ishizaka, K. (1983): Biochemical analysis of initial triggering events of IgE-mediated histamine release from human lung mast cells. *J. Immunol.,* 130:2357–2362.

114. Ishizaka, T., Dvorak, A. M., Conrad, D. H., Niebyl, J. R., Marquette, J. P., and Ishizaka, K. (1985): Morphologic and immunologic characterization of human basophils developed in cultures of cord blood mononuclear cells. *J. Immunol.,* 134:532–540.

115. Ishizaka, T., Foreman, J. C., Sterk, A. R., and Ishizaka, K. (1979): Induction of calcium flux across the rat mast cell membrane by bridging IgE receptors. *Proc. Natl. Acad. Sci. USA,* 76:5858–5862.

116. Ishizaka, T., Helm, B., Hakimi, J., Niebyl, J., Ishizaka, K., and Gould, H. (1986): Biological properties of a recombinant human immunoglobulin epsilon-chain fragment. *Proc. Natl. Acad. Sci. USA,* 83:8323–8327.

117. Ishizaka, T., Hirata, F., Ishizaka, K., and Axelrod, J. (1980): Stimulation of phospholipid methylation, Ca^{2+} influx, and histamine release by bridging of IgE receptors on rat mast cells. *Proc. Natl. Acad. Sci. USA,* 77:1903–1906.

118. Ishizaka, T., Hirata, F., Sterk, A. R., Ishizaka, K., and Axelrod, J. A. (1981): Bridging of IgE receptors activates phospholipid methylation and adenylate cyclase in mast cell plasma membranes. *Proc. Natl. Acad. Sci. USA,* 78:6812–6816.

119. Ishizaka, T., and Ishizaka, K. (1975): Cell surface IgE on human basophil granulocytes. *Ann. NY Acad. Sci.,* 254:462–470.

120. Ishizaka, T., and Ishizaka, K. (1978): Triggering of histamine release from rat mast cells by divalent antibodies against IgE-receptors. *J. Immunol.,* 120:800–805.

121. Ishizaka, T., and Ishizaka, K. (1984): Activation of mast cells for mediator release through IgE receptors. *Prog. Allergy,* 34:188–235.

122. Ishizaka, T., Sterk, A. R., Daeron, M., Becker, E. L., and Ishizaka, K. (1985): Biochemical analysis of desensitization of mouse mast cells. *J. Immunol.,* 135:492–501.

123. Ishizaka, T., Sterk, A. R., and Ishizaka, K. (1979): Demonstration of Fc gamma receptors on human basophil granulocytes. *J. Immunol.,* 123:578–583.

124. Ishizuka, Y., Imai, A., Nakashima, S., and Nozawa, Y. (1983): Evidence for *de novo* synthesis of phosphatidylinositol coupled with histamine release in activated rat mast cells. *Biochem. Biophys. Res. Commun.,* 111:581–587.

125. Ishizuka, Y., Imai, A., and Nozawa, Y. (1984): Polyphosphoinositide turnover in rat mast cells stimulated by antigen: Rapid and preferential breakdown of phosphatidylinositol 4-phosphate (DPI). *Biochem. Biophys. Res. Commun.,* 123:875–881.

126. Ishizuka, Y., and Nozawa, Y. (1983): Concerted stimulation of PI-turnover, Ca^{2+}-influx and histamine release in antigen-activated rat mast cells. *Biochem. Biophys. Res. Commun.,* 117:710–717.

127. Johansen, T. (1980): Further observations on the utilization of adenosine triphosphate in rat mast cells during histamine release induced by the ionophore A23187. *Br. J. Pharmacol.,* 69:657–662.

128. Johansen, T. (1981): Dependence of anaphylactic histamine release from rat mast cells on cellular energy metabolism. *Eur. J. Pharmacol.,* 72:281–286.

129. Kagey-Sobotka, A., Dembo, M., Goldstein, B., Metzger, H., and Lichtenstein, L. M. (1981): Qualitative characteristics of histamine release from human basophils by covalently cross-linked IgE. *J. Immunol.,* 127:2285–2291.

130. Kanner, B. I., and Metzger, H. (1983): Crosslinking of the receptors for immunoglobulin E depolarizes the plasma membrane of rat basophilic leukemia cells. *Proc. Natl. Acad. Sci. USA,* 80:5744–5748.

131. Kanner, B. I., and Metzger, H. (1984): Initial characterization of the calcium channel activated by the cross-linking of the receptors for immunoglobulin E. *J. Biol. Chem.,* 259:10188–10193.

132. Katz, H. R., Stevens, R. L., and Austen, K. F. (1985): Heterogeneity of mammalian mast cells differentiated *in vivo* and *in vitro. J. Allergy Clin. Immunol.,* 76:250–259.

133. Kazimierczak, W., and Diamant, B. (1978): Mechanisms of histamine release in anaphylactic and anaphylactoid reactions. *Prog. Allergy,* 24:295–365.

134. Kazimierczak, W., Meier, H. L., MacGlashan, D. W., Jr., and Lichtenstein, L. M. (1984): An antigen-activated DFP-inhibitable enzyme controls basophil desensitization. *J. Immunol.,* 132:399–405.

135. Kennerly, D. A., Secosan, C. J., Parker, C. W., and Sullivan, T. J. (1979): Modulation of stimulated phospholipid metabolism in mast cells by pharmacologic agents that increase cyclic 3',5' adenosine monophosphate levels. *J. Immunol.,* 123:1519–1524.

136. Kennerly, D. A., Sullivan, T. J., and Parker, C. W. (1979): Activation of phospholipid metabolism during mediator release from stimulated rat mast cells. *J. Immunol.,* 122:152–159.

137. Kennerly, D. A., Sullivan, T. J., Sylwester, P., and Parker, C. W. (1979): Diacylglycerol metabolism in mast cells: A potential role in membrane fusion and arachidonic acid release. *J. Exp. Med.,* 150:1039–1044.

138. Kenten, J., Helm, B., Ishizaka, T., Cattini, P., and Gould, H. (1984): Properties of a human immunoglobulin epsilon-chain fragment synthesized in *Escherichia coli. Proc. Natl. Acad. Sci. USA,* 81:2955–2959.

139. Kido, H., Izumi, K., Otsuka, H., Fukusen, N., Kato, Y., and Katunuma, N. (1986): A chymotrypsin-type serine protease in rat basophilic leukemia cells: Evidence for its immunologic identity with atypical mast cell protease. *J. Immunol.,* 136:1061–1065.

140. Kikkawa, U., and Nishizuka, Y. (1986): The role of protein kinase C in transmembrane signalling. *Annu. Rev. Cell Biol.,* 2:149–178.

141. Kikutani, H., Inui, S., Sato, R., Barsumian, E. L., Owaki, H., Yamasaki, K., Kaisho, T., Uchibayashi, N., Hardy, R. R., Hirano, T., et al. (1986): Molecular structure of human lymphocyte receptor for immunoglobulin E. *Cell,* 47:657–665.

142. Kitamura, Y., Sonoda, T., Nakano, T., and Kanayama, Y. (1986): Probable dedifferentiation of mast cells in mouse connective tissues. *Curr. Top. Dev. Biol.,* 20:325–332.

143. Kobayashi, T., Nakano, T., Nakahata, T., Asai, H., Yagi, Y., Tsuji, K., Komiyama, A., Akabane, T., Kojima, S., and Kitamura, Y. (1986): Formation of mast cell colonies in methylcellulose by mouse peritoneal cells and differentiation of these cloned cells in both the skin and the gastric mucosa of W/W^v mice: Evidence that a common precursor can give rise to both "connective" tissue-type and "mucosal" mast cells. *J. Immunol.,* 136:1378–1384.

144. Kulczycki, A., Jr., and Metzger, H. (1974): The interaction of IgE with rat basophilic leukemia cells. II. Quantitative aspects of the binding reaction. *J. Exp. Med.,* 140:1676–1695.

145. Kulczycki, A., Jr., Isersky, C., and Metzger, H. (1974): The interaction of IgE with rat basophilic leukemia cells. I. Evidence for specific binding of IgE. *J. Exp. Med.,* 139:600–616.

146. Lagunoff, D., and Chi, E. Y. (1980): Cell biology of mast cells and basophils. In: *The Cell Biology of Inflammation. Handbook of Inflammation,* edited by L. E. Glynn, J. C. Houck, and G. Weissman, pp. 217–265. Elsevier/North-Holland, New York.

147. Lawson, D., Fewtrell, C., and Raff, M. C. (1978): Localized mast cell degranulation induced by concanavalin A-sepharose beads. Implications for the Ca^{2+} hypothesis of stimulus-secretion coupling. *J. Cell Biol.,* 79:394–400.

148. Lawson, D., Raff, M. C., Gomperts, B., Fewtrell, C., and Gilula, N. B. (1977): Molecular events during membrane fusion. A study of exocytosis in rat peritoneal mast cells. *J. Cell Biol.,* 72:242–259.

149. Levi-Schaffer, F., Austen, K. F., Caulfield, J. P., Hein, A., Bloes, W. F., and Stevens, R. L. (1985): Fibroblasts maintain the phenotype and viability of the rat heparin-containing mast cell *in vitro. J. Immunol.,* 135:3454–3462.

150. Levi-Schaffer, F., Austen, K. F., Gravallese, P. M., and Stevens, R. L. (1986): Coculture of interleukin 3-dependent mouse mast cells with fibroblasts results in a phenotypic change of the mast cells. *Proc. Natl. Acad. Sci. USA,* 83:6485–6488.

151. Lewis, R. A., and Austen, K. F. (1984): The biologically active leukotrienes. Biosynthesis, metabolism, receptors, functions, and pharmacology. *J. Clin. Invest.,* 73:889–897.

152. Lewis, R. A., Holgate, S. T., Roberts, L. J., 2nd, Maguire, J. F., Oates, J. A., and Austen, K. F. (1979): Effects of indomethacin on cyclic nucleotide levels and histamine release from rat serosal mast cells. *J. Immunol.,* 123:1663–1668.

153. Lewis, R. A., Soter, N. A., Diamond, P. T., Austen, K. F., Oates, J. A., and Roberts, L. J., 2nd (1982): Prostaglandin D_2 generation after activation of rat and human mast cells with anti-IgE. *J. Immunol.,* 129:1627–1631.

154. Lichtenstein, L. M., and Gillespie, E. (1973): Inhibition of histamine release by histamine controlled by H_2 receptor. *Nature,* 244:287–288.

155. Lichtenstein, L. M., Sobotka, A. K., Malveaux, F. J., and Gillespie, E. (1978): IgE-induced changes in human basophil cyclic AMP levels. *Int. Arch. Allergy Appl. Immunol.,* 56:473–478.

156. Lindau, M., and Fernandez, J. M. (1986): IgE-mediated degranulation of mast cells does not require opening of ion channels. *Nature,* 319:150–153.

157. Liu, F. T., Albrandt, K. A., Bry, C. G., and Ishizaka, T. (1984): Expression of a biologically active fragment of human IgE epsilon chain in *Escherichia coli. Proc. Natl. Acad. Sci. USA,* 81:5369–5373.

158. Liu, F. T., Albrandt, K., Mendel, E., Kulczycki A., Jr., and Orida, N. K. (1985): Identification of an IgE-binding protein by molecular cloning. *Proc. Natl. Acad. Sci. USA,* 82:4100–4104.

159. Liu, F. T., and Orida, N. (1984): Synthesis of surface immunoglobulin E receptor in Xenopus oocytes by translation of mRNA from rat basophilic leukemia cells. *J. Biol. Chem.,* 259:10649–10652.

160. Liu, M. C., Proud, D., Lichtenstein, L. M., MacGlashan, D. W., Jr., Schleimer, R. P., Adkinson, N. F., Jr., Kagey-Sobotka, A., Schulman, E. S., and Plaut, M. (1986): Human lung macrophage-derived histamine-releasing activity is due to IgE-dependent factors. *J. Immunol.,* 136:2588–2595.

161. MacGlashan, D. W., Jr., and Lichtenstein, L. M. (1983): Studies of antigen binding on human basophils. I. Antigen binding and functional consequences. *J. Immunol.,* 130:2330–2336.

162. MacGlashan, D. W., Jr., Mogowski, M., and Lichtenstein, L. M.

(1983): Studies of antigen binding on human basophils. II. Continued expression of antigen-specific IgE during antigen-induced desensitization. *J. Immunol.,* 130:2337–2342.

163. MacGlashan, D. W., Jr., and Lichtenstein, L. M. (1980): The purification of human basophils. *J. Immunol.,* 124:2519–2521.

164. MacGlashan, D. W., Jr., and Lichtenstein, L. M. (1981): The transition from specific to nonspecific desensitization in human basophils. *J. Immunol.,* 127:2410–2414.

165. MacGlashan, D. W., Jr., Peters, S. P., Warner, J., and Lichtenstein, L. M. (1986): Characteristics of human basophil sulfidopeptide leukotriene release: Releasability defined as the ability of the basophil to respond to dimeric cross-links. *J. Immunol.,* 136:2231–2239.

166. MacGlashan, D. W., Jr., Schleimer, R. P., and Lichtenstein, L. M. (1983): Qualitative differences between dimeric and trimeric stimulation of human basophils. *J. Immunol.,* 130:4–6.

167. MacGlashan, D. W., Jr., Schleimer, R. P., Peters, S. P., Schulman, E. S., Adams, G. K., Sobotka, A. K., Newball, H. H., and Lichtenstein, L. M. (1983): Comparative studies of human basophils and mast cells. *Fed. Proc.,* 42:2504–2509.

168. Maeyama, K., Hohman, R. J., Metzger, H., and Beaven, M. A. (1986): Quantitative relationships between aggregation of IgE receptors, generation of intracellular signals, and histamine secretion in rat basophilic leukemia (2H3) cells. Enhanced responses with heavy water. *J. Biol. Chem.,* 261:2583–2592.

169. Majerus, P. W., Connolly, T. M., Deckmyn, H., Ross, T. S., Bross, T. E., Ishii, H., Bansal, V. S., and Wilson, D. B. (1986): The metabolism of phosphoinositide-derived messenger molecules. *Science,* 234:1519–1526.

170. Malveaux, F. J., Conroy, M. C., Adkinson, N. F., Jr., and Lichtenstein, L. M. (1978): IgE receptors on human basophils. Relationship to serum IgE concentration. *J. Clin. Invest.,* 62:176–181.

171. Marone, G., Kagey-Sobotka, A., and Lichtenstein, L. M. (1979): Effects of arachidonic acid and its metabolites on antigen-induced histamine release from human basophils *in vitro. J. Immunol.,* 123:1669–1677.

172. Marone, G., Poto, S., Celestino, D., and Bonini, S. (1986): Human basophil releasability. III. Genetic control of human basophil releasability. *J. Immunol.,* 137:3588–3592.

173. May, W. S., and Ihle, J. N. (1986): Affinity isolation of the interleukin-3 surface receptor. *Biochem. Biophys. Res. Commun.,* 135:870–879.

174. Mazurek, N., Bashkin, P., Loyter, A., and Pecht, I. (1983): Restoration of Ca²⁺ influx and degranulation capacity of variant RBL-2H3 cells upon implantation of isolated cromolyn binding protein. *Proc. Natl. Acad. Sci. USA,* 80:6014–6018.

175. Mazurek, N., Bashkin, P., and Pecht, I. (1982): Isolation of a basophilic membrane protein binding the anti-allergic drug cromolyn. *EMBO J.,* 1:585–590.

176. Mazurek, N., Bashkin, P., Petrank, A., and Pecht, I. (1983): Basophil variants with impaired cromoglycate binding do not respond to an immunological degranulation stimulus. *Nature,* 303:528–530.

177. Mazurek, N., Berger, G., and Pecht, I. (1980): A binding site on mast cells and basophils for the anti-allergic drug cromolyn. *Nature,* 286:722–723.

178. Mazurek, N., Dulic, V., Pecht, I., Schindler, H. G., and Rivnay, B. (1986): The role of the Fc epsilon receptor in calcium channel opening in rat basophilic leukemia cells. *Immunol. Lett.,* 12:31–35.

179. Mazurek, N., Geller-Bernstein, C., and Pecht, I. (1980): Affinity of calcium ions to the anti-allergic drug, dicromoglycate. *FEBS Lett.,* 111:194–196.

180. Mazurek, N., Schindler, H., Schürholz, T., and Pecht, I. (1984): The cromolyn binding protein constitutes the Ca²⁺ channel of basophils opening upon immunological stimulus. *Proc. Natl. Acad. Sci. USA,* 81:6841–6845.

181. McCloskey, M. A., Liu, Z. Y., and Poo, M. M. (1984): Lateral electromigration and diffusion of Fc epsilon receptors on rat basophilic leukemia cells: Effects of IgE binding. *J. Cell Biol.,* 99:778–787.

182. McGivney, A., Crews, F. T., Hirata, F., Axelrod, J., and Siraganian, R. P. (1981): Rat basophilic leukemia cell lines defective in phos-

pholipid methyltransferase enzymes, Ca²⁺ influx, and histamine release: Reconstitution by hybridization. *Proc. Natl. Acad. Sci. USA,* 78:6176–6180.

183. McGivney, A., Morita, Y., Crews, F. T., Hirata, F., Axelrod, J., and Siraganian, R. P. (1981): Phospholipase activation in the IgE-mediated and Ca²⁺ ionophore A23187-induced release of histamine from rat basophilic leukemia cells. *Arch. Biochem. Biophys.,* 212:572–580.

184. Mendoza, G., and Metzger, H. (1976): Distribution and valency of receptor for IgE on rodent mast cells and related tumour cells. *Nature,* 264:548–550.

185. Mendoza, G. R., and Metzger, H. (1976): Disparity of IgE binding between normal and tumor mouse mast cells. *J. Immunol.,* 117:1573–1578.

186. Menon, A. K., Holowka, D., and Baird, B. (1984): Small oligomers of immunoglobulin E (IgE) cause large-scale clustering of IgE receptors on the surface of rat basophilic leukemia cells. *J. Cell Biol.,* 98:577–583.

187. Menon, A. K., Holowka, D., Webb, W. W., and Baird, B. (1986): Cross-linking of receptor-bound IgE to aggregates larger than dimers leads to rapid immobilization. *J. Cell Biol.,* 102:541–550.

188. Menon, A. K., Holowka, D., Webb, W. W., and Baird, B. (1986): Clustering, mobility, and triggering activity of small oligomers of immunoglobulin E on rat basophilic leukemia cells. *J. Cell Biol.,* 102:534–540.

189. Metcalfe, D. D., Kaliner, M., and Donlon, M. A. (1981): The mast cell. *CRC Crit. Rev. Immunol.,* 3:23–74.

190. Metzger, H., Alcaraz, G., Hohman, R., Kinet, J. P., Pribluda, V., and Quarto, R. (1986): The receptor with high affinity for immunoglobulin E. *Annu. Rev. Immunol.,* 4:419–470.

191. Meyer, C., Wahl, L. M., Stadler, B. M., and Siraganian, R. P. (1983): Cell cycle associated changes in histamine release from rat basophilic leukemia cells separated by counterflow centrifugal elutriation. *J. Immunol.,* 131:911–914.

192. Moore, J. P., Johannsson, A., Hesketh, T. R., Smith, G. A., and Metcalfe, J. C. (1984): Calcium signals and phospholipid methylation in eukaryotic cells. *Biochem. J.,* 221:675–684.

193. Morita, Y., Chiang, P. K., and Siraganian, R. P. (1981): Effect of inhibitors of transmethylation on histamine release from human basophils. *Biochem. Pharmacol.,* 30:785–791.

194. Morita, Y., and Siraganian, R. P. (1981): Inhibition of IgE-mediated histamine release from rat basophilic leukemia cells and rat mast cells by inhibitors of transmethylation. *J. Immunol.,* 127:1339–1344.

195. Morita, Y., Siraganian, R. P., Tang, C. K., and Chiang, P. K. (1982): Inhibition of histamine release and phosphatidylcholine metabolism by 5'-deoxy-5'-isobutylthio-3-deazaadenosine. *Biochem. Pharmacol.,* 31:2111–2113.

196. Nagao, K., Yokoro, K., and Aaronson, S. A. (1981): Continuous lines of basophil/mast cells derived from normal mouse bone marrow. *Science,* 212:333–335.

197. Nakamura, T., and Ui, M. (1983): Suppression of passive cutaneous anaphylaxis by pertussis toxin, an islet-activating protein, as a result of inhibition of histamine release from mast cells. *Biochem. Pharmacol.,* 32:3435–3441.

198. Nakamura, T., and Ui, M. (1984): Islet-activating protein, pertussis toxin, inhibits Ca²⁺-induced and guanine nucleotide-dependent releases of histamine and arachidonic acid from rat mast cells. *FEBS Lett.,* 173:414–418.

199. Nakamura, T., and Ui, M. (1985): Simultaneous inhibitions of inositol phospholipid breakdown, arachidonic acid release, and histamine secretion in mast cells by islet-activating protein, pertussis toxin. A possible involvement of the toxin-specific substrate in the Ca²⁺-mobilizing receptor-mediated biosignaling system. *J. Biol. Chem.,* 260:3584–3593.

200. Nakano, T., Sonoda, T., Hayashi, C., Yamatodani, A., Kanayama, Y., Yamamura, T., Asai, H., Yonezawa, T., Kitamura, Y., and Galli, S. J. (1985): Fate of bone marrow-derived cultured mast cells after intracutaneous, intraperitoneal, and intravenous transfer into genetically mast cell-deficient W/Wᵛ mice. Evidence that cultured mast cells can give rise to both connective tissue type and mucosal mast cells. *J. Exp. Med.,* 162:1025–1043.

201. Nemeth, E. F., and Douglas, W. W. (1982): Lipoxygenase inhibitors exert secretagogue-specific effects on mast cell exocytosis. *Eur. J. Pharmacol.*, 79:315–318.

202. Newball, H. H., Berninger, R. W., Talamo, R. C., and Lichtenstein, L. M. (1979): Anaphylactic relase of a basophil kallikrein-like activity. I. Purification and characterization. *J. Clin. Invest.*, 64:457–465.

203. Newball, H. H., Talamo, R. C., and Lichtenstein, L. M. (1979): Anaphylactic relase of a basophil kallikrein-like activity. II. A mediator of immediate hypersensitivity reactions. *J. Clin. Invest.*, 64:466–475.

204. Nishizuka, Y. (1986): Studies and perspectives of protein kinase C. *Science*, 233:305–312.

205. Ogawa, M., Nakahata, T., Leary, A. G., Sterk, A. R., Ishizaka, K., and Ishizaka, T. (1983): Suspension culture of human mast cells/basophils from umbilical cord blood mononuclear cells. *Proc. Natl. Acad. Sci. USA*, 80:4494–4498.

206. Oliver, J. M., Seagrave, J. C., Pfeiffer, J. R., Feibig, M. L., and Deanin, G. G. (1985): Surface functions during mitosis in rat basophilic leukemia cells. *J. Cell Biol.*, 101:2156–2166.

207. Pearce, F. L. (1982): Calcium and histamine secretion from mast cells. *Prog. Med. Chem.*, 19:59–109.

208. Perez-Montfort, R., Fewtrell, C., and Metzger, H. (1983): Changes in the receptor for immunoglobulin E coincident with receptor-mediated stimulation of basophilic leukemia cells. *Biochemistry*, 22:5733–5737.

209. Perez-Montfort, R., and Metzger, H. (1982): Proteolysis of soluble IgE-receptor complexes: Localization of sites on IgE which interact with the Fc receptor. *Mol. Immunol.*, 19:1113–1125.

210. Peters, S. P., Kagey-Sobotka, A., MacGlashan, D. W., Jr., Siegel, M. I., and Lichtenstein, L. M. (1982): The modulation of human basophil histamine release by products of the 5-lipoxygenase pathway. *J. Immunol.*, 129:797–803.

211. Petty, H. R., Ware, B. R., and Wasserman, S. I. (1980): Alterations of the electrophoretic mobility distribution of rat mast cells after immunologic activation. *Biophys. J.*, 30:41–50.

212. Pfeiffer, J. R., Seagrave, J. C., Davis, B. H., Deanin, G. G., and Oliver, J. M. (1985): Membrane and cytoskeletal changes associated with IgE-mediated serotonin release from rat basophilic leukemia cells. *J. Cell Biol.*, 101:2145–2155.

213. Pure, E., Luster, A. D., and Unkeless, J. C. (1984): *Cell* surface expression of murine, rat, and human Fc receptors by Xenopus oocytes. *J. Exp. Med.*, 160:606–611.

214. Quarto, R., Kinet, J. P., and Metzger, H. (1985): Coordinate synthesis and degradation of the alpha-, beta- and gamma-subunits of the receptor for immunoglobulin E. *Mol. Immunol.*, 22:1045–1051.

215. Razin, E., Ihle, J. N., Seldin, D., Mencia-Huerta, J. M., Katz, H. R., LeBlanc, P. A., Hein, A., Caulfield, J. P., Austen, K. F., and Stevens, R. L. (1984): Interleukin 3: A differentiation and growth factor for the mouse mast cell that contains chondroitin sulfate E proteoglycan. *J. Immunol.*, 132:1479–1486.

216. Razin, E., Mencia-Huerta, J. M., Stevens, R. L., Lewis, R. A., Liu, F. T., Corey, E., and Austen, K. F. (1983): IgE-mediated release of leukotriene C4, chondroitin sulfate E proteoglycan, beta-hexosaminidase, and histamine from cultured bone marrow-derived mouse mast cells. *J. Exp. Med.*, 157:189–201.

217. Razin, E., Romeo, L. C., Krilis, S., Liu, F. T., Lewis, R. A., Corey, E. J., and Austen, K. F. (1984): An analysis of the relationship between 5-lipoxygenase product generation and the secretion of preformed mediators from mouse bone marrow-derived mast cells. *J. Immunol.*, 133:938–945.

218. Rivera, J., Mullins, J. M., Furuichi, K., and Isersky, C. (1986): Endocytosis of aggregated immunoglobulin G by rat basophilic leukemia cells; rate, extent, and effects on the endocytosis of immunoglobulin E. *J. Immunol.*, 136:623–627.

219. Robertson, D., Holowka, D., and Baird, B. (1986): Cross-linking of immunoglobulin E-receptor complexes induces their interaction with the cytoskeleton of rat basophilic leukemia cells. *J. Immunol.*, 136:4565–4572.

220. Robin, J. L., Seldin, D. C., Austen, K. F., and Lewis, R. A. (1985): Regulation of mediator release from mouse bone marrow-derived mast cells by glucocorticoids. *J. Immunol.*, 135:2719–2726.

221. Rossi, G., Newman, S. A., and Metzger, H. (1977): Assay and partial characterization of the solubilized cell surface receptor for immunoglobulin E. *J. Biol. Chem.*, 252:704–711.

222. Sagi-Eisenberg, R., Lieman, H., and Pecht, I. (1985): Protein kinase C regulation of the receptor-coupled calcium signal in histamine-secreting rat basophilic leukaemia cells. *Nature*, 313:59–60.

223. Sagi-Eisenberg, R., Mazurek, N., and Pecht, I. (1984): Ca^{2+} fluxes and protein phosphorylation in stimulus-secretion coupling of basophils. *Mol. Immunol.*, 21:1175–1181.

224. Sagi-Eisenberg, R., and Pecht, I. (1983): Membrane potential changes during IgE-mediated histamine release from rat basophilic leukemia cells. *J. Membr. Biol.*, 75:97–104.

225. Sagi-Eisenberg, R., and Pecht, I. (1984): Protein kinase C, a coupling element between stimulus and secretion of basophils. *Immunol. Lett.*, 8:237–241.

226. Sagi-Eisenberg, R., and Pecht, I. (1984): Resolution of cellular compartments involved in membrane potential changes accompanying IgE-mediated degranulation of rat basophilic leukemia cells. *EMBO J.*, 3:497–500.

227. Schellenberg, R. R. (1980): Enhanced phospholipid metabolism in rat mast cells stimulated to release histamine. *Immunology*, 41:123–129.

228. Schleimer, R. P., Davidson, D. A., Lichtenstein, L. M., and Adkinson, N. F., Jr. (1986): Selective inhibition of arachidonic acid metabolite release from human lung tissue by antiinflammatory steroids. *J. Immunol.*, 136:3006–3011.

229. Schleimer, R. P., Gillespie, E., Daiuta, R., and Lichtenstein, L. M. (1982): Release of histamine from human leukocytes stimulated with the tumor-promoting phorbol diesters. II. Interaction with other stimuli. *J. Immunol.*, 128:136–140.

230. Schleimer, R. P., Gillespie, E., and Lichtenstein, L. M. (1981): Release of histamine from human leukocytes stimulated with the tumor-promoting phorbol diesters. I. Characterization of the response. *J. Immunol.*, 126:570–574.

231. Schleimer, R. P., Lichtenstein, L. M., and Gillespie, E. (1981): Inhibition of basophil histamine release by anti-inflammatory steroids. *Nature*, 292:454–455.

232. Schleimer, R. P., MacGlashan, D. W., Jr., Gillespie, E., and Lichtenstein, L. M. (1982): Inhibition of basophil histamine release by anti-inflammatory steroids. II. Studies on the mechanism of action. *J. Immunol.*, 129:1632–1636.

233. Schrader, J. W. (1986): The panspecific hemopoietin of activated T lymphocytes (interleukin-3). *Annu. Rev. Immunol.*, 4:205–230.

234. Schulman, E. S., Kagey-Sobotka, A., MacGlashan, D. W., Jr., Adkinson, N. F., Jr., Peters, S. P., Schleimer, R. P., and Lichtenstein, L. M. (1983): Heterogeneity of human mast cells. *J. Immunol.*, 131:1936–1941.

235. Schulman, E. S., MacGlashan, D. W., Jr., Peters, S. P., Schleimer, R. P., Newball, H. H., and Lichtenstein, L. M. (1982): Human lung mast cells: Purification and characterization. *J. Immunol.*, 129:2662–2667.

236. Segal, D. M., Sharrow, S. O., Jones, J. F., and Siraganian, R. P. (1981): Fc (IgG) receptors on rat basophilic leukemia cells. *J. Immunol.*, 126:138–145.

237. Segal, D. M., Taurog, J. D., and Metzger, H. (1977): Dimeric immunoglobulin E serves as a unit signal for mast cell degranulation. *Proc. Natl. Acad. Sci. USA*, 74:2993–2997.

238. Seldin, D. C., Adelman, S., Austen, K. F., Stevens, R. L., Hein, A., Caulfield, J. P., and Woodbury, R. G. (1985): Homology of the rat basophilic leukemia cell and the rat mucosal mast cell. *Proc. Natl. Acad. Sci. USA*, 82:3871–3875.

239. Sieghart, W., Theoharides, T. C., Alper, S. L., Douglas, W. W., and Greengard, P. (1978): Calcium-dependent protein phosphorylation during secretion by exocytosis in the mast cell. *Nature*, 275:329–331.

240. Sieghart, W., Theoharides, T. C., Douglas, W. W., and Greengard, P. (1981): Phosphorylation of a single mast cell protein in response to drugs that inhibit secretion. *Biochem. Pharmacol.*, 30:2737–2738.

241. Siraganian, P. A., and Siraganian, R. P. (1974): Basophil activation by concanavalin A: Characteristics of the reaction. *J. Immunol.,* 112:2117–2125.

242. Siraganian, R. P. (1981): Immediate hypersensitivity reactions. In: *Cellular Functions in Immunity and Inflammation,* edited by J. J. Oppenheim, D. R. Rosenstrich, and M. Potter, pp. 323–354. Elsevier/North-Holland, New York.

243. Siraganian, R. P. (1983): Histamine secretion from mast cells and basophils. *Trends Pharmacol. Sci.,* 4:432–437.

244. Siraganian, R. P. (1985): Biochemical events in basophil/mast cell activation and mediator secretion. In: *Allergy,* edited by A. P. Kaplan, pp. 31–51. Churchill Livingstone, New York.

245. Siraganian, R. P., and Hazard, K. A. (1979): Mechanisms of mouse mast cell activation and inactivation for IgE-mediated histamine release. *J. Immunol.,* 122:1719–1725.

246. Siraganian, R. P., and Hook, W. A. (1976): Complement-induced histamine release from human basophils. II. Mechanism of the histamine release reaction. *J. Immunol.,* 116:639–646.

247. Siraganian, R. P., and Hook, W. A. (1977): Mechanism of histamine release by formyl methionine-containing peptides. *J. Immunol.,* 119:2078–2083.

248. Siraganian, R. P., and Hook, W. A. (1986): Histamine release and assay methods for the study of human allergy. In: *Manual of Clinical Laboratory Immunology,* edited by N. R. Rose, M. Friedman, and J. L. Fahey, pp. 675–684. American Society for Microbiology, Washington, D.C.

249. Siraganian, R. P., Hook, W. A., and Levine, B. B. (1975): Specific *in vitro* histamine release from basophils by bivalent haptens: Evidence of activation by simple bridging of membrane bound antibody. *Immunochemistry,* 12:149–157.

250. Siraganian, R. P., McGivney, A., Barsumian, E. L., Crews, F. T., Hirata, F., and Axelrod, J. (1982): Variants of the rat basophilic leukemia cell line for the study of histamine release. *Fed. Proc.,* 41:30–34.

251. Siraganian, R. P., and Siraganian, P. A. (1975): Mechanism of action of concanavalin A on human basophils. *J. Immunol.,* 114:886–893.

252. Slattery, J., Holowka, D., and Baird, B. (1985): Segmental flexibility of receptor-bound immunoglobulin E. *Biochemistry,* 24:7810–7820.

253. Sobotka, A. K., Dembo, M., Goldstein, B., and Lichtenstein, L. M. (1979): Antigen-specific desensitization of human basophils. *J. Immunol.,* 122:511–517.

254. Sonoda, S., Sonoda, T., Nakano, T., Kanayama, Y., Kanakura, Y., Asai, H., Yonezawa, T., and Kitamura, Y. (1986): Development of mucosal mast cells after injection of a single connective tissue-type mast cell in the stomach mucosa of genetically mast cell-deficient W/W^v mice. *J. Immunol.,* 137:1319–1322.

255. Sonoda, T., Kanayama, Y., Hara, H., Hayashi, C., Tadokoro, M., Yonezawa, T., and Kitamura, Y. (1984): Proliferation of peritoneal mast cells in the skin of W/W^v mice that genetically lack mast cells. *J. Exp. Med.,* 160:138–151.

256. Spiegelberg, H. L. (1984): Structure and function of Fc receptors for IgE on lymphocytes, monocytes, and macrophages. *Adv. Immunol.,* 35:61–88.

257. Stanworth, D. R. (1971): Immunoglobulin E (reagin) and allergy. *Nature,* 233:310–316.

258. Stanworth, D. R., Humphrey, J. H., Bennich, H., and Johansson, S. G. O. (1968): Inhibition of Prausnitz-Küstner reaction by proteolytic-cleavage fragments of a human myeloma protein of immunoglobulin class E. *Lancet,* 2:17–18.

259. Stenson, W. F., Parker, C. W., and Sullivan, T. J. (1980): Augmentation of IgE-mediated release of histamine by 5-hydroxyeicosatetraenoic acid and 12-hydroxyeicosatetraenoic acid. *Biochem. Biophys. Res. Commun.,* 96:1045–1052.

260. Sterk, A. R., and Ishizaka, T. (1982): Binding properties of IgE receptors on normal mouse mast cells. *J. Immunol.,* 128:838–843.

261. Stevens, R. L., Otsu, K., and Austen, K. F. (1985): Purification and analysis of the core protein of the protease-resistant intracellular chondroitin sulfate E proteoglycan from the interleukin 3-dependent mouse mast cell. *J. Biol. Chem.,* 260:14194–14200.

262. Stracke, M. L., Basciano, L. K., and Siraganian, R. P. (1987): Binding properties and histamine release in variants of rat basophilic leukemia cells with changes in the IgE receptor. *Immunol. Lett.,* 14:287–292.

263. Stryer, L., and Bourne, H. R. (1986): G proteins: A family of signal transducers. *Annu. Rev. Cell Biol.,* 2:391–419.

264. Sullivan, A. L., Grimley, P. M., and Metzger, H. (1971): Electron microscopic localization of immunoglobulin E on the surface membrane of human basophils. *J. Exp. Med.,* 134:1403–1416.

265. Sullivan, T. J., Parker, K. L., Eisen, S. A., and Parker, C. W. (1975): Modulation of cyclic AMP in purified rat mast cells. II. Studies on the relationship between intracellular cyclic AMP concentrations and histamine release. *J. Immunol.,* 114:1480–1485.

266. Sullivan, T. J., Parker, K. L., Kulczycki, A., Jr., and Parker, C. W. (1976): Modulation of cyclic AMP in purified rat mast cells. III. Studies on the effects of concanavalin A and anti-IgE on cyclic AMP concentrations during histamine release. *J. Immunol.,* 117:713–716.

267. Sullivan, T. J., Parker, K. L., Stenson, W., and Parker, C. W. (1975): Modulation of cyclic AMP in purified rat mast cells. I. Responses to pharmacologic, metabolic, and physical stimuli. *J. Immunol.,* 114:1473–1479.

268. Sydbom, A., and Fredholm, B. B. (1982): On the mechanism by which theophylline inhibits histamine release from rat mast cells. *Acta Physiol. Scand.,* 114:243–251.

269. Sydbom, A., Fredholm, B., and Uvnäs, B. (1981): Evidence against a role of cyclic nucleotides in the regulation of anaphylactic histamine release in isolated rat mast cells. *Acta Physiol. Scand.,* 112:47–56.

270. Tadokoro, K., Stadler, B. M., and De Weck, A. L. (1983): Factor-dependent *in vitro* growth of human normal bone marrow-derived basophil-like cells. *J. Exp. Med.,* 158:857–871.

271. Takaishi, T., and Siraganian, R. P. (1985): Changes in ^{45}Ca^{2+} flux following the activation of rat basophilic leukemia cells for histamine release. *Ann. Allergy,* 55:353.

272. Takatsu, K., Ishizaka, T., and Ishizaka, K. (1975): Biologic significance of disulfide bonds in human IgE molecules. *J. Immunol.,* 114:1838–1845.

273. Teshima, R., Ikebuchi, H., and Terao, T. (1984): Ca^{2+}-dependent and phorbol ester activating phosphorylation of a 36K-dalton protein of rat basophilic leukemia cell membranes and immunoprecipitation of the phosphorylated protein with IgE-anti IgE system. *Biochem. Biophys. Res. Commun.,* 125:867–874.

274. Theoharides, T. C., and Douglas, W. W. (1978): Secretion in mast cells induced by calcium entrapped within phospholipid vesicles. *Science,* 201:1143–1145.

275. Theoharides, T. C., Sieghart, W., Greengard, P., and Douglas, W. W. (1980): Antiallergic drug cromolyn may inhibit histamine secretion by regulating phosphorylation of a mast cell protein. *Science,* 207:80–82.

276. Thomas, L. L., Findlay, S. R., and Lichtenstein, L. M. (1979): Augmentation of antigen-stimulated histamine release from human basophils by serum-treated zymosan particles. II. Dependence on IgE-mediated release. *J. Immunol.,* 123:1468–1472.

277. Thomas, L. L., and Lichtenstein, L. M. (1979): Augmentation of antigen-stimulated histamine release from human basophils by serum-treated zymosan particles. I. Characteristics of enhancement. *J. Immunol.,* 123:1462–1467.

278. Thueson, D. O., Speck, L. S., Lett-Brown, M. A., and Grant, J. A. (1979): Histamine-releasing activity (HRA). I. Production by mitogen- or antigen-stimulated human mononuclear cells. *J. Immunol.,* 123:626–632.

279. Thueson, D. O., Speck, L. S., Lett-Brown, M. A., and Grant, J. A. (1979): Histamine-releasing activity (HRA). II. Interaction with basophils and physicochemical characterization. *J. Immunol.,* 123:633–639.

280. Urata, C., and Siraganian, R. P. (1985): Pharmacologic modulation of the IgE or Ca^{2+} ionophore A23187 mediated Ca^{2+} influx, phos-

pholipase activation, and histamine release in rat basophilic leukemia cells. *Int. Arch. Allergy Appl. Immunol.,* 78:92–100.

281. Usdin, E., Borchardt, R. T., and Creveling, C. R., editors (1982): *Biochemistry of S-adenosylmethionine and Related Compounds,* pp. 1–760. Macmillan, London.

282. Uvnäs, B. (1978): Chemistry and storage function of mast cell granules. *J. Invest. Dermatol.,* 71:76–80.

283. Wank, S. A., DeLisi, C., and Metzger, H. (1983): Analysis of the rate-limiting step in a ligand-cell receptor interaction: The immunoglobulin E system. *Biochemistry,* 22:954–959.

284. Warner, J. A., Pienkowski, M. M., Plaut, M., Norman, P. S., and Lichtenstein, L. M. (1986): Identification of histamine releasing factor(s) in the late phase of cutaneous IgE-mediated reactions. *J. Immunol.,* 136:2583–2587.

285. White, J. R., Ishizaka, T., Ishizaka, K., and Sha'afi, R. (1984): Direct demonstration of increased intracellular concentration of free calcium as measured by quin-2 in stimulated rat peritoneal mast cell. *Proc. Natl. Acad. Sci. USA,* 81:3978–3982.

286. White, J. R., Pluznik, D. H., Ishizaka, K., and Ishizaka, T. (1985): Antigen-induced increase in protein kinase C activity in plasma membrane of mast cells. *Proc. Natl. Acad. Sci. USA,* 82:8193–8197.

287. Winslow, C. M., and Austen, K. F. (1982): Enzymatic regulation of mast cell activation and secretion by adenylate cyclase and cyclic AMP-dependent protein kinases. *Fed. Proc.,* 41:22–29.

288. Winslow, C. M., and Austen, K. F. (1984): Role of cyclic nucleotides in the activation-secretion response. *Prog. Allergy,* 34:236–270.

289. Winslow, C. M., Lewis, R. A., and Austen, K. F. (1981): Mast cell mediator release as a function of cyclic AMP-dependent protein kinase activation. *J. Exp. Med.,* 154:1125–1133.

290. WoldeMussie, E., Ali, H., Takaishi, T., Siraganian, R. P., and Beaven, M. A. (1987): Identification of variants of the basophilic leukemia (RBL-2H3) cells that have defective phosphoinositide responses to antigen and stimulants of GTP-regulatory proteins. *J. Immunol.* (in press).

291. Yang, Y. C., Ciarletta, A. B., Temple, P. A., Chung, M. P., Kovacic, S., Witek-Giannotti, J. S., Leary, A. C., Kriz, R., Donahue, R. E., Wong, G. G., et al. (1986): Human IL-3 (multi-CSF): identification by expression cloning of a novel hematopoietic growth factor related to murine IL-3. *Cell,* 47:3–10.

292. Zheutlin, L. M., Ackerman, S. J., Gleich, G. J., and Thomas, L. L. (1984): Stimulation of basophil and rat mast cell histamine release by eosinophil granule-derived cationic proteins. *J. Immunol.,* 133:2180–2185.

293. Zidovetzki, R., Bartholdi, M., Arndt-Jovin, D., and Jovin, T. M. (1986): Rotational dynamics of the Fc receptor for immunoglobulin E on histamine-releasing rat basophilic leukemia cells. *Biochemistry,* 25:4397–4401.

Inflammation: Basic Principles and Clinical Correlates.
Edited by J. I. Gallin, I. M. Goldstein, and R. Snyderman.
Raven Press, Ltd., New York © 1988.

CHAPTER 28

Platelets

Babette B. Weksler

Human blood platelets, cells highly adapted for hemostasis and wound healing, often participate in other cellular responses to injury, reflecting their evolutionary heritage as inflammatory cells. In primitive organisms, a single type of mobile cell serves multiple inflammatory functions: It serves to staunch wounds, repel invading microbes, and initiate tissue repair after injury. In higher organisms, it has been found that separate cell types, thrombocytes, and leukocytes subtend the separate functions of hemostasis and inflammation, although overlap is maintained. In mammals, thrombocytes have further evolved into anucleate fragments, the platelets, with functions mainly directed toward the initiation of hemostasis. Despite this functional specialization, platelets display numerous inflammatory capacities (Table 1).

Platelets retain many aspects of evolutionarily primitive all-purpose inflammatory cells: They contain and release adhesive proteins, activate complement, supply tissue proteases, interact with bacteria and viruses, enhance vascular permeability, alter vascular tone, and take up, store, or metabolize vasoactive substances (77). Platelets provide a major source of growth factors for mesenchymal cells, particularly vascular cells (24). In addition, platelets interact with circulating leukocytes as well as with vascular endothelium to modulate inflammatory activities of the major phagocytes and of the vascular surface.

The platelets circulate as unactivated packets of vasoactive materials sequestered in granules dispersed within the platelet disc. Under normal conditions of blood flow, platelets do not interact with, or adhere to, the vascular endothelium. Platelets possess a highly activatable plasma membrane that is responsive to many types of injurious or inflammatory stimuli. Consequently, contact with surfaces other than normal endothelium, with turbulent blood flow, or with pathologic changes in the vascular surface trigger rapid, profound changes in platelet morphology and metabolism—the process of platelet "activation."

Platelet activation involves changes in the plasma membrane that lead to platelet adhesion to surfaces, followed by aggregation of platelets into fused masses (formation of the primary hemostatic plug; see Fig. 1), the acceleration of the fluid phase of coagulation at the altered platelet surface, the initiation of synthesis of prostanoids, hydroxy acids and platelet-activating factor (PAF), and the release of preformed vasoactive substances. These activities occur within seconds after stimulation and involve many feedbacks that promote hemostasis at a wound site, localize the hemostatic plug, and initiate subsequent repair of injury, a process that involves leukocyte activation, fibrinolysis, and proliferation of cells within the injured blood vessel wall (55,112).

TABLE 1. *Inflammatory functions of platelets*

Release of adhesive proteins
Complement activation and regulation
Binding to microorganisms
Alteration of vascular permeability
Production of chemotactic factors
Uptake, release, metabolism of vasoactive substances
Release of eicosanoid mediators
Release of growth factors
Acceleration of coagulation and fibrinolysis

NORMAL HEMOSTASIS: A SPECIALIZED INFLAMMATORY RESPONSE

Hemostasis can be considered as a specialized type of inflammatory response (112), and platelets can be regarded as cells with functions parallel to those of leukocytes, albeit more limited in scope. Indeed, platelets and polymorphonuclear leukocytes contribute directly to each other's activation during inflammatory responses, and platelet products can modulate leukocyte behavior and vice versa. Moreover, platelets and polymorphonuclear leukocytes can jointly contribute to the synthesis of novel products with inflammatory activity (see Chapter 9, *this volume*).

Normal hemostasis consists of three interacting stages, with platelets most closely involved in the first stage in arteries, where vascular injury is the major inciting event (in veins, where stasis is more likely, platelets have a lesser initiating role in the coagulation process). As soon as the vascular endothelium is injured, platelets adhere to the exposed subendothelial surface via glycoprotein-Ib receptors for von Willebrand factor bound to the subendothelium. This interaction, plus contact with subendothelial collagen, initiates marked changes in the platelet plasma membrane that render the surface pro-coagulant. Among these early changes is a shape change from discs to spread

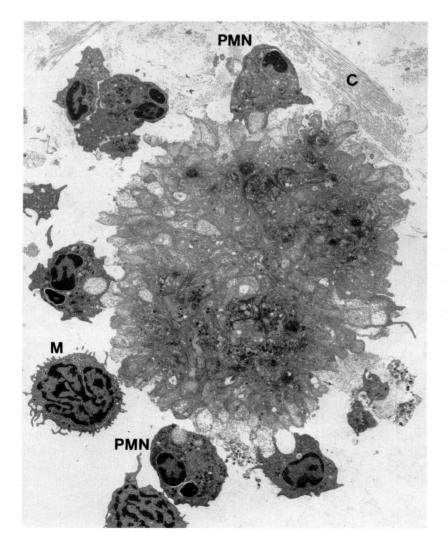

FIG. 1. Platelet aggregate formed upon contact of platelets with collagen (C) during addition of collagen to a mixture of platelets and leukocytes. The platelets are mostly degranulated, and the aggregate is beginning to be digested by polymorphonuclear neutrophils (PMN) which, however, have not been incorporated into the platelet aggregate. (M) Monocyte. (Photograph by D. Zucker-Franklin, from ref. 114.)

forms bearing numerous filapodia. Either platelet adhesion or platelet contact in the fluid phase with activating stimuli, such as adenosine diphosphate, epinephrine, or thrombin, exposes the glycoprotein receptor complex GPIIb-IIIa on the platelet surface and permits platelet-platelet association through fibrinogen bridging between these complexes. During this process of platelet aggregation, a primary hemostatic plug is formed.

Another manifestation of the marked changes in platelet surface properties that accompany vascular injury is the binding and activation of coagulation factors at the platelet surface. Concomitant with the platelet shape change, there is a rearrangement of membrane phospholipids that permits the binding of Factor X to Factor Va on the platelet membrane in the presence of calcium ions, yielding a membrane-bound prothrombinase complex that accelerates local thrombin generation many thousandfold. This mechanism ensures that fibrin is formed locally to stabilize the primary hemostatic plug. It also ushers in the second phase of hemostasis, namely the activation of plasma procoagulant factors to form fibrin strands that then trap erythrocytes to form a bulkier, stable clot. In clot stabilization, platelets contribute the fibrin-cross-linking enzyme, Factor XIII, as well as contraction of smooth muscle actomyosin (thrombasthenin), which mediates clot retraction.

During this process, the same stimuli that activate platelet adhesion and aggregation also trigger the release of arachidonic acid from platelet membrane phospholipids, initiating synthesis of eicosanoids such as thromboxane A_2 and 12-hydroxytetraenoic acid (12-HETE). Thromboxane A_2 (TXA_2) is a potent vasoconstricting agent; together with its immediate precursors, the prostaglandin endoperoxides, TXA_2 further triggers platelet aggregation and the release of vasoactive substances from platelet granules. The synthesis and release of TXA_2 is virtually complete within 30 to 60 sec after platelet activation, whereas production of 12-HETE can continue for many minutes. Activated platelets also release prostaglandin endoperoxides, intermediates in TXA_2 formation; these may be utilized by other cells or may be isomerized in plasma to biologically active prostaglandins. Thus, the initiation of platelet aggregation normally leads to further platelet activation, partly through the release of newly synthesized compounds like TXA_2 and partly through the generation of platelet-activating substances such as thrombin at the platelet surface. Thrombin is one of the most potent activators of platelets.

The release reaction serves to bridge the processes of primary hemostasis and the eventual repair of vascular injury, by reinforcing the hemostatic sequence and by supplying factors that initiate vascular repair (Table 2). Platelets contain two types of storage granules filled with vasoactive materials, as well as containing lysosomal

TABLE 2. *Platelet constituents with inflammatory potential*[a]

Alpha granule	Dense granule	Other
Fibronectin	Serotonin	TXA_2
Fibrinogen	ADP	12-HETE
Thrombospondin	Calcium	
von Willebrand factor		
Plasminogen		
α_2-Plasmin inhibitor		
PDGF		
PF4		
TGF-α and β		
β-Lysin		
Permeability factor		
Factors D and H		
Decay-acclerating factor		
Basic FGF		

[a] TXA_2, thromboxane A_2; ADP, adenosine diphosphate; 12-HETE, 12-hydroxytetraenoic acid; PDGF, platelet-derived growth factor; PF4, platelet factor 4; TGF, transforming growth factor.

granules. The dense granules contain serotonin, the adenine nucleotides adenosine diphosphate (ADP) and triphosphate (ATP), and calcium. Released ADP, itself, induces platelet aggregation and enhances the effects of other platelet agonists; calcium is necessary for both platelet aggregation and coagulation, and serotonin affects vascular tone, potentiates aggregation, and alters interactions between leukocytes and the vascular wall.

The alpha granules contain a large number of adhesive proteins that participate in cell-cell interactions, procoagulants, and growth factors. Thus, platelet alpha granules contain von Willebrand factor, thrombospondin, fibronectin, histidine-rich glycoprotein, fibrinogen, factor V, α_2-antiplasmin, antiheparin PF4, platelet-derived growth factor (PDGF), transforming growth factors alpha and beta, basic fibroblast growth factor (FGF), and a heat-labile endothelial cell growth factor. The substances contained in both dense granules and alpha granules are released when platelets are acted upon by either weaker stimuli, such as epinephrine and ADP, or (in greater amounts) by strong stimuli, such as collagen and thrombin. The contents of platelet lysosomal granules, mainly acyl hydrolases, are only released in response to strong stimuli. Release of all these substances occurs via exocytosis into the surface-connected canalicular system, following centralization of granules by contraction of the peripheral band of microtubules, rather than via fusion of individual granules with the surface membrane as occurs in leukocytes.

Activation of membrane phospholipases is usually accompanied by synthesis of eicosanoids from arachidonic acid but is not irrevocably tied to it. Platelets rendered incapable of producing thromboxane (as after aspirin treatment) or other eicosanoids still undergo the release reaction on contact with appropriate strong stimuli such as collagen and thrombin, as a result of direct phospholipase-C activation. Similarly, platelet aggregation is not necessary for release to occur, and it has been well demonstrated that a single layer of adherent platelets can release alpha-granule proteins onto adjacent vessel walls (55).

ALTERED HEMOSTASIS IN INFLAMMATION

It is a common clinical observation that the incidence of thrombosis is increased during inflammatory states. The function of the hemostatic system tends to be enhanced. Increased levels of fibrinogen and factor VIII, as well as elevated platelet counts, often accompany systemic inflammatory reactions and can contribute to enhanced platelet activation. Much effort has been devoted to attempts to demonstrate that platelet function is "hyperactive" in prethrombotic states, leading to the increased thrombotic tendency. Recent information on the systemic effects of inflammatory mediators such as interleukin-1, tumor necrosis factor, or bacterial lipopolysaccharide suggest that the vascular endothelium, rather than platelets per se, is primarily altered by contact with these inflammatory lymphokines, resulting in the generation of thrombin at the endothelial surface (72,94). Platelets, therefore, are secondarily activated by contact with a locally thrombogenic surface.

During inflammation, the endothelial surface begins to display characteristics similar to those of the activated platelet surface, so that the endothelial cells offer an alternative route to the initiation of coagulation (Table 3). Indeed, the membrane glycoproteins GPIb and GPIIb-IIIa that mediate platelet reactivity and previously considered platelet-specific have now been identified in the endothelial cell surface membrane (10). The same gene codes for adhesive proteins found on platelets, endothelium and leukocytes (21). Exposure of endothelial cells to interleukin-1 or tumor necrosis factor (TNF) results

TABLE 3. *Functional similarities between platelets and activated leukocytes or endothelium*

Membrane expression of GPIIb-IIIa receptors for fibrinogen
Membrane binding of adhesive proteins
Complement binding
Fc-receptor expression
Immune complex binding
Binding and activation of coagulation factors
Eicosanoid secretion
Adherence to microorganisms
Acceleration of coagulation
Enzyme secretion

in membrane changes leading to the binding and activation of plasma coagulation factors IX and X, synthesis and display of tissue factor, down-regulation of the uptake and inactivation of thrombin, production of platelet-activating factor, and release of an inhibitor of plasminogen activation (11,94). Platelets then react with small amounts of thrombin generated on the altered endothelial surface during inflammation, become activated, and secondarily contribute to a thrombotic tendency. Therefore, during inflammation, both platelets and the altered endothelial surface may initiate hemostasis and its pathologic counterpart, thrombosis.

PLATELET INTERACTIONS WITH INFLAMMATORY CELLS

Since hemostasis represents a special form of response to tissue injury, both the development and resolution of the hemostatic process involve participation of inflammatory cells, namely, leukocytes. Considerable evidence indicates that platelets or platelet products can contribute to the accumulation of leukocytes in the clot and to their activation. Conversely, activated leukocytes can alter platelet function. Such interactions of platelets with polymorphonuclear leukocytes and monocytes are characterized below. Whenever possible, studies cited in this chapter refer to human systems.

Platelet Interactions with Monocytes

Factors released from platelets are chemotactic for blood monocytes and for polymorphonuclear (PMN) leukocytes. These factors include PDGF, PF4, 12-HETE, and probably PAF (25,26). Direct cell-cell interactions between monocytes and platelets also occur, resulting in changes in function of either the monocytes or the platelets. For example, thrombin-stimulated platelets bind to blood monocytes, whereas unstimulated platelets do not bind (49). The ligand for this interaction appears to be thrombospondin, which is released by, and becomes bound to, the platelets during activation of the latter by thrombin or other stimuli that initiate the release reaction (88). Monocytes carry receptors for thrombospondin (88). Neither fibronectin nor immunoglobulin G appear to be involved in the association of platelets with monocytes, although monocytes bear both fibronectin receptors and Fc receptors.

In the presence of serum, platelets also augment the adherence of monocytes to surfaces. The glycoprotein complex IIb-IIIa, which is the fibrinogen receptor on the activated platelet membrane, is directly implicated in the adhesion of monocytes to surfaces (10). The glycoprotein complex becomes exposed on the plasma membrane of monocytes following their contact with inflammatory stimuli. This receptor serves as the binding site for fibronectin on the monocyte surface. Monoclonal antibodies to the glycoprotein IIb-IIIa complex block fibronectin binding to monocytes, preventing monocyte adhesion and inhibiting phagocytosis of fibronectin-coated particles (10). Similar glycoprotein IIb-IIIa complexes, originally thought to be restricted to platelets, have been identified as adhesion receptors on the surface membranes of large granular lymphocytes, endothelial cells, megakaryocytes, PMN leukocytes, K562 cells, and neuroblastoma cells.

When human monocytes are exposed to bacterial lipopolysaccharide, tissue factor activity develops on the monocyte surface, with generation of small amounts of thrombin and subsequent platelet aggregation (85). The activation of monocytes during bacterial sepsis, accompanied by consequent local aggregation of platelets with monocytes, may be one of the mechanisms underlying the thrombocytopenia that often accompanies sepsis, even in the absence of disseminated intravascular coagulation. This localized platelet-monocyte aggregation may result in the elevated blood levels of the platelet-specific protein, beta thromboglobulin, observed during sepsis.

Platelets, or their lipoxygenase products, directly stimulate the production of procoagulant activity by monocytes. In the presence of platelets or of platelet membranes, blood monocytes show a threefold increase in endotoxin-induced tissue factor activity (61,74). Aspirin-treated platelets, which have increased lipoxygenase activity, induce more tissue factor activity in monocytes than do untreated platelets (61). Conversely, lipoxygenase inhibitors impede generation of monocyte procoagulant activity (23). Monocytes respond to 12-HETE, the major lipoxygenase product of platelets, by enhanced activity of tissue factor. Arachidonic acid enhances tissue factor activity in monocytes when platelets are present but not when they are absent, indicating that the effect of this fatty acid is platelet-dependent (61). Other polyunsaturated fatty acids lacked this effect on procoagulant activity, as did other lipoxygenase products including leukotrienes. Although endotoxin, immune complexes, lipoproteins, C5a, and activated T-cells have previously been reported to induce monocyte expression of tissue factor activity, induction of such procoagulant activity by platelet-monocyte interaction represents a new mechanism that may contribute to the severity of endotoxin-induced disseminated intravascular coagulation.

Both activated platelets and monocytes release the enzyme galactosyltransferase, which digests components of the extracellular matrix and therefore may modulate the properties of that structure during inflammatory reactions (44).

Pure suspensions of human monocytes, prepared so as to be free of platelets, synthesize thromboxane A_2 as the major eicosanoid product when these suspensions are stimulated with particles such as opsonized zymosan or immunoglobulin complexes (78). Platelets can modify fatty acid oxidation by monocytes. In the presence of platelets, monocytes synthesize a different spectrum of eicosanoids, including 12-HETE, suggesting that the balance of cyclooxygenase and lipoxygenase activity has been shifted by the cell-cell interaction (35).

Platelet Interactions with PMN Leukocytes

Platelet interactions with PMN leukocytes occur at many steps in the inflammatory response, including chemotaxis, secretion, degranulation, and oxidative metabolism.

Platelet Role in Chemotaxis of Leukocytes

The observation that leukocytes are attracted to blood clots and participate in their eventual dissolution is a venerable one in the history of pathology. Several components in the coagulation process including kallikrein, fibrin fragments, Hageman factor fragments, and plasminogen activator, are reported to be chemotactic in vitro for leukocytes. The physiologic role of these substances as chemotaxins is, however, unclear. Platelets themselves may contribute a variety of chemotactic mediators of inflammation when they release preformed vasoactive substances, synthesize lipid chemotaxins, or enzymatically cleave complement to form peptide chemotaxins (97,105,34). Thus, both immediately acting and more slowly produced chemotactic substances are derived from platelets.

Serum is strongly chemotactic for PMN leukocytes and monocytes when blood is clotted in the presence of platelets (43). Sources of this chemotactic activity include the complement peptide C5a as well as lipid mediators 12-HETE and PAF. Released alpha granule proteins PDGF and PF4 are also chemotactic (24,26,36) (see below).

The complement-related chemotactic activity generated by platelets depends on cleavage of C5 by neutral proteases released from activated platelets during aggregation (105). The anaphylatoxin C5a, which also can be produced by leukocyte proteases, is rapidly inactivated by the heat-labile carboxypeptidase inhibitors of plasma; however, generation of C5a within platelet aggregates or blood clots may permit a more protected local environment for protracted effects.

Conversely, both C3 and C5 interact with platelets to enhance their aggregation by arachidonic acid and by thrombin, as well as to augment the release reaction (see below).

Platelet lipoxygenase acting on arachidonic acid liberated during platelet activation forms unstable 12-hydroperoxyeicosatetraenoic acid (12-HPETE), which is reduced to 12-HETE, a weak chemotactic factor for neutrophils, monocytes, and eosinophils (active in low microgram-per-milliliter concentrations). The precursor 12-HPETE can also be transformed by nearby neutrophils into 12,20-diHETE, another chemotaxin (65). Since platelet lipoxygenase, unlike cyclooxygenase, is not rapidly inactivated by its enzymatic products, the production of 12-HETE within a platelet plug can continue for many hours and can maintain a well-localized chemotactic stimulus in a wound.

One reported biologic activity of PDGF is the induction of chemotaxis of PMN leukocytes and monocytes, as well as chemotaxis of smooth muscle cells and fibroblasts (24,26). PDGF is better known as a competence factor for the proliferation of fibroblasts and vascular smooth muscle cells, but at low picomolar concentrations (less than the amount required for cell proliferation) it acts as a powerful chemotaxin. The chemotactic effect of PDGF involves a cellular receptor that is different from the receptor for C5a or PF4. It is postulated that the major function of such chemotaxis is the recruitment of cells to a site of healing. PDGF, which binds avidly to the extracellular matrix, is extremely stable and therefore may produce very protracted biologic effects.

The platelet alpha-granule protein, platelet factor 4 (PF4), is a highly cationic protein that antagonizes heparin. On release from platelets, it rapidly is taken up by endothelium and enters the vascular wall (36). PF4 is chemotactic both for PMN leukocytes and for monocytes and may help to direct these cells into the vessel wall following tissue injury (25,87). In addition, PF4 has been found to stimulate histamine release from human basophils (8). Both the chemotactic and the histamine-releasing activity of PF4 reside in the carboxy-terminal fragment of that molecule, PF4 (8,25,59–70).

Platelet Stimulation of PMN-Leukocyte Activation

Platelets enhance leukocyte adhesion to the vascular wall, provide substrate for the synthesis of novel cellular products, augment release of leukocytic enzymes, modulate the activity of the enzymes, and stimulate the production of leukocytic inflammatory mediators. Mixed aggregates of platelets and leukocytes form in response to inflammatory stimuli. In addition, mediators released by platelets can augment or decrease leukocyte-mediated vascular injury.

The release of chemotactic factors by platelets contained in a hemostatic plug may stimulate the influx of PMN leukocytes into a site of local thrombosis (7). This mechanism, as well as release of other chemotactic materials, such as fragments of fibrin released during blood clotting, probably has a role in initiating healing in a wound. Conversely, a number of inflammatory stimuli cause rapid local simultaneous accumulation of PMN leukocytes and platelets prior to the occurrence of hemorrhage or thrombosis. Thus, intradermal injection of C5a, zymosan-treated plasma, *Escherichia coli,* endotoxin, or conjugates of *N*-formyl-methionyl-leucyl-phenylalanine with bovine serum albumin into rabbits induces a rapid accumulation of both PMN and platelets, independent of changes in vascular permeability, peaking at 1 to 3 hr after application of the stimulus (45). The time course of ^{111}In-labeled platelet influx exactly parallels that of ^{51}Cr-labeled PMN leukocytes (47). The appearance of platelets precedes the development of hemorrhagic or thrombotic lesions, which appear only after 7 hr as measured by accumulation of ^{59}Fe-labeled erythrocytes (45,47). In this setting, the influx of PMN leukocytes appears responsible for the simultaneous influx of platelets, because neutropenic animals show neither PMN-leukocyte nor platelet responses. The factor responsible for the cellular response is probably PAF, since the accumulation of both types of cells is inhibited after pretreatment with CV3988, a PAF antagonist, whereas aspirin pretreatment had no effect (46). In addition, this antagonist abolished the platelet and PMN-leukocyte response but not the hyperemia, caused by direct injection of PAF itself (1). An additional possible role for leukotriene B$_4$ (LTB$_4$) has not been clearly established.

Activated platelets release several other products that enhance leukocyte adhesion and enzyme activities. Serotonin, released from dense granules of activated platelets, enhances the adherence of human PMN leukocytes to vascular endothelial cells (6). When either stimulated platelets or supernatant fluid derived from suspensions of aggregating platelets was incubated with complement-activated PMN leukocytes, adherence of the PMN leukocytes to endothelial cells was enhanced twofold, and ^{51}Cr release from the endothelial cells was significantly augmented, documenting a serotonin-dependent increase in endothelial injury (6). Antagonists of serotonin uptake or activity prevented this augmenting effect of platelets. Adenosine, which can be formed from adenine nucleotides released by platelets, endothelial cells, or erythrocytes, has recently been proposed as an inhibitor of PMN-leukocyte-induced endothelial injury. The endothelial cell ectoenzyme, 5'-nucleotidase, converts adenine nucleotides to adenosine. Thus, a stable adenosine analog, 2-chloroadenosine, has been observed to (a) decrease PMN leukocyte adherence to endothelial cells, (b) block ^{51}Cr release from endothelial cells in contact with activated PMN leukocytes, and (c) inhibit the release of superoxide and H$_2$O$_2$

from PMN leukocytes through an action requiring binding to A2 adenosine sites on PMN leukocytes (22). Adenosine is well known as a vasodilator and as a strong inhibitor of platelet activation; the possibility that it also acts to modify PMN-leukocyte behavior at the vascular wall is a newly described function. During interactions of platelet-release products with PMN leukocytes, neither serotonin nor adenosine seems to alter the release of lysosomal enzymes from PMN leukocytes (6,22).

The platelet alpha granule protein PF4, also released during platelet activation, enhances the enzymatic activity of human leukocyte elastase by inducing a conformational change in the elastin molecule such that additional elastase-sensitive sites are exposed for enzymatic degradation (62). Diseases in which levels of leukocyte elastase are increased (e.g., chronic obstructive pulmonary disease, cigarette smoking, and pneumonia) are conditions in which platelet activation is also enhanced. Local release of platelet products within inflammatory foci could therefore contribute to the breakdown of lung elastin in these diseases, where oxidative inhibition of alpha-1-antiprotease, the major inhibitor of elastase, is also enhanced (see Chapter 45, *this volume*).

Thromboxane A2, the major eicosanoid released from activated platelets, has also been found to enhance PMN-leukocyte adhesiveness (90). Endotoxin-induced adhesion of PMN leukocytes to endothelium is preventable by indomethacin or imidazole, inhibitors of TXA_2 synthesis.

The major lipoxygenase product of platelets, 12-HETE, is reported to be chemotactic for PMN. Moreover, 12-HETE at even lower concentrations stimulates oxidative metabolism in neutrophils, enhances their adhesion to the vascular endothelium, and stimulates chemokinesis (34). At the same time, 12-HETE enhances prostacyclin (PGI2) production by endothelium (84), a double action that further modulates the interaction of PMN leukocytes with the vascular surface, since PGI2 has been found to decrease PMN-leukocyte adhesion and can act as a scavenger for toxic oxygen metabolites such as superoxide, produced by stimulated PMN leukocytes. The PGI2 is inactivated by oxygen free radicals during this process. Platelet-derived 12-HETE is acted upon by PMN lipoxygenase to form 12,20-diHETE, a compound that has moderate chemotactic activity (66). Moreover, the precursor of 12-HETE, 12-HPETE, has been reported to stimulate leukotriene-B4 synthesis in human PMN leukocytes (67). High shear stresses that occur in turbulent flow, such as across artificial heart valves or during extracorporeal perfusion, stimulate lipoxygenase activity in blood. At physiologic platelet/PMN-leukocyte ratios, shear-induced activation of platelets releases platelet 12-HPETE, which subsequently activates PMN-leukocyte 5-lipoxygenase to form leukotrienes that induce PMN-

leukocyte aggregation (83). It is of interest that the lipoxygenase-deficient platelets of patients with myeloproliferative disease are poor activators of LTB4 synthesis in PMN leukocytes (50).

Experimental subcutaneous injections of platelets or platelet homogenates induce marked edema and infiltration by PMN leukocytes and later induce the accumulation of "myofibroblasts" that form a fibroblastic reaction. Similar injection of homogenates from other tissues, such as brain, heart, or kidney, produce milder inflammatory reactions and little fibrosis. The influx of PMN leukocytes appears to be necessary for subsequent fibroblast proliferation, with the role of platelets being that of initiator of the entire sequence. Cationic proteins released from the granules of activated platelets can produce edema and PMN-leukocyte accumulation by several mechanisms (70,71). An immediate permeability response is induced by degranulation of mast cells and release of mast-cell histamine (70,75); it is blocked by histamine pretreatment. A second permeability increase requires several hours, is unrelated to histamine release, and involves neutrophil infiltration; this may involve PAF release from platelets and/or activation of the terminal components of complement by platelet proteases (105).

Platelet Interactions with PMN-Leukocyte Products

Substances that are released by PMN leukocytes and that affect platelet behavior (Table 4) include oxygen radicals, enzymes, arachidonic acid metabolites, and PAF. Indeed, the acidic pH characteristic of an inflammatory focus has been shown to increase platelet sensitivity to aggregation by arachidonic acid, suggesting that local pH might itself contribute to thrombosis accompanying inflammation (54).

Active oxygen metabolites produced by activated PMN leukocytes alter platelet function. When platelets are exposed to phagocytizing PMN leukocytes, they exhibit decreased aggregation responses. Because catalase reversed the inhibitory effect of the leukocytes on aggregation, H_2O_2 release from the leukocytes appears to be the soluble effector (60). Hydrogen peroxide alone is an inefficient inducer of the platelet release reaction and may cause platelet lysis. In the presence of myeloperoxidase and a halide,

TABLE 4. *Leukocyte products affecting platelet function*

Active oxygen metabolites: H_2O_2, superoxide, hydroxyl radical
Enzymes: elastase, myeloperoxidase
Eicosanoids: LTB4, 5-HETE
Platelet-activating factor
Tissue factor

very low concentrations of H_2O_2 induce release of serotonin from platelets without lysis; this reaction requires intact platelet metabolism and is blocked by inhibitors of peroxidase (17). These findings suggest that other oxygen products of leukocytes, such as hydroxyl ion, can induce platelet activation. Superoxide also induces serotonin release and acts synergistically with thrombin to activate platelets (38). Thus, several active oxygen intermediates produced by activated PMN leukocytes may alter the function of platelets in their immediate vicinity.

Enzymes released from PMN leukocytes affect hemostasis by several mechanisms, including proteolysis of coagulation factors, inactivation of plasma inhibitors for activated coagulation and complement components, and direct effects on platelets. Proteolytic enzymes are known to alter platelet reactivity and can affect the biological activity of products released by platelets. Exposure of fibrinogen receptors on the platelet membrane is requisite for fibrinogen binding and subsequent platelet aggregation in response to platelet-activating stimuli. Platelets treated with proteolytic enzymes can aggregate spontaneously. This may be one route to thrombocytopenia in sepsis and in acute leukemia, two clinical conditions in which high levels of circulating leukocyte proteases are detected. In particular, low concentrations of leukocyte elastase have been shown to expose (irreversibly) fibrinogen receptors on platelets and to produce spontaneous aggregation in the presence of fibrinogen (58). This aggregation could not be inhibited by prostacyclin or other agents that raise platelet cyclic adenosine monophosphate (cAMP) levels (despite an intact adenylate cyclase system), unlike the situation in intact platelets where exposure of fibrinogen receptors by physiologic agonists is reversible, suggesting that platelets exposed to elastase had lost a major regulatory function. Moreover, human leukocyte elastase at physiologically relevant concentrations has been observed to inhibit thrombin-stimulated platelet aggregation and serotonin release as well as ristocetin-mediated platelet agglutination. This loss of function is related to proteolytic inactivation of high-affinity thrombin receptors and cleavage of glycoprotein Ib on the platelet membrane, respectively (9).

Platelet-activating factor (1-O-alkyl-12-acetyl-*sn*-glycero-3-phosphorylcholine, also called PAF, AGEPC, or PAF-acether), a family of ether-linked phospholipid derivatives, is known to be released by human neutrophils, monocytes, mast cells, and platelets (14,15,42,102). Platelets, like leukocytes, have specific membrane receptors for PAF (100). Although named "platelet-activating factor" because of its powerful effect on rabbit platelets (active at 10^{-10} *M*), PAF is a much weaker direct agonist for human platelets (64). The effects of PAF on human platelets are potentiated by epinephrine, ADP, arachidonic acid, or aggregated IgG, suggesting synergy-requiring re-

lease of ADP (101). However, PAF is a strong activating agent for human neutrophil aggregation, chemotaxis, granule secretion, and superoxide production (102). In addition, PAF induces vascular permeability, contracts bronchial and vascular smooth muscle, and produces pain (46).

Arachidonic acid metabolites released by PMN leukocytes can be transformed by platelets into novel products during cell-cell interactions. For example, leukocyte-derived 5-HETE reacts with platelet 12-lipoxygenase to form 5,12-diHETE (64). Leukotrienes potentiate the effects of platelet agonists on platelet aggregation (63). Leukotriene C_4 (LTC$_4$), LTD$_4$, and LTE$_4$, which have no direct aggregating effect on human platelets, strongly enhance platelet aggregation and thromboxane release when combined with subthreshold concentrations of epinephrine or thrombin. This synergy suggests another rationale for the increased incidence of thrombotic phenomena associated with inflammatory lesions (64).

PLATELET INTERACTIONS WITH FIBROBLASTS

Release of peptide growth factors from activated platelets has an important role in the initiation of tissue repair after inflammatory responses, just as the release of other mediators has a role in earlier stages of the inflammatory response. Platelets contain and release not only PDGF but also TGF-α (transforming growth factor alpha) TGF-β, and basic FGF (fibroblast growth factor) (92). Platelets represent a major reservoir for these factors and are the source of their presence in serum. Other mesenchymal cells, such as activated macrophages and dividing fibroblasts and smooth muscle cells, may also synthesize these growth factors (93).

The PDGF released by platelets is reported to be strongly chemotactic for fibroblasts, neutrophils, monocytes, and vascular smooth muscle cells (24,86,87) and is mitogenic for fibroblasts in the presence of TGF-α or EGF (epidermal growth factor, a structural homolog of TGF-β) (92). The mitogenic activity of PDGF for fibroblasts is lost when the molecule undergoes reduction, but chemotactic activity is said to be retained (107). Moreover, PDGF stimulates the production of collagenase by fibroblasts (24), an essential part of tissue remodeling during resolution of inflammation. Phospholipid metabolism and the production of arachidonic acid metabolites by fibroblasts is also stimulated by PDGF, as is the synthesis of cyclooxygenase, a key enzyme in prostaglandin synthesis (37). TGF-β appears to be a regulatory substance in tissue repair: It stimulates the formation of collagen by fibroblasts and causes an angiogenic response (92). In addition to direct effects, TGF-beta enhances or inhibits the effects of PDGF, EGF, or FGF on different cell types, including fibroblasts (3). Current interpretation is that combinations of growth factors act together to integrate normal (or pathologic) responses to tissue injury.

PLATELET INTERACTIONS WITH MICROORGANISMS

Platelets and Bacteria

Many types of bacteria aggregate platelets, forming mixed aggregates that may, on the one hand, enhance killing of the bacteria by phagocytes, or, on the other hand, protect the bacteria sequestered in the aggregates (often reinforced with fibrin) from destruction (18). An example of the latter situation is subacute bacterial endocarditis, where bacteria trapped within platelet-fibrin vegetations on the heart valve may remain viable, protected against the bactericidal effects of antibiotics, and continue to act as sources of infection (30). The aggregation of platelets by bacteria stimulates the platelet release reaction, but platelet lysis does not occur (19). Staphylococci and streptococci actively aggregate platelets, but *S. pneumoniae* does so only in the presence of anti-pneumococcal antibody (110).

At least three mechanisms underlie the interaction between staphylococci and human platelets, all of which require plasma components. First, fibrinogen is necessary for the aggregation of platelets in the presence of *S. aureus;* fibrinogen has a specific binding site for this organism (20). Second, protein-A-bearing *S. aureus* (about 40% of coagulase-positive strains) aggregate platelets in the presence of IgG via the Fc-binding activity of protein A present in the bacterial wall (40). The IgG acts as a bridge, binding simultaneously to the platelet Fc receptor and to protein A on the staphylococci. Both aggregation and serotonin release are induced. Complement activation is not required. Third, the peptidoglycan present in the staphylococcal cell wall also may activate platelets and contribute to the cytopenias and complement activation that characterize certain staphylococcal bacteremias by complement-independent, as well as complement-dependent, mechanisms (91).

Endotoxemia is frequently characterized by thrombocytopenia. Many mechanisms are involved, including endotoxin-induced vascular damage and thrombogenicity (as detailed above), release of PAF, and disseminated intravascular coagulation. In addition, the interaction between platelets and aggregated IgG is enhanced, in general, by lipid-A-rich lipopolysaccharides, indicating that binding of endotoxin augments antibody-dependent platelet aggregation (33).

Platelets contain a heat-stable bactericidal protein, first detected in the nineteenth century as a plasma "beta-lysin"

active against gram-positive microorganisms such as *Bacillus* species (including *B. anthracis*) and streptococcus but not staphylococci (28,71). Demonstration that serum β-lysin levels were higher than plasma levels suggested that this bactericidal activity was cell-derived (43), and platelets rather than leukocytes were identified as the specific source (104). Serum levels were shown to be elevated during pneumonia and in myocardial infarction and cancer. β-lysin is released from platelets during their aggregation by strong stimuli (28,104), including thrombin, immune complexes, and collagen. It has been identified as a cationic, heat-stable peptide of molecular weight 6,000, and its bactericidal activity is blocked by DNA and acidic phospholipids (28). Its mode of action is directly on the cell membrane, not on the bacterial cell wall. The biologic importance of platelet beta-lysin in the killing of pathogenic microorganisms, however, is minimal compared to the effects of immunoglobulins and complement, and this protein probably represents a vestigial marker of the inflammatory potential of platelets.

Platelets and Viruses

Thrombocytopenia is a feature of many acute viral infections, and direct platelet-virus interactions have been implicated as the cause. Mechanisms proposed include decreased platelet production by virus-infected megakaryocytes, disseminated intravascular coagulation with platelet consumption, and platelet aggregation and lysis by virus, immune complexes, or cross-reacting antibodies directed at platelet surface antigens. Myxoviruses (such as influenza virus) have been shown to shorten platelet survival, associated with removal of platelet membrane sialic acid by viral neuraminidase (96,98). During influenza infection, membrane-bound viral hemagglutinin appears on the platelet surface membrane. In the presence of specific antibody and complement, immune lysis of platelets occurs (51). Other myxoviruses, such as measles virus, may have similar interactions with platelets, as can vaccinia and herpesviruses. Vaccinia virus, which lacks neuraminidase, has been shown to bind to human platelets in a specific manner via electrostatic interactions, as well as to cause serotonin release, but it has also been found to inhibit platelet aggregation (5). It is proposed that either viral proteolysis of surface components or induction of a calcium leak mediates these effects of vaccinia virus on platelets.

Platelets and Parasites

Malarial plasmodia have been observed within platelets, and thrombocytopenia is a characteristic of severe malarial infection (32). As in viral and bacterial infections, the major mechanism of thrombocytopenia in malaria appears to involve immune complexes that interact with platelet Fc receptors, leading to enhanced platelet clearance (52).

Platelets have cytotoxic effects on schistosomal and filarial parasites through an IgE-mediated mechanism (13). Human platelets display on their surfaces a low-affinity receptor for IgE that is associated with the GPIIb-IIIa glycoprotein complex on the platelet membrane (13,16). Binding of IgE does not require platelet activation and is not affected by ADP or the presence or absence of calcium. The IgE receptors are different from IgG or Fc receptors on the platelet membrane, and binding of IgG does not interfere with binding of IgE or vice versa. However, binding of fibrinogen to the GPIIb-IIIa complex inhibits IgE binding, suggesting possible steric hindrance. Thrombasthenic platelets that completely lack the GPIIb-IIIa glycoproteins fail to bind IgE, and platelets from mild thromboasthenic patients, showing a decreased concentration of GPIIb-IIIa, bind reduced amounts of IgE (13). Antibodies to the GPIIb-IIIa complex block IgE binding to platelets. Only a fraction (20–30%) of the platelets from normal individuals bind IgE, but more than 50% of the platelets from patients with aspirin-induced asthma, as well as patients with schistosomiasis or filariasis, bind IgE (13,48).

Monoclonal (myeloma) IgE also binds to about 25% of normal platelets in a similar way; its binding is also blocked by antibodies to GPIIb-IIIa but not by antibodies to GPIb or by IgG. In the presence of anti-IgE, the IgE-sensitized platelets undergo aggregation and the release reaction (16).

A series of recent investigations in both rat and human systems suggests that platelets can participate in a specific type of antibody-dependent cellular cytotoxicity (ADCC) mechanism against metazoan parasites, reactions usually attributed to mononuclear cells (48). Whereas normal platelets (IgE binding or not) are not cytotoxic for *Schisotosoma mansoni* larvae, the platelets from patients with schistosomiasis or from patients with aspirin-inducible asthma were reported to be cytotoxic; incubation of normal platelets in IgE-rich immune serum from patients with *S. mansoni* infection led to killing of schistosome larvae in proximity to the platelets. Contamination of the platelet preparations by mononuclear cells was excluded as a cytotoxic source.

Immune serum alone does not kill the larvae. A cytotoxic factor that is heat-labile and adsorbed on an anti-IgE column has been isolated; its effect is duplicated by a monoclonal anti-schistosomal IgE antibody. In the presence of schistosomal antigen or of anti-IgE antibodies, IgE-dependent platelet activation occurs and leads to the release of cytocidal mediators that kill the parasites. These mediators were reported to be active oxygen metabolites

rather than granule constituents, since platelets from patients congenitally lacking platelet alpha granules (gray platelet syndrome) normally kill schistosomal larvae (13). Moreover, platelets from aspirin-sensitive asthmatics, when treated *in vitro* with cyclooxygenase inhibitors, were found to generate oxygen metabolites and to kill parasites by an IgE-independent mechanism, whereas platelets from normal subjects or extrinsic asthmatics were not cytotoxic. Salicylate pretreatment of the platelets from aspirin-sensitive asthmatics could block the cytotoxic effect induced by aspirin or other nonsteroidal anti-inflammatory drugs.

Platelets may also augment IgE-dependent histamine release from human basophils and mast cells, most likely through a PAF-mediated pathway (56) or by release of protein mediators (70,75). During antigen challenge of allergic asthmatic subjects, platelet activation can be documented by a rise in plasma levels of PF4 and β-thromboglobulin (57), presumably through the release from basophils of PAF. In turn, platelets augment histamine release in a concentration-dependent manner through release of a soluble, nondialyzable, heat- and acid-stable material. This mediator has not yet been characterized but is clearly not PDGF (56). Purified PF4 and its carboxy-terminal peptide have been observed to release histamine from purified human basophils in a calcium-independent and IgE-independent manner (8). Basophil granules rapidly bind PF4, which appears to displace histamine; there is no cytotoxic reaction. (8) Thus platelet interactions with basophils may represent a double, positive-feedback mechanism for augmenting immediate hypersensitivity reactions, irrespective of IgE sensitization.

PLATELETS AND ACUTE-PHASE REACTANTS

Platelet function can be modulated by acute-phase reactants, such as fibrinogen, complement, and immunoglobulins, which are plasma components involved in inflammatory processes. Fibrinogen is required for platelet aggregation, and the exposure of the fibrinogen receptor (the glycoprotein IIb-IIIa complex) on the platelet membrane is one of the earliest markers of platelet activation (58). Platelets secrete fibrinogen during the release reaction; fibrinogen comprises 20% of the platelet weight and is one of the four adhesive proteins present in platelet alpha granules. Platelet reactivity is increased during inflammatory states when plasma fibrinogen is elevated, but platelet fibrinogen content rises much more slowly than does plasma fibrinogen content during inflammation, since platelet fibrinogen represents that synthesized in megakaryocytes (106). Platelet aggregation can be induced by derivatives of C-reactive protein (CRP), another acute-phase reactant (88a). Heat-aggregated C-reactive protein, like aggregated immunoglobulin, aggregates platelets and induces the platelet release reaction and thromboxane synthesis. In this function, heated CRP is 10- to 20-fold more active than aggregated IgG (88a). CRP complexed to the cationic compound poly-L-lysine, or adsorbed onto latex beads, also activates platelets. These reactions are only partly inhibited by cyclooxygenase blockade, suggesting the CRP may activate platelets, in part, by the "third pathway" shared by thrombin and PAF, probably by a direct activation of phospholipase C.

PLATELETS AND IMMUNE COMPLEXES

The human platelet membrane normally adsorbs IgG in a nonspecific manner but also displays specific receptors for the Fc portion of immunoglobulins and thus binds immune complexes (42). The binding of immune complexes by human platelets is independent of complement binding. An alteration in the density and reactivity of platelet Fc receptors has been observed in platelets from patients with myeloproliferative disease; these platelets show a marked increase in Fc binding (68). Thus, platelets coated with immune complexes may become involved as "innocent bystanders" during immunologic reactions, being removed from the circulation prematurely in the spleen. This is felt to be a major mechanism in drug-induced thrombocytopenias (in some of which there is nonspecific drug adsorption to the platelet surface, with secondary antibody binding to the drug) and in the thrombocytopenia associated with a number of immunologic disorders such as systemic lupus erythematosus (42). In idiopathic (autoimmune) thrombocytopenic purpura, in contrast, it is generally considered that specific antibody to particular platelet surface antigens is bound to the platelets, although the nature of the antigens is often elusive. In both drug-induced and idiopathic immune thrombocytopenias, antibodies with specificity for platelet membrane glycoproteins such as GP1b, GPIIb-IIIa, and GPV have been described (4,59,95). In addition, monoclonal DNA-binding antibodies derived from patients with systemic lupus erythematosus apparently bind to platelet-membrane lipid components but not to platelet-membrane proteins (2).

Surface-bound IgG is a strong stimulus for platelet aggregation, so that opsonized microorganisms or aggregated IgG initiate platelet aggregation and the release reaction (79,110). This may be a complement-dependent mechanism in human platelets (113). Lipopolysaccharide enhances the platelet response to IgG aggregates (33). Human platelets contain very little histamine, so that histamine release by immune complex-stimulated platelets is *not* an important pathogenic mechanism in human immunologic disease, although it is a key mechanism in the rabbit, where the platelets are the major reservoir of blood histamine (42). However, aggregated IgG may potentiate platelet responses to other agonists, such as PAF (101). Since aggregated IgG may also activate complement, bind Fc receptors, and induce production of PAF by leukocytes during immune complex-mediated reaction, this synergy may represent another type of augmentation of inflammatory responses by leukocyte-platelet interactions (102). It is interesting that normal female platelets display greater serotonin secretion than do normal male platelets upon activation with aggregated IgG (69).

Platelet participation in immunologic injury in humans has been documented in renal transplant rejection, where platelet accumulation in the rejecting graft can be detected by gamma scanning after injection of ^{111}In-labeled platelets (103) and by a rise in urine thromboxane values (12). Since platelets bear HLA antigens on their surface, this phenomenon appears to involve an immune-complex mechanism leading to microvascular thrombosis. In chronic glomerulonephritis, platelet-related antigens are found within glomeruli and might indicate that platelet aggregation and the release of chemotactic substances, permeability factors, and growth factors could locally contribute to nephritic pathology (12,29). Serotonin depletion of circulating platelets has been demonstrated in glomerulonephritis and in collagen vascular disease (12,109). In the nephrotic syndrome, platelets are hyperaggregable in response to alterations of plasma proteins (12).

Platelet activation may also accompany antigenic stimulation in extrinsic asthma. Inhalation of ragweed antigens in patients with documented ragweed-induced asthma produces a prompt increase in plasma PF4 in association with decreased FEV, indicating airway obstruction (55). The specificity of this reaction is indicated by the fact that methacholine-induced bronchoconstriction in the same patients is not accompanied by any rise in plasma PF4. A less well understood form of vascular inflammation involving platelet obstruction of the microvasculature is erythromelalgia, a condition in which attacks of burning pain, warmth, and erythema in hands or feet is associated with an elevated platelet count in patients with myeloproliferative disease, especially primary thrombocythemia (66). This condition represents platelet plugging of small arterioles with acute inflammatory infiltration and microthrombosis. It responds promptly to aspirin and is alleviated by lowering of the platelet count.

PLATELETS AND THE COMPLEMENT SYSTEM

Platelets participate in a variety of complement-mediated reactions. As noted earlier, a granule-derived platelet protease can cleave plasma C5 to C5a, forming a potent chemotaxin for PMN leukocytes and monocytes (105). The lysis of virus-infected platelets requires the participation of both antibody and complement, as does lysis of "innocent bystander" platelets bearing immune complexes. Human platelets interact with many, but not all, of the components of the complement system. The early component C1q inhibits collagen-induced platelet adhesion and aggregation. Platelets from persons with deficiencies in C3, C5, C6, or C7 show impaired platelet aggregation to zymosan, which aggregates normal platelets in the presence of plasma (113). Human platelets appear to lack the capacity to bind C3b (the "immune adherence" receptor characteristic of platelets of many animal species) (31,42). Recently, a C3-binding protein that is similar to a leukocyte-C3-binding protein known as gp45-70 has been isolated from human platelets (108). This protein has cofactor activity for the Factor-I-mediated cleavage of C3 and may act to limit lytic complement activation on platelets in a manner supplementary to decay-accelerating factor. Zymosan-activated human platelets exhibit C3d binding and display increased prothrombin-converting activity and augmented binding of Factor Xa; these enhanced procoagulant effects are mediated by the alternative pathway of complement activation (76).

Human platelets initiate the formation of the C5-C9 complex and bind this terminal complex of complement activation (80,111). Ultrastructural changes in the platelet membrane accompany such binding (80). Depolarization of the membrane potential occurs which can be spontaneously restored in metabolically active platelets with exocytic vesiculation (shedding) of the C5-9 pores that have formed (89). The depolarization also triggers a rise in cytoplasmic Ca^{2+} concentration (89). Thrombin-induced platelet aggregation, thromboxane formation, and serotonin release are augmented by binding of C5b-9 (81). This augmentation of platelet activation by the terminal complement complex is abolished by pretreatment of the platelets with aspirin or indomethacin, or by specific antisera to C5, C6, or C9 (80,81). Prostanoid synthesis in platelets may be induced by the action of the late complement components C5b-9 via the induction of ion channels and simultaneous inhibition of the reacylation of liberated arachidonic acid (39). Thus, treatment of platelets with C5b-9 produces a dose- and time-related inhibition of acyl-CoA:lysolecithin acyl transferase, resulting in release of both TXB_2 and prostaglandin E_2 (PGE_2). This specific inhibition of fatty acid reacylation, rather than direct enhancement of arachidonate release by C5b-9 complex binding, can be demonstrated by measuring conversion by platelets of labeled lyso-phosphatidyl choline to phosphatidylcholine in the presence of a suitable acyl-CoA substrate. A similar effect is produced by the antibiotic nystatin (39).

Platelets may also directly participate in the alternative pathway of complement activation. Factor D is present in platelet alpha granules and is secreted during thrombin-induced activation (53). Factor D is a serine protease that binds to the platelet membrane and inhibits subsequent binding of thrombin and thrombin-mediated activation. Its secretion from the alpha granules suggests a mechanism for regulation of thrombin-platelet interaction. Factor H (previously known as beta-1 H) is also present in platelet alpha granules and appears to inhibit alternative pathway C3 convertase (53). Usually, a regulatory protein, decay-accelerating factor (DAF), modulates active C3 convertase activity. In paroxysmal nocturnal hemoglobinuria, the platelets lack DAF, so that C3 convertase activity is unregulated and complement activation proceeds at an accelerated pace (73). In some patients with paroxysmal nocturnal hemoglobinuria, elevated C3 convertase activity is not demonstrated. Factor-H release from these platelets, triggered by thrombin, blocks C3 convertase even in the absence of DAF (27). Thus platelets possess a novel mechanism for modulating the alternative pathway of complement activation that is not present in other cell types.

In addition to interactions with the classical and alternative pathways of complement activation, platelets demonstrate specific interactions with complement-derived anaphylatoxins. Human C3a induces platelet aggregation and potentiates aggregation, serotonin release, and thromboxane production induced by low concentrations of ADP (82). Similar effects were produced by C3a des-Arg at picomolar concentrations. Binding of C3a was demonstrable on the platelet membrane subsequent to interaction of platelets to C3a. Thrombin-induced platelet activation was not affected by C3a, although it was markedly enhanced when washed platelets were exposed to C5-C9, as described above. The enhancement was abolished by inhibition of cyclooxygenase in the platelets by aspirin or indomethacin, indicating that the thrombin-complement synergy was mediated by the arachidonic acid pathway. Similarly, in the presence of C5a des-Arg, but without participation of other components of the complement system, platelet aggregation to ADP, arachidonic acid, or thrombin is augmented. These effects may represent another mechanism by which complement activation during blood clotting participates in hemostasis.

REFERENCES

1. Archer, C. B., Page, C. P., Morley, J., MacDonald, D. M. (1985): Accumulation of inflammatory cells in response to intracutaneous platelet activating factor (PAF-acether) in man. *Br. J. Derm.*, 112: 285–290.
2. Asano, T., Furie, B. C., and Furie, B. (1985): Platelet-binding prop-

erties of monoclonal lupus autoantibodies produced by human hybridomas. *Blood,* 66:1254–1260.

3. Assoian, R. K., Grotendorst, G. R., Miller, D. M., and Sporn, M. B. (1984): Cellular transformation by coordinated action of three peptide growth factors from human platelets. *Nature,* 309: 804–806.

4. Berndt, M. C., Chong, B. H., Bull, H. A., Zola, H., and Castaldi, P. (1985): Molecular characterization of quinine/quinidine drug-dependent antibody-platelet interaction using monoclonal antibodies. *Blood,* 66:1292–1301.

5. Bik, T., Sarow, I., and Livne, A. (1982): Interaction between virus and human blood platelets. *Blood,* 59:482.

6. Boogaerts, M. A., Yamada, O., Jacob, H. S., and Moldow, C. F. (1982): Enhancement of granulocyte-endothelial cell adherence and granulocyte-induced cytotoxicity by platelet release products. *Proc. Natl. Acad. Sci. USA,* 79:7019–7023.

7. Braunstein, P. W., Cuenard, H. F., Joris, I., and Majno, G. (1980): Platelets, fibroblasts and inflammation. Tissue reactions to platelets injected subcutaneously. *Am. J. Pathol.,* 99:53–66.

8. Brindley, L. L., Sweat, J. M., and Goetzl, B. J. (1983): Stimulation of histamine release from human basophils by human PF4. *J. Clin. Invest.,* 72:1218–1223.

9. Brower, M. S., Levin, R. I., and Garry, K. (1985): Human neutrophil elastase modulates platelet function by limited proteolysis of membrane glycoproteins. *J. Clin. Invest.,* 75:657–666.

10. Burns, G. F., Cosgrove, L., Triglia, T., Beall, J. A., Lopez, A. F., Werkmeister, J. A., Begley, C. G., Haddad, A. P., Apice, A. J., Vadus, M. A., and Cawley, J. C. (1986): The IIb-IIIa glycoprotein complex that mediates platelet aggregation is directly implicated in leukocyte adhesion. *Cell,* 45:269–280.

11. Bussolino, F., Breviario, F., Tetta, C., Aglietta, M., Mantovani, A., and Dejana, E. (1986): Interleukin 1 stimulates platelet-activating factor production in cultured human endothelial cells. *J. Clin. Invest.,* 77:2020–2023.

12. Cameron, J. S. (1984): Platelets in glomerular disease. *Annu. Rev. Med.,* 35:175–180.

13. Capron, J., Ameisen, J. C., Joseph, M., Aurialt, C., Tonnel, A. B., and Caen, J. (1985): New functions for platelets and their pathologic implications. *Int. Arch. Allergy Appl. Immunol.,* 77:107–114.

14. Chignard, M., Le Couedic, J. P., Tence, M., Vargaftig, B. B., and Benveniste, J. (1979): The role of platelet-activating factor in platelet aggregation. *Nature,* 279:799–800.

15. Chignard, M., Le Couedic, J. P., Vargaftig, J. P., and Benveniste, J. (1980). Platelet activating factor (PAF acether) secretion from platelets: effects of aggregating agents. (1980): *Br. J. Haematol.,* 46:455–464.

16. Cines, D. B., vanderKeyl, H., and Levinson, A. Z. (1986): *In vitro* binding of an IgE protein to human platelets. *J. Immunology,* 136: 3433–3440.

17. Clark, R. A., and Klebanoff, S. J. (1979): Myeloperoxidase-mediated platelet release reaction. *J. Clin. Invest.,* 63:177–183.

18. Clawson, C. C. (1971): Platelet interaction with bacteria. II. Fate of the bacteria. *Am. J. Pathol.,* 65:381–398.

19. Clawson, C. C., Rao, G. H., and White, J. G. (1975): Platelet interaction with bacteria. IV. Stimulation of the release reaction. *Am. J. Pathol.,* 81:411–420.

20. Clawson, C. C., White, J. G., and Herzberg, M. C. (1980): Platelet interaction with bacteria VI. Contrasting the role of fibrinogen and fibronectin. *Am. J. Hematol.,* 9:43–53.

21. Cosgrove, L., Sandrin, M., Rajasekariah, P., and McKenzie, I. F. (1986): Description of a genomic clone coding for the chain of OKM1, LFA-1 and platelet IIb-IIIa molecules. *Proc. Natl. Acad. Sci. USA,* 83:752–756.

22. Cronstein, B. N., Levin, R. I., Belanoff, J., Weissman, G., and Hirschhorn, R. (1986): Adenosine: An endogenous inhibitor of neutrophil-mediated injury to endothelial cells. *J. Clin. Invest.,* 78: 760–770.

23. Crutchley, D. J. (1984): Effect of inhibitors of arachidonic acid metabolism on thromboplastic activity in human monocytes. *Biophys. Res. Commun.,* 119:179–184.

24. Deuel, T. F., and Huang, J.-S. (1984): Platelet-derived growth factor: Structure, function and roles in normal and transformed cells. *J. Clin. Invest.,* 74:669–676.

25. Deuel, T. F., Senior, K. M., Chang, D., Griffin, G. L., Heinrickson, R. L., and Kaiser, E. T. (1981): Platelet factor 4 is chemotactic for neutrophils and monocytes. *Proc. Natl. Acad. Sci. USA,* 78:4584–4587.

26. Deuel, T. F., Senior, R. M., Huang, J. S., et al. (1982): Chemotaxis of monocytes and neutrophils to platelet derived growth factor. *J. Clin. Invest.,* 69:1046–1049.

27. Devine, D. V., Siegel, R. S., and Rosse, W. F. (1987): Interactions of the platelets in paryoxysmal nocturnal hemoglobinuria with complement. *J. Clin. Invest.,* 79:131–137.

28. Donaldson, D. M., and Tew, J. G. (1977): Beta lysin of platelet origin. *Bacteriol. Rev.,* 41:501–513.

29. Duffus, P., Parbtani, A., Frampton, G., and Cameron, J. S. (1982): Intraglomerular localization of platelet-released antigens, platelet factor 4 and beta thromboglobulin in glomerulonephritis. *Clin. Nephrol.,* 18:298–302.

30. Durack, D. (1975): Experimental bacterial endocarditis. Structure and evolution of very early lesions. *J. Pathol.,* 115:81–90.

31. Endresen, G. K. M., and Mellbye, O. J. (1984): Studies on the binding of complement factor C3 to the surface of human blood platelets. *Haemostasis,* 14:269–280.

32. Fajardo, L. F. (1973): Malarial parasites in mammalian platelets. *Nature,* 243:298–299.

33. Ginsberg, M. H., and Henson, P. M. (1978): Enhancement of platelet response to immune complexes and IgG aggregates by lipid A-rich bacterial lipopolysaccharides. *J. Exp. Med.,* 147:207–218.

34. Goetzl, E. J., Woods, J. M., and Gorman, R. R. (1977): Stimulation of human eosinophil and neutrophil PMN leukocyte chemotaxis and random migration by 12-L-hydroxy-5,8,10,14-eicosatetraenoic acid (HETE). *J. Clin. Invest.,* 59:179–183.

35. Goetzl, E. J., Brash, A. R., Tauber, A. L., Oates, J. A., and Hubbard, W. C. (1980): Modulation of human neutrophil function by monohydroxy-eicosatetraenoic acids. *Immunology,* 39:491–501.

36. Goldberg, I. D., Stemerman, M. B., and Handin, R. I. (1980): Vascular permeation of platelet factor 4 alters endothelial injury. *Science,* 209:611–612.

37. Habenicht, A. J., Goerig, M., Grulich, J., Rothe, D., Gronwald, R., Loth, U., Schettler, G., Kommerell, B., and Ross, R. (1985): Human platelet-derived growth factor stimulates prostaglandin synthesis by activation and by rapid *de novo* synthesis of cyclooxygenase. *J. Clin. Invest.,* 75:1381–1387.

38. Handin, R. I., Karabin, R., and Boxer, G. J. (1977): Enhancement of platelet function by superoxide anion. *J. Clin. Invest.,* 59:959–963.

39. Hansch, G. M., Gemsa, D., and Resch, K. (1985): Induction of prostanoid synthesis in human platelets by the late complement components C5b-9 and channel forming antibiotic nystatin: Inhibition of the reacylation of liberated arachidonic acid. *J. Immunol.,* 135:1320–1324.

40. Hawiger, J., Streackley, S., Hammond, D., Chang, C., Timmons, S., Glick, A., and desPrez, R. M. (1979): Staphylocase-induced human platelet injury mediated by protein A and immunoglobulin G Fc fragment receptor. *J. Clin. Invest.,* 64:931–937.

41. Henson, P. M. (1981): Platelet-activating factor (PAF) as a mediator of neutrophil-platelet interactions in inflammation. *Agents Actions,* 11:545–547.

42. Henson, P. M., and Ginsberg, M. H. (1981): Immunologic reactions of platelets. In: *Platelets in Biology and Pathology, Vol 2,* edited by J. L. Gordon, pp. 265–308. Elsevier/North-Holland, New York.

43. Hirsch, J. G. (1960): Comparative bactericidal activities of blood serum and plasma serum. *J. Exp. Med.,* 112:15–22.

44. Hopper, K. E., Semler, A. D., Chapman, V. V., and Davey, R. A. (1986): Release of galactosyltransferase from human platelets and a subset of monocytes in culture. *Blood,* 68:167–172.

45. Issekutz, A. C., Ripley, M., and Jackson, J. R. (1983): Role of neutrophils in the deposition of platelets during acute inflammation. *Lab. Invest.,* 49:716–724.

46. Issekutz, A. C., and Szpejda, M. (1986): Evidence that platelet activating factor may mediate some acute inflammatory responses. Studies with the platelet-activating factor antagonist, CV3988. *Lab Invest.*, 54:275–281.

47. Jeynes, B. J., Issekutz, A. C., Issekutz, T. B., and Movatt, H. Z. (1980): Quantitation of platelets in the microcirculation measurement of indium-111 in microthrombi induced in rabbits by inflammatory lesions and related phenomena. *Proc. Soc. Exp. Biol. Med.*, 165:445–452.

48. Joseph, M., and Aarialt, C. (1983): A new function for platelets: IgE-dependent killing of schistosomes. *Nature*, 303:810.

49. Jungi, T. W., Spycher, M. O., Nydegger, V. E., and Barandun, S. (1986): Platelet-leukocyte interaction: Selective binding of thrombin-stimulated platelets to human monocytes, polymorphonuclear leukocytes and related cell lines. *Blood*, 67:629–636.

50. Kanaji, K., Okuma, M., and Uchino, H. (1986): Deficient induction of leukotriene synthesis in human neutrophils by lipoxygenase-deficient platelets. *Blood*, 67:903–908.

51. Kazatchkine, M. D., Lambre, Claude, R., Kieffer, N., Mailler, F., and Nurden, A. T. (1984): Membrane-bound hemagglutinin mediates antibody and complement dependent lysis of influenza virus-treated human platelets in autologous serum. *J. Clin. Invest.*, 74:976–984.

52. Kelton, J. G., Keystone, J., Moore, J., Denomme, G., Tozman, E., Glynn, M., Neame, P. B., Gauldie, J., and Jensen, J. (1983). Immune-mediated thrombocytopenia of malaria. *J. Clin. Invest.*, 71:832–836.

53. Kenney, D. M., and Davis, A. E., III (1981): Association of alternative complement pathway components with human blood platelets: secretion and localization of Factor D and beta 1H globulin. *Clin. Immunol. Immunopath.*, 21:351–363.

54. Kerry, P. J., and Paton, C. J. (1984): Increased sensitivity of arachidonic-acid induced platelet aggregation in the presence of carbon dioxide. *Br. J. Pharmacol.*, 81:125–130.

55. Kinlough-Rathbone, R. L., Packham, M. A., and Mustard, J. F. (1983): Vessel injury, platelet adherence and platelet survival. *Arteriosclerosis*, 3:529–546.

56. Knauer, K. A., Ogey-Sobstke, A., Adkinson, N. F., Lichlenstein, L. M. (1984): Platelet augmentation of IgE-dependent histamine release from human basophils and mast cells. *Int. Arch. Allergy Appl. Immunol.*, 74:2935.

57. Knauer, K. A., Lichtenstein, L. M., Adkinson, N. F., and Fish, J. E. (1984): Platelet activation during antigen-induced airway reactions in asthmatic subjects. *N. Engl. J. Med.*, 304:1404–1407.

58. Kornecki, E., Ehrlich, Y. H., DeMars, D., and Lenox, R. H. (1986): Exposure of fibrinogen receptors in human platelets by proteolysis with elastase. *J. Clin. Invest.*, 77:750–756.

59. Kunicki, T. J., Russel, J., Nurden, A. T., Aster, R. H., and Caen, J. P. (1981): Further studies of the human platelet receptor for quinine and quinidine-dependent antibodies. *J. Immunol.*, 126:398–403.

60. Levine, P. H., Weinger, R. S., Simon, J., Scoon, K. L., and Krinsky, H. I. (1976): Leukocyte-platelet interaction. Release of hydrogen peroxide by granulocytes as a modulator of platelet reactions. *J. Clin. Invest.*, 57:955–963.

61. Lorenzet, R., Niemetz, J., Marcus, A. J., and Broekman, M. J. (1986): Enhancement of mononuclear procoagulant activity by platelet 12-hydroxyeicosatetraenoic acid. *J. Clin. Invest.*, 78:418–423.

62. Lonky, S. A., and Wohl, H. (1981): Stimulation of human leukocyte elastase by platelet factor 4. Physiologic, morphologic and biochemical effects on hamster lungs *in vitro*. *J. Clin. Invest.*, 67:817–826.

63. Mehta, P., Mehta, J., and Lawson D. (1986): Leukotrienes potentiate the effects of epinephrine and thrombin on human platelet-aggregation. *Thromb. Res.*, 41:731–738.

64. Marcus, A. J., Safier, L. B., Ullman, H. L., Wong, K. T., Broekman, M. J., Weksler, B. B., and Kaplan, K. L. (1981): Effects of acetyl glyceryl ether phosphorylcholine on human platelet function *in vitro*. *Blood*, 58:1027–1031.

65. Marcus, A. J., Safier, L. B., Ullman, H. L., Broekman, M. J., Islam, N., Oglesby, T., and Gorman, R. R. (1984): 12S,20-dihydroxyicosatetraenoic acid: A new icosanoid synthesized by neutrophils from 12S-hydroxyicosatetraenoic acid produced by thrombin- or collagen-stimulated platelets. *Proc. Natl. Acad. Sci. USA*, 81:903–907.

66. Michiels, J. J., Abels, J., Stektee, J., Vanvliet, H. H., and Vuzevski, V. D. (1985): Erythromelalgia caused by platelet-mediated arteriolar inflammation and thrombosis in thrombocythemia. *Ann. Intern. Med.*, 102:466–471.

67. Maclouf, J., Lados, B. F., and Borgeat, P. (1982): Stimulation of leukotriene biosynthesis in human blood leukocytes by platelet derived 12-hydroperoxy-icosatetraenoic acid. *Proc. Natl. Acad. Sci. USA*, 79:6042–6046.

68. Moore, A., and Nachman, R. L. (1981): Platelet Fc-receptor increased expression in myeloproliferative diseases. *J. Clin. Invest.*, 67:1064–1069.

69. Moore, A., Weksler, B. B., and Nachman, R. L. (1981): Platelet Fc-IgG receptor. Increased expression in female platelets. *Thromb. Res.*, 21:469–474.

70. Nachman, R. L., Weksler, B. B., and Ferris, B. (1972): Characterization of human platelet vascular permeability enhancing activity. *J. Clin. Invest.*, 51:549–556.

71. Nachman, R. L., and Weksler, B. B. (1980): The platelet as an inflammatory cell. In: *The Cell Biology of Inflammation*, edited by G. Weissman, pp. 145–162. Elsevier, Amsterdam.

72. Nawroth, P., and Stern, D. (1986): Modulation of endothelial cell hemostatic properties by tumor necrosis factor. *J. Exp. Med.*, 164:740–749.

73. Nicholson-Weller, A., Spicer, D. B., and Austen, K. F. (1985): Deficiency of the complement regulatory protein "decay-accelerating factor" on membranes of granulocytes monocytes and platelets in paroxysmal nocturnal hemoglobinemia. *N. Engl. J. Med.*, 312:1091–1097.

74. Niemetz, J., and Marcus, A. J. (1974): The stimulatory effect of platelets and platelet membranes on the procoagulant activity of leukocytes. *J. Clin. Invest.*, 54:1437–1443.

75. Orchard, M. A., Kagey-Sobotka, A., Proud, D., and Lichtenstein, L. M. (1986): Basophil histamine release induced by a substance from stimulated human platelets. *J. Immunol.*, 136:2240–2244.

76. Ozge-Anwar, A. H., Freedman, J. J., Senyi, A. F., Cerskus, A. L., Blajchman, M. A. (1984): Enhanced prothrombin converting activity and factor Xa binding of platelets activated by the alternative complement pathway. *Br. J. Haematol.*, 57:221–228.

77. Packham, M. A., Nishizawa, E., and Mustard, J. F. (1968): Response of platelets to tissue injury. *Biochem. Pharmacol.*, 17(Suppl):171–184.

78. Pawloski, N., Abraham, E., Hamill, A., and Scott, W. A. (1984): The cyclooxygenase and lipoxygenase activities of platelet-depleted human monocytes. *J. Allergy Clin. Immunol.*, 74:324–330.

79. Pfueller, S. L., Weber, S., and Luscher, E. F. (1977): Studies of the mechanism of the human platelet release reaction induced by immunologic stimuli: III. Relationship between the binding of soluble IgG aggregates to the Fc receptor and cell response in the presence and absence of plasma. *J. Immunol.*, 118:514–524.

80. Polley, M. J., and Nachman, R. L. (1979): Human complement in thrombin-mediated platelet function. Uptake of the C5b-9 complex. *J. Exp. Med.*, 150:633–645.

81. Polley, M. J., Nachman, R. L., and Weksler, B. B. (1981): Human complement in the arachidonic acid transformation pathway in platelets. *J. Exp. Med.*, 153:257–268.

82. Polley, M. J., and Nachman, R. L. (1983): Human platelet activation by C3a and C3a des-arg. *J. Exp. Med.*, 158:603–615.

83. Rhee, B. G., Hall, E. R., and McIntire, L. V. (1986): Platelet modulation of polymorphonuclear leukocyte shear induced aggregation. *Blood*, 67:240–246.

84. Schafer, A. L., Takanyewa, H., Farrell, S., and Gimbrone, M. A. (1986): Incorporation of platelet and leukocyte lipoxygenase metabolites by cultured vascular cells. *Blood*, 67:373–378.

85. Schwartz, B. F., and Monroe, M. C. (1986): Human platelet aggregation is initiated by peripheral blood mononuclear cells exposed to bacterial lipopolysaccharide *in vitro*. *J. Clin. Invest.*, 78:1136–1141.

86. Seppa, H., Grotendorst, G., Seppa, S., Schiffman, E., and Martin,

G. R. (1982): Platelet derived growth factor is chemotactic for fibroblasts. *J. Cell. Biol.*, 92:584–588.

87. Senior, R. M., Griffin, G. L., Huang, J.-S., Walz, D. A., and Deuel, T. F. (1983): Chemotactic activity of platelet alpha granule proteins for fibroblasts. *J. Cell. Biol.*, 96:382–385.

88. Silverstein, R., and Nachman, R. L. (1987): Thrombospondin mediates the interaction of stimulated platelets with monocytes. *J. Clin. Invest.*, 79:867–874.

88a. Simpson, R. M., Prancan, A., Izzi, J. M., and Fiedel, B. A. (1982): Generation of thromboxane A_2 and aorta-contracting activity from platelets stimulated with modified C-reactive protein. *Immunology*, 47:193–202.

89. Sims, P. J., and Wiedmer, T. (1986): Repolarization of the membrane potential of blood platelets after complement damage: Evidence for a Ca^{++}-dependent exocytic elimination of C5b-9 pores. *Blood*, 68:556–561.

90. Spagnuolo, P. J., Ellner, J. J., and Hassid, A. (1980): Thromboxane A_2 mediates augmented polymorphonuclear leukocyte adhesiveness. *J. Clin. Invest.*, 66:406–414.

91. Spika, J. S., Peterson, P. K., Wilkinson, B. J., Hammerschmidt, D. E., Varbrugh, H. A., Varhoef, J., and Quie, P. G. (1982): Role of peptidoglycan from staphylococcus aureus in leukopenia, thrombocytopenia and complement activation associated with bacteremia. *J. Infect. Dis.*, 146:227–234.

92. Sporn, M. B., and Roberts, A. B. (1986): Peptide growth factors and inflammation, tissue repair and cancer. *J. Clin. Invest.*, 78:329–332.

93. Sporn, M. B., Roberts, A. B., Wakefield, L. M., and Assoian, R. K. (1986): Transforming growth factor-beta: Biologic function and chemical structure. *Science*, 233:532–534.

94. Stern, D., Bank, I., Nawroth, P., Cassimeris, J., Kisiel, W., Fenton, J. W., Dinarello, C., Chess, L., and Jaffe, E. A. (1985): Self-regulation of procoagulant events on the endothelial cell surface. *J. Exp. Med.*, 162:1223–1228.

95. Stricker, R. B., and Shuman, M. (1986): Quinidine purpura. Evidence that glycoprotein V is a target platelet antigen. *Blood*, 67:1377–1381.

96. Terada, H., Baldini, M., Ebbe, S., and Madoff, M. A. (1966): Interaction of influenza virus with blood platelets. *Blood*, 28:213–228.

97. Turner, S. R., Tainer, J. A., and Lynn, W. S. (1977): Biogenesis of chemotactic molecules by the arachidonate lipoxygenase system of platelets, *Nature*, 257:680–682.

98. Turpie, A. G., Chernesky, M. A., Larke, R. P., Packham, M. A., and Mustard, J. F. (1973): Effect of newcastle disease virus on human or rabbit platelets. Aggregation and loss of constituents. *Lab. Invest.*, 28:575–580.

99. Tzeng, D. Y., Deuel, T. F., Huang, J. S., Senior, R. M., Boxer, L. A., and Baehner, R. L. (1984): Platelet-derived growth factor promotes polymorphonuclear leukocyte activation. *Blood*, 64:1123–1128.

100. Valone, F. H., Coles, E., Reinhold, V. R., and Goetzl, E. J. (1982): Specific binding of phospholipid platelet-activating factor by human platelets. *J. Immunol.*, 129:1637–1641.

101. Valone, F. H. (1986): Synergistic platelet activation by aggregates of IgG and the phospholipid platelet-activating factor, 1-*O*-alkyl-2-acetyl-*sn*-glycero-3-phosphorylcholine. *J. Clin. Immunol.*, 6:57–64.

102. Vargaftig, B. B., Chignard, M., Lefort, J., and Benveniste, J. (1981): Platelet-tissue interaction: Role of PAF-acether. *Agents Actions*, 10:502–505.

103. von Willebrand, E., Zola, H., and Hayry, P. (1985): Thrombocyte aggregates in renal allografts. *Transplantation*, 39:258–262.

104. Weksler, B. B., and Nachman, R. L. (1970): Rabbit platelet bactericidal protein. *J. Exp. Med.*, 134:1114–1130.

105. Weksler, B. B., and Coupal, C. E. (1973): Platelet dependent generation of chemotactic activity in serum. *J. Exp. Med.*, 137:1419–1429.

106. Williams, J. E., Cypher, J. J., and Mosesson, M. W. (1985): Evidence that production of platelet fibrinogen is synchronous with platelet production in the turpentine-induced acute phase response. *J. Lab. Clin. Med.*, 106:343–348.

107. Williams, L. T., Antoniades, H. N., and Goetzl, E. J. (1983): Platelet derived growth factor stimulates mouse 3T3 cell mitogenesis and leukocyte chemotaxis through different structural determinants. *J. Clin. Invest.*, 72:1759–1763.

108. Yu, G. H., Holers, V. M., Seya, T., Ballard, L., and Atkinson, J. P. (1986): Identification of a third component of complement-binding glycoprotein of human platelets. *J. Clin. Invest.*, 78:494–501.

109. Zeller, J., Weissbarth, E., Barrith, B., Miekle, H., and Deicher, H. (1983): Serotonin content of platelets in inflammatory rheumatic diseases. Correlation with clinical activity *Arth. Rheum.*, 26:532–540.

110. Zimmerman, T. S., and Spregelberg, H. L. (1975): Pneumococcus-induced serotonin release from human platelets. *J. Clin. Invest.*, 56:828–834.

111. Zimmerman, T. S., and Kolb, W. P. (1976): Human platelet-initiated formation and uptake of the C5-9 complex of human complement. *J. Clin. Invest.*, 57:203–211.

112. Zimmerman, T. S., Fierer, J., and Rothberger, H. (1977): Blood coagulation and the inflammatory response. *Semin. Hematol.*, 14:391–408.

113. Zucker, M. B., Grant, R. A., Alper, C. A., Goodkoflky, I., and Lepow, I. H. (1974): Requirement for complement components and fibrinogen in the zymosan-induced release reaction of human blood platelets. *J. Immunol.*, 113:1744–1755.

114. Zucker-Franklin, D., Graves, M. F., Gossi, C. E., Marmont, A. M., editors (1981): *Atlas of Blood Cells: Function and Pathology*. Ermes, Milan. Also published by Lea & Feibiger, Philadelphia.

Inflammation: Basic Principles and Clinical Correlates.
Edited by J. I. Gallin, I. M. Goldstein, and R. Snyderman.
Raven Press, Ltd., New York © 1988.

CHAPTER 29

Endothelial Cells

Eric A. Jaffe

Endothelial cells (EC) line the insides of all blood vessels; in a normal 70-kg adult, EC occupy a surface area of more than 1000 m^2 and weigh in excess of 100 g. Because of their location and contact with the flowing blood stream, endothelial cells interact with, as well as modulate, the activities of the various biologic systems in blood, particularly circulating white cells. In the early 1970s the development of methods for culturing EC (170,175) made possible the study of EC cell biology. In this chapter, I will review the normal physiologic functions of EC.

SYNTHESIS OF CONNECTIVE TISSUE COMPONENTS

In vivo, EC are attached to the blood vessel wall by their interaction with the underlying basement membrane, which also forms a secondary barrier to the passage of fluid and formed elements into the extravascular compartment. EC basement membranes contain collagen, glycosaminoglycans, elastin, microfibrils, laminin, and some fibronectin and thrombospondin.

Collagen

Cultured human umbilical vein and vena cava EC secrete types IV and V collagen into the underlying extracellular matrix as well as secreting type IV collagen into the culture medium (304). In contrast, bovine aortic, pulmonary artery, and mesenteric vein EC secrete types III, IV, V, and VIII (a newly described collagen type) collagen into the underlying extracellular matrix as well as secreting types III and VIII collagen into the postculture medium (305–309). Bovine adrenal capillary EC secrete types I, III, and V collagen into the extracellular matrix as well as secreting types I and III collagen into the postculture medium (308). In contrast, human microvascular EC secrete type IV collagen into both the postculture medium and extracellular matrix (191). The origin of these differences is unclear but may be due to species differences and/or differences in sites of cell origin within one species. This subject has recently been reviewed in detail (303).

Thrombospondin and Fibronectin

Thrombospondin and fibronectin are present in only small amounts in the basement membrane *in vivo* as compared to other basement membrane proteins, whereas they are two of the major proteins secreted by cultured EC. In human EC, thrombospondin comprises about 14%, and fibronectin about 17%, of the protein secreted into the postculture medium (173,260,304). Both proteins are incorporated into the EC extracellular matrix and form fibrillar meshworks. These proteins are also synthesized by bovine aortic endothelial cells (218,242).

Elastin

Elastin exists as a highly cross-linked protein *in vivo* but is initially synthesized by EC *in vitro* as a single chain molecule, tropoelastin, which has a molecular mass of 75 kilodaltons (kD) (49,243). After secretion, tropoelastin becomes cross-linked as shown by the appearance of the elastin cross-link specific amino acids desmosine and iso-desmosine (48).

Glycosaminoglycans

Glycosaminoglycans are present in EC extracellular matrix and on EC membranes. The cell-surface pool is predominantly heparan sulfate, whereas the extracellular pool contains heparan sulfate, dermatan sulfate, and chondroitin sulfate (21,40,41,122,225,272,312,371). The heparan sulfate synthesized by bovine aortic EC has significant anticoagulant activity (225) and plays a major role in the activation of antithrombin III (see below). In addition, heparan sulfate is involved in initiating cell attachment, although it is not necessary for maintaining attachment (127).

Laminin

Laminin, another component of basement membrane, is also secreted by EC. However, its production rate varies markedly with cell confluency, being secreted in greatest quantities when the EC are subconfluent. In confluent cultures, laminin is associated primarily with the extracellular matrix and co-distributes with type IV collagen (135).

Collagenase

EC can also remodel basement membranes because, when stimulated, they release and/or contain collagenases that can digest types I, II, III, IV, and V collagen (139,183,258). The cells also simultaneously secrete potent inhibitors of collagenase that modulate collagenolytic activity (159,160).

Neutrophils and macrophages contain collagenase, elastase, and a variety of other proteolytic enzymes (116,154,221–223,329,353,380) and presumably digest the basement membrane in the course of migrating from the blood into the extravascular tissue. The subject of neutrophil collagenolytic metalloenzymes has recently been reviewed (375). Interestingly, neutrophil elastase can degrade subendothelial matrices even in the presence of α_1-proteinase inhibitor, and it appears that the neutrophils use oxygen metabolites and lysosomal proteases to inactivate the inhibitor (376).

PROCOAGULANT PROPERTIES OF EC

Subendothelium

The subendothelium is ordinarily covered by EC, and unstimulated platelets do not adhere to intact EC. However, removal or contraction of EC with the subsequent development of intercellular gaps exposes the subendothelium, which rapidly becomes covered with a layer of platelets that soon degranulate (334,370). Collagen types IV and V and microfibrils which are found in the subendothelium cause platelet aggregation and thromboxane A_2 release (11,58,104,198,199,351), whereas laminin, elastin, and heparan sulfate proteoglycan do not (334,351).

von Willebrand Factor

Adhesion of platelets to the subendothelium is dependent on von Willebrand factor (vWF) (246). EC synthesize and secrete functionally active, 220- to 225-kilodalton (kD) vWF (171,172,174). vWF is synthesized intracellularly in a 240- to 260-kD "pro" form (215,361). This "pro" form is glycosylated and dimerized into an intermediate form composed of 275-kD subunits (362). In turn, these 275-kD subunits are cleaved to 220-kD fragments and aggregate into large-molecular-weight disulfide-linked multimers that are stored in Weibel-Palade bodies (294,360,365,369). vWF secreted constitutively by EC is dimeric and contains both provWF and mature subunits (331). In contrast, vWF secreted by EC in response to stimulation with either the calcium ionophore A23187 or thrombin consists of only very large multimers of mature subunits (331). These large multimers are released from the Weibel-Palade bodies and are active in supporting platelet adhesion (217,362–364). Their release markedly depletes the store in the Weibel-Palade body of vWF (209,331). These large multimers bind *in vitro* to types I, III, IV, and V collagen (246) and are found *in vivo* in the subendothelium (25,290). Since platelets contain a surface receptor for vWF (115,184,185,256), it is likely that platelets adhere to the subendothelium via vWF. This concept is consistent with findings that platelet adhesion to the subendothelium is decreased in von Willebrand's disease (352,373) and is corrected by the administration of exogenous vWF (373).

During studies of patients with von Willebrand's disease, it was noted that a second protein, vWFII, was also deficient or absent from the patients' plasma (253). Further studies demonstrated that vWFII was not antigenically related to vWF (252,253), although their levels in plasma were linearly associated (239). In addition, both vWF and vWFII were synthesized by cultured human endothelial cells and released after *in-vivo* stimulation with 1-desamino-8-D-arginine-vasopressin (238). Lastly, vWFII, like vWF, was present in Weibel-Palade bodies (237). Recent amino acid and complementary DNA (cDNA) sequencing studies (see below) have demonstrated that vWFII represents the polypeptide that is cleaved from provWF during intracellular processing and then released into plasma (105).

vWF derived from human plasma has been purified and characterized, its amino acid and cDNA sequences have been determined (61,129,131,197,216,224,302, 322,323,349), and the gene for VIII:vWF has been localized to chromosome 12 (129). Analysis of vWF cDNA sequences derived from an endothelial cell λgt^{11} library has shown that vWF contains five types of repeated domains (A-E); the A domains appear to be homologous to a 225-residue segment of complement factor B. Otherwise, vWF is not related to any other protein in the National Biomedical Research Foundation Protein Sequence Database (323). All of domain A1 lies within a 50-kD tryptic fragment of vWF that binds to membrane surface glycoprotein I_b (GPI_b) of resting platelets (323). Since vWF can be expressed by other types of mammalian cells transfected with a full-length vWF cDNA, the information for assembly of this complex molecule resides largely within its primary structure (26).

The factors that regulate the synthesis and release of vWF by EC *in vitro,* and that therefore play the same role *in vivo,* are poorly understood. Recent work has shown that estradiol, glucose, fibrin, ticlopidine, shear stress, and irradiation increase, but that dexamethasone decreases, the synthesis and secretion of vWF by EC (149,190, 255,280,295,332). Thrombin, the calcium ionophore A23187, phorbol myristate acetate (PMA), interleukin-1

(IL-1), and endotoxin all have been shown to stimulate EC to release vWF (80,205,209,318,331). Since the release of vWF is not blocked by cycloheximide, it probably represents release of vWF from preformed stores in the Weibel-Palade body (see above).

Tissue Factor

Tissue factor reacts with factor VII and calcium and markedly accelerates the ability of factor VII to activate factor X. Intact EC possess little or no tissue factor activity (66,236,297). However, when EC are exposed to thrombin or endotoxin (or lipid A), their tissue factor activity increases 10- to 40-fold (36,66,319). The additional presence of washed platelets enhances tissue factor activity by up to 170-fold (36,181). The presence of either lymphocytes, granulocytes, or macrophages also markedly stimulates tissue factor activity (214) as does IL-1 (17,18,263) and tumor necrosis factor-alpha (TNF-α) (18,265). Since thrombin, endotoxin, and TNF-α all stimulate EC to synthesize and release IL-1 (206,249,262,336,359), these agents may induce tissue factor expression by stimulating IL-1 synthesis. Immune complexes also induce tissue factor production by EC (346).

Factor V

Factor V functions to accelerate the activation of prothrombin by factor X_a. Recently, EC have been shown to synthesize factor V (53), whereas other studies have also demonstrated synthesis of factor V by hepatocytes (382). In addition, EC bind exogenous factor V with a dissociation constant (K_d) = 2 nM. Each cell binds about 20,000 to 25,000 factor V molecules, and this factor V is active in coagulation assays (233). The expression of factor V on the EC surface can be enhanced by mechanical injury (2); also, homocysteine-treated EC develop an activator of endogenously released factor V (298).

Factors IX and X

Recently, factors IX_a and X_a have been shown to bind to EC. Factor IX_a binds to EC with a K_d of 2.3 nM and a B_{max} of 20,000 molecules/cell (155,338). Binding is calcium-dependent and is blocked by unlabeled factors IX or IX_a but not by factor X, prothrombin, or thrombin. Binding and activity of factor IX_a are markedly enhanced in the presence of factors VIII, X, and factor V (341,342). Cell-bound factor IX_a is at least threefold more active than factor IX_a in solution (338), and EC bound factor IX can be activated (337). Similar studies have shown that factors X and X_a also bind to EC (Factor X_a binds to EC with a K_d of 0.5 nM) (337) and that binding is up to sixfold greater in sparse EC (155,299). The bound factor X is endocytosed but not degraded and reappears on the cell surface, whereas the bound factor X_a is both endocytosed and degraded by a lysosomal pathway (264). Similar binding of factor IX and X have been observed in cultured capillary EC (266) and on EC *in situ* in bovine aortic segments (340). Binding of these two coagulation proteins probably serves to localize the coagulation process to the EC surface and to suppress circulation of activated coagulation factors.

Factor XII

The mechanism of the initial activation of Hageman factor (factor XII) *in vivo* is still not clear, but rabbit EC have been shown to activate factor XII by proteolytic cleavage (381). The enzyme responsible for the activation is apparently membrane-bound and does not directly cleave either factor XI or prekallikrein, although the factor XII_a produced will cleave both factor XI and prekallikrein (381).

ANTICOAGULANT PROPERTIES OF EC

Antithrombin III

In vivo, plasma antithrombin III rapidly inactivates thrombin by forming a covalent thrombin-antithrombin complex that is cleared by the liver (210). The inactivation of thrombin by antithrombin III proceeds slowly but is dramatically accelerated by heparin, heparan sulfate, or EC (44,226,343). The acceleratory effect of EC is probably due to anticoagulantly active heparan sulfate on the cell membrane (40,41,44,210,225,227,228). EC may also support the ability of antithrombin III to inactivate factors IX_a, X_a, and XII_a. During aggregation, platelets release both an endoglycosidase that degrades EC surface heparan sulfate (271,371) and platelet factor 4, which blocks the ability of EC to accelerate the inactivation of thrombin by antithrombin III (44). Exogenous heparin also binds to EC (132,161) and appears to promote the inactivation of thrombin by antithrombin III (22).

Protein C

Protein C is a vitamin-K-dependent protein synthesized in the liver that, in its activated form, inactivates factors V_a and VIII_a by proteolysis (96) and is itself inactivated by a protein-C inhibitor circulating in plasma (344). Protein C is activated only by thrombin, and this activation proceeds very slowly unless it takes place in the presence of thrombomodulin, an EC surface protein that binds thrombin and markedly enhances the ability of thrombin

to activate protein C (98,100,273). Thrombomodulin is present on all EC except sinusoidal lining cells in the liver, postcapillary high endothelial cell venules of lymph node, and all vessels in the brain (231). EC contain 30,000 to 55,000 molecules of thrombomodulin per cell, and thrombomodulin accounts for about 50% to 60% of thrombin-binding sites on EC (232). The thrombin-thrombomodulin complex is internalized by endocytosis, and the attached thrombin is degraded; the thrombomodulin then returns to the surface (231). Endotoxin, IL-1, and tumor necrosis factor suppress thrombomodulin activity (254,263,265), in marked contrast to the stimulatory effect of these agents on tissue factor activity (see above). The activity of activated protein C is markedly potentiated by protein S (339,366), which is synthesized and secreted by EC (101,335). Protein S (339,366) binds to the EC membrane and itself binds protein C, forming a cell-surface-bound complex. Thrombin bound to thrombomodulin cannot activate platelets or cleave fibrinogen (97,99). Unlike the antithrombin III-EC interaction, the acceleration of protein-C activation by EC is not blocked by platelet factor 4 (273). Factor V_a binds to the EC surface and accelerates protein-C activation (233). Protein C probably plays an important role *in vivo* because congenital protein-C deficiency is associated with thrombotic disease (31,33,137,321).

Protease Nexin

EC secrete protease nexin, a 40-kD protein which inactivates thrombin by forming a covalent complex at its active site and which is unrelated to antithrombin III (169,188). The thrombin-protease nexin complex then binds to the EC, is internalized, and is degraded by lysosomal enzymes (188). Protease nexin also binds and inactivates trypsin, urokinase, and plasmin (188). Since almost all the thrombin injected into animals rapidly complexes with antithrombin III (210), the role of protease nexin in inhibiting thrombin *in vivo* is unclear.

ANTIPLATELET PROPERTIES OF EC

EC are intrinsically *nonthrombogenic*, and unstimulated platelets do not adhere to the surface of intact confluent monolayers of endothelial cells *in vivo* (83,334) and adhere only minimally to intact monolayers *in vitro* (29,73, 74,114). *In vitro*, platelets that appear to adhere to EC actually adhere to exposed subendothelium and not to the cells themselves (29). This nonthrombogenic property seems to be intrinsic to the EC plasma membrane and is unrelated to prostacyclin production, since inhibition of prostacyclin production does not increase the adhesion of unstimulated platelets (73,74,83,114). In contrast, the inhibition of adhesion of stimulated platelets to EC is highly prostacyclin-dependent (74,75,114).

Prostacyclin

Prostacyclin (prostaglandin I_2 or PGI_2) is a potent vasodilator and inhibitor of platelet function (39,140, 192,250,292). EC synthesize PGI_2 from arachidonic acid, an essential fatty acid, and secrete it into the adjacent fluid (75,229,379). PGI_2 has a short half-life (6 min in whole blood), and its synthesis and secretion can be modulated by a variety of physiologic agonists. PGI_2 synthesis is markedly stimulated by thrombin and trypsin (378), histamine (4,5), bradykinin (164,277), lipoproteins [especially high-density lipoproteins (HDL) (111,286)], serum factors produced during coagulation (296), selenium (316), immunologic injury (133), kallikrein (257), IL-1 (300), α-interferon (90), changes in shear stress (136), ethanol (195), and activated neutrophils (248). Other stimulators of EC PGI_2 synthesis include adenine nucleotides, particularly ATP and ADP (279), enkephalins (27), leukotrienes C_4 and D_4 (69,285), and $MgSO_4$ (372). Synthesis of PGI_2 is inhibited by aspirin (176) and several nonsteroidal anti-inflammatory agents such as indomethacin (379); both types of agents inhibit the enzyme cyclooxygenase. Nicotine and cigarette smoke (293) inhibit the release of PGI_2 (43) as does feeding the cells linoleic acid, the predominant fatty acid in diets high in polyunsaturated fats (330). Factor X_a, 12-hydroxy-eicosatetraenoic acid (12-HETE), and dexamethasone inhibit prostacyclin release (82,141,328). Platelet-calcium-activated protease can also inhibit thrombin-induced EC prostacyclin production (384), suggesting that activated platelets have a mechanism for modulating EC PGI_2 synthesis. EC can also convert prostaglandin endoperoxides secreted by platelets into PGI_2 (230); this mechanism is probably most important in the microvasculature, where the EC/platelet ratio is $\geq 1:1$. Both 6-keto-$PGF_{1\alpha}$ (the stable but inactive end-product of PGI_2) and PGI_2 itself can be converted to 6-keto-PGE_1, a stable and active vasodilator and inhibitor of platelet function (383). Although measurable levels of 6-keto-PGE_1 are found in normal plasma, it is unclear what role, if any, 6-keto-PGE_1 plays *in vivo*. Interestingly, not all EC synthesize PGI_2 as their major arachidonic acid metabolite, since recent studies have demonstrated that human foreskin capillary EC synthesize mainly PGE_2 and $PGF_{2\alpha}$ (54).

Adenosine Nucleotides

Aggregating platelets release adenosine diphosphate (ADP), which recruits nearby platelets into the developing platelet plug, and adenosine triphosphate (ATP), a vasodilator. EC can modulate the effects of the released ADP and ATP because they possess ectoenzymes that rapidly metabolize ADP and ATP to adenosine monophosphate (AMP) and adenosine, a strong inhibitor of platelet func-

tion. EC can take up exogenous adenosine and convert it to ATP and can also release ATP (72,87–89,276,278). However, the conversion of ATP to adenosine is not straightforward, since 5'-nucleotidase is inhibited by ADP (134). This creates a time gap proportional to the size of the initial release between release of ADP (proaggregatory) and the appearance of adenosine (antiaggregatory) (134). Adenosine is a vasodilator and is considered to be a local hormone that can regulate blood flow.

FIBRINOLYTIC PROPERTIES OF EC

Plasminogen activator (PA) exists in two forms; the urokinase type (UK) activates plasminogen in the fluid phase, whereas the tissue type (tPA) is active only when bound to fibrin. *In vivo,* EC contain only tPA (46), whereas *in vitro* EC secrete both tPA and UK (30,46,71,203,212). EC also secrete a 50-kD inhibitor of PA (212,213). In tissue cultures with low cell densities, EC secrete small amounts of PA and high amounts of PA inhibitor, whereas at confluency the secretion of PA by the cells rises and that of the PA inhibitor activity falls (202). Thrombin stimulates the release of tPA by human EC (123,204) but also induces an even larger increase in PA inhibitor (123), causing a net decrease in overall PA activity (123,211). Endotoxin and IL-1 also stimulate PA inhibitor synthesis (20,67,71,91,261). The PA inhibitor from EC has been purified, has a molecular weight of $\sim$50,000, and inhibits both tPA and UK (355). The PA inhibitor secreted by EC is immunologically and biochemically related to the PA inhibitor present in platelets, serum, and plasma (94,95,157). The PA inhibitor has been cloned and sequenced and has extensive homology with other members of the serine protease inhibitor superfamily (130,269). The gene for the PA inhibitor is located on chromosome 7 (130). Activated protein C also stimulates fibrinolysis by complexing with, and thus decreasing, the activity of PA inhibitor secreted by human EC (310,311,354). Plasmin, plasminogen, and tPA all bind to EC (13,142,143), and activation of bound plasminogen is more efficient than that of fluid-phase plasminogen (142). Lastly, purified basic fibroblast growth factor, which induces angiogenesis *in vivo* (251), also stimulates EC to synthesize UK and collagenase (251,259).

EC-DERIVED AND EC-TARGETED GROWTH REGULATORS

Platelet-Derived Growth Factor

EC secrete a platelet-derived growth-factor-like protein (PDGF) that binds to PDGF receptors on both 3T3 cells and smooth muscle cells (84). Binding of EC-derived

PDGF to cells is blocked by incubation with antiserum to human PDGF (84). EC *in vivo* express the mRNA that encodes PDGF (c-*sis*) at low levels, but its expression is elevated when EC are placed in culture (12). Although cultured EC contain mRNA for both the A and B chain of PDGF, they appear to secrete PDGF that is an A-chain homodimer (63,65). Thrombin stimulates c-*sis* expression in EC (77), and both thrombin and factor X_a induce the release of PDGF (117,148). When EC start to form microvessels, c-*sis* mRNA levels decrease and those for fibronectin increase (180). Acetyl-LDL suppresses EC PDGF production, and the cell distribution parallels that of the scavenger receptor as measured using acetyl-LDL (112). PDGF has recently been shown to be a potent vasoconstrictor, and thus platelet release of PDGF may be able to alter regional blood flow (15).

Heparin-like Inhibitor of Smooth Muscle Cell Growth

EC also secrete a heparin-like inhibitor of smooth muscle cell growth that is active at concentrations as low as 10 ng/ml (50). Secreting platelets release an endoglycosidase that can cleave EC-surface heparan-like species from cultured EC (51).

Endothelial Cell Growth Factor

Human EC are usually cultured using endothelial cell growth factor (ECGF) and heparin (220,348). Recently, a variety of factors that stimulate EC growth have been isolated from different tissues and cells and purified using heparin-Sepharose. The purified factors can be divided into two classes: Those in class I have a molecular weight of 15,000 to 17,000, are anionic, and include acidic brain fibroblast growth factor; those in class II have a molecular weight of 18,000 to 20,000, are cationic, and include basic-FGF (208). It now appears that ECGF and acidic fibroblast growth factor are derived from a common precursor (42). ECGF interacts with EC by binding to a cell-surface receptor of molecular weight ~150,000 (113). In addition, EC secrete a factor that can support the growth of other EC and that is different from the PDGF-like material described above (118). This activity may well be the basic fibroblast growth factor that capillary EC have been shown to secrete and that will stimulate the growth of EC (320).

Inhibitors of EC Growth

β-Transforming growth factor derived from platelets transiently inhibits EC growth (156).

METABOLIC PROPERTIES OF EC

Lipoprotein Lipase

Lipoprotein lipase hydrolyzes the di- and triacylglycerol constituents of very low density lipoproteins (VLDL) and chylomicrons. Several groups have demonstrated that although EC do not synthesize lipoprotein lipase, they do bind the enzyme avidly to heparan sulfate or heparan-sulfate-like molecules on their surfaces (57,324). Lipoprotein lipase, itself, is synthesized by macrophages and smooth muscle cells and presumably is transferred from these cell types to EC (186).

Lipoprotein Receptors

EC possess receptors for β-LDL, HDL, acetyl-LDL (the scavenger receptor), and chylomicrons (8,32,107). Whereas rapidly growing EC bind and internalize LDL, confluent EC bind, but do not internalize, LDL (108). EC also can modify LDL molecules and generate a form that is more rapidly degraded by macrophages and that is recognized by the macrophage receptor for acetylated LDL (158).

Insulin

Like many other cells, EC also bind insulin (9). Arterial EC bind 2.5-fold more insulin per cell than do venous EC (10). In addition, there is a difference in the insulin effect among EC from different anatomical locations. Insulin increases glucose incorporation into glycogen and thymidine incorporation into DNA in retinal EC but not in aortic EC (187). These data suggest that a differential response to insulin may exist between the endothelium of large and small vessels.

Angiotensin-Converting and -Related Enzymes

EC contain, on their surface, angiotensin-converting enzyme (ACE), which converts vasoinactive angiotensin I to the vasoconstrictor angiotensin II and inactivates the vasodilator bradykinin (182,270). EC also contain angiotensinases A and C, which inactivate angiotensin II (182,193). EC secrete renin, which converts angiotensinogen to angiotensin I (207).

Atrial Peptides

Atrial natriuretic factor (ANF) binds to two receptors on EC (314). The receptor with a molecular weight of 130,000 is coupled to guanylate cyclase, and treatment of EC with ANF induces a marked elevation in cyclic guanosine monophosphate (cGMP) (200,315).

INTERACTION OF EC WITH LEUKOCYTES

Polymorphonuclear Leukocytes

Polymorphonuclear (PMN) leukocytes adhere to the surfaces of EC *in vivo* (50% of PMN leukocytes are in the marginal pool) and must traverse across the EC barrier before reaching the extravascular space. *In vitro,* PMN leukocytes adhere to monolayers of EC to a much greater degree than to either smooth muscle cells or fibroblasts (165,194,219,275). The extent of adhesion is inversely proportional to both EC density and to time since the culture reached confluency (81). PMN leukocytes move about on the surface of EC and migrate through intercellular junctions as they do *in vivo* (14). PMN-leukocyte adhesion is increased by preincubating the EC with IL-1 (19,284,317), tumor necrosis factor (121,284), endotoxin (121,284,317), or leukotriene B$_4$ (128,166) but not by IL-2 or γ-interferon (317,390). IL-1, tumor necrosis factor, and endotoxin appear to induce synthesis of an EC-surface protein(s) that promotes PMN-leukocyte adherence by a mechanism involving the CDw18 complex present on PMN leukocytes (19,121,284,317). Thrombin and leukotrienes C$_4$ and D$_4$ also act on EC to increase PMN-leukocyte adhesion (240,388). Since thrombin, leukotrienes C$_4$ and D$_4$, and IL-1 also stimulate EC to synthesize platelet-activating factor (PAF), a potent activator of PMN leukocytes which remains bound to EC, these agonists may induce the adherence to EC of previously unstimulated PMN leukocytes via stimulation of PAF production (45,240,287). EC also can convert leukotriene A$_4$ released by PMN leukocytes to leukotriene C$_4$ (106). C5a and C5a des Arg, *N*-formyl-Met-Leu-Phe (FMLP), and immune complexes enhance PMN-leukocyte adhesion to EC primarily by acting on PMN leukocytes (55,150,350,387). Platelet products also stimulate PMN-leukocyte adherence (28,109,275). Serum from patients with Felty's syndrome or systemic lupus erythematosis increases PMN-leukocyte adherence to EC (151). Inhibition of the lipoxygenase pathways inhibits PMN-leukocyte adhesion (38). Although prostacyclin can also inhibit PMN-leukocyte adherence and chemotaxis (390), prostacyclin production is actually a late event in PMN-leukocyte migration into the vessel wall (247). Thus, PMN leukocytes may suppress prostacyclin production perhaps by release of elastase (201), which desensitizes EC to several agonists that induce prostacyclin synthesis. However, hydrogen peroxide, another PMN-leukocyte product, stimulates rapid prostacyclin release by EC (144) so that the reason for the lack of prostacyclin synthesis early in the process of PMN-leukocyte migration is not clear.

Since PMN-leukocyte adherence to EC is inhibited by antibodies to the CDw18 complex on PMN leukocytes (contains LFA-1, Mac-1 or OKM1, and p150/95), these PMN-leukocyte-surface proteins are thought to play a role in PMN-leukocyte–EC interaction (37,146,284,368). It is of great interest that this family of proteins has recently been shown to have a significant degree of structural and immunological homology with the platelet glycoproteins II$_b$/III$_a$ (56,68), which are also present on EC (110,196,268,281,347).

Uptake of unopsonized *Staphylococcus aureus* by PMN leukocytes is much higher on an EC surface than on plastic (356), suggesting that EC support PMN leukocytes in killing bacteria, although the mechanism is not understood.

Unstimulated EC release two factors that are chemotactic for PMN leukocytes. One is a protein of ~35 kD, and the other is a lipid of ~1.5 kD (245). Leukotriene B$_4$ and PAF both stimulate PMN-leukocyte chemotaxis through monolayers of EC (167); the effect of PAF, but not leukotriene B$_4$, is suppressed by an inhibitor of 5-lipoxygenase (167). In contrast, leukotrienes C$_4$ and D$_4$ are inactive, and leukotriene A$_4$ is only weakly active (167). Histamine and angiotensin II, but not angiotensin I or bradykinin, also stimulate the generation by EC of a lipid neutrophil chemoattractant, and these effects are also blocked by a lipoxygenase inhibitor, although the active components are neither PAF nor leukotriene B$_4$ (102,103).

PMN leukocytes contain a number of components that can cause EC injury or detachment *in vitro*. Activation of PMN leukocytes on EC monolayers causes EC detachment that is due to release of elastase from PMN leukocytes (145,329). Normal PMN leukocytes can protect released elastase from α_1-protease inhibitor by releasing oxidants; however, other nonoxidant mechanisms must exist because PMN leukocytes from patients with chronic granulomatous disease also can protect their released elastase (374). PMN leukocytes contain heparanase, which can digest heparan sulfate in the basement membrane; this degradation is facilitated by serine proteases (235). PMN leukocytes also release hydrogen peroxide and oxygen radicals, which can cause EC lysis (301,377). Although EC lack catalase (325), the glutathione redox cycle is an important defense mechanism against oxidant damage (147). The extent of EC damage is increased by the presence of platelet products (28). Since the interaction of PMN leukocytes with EC is mediated by the CDw18 complex (see above), this complex is required for EC detachment by activated PMN leukocytes (86). These reactions can be inhibited using 2-chloroadenosine, an analog of adenosine that is known to prevent PMN leukocytes from generating superoxide anions (70). *In vivo*, PMN leukocytes secrete acid and neutral proteases that digest the basement membrane (62,179). Leukotrienes C$_4$ and D$_4$ (76) and PAF (168) directly increase microvascular permeability.

Lymphocytes

The circulation of lymphocytes through the body appears to be controlled by the specific interaction of lymphocytes with specialized high endothelial venules (HEV) at the various locations where lymphocytes leave the blood and enter the tissues. There appear to be at least three independent receptor systems: one in the lymph nodes, one in the mucosa-associated lymphoid tissue, and one in inflamed synovium (119,177). *In-vitro* studies using EC have shown that lymphocytes adhere to EC (78,79). γ-Interferon increases the binding of T lymphocytes to EC (386) as do endotoxin (385), phorbol esters (153), and IL-1 (52). IL-1 also increases the adhesion of B lymphocytes (52). The interaction of T lymphocytes with EC appears to mediated, at least partially, by HLA-DR antigens on EC (234) and by the Leu-3 (T4) and LFA-1 molecules on lymphocytes (152,244). However, the involvement of these proteins is not really well understood, since the degree of inhibition of lymphocyte adhesion obtained with antisera to LFA-1 depends on the agent used to stimulate adhesion; phorbol ester-stimulated adhesion is inhibited, whereas endotoxin- and IL-1-stimulated adhesion is not altered (152). LFA-1 and HLA-DR also play a role in the interaction of cytolytic T lymphocytes with EC (64). Other studies have shown that one purified lymphocyte homing receptor appears to be a core protein that is complexed to ubiquitin (120,327,333) and that others have molecular weights that vary from 40,000 to 135,000 (59,60,178,291). Once attached to EC, activated T lymphocytes can invade through the EC monolayer and degrade the basement membrane (313).

Monocytes

Monocytes also adhere to EC (19,85,274), and pretreatment of the EC with IL-1 increases monocyte adhesion (19). Similarly to lymphocytes and PMN leukocytes, adhesion of monocytes to EC appears to be mediated by monocyte surface proteins that are part of the CDw18 complex (367). Monocyte adherence to EC is increased by β-VLDL (92) and cholesterol- and triglyceride-rich LDL, whereas lipid-poor LDL reduces adhesion (1). EC release a protein that is chemotactic for monocytes but not for PMN, and production of the factor is increased in EC exposed to β-VLDL (16,289). The anti-inflammatory drug benoxaprofen inhibits monocyte adhesion to EC and acts on the monocytes (35).

Colony-Stimulating Factor

EC release granulocyte/macrophage colony-stimulating factor (GM-CSF) (3,189,288). The release of GM-CSF is markedly enhanced by endotoxin, IL-1, and TNF, whereas IL-2 and γ-interferon are ineffective (6,34, 288,326). The synthesis of GM-CSF is apparently suppressed by lactoferrin (7). Thus there seems to be a circular control mechanism for regulating the production of PMN leukocytes and colony-stimulating activity. In addition, EC released material that stimulated the growth of erythroid precursors (3).

Platelet-Activating Factor

Platelet-activating factor (PAF) is a potent inducer of both platelet and PMN-leukocyte aggregation. Thrombin (47,287), vasopressin (47), angiotensin II (47), IL-1 (45), leukotrienes C$_4$ and D$_4$ (240), histamine, bradykinin, and ATP (241) all stimulate EC to synthesize PAF. Most of the PAF remains cell-associated (241,247). Prostacyclin inhibits PAF production (389). PAF increases microvascular permeability and increases PMN-leukocyte adherence to the vessel wall (23). EC metabolize PAF by removing the acetyl group; the lyso-PAF is then further metabolized (24,345).

IMMUNOLOGIC PROPERTIES OF EC

Human EC contain ABO blood group and HLA-A, B antigens (126,175). In contrast, only a few or no unstimulated EC contain Ia, HLA-DP, DQ, or DRW antigens (267,282). However, when human EC are stimulated with γ-interferon or by activated T cells, Ia antigens are induced on the surface of all EC exposed to the stimulus after an exposure of 72 hr (283) as are HLA-DP antigens, although at a lower density (124). This observation is compatible with, and supports, the observation that EC can act as antigen-presenting cells (93,138,162,163,357,358). Interestingly, antibodies to components of the CDw18 complex inhibited OKT3-induced T4 cell proliferation supported by EC, suggesting that the CDw18 complex is necessary for the interaction of T lymphocytes and accessory cells (125).

REFERENCES

1. Alderson, L. M., Endemann, G., Lindsey, S., Pronczuk, A., Hoover, R. L., and Hayes, K. C. (1986): LDL enhances monocyte adhesion to endothelial cells *in vitro. Am. J. Pathol.,* 123:334–342.
2. Annamalai, A. E., Stewart, G. J., Hansel, B., Memoli, M., Chiu, H. C., Manuel, D. W., Doshi, K., and Colman, R. W. (1986): Expression of factor V on human umbilical vein endothelial cells is modulated by cell injury. *Arteriosclerosis,* 6:196–202.
3. Ascensao, J. L., Vercellotti, G. M., Jacob, H. S., and Zanjani, E. D. (1984): Role of endothelial cells in human hematopoiesis: Modulation of mixed colony growth *in vitro. Blood,* 63:553–558.
4. Baenziger, N. L., Fogerty, F. J., Mertz, L. F., and Chernuta, L. F. (1981): Regulation of histamine-mediated prostacyclin synthesis in cultured human vascular endothelial cells. *Cell,* 24:915–923.

5. Baenziger, N. L., Force, L. E., and Becherer, P. R. (1980): Histamine stimulates prostacyclin synthesis in cultured human endothelial cells. *Biochem. Biophys. Res. Commun.*, 92:1435–1440.

6. Bagby, G. C., Jr., Dinarello, C. A., Wallace, P., Wagner, C., Hefeneider, S., and McCall, E. (1986): Interleukin 1 stimulates granulocyte macrophage colony-stimulating activity release by vascular endothelial cells. *J. Clin. Invest.*, 78:1316–1323.

7. Bagby, G. C., Jr., McCall, E., Bergstrom, K. A., and Burger, D. (1983): A monokine regulates colony-stimulating activity production by vascular endothelial cells. *Blood*, 62:663–668.

8. Baker, D. P., Van Lenten, B. J., Fogelman, A. M., Edwards, P. A., Kean, C., and Berliner, J. A. (1984): LDL, scavenger, and b-VLDL receptors on aortic endothelial cells. *Arteriosclerosis*, 4:248–255.

9. Bar, R. S., Hoak, J. C., and Peacock, M. L. (1978): Insulin receptors in human endothelial cells: Identification and characterization. *J. Clin. Endocrinol. Metabol.*, 47:699–702.

10. Bar, R. S., Peacock, M. L., Spanheimer, R. G., Veenstra, R., and Hoak, J. C. (1980): Differential binding of insulin to human arterial and venous endothelial cells in primary culture. *Diabetes*, 29:991–995.

11. Barnes, M. J., Bailey, A. J., Gordon, J. L., and MacIntyre, D. E. (1980): Platelet aggregation by basement membrane-associated collagens. *Thromb. Res.*, 18:375–388.

12. Barrett, T. B., Gajdusek, C. M., Schwartz, S. M., McDougall, J. K., and Benditt, E. P. (1984): Expression of the sis gene by endothelial cells in culture and *in vivo*. *Proc. Natl. Acad. Sci. USA*, 81:6772–6774.

13. Bauer, P. I., Machovich, R., Buki, K. G., Csonka, E., Koch, S. A., and Horvath, I. (1984): Interaction of plasmin with endothelial cells. *Biochem. J.*, 218:119–124.

14. Beesley, J. E., Pearson, J. D., Hutchings, A., Carleton, J. S., and Gordon, J. L. (1979): Granulocyte migration through endothelium in culture. *J. Cell Sci.*, 38:237–248.

15. Berk, B., Alexander, R. W., Brock, T. A., Gimbrone, M. A., Jr., and Webb, R. C. (1986): Vasoconstriction: A new activity for platelet-derived growth factor. *Science*, 232:87–90.

16. Berliner, J. A., Territo, M., Almada, L., Carter, A., Shafonsky, E., and Fogelman, A. M. (1986): Monocyte chemotactic factor produced by large vessel endothelial cells *in vitro*. *Arteriosclerosis*, 6:254–258.

17. Bevilacqua, M. P., Pober, J. S., Majeau, G. R., Cotran, R. S., and Gimbrone, M. A., Jr. (1984): Interleukin-1 (IL-1) induces biosynthesis and cell surface expression of procoagulant activity in human vascular endothelial cells. *J. Exp. Med.*, 160:618–623.

18. Bevilacqua, M. P., Pober, J. S., Majeau, G. R., Fiers, W., Cotran, R. S., and Gimbrone, M. A., Jr. (1986): Recombinant tumor necrosis factor induces procoagulant activity in cultured human vascular endothelium: Characterization and comparison with the actions of interleukin 1. *Proc. Natl. Acad. Sci. USA*, 83:4533–4537.

19. Bevilacqua, M. P., Pober, J. S., Wheeler, M. E., Cotran, R. S., and Gimbrone, M. A., Jr. (1985): Interleukin 1 acts on cultured human vascular endothelium to increase the adhesion of polymorphonuclear leukocytes, monocytes, and related leukocyte cell lines. *J. Clin. Invest.*, 76:2003–2011.

20. Bevilacqua, M. P., Schleef, R. R., Gimbrone, M. A., Jr., and Loskutoff, D. J. (1986): Regulation of the fibrinolytic system of cultured human vascular endothelium by interleukin 1. *J. Clin. Invest.*, 78:587–591.

21. Bihari-Varga, M., Csonka, E., and Jellinek, H. (1980): Endothelial glycosaminglycans—*In vitro* studies. *Artery*, 8:355–361.

22. Bjorck, C., Larsson, R., Olsson, P., and Rothman, U. (1981): Uptake and inactivation of thrombin by the fresh, glutardialdehyde or heparin treated human umbilical cord. *Thromb. Res.*, 21:603.

23. Bjork, J., Lindbom, L., Gerdin, B., Smedegard, G., Arfors, K. E., and Benveniste, J. (1983): Paf-acether (platelet-activating factor) increases microvascular permeability and affects endothelium-granulocyte interaction in microvascular beds. *Acta Physiol. Scand.*, 119:305–308.

24. Blank, M. L., Spector, A. A., Kaduce, T. L., Lee, T. C., and Snyder, F. (1986): Metabolism of platelet activating factor (1-alkyl-2-acetyl-sn-glycero-3-phosphocholine) and 1-alkyl-2-acetyl-sn-glycerol by human endothelial cells. *Biochim. Biophys. Acta*, 876:373–378.

25. Bloom, A. L., Giddings, J. C., and Wilks, C. J. (1973): Factor VIII on the vascular intima: Possible importance in haemostasis and thrombosis. *Nature (New Biol.)*, 241:217–219.

26. Bonthron, D. T., Handin, R. I., Kaufman, R. J., Wasley, L. C., Orr, E. C., Mitsock, L. M., Ewenstein, B., Loscalzo, J., Ginsburg, D., and Orkin, S. H. (1986): Structure of pre-pro-von Willebrand factor and its expression in heterologous cells. *Nature*, 324:270–273.

27. Boogaerts, M. A., Vermylen, J., Deckmyn, H., Roelant, C., Verwilgen, R. L., Jacob, H. S., and Moldow, C. F. (1983): Enkephalins modify granulocyte-endothelial interactions by stimulating prostacyclin production. *Thromb. Haemost.*, 50:572–575.

28. Boogaerts, M. A., Yamada, O., Jacob, H. S., and Moldow, C. F. (1982): Enhancement of granulocyte-endothelial cell adherence and granulocyte-induced cytotoxicity by platelet release products. *Proc. Natl. Acad. Sci. USA*, 79:7019–7023.

29. Booyse, F. M., Bell, S., Sedlak, B., and Rafelson, M. E. (1975): Development of an *in vitro* vessel wall model for studying certain aspects of platelet-vessel (endothelial) interactions. *Artery*, 1:518–539.

30. Booyse, F. M., Osikowicz, G., Feder, S., and Scheinbuks, J. (1984): Isolation and characterization of a urokinase-type plasminogen activator (Mr = 54,000) from cultured human endothelial cells indistinguishable from urinary urokinase. *J. Biol. Chem.*, 259:7198–7205.

31. Branson, H. E., Katz, J., Marble, R., and Griffin, J. H. (1983): Inherited protein C deficiency and coumarin-responsive chronic relapsing purpura fulminans in a newborn infant. *Lancet*, 2:1165–1168.

32. Brinton, E. A., Kenagy, R. D., Oram, J. F., and Bierman, E. L. (1984): Up-regulation of high-density lipoprotein receptor activity of bovine endothelial cells by acetylated low-density lipoproteins. *Clin. Res.*, 31:170A.

33. Broekmans, A. W., Veltkamp, J. J., and Bertina, R. M. (1983): Congenital protein C deficiency and venous thromboembolism. *N. Engl. J. Med.*, 309:340–344.

34. Broudy, V. C., Kaushansky, K., Segal, G. M., Harlan, J. M., and Adamson, J. W. (1986): Tumor necrosis factor type alpha stimulates human endothelial cells to produce granulocyte/macrophage colony-stimulating factor. *Proc. Natl. Acad. Sci. USA*, 83:7467–7471.

35. Brown, K. A., Ferrie, J., Wilbourn, B., and Dumonde, D. C. (1984): Benoxaprofen, a potent inhibitor of monocyte/endothelial-cell interaction. *Lancet*, 2:643 (letter).

36. Brox, J. H., Osterud, B., Bjorklid, E., and Fenton, J. W. II, (1984): Production and availability of thromboplastin in endothelial cells: The effects of thrombin, endotoxin and platelets. *Br. J. Haematol.*, 57:239–246.

37. Buchanan, M. R., Crowley, C. A., Rosin, R. E., Gimbrone, M. A., Jr., and Babior, B. M. (1982): Studies on the interaction between GP-180-deficient neutrophils and vascular endothelium. *Blood*, 60:160–165.

38. Buchanan, M. R., Vazquez, M. J., and Gimbrone, M. A., Jr. (1983): Arachidonic acid metabolism and the adhesion of human polymorphonuclear leukocytes to cultured vascular endothelial cells. *Blood*, 62:889–895.

39. Bunting, S., Gryglewski, R. J., Moncada, S., and Vane, J. R. (1976): Arterial walls generate from prostaglandin endoperoxides a substance which relaxes strips of mesenteric and coeliac arteries and inhibits platelet aggregation. *Prostaglandins*, 12:897–913.

40. Buonassisi, V. (1973): Sulfated mucopolysaccharide synthesis and secretion in endothelial cell cultures. *Exp. Cell Res.*, 76:363–368.

41. Buonassisi, V., and Root, M. (1975): Enzymatic degradation of heparin-related mucopolysaccharides from the surface of endothelial cell cultures. *Biochim. Biophys. Acta*, 385:1–10.

42. Burgess, W. H., Mehlman, T., Marshak, D. R., and Fraser, B. A. (1986): Structural evidence that endothelial cell growth factor beta is the precursor of both endothelial cell growth factor and acidic fibroblast growth factor. *Proc. Natl. Acad. Sci. USA*, 83:7216–7220.

43. Busacca, M., Dejana, E., Balconi, G., Olivieri, S., Pietra, A., Vergara-Dauden, M., and De Gaetano, G. (1982): Reduced prostacyclin production by cultured endothelial cells from umbilical arteries of babies born to women who smoke. *Lancet*, 2:609–610.

44. Busch, C., and Owen, W. G. (1982): Identification *in vitro* of an endothelial cell surface cofactor for antithrombin III. Parallel studies with isolated perfused rat hearts and microcarrier cultures of bovine endothelium. *J. Clin. Invest.,* 69:726–729.

45. Bussolino, F., Breviaro, F., Tetta, C., Aglietta, M., Mantovani, A., and Dejana, E. (1986): Interleukin 1 stimulates platelet-activating factor production in cultured human endothelial cells. *J. Clin. Invest.,* 77:2027–2033.

46. Bykowska, K., Levin, E. G., Rijken, D. C., Loskutoff, D. J., and Collen, D. (1982): Characterization of a plasminogen activator secreted by cultured bovine aortic endothelial cells. *Biochim. Biophys. Acta,* 703:113–115.

47. Camussi, G., Aglietta, M., Malavasi, F., Tetta, C., Piacibello, W., Sanavio, F., and Bussolino, F. (1983): The release of platelet-activating factor from human endothelial cells in culture. *J. Immunol.,* 131:2397–2403.

48. Cantor, J. O., Keller, S., Parshley, M. S., Darnule, T. V., Darnule, A. T., Cerreta, J. M., Turino, G. M., and Mandl, I. (1980): Synthesis of crosslinked elastin by an endothelial cell culture. *Biochem. Biophys. Res. Commun.,* 95:1381–1386.

49. Carnes, W. H., Abraham, P. A., and Buonassisi, V. (1979): Biosynthesis of elastin by an endothelial cell culture. *Biochem. Biophys. Res. Commun.,* 90:1393–1399.

50. Castellot, J. J., Jr., Addonizo, M. L., Rosenberg, R., and Karnovsky, M. J. (1981): Cultured endothelial cells produce a heparinlike inhibitor of smooth muscle cell growth. *J. Cell Biol.,* 90:372–379.

51. Castellot, J. J., Jr., Favreau, L. V., Karnovsky, M. J., and Rosenberg, R. D. (1982): Inhibition of vascular smooth muscle cell growth by endothelial cell-derived heparin. Possible role of a platelet endoglycosidase. *J. Biol. Chem.,* 257:11256–11260.

52. Cavender, D. E., Haskard, D. O., Joseph, B., and Ziff, M. (1986): Interleukin 1 increases the binding of human B and T lymphocytes to endothelial cell monolayers. *J. Immunol.,* 136:203–207.

53. Cerveny, T. J., Fass, D. N., and Mann, K. G. (1984): Synthesis of coagulation factor V by cultured aortic endothelium. *Blood,* 63:1467–1474.

54. Charo, I. F., Shak, S., Karasek, M. A., Davison, P. M., and Goldstein, I. M. (1984): Prostaglandin I2 is not a major metabolite of arachidonic acid in cultured endothelial cells from human foreskin microvessels. *J. Clin. Invest.,* 74:914–919.

55. Charo, I. F., Yuen, C., Perez, H. D., and Goldstein, I. M. (1986): Chemotactic peptides modulate adherence of human polymorphonuclear leukocytes to monolayers of cultured endothelial cells. *J. Immunol.,* 136:3412–3419.

56. Charo, I., Fitzgerald, L. A., Steiner, B., Rall, S. C., Jr., Bekeart, L. S., and Phillips, D. R. (1986): Platelet glycoproteins IIb/IIIa: Evidence for a family of immunologically and structurally related glycoproteins in mammalian cells. *Proc. Natl. Acad. Sci. USA,* 83:8351–8355.

57. Cheng, C.-F., Oosta, G. M., Bensadoun, A., and Rosenberg, R. D. (1981): Binding of lipoprotein lipase to endothelial cells in culture. *J. Biol. Chem.,* 256:12893–12898.

58. Chiang, T. M., Mainardi, C. L., Seyer, J. M., and Kang, A. H. (1980): Collagen platelet interaction. Type V (A-B) collagen induces platelet aggregation. *J. Lab. Clin. Med.,* 95:99–107.

59. Chin, Y. H., Carey, G. D., and Woodruff, J. J. (1983): Lymphocyte recognition of lymph node high endothelium. V. Isolation of adhesion molecules from lysates of rat lymphocytes. *J. Immunol.,* 131:1368–1374.

60. Chin, Y. H., Rasmussen, R. A., Woodruff, J. J., and Easton, T. G. (1986): A monoclonal anti-HEBFPP antibody with specificity for lymphocyte surface molecules mediating adhesion to Peyer's patch high endothelium of the rat. *J. Immunol.,* 136:2556–2561.

61. Chopek, M. W., Girma, J.-P., Fujikawa, K., Davie, E. W., and Titani, K. (1986): Human von Willebrand factor: A multivalent protein composed of identical subunits. Biochemistry, 25:3146–3155.

62. Cochrane, C. G., and Aikin, B. S. (1966): Polymorphonuclear leukocytes in immunologic reactions. The destruction of vascular basement membrane *in vivo* and *in vitro. J. Exp. Med.,* 124:733–752.

63. Collins, T., Ginsburg, D., Boss, J. M., Orkin, S. H., and Pober, J. S. (1985): Cultured human endothelial cells express platelet-derived growth factor B chain: cDNA cloning and structural analysis. *Nature,* 316:748–750.

64. Collins, T., Krensky, A. M., Clayberger, C., Fiers, W., Gimbrone, M. A., Jr., Burakoff, S. J., and Pober, J. S. (1984): Human cytolytic T lymphocyte interactions with vascular endothelium and fibroblasts: Role of effector and target cell molecules. *J. Immunol.,* 133:1878–1884.

65. Collins, T., Pober, J. S., Gimbrone, M. A., Jr., Hammacher, A., Betsholtz, C., Westermark, B., and Heldin, C.-H. (1987): Cultured human endothelial cells express platelet-derived growth factor A chain. *Am. J. Pathol.,* 126:7–12.

66. Colucci, M., Balconi, G., Lorenzet, R., Pietra, A., Locati, D., Donati, M. B., and Semararo, N. (1983): Cultured human endothelial cells generate tissue factor in response to endotoxin. *J. Clin. Invest.,* 71:1893–1896.

67. Colucci, M., Paramo, J. A., and Collen, D. (1985): Generation in plasma of a fast-acting inhibitor of plasminogen activator in response to endotoxin stimulation. *J. Clin. Invest.,* 75:818–824.

68. Cosgrove, L. J., Sandrin, M. S., Rajasekariah, P., and McKenzie, I. F. C. (1986): A genomic clone encoding the alpha chain of the OKM1, LFA-1, and platelet glycoprotein IIb-IIIa molecule. *Proc. Natl. Acad. Sci. USA,* 83:752–756.

69. Cramer, E. B., Pologe, L., Pawlowski, N. A., Cohn, Z. A., and Scott, W. A. (1983): Leukotriene C promotes prostacyclin synthesis by human endothelial cells. *Proc. Natl. Acad. Sci. USA,* 80:4109–4113.

70. Cronstein, B. N., Levin, R. I., Belanoff, J., Weissmann, G., and Hirschhorn, R. (1986): Adenosine: An endogenous inhibitor of neutrophil-mediated injury to endothelial cells. *J. Clin. Invest.,* 78:760–770.

71. Crutchley, D. J., and Conanan, L. B. (1986): Endotoxin induction of an inhibitor of plasminogen activator in bovine pulmonary artery endothelial cells. *J. Biol. Chem.,* 261:154–159.

72. Crutchley, D. J., Ryan, U. S., and Ryan, J. W. (1980): Effects of aspirin and dipyridamole on the degradation of adenosine diphosphate by cultured cells derived from bovine pulmonary artery. *J. Clin. Invest.,* 66:29–35.

73. Curwen, K. D., Gimbrone, Jr., M. A., and Handin, R. I. (1980): *In vitro* studies of thromboresistance. The role of prostacyclin (PGI2) in platelet adhesion to cultured normal and virally transformed human vascular endothelial cells. *Lab. Invest.,* 42:366–374.

74. Czervionke, R. L., Hoak, J. C., and Fry, G. L. (1978): Effect of aspirin on thrombin-induced adherence of platelets to cultured cells from the blood vessel wall. *J. Clin. Invest.,* 62:847–856.

75. Czervionke, R. L., Smith, J. B., Fry, G. L., Hoak, J. C., and Haycraft, D. L. (1979): Inhibition of prostacyclin by treatment with aspirin. Correlation with platelet adherence. *J. Clin. Invest.,* 63:1089–1092.

76. Dahlen, S. E., Bjork, J., Hedqvist, P., Arfors, K. E., Hammarstrom, S., Lindgren, J. A., and Samuelsson, B. (1981): Leukotrienes promote plasma leakage and leukocyte adhesion in postcapillary venules: *In vivo* effects with relevance to the acute inflammatory response. *Proc. Natl. Acad. Sci. USA,* 78:3887–3891.

77. Daniel, T. O., Gibbs, V. C., Milfay, D. F., Garovey, M. R., and Williams, L. T. (1986): Thrombin stimulates c-sis gene expression in microvascular endothelial cells. *J. Biol. Chem.,* 261:9579–9582.

78. de Bono, D. (1976): Endothelial-lymphocyte interactions *in vitro.* I. Adherence of nonallergised lymphocytes. *Cell. Immunol.,* 26:78–88.

79. de Bono, D. (1979): Endothelium-lymphocyte interactions *in vitro.* II. Adherence of allergised lymphocytes. *Cell. Immunol.,* 44:64–70.

80. de Groot, P. G., Gonsalves, M. D., Loesberg, C., van Buul-Wortelboer, M. F., van Aken, W. G., and van Mourik, J. A. (1984): Thrombin-induced release of von Willebrand factor from endothelial cells is mediated by phospholipid methylation. Prostacyclin synthesis is independent of phospholipid methylation. *J. Biol. Chem.,* 259:13329–13333.

81. de Bono, D. P., and Green, C. (1984): The adhesion of different cell types to cultured vascular endothelium: Effects of culture density and age. *Br. J. Exp. Pathol.,* 65:145–154.

82. De Caterina, R., and Weksler, B. B. (1986): Modulation of arachidonic acid metabolism in human endothelial cells by glucocorticoids. *Thromb. Haemost.,* 55:369–374.

83. Dejana, E., Cazenave, J.-P., Groves, H. M., Kinlough-Rathbone, R. L., Packham, M. A., and Mustard, J. F. (1980): The effect of aspirin inhibition of PGI2 production on platelet adherence to normal and damaged rabbit aortae. *Thromb. Res.,* 17:453–464.

84. DiCorleto, P. E., and Bowen-Pope, D. F. (1983): Cultured endothelial cells produce a platelet-derived growth factor-like protein. *Proc. Natl. Acad. Sci. USA,* 80:1919–1923.

85. DiCorleto, P. E., and de la Motte, C. A. (1985): Characterization of the adhesion of the human monocytic cell line U937 to cultured endothelial cells. *J. Clin. Invest.,* 75:1153–1161.

86. Diener, A. M., Beatty, P. G., Ochs, H. D., and Harlan, J. M. (1985): The role of neutrophil membrane glycoprotein 150 (Gp-150) in neutrophil-mediated endothelial cell injury *in vitro. J. Immunol.,* 135:537–543.

87. Dieterle, Y., Ody, C., Ehrensburger, A., Stalder, H., and Junod, A. F. (1978): Metabolism and uptake of adenosine triphosphate and adenosine by porcine aortic and pulmonary endothelial cells and fibroblasts in culture. *Circ. Res.,* 42:869–876.

88. Dosne, A. M., Escoubet, B., Bodevin, E., and Caen, J. P. (1979): Adenosine diphosphate metabolism by cultured human endothelial cells. *FEBS Lett.,* 105:286–290.

89. Dosne, A. M., Legrand, C., Bauvois, B., Bodevin, E., and Caen, J. P. (1978): Comparative degradation of adenyl-nucleotides by cultured endothelial cells and fibroblasts. *Biochem. Biophys. Res. Commun.,* 85:183–189.

90. Eldor, A., Fridman, R., Vlodavsky, I., Hy-Am, E., Fuks, Z., and Panet, A. (1984): Interferon enhances prostacyclin production by cultured vascular endothelial cells. *J. Clin. Invest.,* 73:251–257.

91. Emeis, J. J., and Kooistra, T. (1986): Interleukin 1 and lipopolysaccharide induce an inhibitor of tissue-type plasminogen activator *in vivo* and in cultured endothelial cells. *J. Exp. Med.,* 163:1260–1266.

92. Endemann, G., Pronczuk, A., Friedman, G., Lindsey, S., Alderson, L., and Hayes, K. C. (1987): Monocyte adherence to endothelial cells in vitro is increased by beta-VLDL. *Am. J. Pathol.,* 126:1–6.

93. Ercolani, L., Parsons, T. J., Hoak, J. C., Fry, G. L., and Nghiem, D. D. (1984): Induction and amplification of T-lymphocyte proliferative responses to periodate and soybean agglutinin by human adult vascular endothelial cells. *Cell. Immunol.,* 85:225–234.

94. Erickson, L. A., Hekman, C. M., and Loskutoff, D. J. (1985): The primary plasminogen-activator inhibitors in endothelial cells, platelets, serum, and plasma are immunologically related. *Proc. Natl. Acad. Sci. USA,* 82:8710–8714.

95. Erickson, L. A., Hekman, C. M., and Loskutoff, D. J. (1986): Denaturant-induced stimulation of the beta-migrating plasminogen activator inhibitor in endothelial cells and serum. *Blood,* 68:1298–1305.

96. Esmon, C. T. (1983): Protein-C: biochemistry, physiology, and clinical implications. *Blood,* 62:1155–1158.

97. Esmon, C. T., Esmon, N. L., and Harris, K. W. (1982): Complex formation between thrombin and thrombomodulin inhibits both thrombin-catalyzed fibrin formation and factor V activation. *J. Biol. Chem.,* 257:7944–7947.

98. Esmon, C. T., and Owen, W. G. (1981): Identification of an endothelial cell cofactor for thrombin-catalyzed activation of protein C. *Proc. Natl. Acad. Sci. USA,* 78:2249–2252.

99. Esmon, N. L., Carroll, R. C., and Esmon, C. T. (1983): Thrombomodulin blocks the ability of thrombin to activate platelets. *J. Biol. Chem.,* 258:12238–12242.

100. Esmon, N. L., Owen, W. G., and Esmon, C. T. (1982): Isolation of a membrane-bound cofactor for thrombin-catalyzed activation of protein C. *J. Biol. Chem.,* 257:859–864.

101. Fair, D. S., Marlar, R. A., and Levin, E. G. (1986): Human endothelial cells synthesize protein S. *Blood,* 67:1168–1171.

102. Farber, H. W., Center, D. M., and Rounds, S. (1985): Bovine and human endothelial cell production of neutrophil chemoattractant activity in response to components of the angiotensin system. *Circ. Res.,* 57:898–902.

103. Farber, H. W., Weller, P. F., Rounds, S., Beer, D. J., and Center,

D. M. (1986): Generation of, lipid neutrophil chemoattractant activity by histamine-stimulated cultured endothelial cells. *J. Immunol.,* 137:2918–2924.

104. Fauvel, F., Grant, M. E., Legrand, Y. J., Souchon, H., Tobelem, G., Jackson, D. S., and Caen, J. P. (1983): Interaction of blood platelets with a microfibrillar extract from adult bovine aorta: Requirement for von Willebrand factor. *Proc. Natl. Acad. Sci. USA,* 80:551–554.

105. Fay, P. J., Kawai, Y., Wagner, D. D., Ginsburg, D., Bonthron, D., Ohlsson, Wilhelm, B. M., Chavin, S. I., Abraham, G. N., Handin, R. I., Orkin, S. H., et al. (1986): Propolypeptide of von Willebrand factor circulates in blood and is identical to von Willebrand antigen II. *Science,* 232:995–998.

106. Feinmark, S. J., and Cannon, P. J. (1986): Endothelial cell leukotriene C4 synthesis results from intercellular transfer of leukotriene A4 synthesized by polymorphonuclear leukocytes. *J. Biol. Chem.,* 261:16466–16472.

107. Fielding, C. J., Vlodavsky, I., Fielding, P. E., and Gospodarowicz, D. (1979): Characteristics of chylomicron binding and lipid uptake by endothelial cells in culture. *J. Biol. Chem.,* 254:8861–8868.

108. Fielding, P. E., Vlodavsky, I., Gospodarowicz, D., and Fielding, C. J. (1979): Effect of contact inhibition on the regulation of cholesterol metabolism in cultured vascular endothelial cells. *J. Biol. Chem.,* 254:749–755.

109. Fischer, D. G., Pike, M. C., Koren, H. S., and Snyderman, R. (1980): Chemotactically responsive and nonresponsive forms of a continuous human monocyte cell line. *J. Immunol.,* 125:463–465.

110. Fitzgerald, L. A., Charo, I. F., and Phillips, D. R. (1985): Human and bovine endothelial cells synthesize membrane proteins similar to human platelet glycoproteins IIb and IIIa. *J. Biol. Chem.,* 260:10893–10896.

111. Fleisher, L. N., Tall, A. R., Witte, L. D., Miller, R. W., and Cannon, P. J. (1982): Stimulation of arterial endothelial cells prostacyclin synthesis by high density lipoproteins. *J. Biol. Chem.,* 257:6653–6655.

112. Fox, P. L., and DiCorleto, P. E. (1986): Modified low density lipoproteins suppress production of a platelet-derived growth factor-like protein by cultured endothelial cells. *Proc. Natl. Acad. Sci. USA,* 83:4774–4778.

113. Friesel, R., Burgess, W. H., Mehlman, T., and Maciag, T. (1986): The characterization of the receptor for endothelial cell growth factor by covalent ligand attachment. *J. Biol. Chem.,* 261:7581–7584.

114. Fry, G. L., Czervionke, R. L., Hoak, J. C., Smith, J. B., and Haycraft, D. L. (1980): Platelet adherence to cultured vascular cells: influence of prostacyclin (PGI2). *Blood,* 55:271–275.

115. Fujimoto, T., Ohara, S., and Hawiger, J. (1982): Thrombin-induced exposure and prostacyclin inhibition of the receptor for factor VIII/von Willebrand factor on human platelets. *J. Clin. Invest.,* 69:1212–1222.

116. Gadek, J. E., Fells, G. A., Wright, D. G., and Crystal, R. G. (1980): Human neutrophil elastase functions as a type III collagen "collagenase." *Biochem. Biophys. Res. Commun.,* 95:1815–1822.

117. Gajdusek, C. M., Carbon, S., Ross, R., Nawroth, P., and Stern, D. (1986): Activation of coagulation releases endothelial cell mitogens. *J. Cell Biol.,* 103:419–428.

118. Gajdusek, C. M., and Schwartz, S. M. (1982): Ability of endothelial cells to condition culture medium. *J. Cell. Physiol.,* 110:35–42.

119. Gallatin, M., St. John, T. P., Siegelman, M., Reichert, R., Butcher, E. C., and Weissman, I. L. (1986): Lymphocyte homing receptors. *Cell,* 44:673–680.

120. Gallatin, W. M., Weissman, I. L., and Butcher, E. C. (1983): A cell-surface molecule involved in organ-specific homing of lymphocytes. *Nature,* 304:30–34.

121. Gamble, J. R., Harlan, J. M., Klebanoff, S. J., and Vadas, M. A. (1985): Stimulation of the adherence of neutrophils to umbilical vein endothelium by human recombinant tumor necrosis factor. *Proc. Natl. Acad. Sci. USA,* 82:8667–8671.

122. Gamse, G., Fromme, H. G., and Kresse, H. (1978): Metabolism of sulfated glycosaminoglycans in cultured endothelial cells from bovine aorta. *Biochim. Biophys. Acta,* 544:514–528.

123. Gelehrter, T. D., and Sznycer, Laszuk, R. (1986): Thrombin in-

duction of plasminogen activator-inhibitor in cultured human endothelial cells. *J. Clin. Invest.,* 77:165–169.

124. Geppert, T. D., and Lipsky, P. E. (1985): Antigen presentation by interferon-gamma-treated endothelial cells and fibroblasts: Differential ability to function as antigen-presenting cells despite comparable Ia expression. *J. Immunol.,* 135:3750–3762.

125. Geppert, T. D., and Lipsky, P. E. (1986): Accessory cell-T cell interactions involved in anti-CD3-induced T4 and T8 cell proliferation: Analysis with monoclonal antibodies. *J. Immunol.,* 137:3065–3073.

126. Gibofsky, A., Jaffe, E. A., Fotino, M., and Becker, C. G. (1975): The identification of HL-A antigens on fresh and cultured human endothelial cells. *J. Immunol.,* 115:730–733.

127. Gill, P. J., Silbert, C. K., and Silbert, J. E. (1986): Effects of heparan sulfate removal on attachment and reattachment of fibroblasts and endothelial cells. *Biochemistry,* 25:405–410.

128. Gimbrone, M. A., Jr., Brock, A. F., and Schafer, A. I. (1984): Leukotriene B4 stimulates polymorphonuclear leukocyte adhesion to cultured vascular endothelial cells. *J. Clin. Invest.,* 74:1552–1555.

129. Ginsburg, D., Handin, R. I., Bonthron, D. T., Donlon, T. A., Bruns, G. A. P., Latt, S. A., and Orkin, S. H. (1985): Human von Willebrand factor (vWF): Isolation of complementary DNA (cDNA) clones and chromosomal localization. *Science,* 228:1401–1406.

130. Ginsburg, D., Zeheb, R., Yang, A. Y., Rafferty, U. M., Andreasen, P. A., Nielsen, L., Dano, K., Lebo, R. V., and Gelehrter, T. D. (1986): cDNA cloning of human plasminogen activator-inhibitor from endothelial cells. *J. Clin. Invest.,* 78:1673–1680.

131. Girma, J.-P., Chopek, M. W., Titani, K., and Davie, E. W. (1986): Limited proteolysis of human von Willebrand factor by *Staphylococcus aureus* V-8 protease: Isolation and partial characterization of a platelet-binding domain. *Biochemistry,* 25:3156–3163.

132. Glimelius, B., Busch, C., and Hook, M. (1978): Binding of heparin on the surface of cultured endothelial cells. *Thromb. Res.,* 12:773–782.

133. Goldsmith, J. C., and McCormick, J. J. (1984): Immunologic injury to vascular endothelial cells: Effects on release of prostacyclin. *Blood,* 63:984–989.

134. Gordon, E. L., Pearson, J. D., and Slakey, L. L. (1986): The hydrolysis of extracellular adenine nucleotides by cultured endothelial cells from pig aorta. Feed-forward inhibition of adenosine production at the cell surface. *J. Biol. Chem.,* 261:15496–15504.

135. Gospodarowicz, D., Greenburg, G., Foidart, J. M., and Savion, N. (1981): The production and localization of laminin in cultured vascular and corneal endothelial cells. *J. Cell. Physiol.,* 107:171–183.

136. Grabowski, E. F., Jaffe, E. A., and Weksler, B. B. (1985): Prostacyclin production by cultured endothelial cell monolayers exposed to step increases in shear stress. *J. Lab. Clin. Med.,* 105:36–43.

137. Griffin, J. H., Evatt, B., Zimmerman, T. S., Kleiss, A. J., and Wideman, C. (1981): Deficiency of protein C in congenital thrombotic disease. *J. Clin. Invest.,* 68:1370–1373.

138. Groenewegen, G., and Buurman, W. A. (1984): Vascular endothelial cells present alloantigens to unprimed lymphocytes. *Scand. J. Immunol.,* 19:269–273.

139. Gross, J. L., Moscatelli, D., Jaffe, E. A., and Rifkin, D. B. (1982): Plasminogen activator and collagenase production by cultured capillary endothelial cells. *J. Cell Biol.,* 95:974–981.

140. Gryglewski, R., Bunting, S., Moncada, S., and Vane, J. R. (1976): Arterial walls are protected against deposition of platelet thrombi by a substance (prostaglandin X) which they make from prostaglandin endoperoxides. *Prostaglandins,* 12:685–714.

141. Hadjiagapiou, C., and Spector, A. A. (1986): 12-Hydroxyeicosatetraenoic acid reduces prostacyclin production by endothelial cells. *Prostaglandins,* 31:1135–1144.

142. Hajjar, K. A., Harpel, P. C., Jaffe, E. A., and Nachman, R. L. (1986): Binding of plasminogen to cultured human endothelial cells. *J. Biol. Chem.,* 261:11656–11662.

143. Hajjar, K. A., Harpel, P. C., and Nachman, R. L. (1987): Binding of tissue plasminogen activator to cultured human endothelial cells. *J. Clin. Invest.,* (in press).

144. Harlan, J. M., and Callahan, K. S. (1984): Role of hydrogen peroxide in the neutrophil-mediated release of prostacyclin from cultured endothelial cells. *J. Clin. Invest.,* 74:442–448.

145. Harlan, J. M., Killen, P. D., Harker, L. A., Striker, G. E., and Wright, D. G. (1981): Neutrophil-mediated endothelial injury *in vitro* mechanisms of cell detachment. *J. Clin. Invest.,* 68:1394–1403.

146. Harlan, J. M., Killen, P. D., Senecal, F. M., Schwartz, B. R., Yee, E. K., Taylor, R. F., Beatty, P. G., Price, T. H., and Ochs, H. D. (1985): The role of neutrophil membrane glycoprotein GP-150 in neutrophil adherence to endothelium *in vitro. Blood,* 66:167–178.

147. Harlan, J. M., Levine, J. D., Callahan, K. S., Schwartz, B. R., and Harker, L. A. (1984): Glutathione redox cycle protects cultured endothelial cells against extracellularly generated hydrogen peroxide. *J. Clin. Invest.,* 73:706–713.

148. Harlan, J. M., Thompson, P. J., Ross, R. R., and Bowen-Pope, D. F. (1986): Alpha-thrombin induces release of platelet-derived growth factor-like molecule(s) by cultured human endothelial cells. *J. Cell Biol.,* 103:1129–1133.

149. Harrison, R. L., and McKee, P. A. (1984): Estrogen stimulates von Willebrand factor production by cultured endothelial cells. *Blood,* 63:657–664.

150. Hashimoto, Y., and Hurd, E. R. (1981): Human neutrophil aggregation and increased adherence to human endothelial cells induced by heat-aggregated IgG and immune complexes. *Clin. Exp. Immunol.,* 44:538–547.

151. Hashimoto, Y., Ziff, M., and Hurd, E. R. (1982): Increased endothelial cell adherence, aggregation, and superoxide generation by neutrophils incubated in systemic lupus erythematosus and Felty's syndrome sera. *Arthritis Rheum.,* 25:1409–1418.

152. Haskard, D., Cavender, D., Beatty, P., Springer, T., and Ziff, M. (1986): T lymphocyte adhesion to endothelial cells: Mechanisms demonstrated by anti-LFA-1 monoclonal antibodies. *J. Immunol.,* 137:2901–2906.

153. Haskard, D., Cavender, D., and Ziff, M. (1986): Phorbol ester-stimulated T lymphocytes show enhanced adhesion to human endothelial cell monolayers. *J. Immunol.,* 137:1429–1434.

154. Hasty, K. A., Hibbs, M. S., Kang, A. H., and Mainardi, C. L. (1986): Secreted forms of human neutrophil collagenase. *J. Biol. Chem.,* 261:5645–5650.

155. Heimark, R. L., and Schwartz, S. M. (1983): Binding of coagulation factors IX and X to the endothelial surface. *Biochem. Biophys. Res. Commun.,* 111:723–731.

156. Heimark, R. L., Twardzik, D. R., and Schwartz, S. M. (1986): Inhibition of endothelial regeneration by type-beta transforming growth factor from platelets. *Science,* 233:1078–1080.

157. Hekman, C. M., and Loskutoff, D. J. (1985): Endothelial cells produce a latent inhibitor of plasminogen activators that can be activated by denaturants. *J. Biol. Chem.,* 260:11581–11587.

158. Henriksen, T., Mahoney, E. M., and Steinberg, D. (1981): Enhanced macrophage degradation of low density lipoprotein previously incubated with cultured endothelial cells: Recognition by receptors for acetylated low density lipoproteins. *Proc. Natl. Acad. Sci. USA,* 78:6499–6503.

159. Herron, G. S., Banda, M. J., Clark, E. J., Gavrilovic, J., and Werb, Z. (1986): Secretion of metalloproteinases by stimulated capillary endothelial cells. II. Expression of collagenase and stromelysin activities is regulated by endogenous inhibitors. *J. Biol. Chem.,* 261:2814–2818.

160. Herron, G. S., Werb, Z., Dwyer, K., and Banda, M. J. (1986): Secretion of metalloproteinases by stimulated capillary endothelial cells. I. Production of procollagenase and prostromelysin exceeds expression of proteolytic activity. *J. Biol. Chem.,* 261:2810–2813.

161. Hiebert, L. M., and Jacques, L. B. (1976): The observation of heparin on endothelium after injection. *Thromb. Res.,* 8:195–204.

162. Hirschberg, H., Bergh, O. J., and Thorsby, E. (1980): Antigen-presenting properties of human vascular endothelial cells. *J. Exp. Med.,* 152:249s–255s.

163. Hirschberg, H., Hirschberg, T., Jaffe, E., and Thorsby, E. (1981): Antigen-presenting properties of human vascular endothelial cells: Inhibition by anti-HLA-DR antisera. *Scand. J. Immunol.,* 14:545–553.

164. Hong, S. L. (1980): Effect of bradykinin and thrombin on prostacyclin synthesis in endothelial cells from calf and pig aorta and human umbilical vein. *Thromb. Res.*, 18:787–795.

165. Hoover, R. L., Folger, R., Haering, W. A., Ware, B. R., and Karnovsky, M. J. (1980): Adhesion of leukocytes to endothelium: Roles of divalent cations, surface charge, chemotactic agents and substrate. *J. Cell Sci.*, 45:73–86.

166. Hoover, R. L., Karnovsky, M. J., Austen, K. F., Corey, E. J., and Lewis, R. A. (1984): Leukotriene B4 action on endothelium mediates augmented neutrophil/endothelial adhesion. *Proc. Natl. Acad. Sci. USA*, 81:2191–2193.

167. Hopkins, N. K., Schaub, R. G., and Gorman, R. R. (1984): Acetyl glyceryl ether phosphorylcholine (PAF-acether) and leukotriene B4-mediated neutrophil chemotaxis through an intact endothelial cell monolayer. *Biochim. Biophys. Acta*, 805:30–36.

168. Humphrey, D. M., McManus, L. M., Hanahan, D. J., and Pinckard, R. N. (1984): Morphologic basis of increased vascular permeability induced by acetyl glyceryl ether phosphorylcholine. *Lab. Invest.*, 50:16–25.

169. Isaacs, J., Savion, N., Gospodarowicz, D., and Shuman, M. A. (1981): Effect of cell density on thrombin binding to a specific site on bovine vascular endothelial cells. *J. Cell Biol.*, 90:670–674.

170. Jaffe, E. A. (1984): Culture and identification of large vessel endothelial cells. In: *Biology of Endothelial Cells*, edited by E. A. Jaffe, pp. 1–13. Martinus Nijhoff, Boston.

171. Jaffe, E. A., Hoyer, L. W., and Nachman, R. L. (1973): Synthesis of antihemophilic factor antigen by cultured human endothelial cells. *J. Clin. Invest.*, 52:2757–2764.

172. Jaffe, E. A., Hoyer, L. W., and Nachman, R. L. (1974): Synthesis of von Willebrand factor by cultured human endothelial cells. *Proc. Natl. Acad. Sci. USA*, 71:1906–1909.

173. Jaffe, E. A., and Mosher, D. F. (1978): Synthesis of fibronectin by cultured human endothelial cells. *J. Exp. Med.*, 147:1779–1791.

174. Jaffe, E. A., and Nachman, R. L. (1975): Subunit structure of factor VIII antigen synthesized by cultured human endothelial cells. *J. Clin. Invest.*, 56:698–702.

175. Jaffe, E. A., Nachman, R. L., Becker, C. G., and Minick, C. R. (1973): Culture of human endothelial cells derived from umbilical cord veins. Identification by morphologic and immunologic criteria. *J. Clin. Invest.*, 52:2745–2756.

176. Jaffe, E. A., and Weksler, B. B. (1979): Recovery of endothelial cell prostacyclin production after inhibition by low doses of aspirin. *J. Clin. Invest.*, 63:532–535.

177. Jalkanen, S., Reichert, R. A., Gallatin, W. M., Bargatze, R. F., Weissman, I. L., and Butcher, E. C. (1986): Homing receptors and the control of lymphocyte migration. *Immunol. Rev.*, 91:39–60.

178. Jalkanen, S. T., Bargatze, R. F., Herron, L. R., and Butcher, E. C. (1986): A lymphoid cell surface glycoprotein involved in endothelial cell recognition and lymphocyte homing in man. *Eur. J. Immunol.*, 16:1195–1202.

179. Janoff, A., and Zeligs, J. D. (1968): Vascular injury and lysis of basement membrane *in vitro* by neutral protease of human leukocytes. *Science*, 161:702–704.

180. Jaye, M., McConathy, E., Drohan, W., Tong, B., Deuel, T., and Maciag, T. (1985): Modulation of the sis gene transcript during endothelial cell differentiation *in vitro*. *Science*, 228:882–885.

181. Johnsen, U. L. H., Lyberg, T., Galdal, K. S., and Prydz, H. (1983): Platelets stimulate thromboplastin synthesis in human endothelial cells. *Thromb. Haemost.*, 49:69–72.

182. Johnson, A. R., and Erdos, E. G. (1977): Metabolism of vasoactive peptides by human endothelial cells in culture. Angiotensin I converting enzyme (kininase II) and angiotensinase. *J. Clin. Invest.*, 59:684–695.

183. Kalebic, T., Garbisa, S., Glaser, B., and Liotta, L. A. (1983): Basement membrane collagen: degradation by migrating endothelial cells. *Science*, 221:281–283.

184. Kao, K. J., Pizzo, S. V., and McKee, P. A. (1979): Demonstration and characterization of specific binding sites of factor VIII/von Willebrand factor on human platelets. *J. Clin. Invest.*, 63:656–664.

185. Kao, K. J., Pizzo, S. V., and McKee, P. A. (1979): Platelet receptor for human factor VIII/von Willebrand protein: Functional correlation of receptor occupancy and ristocetin-induced platelet aggregation. *Proc. Natl. Acad. Sci. USA*, 76:5317–5320.

186. Khoo, J. C., Mahoney, E. M., and Witztum, J. L. (1981): Secretion of lipoprotein lipase by macrophages in culture. *J. Biol. Chem.*, 256:7105–7108.

187. King, G. L., Buzney, S. M., Kahn, C. R., Hetu, N., Buchwald, S., Macdonald, S. G., and Rand, L. I. (1983): Differential responsiveness to insulin of endothelial and support cells from micro- and macrovessels. *J. Clin. Invest.*, 71:974–979.

188. Knauer, D. J., and Cunningham, D. D. (1984): Protease nexins: Cell-secreted proteins which regulate extracellular serine proteases. *Trends Biochem. Sci.*, 9:231–233.

189. Knudtzon, S., and Mortensen, B. T. (1975): Growth stimulation of human bone marrow cells in agar culture by vascular cells. *Blood*, 46:937–943.

190. Koslow, A., Stromberg, R., Gritsman, H., Friedman, L., and Batra, K. (1984): Response of endothelial cells grown on microcarrier beads to shear stress. *Fed. Proc.*, 43:783.

191. Kramer, R. H., Fuh, G. M., Bensch, K. G., and Karasek, M. A. (1985): Synthesis of extracellular matrix glycoproteins by cultured microvascular endothelial cells isolated from the dermis of neonatal and adult skin. *J. Cell. Physiol.*, 123:1–9.

192. Kulkarni, P. S., Roberts, R., and Needleman, P. (1976): Paradoxical endogenous synthesis of a coronary dilating substance from arachidonate. *Prostaglandins*, 12:337–353.

193. Kumamoto, K., Stewart, T. A., Johnson, A. R., and Erdos, E. G. (1981): Prolylcarboxypeptidase (angiotensinase C) in human lung and cultured cells. *J. Clin. Invest.*, 67:210–215.

194. Lackie, J. M., and DeBono, D. (1977): Interactions of neutrophil granulocytes (PMNs) and endothelium *in vitro*. *Microvasc. Res.*, 13:107–112.

195. Landolfi, R., and Steiner, M. (1984): Ethanol raises prostacyclin *in vivo* and *in vitro*. *Blood*, 64:679–682.

196. Leeksma, O. C., Zandbergen-Spaargaren, J., Giltay, J. C., and van Mourik, J. A. (1986): Cultured human endothelial cells synthesize a plasma membrane protein complex immunologically related to the platelet glycoprotein IIb/IIIa complex. *Blood*, 67:1176–1180.

197. Legaz, M., Schmer, G., Counts, R. B., and Davie, E. W. (1973): Isolation and characterization of human factor VIII (antihemophilic factor). *J. Biol. Chem.*, 248:3946–3955.

198. Legrand, Y., Fauvel, F., Gutman, N., Muh, J. P., Tobelem, G., Souchon, H., Karniguian, A., and Caen, J. P. (1980): Microfibrils (MF) platelet interaction: Requirement of von Willebrand factor. *Thromb. Res.*, 19:737–739.

199. Legrand, Y. J., Fauvel, F., Arbeille, B., Leger, D., Mouhli, H., Gutman, N., and Muh, J. P. (1986): Activation of platelets by microfibrils and collagen. A comparative study. *Lab. Invest.*, 54:566–573.

200. Leitman, D. C., Andresen, J. W., Kuno, T., Kamisaki, Y., Chang, J.-W., and Murad, F. (1986): Identification of multiple binding sites for atrial natriuretic factor by affinity cross-linking in cultured endothelial cells. *J. Biol. Chem.*, 261:11650–11655.

201. LeRoy, E. C., Ager, A., and Gordon, J. L. (1984): Effects of neutrophil elastase and other proteases on porcine aortic endothelial prostaglandin I2 production, adenine nucleotide release, and responses to vasoactive agents. *J. Clin. Invest.*, 74:1003–1010.

202. Levin, E. G., and Loskutoff, D. J. (1979): Comparative studies of the fibrinolytic activity of cultured vascular cells. *Thrombos. Res.*, 15:869–878.

203. Levin, E. G., and Loskutoff, D. J. (1982): Cultured bovine endothelial cells produce both urokinase and tissue-type plasminogen activators. *J. Cell Biol.*, 94:631–636.

204. Levin, E. G., Marzec, U., Anderson, J., and Harker, L. A. (1984): Thrombin stimulates tissue plasminogen activator release from cultured human endothelial cells. *J. Clin. Invest.*, 74:1988–1995.

205. Levine, J. D., Harlan, J. M., Harker, L. A., Joseph, M. L., and Counts, R. B. (1982): Thrombin-mediated release of factor VIII antigen from human umbilical vein endothelial cells in culture. *Blood*, 60:531–534.

206. Libby, P., Ordovas, J. M., Auger, K. R., Robbins, A. H., Birinyi, L. K., and Dinarello, C. A. (1986): Endotoxin and tumor necrosis

factor induce interleukin-1 gene expression in adult human vascular endothelial cells. *Am. J. Pathol.,* 124:179–185.

207. Lilly, L. S., Pratt, R. E., Alexander, R. W., Larson, D. M., Ellison, K. E., and Gimbrone, M. A., Jr. (1985): Renin expression by vascular endothelial cells in culture. *Circ. Res.,* 57:312–318.

208. Lobb, R., Sasse, J., Sullivan, R., Shing, Y., D'Amore, P., Jacobs, J., and Klagsbrun, M. (1986): Purification and characterization of heparin-binding endothelial cell growth factors. *J. Biol. Chem.,* 261:1924–1928.

209. Loesberg, C., Gonsalves, M. D., Zandbergen, J., Willems, C., van Aken, W. G., Stel, H. V., van Mourik, J. A., and de Groot, P. G. (1983): The effect of calcium on the secretion of factor VIII-related antigen by cultured human endothelial cells. *Biochim. Biophys. Acta,* 763:160–168.

210. Lollar, P., and Owen, W. G. (1980): Clearance of thrombin from circulation in rabbits by high-affinity binding sites on endothelium. Possible role in the inactivation of thrombin by antithrombin III. *J. Clin. Invest.,* 66:1222–1230.

211. Loskutoff, D. J. (1979): Effect of thrombin on the fibrinolytic activity of cultured bovine endothelial cells. *J. Clin. Invest.,* 64:329–332.

212. Loskutoff, D. J., and Edgington, T. S. (1977): Synthesis of a fibrinolytic activator and inhibitor by endothelial cells. *Proc. Natl. Acad. Sci. USA,* 74:3903–3907.

213. Loskutoff, D. J., van Mourik, J. A., Erickson, L. A., and Lawrence, D. (1983): Detection of an unusually stable fibrinolytic inhibitor produced by bovine endothelial cells. *Proc. Natl. Acad. Sci. USA,* 80:2956–2960.

214. Lyberg, T., Galdal, K. S., Evensen, S. A., and Prydz, H. (1983): Cellular cooperation in endothelial cell thromboplastin synthesis. *Br. J. Haematol.,* 53:85–95.

215. Lynch, D. C., Williams, R., Zimmerman, T. S., Kirby, E. P., and Livingston, D. M. (1983): Biosynthesis of the subunits of factor VIIIR by bovine aortic endothelial cells. *Proc. Natl. Acad. Sci. USA,* 80:2738–2742.

216. Lynch, D. C., Zimmerman, T. S., Collins, C. J., Brown, M., Morin, M. J., Ling, E. H., and Livingston, D. M. (1985): Molecular cloning of cDNA for human von Willebrand factor: Authentication by a new method. *Cell,* 41:49–56.

217. Lynch, D. C., Zimmerman, T. S., Kirby, E. P., and Livingston, D. M. (1983): Subunit composition of oligomeric human von Willebrand factor. *J. Biol. Chem.,* 258:12757–12760.

218. Macarak, E. J., Kirby, E., Kirk, T., and Kefalides, N. A. (1978): Synthesis of cold-insoluble globulin by cultured calf endothelial cells. *Proc. Natl. Acad. Sci. USA,* 75:2621–2625.

219. MacGregor, R. R., Macarak, E. J., and Kefalides, N. A. (1978): Comparative adherence of granulocytes to endothelial monolayers and nylon fiber. *J. Clin. Invest.,* 61:697–702.

220. Maciag, T., Hoover, G. A., Stemerman, M. B., and Weinstein, R. (1981): Serial propagation of human endothelial cells *in vitro. J. Cell Biol.,* 91:420–426.

221. Mainardi, C. L., Dixit, S. N., and Kang, A. H. (1980): Degradation of type IV (basement membrane) collagen by a proteinase isolated from human polymorphonuclear leukocyte granules. *J. Biol. Chem.,* 255:5435–5441.

222. Mainardi, C. L., Hasty, D. L., Seyer, J. M., and Kang, A. H. (1980): Specific cleavage of human type III collagen by human polymorphonuclear leukocyte elastase. *J. Biol. Chem.,* 255:12006–12010.

223. Mainardi, C. L., Seyer, J. M., and Kang, A. H. (1980): Type-specific collagenolysis: A type V collagen-degrading enzyme from macrophages. *Biochem. Biophys. Res. Commun.,* 97:1108–1115.

224. Marchesi, S., Shulman, N. R., and Gralnick, H. R. (1972): Studies on the purification and characterization of human factor VIII. *J. Clin. Invest.,* 51:2151–2161.

225. Marcum, J. A., Atha, D. H., Fritze, L. M., Nawroth, P., Stern, D., and Rosenberg, R. D. (1986): Cloned bovine aortic endothelial cells synthesize anticoagulantly active heparan sulfate proteoglycan. *J. Biol. Chem.,* 261:7507–7517.

226. Marcum, J. A., McKinney, J. B., and Rosenberg, R. D. (1984): Acceleration of thrombin-antithrombin complex formation in rat hindquarters via heparinlike molecules bound to the endothelium. *J. Clin. Invest.,* 74:341–350.

227. Marcum, J. A., and Rosenberg, R. D. (1984): Anticoagulantly active heparin-like molecules from vascular tissue. *Biochemistry,* 23:1730–1737.

228. Marcum, J. A., and Rosenberg, R. D. (1985): Heparin-like molecules with anticoagulant activity are synthesized by cultured endothelial cells. *Biochem. Biophys. Res. Commun.,* 126:365–372.

229. Marcus, A. J., Weksler, B. B., and Jaffe, E. A. (1978): Enzymatic conversion of prostaglandin endoperoxide H2 and arachidonic acid to prostacyclin by cultured human endothelial cells. *J. Biol. Chem.,* 253:7138–7141.

230. Marcus, A. J., Weksler, B. B., Jaffe, E. A., and Broekman, M. J. (1980): Synthesis of prostacyclin from platelet-derived endoperoxides by cultured human endothelial cells. *J. Clin. Invest.,* 66:979–986.

231. Maruyama, I., Bell, C. E., and Majerus, P. W. (1985): Thrombomodulin is found on endothelium of arteries, veins, capillaries, and lymphatics, and on syncytiotroblast of human placenta. *J. Cell Biol.,* 101:363–371.

232. Maruyama, I., and Majerus, P. W. (1985): The turnover of thrombin-thrombomodulin complex in cultured human umbilical vein endothelial cells and A549 lung cancer cells. Endocytosis and degradation of thrombin. *J. Biol. Chem.,* 260:15432–15438.

233. Maruyama, I., Salem, H. H., and Majerus, P. W. (1984): Coagulation factor Va binds to human umbilical vein endothelial cells and accelerates protein C activation. *J. Clin. Invest.,* 74:224–230.

234. Masuyama, J., Minato, N., and Kano, S. (1986): Mechanisms of lymphocyte adhesion to human vascular endothelial cells in culture. T lymphocyte adhesion to endothelial cells through endothelial HLA-DR antigens induced by gamma interferon. *J. Clin. Invest.,* 77:1596–1605.

235. Matzner, Y., Bar, Ner, M., Yahalom, J., Ishai, Michaeli, R., Fuks, Z., and Vlodavsky, I. (1985): Degradation of heparan sulfate in the subendothelial extracellular matrix by a readily released heparanase from human neutrophils. Possible role in invasion through basement membranes. *J. Clin. Invest.,* 76:1306–1313.

236. Maynard, J. R., Dreyer, B. E., Stemerman, M. B., and Pitlick, F. A. (1977): Tissue-factor coagulant activity of cultured human endothelial and smooth muscle cells and fibroblasts. *Blood,* 50:387–396.

237. McCarroll, D. R., Levin, E. G., and Montgomery, R. R. (1985): Endothelial cell synthesis of von Willebrand antigen II, von Willebrand factor, and von Willebrand factor/von Willebrand antigen II complex. *J. Clin. Invest.,* 75:1089–1095.

238. McCarroll, D. R., Ruggeri, Z. M., and Montgomery, R. R. (1984): The effect of DDAVP on plasma levels of von Willebrand antigen II in normal individuals and patients with von Willebrand's disease. *Blood,* 63:532–535.

239. McCarroll, D. R., Ruggeri, Z. M., and Montgomery, R. R. (1984): Correlation between circulating levels of von Willebrand's disease antigen II and von Willebrand factor: Discrimination between Type I and Type II von Willebrand's disease. *J. Lab. Clin. Med.,* 103:704–711.

240. McIntyre, T. M., Zimmerman, G. A., and Prescott, S. M. (1986): Leukotrienes C4 and D4 stimulate human endothelial cells to synthesize platelet-activating factor and bind neutrophils. *Proc. Natl. Acad. Sci. USA,* 83:2204–2208.

241. McIntyre, T. M., Zimmerman, G. A., Satoh, K., and Prescott, S. M. (1985): Cultured endothelial cells synthesize both platelet-activating factor and prostacyclin in response to histamine, bradykinin, and adenosine triphosphate. *J. Clin. Invest.,* 76:271–280.

242. McPherson, J., Sage, H., and Bornstein, P. (1981): Isolation and characterization of a glycoprotein secreted by aortic endothelial cells in culture. Apparent identity with platelet thrombospondin. *J. Biol. Chem.,* 256:11330–11336.

243. Mecham, R. P., Madaras, J., McDonald, J. A., and Ryan, U. (1983): Elastin production by cultured calf pulmonary artery endothelial cells. *J. Cell. Physiol.,* 116:282–288.

244. Mentzer, S. J., Burakoff, S. J., and Faller, D. V. (1986): Adhesion of T lymphocytes to human endothelial cells is regulated by the LFA-1 membrane molecule. *J. Cell. Physiol.,* 126:285–290.

245. Mercandetti, A. J., Lane, T. A., and Colmerauer, M. E. (1984):

Cultured human endothelial cells elaborate neutrophil chemoattractants. *J. Lab. Clin. Med.*, 104:370–380.

246. Meyer, D., and Baumgartner, H. R. (1983): Role of von Willebrand factor in platelet adhesion to the subendothelium. *Br. J. Haematol.*, 54:1–9.

247. Meyrick, B., Workman, R. J., Frazer, M. G., Okamoto, M., Hazlewood, J. E., and Brigham, K. L. (1985): Endothelial prostacyclin production is a late event in granulocyte migration into bovine pulmonary artery intimal explants. *Blood*, 66:1379–1383.

248. Miller, D. K., Sadowski, S., Soderman, D. D., and Kuehl, F. A., Jr. (1985): Endothelial cell prostacyclin production induced by activated neutrophils. *J. Biol. Chem.*, 260:1006–1014.

249. Miossec, P., Cavender, D., and Ziff, M. (1986): Production of interleukin 1 by human endothelial cells. *J. Immunol.*, 136:2486–2491.

250. Moncada, S., Gryglewski, R., Bunting, S., and Vane, J. R. (1976): An enzyme isolated from arteries transforms prostaglandin endoperoxides to an unstable substance that inhibits platelet aggregation. *Nature*, 263:663–665.

251. Montesano, R., Vassalli, J. D., Baird, A., Guillemin, R., and Orci, L. (1986): Basic fibroblast growth factor induces angiogenesis *in vitro*. *Proc. Natl. Acad. Sci. USA*, 83:7297–7301.

252. Montgomery, R. R., and Johnson, J. (1982): Specific factor VIII-related antigen fragmentation: An *in vivo* and *in vitro* phenomenon. *Blood*, 68:930–939.

253. Montgomery, R. R., and Zimmerman, T. S. (1978): von Willebrand's disease antigen II: A new plasma and platelet antigen deficient in severe von Willebrand's disease. *J. Clin. Invest.*, 61:1498–1507.

254. Moore, K. L., Andreoli, S. P., Esmon, N. L., Esmon, C. T., and Bang, N. U. (1987): Endotoxin enhances tissue factor and suppresses thrombomodulin expression of human vascular endothelium *in vitro*. *J. Clin. Invest.*, 79:124–130.

255. Mordes, D. B., Lazarchick, J., Colwell, J. A., and Sens, D. A. (1983): Elevated glucose concentrations increase factor VIIIR: Ag levels in human umbilical vein endothelial cells. *Diabetes*, 32:876–878.

256. Morisato, D. K., and Gralnick, H. R. (1980): Selective binding of the factor VIII/von Willebrand factor protein to human platelets. *Blood*, 55:9–15.

257. Morita, I., Kanayasu, T., and Murota, S. I. (1984): Kallikrein stimulates prostacyclin production in bovine vascular endothelial cells. *Biochim. Biophys. Acta*, 792:304–309.

258. Moscatelli, D., Jaffe, E., and Rifkin, D. B. (1980): Tetradecanoyl phorbol acetate stimulates latent collagenase production by cultured human endothelial cells. *Cell*, 20:343–351.

259. Moscatelli, D., Presta, M., and Rifkin, D. B. (1986): Purification of a factor from human placenta that stimulates capillary endothelial cell protease production, DNA synthesis, and migration. *Proc. Natl. Acad. Sci. USA*, 83:2091–2095.

260. Mosher, D. F., Doyle, M. J., and Jaffe, E. A. (1982): Synthesis and secretion of thrombospondin by cultured endothelial cells. *J. Cell Biol.*, 93:343–348.

261. Nachman, R. L., Hajjar, K. A., Silverstein, R. L., and Dinarello, C. A. (1986): Interleukin 1 induces endothelial cell synthesis of plasminogen activator inhibitor. *J. Exp. Med.*, 163:1595–1600.

262. Nawroth, P. P., Bank, I., Handley, D., Cassimeris, J., Chess, L., and Stern, D. (1986): Tumor necrosis factor/cachectin interacts with endothelial cell receptors to induce release of interleukin 1. *J. Exp. Med.*, 163:1363–1375.

263. Nawroth, P. P., Handley, D. A., Esmon, C. T., and Stern, D. M. (1986): Interleukin 1 induces endothelial cell procoagulant while suppressing cell-surface anticoagulant activity. *Proc. Natl. Acad. Sci. USA*, 83:3460–3464.

264. Nawroth, P. P., McCarthy, D., Kisiel, W., Handley, D., and Stern, D. M. (1985): Cellular processing of bovine factors X and Xa by cultured bovine aortic endothelial cells. *J. Exp. Med.*, 162:559–572.

265. Nawroth, P. P., and Stern, D. M. (1986): Modulation of endothelial cell hemostatic properties by tumor necrosis factor. *J. Exp. Med.*, 163:740–745.

266. Nawroth, P. P., Stern, D. M., Kisiel, W., and Dietrich, M. (1986): A pathway of coagulation on bovine capillary endothelial cells. *Br. J. Haematol.*, 63:309–320.

267. Neppert, J., Nunez, G., and Stastny, P. (1984): HLA-A, B, C; -DR; -MT, -MB, and SB antigens on unstimulated human endothelial cells. Tissue. *Antigens*, 24:40–47.

268. Newman, P. J., Kawai, Y., Montgomery, R. R., and Kunicki, T. J. (1986): Synthesis by cultured human umbilical vein endothelial cells of two proteins structurally and immunologically related to platelet membrane glycoproteins IIb and IIIa. *J. Cell Biol.*, 103:81–86.

269. Ny, T., Sawdey, M., Lawrence, D., Millan, J. L., and Loskutoff, D. J. (1986): Cloning and sequence of a cDNA coding for the human beta-migrating endothelial-cell-type plasminogen activator inhibitor. *Proc. Natl. Acad. Sci. USA*, 83:6776–6780.

270. Ody, C., and Junod, A. F. (1977): Converting enzyme activity in endothelial cells isolated from pig pulmonary artery and aorta. *Am. J. Physiol.*, 232:C95–C98.

271. Oldberg, A., Heldin, C.-H., Wasteson, A., Busch, C., and Hook, M. (1980): Characterization of a platelet endglycosidase degrading heparin-like polysaccharides. *Biochemistry*, 19:5755–5762.

272. Oohira, A., Wight, T. N., and Bornstein, P. (1983): Sulfated proteoglycans synthesized by vascular endothelial cells in culture. *J. Biol. Chem.*, 258:2014–2021.

273. Owen, W. G., and Esmon, C. T. (1981): Functional properties of an endothelial cell cofactor for thrombin-catalyzed activation of protein C. *J. Biol. Chem.*, 256:5532–5535.

274. Pawlowski, N. A., Scott, W. A., Pontier, S., Scott, W. A., and Cohn, Z. A. (1985): Human monocyte-endothelial cell interaction *in vitro*. *Proc. Natl. Acad. Sci. USA*, 82:8208–8212.

275. Pearson, J. D., Carleton, J. S., Beesley, J. E., Hutchings, A., and Gordon, J. L. (1979): Granulocyte adhesion to endothelium in culture. *J. Cell Sci.*, 38:225–235.

276. Pearson, J. D., Carleton, J. S., and Gordon, J. L. (1980): Metabolism of adenosine nucleotides by ectoenzymes of vascular endothelial and smooth muscle cells in culture. *Biochem. J.*, 190:421–429.

277. Pearson, J. D., Carleton, J. S., and Hutchings, A. (1983): Prostacyclin release stimulated by thrombin or bradykinin in porcine endothelial cells cultured from aorta and umbilical vein. *Thromb. Res.*, 29:115–124.

278. Pearson, J. D., and Gordon, J. L. (1979): Vascular endothelial and smooth muscle cells in culture selectively release adenine nucleotides. *Nature*, 281:384–386.

279. Pearson, J. D., Slakey, L. L., and Gordon, J. L. (1983): Stimulation of prostaglandin production through purinergic receptors on endothelial cells and macrophages. *Biochem. J.*, 214:273–276.

280. Piovella, F., Giddings, J. C., Almasio, P., Ricetti, M. M., and Thomas, J. E. (1983): Effects of ticlopidine and dexamethasone on fibronectin and factor VIII-related antigen synthesis by cultured endothelial cells. *Thromb. Res. (Suppl.)*, IV:69–73.

281. Plow, E. F., Loftus, J. C., Levin, E. G., Fair, D. S., Dixon, D., Forsyth, J., and Ginsberg, M. H. (1986): Immunologic relationship between platelet membrane glycoprotein GPIIb/IIIa and cell surface molecules expressed by a variety of cells. *Proc. Natl. Acad. Sci. USA*, 83:6002–6006.

282. Pober, J. S., and Gimbrone, M. A. Jr. (1982): Expression of Ia-like antigens by human vascular endothelial cells is inducible *in vitro*: Demonstration by monoclonal antibody binding and immunoprecipitation. *Proc. Natl. Acad. Sci. USA*, 79:6641–6645.

283. Pober, J. S., Gimbrone, M. A., Jr., Cotran, R. S., Reiss, C. S., Burakoff, S. J., Fiers, W., and Ault, K. A. (1983): Ia expression by vascular endothelium is inducible by activated T cells and by human gamma interferon. *J. Exp. Med.*, 157:1339–1353.

284. Pohlman, T. H., Stanness, K. A., Beatty, P. G., Ochs, H. D., and Harlan, J. M. (1986): An endothelial cell surface factor(s) induced *in vitro* by lipopolysaccharide, interleukin 1, and tumor necrosis factor-alpha increases neutrophil adherence by a CDw18-dependent mechanism. *J. Immunol.*, 136:4548–4553.

285. Pologe, L. G., Cramer, E. B., Pawlowski, N. A., Abraham, E., Cohn, Z. A., and Scott, W. A. (1984): Stimulation of human endothelial cell prostacyclin synthesis by selected leukotrienes. *J. Exp. Med.*, 160:1043–1053.

286. Pomerantz, K. B., Fleisher, L. N., Tall, A. R., and Cannon, P. J. (1985): Enrichment of endothelial cell arachidonate by lipid transfer from high density lipoproteins: Relationship to prostaglandin I2 synthesis. *J. Lipid Res.*, 26:1269–1276.

287. Prescott, S. M., Zimmerman, G. A., and McIntyre, T. M. (1984): Human endothelial cells in culture produce platelet-activating factor (1-alkyl-2-acetyl-*sn*-glycero-3-phosphocholine) when stimulated with thrombin. *Proc. Natl. Acad. Sci. USA*, 81:3534–3538.

288. Quesenberry, P. J., and Gimbrone, M. A., Jr. (1980): Vascular endothelium as a regulator of granulopoiesis: Production of colony-stimulating activity by cultured human endothelial cells. *Blood*, 56:1060–1067.

289. Quinn, M. T., Parthasarathy, S., and Steinberg, D. (1985): Endothelial cell-derived chemotactic activity for mouse peritoneal macrophages and the effects of modified forms of low density lipoprotein. *Proc. Natl. Acad. Sci. USA*, 82:5949–5953.

290. Rand, J. H., Gordon, R. E., Sussman, I. I., Chu, S. V., and Solomon, V. (1982): Electron microscopic localization of factor-VIII-related antigen in adult human blood vessels. *Blood*, 60:627–634.

291. Rasmussen, R. A., Chin, Y. H., Woodruff, J. J., and Easton, T. G. (1985): Lymphocyte recognition of lymph node high endothelium. VII. Cell surface proteins involved in adhesion defined by monoclonal anti-HEBFLN (A.11) antibody. *J. Immunol.*, 135:19–24.

292. Raz, A., Isakson, P. C., Minkes, M. S., and Needleman, P. (1977): Characterization of a novel metabolic pathway of arachidonate in coronary arteries which generates a potent coronary vasodilator. *J. Biol. Chem.*, 252:1123–1126.

293. Reinders, J. H., Brinkman, H. J., van Mourik, J. A., and de Groot, P. G. (1986): Cigarette smoke impairs endothelial cell prostacyclin production. *Arteriosclerosis*, 6:15–23.

294. Reinders, J. H., de Groot, P. G., Gonsalves, M. D., Zandbergen, J., Loesberg, C., and van Mourik, J. A. (1984): Isolation of a storage organelle containing von Willebrand protein from cultured human endothelial cells. *Biochim. Biophys. Acta*, 804:361–369.

295. Ribes, J. A., Francis, C. W., and Wagner, D. D. (1987): Fibrin induces release of von Willebrand factor from endothelial cells. *J. Clin. Invest.*, 79:117–123.

296. Ritter, J. M., Ongari, M.-A., Orchard, M. A., and Lewis, P. J. (1983): Prostacyclin synthesis is stimulated by a serum factor formed during coagulation. *Thromb. Haemost.*, 49:58–60.

297. Rodgers, G. M., Greenberg, C. S., and Shuman, M. A. (1983): Characterization of the effects of cultured vascular cells on the activation of blood coagulation. *Blood*, 61:1155–1162.

298. Rodgers, G. M., and Kane, W. H. (1986): Activation of endogenous factor V by a homocysteine-induced vascular endothelial activator. *J. Clin. Invest.*, 77:1909–1916.

299. Rodgers, G. M., and Shuman, M. A. (1983): Prothrombin is activated on vascular endothelial cells by factor Xa and calcium. *Proc. Natl. Acad. Sci. USA*, 80:7001–7005.

300. Rossi, V., Breviario, F., Ghezzi, P., Dejana, E., and Mantovani, A. (1985): Prostacyclin synthesis induced in vascular cells by interleukin-1. *Science*, 229:174–176.

301. Sacks, T., Moldow, C. F., Craddock, P. R., Bowers, T. K., and Jacob, H. S. (1978): Oxygen radicals mediate endothelial cell damage by complement-stimulated granulocytes. *J. Clin. Invest.*, 61:1161–1167.

302. Sadler, J. E., Shelton-Inloes, B. B., Sorace, J. M., Harlan, J. M., Titani, K., and Davie, E. W. (1985): Cloning and characterization of two cDNAs coding for human von Willebrand factor. *Proc. Natl. Acad. Sci. USA*, 82:6394–6398.

303. Sage, H. (1984): Collagen synthesis by endothelial cells in culture. In: *Biology of Endothelial Cells*, edited by E. A. Jaffe, pp. 161–177. Martinus Nijhoff, Boston.

304. Sage, H., and Bornstein, P. (1982): Endothelial cells from umbilical vein and a hemangioendothelioma secrete basement membrane largely to the exclusion of interstitial collagens. *Arteriosclerosis*, 2:27–36.

305. Sage, H., Crouch, E. C., and Bornstein, P. (1979): Collagen synthesis by bovine aortic endothelial cells in culture. *Biochemistry*, 18:5433–5442.

306. Sage, H., Pritzl, P., and Bornstein, P. (1980): A unique, pepsin-sensitive collagen synthesized by aortic endothelial cells in culture. *Biochemistry*, 19:5747–5755.

307. Sage, H., Pritzl, P., and Bornstein, P. (1981): Characterization of cell matrix-associated collagens synthesized by aortic endothelial cells in culture. *Biochemistry*, 20:436–442.

308. Sage, H., Pritzl, P., and Bornstein, P. (1981): Secretory phenotypes of endothelial cells in culture: Comparison of aortic, venous, capillary, and corneal endothelium. *Arteriosclerosis*, 1:427–442.

309. Sage, H., Trueb, B., and Bornstein, P. (1983): Biosynthetic and structural properties of endothelial cell type VIII collagen. *J. Biol. Chem.*, 258:13391–13401.

310. Sakata, Y., Curriden, S., Lawrence, D., Griffin, J. H., and Loskutoff, D. J. (1985): Activated protein C stimulates the fibrinolytic activity of cultured endothelial cells and decreases antiactivator activity. *Proc. Natl. Acad. Sci. USA*, 82:1121–1125.

311. Sakata, Y., Loskutoff, D. J., Gladson, C. L., Hekman, C. M., and Griffin, J. H. (1986): Mechanism of protein C-dependent clot lysis: Role of plasminogen activator inhibitor. *Blood*, 68:1218–1223.

312. Sampson, P., Parshley, M. S., Mandl, I., and Turino, G. M. (1975): Glycosaminoglycans produced in tissue culture by rat lung cells. Isolation from a mixed cell line and a derived endothelial clone. *Connect. Tissue Res.*, 4:41–49.

313. Savion, N., Vlodavsky, I., and Fuks, Z. (1984): Interaction of T lymphocytes and macrophages with cultured vascular endothelial cells: Attachment, invasion, and subsequent degradation of the subendothelial extracellular matrix. *J. Cell. Physiol.*, 118:169–178.

314. Schenk, D. B., Johnson, L. K., Schwartz, K., Sista, H., Scarborough, R. M., and Lewicki, J. A. (1985): Distinct atrial natriuretic factor receptor sites on cultured bovine aortic smooth muscle and endothelial cells. *Biochem. Biophys. Res. Commun.*, 127:433–442.

315. Schenk, D. B., Phelps, M. N., Porter, J. G., Scarborough, R. M., McEnroe, G. A., and Lewicki, J. A. (1985): Identification of the receptor for atrial natriuretic factor on cultured vascular cells. *J. Biol. Chem.*, 260:14887–14890.

316. Schiavon, R., Freeman, G. E., Guidi, G. C., Perona, G., Zatti, M., and Kakkar, V. V. (1984): Selenium enhances prostacyclin production by cultured endothelial cells: Possible explanation for increased bleeding times in volunteers taking selenium as a dietary supplement. *Thromb. Res.*, 34:389–396.

317. Schleimer, R. P., and Rutledge, B. K. (1986): Cultured human vascular endothelial cells acquire adhesiveness for neutrophils after stimulation with interleukin 1, endotoxin, and tumor-promoting phorbol diesters. *J. Immunol.*, 136:649–654.

318. Schorer, A. E., Moldow, C. F., and Rick, M. E. (1985): Release of von Willebrand factor antigen (factor VIII-related antigen) from human endothelial cells by interleukin 1 or endotoxin. *Blood*, 66(Suppl. 1):358a.

319. Schorer, A. E., Rick, P. D., Swaim, W. R., and Moldow, C. F. (1985): Structural features of endotoxin required for stimulation of endothelial cell tissue factor production; exposure of preformed tissue factor after oxidant-mediated endothelial cell injury. *J. Lab. Clin. Med.*, 106:38–42.

320. Schweigerer, L., Neufeld, G., Friedman, J., Abraham, J. A., Fiddes, J. C., and Gospodarowicz, D. (1987): Capillary endothelial cells express basic fibroblast growth factor, a mitogen that promotes their own growth. *Nature*, 325:257–259.

321. Seligsohn, U., Berger, A., Abend, M., Rubin, L., Attias, D., Zivelin, A., and Rapaport, S. I. (1984): Homozygous protein C deficiency manifested by massive venous thrombosis in the newborn. *N. Engl. J. Med.*, 310:559–562.

322. Shapiro, G. A., Andersen, J. L., Pizzo, S. V., and McKee, P. A. (1973): The subunit structure of normal and hemophilic factor VIII. *J. Clin. Invest.*, 52:2198–2210.

323. Shelton-Inloes, B. B., Titani, K., and Sadler, J. E. (1986): cDNA sequences for human von Willebrand factor reveal five types of repeated domains and five possible protein sequence polymorphisms. *Biochemistry*, 25:3164–3171.

324. Shimada, K., Gill, P. J., Silbert, J. E., Douglas, W. H., and Fanburg, B. L. (1981): Involvement of cell surface heparin sulfate in the binding of lipoprotein lipase to cultured bovine endothelial cells. *J. Clin. Invest.*, 68:995–1002.

325. Shingu, M., Yoshioka, K., Nobunaga, M., and Yoshida, K. (1985): Human vascular smooth muscle cells and endothelial cells lack catalase activity and are susceptible to hydrogen peroxide. *Inflammation,* 9:309–320.

326. Sieff, C. A., Tsai, S., and Faller, D. V. (1987): Interleukin 1 induces cultured human endothelial cell production of granulocyte-macrophage colony-stimulating factor. *J. Clin. Invest.,* 79:48–51.

327. Siegelman, M., Bond, M. W., Gallatin, W. M., St. John, T., Smith, H. T., Fried, V. A., and Weissman, I. L. (1986): Cell surface molecule associated with lymphocyte homing is a ubiquitinated branched-chain glycoprotein. *Science,* 231:823–829.

328. Sinha, A. K., Dutta-Roy, A. K., Chiu, H. C., Stewart, G. J., and Colman, R. W. (1985): Coagulant factor Xa inhibits prostacyclin formation in human endothelial cells. *Arteriosclerosis,* 5:244–249.

329. Smedly, L. A., Tonnesen, M. G., Sandhaus, R. A., Haslett, C., Guthrie, L. A., Johnston, R. B., Jr., Henson, P. M., and Worthen, G. S. (1986): Neutrophil-mediated injury to endothelial cells. Enhancement by endotoxin and essential role of neutrophil elastase. *J. Clin. Invest.,* 77:1233–1243.

330. Spector, A. A., Hoak, J. C., Fry, G. L., Denning, G. M., Stoll, L. L., and Smith, J. B. (1980): Effect of fatty acid modification on prostacyclin production by cultured human endothelial cells. *J. Clin. Invest.,* 65:1003–1012.

331. Sporn, L. A., Marder, V. J., and Wagner, D. D. (1986): Inducible secretion of large, biologically potent von Willebrand factor multimers. *Cell,* 46:185–190.

332. Sporn, L. A., Rubin, P., Marder, V. J., and Wagner, D. D. (1984): Irradiation induces release of von Willebrand protein from endothelial cells in culture. *Blood,* 64:567–570.

333. St. John, T., Gallatin, W. M., Siegelman, M., Smith, H. T., Fried, V. A., and Weissman, I. L. (1986): Expression cloning of a lymphocyte homing receptor cDNA: Ubiquitin is the reactive species. *Science,* 231:845–850.

334. Stemerman, M. B. (1974): Vascular intimal components: Precursors of thrombosis. In: *Progress in Hemostasis and Thrombosis, Vol. 2,* edited by T. H. Spaet, pp. 1–47. Grune & Stratton, New York.

335. Stern, D., Brett, J., Harris, K., and Nawroth, P. (1986): Participation of endothelial cells in the protein C—Protein S anticoagulant pathway: The synthesis and release of protein S. *J. Cell Biol.,* 102: 1971–1978.

336. Stern, D. M., Bank, I., Nawroth, P. P., Cassimeris, J., Kisiel, W., Fenton, J. W., 2d, Dinarello, C., Chess, L., and Jaffe, E. A. (1985): Self-regulation of procoagulant events on the endothelial cell surface. *J. Exp. Med.,* 162:1223–1235.

337. Stern, D. M., Drillings, M., Kisiel, W., Nawroth, P., Nossel, H. L., and LaGamma, K. S. (1984): Activation of factor IX bound to cultured bovine aortic endothelial cells. *Proc. Natl. Acad. Sci. USA,* 81:913–917.

338. Stern, D. M., Drillings, M., Nossel, H. L., Hurlet-Jensen, A., LaGamma, K., and Owen, J. (1983): Binding of factors IX and IXa to cultured vascular endothelial cells. *Proc. Natl. Acad. Sci. USA,* 80:4119–4123.

339. Stern, D. M., Nawroth, P. P., Harris, K., and Esmon, C. T. (1986): Cultured bovine aortic endothelial cells promote activated protein C-protein S-mediated inactivation of factor Va. *J. Biol. Chem.,* 261:713–718.

340. Stern, D. M., Nawroth, P. P., Kisiel, W., Handley, D., Drillings, M., and Bartos, J. (1984): A coagulation pathway on bovine aortic segments leading to generation of Factor Xa and thrombin. *J. Clin. Invest.,* 74:1910–1921.

341. Stern, D. M., Nawroth, P. P., Kisiel, W., Vehar, G., and Esmon, C. T. (1985): The binding of factor IXa to cultured bovine aortic endothelial cells. Induction of a specific site in the presence of factors VIII and X. *J. Biol. Chem.,* 260:6717–6722.

342. Stern, D., Nawroth, P., Handley, D., and Kisiel, W. (1985): An endothelial cell-dependent pathway of coagulation. *Proc. Natl. Acad. Sci. USA,* 82:2523–2527.

343. Stern, D., Nawroth, P., Marcum, J., Handley, D., Kisiel, W., Rosenberg, R., and Stern, K. (1985): Interaction of antithrombin III with bovine aortic segments: Role of heparin in binding and enhanced anticoagulant activity. *J. Clin. Invest.,* 75:272–279.

344. Suzuki, K., Nishioka, J., and Hashimoto, S. (1983): Protein C inhibitor: Purification from human plasma and characterization. *J. Biol. Chem.,* 258:163–168.

345. Tan, E. L., and Snyder, F. (1985): Metabolism of platelet activating factor (1-alkyl-2-acetyl-*sn*-glycero-3-phosphocholine) by capillary endothelial cells isolated from rat epididymal adipose tissue. *Thromb. Res.,* 38:713–717.

346. Tannenbaum, S. H., Finko, R., and Cines, D. B. (1986): Antibody and immune complexes induce tissue factor production by human endothelial cells. *J. Immunol.,* 137:1532–1537.

347. Thiagarajan, T., Shapiro, S. S., Levine, E., DeMarco, L., and Yalcin, A. (1985): A monoclonal antibody to human platelet glycoprotein IIIa detects a related protein in cultured human endothelial cells. *J. Clin. Invest.,* 75:896–901.

348. Thornton, S. C., Mueller, S. N., and Levine, E. M. (1983): Human endothelial cells: Use of heparin in cloning and long-term serial cultivation. *Science,* 222:623–625.

349. Titani, K., Kumar, S., Takio, K., Ericsson, L. H., Wade, R. D., Ashida, K., Walsh, K. A., Chopek, M. W., Sadler, J. E., and Fujikawa, K. (1986): Amino acid sequence of human von Willebrand factor. *Biochemistry,* 25:3171–3183.

350. Tonneson, M. G., Smedley, L. A., and Henson, P. M. (1984): Neutrophil-endothelial cell interactions. Modulation of neutrophil adhesiveness induced by complement fragments C5a and C5a des arg and formyl-methionyl-leucyl-phenylalanine *in vitro. J. Clin. Invest.,* 74:1581–1592.

351. Tryggvason, K., Oikarinen, J., Viinikka, L., and Ylikorkala, O. (1981): Effects of laminin, proteoglycan and type IV collagen, components of basement membranes, on platelet aggregation. *Biochem. Biophys. Res. Commun.,* 100:233–239.

352. Tschopp, T. B., Weiss, H. J., and Baumgartner, H. R. (1974): Decreased adhesion of platelets to subendothelium in von Willebrand's disease. *J. Lab. Clin. Med.,* 83:296–300.

353. Uitto, V. J., Schwartz, D., and Veis, A. (1980): Degradation of basement-membrane collagen by neutral proteases from human leukocytes. *Eur. J. Biochem.,* 105:409–417.

354. van Hinsbergh, V. W. M., Bertina, R. M., van Wijngaarden, A., van Tilburg, N. H., Emeis, J. J., and Haverkate, F. (1985): Activated protein C decreases plasminogen activator-inhibitor activity in endothelial cell-conditioned medium. *Blood,* 65:444–451.

355. van Mourik, J. A., Lawrence, D. A., and Loskutoff, D. J. (1984): Purification of an inhibitor of plasminogen activator (antiactivator) synthesized by endothelial cells. *J. Biol. Chem.,* 259:14914–14921.

356. Vandenbroucke, Grauls, C. M., Thijssen, H. M., and Verhoef, J. (1985): Phagocytosis of staphylococci by human polymorphonuclear leukocytes is enhanced in the presence of endothelial cells. *Infect. Immun.,* 50:250–254.

357. Wagner, C. R., Vetto, R. M., and Burger, D. R. (1984): The mechanism of antigen presentation by endothelial cells. *Immunobiology,* 168:453–469.

358. Wagner, C. R., Vetto, R. M., and Burger, D. R. (1985): Subcultured human endothelial cells can function independently as fully competent antigen-presenting cells. *Hum. Immunol.,* 13:33–47.

359. Wagner, C. R., Vetto, R. M., and Burger, D. R. (1985): Expression of I-region-associated antigen (Ia) and interleukin 1 by subcultured human endothelial cells. *Cell Immunol.,* 93:91–104.

360. Wagner, D. D., Lawrence, S. O., Ohlsson-Wilhelm, B. M., Fay, F. J., and Marder, V. J. (1987): Topology and order of formation of interchain disulfide bonds in von Willebrand factor. *Blood,* 69: 27–32.

361. Wagner, D. D., and Marder, V. J. (1983): Biosynthesis of von Willebrand protein by human endothelial cells. Identification of a large precursor polypeptide chain. *J. Biol. Chem.,* 258:2065–2067.

362. Wagner, D. D., and Marder, V. J. (1984): Biosynthesis of von Willebrand protein by human endothelial cells: Processing steps and their intracellular localization. *J. Cell Biol.,* 99:2123–2130.

363. Wagner, D. D., Mayadas, T., and Marder, V. J. (1986): Initial glycosylation and acidic pH in the Golgi apparatus are required for multimerization of von Willebrand factor. *J. Cell Biol.,* 102: 1320–1324.

364. Wagner, D. D., Mayadas, T., Urban-Pickering, M., Lewis, B. H.,

and Marder, V. J. (1985): Inhibition of disulfide bonding of von Willebrand protein by monensin results in small, functionally defective multimers. *J. Cell Biol.,* 101:112–120.

365. Wagner, D. D., Olmsted, J. B., and Marder, V. J. (1982): Immunolocalization of von Willebrand protein in Weibel-Palade bodies of human endothelial cells. *J. Cell Biol.,* 95:355–360.

366. Walker, F. J. (1980): Regulation of activated protein C by a new protein. A possible function for bovine protein S. *J. Biol. Chem.,* 255:5521–5524.

367. Wallis, W. J., Beatty, P. G., Ochs, H. D., and Harlan, J. M. (1985): Human monocyte adherence to cultured vascular endothelium: Monoclonal antibody-defined mechanisms. *J. Immunol.,* 135:2323–2330.

368. Wallis, W. J., Hickstein, D. D., Schwartz, B. R., June, C. H., Ochs, H. D., Beatty, P. G., Klebanoff, S. J., and Harlan, J. M. (1986): Monoclonal antibody-defined functional epitopes on the adhesion-promoting glycoprotein complex (CDw18) of human neutrophils. *Blood,* 67:1007–1013.

369. Warhol, M. J., and Sweet, J. M. (1984): The ultrastructural localization of von Willebrand factor in endothelial cells. *Am. J. Pathol.,* 117:310–315.

370. Warren, B. A., and Vales, O. (1972): The release of vesicles from platelets following adhesion to vessel walls *in vitro. Br. J. Exp. Pathol.,* 53:206–215.

371. Wasteson, A., Glimelius, B., Busch, C., Westermark, B., Heldin, C.-H., and Norling, B. (1977): Effect of platelet endoglycosidase on cell surface associated heparan sulfate of human cultured endothelial and glial cells. *Thromb. Res.,* 11:309–321.

372. Watson, K. V., Moldow, C. F., Ogburn, P., and Jacob, H. S. (1986): Magnesium sulfate: Rationale for its use in preeclampsia. *Proc. Natl. Acad. Sci. USA,* 83:1075–1078.

373. Weiss, H. J., Baumgartner, H. R., Tschopp, T. B., Turitto, V. T., and Cohen, D. (1978): Correction by factor VIII of the impaired platelet adhesion to subendothelium in von Willebrand's disease. *Blood,* 51:267–279.

374. Weiss, S. J., Curnutte, J. T., and Regiani, S. (1986): Neutrophil-mediated solubilization of the subendothelial matrix: Oxidative and nonoxidative mechanisms of proteolysis used by normal and chronic granulomatous disease phagocytes. *J. Immunol.,* 136:636–641.

375. Weiss, S. J., and Peppin, G. J. (1986): Collagenolytic metalloenzymes of the human neutrophil. Characteristics, regulation and potential function *in vivo. Biochem. Pharmacol.,* 35:3189–3197.

376. Weiss, S. J., and Regiani, S. (1984): Neutrophils degrade subendothelial matrices in the presence of alpha-1-proteinase inhibitor. Cooperative use of lysosomal proteinases and oxygen metabolites. *J. Clin. Invest.,* 73:1297–1303.

377. Weiss, S. J., Young, J., LoBuglio, A. F., Slivka, A., and Nimeh, N. (1981): Role of hydrogen peroxide in neutrophil-mediated destruction of cultured endothelial cells. *J. Clin. Invest.,* 68:714–721.

378. Weksler, B. B., Ley, C. W., and Jaffe, E. A. (1978): Stimulation of endothelial prostacyclin production by thrombin, trypsin, and the ionophore A23187. *J. Clin. Invest.,* 62:923–930.

379. Weksler, B. B., Marcus, A. J., and Jaffe, E. A. (1977): Synthesis of prostaglandin I2 (prostacyclin) by cultured human and bovine endothelial cells. *Proc. Natl. Acad. Sci. USA,* 74:3922–3926.

380. Werb, Z., Banda, M. J., and Jones, P. A. (1980): Degradation of connective tissue matrices by macrophages. I. Proteolysis of elastin, glycoproteins, and collagen by proteinases isolated from macrophages. *J. Exp. Med.,* 152:1340–1357.

381. Wiggins, R. C., Loskutoff, D. J., Cochrane, C. G., Griffin, J. H., and Edgington, T. S. (1980): Activation of rabbit Hageman factor by homogenates of cultured rabbit endothelial cells. *J. Clin. Invest.,* 65:197–206.

382. Wilson, D. B., Salem, H. H., Mruk, J. S., Maruyama, I., and Majerus, P. W. (1984): Biosynthesis of coagulation factor V by a human hepatocellular carcinoma cell line. *J. Clin. Invest.,* 73:654–658.

383. Wong, P. Y.-K., Lee, W. H., Chao, P. H.-W., Reiss, R. F., and McGiff, J. C. (1980): Metabolism of prostacyclin by 9-hydroxy-prostaglandin dehydrogenase in human platelets. *J. Biol. Chem.,* 255:9021–9024.

384. Yoshida, N., Weksler, B., and Nachman, R. (1983): Purification of human platelet calcium-activated protease. Effect on platelet and endothelial function. *J. Biol. Chem.,* 258:7168–7174.

385. Yu, C. L., Haskard, D., Cavender, D., and Ziff, M. (1986): Effects of bacterial lipopolysaccharide on the binding of lymphocytes to endothelial cell monolayers. *J. Immunol.,* 136:569–573.

386. Yu, C. L., Haskard, D. O., Cavender, D., Johnson, A. R., and Ziff, M. (1985): Human gamma interferon increases the binding of T lymphocytes to endothelial cells. *Clin. Exp. Immunol.,* 62:554–560.

387. Zimmerman, G. A., and Hill, H. R. (1984): Inflammatory mediators stimulate granulocyte adherence to cultured endothelial cells. *Thromb. Res.,* 35:203–217.

388. Zimmerman, G. A., McIntyre, T. M., and Prescott, S. M. (1985): Thrombin stimulates the adherence of neutrophils to human endothelial cells *in vitro. J. Clin. Invest.,* 76:2235–2246.

389. Zimmerman, G. A., McIntyre, T. M., and Prescott, S. M. (1985): Production of platelet-activating factor by human vascular endothelial cells: Evidence for a requirement for specific agonists and modulation by prostacyclin. *Circulation,* 72:718–727.

390. Zimmerman, G. A., Wiseman, G. A., and Hill, H. R. (1985): Human endothelial cells modulate granulocyte adherence and chemotaxis. *J. Immunol.,* 134:1866–1874.

Inflammation: Basic Principles and Clinical Correlates.
Edited by J. I. Gallin, I. M. Goldstein, and R. Snyderman.
Raven Press, Ltd., New York © 1988.

CHAPTER 30

Fibroblasts

Arnold E. Postlethwaite and Andrew H. Kang

Fibroblasts are specialized cells that develop from embryonic mesenchyme. They play a critical role in morphogenesis, dictating the structure of the skeleton, locations of muscle cells, routes taken by nerve fibers, and organization of the skin (87,152,169). In the embryo, fibroblasts not only synthesize matrix components, but also direct organization of the resulting connective tissue. For example, fibroblasts are capable of compressing secreted collagen fibrils into sheets and stretching them out into cables (167). By attaching the fibrils to other embryonic cells, fibroblasts can pull them into proper position to form parts of the developing organism (167).

In the mature animal, fibroblasts continue to synthesize and maintain elements of the connective tissue matrix (e.g., collagens, fibronectin, proteoglycans, and other proteins). The matrix is constantly being turned over and remodeled by fibroblasts and the degradative enzymes that they secrete (e.g., collagenases, proteoglycanases, glycosaminodases, and other proteases). When connective tissue sustains an immunological, mechanical, or chemical injury, fibroblasts are called upon to repair the damage. Chemotactic signals direct their migration from neighboring connective tissue into the site of injury, where they

proliferate and synthesize and remodel new matrix that will comprise the scar tissue (5,29,149).

Studies conducted by a number of different investigators have established that fibroblasts do not function autonomously but, instead, are modulated by distinct molecular signals from T lymphocytes, platelets, tumor cells, neutrophils, macrophages, the complement system, elements comprising the connective tissue matrix, and perhaps other sources (115).

BIOSYNTHESIS OF MATRIX COMPONENTS

The extracellular connective tissue matrix consists of fibrillar proteins (collagen, elastin, and reticulin) and an amorphous ground substance that fills intercellular and interfibrillar spaces. The amorphous ground substance is composed of acidic proteoglycans, glycoproteins (fibronectin, laminin, and chondronectin), and less well characterized minor components. Fibroblasts and other specialized connective tissue cells synthesize various proportions of these matrix constituents and thus give connective tissue unique characteristics in different organs and structures of the body. This chapter will focus on those matrix elements and how their synthesis by fibroblasts is controlled.

Collagens

Of all animal proteins, collagen is the most abundant and ubiquitous. In humans and most other vertebrates, it accounts for approximately one-third of the total body proteins. It is the major protein that holds cells together to give organs their characteristic structure.

Eleven distinct types of collagen have now been identified in connective tissue or cultures of cells from mammals (Table 1). These collagens are composed of constituent polypeptide chains termed α chains. Three α chains come together to form a single collagen molecule or monomer. A feature common to all of the collagens is that they contain triple-helical and globular domains (Fig. 1 and ref. 13). The triple-helical regions are attributed to the fact that stretches of repeating triplet amino acid sequences, Gly-X-Y, where X and Y can be any amino acid but are often the imino acids proline and hydroxyproline, respectively, exist in each α chain. The stereochemical configuration of the imino acids causes each α chain to assume a left-handed helical confirmation (minor helix), with a residue repeat distance of 0.291 nm and a relative twist of 110°, making 3.27 residues per turn of the helix and the distance between each third glycine 0.87 nm (133). Another feature of the α chains necessary to allow the helical structure is the presence of glycine at every third residue. Since there are no bulky side chains on the α carbon atom of glycine, the three α chains can wind around a common axis to form a right-handed super helix. If one were to view a cross section of the triple-helical regions of a collagen molecule, one would see only glycine in the central core, with X and Y amino acid side-chains radiating away from the core. Interchain hydrogen bonds, especially with the hydroxyl groups of hydroxyproline, stabilize the triple-helical structure.

Collagens can be subclassified into fibrillar and nonfibrillar types. It is the fibrillar collagens that form distinctive fibrils that have characteristic cross striations visible by electron microscopy. These fibrils have a high tensile strength necessary to hold tissues and cells together. The nonfibrillar collagens form filtration barriers and scaffolding for binding of tissue cells (e.g., epithelial and endothelial cells). Differences in the primary structure of fibrillar and nonfibrillar collagens are responsible for their different physical properties. The fibrillar collagens lose most of their N-terminal and C-terminal globular domains through posttranslational modification but maintain the repeating triplet sequence throughout each constituent polypeptide chain, whereas the nonfibrillar collagens have globular domains interposed between stretches of the repeating triple sequences (133). These globular domains allow the constituent chains to self-assemble into larger molecules that are more complex than the ordered structure of fibrillar collagens.

The major fibrillar collagens are types I, II, and III (Table 1 and refs. 11,131, and 132). Type I collagen is found in most connective tissues (skin, bone, tendons, and ligaments) and is the most abundant collagen in the body (158). Type III is present in most tissues that contain type I but in less amounts. The aorta, synovial membranes, and uterus contain large amounts of type III collagen, whereas bone contains type I but no type III (158). Types I and III are the major collagens produced by fibroblasts *in vivo* and in culture. Type-II collagen is present in hyaline cartilage and is synthesized by chondrocytes (158).

Types I and III collagens have been most thoroughly studied. Type I collagen is composed of two identical

TABLE 1. *Classification of the collagens*[a]

Group	Characteristics	Common name	Function
1	Chain ≥ 95 kilodaltons, with continuous 300-nm-long helical domain	Type I	Structure, skin, bone, organs
		Type II	Structure, cartilage
		Type III	Structure, skin, organs
		Type V	Cytoskeleton
		Type XI	Chondrocyte cytoskeleton
		(K or 1α, 2α, 3α)	
2	Chain ≥ 95 kilodaltons, with alternating helical and nonhelical domains	Type IV	Structure, basement membrane
		Type VI	Myofibril formation
		Type VII	Anchoring fibril
		Type VIII	Endothelial cell product function unknown
3	Chain < 95 kilodaltons	Type IX	Unknown
		Type X	Structure, hypertrophic cartilage

[a] Adapted from ref. 96.

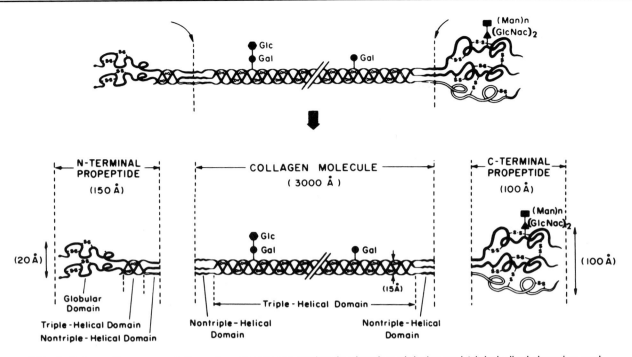

FIG. 1. Schematic representation of a procollagen molecule showing globular and triple-helical domains and cleavage sites of the N- and C-terminal proteases. (From ref. 70.)

polypeptide chains, designated $\alpha 1(I)$, and a structurally different chain, $\alpha 2(I)$. Chains $\alpha 2(I)$ and $\alpha 1(I)$ differ from each other in amino acid composition and chromatographic behavior' (158). The formula for type I collagen can be written as $[\alpha 1(I)]_2 \alpha 2(I)$ (158). Type III collagen is composed of three identical α chains, $[\alpha 1(III)]_3$ (158). The amino acid composition of $\alpha 1(III)$ differs from that of the α chains of type I collagen.

The nonfibrillar collagens (types IV–XI) are normally produced in trace amounts or not at all by fibroblasts *in vitro*. The molecular structure and composition of these collagens are listed in Table 1 and will not be discussed further. The reader can find an excellent discussion of all 11 types of collagen in ref. 38.

Recombinant DNA technology has made possible the characterization of the genes coding for the fibrillar and several of the nonfibrillar collagens (26–28,51,59,103,147). The genes that code for types I and III procollagen have some unusual features. For example, the exons (coding sequences) of the genes are separated by approximately 50 intervening noncoding sequences (introns). This results in a very elaborate structure that is many times larger than the mature messenger RNA (mRNA) transcript and implies that at least 50 splicing events occur to form mature translatable mRNAs. The majority of exons coding for the α-chain domains are either 54 or 108 bases in length (134). Each exon is a multiple of nine base pairs, the number required to code a single Gly-X-Y triplet, and

begins by coding for Gly. The gene for pro $\alpha 1(I)$ is located on human chromosome 17, the gene for pro $\alpha 2(I)$ is on chromosome 7, and the gene for pro $\alpha 1(III)$ is located on chromosome 2 (134).

Several varieties of mRNA of differing length for pro $\alpha 1(I)$ and pro $\alpha 1(I)$ chains have been described in fibroblasts actively synthesizing type I procollagen (102,103,134). It is thought that different varieties of mRNA arise because signals for the termination of transcription and polyadenylation at the 3' end of RNA transcripts are somewhat inefficient. The genes for pro $\alpha 1(I)$ and pro $\alpha 2(I)$ are apparently present as single copies per haploid genome (134). Since the steady-state levels of mRNA for pro $\alpha 1(I)$ and pro $\alpha 2(I)$ chains are 2:1, there appear to be differences either in the rates at which each gene is transcribed or the rates at which initial RNA transcripts are processed (32). The pro α chains are synthesized in the same ratio of 2:1, indicating that the mRNAs for pro $\alpha 1(I)$ and pro $\alpha 2(I)$ are translated at the same rate (32).

The biosynthesis of collagen is accompanied by an unusually large number of cotranslational and posttranslational modifications of the molecule (Fig. 2). Some of these modifications are unique to collagen and other proteins with collagenous (Gly-X-Y) sequences. The modifications occur intracellularly and extracellularly. The synthesis of the polypeptide α chains and intracellular modifications result in the formation of a triple-helical

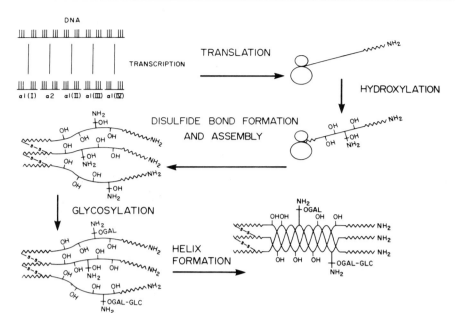

FIG. 2. Biosynthesis of collagen. Each pro-α chain is a distinct gene product. Messenger RNA is translated on membrane-bound ribosomes. As the pro-α chains are being assembled and fed into the cisternae of the rough endoplasmic reticulum, certain prolyl and lysyl hydroxylases, and some of the susceptible hydroxylysyl residues are glycosylated by the action of glycosyl transferases. Following completion of the chain synthesis, chains align and disulfide bonds form at the COOH-terminal extension peptides. Helix formation then follows, and the assembled procollagen molecules are secreted to the extracellular space. (From ref. 158.)

procollagen molecule. Extracellular processing converts the procollagen molecules into fibrillar collagens (e.g., types I, II, and III) or supramolecular structures (e.g., network array of type IV collagen).

The intracellular enzymic modifications of the procollagen polypeptide chains likely take place in the rough endoplasmic reticulum. The NH_2-terminal end of the nascent procollagen polypeptide chains contains a pre-pro segment (signal peptide) that is cleaved either during or shortly after the translocation of the chains across the membrane of the endoplasmic reticulum into the cisternae (51). Since the two characteristic amino acids of collagen (hydroxyproline and hydroxylysine) are not genetically coded, they must be formed from precursor residues of proline and lysine by the action of two specific oxygenases, namely protocollagen proline hydroxylase and protocollagen lysine hydroxylase (17,50). These have absolute and specific enzyme requirements for molecular oxygen ($K_m = 1 \times 10^{-5} M$), Fe^{2+} ions ($K_m = 1 \times 10^{-6} M$), and α-ketoglutarate ($K_m = 5 \times 10^{-6} M$). The enzymes also require a reducing agent, most often ascorbic acid. The specificity of the enzyme is such that hydroxylation is limited to the prolyl and lysyl residues located at the Y position of the triplet sequence (Gly-X-Y) and never at the X position (17,50). Prolyl 4-hydroxylase and prolyl 3-hydroxylase convert prolyl residues to 4-hydroxyproline and 3-hydroxyproline, respectively (17,50). 3-Hydroxyproline is very rare. The only incidence in which it occurs in type I collagen is between glycine and 4-hydroxyproline (58). No 3-hydroxyproline is present in type III collagen. Triple-helix formation cannot occur until after most of the proline residues present in the Y position have been 4-hydroxylated (70).

Collagens are known to contain hexoses. The amounts vary with different types and sources of collagen. In human and other vertebrates, the carbohydrate content is 1% or less in types I and III collagens. Glycosylation of hydroxylysine in the collagen domains and of asparagine in the propeptide sequences occur. In types I, II, and III collagens, the carbohydrates are either the monosaccharide galactose or the disaccharide glycosylgalactose bound by O-glycosidic linkage to the delta-hydroxy group of hydroxylysine (71). Hydroxylysyl-galactosyl-transferase transfers galactose to some of the hydroxylysines, and then galactosyl-hydroxylysyl-glucosyl-transferase transfers glucose to some of the galactosyl-hydroxylysine residues. The sugars are donated in both reactions by the corresponding UDP-glycoside. Both enzymes require a divalent cation, which is usually manganese. The propeptides of procollagen contain asparagine-linked sugars. The carbohydrate units are first synthesized on a carrier lipid and then transferred as a whole to an asparagine residue in the sequence Asn-Ile-Thr in human pro α1(I) and pro α2(I) chains as well as chick pro-α2(I) and pro α1(III) chains (70). It is not apparent whether the glycosyl transferases are located in the cytoplasm or plasma membrane of cells.

The formation of intrachain and interchain disulfide bonds are important events that serve to stabilize and facilitate rapid triple-helix formation. It is thought that the COOH-terminal propeptides direct association of the three pro-α chains of a procollagen molecule and act as a point of initiation for triple-helix formation, since these disulfide bonds will form even if triple-helix formation is prevented (70). The disulfide bonds located in the NH_2-terminal propeptides of types III and IV procollagens form after triple-helix formation (37,70). The enzyme responsible for intracellular formation of disulfide bonds is thought to be protein disulfide isomerase (39,40). This enzyme catalyzes disulfide bond formation in other proteins and is present in fibroblasts and other cells that synthesize collagen (39,40).

The next step in collagen biosynthesis is secretion of the completed triple-helical procollagen molecule into the extracellular space where the NH_2- and COOH-terminal extension peptides are proteolytically removed by the action of specific procollagen peptidases. After the propeptides have been cleaved off procollagen, the resulting collagen molecules have a remarkable tendency for self-assembly and spontaneous formation of fibrils (types I, II, and III) or other ordered structures in the cases of nonfibrillar collagens, and enzyme catalysts or other factors are not required. Although the exact mechanism for the formation of fibrils is not understood at present, the process appears to involve the formation of smaller aggregates from the triple-helical molecules, with subsequent growth to intermediate-sized aggregates (177). The monomeric procollagen molecules begin to aggregate in the secretory vacuoles of fibroblasts, where other macromolecules such as glycoproteins and proteoglycans exert influence on the aggregation state and fibrillogenesis. Thus, fibroblasts may control the different morphologies of collagen fibrils by mixing various connective tissue components (177). The smallest aggregate is most likely formed by the amino-terminal–carboxyl-terminal attachment of monomeric units by charge-charge interactions, giving rise to the $4D$ (D = 67 nm) staggered dimers and trimers. Lateral aggregation occurs afterwards by means of both hydrophobic and electrostatic interactions, giving rise to a basic five membered lateral fibril packing assembly unit. Further lengthening occurs by the addition of other intermediate aggregates at the end of the subfibril. Fibrils grow in width by lateral wrapping of subfibrils. Later, assembly and fibril growth takes place near the cell surface within its indentations, where fibrils are influenced by the microenvironment of the cell surface.

Fibroblast synthesis of type I collagen is thought to be especially inefficient, since 10% to 60% of the newly synthesized collagen may be degraded intracellularly prior to secretion (136). This degraded collagen may arise from two sources. One is the removal of abnormal collagen molecules or errors during synthesis, and the other may be from an attempt by the cells to regulate the amount and type of collagen they secrete. Agents that raise levels of intracellular cyclic adenosine monophosphate (cAMP) can increase the intracellular degradation of newly synthesized type I collagen to a greater extent than they stimulate degradation of type III collagen (136).

Final maturational changes by a process of cross-linking occur when collagen fibrils are deposited in the extracellular matrix (42). Covalent bridges among the polypeptide α chains form both within the molecule and between adjacent molecules. The initial event in the formation of cross-links is the oxidative deamination of the ϵ-amino group in certain lysine and hydroxylysine residues to the corresponding aldehyde by the action of lysyl oxidase (159). The reactive aldehydes formed then participate in the formation of cross-links. The aldehydes can form two major types of cross-links: (i) by aldol condensation of two of the aldehydes or (ii) by condensation between an aldehyde and a hydroxylysine, or a glycosylated hydroxylysine residue (77,159,168). The reader is referred to ref. 94 for a detailed discussion of all the possible compounds formed by cross-linking. Lysyl oxidase requires molecular oxygen and probably pyridoxal also (159). There is considerable charge heterogeneity of lysyl oxidase, but all forms appear to have the same molecular weight; also, no structural, catalytic, or immunological differences have been observed (77,168). Lysyl oxidase can use both collagen and elastin as substrates but require a fibrillar form of collagen (159). The enzyme will not react with procollagen, suggesting that at least one of the two propeptides must be cleaved before cross-linking can occur (77). The degree of cross-linking varies widely, depending on the tissue and age of the organism, with more cross-linking occurring with advancing age (94).

Since various tissues are made up of different collagen polypeptide chains, mechanisms must exist to alter collagen gene expression. Cortisol, anti-inflammatory steroids, and parathyroid hormone cause a specific decrease in the cellular concentration of translatable type I procollagen mRNA (83,108). It is not clear whether this is due to a decrease in the transcription rate of the corresponding genes or an increase in mRNA degradation. Other hormones affect the amounts of cotranslational and posttranslational enzymes and the rate of collagen degradation (71,72). Transformation of cultured fibroblasts with RNA tumor viruses, DNA viruses, or chemical carcinogens lead to a marked reduction in the amount of collagen synthesized and in the levels of type I procollagen mRNAs (3,131,144,145). The detailed mechanisms involved in regulating collagen gene expression are unknown.

Collagen synthesis can also be regulated at the level of translation. For example, during development of fetal sheep skin, the synthesis of collagen falls approximately 10-fold during the last half of fetal life, but the concentration of type I procollagen mRNAs remain constant (172). Also, the N-terminal propeptides of procollagen act as feedback regulators of collagen translation (111). When the N-terminal propeptides of types I or III procollagen are incubated with cultured fibroblasts, there is a specific decrease in the rate of collagen synthesis (187). The N-terminal propeptides influence the efficiency with which the procollagen mRNAs are translated, but it is not known whether the peptides are actually taken up by the cells and transported to the translation site.

Proteoglycans

Proteoglycans are macromolecules that are present in all connective tissues in varying amounts. They largely comprise the amorphous ground substance present in intercellular and interfibrillar spaces. Although proteoglycans are mostly extracellular, there are both intracellular and cell-membrane forms. Proteoglycans are complex molecules in which glycosaminoglycan (GAG) chains are linked covalently to a protein core by an intercalated specific linkage region that involves the terminal reducing sugar of the chain (Fig. 3). GAGs (hyaluronic acid, chondroitin sulfate, dermatan sulfate, heparan sulfate, heparin, and keratan sulfate) are long-chain, unbranched, linear carbohydrate polymers (-glycans) that are composed of repeating disaccharide units (Table 2). One constituent of the unit is an amino sugar (glycosamino-), and the other is a hexuronic acid (glycurono-), with the exception of keratan sulfate, which contains galactose instead of

hexuronic acid. The number of repeat disaccharides varies but is typically on the order of 50. Each proteoglycan molecule is composed of one or two different types of GAG, and the total number of glycosaminoglycan chains may vary from one or two to more than 100, with a potential of giving as many as 10,000 negatively charged groups per proteoglycan molecule. The protein core is also substituted, with a number of oligosaccharides similar to those found in glycoproteins. The molecular weights of proteoglycans are in the range of 50,000 to several million. A still higher level of organization can be attained by the ability of some types of proteoglycans to form aggregates having molecular weights greater than 100 million.

Hyaluronic Acid

Hyaluronic acid (HA) is the largest glycosaminoglycan. Its molecular weight can vary from a few hundred thousand to several million. It is thought to be an unbranched molecule containing from 500 to several thousand of the repeat disaccharide subunits, β-D-glucuronic acid linked to β-D-N-acetylglucosamine. HA is the only GAG that does not contain a sulfated ester group. It still remains to be determined whether HA is covalently bound to protein and has a specific oligosaccharide linkage region. The structural conformation of HA is largely dependent on whether the counter-ion is monovalent or divalent. Data obtained by X-ray crystallography and nuclear magnetic resonance suggest that the HA molecule contains stiff segments and that various parts of the molecule may interact with one another, giving rise to an extended structure in solution that occupies a large domain and produces a solution with a high viscosity (97).

HA is present in all connective tissues, being the major GAG in rooster comb, umbilical cord, and vitreous body. Of the GAGs in skin and aorta, HA represents 10% to 20%. Fibroblasts in culture produce more HA than any other species of GAG (usually >50% of the total GAGs synthesized). Hyaluronic acid has been found to be bound to the surfaces of several types of cells in culture, and specific receptors have been found on liver cells, transformed fibroblasts, and chondrocytes (90,162,178). Hyaluronic acid is thought to play a central role in regulating the flow and content of water in some tissues. It is also involved in the formation of proteoglycan aggregates in that it forms a "backbone" onto which other proteoglycans attach. Furthermore, hyaluronic acid regulates the biosynthesis by chondrocytes of other GAGs by acting as a feedback inhibitor and affects phagocytosis by neutrophils and immune functions of lymphocytes (162). During embryogenesis, HA appears to play a critical role in modulating cell differentiation (174,175). HA can facilitate

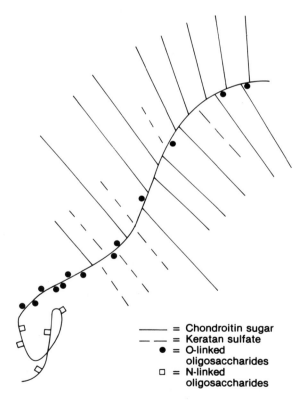

= Chondroitin sugar
= Keratan sulfate
● = O-linked oligosaccharides
□ = N-linked oligosaccharides

FIG. 3. Proteoglycan molecule, depicting bottle-brush configuration and heterogeneity of the core protein with respect to attachment sites for chondroitin sulfate and keratan sulfate; also shown is hyalurate-binding region. (From ref. 12.)

TABLE 2. *The repeating disaccharide units of the glycosaminoglycans*[a]

Glycosaminoglycan	Function	Number of disaccharide units	Disaccharide units
Hyaluronic acid	Retains water and regulates water flow in tissue; participates in proteoglycan aggregation	50–10,000	β-D-Glucuronic acid β-D-*N*-Acetylglucosamine
Chondroitin sulfate	Proteoglycan structure in cartilage, nucleus pulposus, and bone	20–60	β-D-Glucuronic acid β-D-*N*-Acetylgalactosamine
Dermatan sulfate	Proteoglycan structure in loose connective tissue (skin, sclera, cornea)	30–80	β-D-Glucuronic acid β-D-*N*-Acetylgalactosamine and α-L-Iduronic acid β-D-*N*-Acetylgalactosamine
Heparin sulfate	Proteoglycan structure in basement membranes; binds to fibronectin; heparin proteoglycan from mast cells	10–60	β-D-Glucuronic acid α-D-*N*-Acetylglucosamine and α-L-Iduronic acid α-D-*N*-Acetylglucosamine
Keratan sulfate	Proteoglycan structure, cartilage, nucleus pulposus	5–40	β-D-*N*-Acetylglucosamine β-D-Galactose

[a] Compiled from information given in ref. 56.

movement of cells by preventing cell-cell and cell-substrate interactions that would immobilize the cells (90,173,180).

Chondroitin Sulfate

Chondroitin sulfate is a sulfated galactosaminoglycan and contains ester sulfate groups that reside on carbon 4 or 6 of the *N*-acetylgalactosamine residue. It contains only one type of uronic acid, namely glucuronic acid. The number of repeat disaccharides within a preparation of chondroitin sulfate varies from 20 to 60. The average molecular weight of chondroitin sulfate is approximately 20,000. Chondroitin sulfate is attached to a core protein by an *O*-glycosidic bond between serine and a xylose residue that is part of a specific linkage region sequence consisting of xylose-galactose-galactose-glucuronic acid (137). This type of linkage is common to most glycosaminoglycans.

Chondroitin sulfate is found in cartilage and intervertebral discs. Nasal and epiphyseal cartilages have a high content of chondroitin-4-sulfate, whereas articular cartilage and the nucleus pulposus have a higher content of chondroitin-6-sulfate. Very little chondroitin sulfate is found in fibrous connective tissue.

Dermatan Sulfate

Dermatan sulfate is structurally related to chondroitin sulfate. It contains an additional type of monosaccharide, L-iduronic acid (56). This gives rise to a dissaccharide

unit consisting of α-L-iduronic acid, β-D-*N*-acetylgalactosamine. L-Iduronic acid contains an ester sulfate at position 4 and sometimes at position 2 (137). The α-L-iduronic acid and D-glucuronic acid disaccharide units are distributed in a copolymeric fashion. The number of disaccharide units can vary in a dermatan sulfate molecule but is usually on the order of 50 to 60 (56,137). Likewise, the proportion of L-iduronic acid disaccharides in a single molecule varies widely (137).

Dermatan sulfate is found in fibrous connective tissues such as tendon, skin, aorta, sclera, joint capsule, and cornea but is not present in articular cartilage, except in the meniscus (56). The exact functional significance of dermatan sulfate remains to be defined, but it can bind to, and interact with, several matrix components, including collagen (91,176). Since dermatan sulfate can precipitate tropocollagen from solution causing fibril formation *in vitro*, it has been postulated that a main function *in vivo* may be to facilitate collagen fiber formation (91,176).

Heparan Sulfate and Heparin

Heparan sulfate and heparin have similar structures. However, since they are synthesized on different protein acceptors, they are distinct molecular entities. Heparan sulfate is synthesized by fibroblasts and other connective tissue cells, whereas heparin is synthesized by mast cells. Heparin and heparan sulfate are composed of copolymers of β-D-glucuronic acid linked to α-D-*N*-acetylglucosamine as well as α-L-iduronic acid linked to αD-*N*-acetylglucosamine. The chains of these GAGs usually contain 10 to 60 such disaccharide units. Ester sulfate groups are present at positions 3 or 6 in glucosamine residues and at position 2 in L-iduronic acid residues (56). Heparan sulfate, like chondroitin sulfate, contains an *O*-glycosidic bond between xylose and serine (137). Heparan sulfate is located on many cell surfaces and in certain fibrous connective tissues such as lung, aorta, and basement membrane. Although its true physiologic functions are not known, it probably interacts with other matrix constituents, especially collagen. Heparin is found especially in the lungs and intestine. It is an efficient inhibitor of blood coagulation, but it also binds to a specific region of the fibronectin molecule and to a basic protein in granules of mast cells (56).

Keratan Sulfate

Keratan sulfate is composed of the repeating disaccharide unit, β-D-*N*-acetylglucosamine linked to β-D-galactose. Sulfate may be present at position 6 in glucosamine. Two types of keratan sulfate have been found. These are referred to as type I and type II (104,156). Type I occurs in the cornea and has an *N*-glycosidic linkage involving *N*-acetylglucosamine and asparagine (104). Type II is found in cartilage and nucleus pulposus (156). It has an *O*-glycosidic linkage that involves *N*-acetylgalactosamine and the hydroxy amino acids threonine or serine (156). Fibrous connective tissue is not thought to contain keratan sulfate. The physiological function of keratan sulfate is unknown but may be responsible for the transparent characteristics of corneal tissue.

Most connective tissue polysaccharides and GAGs (with the possible exception of HA) are synthesized as proteoglycans. The protein core is the precursor for the proteoglycan and is synthesized in the conventional manner on a ribosomal template, and the carbohydrate chains are assembled posttranslationally. One sugar is added at a time, starting with the attachment of xylose to serine in a structurally specific region of the protein core (56,176). In sulfated GAGs, sulfation takes place after the appropriate monosaccharide has been linked to the growing polysaccharide chain. The addition of sugar and sulfate groups is catalyzed by transferases. Energy for the glycosidic bonds between the monosaccharides is derived from nucleotide sugar precursors [i.e., uridine (UDP) sugar nucleotides]. The sulfate residues are derived from phosphoadenosine-5-phosphate. GAG chains are elongated and sulfated in the endoplasmic reticulum and Golgi complex as the core protein progresses from the polyribosomes to the exterior of the cell. Postsynthetic modifications may occur to yield single-polysaccharide chains that may or may not be linked to peptide.

The levels of the UDP-sugars apparently play an important role in regulatory biosynthesis of GAGs. For example, elevated levels of UDP-xylose inhibit UDP-glycose dehydrogenase, which connects UDP-glycose to UDP glucuronic acid, the immediate precursor of UDP-xylose (91). Also, high concentrations of UDP-*N*-acetylglucosamine inhibit formation of glucosamine-6-phosphate from fructose-6-phosphate and glutamine (91). A deficiency of acceptor protein can result in inhibition of GAG synthesis by causing UDP-xylose to accumulate, which, by negative feedback, can suppress formation of UDP-glucuronic acid.

A detailed discussion of the steps involved in GAG biosynthesis is beyond the scope of this chapter; these are reviewed in detail in ref. 56.

EXTRACELLULAR GLYCOPROTEINS

Most extracellular proteins, be they structural and/or functional, are glycosylated and are technically glycoproteins. There are four types of carbohydrate linkage to proteins among the vertebrates: (i) proteoglycans, with polysaccharide (glycosaminoglycan) *O*-glycosidically linked through xylose to serine or threonine; (ii) the collagens, with glycose and galactose *O*-glycosidically linked to hydroxylysine; (iii) the mucins, with oligosaccharide *O*-glycosidically linked to serine or threonine; and (iv) the large body of glycoproteins in which oligosaccharide with a mannose core is *N*-glycosidically linked to asparagine. In this section we will focus attention mostly on fibronectin, the major glycoprotein synthesized by fibroblasts.

Fibronectin

The fibronectins are multifunctional high-molecular-weight glycoproteins. They are found on cell surfaces and in the pericellular and intercellular matrix, basement membranes, and a variety of body fluids. Fibronectin and other glycoproteins are intimately involved in the interactions of cells with one another and with their extracellular environment. Fibronectin is synthesized by a variety of cells and is closely associated with fibroblasts, endothelial cells, chondrocytes, glial cells, amniotic cells, myocytes, platelets, and monocytes (139). Plasma, amniotic fluid, and seminal fluid contain high concentrations (100–300 μg/ml) of fibronectin (139). Lesser amounts (1–10 μg/ml) are present in cerebrospinal fluid and urine (139).

Fibronectin is composed of two 250-kilodalton subunits that are similar but not identical. The subunits are joined near their C-termini by disulfide bonds. Each subunit has a series of tightly folded globular domains that have specialized binding characteristics (Fig. 4). Starting from the N-termini, globular domain I binds to fibrin, heparin,

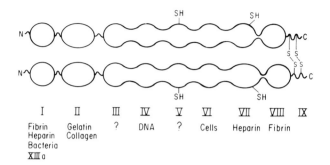

I   II   III   IV   V   VI   VII   VIII   IX
Fibrin Gelatin ? DNA ? Cells Heparin Fibrin
Heparin Collagen
Bacteria
XIII a

FIG. 4. Domain structure of fibronectin. The two subunits of the dimers are attached via a pair of disulfide bonds near the C-terminus. Each subunit is about 250 kilodaltons and consists of a series of globular domains connected by flexible polypeptide segments, some of which are very readily cleaved by proteases (thin lines). Individual domains are specialized for specific binding to other moities, as shown. Different subunits have different structures in the region of domain VII. (From ref. 60.)

bacteria, and Factor XIII (60). The adjacent domain II binds to gelatin and collagen, III has no known binding function, IV binds to DNA, V has no binding function, VI binds to cells, VII binds to heparin, and VIII binds to fibrin (60).

Data obtained from primary sequence information of plasma fibronectin and sequencing of complementary DNA (cDNA) and genomic clones of cellular fibronectin have revealed that they consist of a series of homologous repeats termed types I, II, and III homologies (79–81,113,160,161). Types I and II homologies are 45 to 50 amino acids in length and have a disulfide-bonded loop structure. Type III homologies contain approximately 90 amino acids and do not contain disulfide bonds. Fibronectin is composed of 12 type I, 2 type II, and 15 to 16 type III homologies. These three homologies are responsible for over 90% of fibronectin's sequence.

Earlier observations with plasma and cellular fibronectin indicated that each of the two subunits within a fibronectin molecule were different (112,170,193). Studies with fibronectin cDNA clones have shown that there are at least two positions of subunit variations in rat and human fibronectins. The first is located in the sequence between the penultimate and final type III repeats in the central region of fibronectin (79,81,151). This intervening sequence can be present or absent. The second subunit variation arises by virtue of the fact that a whole type III repeat can be omitted from fibronectin cDNA clones (51).

Analysis of genomic Southern blots probed with cDNA clones of both human and rat fibronectin have indicated that only a single fibronectin gene exists (80,171). The fibronectin gene is complex, being approximately 50 kilobases (kb) long and containing about 50 exons (80,171). The differences in cDNA clones of fibronectins arise by

alternative splicing of the primary transcript. Exon skipping leads to fibronectin with or without the extra type III segment (181). Differences in fibronectins in non-type-III segments are attributed to exon subdivision.

A variety of functions have been assigned to fibronectin by virtue of its cellular and molecular interactions. Fibronectin in plasma and other body fluids may promote cell movement, attachment, spreading, and proliferation (54). Phagocytosis by macrophages, monocytes, and liver Kupffer cells, as well as clearance of cellular debris by the mononuclear phagocyte system, is facilitated by the non-specific opsonic activity of fibronectin. This nonspecific opsonic activity of fibronectin is important in host defense and wound healing and is presumably mediated by its ability to interact with fibrin, C1q component of complement, bacteria, actin, and DNA (30,69,84,93,140,196).

Fibronectin is thought to play a major role in the organization of pericellular and intercellular matrices and basement membranes, although the specific mechanisms by which it performs this function are not completely understood but no doubt involves its ability to bind to collagens, proteoglycan (heparin, heparan sulfate, and hyaluronic acid), and cell surfaces (74,75,165,194). Formation of stable connective tissue structure may be mediated by the ability of fibronectin to form disulfide-stabilized self-aggregates (perhaps involving other macromolecules) and by transglutaminase-mediated covalent cross-linking to collagens, fibrin, and other macromolecules (22,62,100).

The differentiation and morphogenesis of certain types of cells is influenced by fibronectin. Malignant and virus-transformed cells in culture contain greatly reduced cell-surface fibronectin (86). When added exogenously to such cells in culture, there is a reversion to a normal appearing phenotype (4). Myoblasts, before fusing to form myotubules, lose their ability to produce fibronectin (139). Chondrocytes do not synthesize fibronectin; when it is added to cultures of chondrocytes, they dedifferentiate into fibroblastic cells (75). Pericellular fibronectin changes with cell cycle. It is expressed maximally during the G1 phase and decreases through the S and G2 phases and is almost totally absent from cells during the M phase (61).

Additional Matrix Glycoproteins

In addition to fibronectin, other cell-surface glycoproteins have been identified in cultures of fibroblasts. These, on the basis of their molecular weights (in thousands) after denaturation and reduction, are Gp250, Gp190, Gp170, and Gp140 (19–22). These glycoproteins are insoluble in nonionic or zwitterionic detergents and form a multimeric disulfide-bonded structure (19–22). Gp140 is suspected to be a type of pericellular collagen because it contains hydroxylysine and, in secreted form in fibroblast culture medium, is collagenase-sensitive (20). Similarly, Gp170 and 190 from human fibroblasts are both sensitive to bacterial collagenase and are pro α1(I) and pro α2(I), respectively (20). At the cell surface, Gp170 and 190 are organized in the pericellular matrix such that they are resistant to collagenase (20). All of these surface and matrix glycoproteins are greatly reduced when cells are transformed (21,11,54).

Elastin

Elastin, like collagen, is a major fibrous protein constituent of the connective tissue matrix. Elastin is found in high concentrations in specialized ligaments, lung fibrocartilage, and the media of large blood vessels. It is present in relatively small, but important, amounts in the skin, tendon, and bone. The elastic properties of tissue is due to elastin fibers present in the extracellular matrix.

A detailed discussion of the chemistry and mechanical properties will not be covered in this chapter. The reader is referred to several articles that cover these aspects of elastin (49,51,141). However, some salient physicochemical features of elastin deserve to be mentioned. Elastin is very insoluble and is able to resist harsh chemical extraction procedures. This property has been proven to be useful in its purification. Elastin has an unusual amino acid composition. Approximately one-third of its amino acid residues are glycine and 10% to 13% are proline, similar to collagen (51,141). However, there is very little hydroxyproline and no hydroxylysine. Elastin is rich in the nonpolar amino acids alanine, valine, isoleucine, and leucine, but polar amino acids are in the minority (51,141). Another difference between collagen and elastin is the extent to which there is cross-linking, both within and between polypeptide chains. Interstitial collagens contain one or two lysine- or hydroxylysine-derived cross-links per 1,000 residues, whereas elastin can have as many as 40 lysine-derived cross-links per 1,000 residues (41).

The cross-links of elastin are of four basic types: dehydrolysinonorleucine (and its reduced form lysinonorleucine), desmosine, the product of aldol condensation of two allysines, and dehydromerodesmosine (41). The extensive cross-linking of elastin has retarded progress on the study of its primary amino acid sequence. Most of the structural data regarding elastin has been obtained by analyzing tropoelastin (67 kilodaltons), the probable precursor of elastin, which can be obtained from aortas of piglets with copper deficiency, a condition that results in a general inhibition of cross-linking of elastin (143). Sequence analysis of purified tryptic peptides from porcine tropoelastin has revealed that there are long segments of hydrophobic amino acid residues that are interrupted with shorter segments of polyalanine sequences with clusters of lysines. These shorter segments are in alpha-helix conformation, whereas the larger hydrophobic sequences comprise a beta-spiral structure with elastomeric properties (142).

An interacting repeating pentapeptide (Pro-Gly-Val-Gly-Val) is present in the hydrophobic regions and apparently confers some unusual folding properties on elastin (142). Genomic elastin clones have been obtained from chick embryo aortas and have been used to study mechanisms involved in elastin synthesis (14,15). These studies indicate that the rate of elastin synthesis is controlled at the level of elastin mRNA.

THE ROLE OF MATRIX COMPONENTS IN INFLAMMATION AND TISSUE REPAIR

Several matrix components have been found to possess interesting biological properties in addition to their time-honored structural properties that may influence inflammatory reactions and associated tissue repair processes. Matrix components are degraded at sites of tissue injury, and such degradation products might provide important signals to inflammatory cells.

Collagen

Type I collagen and α1(I), α2(I), and α1 CB5 peptide, as well as types II, III, and IV collagen, are all able to induce platelet aggregation in vitro (6,25). In inflammatory reactions in vivo, type I collagen fibers would be degraded by the action of collagenase on matrix glycoproteins, and proteoglycans would be degraded by proteases and proteoglycanases. This could expose type I collagen fibrils so that platelets released from damaged capillaries and blood vessels could be aggregated by interaction with the exposed collagen, α chains, and perhaps smaller collagenous peptides containing the α1 CB5 sequence.

The interstitial collagens, constituent α chains, and small peptides generated by degradation by bacterial collagenase are chemoattractants in vitro for human peripheral blood monocytes and for dermal fibroblasts (115,126). These observations suggest that solubilized collagens, α chains, and collagenous peptides generated by the action of collagenase and proteinases could function to provide chemotactic signals for peripheral blood monocytes and neighboring connective tissue fibroblasts to migrate into the area of tissue inflammation and injury in vivo.

Elastin

Tropoelastin and peptides generated by degrading elastin with pancreatic elastase are chemotactic for fibroblasts

(153). The synthetic elastin pentopeptide, Pro-Gly-Val-Gly-Val, also induces the chemotactic migration of fibroblasts in a dose-dependent manner (154).

Fibronectin

Both plasma and cellular fibronectin are potent chemoattractants for fibroblasts *in vitro* (120,157). The chemotactic property resides in the non-gelatin-binding region of the molecule that is contained in a 140-kilodalton fragment generated by cathepsin D cleavage of plasma fibronectin (120). Other properties of fibronectin already mentioned in this chapter, such as its ability to promote attachment, spreading, and proliferation of fibroblasts and phagocytosis by cells of the reticuloendothelial cell system, may also facilitate repair to damaged connective tissue. The promotion of adhesion to, and spreading of, platelets on exposed collagen fibers and binding of circulating cells to fibrin clots and exposed collagen are probably important functions of fibronectin in homeostasis and wound repair processes (75,76).

Hyaluronic Acid

Studies of wound healing in laboratory animals have shown that hyaluronic acid is produced in the early phases of the repair process and probably serves to promote the migration of inflammatory cells and fibroblasts by interfering with cell-cell and cell-substrate interactions. In both cell-mediated and antibody-mediated immune inflammation, hyaluronic acid may curtail the intensity of the reaction by inhibiting the functions of T and B lymphocytes, since it has been demonstrated *in vitro* to inhibit mitogen-stimulated T-cell proliferation and B-cell immunoglobulin production (57).

MATRIX DEGRADING ENZYMES

Enzymes exist that are capable of degrading all matrix components. Some of these enzymes are synthesized by fibroblasts themselves, whereas others are secreted by inflammatory or organ-specific cells.

Collagenase

Collagens comprising the extracellular matrix are degraded by intracellular and extracellular pathways. Fragments of collagen small enough to be ingested have to be generated first, undoubtedly by the action of collagenase (36). The collagen fragments are then phagocytosed and taken up in phagolysosomes where, at acid pH, cathepsins B and N are thought to degrade the collagen fibrils (36).

Collagenases have been found by immunolocalization studies in a variety of wound and diseased tissue, including human skin, skin fibroblasts, middle ear cholesteotoma, basal cell carcinoma, human cornea, rheumatoid joint tissue, adherent rheumatoid synovial cells, bone, skin melanomas, gingival tissue, involuting rat uterus, rat liver, cirrhotic tissues, and mouse peritoneal macrophages (188). The extracellular collagenases all have optimal activity at neutral pH and are metalloproteases requiring both Ca^{2+} and Zn^{2+} (188). The first event in degradation of collagenase is probably the depolymerization of collagen fibrils. Polymorphonuclear leukocyte elastase and cathepsin G are able to depolymerize fibrillar collagen by degrading the nonhelical ends of collagen molecules (164). Mammalian collagenases themselves can also degrade cross-linked collagen fibrils by attacking the collagen molecule at one specific locus one-quarter of the distance from the carboxy-terminus (130). The larger, three-quarter, fragment is called TC_A; the smaller, one-quarter, carboxy fragment is called TC_B (Fig. 5). Types I, II, and III collagens are all cleaved in this manner (188). At 25°C the TC_A and TC_B fragments will retain the triple-helical structure, but at temperatures greater than 33°C they spontaneously denature and form random coil fragments that can then be further degraded by a variety of tissue and cell-secreted proteinases (188). Collagenases cleave at Gly-Leu or Gly-Ile bonds (52,95).

Types IV and V collagen are resistant to degradation by mammalian collagenases that degrade types I, II and

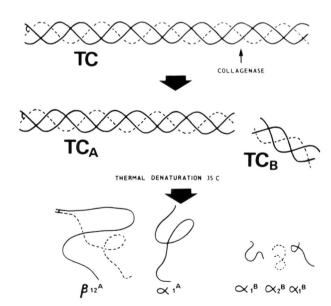

FIG. 5. Diagrammatic illustration showing cleavage of the type I collagen molecule (TC) by collagenase at 35°C. Two helical fragments, TC_A and TC_B, three-quarters and one-quarter the length of the original molecule, respectively, are produced. (From ref. 188.)

III collagen (188). However, enzymes have been identified that will degrade type IV (e.g., chymotrypsin-like enzyme from mast cells, neutrophil elastase, cathepsin G and B, metalloproteases from bone culture) and type V (e.g., metalloprotease from bone culture and metalloproteases from macrophages) collagens (31,88,89,188).

The collagenases that degrade types I, II, and III (interstitial) collagens from human skin, monocytes, gingiva, and synovium appear to be similar and are probably identical. The collagenase from human neutrophils that degrade interstitial collagens is different from skin collagenase with regard to immunologic reactivity, substrate preference, and molecular weight. The cDNA clone representing human skin collagenase mRNA has been isolated and sequenced (46). Human skin collagenase is synthesized as a preproenzyme, with a molecular weight (MW) of 54,092 and a 19-amino-acid-long signal peptide (46). The enzyme is secreted in both glycosylated (MW 57,000) and unmodified (MW 51,929) forms (46). When the procollagenase is activated by proteases, an 81-amino-acid residue from the amino-terminal portion of the molecule is cleaved off (46).

Collagenase activity is not only regulated by proteolytic activation of procollagenase but also by inhibitors that complex with the collagenase. These inhibitors can be removed by certain organic mercurials or chaotropic agents (188). Various inhibitors have been identified in the following: plasma (α_2-macroglobulin, β_1-anticollagenase); cultured mammalian tissues such as rabbit bone, skin, and uterus (tissue inhibitors of metalloprotease, TIMP); human tendon; bovine aorta; chick cartilage and bone; cultured fibroblasts; synovial cells; smooth muscle cells; epithelial cells; gingival fibroblasts; and human amniotic fluid (188). The degradation of collagen in normal and inflamed tissues likely depends on upsetting the balance between collagenase and its inhibitors (198).

Elastase

Elastin is degradable by only a few enzymes, which, because of this property, are called *elastases*. Unlike mammalian collagenases, elastases lack specificity and are general and powerful proteases. Pancreatic and neutrophil elastases are serine proteases and are inhibited by α_1-antiprotease in plasma (49). Macrophage elastase is inhibited by α_2-macroglobulin but not by α_1-antiprotease (49). These three elastases all cleave elastin at different sites (49). The pancreatic elastase probably largely serves a digestive function but in the setting of pancreatitis can contribute to tissue destruction. The neutrophil and macrophage elastases are probably important in degrading elastin and perhaps other proteins at sites of inflammatory reactions.

Proteoglycanases and Glycosaminoglycanases

Proteoglycans are thought first to be partially degraded in the matrix by proteases (146). The core protein and link proteins are attacked by the proteases, allowing fragments to diffuse out of the immediate location or be further degraded in the pericellular area by proteases such as cathepsin B (179). Glycosaminoglycan peptides and free proteoglycans are then pinocytosed by cells, where they are further degraded in the lysosomes by cathepsins with acid pH-optima of about 3, such as cathepsin D. The glycosaminoglycans are depolymerized by endoglycosidases and further degraded by a number of different exoenzymes (184). Sulfate groups are removed first by sulfatases, each specific for a given sulfate group, followed by N-acetylation, and monosaccharides are removed by the alternating action of specific iduronidases or glucuronidases and specific N-acetylglucosaminidases, which together degrade glycosaminoglycans to free sulfate and respective monosaccharide residues.

Glycoproteinases

Fibronectin and other extracellular glycoproteins are quite susceptible to degradation by a wide variety of tissue- and cell-associated proteases, including chymotrypsin, thrombin, pepsin, elastases, trypsin, plasmin, and cathepsin G and D (54). It would appear that glycoproteins could be readily degraded at sites of inflammatory reactions by the concerted action of several different proteases from neutrophils, macrophages, and fibroblasts. Some intermediate fragments from fibronectin degradation could retain biologic activity, such as binding characteristics and the chemotactic property for fibroblasts, which could serve useful functions in promoting tissue repairs.

REGULATORS OF FIBROBLAST GROWTH

Studies with 3T3 cells and human fibroblasts have suggested that fibroblasts require two signals for DNA synthesis to be affected. Scher et al. have called these "competence" and "progression" signals (148). The "competence factors" do not stimulate DNA synthesis but render cells in G_0 or G_1 phase "competent" to do so (148). "Progression factors" stimulate DNA synthesis in competent cells (148). Growth factors can be classified into one of these two groups by a "complementation test" in which fibroblasts are rendered quiescent by reducing serum concentration in medium so that the fibroblasts are growth-arrested (166). The growth factor being tested is then added before and after known progression factors to determine under which conditions fibroblast DNA synthesis is stimulated. Some of the known fibroblast growth factors have been classified as being either competence or progression factors, whereas others remain to be classified (Table 3).

Although the concept of competence and progression factors has proven to be useful in our understanding of fibroblast growth, some factors may well trigger fibroblast growth by stimulating release of platelet-derived growth-factor(PDGF)-like proteins from fibroblasts. Transforming growth factor beta (TGFβ) is such a factor (68). TGFβ will trigger growth of serum-starved fibroblasts but with delayed kinetics (68). This delayed stimulation of fibroblast growth is associated with the release of a PDGF-like protein from fibroblasts (68). It is unclear whether TGFβ then acts as a progression factor after PDGF confers competence on the fibroblasts.

The mechanisms involved in the transmission of mitogenic signals to fibroblasts are not completely understood. Specific receptors have been identified on fibroblasts for several of the growth factors [e.g., epidermal growth factor (EGF); TGFβ, interleukin-1 (IL-1), and PDGF] listed in Table 3. The receptor on murine fibroblasts for PDGF has recently been cloned (195). The primary deduced structure for the PDGF receptor is similar to that of the v-kit oncogene product and the receptor for macrophage-stimulating factor (CSF-1) (195). Its overall structure has properties consistent with a receptor and include transmembrane and tyrosinase kinase domains (195). There is a potential site for N-linked glycosylation in the extracellular domain (195). The protein encoded by the cDNA clone would have an apparent MW of

120,000 after the signal sequence is removed (195). The MW of the native receptor for PDGF is 180,000, and the increase in MW from the predicted figure may be explained by extensive glycosylation as well as by the covalent linking of ubiquitin and phosphate groups (195).

PDGF and other growth factors stimulate cytoskeletal rearrangement and turnover of phosphatidylinositol as well as enhance expression of a family of genes, including c-myc and c-fos proto-oncogenes. These effects are believed to be important in the eventual mitosis of fibroblasts and other targets of various growth factors, although exactly how these events are related to mitosis remains to be established.

FIBROBLAST MIGRATION AND CHEMOTAXIS

It has been widely observed that fibroblasts are capable of substantial migration during their growth *in vitro* on plastic or glass surfaces (1,2,55). As fibroblasts migrate they send out lamellipodia, which adhere to surfaces and allow the body of the fibroblast to be drawn up to the new adhesion site by activation of the contractile filaments within the cell (1,2,55). Using a corneal injury model in the rabbit, Baum was able to show that new fibroblasts migrated into the injury site from neighboring connective tissue (5).

These studies demonstrating the migratory potential of fibroblasts *in vitro* and *in vivo* suggested to us that fibroblasts, like monocytes, T cells, and polymorphonuclear leukocytes, might be capable of directed migration toward specific chemoattractants. We were able to develop an *in-vitro* assay, based on the Boyden technique, that measured fibroblast chemotaxis (129). The assay utilizes gelatin-coated polycarbonate filters with 8-μm pores to separate the lower test compartment from the upper cell compartment (129). Fibroblasts from monolayer cultures are used as target cells in the assay (129). By employing this assay, we and others have identified at least 10 different classes of fibroblast chemoattractants. They can be classified as to their origin, as shown in Table 4.

T Cells

When human or guinea-pig T-cells are stimulated by antigens or mitogens, they produce a specific chemotactic protein (LDCF-F) for fibroblasts (116,129). The human T-cell factor has an MW of approximately 22,000, whereas the guinea-pig factor is larger (approximately 80,000). When macrophages are depleted from cultures of human T cells, LDCF-F is produced as a higher-MW inactive precursor molecule (119). The latent LDCF-F can be converted to active form by trypsin or extracts from son-

TABLE 3. *Classification of fibroblast growth factors*

Growth factor	Reference
Competence factors	
Platelet-derived growth factor	148,166
Fibroblast growth factor	148,166
Calcium-containing crystals	138
Calcium phosphate precipitates	24
Progression factors	
Multiplication-stimulating activity	98
Somatomedins A and C	148,166
Insulin and insulin-like growth factors	98
Epidermal growth factor	101
Alveolar macrophage-derived growth factor	9
Unclassified factors	
Interleukin-1 α and β	124,150
Transforming growth factor β	68
T-cell-derived fibroblast growth factor	118,183
Schistosomal granuloma macrophage-derived growth factor	191
Vanadate	18

TABLE 4. *Chemoattractants for fibroblasts*

Chemoattractant	Reference
T cells	
Lymphocyte-derived chemotactic factor (LDCF-F)	129,116
Complement system	
Serum(C5)-derived chemotactic factor	130
Connective tissue matrix	
Collagen types I, II, and III; α chains; and hydroxyproline peptides	126
Fibronectin	120,157
Tropoelastin and elastin peptides	153,154
Leukocytes	
Leukotriene B$_4$	92
Platelets	
Platelet-derived growth factor (PDGF)	157
Transforming growth factor β (TGFβ)[a]	121
Transformed and neoplastic cells	
PDGF-like factor from SV40/NIH/3T3	10
Breast carcinoma cell line factor	45

[a] TGFβ is produced by a variety of cells, including T cells, macrophages, platelets, and tumor cells.

icated macrophages (119). LDCF-F may be released *in vivo* at sites of cell-mediated immune reactions and could provide a chemotactic signal for fibroblasts.

Complement

Activation of serum complement by the classical or alternative pathways generates an 80,000 MW C5-derived fragment that is chemotactic for fibroblasts (130). Monocytes and neutrophils do not respond to this C5 fragment, and C5a which is chemotactic for neutrophils and monocytes is not chemotactic for fibroblasts (130). This 80,000-MW C5-complement fragment could provide a chemotactic stimulus to fibroblasts in a variety of inflammatory reactions in which complement is activated.

Matrix

Three components (collagens, fibronectin, and elastin) of the connective tissue matrix provide chemotactic signals for fibroblasts (120,126,153,154). Some of the degradation peptides from these components are also chemotactic for fibroblasts, suggesting that they could provide chemotactic

signals for fibroblasts at sites of virtually all types of inflammatory reactions occurring in connective tissue. The collagens are also chemotactic for monocytes (115).

Leukocytes

Leukocytes are a major source of leukotriene B$_4$, and this compound has the ability to induce chemotactic migration of fibroblasts at 10^{-8} M (92). Leukotriene B$_4$ is also chemotactic for monocytes, neutrophils, and eosinophils (92). It is generated in a wide spectrum of inflammatory reactions.

Platelets

Platelets are a source of two potent fibroblast chemoattractants, PDGF and TGFβ (121,157). The aggregation of platelets at sites of different classes of inflammatory reactions would be expected to release PDGF and TGFβ, providing powerful chemotactic signals for fibroblasts. Senior et al. (155) were able to show that treatment of PDGF with neutrophil elastase and reduction and alkylation yielded some peptides that stimulated fibroblast chemotaxis, whereas others stimulated mitogenesis of fibroblasts. TGFβ is produced by a variety of inflammatory, normal, and neoplastic cells and is thus an almost ubiquitous chemoattractant for fibroblasts (121). It is very potent in its chemotactic effect, inducing migration in the 10- to 50-pg/ml concentration range (121). The fibrotic response to certain tumors could be related to TGFβ production by such tumors.

Transformed and Neoplastic Cells

At least two different chemotactic factors for fibroblasts have been reported to be produced by transformed and neoplastic cells (10,45). The relationship of these factors to TGFβ remains to be established.

It is evident from the many different fibroblast chemoattractants in existence that nature has produced a certain degree of redundancy in the chemotactic response of fibroblasts, and this probably speaks for the importance of fibroblast chemotaxis in survival of multicellular organisms.

Serum Inhibitor of Fibroblast Migration

Since so many chemoattractants exist for fibroblasts, we began to wonder whether the body contained an inhibitor that would stop the chemotactic migration of fibroblasts. We found that serum from normal human donors contains a high-MW (~210,000) trypsin-sensitive protein that inhibits fibroblast migration to all known chemoattractants (107). This inhibitor is not cytotoxic to fibroblasts and does not alter collagen or protein synthesis (107). This serum inhibitor may function to control and modulate fibroblast chemotactic responses in general.

FIBROBLAST ADHERENCE

Fibroblasts *in vivo* adhere to, and grow in, a complex extracellular matrix. They are surrounded by the matrix and are thus in vastly different surroundings compared to monolayer cultures on glass or plastic surfaces *in vitro*. It is not possible to know exactly how fibroblast functions are influenced by components in the matrix surrounding them *in vivo*. Adhesion of fibroblasts to various substrate-coated surfaces has been studied *in vitro*. The pseudopodia of fibroblasts attach to substrates at loci called *adhesion plaques*. Examination of adhesion plaques by electron microscopy shows that many actin cables terminate at the locus in the plasma membrane that corresponds to the adhesion plaque (43). A specific actin-binding protein, called *vinculin*, plus alpha-actinin are located at the locus (43). Vinculin may serve to regulate actin attachment and organization at the junction between actin and an as-yet unidentified plasma membrane protein (8). Fibronectin is not located exactly at the locus of the adhesion plaque but is present adjacent to the adhesion plaque (7).

Membrane-intercalated heparan sulfate proteoglycans have been demonstrated to be present on a variety of cells such as fibroblasts, glial cells, endothelial cells, hepatocytes, and mouse mammary epithelial cells that interact with the matrix (73,105,135). The functions of the intercalated heparan sulfate proteoglycans have not yet been determined but may serve as a link between the intracellular and extracellular fibers by interacting with actin microfilaments on the cytoplasmic side of the membrane and with fibronectin, laminin (a high-MW glycoprotein of basement membranes), or collagen fibers in the extracellular space (see Chapter 29, *this volume*). Small chondroitin sulfate proteoglycans may also be intercalated in the plasma membrane, but their function is even less well defined than that of heparan sulfate proteoglycans (105).

In vitro, fibronectin promotes cell attachment and spreading and is thought to play a pivotal role in directing and mediating the organizations of pericellular and intercellular matrices and basement membranes *in vivo*. These matrices bind fibroblasts and other cell types and may regulate functions of cells. The major binding capabilities of fibronectin to collagen, to proteoglycan (heparin, heparan sulfate, and hyaluronic acid), and to the surfaces of fibroblasts and other cells presumably allow it to play a central role in matrix organization (74,76,85,109,194).

MODULATION OF FIBROBLAST FUNCTIONS BY CELLS AND COMPONENTS OF IMMUNE AND INFLAMMATORY REACTIONS

Pathologists have been aware of the association of fibrotic reactions with certain types of immune reactions for many years. Some of the best examples of fibrotic reactions accompanying cell-mediated immune reactions are seen with human infections caused by certain mycobacteria, fungi, and parasites (23,47,114). Over the past decade, more definite links have been established between the immune system and the connective tissue fibroblasts. In this section, we will review how various cells and components of immune and inflammatory reactions might modulate fibroblast functions (see Table 5).

Lymphokines

When T cells, and under certain circumstances B cells, are stimulated *in vitro* with specific antigen or mitogen, they release soluble protein mediators collectively called *lymphokines*. Several fibroblast functions have been shown to be influenced by lymphokines. In 1976, the first

TABLE 5. *Fibroblast functions modulated by products of the immune system and inflammatory cells*

Collagen production

100,000–170,000-MW lymphokine (stimulates)
Transforming growth factor β (stimulates)
Interleukin-1 α and β (stimulate)
Gamma-interferon (inhibits)

Collagenase production

Interleukin-1 α and β (stimulate)

Hyaluronic acid production

60,000-MW lymphokine (stimulates)
Interleukin-1 α and β (stimulate)
Transforming growth factor β (stimulates)

Proliferation

40,000–60,000-MW lymphokines (stimulates)
Interleukin-1 α and β (stimulate)
Transforming growth factor β (stimulates)
Platelet-derived growth factor (stimulates)
Gamma-interferon (inhibits and stimulates)
Prostaglandin E_2 (inhibits)

Chemotaxis

22,000-MW lymphokine (LDCF-F) (stimulates)
Transforming growth factor β (stimulates)
Platelet-derived growth factor (stimulates)
Macrophage-derived fibronectin (stimulates)
Leukotriene B_4 (stimulates)

lymphokine effects on fibroblast collagen production and chemotaxis were reported (66,129). We have already discussed the chemotactic lymphokine in the section dealing with fibroblast migration. The nature of the lymphokine-stimulating collagen production was not further characterized until 1984 (128). The collagen production factor is a heat-labile protein of approximately 100,000 to 170,000 MW (128). It stimulates fibroblasts to produce both type I and III collagens but does not stimulate growth or chemotaxis of fibroblasts (128; A. Postlethwaite, *personal observation*). Supernatants from cultures of stimulated T cells also contain a factor that inhibits collagen production (65,128). This factor has an MW of approximately 55,000 on Sephadex G-150 and has recently been shown to be gamma-interferon (34,64,65,128). Gamma-interferon (natural and recombinant) has been shown to reduce levels of fibroblast type I collagen mRNA (64).

T cells also produce a 40,000- to 60,000-MW protein that stimulates fibroblast growth (117,118,183). Gamma interferon (recombinant) has been reported to both stimulate and suppress fibroblast growth, depending on culture conditions (16,34). A 50,000 to 100,000-MW factor from lymphocytes or monocytes (source unclear) that inhibits fibroblast growth in the presence or absence of indomethacin has also been described (82).

Hyaluronic acid production by fibroblasts has recently been shown to be stimulated by a factor from T cells stimulated with concanavalin A (198). This factor has an MW of approximately 60,000 (186).

Transforming growth factor beta (TGFβ) exerts a variety of effects on fibroblasts. It stimulates chemotaxis (see section on fibroblast migration) as well as collagen and fibronectin production and is a growth factor for fibroblasts (63,67,99,121). TGFβ has recently been found to be produced by antigen- or mitogen-stimulated human T cells in culture (67). Future studies need to examine the relationship of TGFβ to any of the previously described lymphokines that modulate fibroblast chemotaxis, proliferation, and production of collagen and hyaluronic acid.

Monokines

Interleukin-1 (IL-1) is the most completely described and characterized soluble mediator from stimulated monocytes. It is synthesized and released from monocytes in response to a wide variety of stimulants, including lymphokines, phagocytosis of particles, lipopolysaccharide, immune complexes, and gamma interferon (110). Natural and recombinant human IL-1 α and β have been shown to exert a variety of effects on fibroblasts *in vitro*. Proliferation and production of prostaglandin E_2, collagen, collagenase, and hyaluronic acid are all stimulated by IL-1 α and β (35,122,123,125,150). Fibroblast chemotaxis is not stimulated by IL-1 α or β (A. Postlethwaite, *personal observation*). Several reports have emphasized that macrophages also secrete non-IL-1-related fibroblast growth factors (9,35,185). The relationship of these factors to TGFβ, which is also produced by stimulated macrophages, needs to be assessed.

Although not a monokine in the true sense of the word, macrophage-derived fibronectin is also chemotactic for fibroblasts and is the major fibroblast chemoattractant produced by adherent cells (macrophages) from schistosomal granulomas (191). Macrophages also secrete prostaglandin E_2 (which inhibits fibroblast proliferation) and leukotriene B_4 (which stimulates fibroblast chemotaxis) (78,92).

Cytokines

Various tumors have been shown to produce TGFβ-, IL-1-, and PDGF-like factors that can exert similar effects on fibroblasts as the authentic molecules (10,57,78,163,192). These cytokines may modulate fibroblast activities, for example, *in vivo* adjacent to tumors.

Platelets

As we have discussed in previous sections, platelets are the source of PDGF and TGFβ. PDGF stimulates fibroblast chemotaxis and proliferation, whereas TGFβ also stimulates collagen, fibronectin, and hyaluronic acid production.

Complement

We have fractionated, on Sephadex G-200, fresh human serum before and after activation of complement by zymosan particles and have analyzed column fractions for their ability to modulate fibroblast proliferation and production of collagen, glycosaminoglycans, and collagenase (A. Postlethwaite, and A.H. Kang, *personal observation*). We have not found any effects of activated complement on these parameters of fibroblast functions. As described above, activation of complement does generate a unique C5-derived fibroblast chemoattractant (130). It appears from these studies that activation of complement only leads to generation of a fibroblast chemoattractant, whereas other complement components are unable to modulate additional fibroblast activities.

ACKNOWLEDGMENTS

This work was supported, in part, by grants AM16506 and AM26034 from the National Institutes of Health as well as by research funds from the Veterans Administration.

REFERENCES

1. Abercrombie, M., Heaysman, J. E. M., and Pegrum, S. M. (1971): The locomotion of fibroblasts in culture. IV. Electron microscopy of the leading lamella. *Exp. Cell Res.*, 67:359–367.
2. Abercrombie, M., Heaysman, J. E. M., and Pegrum, S. M. (1972): Locomotion of fibroblasts in culture. V. Surface marking with concanavalin A. *Exp. Cell Res.*, 73:536–539.
3. Adams, S. L., Alwine, J. C., de Crombrugghe, B., and Pastan, I. (1979): Use of recombinant plasmids to characterize collagen RNAs in normal and transformed chick embryo fibroblasts. *J. Biol. Chem.*, 254:4935–4938.
4. Ali, I. U., Mautner, V. M., Lanza, R., and Hynes, R. O. (1977): Restoration of normal morphology: Adhesion and cytoskeleton in transformed cells by addition of a transformation sensitive surface protein. *Cell*, 11:115–128.
5. Baum, J. L. (1971): Source of the fibroblast in central corneal wound healing. *Arch. Ophthalmol.*, 85:473–477.
6. Beachey, E. H., Chiang, T. M., and Kang, A. H. (1979): Collagen platelet interaction. *Int. Rev. Connect. Tissue Res.*, 8:1–21.
7. Birchmeier, C., Kreis, T. E., Eppenberger, H. M., Winterhalter, K. H., and Birchmeier, W. (1980): Corrugated attachment membrane in WI-38 fibroblasts: Alternating fibronectin fibers and actin-containing focal contacts. *Proc. Natl. Acad. Sci. USA*, 77:4108–4112.
8. Birchmeier, W. (1981): Fibroblast focal contacts. *Trends Biochem. Sci.*, 6:234–237.
9. Bitterman, P. B., Rennard, S. I., Hunninghake, G. W., and Crystal, R. B. (1982): Human alveolar macrophage growth factor: Regulation and partial characterization. *J. Clin. Invest.*, 70:806–822.
10. Bleiberg, I., Harvey, A. K., Smale, G., and Grotendorst, G. R. (1985): Identification of a PDGF-like mitoattractant produced by NIH/3T3 cells after transformation with SV40. *J. Cell Biol.*, 123:161–166.
11. Bornstein, P., and Traub, W. (1979): The chemistry and biology of collagen. In: *The Proteins, Vol. 4*, edited by H. Newrath and R. L. Hill, pp. 411–632. Academic Press, New York.
12. Brandt, K. D. (1985): Glycosaminoglycans. In: *Textbook of Rheumatology*, edited by W. N. Kelley, E. D. Harris, Jr., S. Ruddy, and C. B. Sledge, pp. 237–253. W. B. Saunders, Philadelphia.
13. Burgeson, R. E., Morris, N. P., Murray, L. W., Duncan, K. G., Keene, D. R., and Sakai, L. Y. (1985): The structure of type VII collagen. *Ann. NY Acad. Sci.*, 460:47–57.
14. Burnett, W., Eichner, R., and Rosenbloom, J. (1980): Correlation of functional elastin messenger ribonucleic acid levels and rate of elastin synthesis in the developing chick aorta. *Biochemistry*, 19:1106–1111.
15. Burnett, W., Finnigan-Bunick, A., Yoon, K., and Rosenbloo, J. (1982): Analysis of elastin gene expression in the developing chick aorta using cloned elastin cDNA. *J. Biol. Chem.*, 257:1569–1572.
16. Brinkerhoff, C. E., and Guyre, P. M. (1985): Increased proliferation of human synovial fibroblasts treated with recombinant immune interferon. *J. Immunol.*, 134:3142–3146.
17. Cardinale, G. J., and Udenfriend, S. (1974): Prolylhydroxylase. *Adv. Enzymol.*, 41:245–300.
18. Carpenter, G. (1981): Vandate, epidermal growth factor and the stimulation of DNA synthesis. *Biochem. Biophys. Res. Commun.*, 102:1115–1121.
19. Carter, W. B. (1982): The cooperative role of the transformation sensitive glycoproteins. GP140 and fibronectin, in cell attractant and spreading. *J. Biol. Chem.*, 257:3249–3259.
20. Carter, W. B. (1982): Transformation-dependent alterations in glycoproteins of the extracellular matrix of human fibroblasts: Characterization of GP250 and the collagen-like GP140. *J. Biol. Chem.*, 257:13805–13815.
21. Carter, W. B., and Hakomor, S. (1978): A protease resistant, transformation-sensitive membrane glycoprotein ("170 Gp") and an

22. Carter, W. B., and Hakomori, S. (1981): A new cell surface, detergent-insoluble glycoproteins matrix of human and harvested fibroblasts. *J. Biol. Chem.*, 256:6953–6960.
23. Cheever, A. W. (1965): A comparative study of *Schistosoma mansoni* infections in mice, gerbils, multimammate rats and hamsters. II. Qualitative pathological differences. *Am. J. Trop. Med. Hyg.*, 14:227–245.
24. Cheung, H. S., Story, M. T., and McCarty, D. J. (1984): Mitogenic effects of hydroxyopatite and calcium pyrophosphate dihydrate crystals on cultured mammalian cells. *Arthritis Rheum.*, 27:668–674.
25. Chiang, T. M., Beachey, E. H., and Kang, A. H. (1975): Interaction of a chick skin collagen fragment (alpha 1–CB 5) with human platelets. Biochemical studies during the aggregation and release reaction. *J. Biol. Chem.*, 250:6916–6922.
26. Chu, M. L., De Wet, W., Bernard, M., Ding, J. F., Morabito, M., Myers, J., Williams, C., and Ramirez, F. (1984): Human pro alpha 1 (I) collagen gene structure reveals evolutionary conservation of a pattern of introns and exons. *Nature*, 310:337–340.
27. Chu, M. L., De Wet, W., Bernard, M., and Ramirez, F. (1985): Isolation of cDNA and genomic clones encoding human pro-alpha 1 (III) collagen. *J. Biol. Chem.*, 260:2315–2320.
28. Chu, M. L., Weil, D., De Wet, W., Bernard, M., Sippola, M., and Ramirez, F. (1985): Isolation of cDNA and genomic clones encoding human pro-alpha 1 (III) collagen. Partial characterization of the 3′ end region of the gene. *J. Biol. Chem.*, 260:4357–4363.
29. Cohen, I. K., Moore, C. D., and Diegelmann, R. F. (1979): Onset and localization of collagen synthesis during wound healing in open rat skin wounds. *Proc. Soc. Exp. Bio. Med.*, 160:458–462.
30. Courtney, H. S., Simpson, W. A., and Beachey, E. H. (1983): Binding of streptococcal lipoteichoic acid to fatty acid-binding sites on human plasma fibronectin. *J. Bacteriol.*, 153:763–770.
31. Davies, M., Barrett, A. J., Travis, J., Sanders, E., and Coles, G. A. (1977): The degradation of human glomerular basement membrane with purified lysosomal proteinases. *Clin. Sci. Mol. Med.*, 54:233–240.
32. De Wet, W. J., Chu, M. L., and Prockop, D. J. (1983): The mRNAs for the pro $\alpha 1$ (I) and pro $\alpha 2$ (I) chains of type I procollagen are translated at the same rate in normal human fibroblasts and in fibroblasts from two varients of osteogenesis imperfecta with altered steady-state rations of the two mRNAs. *J. Biol. Chem.*, 258:14385–14389.
33. Dinarello, C. A., Cannon, J. G., Mier, J. W., Bernheim, H. A., LoPreste, G., Lynn, D. L., Love, R. N., Webb, A. C., Auron, P. E., Reuben, R. C., Rich, A., Wolff, S. M., and Putney, S. D. (1986): Multiple biological activities of human recombinant interleukin 1. *J. Clin. Invest.*, 77:1734–1739.
34. Duncan, M. R., and Berman, D. (1985): Gamma interferon is the lymphokine and beta interferon the monokine responsible for inhibition of fibroblast collagen production and late but not early fibroblast proliferation. *J. Exp. Med.*, 162:516–527.
35. Estes, J. E., Pledger, W. J., and Gillespie, G. Y. (1984): Macrophage-derived growth factor for fibroblasts and interleukin-1 are distinct entities. *J. Leukocyte Biol.*, 35:115–129.
36. Ehterington, D. J. (1980): Proteinases in connective tissue breakdown. *Ciba Found. Symp.*, 75:87–103.
37. Fessler, L. I., and Fessler, J. H. (1982): Identification of the carboxyl peptides of mouse procollagen IV and its implications for the assembly and structure of basement membrane procollagen. *J. Biol. Chem.*, 257:9804–9810.
38. Fleischmajer, R., Olsen, B. R., and Kuhn, K., editors (1985): Biology, chemistry and pathology of collagen. *Ann. NY Acad. Sci.*, 460:1–537.
39. Forster, S. J., and Freedman, R. B. (1984): Catalysis by protein disulfide-isomerase of the assembly of trimeric procollagen from procollagen polypeptide chains. *Biosci. Rep.*, 4:223–229.
40. Freedman, R. B., and Hillson, D. A. (1980): Formation of disulfide bonds. In: *Enzymology of Post-Translational Modifications of Proteins, Vol. 1*, edited by R. B. Freedman and H. C. Hawkins, pp. 157–212. Academic Press, London.

41. Gallop, P. M., Blumenfeld, O. O., and Seifter, S. (1972): Structure and metabolism of connective tissue proteins. *Annu. Rev. Biochem.*, 41:617–645.

42. Gallop, P. M., and Paz, M. A. (1975): Post-translational protein modifications with special attention to collagen and elastin. *Physiol. Rev.*, 55:418–487.

43. Geiger, B. (1979): A 130 K protein from chicken gizzard: Its localization at the termini of microfilament bundles in cultured chicken cells. *Cell*, 18:193–205.

44. Glaser, J. H., and Conrad, H. E. (1979): Chondroitin SO₄ catabolism in chick embryo chondrocytes. *J. Biol. Chem.*, 254:2316–2325.

45. Gleiber, W. E., and Schiffmann, E. (1984): Identification of a chemoattractant for fibroblasts produced by human breast carcinoma cell lines. *Cancer Res.*, 44:3398–3402.

46. Goldberg, G. I., Wilhelm, S. M., Kronberger, A., Bauer, E. A., Grant, B. A., and Eisen, A. Z. (1986): Human fibroblast collagenase: Complete primary structure and homology to an oncogene transformation-induced rat protein. *J. Biol. Chem.*, 261:6600–6605.

47. Goodwin, R. A., Nickell, J. A., and DesPrez, R. M. (1972): Mediastinal fibrosis complicating healed primary histoplasmosis and tuberculosis. *Medicine*, 51:227–246.

48. Gosline, J. M., and French, C. J. (1979): Dynamic mechanical properties of elastin. *Biopolymers*, 18:2091–2103.

49. Gosline, J. M., and Rosenbloom, J. (1984): Elastin. In: *Extracellular Matrix Biochemistry*, edited by K. A. Piez and A. H. Reddi, pp. 191–227. Elsevier, New York.

50. Grant, M. E., and Prockop, D. J. (1972): The biosynthesis of collagen. *N. Engl. J. Med.*, 286:194–199.

51. Graves, P. N., Olsen, B. R., Fietzek, P. P., Prockop, D. J., and Monson, J. M. (1981): Comparison of the NH₂-terminal sequence of chick type I preprocollagen chains synthesized in an mRNA-dependent reticulocyte lysate. *Eur. J. Biochem.*, 118:363–372.

52. Gross, J., Highberger, J. H., Johnson-Wint, B., and Biswas, C. (1980): Mode of action and regulation of tissue collagenases. In: *Collagenase in Normal and Pathological Connective Tissue*, edited by D. E. Woolley and J. M. Evanson, pp. 11–35. John Wiley & Sons, Chichester, U.K.

53. Gross, J., and Lapiere, C. M. (1982): Collagenolytic activity in amphibian tissues: A tissue culture assay. *Proc. Natl. Acad. Sci. USA*, 48:1014–1022.

54. Hakomori, S., Fukuda, M., Sekiguchi, K., and Carter, W. B. (1984): Fibronectin, laminin, and other extracellular glycoproteins. In: *Extracellular Matrix Biochemistry*, edited by K. A. Piez and A. H. Reddi, pp. 229–275. Elsevier, New York.

55. Harris, A., and Dunn, G. (1972): Centripetal transport of attached pastides on both surfaces of moving fibroblasts. *Exp. Cell Res.*, 73:519–523.

56. Heinegard, D., and Paulson, M. (1984): Structure and metabolism of proteoglycans. In: *Extracellular Matrix Biochemistry*, edited by K. A. Piez and A. H. Reddi, pp. 277–328. Elsevier, New York.

57. Hernandez, A., Hibbs, M., and Postlethwaite, A. E. (1985): Establishment of basal cell carcinoma in culture: Evidence for a basal cell carcinoma-derived factor(s) which stimulates fibroblasts to proliferate and produce collagenase. *J. Invest. Dermatol.*, 85:470–475.

58. Highberger, J. H., Corbett, C., Dixit, S. N., Yu, W., Seyer, J. M., Kang, A. H., and Gross, J. (1982): The amino acid sequence of chick skin collagen α1 (I)-CB8 and the complete primary structure of the helical portion of the chick skin collagen α1 (I) chain. *Biochemistry*, 21:2048–2055.

59. Huerre, C., Junien, C., Weil, D., Chu, M. C., Morabito, M., Foubert, C., Myers, J. C., Van Cong, N., Gross, M. S., Prockop, D. J., Boue, A., Kaplan, J. C., De La Chapelle, A., and Ramirez, F. (1982): Human type I procollagen genes are located on different chromosomes. *Proc. Natl. Acad. Sci. USA*, 79:6627–6630.

60. Hynes, R. (1985): Molecular biology of fibronectin. *Annu. Rev. Cell Biol.*, 1:67–90.

61. Hynes, R. O., and Bye, J. M. (1974): Density and cell cycle dependence of cell surface proteins in hamster fibroblasts. *Cell*, 3:113–120.

62. Hynes, R. O., and Destree, A. (1981): Extensive disulfide bonding

at the mammalian cell surface. *Proc. Natl. Acad. Sci. USA*, 74:2844–2859.

63. Ignotz, R. A., and Massaque, J. (1986): Transforming growth factor β stimulates the expression of fibronectin and collagen and their incorporation into the extracellular matrix. *J. Biol. Chem.*, 261:4337–4345.

64. Jimenez, S. A., Freundlich, B., and Rosenbloom, J. (1984): Selective inhibition of human diploid fibroblast collagen synthesis by interferons. *J. Clin. Invest.*, 74:1112–1116.

65. Jimenez, S. A., McArthur, W., and Rosenbloom, J. (1979): Inhibition of collagen synthesis by mononuclear cells supernatants. *J. Exp. Med.*, 150:1421–1431.

66. Johnson, R. L., and Ziff, M. (1976): Lymphokine stimulation of collagen accumulation. *J. Clin. Invest.*, 58:240–252.

67. Kehrl, J. H., Wakefield, L. M., Roberts, A. B., Jakowlew, S., Alvarez-Mon, M., Derynck, R., Sporn, M. B., and Fauci, A. S. (1986): Production of transforming growth factor β by human T lymphocytes and its potential role in the regulation of T cell growth. *J. Exp. Med.*, 163:1037–1050.

68. Keski-Oja, J., Leof, E. B., Lyons, R. M., Coffey, R. J., Jr., and Moses, H. L. (1986): Transforming growth factors and control of neoplastic cell growth. *J. Cell Biochem.* (in press).

69. Keski-Oja, J., Sen, A., and Todaro, G. H. (1980): Direct association of fibronectin and actin molecules *in vitro*. *J. Cell Biol.*, 85:527–533.

70. Kivirikko, K. I., and Myllyla, R. (1984): Biosynthesis of collagens. In: *Extracellular Matrix Biochemistry*, edited by K. A. Piez and A. H. Reddi, pp. 83–118. Elsevier, New York.

71. Kivirikko, K. I., and Myllyla, R. (1979): Collagen glycosyltransferases. *Int. Rev. Connect. Tissue Res.*, 8:23–72.

72. Kivirikko, K. I., and Myllyla, R. (1980): The hydroxylation of prolyl and lysyl residues. In: *Enzymology of Post-Translational Modifications of Proteins, Vol. 1*, edited by R. B. Freedman and H. C. Hawkins, pp. 53–104. Academic Press, London.

73. Kjellen, L., Oldberg, A., and Hook, M. (1980): Cell-surface heparan sulfate. Mechanisms of proteoglycan-cell association. *J. Biol. Chem.*, 255:10407–10413.

74. Klebe, R. U. (1974): Isolation of a collagen-dependent cell attachment factor. *Nature*, 250:248–251.

75. Kleinman, H. K., Klebe, R. J., and Martin, G. R. (1981): Role of collagenous matrices in adhesion and growth of cells. *J. Cell Biol.*, 88:473–485.

76. Kleinman, H. K., McGoodwin, E. B., and Klebe, R. J. (1976): Localization of the cell attachment region in types I and II collagen. *Biochem. Biophys. Res. Commun.*, 72:426–432.

77. Knivaniemi, H., Savolainen, E. R., and Kivirikko, K. I. (1984): Human placental lysyl oxidase. Purification, partial characterization and preparation of two specific antisera to the enzyme. *J. Biol. Chem.*, 259:6996–7002.

78. Korn, J. H., Halushka, P. V., and LeRoy, E. C. (1980): Mononuclear cell modulation of connective tissue function: suppression of fibroblast growth by stimulation of endogenous prostaglandin production. *J. Clin. Invest.*, 65:543–554.

79. Kornblihtt, A. R., Vibe-Pedersen, K., and Baralle, F. E. (1984): Human fibronectin: Cell specific alternative mRNA splicing generates polypeptide chains differing in the number of internal repeats. *Nucleic Acids Res.*, 12:5853–5868.

80. Kornblihtt, A. R., Vibe-Pedersen, K., and Baralle, F. E. (1983): Isolation and characterization of cDNA clones for human and bovine fibronectins. *Proc. Natl. Acad. Sci. USA*, 80:3218–3222.

81. Kornblihtt, A. R., Vibe-Pedersen, K., and Baralle, F. E. (1984): Human fibronectin: Molecular cloning evidence for two mRNA species differing by an internal segment coding for a structural domain. *EMBO J.*, 3:221–226.

82. Korotzer, T. I., Page, R. C., Granger, G. A., and Rabinowitch, P. S. (1982): Regulation of growth of human diploid fibroblasts by factors elaborated by activated lymphoid cells. *J. Cell. Physiol.*, 111:247–254.

83. Kream, B. E., Rowe, D. W., Gworek, S. C., and Raiz, L. G. (1980): Parathyroid hormone alters collagen synthesis and procollagen

mRNA levels in fetal rat calvaria. *Proc. Natl. Acad. Sci. USA,* 77: 5654–5658.

84. Kuusela, P. (1978): Fibronectin binds to *Staphylococcus aureus. Nature,* 276:719–720.

85. Laterra, J., and Culp, L. A. (1982): Differences in hyaluronate binding to plasma and cell surface fibronectin. *J. Biol. Chem.,* 257: 719–726.

86. Levinson, W., Bhatnagar, R. S., and Liu, T. A. (1975): Loss of ability to synthesize collagen in fibroblasts transformed by Rous sarcoma virus. *J. Natl. Cancer Inst.,* 55:807–810.

87. Lewis, J., Chevallier, A., Kieny, M., and Wolpert, I. (1981): Muscle nerve branches do not develop in chick wings devoid of muscle. *J. Embryol. Exp. Morphol.* 64:211–232.

88. Mainardi, C. L., Dixit, S. N., and Kang, A. H. (1980): Degradation of type IV (basement membrane) collagen by a proteinase isolated from human polymorphonuclear leukocyte granules. *J. Biol. Chem.,* 255:5435–5441.

89. Mainardi, C. L., Seyer, J. M., and Kang, A. H. (1980): Type specific collagenolysis: A type V collagen-degrading enzyme from macrophages. *Biochem. Biophys. Res. Commun.,* 97:1108–1115.

90. Mason, M. R. (1981): Recent advances in the biochemistry of hyaluronic acid in cartilage. In: *Connective Tissue Research: Chemistry, Biology, and Physiology,* edited by Z. Dyl and M. Adam, pp. 87–112. Alan R. Liss, New York.

91. Mathews, M. B., and Deckers, L. (1969): The effect of acid mucopolysaccharide proteins on fibril formation from collagen solutions. *Biochem. J.,* 109:517–526.

92. Mensing, H., and Czarnetozki, B. M. (1984): Leukotriene B$_4$ induces *in vitro* fibroblast chemotaxis. *J. Invest. Dermatol.,* 82:9–12.

93. Menzel, E. J., Smolen, J. S., Liotta, L., and Reid, K. B. M. (1981): Interaction of fibronectin with C1q and its collagen-like fragment. *FEBS Lett.,* 129:188–192.

94. Miller, E. J. (1984): Chemistry of the collagens and their distribution. In: *Extracellular Matrix Biochemistry,* edited by K. A. Piez and A. H. Reddi, pp. 41–78. Elsevier, New York.

95. Miller, E. J., Harris, E. D., Jr., Chung, E., Finch, J. E., Jr., Mc-Croskery, P. A., and Butler, W. I. (1976): Cleavage of type II and II collagens with mammalian collagenase: Site of cleavage and primary structure at the NH$_2$-terminal portion of the smaller fragment released from both collagens. *Biochemistry,* 15:787–792.

96. Miller, J. M. (1985): The structure of fibril-forming collagens. *Ann. NY Acad. Sci.,* 460:1–13.

97. Morris, E. R., Rees, D. A., and Welsh, E. J. (1980): Conformation and dynamic interactions in hyaluronate solution. *J. Mol. Biol.,* 138:383–400.

98. Moses, A. C., Nissley, S. P., Rechler, M. M., Short, A., and Podskalny, J. M. (1979): The purification and characterization of multiplication stimulating activity (MSA) from media conditioned by a rat liver cell line. In: *Somatomedins and Growth,* edited by G. Geordano, J. J. Van Wyk, and F. Minuto, pp. 45–49. Academic Press, New York.

99. Moses, H. L., Tucker, R. F., Leof, R. J., Coffey, R. J., Jr., Hulper, J., and Shipley, G. D. (1985): Type-β transforming growth factor is a growth stimulator and a growth inhibitor. In: *Cancer Cells,* edited by J. Feramisco, B. Ozanne, and C. Stiles, pp. 65–71. Cold Spring Harbor Press, New York.

100. Mosher, D. F. (1975): Cross-linking of cold insoluble globulin by fibrin stabilizing factor. *J. Biol. Chem.,* 245:6614–6621.

101. Muller, R., Bravo, R., Burckhardt, J., and Curran, T. (1984): Induction of C-fos gene and protein by growth factors precedes activation of C-myc. *Nature,* 312:716–720.

102. Myers, J. C., Chu, M. L., Faro, S. H., Clark, W. J., Prockop, D. J., Ramirez, F. (1981): Cloning a cDNA for the pro-α2 chain of human type I collagen. *Proc. Natl. Acad. Sci. USA,* 78:3516–3520.

103. Myers, J. C., Dickson, L., De Wet, W., Bernard, M. P., Chu, M. L., Di Liberto, M., Pepe, G., Sangiorgi, F. O., and Ramirez, F. (1983): Analysis of the end of the human pro α2 (I) collagen gene: Utilization of multiple polyadenylation sites in cultured fibroblasts. *J. Biol. Chem.,* 258:10128–10135.

104. Nilsson, B., Nakazawa, K., Hassell, J. R., Newsome, D. A., and Hascall, V. G. (1983): Structure of oligosaccharides and the linkage region between karatan sulfate and the core protein on proteoglycans from monkey cornea. *J. Biol. Chem.,* 258:6056–6062.

105. Norling, B., Glimelius, B., and Wasteson, A. (1981): Heparan sulfate proteoglycan of cultured cells: Demonstration of a lipid—and a matrix-associated form. *Biochem. Biophys. Res. Commun.,* 103: 1265–1272.

106. Noro, A., Kimata, K., Oike, Y., Shinomura, T., Maeda, N., Yano, S., Tahahashi, N., and Suzuki, S. (1983): Isolation and characterization of a third proteoglycan (PG-Lt) from chick embryo cartilage which contains disulfide-bonded collagenous polypeptide. *J. Biol. Chem.,* 258:9323–9331.

107. Ochs, M. E., Postlethwaite, A. E., and Kang, A. H. (1987): Identification of a protein in sera of normal individuals that inhibits fibroblast chemotactic and random migration *in vitro. J. Invest. Dermatol.* (*in press*).

108. Oikasinen, J., and Ryhanen, L. (1981): Cortisol decreases the concentration of translatable type-I procollagen mRNA species in the developing chick-embryo calvaria. *Biochem. J.,* 198:519–524.

109. Oldberg, A., and Ruoslahti, E. (1982): Interaction between chondroitin sulfate proteoglycan, fibronectin and collagen. *J. Biol. Chem.,* 257:4859–4863.

110. Oppenheim, J. J., Kovacs, E. J., Matsushima, K., and Durum, S. K. (1986): There is more than one interleukin-1. *Immunol. Today,* 7:45–56.

111. Paglia, L. M., Wilczek, J., de Leon, L. D., Martin, G. R., Horlein, D., and Muller, P. (1979): Inhibition of procollagen cell-free synthesis by amino-terminal extension peptides. *Biochemistry,* 18: 5030–5034.

112. Paul, J. I., and Hynes, R. O. (1984): Multiple fibronectin subunits and their posttranslational modification. *J. Biol. Chem.,* 259:13477–13488.

113. Petersen, T. E., Thogersen, H., Skorstengaard, K., Vibe-Pedersen, K., Sottrup-Jensen, L., and Magnusson, S. (1983): Partial primary structure of bovine plasma fibronectin, three types of internal homology. *Proc. Natl. Acad. Sci. USA,* 80:137–141.

114. Poole, J. C. (1970): Chronic inflammation and tuberculosis. In: *General Pathology,* edited by H. W. Florey, pp. 1194–1217. W. B. Saunders, Philadelphia.

115. Postlethwaite, A. E. (1983): Cell-cell interaction in collagen biosynthesis and fibroblast migration. In: *Advances in Inflammation Research,* edited by G. Weissmann, pp. 27–55. Raven Press, New York.

116. Postlethwaite, A. E., and Kang, A. H. (1980): Characterization of guinea pig lymphocyte-derived chemotactic factor for fibroblasts. *J. Immunol.,* 124:1462–1466.

117. Postlethwaite, A. E., and Kang, A. H. (1982): Characterization of fibroblast proliferation factors elaborated by antigen- and mitogen-stimulated guinea pig lymph node cells: Differentiation from lymphocyte-derived chemotactic factor for fibroblasts, lymphocyte mitogenic factor and interleukin 1. *Cell. Immunol.,* 73:169–178.

118. Postlethwaite, A. E., and Kang, A. H. (1983): Induction of fibroblast proliferation by human mononuclear derived proteins. *Arthritis Rheum.,* 26:22–27.

119. Postlethwaite, A. E., and Kang, A. H. (1983): Latent lymphokines: Isolation of human latent lymphocyte-derived chemotactic factor for fibroblasts. In: *Interleukin Lymphokines and Cytokines. Proceedings of the Third International Lymphokine Workshop,* edited by J. J. Oppenheim and S. Cohen, pp. 535–541. Academic Press, New York.

120. Postlethwaite, A. E., Keski-Oja, J., and Kang, A. H. (1981): Induction of fibroblast chemotaxis by fibronectin. Localization of the chemotactic region to a 140,000 molecular weight fragment. *J. Exp. Med.,* 153:494–499.

121. Postlethwaite, A. E., Keski-Oja, J., Moses, H. L., and Kang, A. H. (1987): Stimulation of the chemotactic migration of human fibroblasts by transforming growth factor β. *J. Exp. Med.,* 165:251–256.

122. Postlethwaite, A. E., Keski-Oja, J., Moses, H., and Kang, A. H.

(1987): Stimulation of fibroblast hyaluronic acid production by transforming growth factor (TGF)β. *Submitted for publication.*

123. Postlethwaite, A. E., Lachman, L., Mainardi, C. L., and Kang, A. H. (1983): Stimulation of fibroblast collagenase production by human interleukin 1. *J. Exp. Med.,* 157:801–806.

124. Postlethwaite, A. E., Lachman, L. B., and Kang, A. H. (1984): Induction of fibroblast proliferation by interleukin-1 derived from human monocytic leukemia cells. *Arthritis Rheum.,* 27:995–1001.

125. Postlethwaite, A. E., Raghow, R., Stricklin, G. P., Poppleton, H., and Kang, A. H. (1987): Modulation of fibroblast functions by human recombinant interleukin 1 α and β. *Submitted for publication.*

126. Postlethwaite, A. E., Seyer, J. M., and Kang, A. H. (1978): Chemotactic attraction of human fibroblasts to type I, II and III collagens and collagen-derived peptides. *Proc. Natl. Acad. Sci. USA,* 75:871–875.

127. Postlethwaite, A. E., Smith, G. N., Lachman, L. B., Endres, R. O., Poppleton, H. M., Hasty, K. A., and Kang, A. H. (1987): Modulation of fibroblast glycosaminoglycans by mononuclear phagocytes: Stimulation of hyaluronic acid production by natural and recombinant interleukin 1. *Submitted for publication.*

128. Postlethwaite, A. E., Smith, G. N., Mainardi, C. L., Seyer, J. M., and Kang, A. H. (1984): Lymphocyte modulation of fibroblast functions *in vitro:* Stimulation and inhibition of collagen production by different effector molecules. *J. Immunol.,* 132:2470–2477.

129. Postlethwaite, A. E., Snyderman, R., and Kang, A. H. (1976): The chemotactic attraction of human fibroblasts to a lymphocyte-derived factor. *J. Exp. Med.,* 144:1188–1203.

130. Postlethwaite, A. E., Snyderman, R., and Kang, A. H. (1979): Generation of a fibroblast chemotactic factor in serum by activation of complement. *J. Clin. Invest.,* 64:1379–1385.

131. Prockop, D. J., Kivirikko, K. I., Tuderman, L., and Guzman, N. A. (1979): The biosynthesis of collagen and its disorders. *N. Engl. J. Med.,* 301:13–23, 77–85.

132. Prockop, D. J., and Kivirikko, K. I. (1984): The lessons from rare maladies provide a basis for understanding common diseases. *N. Engl. J. Med.,* 311:376–386.

133. Ramachandran, G. N. (1976): Molecular structure (of collagen). In: *Biochemistry of Collagen,* edited by G. N. Ramachandran and A. H. Reddi, pp. 45–84. Plenum, New York.

134. Ramirez, F., Bernard, M., Chu, M. L., Dickson, L., Sangiorgi, F., Weil, D., De Wet, W., Junien, C., and Sobel, M. (1985): Isolation and characterization of the human fibrillar collagen genes. *Ann. NY Acad. Sci.,* 460:117–129.

135. Rapraeger, A. C., and Bernfield, J. (1983): Heparan sulfate proteoglycans from mouse mammary epithelial cells. Putative membrane proteoglycan associates quantitatively with lipid vesicles. *J. Biol. Chem.,* 258:3632–3636.

136. Rennard, S. I., Stein, L. E., and Crystal, R. G. (1982): Intracellular degradation of newly synthesized collagen. *J. Invest. Dermatol.,* 79:77–82.

137. Roden, L. (1980): Structure and metabolism of connective tissue proteoglycans. In: *The Biochemistry of Glycoproteins and Proteoglycans,* edited by W. J. Lennarz, pp. 267–371. Plenum, New York.

138. Rubin, H., and Sanui, H. (1977): Complexes of inorganic pyrophosphate, orthophosphate and calcium: stimulants of 3T3 cell multiplication. *Proc. Natl. Acad. Sci. USA,* 74:5026–5030.

139. Ruoslahti, E., Engvall, E., and Hayman, E. (1981): Fibronectin: Current concepts of its structure and function. *Collagen Res.* 1: 95–128.

140. Ruoslahti, E., and Vaheri, A. (1975): Interaction of soluble fibroblast surface antigen with fibrinogen and fibrin. Identity with cold insoluble globulin of human plasma. *J. Exp. Med.,* 141:497–501.

141. Sandberg, L. B., Gray, W. R., and Franzblau, C., editors (1977): *Elastin and Elastic Tissue.* Plenum, New York.

142. Sandberg, L. B., Soskel, N. J., and Walt, M. S. (1982): Structure of the elastic fiber: An overview. *J. Invest. Dermatol.,* 79:128–140.

143. Sandberg, L. B., Weissman, N., and Smith, D. W. (1969): The purification and partial characterization of a soluble elastin like protein from copper-deficient porcine aorta. *Biochemistry,* 8:2940–2949.

144. Sandmeyer, S., and Bornstein, P. (1979): Declining procollagen mRNA sequences in chick embryo fibroblasts infected with Rous sarcoma virus. Correlation with procollagen synthesis. *J. Biol. Chem.,* 254:4950–4953.

145. Sandmeyer, S., Smith, R., Kiehn, D., and Bornstein, P. (1981): Correlation of collagen synthesis and procollagen messenger RNA levels with transformation in rat embryo fibroblasts. *Cancer Res.,* 41:830–838.

146. Sandy, J. D., Brown, H. L. G., and Lowther, D. A. (1978): Degradation of proteoglycan in articular cartilage. *Biochem. Biophys. Acta,* 543:536–544.

147. Sangiorgi, F. O., Benson-Chanda, V., De Wet, W., Sobel, M., Tsipouras, P., and Ramirez, F. (1985): Isolation and partial characterization of the entire human pro alpha 1 (II) collagen gene. *Nucleic Acids Res.,* 13:2207–2225.

148. Scher, C. D., Shepard, R. C., Antoniades, H. N., and Stiles, C. D. (1979): Platelet-derived growth factor and the regulation of the mammalian fibroblast cell cycle. *Biochem. Biophys. Acta,* 560:212–241.

149. Schilling, J. A. (1968): Wound healing. *Physiol. Rev.,* 48:374–423.

150. Schmidt, J. A., Mizel, S. B., Cohen, D., and Green, I. (1982): Interleukin 1, a potential regulator of fibroblast proliferation. *J. Immunol.,* 128:2177–2182.

151. Schwartzbauer, J. E., Tamkun, J. W., Lemischka, I. R., and Hynes, R. O. (1983): Three different fibronectin mRNAs arise by alternative splicing within the coding region. *Cell,* 35:421–431.

152. Sengel, P. (1976): *Morphogenesis of Skin.* Cambridge University Press, Cambridge, U.K.

153. Senior, R. M., Griffin, G. L., and Mecham, R. P. (1982): Chemotactic responses of fibroblasts to tropoelastin and elastin-derived peptides. *J. Clin. Invest.,* 70:614–618.

154. Senior, R. M., Griffin, G. L., Mecham, R. P., Wrenn, D. S., Prasad, K. U., and Urry, D. W. (1984): Val-Gly-Val-Ala-Pro-Gly, a repeating peptide in elastin, is chemotactic for fibroblasts and monocytes. *J. Cell Biol.,* 99:870–874.

155. Senior, R. M., Huang, J. S., Griffin, G. L., and Deuel, T. F. (1985): Dissociation of the chemotactic and mitogenic activities of platelet-derived growth factor by human neutrophil elastase. *J. Cell Biol.,* 100:351–356.

156. Seno, N., Meyer, K., Anderson, B., and Hoffman, P. (1965): Variations in keratosulfates. *J. Biol. Chem.,* 240:1005–1010.

157. Seppa, H., Seppa, S., and Yamada, K. M. (1980): The cell binding fragment of fibronectin and platelet-derived growth factor are chemoattractants for fibroblasts. *J. Cell Biol.,* 87:323a.

158. Seyer, J. M., and Kang, A. H. (1985): Structural proteins: Collagen, elastin and fibronectin. In: *Textbook of Rheumatology,* edited by W. N. Kelley, E. D. Harris, Jr., S. Ruddy, and C. B. Sledge, pp. 211–237. W. B. Saunders, Philadelphia.

159. Siegel, R. C. (1979): Lysyl oxidase. *Int. Rev. Connect. Tissue Res.,* 8:73–118.

160. Skorstengaard, J., Thogersen, H. C., and Petersen, T. E. (1984): Complete primary structure of the collagen-binding domain of bovine fibronectin. *Eur. J. Biochem.,* 140:235–243.

161. Skorstengaard, K., Thogersen, H. C., Vibe-Pedersen, K., Petersen, T. E., and Magnusson, S. (1982): Purification of twelve cyanogen bromide fragments from bovine plasma fibronectin and the amino acid sequence of eight of them. *Eur. J. Biochem.,* 128:605–623.

162. Solursh, M., Vaerewyck, S. A., and Reiter, R. S. (1974): Depression by hyaluronic acid of glycosaminoglycan synthesis by chick cultured embryo chondrocytes. *Dev. Biol.,* 41:233–240.

163. Sporn, M. B., and Roberts, A. B. (1986): Peptide growth factors and inflammation, tissue repair and cancer. *J. Clin. Invest.,* 78: 329–332.

164. Startex, P. M., Barratt, A. J., and Burleigh, M. C. (1977): The degradation of articular collagen by neutrophil proteinases. *Biochem. Biophys. Acta,* 183:386–397.

165. Stathakis, N. E., and Mosesson, M. W. (1977): Interaction among heparin, cold-insoluble globulin, and fibrinogen in formation on the heparin-precipitable fraction of plasma. *J. Clin. Invest.,* 60: 855–865.

166. Stiles, C. D., Capone, G. T., Scher, C. D., Antoniades, H. N., Van

Wyk, J. J., and Pledger, W. J. (1979): Dual control of cell growth by somatomedins and platelet-derived growth factor. *Proc. Natl. Acad. Sci. USA,* 76:L279–L283.

167. Stopak, D., and Harris, A. K. (1982): Connective tissue morphogenesis by fibroblast traction. *Dev. Biol.,* 90:383–398.

168. Sullivan, K. A., and Kagan, H. M. (1982): Evidence for structural similarities in the multiple forms of aortic and cartilage lysyl oxidase and a catalytically quiescent aortic protein. *J. Biol. Chem.,* 257:13520–13526.

169. Sumnerbell, D., Lewis, J. H., and Walpert, I. (1973): Positional information in chick morphogenesis. *Nature,* 244:492–496.

170. Tamkun, J. W., and Hynes, R. O. (1983): Plasma fibronectin is synthesized and secreted by hepatocytes. *J. Biol. Chem.,* 258:4641–4647.

171. Tamkun, J. W., Schwarzbauer, J. E., and Hynes, R. O. (1984): A single rat fibronectin gene generates three different mRNAs by alternative splicing of a complex exon. *Proc. Natl. Acad. Sci. USA,* 81:5140–5144.

172. Tolstoshev, P., Haber, R., Trapne, B. C., II, and Crystal, R. B. (1981): Procollagen messenger RNA levels and activity and collagen synthesis during fetal development of sheep lung, tendon and skin. *J. Biol. Chem.,* 256:9672–9679.

173. Toole, B. P. (1982): Developmental role of hyaluronate. *Connect. Tissue Res.,* 10:93–101.

174. Toole, B. P. (1982): Hyaluronate turnover during chondrogenesis in the developing chick limb and axial skeleton. *Dev. Biol.,* 29:321–330.

175. Toole, B. P., Jackson, G., and Gross, J. (1972): Hyaluronate in morphogenesis: Inhibition of chondrogenesis *in vitro. Proc. Natl. Acad. Sci. USA,* 69:1384–1389.

176. Toole, B. P., and Lowther, D. (1968): Dermatan sulfate protein: Isolation from and interaction with collagen. *Arch. Biochem.,* 128:567–575.

177. Trelstad, R. L., Birk, D. E., and Silver, F. H. (1982): Collagen fibrillogenesis in tissues, in solution, and from modeling: A synthesis. *J. Invest. Derm.,* 79:109–112.

178. Truppe, W., Basner, R., Von Figura, K., and Kresse, H. (1977): Uptake of hyaluronate by cultured cells. *Biochem. Biophys. Res. Commun.,* 78:713–719.

179. Truppe, W., and Kresse, H. (1978): Uptake of proteoglycans and sulfated glycosaminoglycans by culture skin fibroblasts. *Eur. J. Biochem.,* 85:351–356.

180. Underhill, C. B., and Dorfman, A. (1978): The role of hyaluronic acid in intercellular adhesion of cultured mouse cells. *Exp. Cell Res.,* 117:155–163.

181. Vibe-Pedersen, K., Kornblihtt, A. R., and Petersen, T. E. (1984): Expression of a human α-globulin/fibronectin gene hybrid generates two mRNA by alternative splicing. *EMBO J.,* 3:2511–2516.

182. Tsukameto, Y., Helsel, W. E., and Wahl, S. M. (1981): Macrophage production of fibronectin, a chemoattractant for fibroblasts. *J. Immunol.,* 127:673–678.

183. Wahl, S. M., Wahl, L. M., and McCarthy, J. B. (1978): Lymphocyte-mediated activation of fibroblast proliferation and collagen production. *J. Immunol.,* 121:942–946.

184. Wateson, A., Amado, R., Ingmar, B., and Heldin, C. H. (1975): Degradation of chondroitin sulphate by lysosomal enzymes from embryonic chick cartilage. *Protides Biol. Fluids Proc. Colloq. Bruges,* 22:431–435.

185. Wharton, W., Gillespie, G. Y., Russell, S. W., and Pledger, W. J. (1982): Mitogenic activity elaborated by macrophage-like cell lines acts as competence factor(s) for BALB/c 3T3 cells. *J. Cell Physiol.,* 110:93–100.

186. Whiteside, T. L., Worrall, J. G., Prince, R. K., Buckingham, R. B., and Rodnan, G. P. (1986): Soluble mediators from mononuclear cells increase the synthesis of glycosaminoglycan by dermal fibroblast cultures derived from normal subjects and progressive systemic sclerosis patients. *Arthritis Rheum.,* 28:188–197.

187. Wiestner, M., Krieg, T., Horlein, D., Glanville, R. W., Fietzek, P., and Muller, P. K. (1979): Inhibiting effect of procollagen peptides on collagen biosynthesis in fibroblast cultures. *J. Biol. Chem.,* 254:7016–7023.

188. Woolley, D. E. (1984): Mammalian collagenases. In: *Extracellular Matrix Biochemistry,* edited by K. A. Piez and A. H. Reddi, pp. 119–157. Elsevier, New York.

189. Woolley, D. E., Roberts, D. R., and Evanson, J. M. (1976): Correlation of functional elastin messenger ribonucleic acid levels and rate of elastin synthesis in the developing chick aorta. *Biochemistry,* 19:1106–1111.

190. Wyler, D. J., and Postlethwaite, A. E. (1983): Fibroblast stimulation in schistosomas. IV. Isolated egg granulomas elaborate a fibroblast chemoattractant *in vitro. J. Immunol.,* 130:1371–1375.

191. Wyler, D. J., and Rosenwasser, L. J. (1982): Fibroblast stimulation in schistosomiasis. II. Functional and biochemical characteristics of egg granuloma-derived fibroblast stimulating factor. *J. Immunol.,* 129:1706–1710.

192. Wyler, D. J., Stadecker, M. J., Dinarell, C. A., and O'Dea, J. F. (1984): Fibroblast stimulation in schistosomiasis. V. Egg granuloma macrophages spontaneously secrete a fibroblast-stimulating factor. *J. Immunol.,* 132:3142–3148.

193. Yamada, K. M., and Kennedy, D. W. (1979): Fibroblast cellular and plasma fibronectin are similar but not identical. *J. Cell Biol.,* 80:492–498.

194. Yamada, K. M., Kennedy, D. W., Kimata, K., and Pratt, P. M. (1980): Characteristics of fibronectin interactions with glycosaminoglycans and identification of active proteolytic fragments. *J. Biol. Chem.,* 255:6055–6063.

195. Yarden, Y., Escobedo, J. A., Kuang, W. J., Yang-Feng, T. L., Daniel, T. O., Tremble, P. M., Chen, E. I., Ando, M. E., Harkins, R. N., Francke, U., Fried, V. A., Ullrich, A., and Williams, L. T. (1986): Structure of the receptor for platelet-derived growth factor helps define a family of closely related growth factor receptors. *Nature,* 323:226–232.

196. Zardi, L., Siri, A., Carnemolla, B., Santi, L., Bardner, W. D., and Hoch, S. O., (1979): Fibronectin: A chromatrin-associated protein? *Cell,* 18:649–657.

Inflammation: Basic Principles and Clinical Correlates.
Edited by J. I. Gallin, I. M. Goldstein, and R. Snyderman.
Raven Press, Ltd., New York © 1988.

CHAPTER 31

Lymphocytes: Development and Function

John D. Stobo

The integrity of the immune system is crucially dependent on a complex series of interactions between its constituent functional units and, in particular, lymphocytes. In the past two decades the increase in knowledge of the biology, biochemistry, and molecular biology of lymphocyte function has been exponential. In the 1960s, it became clear that not all lymphocytes were the same. They could be divided into two broad populations based on differences in their ontogeny, display of certain surface molecules, and function. Thymus-derived lymphocytes (T cells) undergo initial differentiation in the thymus, display a receptor binding to sheep red blood cells, and function as effector cells for cell-mediated immunity. Bone-marrow-derived lymphocytes (B cells) undergo their differentiation in the fetal liver or adult bone marrow, display surface immunoglobulin molecules, and are the precursors of antibody-secreting plasma cells necessary for humoral immunity. In the 1970s, T and B cells were further categorized into discrete populations that serve effector and regulatory functions, and discrete effector functions were assigned to phenotypically distinct populations within T and B cells. In the 1980s, advances in molecular biology spawned a description of the genetic events allowing for the tremendous antigen diversity within T and B cells and provided techniques for determining how, at the single-cell level, activation is translated

into function. This progression of knowledge has been characterized by reductionism. In other words, in order to understand how the whole system works it is first necessary to understand the function of the individual parts. This chapter follows this principle in its organization. The development, structure, and function of T and B cells will be discussed individually.

One observation that fosters this reductionist mode is that surface molecules play an important role in lymphocyte differentiation and function. This is especially true for T cells, where phenotypic heterogeneity can correlate with functional heterogeneity. Recent terminology has designated these surface molecules as differentiation clusters (CD). The old terminology, OKT and LEU, refers to epitopes depicted by specific monoclonal antibodies. The CD determination refers to the whole molecule.

T-CELL SURFACE MOLECULES (TABLE 1)

CD2

CD2 is a 50-kilodalton (kD) structure present on 95% of thymocytes and 100% of peripheral-blood T lymphocytes. This molecule is the receptor by which T cells bind to sheep red blood cells. Monoclonal antibodies can detect

TABLE 1. *T-cell markers*

Designation	Molecular weight	Cell-surface expression (%)	
		Thymocytes	T cells
CD2	50 kD	95	100
CD3	T3-γ (25-kD glycoprotein) T3-δ (20-kD glycoprotein) T3-ϵ (20-kD protein)	93	100
CD4	65 kD	90	60
CD8	33–43-kD heterodimer on thymocytes 33-kD homodimer on peripheral T cells 27-kD secreted molecule	90	30
TCR[a]			
α	50-kD } disulfide-linked heterodimer	90	95
β	42-kD		
γ	55-kD } disulfide-linked heterodimer	3	<10
δ	40-kD		

[a] TCR, T-cell receptor.

three distinct epitopes in the molecule: $CD2_1$, $CD2_2$, and $CD2_3$ (26). The $CD2_1$ and $CD2_2$ epitopes are expressed on nearly all thymocytes and on all peripheral blood T cells, and the $CD2_1$ epitope is closely linked to the region binding to the sheep red blood cells. $CD2_3$ is expressed only when T cells are activated. Addition of antibodies to the $CD2_2$ epitope can induce expression of the $CD2_3$ epitope. Recently, the CD2 molecule has been implicated in a pathway of T-cell activation that does not involve direct signaling through the antigen receptor/T3 complex (31). Simultaneous addition of anti-$CD2_2$ and $CD2_3$ antibody can induce T-cell proliferation. The mitogen, phytohemagglutinin (PHA), may bind to the $CD2_2$ epitope, induce expression of $CD2_3$, and then bind to this epitope (29). The CD2 molecule, therefore, appears to be crucial in transmembrane signaling necessary for PHA-induced mitogenesis.

CD3

The CD3 (T3) complex is a heterotrimer expressed on approximately 93% of thymocytes and on 100% of peripheral blood T cells (42). The three CD3 peptides are called CD3/γ (a 25-kD glycoprotein), CD3/δ (a 20-kD glycoprotein), and CD3/ϵ (a 20-kD protein). Each of the T3 molecules spans the plasma membrane and have substantial cytoplasmic tails. The genes for the T3/δ chain have been cloned and been shown to reside on the distal portion of the long arm of chromosome 11.

The CD3 molecules have been shown to be linked, noncovalently, to the α/β antigen receptor heterodimer as well as a γ/δ heterodimer expressed on a small portion of thymocytes and peripheral T cells (42). The hydrophobic region of the transmembrane segment of the CD3/δ chain contains an aspartic acid residue, which can form a salt bridge with a lysine residue present in the transmembrane segment of the α or β chain (42). The relatively longer cytoplasmic tails of the T3 molecules, when compared with the α/β chain, suggests that, while the antigen-receptor molecules (α, β) play a crucial role in antigen recognition, the CD3 molecules may function to transmit signals across the plasma membrane into the interior of the cell (42).

CD4

The CD4 molecule exists as a 65-kD single-polypeptide chain displayed by approximately 90% of thymocytes and by 60% of peripheral-blood T cells. CD4 marks cells whose activation is dependent on the recognition of class II major histocompatibility complex (MHC) gene products (32). Antibodies with specificity for CD4 can block priming of cells by antigen recognized in conjunction with class II MHC gene products but does not block activation of cells that have already been primed (23). Based on this, it has been hypothesized that the CD4 complex serves as an adhesion molecule necessary to provide extra "glue" for priming T cells (Fig. 1). This glue is not necessary for cells that have been previously activated. The CD4 phenotype indicates cells that function predominately as helper cells for B-cell differentiation and as effector cells for delayed hypersensitivity (32).

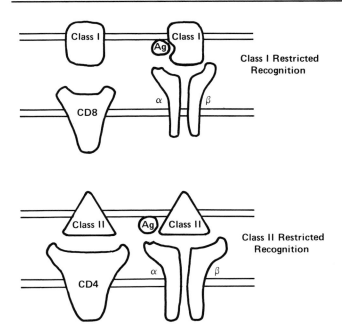

FIG. 1. Class I and class II restricted interactions with T cells. The proposed role of CD8 and CD4 molecules in MHC restriction is shown. In cells that recognize antigen in conjunction with class I MHC molecules, the CD8 molecule provides extra adhesion by reacting with the class I molecule. In situations where antigen is recognized in conjunction with class II MHC molecules, the CD4 molecule serves as an adhesion molecule by interacting with class II determinants alone. α and β refer to the α and β chains of the T-cell antigen receptor.

The CD4 molecule also serves as a receptor by which the HTLV-III virus infects mononuclear cells (24). Antibodies against the CD4 molecule can block HTLV-III infectivity, and transfection of CD4 genes into cells that previously could not be infected by HTLV-III renders them permissive for infection.

CD8

The CD8 epitope is expressed on approximately 90% of thymocytes and 30% of peripheral-blood T cells (7,36,37). On thymocytes, the CD8 molecule exists as a heterodimer of 33-kD and 43-kD polypeptides. On peripheral-blood T cells it exists as a 33-kD disulfide-linked homodimer. The molecule marks T cells whose activation is dependent on the recognition of antigen in conjunction with class I MHC gene products. Just as the CD4 complex appears to represent an adhesion molecule necessary for activation by antigen plus MHC class II gene products, the CD8 molecule appears to represent an adhesion molecule necessary for activation of cells by antigen seen in conjunction with class I MHC gene products (Fig. 1). The CD8 phenotype indicates cells that function predominately as killer cells for virally infected cells.

T-CELL RECEPTOR (TCR)

One of the most important advances in immunology has been the delineation of the molecules that constitute the T-cell receptor for antigen, coupled with the delineation of the genes that encode these molecules (4,12,25). From studies performed in the 1960s, it was clear that T cells demonstrated antigen specificity and immunologic memory. For example, immunization of an animal with a given antigen led to the generation of T cells primed to respond to that specific antigen and not others. Since the immune system must distinguish among a million different antigens to which it potentially can be exposed, it is necessary that T cells display an antigen receptor capable of exhibiting tremendous diversity. Since the only antigen recognition system known to exhibit such diversity involves immunoglobulins, it was fully expected that the antigen receptor on T cells would indeed be some form of immunoglobulin molecule. Initial studies failed to demonstrate these molecules on the surface of T cells; also, immunoglobulin genes in T cells were not rearranged, indicating that this mechanism of diversity was not used in these cells for antigen recognition. Two approaches proved crucial for demonstrating that the structure of the T-cell receptor was different from that of immunoglobulins. The first involved the generation of monoclonal antibodies capable of reacting only with T-cell clones reactive with a specific antigen (12). Animals were immunized with clones of antigen-specific T cells, and monoclonal antibodies generated by somatic cell hybridization were tested for their ability to react to the immunizing clone as compared to other clones of T cells reactive to other antigens. The assumption was that the antibodies reacting only to the immunizing clone would have specificity for epitopes in that T-cell receptor. The antibody then could be used to isolate the T-cell receptor from that specific clone and determine its structure. These studies demonstrated that such monoclonal antibodies can immunoprecipitate, from solubilized T cells, a disulfide-linked heterodimer made up of an $\sim$50,000-kD acidic α chain and an $\sim$42,000-kD basic β chain (Fig. 2). A second approach to determine the structure of the antigen receptor utilized techniques of recombinant DNA (4). This approach, termed *subtraction hybridization,* was based on the assumption that RNA expressed in T cells, but not B cells, could represent RNA that translates the antigen receptor. For example, a complementary DNA (cDNA) library was constructed from the mRNA of T cells and then hybridized against a cDNA library generated from the messenger RNA (mRNA) of B cells to assay for RNA that was specific for T cells and not present in B cells. Approximately 10 to 20 T-cell-specific clones could be demonstrated; only two of these were of the size that could encode for the α and β chain depicted by the monoclonal

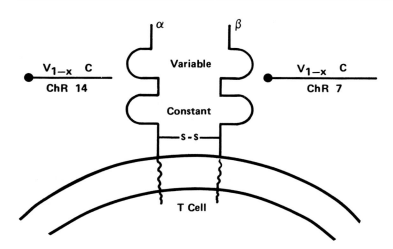

FIG. 2. T-cell receptors for antigen. Genes encoding the α chain of the T-cell receptor for antigen can be broadly divided into variable(V)- and constant(C)-region genes residing on chromosome (CHR) 14, whereas genes encoding the β chain can be broadly divided into variable and constant region genes located on chromosome 7. The basic structure of the antigen-receptor heterodimer can also be divided into variable and constant regions encoded by the respective genes.

antibody studies. Molecular analysis of the genes encoding for the RNA demonstrated that they had a structure very similar to immunoglobulin genes (see Fig. 2 and Table 2). That is, they contained variable (V), diversity (D), joining (J), and constant region genes. Moreover, it was the rearrangement of these genes which could account for tremendous diversity in the antigen receptor, just as rearrangement among immunoglobulin genes could account for the tremendous diversity of immunoglobulin molecules. Analysis of the structure of the α and β chains of the T-cell receptor confirmed the genetic organization and demonstrated that, like immunoglobulin molecules, the α and β chains could be divided into variable and constant region domains (Fig. 2). The variable region of each chain isolated from T-cell clones reactive with distinct antigens was different, whereas the constant region was quite similar. As indicated in Table 2, there are approximately 60 different V regions for the α chain and approximately 30 different V regions for the β chain. The V regions, by themselves, are not sufficient to account for the antigenic diversity present in the T-cell repertoire (approximately one million different specificities). Antigenic diversity is accounted for by three different mechanisms. First, each different V region gene can code for an α or β chain that has a different antigen specificity. Therefore, there are approximately 60 different specificities encoded for by the V region of the α and approximately 30 different specificities encoded for by the V region of the β chain. Second, junctional diversity is created when a single V region is joined to a different D or J region. For example, interaction of a single V region gene of the β chain gene with two different D regions results in two β chains that have different antigen specificities. Therefore, specificity encoded for by the α and β chains is represented by the total number of V regions multiplied by the total number of D regions multiplied by the total number of J regions. There are no D-region genes in the α chain, but there are 40 J regions. This results in 2,400 (60 × 40) different specificities that can be accounted for by differential V-J joining. In the case of the β chain, the 30 different V regions can combine with any of the two different D regions and any of the 12 different J regions, leading to a total diversity of 720 (30 × 2 × 12). Third, the antigen specificity of the α-β heterodimer is not simply inherent in the primary amino acid sequence of the α and β chains but, instead, can also be dictated by interactions between the two chains. A single α chain interacting with two different β chains will give rise to a receptor having two distinct antigen specificities. The repertoire of the α-β heterodimer is, therefore, a multiple of the diversity generated by each chain (720 × 2,400), leading to a structure capable of manifesting 1.7 million different specificities. This is consistent with the total amount of diversity necessarily present in the T-cell repertoire.

The approach of subtractive hybridization to look for genes whose expression is unique to T cells demonstrated a gene which was distinct from the genes encoding the α and β chain but which was rearranged in mature, cytotoxic T cells (16). Based on the nucleotide sequence, the gene could code for a protein of approximately 55,000 molecular weight. Initially, all rearrangements of this gene were shown to be nonproductive, in that they could not transcribe RNA. Moreover, no product of this gene, called the γ gene, could be detected in the cytoplasm or on the

TABLE 2. *Organization of the genes coding the human T-cell receptor for antigen*

α Chain, chromosome 14:	$V_{1-60}\ J_{1-40}\ C_{\alpha}$
β Chain, chromosome 7 (long arm):	$V_{1-30}\ D_{\beta_1}\ J_{\beta_1,1-6}\ C_{\beta_1}\ D_{\beta_2}\ J_{\beta_2,1-6}\ C_{\beta_2}$
γ Chain, chromosome 7 (short arm):	$V_{\gamma_1,1-10}\ V_{\gamma_2,1-4}\ V_{\gamma_3}\ J_{\gamma_1}\ C_{\gamma_1}\ J_{\gamma_2}\ C_{\gamma_2}$

surface of T cells. Unfortunately, the terminology can be confusing. The designation γ here and the designation δ further on in this paragraph refer to polypeptide chains that are distinct from the γ and δ polypeptides that comprise two of the three molecules in the CD3 complex. In an attempt to clarify this, the designation TCR will precede γ and δ to distinguish these molecules from the γ and δ molecules of the CD3 complex. Very recently, TCR-γ chains have been demonstrated on the surface of a small proportion (less than 5%) of thymocytes and peripheral T cells (2,3,18,19,20,43). The TCR-γ chain is linked by a disulfide bond to another chain (42,000 molecular weight), termed TCR-δ, which is also distinct from TCR-α and -β chains. The TCR-γ-δ heterodimer is expressed in conjunction with CD3 molecules both in the thymus and in the periphery and is found only on cells that lack the CD4 and CD8 molecules (Table 3). To date, clones of T cells expressing the TCR-γ-δ heterodimer have been generated, and antibodies to the heterodimer can induce T-cell activation, suggesting that the complex is capable of transmitting activation signals. Mice that lack a thymus have circulating T cells displaying the TCR-γ-δ heterodimer but not T cells displaying the α-β heterodimer. This finding suggests that whereas thymic maturation is necessary for expression of TCR-α-β, it is not necessary for expression of TCR-γ-δ. Transfection experiments demonstrate that antigen specificity can be accounted for entirely by the α-β heterodimer (5). Therefore, the TCR-γ-δ heterodimer does not appear to be required to recognize antigen. What function is served by TCR-γ-δ is not known.

T-CELL RECOGNITION OF ANTIGEN

It is clear that the α-β heterodimer clearly serves as a T-cell receptor for antigen and can determine its specificity, whether the antigen is a soluble one or a particle such as a virus. Transfection of genes encoding for the α and β chains into cytotoxic T cells, for example, results in cells that have the antigen specificity dictated by the transfected

α and β chains. It is equally clear that the α-β heterodimer does not recognize antigen alone, but instead must view antigen in conjunction with either class I or class II MHC gene products. In the case of soluble antigen, recognition is restricted by class II MHC molecules, whereas for replicating intracellular organisms such as viruses, recognition is restricted by class I MHC gene products (38). For soluble antigens, the antigen is taken up, degraded, and expressed in conjunction with class II MHC gene products on the surface of antigen-presenting cells such as macrophages. The process of antigen degradation and expression is energy dependent and can be further inhibited by the drug chloroquine (38). Expression of viral antigens can occur in any cell bearing class I molecules. The metabolic process by which viral antigens are expressed appears to be different than that required for the expression of soluble antigens. Although the viral antigens are degraded, expression is not inhibited by chloroquin.

It has been hypothesized that there is a physical interaction between antigen and other class I or class II MHC molecules. However, with only one or two exceptions, it has not been possible to demonstrate physical association between antigen alone and either class I or class II MHC molecules (14). However, in the presence of a T-cell clone specific for the antigen under study, it appears that the strength of the bond between the antigen and MHC gene product is markedly increased and that the binding of the antigen to the MHC determinant can be detected (1,28,40). Therefore, it appears that an antigen-specific T cell can stabilize the association between the specific antigen and the surface MHC gene product. It is the combination of antigen plus MHC gene product which is best recognized by the T-cell α-β heterodimer. Neither antigen alone nor autologous MHC bearing cells alone can activate antigen-specific T cells.

The fact that the antigen receptor contains two chains and that the heterodimer recognizes two structures (antigen plus MHC molecules) suggest that one chain of the antigen-receptor heterodimer might recognize antigen and that the other chain might recognize MHC. To investigate this, the structures of the α and β chains from different

TABLE 3. T-cell ontogeny

	TCR gene rearrangement[a]				Surface phenotype					
	T_γ	T_δ	T_α	T_β	CD2	CD3	CD4	CD8	TCR-$\gamma\delta$	TCR-$\alpha\beta$
Thymic cortex	−	−	−	−	+	−	−	−	−	−
	+	+	−	−	+	+	−	−	+	−
	+	+	−	+	+	+	−	−	+	−
	+	+	+	+	+	+	+	+	+	+
Thymic medulla	+	+	+	+	+	+	+	+	+	+

[a] The indicated rearrangements for the δ gene are implied from the phenotypic expression of $T_{\gamma\delta}$. The δ gene has not yet been cloned.

clones that recognize the same antigen in conjunction with different MHC molecules have been compared. The structure of both the α and β chains from each of the clones is different, suggesting that the simplistic situation in which one chain recognizes antigen and the other chain recognizes MHC, or vice versa, does not exist. Instead, the α-β heterodimer most likely recognizes an associated determinant generated by interactions between antigen plus MHC. This recognition requires interaction between the α and β chain. This is very similar to the situation demonstrated for antibody molecules, in which it can be shown that the combination of light and heavy chains binds best to antigen when compared to the binding of isolated light and heavy chains.

T-CELL ONTOGENY

The appearance of mature T cells in the periphery represents the culmination of a series of differentiation steps initiated when stem cells enter the thymic cortex. From the cortex, cells traverse the medulla and pass out into the peripheral lymphoid tissue, a process that takes approximately 3 days. During intrathymic development, T cells acquire functional maturity that is reflected by gene expression and changes in the cell surface phenotype (31,33; Table 3). The first T-cell marker expressed is the CD2 determinant, followed by expression of CD3. The first cells found to express CD3 do so in conjunction with the TCR-γ-δ heterodimer. These cells are CD4 and CD8 negative. Subsequently, the TCR-α-β heterodimer is expressed in conjunction with CD3, and thymocytes diverge to two distinct lineages; 65% of the T cells are CD4 positive and CD8 negative, whereas the remaining 35% are CD4 negative and CD8 positive.

The fact that the TCR-γ-δ heterodimer is found to be expressed before the TCR-α-β heterodimer does not mean that a single lineage of cells exists with cells displaying the latter developing from those expressing the former. There may be two distinct populations of cortical T cells: CD2+, TCR-γ-δ+, CD4−, CD8−; and CD2+, TCR-α-β+, CD4+,

CD8+. It appears that the CD3-positive cells, which express the TCR-γ-δ heterodimer and which are CD4 and CD8 negative, may represent a distinct, minor subpopulation of thymocytes. When these cells are grown *in vitro*, they do not develop CD4 or CD8 expression, nor do they develop into cells that express the TCR-α-β heterodimer.

The thymus plays a major function in determining the repertoire of antigen reactivity among T cells. It is within the thymus that T cells acquire the ability to recognize self-MHC gene products. As discussed, recognition of antigen by peripheral T cells requires that they see antigen in conjunction with MHC gene products. In the case of helper T cells, the antigen is viewed in conjunction with class II MHC gene products or Ia molecules. Cytotoxic T cells see antigen in conjunction with class I MHC gene products. Expression of MHC antigens on thymus epithelial cells is important in this learning process (thymus epithelial cells express both class I and class II MHC gene products). This process of MHC recognition is exemplified by the following experiment (21; Fig. 3). MHC heterozygote (A × B stem cells) were allowed to develop into T cells in the presence of epithelium expressing both A and B MHC molecules (A × B) or in the presence of epithelium bearing only A or only B MHC molecules. In the presence of A × B epithelium, the ratio of T cells restricted to recognize antigen in conjunction with A or B MHC molecules was 1:1. In the presence of the A epithelium, the ratio of A-restricted to B-restricted T cells was 10:1; in the case of the B epithelium, the ratio was 1:10. Therefore, the interaction between stem cells and thymic epithelium bends the thymic repertoire to recognize self-MHC gene products. These cells, however, do not recognize self-MHC gene products alone but, instead, are restricted to recognize self-MHC in conjunction with antigen. Presumably, T cells that can recognize self-MHC gene products alone are deleted during interthymic development. This is consistent with the observation that only 10% of T cells that enter the thymus ever exit to the periphery (34).

Thymic epithelial cells clearly play an important role in MHC restriction (13,17). Just how this is accomplished

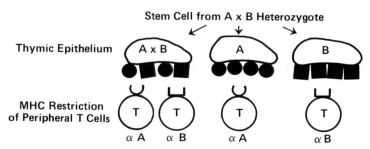

FIG. 3. Thymic epithelium determines T-cell MHC restriction. Diagrammed is an experiment in which stem cells from an MHC heterozygous animal (A × B) were incubated with thymic epithelial cells bearing both A and B MHC determinants (A × B), thymic epithelial cells bearing only A MHC determinants (A), and thymic epithelial cells bearing only B MHC determinants (B). In the presence of A × B thymic epithelium, the developed T cells were restricted to recognize antigen in conjunction with either A or B MHC determinants. In the case of thymic epithelium bearing only A MHC, the developed T cells could recognize antigen only when seen in conjunction with A MHC determinants. In the case of B thymic epithelium, the T cells could recognize antigen only in conjunction with B MHC determinants.

is not clear. It is possible to isolate, from the thymus, epithelial cells that engulf anywhere from 10 to 100 thymocytes. These "thymic nurse cells" presumably function to determine MHC restriction. These "nurse cells" do display both class I and class II MHC molecules.

Immunocompetent T cells leave the thymus through the walls of postcapillary venules in the medulla and enter the blood stream. They subsequently distribute among the peripheral lymphoid tissue. Once there, the cells localize in the thymus-dependent regions (the inner cortex) of lymph nodes, periarterial sheaths of the spleen, or intranodular areas and Peyer's patches. In less than 24 hr, the T cells leave by efferent lymphatics, move into the large lymphatics, and then travel into the thoracic duct and return to the blood stream. The movement of lymphocytes from the circulation into lymphoid organs occurs through specialized areas in the blood vessels called *postcapillary high endothelial venules.* The lymphocytes bind to these venules by means of specific receptors, and there is a strong preference to binding to venules of those lymphoid organs from which the lymphocytes were originally isolated. For instance, if peripheral lymph node cells are injected back into an animal from which they are removed, they preferentially localize to the peripheral lymph nodes, not to the spleen or the Peyer's patches. Identical preferential tracking of Peyer's patch lymphocytes can be demonstrated. Evidence that the lymphoid organ localization of lymphocytes is due to binding to cell-surface recognition units comes from studies in which cell-surface molecules are proteolytically removed by digestion with enzymes. Lymphocytes so treated lose their homing pattern, and their tissue distribution becomes random. One

molecule that is involved in directing migration to peripheral lymph nodes, as opposed to Peyer's patches, has a molecular weight of 80,000 and is detected by monoclonal antibody MEL-14 (8). Treatment of peripheral T cells with this antibody inhibits their migration into lymph nodes but does not affect their migration into Peyer's patches.

T-CELL ACTIVATION

Two advances have facilitated our understanding of the biochemical and molecular events involved in T-cell activation. The first advance is the finding that large numbers of T cells can be cloned in culture using the T-cell growth factor, interleukin-2 (IL-2). This provides large numbers of cells for study. The second advance is the finding that monoclonal antibodies with specificity for molecules on the cell surface can serve as agonists for the physiologic activation of T cells by antigen. For example, monoclonal antibodies with specificity for the TCR-α-β heterodimer or for CD3 can substitute for antigen and serve as stimuli for T-cell activation. These antibodies then can be used to induce activation of cloned T-cell lines and obviate the need to use specific antigen (42).

The events involved in T-cell activation are summarized in Fig. 4 (15,42). Activation of resting T cells requires two stimuli. One is represented by antigen seen in conjunction with MHC gene products on the surface of accessory cells. A signal transmitted to the antigen-receptor-heterodimer/CD3 complex activates a phosphodiesterase, phospholipase C, which cleaves an important metabolite of mem-

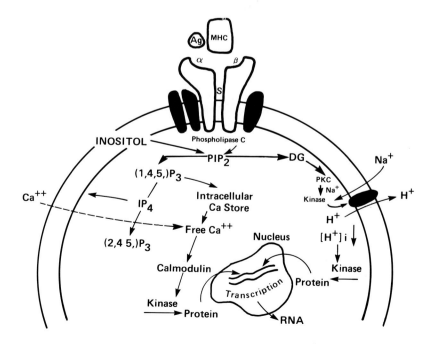

FIG. 4. T-cell activation. Signals transmitted to the antigen-receptor/CD3 complex begin with activation of the enzyme phospholipase C, which converts phosphatidylinositol-bisphosphate (PIP$_2$) into two important intermediaries, namely (1,4,5)-P$_3$ and diacylglycerol (DG). The IP$_3$ increases cytoplasmic free calcium by mobilizing calcium from bound intracellular stores. Conversion of IP$_3$ to IP$_4$ can cause sustained increase in cytoplasmic free calcium by opening calcium channels and allowing the influx of extracellular calcium. This increase in calcium may activate a kinase that phosphorylates proteins, which can then shuttle into the nucleus and turn on transcription of important genes. Diacylglycerol can activate protein kinase C, which then may phosphorylate a sodium proton exchanger that pumps hydrogen ions out of the cell, thus raising the pH. This, in turn, may activate a kinase that again phosphorylates a protein capable of regulating transcription of genes important for the function of the activated cell.

brane inositol, phosphatidylinositol-bisphosphate (PIP_2), into two crucial products. The first is 1,4,5-inositol-tris-phosphate ($1,4,5-IP_3$). This product binds to receptors present on the endoplasmic reticulum and mobilizes calcium from bound intracellular stores. Resulting increases in cytoplasmic free calcium constitute a crucial intracellular signal necessary for activation. Recently, it has been suggested that a kinase generates IP_4 from $1,4,5-IP_3$ (27). This product can open calcium channels in the cell membrane, thus sustaining increases in cytoplasmic free calcium.

A second major product generated from PIP_2 is diacylglycerol (DG). DG is a physiologic activator of an intracellular kinase, protein kinase C (PKC) (41). Activation of PKC constitutes a crucial second signal for T-cell activation. Following activation of kinase C, there occurs a drop in intracellular hydrogen ion concentration reflected by an increase in intracellular pH of 0.1 to 0.15 pH units. This export of hydrogen ions presumably occurs through activation of a sodium proton exchanger, activation which may involve phosphorylation of the exchanger by PKC.

The importance of increases in cytoplasmic free calcium and activation of PKC in T-cell activation is demonstrated by the finding that it is possible to by-pass requirements for the antigen-receptor/T3 complex in T-cell activation by adding calcium ionophores and phorbol esters to T cells. Calcium ionophores increase cytoplasmic free calcium, both by directly mobilizing calcium from bound intracellular stores and by opening channels in the cell membrane which allow influx of extracellular calcium. Phorbol esters penetrate into the cell and directly activate PKC (42).

For resting T cells, it appears that a third signal is also required for cell activation. Physiologically, this third stimulus can be represented by interleukin-1 (IL-1), a lymphokine released by accessory cells (Fig. 5). Precisely how IL-1 contributes to the biochemical events required for T-cell activation is not clear. It is interesting that in addition to activating PKC, phorbol esters also mimic the events mediated by IL-1 (6,30,41).

During physiologic activation of T cells, the three signals required for activation, i.e., increases in cytoplasmic free calcium, activation of PKC, and events mediated by IL-1, are mediated by two stimuli. The first stimulus is an interaction between the antigen-receptor-heterodimer/T3 complex and antigen presented by accessory cells. This stimulus is sufficient to cause cleavage of PIP_2 into the two metabolic products, which increase cytoplasmic free calcium and activate PKC. IL-1, which is released by the accessory cell, then provides the second stimulus and, thereby, the third signal necessary for T-cell activation.

Movement of the antigen-receptor-heterodimer/CD3 complex on the cell surface is important in activation. Under conditions where soluble antibodies to the antigen-

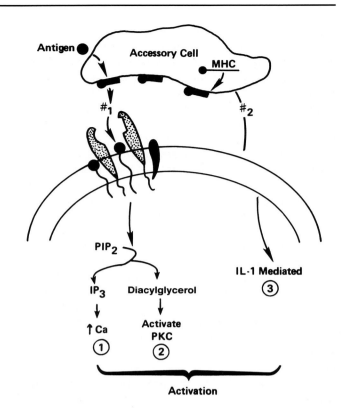

FIG. 5. Two stimuli and three signals are required for T-cell activation. Activation of resting T cells requires two stimuli, which consequently mediate three signals. The first stimulus is transmitted to the antigen-receptor/CD3 complex and is represented by recognition of antigen in conjunction with MHC gene products. This stimulus initiates the two signals represented by the generation of inositol-trisphosphate (IP_3) and diacylglycerol. The increase in cytoplasmic free calcium and activation of protein kinase C, which occur in response to each of these signals, respectively, is not sufficient to activate resting T cells. A third signal, which is mediated by the lymphokine interleukin-1 (IL-1), is also required. The biochemical pathway by which IL-1 participates in activation is unknown.

receptor/T3 complex are utilized, the complex is removed from the cell surface. More importantly, whereas sufficient amounts of IP_3 are generated to increase cytoplasmic free calcium, there is not sufficient activation of PKC to provide a second signal for T-cell activation. Immobilization of antibodies to the antigen-receptor/CD3 complex recapitulates the events occurring when antigen is seen on the surface of a cell in conjunction with MHC gene products (42). That is to say, the immobilized antibodies do not result in the clearing of the antigen-receptor/T3 complex from the cell surface, and activation of PKC is such that a sufficient second signal is generated.

The culmination of these biochemical events is the appearance of proteins not previously synthesized in the cell. For most of these proteins, such as IL-2 and gamma interferon, this increased synthesis represents events occurring at the level of gene transcription (9,42). The cascade of events initiated at the cell surface induce the appearance of new gene products by initiating gene transcription rather than by affecting the processing of transcribed RNA, translation of RNA into protein, or posttranslational events. It is possible that the initial biochemical events generate proteins which then bind to regulatory regions of genes, causing their activation.

Two genes whose expression is initiated during T-cell activation are crucial for the growth of stimulated T cells. These are genes coding for the IL-2 receptor and genes coding for the synthesis of IL-2 (10; Fig. 6) (see also Chapter 14, *this volume*). Activation of these genes occurs in response to independent signals. For example, addition of phorbol esters can result in increased expression of the receptor for IL-2 but does not influence synthesis of IL-2. Calcium ionophores may increase IL-2 synthesis but do not influence IL-2 receptor expression (41). In the presence of increased expression of IL-2 receptors, IL-2 acts in an autocoid fashion to expand growth of the activated T cell. Subsequently, IL-2 receptors are down-regulated so that autonomous T-cell proliferation does not ensue.

As indicated, the CD3 heterotrimer is noncovalently linked to the TCR-α-β heterodimer on the T-cell surface. Antibodies to CD3, as well as antibodies to TCR-α-β, can

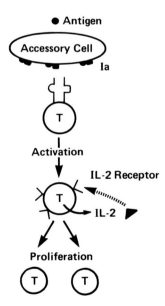

FIG. 6. T-cell activation. T-cell activation culminates in the expression of several genes that previously were not transcribed. Two of these are crucial for T-cell development and include a gene that encodes a receptor for interleukin-2 (IL-2) and a gene that encodes for IL-2. IL-2 then acts in an autocoid reaction stimulating the proliferation of T cells that have been activated. Subsequently, there is down-regulation of the IL-2 receptor so that autonomous proliferation does not ensue.

trigger T-cell activation. Therefore, activation of T cells by antigen plus MHC occurs through a five-chain structure. How each of these five chains contribute to activation is not known. It is possible that the CD3 complex simply serves to stabilize the α-β heterodimer on the cell surface. The finding that the α-β heterodimer is never expressed in the absence of the CD3 complex supports this possibility. Alternatively, the CD3 complex may play an important role in signal transduction. In this model, the α-β heterodimer would confer antigen recognition and, thus, specificity. Transduction of signals from the outside to the inside of the cell might occur via the CD3 complex in response to perturbations of the α-β chain complex. The finding that activation of T cells results in phosphorylation of one of the CD3 chains supports this possibility. Phosphorylation is a hallmark of signal transduction mediated by other receptors.

T-CELL FUNCTION

There are two major functions of T cells: effector and regulatory. Effector functions include graft versus host reactivity, cytotoxicity, and delayed hypersensitivity. Regulatory function includes modulation of both cell mediated and humoral immunity.

Cell-mediated cytotoxicity is discussed elsewhere in this volume. The effector function of T cells in delayed hypersensitivity will be discussed here as a prototype of T-cell function. The number of T cells specific for a single antigenic determinant is exceedingly small: approximately one of every 100,000. Therefore, reactivity of T cells to a foreign antigen containing, for example, 10 different antigenic determinants would not result in substantial immune reactivity unless there was some way by which the small number of T cells activated could enhance their reactivity. This is accomplished through the liberation of soluble material, lymphokines. Lymphokines act on other lymphocytes and macrophages in an antigen-nonspecific fashion, thus augmenting, by recruitment, the number of T cells reactive to the initial antigen.

Delayed hypersensitivity is crucially required for host defense against infection with organisms that replicate intracellularly, such as viruses, fungi, and mycobacteria. Activation of reactive T cells is not initiated by interactions between these organisms in the circulation and the T cell but, instead, are initiated only when these organisms are presented to a T cell in conjunction with products of genes in the MHC. For example, circulating virus cannot activate T cells potentially reactive to that virus. Instead, the virus must encounter a macrophage or infect a cell and replicate. Viral antigens are then expressed on the cell surface, in conjunction with MHC gene products. Recognition of the viral antigens in conjunction with the

MHC gene product then can activate the T cell of the appropriate specificity. As mentioned previously, in the case of replicating virus, it is class I MHC gene products that are recognized in association with viral antigens.

Activation of the appropriate T cell by the virus plus MHC can result in the synthesis of lymphokines listed in Table 4. Release of IL-2 serves to expand the population of T cells whose activation was initiated by the specific viral antigen, as well as T cells in the immediate vicinity which are expressing IL-2 receptors as a consequence of reactivity to some other antigen. This can account for the nonspecific activation of T cells in an area of T-cell reactivity initiated by a specific antigen. Interferons released during T-cell activation can directly act to inhibit viral replication among infected cells.

One of the strongest amplifiers in T-cell reactivity is the activation of monocytes/macrophages. Lymphokines such as macrophage inhibition factor (MIF) result in the accumulation of macrophages in the area of activation by inhibiting the random migration of macrophages through tissues. Release of lymphokines such as macrophage-activating factor (MAF) (probably IFN-γ) can "arm" these accumulated macrophages to destroy, by phagocytosis or cytolytic mechanisms, the antigen under attack. The formation of granulomas in response to foreign antigen may also be a consequence of a delayed T-cell-mediated reaction. T cells release factors that cause macrophages to fuse forming giant cells. The effector cells that serve to initiate such reactions as delayed hypersensitivity have the phenotype of CD4$^+$ and CD8$^-$.

T cells also play an important role in regulating immune reactivity. For example, T cells are required to help B cells develop into antibody-secreting plasma cells (see next section), and T cells play an important role in helping other T cells develop their full cytotoxic potential. In addition, it has been postulated that T cells can suppress immune reactivity. This postulate is based on experiments in which the transfer of T cells can blunt delayed hypersensitivity responses or antibody production occurring in response to challenges with specific antigen. However, it has been difficult to isolate numbers of suppressor cells sufficient to clearly and convincingly establish their existence and mechanism of action. For suppressor cells that have been isolated, there have been no noted rearrangements of genes encoding the TCR-α or -β chain. Therefore, if they truly exist, these cells must use an antigen receptor that is distinct from the α or β chain. These cells also fail to express λ or δ chains. Therefore, if these cells exist, it is not clear exactly how they could function in an antigen-specific function. Presently, there is growing skepticism concerning the existence of suppressor T cells.

B LYMPHOCYTES

B cells represent the effector cells of the humoral limb of immunity. Under the appropriate conditions, they develop into plasma cells that secrete abundant amounts of immunoglobulin into the interstitial and intervascular spaces. As noted for T-cell activation, advances in recombinant DNA technology have enhanced our knowledge of the events involved in the development and function of B cells. In fetal life, stem cells destined to become B cells migrate from the yolk sac to the liver. Within this microenvironment, they express genes that characterize and distinguish B cells from other lymphoid elements. In adult life, B cells are continually produced in the bone marrow. The factors in the microenvironment which are important for the development and differentiation of B cells within the fetal liver and adult bone marrow microenvironment are not clear. Fetal liver does contain a population of nonadherent cells; it also contains bone marrow, a population of adherent cells that are necessary for B-cell development.

The hallmark of the B-cell/plasma-cell lineage is immunoglobulin. Surface immunoglobulin serves as the antigen receptor on B cells transmitting at least one signal necessary for activation (11). Plasma cells secrete immunoglobulin that is of the same specificity and isotype as the surface immunoglobulin on the B-cell receptor. The development of B cells into plasma cells can be best explained by examining the genetic events that occur among immunoglobulin genes (Fig. 7). Like genes for the T-cell receptor, immunoglobulin genes consist of V-, D-, J-, and C-region genes. Genes encoding the constant region of the heavy chain consist of CμCδCγCϵCα, representing the corresponding immunoglobulin isotype. In humans, genes encoding the κ chain are on chromosome 2, genes encoding the λ chain are on chromosome 22, and genes encoding the heavy chain are on chromosome 14. During the development of B cells, there is an orderly, sequential rearrangement in each of these genes, and the translated light and heavy chains join to form an intact

TABLE 4. *Lymphokines synthesized by T cells which are important for their effector function*

Lymphokine	Function
IL-2	T-cell growth factor
IL-3	Hematopoietic growth factor
Interferons	Inhibit viral growth
Macrophage-activation factor (interferon-γ and others?)	Activates several metabolic processes by macrophages, including cytotoxicity
B-cell growth factor	Stimulates B-cell proliferation
B-cell differentiation factor	Stimulates B-cell differentiation into plasma cells

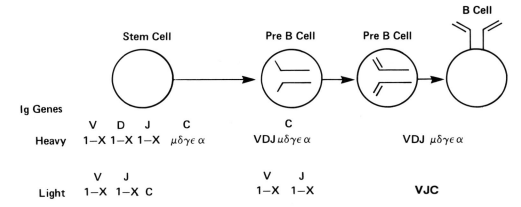

FIG. 7. B-cell development and Ig rearrangement. The development of B cells from stem cells proceeds through an orderly series of events characterized by rearrangements in immunoglobulin genes. First, there occurs rearrangement in immunoglobulin heavy-chain genes in which a VDJ complex rearranges and links to a new heavy-chain gene. This results in the synthesis and presence of IgM heavy chains in the cytoplasm. Subsequently, a rearrangement in light-chain genes occurs, characterized by the linking of a VJ complex to a constant-region gene. This is followed by a synthesis of light chains, which then combine with the heavy chains, thus forming an intact, monomeric IgM molecule in the cytoplasm. Finally, as the cell moves from the pre-B cell into the B-cell stage, the IgM is inserted in the cell membrane and serves as a receptor for antigen.

immunoglobulin molecule. At the stem-cell level, none of the immunoglobulin genes are rearranged; also, they exist in the germ-like configuration and are not transcribed. The earliest stage of development, in which a cell can be defined as committed to the B-cell lineage, is the pre-B-cell stage. At this stage, the first immunoglobulin gene rearrangement is represented by a joining of genes in the D and J region of the heavy chain on one allele. This is followed by the joining of one V-region gene to the D-J complex, and finally the VDJ complex is linked to a $C\mu$ gene. At this point, the heavy chains of IgM are present in the cytoplasm of the pre-B cell. Next, rearrangement occurs among the light-chain genes. First, an allele of the κ chain rearranges. If this results in a normal VJC segment, the gene is transcribed and the κ chains associate with μ heavy chains in the cytoplasm. If the rearrangement is aberrant or truncated, then rearrangement involving the other κ-chain allele occurs. If this is a normal gene rearrangement, then this transcribes a κ chain that can associate with μ heavy chains. If neither of the κ-chain rearrangements are functional, then rearrangements occur first at one and then at another of the λ-chain alleles. If these rearrangements result in a functional VJC, then transcription occurs and λ heavy chains are associated with the μ heavy chains of the cytoplasm. If neither of these rearrangements are productive, B-cell development terminates.

At the B-cell stage, the immunoglobulin synthesized in the cytoplasm moves to the cell membrane, and the IgM becomes a receptor important in B-cell activation. Further maturation along the B-cell line is represented by the rearrangement of heavy-chain constant-region genes.

However, there is no further rearrangement among the VDJ genes so that antigen specificity of the immunoglobulin does not change, even though there is a change in the isotype. Next, an IgD molecule appears on the cell surface in conjunction with IgM. The appearance of this surface IgD is an important event and allows B cells to move forward into distinct differentiation pathways where they could display IgD only, IgE only, or IgA only.

Development to the stage where a cell expresses IgM and IgD occurs independently of stimulation with antigen. From here, further differentiation is dependent on antigen stimulation and can occur in one of several pathways. First, the B cell can be activated to express only surface IgM and then develop into a plasma cell that secretes IgM. Second, the B cell can be activated to a stage where it expresses one of the subclasses of IgG and then can develop into a plasma cell that secretes that IgG subclass. Third, it could develop into a B cell that displays IgA and then into a plasma cell that secretes IgA. Finally, it could develop into a B cell that expresses IgE and into a plasma cell that secretes IgE (Fig. 8). Recently, there have been many studies to delineate the biochemical events involved in B-cell activation as well as to explore the cell-to-cell interactions and the soluble materials involved in this process. Activation steps required to drive B cells into antibody-secreting plasma cells can be divided into three stages (Fig. 9). The first stage is represented by interactions between antigen and surface immunoglobulin receptors. This induces the expression of receptors for specific growth factors. The second stage is represented by interactions between T cells specific for the same antigen and antigen-presenting cells. This interaction results in the release of

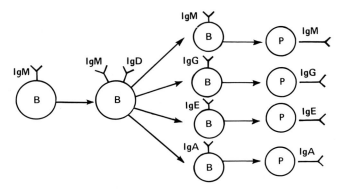

FIG. 8. B-cell–plasma-cell development. B cells initially display IgM on the surface. At this stage, interaction between the IgM antigen receptor and antigen leads to inactivation of the cell. Activation does not occur until the cell expresses both IgM and IgD. From this point, the B cell can move forward to produce cells expressing only IgM, only IgG, only IgE, or only IgA. From here, the B cells can develop into plasma cells that secrete an immunoglobulin corresponding to the isotype expressed on the surface.

growth factors such as B-cell growth factor (BCGF), which causes proliferation of B cells but does not induce their differentiation into plasma cells. The third stage is represented by the action of a group of factors called B-cell differentiation factors (BCDF), also released from T cells that cause a differentiation of B cells into immunoglobulin-secreting plasma cells.

REGULATION OF IMMUNE REACTIVITY

It is clear that T cells can play a crucial role in amplifying both cell-mediated and humoral immunity. It is equally clear that circulating antibodies can modulate

these same reactivities. The most direct demonstration of this is an experiment in which, following immunization of an animal, specific antibody is removed and replaced with normal serum. When compared to control animals, the amount of antibody produced in response to a single antigenic challenge is dramatically increased. In other words, there is antibody-mediated feedback inhibition that modulates the humoral response to a specific antigen.

There are three mechanisms by which antibodies can modulate immune reactivity (Fig. 10). In the first mechanism, the antibody competes with receptors on T and B cells for the antigen and, thus, prevents activation. In this situation, the inhibitory effects of antibody are concentration-dependent. In the second mechanism, the Fc portion of the antibody is important and, presumably, mediates its effects by binding to Fc receptors on the surface of B and T cells. In this situation, the Fc region of the antibody binds to the Fc receptor. The antigen-combining region of the antibody then cross-links antigen receptors on the surface of the cell and can either inhibit or augment immune reactivity. The third mechanism by which antibodies can modulate immune reactivity occurs through the idiotypic network in which antibodies react with determinants present in receptors for antigen. *Idiotype* refers to an antigenic determinant present in the variable region of an immunoglobulin or T-cell receptor which can react with antigens (Fc antibodies, antigen receptors). Since these antigenic determinants are limited to the variable region, each immunoglobulin molecule or T-cell receptor specific for a given antigen will have an idiotypic determinant which is specific for that immunoglobulin or receptor and which is distinct for immunoglobulin molecules or T-cell receptors reactive with other antigens. According to Jerne's network hypothesis, antibody produced in response to antigen stimulates production of anti-

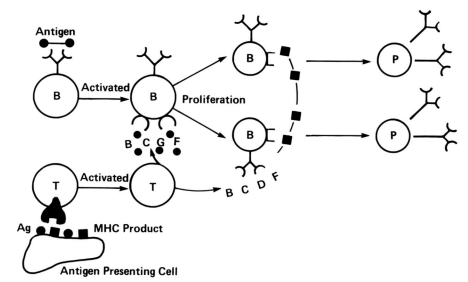

FIG. 9. B-cell development into plasma cells. Development of plasma cells from B cells involves three major steps. In the first step, the immunoglobulin receptor on B cells interacts with antigen, leading to activation and expression of receptors for growth factors, such as B-cell growth factor (BCGF). In the second step, T cells activated by antigen seen in conjunction with MHC determinants release BCGF, thus allowing the proliferation of B cells and expression of receptors for other differentiating factors such as B-cell differentiation faction (BCDF). In the third step, activated T cells release BCDF, which allow the B cells to differentiate into plasma cells. These then secrete immunoglobulin having the same antigen specificity as the immunoglobulin receptor displayed on the B cell.

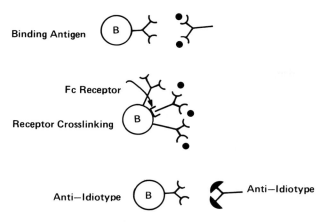

FIG. 10. Three mechanisms by which antibody regulates immune reactivity. In the first mechanism, high concentrations of circulating antibody compete with receptors on immunocompetent cells, such as B cells, for circulating antigen. In this mechanism the antibody simply acts as a sponge to sop up antigen, thus preventing activation of antigen-specific cells. In the second mechanism, the antibody binds to an Fc receptor present on the surface of cells, binds to antigen present in antigen receptors, and cross-links the receptors. This cross-linking can result either in inactivation or activation. In the third mechanism, an antibody is made against epitopes present in circulating antibodies. This anti-idiotype can react with cellular receptors to that antigen and, depending on the concentration and isotype of the anti-idiotype, can either cause inactivation or activation of B cells and T cells.

idiotypes, which then regulate the production of antibody to that antigen. Since the antibody initially formed in response to the antigen carries the specificity of the immunoglobulin antigen receptor on B cells, the anti-idiotype antibody can directly react with the B-cell receptor. Whether or not this interaction augments or suppresses immune reactivity depends on several factors, including the amount of anti-idiotype formed and the isotype of the antibody. Anti-idiotypes can also react with the antigen receptor on T cells and can modulate T-cell effector functions, such as delayed hypersensitivity.

Antigen can also modulate immune reactivity. Whether antigen enhances or inhibits an immune response (tolerance) is related to three factors. The first one is the concentration of antigen used for immunization. Very high concentrations or low concentrations of antigen fail to generate a significant immune response and can inhibit reactivity or can render an animal tolerant to subsequent challenge with the same antigen. This is referred to as *high-zone* and *low-zone tolerance,* respectively. In both high-zone and low-zone tolerance, the lack of reactivity resides at the level of the T cell. In other words, the T cell has become tolerant to subsequent challenge. In high-zone tolerance, B cells are also paralyzed. In some cases, this paralysis is reflected by deletion of the clone of T or B

cells responsive to the particular antigen; in other situations, however, clones of antigen-reactive cells are present but cannot be activated.

A second factor related to antigen-induced regulation depends on when, during the development of an organism, the antigen is encountered. Immunization during embryonic life can result in tolerance. This was demonstrated by the classic experiment in which injection of spleen cells from strain-B mice into neonatal strain-A mice rendered the strain-A mice tolerant to subsequent skin grafts obtained from strain-B mice.

The third factor related to the ability of antigen to induce tolerance is the chemical characteristics of the antigen. For example, one isomer of a compound can be immunogenic, whereas another can produce unresponsiveness to subsequent challenge with the immunogenic compound.

SUMMARY

Advances in our basic understanding of lymphocyte differentiation and function have already had a tremendous impact in devising strategies to beneficially manipulate immune reactivity and have contributed to our understanding of how rearrangements of immune reactivity may occur. Two examples of this are: (i) the use of monoclonal antibodies to CD3 and CD4 to inhibit cell-mediated reactivity that contributes to graft rejection and autoimmune states; (ii) our increased understanding of how the HIV virus inhibits T-cell function. Given the rate of the generation of new knowledge in this area, further advances in understanding and manipulating the immune system are to be expected in the foreseeable future.

REFERENCES

1. Ashwell, J. D., and Schwartz, R. H. (1986): T-cell recognition of antigen and the Ia molecule as a ternary complex. *Nature,* 320:176–179.
2. Bank, I., DePinho, R. A., Brenner, M. B., Cassimeris, J., Alt, F. W., and Chess, L. (1986): A functional T3 molecule associated with a novel heterodimer on the surface of immature human thymocytes. *Nature,* 322:179–181.
3. Brenner, M. B., McLean, J., Dialynas, D. P., Strominger, J. L., Smith, J. A., Owen, F. L., Seidman, J. G., Ip, S., Rosen, F., and Krangel, M. S. (1986): Identification of a putative second T-cell receptor. *Nature,* 322:145–149.
4. Davis, M. M. (1985): Molecular genetics of the T cell-receptor beta chain. *Annu. Rev. Immunol.,* 3:537–560.
5. Dembic, Z., Von Boehmer, H., and Steinmetz, M. (1986): The role of T-cell receptor and α and β genes in MHC-restricted antigen recognition. *Immunol. Today,* 7(10):308–311.
6. Durum, S. K., Schmidt, J. A., and Oppenheim, J. J. (1985): Interleukin 1: An Immunological Perspective. *Annu. Rev. Immunol.,* 3:263–287.
7. Fujimoto, J., Stewart, S. J., and Levy, R. (1984): Immunochemical analysis of the released Leu-2 (T8) molecule. *J. Exp. Med.,* 160:116–124.
8. Gallatin, W. M., Weissman, I. L., and Butcher, E. C. (1983): A cell-

surface molecule involved in organ-specific homing of lymphocytes. *Nature,* 304:30–34.

9. Granelli-Piperno, A., Andrus, L., and Steinman, R. M. (1986): Lymphokine and nonlymphokine mRNA levels in stimulated human T cells. *J. Exp. Med.,* 163:922–937.

10. Greene, W. C. (1986): The human interleukin-2 receptor. *Annu. Rev. Immunol.,* 4:69–95.

11. Hamaoka, T., and Ono, S. (1986): Regulation of B-cell differentiation: Interactions of factors and corresponding receptors. *Annu. Rev. Immunol.,* 4:167–204.

12. Haskins, K., Kappler, J., and Marrack, P. (1984): The major histocompatibility complex-restricted antigen receptor on T cells. *Annu. Rev. Immunol.,* 2:51–66.

13. Haynes, B. F. (1984): Phenotypic characterization and ontogeny of components of the human thymic microenvironment. *Clin. Res.,* 500–507.

14. Inada, T., and Mims, C. A. (1984): Mouse Ia antigens are receptors for lactate dehydrogenase virus. *Nature,* 309:59–61.

15. Isakov, N., Wolfgang, S., and Altman, A. (1986): Signal transduction and intracellular events in T-lymphocyte activation. *Immunol. Today,* 7(9):271–275.

16. Kranz, D. M., Saito, H., Heller, M., Takagaki, Y., Haas, W., Eisen, H. N., and Tonegawa, S. (1985): Limited diversity of the rearranged T-cell gene. *Nature,* 313:752–755.

17. Kyewski, B. A. (1986): Thymic nurse cells: Possible sites of T-cell selection. *Immunol. Today,* 7(12):374–379.

18. Lanier, L. L., Federspiel, N. A., Ruitenberg, J. J., Phillips, J. H., Allison, J. P., Littman, D., and Weiss, A. The T cell antigen receptor complex expressed on normal peripheral blood CD4-, CD8-T lymphocytes: A CD3-associated disulfide-linked-chain heterodimer. *J. Exp. Med. (in press).*

19. Lanier, L. L., and Weiss, A. (1986): Presence of Ti (WT31) negative T lymphocytes in normal blood and thymus. *Nature,* 324:268–270.

20. Littman, D., Newton, M., Crommie, D., Siew-Lan, A., Seidman, J. G., Gettner, S., and Weiss, A. Characterization of an expressed CD3-associated Ti chain reveals C domain polymorphism. *Nature (in press).*

21. Lo, D., and Sprent, J. (1986): Identity of cells that imprint H-2-restricted T-cell specificity in the thymus. *Nature,* 319:672–675.

22. Majerus, Ph. W., Connolly, T. M., Deckmyn, H., Ross, T. S., Bross, T. E., Ishii, H., Bansal, V. S., and Wilson, D. B. (1986): The metabolism of phosphoinositide-derived messenger molecules. *Science,* 234:1519–1526.

23. Marrack, P., Endres, R., Shimonkevitz, R., Zlotnik, A., Dialynas, D., Fitch, F., and Kappler, J. (1983): The major histocompatibility complex-restricted antigen receptor on T cells. *J. Exp. Med.,* 158:1077–1091.

24. McDougal, J. S., Mawle, A., Cort, S. P., Nicholson, J. K. A., Cross, G. D., Scheppler-Campbell, Hicks, D., and Sligh, J. (1985): Cellular tropism of the human retrovirus HTLV-III/LAV. *J. Immunol.,* 5:3151–3162.

25. Meuer, S. C., Acuto, O., Hercent, T., Schlossman, S. F., and Reinherz, E. L. (1984): The human T-cell receptor. *Annu. Rev. Immunol.,* 2:23–50.

26. Meuer, S. C., Hussey, R. E., Fabbi, M., Fox, D., Acuto, O., Fitzgerald, K. A., Hodgdon, J. C., Protentis, J. P., Schlossman, S. F., and Rein-

herz, E. L. (1984): An alternative pathway of T-cell activation: A functional role for the 50 kd T11 sheep erythrocyte receptor protein. *Cell,* 36:897–906.

27. Michell, B. (1986): Cellular signalling: A second messenger function for inositol tetrakisphosphate. *Nature,* 324:613.

28. Mitchison, N. A. (1986): Antigen binding and T cells. *Nature,* 320:106–107.

29. O'Flynn, K., Krensky, A. M., Beverley, P. C. L., Burakoff, S. J., and Linch, D. C. (1985): Phytohaemagglutinin activation of T cells through the sheep red blood cell receptor. *Nature,* 313:686–687.

30. Oppenheim, J. J., Kovacs, E. J., Matsushima, K., and Durum, S. K. (1986): There is more than one interleukin 1. *Immunol. Today,* 7(2):45–56.

31. Reinherz, E. L. (1985): A molecular basis for thymic selection: Regulation of T11 induced thymocyte expansion by the T3-Ti antigen/MHC receptor pathway. *Immunol. Today,* 6(3):75–79.

32. Reinherz, E. L., and Schlossman, S. F. (1981): The characterization and function of human immunoregulatory T lymphocyte subsets. *Immunol. Today,* 2:69–75.

33. Royer, H. D., Acuto, O., Fabbi, M., Tizard, R., Ramachandran, K., Smart, J. E., and Reinherz, E. L. (1984): Genes encoding the Ti subunit of the antigen/MHC receptor undergo rearrangement during intrathymic ontogeny prior to surface T3-Ti expression. *Cell,* 39:261–266.

34. Schrader, J. W. (1986): The panspecific hemopoietin of activated T lymphocytes (interleukin-2). *Annu. Rev. Immunol.,* 4:205–230.

35. Signas, C., Katze, M. G., Persson, H., and Philipson, L. (1982): An adenovirus glycoprotein binds heavy chains of class I transplantation antigens from man and mouse. *Nature,* 299:175–178.

36. Snow, P. M., and Terhorst, C. (1983): The T8 antigen is a multimeric complex of two distinct subunits on human thymocytes but consists of homomultimeric forms on peripheral blood T lymphocytes. *J. Biol. Chem.,* 258(23):14675–14681.

37. Sukhatme, V. P., Vollmer, A. C., Erikson, J., Isobe, M., Croce, C., and Parnes, J. R. (1985): Gene for the human T cell differentiation antigen Leu-2/T8 is closely linked to the κ light chain locus on chromosome 2. *J. Exp. Med.,* 161:429–434.

38. Towsend, A. R. M., Rothbard, J., Gotch, F. M., Bahadur, G., Wraith, D., and McMichael, A. J. (1986): The epitopes of influenza nucleoprotein recognized by cytotoxic T lymphocytes can be defined with short synthetic peptides. *Cell,* 44:959–968.

39. Von Boehmer, H. (1986): The selection of the α,β heterodimeric T-cell receptor for antigen. *Immunol. Today,* 7(11).

40. Watts, T. H., Gaub, H. E., and McConnell, H. M. (1986): T-cell-mediated association of peptide antigen and major histocompatibility complex protein detected by energy transfer in an evanescent wave-field. *Nature,* 320:179–181.

41. Weinstein, I. B. (1983): Tumour promoters: Protein kinase, phospholipid and control of growth. *Nature,* 302:750.

42. Weiss, A., Imboden, J., Hardy, K., Manger, B., Terhorst, C., and Stobo, J. (1986): The role of the T3/antigen receptor complex in T-cell activation. *Annu. Rev. Immunol.,* 4:593–619.

43. Weiss, A., Newton, M., and Crommie, D. Immunology: Expression of T3 in association with a molecule distinct from the T cell antigen receptor heterodimer *(in press).*

Inflammation: Basic Principles and Clinical Correlates.
Edited by J. I. Gallin, I. M. Goldstein, and R. Snyderman.
Raven Press, Ltd., New York © 1988.

CHAPTER 32

Lymphocytes: Cytotoxic Activities

Ronald B. Herberman

One of the major mechanisms by which the immune response deals with foreign or abnormal cells is to damage or destroy them. Such immunologic cytotoxicity may lead to complete loss of viability of the target cells (cytolysis) or an inhibition of the ability of the cells to continue growing (cytostasis). Immunologic cytotoxicity can be manifested against a wide variety of target cells. These include malignant cells, normal cells from individuals unrelated to the responding host, and normal cells of the host that are infected with viruses or other microorganisms. In addition, the immune system can cause direct cytotoxic effects on some microorganisms, including bacteria, parasites, and fungi. Immunologic cytotoxicity is a principal mechanism by which the immune response copes with, and often eliminates, foreign materials or abnormal cells. Cytotoxic reactions are frequently observed as a major component of an immune response that develops following exposure to foreign cells or microorganisms. In addition, there is increasing recent evidence that cytotoxic reactions represent a major mechanism for natural immunity and resistance to such materials. In most instances, cytotoxicity by immune components involves the recognition of particular structures on the target cells; in addition, the targets need to be susceptible to attack by the immune components. Some cells are quite resistant to immunologic cytotoxicity, and this appears to represent a major mechanism by which they can escape control by the immune system.

There are a variety of mechanisms for immunologic cytotoxicity. The two main categories are antibody- and cell-mediated cytotoxicity. Within cell-mediated cytotoxicity, there is a multiplicity of effector cell types and mechanisms that can be involved. In this review, I will focus only on cytotoxicity by lymphocytes. Furthermore, since my own expertise is largely restricted to natural killer (NK) cells and related effector cells, and since the characteristics and functions of cytotoxic T lymphocytes (CTL) have been extensively reviewed elsewhere (6), I will primarily emphasize information related to NK cells and will discuss their similarities and differences with regard to CTL. Also, to reduce the number of references cited, I will frequently refer to review articles or books rather than to the primary publications.

TYPES OF LYMPHOCYTIC EFFECTOR CELLS AND THEIR CHARACTERISTICS

Cytotoxic T Lymphocytes

Immune T cells are important effectors of cell-mediated cytotoxicity. Upon immunization with cells that differ from the host in their major histocompatibility antigens and thereby recognized as foreign, cytotoxic T cells are generated which have a potent ability to lyse a variety of target cells bearing the foreign histocompatibility antigens.

In addition, cytotoxic T cells can be generated against a variety of other foreign antigenic structures on the surface of cells. This can include antigens associated with tumors of the host and also host cells infected with various microorganisms, particularly viruses. In general, cytotoxicity against cells with these other antigens is only displayed when the cells share the same major histocompatibility antigens with the responding host.

A summary of some of the general characteristics of cytotoxic T cells is given in Table 1. CTL usually are typical small lymphocytes, although they may be larger and blastic in appearance during the early phases of induction *in vitro* or *in vivo*. They lack readily detectable azurophilic granules in their cytoplasm, although occasional small numbers of such granules have been described, especially upon electron microscopic examination (147). In contrast, some clones of CTL, maintained in culture in the presence of interleukin-2 (IL-2), have been found to have prominent azurophilic granules in their cytoplasm, very similar to those observed in large granular lymphocytes. Also, it has recently been reported that during the early phase of *in vivo* generation of mouse CTL

reactive with virus-associated antigens, at least some of the CTL have the morphologic characteristics of large granular lymphocytes (10). CTL are characteristically nonadherent and can be enriched from other cell types by passage over nylon wool columns. They have no detectable Fc receptors for IgG and, consequently, seem to be incapable of mediating antibody-dependent cell-mediated cytotoxicity (ADCC). Most CTL have a characteristic cell-surface phenotype, expressing considerable amounts of T-cell lineage markers (CD3 in human or Thy-1 in mouse) and being associated with a particular subset of T cells. Human CTL are characteristically within the CD4$^-$/CD8$^+$ subpopulation, and mouse CTL usually express Lyt-2 and have low expression of Lyt-1. This phenotype is also characteristic of suppressor T cells, and it seems likely that CTL represent only a portion of T cells with these markers. However, as yet there have been no cell-surface antigens identified which are entirely selective for the CTL.

In regard to functional characteristics, CTL are generally not detectable in the lymphoid organs of normal individuals. They must be induced by *in-vitro* stimulation

TABLE 1. *General characteristics of cytotoxic T cells and natural killer (NK) cells*

Characteristic	Cytotoxic T cells	NK cells
Morphologic		
Size (diameter)	9–12 μm	16–20 μm
Cytoplasmic:nuclear ratio	Low	High
Nuclear shape	Round	Slightly indented
Azurophilic cytoplasmic granules	Usually −	+
General features		
Adherence to surfaces	−	Some after activation
Phagocytosis	−	−
Cell-surface markers		
Fc receptors for IgG	−	+ (>90% of cells)
Human receptors for sheep erythrocytes	+ (100% of cells), high affinity	+ (50% of cells), low affinity
Human antigens	CD3$^+$, CD2$^+$, CD8$^+$, CD4$^-$, CD16$^-$, NKH1 (Leu-19)$^-$	CD3$^-$, CD2 (majority$^+$), CD4$^-$, CD16$^+$, NKH1 (Leu-19)$^+$
Mouse antigens	Thy-1$^+$, Lyt-2$^+$, NK-1.1$^-$, NK-2.1$^-$, asialo-GM$_1$ low or negative	Thy-1 (low on 50%), Lyt-2$^-$, NK-1.1$^+$, NK-2.1$^+$, asialo-GM$_1^+$
Functional features		
Spontaneous reactivity	−	+
Period to develop augmented activity	Long (primary: 7–10 days; secondary: 3–5 days)	Short (minutes to hours)
Memory response	+	−
Antibody-dependent cellular cytotoxicity	−	+
Responses to IL-2		
Growth	+	+
Rapid activation of reactivity	−	+
Responses to IFN		
Rapid activation of reactivity	−	+
Increased generation of reactivity	+	+

with the appropriate antigens or mitogens or by *in-vitro* immunization. In most instances, the development of CTL activity takes considerable time, with primary responses, even to alloantigens or other strong antigens, becoming detectable only after about 1 week. A characteristic feature of CTL as well as other immune T cells is to manifest memory, with more rapid induction of cytolytic activity in cells that have been previously exposed to the antigen.

NK Cells

NK cells were discovered about 15 years ago (41,114), during studies of cell-mediated cytotoxicity. Although investigators expected to find specific cytotoxic activity of tumor-bearing individuals against autologous tumor cells or against allogeneic tumors of similar or the same histologic type, appreciable cytotoxic activity was observed with lymphocytes from normal individuals. With the wide array of recent studies related to natural cell-mediated cytotoxicity, there has been considerable diversity in the terminology related to the effector cells, and consequently there has been confusion in the literature. However, at a recent workshop devoted to the study of NK cells, a consensus definition for these effector cells was developed (61). NK cells were defined as effector cells with spontaneous cytotoxicity against various target cells; these effector cells lack the properties of classical macrophages, granulocytes, or CTL; and the observed cytotoxicity does not show restriction related to the major histocompatibility complex (MHC). This definition is sufficiently broad to include not only "classical" NK cells but also other natural effector cells such as natural cytotoxic (NC) cells (see section on NK cytotoxic factors). The workshop participants agreed that the observations relating to the development of cytotoxic cells in culture [e.g., lymphokine-activated killers (LAK), anomalous killers (AK)] were difficult to interpret. However, more recently it has become rather clear that most LAK activity of blood or splenic lymphocytes can be attributed to IL-2-stimulated NK cells (see section on LAK cells).

Until recently, the cells responsible for NK activity could be defined only in a negative way, i.e., by distinguishing them from typical T cells, B cells, or macrophages. However, it is now possible to isolate highly enriched populations and show that the NK activity is closely associated with a subpopulation of lymphocytes, morphologically identified as large granular lymphocytes (LGL) (125), that compromise about 5% of peripheral blood lymphocytes and 1% to 3% of total mononuclear cells. LGL have been found in all vertebrates tested, e.g., human, mouse, hamster, rat, chicken, guinea pig, and miniature swine. Cells with similar morphology and with spontaneous cytotoxic reactivity have also been identified in several invertebrate species, suggesting that NK cells represent a phylogenetically ancient effector mechanism (117). LGL, which contain azurophilic cytoplasmic granules, can be isolated by discontinuous density gradient centrifugation on Percoll. LGL are nonphagocytic, nonadherent cells that lack surface immunoglobulin or receptors for the third component of complement but contain cell-surface receptors for the Fc portion of IgG (125). This latter quality allows them to bind antibody-coated target cells and to mediate the phenomenon termed *antibody-dependent cellular cytotoxicity* (ADCC) (57), a function previously attributed to the K (killer) cell. Hence, the same cells (i.e., NK/K cells) seem able to mediate both forms of cytotoxicity, with NK activity due to NK receptors being discrete from the Fc receptors that interact with target-cell-bound antibody (57,62).

The levels of NK activity have a characteristic organ distribution. Studies first performed with mouse and rat cells (36,41), and more recently with human cells (36,37,125), have demonstrated high levels of NK activity in the peripheral blood and spleen, with intermediate to low levels of activity present in the lymph nodes, peritoneal cavity, and bone marrow, as well as undetectable levels present in the tonsil or thymus. Recently, studies in the rat (36,37) have demonstrated a high degree of association of LGL with mucosal epithelial tissues, especially with the bronchial-associated lymphoid tissue and epithelium of the gut. Mucosal LGL have been isolated from the small intestine of mice and have been shown to possess intermediate to high levels of NK activity. In addition, precursors of NK cells have been shown, by transplantation experiments, to be derived from the bone marrow.

NK cells have been found to be mainly nonadherent, nonphagocytic, surface immunoglobulin-negative cells that are positive for β-glucuronidase and acid phosphatase and negative for nonspecific esterases (36,37). No diversity in the cytochemical features of these cells has been reported, with virtually all cells in the population showing the same pattern of cytoplasmic enzymes.

Although LGL appear to account for most NK activity in humans, other primates, and rodents, not all LGL possess measurable NK activity (36,37,125). One possible explanation for the lack of detectable cytotoxic activity in some LGL is that the array of target cells tested has not been sufficient to reflect the entire repertoire and that some LGL may recognize and lyse only a limited variety of target cells. Despite this potential limitation, tests of human LGL against several NK-susceptible target cell lines in a single-cell cytotoxicity assay enable us to estimate that in most normal individuals, after activation of the cells with interferon, 75% to 85% (126) of the LGL are capable of killing at least one NK-susceptible target cell line. The nature of the other 15% or 20% of the LGL, with no detectable cytolytic activity, is unclear. A recent report indicates that at least some of these LGL are CD3[+] T cells, also with the potential for mediating cytotoxic activity (91).

Most LGL have surface receptors for the Fc portion of IgG, and both NK activity and K-cell-mediated ADCC have been closely associated with LGL (36,37,125). Approximately one-half of human NK cells and LGL express detectable receptors for sheep erythrocytes, as measured by rosette formation at 4°C. However, some monoclonal antibodies to the sheep erythrocyte receptor react with a considerably higher proportion of LGL (89). Analogously, a proportion of mouse NK cells express Thy-1 antigens (70), and most rat NK cells express OX-8 and some other T-cell-associated markers (99).

Thus, although NK cells are clearly not thymus-dependent [since high levels of activity have been detected in athymic nude mice or in neonatally thymectomized mice (36,37,41)], they share many characteristics associated with CTL and other T cells.

In both rat and human spleens, and to a lesser extent in other organs, large agranular lymphocytes (LAL) have been detected that possess morphological characteristics similar to those of LGL but that lack detectable azurophilic granules (36,37). Aside from their lack of cytoplasmic granules, LAL have been indistinguishable from LGL. They copurify in the lower-density fractions of Percoll density gradients, they have the same morphology, and their cytoplasm has the same appearance with Wright's-Giemsa stain. Also, no cell-surface markers have been found to distinguish between LGL and LAL. In studies with purified populations of human LGL plus LAL, a high proportion of both LAL and LGL binds to NK-susceptible target cells. However, because it has not been possible to separate these cells or distinguish them adequately in a cytolytic assay, it has not as yet been documented whether LAL have NK activity similar to that of LGL. Thus, the precise relationship of LAL with LGL or with NK cells remains unclear. One possibility is that LGL and LAL are directly related and differ only in their stages of granule maturation. A range of granule development has been reported in LGL, detectable by electron microscopy (36,37). It has been suggested that the earliest forms of LGL are in the bone marrow, with immature granules, and that differentiation of this cell population is reflected by increasing development of mature, typical granules. According to this hypothesis, LGL in the peripheral blood, with high NK activity and usually few cells without readily detectable granules, would represent the most differentiated cells in this lineage. Cells in the spleen and lymph nodes, with lower NK activity and less prominent granules, might be at an intermediate stage of differentiation. It is possible that the cytoplasmic granules are more directly related to cytolytic capability and that

LAL are pre-NK cells, with the ability to bind, but not lyse, NK-susceptible targets. This hypothesis is consistent with a body of evidence for the existence of pre-NK cells (37), which can be induced to develop NK activity after treatment with interferon or other activating stimuli.

Overall, the results to date indicate that a discrete, small subpopulation of lymphoid cells (i.e., LGL) are responsible for most NK activity (at least 90%). These findings seem to rule out the possibility that diverse cell types share the NK function. Rather, the observed heterogeneity remains mainly within the LGL and related populations.

Some cell-surface antigens, particular those detected by monoclonal antibodies, have been found on virtually all NK cells. They therefore help to characterize the phenotype of these effector cells. For example, most human NK cells react with the following antibodies: (a) monoclonal antibodies (B73.1, 3G8, Leu-11) (90) reactive with the CD16 Fc receptors for IgG on LGL (3G8 and Leu-11 also are strongly expressed on granulocytes); (b) rabbit antisera to the glycolipid asialo-GM$_1$, which also reacts with monocytes and granulocytes (89); (c) OKT10, which also reacts with most thymocytes and activated lymphocytes (89); (d) OKM1, which also reacts with monocytes/macrophages, neutrophils, and platelets (89); and (e) NKH1 or Leu-19, which is quite selective for NK cells but also recognizes a small percentage of T cells (45). Removal of cells bearing any of these markers, either by treatment with antibody plus complement or by negative selection immunoaffinity procedures, results in a depletion of most or all detectable NK activity.

In the rat, a monoclonal antibody, OX-8, which also reacts with the subpopulation of T cells with suppressor activity (similar to the human T8 subpopulation of T cells with cytotoxic and suppressor activities) (99), reacts with most NK cells and LGL. Antisera to asialo-GM$_1$ also react with virtually all rat and mouse NK cells (99). NK cells can also be characterized by a lack of expression of certain cell-surface markers. For example, human NK cells have no detectable surface reactivity with monoclonal antibodies to pan-T-cell antigens such as CD5 and CD3 or to the CD4 T-helper antigen (37,89). Human NK cells also do not express surface antigens detected by a number of monocyte-specific reagents such as MO2 and Leu-M1 (37,89).

In contrast to a pattern of features common to most or all CTL, NK cells and also LGL in general are rather heterogeneous with respect to other monoclonal antibody-defined markers. Human NK cells react, to a variable extent, with monoclonal antibodies directed against the sheep erythrocyte receptor, CD2 (Lyt-3, OKT11, Leu-5) (89), with only about half of the NK cells in some experiments giving positive results. Only a portion of human NK cells have been shown to react with a variety of other monoclonals, including 3A1 (on most CTL and other T cells and 50–60% of LGL) HNK1 (or Leu-7 on 40–60% of NK cells), and CD8 (on suppressor/cytotoxic T lymphocytes and 10–30% of LGL); also, about 25% of LGL react with monoclonal antibodies against Ia framework (HLA-DR) determinants (89).

Similarly, in the mouse, only about half of the NK cells (70) express Thy-1, and only 20% express readily detectable Lyt-1 (36,37). In addition, the allelic markers NK1.1 and NK2.1 (36,37) are expressed on at least 50% to 60% of mouse NK cells.

In contrast to classical mouse NK cells, natural cytotoxicity (NC) cells appear to be devoid of most lymphoid surface markers, namely Lyt-1$^-$, Thy-1$^-$, asialo-GM$_1^-$, and H$_2$K$^-$D$^-$ (36,37). All attempts to phenotype NC cells have failed to define a characteristic marker on these cells. However, despite such indications that NC cells might be completely distinct from typical NK cells, it has been found that NC cells and typical mouse NK cells copurify in Percoll density gradients (40). Thus NC cells may also be LGL—either a subset of NK cells or at a stage of differentiation associated with poor expression of cell-surface markers and altered receptors for target cells.

Although most NK cells and LGL are nonadherent to plastic or nylon wool, a subset of these cells shows some adherence. For instance, when isolating human myelomonocytic cells by means of their adherence to plastic, the small percentage of contaminating cells is disproportionately comprised of LGL (16). In addition, after *in vivo* stimulation of NK cells with microbial agents such as *Corynebacterium parvum* or with interferon after *in vitro* stimulation with allogeneic cells or lectins, a substantial proportion of NK cells adheres either to plastic or to nylon-wool columns (36,37). Although this subpopulation of cells shares the adherence property with myelomonocytic cells, it retains the morphology and cell-surface characteristics of LGL. The phenotype of human adherent NK cells has been shown to be OKT3$^-$, OKT10$^+$, OKT11$^+$, OKM1$^+$, Leu-M1$^-$, B73.1$^+$ (16). Such cells thus contrast with typical adherent monocytes, which only react with OKM1 and Leu-M1.

In summary, NK cells have a characteristic phenotype. For example, most human NK cells and LGL can be described at CD3$^-$, CD4$^-$, OKT10$^+$, CD16$^+$, NKH1$^+$, OKM1$^+$, Leu-M1$^-$. Thus, these cells have a readily definable and general phenotype, which sets them apart from all other lymphoid cell types. The heterogeneity in cell-surface phenotypes extends to only a few markers (e.g., with human NK cells: CD8, HNK1, Ia, and CD2).

The observed heterogeneity in surface-marker expression on NK cells has not been explained. However, recent studies using a new method to examine intracellular expression of monoclonal antibody-defined markers in NK and T cells have indicated the need for caution in conclusions about the ability of lymphoid-cell subpopulations to express particular antigens (76). By means of this new procedure, all human T cells have been shown to express CD4 (only on the surface of the helper-T-cell subset), B$_2$ (considered to be B-cell-associated), and MO2 (expressed on the surface of only myelomonocytic cells). Most LGL were also found to have internal MO2 and B$_2$ and to contain CD5 (pan-T) antigen. Although the mechanisms responsible for expression of markers intracellularly and/or on the cell surface remain to be determined, expression of a variety of markers may depend on many factors. One must be cautious in using marker data to draw conclusions about the degree of divergence among subsets of NK cells or other lymphoid cells.

Taken together, the above data indicate that there may be discrete subsets of NK cells that vary in their cell-surface markers and adherence properties. However, an alternative explanation for such data is that cell-surface markers and adherence properties of NK cells vary with the stage of activation or maturation of the cells. In regard to this possibility, one notes that most of these markers do not change after stimulation with interferon (126) or other NK stimulators such as IL-2 or *C. parvum*. In contrast, such treatments induce substantial changes in the levels of expression of Fc receptors and β_2-microglobulin on a variety of lymphoid cells.

REGULATION OF CYTOTOXIC ACTIVITY OF EFFECTOR CELLS

Interferon

In vivo treatment of allosensitized mice with interferon (IFN) has been reported to augment the reactivity of CTL (65). However, studies in my laboratory have failed to confirm these results (*unpublished observation*); also, the activity of human CTL, after *in vitro* sensitization in mixed lymphocyte cultures, was not boosted by IFN (42). In contrast, the NK-like activity that develops in such cultures was augmented by IFN (42). Thus it appears that the human-CTL-mediating alloimmune cytotoxicity is resistant to augmentation by IFN.

In contrast to the largely negative results with CTL, all three types of IFN (α, β, γ), have been shown to potently augment the activity of NK cells (42,100,126). *In vivo* administration, to mice or rats, of a variety of IFN inducers (81), or of IFN itself, led to rapid boosting of NK activity. Similarly, incubation *in vitro* of lymphoid cells or of purified LGL with IFN induced considerable augmentation of NK activity (42,100,126).

To determine the role of IFN more definitively, experiments were performed with a variety of IFN species, most of which were purified to homogeneity. Almost all of the proteins with antiviral activity that have been studied, including various species of IFN-α, IFN-β, and IFN-γ, have had the ability to increase NK activity significantly (43). The one exception found to date has been IFN-αJ, which, although apparently able to bind to LGL, induced no boosting of NK activity after treatment of human NK cells for several hours and induced low levels of boosting after overnight incubation (84). In addition, there have been considerable quantitative differences in the efficacy of boosting by the various species (43). Some species have been shown to be high-level boosters, with greater than 50% increase in NK activity by less than 50 units of IFN, whereas other interferon species have been found to have low-level boosting activity, with an NK-activity increase of only 50% by 500 units or more of IFN.

Several groups of investigators have been very interested in determining the mechanisms by which IFN augments NK activity. Such studies have been considerably facilitated by the ability to identify morphologically, as well as purify, human and rat NK cells. One question was whether purified LGL, after pretreatment with IFN, acquire an increased ability to recognize and bind to NK-susceptible target cells (126). When such studies were done with K562 or other suspension target cells, pretreatment with IFN was not found to result in an increased percentage of LGL-forming conjugates. In contrast, when various monolayer target cells were studied, IFN pretreatment of LGL resulted in an increased proportion of binding cells. Thus, with some target cells but not with others, one action of IFN is to convert pre-NK cells into cells able to recognize and bind to the targets. To determine the possible effects of IFN on postbinding interactions with target cells, a single-cell agarose cytotoxicity assay was utilized (126). With K562 targets, pretreatment of LGL with interferon was shown to result primarily in an accelerated rate of lysis of bound target cells. In contrast, with G-11 monolayer target cells, IFN pretreatment of LGL resulted in a substantial increase in the proportion of bound targets that were lysed. In addition, IFN pretreatment caused an acceleration in the kinetics of lysis. IFN has also been shown to increase interactions with target cells by increasing the degree of recycling, i.e., facilitating the interaction with, and lysis of, multiple target cells during the cytotoxicity assay. IFN-induced augmentation of recycling was demonstrated directly by observation of the dissociation of LGL from bound targets and their subsequent rebinding (126). When LGL were pretreated with IFN, the dissociation was decreased and rebinding occurred considerably more rapidly. Yet another aspect of the effect of IFN on the interactions between NK cells and targets has been the demonstration of the ability of IFN to protect certain target cells from lysis by NK cells (54). Thus, IFN can have opposite effects on effector-cell–target-cell interactions, depending on the cells exposed to the IFN.

It should be noted that IFN or IFN inducers may not be able to augment all forms of natural cell-mediated cytotoxicity. Lattime et al. (64) have reported that IFN treatment in vitro or various IFN inducers (poly I:C, tilorone, C. parvum) in vivo failed to induce detectable augmentation of mouse NC activity, under conditions in which NK activity was boosted well. It appears that NC cells and NK cells are regulated by different cytokines, with the growth and activation of NC cells being influenced primarily by interleukin-3 (64).

Although IFN does not appear to affect the activity of CTL, as discussed above, it can influence the levels of CTL activity which are generated from their precursors. The addition of IFN at the time of initiation of human mixed lymphocyte cultures resulted in the generation of considerably higher levels of CTL activity than those observed in cultures without IFN (148). However, the mechanism responsible for this more efficient generation of CTL has not been determined.

Interleukin-2

Since the discovery of Morgan et al. (77) that human T cells could be maintained in continuous culture in the presence of T-cell growth factor, (TCGF), an extensive amount of research has been performed on the role of this factor in the growth and regulation of T cells. T-cell growth factor, now known as *interleukin-2* (IL-2), has been demonstrated to be a key intermediary for the lympho-proliferative responses of T cells (12) and for the generation of CTL (23) (also see Chapter 13, *this volume*). The responses of T cells to IL-2 have been shown to be dependent on the activation of the cells to express cell-surface receptors for IL-2 (12). The human IL-2 receptor on T cells has been found to react with a monoclonal antibody, anti-Tac (109). The anti-Tac antibody has been found to inhibit the binding of radiolabeled IL-2 to T-cell lines or to activated T cells expressing Tac (109), and it thereby strongly inhibits the proliferative responses to IL-2.

Lymphocytes sensitized in mixed lymphocyte cultures (MLC) represent primed cells that undergo rapid proliferation in response to the specific alloantigens during a secondary culture period, referred to as the *primed lymphocyte test*. By the addition of IL-2 at the end of the MLC, cultured T cells (MLC-CTC) that retained specific proliferative reactivity in primed lymphocyte tests could be generated (118). In most cases, the MLC-CTC also retained strong cytotoxic activity against the priming antigens, raising the possibility of growing large quantities of CTL, with reactivity to well-defined alloantigens (118).

IL-2 also has been shown to have two types of effects on NK cells: the stimulation of both proliferation and augmentation of cytotoxicity. In parallel with the potent ability of IL-2 to act as a growth factor for T cells, it has also been shown to promote the growth of NK cells (127). As with T cells, this proliferative effect of IL-2 on NK cells has been shown to be dependent on an interaction of the lymphokine with receptors for IL-2, as detected by anti-Tac monoclonal antibodies (144). Proliferating LGL have been shown to express Tac, and anti-Tac completely interfered with the growth of the cells and their maintenance of cytotoxic activity. However, as a major divergence from the data obtained with T cells, in which IL-2 receptors had to be induced by mitogens or antigens in order for the cells to become responsive to IL-2 (12), IL-2 alone has been shown to promote the growth of human or murine NK cells (124,144). Quite unexpectedly, fresh IL-2-responsive human LGL have been found to have no detectable IL-2 receptors, as measured either by flow cytometry with anti-Tac or by binding studies with radio-labeled anti-Tac (144). In addition, messenger RNA for IL-2 receptors was not detectable in fresh human LGL (144). However, upon exposure of such LGL to IL-2 alone, message for the receptor became detectable within 2 days of culture, and this was accompanied by detectable expression of IL-2 receptors on the cells and the onset of proliferation. Thus, it appears that IL-2 alone can induce the up-regulation of IL-2 receptors at the transcriptional level (144), and this appears to account for the ability of this lymphokine by itself to promote the growth of NK cells.

In contrast to the dependence of NK cell proliferation on the expression of detectable levels of IL-2 receptors, the ability of IL-2 to rapidly induce augmented levels of cytolytic activity has been found to be independent of entry into the cell cycle or the detectable expression of Tac (86). Overnight incubation of LGL with IL-2 could strongly stimulate NK activity, despite the presence, in the culture medium, of high concentrations of antibodies to Tac. Thus, it appears that LGL express some non-Tac receptors for IL-2, which allow their cytotoxic reactivity to be stimulated. In addition, such interaction of IL-2 with Tac-independent receptors for IL-2 may provide the signal for induction of expression of Tac and the consequent proliferative response to IL-2.

In addition to clear-cut situations in which cell cultures are initiated with highly purified LGL that retain their morphologic and cytotoxic characteristics (3), cultures have usually been initiated with unseparated lymphoid populations, and cytolytic activity has been observed against NK-susceptible target cells (59). Since the relationship of the generated cytotoxic effector cells to NK cells has been difficult to determine, such activities have been referred to as *NK-like* or are considered to be caused by activated killer cells. Under some conditions, cells with broad, NK-like reactivity can be generated in cultures from precursors lacking NK activity and having a somewhat different phenotype than NK cells (83). Furthermore,

NK-like cytotoxic activity has developed in culture of thymocytes or highly purified T cells or T-cell clones, in the presence of IL-2, especially when the concentrations of IL-2 have been high (14,26,50,123,128).

Lymphokine-Activated Killer (LAK) Cells

Recently, LAK cells have been described (27) that share many of the characteristics of the above-mentioned culture-activated NK-like cells. LAK cells have been activated after a short period of culture *in vitro* with highly purified IL-2 and display cytotoxic activity against a variety of autologous, allogeneic, and xenogeneic tumors. These cells were initially thought to lack markers typical of fresh NK cells, to be devoid of cytolytic activity prior to culture, and to develop T-cell markers upon activation (28). However, more recent studies in several laboratories have indicated that most LAK activity developing from blood or splenic lymphocytes is attributable to IL-2-stimulated NK cells; in fact, most LAK cells and their progenitors have a phenotype characteristic of NK cells but not of T cells (38).

In the initial descriptions of LAK cells, much emphasis was placed on the observations that fresh solid tumor target cells appeared to be resistant to lysis by NK cells (27). However, susceptibility or resistance of target cells to lysis by NK cells appears to be a relative rather than an absolute distinction. Under some circumstances, "NK-resistant" targets can be lysed to a significant extent by unstimulated NK cells. Regarding the possibility of NK activity against fresh noncultured tumor cells, low but significant levels of cytotoxic activity against fresh human leukemia cells were observed in the earliest studies of human NK cells (114). Similarly, some of the "NK-resistant" cultured cell lines that are being used as good targets for assessing LAK activity, particularly the Raji cell line, were used in early studies of NK activity (71,115), prior to the discovery of more sensitive targets such as K562. Clearly, the increase of NK activity by various agents, including interferon as well as IL-2, does not only increase the levels of reactivity against NK-sensitive target cells but also can induce detectable levels of lysis of targets that seemed refractory to unstimulated NK cells. The artificiality of the distinction between NK-sensitive and NK-resistant target cells has been emphasized by a series of *in-vivo* studies of the role of NK cells in resistance to metastatic spread of tumors. Much of the strong evidence for the potent ability of NK cells *in vivo* to rapidly eliminate tumor cells from the circulation and to prevent the subsequent development of metastases in the lungs and other organs has come from studies with tumor cell lines that appear to be highly resistant to NK activity *in vitro* (4,5,25).

Even when it has not been possible to detect lysis of

fresh leukemia or solid tumor target cells by unseparated blood or splenic lymphocytes, significant levels of NK activity could be detected simply after purification of the effector cells. Human LGL, purified by Percoll density gradient centrifugation, have been shown to have significant cytotoxic activity against the majority of fresh solid tumor cells and fresh leukemia cells, whereas LGL-depleted populations had significantly lower, or undetectable, activity. The effector cells for solid tumor targets appeared to be a subset of LGL (130), but in conjugate assays with two target cells it was shown that the effector cells lysing autologous tumor cells could also lyse the NK-sensitive K562 cell line (134). The effector cells reactive against human leukemia targets were further shown to be CD16$^+$ and NKH1$^+$ (Leu-19$^+$) (67,68). In contrast to such lytic activity of LGL against fresh human "NK-resistant" targets, LGL-depleted populations of small T cells were without detectable activity.

In addition to the above evidence that unstimulated NK cells as well as cells with LAK activity can have cytotoxic activity against fresh tumor cells and other "NK-resistant" targets, there are some indications that NK cells and cells with LAK activity may recognize the same target structures. In cold target inhibition experiments, NK-susceptible targets such as K562 could efficiently inhibit human LAK activity against an NK-resistant target. Similarly, NK-sensitive target cells were found to adsorb cells with LAK activity more efficiently in monolayer depletion experiments than did NK-resistant cells. Further, after exposure of NK-susceptible target cells to cells with LAK activity, the surviving target cells were found to be transiently resistant to both NK cells and cells with LAK activity (20). One might explain such data by postulating that NK-sensitive target cells simply express NK target structures better or in higher concentration than NK-resistant targets. However, to satisfactorily settle this question, it will be necessary to directly characterize the target structures recognized by NK cells and cells with LAK activity and, in a complementary way, characterize the recognition structures on each type of effector cells.

Extensive studies have now been done on the phenotype of both the lymphocytes that develop LAK activity after culture with IL-2 (i.e., progenitors of cells with LAK activity) and the effector cells themselves, after culture in the presence of IL-2. Although the initial studies on LAK activity suggested a shift in phenotype, from progenitors lacking T-cell as well as NK-cell markers (28) to effector cells with T-cell markers, subsequent studies have indicated the expression of a very similar pattern of markers on both the progenitors and effector cells. Data on the phenotype of cells with LAK activity have now been obtained in three species (mouse, rat, and human), and these are summarized below.

Phenotype of Progenitors of LAK Activity

Table 2 provides a summary of the characteristics that have been associated with the blood or splenic lymphocytes that developed LAK activity after culture in the presence of IL-2. The most extensive studies have been performed with human lymphocytes, and it seems clear that most of the LAK activity from blood lymphocytes is generated from cells with the same characteristics as NK cells. As summarized in Table 2, the progenitors of LAK activity in human peripheral blood have been shown to be mainly LGL with the CD3$^-$ CD16$^+$ NKH1$^+$ phenotype. Some of the progenitors appear to be low-density lymphocytes that lack the characteristic granules of LGL and are thereby resistant to the lysosomotropic agent, L-leucine methyl ester (122). The finding of low levels of LAK activity generated from CD3$^+$ blood lymphocytes represents somewhat divergent data. CD3$^+$ NKH1$^+$ lymphocytes have been detected in low concentrations in peripheral blood, have been associated with some MHC-unrestricted cytotoxicity, and have been shown to give rise to some clones with "NK-like" activity (46,119). More strongly divergent results have come from a recent study (18), indicating that appreciable LAK activity could be generated from a wide variety of lymphocyte subpopulations, including CD4$^+$ and CD8$^+$ T cells and also B cells. The explanation for these divergent results is not

TABLE 2. *Characteristics of the predominant type of blood or splenic progenitors of LAK activity*

Characteristic	References
Human	
Mainly associated with LGL	26,28,66–69,91,122
Mainly CD16 (Leu-11)$^+$	66–69,91
Mainly CD3 (T3)$^-$	66–69,91
NKH1 (Leu-19)$^+$	66–69,91
Some are resistant to L-leucine methyl ester	26,122
Mouse	
Asialo-GM$_1^+$	72–74,101–107,116
L3T4$^-$ and Lyt-2$^-$	
Some Thy-1$^+$ and Thy-1$^-$	
Rat	
Mostly associated with LGL	50
Asialo-GM$_1^+$	
OX8$^+$	
Negative for pan-T-cell markers or helper-T-cell markers	
Laminin$^+$	
Sensitive to L-leucine methyl ester	

clear but may be attributable to some technical limitations of the panning technique utilized for cell separations.

The LAK activity generated from mouse or rat spleen cells or peripheral blood cells has been associated with progenitors with characteristics virtually identical to those associated with NK cells (Table 2). For example, rat NK cells have been closely associated with LGL and the asialo-GM$_1$ and OX8 cell-surface antigens (99). In addition, cell-surface molecules reactive with polyclonal and monoclonal antibodies to laminin have been found to be selectively expressed on rat NK cells (49). These same markers are also expressed on the progenitors of rat LAK cells. Furthermore, high levels of LAK activity were generated from highly purified populations of blood or splenic LGL, whereas little or no activity was generated from purified populations of T cells. Most studies with mouse lymphocytes have also indicated that the splenic progenitors of LAK activity have a phenotype compatible with NK cells, with expression of asialo-GM$_1$, some positivity for Thy-1, and absence of L3T4 or Lyt-2. However, Shortman et al. (123) have depicted the generation of some mouse strains from Lyt-2$^+$ cells by a limiting dilution technique of cells with lytic activity against NK-resistant targets. However, these cultures have been performed in the presence of Con A and irradiated feeder cells, and those conditions may account for the divergent results.

Phenotype of Effector Cells with LAK Activity

Table 3 summarizes the characteristics of cells with LAK activity, generated from blood or splenic lymphocytes upon culture in the presence of IL-2. These char-acteristics indicate that the phenotype of most of the progenitor cells and of most of the effectors for LAK activity is very similar, each quite compatible with the phenotype of NK cells but divergent from that of typical T cells. As with the progenitors of LAK activity, some effector cells with LAK activity have been shown to have T-cell markers. However, under the usual conditions of generating LAK activity from blood or splenic lymphocytes, such effector cells appear to be very infrequent. Also, such T cells with LAK activity appear to have been derived from T-cell progenitors. It is of interest that the CD3$^+$ human lymphocytes with LAK activity appear to be, at least in part, atypical T cells expressing NKH1 (48,119) but lacking expression of either CD4 or CD8 (135).

Thus, LAK should be considered a phenomenon rather than a new or distinct effector cell, with most of the blood or splenic activity attributable to NK cells. The LAK phenomenon appears to be of particular interest because of the potent ability of IL-2 to both stimulate cytotoxic activity and to promote the expansion of the effector-cell population. With regard to the major therapeutic effects of LAK cells, this should now be viewed as an outgrowth of the extensive studies over the last several years on the role of natural effector cells in host resistance against tumors. Most of the results in animal models have indicated a predominant involvement of NK cells in prevention of metastases (140), and there have been less data supporting a role for these effector cells in therapy. However, the recent experience with the LAK phenomenon suggests that this distinction is not complete and that highly activated NK cells, when given in sufficient numbers, can have therapeutic as well as prophylactic antitumor effects.

TABLE 3. *Characteristics of blood or spleen cells with LAK activity*

Characteristics	References
Human	
Mainly associated with LGL	66–69,91,122
Mainly CD3$^-$	66–69,91
Mainly NKH1 (Leu-19)$^+$	66–69,91
Mainly CD16$^+$	66–69
Mouse	
Asialo-GM$_1^+$	72–74,100–107
L3T4$^-$, Lyt-1$^-$ and Lyt-2$^-$	
Mainly Thy-1$^+$	
Rat	
Asialo-GM$_1^+$	50
OX8$^+$	
OX6 (Ia)$^+$	
Negative for pan-T-cell markers or helper-T-cell markers	
Laminin$^+$	

INTERACTIONS BETWEEN EFFECTOR AND TARGET CELLS WHICH LEAD TO CYTOTOXICITY

As a result of efforts to closely study the mechanisms involved in the interactions between cytotoxic effector cells and target cells, it has been possible to define a sequence of events that appear to be required for the lytic process (17). These steps were first described for CTL (6), and subsequently a similar sequence has been shown to be involved in NK activity (37). The main stages can be identified as: (a) recognition of target cells by effector cells; (b) binding of effectors to targets; (c) activation of lytic machinery of effector cells; (d) lytic effects on target cells, often referred to as the *lytic hit;* and (e) effector-cell-in-dependent dissolution of the targets. In the following discussion, some of the main features of each of these stages will be summarized, with particular emphasis on the similarities and differences between CTL and NK cells.

Recognition of Target Cells by Effector Cells

The recognition event appears to be dependent on two types of structures: (i) the cell-surface recognition receptors on the effector cells; (ii) the antigens or other structures on the target cells which need to be recognized.

Recognition Structures on Effector Cells

Much attention has been devoted to the nature of the T-cell receptor, and there has been some recent exciting advances in our understanding of the biochemical and molecular biologic features of this receptor (139). In contrast, there has been little documentation of the nature of the recognition receptors on NK cells. The binding of NK cells to target cells is clearly required to activate the lytic process of these cells. Most of the data regarding the NK-recognition receptor only serve to show what it is not. For instance, although NK and antibody-dependent cellular cytotoxic (ADCC) activities may be mediated by the same effector cell, blocking of the receptor for the Fc portion of immunoglobulin G (IgG) inhibits only ADCC activity and has little or no effect on NK activity (90). This demonstrates that the NK receptor is not simply the Fc receptor binding to cell-bound antibody on the target. Similarly, the NK-recognition receptor is unlikely to be Ig, since Ig-like molecules are absent from the surface membrane of LGL (89,99); also, treatment of lymphocytes with anti-Ig and complement has no effect on their NK activity (60).

It has been suggested that the recognition of NK-susceptible target cells by NK cells is via a laminin-like structure (49,50). NK cells and cells with LAK activity selectively express surface structures that react with polyclonal and some monoclonal antibodies to laminin. Such antibodies have been found to inhibit NK activity. However, it is presently unclear whether the laminin-like molecules on NK cells represent primary recognition structures or are needed for secondary binding interactions with target cells.

It has also been suggested that murine NK cells and cytotoxic T lymphocytes (CTL) and other clones with NK-like activity express mRNA as well as rearrangements of the genes coding for the β-chain of the T-cell receptor (145). In experiments in the human cells using T3$^+$ but not T3$^-$, lymphocyte clones with NK-like activity have produced similar data (108). The authors suggest that the T-cell receptor on such cells acts as the recognition receptor for NK-like activity, since antibodies to the idiotypic determinants of the T-cell receptor blocked cytotoxic activity against K562 (46). However, even in those studies, some clones with NK-like activity had no detectable expression of T-cell receptors, indicating that other structures can recognize NK-susceptible targets. In addition,

much data now indicate that the NK-recognition receptor is different from the T-cell receptor. First, in the rat, LGL tumor lines with high NK activity have no genomic rearrangement of the T-cell receptor β-chain and no detectable complete 1.3-kilobase (kb) mRNA for this structure (97). Second, freshly isolated, highly purified populations of rat, mouse, and human LGL have no detectable 1.3-kb mRNA or β-chain gene rearrangement, in spite of very high NK activity (146). Third, the addition of anti-T3 antibody, which recognizes a portion of the human T-cell-receptor complex, has no effect on the NK activity of freshly isolated human LGL or T3$^+$ cytotoxic clones with NK-like activity (44). Finally, Binz et al. (9) have reported that addition of anti-idiotype antibodies to CTL lines with both antigen-specific and NK-like activity inhibited only the antigen-specific cytotoxicity but did not affect the NK-like activity of these clones.

The likely reason for divergent results regarding fresh mouse NK cells (145,146) is related to the difficulty in obtaining highly purified NK cells without appreciable contamination by T cells (i.e., <5% T cells) from mouse spleen, and the previous positive report (145) is probably due to insufficient purification of the effector-cell population. The detection of T-cell-receptor gene rearrangement and/or expression in cells *in vitro* is more likely due to the development of NK-like activity in typical T cells when cultured in IL-2 (14). However, the expression of the T-cell receptor is unlikely to be related to the expression of NK-like receptors on these cells.

Taken together, these results indicate that the NK-cell recognition receptor is not identical to the previously described T-cell-receptor complex, and its molecular nature remains elusive. Perhaps use of a molecular biological approach similar to that successfully used for the T-cell receptor will lead to elucidation of the structure(s) by which NK cells recognize target cells.

Target Structures Recognized by Effector Cells

In most instances, the recognition of target cells by CTL is restricted by the major histocompatibility complex (MHC), and the target structures themselves seem to be closely associated with the MHC (6). It has been proposed that MHC proteins on target cells are critical molecular mediators by which the CTL receptors transmit signals that are required for the subsequent lysis of the target cells (6).

In contrast to the extensive studies on the target structures recognized by CTL, little definitive information exists about the nature of the target structures recognized by NK cells.

NK cells react against a wide variety of syngeneic, allogeneic, and xenogeneic tumor cells. Susceptibility to cytotoxic activity is not restricted to malignant cells, with fetal cells, virus-infected cells, and subpopulations of normal lymphoid or hematopoietic stem cells (thymus cells, bone marrow cells) being susceptible to lysis by NK cells. In contrast to cytolytic T lymphocytes, NK cells demonstrate no known MHC restriction (36,37). In fact, they have strong reactivity against MHC-deficient targets (e.g., K562), and their activity is not inhibited by antibodies against MHC determinants. Differentiation antigens may be a major type of target-cell structure recognized by NK cells. Studies with maturational agents (37) and with a wide variety of target cells (36,37) indicate that undifferentiated cells are generally more susceptible NK targets. In further support of this possibility, normal lymphoid cells are totally insensitive to NK lysis, whereas a subpopulation of relatively immature hematopoietic cells, particularly thymus and bone marrow cells (13,31), are susceptible to cytolysis.

A central issue in the study of the specificity of NK cells is whether one common target structure is recognized by all NK cells or whether subsets of NK cells recognize a variety of target-cell structures. If multiple structures exist, attention must be focused on the extent or size of the repertoire and on whether discrete subpopulations of NK cells each have restricted reactivity against one or a few of these target structures.

From studies using adsorption procedures (53,92) or cloning of effector cells (3,11,47), the evidence favors the existence of at least several subsets of NK cells, some with broad reactivity and others with narrower patterns of cytotoxic effects.

Insight into the nature of the NK target structure and its heterogeneity would be much increased by determination of the biochemical nature of the target-cell determinant. However, very few studies have directly addressed this question. The paucity of biochemical studies on the NK target structure can be attributed (a) to limitations, at least until recently, in the methodology to isolate and purify large numbers of NK cells and (b) to unavailability of a rapid quantitative method to assess the interaction of NK cells with soluble membrane-derived materials.

A number of indirect approaches have been used to investigate NK target structure(s). Treatment of targets with various enzymes (e.g., proteases and lipases) and agents such as tunicamycin have led to the suggestion of a role for a glycoprotein or glycolipid structure (82). A second, more indirect, approach used specific reagents such as antitransferrin receptor (2,80,120,137), antilaminin (49), or antitarget antibodies (138). However, none of these studies yielded information that accounts for NK activity against an array of susceptible target cells; of more concern, most such inhibitory agents block NK activity at step(s) subsequent to binding of the effector cells to target cells. However, digestion of target cells with pro-

teases can result in the loss of recognition by NK cells (19), implying that surface proteins are a part of the target structure that is recognized.

A more direct approach would be to isolate membrane components from NK-susceptible targets and to measure their effects on the binding of NK cells to targets. Roder et al. (110,113) reported that high-molecular-weight (140–200 kilodaltons) glycoproteins can inhibit conjugate formation of normal mouse spleen cells with NK-susceptible targets, but a more detailed characterization of the target-cell molecules and the determinants recognized by mouse NK cells has not been reported. The ability to isolate highly purified NK cells, using discontinuous Percoll gradients, prompted a biochemical characterization of NK target-cell molecules involved in binding of human NK cells to the highly NK-susceptible target K562 (85).

The use of highly purified effector cells was important, since the previous study by Roder et al. (113) used unfractionated mouse spleen cells, which have been shown to contain a high percentage of cells that bind to NK-susceptible targets but that lack any detectable cytolytic activity (93). A detection system using highly purified NK cells avoids inhibition by non-NK-cell binders, since the majority (>80%) of binders have lytic activity against the target cells (126). Solubilized membrane proteins from K562 target cells were purified by various chromatographic procedures, reconstituted with exogenous lipid, and were then tested for their ability to inhibit formation of conjugates of LGL and target cells (85). The evidence that the inhibitory material was the target-cell molecule(s) recognized by NK cells was provided by the specificity of the inhibition. Membrane material from the human NK-susceptible target K562 inhibited conjugate formation between human LGL and several human NK-susceptible target cells but did not affect binding between human LGL and antibody-coated targets nor between rat NK cells and their NK-susceptible mouse or rat targets. Results from the studies with human target cells indicate that the target-cell structures are protein in nature (85). The inhibitory material was sensitive to trypsin, and it lost activity after incubation at 65°C for 40 min but not after incubation at 56°C. The material could be purified by a variety of lectins, with strong binding to concanavalin A and weak binding to peanut agglutinin. The size of the inhibitory molecules appeared to cover a broad range of molecular weights: In the human, the range was between 30 and 165 kilodaltons; in the mouse, it was between 140 and 240 kilodaltons. Collectively these studies indicate that inhibition of binding of effector cells to target cells by materials that have been separated by standard biochemical methods can be used to elucidate the structure recognized by NK cells. The available evidence regarding the detailed characteristics of the molecule(s) remains limited with regard to (a) the relationship of binding structures from one target to the next, (b) what regulates the expression of these target-cell structures, and (c) whether they are associated with viral or oncogene products. Current data do not indicate the nature of the determinant(s) recognized by NK cells; they only indicate the characteristics of molecules bearing these determinants. It is possible that the determinants recognized by NK cells may be protein and/or carbohydrate in nature. That treatment with trypsin destroyed the inhibitory activity does not exclude a carbohydrate determinant, since the protein may be required for efficient interaction of the soluble inhibitory material with lipid. Evidence for such a requirement exists for the human T-cell receptor that has a transmembrane lipophilic sequence (33,139). Likewise, the heat inactivation of the target structure may be attributable to a requirement for tertiary protein conformation for its reconstitution into lipid vesicles or for presentation to the effector cell; it does not necessarily imply a protein determinant. As discussed below, initial binding is only one step in these cytolytic mechanisms. A number of systems have been defined in which inhibition of lysis is due to postbinding events. Also, some mutant NK-resistant target cells are not deficient in their binding to NK cells, but rather in their ability to activate NK-cell cytolytic mechanisms (56,143), indicating that some postbinding activation structures or signals are not recognized by the effector cell. Therefore, a target cell may be easily recognized by the effector cells but may be unable to activate the lytic machinery or, alternatively, may possess molecules that interfere with subsequent events required to lyse the target cell.

Postrecognition Steps Leading to Lysis of Target Cells

After the requisite recognition of target cells by effectors and their binding together to form conjugates, a complex series of events is initiated which leads to the lysis of the target cells. Many of the early biochemical changes in the effector cells and the clear definition of a Ca^{2+}-dependent step have been found to be similar for CTL and NK cells (6,15). However, the actual mechanism underlying the lethal hit has been difficult to identify. There have been some suggestions that both CTL activity and NK activity are dependent on the generation of reactive oxygen intermediates (112). However, subsequent studies have essentially ruled out an involvement of this mechanism (58).

Recently, an appreciable amount of experimental evidence has accumulated for a mechanism of NK activity involving secretion of cytolytic molecules. This evidence includes: (a) rearrangement of cytoplasmic organelles and release of granules from NK cells following their binding to target cells (15,34); (b) decreased NK activity in Chediak-Higashi patients (1,30,55) and beige (bg/bg) mice (111) that bear mutations leading to abnormal formation

of lysosomal granules; (c) the reported inability of agranular lymphocytes to kill after they contact tumor cells (52); (d) a reduction in NK activity by strontium (78), which promotes leukocyte degranulation (24); (e) a requirement for lipid metabolism (transmethylation and phospholipase-A_2 activity) for both secretion of lysosomal enzymes and NK-cell activity (32,51); and (f) the inhibition of NK activity by lysosomotropic amines that interfere with lysosomal function (136). Demonstrations that NK cells release soluble cytolytic factors (NKCF) upon incubation with NK-susceptible target cells or lectins (141,142) provide further evidence that a secretory process is involved.

LGL-Granule Cytolysin

To evaluate directly the role of LGL granules in the lysis of tumor cells, the cytoplasmic granules from rat LGL tumors have been purified (35,75). These cells provide a convenient and uniform source of highly active cytolytic cells with NK specificity (96). The granules contain a potent, calcium-dependent cytolytic material, termed *LGL-granule cytolysin,* not present in the cytoplasmic granules of other noncytolytic leukocytes (35). LGL cytolysin is an approximately 60-kilodalton protein that lyses a wide range of target cells in a rapid and Ca^{2+}-dependent manner. When tested on liposomes, LGL cytolysin induced a rapid release of internalized carboxyfluorescein. As previously seen on lysed NK or ADCC targets, characteristic ring-like structures appeared, inserted into the lipid membrane. Penetration of negative stain into the liposomes correlated well with the presence of these pore structures. Together these data provide strong support for the model that assumes LGL-granule-derived pore insertion into the lipid layer as a mechanism of cytolysin activity.

The activity of LGL cytolysin clearly supports the model for lymphocyte cytotoxicity involving granule exocytosis after target-cell recognition. However, it is not easy to design definitive experiments to test whether granule cytolysins are responsible for the lethal damage inflicted by cytotoxic lymphocytes. One approach is to use rabbit antibodies against the purified LGL tumor granules. Fluorescence microscopy shows that such rabbit antibodies stain cytoplasmic granules in LGL tumor cells, LGL, and CTL but not in normal splenocytes, thymocytes, or peripheral T cells (98). The antibodies do not stain the plasma membranes of LGL, and granule staining can be detected only after permeabilization of the membrane. By Western blots, antigranule antibodies react with four of the five major granule proteins, and IgG from the antigranule sera specifically block granule cytolysin activity (98). Importantly, F(ab')$_2$ fragments of these antibodies specifically block the lytic activity of purified rat LGL in NK and ADCC assays in addition to the cytolysin activity. The antibodies do not interfere with binding of LGL to target cells, an expected result for antibodies to cytoplasmic granules. Presumably the antibodies have access to the granule cytolysin upon its release from the NK cells and prior to its effective interaction with target cells bound to the effector cells.

The LGL-granule cytolysin has much broader specificity for target cells than that seen with NK cells. NK-resistant tumor cell lines and even LGL themselves are lysed by the cytolysin, and sheep erythrocytes—not susceptible to NK activity—are particularly sensitive indicators of cytolysin activity (35). This major difference in specificity of NK cells and cytolysin, as well as the lack of lysis of NK-resistant third-party cells during an NK assay, needs to be explained to postulate a central role for LGL-granule cytolysin in the lytic process of NK cells. It is likely that during the interaction between NK cells and targets, the granule cytolysin is released mainly in the small intercellular space at the point of conjugate formation. Extracellular Ca^{2+} should rapidly inactivate the cytolysin that escapes into the surrounding medium before it reaches other target cells. Thus, the specificity of the NK reaction would be defined mainly by the initial recognition of susceptible targets, with cytolysin released only upon an effective interaction. According to this model, it would not be necessary to have specificity at the lytic molecule phase as well.

Essentially the same cytolytic molecule, termed *perforin,* has been isolated from some murine cloned CTL lines (21,95). Thus, it has been proposed that granule cytolysin or perforin is responsible for the lytic damage by both NK cells and CTL (94). However, as noted above, in many instances azurophilic granules have not been detected in CTL; also, some recent studies have failed to detect any involvement of a granule-dependent lytic molecule in the potent cytolysis produced by some preparations of CTL (7,8). These studies have included attempts to block cytotoxicity by anti-cytolysin antibodies; under conditions in which inhibition of NK activity had been observed, no inhibition of lysis by CTL was seen. Thus, it seems quite possible that these molecules contribute to the lytic process but may not be essential for cytotoxicity.

NK Cytotoxic Factors

Another somewhat similar pathway for the mechanism of cytotoxicity by NK cells has been described involving the release of a soluble cytotoxic factor, termed *NK cytotoxic factor* (NKCF), from NK cells upon stimulation by NK-susceptible target cells or lectins (39). NKCF has been shown to bind selectively to NK-susceptible target cells and then cause their lysis, but with kinetics considerably slower than those observed with intact NK cells or the LGL granule cytolysin. Although the difference in kinetics stands out as a major divergent point, most other characteristics related to NKCF have been very similar to those associated with NK activity. For example, a variety of inhibitors that were previously demonstrated to inhibit NK activity were also shown to inhibit the activity of NKCF. Initial attempts at purification have indicated that NKCF has apparent molecular weights of 18,000 and 36,000. The possible relationship between NKCF and the granule cytolysin is currently unclear. However, they may represent alternative pathways of a common mediator, since the anti-LGL granule antibodies have been found to interfere with the cytotoxic activity of human NKCF. It is possible that NKCF represents an altered or considerably more diluted version of the cytolysin in granules, and direct studies on the possible relationship between their physicochemical properties and amino acid sequences will be needed to settle this question.

Recently, studies have been performed to determine the possible relationship of NKCF to other, known, cytotoxic molecules. It has been possible to demonstrate that NKCF is distinct from tumor necrosis factor, lymphotoxin, or leukoregulin (44,88), and thus NKCF appears to be a quite novel cytotoxic molecule. In contrast, mouse NC activity has been found to be dependent on the release of tumor necrosis factor upon interaction of NC cells with their target cells (87).

In contrast to the rather extensive studies on release of NKCF from NK cells upon interactions with their targets and on their role for this factor in NK activity, there have been virtually no reports on the possible involvement of this or an analogous factor in cytotoxicity by CTL. Thus, it remains unclear as to whether NK cells and CTL indeed have essentially the same mechanisms for cytolysis or whether they diverge appreciably, if not fundamentally, with regard to their lytic machinery. As soon as NKCF is characterized, it will be important to directly look for an analogous protein in CTL.

CONCLUSIONS

Many of the features of CTL and NK cells and their lytic activity appear to be very similar. The main aspect of divergence appears to be related to their recognition receptors. It is possible that they are derived from two distinct lineages of effector cells, which simply share some properties. However, an alternative possibility is that NK cells represent an alternative thymic-independent pathway of T-cell differentiation and that they are basically the same as CTL but operate with different recognition receptors for non-MHC-associated target structures (29).

Further, detailed studies on the ontogeny and pathways of differentiation of NK cells and on possible similarities in their lytic mechanisms may help to distinguish between these possibilities.

REFERENCES

1. Abo, T., Cooper, M., and Balch, C. (1982): NK (HNK-1⁺) cells in Chediak-Higashi patients are present in normal numbers but are abnormal in function and morphology. *J. Clin. Invest.*, 70:193–200.
2. Alarcon, B., and Fresno, M. (1985): Specific effect of anti-transferrin antibodies on natural killer cells directed against tumor cells. Evidence for the transferrin receptor being one of the target structures recognized by NK cells. *J. Immunol.*, 134:1286–1291.
3. Allavena, P., and Ortaldo, J. R. (1983): Specificity and phenotype of IL-2 expanded clones and human large granular lymphocytes. *Diagn. Immunol.*, 1:162–167.
4. Barlozzari, T., Leonhardt, J., Wiltrout, R., Herberman, R., and Reynolds, C. (1985): Direct evidence for the role of LGL in the inhibition of experimental tumor metastases. *J. Immunol.*, 134: 2783–2789.
5. Barlozzari, T., Reynolds, C. W., and Herberman, R. B. (1983): *In vivo* role of natural killer cells: Involvement of large granular lymphocytes in the clearance of tumor cells in anti-asialo GM₁-treated rats. *J. Immunol.*, 131:1024–1027.
6. Berke, G. (1980): Interaction of cytotoxic T lymphocytes and target cells. *Prog. Allergy*, 27:69–95.
7. Berke, G., and Rosen, D. (1987): Circular lesions detected on membranes of target cells lysed by antibody and complement or natural killer (spleen) cells but not by *in vivo* primed cytolytic T lymphocytes. In: *Membrane Mediated Cytotoxicity*, UCLA Symposia (*in press*).
8. Berke, G., and Rosen, D. (1987): Are lytic granules and perforin 1 thereof involved in lysis induced by *in vivo* primed peritoneal exudate CTL *Transpl. Proc.* (*in press*).
9. Binz, H., Fenner, M., Frei, D., and Wigzell, H. (1983): Two independent receptors allow selective target lysis by T cell clones. *J. Exp. Med.*, 157:1252–1260.
10. Biron, C. A., Natuk, R. J., and Welsh, R. M. (1986): Generation of large granular T lymphocytes *in vivo* during viral infection. *J. Immunol.*, 136:2280–2286.
11. Bolhuis, R. L., van de Griend, R. J., and Ronteltap, C. P. (1983): Clonal expansion of human B73.1-positive natural killer cells or large granular lymphocytes exerting strong antibody-dependent and independent cytotoxicity and occasionally lectin-dependent cytotoxicity. *Nat. Immun. Cell Growth Regul.*, 3:61–72.
12. Bonnard, G. D., Yasaka, K., and Jacobson, D. (1979): Ligand-activated T cell growth factor-induced T-cell proliferation. Absorption of T cell growth factor factor by activated T cells. *J. Immunol.*, 123:2704–2708.
13. Bordignon, C., Daily, J. P., and Nakamura, I. (1983): NK-like effectors regulate hemopoietic colony formation *in vitro*: A model for hybrid resistance to bone marrow grafts? *J. Reticuloendothel. Soc.*, 34:75–76.
14. Brooks, C. G. (1983): Reversible induction of natural killer cell activity in clonal murine cytotoxic T lymphocytes. *Nature*, 305: 155–158.
15. Carpen, O., Virtanen, I., and Saksela, E. (1982): Ultrastructure of human natural killer cells: Nature of the cytolytic contacts in relation to cellular secretion. *J. Immunol.*, 128:2691–2697.
16. Chang, Z. L., Hoffman, T., Bonvini, E., Stevenson, H. C., and Herberman, R. B. (1983): Spontaneous cytotoxicity by monocyte-enriched subpopulations of human peripheral blood mononuclear cells against human or mouse anchorage-dependent tumor cell lines: Contribution of NK-like cells. *Scand. J. Immunol.*, 18:439–449.
17. Clark, W. R., and Golstein, P., editors (1982): *Mechanisms of Cell-Mediated Cytotoxicity*, Plenum Press, New York.
18. Damle, N. K., Doyle, L. V., and Bradley, E. C. (1986): Interleukin-2-activated human killer cells are derived from phenotypically heterogeneous precursors. *J. Immunol.*, 137:2814–2822.
19. Decker, J. M., Hinson, A., and Ades, E. W. (1984): Inhibition of human NK cell cytotoxicity against K562 cells with glycopeptides from K562 plasma membranes. *J. Clin. Lab. Immunol.*, 15:137–143.
20. DeFries, R., and Golub, S. (1986): Target recognition by human NK cells and lymphokine activated killer cells. *Fed. Proc.*, 45:a2760.
21. Dennert, G., and Podack, E. R. (1983): Cytolysis by H-2 specific T killer cells. *J. Exp. Med.*, 157:1483–1495.
22. Domzig, W., Stadler, B. M., and Herberman, R. B. (1983): Interleukin-2 dependence of human natural killer (NK) cell activity. *J. Immunol.*, 130:1970–1973.
23. Farrar, W. L., Johnson, H. M., and Farrar, J. J. (1981): Regulation of the production of immune interferon and cytotoxic T lymphocytes by interleukin 2. *J. Immunol.*, 126:1120–1125.
24. Foreman, J. C. (1977): Spontaneous histamine secretion from mast cells in the presence of strontium. *J. Physiol.*, 271:215–232.
25. Gorelik, E., Wiltrout, R. H., Okomura, K., Habu, S., and Herberman, R. B. (1982): Role of NK cells in the control of metastatic spread and growth of tumor cells in mice. *Int. J. Cancer*, 30:107–112.
26. Gray, J. D., Torten, M., and Golub, S. H. (1983): Generation of natural killer-like cytotoxicity from human thymocytes with interleukin-2. *Nat. Immun. Cell Growth Regul.*, 3:124–133.
27. Grimm, E. A., Mazumder, A., Zhang, H. Z., and Rosenberg, S. A. (1982): Lymphokine-activated killer cell phenomenon, lysis of natural killer cell resistant fresh solid tumor cells by interleukin-2-activated autologous human peripheral blood lymphocytes. *J. Exp. Med.*, 155:823–830.
28. Grimm, E. A., Ramsey, K. M., Mazumder, A., Wilson, D. J., Djeu, J. Y., and Rosenberg, S. A. (1983): Lymphokine activated killer cell phenomenon. II. Precursor phenotype is serologically distinct from peripheral T lymphocytes, memory cytotoxic thymus-derived lymphocytes and natural killer cells. *J. Exp. Med.*, 157:884–897.
29. Grossman, Z., and Herberman, R. B. (1986): Natural killer cells and their relationship to T cells: Hypothesis on the role of T cell receptor gene rearrangement on the course of adoptive differentiation. *Cancer Res.*, 46:2651–2658.
30. Haliotis, R., Roder, J., Klein, M., Ortaldo, J. R., Fauci, A. S., and Herberman, R. B. (1980): Chediak-Higashi gene in humans. I. Impairment of natural killer function. *J. Exp. Med.*, 151:1039–1048.
31. Hansson, M., Karre, K., Kiessling, R., Roder, J., Anderson, B., and Hayry, P. (1979): Natural NK cell targets in the mouse thymus: Characteristics of the sensitive cell population. *J. Immunol.*, 123: 765–771.
32. Hattori, T., Hirata, F., Hoffman, T., Hizuta, A., and Herberman, R. B. (1983): Inhibition of human natural killer (NK) activity and antibody-dependent cellular cytotoxicity (ADCC) by lipomodulin, a phospholipase inhibitory protein. *J. Immunol.*, 131:662–665.
33. Hedrick, S. M., Nielsen, E. A., Kavaler, J., Cohen, D. I., and Davis, M. M. (1984): Sequence relationships between putative T-cell receptor polypeptides and immunoglobulins. *Nature*, 308:153–158.
34. Henkart, M. P., and Henkart, P. A. (1982): Lymphocyte mediated cytolysis as a secretory process. In: *Mechanisms of Cell Mediated Cytotoxicity*, edited by W. R. Clark and P. Goldstein, p. 227. Plenum Press, New York.
35. Henkart, P. A., Millard, P. J., Reynolds, C. W., and Henkart, M. P. (1984): Cytolytic activity of purified cytoplasmic granules from cytotoxic rat lymphocyte tumors. *J. Exp. Med.*, 160:75–93.
36. Herberman, R. B. (1980): *Natural Cell-Mediated Immunity Against Tumors*. Academic Press, New York.
37. Herberman, R. B. (1982): *NK Cells and Other Natural Effector Cells*. Academic Press, New York.
38. Herberman, R. B. (1987): Adoptive therapy of cancer with interleukin 2 (IL-2) activated killer cells. *Cancer Bulletin*, 39:6–13.
39. Herberman, R. B., and Callewaert, D., editors (1985): *Mechanisms of Cytotoxicity by NK Cells*. Academic Press, Orlando, Fla.
40. Herberman, R. B., Mason, L., and Ortaldo, J. R. (1984): Studies on the possible relationship of NC cells to mouse NK cells. In: *Natural Killer Activity and Its Regulation*, edited by T. Hoshino, H. S. Koren, and A. Uchida, pp. 16–21. Excerpta Medica, Tokyo.

41. Herberman, R. B., Nunn, M. E., and Lavrin, D. H. (1975): Natural cytotoxic reactivity of mouse lymphoid cells against syngeneic and allogeneic tumors I. Distribution of reactivity and specificity. *Int. J. Cancer,* 16:216–229.

42. Herberman, R. B., Ortaldo, J. R., Djeu, J. Y., Holden, H. T., Jett, J., Lang, N. P., Rubinstein, M., and Pestka, S. (1980): Role of interferon in regulation of cytotoxicity by natural killer cells and macrophages. *Ann. NY Acad. Sci.,* 350:63–71.

43. Herberman, R. B., Ortaldo, J. R., Riccardi, C., Timonen, T., Schmidt, A., Maluish, A., and Djeu, J. (1982): Interferon and NK cells. In: *Interferons, UCLA Symposium on Molecular and Cellular Biology, Vol. XXV,* edited by T. C. Merigan and R. M. Friedman, pp. 287–293. Academic Press, New York.

44. Herberman, R. B., Reynolds, C. W., and Ortaldo, J. R. (1986): Mechanism of cytotoxicity by natural killer (NK) cells. In: *Annual Review of Immunology,* edited by W. E. Paul, C. G. Fathman, and H. Metzger, pp. 651–680. Annual Reviews, Palo Alto, Cal.

45. Hercend, T., Griffin, J. D., Bensussan, A., Schmidt, R. E., Edson, M. A., Brennan, A., Murray, C., Daley, J. F., Schlossman, S. F., and Ritz, J. (1985): Generation of monoclonal antibodies to a human natural killer clone characterization of 2 natural killer-associated antigens, NKH1A and NKH2, expressed on subsets of large granular lymphocytes. *J. Clin. Invest.,* 75:932–943.

46. Hercend, T., Meuer, S. C., Brennan, A., Edson, M. A., Acuto, O., Reinherz, E. L., Schlossman, S. F., and Ritz, J. (1983): Identification of a clonally restricted 90 KD heterodimer on two cloned natural killer cell lines: Its role in cytotoxic effector function. *J. Exp. Med.,* 158:1547–1560.

47. Hercend, T., Meuer, S., Reinherz, E. L., Schlossman, S. F., and Ritz, J. (1982): Generation of a cloned NK cell line derived from the "null cell" fraction of human peripheral blood. *J. Immunol.,* 129:1299–1305.

48. Hercend, T., Reinherz, E. L., Meuer, S. C., Schlossman, S. F., and Ritz, J. (1983): Phenotypic and functional heterogeneity of human cloned natural killer cell lines. *Nature,* 30:158–160.

49. Hiserodt, J. C., Laybourn, K. A., and Varani, J. (1985): Expression of a laminin-like substance on the surface of murine natural killer (NK) lymphocytes and its role in NK recognition of tumor target cells. *J. Immunol.,* 135:1481.

50. Hiserodt, J. C., Vujanovic, N. L., Reynolds, C. V., Herberman, R. B., and Cramer, D. V. (1987): Studies on lymphokine activated killer cells in rats: Analysis of precursor and effector cell phenotype and relationship to natural killer cells. In: *Cellular Immunotherapy of Cancer,* edited by R. L. Truitt, R. P. Gale, and M. M. Bortin. Alan R. Liss, New York (in press).

51. Hoffman, T., Hirata, F., Bougnoux, P., Fraser, B. A., Goldfarb, R. H., Herberman, R. B., and Axelrod, J. (1981): Phospholipid methylation and phospholipase A$_2$ activation in cytotoxicity by human natural killer cells. *Proc. Natl. Acad. Sci. USA,* 78:3839–3843.

52. Itoh, K., Suzuki, R., Umezu, Y., Hanaumi, K., and Kumagai, K. (1982): Studies on murine large granular lymphocytes. II. Tissue, strain, and age distributions of LGL and LAL. *J. Immunol.,* 129:395–405.

53. Jensen, P. J., and Koren, H. S. (1979): Depletion of NK by cellular immunoadsorption. *J. Immunol.,* 123:1127–1132.

54. Karre, K., Ljunggren, H., Piontek, G., Kiessling, R., Klein, G., Taniguchi, K., and Gronberg, A. (1984): Activation of cell mediated immunity by absence or deleted expression of normal cellular gene products, i.e. by "no-self" rather than "nonself". *Immunobiology,* 167:43–44.

55. Katz, P., Zaytoun, A. M., and Fauci, A. S. (1982): Deficiency of active natural killer cells in the Chediak-Higashi syndrome: Localization of the defect using a single cell cytotoxicity assay. *J. Clin. Invest.,* 69:1231–1238.

56. Kawase, I., Urdal, D. L., Brooks, C. G., and Henney, C. S. (1982): Selective depletion of NK cell activity *in vivo* and its effect on the growth of NK-sensitive and NK-resistant tumor cell variants. *Int. J. Cancer,* 29:567–574.

57. Kay, H. D., Bonnard, G. D., and Herberman, R. B. (1979): Evaluation of the role of IgG antibodies in human natural cell-mediated cytotoxicity against the myeloid cell line K562. *J. Immunol.,* 122:675–685.

58. Kay, H. D., Goldfarb, R. H., Wayner, E. A., and Brooks, C. G. (1985): No confirmed role for reactive oxygen intermediates in natural killer (NK) cell-mediated cytolysis. In: *Mechanisms of Cytotoxicity by NK Cells,* edited by R. B. Herberman and D. M. Callewart, pp. 263–286. Academic Press, Orlando, Fla.

59. Kedar, B. L., Ikerjiri, B., Sredni, B., Bonavida, B., and Herberman, R. B. (1982): Propagation of mouse cytotoxic clones with characteristics of natural killer (NK) cells. *Cell Immunol.,* 69:305–329.

60. Kiessling, R., Klein, R., and Wigzell, H. (1975): Natural killer cells in the mouse. I. Cytotoxic cells with specificity for mouse Moloney leukemia cells. Specificity and distribution according to genotype. *Eur. J. Immunol.,* 5:112–117.

61. Koren, H. S., and Herberman, R. B. (1983): Natural killing-present and fugure (summary of workshop on natural killer cells). *JNCI,* 70:785–786.

62. Landazuri, M. D., Silva, A., Alvarez, J., and Herberman, R. B. (1979): Evidence that natural cytotoxicity and antibody dependent cellular cytotoxicity are mediated in humans by the same effector cell populations. *J. Immunol.,* 123:252–258.

63. Lanier, L. L., Le, A. M., Phillips, J. H., Warner, N. L., and Babcock, G. F. (1983): Subpopulations of human natural killer cells defined by expression of the Leu-7 (HNK-1) and Leu-11 (NKP-15) antigens. *J. Immunol.,* 131:1789–1795.

64. Lattime, E. C., MacPhail, S., and Stutman, O. (1985): Lymphokines involved in the generation and regulation of NK and NC cells. In: *Mechanisms of Cytotoxicity by NK Cells,* edited by R. B. Herberman and D. M. Callewart, pp. 409–420. Academic Press, Orlando, Fla.

65. Lindahl, P., Leary, P., and Gresser, I. (1972): Enhancement by interferon of the specific cytotoxicity of sensitized lymphocytes. *Proc. Natl. Acad. Sci. USA,* 69:721–725.

66. Lotzova, E., Savary, C. A., and Herberman, R. B., editors (1986): *Natural Immunity, Cancer and Biological Response Modification.* Karger, Basel.

67. Lotzova, E., Savary, C. A., and Herberman, R. B. (1987): Induction of NK cell activity against fresh human leukemia in culture with interleukin-2. *J. Immunol. (in press).*

68. Lotzova, E., Savary, C. A., Herberman, R. B., and Dicke, K. A. (1986): Brief research news: Can NK cells play a role in therapy of leukemia? *Nat. Immun. Cell Growth Regul.,* 5:61–63.

69. Lotzova, E., Savary, C. A., Herberman, R. B., McCredie, K. B., and Barlogie, B. (1987): The role of natural killer cells in resistance to leukemia: Generation of antileukemia activity in NK-deficient leukemic patients. In: *Proceedings of the International Cancer Congress (in press).*

70. Mattes, M. J., Sharrow, S. O., Herberman, R. B., and Holden, H. T. (1979): Identification and separation of thy-1 positive mouse spleen cells active in natural cytotoxicity and antibody-dependent cell-mediated cytotoxicity. *J. Immunol.,* 123:2851–2860.

71. McCoy, J. L., Herberman, R. B., Rosenberg, E. E., Donnelly, F. C., Levine, P. H., and Alford, C. (1973): ^{51}Chromium release assay for cell-mediated cytotoxicity of human leukemia and lymphoid tissue culture cells. *Natl. Cancer Inst. Monogr.,* 37:59–67.

72. Migliorati, G., Cannarile, L., Herberman, R. B., Bartocci, A., Stanley, R., and Riccardi, C. (1987): Role of interleukin-2 (IL-2) and hemopoietin-1 (H-1) in the generation of mouse natural killer (NK) cells from primitive bone marrow precursors. *J. Immunol.,* 138:3618–3625.

73. Migliorati, G., Herberman, R. B., and Riccardi, C. (1986): Low frequency of NK cell progenitors and development of suppressor cells in IL-2 dependent cultures of spleen cells from low NK reactive SJL/J mice. *Int. J. Cancer,* 38:117–125.

74. Migliorati, G., Riccardi, C., Cannarile, L., Ayroldi, E., and Herberman, R. B. (1985): Development of large granular lymphocytes from mouse bone marrow cells cultured *in vitro* in the presence of recombinant IL-2. *Nat. Immun. Cell Growth Regul.,* 4:264–265.

75. Millard, P., Henkart, P., Reynolds, and C. W., Henkart, P. A. (1984): Purification and properties of cytoplasmic granules from cytotoxic rat LGL tumors. *J. Immunol.,* 132:3197–3204.

76. Morgan, A. C., Schroff, R. W., Klein, R. A., McIntyre, R. F., Mason, A., Herberman, R. B., and Ortaldo, J. (1987): Occult (non-surface

expression) of T, B and monocyte markers in human large granular lymphocytes. *Mol. Immunol.*, 24:117–125.

77. Morgan, D. A., Ruscetti, F. W., and Gallo, R. (1976): Selective *in vitro* growth of T lymphocytes from normal human bone marrows. *Science*, 193:1007–1008.

78. Neighbour, P. A., and Huberman, H. S. (1982): Sr^{+2}-induced inhibition of human natural killer (NK) cell-mediated cytotoxicity. *J. Immunol.*, 128:1236–1240.

79. Neighbour, P. A., Huberman, H. S., and Kress, Y. (1982): Human large granular lymphocytes and natural killing ultrastructural studies of strontiuminduced degranulation. *Eur. J. Immunol.*, 12:588–595.

80. Newman, R. A., Warner, J. F., and Dennert, G. (1984): NK recognition of target structures: Is the transferrin receptor the NK target structure? *J. Immunol.*, 133:1841–1845.

81. Oehler, J. R., Lindsay, L. R., Nunn, M. E., Holden, H. T., and Herberman, R. B. (1978): Natural cell-mediated cytotoxicity in rats. II. *In vivo* augmentation of NK-cell activity. *Int. J. Cancer*, 21:210–220.

82. Ortaldo, J. R., Blanca, I., and Herberman, R. B. (1985): Studies of human natural killer cytotoxic factor (NKCF): Characterization and analysis of its mode of action. In: *Mechanisms of Cell-Mediated Cytotoxicity*, edited by P. Henkart and E. Martz, pp. 203–220. Plenum Press, New York.

83. Ortaldo, J. R., Bonnard, G. D., Kind, P. D., and Herberman, R. B. (1979): Cytotoxicity by cultured human lymphocytes: Characteristics of effector cells and specificity of cytotoxicity. *J. Immunol.*, 122:1489–1494.

84. Ortaldo, J. R., Herberman, R. B., Harvey, C., Osheroff, P., Pan, Y., C. E., Kelder, B., and Pestka, S. (1984): A species of human-interferon which lacks the ability to boost human natural killer (NK) activity. *Proc. Natl. Acad. Sci. USA*, 81:4926–4929.

85. Ortaldo, J. R., Lewis, J. T., Braatz, J., Mason, A., and Henkart, P. (1982): Isolation of target antigens from NK-susceptible targets. In: *Intracellular Communication in Leukocyte Functions*, edited by J. W. Parker and R. L. O'Brien. John Wiley & Sons, New York.

86. Ortaldo, J. R., Mason, A. T., Gerard, J. P., Henderson, L. E., Farrar, W., Hopkins, R. F., III, Herberman, R. B., and Rabin, H. (1984): Effects of natural and recombinant IL-2 on regulation of IFN production and natural killer activity: Lack of involvement of the Tac antigen for these immunoregulatory effects. *J. Immunol.*, 133:779–783.

87. Ortaldo, J. R., Mason, L. H., Mathieson, B. J., Liang, S. M., Flick, D. A., and Herberman, R. B. (1986): Mediation of mouse natural cytotoxic (NC) activity by tumor necrosis factor (TNF). *Nature*, 321:700–702.

88. Ortaldo, J. R., Ransom, J. R., Sayers, T. J., and Herberman, R. B. (1986): Analysis of cytostatic/cytolytic lymphokines: Relationship of natural killer cytotoxic factor to recombinant lymphotoxin, recombinant tumor necrosis factor, and leukoregulin. *J. Immunol.*, 137:2857–2863.

89. Ortaldo, J. R., Sharrow, S. O., Timonen, T., and Herberman, R. B. (1981): Determination of surface antigens on highly purified human NK cells by flow cytometry with monoclonal antibodies. *J. Immunol.*, 127:2401–2409.

90. Perussia, B., Acuto, O., Terhorst, C., Faust, J., Lazaruz, R., Fanning, V., and Trinchiesi, G. (1983): Human natural killer cells analyzed by B731.1, a monoclonal antibody blocking Fc receptor functions. *J. Immunol.*, 130:2142–2148.

91. Phillips, J. H., and Lanier, L. L. (1986): Dissection of the lymphokine-activated killer phenomenon. Relative contribution of peripheral blood natural killer cells and T lymphocytes to cytolysis. *J. Exp. Med.*, 164:814–825.

92. Phillips, W. H., Ortaldo, J. R., and Herberman, R. B. (1980): Selective depletion of human natural killer cells on monolayers of target cells. *J. Immunol.*, 125:2322–2327.

93. Piontek, G. E., Gronberg, A., Ahrlund-Richter, L., Kiessling, R., and Hengartner, H. (1982): NK-patterned binding expressed by non-NK mouse leukocytes. *Int. J. Cancer*, 30:225–229.

94. Podack, E. R. (1985): The molecular mechanism of lymphocyte-mediated tumor cell lysis. *Immunol. Today*, 6:21–27.

95. Podack, E. R., Young, J. D. E., and Cohn, Z. A. (1985): Isolation and biochemical and functional characterization of perforin 1 from cytolytic T-cell granules. *Proc. Natl. Acad. Sci. USA*, 82:8629–8633.

96. Reynolds, C. W., Bere, E. W., and Ward, J. M. (1984): Natural killer activity in the rat. III. Characterization of transplantable large granular lymphocyte (LGL) leukemias in the F344 rat. *J. Immunol.*, 132:534–540.

97. Reynolds, C. W., Bonyhadi, M., Herberman, R. B., Young, H. A., and Hedrick, S. M. (1985): Lack of gene rearrangement and mRNA expression of the beta chain of the T cell receptor in spontaneous rat large granular lymphocyte leukemia lines. *J. Exp. Med.*, 161:1249–1254.

98. Reynolds, C. W., Reichardt, D., Henkart, M., Millard, P., and Henkart, P. (1987): Inhibition of NK and ADCC activity by antibodies against purified cytoplasmic granules from rat LGL tumors. *J. Leukocyte Biol. (in press)*.

99. Reynolds, C. W., Sharrow, S. O., Ortaldo, J. R., and Herberman, R. B. (1981): Natural killer (NK) activity in the rat. II. Analysis of surface antigens on LGL by flow cytometry. *J. Immunol.*, 127:2204–2208.

100. Reynolds, C. W., Timonen, T. T., Holden, H. T., Hansen, C. T., and Herberman, R. B. (1982): Natural killer (NK) cell activity in the rat: Analysis of effector cell morphology and effects of interferon on NK cell function in the athymic (nude) rat. *Eur. J. Immunol.*, 12:577–582.

101. Riccardi, C., Cannarile, L., D'Adamio, L., and Migliorati, G. (1986): NK cell generation from bone marrow stem cells. *Nat. Immun. Cell Growth Regul.*, 5:155–156.

102. Riccardi, C., Giampietri, A., Migliorati, G., Ayroldi, E., Cannarile, L., and Herberman, R. B. (1985): Pathways of differentiation of natural effector cells. *Nat. Immun. Cell Growth Regul.*, 4:273.

103. Riccardi, C., Giampietri, A., Migliorati, G., Cannarile, L., D'Adamio, L., and Herberman, R. B. (1986): Generation of mouse natural killer (NK) cell activity: Effect of interleukin-2 (IL-2) and interferon (IFN) on the *in vivo* development of natural killer cells from bone marrow prevention cells. *Int. J. Cancer*, 38:553–562.

104. Riccardi, C., Migliorati, G., Giampietri, A., Ayroldi, E., Cannarile, L., D'Adamio, L., and Herberman, R. B. (1986): Regulation of differentiation of bone marrow precursors into natural killer effector cells. In: *Natural Immunity, Cancer and Biological Response Modification*, edited by E. Lotzova and R. B. Herberman, pp. 34–39, Karger, Basel.

105. Riccardi, C., Migliorati, G., Giampietri, A., Ayroldi, E., and Herberman, R. B. (1985): Regulation of mouse NK activity. In: *Mechanisms of Cytotoxicity by NK Cells*, edited by R. B. Herberman and D. Callewaert, pp. 421–431. Academic Press, New York.

106. Riccardi, C., Migliorati, G., and Herberman, R. B. (1983/84): Partially restorative role of T cells for low interleukin-2 dependent growth of NK cell progenitors from nude mice. *Nat. Immun. Cell Growth Regul.*, 3:7–21.

107. Riccardi, C., Vose, B., and Herberman, R. B. (1983): Modulation of IL-2-dependent growth of mouse NK cells by interferon and T lymphocytes. *J. Immunol.*, 150:228.

108. Ritz, J., Campen, T. J., Schmidt, R. E., Royer, H. D., Hercend, T., Hussey, R. E., and Reinherz, E. L. (1985): Analysis of T-cell receptor gene rearrangement and expression in human natural killer clones. *Science*, 228:1540–1543.

109. Robb, R. J., and Greene, W. C. (1983): Direct demonstration of the identity of T cell growth factor binding protein and the Tac antigen. *J. Exp. Med.*, 158:1332–1340.

110. Roder, J. C., Ahrlund-Richter, L., and Jondal, M. (1979): Target-effector interaction in the human and murine natural killer system. Specificity and xenogeneic reactivity of the solubilized natural killer-target structure complex and its loss in a somatic cell hybrid. *J. Exp. Med.*, 150:471–481.

111. Roder, J. C., and Duwe, A. K. (1979): The beige mutation in the mouse selectively impairs NK cell function. *Nature*, 278:451–453.

112. Roder, J. C., Helfand, S. L., Werkmeister, J., McGarry, R., Beumont, T. J., and Duwe, A. (1982): Oxygen intermediates are triggered early in the cytolytic pathway of human NK cells. *Nature*, 298:569–572.

113. Roder, J. C., Rosen, A., Fenyo, E., and Troy, F. (1979): Target effector interaction in the natural killer cell system: Isolation of target structures. *Proc. Natl. Acad. Sci. USA*, 3:1405–1409.

114. Rosenberg, E. B., Herberman, R. B., Levine, P. H., Halterman, R. H., McCoy, J. L., and Wunderlich, J. R. (1972): Lymphocyte

cytotoxicity reactions to leukemia-associated antigens in identical twins. *Int. J. Cancer,* 9:648–658.

115. Rosenberg, E. B., McCoy, J. L., Green, S. S., Donnelly, F. C., Siwarski, D. F., Levine, P. H., and Herberman, R. B. (1974): Destruction of human lymphoid tissue culture cell lines by human peripheral lymphocytes in ^{51}Cr-release cellular cytotoxicity assays. *J. Natl. Cancer Inst.,* 52:345–352.

116. Santoni, A., Velotti, F., Testi, R., Galli, M. C., Piccoli, M., Herberman, R. B., and Frati, L. (1986): Mechanisms for *in vivo* expansion of natural killer cells. In: *Natural Immunity, Cancer and Biological Response Modification,* edited by E. Lotzova and R. B. Herberman, pp. 124–130. Karger, Basel.

117. Savary, C. A., and Lotzova, E. (1986): Phylogeny and ontogeny of NK cells. *Immunobiology of Natural Killer Cells,* edited by E. Lotzova and R. B. Herberman, pp. 45–61. CRC Press, Boca Raton, Fla.

118. Schendel, D. J., Wank, R., and Bonnard, G. D. (1980): Genetic specificity of primary and secondary proliferative and cytotoxic responses of human lymphocytes grown in conditioned culture. *Scand. J. Immunol.,* 11:99–107.

119. Schmidt, R. E., Hercend, T., Fox, D. A., Bensussan, A., Bartley, G., Daley, J. F., Schlossman, S. F., Reinherz, E. L., and Ritz, J. (1985): The role of interleukin-2 and T11-E rosette rosette antigen in activation and proliferation of human NK clones. *J. Immunol.,* 135:672–678.

120. Schuurman, H. J. Kluin, P. M., deGast, R., and Kater, L. (1985): HNK-1$^+$ cells in non-Hodgkin's lymphoma: Lack of relation with transferrin receptor expression on malignant cells. *Br. J. Cancer,* 51:171–177.

121. Serrate, S. A., Vose, B. M., Timonen, T., Ortaldo, J. R., and Herberman, R. B. (1982): Association of human natural killer cell activity against human primary tumors with large granular lymphocytes. In: *NK Cells and Other Natural Effector Cells,* edited by R. B. Herberman, pp. 1055–1060. Academic Press, New York.

122. Shau, H., and Golub, S. H. (1985): Depletion of NK cells with the lysosomotropic agent L-leucine methyl ester and the *in vitro* generation of NK activity from NK precursor cells. *J. Immunol.,* 134:1136–1141.

123. Shortman, K., Wilson, A., and Scollay, R. (1984): Loss of specificity in cytolytic T lymphocyte clones obtained by limit dilution culture of Lyt-2$^+$ T cells. *J. Immunol.,* 132:584–593.

124. Talmadge, J. E., Wiltrout, Counts, D. F., Herberman, R. B., McDonald, T., and Ortaldo, J. (1986): Proliferation of human peripheral blood lymphocytes induced by recombinant human interleukin-2: Contribution of large granular lymphocytes and T lymphocytes. *Cell. Immunol.,* 102:261–272.

125. Timonen, T., Ortaldo, J. R., and Herberman, R. B. (1981): Characteristics of human large granular lymphocytes and relationship to natural killer and K cells. *J. Exp. Med.,* 153:569–584.

126. Timonen, T., Ortaldo, J. R., and Herberman, R. B. (1982): Analysis by a single cell cytotoxicity assay of NK cell frequencies among assay of NK cell frequencies among human large granular lymphocytes and of the effects of interferon on their activity. *J. Immunol.,* 128:2514–2521.

127. Timonen, T., Ortaldo, J. R., Stadler, B. M., Bonnard, G. D., Sharrow, S. O., and Herberman, R. B. (1982): Cultures of purified human natural killer cells: Growth in the presence of interleukin 2. *Cell Immunol.,* 72:178–185.

128. Torten, M., Sidell, N., and Golub, S. H. (1982): Interleukin-2 and stimulator lymphoblastoid thymocytes to bind and kill K562 targets. *J. Exp. Med.,* 156:1545–1550.

129. Uchida, A., and Micksche, M. (1983): Lysis of fresh human tumor cells by autologous large granular lymphocytes from peripheral blood and pleural effusions. *Int. J. Cancer,* 32:37–44.

130. Uchida, A., and Micksche, M. (1983): Lysis of fresh human tumor cells by autologous peripheral blood lymphocytes and pleural effusion lymphocytes activated by OK-432. *JNCI,* 71:673–680.

131. Uchida, A., Micksche, M., and Hoshino, T. (1984): Intrapleural administration of OK-432 in cancer patients: Augmentation of autologous tumor killing activity of tumor-associated large granular lymphocytes. *Cancer Immunol. Immunother.,* 18:5–12.

132. Uchida, A., and Moore, M. (1984): Lysis of fresh human tumor cells by autologous large granular lymphocytes and T-lymphocytes: Two distinct killing activities induced by co-culture with autologous tumor. *JNCI,* 73:1285–1292.

133. Uchida, A., and Moore, M. (1985): Lysis of fresh human tumor cells by autologous tumor-associated lymphocytes: Two distinct types of autologous tumor killer cells induced by co-culture with autologous tumor. *Cancer Immunol. Immunother.,* 20:29–37.

134. Uchida, A., and Yanagawa, E. (1984): Natural killer cell activity and autologous tumor killing activity in cancer patients: Overlapping involvement of effector cells as determined in two-target conjugate cytotoxicity assay. *JNCI,* 73:1093–1100.

135. Van de Griend, R. J., Tax, W. J. M., van Krimpen, B. A., Vreugdenhil, R. J., Ronteltap, C. P. M., and Bolhuis, R. L. H. (1987): Lysis of tumor cells by CD3$^+$4$^-$8$^-$16$^+$ T cell receptor $\alpha\beta$ clones, regulated via CD3 and CD16 activation sites, REC interleukin 2 and interferon β_1. *J. Immunol.,* 138:1627–1633.

136. Verhoef, J., and Sharma, S. D. (1983): Inhibition of human natural killer activity by lysosomatropic agents. *J. Immunol.,* 131:125–131.

137. Vodinelich, L., Sutherland, R., Schneider, C., Newman, R., and Greaves, M. (1983): Receptor for transferrin may be a "target" structure for natural killer cells. *Proc. Natl. Acad. Sci. USA,* 80:835–839.

138. Werkmeister, J. A., Burns, G. F., and Triglia, T. (1984): Antiidiotype antibodies to the 9.1C3 blocking antibody used to probe the lethal hit stage of NK cell-mediated cytolysis. *J. Immunol.,* 133:1385–1391.

139. Williams, A. F. (1984): The T-lymphocyte antigen (T cell receptor)-elusive no more. *Nature,* 308:108–109.

140. Wiltrout, R. H., Talmadge, J. E., and Herberman, R. B. (1987): Role of NK cells in prevention and treatment of metastases by biological response modifiers. In: *Immune Responses to Metastases,* edited by R. B. Herberman, R. H. Wiltrout, and E. Gorelik. CRC Press, Boca Raton, Fla. *(in press).*

141. Wright, S. C., and Bonavida, B. (1981): Selective lysis of NK-sensitive target cells by a soluble mediator released from murine spleen cells and human peripheral blood lymphocytes. *J. Immunol.,* 125:1516–1521.

142. Wright, S. C., and Bonavida, B. (1982): Studies on the mechanism of natural killer (NK) cell mediated cytotoxicity (CMC). I. Release of cytotoxic factors specific for NK-sensitive target cells (NKCF) during coculture of NK effector cells with NK target cells. *J. Immunol.,* 129:433–439.

143. Wright, S. C., and Bonavida, B. (1983): YAC-1 variant clones selected for resistance to natural killer cytotoxic factors are also resistant to natural killer cell-mediated cytotoxicity. *Proc. Natl. Acad. Sci. USA,* 80:1688–1692.

144. Yamada, S., Ruscetti, F. W., Overton, W. R., Herberman, R. B., Birchenall-Sparks, M. C., and Ortaldo, J. R. (1987): Regulation of human large granular lymphocytes and T cell growth and function by recombinant interleukin 2. I. Induction of interleukin 2 receptor and promotion of growth of cells with enhanced cytotoxicity. *J. Leukocyte Biol.,* 41:505–517.

145. Yanagi, Y., Caccia, N., Kronenberg, M., Chin, B., Roder, J., Rohel, D., Kiyohara, T., Lauzon, R., Toyanaga, B., Rosenthal, O. K., Dennert, G., Acha-Orbea, H., Hengartner, H., Hood, L., and Mak, T. W. (1985): Gene rearrangement in cells with natural killer activity and expression of the β-chain of the T-cell antigen receptor. *Nature,* 314:631.

146. Young, H. A., Ortaldo, J. R., Herberman, R. B., and Reynolds, C. W. (1986): Analysis of T cell receptors in highly purified human and rat large granular lymphocytes (LGL); lack of functional 1.3 kb β-chain mRNA. *J. Immunol.,* 136:2701–2704.

147. Zagury, D. (1982): Direct analysis of individual killer T cells. Susceptibility of target cells to lysis and secretion of hydrolytic enzymes by CTL. In: *Mechanisms of Cell-Mediated Cytotoxicity,* edited by W. R. Clark and P. Golstein, pp. 149–156. Plenum Press, New York.

148. Zarling, J. M., Eskra, L., Borden, E. C., Horoszewicz, J., and Carter, W. A. (1979): Activation of human natural killer cells cytotoxic for human leukemia cells by purified interferon. *J. Immunol.,* 123:63–70.

Inflammation: Basic Principles and Clinical Correlates.
Edited by J. I. Gallin, I. M. Goldstein, and R. Snyderman.
Raven Press, Ltd., New York © 1988.

CHAPTER 33

Lymphocytes: Interaction with Macrophages

Harley Y. Tse and Alan S. Rosenthal

The Cell Biology of Lymphocyte-Macrophage Interaction
    Lymphoid Subpopulations • Effector and Regulatory Functions of Macrophages • Heterogeneity of Antigen-Presenting Cells • Macrophage–B-Lymphocyte Interactions
The Genetic Regulation of Lymphocyte-Macrophage Interaction
    Genes of the Major Histocompatibility Complex • Immune Response Genes (Ir Genes) and I-Region-Restricted Lymphocyte-Macrophage Interaction • Ia as Ir Gene Product and Restriction Element in T-Cell–

Macrophage Interaction • Mechanisms of Ir Gene Function • Macrophage Functions in the Induction of Suppressor T Cells
The Biochemistry and Pharmacology of Lymphocyte-Macrophage Interaction
    Regulation of Ia Expression on Macrophage • Macrophage Handling of Antigens • Macrophage Presentation of Antigens • Cytokine Regulation of Lymphocyte-Macrophage Interactions
Summary
References

Although vaccination had been in practice for several centuries, the cellular events occurring between the point of immunization and the manifestation of immunity remained an enigma for a long period of time. The mechanisms of antigen recognition are beginning to be understood in large measure because of the application of biochemical and molecular biologic techniques. Figure 1 depicts a glimpse of the contents of this black box as we currently understand it. It is immediately apparent that an immune response is the result of a complex network of cellular interactions. The afferent limb of the immune response involves the recognition of an inflammatory stimulus by the host as being foreign. Under normal circumstances, such stimuli are derived from exogenous sources. Occasionally, an endogenous protein may also be rendered immunogenic. When this occurs, autoimmunity ensues. The net result of recognition of an immunogen is either the production and release of antibodies by B lymphocytes or the release of pro-inflammatory mediators by T lymphocytes and macrophages. It is important to note that an immunogen is first handled by a class

of antigen-presenting cells exemplified by the macrophages or closely related cells that render the immunogen to a form recognizable by the T lymphocytes. T lymphocytes so activated may release a variety of mediators (lymphokines) that, when appropriately delivered to their prospective target populations, institute broad protective measures by the host. The efferent limb of the immune response concerns the mechanisms by which the host attempts to neutralize the stimulus by the combined activity of the products of the afferent limb and phagocytic cells aided by activation of a series of humoral mediator systems. Since an immune response is a continuous process and in some cases is regulated by feedback mechanisms, the division between the afferent limb and the efferent limb is by no means absolute. This distinction, however, helps our understanding of the cause-and-effect relationship in certain inflammatory responses that have an immune origin.

Obviously, the complexity of this cellular network requires that each component of the system be tightly regulated. Intrinsic functional aberrations of the system often

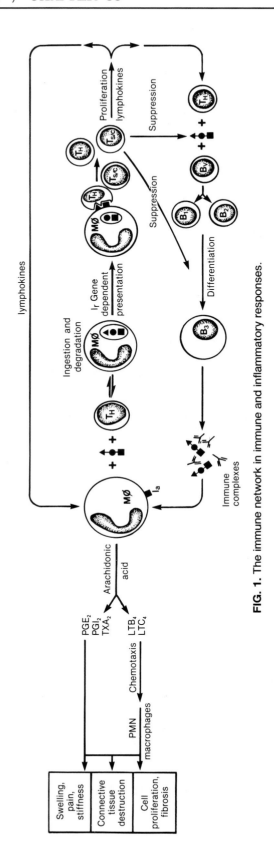

FIG. 1. The immune network in immune and inflammatory responses.

lead to subsequent expression of diseases. The involvement of immunoglobulins, complement, histamine, and other mediators in the efferent limb of the immune system has been described in great length by other authors. In this chapter, we provide an overview of the early events in the initiation of an immune response. Emphasis is placed on the interactions between T lymphocytes and macrophages and their roles in the subsequent manifestation of an inflammatory response.

THE CELL BIOLOGY OF LYMPHOCYTE-MACROPHAGE INTERACTION

Lymphoid Subpopulations

Major players of the afferent limb include the T lymphocytes, B lymphocytes, and macrophages. The T lymphocyte is pivotal in the system and is capable of both regulatory and effector functions. Since the T lymphocyte is the primary lymphoid subpopulation that has a close functional relationship with the macrophages, it is essential to have a basic understanding of its activities.

The first direct evidence for the regulatory role of T cells in the humoral response was provided by the now-famous three-mouse experiment of Claman et al. (1). It was shown that the injection of either donor thymus or bone marrow cells together with sheep erythrocytes as antigen into irradiated recipients gave only poor antibody production. However, when both thymus and bone marrow cells were injected into the same recipient, a marked synergism could be directly related to the number of cells injected. At the molecular level, experiments using hapten-carrier conjugates as antigens indicated that T cells and B cells may recognize distinct epitopes on the antigen (2,3), and maximum production of anti-hapten antibody by hapten-specific B cells required helper effects provided by the carrier-specific T cells. In this situation, the hapten-carrier antigen served as an "antigen bridge" between the T and B cells. Besides specific help, T cells can also provide nonspecific enhancement of B-cell antibody production. The so-called "allogeneic effect" (4) can be achieved through stimulation of T cells by alloantigen recognition or even mitogens.

It was in 1972 that Gershon and Kondo (5) first suggested that T cells could also negatively regulate B-cell antibody production. These investigators injected a very large number of sheep erythrocytes into mice that were previously thymectomized, lethally irradiated, and reconstituted with syngeneic bone marrow cells together with a small number of thymocytes. They found that these mice were no longer able to give an anti-sheep-erythrocyte response. Transfer of cells from "tolerant" mice to normal mice conferred tolerance on the recipient. This "infectious tolerance" was due to T cells because T cells had to be present for the induction of tolerance. The term "suppressor T cell" was eventually used for this functional activity.

Delayed cutaneous hypersensitivity responses and rejection of foreign tissue graft and tumor are the effector functions of T cells. Delayed hypersensitivity is an inflammatory reaction at the site of antigen deposition characterized by an influx of mononuclear cells as well as neutrophils. Although the mechanisms of delayed hypersensitivity are not yet fully understood, it is believed that a helper T cell is necessary to provide the stimulatory signals to a delayed-hypersensitivity effector T cell. On the other hand, regulation of delayed hypersensitivity through generation of suppressor cells has also been demonstrated. A great deal of effort has been directed to understand the mechanisms of suppression of delayed hypersensitivity. It is now well documented that this involves a cascade of three suppressor-T-cell subsets appropriately named first order (Ts_1), second order (Ts_2), and third order (Ts_3) (6). Ts_1 and Ts_3 are antigen-specific, whereas Ts_2 is idiotype-specific (7). Although tissue graft and tumor rejections are primarily *in vivo* phenomena, a variety of *in vitro* assays that are thought to mimic *in-vivo* cell-mediated responses have been developed. The *in vitro* mixed lymphocyte reaction reflects the clonal expression of T helper cells upon stimulation with allogeneic antigens, and cell-mediated lympholysis represents the final step of tissue destruction by cytotoxic T cells (8,9). T-cell-mediated tissue destruction is independent of both antibody and the complement system.

The identification of separate subpopulations of functional T cells has been achieved through the discovery of selective expression of specific cell-surface antigens on lymphoid cells. In 1975, Shiku et al. (10) generated a series of antisera against specific cell-surface antigens of the murine T-cell lineage (the Ly antisera). Using these antisera, Cantor and Boyse (11,12) demonstrated correlation between T-cell functions and expression of the Ly antigens. Helper T cells were found to be Ly-$1^+2^-3^-$ (later designated Lyt-1^+2^-), whereas suppressor and cytotoxic T cells were Ly-$1^-2^+3^+$ (later designated Lyt-1^-2^+). The T cells responsible for delayed hypersensitivity, as well as those participating the mixed lymphocyte reaction, have also been shown to be Lyt-1^+2^- (13). More recently, the development of the hybridoma technology (14) has enabled us to use monoclonal antibodies to define a functional subset of T cells in the human. The helper/inducer-T-cell subset, as defined by anti-Leu-3 or OKT4 monoclonal antibodies, is now designated CD4$^+$ T cells (15–18). This subset represents approximately 60% of peripheral T cells in healthy individuals. CD4$^+$ T cells include effector cells for delayed-type hypersensitivity and the responder cells in mixed lymphocyte reactions (19). The reciprocal sup-

pressor/cytotoxic T cells are CD8$^+$ and are defined by the monoclonal antibodies anti-Leu-2 or OKT8. As in the murine system, the helper-T-cell population can also serve as inducer cells for other T cells and B cells. The CD4$^+$ subset can further be separated into functionally distinct subpopulations with monoclonal antibodies such as anti-OKT17 and anti-Leu-8. Anti-OKT17 detected an antigen on the majority of resting T cells (20). Upon pokeweed mitogen stimulation, the OKT17 antigen was lost from a subset of the CD4$^+$ population so that CD4$^+$ OKT17$^-$ T cells exhibited solely helper activity, whereas CD4$^+$ OKT17$^+$ cells contained both helper and suppressor cells. Another marker, Leu-8, as described by Kansas and co-workers (21,22), is present on 75% to 90% of CD4$^+$ cells and 50% to 65% of CD8$^+$ cells. When mixed-lymphocyte-reaction cultures were established in the presence of cyclosporine A and the subsequent cultures were fractionated into Leu-8$^+$ and Leu-8$^-$ cells, it was shown that only CD4$^+$ Leu-8$^-$ T cells provided major helper activity for B-cell antibody synthesis. The fraction that contained CD4$^+$ cells that also expressed the Leu-8 marker was capable of inducing antigen-specific suppressor function of CD8$^+$ cells. Interestingly, helper function for the differentiation of CD8$^+$ cytotoxic T cells, on the other hand, could be provided by both subpopulations (23). Although most suppressor and cytotoxic T cells are of the CD8$^+$ phenotype, the recent experiments of Damle and Engleman (24), utilizing the monoclonal antibody designated 9.3, demonstrated the possibility of separating these two functions. Upon stimulation with alloantigen, activated CD4$^+$ 9.3$^-$ subpopulation proliferated and developed into suppressor cells that inhibited the mixed-lymphocyte-reaction responses of fresh autologous CD4$^+$ cells. The CD8$^+$ 9.3$^+$ subpopulation remained nonproliferative and contained the precursors of cytotoxic T cells.

Effector and Regulatory Functions of Macrophages

The effector functions of macrophages in inflammatory processes and tumoricidal activities have been treated in detail in previous chapters (17 and 25) and will not be repeated here. The first demonstrations that macrophages play a regulatory role in the afferent limb of the immune system came from the work of Mosier and Coppleson (25). These investigators first separated mouse spleen cells into adherent and nonadherent cell populations in plastic petri dishes. The vast majority of the adherent cells were identified to be macrophages, both morphologically and functionally. The sheep-erythrocyte antigen was incubated with the adherent cell population for 30 min and then washed thoroughly. In the first set of experiments, the number of nonadherent cells was held constant and varying numbers of adherent cells were added to the cultures without further addition of sheep erythrocytes. Responses to sheep erythrocytes were measured in a plaque assay. In the second set of experiments, the number of nonadherent cells was varied while the number of adherent cells was held constant. Based on a statistical analytical technique employed previously by Coppleson and Michie (26), who estimated the number of cell types interacting in a graft-versus-host reaction from the slope of the log-cell-dose–log-response line, Mosier and Coppleson showed that the slope for the first set of experiments was 1 and that the slope of the second set was 2. It was concluded that an adherent cell population, probably consisting of macrophages, was required in addition to two nonadherent cell populations (T and B cells) for the generation of a primary antibody response to sheep erythrocytes. It is interesting to note that the design of the experiments called for exposure of the antigen to the adherent cell population only. It was interpreted to suggest that interaction between cells and antigen must have occurred at the level of the macrophage. The functional significance of macrophages in humoral responses was also investigated by Kunin et al. (27). In these experiments, thioglycolate-induced peritoneal exudate cells preincubated with the rabbit serum albumin antigen were used to immunize mice and then to assay spleen cells for in-vitro antibody responses to dinitrophenol–rabbit serum albumin. It was shown that antigen-bound macrophages could successfully prime T cells to provide carrier effects for antibody synthesis by B cells. If recipient mice were irradiated and then repopulated with thymus cells followed 8 days later by bone marrow cells or if the order of injecting thymus and bone marrow cells was reversed, it was observed that rabbit-serum-albumin-pulsed macrophages only triggered a carrier effect on recipients given thymus cells first but not in those in which bone marrow cells were given before thymus cells. Kunin et al. (27) concluded that priming involved an initial interaction between macrophages and T cells. The conclusions were basically confirmed in in-vitro systems by other investigators (28–30).

One of the difficulties in studying macrophage functions in in-vitro systems is the inability to achieve complete depletion of adherent cells in target populations. In fact, when investigating the requirement of accessory cell functions in the primary and secondary antibody responses to sheep erythrocytes, Pierce et al. (31) noted that although the primary responses were readily abrogated by the removal of adherent cells on plastic plates, secondary responses were only reduced by 50% with the same depletion procedures. It appeared that secondary responses were less dependent on macrophage functions. However, using more stringent depletion methods such as anti-macrophage antibodies (32) or Sephadex G10 columns (33), other investigators were able to reduce secondary antibody responses by 90%.

What finally settled the matter came from the work of Rosenthal and co-workers (35–37), whose genetic analysis of the macrophage–T-cell interaction phenomenon led to an explosion of experimentation that firmly established the central role of the macrophage in the initiation of an immune response in both rodents and humans. These genetic studies will be discussed in a later section. At the cellular level, one approach taken by the Rosenthal group was to examine direct physical interaction between macrophage and T cells in binding assays, electron micrography, and in-vitro induction of T-cell proliferation. Following up on the previous observation of Siegel (34) that thymocyte "rosettes" developed about fresh guinea-pig peritoneal mononuclear cells when the two cell types were mixed in suspension, Lipsky and Rosenthal (35) prepared glass-adherent spleen cells and added thymocytes to the monolayer. They observed at least two types of physical interactions occurring between macrophages and lymphocytes. The first was not dependent on the presence of antigen and was without immunologic commitment. This step required active macrophages (but not lymphocytes), metabolism, divalent cations, and a trypsin-sensitive macrophage site. This binding did not distinguish T or B cells and was reversible so that binding represented an equilibrium between cellular association and dissociation. When this step had brought specifically immune lymphocytes into opposition with antigen-bearing macrophages, a second type of binding resulted. This latter phenomenon was dependent upon the presence of antigen. This association was not easily reversed and resulted in proliferation of the bound lymphocyte (36). An electron micrograph of this antigen-specific macrophage-lymphocyte interaction is presented in Fig. 2. Furthermore, a linkage between physical and functional macrophage-lymphocyte interaction in the antigen recognition process was also established by using cytochalasin B (37). Cytochalasin B is a reagent that inhibits recognition of antigen-specific signals by T cells but does not affect mitogenic signals such as phytohemagglutinin (PHA). It was found that cytochalasin B inhibited antigen-initiated lymphocyte proliferation and antigen-dependent lymphocyte-macrophage interaction when added immediately to culture, but it was progressively less effective when added later in the culture period. This suggested that cytochalasin B acts selectively on an early event in antigen-specific proliferation. Since it neither interferes with uptake of antigen by macrophages nor inhibits PHA-induced proliferation, antigen recognition itself is disrupted, not the machinery of DNA synthesis. The effects of cytochalasin B are thus likely to result from its inhibition of antigen-independent phase of macrophage-lymphocyte interaction.

As a result of the antigen-dependent specific interaction phase, T cells may proceed to clonal expansion through proliferation. This response is usually measured by an in-

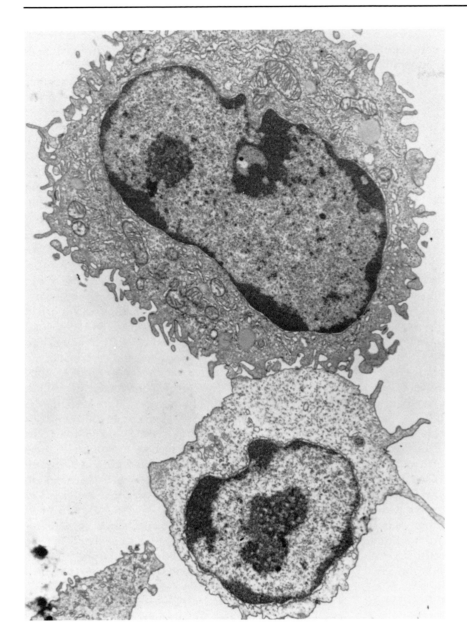

FIG. 2. Electron micrograph of antigen-specific macrophage-lymphocyte interaction. Note the close physical contact between macrophage and blast-transformed lymphocyte. From Rosenthal (162).

vitro T-cell–tritiated-thymidine incorporation assay. Because the assay is simple to perform, a substantial amount of our present knowledge regarding macrophage–T-lymphocyte interaction has been derived using these procedures (38–41). The general scheme involves mixing nylon-wool-column-purified T cells (42) and plastic adherent cells or simply irradiated spleen cells (43) in a 3- to 4-day *in-vitro* culture. In some instances, the antigen is directly pulsed onto the macrophages and washed before the T cells are added. Tritiated thymine as radioactive tracer of cell division is usually added several hours before the termination of culture, and the amount of radioactivity in-

corporated is a measure of the proliferative activities of the T cells.

It may be a good place here to point out that, over the years, a number of terms have been used to describe this population of cells that induce T cells in an antigen-specific manner. The term *adherent cell* is used almost as a synonym for macrophage because of the adherent properties of macrophages. Investigators who have not attempted to characterize their adherent cell population may feel more comfortable using the term *accessory cell.* This is especially true in studies involving antibody responses. More recently, it has been shown that antigen presentation is not the unique function of macrophages, since other cell types have been shown to be capable of stimulating antigen-specific T cells. The term *antigen-presenting cells* has become very popular. It is our preference that since a large amount of the work to be described used macrophages as the presenting cells, we will continue to use this term as long as it is noted that these functions are shared with other cell types as well.

Heterogeneity of Antigen-Presenting Cells

As will be detailed in a later section (on the genetic regulation of lymphocyte-macrophage interaction), macrophages present antigens to T cells through a cell-surface molecule referred to as Ia (I-region-associated) (39). Ia is a gene product of the major histocompatibility complex (MHC) and serves as a recognition molecule among cells of the immune system. Once it was demonstrated that Ia is instrumental in antigen presentation, questions were asked as to whether other Ia-bearing cell types besides macrophages have antigen-presenting capability. Indeed, Kupffer cells (which are resident macrophages of the liver) and alveolar macrophages (which line the alveoli of the lung) are capable of functioning as accessory cells in a number of distinct assays of T-cell activation (44,45). One of the early nonphagocytic cell types reported to serve in antigen presentation is the Langerhans cells. Langerhans cells are epidermal dendritic cells of the bone marrow derivation and have been shown to express Ia (46). These cells have been used in the initiation of both proliferative and cytotoxic T-cell responses toward soluble protein antigens, hapten, and alloantigens (47–49). A more potent dendritic cell population has been purified from spleen by Steinman and co-workers (50,51). It constitutes less than 1% of all the cells in the lymphoid organs and can be differentiated from the conventional mononuclear phagocytes by its morphology. Dendritic cells lack Fc receptors and do not stain for nonspecific esterase activity. Splenic dendritic cells are potent stimulators in mixed lymphocyte cultures, both allogeneic and syngeneic (52). In fact, a monoclonal antibody that specifically recognizes these splenic dendritic cells (53), when added together with complement, depleted 75% to 90% of the mixed-lymphocyte-reaction responses. It has also been shown that dendritic cells participate in the generation of trinitrophenyl (TNP)-specific cytotoxic T cells and antigen-specific T-cell proliferation. A third potential candidate of antigen-presenting cell is the B cell itself because B cells are highly Ia positive. The early experiments of Mosier and Coppleson (25) would have precluded the B cell as an antigen-presenting cell because an additional adherent cell population is necessary to effect B-cell antibody synthesis. Nevertheless, Chestnut and Grey (56) ingeniously

primed murine T cells to rabbit immunoglobulins and showed that purified B cells could indeed stimulate a T-cell proliferative response in the presence of rabbit anti-mouse antibodies. The rabbit anti-mouse antibodies served both as an antigen and as a means of anchoring onto the surface of the B cells (or antigen-presenting cell) to facilitate presentation. It is worth noting that this situation is not unlike that of the classical "antigen bridge" in the interaction between T and B cells; however, in the latter case, an adherent cell is obviously necessary to activate the T cells. In the experiments of Chestnut and Grey, the extra "push" may have come from the use of the rabbit anti-mouse antibodies, which effectively bind to all B cells. Besides increasing the number of effector antigen-presenting cells, these antibodies may also have stimulatory effects on the cells. It is thus not surprising that normal rabbit immunoglobulins would not work in their system. Another factor that determines the ability of B cells to present antigen is the differentiation stage of the B cells. Whereas resting B cells have not been good antigen presenters, B-cell lymphomas and mitogen-activated B cells have been shown by several investigators to present a wide variety of antigens (57–60). These cells, by virtue of their larger size and being at an activated stage, may have taken up larger quantities of antigens than did resting B cells and may be able to elaborate soluble factors essential for the activation of T cells. The ability of B cells to present antigens to T cells has been taken as a logical explanation for the classical observation that B-cell antibodies recognize native tertiary structure of protein antigens, whereas T cells can react with denatured peptides (61). B cells thus nonspecifically bind the antigen in its native configuration and, following some yet unclear mechanisms of processing or unfolding of the protein molecule (see section on the biochemistry and pharmacology of lymphocyte-macrophage interaction), present a sequential peptide to the T cells (62).

The list of potential antigen-presenting cells is still growing. Many of these are specialized cells in tissues and organs. In the human, monocytes and macrophages exhibit functions that are similar to those of their counterparts in the mouse (63). The main source of human monocytes is from the peripheral blood in which they constitute 10% to 20% of the mononuclear cells. Recently, antigen presentation functions have been demonstrated for human dendritic cells from tonsils and thymus (64), cells from human decidual tissues (65), and endothelial cells from umbilical veins (66,67). The last example represents an important and extremely interesting study, since the vascular endothelial cell plays a key role in separating circulating T cells from extravascular tissues. During acute inflammatory reactions, small chemicals are released; these substances may cause endothelial cell contraction, resulting in increased microvascular permeability to plasma protein. The interaction between antigen-specific T cells and the prospective antigen present on the surface of the endothelial cells is thought to have a regulatory function in these inflammatory processes. One immediate question that arises from studies of this diverse variety of antigen-presenting cells is whether all of these cells present antigens to T cells through the same mechanism. Because dendritic cells lack phagocytic activities and hence cannot internally degrade complex molecules, Lee et al. (68) suggested that dendritic cells are limited to presentation of small molecules not requiring extensive degradation. This conclusion, however, has not been confirmed in the studies of other investigators (69–72). In fact, the Feldmann group found that dendritic cells presented mycobacteria and complex molecules such as keyhole limpet hemocyanin (KLH) as efficiently as macrophages and suggested that dendritic cells may possess "ectoenzyme" systems on the surface for the degradation of complex molecules. It is interesting to note that except for macrophages, most experiments testing for antigen-presenting activities were done in proliferative assays or T-cell cytotoxic functions. Ramila et al. (73) pointed out that although B-cell tumor lines were able to reconstitute the anti-dinitrophenol response of adherent cell-depleted B cells in the presence of helper T cells and antigen and were able to activate T cells for lymphokine production, these cells were unable to induce helper cells required to cooperate with B cells by linked recognition. This was shown by the failure of T cells preincubated with the tumor lines TA3 or BC3A plus antigen to cooperate with B cells in the presence of concanavalin-A supernatants. These observations underscore the unique role of macrophages that is not shared with other antigen-presenting cells in their interaction with lymphocytes; also stressed is that macrophages have more than one antigen-presenting function. Obviously, many issues still have to be resolved. The intense interest in the biology of macrophage–T-lymphocyte interaction in recent years will undoubtedly yield answers to some of these questions.

Macrophage–B-Lymphocyte Interactions

Since the major function in their interaction with lymphocytes is to present antigen to and activate T cells, it would appear that macrophages would have no function in the activation process of B cells. This issue is still not fully resolved. The responses of macrophage-depleted B-cell populations to T-independent antigens and B-cell mitogens have been shown not to be affected by such depletion procedures (74,75). On the other hand, there are reports that anti-immunoglobulin stimulation of murine B-cell proliferation and B-cell responses to certain T-independent type-2 antigens do require the presence of accessory cells (76,77). Similar to studies of accessory cell functions in T-cell activation, one of the difficulties in these experiments is to demonstrate complete depletion of macrophages. A few contaminating macrophages may make all the difference between a response and the lack of a response. At this stage, answers to many of these issues still await further experimentation.

THE GENETIC REGULATION OF LYMPHOCYTE-MACROPHAGE INTERACTION

Genes of the Major Histocompatibility Complex

The major histocompatibility complex (MHC) occupies a stretch of 0.5 map unit or centimorgan (cM) on chromosome 17 and 1.7 cM on chromosome 6 of the mouse and the human, respectively. The mouse MHC is often referred to as the H-2, and the human MHC is often called the HLA. Equivalent genetic complexes have also been identified in other species such as the guinea pig (GPLA), rabbit (RLA), rat (RT1), dog (DLA), pig (SLA), and chimpanzee (ChLA). The bulk of the information gathered on the genetics of the MHC, however, has come from the H-2 because of the feasibility in that species for the construction of inbred, congenic, and recombinant strains for analysis. The importance of the H-2 was originally recognized by its association with allograft rejection. It is now established that the H-2 complex consists of four regions, namely, the K, I, S, and D. The I region is further divisible into three subregions, namely, the A, J, and E (Fig. 3). Gene products of the K and D regions are generally referred to as class I antigens. Class I antigens are the principal antigens recognized by the host during tissue graft rejection. In cell-mediated lympholysis, class I antigens are the surface molecules on the target cells recognized by cytotoxic T cells. The true physiologic role of the class I antigens is related to the mechanisms of self-nonself discrimination. In virus infection, killing of virus-infected cells requires that the target cells express both the viral antigens and class I antigens compatible to those on the cytotoxic T cells. This phenomenon is termed "MHC restriction" of cellular recognition. Gene products of the I region are designated class II antigens. For historic reasons, these have also been referred to as Ia antigens (for Ir-associated antigens). These two terms will be used interchangeably throughout this chapter. Of the I-region genes, two products have been identified, namely, the I-A and I-E molecules. These are cell-surface glycoprotein heterodimers consisting of an alpha chain with a molecular weight of approximately 32,000 and a beta chain with a molecular weight of about 28,000. Each of these polypeptide chains consists of two extracellular domains β_1 and β_2 encoded by separate exons. Ia antigens are ex-

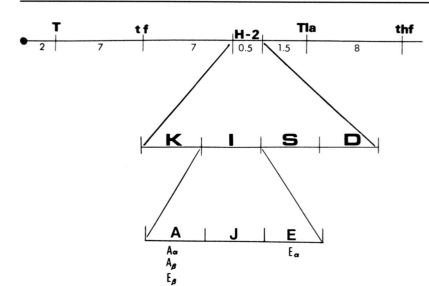

FIG. 3. A graphic map of the murine H-2 complex on chromosome 17.

pressed predominantly by B cells and mononuclear phagocytic cells such as macrophages.

Much of what we know regarding the functions of the HLA antigens is based on those already described for the H-2 complex. Numerous components of the HLA complex are homologous to loci of the H-2 complex. As shown in Fig. 4, the three class I HLA loci have been named A, B, and C. The human analog of the mouse H-2 I region is generally accepted to be the HLA-D/DR region. The HLA-D antigens are defined and typed by mixed leukocyte reactions, whereas the HLA-DR specificities are defined by serologic means and are found to map to the same, or very closely linked, HLA-D locus (DR stands for D-region-related). Interestingly, amino acid sequences reveal that there is greater homology between DR and I-E products than between DR and I-A products. Only recently have Goyert et al. (78) identified a human class II molecule designated DS, which showed sequence homology with the murine I-A alpha and beta chains at the amino-terminal end.

Immune Response Genes (Ir Genes) and I-Region-Restricted Lymphocyte-Macrophage Interaction

Two important discoveries of the late 1960s early 1970s shaped the course of immunology in the 10 years that followed. The first was the observation, by McDevitt and Sela (79) in mice and Benacerraf et al. (80) in guinea pigs, that outbred animals showed marked quantitative differences in their ability to develop humoral and cellular immune responses to certain antigens. Subsequent uses of inbred strains of animals and simple synthetic antigens led to the conclusion that responses to these peptides were indeed under genetic control. The two prototype strains used in the experiments of McDevitt and Sela were C57BL/6 and CBA. C57BL/6 mice were good producers of antibodies to the antigen (T,G)-A-L (high responders), and CBA were poor producers (low responders). Breeding experiments further showed that responsiveness was controlled by a single, autosomal dominant gene located within the H-2 complex (81). Detailed investigation using

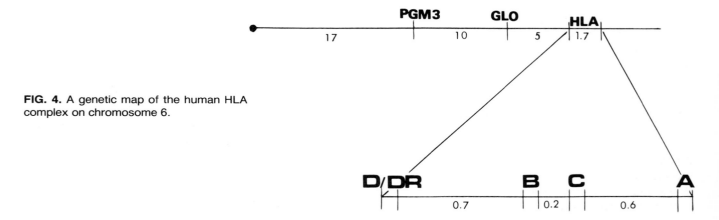

FIG. 4. A genetic map of the human HLA complex on chromosome 6.

recombinant strains mapped the gene to a region between K and D and was denoted by the letter I for immune response genes (Ir-1) (82). Subsequently, a large number of antigens were found to be under Ir gene control. One common characteristic of these antigens was their T-cell dependency. Relevant Ir genes were required for the development of cellular immunity as well as antibody production. Comparison of the responses of a number of these antigens revealed that some antigen responsiveness mapped to I-A and some mapped to I-E.

Although the I region was originally established for immune response genes, a number of other traits were also found to be associated with this region. Among these was the mixed lymphocyte reaction. As pointed out earlier, a mixed lymphocyte reaction occurs when the lymphocytes from two I-region disparate strains are mixed together *in vitro*. This immediately raised hope that an antisera to these mixed-lymphocyte-reaction determinants could be produced because these antigens were apparently expressed on the cell surface. Indeed, several laboratories vigorously searched for such a product by immunizing K,D-region compatible, but I-region disparate, strains against each other. Antibodies raised against I-region gene products are referred to as anti-Ia antibodies (83). These antisera became powerful tools for the study of cellular recognition and interactions.

Although macrophages had been shown to be necessary for T-cell activation in previous studies (84), it was not until the demonstration that their interaction was also restricted by Ir genes and Ia expression that the roles of macrophages to act as antigen-presenting cells began to be understood. The original studies of Shevach and Rosenthal (39) used two strains of guinea pigs, namely, strain 2 and strain 13, that differed at the I region. To study Ir-gene functions, they measured the *in vitro* T-cell proliferative response to the antigens GL (copolymers composed of L-glutamic acid and L-lysine) and GT (copolymers composed of L-glutamic acid and L-tyrosine), which were under Ir gene control. In their experiments, it was shown that $(2 \times 13)F_1$ T cells proliferated to GT only in the presence of GT-pulsed F_1 or strain-13 macrophages. GT-pulsed strain-2 macrophages failed to stimulate the F_1 T cells. In contrast, F_1 T cells responded to the antigen dinitrophenol-GL pulsed onto the macrophages of F_1 and strain 2 but not strain 13. Taken together, these experiments demonstrated that although the F_1 T cells were able to respond to these Ir-gene-controlled antigens, they did so only if the antigen-presenting macrophages possessed the responder Ir-gene alleles. In another series of experiments to test for I-region compatibility requirements for the activation of T cells, Rosenthal and Shevach (85) used the antigen PPD, to which both strain-2 and strain-13 guinea pigs were responders. PPD was pulsed on the macrophages of strain 2 and strain 13, which

were then tested for their ability to stimulate T-cell proliferation. As shown in Table 1, PPD-pulsed strain-2 macrophages only stimulated proliferation of strain-2 T cells and not strain-13 T cells. Conversely, strain-13 macrophages only interacted with strain-13 T cells and not strain-2 T cells. F_1 macrophages, by virtue of their expression of both strain-2 and strain-13 Ir-region gene products, were stimulatory to both strain-2 and strain-13 T cells. These observations have profound implications in our understanding of the interaction between T cells and macrophages. For effective interaction with T cells, macrophages must (a) possess a responder status to the antigen concerned and (b) possess an Ia allele compatible with the T cells. The relationship between Ir gene and Ia have since become an important issue in explaining the mechanism of Ir-gene regulation. The observations of Shevach and Rosenthal have also been confirmed in other species, including mice (86) and human (87).

The question of whether B-cell responses to antigens also require corecognition of I-region gene products by T cells has been debated for a long period of time and still has no resolution. I-region restriction in the interaction between T cells and B cells was first demonstrated by Katz and Benacerraf (88). However, it has not been resolved whether this restriction merely reflects the restriction of T-macrophage interaction which precedes the T-B interaction. One suggestion is that there are subsets of B cells with different activation requirements. Cells expressing the Lyb5 surface antigen are capable of accepting activation signals from nonspecific T-cell-soluble mediators, thus bypassing the genetic requirements. Lyb5⁻ cells, on the other hand, can only be activated through recognition of both antigen and Ia (89).

TABLE 1. *The requirement for histocompatible macrophages in antigen-mediated DNA synthesis in immune guinea-pig lymph node lymphocytes*[a]

Macrophages		Lymphocyte DNA synthesis (cpm $\times 10^{-3}$)		
Strain	Antigen pulse	Strain 2	Strain 13	$(2 \times 13)F_1$
2	0	0.92	5.68	1.60
2	+	26.38	8.61	6.98
13	0	4.63	1.66	1.78
13	+	3.12	19.89	7.81
$(2 \times 12)F_1$	0	1.91	4.27	1.66
$(2 \times 13)F_1$	+	12.42	11.81	12.57

[a] Macrophage-rich peritoneal exudate cells from nonimmunized strain-2, -13, or -$(2 \times 13)F_1$ guinea pigs were incubated with mitomycin C and/or PPD for 60 min at 37°C and washed, and then each were mixed with column-purified immune lymph-node cells. From Rosenthal and Shevach (85).

MHC-restricted T-cell recognition is also required for cytotoxic T-cell killing of target cells. In this case, the restriction elements are the class I (K and D) antigens (90,91).

Ia as Ir Gene Product and Restriction Element in T-Cell–Macrophage Interaction

As noted earlier, both Ir genes and I-region restriction in the interaction between T cells and macrophages are mapped to the same genetic region. Several lines of evidence now suggest that Ia is the molecule that exerts Ir gene function in the response of T cells to certain antigens. Shevach et al. (92) earlier showed that guinea-pig alloantisera inhibited the antigen-specific proliferative responses of responder T cells. However, more direct demonstration equating Ia to Ir genes came from the analysis of an IA mutant strain of mouse, B6.C-H-2^{bm12} (bm12). The bm12 strain was originally detected as a gain/loss mutation by Melvold and Kohn (93) in skin-graft studies employing (B6 × Balb/c)F_1 mice. Breeding experiments demonstrated that the mutation occurred in the H-2^b haplotype of the B6 strain. The mutant haplotype was rendered homozygous and congenic with B6, establishing a new mutant line B6.C-H-2^{bm12} coisogenic with B6. Skin-graft complementation studies by McKenzie et al. (94) and Hansen et al. (95), using recombinant strains separating the K, IA, and IE regions, demonstrated that the bm12 mutation mapped to the IA region. The precise bm12 mutation site was analyzed by using molecular biological techniques (96). The Aβ genes of bm12 and B6 mice were found to differ by three productive nucleotides within a stretch of 14 nucleotides in the exon encoding the first extracellular domain (β_1). To test whether these changes in the resultant Ia molecule caused corresponding changes in the immune response patterns between the wild-type B6 and the mutant bm12, Lin et al. (97) compared the responses of these two strains to several soluble protein antigens. In their experiments, B6, bm12, and their F_1 were immunized to several antigens, including beef insulin *in vivo*. T cells were isolated by nylon-wool-column purification and were tested for proliferative responses in the presence of irradiated spleen cells and antigen. As shown in Table 2, while B6 responded to the Ir-gene-controlled antigens, beef insulin, (TG)-AL, and collagen nicely, bm12 only responded to (TG)-AL and collagen but not to beef insulin. The response of the F_1's to beef insulin was intermediate. The results of this study showed that limited alteration of the Ia molecule concomitantly led to changes in the immune response pattern of T cells to soluble antigens. The changes are selective, since bm12 responded to other antigens such as (TG)-AL and collagen at levels comparable to those of B6. Mutant bm12 was also found to be defective in its responses to the H-Y antigens (98). It is concluded that Ia is the long-sought-after immune response gene product and that the nonresponder defect is related to Ia function.

Initial evidence that Ia is also the restriction molecule governing the interaction between T cells and macrophages was inferred from inhibition studies of antigen-specific T-cell responses with anti-Ia antibodies (99). Macrophage stimulation of T-cell proliferation to antigens was abolished when the appropriate anti-Ia antisera were included in the cultures. More direct evidence was again provided by studies of the IA mutant bm12. The question asked was whether bm12 macrophages, which had limited structural alteration in Ia, could interact with B6 T cells. To avoid allogeneic stimulation masking true cooperation between T cells and macrophages, Kanamori et al. (100) generated antigen-specific T-cell clones from B6 and demonstrated that the majority of the clones would respond to antigen only if it was presented by B6 macrophages and not by bm12 macrophages. Thus there is a direct link between Ia and genetic restriction in the interaction between T cells and macrophages. The picture

TABLE 2. *Proliferative response of (B6 × B6.C-H-2^{bm12})F_1 T cells in the presence of antigen-presenting cells from F_1 hybrid or parental strains*[a]

Source of spleen cells	[³H]Thymidine incorporation (Δcpm)					
	Beef insulin (100 µg/ml)	(TG)AL (100 µg/ml)	Collagen (100 µg/ml)	Ovalbumin (100 µg/ml)	PPD (100 µg/ml)	Medium control (cpm)
F_1	28,746	43,294	10,654	33,813	51,279	9,120
B6	38,527	39,458	8,213	33,184	50,045	5,362
B6.C–H–2^{bm12}	8,935	26,537	8,986	27,454	49,750	8,400

[a] (B6 × B6.C–H–2^{bm12})F_1 mice were immunized with 50 µg each of beef insulin, (TG)AL, type II collagen, and ovalbumin in complete Freund's adjuvant. T-cell proliferation was measured by tritiated thymidine incorporation. Δcpm was calculated by subtracting medium control from values for antigen-stimulated cultures. Each experimental point represents the mean of triplicate cultures. From Lin et al. (97).

that emerges from studies of Ir gene function and MHC restriction indicates that the basic requirement for T-cell–macrophage interaction is Ia compatibility. The Ir gene phenomenon is only a special situation of this restricted recognition, so that in the nonresponders a particular combination of antigen and Ia is either not properly formed or not properly recognized.

Mechanisms of Ir Gene Function

Over the past 10 years, interest in understanding why recognition fails in nonresponders has generated a great deal of excitement and controversy. There are currently three different views as to how this can occur. First, a hypothesis proposed by Rosenthal et al. (101) and by Benacerraf (102) placed Ir-gene regulation at the level of the macrophage. It was suggested that macrophage Ia, by virtue of its specificity polymorphism, selectively associated with a given antigenic determinant, the pairing of which ultimately determined the outcome of its interaction with the T cells. In a series of experiments carried out by Rosenthal et al. (101), it was established that guinea-pig and mouse T-cell responses to insulin were strain- and determinant-specific. For example, strain-2 guinea pigs recognized the A-chain loop of insulin because the T-cell response was sensitive to amino acid changes in positions A8, A9, and A10 (103). Species of insulin with total identity in this area completely cross-reacted in T-cell proliferation and T-helper-cell activity. Insulin with partial or no identity in these amino acid residues showed partial or no cross-reactivity, respectively. The responses of strain-13 T cells, on the other hand, were independent of their A-chain loop constitution. The determinant recognized by this strain resided in the B-chain region of the insulin molecule, as evidenced by the capacity of immune strain 13, but not strain 2, to respond to isolated oxidized B chain. When strain-2, -13, and -(2 × 13)F$_1$ guinea pigs were immunized with oxidized B chain, strain 13 and F$_1$ (but not strain 2) responded to either isolated B chain or native insulin. In the mouse, the immune T-cell proliferative response to insulin in the responder strains, H-2^b and H-2^d, was also governed by two distinct determinants, the H-2^b by the A-chain determinant and H-2^d by the B-chain determinant. The pattern of recognition of determinants in H-2^b and H-2^d mice was remarkably similar to the determinant specificity exhibited by strain-2 and strain-13 guinea pigs, respectively. It was therefore suggested that the function of Ir genes at the level of macrophage Ia was an intramolecular selection of discrete regions within the antigen for recognition by T cells (the Determinant Selection Hypothesis). The defect in nonresponders would consist of a failure of the nonresponder macrophage to select the stimulatory determinant for presentation to T cells.

A completely different view was taken by Schwartz (104), Ishii et al. (105), and Dos Reis and Shevach (106). In the Clonal Deletion Model, emphasis of Ir-gene function was placed at the level of the T cells. It was argued that nonresponder macrophages did not handle the antigen differently than responder macrophages. Rather, the failure of responsiveness was due to a lack in nonresponders of a T cell with receptors capable of recognizing such a macrophage–Ia-antigen combination. Such a "hole" in the T-cell repertoire could be due to a clonal deletion mechanism of tolerance to self during ontogeny. Support for such a concept was derived from experiments demonstrating the priming of responder T cells to antigen by responder macrophages in vitro after elimination of alloreactive T cells. In the guinea-pig system, Dos Reis and Shevach (106) were able to show presentation of insulin B chain by strain-2 macrophages to strain-13 T cells, thus eliminating the objection that allogeneic macrophages might be presenting different antigenic determinants from syngeneic macrophages. It must be noted, however, that the success of these experiments depends on the elimination of allogeneic cells by BudR and light. Any trace of these cells may evoke a weak allogeneic effect and thus obscure the interpretation of the experiment.

The third possibility of Ir-gene-controlled unresponsiveness is the activation of suppressor cells specific for a certain combination of antigen and Ia. The existence of suppressor cells in nonresponder strains to the antigen GAT has been demonstrated by Pierce and Kapp (107) and has been shown more recently in LDH$_B$ by Nagy et al. (108). One still unresolved question in this model is the nature of the restriction element in the induction of suppressor T cells. Without knowledge of this restriction element, it is difficult to envisage how suppression can be specific for a given pair of Ia and antigenic determinants.

One of the facets of the Determinant Selection Model is the requirement of pairing of a given set of Ia and antigenic determinant. Previously, the concept of an antigen-Ia interaction has not been widely accepted because macrophages have never been thought to discriminate antigenic specificities. However, evidence has accumulated in recent years indicating that specific antigen-Ia associations do occur. The most persuasive support is derived from the studies of Babbitt et al. (152), who used biochemical methods and demonstrated a weak, but measurable, physical association between a hen-egg lysozyme antigenic fragment and purified Ia molecules (see section on biochemistry and pharmacology of lymphocyte-macrophage interaction). This association was demonstrated for Ia derived from a responder strain but not that from a nonresponder strain. Another line of evidence came from analysis of a B10.A T cell clone responding to the antigen cytochrome c (163). It was shown that presentation required recognition of cytochrome c in association with the $E_\beta^k:E_\alpha^k$ molecule, and a lower concentration of moth cytochrome c than of pigeon cytochrome c was required to stimulate a given level of T-cell response. In addition, macrophages from another strain B10.S (9R) that possessed the $E_\beta^s:E_\alpha^k$ molecule were also capable of presenting antigen to this clone except that in this case, pigeon cytochrome c was more stimulatory than moth cytochrome c. This series of experiments suggest that both antigen and Ia contribute to the complex recognized by T cells and that a given T-cell receptor can be triggered by different combinations of antigen and Ia specificities. This different combination apparently has to involve changes in both antigen and Ia, since changes in the Ia molecule alone in the case of bm12 abrogated the response (97).

The HLA-D/DR region is generally considered to be the human counterpart of the I region of the murine MHC. HLA-D/DR restriction in T-cell–macrophage interactions (109–111) and anti-DR antisera blocking of T-cell proliferative responses have been demonstrated for several antigens (112,113). Precise analysis of Ir-gene functions in humans is naturally difficult. Over the past decade, numerous reports have demonstrated strong association between diseases and certain HLA alleles (114,115). For example, multiple sclerosis, insulin-dependent diabetes mellitus (IDDM), and Graves' disease are shown to be strongly associated with D/DR3 (116). Numerous attempts have also been made to demonstrate the existence of Ir-gene functions in humans. Analysis of immune responses to measles (117), streptococcal antigen (118), and synthetic antigen TGAL (119) has led several groups to believe that responsiveness to these antigens are indeed under HLA genetic control. Studies of this nature, however, are far from complete, especially since the HLA-D/DR region is not yet fully characterized.

Macrophage Functions in the Induction of Suppressor T Cells

Discussion of lymphocyte-macrophage interactions cannot be complete without mention of the induction of suppressor T cells by macrophages. Previously, it was thought that the suppressor cell pathway was preferentially stimulated when antigen escaped "processing" by macrophages and activated the T cell directly (120). More recently, it has been demonstrated that induction of antigen-specific T cells in many ways resembles the induction of antigen-specific helper cells, i.e., the antigen has to be presented, the presenting cell has to express Ia, and the H-2 alleles expressed on the presenting cell determine the genetic restriction of the suppressor T cells (121). In addition, functional expression of I-J determinants is also required for this form of macrophage-suppressor T-cell

interactions (122). Perhaps one of the best characterized systems for the study of the suppressor-T-cell cascade is the contact sensitivity responses of the hapten 4-hydroxy-3-nitrophenyl acetyl (NP). In this system, three operationally distinct T-cell subsets, namely, Ts_1 (inducer), Ts_2 (transducer), and Ts_3 (effector), have been identified (123). It has been shown that induction of Ts_1 and Ts_3 requires accessory cells that functionally express I-J determinants. The propagation of the suppressor-cell cascade is mediated by the generation of suppressor factors at each stage. An additional function for the accessory cell is that of a target cell for the suppressor factor TsF_3, which eventually asserts the suppression. Analysis of macrophage functions in suppressor cell induction has recently been carried out using cloned macrophage hybridomas (124).

THE BIOCHEMISTRY AND PHARMACOLOGY OF LYMPHOCYTE-MACROPHAGE INTERACTION

Regulation of Ia Expression on Macrophage

The obligatory requirement of Ia in T-cell activation predicts that regulation of Ia expression has profound effects on the outcome of an immune response. Cowing et al. (125) demonstrated that normal tissues varied extensively in the percentage of Ia-positive cells in the macrophage population. For example, whereas only 10% to 15% of peritoneal macrophages are Ia positive, as much as 60% of the splenic adherent cell population expressed Ia. That immune T cells played a role in inducing Ia expression in macrophages was first shown by the experiments of Beller et al. (126). It was demonstrated that the percentages of Ia-positive peritoneal exudate macrophages derived from thioglycollate- or peptone-injected animals were not different from those of normal animals, whereas *Listeria monocytogenes*-infected exudates showed a marked increase in Ia-positive macrophages. Two pieces of evidence indicated that this increase was immune-based. First, the T cells from such immunized animals could be transferred to normal recipients to achieve the same effect; second, soluble mediators from T cells also induce macrophage Ia *in vivo* and *in vitro* (127,128). A more readily detectable class of molecules that induces macrophage cell-surface antigen expression is the interferons (IFN). Interferons are polypeptides with anti-viral and immunoregulatory functions (see Chapter 14, *this volume*). α-IFN (leukocyte-derived) and β-IFN (fibroblast-derived) are released when cells are infected with virus and are both biologically and physiochemically distinct from γ-IFN (immune interferon), which is produced by lymphocytes upon antigenic and mitogenic activation (129,130). The ability to positively regulate Ia expression on macrophages appears to be the exclusive property of γ-IFN, since other IFN types are found to have little or no effect on Ia expression in the various types of cells that have been examined. Steeg et al. (131) and Wong et al. (132) reported that natural γ-IFN contained in concanavalin-A-activated murine spleen-cell culture supernatants as well as recombinant γ-IFN induced Ia expression in several macrophage cell lines. Analogous results have been obtained for the human. Basham and Merigan (133) showed that pure recombinant γ-IFN augmented class II antigen expression by about twofold in normal human monocytes. γ-IFN was apparently produced by a subset of T cells reactive with OKT4 monoclonal antibodies in the presence of human monocytes (134). Although the mechanism of γ-IFN induction of Ia expression is far from clear, it is conceivable that the cyclic effects of antigen presentation to T cells and T-cell release of γ-IFN together with the monokine IL-1 and lymphokine IL-2 (see below) form the major regulatory circuit in the interaction between T cells and macrophages.

The importance of Ia expression in T-cell regulation ensures that it should also be down-regulated. Under normal circumstances, Ia expression is a transient phenomenon lasting 12 to 48 hr, after which the cells rapidly become Ia negative and lose their antigen-presentation functions (135). Ia expression can also be inhibited by such agents as prostaglandin E (PGE), alpha-fetoprotein, and glucocorticoid (136–138). These inhibitory mechanisms are probably reflected in the local environment of the peritoneal cavity and in the neonates. Alpha and beta interferons have also been shown to reverse the effects of gamma interferon in Ia induction (139). Since inflammatory stimuli involve an influx of interferons and high levels of Ia expression, it has been suggested that β-IFN represents a naturally occurring antagonist of γ-IFN-induced Ia at sites of inflammation.

Macrophage Handling of Antigens

The fate of the antigen after it is taken up by the macrophage has been the subject of intense research in the last 15 years. Two classical observations have been interpreted to suggest that macrophages played a major role in the handling of antigens. First, Gell and Benacerraf (61) in 1959 demonstrated that delayed-type hypersensitivity (which is a T-cell function) could be elicited either with native or denatured forms of antigen, whereas anaphylaxis (which involves recognition of antigen by antibodies) was triggered only by the native antigen. Interpreted in contemporary terms it can be said that B cells recognize the tertiary structure of antigen, whereas T cells recognize linear sequences. This observation was confirmed in many other studies (140–142). The differences in T- and B-cell recognition of antigen were attributed to

the requirement for "antigen processing" by macrophages before recognition of antigen by T cells. The second observation related to the consistent failure of antibodies specific for the antigen to inhibit the antigen-specific T-cell proliferative responses (143). The implication is that the antigen must have been altered from its native state so that it is no longer recognizable by immunoglobulins. The concept of antigen processing also arises from attempts to explain the time that lags between antigen uptake and the earliest point of stimulation of T cells (144). In these experiments, macrophages were allowed to take up antigen at 4°C. The cells were then incubated at 37°C for various periods of time and then fixed in paraformaldehyde or glutaraldehyde to prevent further processing of the antigen. The ability of the antigen-pulsed and fixed macrophages to induce an antigen-specific T-cell response was then assessed. It was found that a lag period of at least an hour was required before cells could be fixed and still be unaffected in their ability to present antigen. It was interpreted that this lag period was necessary for the macrophage to process the antigen.

Perhaps the most cited examples implicating a requirement for antigen processing by macrophages are from the use of pharmacological agents that interfere with macrophage metabolic processes. As alluded to in the previous paragraph, paraformaldehyde- or glutaraldehyde-fixed macrophages are rendered metabolically inactive; also, their ability to present antigen depends on the time of antigen exposure relative to the time of fixation. It has been demonstrated (144,145) that exposure of macrophages to antigen prior to fixation allowed full function of the macrophages to present antigen. However, if macrophages were fixed before antigen treatment, the presentation function was completely abrogated. Interestingly, Schmonkevitz et al. (146) further demonstrated that although fixed macrophages failed to present native or denatured ovalbumin, such cells were able to present proteolytic fragments or CNBr-derived fragments of ovalbumin. These experiments directly implied that antigen processing involved fragmentation of antigen so that if biochemically fragmented peptides were used, no further processing was required from the macrophages. The first evidence that proteolysis might be important came from studies using lysosomotropic agents such as chloroquine or ammonium chloride (147,148). Among other properties, these agents accumulate in their protonated form in lysosomal vesicles and raise the normally acidic pH environment to 6 or 7, resulting in inhibition of protein degradation by lysosomal acid hydrolases. Similar to paraformaldehyde, chloroquine incubated with macrophages and antigen completely inhibited the ability of the macrophages to present antigen. To ensure that chloroquine inhibited only the antigen-processing steps and not the subsequent presentation of antigen, Chestnut et al.

(148) used macrophages that were previously pulsed to ovalbumin, added chloroquine to these macrophages, and then pulsed with a second antigen KLH in the presence of chloroquine. It was shown that although the presentation of ovalbumin was not affected, KLH was not presented by the macrophages.

Taken collectively, the aforementioned experiments depict a four-stage process in the handling of antigen by macrophages, involving: (a) binding of antigen to the surface of macrophages; (b) endocytosis of antigen; (c) proteolytic cleavage of antigen in lysosomal vesicles; and (d) reinsertion of cleaved antigenic fragments onto the surface of the macrophages for further presentation to T cells. Over the past couple of years, however, many of these premises have been challenged. There is no debate that antigen processing does occur. The question is whether antigen processing is required for subsequent antigen presentation. As mentioned earlier, lysosomotropic agents that appear to block antigen degradation may also affect other intracellular processes associated with subsequent antigen presentation. For example, Nowell and Quaranta (149) showed that the intracellular biosynthesis of Ia during a process converting the Ia oligomers from a three-chain structure (α, β, γ) into a two-chain structure (α, β) was inhibited by the presence of chloroquine. More recently, Walden et al. (150) were able to covalently bind Ia molecules and antigen to lipids and then incorporate this complex into liposomes. These investigators showed that liposomes so created could present antigens to T cells. More importantly, presentation could be inhibited with antibodies against the antigen itself. Klein et al. (151) also raised the issue that since not all antigen presenting cells had the ability to phagocytose particles, antigen processing through phagocytosis was probably not a general property of all antigen-presenting cells.

Macrophage Presentation of Antigens

Regardless of how the antigen is handled by the macrophage, it is ultimately presented to T cells. The mechanism of antigen presentation is even less understood. One of the early events subsequent to antigen fragmentation is probably the association of the antigen fragment with surface Ia molecules. The biochemical feasibility of this association has recently been demonstrated experimentally by Babbitt et al. (152). It was first shown that the antigenic epitope of the hen-egg lysozyme protein (HEL) lied in a sequence of 15 amino acids between residue number 46 and 61. This peptide was fluorescently labeled by coupling it to 7-fluoro-4-nitrobenzo-2-oxa-1,3-diazole (NBD-F). After assuring that the resulting molecule NBD-HEL (46–61) retained its antigenic specificity, an attempt was made to measure its association with purified IA molecules from H-2^k and H-2^d by equilibrium dialysis. Results indicated that NBD-HEL (46–61) could

indeed bind to IA^k but not to IA^d, with a dissociation constant of approximately 2 μM. This binding was also inhibitable by native HEL (46–61). More recent data (153) further showed that the IA molecules did not discriminate between autologous and foreign epitopes, since binding affinities to these determinants appeared to be similar. It was also suggested that separate IA sites were utilized in binding of different antigenic determinants.

The second step probably involves receptor-ligand interaction between the T-cell antigen receptor and the antigen:Ia complex. Although the basic structure of the T-cell receptor is now known and some of the receptor genes cloned (154–157), the nature of this receptor-ligand interaction remains largely unclear. The basic structure of the T-cell receptor is comprised of an alpha chain (40–45 kilodaltons) and a beta chain (42–44 kilodaltons). Complementary DNA (cDNA) clones encoding for the beta chains of both human and mouse T-cell receptors have been isolated. Restriction maps and sequence analysis reveal that the genomic organization of the beta chain is very similar to that of the B-cell immunoglobulin genes. There are variable (V), constant (C), joining (J), and diversity (D) segments (see Chapter 31, *this volume*). It is interesting to note that although the murine T-cell-surface molecule, L3T4, is not considered part of the T-cell receptor, antibodies against these cell-surface markers strongly inhibited antigen-specific T-cell activation (158). In a recent report, Janeway et al. (159) offered a number of interesting conjectures related to the binding of ligand to the receptor for this phase of the lymphocyte-macrophage interaction. It was postulated that the initial step involved binding of T-cell L3T4 to the nonpolymorphic portion of the macrophage Ia molecule. This brought the antigen fragment associated with the Ia molecule in juxtaposition with the T-cell receptor, the binding of which resulted in aggregation of the T-cell receptors and T-cell activation. Activated T cells could then secrete the lymphokine IL-2 and express cell-surface receptors for IL-2 molecules. A novel lymphokine that could inhibit IL-2-sensitive T-cell growth was also secreted by these cells. The function of this inhibitor was to limit third-party bystander effects. The role of IL-2 was seen as that of a molecule which, in conjunction with the antigen:Ia complex, stimulated enhanced expression of IL-2 receptors on T cell and minimized the effect of the putative inhibitor.

Cytokine Regulation of Lymphocyte-Macrophage Interactions

Although our knowledge of the mechanism of T-cell induction is still not complete, research into the biology of cytokines that directly or indirectly affect T-cell growth and functions has advanced rapidly in the past several years. The sources and structures of these growth factors, as well as their pathology related to inflammation, have been extensively discussed in other chapters of this volume and will not be repeated here. One final point to be emphasized here is the interplay of these molecules in relation to the interaction between T cells and macrophages. IL-1, a product of activated macrophages whose activity is defined by a thymocyte proliferative assay, is believed to be one of the activation signals delivered to the T cells resulting in the release of IL-2 and expression of IL-2 receptors. Although it was demonstrated that IL-1 and PHA could activate T cells to produce IL-2 in the absence of macrophages (160), IL-1 alone could not reconstitute an antigen-specific immune response that was found to be totally dependent on the presence of macrophages (161). However, it remains unclear as to whether T cells have to be triggered first by antigen to be responsive to IL-1 or whether IL-1 can stimulate resting T cells. Nevertheless, besides IL-2, activated T cells also elaborate other lymphokines such as colony-stimulating factor and gamma interferon. These agents, in turn, can induce further production of IL-1 by macrophages and thus complete the reciprocal stimulation loop. Recent data (139) further suggest that the induction of Ia expression on macrophages by γ-IFN is regulated by another member of the interferon family, namely, β-IFN.

SUMMARY

We have broadly reviewed the cellular and molecular basis of macrophage-lymphocyte interaction as a critical early event in the immune response. This critical event provides for the primary inductive signal in T-cell antigen recognition as well as providing a regulatory step which, in the final analysis, appears to be the genetically controlled step in immune competence. At the molecular level, protein antigens, whether self or nonself, are processed by antigen-presenting cells and are associated with cell-surface Ia molecules in a manner such that activation of the T cell to a given epitope is dependent upon a physical interaction of macrophage and T cell. Antigen-Ia-complex recognition takes place only in those lymphocytes that bear receptors specific for the macrophage and its displayed antigen complex. This mechanistic process has been termed *determinant selection*. The events described have been shown to operate in humans as well as rodents; these events provide the cellular basis for normal immune defense and will undoubtedly be an important step in expression of pathological processes such as immune-based chronic inflammatory diseases.

REFERENCES

1. Claman, H. N., Chaperon, E. A., and Triplett, R. F. (1966): Thymus-marrow cell combination. Synergy in antibody production. *Proc. Soc. Exp. Biol. Med.*, 122:1167.

2. Mitchison, N. A. (1969): Cell populations involved in immune responses. In: *Immunological Tolerance*, edited by M. Landy and W. Braun, pp. 149–155. Academic Press, New York.

3. Melchers, I., Rajewsky, K., and Shreffler, D. C. (1973): Ir-LDH$_B$: Map position and functional analysis. *Eur. J. Immunol.*, 3:754.

4. Katz, D. H. (1972): The allogeneic effect on the immune response: Model for regulatory influence to T lymphocytes on the immune system. *Transplant. Rev.*, 12:141.

5. Gershon, R. K., and Kondo, K. (1972): Tolerance to sheep red cells: Breakage with thymocytes and horse red cells. *Science*, 175:996.

6. Greene, M. I., Nelles, M. J., Sy, M.-S., and Nisonoff, A. (1982): Regulation of immunity to the azobenzenearsonate hapten. *Adv. Immunol.*, 32:253.

7. Sherr, D. H., Ju, S-T., and Dorf, M. E. (1981): Hapten-specific T cell responses to 4-hydroxy-3-nitrophenyl acetyl. XII. Fine specificity of anti-idiotypic suppressor T cells (Ts2). *J. Exp. Med.*, 153:640.

8. Bach, F. H., Segall, M., Zier, K. S., Sondel, P. M., and Alter, B. J. (1973): Cell mediated immunity: Separation of cells involved in recognitive and destructive phase. *Science*, 180:403.

9. Pilarski, L. M. (1977): A requirement of antigen-specific helper T cells in the generation of cytotoxic T cells from thymocyte precursors. *J. Exp. Med.*, 145:709.

10. Shiku, H., Kisielow, P., Bean, M. A., Takahashi, T., Boyse, E. A., Oettgen, H. F., and Old, L. J. (1975): Expression of T-cell differentiation antigen on effector cells in cell-mediated cytotoxicity *in vitro*. Evidence for functional heterogeneity related to the surface phenotype of T cells. *J. Exp. Med.*, 141:227.

11. Cantor, H., and Boyse, E. A. (1975): Functional subclasses of T lymphocytes bearing different Ly antigens. I. The generation of functionally distinct T cell classes is a differentiative process independent of antigen. *J. Exp. Med.*, 141:1376.

12. Cantor, H., and Boyse, E. A. (1975): Functional subclasses of T lymphocytes bearing different Ly antigens. II. Cooperation between subclasses of Ly cells in the generation of killer activity. *J. Exp. Med.*, 141:1390.

13. Vadas, M. A., Miller, J. F. A. P., McKenzie, I. F. C., Chism, S. E., Shen, F. W., Boyse, E. A., Gamble, J. R., and Whitelaw, A. M. (1976): Ly and Ia antigen phenotypes of T cells involved in delayed-type hypersensitivity and in suppression. *J. Exp. Med.*, 144:10.

14. Kohler, G., and Milstein, C. (1975): Continuous cultures of fused cells secreting antibody of predefined specificity. *Nature*, 256:495.

15. Engleman, E. G., Benike, C. J., Grumet, F. C., and Evans, R. L. (1981): Activation of human T lymphocyte subsets: Helper and suppressor/cytotoxic T cells recognize and respond to distinct histocompatibility antigens. *J. Immunol.*, 127:2124.

16. Reinherz, E. L., and Schlossman, S. F. (1980): The differentiation and function of human T lymphocytes. *Cell*, 19:821.

17. Evans, R. L., Wall, D. W., Platsoucas, C. D., Siegal, F. P., Fikrig, S. M., Testa, C. M., and Good, R. A. (1981): Thymus-dependent membrane antigens in man: Inhibition of cell-mediated lympholysis by monoclonal antibodies to TH2 antigen. *Proc. Natl. Acad. Sci. USA*, 78:544.

18. Gatenby, P. A., Kotzin, B. L., and Engleman, E. G. (1981): Induction of immunoglobulin secreting cells in the human autologous mixed lymphocyte subsets defined with monoclonal antibodies. *J. Immunol.*, 127:2130.

19. Rich, R. R., and Rich, S. S. (1983): T-T cell interactions in cell-mediated immune responses to major histocompatibility complex antigens. *Crit. Rev. Immunol.*, 4:129.

20. Thomas, Y., Rogozinski, L., Irigoyen, O. H., Shen, H. H., Talle, M. A., Goldstein, G., and Chess, L. (1982): Functional analysis of human T cell subsets defined by monoclonal antibodies. V. Suppressor cells within the activated OKT$_4^+$ population belong to a distinct subset. *J. Immunol.*, 128:1386.

21. Mohagheghpour, N., Benike, C. J., Kansas, G., Bieber, C., and Engleman, E. G. (1983): Activation of antigen-specific suppressor T cells in the presence of cyclosporin requires interactions between T cells of inducer and suppressor lineage. *J. Clin. Invest.*, 72:2092.

22. Gatenby, P. A., Kansas, G. S., Yian, C. Y., Evans, R. L., and Engleman, E. G. (1982): Dissection of immunoregulatory subpop-

ulations of T lymphocytes within the helper and suppressor sublineages in man. *J. Immunol.,* 129:1997.

23. Kansas, G. S., Wood, G. S., Fishwild, D. M., and Engleman, E. G. (1985): Functional characterization of human T lymphocyte subsets distinguished by monoclonal anti-Leu-8. *J. Immunol.,* 134:2995.
24. Damle, N. K., and Engleman, E. G. (1983): Immunoregulatory T cell circuits in man: Alloantigen-primed inducer T cells in the alloantigen-specific suppressor T cells in the absence of the initial antigenic stimulus. *J. Exp. Med.,* 158:159.
25. Mosier, D. E., and Coppleson, L. W. (1968): The three-cell interaction required for the induction of the primary immune response. *Proc. Natl. Acad. Sci. USA,* 61:542.
26. Coppleson, L. W., and Michie, D. (1966): A quantitative study of the chorioallantoic membrane reaction in the chick embryo. *Proc. R. Soc. Lond. (Biol).,* B163:555.
27. Kunin, S., Shearer, G. M., Globerson, A., and Feldman, M. (1972): Immunologic function of macrophages: *In vitro* production of antibodies to a hapten-carrier conjugate. *Cell. Immunol.,* 5:288.
28. Katz, D. H., and Unanue, E. R. (1973): Critical role of determinant presentation in the induction of specific response in immunocompetent lymphocytes. *J. Exp. Med.,* 137:967.
29. Erb, P., and Feldman, M. (1975): The role of macrophages in the generation of T-helper cells. I. The requirement for macrophages in helper cell induction and characteristics of macrophage-T cell interaction. *Cell. Immunol.,* 19:356.
30. Hodes, R. J., and Singer, A. (1977): Cellular and genetic control of antibody responses *in vitro.* I. Cellular requirements for the generation of genetically controlled primary IgM responses to soluble antigens. *Eur. J. Immunol.,* 7:892.
31. Pierce, C. W., Kapp, J. A., and Benacerraf, B. (1976): Regulation by the H-2 gene complex of macrophage-lymphoid cell interactions in secondary antibody response *in vitro. J. Exp. Med.,* 144:371.
32. Feldman, M., and Palmer, J. (1971): The requirement for macrophages in the secondary immune response to antigens of small and large size *in vitro. Immunology,* 21:685.
33. Ly, I. A., and Mishell, R. A. (1974): Separation of mouse spleen cells by passage through columns of Sephadex G-10. *J. Immunol. Methods,* 5:239.
34. Siegel, I. (1970): Autologous macrophage-thymocyte interactions. *J. Allergy,* 46:190.
35. Lipsky, P. E., and Rosenthal, A. S. (1973): Macrophage-lymphocyte interaction. I. Characteristics of the antigen-independent-binding of guinea pig thymocytes and lymphocytes to syngeneic macrophages. *J. Exp. Med.,* 138:900.
36. Lipsky, P. E., and Rosenthal, A. S. (1975): Macrophage-lymphocyte interaction. II. Antigen-mediated physical interactions between immune guinea pig lymph node lymphocytes and syngeneic macrophages. *J. Exp. Med.,* 148:138.
37. Rosenthal, A. S., Blake, J. T., and Lipsky, P. E. (1975): Inhibition of macrophage-lymphocyte interaction by cytochalasin B during antigen recognition by T lymphocytes. *J. Immunol.,* 115:1135.
38. Waldron, J. A., Horn, R. G., and Rosenthal, A. S. (1973): Antigen-induced proliferation of guinea pig lymphocytes *in vitro:* Obligatory role of macrophages in the recognition of antigen by immune T-lymphocytes. *J. Immunol.,* 111:58.
39. Shevach, E. M., and Rosenthal, A. S. (1973): Function of macrophages in antigen recognition by guinea pig T lymphocytes. II. Role of the macrophage in the regulation of genetic control of the immune response. *J. Exp. Med.,* 138:1213.
40. Schwartz, R. H., Jackson, L., and Paul, W. E. (1975): T lymphocyte-enriched murine peritoneal exudate cells. I. A reliable assay for antigen-induced T lymphocyte proliferation. *J. Immunol.,* 115:1330.
41. Corradin, G., Etlinger, H. M., and Chiller, J. M. (1977): Lymphocyte specific to protein antigen. I. Characterization of the antigen induced *in vitro* T cell-dependent proliferative response with lymph node cells from primed mice. *J. Immunol.,* 119:1048.
42. Julius, M., Simpson, H. E., and Herzenberg, L. A. (1973): A rapid method for the isolation of functional thymus-derived lymphocytes. *Eur. J. Immunol.,* 3:645.
43. Cowing, C., Pincus, S. H., Sachs, D. H., and Dickler, H. B. (1978): A subpopulation of adherent accessory cells bearing both I-A and I-E or C subregion antigens is required for antigen-specific murine T lymphocyte proliferation. *J. Immunol.,* 121:1680.
44. Rogoff, T. M., and Lipsky, P. E. (1980): Antigen presentation by isolated guinea pig Kupffer cells. *J. Immunol.,* 124:1740.
45. Lipscomb, M. R., Toews, G. R., Lyons, C. R., and Uhr, J. W. (1981): Antigen presentation by guinea pig alveolar macrophages. *J. Immunol.,* 126:286.
46. Stingl, G., Katz, S. I., Shevach, E. M., Wolff-Schreiner, E., and Green, I. (1978): Detection of Ia antigens on Langerhans cells in guinea pig skin. *J. Immunol.,* 120:570.
47. Pehamberger, H., Stingl, L. A., Pogantsch, S., Steiner, G., Wolff, K., and Stingl, G. (1973): Epidermal cell-induced generation of cytotoxic T-lymphocyte responses against alloantigens or TNP-modified syngeneic cell-requirements for Ia-positive Langerhans cells. *J. Invest. Dermatol.,* 81:208.
48. Stingl, G., Katz, S. I., Clement, K., Green, I., and Shevach, E. M. (1978): Immunologic functions of Ia-bearing epidermal Langerhans cells. *J. Immunol.,* 121:2005.
49. Braathen, L. R., and Thorsby, E. (1980): Studies on human epidermal Langerhans cells. I. Allo-activating and antigen-presenting capacity. *Scand. J. Immunol.,* 11:401.
50. Steinman, R., and Cohn, Z. (1974): The identification of a novel cell type in peripheral organs of the mouse. II. Functional properties. *J. Exp. Med.,* 139:380.
51. Steinman, R. M., Kaplan, G., Witmer, M. D., and Cohn, Z. A. (1979): Identification of a novel cell type in peripheral lymphoid organs of mice. V. Purification of spleen dendritic cells, new surface markers, and maintenance *in vitro. J. Exp. Med.,* 149:1.
52. Steinman, R. M., and Witmer, M. D. (1978): Lymphoid dendritic cells are potent stimulators of the primary mixed leukocyte reaction in mice. *Proc. Natl. Acad. Sci. USA,* 75:5132.
53. Nussenzweig, M. C., Steinman, R. M., Witmer, M. D., and Gutchinov, B. (1982): A monoclonal antibody specific for mouse dendritic cells. *Proc. Natl. Acad. Sci. USA,* 79:161.
54. Nussenzweig, M. C., Steinman, R. M., Gutchinov, B., and Cohn, Z. A. (1980): Dendritic cells are accessory cells for the development of anti-trinitrophenyl cytotoxic T lymphocytes. *J. Exp. Med.,* 152:1070.
55. Sunshine, G. H., Katz, D. R., and Feldman, M. (1980): Dendritic cells induce T cell proliferation to synthetic antigens under Ir gene control. *J. Exp. Med.,* 152:1817.
56. Chestnut, R. W., and Grey, W. H. (1981): Studies on the capacity of B cells to serve as antigen-presenting cells. *J. Immunol.,* 126:1075.
57. Glimcher, L. H., Kim, Kyung-Jin, Green, I., and Paul, W. E. (1982): Ia antigen-bearing B cell tumor line can present protein antigen and alloantigen in a major histocompatibility complex-restricted fashion to antigen-reactive T cells. *J. Exp. Med.,* 155:445.
58. McKean, D. J., Infante, A. J., Nilson, A., Kimoto, M., Fathman, C. G., Walker, E., and Warner, N. (1981): Major histocompatibility complex-restricted antigen presentation to antigen-reactive T cells by B lymphocyte tumor cells. *J. Exp. Med.,* 154:1419.
59. Issekutz, T., Chu, E., and Geha, R. S. (1982): Antigen-presentation by human B cells: T cell proliferation induced by Epstein-Barr virus B lymphoblastoid cells. *J. Immunol.,* 129:1446.
60. Chestnut, R. W., Colon, S. M., and Grey, H. M. (1982): Antigen presentation by normal B cells, B cell tumors and macrophages: Functional and biochemical comparison. *J. Immunol.,* 128:1764.
61. Gell, P. G. H., and Benacerraf, B. (1959): Studies on hypersensitivity. II. Delayed hypersensitivity to denatured protein in guinea pigs. *Immunol.,* 2:64.
62. Unanue, E. R., Beller, D. I., Lu, C. Y., and Allen, P. M. (1984): Antigen presentation: Comments on its regulation and mechanism. *J. Immunol.,* 132:1.
63. Treves, A. J., Tal, T., Barak, V., and Fuks, Z. (1981): Antigen presentation and regulatory functions of human monocytes. *Eur. J. Immunol.,* 11:487.
64. Le, J., Yao, J. S., Knowles, D. M., and Vilcek, J. (1986): Accessory function of thymic and tonsillar dendritic cells in interferon gamma production by T lymphocytes. *Lymphokine Res.,* 5:205.
65. Oksenberg, J. R., Mor-Yousef, S., Persitz, E., Schenker, Y., Mozes,

E., and Brautbar, C. (1986): Antigen-presenting cells in human decidual tissue. *Am. J. Reprod. Immunol. Microbiol.*, 11:82.

66. Geppert, T. D., and Lipsky, P. E. (1985): Antigen presentation by interferon-treated endothelial cells and fibroblasts: Differential ability to function as antigen-presenting cells despite comparable Ia expression. *J. Immunol.*, 135:3750.

67. Burger, D. R., Ford, D., Vetto, R. M., Hamblin, A., Goldstein, A., Hubbard, M., and Dumonde, D. C. (1981): Endothelial cell presentation of antigen to human T cells. *Hum. Immunol.*, 3:209.

68. Lee, K. C., Wong, M., and Spiltzer, D. (1982): Chloroquine as a probe for antigen processing by accessory cells. *Transplantation*, 34:150.

69. Streicher, H. Z., Berkower, I. J., Bush, M., Gurd, F. R. N., and Berzofsky, J. A. (1984): Antigen confirmation determines processing requirements for T cell activation. *Proc. Natl. Acad. Sci. USA*, 81:6831.

70. Katz, D. R., Feldmann, M., Tees, R., and Schreier, M. H. (1986): Heterogeneity of accessory cells interacting with T-helper clones. *Immunology*, 58:167.

71. Chain, B. M., Kaye, P. M., and Feldmann, M. (1986): The cellular pathway of antigen presentation: Biochemical and functional analysis of antigen processing in dendritic cells and macrophages. *Immunology*, 58:271.

72. Kaye, P. M., Chain, B. M., and Feldmann, M. (1985): Non-phagocytic dendritic cells are effective accessory cells for anti-mycobacterial response *in vitro*. *J. Immunol.*, 134:1920.

73. Ramila, G., Studer, S., Kennedy, M., Sklenar, I., and Erb, P. (1985): Evaluation of accessory cell heterogeneity. I. Differential accessory cell requirement for T helper cell activation and for T-B cooperation. *Eur. J. Immunol.*, 15:1.

74. Wetzel, G. D., and Kettman, J. R. (1981): Activation of murine B lymphocytes. III. Stimulation of B lymphocyte clonal growth with lipopolysaccharide and dextran sulfate. *J. Immunol.*, 126:723.

75. Sieckmann, D. G., Scher, I., Asofsky, R., Moiser, D. E., and Paul, W. E. (1978): Activation of mouse lymphocytes by anti-immunoglobulin. II. A thymus-independent response by a mature subset of B lymphocyte. *J. Exp. Med.*, 148:1628.

76. Mongini, P., Friedman, S., and Wortis, H. (1978): Accessory cell requirement for anti-IgM-induced proliferation of B lymphocytes. *Nature*, 276:709.

77. Morrissey, P. J., Boswell, H. S., Scher, I., and Singer, A. (1981): Role of accessory cells in B cell activation. IV. Ia⁺ accessory cells are required for the *in vitro* generation of thymus independent type 2 antibody responses to polysaccharide antigens. *J. Immunol.*, 127:1345.

78. Goyert, S. M., Shively, J. E., and Silver, J. (1982): Biochemical characterization of a second family of human Ia molecules, HLA-DS, equivalent to murine I-A subregion molecules. *J. Exp. Med.*, 156:550.

79. McDevitt, H. O., and Sela, M. (1965): Genetic control of the antibody response. I. Demonstration of determinant-specific differences in response to synthetic polypeptide antigens in two strains of inbred mice. *J. Exp. Med.*, 122:517.

80. Benacerraf, B., Green, I., and Paul, W. E. (1967): The immune response of guinea pig to hapten-poly-L-lysine conjugates as an example of the genetic control of the recognition of antigenicity. *Cold Spring Harbor Symp. Quant. Biol.*, 32:569.

81. McDevitt, H. O., and Benacerraf, B. (1969): Genetic control of specific immune respones. *Adv. Immunol.*, 11:31.

82. McDevitt, H. O., Deak, B. D., Shreffler, D. C., Klein, J., Stimpfling, J. H., and Snell, G. D. (1972): Genetic control of the immune response. Mapping of the *Ir-1* locus. *J. Exp. Med.*, 135:1259.

83. Shreffler, D. C., and David, C. S. (1975): The H-2 major histocompatibility complex and the I immune response region: Genetic variation, function and organization. *Adv. Immunol.*, 20:125.

84. Unanue, E. (1972): The regulatory role of macrophages in antigenic stimulation. *Adv. Immunol.*, 15:95.

85. Rosenthal, A., and Shevach, E. (1973): Function of macrophages in antigen recognition by guinea pig T lymphocytes. I. Requirement for histocompatible macrophages and lymphocytes. *J. Exp. Med.*, 138:1194.

86. Schwartz, R. H., Yano, A., and Paul, W. E. (1978): Interaction between antigen-presenting cells and primed T lymphocytes: An assessment of Ir gene expression in the antigen-presenting cell. *Immunol. Rev.*, 40:153.

87. Bergholz, B., and Thorsby, E. (1979): Macrophage/T-lymphocyte interaction in the immune response to PPD in humans. *Scand. J. Immunol.*, 9:511.

88. Katz, D. H., and Benacerraf, B. (1972): The regulatory influence of activated T cells on B cell response to antigen. *Adv. Immunol.*, 15:1.

89. Singer, A., Morrissey, P. J., Hathcock, K. S., Ahmed, A., Scher, I., and Hodes, R. J. (1981): Role of the major histocompatibility complex in T cell activation of B cell subpopulations Lyb5⁺ and Lyb5⁻ B cell subpopulations differ in their requirement for major histocompatibility complex-restricted T cell recognition. *J. Exp. Med.*, 154:501.

90. Shearer, G. M., Rehn, T. G., and Garbarino, C. A. (1975): Cell-mediated lympholysis of trimtrophenyl-modified autologous lymphocytes. Effector cell specificity to modified cell surface components controlled by the H-2K and H-2D serological regions of the murine major histocompatibility complex. *J. Exp. Med.*, 141:591.

91. Zinkernagel, R. M., and Doherty, P. C. (1975): Restriction of *in vitro* T cell-mediated cytotoxicity in lymphocytic choriomeningitis within a syngeneic or semiallogeneic system. *Nature*, 248:701.

92. Shevach, E. M., Paul, W. E., and Green, I. (1972): Histocompatibility-linked immune response gene function in guinea pig: Specific inhibition of antigen induced lymphocyte proliferation by alloantisera. *J. Exp. Med.*, 136:1207.

93. Melvold, R. W., and Kohn, H. I. (1976): Eight new histocompatibility mutations associated with the H-2 complex. *Immunogenetics*, 3:185.

94. McKenzie, I. F. C., Morgan, G. M., Sandrin, M. S., Michaelides, M. M., Melvold, R. W., and Kohn, H. I. (1979): B6.C-*H-2*ᵇᵐ¹², a new *H-2* mutation in the I region in the mouse. *J. Exp. Med.*, 150:1323.

95. Hansen, T. H., Melvold, R. W., Arn, J. S., and Sachs, D. H. (1980): Evidence for mutation in an I-A gene. *Nature*, 285:340.

96. MyIntyre, K. R., and Seidman, J. G. (1984): Nucleotide sequence of mutant I-Aᵇᵐ¹² gene is evidence for genetic exchange between mouse immune response genes. *Nature*, 308:551.

97. Lin, C-C. S., Rosenthal, A. S., Passmore, H. C., and Hansen, T. H. (1981): Selective loss of antigen-specific Ir gene function in *I-A* mutant B6.C-*H-2*ᵇᵐ¹² is an antigen-presenting cell defect. *Proc. Natl. Acad. Sci. USA*, 78:6406.

98. Michaelides, M., Sandrin, M., Morgan, G., McKenzie, I. F. C., Ashman, R., and Melvold, R. W. (1981): Ir gene function in an I-A subregion mutant B6.C-*H-2*ᵇᵐ¹². *J. Exp. Med.*, 153:464.

99. Schwartz, R. H., David, C. S., Sachs, D. H., and Paul, W. E. (1976): T lymphocyte-enriched murine peritoneal exudate cells. III. Inhibition of antigen-induced T lymphocyte proliferation with anti-Ia antisera. *J. Immunol.*, 117:531.

100. Kanamori, S., Walsh, W. D., Hansen, T. H., and Tse, H. Y. (1984): Assessment of antigen-specific restriction sites on Ia molecules as defined by the bm12 mutation. *J. Immunol.*, 133:2811.

101. Rosenthal, A. S., Barcinski, M. A., and Blake, J. T. (1977): Determinant selection is a macrophage dependent immune response gene function. *Nature*, 267:156.

102. Benacerraf, B. (1978): A hypothesis to relate the specificity of T-lymphocytes and the activity of I-region-specific Ir gene in macrophages and B lymphocytes. *J. Immunol.*, 120:1809.

103. Barcinski, M. A., and Rosenthal, A. S. (1977): Immune response gene control of determinant selection. I. Intramolecular mapping of the immunogenic sites on insulin recognized by guinea pig T and B cells. *J. Exp. Med.*, 145:726.

104. Schwartz, R. H. (1978): A clonal deletion model for Ir gene control of the immune response. *Scand. J. Immunol.*, 7:3.

105. Ishii, N., Nagy, Z. A., and Klein, J. (1982): Absence of Ir gene control of T cells recognizing foreign antigen in the context of alogeneic MHC molecules. *Nature*, 295:531.

106. Dos Reis, G. A., and Shevach, E. M. (1983): Antigen presenting cells from nonresponder strain 2 guinea pigs are fully competent to presenting bovine insulin B chain to responder strain 13 T cells: Evidence against a determinant selection model and in favor of a

clonal deletion model of immune response gene function. *J. Exp. Med.*, 157:1287.

107. Pierce, C. A., and Kapp, J. A. (1978): Suppressor T cell activity in responder × nonresponder (C57BL/10 × DBA/1)F₁ spleen cells responsive to L-glutamic acid⁶⁰-L-alanine³⁰-L-tyrosine¹⁰. *J. Exp. Med.*, 148:1282.

108. Nagy, Z. A., Baxevenis, C. N., and Klein, J. (1982): Hapltype-specific suppression of T cell response to lactate dehydrogenase B in (responder × nonresponder)F₁ mice. *J. Immunol.*, 129:2608.

109. Rodey, G. E., Luchrman, L. K., and Thomas, D. W. (1979): *In vitro* primary immunization of human peripheral blood lymphocytes to KLH: Evidence for HLA-D region restriction. *J. Immunol.*, 123:2250.

110. Berle, E. J., and Thorsby, E. (1980): The proliferative T cell response to herpes simplex virus (HSV) antigen is restricted by self HLA-D. *Clin. Exp. Immunol.*, 39:668.

111. Koide, Y., Awashima, F., Akaza, T., and Yoshida, T. O. (1981): Human antigen-presenting cells: Characterization of the cells in T lymphocyte proliferative response. *Microbiol. Immunol.*, 25:489.

112. Geha, R. S., Milgrow, H., Briff, M., Alpert, S., Martin, S., and Yupis, E. G. (1979): Effect of anti-HLA antisera on macrophage-T cell interaction. *Proc. Natl. Acad. Sci. USA*, 76:4038.

113. Bergholtz, B. O., and Thorsby, E. (1978): HLA-D restriction of the macrophage-dependent response of immune human T lymphocytes to PPD *in vitro:* Inhibition by anti-HLA-D antisera. *Scand. J. Immunol.*, 8:63.

114. Brewerton, D. A., Caffrey, M., Hart, F. D., James, D. C. O., Nocholls, A., and Sturrock, R. D. (1973): Ankylosing spondylitis and HL-A27. *Lancet*, i:904.

115. Moller, G., editor (1975): HL-A and disease. *Transplant. Rev.*, 22.

116. Svejgaard, A., Platz, P., and Ryder, L. P. (1983): HLA and Disease 1982—A survey. *Immunol. Rev.*, 70:193.

117. Haverkern, M. J., Hoffman, B., Masural, N., and van Rood, J. J. (1975): HLA-linked genetic control of immune response in man. *Transplant. Rev.*, 22:120.

118. Greenberg, L. J., Bradkey, P. W., Chopyk, R. L., and Lalovel, J. M. (1980): Immunogenetics of response to a purified antigen from group A streptococci. II. Linkage of response to HLA. *Immunogenetics*, 11:161.

119. Hsu, S. H., Chan, M. M., and Bias, W. B. (1981): Genetic control of major histocompatibility complex-linked immune responses to synthetic polypeptides in man. *Proc. Natl. Acad. Sci. USA*, 78:440.

120. Ishizaka, K., and Adachi, T. (1976): Generation of specific helper cells and suppressor cells *in vitro* for IgE and IgG antibody response. *J. Immunol.*, 117:40.

121. Usui, M., Aoki, I., Sunshine, G. H., and Dorf, M. E. (1984): A role for macrophages in suppressor cell induction. *J. Immunol.*, 132:1728.

122. Dorf, M. E., and Benacerraf, B. (1985): I-J as a restriction element in the suppressor T cell system. *Immunol. Rev.*, 83:23.

123. Dorf, M. E., and Benacerraf, B. (1984): Suppressor cells and immunoregulation. *Annu. Rev. Immunol.*, 2:127.

124. Kawasaki, H., Martin, C. A., Uchide, T., Usui, M., Noma, T., Minami, M., and Dorf, M. E. (1986): Functional analysis of cloned macrophage hybridomas. V. Induction of suppressor T cell responses. *J. Immunol.*, 137:2145.

125. Cowing, C., Schwartz, B. D., and Dickler, H. B. (1978): Macrophage Ia antigens. I. Macrophage populations differ in their expression of Ia antigens. *J. Immunol.*, 120:378.

126. Beller, D. I., Kiely, J.-M., and Unanue, E. R. (1980): Regulation of macrophage populations. I. Preferential induction of Ia-rich peritoneal exudates by immunological stimuli. *J. Immunol.*, 124:1426.

127. Scher, M. G., Beller, D. I., and Unanue, E. R. (1980): Demonstration of a soluble mediator that induces exudates rich in Ia-positive macrophages. *J. Exp. Med.*, 152:1684.

128. Beller, D. I., and Ho, K. (1982): Regulation of macrophage populations. VI. Evaluation of control of macrophage Ia expression *in vitro. J. Immunol.*, 129:971.

129. De Maeyer, E., and De Maeyer-Gluignard, J. (1979): Interferons. *J. Comprehens. Virology*, 15:205.

130. McKimma-Breschkin, J. L., Mottram, P. L., Thomas, W. R., and Miller, J. F. A. P. (1982): Antigen-specific production of immune interferon by T cell lines. *J. Exp. Med.*, 155:1204.

131. Steeg, R. S., Moore, R. N., Johnson, H. M., and Oppenheim, J. J. (1982): Regulation of murine macrophage Ia antigen expression by a lymphokine with immune interferon activity. *J. Exp. Med.*, 156:1780.

132. Wong, G. H. W., Clark-Lewis, I., McKimma-Breschkin, J. L., Harris, A. W., and Schrader, J. W. (1983): Interferon-γ induces enhanced expression of Ia and H-2 antigens on B lymphoid, macrophage and myeloid cell lines. *J. Immunol.*, 131:788.

133. Basham, T. Y., and Merigan, T. C. (1983): Recombinant interferon-γ increases HLA-DR synthesis and expression. *J. Immunol.*, 130:1492.

134. Wang, T. W., Testa, D., Kung, P., Perry, L., Dreskin, H. J., and Goldstein, G. (1982): Cellular origin and interactions involved in γ-interferon production induced by OKT3 monoclonal antibody. *J. Immunol.*, 128:585.

135. Beller, D. I., and Unanue, E. R. (1981): Regulation of macrophage population. II. Synthesis and expression of Ia antigen by peritoneal exudate macrophage is a transient event. *J. Immunol.*, 126:263.

136. Snyder, D. S., Beller, D. I., and Unanue, E. R. (1982): Prostaglandins modulate macrophage Ia expression. *Nature*, 299:163.

137. Lu, C. Y., Changelian, P. S., and Unanue, E. R. (1984): Alpha-fetoprotein inhibits macrophage expression of Ia antigen. *J. Immunol.*, 132:1722.

138. Snyder, D. S., and Unanue, E. R. (1982): Corticosteroids inhibit murine macrophage Ia expression and interleukin-1 production. *J. Immunol.*, 129:1803.

139. Ling, P. D., Warren, M. K., and Vogel, S. N. (1985): Antagonistic effect of interferon-β on the interferon-γ-induced expression of Ia antigen in murine macrophages. *J. Immunol.*, 135:1857.

140. Schirrmacher, V., and Wigzell, H. (1972): Immune responses against native and chemically modified albumins in mice. *J. Exp. Med.*, 136:1616.

141. Ishizaka, K., Okudaira, H., and King, T. (1975): Immunogenic properties of modified antigen E. II. Ability of urea-denatured antigen and E-polypeptide chain to prime T cells specific for antigen E. *J. Immunol.*, 114:110.

142. Chestnut, R., Endres, R., and Grey, H. M. (1980): Antigen recognition by T cells and B cells: Recognition of cross-reactivity between native and denatured forms of globular antigens. *Clin. Immunol. Immunopathol.*, 15:397.

143. Ellner, J., and Rosenthal, A. (1975): Quantitative and immunogenic aspects of the handling of 2,4 dinitrophenyl guinea pig albumin by macrophages. *J. Immunol.*, 114:1563.

144. Ziegler, H., and Unanue, E. (1981): Identification of a macrophage antigen-processing event required for I-region-restricted antigen presentation to T lymphocytes. *J. Immunol.*, 127:1869.

145. Scalla, G., and Oppenheim, J. (1983): Antigen presentation by human monocytes: Evidence for stimulated processing and requirement of interleukin 1. *J. Immunol.*, 131:1160.

146. Schmonkevitz, R., Kappler, J., Marrack, P., and Grey, H. (1983): Antigen recognition by H-2 restricted T cells. I. Cell free antigen processing. *J. Exp. Med.*, 158:303.

147. Ziegler, H. K., and Unanue, E. R. (1982): Decrease in macrophage antigen catabolism by ammonia and chloroquine is associated with inhibition of antigen presentation to T cells. *Proc. Natl. Acad. Sci. USA*, 79:175.

148. Chestnut, R., Colon, S., and Grey, H. (1982): Requirement for the processing of antigen by antigen-presenting B cells. I. Functional comparison of B cell tumors and macrophages. *J. Immunol.*, 129:2382.

149. Nowell, J., and Quaranta, V. (1985): Chloroquine affects biosynthesis of Ia molecules by inhibiting dissociation of invariant (γ) chains from α-β dimers in B cells. *J. Exp. Med.*, 162:1371.

150. Walden, P., Nagy, Z. A., and Klein, J. (1986): Antigen presentation by liposomes: Inhibition with antibodies. *Eur. J. Immunol.*, 16:717.

151. Klein, J., Walden, P., and Nagy, Z. A. (1985): Antigen processing: A reevaluation. In: *Immune Regulation*, edited by M. Feldman

and N. A. Mitchison, p. 335–344. Humana Press, Clifton, New Jersey.

152. Babbitt, B. P., Allen, P. M., Matsueda, G., Haben, E., and Unanue, E. R. (1985): Binding of immunogenic peptides to Ia histocompatibility molecules. *Nature,* 317:359.

153. Babbitt, B. P., Masueda, G., Haber, E., Unanue, E. R., and Allen, P. M. (1986): Antigenic competition at the level of peptide-Ia binding. *Proc. Natl. Acad. Sci. USA,* 83:4509.

154. Haskins, K., Kappler, J., and Marack, P. (1984): The major histocompatibility complex-restricted antigen receptor on T cells. *Annu. Rev. Immunol.,* 2:51.

155. Mauer, S., Acuto, O., Herund, T., Schlossman, S. F., and Reinherz, E. L. (1984): The human T-cell receptor. *Annu. Rev. Immunol.,* 2: 23.

156. Davis, M., Chien, Y. H., Gascoigne, N. R., and Hedrick, S. M. (1984): A murine T cell receptor gene complex: Isolation, structure and rearrangement. *Immunol. Rev.,* 81:235.

157. Yanagi, Y., Yoshikai, Y., Leggett, K., Clark, S. P., Aleksander, I., and Mak, T. (1984): A human T cell-specific cDNA clone encodes a protein having extensive homology to immunoglobulin chains. *Nature,* 308:145.

158. Wilde, D. B., Marrack, P., Kappler, J., Dialynas, D. P., and Fitch, F. (1983): Evidence implicating L3T4 in class II MHC antigen reactivity; monoclonal antibody GL1.5 (anti-L3T4a) blocks class II MHC antigen-specific proliferation, release of lymphokines, and binding by cloned murine helper T lymphocyte lines. *J. Immunol.,* 131:2178.

159. Janeway, C. A., Jr., Conrad, P. J., Horowitz, J. B., Katz, M. E., Kaye, J., Saizawa, K. M., Smith, L., and Tite, J. P. (1986): Steps in the process of T lymphocyte activation. In: *Mediators of Immune Regulation and Immunotherapy,* edited by S. K. Singhal and T. L. Delovitch, pp. 31–99. Elsevier, New York.

160. Farrar, J. J., Mizel, S. B., Fuller-Farrar, J., Farrar, W. L., and Hilfiker, M. L. (1980): Macrophage-independent activation of helper T cells. I. Production of interleukin 2. *J. Immunol.,* 125:793.

161. Mizel, S. B., and Ben-Zri, A. (1980): Studies on the role of lymphocyte activating factor (interleukin 1) in antigen-induced lymph node lymphocyte proliferation. *Cell. Immunol.,* 54:382.

162. Rosenthal, A. S. (1978): Determinant selection and macrophage function in genetic control of the immune response. *Immunol. Rev.,* 40:136.

163. Heber-Katz, E., Schwartz, R. H., Matis, L. A., Hannum, C., Fairwell, T., Appella, E., and Hansburg, D. (1982): Contribution of antigen-presenting cell major histocompatibility complex gene products to the specificity of antigen induced T cell activation. *J. Exp. Med.,* 155:1086.

Inflammation: Basic Principles and Clinical Correlates.
Edited by J. I. Gallin, I. M. Goldstein, and R. Snyderman.
Raven Press, Ltd., New York © 1988.

CHAPTER 34

Leukocyte Ion Channels and Their Functional Implications

Elaine K. Gallin and Paul A. Sheehy

Leukocytes receive, and respond to, a variety of stimuli as part of their role in host defenses and immune function. In the nervous system, information processing and signal transduction are often initiated by the opening of ion channels (40). Similar processes may be involved in signal transduction in leukocytes, but these cells have been difficult to study using intracellular microelectrodes. With the recent development of the patch-clamp technique (40), such studies are now feasible, and our knowledge of the electrophysiological properties of leukocytes has expanded rapidly in recent years.

This chapter reviews the ion channels (listed in Table 1) that have been described in lymphocytes, macrophages/monocytes, neutrophils, and basophils/mast cells. It focuses on data primarily obtained using patch-clamp techniques and, to the extent that data are available, on ways that these channels may affect leukocyte function. In many cases, these channels have been only cursorily described, and much more information needs to be obtained in order to characterize them adequately.

TERMINOLOGY

Ion channels are integral membrane proteins through which ions passively flow down their electrochemical gradient at rates exceeding 10^6 ions/sec. Channels are characterized according to the following properties: their ionic selectivity (differential permeability), pharmacology (action of specific agents in blocking or changing the flow of ions), gating properties (factors that control their opening and closing), conductance (a measure of the ease with which ions flow), and kinetics (rates at which the channels open and close). Channel gating can be controlled by specific chemical ligands (ligand-gated), voltage (voltage-gated), or other factors (40). In addition, the recent findings that channel gating can be modulated by phosphorylation and dephosphorylation reactions provide an important regulatory link between biochemical events inside the cell and channel activity (49).

Voltage-gated ion channels are usually named in terms of the ion(s) to which they are permeable. A channel that

TABLE 1. *Ionic channels in leukocytes*

Channel	Cell type	Reference	Gating[a]	Blockers	Possible physiological role
K⁺ channels					
Outwardly rectifying K⁺	T-cells	6,14	V	D-600, verapamil, TEA, 4-AP, Ni, Co, quinidine	In T-cells: mitogenesis killing
	Macrophages	98,31			
	B-cells	14,22			
	NK cells	72			
Inwardly rectifying K⁺	Macrophages	30,31	V	Ba, Cs, Rb	Setting membrane potential to E_k
	Basophils	52			
Ca-activated K⁺	Macrophages	27,32	V, Ca	Charybdtoxin	—
Na⁺ channel	T-cells	6	V	Tetrodotoxin	—
Ca²⁺ channel	B-cells	25	V	Mn	Secretion
Cation channel	Mast cells	52	Ca	—	Chemotaxis/secretion
	Neutrophils	89			
Cl⁻ channel	Macrophages	74	V	SITS[b]	—
	Mast cell	52			
	B-cells	4			
Fc-receptor cation channel	Macrophages	96	L (IgG)	—	Phagocytosis
Cromolyn-binding-receptor calcium channel	Basophils	58	L (IgE)	—	Secretion

[a] V, voltage gated; L, ligand gated; Ca, gated by intracellular free calcium.
[b] 4-Acetamido-4'-isothiocyanostilbene-2,2'-disulfonic acid.

is much more permeable to potassium (K⁺) than other ions is designated a K⁺ channel, even though it may have a finite permeability to other ions. Since more than one type of channel in a cell may exist that is permeable to a particular ion, it is often necessary to specify additional properties of the channel in order to uniquely identify it. An important property of some ion currents is that current flows in one direction more easily than in the other, a property called *rectification.* Rectification can be an intrinsic property of a channel or it can result simply from the voltage dependence of the channel gating and the ion gradient across the membrane. For example, if a K⁺ channel is activated (opened) only when the membrane potential of the cell is −40 mV or less negative (more depolarized) and the equilibrium potential for potassium (E_K) is normally −80 mV, then K⁺ only will flow out of the cell through this channel. That is, for K⁺ to flow into the cell the membrane potential across the cell would have to be more negative than −80 mV, and the channels would be closed at those potentials. The K⁺ current that flows through this channel is referred to as an *outward rectifying current,* since the current will flow out of the cell more easily than into the cell.

Ligand-gated ion channels are usually referred to by the specific ligand that opens the channel rather than by the ions that permeate the channel. For example, even though the acetylcholine channel is permeable to Na⁺ and K⁺, it is referred to as the *acetylcholine channel.*

A term used throughout this chapter to describe channels is conductance, *G,* which is a measure of the ease with which current flows through the channel. From Ohm's law, it is equal to the current divided by the potential across the channel. It is expressed in siemens, and its value is the inverse of the resistance.

METHODS

The studies reviewed in this chapter primarily use electrophysiological techniques to monitor current flow or voltage changes induced by current flow across whole cell membranes, patches of membrane, or artificial lipid bilayers. The earliest studies were done using high-resistance ($>30 \times 10^6$ Ω) intracellular microelectrodes; however, this technique is not well suited for use in leukocytes, where microelectrode penetration can damage the cells and produce a significant leak current (43). Patch-clamp techniques are more suitable for studies in leukocytes and other small cells. Low-resistance (5×10^6 Ω) patch electrodes can be used in five recording configurations. Four of these are diagrammed in Fig. 1 (the fifth configuration, the "slow patch clamp," is discussed in the following paragraphs). A recording is initiated by placing a low-resistance electrode against the surface of a cell. When gentle suction is applied, the electrode forms a seal with the cell membrane, isolating the underlying patch of membrane electrically and mechanically. The seal has very high resistance ($>10^9$ Ω), which minimizes leak current and reduces the noise level. In this way, small current fluctuations (on the order of 10^{-12} A) can be recorded, which represent the opening and closing of single-ion

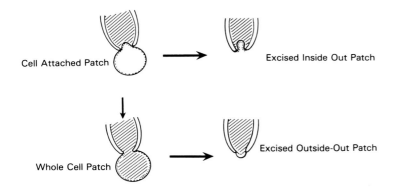

FIG. 1. Schematic of four patch-clamp recording configurations.

channels in the patch of membrane underlying the electrode. Single-channel current fluctuations through inwardly rectifying K⁺ channels recorded in this type of cell-attached configuration are shown in Fig. 2.

Because the seal is mechanically stable, the electrode can be pulled away from the cell, creating an excised patch with the inside of the membrane facing the bathing solution. Single channels similar to those in the cell-attached patch configuration can be recorded while solutions on both sides of the patch membrane are controlled. Alternatively, after formation of a seal, the patch can be destroyed by further suction to gain access to the inside of the cell. Thus, the inside of the cell will become contiguous with the recording electrode, and currents can be measured across the whole-cell membrane. In this recording mode, namely, the whole-cell configuration, the current measured represents the sum of the currents flowing through all open channels, and single-channel events usu-

ally are not evident (unless the cell has a very low conductance). Figure 2 shows whole-cell currents obtained in response to applied voltage steps from a human macrophage before and after the addition of barium. The inward currents, which are barium-inhibitable K⁺ currents, represent the sum of individual channel events similar to those shown on the left side of Fig. 2.

The whole-cell patch technique has the additional disadvantage (or advantage, depending on the purpose of the study) of perfusing the inside of the cell with the solution contained in the patch electrode. It takes approximately 10 min for a whole-cell recording to stabilize, and conductances can disappear during this period, presumably due to the dialysis of critical intracellular constituents. In some cases, as in the secretory response of the mast cell (53), intracellular perfusion also blocks cellular responses. Methods recently have been developed to partially permeabilize the patch of membrane under the elec-

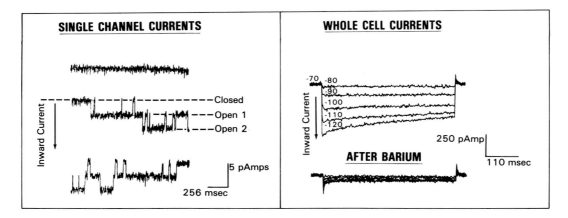

FIG. 2. Data obtained using patch-clamp recording techniques from a human macrophage grown in tissue culture for 2 weeks. (*Left panel*) Continuous current tracing of single-channel current fluctuations recorded in a cell-attached patch. Two channels were present in the patch. Initially (*top tracing*) both channels were closed. (*Right panel*) Currents recorded in a whole-cell recording configuration. Cell was perfused with the contents of the patch electrode (150 mM KCl, 10 mM NaCl, 0.1 mM CaCl$_2$, 1.1 mM EGTA, 1.2 mM MgCl$_2$, 10 mM HEPES, pH 7.2). Membrane potential was held at -70 mV and was stepped to more negative potentials every 3 sec. After the addition of barium chloride (2 mM), another set of voltage steps was recorded. The inward currents were reduced. The barium-inhibitable inward currents in the whole-cell recording configuration are a summation of single-channel events similar to those in the left panel.

trode while in the cell-attached patch configuration and obtain a "slow patch clamp." Using this technique, currents across whole cells can be measured while the intracellular constituents necessary for cell functions are maintained (53).

In addition to electrophysiological techniques, numerous studies have used indirect probes of the membrane potential to monitor membrane potential changes occurring during stimulation in leukocytes (44,75,91). Although these techniques have provided much information, no attempt is made to review that literature in this chapter.

MACROPHAGES

Macrophages are found in virtually every tissue in the body, emigrating as blood monocytes and maturing into tissue macrophages over a period of days (see Chapter 17, *this volume*). Their activation *in situ* is important in both host defenses and immune regulation but, if uncontrolled, can result in chronic inflammation and severe tissue injury. Understanding how events at the surface of the macrophage initiate secretion, phagocytosis, chemotaxis, and other cell functions will provide important information about these processes. Ion channels have been implicated in signal transduction in many different cell types and may play a role in macrophages too.

Recent studies have demonstrated that macrophages exhibit voltage-gated, calcium-gated, and ligand-gated ion channels. The channels described to date include three different potassium (K^+)-selective channels (27,31,98) and a high-conductance anion-selective channel (74). One of the K^+ channels is gated by both intracellular ionized calcium $[Ca]_i$ and voltage (27). $[Ca]_i$ also modulates the activity of a second type of channel, a nonselective cation channel activated following exposure of mouse peritoneal macrophages to IgG (62). This channel is different from the cation-selective channel, demonstrated in lipid bilayers, that results from the binding and cross-linking of ligands to the isolated Fc receptor (97).

The resting membrane potential (RMP) of macrophages or macrophage-like cell lines has been measured with both intracellular microelectrodes and patch-clamp electrodes. Early studies using intracellular microelectrodes gave artificially low values of RMP (-15 to -30 mV) for both cultured human and murine macrophages (18,33). Later studies with both intracellular microelectrodes and patch electrodes indicate that the RMP of macrophages is more negative. Values for mouse peritoneal macrophages (cultured for 24 hr or longer) and adherent J774 cells range from -70 to -90 mV (30,31). Human peripheral blood monocytes cultured for several days have less negative RMPs, ranging from -30 to -70 mV (32,59).

Inwardly Rectifying K^+ Channel

A K^+ channel that activates at voltages negative to -60 mV was first described in mouse spleen and thioglycollate-induced macrophages that had been cultured for several weeks (26,30). This channel is also present in cultured human macrophages (32) and in the mouse-derived macrophage-like cell line J774 (31). Since this channel allows K^+ to move more readily into the cell than out of the cell, it is referred to as an *inwardly rectifying K^+ channel*. It is very similar to a K^+ channel extensively characterized in both muscle and egg cells (37), which has a steep voltage dependence, activating at potentials negative to -50 mV. The probable function of this channel is to set the resting membrane potential of the macrophage near the K^+ equilibrium potential. Addition of barium, cesium, or rubidium to the bathing medium blocks the flow of K^+ through the channel and results in a depolarization of 20 mV or more (30,31).

The gating of this channel is unique in that it depends not only on membrane voltage but also on the $[K^+]_0$ (31,37). That is, increasing $[K^+]_0$ shifts the voltage range in which the channels open so that they open at more depolarized potentials. In addition, the conductance of the channel is proportional to the square root of $[K^+]_0$. Macrophages and other cells exhibiting this conductance can exhibit two stable states of resting membrane potential, i.e., small changes in current can flip a cell between resting potentials of approximately -80 mV and -30 mV (26). The macrophage is present in sites of dead and dying tissue, and it may well be exposed to significant fluctuations in $[K^+]_0$. A rise in $[K^+]_0$ will increase the conductance through inwardly rectifying K^+ channels, thus preserving a steep current-voltage relationship so that the cells remain sensitive to small current fluctuations, which may be triggered by physiological stimuli.

Single-channel current fluctuations, which correspond to the macroscopic inward currents measured across whole cells, have been described recently in both J774 cells (60) and cultured human macrophages (32). The inwardly rectifying channel has a conductance of 29 picosiemens (pS) in symmetric (145 m*M*) K^+. As found with the whole-cell conductance, the single-channel conductance is proportional to the square root of $[K^+]_0$. Similar inwardly rectifying K^+ channels are present in rat basophilic leukemic cells (41).

Not all macrophages exhibit inwardly rectifying K^+ channels. They are absent in freshly isolated human peripheral blood monocytes (Gallin, *unpublished observations*) and also in mouse peritoneal macrophages during the first 4 days in culture (98). However, these channels are present in mouse peritoneal macrophages grown in culture for several weeks (30), adherent J774 cells (31), and some long-term cultured human macrophages (32). The time course of expression of this conductance has been followed in J774 cells, where it has been shown that several hours are required for the channels to be fully expressed (31). The RMP of suspended and adherent J774 cells (estimated using the lipophilic cation tetraphosphonium) was found to be -14 and -70 mV, respectively. The more negative resting potential may correspond to the appearance of this conductance in adherent cells (86). These findings further support the view that this channel, when present, sets the resting potential of the macrophage.

Outwardly Rectifying Potassium Channel

Macrophages exhibit an outwardly rectifying K^+ conductance (98) similar to that described in detail in T-lymphocytes (6). This current activates at potentials positive to -50 mV, inactivates with time, and is blocked by 4-aminopyridine. Ypey and Clapham (98), using resident peritoneal macrophages, reported that this current was absent during the first day following isolation but was present in 96% of the cells cultured for 1 to 4 days. The mouse-derived cell lines J774 (31) and P388D1 (43) also exhibit a similar K^+ conductance. In J774 cells, the channel is present only 1 to 8 hr after adherence and is not present in long-term adherent cultures when the inwardly rectifying potassium channel is the predominant channel (31).

In T-lymphocytes and natural killer cells, this channel may play a role in mitogenesis and cytotoxicity, respectively (see section on lymphocytes). In the macrophage, this conductance is not present in all cells, and little evidence pertaining to its functional relevance is available.

Calcium- and Voltage-Activated K^+ Channel

In 1975 a study using high-resistance intracellular microelectrodes described spontaneous rhythmic membrane hyperpolarizations in human macrophages grown in tissue culture for 2 to 5 weeks (33). The hyperpolarizations involved an increase in permeability, were blocked by addition of a calcium chelator, and could be induced by the calcium ionophore A23187. It was concluded that the hyperpolarizations were due to the activation of a calcium-activated K^+ conductance. Persechini et al. (68) provided further support for the existence of a calcium-activated K^+ channel by demonstrating that injection of calcium into mouse macrophages could trigger hyperpolarization. More recently, patch-clamp experiments have demonstrated (in human macrophages) high-conductance (200 pS in symmetrical K^+) K^+ channels activated both by voltage and $[Ca]_i$ (27). Thus, as the membrane potential became more depolarized and/or the calcium concentration increased (from 10^{-7} to 10^{-4}), the probability of

channel opening increased. These channels are blocked by charybdotoxin (32), a protein purified from scorpion toxin, which blocks calcium-activated K^+ channels in skeletal muscle (63).

Similar large conductance calcium- and voltage-gated channels have been described in a variety of cells (2,69). The sensitivity of these channels to $[Ca]_i$ differs in different tissues. In pancreatic acinar cells, a change in $[Ca]_i$ from 10^{-8} to 10^{-7} M produces a large increase in the probability of channels opening (69). In contrast, in muscle cells (2) and macrophages (27), 10^{-6} M $[Ca]_i$ is needed to increase significantly the opening probability. Thus, $[Ca]_i$ must rise above 10^{-6} M for these channels to be activated at negative membrane potentials. Since the RMP of human macrophages ranges from -30 to -70 mV (27,59), it is likely that only a very small fraction (if any) of these channels are activated during physiological stimulation.

The physiological relevance of the calcium-activated K^+ channel in the macrophage is uncertain. It provides a link between membrane potential and internal calcium concentration, repolarizing the cell to the K^+ equilibrium potential during instances when $[Ca]_i$ rises sufficiently to open channels. By increasing the membrane permeability to K^+, the channel also may regulate volume or modulate the intracellular K^+ concentration. Evidence exists in other cell types to show that changes in intracellular K^+ can influence synthetic processes (55,78) as well as receptor-mediated endocytosis (47). The contractile machinery of the macrophage may be particularly influenced by changes in K^+, since it contains an actin-modulating protein, acumentin, whose activity is modified by changes in K^+ in the physiological range (100–200 mM) (85) (see also Chapter 20, *this volume*).

As is the case for other K^+ conductances present in macrophages, the expression of the calcium-activated K^+ channel is time-dependent. Freshly isolated human peripheral blood monocytes do not exhibit calcium-activated K^+ channels, which are, however, present in macrophages cultured for 2 to 4 days (28). After 7 days in culture, 90% of patches from the human macrophages contained three or more channels. During this time, the monocyte matures into a macrophage. This maturation process involves morphological and functional changes, including increases in protein content and decreases in H_2O_2 production (65). Gallin and Gallin (29) demonstrated that chemotactic factors induce membrane hyperpolarization in long-term cultured human macrophages. It is likely that the hyperpolarization was caused by the activation of calcium-activated K^+ channels. However, the fact that freshly isolated human peripheral blood monocytes (which lack calcium- and voltage-activated K^+ channels) are both phagocytic and chemotactic implies that these channels are not essential for those events.

Chloride Channel

Schwarze and Kolb (74) have described a channel, present in excised patches from mouse peritoneal macrophages, that has a very high conductance (340 pS) as well as several subconductance states. It is poorly selective for chloride (the permeability ratio of Cl to Na [P_{Cl}:P_{Na}] is 5:1). The channel was seen in cell-attached patches only after treatment with the calcium ionophore A23187. In quiescent patches, excision of the membrane activated the channel. The channel is activated by both depolarizing and hyperpolarizing voltage jumps, and it exhibits voltage-dependent inactivation that is consistent with a model of a single channel controlled by two independent voltage-sensitive gates. Similar models have been used to describe the behavior of voltage-dependent gap junctions, and it was suggested that the chloride channel may play a role in intracellular communication (74). A high-conductance anion channel also has been described recently in B-lymphocytes (4).

Fc-Receptor Channel

Ligand binding to the macrophage Fc receptor, as well as its subsequent cross-linking, initiates the ingestion of particles and the secretion of a number of mediators (88). One of the first indications that the ligand–Fc-receptor interaction was linked to the activation of ionic channels came from the observation of Young et al. (94) that membrane potential changes occurred in J774 cells following the binding and cross-linking of the Fc receptor. These studies, done by monitoring membrane potential indirectly with [^{3}H]tetraphenylphosphonium ions, demonstrated a membrane depolarization following addition of IgG or immune complexes. This depolarization required multivalent ligand and was inhibited by substituting choline for sodium. Subsequently, the insertion of partially purified Fc γ2b/γ1 receptor (FcR) into lipid vesicles and lipid bilayers provided an important breakthrough in determining how ligand binding and cross-linking induce membrane-potential changes in the macrophage. It was shown that ligand binding to proteoliposomes containing purified FcR increased cation permeability (97). This observation was extended by demonstrating that the addition of specific ligands induces ion channels in lipid bilayers containing FcR (96). The induced channels were cation-selective, had a conductance of 60 pS in symmetrical 1 M KCl, and decreased in activity within minutes of adding the ligand.

Two studies have been done on intact macrophages or macrophage membranes in which patch-clamp electrodes were used to monitor channel activity before and after the addition of IgG. Nelson et al. (66) recorded whole-cell currents as well as single channels in human alveolar macrophages exposed to heat-aggregated IgG (aIgG). The application of aIgG to cells during whole-cell recording produced an inward current that diminished with successive applications of aIgG, indicating that the response desensitized. In cell-attached patches, channel activity was noted only when the electrode contained aIgG. The channels had a unitary conductance of 350 pS in symmetrical 140 mM NaCl. Changing the permeant cation from Na$^+$ to K$^+$ did not affect the reversal potential of the channel, indicating that if the channel is a cation channel, it is nonselective. Unfortunately, its anion permeability was not examined. The discrepancy between the channel conductance in this study and the data of Young et al. (96) on isolated FcR needs to be investigated further. It may reflect the difference in the ionic conditions, and/or the ligands in the two sets of experiments, or a change in channel behavior following isolation.

Work by Lipton (54) provides evidence that the ligand-FcR complex, in addition to acting as an ion channel itself, may release a second messenger that indirectly activates ion channels. In this study, IgG2b was added to the bath during a cell-attached recording from P388D1 cells (a murine-derived macrophage-like cell line). Following the addition of IgG2b, channels with multiple amplitudes were evident, representing either several different types of channels or a single channel type with different subconductance states; the conductance of the smallest channels was 35 to 45 pS. The channels were cation-selective. Channel activity could be maintained following excision of the patch, and activity was modulated by changes in [Ca]$_i$. Since in this study the ligand was added to the bath, not to the patch electrode, the ligand must be acting indirectly through a second messenger. Thus, it is unlikely that these channels are the same as those described by Nelson et al. (66). Calcium-sensitive (and voltage-insensitive) cation-permeable channels have been reported in a number of other cells, including pancreatic acinar cells and heart cells. Lipton (54) suggests that these channels are activated by increases in [Ca]$_i$ that may occur following binding and cross-linking of the FcR. However, conflicting data exist with regard to what the [Ca]$_i$ actually is during Fc-mediated phagocytosis. Young et al. (95), using the calcium indicator, Quin-2, demonstrated a transient rise in [Ca]$_i$ (from 87 to 400 nM) following addition of 2.4G2 IgG to J774 cells. Similar data have been obtained in the neutrophil, where it was demonstrated that Fc-mediated phagocytosis requires a transient rise in [Ca]$_i$ (measured with Quin-2). In contrast to Fc-mediated phagocytosis, neutrophil iC3b-mediated ingestion does not require a rise in [Ca]$_i$ (50). Conflicting data, measuring no change in [Ca]$_i$ during Fc-mediated phagocytosis, have been reported in a recent study using aequorin to measure [Ca]$_i$ in mouse peritoneal macrophages (62). The aequorin studies led the authors to conclude that either (a) calcium is not involved as a cytoplasmic signal in phagocytosis or (b) changes in calcium occur in very small areas of the cell which are difficult to detect.

It is not known how ion fluxes through ligand-FcR channels or other channels actually mediate phagocytosis and its related events. The ion fluxes and/or the potential changes resulting from FcR-ligand interactions presumably are linked to one or more second messengers connecting the membrane events to ensuing intracellular events.

LYMPHOCYTES

Lymphocytes are responsible for both cell-mediated and humoral immunity. Stimulation of resting lymphocytes causes their clonal expansion and differentiation into competent effector cells such as cytotoxic lymphocytes or plasma cells that are ultimately responsible for host defense. Changes in RMP and/or $[Ca]_i$ (measured with indirect probes of calcium and membrane potential) are among the first detectable events associated with lymphocyte activation or effector cell function. For instance, antibodies directed at either the T3 (42,67,90) or T11 (1) epitopes of T-cells produce a rapid rise in $[Ca]_i$; phytohemagglutin (PHA) stimulation produces a similar rise in $[Ca]_i$ as well as a depolarization of peripheral blood and splenic lymphocytes (20) and a hyperpolarization of thymocytes (87). In B-cells, antigen binding by surface immunoglobulin elicits both a rapid rise in $[Ca]_i$ and membrane depolarization (64). These studies implicate ionic channels in lymphocyte function. Recent findings of the development of an atypical channel in MRL mice concurrent with the development of a lupus-like syndrome (8) suggest a role for ionic channels in lymphocyte dysfunction as well.

Several ionic currents in T-lymphocytes have been described using patch electrodes: Virtually all T-cells studied to date express one or both of two transient K^+ currents, and some T-cells also express Na^+ current (11). Although indirect probes of membrane potential have provided considerable evidence for a K^+ conductance that is sensitive to $[Ca^{2+}]_i$ (34,89,91), no direct (microelectrode) evidence supports these findings. Voltage-dependent calcium currents have not been detected in T-cells, but there is evidence for a voltage-independent calcium channel whose gating is sensitive to application of PHA (46).

Ionic conductances in B-cells have not been studied to the same degree as those in T-cells. Both human and mouse B-cells exhibit time- and voltage-dependent outward K^+ current similar to that of T-cells (14; Sheehy, *unpublished observations*). In contrast, antibody-secreting B-cell hybridomas exhibit a prominent voltage-dependent

calcium current, whereas only 10% of the cells expressed an outward K^+ current (22). A chloride channel is also present in the hybridoma cells (4). No evidence exists at this time for either Na^+ or Ca-dependent K^+ channels in human or mouse B-cells, although substantial evidence for a ligand-gated depolarizing conductance mechanism associated with B-cell activation exists from studies using indirect probes of membrane potential (39,64).

Estimates of the RMP of unstimulated lymphocytes done using indirect probes of membrane potential are in general agreement. Both the distribution of radiolabeled lipophilic ions (17,44) and the distribution of fluorescent dyes (34,87,91) indicate that the RMP ranges from -60 to -70 mV. For $[K]_0 > 10$ mM, RMP is largely determined by the K^+ equilibrium potential; at lower K^+ concentrations, the relative contribution of the sodium permeability increases (34,91).

T-LYMPHOCYTES

Potassium Currents

Voltage-dependent currents were first described in human T-lymphocytes by Matteson and Deutsch (56) and Cahalan et al. (9) and were first reported in a mouse clonal cytotoxic T-lymphocyte (CTL) line by Fukushima et al. (24). In cells exhibiting this current, transient outward currents were activated upon depolarization beyond -50 mV. Investigations of the instantaneous current/voltage relation showed that the current was carried by K^+ (9,24,56). Activation was followed by a voltage- and time-dependent inactivation, reflecting a decrease in the underlying conductance (24). The amount of inactivation present under resting conditions is presently unsettled. Estimates obtained in human T-cells held at -70 mV range from $>50\%$ (6) to 0% (14). In mouse cells the voltage of 50% steady-state inactivation was significantly depolarized; estimates range from -46 (61) to -62 mV (12).

This current has been found in all types of T-cells and does not correlate with expression of the surface markers T1, T3, T4, T8, or 9.6 (11,56,73). Resting mouse T-cells seem to have a low current density (10 channels per cell) as compared to human T-cells, which express several hundred K^+ channels per cell. Upon stimulation by lectin, or in cell lines maintained in an activated state (11,48,61), K^+ current density in mouse T-cells is comparable to that in human T-cells. The expression of the K^+ current in mouse thymocytes and lymph-node T-cells best correlates to the expression of the J11D surface marker (61).

The antagonists of the transient K^+ conductance are particularly diverse. Voltage-dependent outward current is blocked by classical K^+-channel antagonists such as 4-aminopyridine (4AP) and quinine and is blocked less well by tetraethylammonium (TEA) (9,24,56). Significantly, outward current is also blocked by classical calcium-channel antagonists such as diltiazem and verapamil and by the multivalent cations nickel, cobalt, zinc, and lanthanum (9,56). It is nonetheless clear that this current is not the calcium-activated K^+ conductance suggested by membrane potential-sensitive dye observations. Direct manipulations of calcium show either no effect on peak K^+ current (6) or an actual reduction (5). Furthermore, the conductance activates in the virtual absence of $[Ca]_i$ (in the presence of 140 mM fluoride, $[Ca]_i$ <2nM). Raising $[Ca]_0$ in order to increase calcium influx actually reduces voltage-dependent K^+ current as a result of a positive shift in the conductance's activation parameters (5,6,24).

Because the input resistance of these cells is so high, the openings and closings of single K^+ channels can be resolved in the whole-cell recording configuration (6). Step-like current fluctuations that correspond to single-channel events underlying the whole-cell K^+ currents have been recorded in both human and mouse T-cells, and each provides an estimate of the single-channel conductance of about 9 to 16 pS (5,6). However, the K^+ current has not been systematically analyzed at the level of single channels.

T-cells isolated from MRL mice (a strain of mice that develops a disease similar to human systemic lupus erythematosus) exhibit a variant type of K^+ current (8,10). This current activates at more positive potentials, inactivates more slowly, is more sensitive to block by TEA, and is less sensitive to block by cobalt than is the K^+ channel most prevalent in other T-cells. These channels also have a higher unitary conductance (21 pS) than the first type of K^+ channel. MRL mice initially (after birth) have predominantly normal K^+ channels and develop an increasing number of variants concomitant with the onset of splenic enlargement and other prodromal symptoms of lupus.

Several findings support a role for voltage-gated K^+ channels in T-cell activation, although they provide little information regarding how the channel is coupled to activation. For instance, indirect probes indicate that PHA initially depolarizes and then (>10 hr) hyperpolarizes and increases the passive K^+ efflux from T-cells (44). However, direct examinations of the acute effects of PHA on the voltage-gated K^+ current are in conflict: One group reported an increase (6), one reported no change (56), and a third reported a decrease (73). Both lectins (9,56) and phorbol ester (14) produce a transient increase (approximately twofold) in the K^+ current per unit surface.

A more convincing line of evidence supporting the involvement of the transient K^+ current in T-cell physiology comes from pharmacological studies. Agents that block the K^+ current are very effective in blocking many aspects of T-cell activation without affecting cell viability. K^+-channel blockers inhibit T-cell activation induced by allogenic cells, lectins (7), antibody against the T3 receptor (11), and phorbol ester (14). On the other hand, it is clear that K^+ current is not an absolute requirement for mitogenesis. For instance, T-cells respond normally to lectins even while the K^+ channel is closed by prolonged depolarization in 88 mM $[K]_0$ (16); also, the CTLL-2 cell line, which lacks K^+ channels, does respond mitogenically to interleukin-2 (IL-2) (11). In addition to the role of K^+ current in T-cell activation, there is evidence that it may play a role in cell-mediated cytotoxicity. A mouse-derived line of cytotoxic cells exhibits K^+ current which is slightly increased when these cells are conjugated with targets (24). Cytotoxicity is also blocked by K^+-channel blockers. This aspect of the transient K^+ current and leukocyte function will be addressed in greater detail in the section on natural killer cells (see below).

In addition to their effects on mitogenesis and cytotoxicity, K^+-channel antagonists also block PHA-stimulated DNA synthesis and protein synthesis. Yet these effects are not simply nonspecific drug toxicities, since PHA-stimulated expression of the IL-2 receptor is unaffected (7). Furthermore, PHA-stimulated proliferation of CCRF cells, which do not express K^+ current, is insensitive to K^+-channel blockers (11). K^+-channel blockers that concurrently block lymphocyte activation or effector-cell function include 4-aminopyridine, tetraethylammonium, quinine, verapamil, Cd^{2+}, and retinoic acid (11,80). Considering the diverse natures of these drugs it seems unlikely that block of activation and/or function is due to side effects of the drugs.

The mechanism by which K^+ channels are involved in T-cell activation is unknown. The simplest possibility is that T-cell activation is membrane-potential-dependent and thus indirectly coupled to the channel. The data about membrane potential and T-cell activation, although somewhat complex and contradictory, indicate that depolarization is neither a necessary nor sufficient stimulus for T-cell activation. For instance, clamping cells to −15 mV for an hour by raising $[K]_0$ is inhibitory to PHA stimulation of proliferation (35). This is in contrast to the rapid and sustained depolarization that has been reported to occur under physiological conditions following PHA stimulation (44). Consistent with the finding of a sustained depolarization are the results of Deutsch and Price (15), indicating that prolonged depolarization with high $[K]_0$ has no effect on proliferation. The potassium channel also does not appear to facilitate the influx of calcium, since: (a) K^+-channel blockers at concentrations that block both Rb^+ permeability and lectin-induced proliferation do not affect the lectin-induced calcium spike (34); (b) K^+-channel antagonists block calcium-independent phorbol ester-independent proliferation (34); and (c) depolarization to potentials that activate K^+ channels does not lead to a rise in $[Ca]_i$ as it would if calcium entered through these channels (34).

An alternative suggestion is that the K^+ channels are important in T-cell activation because they have a role in volume regulation. Lymphocytes have both cation- and anion-mediated volume regulatory pathways, including some that are electrogenic and that consequently require the movement of counterions (36). At this time no evidence directly links the transient K^+ current with volume regulation, although volume regulatory responses to induced swelling are blocked by quinine and verapamil (16).

Sodium Currents

Small inward currents that have the kinetics and voltage-dependence of Na^+ currents found in nerve and muscle cells have been observed in approximately 3% of human peripheral blood T-cells, 14% of activated mouse T-cells, and, to a variable extent, in a few T-cell lines (11). Sodium current is considerably more prominent in thymocytes, whereas the K^+ conductance in these immature T-cell precursors is similar to the more mature cells (73). Although tetrodotoxin, a specific Na^+-channel blocker, is effective in blocking the Na^+ current, similar concentrations had no effect on mitogenesis (6).

Other Currents

Extensive attempts to demonstrate the presence of voltage-dependent calcium currents in T-cells have failed. In contrast, a cloned helper-T-cell line shows a low density of channels that have the characteristics of a calcium channel but that are voltage-independent. The channel's probability of opening is increased dramatically by PHA and thus may be responsible for the well-documented $[Ca]_i$ increase following PHA stimulation (46).

A slowly developing outward current can be observed at very positive potentials in some human T-cells, indicating the presence of at least one other voltage-dependent current. This current has not been studied in detail but shows little ion selectivity and is not sensitive to K^+-channel blockers (6,76).

NATURAL KILLER CELLS

Natural killer (NK) cells constitute a morphologically and functionally distinct subpopulation of lymphocytes (38). They are also known as *large granular lymphocytes* (LGL) because they are typically larger than other lymphocytes and contain azurophilic granules in their cytoplasm. It should be noted that as many as 90% of NK cells are LGL, whereas fewer than 70% of LGL are killers (38).

LGL isolated from T-cell-depleted (E-rosette-forming) human peripheral blood manifest a time- and voltage-dependent outward K^+ current essentially identical in electrophysiology and pharmacology to that found in human and mouse T-cells (72). There is no evidence for voltage-dependent calcium current or detectable permeability of the K^+ channel to calcium. Agents that block the K^+ current also inhibit LGL-mediated killing of various target cells (72,79). Although the target cells themselves expressed voltage-dependent current, two lines of evidence showed that the agents were acting directly on the killer cells (72): (a) Different cell lines used as targets (U937 and K562) expressed different ionic currents. U937 cells exhibit outward K^+ current similar in electrophysiology and pharmacology to the LGL, but K562 cells exhibit an inward Na^+ current resistant to agents that block outward K^+. Tetrodotoxin block of Na^+ current did not affect LGL-mediated killing of K562 cells. (b) Preincubation of the targets with K^+-channel blockers did not reduce killing.

The precise role of the K^+ current in the lymphocyte cytotolytic mechanism remains unclear at present. The observation that the "binding phase" is associated with increased $^{86}Rb^+$ flux (70) is consistent with increased K^+ conductance reported in mouse CTL when conjugated to targets (24). Quinidine and verapamil reduce somewhat but do not block the formation of LGL:target conjugates; they do inhibit the release (but not production or activity) of NKCF (79), a soluble factor produced by NK cells which has been proposed to mediate target-cell damage (92). On the other hand, it is clear that the conductance mechanism is not used to maintain a "permissive RMP," since cells kill while depolarized by either high external K^+ or gramicidin or while hyperpolarized by valinomycin (Schlicter, *personal communication*). Given that all LGL express K^+ current though not all LGL are killers, it seems reasonable to conclude that the K^+ conductance mechanism is not exclusively coupled to the cytotoxic functions of NK cells.

B-LYMPHOCYTES

Calcium Currents

Fukushima and Hagiwara (22) described inward currents in a mouse myeloma cell line (S194) that required the presence of external calcium, was unaffected by sodium removal, and was blocked by manganese. Strontium and barium could substitute for calcium in carrying the current (22). S194 is a nonsecretory cell line, and the amount of calcium current varied widely from cell to cell. Secretory hybridomas constructed by the fusion of S194 with mouse spleen cells were subsequently characterized because they expressed calcium current more consistently

(25). Calcium current in other tissues is the sum of at least three voltage-dependent conductance mechanisms that are distinguishable by kinetic and pharmacologic criteria. In contrast, B-cells apparently express only one of these subtypes (23).

Peak inward calcium current in hybridomas increases with time in culture. The increase parallels that of the culture's capacity to secrete immunoglobulin, whereas the variation in calcium current in nonsecreting S194 cells was seemingly random (25), suggesting that the development of calcium current is coupled to immunoglobulin secretion. But this suggestion is clouded by studies that show a differential sensitivity of the two processes to pharmacological agents; inward current in these cells is relatively insensitive to calcium-channel antagonists (100 μM D-600 blocks only 37%), whereas the same concentration completely blocked immunoglobulin secretion (25).

Chloride Channel

The S194/spleen-cell hybridoma also expresses a poorly selective anion channel (4). The channel is particularly interesting because its properties change markedly upon excision from the membrane. In cell-attached recordings the conductance of the channel was relatively low (30 pS); the channels are active at rest and over a broad range of voltages. Upon excision, single-channel conductance increases 10-fold, more than one conductance level is observed, and the voltage range over which it is active is reduced. Since the channel is active at rest *in situ*, this conductance probably contributes to the RMP of the cell. The observation that the channel properties change dramatically when removed from the cell suggest that the channel may be coupled to soluble proteins in the cell.

BASOPHILS AND MAST CELLS

Mast cells and basophils initiate inflammatory and allergic reactions by secreting histamine, serotonin, and other mediators. Degranulation in the rat basophilic leukemia cell line RBL-2H3 is associated with both an influx of calcium and a membrane depolarization (19). However, inward calcium currents have not been detected in either mast cells or RBL cells (52). Lindau and Fernandez (53) demonstrated that dialysis of mast cells during whole-cell patch recordings prevented degranulation in response to either 48/80 or antigens. The addition to the pipette of the GTP analog, γ-S-GTP (along with Mg-ATP), induced degranulation, even in the absence of calcium (53). The problems inherent in dialyzing the mast cells were prevented by permeabilizing the cell-attached patch with ATP (added to the patch electrode) and by recording in the slow whole-cell clamp configuration (53). This study demonstrated that degranulation was associated with an increase in membrane capacitance (due to the insertion of new membrane into the plasma membrane) (21) but was not necessarily associated with an increase in membrane conductance. The conductance increase, when present, could be blocked by quinidine and pimozide, without affecting degranulation itself. These data provide excellent evidence that, in mast cells, the opening of ionic channels is not required for degranulation to occur.

Although basophils and mast cells lack voltage-gated calcium channels, other ionic channels have been described in these cells. RBL-2H3 cells have a prominent inward rectifying K^+ conductance (41,52), which is similar to the one described in macrophages (31). Mast cells do not exhibit this K^+ conductance but have both a calcium-activated nonselective cation channel and a large conductance anion channel (52) similar to that described in lymphocytes and macrophages (4,74). In addition to these voltage and/or calcium-activated channels, a cromolyn-binding protein from RBL cells has been shown to form ion channels when cross-linked by antigen (58).

Potassium Channel

RBL 2H3 cells exhibit an inward rectifying K^+ conductance (41,52) similar to that described in macrophages (31). This conductance is increased by raising the external K^+, activated at potentials negative to -60 mV, and is blocked by barium. As in the macrophage, this conductance sets the membrane potential near the equilibrium potential for K^+.

Calcium-Activated Nonselective Cation Channel

The addition of antigen to sensitized mast cells results in the activation of ion channels (52) that are similar to the calcium-activated nonselective cation channels present in other cell types (93). These channels have a unitary conductance of 30 pS and are voltage-independent (52).

Chloride Channel

Excised patches from mast cell display high-conductance (350 pS) channels following dialysis of cells with high $[Ca]_i$ (52). These channels are more permeable to chloride than to sodium ($P_{Cl}:P_{Na}$, 5:1) and are voltage-sensitive, opening when the potential across the membrane is zero and closing as the potential is stepped to either -40 or $+50$ mV. The channels are similar to those described in macrophages (74), lymphocytes (4), and other cell types (3).

Cromolyn-Binding Protein Receptor Channel

The antihistamine cromolyn binds to a specific membrane protein (referred to as the *cromolyn-binding protein* or *CBP*) and blocks mediator-induced calcium influx and secretion in RBL-2H3 cells (57). This protein has been implicated in the secretory response because cells lacking this protein do not degranulate in response to physiological stimuli. Furthermore, the insertion of purified CBP into cells lacking the protein restores their secretory response (57). When the electrical activity of lipid bilayers containing either CBP or plasma membrane isolated from RBL-2H3 cells was monitored following the addition of monoclonal antibody against CBP, ion channels permeable to calcium (and to K^+ and Na^+ in zero calcium) were evident (58). Channel formation required aggregation of CBP. These data demonstrate that binding to, and cross-linking of, the CBP result in the formation of an ion channel. However, the relationship of this channel to the process of degranulation induced by IgE cross-linking is not clear.

NEUTROPHILS

The mechanism(s) of signal transduction in the neutrophil following exposure to chemotactic factors and/or secretagogues has been extensively studied using a variety of techniques. These studies have demonstrated that increases in $[Ca]_i$ (51), activation of a guanine nucleotide (N) regulatory protein (and subsequent activation of phospholipase C) (84), intracellular alkalinization and acidification (82,99), and changes in ion fluxes and membrane potential (45,75,83) occur after stimulation. (For more information on signal transduction see Chapter 19, *this volume*).

The changes in both ion fluxes and membrane potential (assessed using indirect probes) following stimulation (75,83) indicate that ion channels may be involved in signal transduction in the neutrophil. The resting membrane potential of the neutrophil, estimated using the carbocyanine dye diSC$_3$ (5), is −59 mV (83). Following the addition of the chemotactic factor, N-formyl-methionyl-leucyl-phenylalanine (FMLP), neutrophils transiently depolarize and then repolarize (45,75). Unfortunately, the ionic basis of the transient depolarization never has been adequately delineated. For example, although both a calcium and a sodium influx occurs following stimulation with FMLP (100) (an influx of either of these ions would result in a membrane depolarization), the FMLP-induced membrane depolarization occurs in the absence of either calcium and sodium (75). The sodium influx can be accounted for almost entirely by activation of the Na^+/H^+ antiporter (82). Activation of this antiporter results in a pronounced intracellular alkalinization, following stim-

ulation with FMLP (71,82). Ameloride and its analogs, which block Na^+/H^+ exchange, have been found to inhibit chemotaxis, indicating that the control of intracellular pH may be important in regulating chemotaxis (82). Ameloride does not affect the FMLP-induced calcium flux, indicating that calcium and sodium influx are through different pathways (71).

A recent study in neutrophils using patch-clamp techniques to examine ion channels during stimulation with FMLP has provided new insight into the ionic events occurring in these cells (89). The addition of FMLP to the bath during cell-attached patch recordings increased channel activity in 13 of 24 patches. These channels appeared to be calcium-activated, since (a) depleting $[Ca]_i$ levels with Fura-2 prevented channel activation by FMLP and (b) treating cells with saponin, to increase $[Ca]_i$, activated channels in the absence of FMLP. Two types of single-channel currents were identified with conductances of 18 to 25 and 4 to 6 pS, respectively. Ion substitution experiments indicated that these channels were equally permeable to potassium, sodium, and calcium but were impermeable to chloride.

Activation of these channels could account for both the influx of $[Ca]_i$ (84) and the membrane depolarization that occurs following addition of FMLP. However, if the membrane depolarization measured with indirect probes of membrane potential is reliable, then the finding that the depolarization occurs in the absence of calcium and sodium is difficult to reconcile with a model attributing the depolarization solely to these channels. This model also conflicts with the data demonstrating that the Na influx can be accounted for by stimulation of the Na^+/H^+ antiporter (71,82). Future studies using patch-clamp techniques to determine if the potential measurements with indirect probes have been accurate, as well as to determine what role these and other still unknown ion channels play in signal transduction in the neutrophil, will help to resolve these questions.

CONCLUSIONS

Virtually all of the cell types involved in inflammatory responses that have been examined electrophysiologically express either voltage- or ligand-gated ion channels. At this time the nature of the connection of these conductances to leukocyte function remains somewhat ambiguous, although a large and increasing body of evidence links the two. It should be noted that ion channels in leukocytes need not primarily be used as in nerve cells for stimulus/response coupling but may function in other processes such as volume regulation. Our understanding of the role of ion channels in leukocyte function will undoubtedly increase as the connections of channels to the cell's biochemical machinery are described. The prospects of attaining this information are excellent because techniques now exist to address these problems.

ACKNOWLEDGMENTS

The authors thank Dr. Leslie McKinney for critically reading the manuscript; they also thank Ms. Junith Van Deusen and Ms. Marianne Owens for their editorial and secretarial assistance. This work was supported by the Armed Forces Radiobiology Research Institute, Defense Nuclear Agency, under Research Work Unit MJ 00020. The views presented in this chapter are those of the author; no endorsement by the Defense Nuclear Agency has been given or should be inferred.

REFERENCES

1. Alcover, A., Weiss, M. J., Daley, J. F., and Reinherz, E. L. (1986): The T11 glycoprotein is functionally linked to a calcium channel in precursor and mature T-lineage cells. *Proc. Natl. Acad. Sci. USA,* 83:2614–2618.
2. Barrett, J. N., Magleby, K. L., and Pallota, B. S. (1982): Properties of single calcium-activated potassium channels in cultured rat muscle. *J. Physiol.,* 331:211–230.
3. Blatz, A. L., and Magleby, K. L. (1983): Single voltage-dependent chloride-selective channels of large conductance in cultured rat muscle. *Biophys. J.,* 43:237–241.
4. Bosma, M. (1986): Chloride channels in neoplastic B lymphocytes. *Biophys. J.,* 49:413a.
5. Bregestovski, P., Redkosubov, A., and Alexeev, A. (1986): Elevation of intracellular calcium reduces voltage-dependent potassium conductance in human T cells. *Nature,* 319:776–778.
6. Cahalan, M. D., Chandy, K. G., DeCoursey, T. E., and Gupta, S. (1985): A voltage-gated potassium channel in human T lymphocytes. *J. Physiol.,* 358:197–238.
7. Chandy, K. G., DeCoursey, T. E., Cahalan, M. D., McLaughlin, C., and Gupta, S. (1984): Voltage-gated potassium channels are required for human T lymphocyte activation. *J. Exp. Med.,* 160:369–385.
8. Chandy, K. G., DeCoursey, T. E., Fischbach, M., Talal, N., Cahalan, M. D., and Gupta, S. (1986): Altered K$^+$ channel expression in abnormal T lymphocytes from mice with the lpr gene mutation. *Science,* 233:1197–1200.
9. DeCoursey, T. E., Chandy, K. G., Gupta, S., and Cahalan, M. D. (1984): Voltage-gated K$^+$ channels in human T lymphocytes: A role in mitogenesis? *Nature,* 307:465–468.
10. DeCoursey, T. E., Chandy, K. G., Gupta, S., and Cahalan, M. D. (1984): Pharmacology of human T lymphocyte K channels. *Biophys. J.,* 45:144a.
11. DeCoursey, T. E., Chandy, K. G., Gupta, S., and Cahalan, M. D. (1985): Voltage-dependent ion channels in T-lymphocytes. *J. Neuroimmunol.,* 10:71–95.
12. DeCoursey, T. E., Chandy, K. G., Gupta, S., and Cahalan, M. D. (1987): Two types of potassium channels in murine T lymphocytes. *J. Gen. Physiol. (in press).*
13. DeCoursey, T. E., Chandy, K. G., Gupta, S., and Cahalan, M. D. (1987): Mitogen induction of ion channels in murine lymphocytes. *J. Gen. Physiol. (in press).*
14. Deutsch, C., Krause, D., and Lee, S. C. (1986): Voltage-gated potassium conductance in human T lymphocytes stimulated with phorbol ester. *J. Physiol.,* 372:405–423.
15. Deutsch, C., and Price, M. (1982): Role of extracellular Na and K in lymphocyte activation. *J. Cell. Physiol.,* 113:73–79.
16. Deutsch, C., Patterson, J., Lee, S., and Prytowsky, M. B. (1986): Volume regulation in cloned T-lymphocytes. *Biophys. J.,* 49:162a.
17. Deutsch, C., Holian, A., Holian, S. K., Daniele, R. P., and Wilson, D. F. (1979): Transmembrane electrical and pH gradients across human erythrocytes and human peripheral lymphocytes. *J. Cell. Physiol.,* 99:79–94.
18. Dos Reis, G. A. and Oliveira-Castro, G. M. (1977): Potassium-dependent slow membrane hyperpolarizations in mice macrophages. *Biochim. Biophys. Acta,* 469:257–263.
19. Eisenberg, R., and Pecht, I. (1983): Membrane potential changes during IgE mediate and histamine release in rat basophilic leukemia cells. *J. Membrane Biol.,* 75:97–104.
20. Felber, S. M., and Brand, M. D. (1983a): Early plasma-membrane-potential changes during stimulation lymphocytes by concanavalin A. *Biochem. J.,* 210:885–891.
21. Fernandez, J. M., Neher, E., and Gomperts, B. P. (1984): Capacitance measurements reveal fusion events in degranulating mast cells. *Nature,* 312:453–455.
22. Fukushima, Y., and Hagiwara, S. (1983): Voltage-gated Ca^{2+} channel in mouse myeloma cells. *Proc. Natl. Acad. Sci. USA,* 80:2240–2242.
23. Fukushima, Y., and Hagiwara, S. (1985): Currents carried by monovalent cations through calcium channels in mouse neoplastic lymphocytes. *J. Physiol.,* 358:255–284.
24. Fukushima, Y., Hagiwara, S., and Henkart, M. (1984): Potassium current in clonal cytotoxic T Lymphocytes from the mouse. *J. Physiol.,* 351:645–656.
25. Fukushima, Y., Hagiwara, S., and Saxton, R. E. (1984): Variation of calcium current during the cell growth cycle in mouse hybridoma lines secreting immunoglobulins. *J. Physiol.,* 355:313–321.
26. Gallin, E. K. (1981): Voltage clamp studies in macrophages from mouse spleen cultures. *Science,* 214:458–460.
27. Gallin, E. K. (1984): Calcium- and voltage-activated potassium channels in human macrophages. *Biophys. J.,* 46:821–825.
28. Gallin, E. K. (1985): Expression of calcium-activated potassium channels in human monocytes with time after culture. *Biophys. J.,* 47:135a.
29. Gallin, E. K., and Gallin, J. I. (1977): Interaction of chemotactic factors with human macrophages: Induction of transmembrane potential changes. *J. Cell Biol.,* 75:277–289.
30. Gallin, E. K., and Livengood, D. R. (1981): Inward rectification in mouse macrophages: Evidence for a negative resistance region. *Am. J. Physiol.,* 241:C9–C17.
31. Gallin, E. K., and Sheehy, P. A. (1985): Differential expression of inward and outward potassium currents in the macrophage-like cell line J774.1. *J. Physiol.,* 369:475–499.
32. Gallin, E. K., and McKinney, L. (1986): Identification of inward and outward rectifying K conductances in cultured human macrophages. *Neurosci. Abstr.,* 12:1341a.
33. Gallin, E. K., Wiederhold, M., Lipsky, P., and Rosenthal, A. (1975): Spontaneous and induced membrane hyperpolarizations in macrophages. *J. Cell Physiol.,* 86:653–662.
34. Gelfland, E. W., Cheung, R. K., and Grinstein, S. (1986): Mitogen-induced changes in Ca^{2+} permeability are not mediated by voltage-gated K$^+$ channels. *J. Biol. Chem.,* 261:11520–11523.
35. Gelfand, E. W., Cheung, R. K., and Gunstein, S. (1987): Role of membrane potential in the response of human T lymphocytes to phytohemagglutinin. *J. Immunol.,* 138:527–531.
36. Grinstein, S., Rothstein, A., Sarkadi, B., and Gelfland, E. W. (1984): Responses of lymphocytes to anisotonic media: Volume-regulating behavior. *Am. J. Physiol.,* 246:C204–C215.
37. Hagiwara, S., and Jaffe, L. (1979): Electrical properties of egg cell membranes. *Annu. Rev. Biophys. Bioeng.,* 8:385–416.
38. Heberman, R. B. (1986): Natural killer cells. *Annu. Rev. Med.,* 37:347–352.
39. Heilkkila, R., Iversen, J., and Godal, T. (1985): No correlation between membrane potential and increased cytosolic free Ca^{2+} concentration, ^{86}Rb$^+$ influx or subsequent [^{3}H$^+$]-thymidine incorporation in neoplastic human B cells stimulated with antibodies to surface immunoglobulin. *Acta Physiol. Scand.,* 124:107–115.
40. Hille, B. (1984): *Ionic Channels in Excitable Membranes.* Sinauer Association, Sunderland, Mass.
41. Ikeda, S., and Weight, F. (1984): Inward rectifying K$^+$ currents recorded from rat basophilic leukemia cells by whole cell patch clam. *Neurosci. Abstr.,* 10:870a.

42. Imboden, J. B., Weiss, A., and Stobo, J. D. (1985): The antigen receptor on a human T cell line initiates activation by increasing cytoplasmic calcium. *J. Immunol.,* 134:663–665.

43. Ince, C., Leijh, P. C. J., Meijer, J., Van Bavel, E., and Ypey, D. (1984): Oscillatory hyperpolarizations and resting membrane potentials of mouse fibroblast and macrophage cell lines. *J. Physiol.,* 352:625–635.

44. Kiefer, H., Blume, A. J., and Kaback, H. R. (1980): Membrane potential changes during mitogenic stimulation mouse spleen lymphocytes. *Proc. Natl. Acad. Sci. USA,* 77:2200–2204.

45. Korchak, H. M., and Weissmann, G. (1978): Changes in membrane potential of human granulocytes antecede the metabolic responses to surface stimulation. *Proc. Natl. Acad. Sci. USA,* 75:3818–3822.

46. Kuno, M., Goronzy, J., Weyand, C. M., and Gardner, P. (1986): Single-channel and whole-cell recordings of mitogen-regulated inward currents in human cloned helper T lymphocytes. *Nature,* 323:269–273.

47. Larkin, J., Brown, M., Goldstein, J., and Anderson, R. (1983): Depletion of intracellular potassium arrests coated pit formation and receptor-mediated endocytosis in fibroblasts. *Cell,* 33:273–285.

48. Lee, S. E., Sabath, D. E., Deutsch, C., and Prystowsky, M. B. (1986): Increased voltage-gated potassium conductance during interleukin 2-stimulated proliferation of a mouse helper T lymphocyte clone. *J. Cell Biol.,* 102:1200–1208.

49. Levitan, I. B., Lemos, J. R., and Novak-Hofer, I. (1983): Protein phosphorylation and the regulation of ion channels. *Trends Neuroscience,* 6:496–499.

50. Lew, D. P., Anderson, T., Hed, J., DiVirgillo, F., Pozzan, T., and Stendahl, O. (1985): Ca^{++}-dependent and Ca^{++}-independent phagocytosis in human neutrophils. *Nature,* 315:509–511.

51. Lew, D. P., Wollheim, C. B., Waldvogel, F. A., and Pozzan, T. (1984): Modulation of cytosolic-free calcium transients by changes in intracellular calcium-buffering capacity: Correlation with exocytosis and O$_2$—Production in human neutrophils. *J. Cell Biol.,* 99:1212–1220.

52. Lindau, M., and Fernandez, J. M. (1986): A patch-clamp study of histamine-secreting cells. *J. Gen. Physiol.,* 88:349–368.

53. Lindau, M., and Fernandez, J. M. (1986): IgE-mediated degranulation of mast cells does not require opening of ion channels. *Nature,* 319:150–153.

54. Lipton, S. (1986): Antibody activates cation channels via second messenger calcium. *Biochim. Biophys. Acta,* 856:59–67.

55. Lopez-Rivas, A., Adelberg, E., and Rozengurt, E. (1982): Intracellular K$^+$ and the mitogenic response of 3T3 cells to peptide factors in serum-free medium. *Proc. Natl. Acad. Sci. USA,* 79:6275–6279.

56. Matteson, D. R., and Deutsch, C. (1984): K channels in T lymphocytes: A patch clamp study using monoclonal antibody adhesion. *Nature,* 307:468–471.

57. Mazurek, N., Bashkin, P., Loyter, A., and Pecht, I. (1983): Restoration of Ca^{2+} influx and degranulation capacity of variant RBL-2H3 cells upon implantation of isolated cromolyn binding protein. *Proc. Natl. Acad. Sci. USA,* 80:6014–6018.

58. Mazurek, N., Schindler, H., Schurholz, T. H., and Pecht, I. (1984): The cromolyn binding protein constitutes the Ca^{2+} channel of basophils opening upon immunological stimulus. *Proc. Natl. Acad. Sci. USA,* 81:6841–6845.

59. McCann, F., Cole, J., Guyre, P., and Russell, J. (1983): Action potentials in human macrophages derived from human monocytes. *Science,* 219:991–993.

60. McKinney, L., and Gallin, E. K. (1986): Single channel records from the murine macrophage cell line J774.1. *Biophys. J.,* 49:167a.

61. McKinnon, D., and Ceredig, R. (1986): Changes on the expression of potassium channels during mouse T cell development. *J. Exp. Med.,* 164:1846–1861.

62. McNeil, P. L., Swanson, J. A., Wright, S. D., Silverstein, S. C., and Taylor, D. L. (1986): Fc-receptor-mediated phagocytosis occurs in macrophages without an increase in average [Ca^{++}]. *J. Cell Biol.,* 102:1586–1592.

63. Miller, C., Moczydlowski, E., Latorre, R., and Phillips, M. (1985): Charybtoxin, a protein inhibitor of single Ca^{++}-activated K$^+$ channels from mammalian skeletal muscle. *Nature,* 313:316–318.

64. Monroe, J. G., and Cambier, J. C. (1983): B-cell activation I. Anti-immunoglobulin induced receptor crosslinking results in a decrease in the plasma membrane potential of murine B lymphocytes. *J. Exp. Med.,* 157:2073–2086.

65. Nakagawara, A., Nathan, C., and Cohn, Z. (1981): Hydrogen peroxide metabolism in human monocytes during differentiation *in vitro. J. Clin. Invest.,* 68:1243–1252.

66. Nelson, A. D. J., Jacobs, E. R., Tang, J. M., Zeller, J. M., and Bone, R. C. (1985): Immunoglobulin G-induced single ionic channels in human alveolar macrophage membranes. *J. Clin. Invest.,* 76:500–507.

67. Oettgen, H. C., Terhorst, C., Cantley, L., and Rosoff, P. (1985): Stimulation of the T3–T-cell receptor complex induces a membrane-potential-sensitive calcium influx. *Cell,* 40:583–590.

68. Persechini, P. M., Araujo, E. G., and Oliveira-Castro, G. M. (1981): Electrophysiology of phagocytic membranes: Induction of slow membrane hyperpolarizations in macrophages and macrophage polykaryons by intracellular calcium injection. *J. Membrane Biol.,* 61:81–90.

69. Petersen, O. H., and Maruyama, Y. (1984): Calcium-activated potassium channels and their role in secretion. *Nature,* 307:693–696.

70. Russell, J. H., and Dobos, C. B. (1983): Accelerated ^{86}Rb(K$^+$) release from the cytotoxic T lymphocytes is a physiologic event associated with delivery of the lethal hit. *J. Immunol.,* 131:1138–1141.

71. Sha'afi, R., Molski, T. F., and Naccache, P. H. (1981): Chemotactic factors activate differentiable permeation pathways for sodium and calcium in rabbit neutrophils. Effect of ameloride. *Biochem. Biophys. Res. Commun.,* 99:1271–1276.

72. Schlicter, L., Sidell, N., and Hagiwara, S. (1986): Potassium channels mediate killing by human natural killer cells. *Proc. Natl. Acad. Sci. USA,* 83:451–455.

73. Schlicter, L., Sidell, N., and Hagiwara, S. (1986): K channels are expressed early in human T-cell development. *Proc. Natl. Acad. Sci. USA,* 83:5625–5629.

74. Schwarze, W., and Kolb, H. A. (1984): Voltage-dependent kinetics of an ionic channel of large unit conductance in macrophages and myotube membranes. *Pflugers Arch.,* 402:281–291.

75. Seligmann, B. E., and Gallin, J. I. (1983): Comparison of indirect probes of membrane potential utilized in studies of human neutrophils. *J. Cell. Physiol.,* 115:105–115.

76. Sheehy, P. A., Grimm, E. H., and Barker, J. L. (1986): Late outward current in cultured, lymphokine-activated human lymphocytes. *Biophys. J.,* 49:1652a.

77. Sheridan, R. E., and Bayer, B. M. (1986): Ionic membrane currents induced in macrophages during cytolysis. *Fed. Proc.,* 45:1009a.

78. Shinohara, T., and Piatigorsky, J. (1977): Regulation of protein synthesis, intracellular electrolytes and cataract formation *in vitro. Nature,* 270:406–411.

79. Sidell, N., Schlicter, L., Wright, S., Hagiwara, S., and Golub, S. (1986): Potassium channels in human NK cells are involved in discrete stages of the killing process. *J. Immunol.,* 137:1650–1658.

80. Sidell, N., and Schlichter, L. (1986b): Retinoic acid blocks potassium channels in human lymphocytes. *Biochem. Biophys. Res. Commun.,* 138:560–567.

81. Sigworth, F. J., and Neher, E. (1980): Single Na$^+$ channel currents observed in cultured rat muscle cells. *Nature,* 287:447–449.

82. Simchowitz, L. (1985): Intracellular pH modulates the generation of superoxide radicals by human neutrophils. *J. Clin. Invest.,* 76:1079–1089.

83. Simchowitz, L., Spilberg, I., and De Weer, P. (1982): Sodium and potassium fluxes and membrane potential of human neutrophils. *J. Gen. Physiol.,* 79:453–479.

84. Smith, C. D., Cox, C. C., and Snyderman, R. (1986): Receptor-coupled activation of phosphoinositide-specific phospholipase C by an N protein. *Science,* 232:97–100.

85. Southwick, F., Tatsumi, N., and Stossel, T. (1982): Acumentin, an actin-modulating protein of rabbit pulmonary macrophages. *Biochemistry,* 21:6321–6326.

86. Sung, S.-S. J., Young, J. D.-E., Origlio, A. M., Heiple, J. M., Kaback, H. R., and Silverstein, S. C. (1985): Extracellular ATP perturbs transmembrane ion fluxes, elevates cytosolic [Ca^{2+}], and inhibits

phagocytosis in mouse macrophages. *J. Biol. Chem.,* 260(25): 13442–13449.

87. Tsien, R. Y., Pozzan, T., and Rink, T. J. (1982): T-cell mitogens cause early changes in cytoplasmic free Ca^{2+} and membrane potential in lymphocytes. *Nature,* 295:68–70.

88. Unkeless, J. C., Fleit, H., and Mellman, I. S. (1981): Structural aspects and heterogeneity of immunoglobulin Fc receptors. *Adv. Immunol.,* 31:247–257.

89. von Tscharner, V., Prod'hom, B., Baggiolini, M., and Reuter, H. (1986): Ion channels in human neutrophils are activated by a rise in the free cytosolic calcium concentration. *Nature,* 324:369–371.

90. Weiss, A., Imboden, J. B., Shoback, D., and Stobo, J. D. (1984): Role of T3 surface molecules in human T-cell activation: T3-dependent activation results in an increase in cytoplasmic free calcium. *Proc. Natl. Acad. Sci. USA,* 81:4169–4173.

91. Wilson, H. A., and Chused, T. M. (1985): Lymphocyte membrane potential and Ca^{2+}-sensitive potassium channels described by oxonol dye fluorescence measurements. *J. Cell. Physiol.,* 125:72–81.

92. Wright, S. C., and Bonivida, B. (1981): Selective lysis of NK-sensitive target cells by a soluble mediator released from murine cells and human peripheral blood monocytes. *J. Immunol.,* 126:1516–1521.

93. Yellen, G. (1982): Single Ca^+-activated nonselective cation channels in neuroblastoma. *Nature,* 296:357–359.

94. Young, D. J., Unkeless, J. C., Kaback, H. R., and Cohn, Z. A. (1983): Macrophage membrane potential changes associated with $\gamma2b/\gamma1$Fc receptor-ligand binding. *Proc. Natl. Acad. Sci. USA,* 80: 1357–1361.

95. Young, D. J., Ko, S., and Cohn, Z. (1984): The increase in intracellular free calcium associated with IgG $\gamma2b/\gamma$Fc receptor-ligand interactions: Role of phagocytosis. *Proc. Natl. Acad. Sci. USA,* 81: 5430–5434.

96. Young, D. J., Unkeless, J. C., Young, T. M., Mauro, A., and Cohn, Z. A. (1983): Role for mouse macrophage IgG Fc receptor as ligand-dependent ion channel. *Nature,* 306:186–189.

97. Young, D. J., Unkeless, J. C., Kaback, H. R., and Cohn, Z. A. (1983): Mouse macrophage Fc receptor for IgG $\gamma2b/\gamma1$ in artificial and plasma membrane vesicles functions as a ligand-dependent ionophore. *Proc. Natl. Acad. Sci. USA,* 80:1636–1640.

98. Ypey, D. L., and Clapham, D. E. (1984): Development of a delayed outward-rectifying K^+ conductance in cultured mouse peritoneal macrophages. *Proc. Natl. Acad. Sci. USA,* 81:3083–3087.

99. Yuli, I., and Oplatka, A. (1987): Cytosolic acidification as an early transductory signal in human neutrophil chemotaxis. *Science,* 235: 340–342.

100. Zigmond, S. (1978): Chemotaxis by polymorphonuclear leukocytes. *J. Cell Biol.,* 77:269–286.

Clinical Correlates

Inflammation: Basic Principles and Clinical Correlates.
Edited by J. I. Gallin, I. M. Goldstein, and R. Snyderman.
Raven Press, Ltd., New York © 1988.

CHAPTER 35

Urticaria and Angioedema

Allen P. Kaplan

The Physical Urticarias
  Cold-Dependent Disorders • Exercise-Induced Disorders • Other Physically Induced Forms of Urticaria or Angioedema

Acute, Nonphysically Induced Urticaria
Chronic Idiopathic Urticaria and Idiopathic Angioedema
References

Urticaria and angioedema are common disorders affecting approximately 20% of the population at some time during their lifetime. Urticaria (hives) is an intensely pruritic rash that consists of a centrally raised, blanched wheal surrounded by an erythematous flare that is generally circular but can vary greatly in size and shape depending on the particular type. It is caused by inflammation that is localized to the venular plexuses of the superficial dermis. Angioedema has the same causes and pathogenic mechanisms as does urticaria (except hereditary and vibratory angioedema), but the reaction occurs in the deep dermis and subcutaneous tissue and has swelling as the prominent manifestation with a normal external appearance of the skin.

Inflammatory mechanisms operative in urticaria can be divided into two general types, depending on the rate at which hive formation occurs and the length of time it is evident. One form of urticaria has lesions that last 1 to 2 hr and results from degranulation of mast cells. The inciting stimulus is present only briefly, and there is no late component to the urticaria. Biopsy of such lesions reveals little or no cellular infiltrate. The second form has a prominent cellular infiltrate, and individual lesions can last from many hours to as long as 2 days. In this review I will describe the various types of urticarias, ranging from those that are among the most fleeting (and simplest) to those of progressively longer duration. The focus will be on pathogenic mechanisms and the nature of the inflammatory reaction.

THE PHYSICAL URTICARIAS

Physically induced hives and/or swelling share the common property of being reproducibly induced by environmental factors such as a change in temperature or by direct stimulation of the skin by pressure, stroking, vibration, or light (25). These disorders have been the subject of considerable investigation and serve as models (91) from which we have learned a great deal about pathogenic mechanisms leading to hive formation and swelling. A classification of these disorders is given in Table 1, which includes virtually all described types.

Cold-Dependent Disorders

Idiopathic cold urticaria is characterized by the rapid onset of pruritus, erythema, and swelling after exposure to a cold stimulus. The location of the swelling is confined to those parts of the body that have been exposed; in this sense it is a local, rather than a systemic, disorder. However, total body exposure such as occurs with swimming can cause massive release of vasoactive mediators, resulting in hypotension; if the subject "passes out," death by drowning can result. The disease can begin in any age group and has no obvious sex predilection. When suspected, an ice-cube test can be performed in which an ice cube is placed on the subject's forearm for 4 to 5 min. A positive reaction leads to formation of a hive the shape

TABLE 1. *Classification of physically induced urticaria and/or angioedema*

1. Cold-dependent disorders
   a. Idiopathic cold urticaria
   b. Cold urticaria associated with abnormal serum proteins: cold agglutinins, cryoglobulin, cryofibrinogen, Donath-Landsteiner antibody
   c. Systemic cold urticaria
   d. Cold-induced cholinergic urticaria
   e. Cold-dependent dermatographism
   f. Delayed cold urticaria
2. Exercise-induced disorders
   a. Exercise-induced anaphylaxis: idiopathic or food-dependent
   b. Cholinergic urticaria (see item 1d for cold-dependent variant)
   c. Exercise-induced angioedema
3. Local heat urticaria
   a. Familial variant
4. Dermatographism
   a. Urticaria pigmentosa/systemic mastocytosis
   b. Cold-dependent variant (see item 1e)
   c. Delayed dermatographism
5. Pressure-induced urticaria/angioedema (delayed)
   a. Immediate-pressure urticaria
6. Solar urticaria
   a-f. Types I-VI
7. Aquagenic urticaria
8. Vibratory angioedema
   a. Familial
   b. Sporadic

of the ice cube within 10 min *after* the stimulus is removed. The time course of this reaction, i.e., cold challenge followed by hive formation as the area returns to body temperature, demonstrates that a two-step reaction has occurred in which exposure to cold is a prerequisite, but hive formation actually occurs as the temperature increases.

The term "idiopathic" was utilized to indicate that the cause of cold urticaria is unknown and is unassociated with abnormal circulating plasma proteins such as cryoglobulins. However, there is evidence that many of these are nevertheless caused by an immunologic reaction. Within this group, most have been shown to be IgE-dependent, based on passive-transfer studies (37). Serum of the subject is injected intradermally into a normal recipient. After 48 hr, the site is challenged with an ice cube. Although the incidence of positive transfer has varied in different studies, our experience suggests that about 10% clearly are positive. This is undoubtedly an underestimate, since the passive transfer is far less sensitive than doing an ice cube test in the propositus, and only those with sufficient pathogenic IgE in the circulation (rather than those bound to mast cells) are detected. In two cases, an IgM antibody was shown to mediate cold urticaria (98). In these cases, passive transfer was positive after a short

interval of 3 to 6 hr but was negative at 48 hr, in contrast to an IgE-mediated reaction, which remains positive at 48 hr. We have recently reported a similar passive transfer (i.e., positive only after short-term sensitization) that seemed to be caused by an IgG antibody (32).

Studies of the pathogenesis of cold urticaria have demonstrated release of mediators into the circulation upon challenge of patients by placing one hand in ice water for 5 min (Fig. 1) and obtaining serial blood samples for 20 min thereafter. As with the ice-cube test, swelling is usually not evident while the hand is being chilled; instead, swelling appears between 4 and 8 min thereafter and is associated with marked pruritus. In this case, chilling occurs in the deep dermis and subcutaneous tissue in addition to more superficial skin layers; thus the entire hand swells and angioedema results. Studies have documented release of histamine (43), eosinophilotactic peptides (97), high-molecular-weight neutrophil chemotactic factor (NCF) (99), platelet-activating factor (26), and protaglandin D_2 (100) into the circulation with a time course that parallels the manifest swelling. It is envisioned that chilling initiates a reaction mediated by IgE bound to mast cells and that, upon warming, mediators are released into the circulation. When skin biopsy specimens were tested by chilling and warming, histamine release was also demonstrable (42) (Fig. 2); however, chilling and warming basophils of pa-

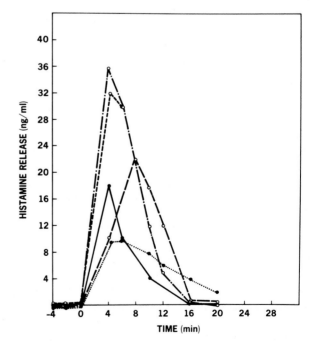

FIG. 1. Time course of histamine release into the venous circulation of five patients with cold urticaria. The patient's hand was placed in ice water for 5 min, and serial blood samples were obtained from the brachial vein draining that arm. Histamine was determined by radioenzyme assay.

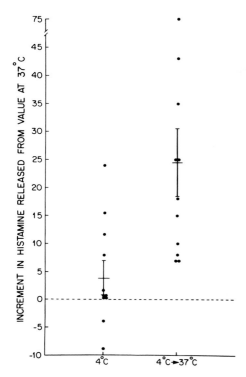

FIG. 2. Histamine release from skin biopsy specimens of patients with cold urticaria. Replicate skin fragments were suspended in phosphate-buffered saline and either (a) chilled for 30 min at 4°C and then maintained for 30 min at 37°C or (b) chilled for 15 min at 4°C and then warmed to 37°C for 15 min. Histamine was determined in the surrounding fluid. Samples that were chilled or chilled and then warmed were compared to those kept at 37°C, and the differences in histamine values were plotted. The mean ±1 standard error is indicated. Samples that are chilled are not significantly different from those maintained at 37°C, whereas those that are chilled and warmed release histamine into the surrounding medium.

tients did not result in histamine release, even in those in whom IgE-mediated disease was documented. Thus it appeared unlikely that the disorder is caused by a circulating IgE cryoglobulin (unless patient basophils are desensitized). Rather, the presence of skin and/or cutaneous mast cells is important.

One proposal to explain such a result is that patients have an IgE autoantibody to a cold-induced skin antigen. Thus sensitization might occur in the cold, and release of mediators proceeds as the cells warm. Studies to test this hypothesis are in progress but have thus far been negative. We have also found high levels of IgM and IgG antibodies directed against the Fc portion of IgE in patients with cold urticaria (32) and, although the clinical significance of such autoantibodies is questionable (75), one such serum causes release of histamine when incubated with normal basophils. However, this reaction is demonstrable at 37°C and does not require chilling followed by warming, so its

relationship to the disease is not yet apparent. Cyproheptadine (Periactin) in divided doses is the drug of choice for cold urticaria. Histamine release, however, is unaffected by doses that completely control symptoms (13). It appears, therefore, to act as a classical antihistamine, i.e., by blockade of H_1 receptors. However, other antihistamines of comparable potency are less effective; the reason for this is uncertain. Although cyproheptadine has antiserotonin activity, serotonin does not appear to be released in cold urticaria. Some patients do not respond well to cyproheptadine either, and it has been reported that symptoms do not always correlate well with histamine release (47). Thus other vasoactive factors may also make a significant contribution for some patients. An experimental cromolyn-like drug, which inhibits mast-cell degranulation, was effective in controlling symptoms and suppressing the ice-cube test in patients who were poorly responsive to cyproheptadine (71).

Cold urticaria has also been described as being associated with the presence of cryoproteins such as cold agglutinins, cryoglobulins, cryofibrinogen, and the Donath-Landsteiner antibody seen in secondary syphilis (paroxysmal cold hemoglobinuria). The only reported studies that address mechanisms of hive formation are those performed in patients with associated cryoglobulins. The isolated proteins appear to transfer cold sensitivity and activate the complement cascade upon *in vitro* incubation with normal plasma (7,8). Thus it is possible that hive formation in these subjects is due to cold-dependent anaphylatoxin release. Therapy in this case is directed toward the underlying disease plus antihistamines. It is clear that a disorder such as cryoglobulinemia can be associated with cutaneous vasculitis as well as cold urticaria, and other associations between these two entities have been reported. Eady and Greaves (17) reported that frequent and repeated cooling of the skin in patients with idiopathic cold urticaria can cause vasculitic lesions. In one case, immune reactants (IgM and C3) deposited in the vessels of such lesions (18). In two other patients, leukocytoclastic vasculitis was seen in association with cold urticaria, and circulating immune complexes were clearly evident (89,97). It appeared that the mediator release caused by cold challenge could localize immune complexes to cutaneous sites where they then caused vasculitis (89). Sites of typical urticarial vasculitis independent of temperature change were also evident (97).

Other cold-dependent syndromes have been reported, but the incidence of such cases is unknown. A delayed form of cold urticaria was described (88) in which swelling appeared 9 to 18 hr after cold exposure. Studies of mediator release were unrevealing, the cold sensitivity could not be passively transferred, and biopsy of a lesion revealed edema and a mononuclear cell infiltrate. Family studies suggested a dominant mode of inheritance. A series of four patients have been described in whom exercise in a cold environment induced hives similar to those seen with cholinergic urticaria; however, hive formation did not occur if exercise was performed in a heated environment. In this disorder the cold exposure is systemic rather than local, and it should be suspected in any patient whose symptoms are suggestive of either cold urticaria or cholinergic urticaria and in whom standard tests for each disorder are negative (41). Exercise in a cold room or running on a winter's day will lead to generalized urticaria and confirm the diagnosis. Because of the visual resemblance of the lesions to those of typical cholinergic urticaria, the disorder has been called *cold-induced cholinergic urticaria.*

Another related disorder called *systemic cold urticaria* yields severe generalized hive formation upon systemic cold challenge occurring over covered or uncovered parts of the body. Symptoms are unrelated to exercise or other activities (39), and the ice-cube test is negative. Histamine release upon cold challenge (with or without exercise as appropriate) has been seen in cold-induced cholinergic urticaria as well as systemic cold urticaria. A treatment regimen of hydroxyzine plus cyproheptadine in high dosage has been utilized successfully.

Finally, a disorder called *cold-dependent dermatographism* has been reported in which prominent hive formation is seen if the skin is scratched and then chilled (39). In this disorder the ice-cube test and systemic cold challenge yield no hives. Simply scratching the skin yields a weakly positive dermatographic response, but dramatic accentuation is seen when the scratched area is chilled. Treatment once again is high-dose antihistamines, e.g., 200 mg of diphenhydramine per day or a combination of hydroxyzine (100–200 mg/day) and cyproheptadine (8–16 mg/day).

Exercise-Induced Disorders

Cholinergic or generalized heat urticaria is characterized by the onset of small punctate wheals surrounded by a prominent erythematous flare associated with exercise, hot showers, sweating, and anxiety (28). Typically, lesions first appear about the neck and upper thorax; and when viewed from a distance, hives may not be perceived and the patient appears flushed (Fig. 3). However, pruritus is a prominent feature of the reaction; upon close inspection, small punctate wheals can be discerned, sometimes as small as 1 mm in diameter, that are surrounded by a prominent flare. Gradually the lesions spread distally to involve the face, back, and extremities, and the wheals increase in size. In some patients the hives become confluent and resemble angioedema (51). Also occasionally seen are symptoms of more generalized cholinergic stim-

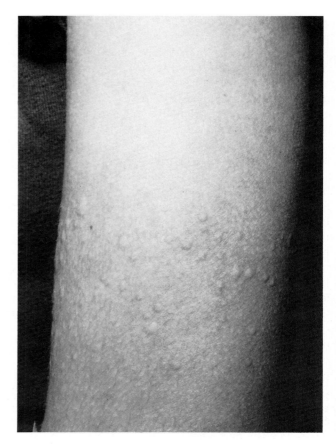

FIG. 3. Urticaria developing about the forearm of a patient with cholinergic urticaria.

ulation such as lacrimation, salivation, and diarrhea. These various stimuli have the common feature of being mediated by cholinergic nerve fibers that innervate the musculature via parasympathetic neurons and innervate the sweat glands by cholinergic fibers that travel with the sympathetic nerves (35). The characteristic lesion of cholinergic urticaria can be reproduced by intradermal injection of 100 μg of methacholine (Mccholyl) in 0.1 ml saline. When positive, the resultant localized hive surrounded by satellite lesions is indistinguishable from the patient's spontaneously induced lesions and confirms the diagnosis. However, we have found that only about one-third of patients give a clearly positive skin test, these generally being the most severe cases. Challenge by exercise (e.g., running in an 85°C warmed room or using a bicycle ergometer for 10–15 min) is a far more sensitive test. Thus the skin test can be used to confirm the diagnosis but cannot be used as a diagnostic test (6). Those patients who have a positive methacholine skin test demonstrate a "hypersensitivity" to cholinergic mediators, but they have no evidence of an immunoglobulin-mediated allergy to acetylcholine. It is possible that the disorder is due to an intrinsic cellular abnormality that results in abnormal mediator release in the presence of cholinergic agents. One study addressing this issue demonstrated an increased number of muscarinic receptors in urticarial sites. These receptors were further augmented when exercise followed patch-testing to copper-containing materials (82). The increased number of acetylcholine binding sites may be an important key to understanding the pathogenesis of cholinergic urticaria. The importance of copper is unclear, but it may affect ligand-receptor affinity.

There is evidence that a reflex consisting of afferent humoral and efferent neurogenic components is involved in this urticarial disorder. When one places a patient's hand in warm water with a tourniquet tied proximal to that hand, there is no urticaria until the tourniquet is released. A generalized eruption then ensues. Thus a central perception of a temperature change transmitted via the circulation appears to be followed by an efferent reflex leading to urticaria. Such a reflex could also account for the association of hives with anxiety (62), although it should be emphasized that in these instances the emotional reaction can be completely appropriate.

Studies of mediator release during attacks of cholinergic urticaria have demonstrated that, in most cases, elevated plasma histamine levels parallel the onset of pruritus and urticaria (Fig. 4). Subsequent studies confirmed the presence of histaminemia in association with cholinergic urticaria (43,84), and release of eosinophilotactic peptides and neutrophil chemotactic factor have also been observed (94). When patients were challenged while wearing a plastic occlusive suit to produce maximal changes in cutaneous and core body temperature, significant falls in 1-sec forced-expiratory volumes, maximal mid-expiratory flow rate, and specific conductance were seen associated with a rise in residual volume. Four of seven patients also had wheezing detected by auscultation. Thus under such conditions, an abnormality in pulmonary function can be detected reflecting either primary pulmonary involvement or altered pulmonary mechanics secondary to circulating mediators. A clinically significant alteration in

pulmonary function is unusual in cholinergic urticaria and has no known association with exercise-induced asthma. Kaplan et al. (46) have also described two cases of typical cholinergic urticaria in whom lesions became confluent and were associated with prominent elevation of plasma histamine as well as being associated with recurrent episodes of hypotension (46). Thus some extreme cases of cholinergic urticaria can resemble the exercise-induced anaphylactic syndrome. One should also point out that combinations of "physical urticarias" can occur in the same patient, e.g., cold urticaria (84) or dermatographism (94) in association with cholinergic urticaria. Furthermore, combined cold and cholinergic urticaria, fulfilling separate criteria for each disorder (84), is to be distinguished from cold-induced cholinergic urticaria (41).

Treatment of cholinergic urticaria generally consists of hydroxyzine (100–200 mg/day) in divided doses (62). Many, but certainly not all, patients respond to this regimen. Anticholinergic agents such as atropine or propantheline bromide (Pro-Banthine) have little effect, perhaps due to an inability to attain a sufficient systemic level; however, injected atropine can reverse the methacholine skin test (84).

The syndrome of exercise-induced anaphylaxis was first described in a series of patients in whom combinations of pruritus, urticaria, angioedema, wheezing, and hypotension occurred as a result of exercise. Symptoms did not occur with each exercise experience, and most described patients were accomplished athletes (84). The disorder is distinguished from cholinergic urticaria by the following criteria. First, although exercise is the precipitating stimulus of each disorder, hot showers, sweating in the absence of exercise, and anxiety do not trigger attacks of exercise-induced anaphylaxis as they do in cholinergic urticaria (28). Second, the hives seen with exercise-induced anaphylaxis are large (10–15 mm), in contrast to the punctate lesions characteristic of cholinergic urticaria. Finally, when patients with exercise-induced anaphylaxis were challenged in an occlusive suit, no change in pulmonary function was seen, although histamine release was

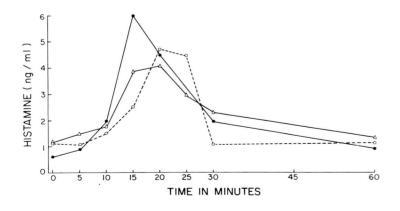

FIG. 4. Time course of histamine release in three patients with cholinergic urticaria who were challenged by running in a heated room (85°F) for 10 min.

documented (81). Optimal therapy for the exercise-induced anaphylactic syndrome is uncertain, and attempts at prophylaxis utilizing H_1 and H_2 antagonists have not generally been effective (52). In contrast, classic cholinergic urticaria is usually responsive to prophylactic use of hydroxyzine.

Subtypes of exercise-induced anaphylaxis have also been described that are food-related. In one case, exercise-induced anaphylaxis occurred if the exercise took place 5 to 24 hr after eating shellfish, whereas exercise alone or eating shellfish alone did not cause any symptoms (58). In five other reported cases, two had symptoms only if exercise followed the ingestion of any food within 2 hr (49,66); in the remaining three cases, symptoms were precipitated by the specific ingestion of celery within 2 hr of exercise (49). The latter patients also had positive skin tests to celery. Thus various forms of food-dependent exercise-induced anaphylaxis are possible, and treatment requires avoiding specific foodstuffs prior to exercising or avoiding exercise within certain time intervals after eating. It is also of interest that one patient with cholinergic urticaria and associated anaphylaxis was successfully treated by vigorous daily exercise such that desensitization occurred within a week (46). The number of patients with cholinergic urticaria or the exercise-induced anaphylactic syndrome that might respond to such treatment is unknown, although it is more likely to be effective in cholinergic urticaria with or without hypotension because symptoms occur reproducibly each time an exercise challenge is done.

Other Physically Induced Forms of Urticaria or Angioedema

The remaining forms of physically induced hives or swelling are, with the exception of dermatographism, relatively rare disorders. These include local heat urticaria, pressure-induced urticaria/angioedema, solar urticaria, aquagenic urticaria, and vibratory angioedema.

Localized Heat Urticaria

A local form of heat urticaria is a rare disorder in which urticaria develops within minutes after exposure to applied heat (30). Sixteen cases have thus far been reported, most of which appear in females. When suspected, it can be tested by application of a test tube of warm water at 44°C to the arm for 4 to 5 min. If positive, a hive is seen a few minutes after the test tube is removed. Studies of mediator release in local heat urticaria resemble those reported in cold urticaria; plasma histamine levels peak 5 to 10 min after heat exposure (3,27), although passive-transfer studies have been negative. Neutrophil chemotactic factor was

also released in one study (3); thus, mast-cell degranulation in response to heat challenge seems likely. In one report, complement abnormalities were reported in the absence of histamine release (10). Association with other forms of physical allergy is also sometimes seen, e.g., combined cold urticaria and local heat urticaria (95). Therapy has been problematic, since antihistamines such as hydroxyzine or cyproheptadine as well as oral disodium cromoglycate have been ineffective. One patient was successfully desensitized by repeated daily immersion in hot baths, but caution is in order as systemic reactions are possible (10).

A variant of this disorder has been described which was familial and in which urticaria occurred 1.5 to 2 hr after application of a warm stimulus (60) and persisted for 6 to 10 hr. Sunbathing with pronounced heating of skin could produce wheals as a result of the temperature effect, whereas sunlight itself could be tolerated. Desensitization of an area could be achieved with repeated challenge every few days. Skin biopsy demonstrated a pronounced inflammatory cell infiltrate in the upper dermis and around hair follicles. The pathogenesis of this form of local heat urticaria is unknown. Partial control could be achieved with oral antihistamines.

Dermatographism

The ability to write on skin, termed *dermatographism,* can occur as an isolated disorder that often presents as traumatically induced urticaria. It can be diagnosed by observing the skin after stroking it with a tongue depressor or fingernail. In such patients, a white line secondary to reflex vasoconstriction is followed by pruritus, erythema, and a linear wheal, as is seen in a classic wheal-and-flare reaction. It is said to be present in 2% to 5% of the population (54,91); however, only a small fraction of these are of sufficient severity to warrant treatment. Biopsy of the skin reveals few changes, but most occur in the epidermis and consist of vacuolation of keratinocytes and basal epidermal-cell pseudopodia, as well as the appearance of typical mast-cell granules (5). In approximately 50% of cases, passive-transfer studies have demonstrated an IgE-dependent mechanism (1,65). Thus, many patients have an abnormal circulating IgE that confers a particular form of pressure sensitivity to dermal mast cells. Such observations further suggest that histamine is one of the mediators of dermatographism, although demonstration of such release has been difficult because of the localized nature of the reaction. Early studies, however, did suggest that: (a) histamine is released into whole blood (77); (b) induced blisters over lesions contain elevated histamine levels (45); (c) 24-hr urine histamine levels are elevated (29); and (d) histamine is increased in the perfusate, as shown by *in vivo* subcutaneous perfusion studies (31). In a single, unusually severe case of IgE-mediated dermatographism, elevation of plasma histamine levels was documented within 1 min of stroking the skin, and the baseline histamine level was abnormal in multiple determinations, suggesting that "leakage" of histamine is on-going at all times (22).

Although the evidence is anecdotal because a formal study has not been performed, dermatographism has been observed as a consequence of drug reactions (54); in one case, dermatographism could be observed only upon challenge with the offending agent—in this instance, penicillin (83). Therapy for dermatographism consists of antihistamines (56,57); for severe symptoms, high doses may be needed. The initial objective of therapy is to decrease pruritus so the stimulation for scratching is diminished; many patients complain of a sensation of itching or "skin crawling" that is readily relieved by antihistamines. At higher doses, one can show that the wheal-and-flare reaction to stroking is also markedly diminished.

Dermatographism also occurs in association with other disorders; for example, a mild form may be seen in some patients with chronic urticaria. Severe dermatographism is also associated with disorders in which a marked increase in dermal mast cells is seen, e.g., urticaria pigmentosa or systemic mastocytosis. Release of histamine in these disorders has been demonstrated (29). It is also possible that other vasoactive agents released from cutaneous mast cells can be implicated in dermatographism and, in fact, all forms of physically induced urticaria. An example is the elevation of PGD_2 metabolites seen in the urine of patients with systemic mastocytosis, which may relate to the hypotension associated with this disorder (76).

Pressure-Induced Urticaria/Angioedema

Pressure-induced urticaria differs from most of the aforementioned types of hives or angioedema in that symptoms typically occur 4 to 6 hr after pressure has been applied. The disorder is clinically heterogeneous in that some patients may complain of swelling secondary to pressure with normal-appearing skin (i.e., no erythema or superficial infiltrating hive) so that the term *angioedema* is more appropriate. Others are predominantly urticarial and may or may not be associated with significant swelling. When urticaria is present, an infiltrative lesion is seen characterized by a perivascular mononuclear-cell infiltrate and dermal edema similar to that seen with chronic idiopathic urticaria (21). Immediate dermatographism is not present, but delayed dermatographism is seen and may represent the same disorder (38,76). Symptoms occur about tight clothing, the hands may swell with activity such as hammering, foot swelling is common after walk-

ing, and buttock swelling may be prominent after sitting for a few hours. Testing for it can be done using a sling (with a 5- to 15-lb weight attached) that is placed over the forearm or shoulder for 10 to 20 min. Gradual pressure applied by devices in grams per square millimeter can also be used (21). There are few available studies regarding pathogenesis; however, mediators that cause pain rather than pruritus (e.g., kinins) have been considered, since the lesions are typically described as burning or painful. Nevertheless, induced blisters over lesions revealed histamine release following the time course of hive formation (45). Antihistamines, however, have little effect on the disorder, and patients with severe disease often have to be treated with corticosteroids.

Although pressure urticaria/angioedema can occur as an isolated disorder, it is most often seen in association with chronic urticaria. Therapy is then usually directed toward the chronic urticaria. Recent data also suggest an increased incidence of food allergy in those patients with chronic urticaria in whom pressure-induced symptoms are also prominent (11).

Immediate-pressure urticaria has been described in patients with the hypereosinophilia syndrome characterized by an acute wheal-and-flare reaction within 1 to 2 min of applied pressure, e.g., pressing on the back with one's thumb. Those patients also were dermatographic, although dermatographics typically do not have immediate-pressure urticaria and require a stroking motion to produce a hive (67).

Solar Urticaria

Solar urticaria is a rare disorder in which brief exposure to light causes the development of urticaria within 1 to 3 min. Typically, pruritus occurs first, in about 30 sec, followed by edema confined to the light-exposed area and surrounded by a prominent erythematous zone caused by an axon reflex. The lesions then usually disappear within 1 to 3 hr. When large areas of the body are exposed, systemic symptoms may occur, including hypotension and asthma. Although most reported patients have been in their third and fourth decades, the disorder can occur in any age group and has no association with other allergic disorders.

Solar urticaria has been classified into six types, depending on the wavelength of light that induces lesions and the ability or inability to passively transfer the disorder with serum (33,36,79). Types I and IV can be passively transferred and may therefore by immunologically (IgE?) mediated; they are associated with wavelengths of 280 to 320 nm and 400 to 500 nm, respectively. The antigen has not been identified. Histamine release, mast-cell degranulation (34), and formation of chemotactic factors for eosinophils and neutrophils (93) have been observed coincident with induction of lesions when ultraviolet light (type I) was shone on skin. Type VI, activated at 400 nm, is clearly an inherited metabolic disorder in which protoporphyrin IX acts as a photosensitizer and is synonymous with erythropoietic protoporphyria. In contrast to other forms of porphyria, the urinary porphyrin excretion is normal; however, red-blood-cell protoporphyrin and fecal protoporphyrin and coproporphyrin levels are elevated. Irradiation of serum samples of such patients resulted in activation of the classic complement pathway and generation of C5a chemotactic activity (53); this activity was proportional to the serum level of protoporphyrin (24). Consistent with these observations is that deposition of C3 and accumulation of neutrophils is seen in the dermis of patients (4,20), and complement fragments can be detected in the serum and suction blister fluid of irradiated skin (4). It responds to oral β-carotene, which absorbs light at the same wavelengths as protoporphyrin IX (63). The mechanism by which urticaria is produced in types II, III, and V is unknown, but these are induced by inciting wavelengths of 320 to 400, 400 to 500, and 280 to 500 nm, respectively. As a simple screen, fluorescent tubes that emit a broad, continuous spectrum can be used to test the patient, and filters can then be used to define the spectrum that causes urticaria. Therapy of this disease requires avoidance of sunlight, protective garments to cover the skin, and use of topical preparations to absorb or reflect light. A 5% solution of paraaminobenzoic acid in ethanol, as in sunscreen lotions, can be helpful in the 280- to 320-nm range; however, it is more difficult to screen out the visible spectrum. The most effective agents for this purpose contain titanium oxide and/or zinc oxide. The efficacy of antihistaminics, antimalarials, and corticosteroids in these disorders is not clear and needs to be evaluated in each case.

Aquagenic Urticaria

Thirteen cases have been reported of patients who developed small wheals after contact with water, regardless of its temperature, and who were distinguishable from patients with cold urticaria or cholinergic urticaria. This disorder has been termed *aquagenic urticaria* (6). Direct application of a compress of tap water or distilled water to the skin is used to test for its presence. The diagnosis should be reserved for those rare cases that test positively for water but that test negatively for all other forms of physical urticaria. Combined cholinergic and aquagenic urticaria has been reported, and histamine release into the circulation has been documented upon challenge with water (12).

Hereditary Vibratory Angioedema

Hereditary vibratory angioedema has been described in a single family in whom it was inherited in an autosomal dominant pattern. It is properly viewed as a physically induced angioedema, since patients complain of intense pruritus and swelling within minutes after vibratory stimuli (68). The patients are not dermatographic and do not have pressure-induced urticaria. Lesions can be reproduced by gently stimulating the patient's forearm with a laboratory vortex for 4 min. Rapid swelling of the entire forearm and a portion of the upper arm ensues, and histamine has been shown to be released secondary to such a vibratory stimulus (59). With care, patients can avoid vibratory stimuli, and their symptoms can otherwise be partially relieved with diphenhydramine (Benadryl). Nonfamilial, sporadic cases have also been described.

ACUTE, NONPHYSICALLY INDUCED URTICARIA

Acute urticaria is a commonly encountered disorder that can be caused by a wide variety of agents. Most prominent are drug reactions, allergy to foods, and urticaria in association with infection or other systemic diseases. Episodes of acute urticaria usually last from a few days to 2 or 3 weeks. When the urticarial episode exceeds 6 weeks, it is arbitrarily designated "chronic."

The hive due to a food or drug reaction differs from that seen with the various physical urticarias because individual lesions can remain prominent from many hours to 1 to 2 days. In this respect, the lesions more closely resemble chronic urticaria rather than the physical urticarias (40). An allergic mechanism, in the strictest sense, requires an interaction of IgE antibody with the allergen (e.g., food or drug) followed by degranulation of cutaneous mast cells. Studies of physical urticarias indicate that a single abrupt degranulation leads to a fleeting lesion with no appreciable delayed component. However, it has been observed that when an allergic person is skin-tested (e.g., intracutaneous administration of ragweed antigen to a person with ragweed-induced rhinitis), the immediate wheal-and-flare reaction lasts a few minutes and disappears; it may then be followed by a swelling, 4 to 6 hr later, which is called a *late-phase reaction* (14). It has been shown that late-phase reactions are dependent upon the prior IgE reaction (13). They consist of a mixed cellular infiltrate containing mononuclear cells, neutrophils, eosinophils, and basophils (86) and are associated with a second wave of secretion of histamine (61) and other vasoactive substances. Cutaneous injection of 48/80, a polypeptide that causes mast-cell degranulation, can also lead to late-phase reactions (15). It appears that the late-phase reaction in the skin requires something besides a single burst of mast-cell degranulation, but no data are available regarding this issue. We can theorize that mast-cell degranulation that persists over time and/or persistence of antigenic stimulation over time is the critical difference. This would be absent in virtually all the physical urticarias except delayed pressure urticaria. Perhaps the persistence of the hive in food or drug reactions is related to this phenomenon.

Urticaria has also been well documented during viral infections such as hepatitis (50) or infectious mononucleosis (9), and a large number of helminthic parasites are associated with hives. Serum sickness reactions (including the prodrome of hepatitis-B infection) can be seen as a manifestation of drug reactions, and upon biopsy one observes evidence of a small vessel cutaneous vasculitis (2). Urticaria in association with systemic lupus erythematosus (69,74) or other vasculitides appears similar. There is necrosis of the vessel wall (most prominent in small venules), infiltration with neutrophils, and deposition of immunoglobulins and complement. It is thought that these disorders are caused by immune complex deposition in the dermal vasculature and release of histamine (and other mediators) from perivenular mast cells caused by local formation of the anaphylatoxins C3a, C5a, and C4a (23). IgE antibody to the initiating antigen may also be contributory.

CHRONIC IDIOPATHIC URTICARIA AND IDIOPATHIC ANGIOEDEMA

This is a common disorder of unknown origin, whose victims are not atopic individuals; that is, they do not have an increased incidence of atopic dermatitis, allergic rhinitis, or asthma compared to the incidence of these disorders in the absence of chronic urticaria. Their IgE level, as a group, is within normal limits. Some patients are dermatographic, although this is usually of milder degree than is seen with the IgE-dependent dermatographism described earlier; curiously, the dermatographism may wax and wane, just as the urticaria may vary from severe to mild or may intermittently subside. These patients have a normal white-blood-cell count and sedimentation rate (ESR) and have no evidence of systemic disease. Thus they do not demonstrate evidence of any of the causes of urticaria or angioedema discussed earlier, i.e., foods, drugs, additives, infection, systemic disease, association with other allergic phenomena, or triggering by physical agents. Chronic urticaria therefore does not appear to be an allergic reaction in the classic sense, since IgE antibody is not involved and no external allergen is needed to initiate or perpetuate the process. It differs from allergen-induced skin reactions or from physically induced urticaria (e.g., dermatographia or cold urticaria) in that histologic studies reveal a cellular infiltrate predominantly about small ven-

ules (40). External examination reveals infiltrative hives with palpably elevated borders, sometimes varying greatly in size and/or shape but generally being rounded.

The typical lesion consists of a non-necrotizing perivascular mononuclear-cell infiltrate (Fig. 5). However, many types of histopathologic processes can occur in the skin and manifest as hives. For example, patients with hypocomplementemia and cutaneous vasculitis can have urticaria (or angioedema), and biopsy of patients with urticaria, arthralgias, myalgias, and an elevated ESR as manifestations of necrotizing venulitis revealed fibrinoid necrosis with a predominant neutrophilic infiltrate (87,90). Yet the urticarial lesions were indistinguishable from those seen in the more typical, nonvasculitis cases.

Other studies (55,61,64,72) have examined the incidence of vasculitis in patients with urticaria, with a wide variety of results. Mathison and colleagues (55) found that 10 of 78 patients had hypocomplementemia, and many patients showed evidence of activation of the classic complement pathway. Six of the 10 had elevated levels of circulating immune complexes. If hypocomplementemia and vasculitis are equated, the incidence of presumed vasculitis was 14%. Monroe and co-workers (61) found neutrophilic leukocytoclastic angiitis in 20% of patients; the other 80% had a perivascular infiltrate of mononuclear cells that was classified as "dense" or "sparse." Interestingly, the "vasculitis," "dense," and "sparse" groups had circulating immune complex levels of 33%, 29%, and 13%, respectively, as measured by multiple assays. Phanuphak et al. (72) used the criterion of significant cellular infiltrate within vessel walls to define vasculitis (rather than that of endothelial damage, nuclear dust, fibrin deposition, or red-blood-cell extravasation) and found a 52% incidence of vasculitis (various types of predominant cells) and a 48% incidence of a perivascular mononuclear-cell infiltrate. Deposition of immune complexes in skin was seen in 18% of the vasculitis group, almost exclusively in those with an abundance of neutrophils.

My colleagues and I have reported results of a study of the histopathology of chronic idiopathic urticaria in 43 consecutive patients (64). All but one in the group had a non-necrotizing perivascular infiltrate consisting primarily of lymphocytes (Table 1). We therefore found vasculitis to be a rare cause of urticaria and believe that our group is comparable to the group without vasculitis in the study of Mathison et al. (55), to the "sparse" and/or "dense" infiltrate groups of Monroe et al. (61), and to the "perivasculitis" group of Phanuphak et al. (72).

We also noted a 10-fold increase in the number of mast cells and a fourfold increase in the number of mononuclear cells in skin biopsy specimens from the patients with chronic urticaria as compared with those from normal controls (Table 2). No increase in basophil number was seen. Thus the increase in mast cells observed may relate

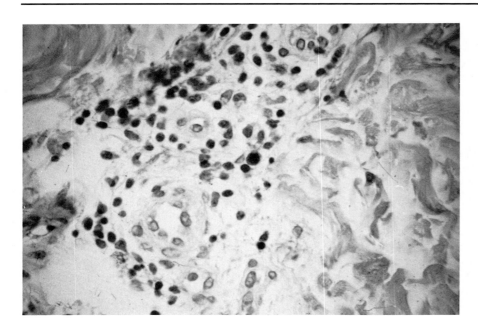

FIG. 5. Skin biopsy of chronic urticaria demonstrating a non-necrotizing perivenular infiltrate consisting primarily of mononuclear cells.

to the increased amount of histamine found in suction blister fluid obtained from patients with chronic urticaria as compared with the amount in such fluid from normal controls (45) as well as the increased level of total skin histamine content reportedly present in such patients (73). Because lymphocytes and mast cells accumulate, we propose that a lymphokine or monokine may be released that causes mast-cell proliferation (or accumulation) and degranulation. An analogous factor that can cause basophil degranulation is released from lymphocytes (44,96). Basophils of chronic urticaria patients are reported to be less responsive to anti-IgE than are cells of normals, suggesting *in-vivo* desensitization (48). Although eosinophils were not prominent in the skin biopsies of our series of patients when considered as a group, an occasional patient had a prominent eosinophil accumulation. In one study, deposition of eosinophil major basic protein in skin specimens of 50% of chronic urticaria patients has been demonstrated, although only a fraction of them had obvious eosinophil infiltration (70). Thus, degranulated eosino-

phils may be present, perhaps more commonly than previously appreciated.

We have concluded that chronic urticaria is characterized by a non-necrotizing perivascular mononuclear-cell infiltrate with an accumulation of mast cells. The etiology is unknown, and we cannot as yet state whether the process is immunologically mediated. We consider patients with vasculitis and urticaria a separate subpopulation in whom the cause and pathogenesis of hive formation probably involves immune complexes, complement activation, anaphylatoxin formation, histamine release, and neutrophil accumulation, activation, and degranulation. Our most recent studies of the pathogenesis of chronic urticaria demonstrates that about 50% of the cells are T-lymphocytes, there are no B-cells, 20% of the cells are monocytes, and 10% are mast cells (19). Twenty percent could not be identified utilizing monoclonal antibodies or enzyme histochemical methods. The infiltrate most closely resembles a cellular immune reaction with a proliferation and/or accumulation of mast cells.

An approach to the therapy of this disorder has been published (40). Antihistamines can control the pruritus but are often ineffective in relieving the hive formation. Thus, other vasoactive mediators may have a role. Aspirin does not ameliorate urticaria (and may worsen it); thus, a prostaglandin or thromboxane mediator is unlikely. However, we have no specific agents that antagonize mediators, such as the leukotrienes, platelet-activating factor, or kinins. Further, the hive has a prominent cellular infiltrate that appears to be an important constituent of the lesion. Corticosteroids are highly effective in treating chronic urticaria (although one must balance efficacy and side effects), and they may act to inhibit the function of the infiltrating mononuclear cells.

TABLE 2. *Infiltrating cells in skin biopsy specimens from patients with chronic urticaria and normal controls*

	No. of cells, mean (range)[a]	
Cell type	Patients (N = 43)	Control (N = 7)
Eosinophils	1.2 (0–12)	0
Basophils	0.35 (0–2)	0
Neutrophils	3.0 (0–50)	0.14 (0–1)
Mononuclear cells	52.4 (16–247)	13.4 (3–25)
Mast cells	7.6 (0–19)	0.71 (0–3)

[a] Number counted per five reticules.

REFERENCES

1. Aoyama, H., Katsumata, Y., and Olzawa, J. (1970): Dermographism-inducing principle of urticaria factitia. *Jpn. J. Dermatol.,* 80:122.

2. Arbesman, C. E., and Reisman, R. E. (1971): Serum sickness and human anaphylaxis. In: *Immunologic Diseases, Vol. 1,* edited by M. Samter, p. 495. Little Brown, Boston, Mass.

3. Atkins, P. C., and Zweiman, B. (1981): Mediator release in local heat urticaria. *J. Allergy Clin. Immunol.,* 68:286.

4. Baart, D. L. F. H., Beerens, E. G. J., Van Weelden, H., and Berens, L. (1978): Complement components in blood serum and suction blister fluid in erythropoietic protoporphyria. *Br. J. Dermatol.,* 99:401.

5. Cauna, N., and Levine, M. I. (1970): The fine morphology of the human skin in dermographism. *J. Allergy Clin. Immunol.,* 45:266.

6. Chalamidas, S. L., and Charles, C. R. (1971): Aquagenic urticaria. *Arch. Dermatol.,* 104:541.

7. Costanzi, J. J., and Coltman, C. A., Jr. (1967): Kappa chain cold precipitable immunoglobulin (IgG) associated with cold urticaria. 1. Clinical observations. *Clin. Exp. Immunol.,* 2:167.

8. Costanzi, J. J., Coltman, C. A., Jr., and Donaldson, V. H. (1969): Activation of complement by a monoclonal cryoglobulin associated with cold urticaria. *J. Lab. Clin. Med.,* 74:902.

9. Cowdry, S. L., and Reynolds, J. S. (1969): Acute urticaria in infectious mononucleosis. *Ann. Allergy,* 27:182.

10. Daman, L., Lieberman, P., Garner, M., and Hashimoto, K. (1978): Localized heat urticaria. *J. Allergy Clin. Immunol.,* 61:273.

11. Davis, K. C., Mekori, Y. A., Kohler, P. F., and Schocket, A. L. (1984): Possible role of diet in delayed pressure urticaria. *J. Allergy Clin. Immunol.,* 73:183 (abstract).

12. Davis, R. S., Remigo, L. K., Schocket, A. L., and Bock, S. A. (1981): Evaluation of a patient with both aquagenic and cholinergic urticaria. *J. Allergy Clin. Immunol.,* 68:479.

13. Dolovich, J., Hargreave, F. E., Chalmers, R., Shier, K. J., Gouldie, J., and Bienenstock, J. (1973): Late cutaneous allergic responses in isolated IgE-dependent reactions. *J. Allergy Clin. Immunol.,* 52:38.

14. Dolovich, J., and Little, D. C. (1972): Correlates of skin test reactions to *Bacillus subtilis* enzyme preparations. *J. Allergy Clin. Immunol.,* 49:43.

15. Dor, P. J., Vervloet, D., Supene, M., Andrac, L., Bonerandi, J. J., and Charpin, J. (1983): Induction of late cutaneous reaction by kallikrein injection: comparison with allergic-like late response to compound 48/80. *J. Allergy Clin. Immunol.,* 71:363.

16. Durham, S. R., Lee, T. H., Cromwell, O., Shaw, R. J., Merrett, T. G., Merret, J., Cooper, P., and Kay, A. B. (1984): Immunologic studies in allergen-induced late-phase asthmatic reactions. *J. Allergy Clin. Immunol.,* 74:49.

17. Eady, R. A., and Greaves, M. W. (1978): Induction of cutaneous vasculitis by repeated cold challenge in cold urticaria. *Lancet,* 1:336.

18. Eady, R. A. J., Keahey, T. M., Sibbald, R. G., and Black, A. K. (1981): Cold urticaria with vasculitis: Report of a case with light and electron microscopic, immunofluorescence, and pharmacological studies. *Clin. Exp. Dermatol.,* 6:355.

19. Elias, J., Boss, E., and Kaplan, A. P. (1987): Studies of the cellular infiltrate of chronic idiopathic urticaria: Prominence of T lymphocytes, monocytes, and mast cells. *J. Allergy Clin. Immunol. (in press).*

20. Epstein, J. H., Tuffanelli, D. L., and Epstein, W. L. (1973): Cutaneous changes in the porphyrias: a microscopic study. *Arch. Dermatol.,* 107:689.

21. Estes, S. A., and Yang, C. W. (1981): Delayed pressure urticaria: An investigation of some parameters of lesion induction. *J. Am. Acad. Dermatol.,* 5:25.

22. Garofalo, J., and Kaplan, A. P. (1981): Histamine release and therapy of severe dermatographism. *J. Allergy Clin. Immunol.,* 68:103.

23. Ghebrehiwet, B. (1985): The complement system: Mechanism of activation, regulation, and biological functions. In: *Allergy,* edited by A. P. Kaplan, pp. 131–152. Churchill Livingstone, New York.

24. Gigli, I., Schothorst, A. A., Soter, N. A., Pathak, M. A. (1980): Erythropoietic protoporphyria: Photoactivation of the complement system. *J. Clin. Invest.,* 66:517.

25. Gorevic, P., and Kaplan, A. P. (1980): The physical urticarias. *Int. J. Dermatol.,* 19:417.

26. Grandel, K. E., Farr, R. S., Wanderer, A. A., Eisenstadt, T. C., and Wasserman, S. I. (1985): Association of platelet-activating factor with primary acquired cold urticaria. *N. Engl. J. Med.,* 313:405.

27. Grant, J. A., Findlay, J. R., Thueson, D. O., et al. (1981): Local heat urticaria/angioedema: Evidence for histamine release without complement activation. *J. Allergy Clin. Immunol.,* 67:75.

28. Grant, R. T., Pearson, R. S. B., and Comeaw, W. J. (1935): Observations on urticaria provoked by emotion, by exercise, and by warming the body. *Clin. Sci.,* 2:253.

29. Greaves, M. W. (1971): Histamine excretion and dermographism in urticaria pigmentosa before and after administration of a specific histidine-decarboxylase inhibitor. *Br. J. Dermatol.,* 85:467.

30. Greaves, M. W., Sneddon, I. B., Smith, A. K., and Stanworth, D. R. (1974): Heat urticaria. *Br. J. Dermatol.,* 90:L289.

31. Greaves, M. W., and Sundergoard, J. (1970): Urticaria pigmentosa and factitious urticaria. *Arch. Dermatol.,* 101:418.

32. Gruber, B. L., Marchese, M., Ballan, D., and Kaplan, A. P. (1986): Anti IgG autoantibodies: Detection in urticarial syndromes and ability to release histamine from basophils. *J. Allergy Clin. Immunol.,* 77:187 (abstract).

33. Harber, L. C., Holloway, R. M., Sheatley, V. R., and Baer, R. L. (1963): Immunologic and biophysical studies in solar urticaria. *J. Invest. Dermatol.,* 41:439.

34. Hawk, J. L. M., Eady, R. A. J., Challiner, A. V. J., et al. (1980): Elevated blood histamine levels and mast cell degranulation in solar urticaria. *Br. J. Clin. Pharmacol.,* 9:183.

35. Herxheimer, A. (1956): The nervous pathway mediating cholinergic urticaria. *Clin. Sci.,* 15:195.

36. Horio, T. (1978): Photoallergic urticaria induced by visible light: Additional cases and further studies. *Arch. Dermatol.,* 114:1761.

37. Houser, D. D., Arbesman, C. E., Ito, K., and Wicher, K. (1970): Cold urticaria: Immunologic studies. *Am. J. Med.,* 49:23.

38. Kalz, F., Bower, C. M., and Prichard, H. (1950): Delayed and persistent dermographia. *Arch. Dermatol.,* 61:772.

39. Kaplan, A. P. (1984): Unusual cold-induced disorders: Cold dependent dermatographism and systemic cold urticaria. *J. Allergy Clin. Immunol.,* 73:453.

40. Kaplan, A. P. (1985): Urticaria and angioedema. In: *Allergy,* edited by A. P. Kaplan, pp. 439–471. Churchill Livingstone, New York.

41. Kaplan, A. P., and Garofalo, J. (1981): Identification of a new physically induced urticaria: Cold induced cholinergic urticaria. *J. Allergy Clin. Immunol.,* 68:438.

42. Kaplan, A. P., Garofalo, J., Sigler, R., and Hauber, T. (1981): Idiopathic cold urticaria: *In vitro* demonstration of histamine release upon challenge of skin biopsies. *N. Engl. J. Med.,* 305:1074.

43. Kaplan, A. P., Gray, L., Shaff, R. E., et al. (1975): *In vivo* studies of mediator release in cold urticaria and cholinergic urticaria. *J. Allergy Clin. Immunol.,* 55:394.

44. Kaplan, A. P., Haak-Frendscho, M., Fauci, A., Dinarello, C., and Halbert, E. (1985): A histamine-releasing factor from activated human mononuclear cells. *J. Immunol.,* 35:2027.

45. Kaplan, A. P., Horakova, Z., and Katz, S. I. (1978): Assessment of tissue fluid histamine levels in patients with urticaria. *J. Allergy Clin. Immunol.,* 6:350.

46. Kaplan, A. P., Natbony, S. F., Tawil, A. P., et al. (1981): Exercise-induced anaphylaxis as a manifestation of cholinergic urticaria. *J. Allergy Clin. Immunol.,* 28:319.

47. Keahey, T. M., and Greaves, M. W. (1980): Cold urticaria: Dissociation of cold-evoked histamine release and urticaria following cold challenge. *Arch. Dermatol.,* 116:174.

48. Kern, F., and Lichtenstein, L. M. (1977): Defective histamine release in chronic urticaria. *J. Clin. Invest.,* 57:1360.

49. Kidd, J. M., III, Cohen, S. H., Sosman, A. J., and Fink, J. N. (1983): Food dependent exercise-induced anaphylaxis. *J. Allergy Clin. Immunol.,* 71:407.

50. Koehn, G. G., and Thorne, E. G. (1972): Urticaria and viral hepatitis. *Arch. Dermatol.,* 106:442.

51. Lawrence, C. M., Jorizzo, J. L., Kobza-Black, A., et al. (1981):

Cholinergic urticaria with associated angioedema. *Br. J. Dermatol.,* 105:543.

52. Lewis, J., Lieberman, P., Treadwell, G., and Erffmeyer, J. (1981): Exercise-induced urticaria, angioedema, and anaphylactoid episodes. *J. Allergy Clin. Immunol.,* 68:432.

53. Lim, H. W., Perez, H. D., Poh-Fitzpatrick, M., et al. (1981): Generation of chemotactic activity in serum from patients with erythropoietic protoporphyria and porphyria cutanea tarda. *N. Engl. J. Med.,* 304:212.

54. Mathews, K. P. (1983): Urticaria and angioedema. *J. Allergy Clin. Immunol.,* 72:11.

55. Mathison, D. A., Arroyave, C. M., Bhat, K. N., et al. (1977): Hypocomplementemia in chronic idiopathic urticaria. *Ann. Intern. Med.,* 86:534.

56. Matthews, C. N. A., Boss, J. M., Warin, R. P., and Storari, F. (1979): The effect of H₁ and H₂ histamine antagonists on symptomatic dermographism. *Br. J. Dermatol.,* 101:57.

57. Matthews, C. N. A., Kirby, J. D., James, J., and Warin, R. P. (1973): Dermographism: Reduction in wheal size by chlorpheniramine and hydroxyzine. *Br. J. Dermatol.,* 88:279.

58. Maulitz, R. M., Pratt, D. S., and Schocket, A. L. (1979): Exercise-induced anaphylactic reaction to shellfish. *J. Allergy Clin. Immunol.,* 63:433.

59. Metzger, W. J., Kaplan, A. P., Beaven, M. A., et al. (1976): Hereditary vibratory angioedema: Confirmation of histamine release in a type of physical hypersensitivity. *J. Allergy Clin. Immunol.,* 57:605.

60. Michaelsson, G., and Ros, A. (1971): Familial localized heat urticaria of delayed type. *Acta Derm. Venereol. (Stockh.),* 51:279.

61. Monroe, E. W., Schulz, C. I., Maize, J. C., and Jordon, R. E. (1981): Vasculitis in chronic urticaria: An immunopathologic study. *J. Invest. Dermatol.,* 76:103.

62. Moore-Robinson, M., and Warin, R. P. (1968): Some clinical aspects of cholinergic urticaria. *Br. J. Dermatol.,* 80:794.

63. Moshell, A. N., and Bjornson, L. (1977): Protection in erythropoietic protoporphyria: Mechanism of photoprotection by B carotene. *J. Invest. Dermatol.,* 68:157.

64. Natbony, S. F., Phillips, M., Elias, J. M., et al. (1983): Histologic studies of chronic idiopathic urticaria. *J. Allergy Clin. Immunol.,* 71:177.

65. Newcomb, R. W., and Nelson, H. (1973): Dermographism mediated by IgE. *Am. J. Med.,* 54:174.

66. Novey, H. S., Fairshter, R. D., Salness, K. et al. (1983): Postprandial exercise-induced anaphylaxis. *J. Allergy Clin. Immunol.,* 71:498.

67. Parrillo, J. E., Lawley, T. J., Frank, M. M., et al. (1979): Immunologic reactivity in the hypereosinophil syndrome. *J. Allergy Clin. Immunol.,* 64:113.

68. Patterson, R., Mellies, C. J., Blankenship, M. L., Pruzansky, J. J. (1972): Vibratory angioedema: A hereditary type of physical hypersensitivity. *J. Allergy Clin. Immunol.,* 50:174.

69. Paver, W. K. (1971): Discoid and subacute systemic lupus erythematosus associated with urticaria. *Aust. J. Dermatol.,* 12:113.

70. Peters, M. S., Schroeter, A. L., Kephart, G. M., and Gleich, G. J. (1983): Localization of eosinophil granule major basic protein in chronic urticaria. *J. Invest. Dermatol.,* 81:39.

71. Petillo, J. J., Natbony, S. K., Zisblatt, M., Vukovich, R. A., Neiss, E. S., and Kaplan, A. P. (1983): Preliminary report of the effects of tiaramide on the ice cube test in patients with idiopathic cold urticaria. *Ann. Allergy,* 51:511.

72. Phanuphak, P., Kohler, P. F., Stanford, R. E., et al. (1980): Vasculitis in chronic urticaria. *J. Allergy Clin. Immunol.,* 65:436.

73. Phanuphak, P., Schocket, A. L., Arroyave, C. M., et al. (1980): Skin histamine in chronic urticaria. *J. Allergy Clin. Immunol.,* 65: 371, 1980.

74. Provost, T. T., Zone, J. J., Synkowski, D., et al. (1980): Unusual clinical manifestations of systemic lupus erythematosus. I. Urticaria-like lesions: Correlations with clinical and serological abnormalities. *J. Invest. Dermatol.,* 75:495.

75. Quinti, I., Brozek, C., Wood, N., Geha, R., and Leung, O. Y. M. (1986): Circulating IgG autoantibodies to IgE in atopic syndromes. *J. Allergy Clin. Immunol.,* 77:586.

76. Roberts, L. J., II, Sweetman, B. J., Lewis, R. A., et al. (1980): Increased production of prostaglandin D₂ in patients with systemic mastocytosis. *N. Engl. J. Med.,* 303:1400.

77. Rose, B. (1941): Studies on blood histamine in cases of allergy. I. Blood histamine during wheal formation. *J. Allergy,* 12:327.

78. Ryan, T. J., Shim-Young, N., and Turk, J. L. (1968): Delayed pressure urticaria. *Br. J. Dermatol.,* 80:485.

79. Sams, W. M., Jr., Epstein, J. H., and Winkelmann, R. K. (1969): Solar urticaria: Investigation of pathogenic mechanisms. *Arch. Dermatol.,* 99:330.

80. Sheffer, A. L., and Austen, K. F. (1980): Exercise-induced anaphylaxis. *J. Allergy Clin. Immunol.,* 66:106.

81. Sheffer, A. L., Soter, N. A., McFadden, E. R., Jr., and Austen, K. F. (1983): Exercise-induced anaphylaxis: A distinct form of physical allergy. *J. Allergy Clin. Immunol.,* 71:3112.

82. Shelley, W. B., Shelley, C. D., and Ho, A. K. S. (1983): Cholinergic urticaria: Acetylcholine-receptor dependent immediate-type hypersensitivity reaction to copper. *Lancet,* 1:843.

83. Smith, J. A., Mansfield, L. E., Fokakis, A., and Nelson, H. S. (1983): Dermographism caused by IgE mediated penicillin allergy. *Ann. Allergy,* 57:30.

84. Sigler, R. W., Leviknson, A. I., Evans, R., III, et al. (1979): Evaluation of a patient with cold and cholinergic urticaria. *J. Allergy Clin. Immunol.,* 63:35.

85. Sigler, R. W., Evans, R., III, Horakova, Z., et al. (1980): The role of cyproheptadine in the treatment of cold urticaria. *J. Allergy Clin. Immunol.,* 65:309.

86. Solley, G. O., Gleich, G. J., Jordon, R. E., and Schroeter, A. L. (1976): The late phase of the immediate wheal and flare skin reaction. *J. Clin. Invest.,* 58:408.

87. Soter, N. A., Austen, K. F., and Gigli, I. (1974): Urticaria and arthralgias as a manifestation of necrotizing angiitis. *J. Invest. Dermatol.,* 63:485.

88. Soter, W. A., Joski, N. P., Twarog, F. J., et al. (1977): Delayed cold-induced urticaria: A dominantly inherited disorder. *J. Allergy Clin. Immunol.,* 54:294.

89. Soter, N. A., Mihm, M. C., Jr., Dvorak, H. F., and Austen, K. F. (1978): Cutaneous necrotizing venulitis: A sequential analysis of the morphological alterations occurring after mast cell degranulation in a patient with a unique syndrome. *Clin. Exp. Immunol.,* 32:46.

90. Soter, N. A., Mihm, M. C., Jr., Gigli, I., et al. (1976): Two distinct cellular patterns in cutaneous necrotizing angiitis. *J. Invest. Dermatol.,* 66:334.

91. Soter, N. A., and Wasserman, S. I. (1980): Physical urticaria/angioedema: An experimental model of mast cell activation in humans. *J. Allergy Clin. Immunol.,* 66:358.

92. Soter, N. A., Wasserman, S. I., and Austen, K. F. (1976): Cold urticaria: Release into the circulation of histamine and eosinophil chemotactic factor of anaphylaxis during cold challenge. *N. Engl. J. Med.,* 294:687.

93. Soter, N. A., Wasserman, S. I., Pathak, M. A., et al. (1979): Solar urticaria: Release of mast cell mediators into the circulation after experimental challenge. *J. Invest. Dermatol.,* 72:282.

94. Soter, N. A., Wasserman, S. I., Austen, K. F., and McFadden, E. R., Jr. (1980): Release of mast-cell mediators and alterations in lung function in patients with cholinergic urticaria. *N. Engl. J. Med.,* 302:604.

95. Tennenbaum, J. I., and Lowney, E. (1973): Localized heat and cold urticaria. *J. Allergy Clin. Immunol.,* 51:57.

96. Thueson, D. O., Speck, L. S., Lett-Brown, M. A., et al. (1979): Histamine releasing activity (HRA). I. Production by mitogen- or antigen-stimulated human mononuclear cells. *J. Immunol.,* 23:626.

97. Wanderer, A. A., Nuss, D. P., Tormey, A. D., and Giclas, P. C. (1983): Urticarial leukocytoclastic vasculitis with cold urticaria: Report of a case and review of the literature. *Arch. Dermatol.,* 119: 145.

98. Wanderer, A. A., Maselli, R., Ellis, E. F., and Ishizaka, K. (1971): Immunologic characterization of serum factors responsible for cold urticaria. *J. Allergy Clin. Immunol.,* 48:13.

99. Wasserman, S. E., Soter, N. A., Center, D. M., and Austen, K. F. (1977): Cold urticaria: Recognition and characterization of a neutrophil chemotactic factor which appears in serum during experimental cold challenge. *J. Clin. Invest.,* 60:189.

100. Weinstock, G., Arbeit, L., and Kaplan, A. P. (1986): Release of prostaglandin D₂ and kinins in cold urticaria and cholinergic urticaria. *J. Allergy Clin. Immunol.,* 77:188 (abstract).

Inflammation: Basic Principles and Clinical Correlates.
Edited by J. I. Gallin, I. M. Goldstein, and R. Snyderman.
Raven Press, Ltd., New York © 1988.

CHAPTER 36

Asthma

Timothy D. Bigby and Jay A. Nadel

Asthma is a disorder characterized by varying degrees of reversible airway obstruction in association with exaggerated airway responsiveness to a wide variety of physical and pharmacologic agents (17,164). Until recently, asthma had been thought of solely as an immunologic disorder involving the release of bronchoactive mediators from mast cells that are triggered by antigen via IgE-dependent mechanisms. However, allergy has been reported in approximately 80% of children, but in as few as 25% of adults, with asthma (202). Thus, allergy is not present in all asthmatics, and, more important, not all asthmatics with demonstrable allergy have bronchospasm provoked by inhalation of antigen. In addition, people with asthma who can be provoked by antigen in the laboratory can, under different conditions, have bronchospasm provoked by other triggers (such as cold air, viral infections, exercise). Therefore, allergically mediated bronchospasm is not a fundamental feature present in all asthmatics and is not the basic pathophysiologic aberration present in all asthma.

Irrespective of the presence or absence of allergy, there are features common to virtually all asthmatics. Exaggerated airway responsiveness to a broad range of stimuli is characteristically found. Recent investigation has also established that airway inflammation is characteristic. The purpose of this chapter will be to examine in detail the relationship between these two features and their relationship to asthma.

CLINICAL EVIDENCE OF INFLAMMATION

The possibility that inflammation is involved in the pathogenesis of asthma was first suggested by indirect ev-

idence. Thus, pathologic findings in patients who had died in status asthmaticus demonstrated airway plugging with an inflammatory exudate and an intense mucosal and submucosal inflammatory infiltrate consisting of neutrophils, eosinophils, lymphocytes, and mononuclear phagocytes (47,80). More recent data obtained from bronchial biopsies from patients with mild asthma reveal similar inflammatory cell infiltrates (113). Examination of sputum (46,163) and bronchoalveolar lavage fluid (40,191) from patients with asthma also demonstrates increased numbers of inflammatory cells present, including eosinophils, neutrophils, macrophages, and lymphocytes.

Clinical data also exist suggesting a relationship between the development of inflammation and airway hyperresponsiveness or asthma. Thus, clinical reports have noted an association between the development or clinical worsening of asthma and viral respiratory tract infection (114) or oxidant pollutant exposure (167). Both viral infection (198) and oxidant pollutant exposure (165) are known to cause an inflammatory cell infiltrate in the airway. Similarly, occupational exposure to agents such as toluene diisocyanate has been associated with the development of airway hyperresponsiveness (104) and has also been shown to be associated with airway inflammation (45).

This clinical information suggests that inflammation might play a role in the pathogenesis. Further investigation into the mechanisms of these responses has involved clinical studies with humans, animal studies, and cell studies. These data will be reviewed here in sequence.

HUMAN EXPERIMENTAL INVESTIGATIONS

Hyperresponsiveness has long been recognized to play an important role in asthma, but many assumed that the defect might be genetic. The first suggestion that increased airway responsiveness could be acquired was the observation that viral respiratory infection caused transient hyperresponsiveness in otherwise healthy individuals (49,112). Because respiratory viruses grow in airway epithelium and cause inflammation (198), Nadel and associates sought other stimuli known to produce epithelial inflammation. They showed that the air pollutant ozone also caused epithelial damage and caused airway hyperresponsiveness (69). Bronchoalveolar lavage after ozone exposure is associated with neutrophil influx (171). Inhalation of antigen in allergic individuals also causes hyperresponsiveness (35), associated with inflammatory cell influx into the airways (138).

Studies in humans are limited in their ability to examine mechanisms; so investigations in animals have also been pursued.

ANIMAL STUDIES

More direct evidence implicating inflammatory mechanisms in the development of asthma and airway hyperresponsiveness has been obtained by studying experimentally induced airway hyperresponsiveness in laboratory animals. Thus, exposure of dogs to oxidant pollutants, such as ozone, causes the development of airway hyperresponsiveness (115). Associated with the development of airway hyperresponsiveness there is an inflammatory cell influx into the airways consisting primarily of neutrophils, as demonstrated by airway biopsy (87) and bronchoalveolar lavage (50). The development of this hyperresponsiveness can be prevented in dogs by granulocyte depletion with hydroxyurea (149). Similar studies in guinea pigs have shown that this species also develops airway hyperresponsiveness and has an influx of neutrophils into the airway after ozone exposure (162).

Exposure of guinea pigs to toluene diisocyanate is likewise associated with the development of airway hyperresponsiveness, an effect that is temporally associated with histologic evidence of an inflammatory cell influx into the conducting airways (71). The inflammatory cell infiltrate consists initially of neutrophils and, subsequently, of eosinophils; however, the development of airway hyperresponsiveness is temporally correlated with the neutrophil influx (71).

Examining the link between hyperresponsiveness and inflammation from the opposite perspective, some investigators have examined the effects on airway responsiveness of agents known to initiate inflammatory responses. Thus, studies in awake, chronically instrumented sheep have revealed that intravenous infusion of endotoxin, a component of bacterial cell walls and a potent stimulus for inflammatory cell recruitment *in vivo*, results in the development of airway hyperresponsiveness to inhaled histamine 5 hr after infusion (93). Subsequent studies of the effects of granulocyte depletion with hydroxyurea on airway responsiveness to inhaled histamine in sheep suggest that the number of circulating granulocytes correlates directly with the degree of airway responsiveness (84), thus indirectly suggesting that granulocytes may also be involved in the development of this form of hyperresponsiveness. Similar experiments performed in rats have shown that inhalation of endotoxin can be associated with the development of airway hyperresponsiveness to 5-hydroxytryptamine 1.5 to 2 hr after exposure and that this hyperresponsiveness is associated with a neutrophil influx into the airways, as assessed by bronchoalveolar lavage (155).

Another potent stimulus to inflammatory cell recruitment *in vivo* is the complement-derived fragment C5a-Des-Arg. Aerosolization of C5a-Des-Arg to rabbits leads to the development of airway hyperresponsiveness and is associated with the influx of neutrophils, as shown by histologic examination of airways (95). This effect can be prevented by granulocyte depletion with nitrogen mustard (95).

Other investigations have begun to examine the role of inflammation in antigen-induced bronchospasm and airway hyperresponsiveness. Antigen challenge of rabbits immunized from birth with *Alternaria* leads to the development of airway hyperresponsiveness and, in some animals, to the development of a late asthmatic response (176). Although these animals generate specific IgG and IgE antibodies to *Alternaria* antigen, the airway response is IgE-specific and is associated with an inflammatory infiltrate of the airways, as demonstrated by morphometric analysis of histopathologic specimens at the time of the late response (10). Similar findings are demonstrated by bronchoalveolar lavage (133). The late asthmatic response, in rabbits passively sensitized with serum containing antiragweed IgE and then challenged with inhaled ragweed antigen, can be blocked by neutrophil depletion and reconstituted with neutrophil repletion (140). Aerosolization of antigen to ragweed-sensitized dogs also results in the development of airway hyperresponsiveness to acetylcholine and is associated with neutrophil and eosinophil influx, as demonstrated by bronchoalveolar lavage (32).

Finally, very provocative recent work has suggested that remote sites of inflammation can result in nonspecific airway hyperresponsiveness. Thus, inflammatory sites in the paranasal sinuses, induced by local injection of C5a-Des-Arg, are associated with airway hyperresponsiveness to inhaled histamine in the rabbit (36).

Together, these studies show that many stimuli, from viruses and air pollutants to antigen, produce airway hyperresponsiveness. Subsequent investigations have revealed that many mediators, when inhaled, are capable of causing reversible hyperresponsiveness. These cannot be reviewed in detail. Suffice it to say that mediators such as prostaglandin $F_{2\alpha}$ ($PGF_{2\alpha}$) (199), platelet-aggregating factor (31), and thromboxane (188) increase the responsiveness of airway smooth muscle. Other mediators (e.g., PGE_2) inhibit airway smooth-muscle activity (199). Thus, an imbalance between relaxant and constrictor effects could cause hyperresponsiveness. These mediators will be discussed further when specific cells and their products are reviewed.

All results of experimental hyperresponsiveness in humans and in animals have one characteristic in common that differs from clinical asthma: They are all transient, lasting for days or, at most, for weeks. It seems reasonable that these mechanisms are important in triggering exacerbations of asthma. In clinical asthma, in which inflammation and hyperresponsiveness are chronic, lasting for years, a key question remains: What causes the chronic, prolonged inflammation?

CELLULAR MECHANISMS

The "classic" concept of asthma was a disease caused by allergens, triggering an IgE-mediated antigen-antibody reaction in mast cells, resulting in the release of mediators that cause asthma: one cell, one disease! However, because many patients do not have evidence of allergy, because asthma is triggered by multiple stimuli at the airway surface, and because multiple cells are involved in asthmatic responses (e.g., smooth-muscle spasm, mucus production, cough, increased capillary permeability), it is reasonable to assume that multiple cells and multiple mechanisms are involved in asthma. Furthermore, because many of the cells that exist in the airways also exist in other epithelial tissues (epithelial cells, mast cells, monocytes, sensory nerves, etc.), we suggest that inflammation in these various epithelial tissues is common. The differences that distinguish airway epithelium from other epithelia are the target cells: cough receptors, smooth muscle, glands.

As mentioned, multiple cells are likely to be involved in asthma, and these cells interact to produce the clinical responses. In this section we shall discuss some of these cells and their actions in relation to asthma.

Nonimmunologic Functions of Mast Cells

The role of the mast cell and basophil in allergically mediated diseases, including allergic asthma, has been studied extensively and has been the topic of multiple volumes of literature. These immunologic functions of the mast cell and their roles in asthma will not be reviewed in this chapter. However, several features of the mast cell and its interaction with other cells are of potential importance in the inflammatory response. Some of these features will be reviewed here.

Although allergic asthmatics are thought of as having

disease mediated by specific antigen triggering release of mediators from mast cells through IgE-dependent mechanisms, the distinction between diseases mediated via immunologic mechanisms and inflammatory mechanisms has become progressively less clear. For many years, clinicians have been aware that diverse agents such as muscle relaxants, opioids, antibiotics, and iodinated contrast material are capable of inducing anaphylactoid responses in people without demonstrable evidence of IgE-mediated allergy (57). Along similar lines, exercise (116) and sleep (8) have been shown to induce histamine release in some asthmatics. Further investigations *in vitro* have revealed that many agents are capable of stimulating mast cells via IgE-independent mechanisms (57).

Likewise, macrophages (168), neutrophils (207), eosinophils (82,209), and platelets (20) can secrete products that stimulate release of histamine and, possibly, other mediators from mast cells. The distinction between mast cells and inflammatory cells becomes more vague when their surface receptors are considered. Thus, macrophages (100), eosinophils (24), and platelets (99) have surface receptors for IgE. Therefore, not only can mast cells be stimulated by nonimmunologic mechanisms, but also immunologic stimulation of the mast cell may be, in fact, an indirect effect mediated by an inflammatory cell.

Investigations examining the late asthmatic response have also raised questions regarding the effector cell of the allergic response. These investigations have shown that symptoms in patients with allergic disease correspond more closely to the late rather than the immediate response to antigen (61,102). Initial observations regarding the histopathology of the late response involved clinical studies of the skin and demonstrated edema, mast cell degranulation, and cellular infiltration with neutrophils and eosinophils (42) or a mixed cellular infiltrate (183). Subsequent studies in the rat have shown early neutrophil influx, followed by a later mononuclear cell infiltration (151,189). In the lower airways of people, as previously stated, neutrophils and eosinophils (138) or eosinophils alone (38) were found in bronchoalveolar lavage during the late-phase response after antigen challenge in asthmatics. Similarly, in a rabbit model, the late-phase response to inhaled antigen led to edema and a mixed cellular infiltrate in the airway, as demonstrated by histopathology (10). This infiltrate included neutrophils, eosinophils, and mononuclear cells and extended to the bronchiolar region. Bronchoalveolar lavage fluid reflects a similar cell composition, with increased neutrophils, eosinophils, and mononuclear cells (133). These data, taken together, suggest that the late response and its symptoms may be associated with and perhaps are results of recruitment of inflammatory cells to the affected area. That is to say, these inflammatory cells may be the effector cells of the late response to antigen.

In support of this hypothesis, neutrophil depletion with

vinblastine diminishes the cutaneous late-phase response in rats (119). This effect is partially reconstituted by neutrophil repletion (119). Along similar lines, the late-phase response to inhaled antigen in rabbits, as measured by change in specific conductance, is prevented by granulocyte depletion with nitrogen mustard; however, the immediate response to inhaled antigen remains unchanged (140). Similar findings have been obtained when animals have been passively sensitized with antigen-specific IgE (140). Likewise, airway hyperresponsiveness to inhaled histamine develops after antigen challenge in directly and passively sensitized rabbits and can be blocked by granulocyte depletion (140). Granulocyte repletion results in reconstitution of the late-phase response of the airway. Therefore, inflammation appears to play an important role in allergically mediated airway disease as well as non-allergic airway disease.

Neutrophils

As mentioned previously, the initial data implicating the neutrophil in asthma and airway hyperresponsiveness were anatomic. Thus, postmortem tissue obtained from patients dying in status asthmaticus (47,80) and bronchial biopsy specimens obtained from patients with relatively mild asthma (113) revealed neutrophilic infiltration of airways. Also as mentioned, airway hyperresponsiveness associated with exposure to ozone (87,171), exposure to toluene diisocyanate (71), inhalation of C5a-Des-Arg (95), and the late asthmatic response to antigen (10) have all been shown to be associated with an influx of neutrophils, as assessed by airway histopathology, bronchial biopsy, and/or bronchoalveolar lavage.

Studies attempting to establish a causative role for the neutrophil in the development of asthma and airway hyperresponsiveness have utilized primarily neutrophil depletion in animals. Thus, dogs depleted of neutrophils with hydroxyurea and then exposed to ozone did not develop airway hyperresponsiveness (149). Similar findings were obtained when rabbits were depleted of neutrophils with nitrogen mustard and then exposed to aerosols of C5a-Des-Arg (95). Depleted animals were less responsive than their C5a-Des-Arg-exposed controls to inhaled histamine. Similarly, sheep depleted of neutrophils with hydroxyurea and infused with bacterial endotoxin did not develop airway hyperresponsiveness to inhaled histamine as did their endotoxin-treated controls (93). However, this latter study has been interpreted as suggesting effects of circulating granulocytes, rather than granulocytes present in the lung.

Further examination of the neutrophil in the development of asthma and airway hyperresponsiveness has involved studies of neutrophil repletion, after depletion with cytotoxic agents, to rule out direct effects of the cytotoxic agents themselves. In these studies, rabbits were depleted of neutrophils with nitrogen mustard and passively sensitized with serum containing antiragweed IgE (140). After depletion, the neutrophil influx into the airway, the late asthmatic response, and hyperresponsiveness to inhaled histamine were prevented. The response to inhaled ragweed antigen could be reconstituted by neutrophil repletion; however, the neutrophil influx into bronchoalveolar lavage fluid was not present at 3 days as it was in passively sensitized controls after inhaled antigen. These results were interpreted as indicating a requirement for neutrophils only at the time of antigen challenge to mediate the airway response (140).

In spite of this substantial data base suggesting a role for the neutrophil in the development of airway hyperresponsiveness and asthma, questions have been raised about this role. For example, exposure of guinea pigs to ozone resulted in the development of airway hyperresponsiveness within 2 hr of exposure, but neutrophil influx into the airways, as assessed histologically, did not occur until 6 hr after exposure (139). Furthermore, the hyperresponsiveness present at 2 hr could not be prevented in animals treated with corticosteroids and depleted of neutrophils with cyclophosphamide (139). This hyperresponsiveness cannot be explained by changes in airway epithelial permeability to the inhaled agonist (162). Additional investigations in guinea pigs have focused on the effects of neutrophil depletion on hyperresponsiveness that develops after exposure to toluene diisocyanate (190). Treatment of animals with hydroxyurea resulted in neutrophil depletion and inhibited the increase in airway responsiveness associated with exposure to toluene diisocyanate. Treatment of animals with cyclophosphamide resulted in neutrophil depletion of the same degree, but did not inhibit the development of airway hyperresponsiveness. These findings suggest that the effect of hydroxyurea was to inhibit the development of hyperresponsiveness through a mechanism other than neutrophil depletion.

Guinea pigs exposed to whole cigarette smoke show an increase in airway epithelial permeability in 30 min and neutrophil migration into the airway epithelium 4 to 6 hr after exposure (90). Airway reactivity to inhaled histamine is increased at 30 min in these animals, but not at 6 hr or 24 hr after exposure (91). These multiple stimuli for hyperresponsiveness cast considerable doubt on a role for the neutrophil in the development of airway hyperresponsiveness in the guinea pig. However, the balance of data in other species studied, including humans, suggests, but does not establish, a role for the neutrophil as an effector cell in hyperresponsive states.

The mechanisms of neutrophil recruitment, stimuli for neutrophil movement in the airway, and the products of the neutrophil in the airway that may mediate effects in asthma are largely unknown. However, because substantial information exists regarding neutrophils and their products in other settings, mechanisms by which neutrophils may modulate airway function can be conjectured.

Neutrophils may be recruited to an inflammatory site by a broad range of agents. These include bacterial cell wall constituents such as lipopolysaccharide, the complement-derived fragment C5a (181), and a high-molecular-weight chemotactic factor presumed to be derived from mast cells (7).

In addition, neutrophils are recruited to the airway after airway epithelial damage, irrespective of the cause of this damage. Although the recruitment of the neutrophil may be mediated by the lung macrophage, mast cell, or other cell types, airway epithelial cells have also been studied for their ability to directly produce mediators chemotactic for neutrophils. Thus, airway epithelial cells acutely isolated from mongrel dogs have been shown to release leukotriene B_4 (LTB_4) and 5-hydroxyeicosatetraenoic acid (5-HETE) in response to exogenous arachidonic acid (86), as well as calcium ionophore and arachidonic acid (12). LTB_4 is one of the most chemotactic agents for neutrophils known (131), and 5-HETE has also been shown to have modest chemotactic effects for neutrophils (64). Furthermore, human airway epithelial cells, isolated post mortem and incubated with exogenous arachidonic acid, have been shown to produce large quantities of 15-lipoxygenase products, including 8,15-dihydroxyeicosatetraenoic acid (8,15-diHETE) (92). This diHETE has also been shown to be chemotactic for human neutrophils (175). Therefore, airway epithelial cells may play a role in recruitment of neutrophils to the airway via generation of chemotactic polar lipids such as leukotrienes.

The range of potential stimuli that neutrophils may be exposed to in the airway is extensive. For example, phagocytosis is a potent stimulus to many neutrophil functions, including secretion of a number of inflammatory mediators (see Chapter 26). Phagocytosis, although it can occur via nonspecific mechanisms, is mediated primarily by cell surface receptors for fragments of C3 or the Fc portions of IgG_3 and IgG_1 (41). In the presence of substances that fix complement or in the presence of antigen that binds specific immunoglobulin, phagocytosis occurs, and thus secretion is initiated. Therefore, inhaled particulate antigens or bacteria can stimulate secretion from neutrophils in the lung.

Additionally, soluble agents present in the airway may stimulate secretion. For example, LTB_4 has been shown to stimulate neutrophil secretion via an ionophore-like effect (172). Likewise, lipopolysaccharide, neuropeptides, and C5a have all been shown to stimulate neutrophil secretion (181) as well as to initiate cell recruitment. All of these materials may be present in the lung.

Direct evidence demonstrating airway effects of products derived from neutrophils present in the airway does not exist. However, attempts have been made to examine this indirectly. Thus, crude neutrophil products have been shown to have airway effects. Supernatants obtained from incubations of human neutrophils with opsonized zymosan resulted in the development of hyperresponsiveness to inhaled histamine when nebulized to rabbits (94).

A vast array of secreted products of neutrophils may be involved in mediating these pathophysiologic events. Available information regarding many of these products will be reviewed here: Neutrophils have been shown to be rich sources of metabolites of arachidonic acid. Specifically, neutrophils are capable of producing thromboxane A_2 (70). The relevance of this product to airway hyperresponsiveness has been examined by demonstrating that treatment with indomethacin prevents the development of airway hyperresponsiveness after ozone exposure in dogs, but not the neutrophil influx into the airways (148). The thomboxane synthetase inhibitor OKY-046 has also been shown to inhibit the development of airway hyperresponsiveness in dogs after ozone exposure (2), and the thomboxane A_2 mimetic U46619 has been shown to increase airway responsiveness (2). Interestingly, similar data have been found in allergic dogs (32), thus strongly suggesting that thromboxane A_2 from the neutrophil is involved in the development of hyperresponsiveness in the dog. Thromboxane A_2 has also been implicated in modulation of cholinergic neurotransmission in the airway by demonstrating that the thromboxane mimetic drug U46619 facilitates cholinergic neurotransmission in the dog airway (33). However, the role of thromboxane A_2 in human asthma is suspect. Asthmatics do not have a dramatic improvement in their disease when treated with drugs that block the cyclooxygenase pathway and, in fact, may have a profound worsening of their disease (1).

Neutrophils also produce large quantities of LTB_4 when stimulated (14). LTB_4 has potent effects on neutrophil and monocyte chemotaxis (131), on neutrophil adherence (37), and on neutrophil stimulation (172). Therefore, LTB_4 may recruit inflammatory cells to the airway and mediate their stimulation. LTB_4 has only weak direct bronchoconstricting effects (179), but it has been shown to induce airway hyperresponsiveness to acetylcholine when administered as an aerosol to dogs (147). The cyclooxygenase and lipoxygenase inhibitor BW755C has been shown to inhibit the airway hyperresponsiveness that develops in dogs after ozone exposure, thus suggesting that LTB_4 may also have a role in this process. However, the effects of LTB_4 on human airways have not been examined, and therefore the function of this product in asthma is unknown.

The neutrophil also has recently been shown to produce trihydroxy metabolites of arachidonic acid, called lipoxins, when incubated in the presence of 15-HETE or 15-hydroperoxyeicosatetraenoic acid (15-HPETE) (173). These compounds have been shown to degranulate neutrophils (173), to generate superoxide from neutrophils (173), to activate protein kinase C (78), and to cause airway smooth-muscle contraction (173). The roles of these compounds in the human airway are unknown at this time; however, the presence of a potent 15-lipoxygenase pathway in the human airway epithelial cell (92) suggests that lipoxin generation in airways is possible and may be of importance when inflammatory cells are present, as is the case in asthma.

Neutrophils also release other products that may be important in airway hyperresponsiveness and asthma. Platelet-activating factor (PAF) is an ether phospholipid produced from lyso-PAF after its generation by the action of phospholipase A_2. PAF is produced in large quantities by the human neutrophil (123). As will be discussed in subsequent sections, this mediator has been shown to have profound bronchoconstricting effects that are platelet-dependent in animals. PAF, when nebulized in dogs, has also been shown to induce the development of airway hyperresponsiveness (30), which in this species may be mediated via effects of thromboxane.

The neutrophil is also a potent source of reactive oxygen intermediates that have well-defined roles in the cell's microbicidal and cytocidal functions. In addition, these reactive compounds may play a role in asthma. In guinea pig trachealis muscle, LTD_4 induces hyperresponsiveness to histamine that can be blocked by pretreatment with superoxide dismutase. This suggests that LTD_4 stimulates the generation of oxygen intermediates and that these compounds mediate the observed hyperresponsiveness (201). Sheep given intravenous phorbol myristate acetate, a potent stimulator of reactive oxygen intermediates, also develop hyperresponsiveness to histamine aerosol, thus indirectly suggesting a role for these compounds (48). Clinical relevance of this effect is suggested by the finding that leukocytes obtained from asthmatic children have an increased capacity to release reactive oxygen intermediates (145).

In summary, the neutrophil can be recruited to the airway in asthma; it can be stimulated by a variety of mechanisms and can release an impressive array of potential mediators that may have direct or indirect effects in the airway. However, other inflammatory cells also may have important roles in the pathogenesis and pathophysiology of asthma.

Eosinophils

The presence of increased numbers of eosinophils in the blood, sputum, and airways of asthmatics has been noted since shortly after discovery of the unique staining characteristics of this cell over 100 years ago (62). Blood and sputum eosinophils have been noted so frequently in asthma that they have been used in the past as diagnostic (56) and prognostic (88) tools. However, the role of the eosinophil in asthma remains largely speculative. Whether this cell represents an inflammatory effector cell, a regulator of the inflammatory response, or an innocent bystander in asthma awaits further investigation. Nevertheless, the association of the eosinophil with asthma is indisputable, and thus available data regarding this association warrant close scrutiny and continued investigation.

Eosinophils are present in sputum obtained from most patients with asthma (44). The airway as a source of these cells is confirmed by the fact that eosinophils are present in the airways of patients dying in status asthmaticus (47,80) and are present in bronchial biopsy material obtained from patients with mild asthma (113). In addition, these cells have been shown to be present in increased numbers in bronchoalveolar lavage fluid obtained from asthmatics (40,191). After antigen challenge, the numbers of eosinophils present in bronchoalveolar lavage fluid obtained from asthmatics are increased (38).

Direct experimentation in humans regarding the effects of eosinophils on airway function has not been performed, and animal models of eosinophil recruitment to the lung, associated with asthma and airway hyperresponsiveness, do not exist. Thus, no in vivo whole-animal model exists, but a number of in vitro observations suggest that eosinophils may be important: Eosinophils can be recruited to the lung by a number of factors. Peripheral blood and tissue eosinophilias are commonly found in disorders thought to be mediated by mast cells (51,124). Thus, the finding that mast cells release a number of factors chemotactic for eosinophils is not surprising. Eosinophil chemotactic factor of anaphylaxis (ECF-A) is in fact a family of acidic peptides present, preformed, in mast cell granules, with molecular weights ranging from 360 to more than 1,000 (106). ECF-A is selectively chemotactic for eosinophils and is released from the mast cell on antigenic and nonantigenic stimulation (21). PAF (177) and PGD_2 (67) also appear to be selectively chemotactic for eosinophils. Other factors, such as LTB_4 (143), histamine (34), mono-HETEs (64), and C5a (105), are also chemotactic for eosinophils, but are not selective.

On arrival in the lung, eosinophils can be stimulated by a variety of agents, including nonspecific phagocytosis of particles, or by receptor-mediated events. As is the case for neutrophils, eosinophils have receptors for complement and immunoglobulin. Thus, eosinophils have surface receptors for fragments of C3 (54) and, possibly, C5a. In addition, eosinophils have receptors for most fractions of IgG (4). Like neutrophils, these cells have also been shown to have receptors for IgE on their surfaces (24). Hypodense eosinophils, presumed to be activated, have increased expression of these receptors on their surfaces, and secretion or phagocytosis may be stimulated via these receptors (25).

Although the role of the eosinophil in killing parasites seems well established (22), the function of the eosinophil in other settings is controversial. Several investigators have suggested that the function of the eosinophil at inflammatory sites, including the lung, is to regulate or limit inflammation (39,203). This interpretation is based largely on observations that the eosinophil is capable of inactivating a number of inflammatory mediators. Thus, eosinophils contain histaminase, which inactivates histamine (208), and they have been suggested to inactivate the slow-reacting substance of anaphylaxis (SRS-A) by arylsulfatase B (200) or eosinophil peroxidase (83). They have also been shown to inactivate heparin by its binding to major basic protein (60), to release an inhibitor of histamine release on antigenic stimulation (subsequently shown to be PGE_1 and PGE_2) (89), and to remove mast cell granules by phagocytosis (132).

In spite of these suggested regulatory roles for the eosinophil, data have accumulated suggesting that eosinophils may have potent inflammatory effects and that some of the mediators of these effects may have roles in airway hyperresponsiveness and asthma. The best studied of these, major basic protein, is the principal protein constituent of eosinophil granules and composes the core in these granules (63,120). Purified major basic protein has been shown to cause desquamation and toxicity to the tracheal epithelium of guinea pigs, very similar to the epithelial desquamation observed in asthma (58). The sputum of patients with asthma has been shown to contain quantities of major basic protein that are known to be toxic to respiratory epithelium (59). These observations have been extended by the finding of deposition of major basic protein at sites of damaged bronchial epithelium in patients dying of asthma. Other biological effects of major basic protein include stimulation of histamine release from mast cells and basophils (150) and increases in ion transport in cultured dog tracheal epithelial cells (97). Other protein products of eosinophils may be important in asthma. For example, eosinophil peroxidase, distinct from the peroxidase present in the neutrophil, is capable of stimulating the mast cell in the presence of hydrogen peroxide and a halide ion (82). Similarly, eosinophil cationic protein has been shown to cause histamine release from basophils and rat mast cells (209).

With respect to lipid mediators, the eosinophil is a rich source of these products. These cells contain both a 5-lipoxygenase pathway and a 15-lipoxygenase pathway of arachidonic acid metabolism. The 5-lipoxygenase pathway is stimulated by transmembrane calcium flux and by a wide variety of receptor-mediated membrane stimuli (204). The principal products of this pathway are the peptide-containing LTC_4 and LTD_4, which have potent bronchoconstricting effects on airway smooth muscle both in animals (43) and in humans (85). In addition, the eosinophil, in the presence of unesterified arachidonic acid, is capable of producing 15-lipoxygenase products, including 8,15-diHETE and large quantities of 15-HETE. 8,15-diHETE has been shown to be chemotactic for neutrophils both *in vitro* (175) and *in vivo* (110). The other principal product, 15-HETE, has been shown to be weakly chemotactic (64), to stimulate histamine release from mast cells (65), and to stimulate leukotriene biosynthesis in a murine mast cell tumor line (194).

In summary, no conclusive data exist demonstrating that the eosinophil has an effector role in airway hyperresponsiveness and asthma. In fact, considerable controversy exists whether this cell functions as a proinflammatory or antiinflammatory cell. Nevertheless, the eosinophil is a potent source of a number of products with profound effects in the lungs and airways. The ability of these products to mimic some of the features of asthma and the strong association of this cell with asthma support a possible effector role, but investigation is still required to delineate the eosinophil's role.

Macrophages

Surprisingly little research has been performed investigating the possible role of macrophages in asthma. This is perhaps because these cells are traditionally thought of as intraalveolar or interstitial cells in the lung, and anatomic studies have not demonstrated striking changes in these cells in asthma. However, there are several reasons to further examine their role and some data to implicate their involvement.

The lung macrophage is the sentinel inflammatory cell of the lung, representing the lung's first line of defense to a broad range of inhaled substances (184). Although poorly recognized, macrophages not only are present in the alveolus and alveolar interstitium but also are present on the airway surface and within the airway wall (19,184). In fact, the movement of macrophages through the airways is substantial and has been reported to be between 1 and 5 million cells per hour in small animals (18). Thus, in addition to its better defined role in the lung's defense against infection, the macrophage is uniquely located within both the airway and the airway wall such that it can respond to inhaled or endogenous stimuli and, through secreted products, have end-organ effects in the airway. Although it is assumed that macrophages are primarily responsible for initiating and regulating inflammatory responses to a wide variety of substances that enter the alveolus, it is likely that this phenomenon likewise occurs in the airway. In addition to the macrophage's location, the fact that it is a resident cell in the lung and has a long half-life, estimated at 30 days, makes this cell appealing as one having a role in the chronic disorder of asthma.

Some of the immunologic functions of the macrophage likewise suggest a role for this cell in asthma. Although not discussed in detail here, the macrophage is the primary antigen-processing cell (27); so all immunologic responses must first involve the macrophage. The macrophage also has receptors for immunoglobulin on its surface. These receptors consist primarily of IgG_3 and IgG_1 receptors (142); IgG_3 has the greatest number of binding sites on the lung macrophage. This is of particular interest because IgG appears to be the predominant immunoglobulin of the lower respiratory tract (161) and will bind in a monomeric or complex form to the macrophage. Evidence has also accumulated that human macrophages have immunoglobulin bound to some of these receptors on their surfaces (142). In addition, the human lung macrophage has been shown to have receptors for IgE on its surface (135). Further evidence of their relevance are studies showing asthmatic subjects to have increased numbers of IgE receptors on their macrophages (100) and to have IgE bound to some of these receptors on lung macrophages (100). Similarly, these cells can be stimulated with specific antigen, via these receptors, both *in vitro* (100) and *in vivo* (192). These data suggest that the macrophage may have a role in immunologic phenomena observed in some patients with asthma, and thus functions traditionally ascribed to the mast cell may, in part, be functions of macrophages. These immunologic functions of the macrophage may be of greater importance because of obvious accessibility of this cell to antigen, as opposed to the mast cell, which is located principally below the epithelial basement membrane (75).

As in the case of the neutrophil, the macrophage also has numerous cell surface receptors by which it can be stimulated (53). Phagocytosis and soluble agents can similarly stimulate secretion via membrane receptors; however, as in neutrophils, nonspecific phagocytosis is relatively unimportant, and phagocytosis proceeds via the IgG receptor and complement receptors primarily (53).

No *in vivo* studies of macrophage function in the lung exist to suggest that this cell may mediate the airway hyperresponsiveness or bronchoconstriction of asthma. However, macrophages obtained from asthmatics have been shown to release factors chemotactic for neutrophils and eosinophils when challenged with specific antigen (72). Similarly, macrophages obtained from allergic patients have been shown to have increased IgE-mediated cytotoxicity (136). The effect of macrophage stimulation on airway smooth muscle has been examined by addition of stimulated dog macrophages to a bronchial ring preparation (186). In this preparation, addition of stimulated macrophages enhanced the contractile response to electric-field stimulation without directly causing contraction. These effects were prevented by indomethacin and by the thromboxane antagonist SQ29548. These physiologic events were correlated with release of thromboxane A_2 from the macrophage, thus suggesting that the dog macrophage enhances cholinergic nerve transmission in the airway by release of thromboxane A_2.

There is a wide range of secreted products from the macrophage that are of potential importance in asthma. As is the case for the neutrophil, the macrophage is a rich source of metabolites of arachidonic acid. The principal cyclooxygenase product of the human macrophage is thromboxane A_2 (53). It has also been shown to produce $PGF_{2\alpha}$ and PGD_2 (129). $PGF_{2\alpha}$ has been shown to increase airway responsiveness to inhaled acetylcholine in dogs (146). PGD_2 has been shown to increase cholinergic neurotransmission in dog bronchial rings (187).

The principal lipoxygenase products of the human macrophage are LTB_4 and 5-HETE (13,52,134). In fact, the human lung macrophage has the most potent 5-lipoxygenase pathway yet described (121). As the human monocyte matures into a macrophage in the lung, the 5-lipoxygenase pathway is enhanced 10- to 20-fold (13), thus making this cell a greater source of these products. Preliminary observations in rat lung macrophages also suggest that these cells can convert 15-HETE and 15-HPETE to lipoxins (109). Human lung macrophages also have the capacity to release PAF (5). More important, lung macrophages obtained from asthmatics have been shown to release PAF on challenge with specific antigen (6).

Although less powerful than the neutrophil or blood monocyte (144), the human lung macrophage also has an oxidative pathway that generates significant quantities of reactive oxygen intermediates (73). However, when the lung macrophage is activated with γ-interferon, the activity of this oxidative pathway increases twofold to threefold (53). Thus, activated macrophages may have a greater capacity to generate reactive oxygen intermediates in the lung. A preliminary observation suggests that lung macrophages obtained from subjects with asthma have a greater spontaneous release of reactive oxygen intermediates than those in normal subjects, as measured by superoxide generation (23). A similar report indicates that macrophages from asthmatics may release greater quantities of superoxide anion with stimulation (26). These studies imply that the increased capacity to produce reactive oxygen intermediates in asthma may reflect macrophage activation, and the spontaneous release of the metabolites may reflect previous cell stimulation. However, the biological relevance of these findings in the airway awaits further investigation.

The lung macrophage is also a rich source of a variety of proteins, including complement components, clotting factors, elastase, collagenase, and other neutral or acid proteases (53,206). The macrophage also produces a number of regulatory proteins, including interleukin-1 and tumor necrosis factor α, with widespread effects on other cells. The roles of these proteins in asthma have not been explored. However, macrophages from the lung have been shown to release a protein capable of causing histamine release from mast cells and basophils (168).

In summary, the macrophage is a powerful phagocytic and secretory cell that is normally resident in the lung, including the airways. It is capable of altering its phagocytic or secretory functions, and there is also evidence that this may be the case in asthma. The macrophage's location in the airway, available to first encounter inhaled materials, and its secretory capabilities, with a number of products known to have airway effects, make this cell an appealing candidate to be involved in airway disease. However, the definition of this role awaits further investigation.

Platelets

The primary hemostatic response, an established function of platelets, in many ways resembles the inflammatory response (141), and this property of platelets, as well as others, has led to examination of platelets for their possible role in inflammation. This role is reviewed in detail elsewhere in this volume and points out that platelets may well be potent inflammatory effector cells that can release products with proinflammatory effects. In addition, there are several reasons to consider platelets as effector cells in the inflammatory process in the airways and some data to suggest that they may be involved in airway hyperresponsiveness and asthma. These concepts and available data will be reviewed later.

The primary clinical evidence suggesting that platelets may have a role in airway disease comes from reports of acute respiratory failure (166) and sudden death (160) associated with platelet aggregation in pulmonary vessels. These clinical reports suggest that platelet aggregation in the lung may be associated with bronchospasm. This is especially interesting because spontaneous aggregation of platelets has been observed in blood samples obtained from asthmatics (154).

Although platelets may spontaneously aggregate in blood obtained from asthmatic subjects, aggregation to a variety of stimuli in these patients appears to be impaired in the setting of known allergy (79,128,182), perhaps representing previous exposure to a stimulus. This impairment in platelet aggregation can be transferred with cell-free plasma obtained from asthmatic patients (182) and

seems to be more frequent in individuals with increased serum IgE (128). Thus, platelet aggregation does seem to be altered in the circulation in asthmatics; however, the specific nature of this alteration remains unclear.

It has been observed that thrombocytopenia can occur in allergic asthmatics challenged with antigen aerosol, suggesting sequestration and possibly stimulation of platelets (185). More direct evidence that platelets may be stimulated during antigen-induced bronchospasm comes from studies examining release of platelet factor 4 (PF4) after antigen challenge (111). In these studies, PF4 was increased in antigen-aerosol-challenged subjects, but not in controls, and was associated with a fall in forced expiratory volume (FEV$_1$). Similarly, β-thromboglobulin and circulating platelet aggregates have been shown to increase after antigen challenge in asthmatics (74). Therefore, platelet abnormalities, possibly representing cell stimulation, may exist in asthma, and in the setting of antigen challenge, platelet products are released that could have biological effects in the airways.

Because investigation in human subjects must be limited by the risk to the subject, the foregoing observations have been extended by animal investigations. Intravenous administration of PAF to guinea pigs has been shown to induce bronchoconstriction and thrombocytopenia (195). Associated with the bronchoconstriction, sequestration of platelets in the lung has been demonstrated by radiolabeling with ^{111}In oxine (153). The bronchoconstricting response, thrombocytopenia, and platelet sequestration in the lung, after administration of PAF, can be abrogated by platelet depletion with antiplatelet antiserum (195). Similarly, sensitized rabbits challenged with an antigen aerosol develop intravascular aggregation of platelets and sequestration in the lung (159). Platelet depletion significantly inhibits these effects (159). Thus, in animals, the bronchoconstricting effects of PAF may be mediated by the platelet, and platelet sequestration and aggregation in the lung can occur after aerosol antigen challenge.

The products of platelets that may mediate the effects described earlier are unknown, but data are available regarding mechanisms of platelet stimulation, and some data exist concerning the biological effects of some platelet-derived products in the lung. These will be reviewed later.

As noted, PAF is released by mast cells (137), basophils (11), monocytes (101), macrophages (5), neutrophils (123), and platelets (28). In addition to PAF, a variety of substances potentially may stimulate platelets in the lung. These include adenosine diphosphate, epinephrine, thromboxane A$_2$, serotonin, thrombin, trypsin, factor VIII, immune complexes, endotoxin, viruses, and collagen (81). Platelets have also been demonstrated to have specific surface receptors for IgG (103) and for IgE (99). These cells can be stimulated via these specific receptors.

The platelet is capable of releasing a number of products on stimulation. Prostaglandins present in the blood are almost exclusively produced by platelets during aggregation and blood clotting (178). The major cyclooxygenase-pathway product of platelets is thromboxane A_2 (76), which has potent effects on airway smooth-muscle contraction (2) and an enhancing effect on cholinergic nerve transmission in the airway (33). Additional cyclooxygenase metabolites produced by platelets, including the cyclic endoperoxides PGH_2 and PGG_2, may further influence platelet aggregation in the lung (77). Lipoxygenation of arachidonic acid in platelets occurs via the 12-lipoxygenase pathway. The principal product of this pathway is 12-hydroxyeicosatetraenoic acid (193), which is chemotactic for neutrophils and eosinophils (68). The platelet is also a source of PAF, which has positive-feedback effects in stimulating additional platelets (29). With respect to protein constituents, PF4 is a preformed protein constituent of platelet alpha granules (141). The role of PF4 in asthma is unknown; however, PF4 is released after antigen challenge in allergic asthmatics (111), as previously mentioned, and is capable of stimulating histamine release from human basophils (20).

In summary, clinical and experimental data suggest that platelets may be abnormal in asthma, may aggregate in the lung after antigenic or nonantigenic stimulation, and may release mediators with potent direct and indirect effects on airways. The intravascular location of the platelet and its central role in hemostasis have directed attention away from this cell in asthma research; however, the foregoing data persuasively suggest that platelets are important cells in asthma and airway hyperresponsiveness.

Sensory Nerves

In addition to the sympathetic and parasympathetic nervous systems, a new nervous system has recently been described. These nerves contain a new class of molecules, the neuropeptides. Among these, the best known is substance P (SP). SP-immunoreactive fibers occur in the sensory nerves of the lower respiratory tract (126). Mechanical, chemical, and pharmacologic stimuli cause these nerves to release neuropeptides (127). SP and the other neuropeptides known as "tachykinins" are interesting in relation to asthma because of their ability to stimulate gland secretion (15), smooth-muscle contraction (170), and manifestations of inflammation such as neutrophil chemotaxis (156), vasodilation (157), and increased capillary permeability (125).

Just as acetylcholine is degraded by acetylcholinesterase, SP is degraded in the airway by an enzyme, enkephalinase (15,170). This enzyme, a membrane-bound peptidase (108,130), has been shown to exist in the lungs of various species (16,98,107,122), including humans (98), and especially in the airways (16,98). This peptidase cleaves SP between the 9 and 10 positions (180), generating the N-terminal fragment SP_{1-9}, which does not contract airway smooth muscle (170) or cause gland secretion (15). Such cleavage results in a decreased amount of SP reaching the smooth muscle or submucosal gland receptors, resulting in less bronchoconstriction or gland secretion. The selectivity of enkephalinase is based not only on this specific site of peptide cleavage (180) but also on its location. Because it is bound to cell membranes, its action is limited to the cells where the enzyme resides. Thus, the presence of enkephalinase in nerve cells where it is released and in cells that contain tachykinin receptors (e.g., glands, smooth muscle) could be key to its ability to modulate certain peptide-induced responses.

The evidence that enkephalinase modulates SP-induced responses is based on the following observations. SP-induced bronchoconstriction (170) and gland secretion (15) are potentiated by inhibitors of enkephalinase, but not by other protease inhibitors. By inhibiting enkephalinase, the inhibitors allow a higher concentration of SP to reach the tissue receptor sites and cause greater tissue responses. This indirect evidence of the presence of enkephalinase in airways is confirmed by the demonstration of enkephalinase-like activity in airway tissue. In the airway, enkephalinase-like activity is found in the epithelium, smooth muscle, glands, and vagus nerves (16). It can also be localized to the airway by immunocytochemical techniques (169).

In summary, SP and other tachykinins have been shown experimentally to cause "neural" inflammation. Endogenous enkephalinase, because of its critical location in airway tissue, modulates tachykinin effects. Up- or down-regulation of enkephalinase activity in specific tissues can be predicted to modify the extent of neural inflammatory responses. No specific method yet exists for examining the role of neural inflammation in human disease, and so it is not surprising that its role in asthma remains enigmatic.

Epithelial Cells

Airway epithelial cells were long believed to constitute an inert integument that acted merely as a physical lining to provide a "zipper" or covering to the airways. It is now evident that the epithelial cells, with their key location at the interface between the environment and the internal milieu, play an important role in defense of the airways. These functions, especially as they relate to inflammation, will be discussed briefly.

Generation of lipoxygenase products of arachidonic acid. Recently, the epithelial cell has been identified as a possible source of mediators. This suggestion first came from observations that respiratory viral infections (49) and inhalation of ozone (69,115), two stimuli that damage airway epithelium, cause increased smooth-muscle responsiveness. When airway epithelial cells were isolated in acute culture conditions, it was found that they were capable of generating potent products of arachidonic acid (86,92). Thus, dog epithelial cells produce LTB_4 and selected HETEs (86), whereas human airway epithelial cells produce 15-HETE and 8,15-diHETEs (92). It is interesting that both LTB_4 and 8,15-diHETEs (175) are chemotactic for neutrophils, and this could be the mechanism for the neutrophil chemotaxis that occurs with viral infection, ozone, and other airway stimuli. The 15-HETEs are also of interest because they have been shown to stimulate mast cell release (158). Thus, epithelial cells, when damaged or otherwise stimulated, produce lipoxygenase products that in turn stimulate other inflammatory cells (neutrophils and mast cells).

Airway epithelium can affect smooth muscle in various ways. First, intact epithelium can inhibit muscle tone by releasing PGE_2. This prostaglandin inhibits tone by inhibiting vagal neural transmission and by a direct effect on the muscle itself (199). Cultured dog and human epithelial cells produce low concentrations of PGE_2, but when stimulated by inflammatory mediators, including bradykinin (117) and leukotrienes (118), or by eosinophil major basic protein (96), epithelial cells produce large amounts of PGE_2, which has profound effects on smooth-muscle tone (9). Removal of airway epithelium is reported to produce an inhibitory effect on airway smooth muscle via an unknown mechanism (55). Finally, 15-HETE produced by the epithelium can be converted to lipoxins, substances that contract airway smooth muscle (174). Thus, the epithelium has the potential of exerting potent tonic and inhibitory effects on airway smooth muscle by direct effects (e.g., release of prostaglandins) and, indirectly, by effects on other (e.g., mast) cells.

Epithelial glycocalyx. The surface of the airway epithelium contains a glycocalyx made up of high-molecular-weight glycoconjugates that contain specific types of carbohydrate chains of the poly(*N*-acetyllactosamine) type (196). There is preliminary evidence that they provide a surface for the binding of inflammatory cells, such as mast cells (197). By adhering, the inflammatory cells have a prolonged opportunity to act at epithelial sites.

Ion transport. Active transport of chloride by epithelial cells (152) and secondary osmotic movement of fluid (205) provide a mechanism for producing the sol layer in which the cilia move in the airways. PGE_2 produced by the epithelial cells stimulates Cl transport (3), and the inflammatory mediators mentioned earlier stimulate PGE_2, thus increasing Cl transport. This autocrine function of the epithelium allows it to dilute inflammatory irritants in its environment and thereby lessen their inflammatory effects.

In summary, airway epithelium may play a potent role in defense of the airways: It regulates the watery environment, produces cell surface molecules that bind to inflammatory cells, modulates smooth-muscle responses, and (by producing arachidonate products) stimulates inflammatory cells. In asthma, there are significant alterations in the epithelium. The pathophysiologic implications of these changes remain to be elucidated.

SUMMARY AND CLINICAL IMPLICATIONS

Recent investigations have shown the importance of increased airway responsiveness in clinical asthma: A decreased threshold for various mechanical, chemical, and pharmacologic stimuli makes asthmatic airways likely to overreact and produce clinical bronchospasm. Subsequent studies of mechanisms responsible for hyperresponsiveness have implicated inflammatory responses.

The emphasis in research on asthma is shifting from a search for a single mediator that will explain all of the manifestations of the disease to a careful examination of the actions and regulation of the resident and migratory cells as well as their interactions and their responses to various stimuli.

It is now clear that various cells in airways are sources of the inflammatory and bronchomotor responses in asthma, and it is likely that multiple cells could be involved in asthmatic responses in different individuals or even within a single asthmatic patient.

The treatment of asthma is still largely symptomatic. Thus, the physician treats bronchospasm with a combination of bronchodilators. When this therapy is inadequate, the inflammatory process is treated (nonspecifically) with steroids. These strategies make no attempt to attack the primary cellular mechanisms that underlie asthma. Investigations must stress an understanding of how the chronic inflammatory process(es) comes about, which cells are involved, and how they interact. Perhaps new drug therapy, by focusing on prevention of inflammation, may eliminate a primary mechanism in this chronic disease, whereas the present state of therapy principally provides symptomatic relief.

ACKNOWLEDGMENTS

The authors thank Beth Cost and Patty Snell for manuscript preparation. This research was supported in part by NIH Program Project Grant HL-24136. T. D. Bigby is the recipient of NIH Clinical Investigator Award 1-K08-HL-01888.

REFERENCES

1. Abrishami, M. A., and Thomas, J. (1977): Aspirin intolerance—a review. *Ann. Allergy*, 39:28–37.
2. Aizawa, H., Chung, K. F., Leikauf, G. D., Ueki, I., Bethel, R. A., O'Byrne, P. M., Hirose, T., and Nadel, J. A. (1985): Significance of thromboxane generation in ozone-induced airway hyperresponsiveness in dogs. *J. Appl. Physiol.*, 59:1918–1923.
3. Al-Bazzaz, F. J., Yadava, V. P., and Westenfelder, C. (1981): Modification of Na and Cl transport in canine tracheal mucosa by prostaglandins. *Am. J. Physiol.*, 240:F101–F105.
4. Anwar, A. R. E., and Kay, A. B. (1977): Membrane receptors for IgG and complement (C4, C3b, and C3d) on human eosinophils and neutrophils and their relationship to eosinophilia. *J. Immunol.*, 119:976–982.
5. Arnoux, B., Duval, D., and Benveniste, J. (1980): Release of platelet-activating factor (PAF-acether) from alveolar macrophages by the calcium ionophore A23187 and phagocytosis. *Eur. J. Clin. Invest.*, 10:437–441.
6. Arnoux, B., Simoes, M. H., Landes, A., Mathieu, M., Duroux, P., and Benveniste, J. (1987): Alveolar macrophages from asthmatic patients release platelet-activating factor (PAF-acether) and lyso-PAF-acether when stimulated with specific allergen. *Am. Rev. Respir. Dis.*, 135:70A (abstract).
7. Atkins, P. C., Norman, M., Weiner, H., and Zweiman, B. (1977): Release of neutrophil chemotactic activity during immediate hypersensitivity reactions in humans. *Ann. Intern. Med.*, 86:415–418.
8. Barnes, P., Fitzgerald, G., Brown, M., and Dollery, C. (1980): Nocturnal asthma and changes in circulating epinephrine, histamine and cortisol. *N. Engl. J. Med.*, 303:263–267.
9. Barnett, K., Jacoby, D. B., Lazarus, S. C., and Nadel, J. A. (1987): Bradykinin stimulates release of an epithelial cell product that inhibits smooth muscle contraction. *Am. Rev. Respir. Dis.*, 135:A274 (abstract).
10. Behrens, B. L., Clark, R. A. F., Feldsein, D. L., Presley, D. M., Glezen, L. S., Graves, J. P., and Larsen, G. L. (1985): Comparison of the histopathology of the immediate and late asthmatic and cutaneous responses in a rabbit model. *Chest*, 87:153S–155S.
11. Benveniste, J., Henson, P. M., and Cochrane, C. G. (1972): Leukocyte-dependent histamine release from rabbit platelets: The role of IgE, basophils, and a platelet-activating factor. *J. Exp. Med.*, 136:1356–1377.
12. Bigby, T. D., Goetzl, E. J., and Holtzman, M. J. (1985): Canine tracheal epithelial cells generate leukotriene B₄ in response to calcium ionophore. *Clin. Res.*, 33:76A (abstract).
13. Bigby, T. D., and Holtzman, M. J. (1987): Enhanced 5-lipoxygenase activity in lung macrophages compared to monocytes from normal subjects. *J. Immunol.*, 138:1546–1550.
14. Borgeat, P., and Samuelsson, B. (1979): Arachidonic acid metabolism in polymorphonuclear leukocytes: Effects of ionophore A23187. *Proc. Natl. Acad. Sci. USA*, 76:2148–2152.
15. Borson, D. B., Corrales, R., Varsano, S., Gold, M., Viro, N., Caughey, G., Ramachandran, J., and Nadel, J. A. (1987): Enkephalinase inhibitors potentiate substance P-induced secretion of ³⁵SO₄-macromolecules from ferret trachea. *Exp. Lung Res.*, 12:21–36.
16. Borson, D. B., Malfroy, B., Gold, M., Ramachandran, J., and Nadel, J. A. (1986): Tachykinins inhibit enkephalinase activity from tracheas and lungs of ferrets. *Physiologist*, 29:174 (abstract).
17. Boushey, H. A., Holtzman, M. J., Sheller, J. R., and Nadel, J. A. (1980): State of the art. Bronchial hyperreactivity. *Am. Rev. Respir. Dis.*, 121:389–413.
18. Brain, J. D. (1970): Free cells in the lungs: Some aspects of their role, quantitation, and regulation. *Arch. Intern. Med.*, 126:477–487.
19. Brain, J. D., Gehr, P., and Kavet, R. I. (1984): Airway macrophages. The importance of the fixation method. *Am. Rev. Respir. Dis.*, 129:823–826.
20. Brindley, L. L., Sweet, J. M., and Goetzl, E. J. (1983): Stimulation of histamine release from human basophils by human platelet factor 4. *J. Clin. Invest.*, 72:1218–1223.
21. Bryant, D. H., and Kay, A. B. (1977): Cutaneous eosinophil accumulation in atopic and non-atopic individuals. The effects of ECF-A tetrapeptide and histamine. *Clin. Allergy*, 7:211–217.
22. Butterworth, A. E., Wassom, D. L., Gleich, G. J., Loegering, D. A., and David, J. R. (1979): Damage to schistosomula of *Schistosoma mansoni* induced directly by eosinophil major basic protein. *J. Immunol.*, 122:221–229.
23. Calhoun, W. J., Salisbury, S. M., Bush, R. K., and Busse, W. W. (1987): Increased superoxide release from alveolar macrophages in symptomatic asthma. *Am. Rev. Respir. Dis.*, 135:224A (abstract).
24. Capron, M., Capron, A., Dessaint, J. P., Torpier, G., Johansson, S. G. O., and Prin, L. (1981): Fc receptors for IgE on human and rat eosinophils. *J. Immunol.*, 126:2087–2092.
25. Capron, M., Spiegelberg, H. L., Prin, L., Bennich, H., Butterworth, A. E., Pierce, R. T., Ouaissi, M. A., and Capron, A. (1984): Role of IgE receptors in effector function of human eosinophils. *J. Immunol.*, 132:462–468.
26. Chanez, P., Damon, M., Loubatiere, J., Cluzel, M., Crastes de Paulet, A., Michel, F. B., and Godard, P. (1987): Superoxide anion release by alveolar macrophages stimulated by FMLP from healthy subjects and asthmatics. *Am. Rev. Respir. Dis.*, 135:393A (abstract).
27. Chesnut, R. W. (1985): Macrophage Ia-dependent antigen presentation. In: *Mononuclear Phagocytes: Physiology and Pathology,* edited by R. T. Dean and W. Jessup, pp. 363–379. Elsevier, New York.
28. Chignard, M., Coeffier, E., and Benveniste, J. (1985): Role of PAF-acether and related ether-lipid metabolism in platelets. In: *Advances in Medicine and Biology. Mechanisms of Stimulus Response Coupling in Platelets,* edited by J. Westwick, M. F. Scully, D. D. McIntyre, and V. V. Kakar, pp. 309–326. Plenum Press, New York.
29. Chignard, M., LeCouedic, J. P., Tence, M., Vargaftig, B. B., and Benveniste, J. (1979): The role of platelet-activating factor in platelet aggregation. *Nature*, 279:799–800.
30. Chung, K. F., Aizawa, H., Becker, A. B., Frick, O., Gold, W. M., and Nadel, J. A. (1986): Inhibition of antigen-induced airway hyperresponsiveness by a thromboxane synthetase inhibitor (OKY-046) in allergic dogs. *Am. Rev. Respir. Dis.*, 134:258–261.
31. Chung, K. F., Aizawa, H., Leikauf, G. D., Ueki, I. F., Evans, T. W., and Nadel, J. A. (1986): Airway hyperresponsiveness induced by platelet-activating factor: Role of thromboxane generation. *J. Pharmacol. Exp. Ther.*, 236:580–584.
32. Chung, K. F., Becker, A. B., Lazarus, S. C., Frick, O. L., Nadel, J. A., and Gold, W. M. (1985): Antigen-induced airway hyperresponsiveness and pulmonary inflammation in allergic dogs. *J. Appl. Physiol.*, 58:1347–1353.
33. Chung, K. F., Evans, T. W., Graf, P. D., and Nadel, J. A. (1985): Modulation of cholinergic neurotransmission in canine airways by thromboxane mimetic U46619. *Eur. J. Pharmacol.*, 117:373–375.
34. Clark, R. A. F., Gallin, J. I., and Kaplan, A. P. (1975): The selective eosinophil leukocyte chemotactic activity of histamine. *J. Exp. Med.*, 142:1462–1476.
35. Cockcroft, D. W., Ruffin, R. E., Dolovich, J., and Hargreave, F. E. (1977): Allergen-induced increase in non-allergic bronchial reactivity. *Clin. Allergy*, 7:503–513.
36. Cummings, N. P., Irvin, C. G., Haslett, C., and Henson, P. M. (1984): C5a-des-arg-induced sinusitis in rabbits: Effect of bronchial reactivity to histamine. *Pediatr. Res.*, 18:389A (abstract).
37. Dahlen, S. E., Bjork, J., Hedqvist, D., Arlors, K.-F., Hammarstrom, S., Lindgren, J. A., and Samuelsson, B. (1981): Leukotrienes promote plasma leakage and leukocyte adhesion in post capillary venules. In vivo effects with relevance to the acute inflammatory response. *Proc. Natl. Acad. Sci. USA*, 78:3887–3891.
38. de Monchy, J. G. R., Kauffman, H. F., Venge, P., Koeter, G. H., Jansen, H. M., Sluiter, H. J., and de Vries, K. (1985): Bronchoalveolar eosinophilia during allergen-induced late asthmatic reactions. *Am. Rev. Respir. Dis.*, 131:373–376.
39. Dessein, A. J., Parker, W., James, S. L., and David, J. R. (1981): IgE antibody in resistance to infections. I. Selective suppression of the IgE antibody response in rats diminishes the resistance and the eosinophil response to *Trichinella spiralis* infection. *J. Exp. Med.*, 153:423–436.
40. Diaz, P., Galleguillas, F. R., Gonzales, M. C., Pantin, C. F. A., and

Kay, A. B. (1984): Bronchoalveolar lavage in asthma: The effect of disodium cromoglycate on leukocyte counts, immunoglobulins and complements. *J. Allergy Clin. Immunol.*, 74:41–48.

41. Dierich, M. P., Mussel, H. H., Scheiner, O., Ehlen, T., Burger, R., Peters, H., Schmitt, M., Trepke, S., and Zimmer, G. (1982): Differentiation of C3b receptors on human lymphocytes, phagocytes, erythrocytes, and renal glomerulus cells by monoclonal antibodies. *Immunology*, 45:85–96.

42. Dolovich, J., Hargreave, F. E., Chalmers, R., Shies, K. J., Gauldie, J., and Bienenstock, J. (1973): Late cutaneous allergic responses in isolated IgE-dependent reactions. *J. Allergy Clin. Immunol.*, 52: 38–46.

43. Drazen, J. M., Lewis, R. A., Wasserman, S. I., Orange, R. P., and Austen, K. F. (1979): Differential effects of a partially purified preparation of slow-reacting substance of anaphylaxis on guinea pig tracheal spirals and parenchymal strips. *J. Clin. Invest.*, 63:1–5.

44. Dulfano, M. J., and Ishikawa, S. (1985): Sputum and bronchial asthma. In: *Bronchial Asthma*, edited by E. B. Weiss, M. S. Segal, and M. Stein, pp. 548–561. Little, Brown, Boston.

45. Duncan, B., Scheel, L. D., Fairchild, E. J., Killens, R., and Graham, S. (1962): Toluene diisocyanate inhalation toxicity: Pathology and mortality. *Am. Ind. Hyg. Assoc. J.*, 23:447–456.

46. Dunnill, M. S. (1971): The identification of asthma. In: *Ciba Foundation Symposium*, edited by R. Porter, and J. Birch, pp. 35–46. Churchill, London.

47. Dunnill, M. S., Massarella, G. R., and Anderson, J. A. (1969): Comparison of the quantitative anatomy of the bronchi in normal subjects, in status asthmaticus, in chronic bronchitis, and in emphysema. *Thorax*, 24:176–179.

48. Dyer, E. L., Lefferts, P. L., and Snapper, J. R. (1986): Phorbol myristate acetate lung injury and airway responsiveness to aerosol histamine in awake sheep. *J. Allergy Clin. Immunol.*, 78:44–50.

49. Empey, D. W., Laitinen, L. A., Jacobs, L., Gold, W. M., and Nadel, J. A. (1976): Mechanisms of bronchial hyperreactivity in normal subjects following upper respiratory tract infection. *Am. Rev. Respir. Dis.*, 113:131–139.

50. Fabbri, L. M., Aizawa, H., Alpert, S. E., Walters, E. H., O'Byrne, P. M., Gold, B. D., Nadel, J. A., and Holtzman, M. J. (1984): Airway hyperresponsiveness and changes in cell counts in bronchoalveolar lavage after ozone exposure in dogs. *Am. Rev. Respir. Dis.*, 129:288–291.

51. Felcara, A. B., and Lowell, F. C. (1967): The total eosinophil count in a nonatopic population. *J. Allergy*, 40:16–20.

52. Fels, A. O., Pawlowski, N. A., Cramer, E. B., King, T. K. C., Cohn, Z. A., and Scott, W. A. (1982): Human alveolar macrophages produce leukotriene B₄. *Proc. Natl. Acad. Sci. USA*, 79:7866–7870.

53. Fels, A. O. S., and Cohn, Z. A. (1986): The alveolar macrophage. *J. Appl. Physiol.*, 60:353–369.

54. Fischer, E., Capron, M., Prin, L., Kusnierz, J. P., and Kazatchkive, M. D. (1986): Human eosinophils express CR1 and CR3 complement receptors for cleavage fragments of C3. *Cell. Immunol.*, 97: 297–306.

55. Flavahan, N. A., Aarhus, L. L., Rimele, T. J., and Vanhoutte, P. M. (1985): Respiratory epithelium inhibits bronchial smooth muscle tone. *J. Appl. Physiol.*, 58:834–838.

56. Franklin, W. (1974): Treatment of severe asthma. *N. Engl. J. Med.*, 290:1469–1472.

57. Friedman, M. M., and Kaliner, M. A. (1987): Symposium on mast cells and asthma: Human mast cells and asthma. *Am. Rev. Respir. Dis.*, 135:1157–1164.

58. Frigas, E., Loegering, D. A., and Gleich, G. J. (1980): Cytotoxic effects of the guinea-pig eosinophil major basic protein on tracheal epithelium. *Lab. Invest.*, 42:35–43.

59. Frigas, E., Loegering, D. A., Solley, G. O., Farrow, G. M., and Gleich, G. J. (1981): Elevated levels of the eosinophil granule major basic protein in the sputum of patients with bronchial asthma. *Mayo Clin. Proc.*, 56:345–353.

60. Gleich, G. J. (1977): The eosinophil: New aspects of structure and function. *J. Allergy Clin. Immunol.*, 60:73–82.

61. Gleich, G. J. (1982): The late phase of the immunoglobulin E-mediated reaction: A link between anaphylaxis and common allergic disease? *J. Allergy Clin. Immunol.*, 70:160–169.

62. Gleich, G. J. (1986): The functions of eosinophils. *Annales de l'Institut Pasteur/Immunologie*, 137D:136–140.

63. Gleich, G. J., Loegering, D. A., and Maldonado, J. E. (1973): Identification of a major basic protein in guinea-pig eosinophil granules. *J. Exp. Med.*, 137:1459–1471.

64. Goetzl, E. J., Brash, A. R., Tauber, A. I., Oates, J. A., and Hubbard, W. C. (1980): Modulation of human neutrophil function by monohydroxyeicosatetraenoic acids. *Immunology*, 39:491–501.

65. Goetzl, E. J., Phillips, M. J., and Gold, W. M. (1983): Stimulus specificity of the generation of leukotrienes by dog mastocytoma cells. *J. Exp. Med.*, 158:731–737.

66. Goetzl, E. J., and Pickett, W. C. (1980): The human PMN leukocyte chemotactic activity of complex hydroxy-eicosatetraenoic acids (HETES). *J. Immunol.*, 125:1789–1791.

67. Goetzl, E. J., Weller, P. F., and Valone, F. H. (1979): Biochemical and functional bases of the regulation and protective roles of the human eosinophil. In: *Advances in Immunology*, edited by G. Weissman, B. Samuelsson, and R. Paoletti, pp. 157–167. Raven Press, New York.

68. Goetzl, E. J., Woods, J. M., and Gorman, R. R. (1977): Stimulation of human eosinophil and neutrophil PMN leukocyte chemotaxis and random migration by 12-L-hydroxy-5,8,10,14-eicosatetraenoic acid (HETE). *J. Clin. Invest.*, 59:179–183.

69. Golden, J. A., Nadel, J. A., and Boushey, H. A. (1978): Bronchial hyperirritability in healthy subjects after exposure to ozone. *Am. Rev. Respir. Dis.*, 118:287–294.

70. Goldstein, I. M., Malmsten, C. L., Kindahl, H., Kaplan, H. B., Radmark, O., Samuelsson, B., and Weissmann, G. (1978): Thromboxane generation by human peripheral blood polymorphonuclear leukocytes. *J. Exp. Med.*, 148:787–792.

71. Gordon, T., Sheppard, D., McDonald, D. M., Distefano, S., and Scypinski, L. (1985): Airway hyperresponsiveness and inflammation induced by toluene diisocyanate in guinea pigs. *Am. Rev. Respir. Dis.*, 132:1106–1112.

72. Gosset, P., Tonnel, A. B., Joseph, M., Prin, L., Mallart, A., Charon, J., and Capron, A. (1984): Secretion of a chemotactic factor for neutrophils and eosinophils by alveolar macrophages from asthmatic patients. *J. Allergy Clin. Immunol.*, 74:827–834.

73. Greening, A. P., and Lowrie, D. B. (1983): Extracellular release of hydrogen peroxide by human alveolar macrophages: The relationship to cigarette smoking and lower respiratory tract infections. *Clin. Sci.*, 65:661–664.

74. Gresele, P., Todisco, T., Merante, F., and Nenci, G. G. (1982): Platelet activation and allergic asthma. *N. Engl. J. Med.*, 306:549.

75. Guerzon, G. M., Pare, P. D., Michoud, M. C., and Hogg, J. C. (1979): The number and distribution of mast cells in monkey lungs. *Am. Rev. Respir. Dis.*, 119:59–66.

76. Hamberg, M., Svensson, J., and Samuelsson, B. (1975): Thromboxanes: A new group of biologically active compounds derived from prostaglandin endoperoxides. *Proc. Natl. Acad. Sci. USA*, 72: 2994–2998.

77. Hamberg, M., Svensson, J., Wakabayashi, T., and Samuelsson, B. (1974): Isolation and structure of two prostaglandin endoperoxides that cause platelet aggregation. *Proc. Natl. Acad. Sci. USA*, 71: 345–349.

78. Hansson, A., Serhan, C. N., Haeggstrom, J., Ingelman-Sundberg, M., and Samuelsson, B. (1986): Activation of protein kinase C by lipoxin A and other eicosanoids. Intracellular action of oxygenation products of arachidonic acid. *Biochem. Biophys. Res. Commun.*, 134:1215–1222.

79. Harwell, W. B., Patterson, J. T., Lieberman, P., and Beachey, E. (1973): Platelet aggregation in atopic and normal patients. *J. Allergy Clin. Immunol.*, 51:274–284.

80. Hayes, J. A. (1976): The pathology of bronchial asthma. In: *Bronchial Asthma*, edited by E. B. Weiss and M. S. Segal, pp. 347–381. Little, Brown, Boston.

81. Heffner, J. E., Sahn, S. A., and Repine, J. E. (1987): The role of platelets in the adult respiratory distress syndrome. *Am. Rev. Respir. Dis.*, 135:482–492.

82. Henderson, W. R., Chi, E. Y., and Klebanoff, S. J. (1980): Eosin-

ophil peroxidase-induced mast cell secretion. *J. Exp. Med.,* 152: 265–279.

83. Henderson, W. R., Jorg, A., and Klebanoff, S. J. (1982): Eosinophil peroxidase-mediated inactivation of leukotrienes B_4, C_4, and D_4. *J. Immunol.,* 128:2609–2613.

84. Hinson, J. M., Hutchison, A. A., Brigham, K. L., Meyrick, B. O., and Snapper, J. R. (1984): Effects of granulocyte depletion on pulmonary responsiveness to aerosol histamine. *J. Appl. Physiol.,* 56: 411–417.

85. Holroyde, M. C., Altounyan, R. E. C., Cole, M., Dixon, M., and Elliott, E. V. (1981): Bronchoconstriction produced in man by leukotrienes C and D. *Lancet,* 2:17–18.

86. Holtzman, M. J., Aizawa, H., Nadel, J. A., and Goetzl, E. J. (1983): Selective generation of leukotriene B_4 by tracheal epithelial cells from dogs. *Biochem. Biophys. Res. Commun.,* 114:1071–1076.

87. Holtzman, M. J., Fabbri, L. M., O'Byrne, P. M., Gold, B. D., Aizawa, H., Walters, E. H., Alpert, S. E., and Nadel, J. A. (1983): Importance of airway inflammation for hyperresponsiveness induced by ozone in dogs. *Am. Rev. Respir. Dis.,* 127:686–690.

88. Horn, B. R., Robin, E. D., Theodore, J., and Van Kessel, A. (1975): Total eosinophil counts in the management of bronchial asthma. *N. Engl. J. Med.,* 292:1152–1155.

89. Hubscher, T. (1975): Role of the eosinophil in the allergic reactions. I. EDI—an eosinophil-derived inhibitor of histamine release. *J. Immunol.,* 114:1379–1388.

90. Hulbert, W., Walker, D. C., Jackson, A., and Hogg, J. C. (1981): Airway permeability to horseradish peroxidase in guinea pigs: The repair phase after injury by cigarette smoke. *Am. Rev. Respir. Dis.,* 123:320–326.

91. Hulbert, W. M., McLean, T., and Hogg, J. C. (1985): The effect of acute airway inflammation on bronchial reactivity in guinea pigs. *Am. Rev. Respir. Dis.,* 132:7–11.

92. Hunter, J. A., Finkbeiner, W. E., Nadel, J. A., Goetzl, E. J., and Holtzman, M. J. (1985): Predominant generation of 15-lipoxygenase metabolites of arachidonic acid by epithelial cells from human trachea. *Proc. Natl. Acad. Sci. USA,* 82:4633–4637.

93. Hutchison, A. A., Hinson, J. M., Jr., Brigham, K. L., and Snapper, J. R. (1983): Effect of endotoxin on airway responsiveness to aerosol histamine in sheep. *J. Appl. Physiol.,* 54:1463–1468.

94. Irvin, C. G., Baltopoulos, G., and Henson, P. (1984): Airway hyperreactivity produced by products from phagocytizing neutrophils. *Am. Rev. Respir. Dis.,* 131:278A (abstract).

95. Irvin, C. G., Berend, N., and Henson, P. M. (1986): Airway hyperreactivity and inflammation produced by aerosolization of human C5a-des-arg. *Am. Rev. Respir. Dis.,* 134:777–783.

96. Jacoby, D. B., Ueki, I. F., Loegering, D. A., Gleich, G. J., Widdicombe, J. H., and Nadel, J. A. (1986): Effect of human eosinophil major basic protein on ion transport in canine tracheal epithelium. *Am. Rev. Respir. Dis.,* 133:A212 (abstract).

97. Jacoby, D. B., Ueki, I. F., Widdicombe, J. H., Loegering, D. A., Gleich, G. J., and Nadel, J. A.: Effect of human eosinophil major basic protein on ion transport in dog tracheal epithelium. *Am. Rev. Respir. Dis.* (in press).

98. Johnson, A. R., Ashton, J., Schulz, W. W., and Erdos, E. G. (1985): Neutral metalloendopeptidase in human lung tissue and cultured cells. *Am. Rev. Respir. Dis.,* 132:564–568.

99. Joseph, M., Capron, A., Ameisen, J. C., Capron, M., Vorng, H., Pancre, V., Kusnierz, J. P., and Auriault, C. (1986): The receptor for IgE on blood platelets. *Eur. J. Immunol.,* 16:306–312.

100. Joseph, M., Tonnel, A.-B., Torpier, G., Capron, A., Arnoux, B., and Benveniste, J. (1983): Involvement of immunoglobulin E in the secretory processes of alveolar macrophages from asthmatic patients. *J. Clin. Invest.,* 71:221–230.

101. Jouvin-Marche, E., Ninio, J., Beaurain, G., Tence, M., Niaudet, P., and Benveniste, J. (1984): Biosynthesis of PAF-acether (platelet activating factor). VII. Precursors of PAF-acether and acetyl-transferase activity in human leukocytes. *J. Immunol.,* 133:892–898.

102. Kaliner, M., Marom, Z., Patow, C., and Shelhamer, J. (1984): Human respiratory mucus. *J. Allergy Clin. Immunol.,* 73:318–323.

103. Karas, S. P., Rosse, W. F., and Kurlander, R. J. (1982): Characterization of the IgG-Fc receptor on human platelets. *Blood,* 60: 1272–1282.

104. Karr, R. M., Davies, R. J., Butcher, B. T., Lehrer, S. B., Wilson, M. B., Dharmarajan, V., and Salvaggio, J. E. (1978): Occupational asthma. *J. Allergy Clin. Immunol.,* 61:54–65.

105. Kay, A. B. (1970): Studies on eosinophil leucocyte migration. II. Factors specifically chemotactic for eosinophils and neutrophils generated from guinea-pig serum by antigen-antibody complexes. *Clin. Exp. Immunol.,* 7:723–737.

106. Kay, A. B., and Austen, K. F. (1971): The IgE-mediated release of an eosinophil leukocyte chemotactic factor from human lung. *J. Immunol.,* 107:899–902.

107. Kenny, A. J., Bowes, M. A., Gee, N. S., and Matsas, R. (1985): Endopeptidase-2411: A cell-surface enzyme for metabolizing regulatory peptides. *Biochem. Soc. Trans.,* 13:293–295.

108. Kerr, M. A., and Kenny, A. J. (1974): The purification and specificity of a neutral endopeptidase from rabbit kidney brush border. *Biochem. J.,* 137:477–488.

109. Kim, S. J., Lam, B., Godfrey, H. P., Wong, P. Y.-K., and Kikkawa, Y. (1987): Generation of lipoxins and short-chain aldehydes by rat alveolar macrophages. *Fed. Proc.,* 46:692A (abstract).

110. Kirsch, C. M., Sigal, E., Holtzman, M. J., Nadel, J. A., and Graf, P. D. (1987): An in vivo chemotaxis assay in the dog trachea: Evidence for chemotactic activity of 8S,15S-dihydroxyeicosatetraenoic acid. *Am. Rev. Respir. Dis.,* 135:A315 (abstract).

111. Knauer, K. A., Lichtenstein, L. M., Adkinson, N. F., and Fish, J. E. (1981): Platelet activation during antigen-induced airway reactions in asthmatic subjects. *N. Engl. J. Med.,* 304:1404–1407.

112. Laitinen, L. A., Elkin, R. B., Empey, D. W., Jacobs, L., Mills, J., Gold, W. M., and Nadel, J. A. (1976): Changes in bronchial reactivity after administration of live attenuated influenza virus. *Am. Rev. Respir. Dis.,* 113:194 (abstract).

113. Laitinen, L. A., Heino, M., Laitinen, A., Kava, T., and Haahtela, T. (1985): Damage of the airway epithelium and bronchial reactivity in patients with asthma. *Am. Rev. Respir. Dis.,* 131:599–606.

114. Lambert, H. P., and Stern, H. (1972): Infective factors in exacerbations of bronchitis and asthma. *Br. Med. J.,* 3:323–326.

115. Lee, L.-Y., Bleecker, E. R., and Nadel, J. A. (1977): Effect of ozone on bronchomotor response to inhaled histamine aerosol in dogs. *J. Appl. Physiol.,* 43:626–631.

116. Lee, T. H., Nagakura, T., Walport, M. J., and Kay, A. B. (1981): Identification and partial characterization of an exercise-induced neutrophil chemotactic factor in bronchial asthma. *J. Clin. Invest.,* 69:889–899.

117. Leikauf, G. D., Ueki, I. F., Nadel, J. A., and Widdicombe, J. H. (1985): Bradykinin stimulates Cl secretion and prostaglandin E_2 release by canine tracheal epithelium. *Am. J. Physiol.,* 248:F48–F55.

118. Leikauf, G. D., Ueki, I. F., Widdicombe, J. H., and Nadel, J. A. (1986): Alteration of chloride secretion across canine tracheal epithelium by lipoxygenase products of arachidonic acid. *Am. J. Physiol.,* 250:F47–F53.

119. Lemanske, R. F., Guthman, D. A., Oertel, H., Barr, L., and Kaliner, M. (1983): The biologic activity of mast cell granules. VI. The effect of vinblastine-induced neutropenia of rat cutaneous late phase reactions. *J. Immunol.,* 130:2837–2842.

120. Lewis, D. M., Lewis, J. C., Loegering, D. A., and Gleich, G. J. (1978): Localization of the guinea pig eosinophil major basic protein to the core of the granule. *J. Cell Biol.,* 77:702–713.

121. Lewis, R. A., and Austen, K. F. (1984): The biologically active leukotrienes. Biosynthesis, metabolism, receptors, function and pharmacology. *J. Clin. Invest.,* 73:889–897.

122. Llorens, C., and Schwartz, J.-C. (1981): Enkephalinase activity in rat peripheral organs. *Eur. J. Pharmacol.,* 69:113–116.

123. Lotner, G. Z., Lynch, J. M., Betz, S. J., and Henson, P. M. (1980): Human neutrophil-derived platelet activating factor. *J. Immunol.,* 124:676–684.

124. Lowell, F. C. (1967): Clinical aspects of eosinophilia in atopic disease. *J.A.M.A.,* 202:875–878.

125. Lundberg, J. M., Brodin, E., Hua, X., and Saria, A. (1984): Vascular permeability changes and smooth muscle contraction in relation to capsaicin-sensitive substance P afferents in the guinea-pig. *Acta Physiol. Scand.,* 120:217–227.

126. Lundberg, J. M., Hokfelt, T., Martling, C.-R., Saria, A., and Cuello, S. (1984): Substance P-immunoreactive sensory nerves in the lower

respiratory tract of various animals including man. *Cell Tissue Res.*, 235:251–261.

127. Lundberg, J. M., and Saria, A. (1983): Capsaicin-induced desensitization of airway mucosa to cigarette smoke, mechanical and chemical irritants. *Nature*, 302:251–253.

128. Maccia, C. A., Gallagher, J. S., Ataman, G., Glueck, H. I., Brooks, S. M., and Bernstein, I. L. (1977): Platelet thrombopathy in asthmatic patients with elevated immunoglobulin E. *J. Allergy Clin. Immunol.*, 59:101–108.

129. MacDermot, J., Kelsey, C. R., Waddell, K. A., Richmond, R., Knight, R. K., Cole, P. J., Dollery, C. T., Landon, D. N., and Blair, I. A. (1984): Synthesis of leukotriene B_4 and prostanoids by human alveolar macrophages: Analysis by gas chromatography/mass spectrometry. *Prostaglandins*, 27:163–177.

130. Malfroy, B., and Schwartz, J.-C. (1985): Comparison of dipeptidyl carboxypeptidase and endopeptidase activities in the three enkephalin-hydrolysing metallopeptidases: "Angiotensin-converting enzyme," thermolysin and "enkephalinase." *Biochem. Biophys. Res. Commun.*, 130:372–378.

131. Malmsten, C. L., Palmblad, J., Uden, A. M., Radmark, O., Engstedt, L., and Samuelsson, B. (1980): A highly potent stereospecific factor stimulating migration of polymorphonuclear leukocytes. *Acta Physiol. Scand.*, 110:449–451.

132. Mann, P. R. (1969): An electron microscope study of the relationship between mast cells and eosinophil leukocytes. *J. Pathol.*, 98:182–186.

133. Marsh, W. R., Irvin, C. G., Murphy, K. R., Behrens, B. L., and Larsen, G. L. (1985): Increases in airway reactivity to histamine and inflammatory cells in bronchoalveolar lavage after the late asthmatic response in an animal model. *Am. Rev. Respir. Dis.*, 131:875–879.

134. Martin, T. R., Altman, L. C., Albert, R. K., and Henderson, W. R. (1984): Leukotriene B_4 production by the human alveolar macrophage: A potential mechanism for amplifying inflammation in the lung. *Am. Rev. Respir. Dis.*, 129:106–111.

135. Melewicz, F. M., Kline, L. E., Cohen, A. B., and Spiegelberg, H. L. (1982): Characterization of Fc receptors for IgE on human alveolar macrophage. *Clin. Exp. Immunol.*, 49:364–370.

136. Melewicz, F. M., Zeiger, R. S., Mellon, M. N., O'Connor, R. D., and Spiegelberg, H. L. (1981): Increased IgE-dependent cytotoxicity by blood mononuclear cells of allergic patients. *Clin. Exp. Immunol.*, 43:526–533.

137. Mencia-Huerta, J. M., Lee, C. W., Lee, T. H., Razin, E., Corey, E. J., Lewis, R. A., and Austen, K. F. (1983): Platelet-activating factor (PAF-acether): Generation from a mast cell subclass by an IgE-dependent mechanism. In: *Platelet-Activating Factor*, edited by J. Benveniste and B. Arnoux, pp. 327–334. Elsevier, Amsterdam.

138. Metzger, W. J., Zavala, D., Richerson, H. B., Moseley, P., Iwamota, P., Monick, M., Sjoerdsma, K., and Hunninghake, G. W. (1987): Local allergen challenge and bronchoalveolar lavage of allergic asthmatic lungs. *Am. Rev. Respir. Dis.*, 135:433–440.

139. Murlas, C. G., and Roum, J. H. (1985): Sequence of pathologic changes in the airway mucosa of guinea pigs during ozone-induced bronchial hyperreactivity. *Am. Rev. Respir. Dis.*, 131:314–320.

140. Murphy, K. R., Wilson, M. C., Irvin, C. G., Clezen, L. S., Marsh, W. R., Haslett, C., Henson, P. M., and Larsen, G. L. (1986): The requirement for polymorphonuclear leukocytes in the late asthmatic response and heightened airways reactivity in an animal model. *Am. Rev. Respir. Dis.*, 134:62–68.

141. Nachman, R. L., and Weksler, B. B. (1980): The platelet as an inflammatory cell. In: *Cell Biology of Inflammation*, edited by G. Weissmann, pp. 145–162. Elsevier, New York.

142. Naegel, G. P., Young, R. K., and Reynolds, H. Y. (1984): Receptors for human IgG subclasses on human alveolar macrophages. *Am. Rev. Respir. Dis.*, 129:413–418.

143. Nagy, L., Lee, T. H., and Kay, A. B. (1982): Neutrophil chemotactic activity in antigen-induced late asthmatic reactions. *N. Engl. J. Med.*, 306:497–501.

144. Nakagawara, A., Nathan, C. F., and Cohn, Z. A. (1981): Hydrogen peroxide metabolism in human monocytes during differentiation in vitro. *J. Clin. Invest.*, 68:1243–1252.

145. Neijens, H. J., Raatgeep, R. E., Degenhart, H. J., Duiverman, E. J., and Kerrebijn, K. F. (1984): Altered leukocyte response in

relation to the basic abnormality in children with asthma and bronchial hyperresponsiveness. *Am. Rev. Respir. Dis.*, 130:744–747.

146. O'Byrne, P. M., Aizawa, H., Bethel, R. A., Chung, K. F., Nadel, J. A., and Holtzman, M. J. (1984): Prostaglandin $F_{2\alpha}$ increases responsiveness of pulmonary airways in dogs. *Prostaglandins*, 28:537–543.

147. O'Byrne, P. M., Leikauf, G. D., Aizawa, H., Bethel, R. A., Ueki, I. F., Holtzman, M. J., and Nadel, J. A. (1985): Leukotriene B_4 induces airway hyperresponsiveness in dogs. *J. Appl. Physiol.*, 59:1941–1946.

148. O'Byrne, P. M., Walters, E. H., Aizawa, H., Fabbri, L. M., Holtzman, M. J., and Nadel, J. A. (1984): Indomethacin inhibits the airway hyperresponsiveness but not the neutrophil influx induced by ozone in dogs. *Am. Rev. Respir. Dis.*, 130:220–224.

149. O'Byrne, P. M., Walters, E. H., Gold, B. D., Aizawa, H. A., Fabbri, L. M., Alpert, S. E., Nadel, J. A., and Holtzman, M. J. (1984): Neutrophil depletion inhibits airway hyperresponsiveness induced by ozone exposure. *Am. Rev. Respir. Dis.*, 130:214–219.

150. O'Donnell, M. C., Ackerman, S. J., Gleich, G. J., and Thomas, L. L. (1983): Activation of basophil and mast cell histamine release by eosinophil granule major basic protein. *J. Exp. Med.*, 157:1981–1991.

151. Oertel, H. L., and Kaliner, M. (1981): The biologic activity of mast cell granules. III. Purification of inflammatory factors of anaphylaxis (IFA) responsible for causing late-phase reactions. *J. Immunol.*, 127:1398–1402.

152. Olver, R. E., Davis, B., Marin, M. G., and Nadel, J. A. (1975): Active transport of Na^+ and Cl^- across the canine tracheal epithelium in vitro. *Am. Rev. Respir. Dis.*, 112:811–815.

153. Page, C. P., Paul, W., and Morley, J. (1983): In vivo aggregation of guinea-pig platelets in response to synthetic platelet activating factor (PAF-acether). *Agents Actions*, 13:506–507.

154. Parker, C. W., Huber, M. G., and Baumann, M. L. (1973): Alterations in cyclic AMP metabolism in human bronchial asthma. III. Leukocyte and lymphocyte responses to steroids. *J. Clin. Invest.*, 52:1342–1348.

155. Pauwels, R., Peleman, R., and Van Der Straeten, M. (1986): Airway inflammation and non-allergic bronchial responsiveness. *Eur. J. Respir. Dis.*, 144:137–162.

156. Pernow, B. (1983): Substance P. *Pharmacol. Rev.*, 35:85–141.

157. Pernow, B. (1985): Role of tachykinins in neurogenic inflammation. *J. Immunol.*, 135:812S–815S.

158. Phillips, M. J., Gold, W. M., and Goetzl, E. J. (1983): IgE-dependent and ionophore-induced generation of leukotrienes by dog mastocytoma cells. *J. Immunol.*, 131:906–910.

159. Pinckard, R. M., Halonen, M., Palmer, J. D., Butler, C., Shaw, J. P., and Henson, P. M. (1977): Intravascular aggregation and pulmonary sequestration of platelets during IgE-induced systemic anaphylaxis in the rabbit: Abrogation of lethal anaphylactic shock by platelet depletion. *J. Immunol.*, 119:2185–2193.

160. Pirkle, H., and Carstens, P. (1974): Pulmonary platelet aggregates associated with sudden death in man. *Science*, 185:1062–1064.

161. Reynolds, H. Y., Fulmer, J. D., Kazierowski, J. A., Roberts, W. C., Frank, M. M., and Crystal, R. G. (1977): Analysis of cellular and protein content of bronchoalveolar lavage fluid from patients with idiopathic pulmonary fibrosis and chronic hypersensitivity pneumonitis. *J. Clin. Invest.*, 59:165–175.

162. Roum, J. H., and Murlas, C. (1984): Ozone-induced changes in muscarinic bronchial reactivity by different testing methods. *J. Appl. Physiol.*, 57:1783–1789.

163. Sanerkin, N. G., and Evans, D. M. D. (1965): The sputum in bronchial asthma: Pathognomonic patterns. *J. Pathol. Bacteriol.*, 89:535–541.

164. Scadding, J. G. (1985): Definition and clinical categorization. In: *Bronchial Asthma*, edited by E. B. Weiss, M. S. Segal, and M. Stein, pp. 3–13. Little, Brown, Boston.

165. Scheel, L. D., Dobrogorski, O. J., Mountain, J. T., Svirbely, J. L., and Stokinger, H. E. (1959): Physiologic, biochemical, immunologic, and pathologic changes following ozone exposure. *J. Appl. Physiol.*, 14:67–80.

166. Schneider, R. C., Zapol, W. M., and Carvalho, A. C. (1980): Platelet

consumption and sequestration in severe acute respiratory failure. *Am. Rev. Respir. Dis.,* 122:445–451.

167. Schoettlin, C. E., and Landau, E. (1961): Air pollution and asthmatic attacks in the Los Angeles area. *Public Health Rep.,* 76:545–550.

168. Schulman, E. J., Liu, R. C., Proud, D., MacGlashan, D. W., Lichtenstein, L., and Plaut, M. (1985): Human lung macrophages induce histamine release from basophils and mast cells. *Am. Rev. Respir. Dis.,* 131:230–235.

169. Sekizawa, K., Tamaoki, J., Graf, P. D., Borson, D. B., and Nadel, J. A. Enkephalinase inhibitor potentiates mammalian tachykinin-induced contraction in ferret trachea. *J. Pharmacol. Exp. Ther.* (in press).

170. Sekizawa, K., Tamaoki, J., Nadel, J. A., and Borson, D. B. Enkephalinase inhibitor potentiates substance P- and electrically induced contraction in ferret trachea. *J. Appl. Physiol.* (in press).

171. Seltzer, J., Bigby, B. G., Stulbarg, M., Holtzman, M. J., Nadel, J. A., Ueki, I. F., Leikauf, G. D., Goetzl, E. J., and Boushey, H. A. (1986): O_3-induced change in bronchial reactivity to methacholine and airway inflammation in humans. *J. Appl. Physiol.,* 60:1321–1326.

172. Serhan, C. N., Fridovich, J., Goetzl, E. J., Dunham, P. B., and Weissman, G. (1982): Leukotriene B_4 and phosphatidic acid are calcium ionophores. *J. Biol. Chem.,* 257:4746–4752.

173. Serhan, C. N., Hamberg, M., and Samuelsson, B. (1984): Lipoxins: Novel series of biologically active compounds formed from arachidonic acid in human leukocytes. *Proc. Natl. Acad. Sci. USA,* 81:5335–5339.

174. Serhan, C. N., Nicolaou, K. C., Webber, S. E., Veale, C. A., Dahlen, S. E., Puustinen, T. J., and Samuelsson, B. (1986): Lipoxin A stereochemistry and biosynthesis. *J. Biol. Chem.,* 261:16340–16345.

175. Shak, S., Perez, H. D., and Goldstein, I. M. (1983): A novel dioxygenation product of arachidonic acid possesses potent chemotactic activity for human polymorphonuclear leukocytes. *J. Biol. Chem.,* 258:14948–14953.

176. Shampain, M. P., Behrens, B. L., Larsen, G. L., and Henson, P. M. (1982): An animal model of late pulmonary responses to *Alternaria* challenge. *Am. Rev. Respir. Dis.,* 126:493–498.

177. Sigal, C. E., Valone, F. H., Holtzman, M. J., and Goetzl, E. J. (1987): Preferential human eosinophil chemotactic activity of the platelet activating factor, 1-*o*-hexadecyl-2-acetyl-*sn*-glycerol-3-phosphocholine (AGEPC). *J. Clin. Immunol.,* 7:179–184.

178. Silver, M. J., Smith, J. B., Ingerman, C., and Kocsis, J. J. (1972): Human blood prostaglandins: Formation during clotting. *Prostaglandins,* 1:429–436.

179. Sirois, P., Borgeat, P., Jeanson, A., Roy, S., and Girard, G. (1980): The action of leukotriene B_4 (LTB$_4$) on the lung. *Prostaglandins Med.,* 5:429–444.

180. Skidgel, R. A., Engelbrecht, A., Johnson, A. R., and Erdos, E. G. (1984): Hydrolysis of substance P and neurotensin by converting enzyme and neutral endoproteinase. *Peptides,* 5:769–776.

181. Snyderman, R., and Goetzl, E. J. (1981): Molecular and cellular mechanisms of leukocyte chemotaxis. *Science,* 213:830–837.

182. Solinger, A., Bernstein, I. L., and Gleuck, H. I. (1973): The effect of epinephrine on platelet aggregation in normal and atopic subjects. *J. Allergy Clin. Immunol.,* 51:29–34.

183. Solley, G. O., Gleich, G. J., Jordan, R. E., and Schroeter, A. L. (1976): The late phase of the immediate wheal and flare skin reaction. *J. Clin. Invest.,* 58:408–420.

184. Sorokin, S. P., and Brain, J. D. (1975): Pathways of clearance in mouse lungs exposed to iron oxide aerosols. *Anat. Rec.,* 181:581–626.

185. Storck, H., Hoigne, R., and Koller, F. (1955): Thrombocytes in allergic reactions. *Int. Arch. Allergy,* 6:372–384.

186. Tamaoki, J., Sekizawa, K., Graf, P. D., and Nadel, J. A. (1987): Prostaglandin D_2 increases cholinergic neurotransmission in canine airway smooth muscle. *Fed. Proc.,* 46:650 (abstract).

187. Tamaoki, J., Sekizawa, K., Graf, P. D., and Nadel, J. A. Cholinergic neuromodulation by prostaglandin D_2 in canine airway smooth muscle. *J. Appl. Physiol.* (in press).

188. Tamaoki, J., Sekizawa, K., Osborne, M. L., Ueki, I. F., Graf, P. D., and Nadel, J. A. Platelet aggregation increases cholinergic neurotransmission in canine airways. *J. Appl. Physiol.* (in press).

189. Tannenbaum, S., Oertel, H., Henderson, W., and Kaliner, M. (1980): The biologic activity of mast cell granules. I. Elicitation of inflammatory responses in rat skin. *J. Immunol.,* 125:325–335.

190. Thompson, J. E., Scypinski, L. A., Gordon, T., and Sheppard, D. (1986): Hydroxyurea inhibits airway hyperresponsiveness in guinea pigs by a granulocyte-independent mechanism. *Am. Rev. Respir. Dis.,* 134:1213–1218.

191. Tomioka, M., Ida, S., Shindoh, Y., Ishihara, T., and Takishima, T. (1984): Mast cells in bronchoalveolar lumen of patients with bronchial asthma. *Am. Rev. Respir. Dis.,* 129:1000–1005.

192. Tonnel, A. B., Joseph, M., Gosset, P., Fournier, E., and Capron, A. (1983): Stimulation of alveolar macrophages in asthmatic patients after local provocation test. *Lancet,* 1:1406–1408.

193. Turner, S. R., Tainer, J. A., and Lynn, W. S. (1975): Biogenesis of chemotactic molecules by the arachidonate lipoxygenase system of platelets. *Nature,* 257:680–681.

194. Vanderhoek, J. Y., Tare, N. S., Bailey, J. M., Goldstein, A. L., and Pluznik, D. H. (1982): New role for 15-hydroxyeicosatetraenoic acid. Activator of leukotriene biosynthesis in PT-18 mast/basophil cells. *J. Biol. Chem.,* 257:12191–12195.

195. Vargaftig, B. B., Lefort, J., Chignard, M., and Benveniste, J. (1980): Platelet-activating factor induces a platelet-dependent bronchoconstriction unrelated to the formation of prostaglandin derivatives. *Eur. J. Pharmacol.,* 65:185–192.

196. Varsano, S., Basbaum, C. B., Forsberg, L. S., Borson, D. B., Caughey, G., and Nadel, J. A. (1987): Dog tracheal epithelial cells in culture synthesize sulfated macromolecular glycoconjugates and release them from the cell surface upon exposure to extracellular proteinases. *Exp. Lung Res.,* 13:157–183.

197. Varsano, S., Rosen, S. D., Lazarus, S. C., Gold, W. M., and Nadel, J. A. (1987): Selective adhesion of mast cells to tracheal epithelial cells. *Fed. Proc.,* 46:992 (abstract).

198. Walsh, J. J., Dietlein, L. F., Low, F. N., Burch, G. E., and Mogabgab, W. J. (1961): Bronchotracheal response in human influenza. *Arch. Intern. Med.,* 108:376–382.

199. Walters, E. H., O'Byrne, P. M., Fabbri, L. M., Graf, P. D., Holtzman, M. J., and Nadel, J. A. (1984): Control of neurotransmission by prostaglandins in canine trachealis smooth muscle. *J. Appl. Physiol.,* 57:129–134.

200. Wasserman, S. I., Goetzl, E. J., and Austen, K. F. (1975): Inactivation of human SRS-A by intact eosinophils and by eosinophil arylsulfatase. *J. Allergy Clin. Immunol.,* 55:72A.

201. Weiss, E. B., and Bellino, J. R. (1986): Leukotriene-associated toxic oxygen metabolites induce airway hyperreactivity. *Chest,* 89:709–716.

202. Weiss, S. T., and Speizer, F. E. (1985): Epidemiology of asthma: Risk factors and natural history. In: *Bronchial Asthma,* edited by E. B. Weiss, M. S. Segal, and M. Stein, pp. 14–23. Little, Brown, Boston.

203. Weller, P. F., and Goetzl, E. J. (1980): The human eosinophil. Roles in host defense and tissue injury. *Am. J. Pathol.,* 100:793–820.

204. Weller, P. F., Lee, C. W., Foster, D. W., Corey, E. J., Austen, K. F., and Lewis, R. A. (1983): Generation and metabolism of 5-lipoxygenase pathway leukotrienes by human eosinophils: Predominant production of leukotriene C_4. *Proc. Natl. Acad. Sci. USA,* 80:7626–7630.

205. Welsh, M. J., Widdicombe, J. H., and Nadel, J. A. (1980): Fluid transport across the canine tracheal epithelium. *J. Appl. Physiol.,* 49:905–909.

206. Werb, Z. (1983): How the macrophage regulates its extracellular environment. *Am. J. Anat.,* 166:237–256.

207. White, M. V., and Kaliner, M. A. (1985): Neutrophil induced mast cell degranulation. *J. Allergy Clin. Immunol.,* 75:175A (abstract).

208. Zeiger, R. S., Yurdin, D. L., and Colten, H. R. (1976): Histamine metabolism: II. Cellular and subcellular localization of the catabolic enzymes, histaminase, and histamine methyl transferase, in human leukocytes. *J. Allergy Clin. Immunol.,* 58:172–179.

209. Zheutlin, L. M., Ackerman, S. J., Gleich, G. J., and Thomas, L. L. (1984): Stimulation of basophil and rat mast cell histamine release by eosinophil granule-derived cationic proteins. *J. Immunol.,* 133:2180–2185.

Inflammation: Basic Principles and Clinical Correlates.
Edited by J. I. Gallin, I. M. Goldstein, and R. Snyderman.
Raven Press, Ltd., New York © 1988.

CHAPTER 37

Pemphigus: An Autoantibody-Mediated Dermatosis

Pamela J. Jensen, Shinji Morioka, Koji Hashimoto,
Kay H. Singer, and Gerald S. Lazarus

CLINICAL, HISTOLOGICAL, AND ULTRASTRUCTURAL CHARACTERISTICS OF PEMPHIGUS LESIONS

Pemphigus is an autoimmune dermatosis characterized by loss of epidermal cell adhesion. The disruption in cell-cell adhesion is manifested clinically as severe blistering of the skin and mucous membranes (40). Frequently, even clinically normal-appearing skin adjacent to a lesion can be induced to blister by the application of gentle pressure (Nikolsky sign), indicating that epidermal cohesion can be abnormal even in clinically uninvolved skin. Autoantibodies directed against molecules of the epithelial cell surface (6) clearly mediate the clinical symptoms and histopathology of pemphigus (64).

Microscopic examination of an early pemphigus lesion reveals a split within the plane of the epidermis resulting from loss of intercellular bridges (Fig. 1). Frequently, some epidermal cells will have totally detached and rounded up and will appear in the intraepidermal cleft; these "acantholytic" cells may show some degenerative changes such as peripheral condensation of the cytoplasm. The characteristic histological picture resulting from loss of epidermal cohesion is referred to as "acantholysis" (41).

Two major forms of pemphigus are differentiated on the basis of the specific location of the intraepidermal cleft and their clinical presentations. In pemphigus vulgaris, the split is deep in the epidermis (Fig. 1A), just above the least differentiated, lowest layer of epidermal cells, called basal cells. Pemphigus vulgaris lesions commonly occur on the trunk and intertriginous areas, such as the axillae and groin, as well as in the mucous membranes of both the oral and genital tracts. Small, flaccid bullae that break easily give rise to large denuded areas that may expand around their periphery without further formation of distinct bullae. These erosions can become secondarily infected, and they heal slowly.

In pemphigus foliaceous (Fig. 1B), the intraepidermal split is high in the plane of the epidermis, between the more differentiated cells that comprise the granular layer; acantholytic cells often are present near the floor and roof of the blister. Mucosal lesions are rare. Bullae are small, flaccid, and fragile and produce shallow erosions; frequently, detachment of the epidermis occurs without formation of distinct bullae. Erythema, scaling, and crusting often are present around blisters and in blister-free areas. Pemphigus foliaceous is less severe than pemphigus vulgaris, probably because of the rather superficial nature of the lesions in the former disease.

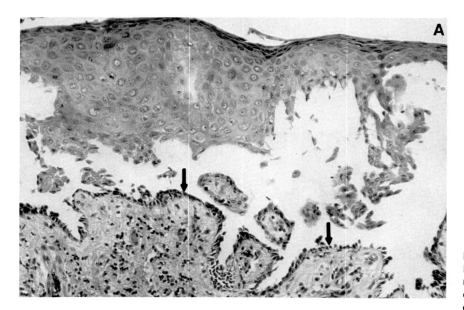

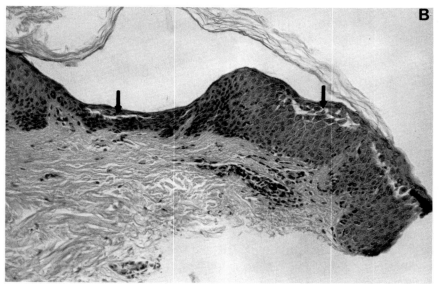

FIG. 1. Histology of pemphigus lesions. Biopsies of involved skin were fixed in formalin and stained with hematoxylin and eosin. **A:** Pemphigus vulgaris lesion. Basal cells (*arrows*) remain attached to the dermal-epidermal junction. ×100. **B:** Pemphigus foliaceous lesion. *Arrows* indicate an early intraepidermal split, initiated high in the epidermis. ×100.

Several variants of pemphigus are also recognized. Pemphigus erythematosus is a localized variant form of pemphigus foliaceous that also has clinical and immunological characteristics of lupus erythematosus. Brazilian pemphigus (pemphigus foliaceous endemicus) is histopathologically indistinguishable from pemphigus foliaceous, but has a unique epidemiology. Its endemic occurrence in parts of South America suggests an arthropod vector, although direct proof of this has not been found. Pemphigus vegetans is a variant of pemphigus vulgaris. Early lesions in these two disorders are identical; however, when pemphigus vegetans lesions heal, they develop hypertrophic, verrucoid granulations (the "vegetations") that become papillomatous and hyperkeratotic.

Studies of early lesions of pemphigus vulgaris at the ultrastructural level revealed that dilatation of the intercellular space and dissolution of the intercellular substance were the earliest recognizable alterations in affected skin (24). Desmosomal plaques, which are regions of close contact and cohesion between epidermal cells, frequently remained intact during the first stages of acantholysis (24). The basal cells remained tightly attached to the basement membrane of the dermis, even when serum exudate filled the intercellular spaces between the basal cells; this distinctive pattern has been compared to a "row of tombstones" (17). As the lesions progressed, tonofilaments began to retract, and the desmosomes eventually disappeared. These findings demonstrate that microscopically and ultrastructurally there is considerable specificity to the loss of cohesion induced by pemphigus autoantibody.

PEMPHIGUS AUTOANTIBODY

Specificity

Biopsies of perilesional skin have revealed the deposition of antibody, primarily of the IgG class, distributed in a characteristic pattern around the plasma membranes of epidermal cells (6). Deposition of IgA and IgM is also sometimes observed, particularly in oral lesions (34,37). In addition, sera from pemphigus patients contain autoantibodies that can bind to normal human or other mammalian stratified squamous epithelium (6,7).

The specificities of vulgaris- and foliaceous-type antibodies differ, although both classes appear to recognize normal epidermal cell surface molecules. Pemphigus vulgaris sera immunoprecipitated a single glycoprotein synthesized by cultured human epidermal cells (66). The glycoprotein had a molecular weight of 210,000 when determined by nonreduced sodium dodecylsulfate/polyacrylamide-gel electrophoresis (SDS-PAGE); under reducing conditions, two chains with molecular weights of 130,000 and 80,000 were formed. Pemphigus foliaceous sera, on the other hand, were more heterogeneous. Six of 13 foliaceous sera tested in one study (39) recognized a desmosomal core glycoprotein called desmoglein I; this molecule was extractable from human epidermis and had a molecular weight of 160,000 when analyzed by SDS-PAGE. None of the vulgaris sera recognized desmoglein I, although one pemphigus foliaceous serum also recognized the pemphigus vulgaris antigen described earlier (66). Reactivity of pemphigus antisera with murine keratinocyte desmosomes was also reported, although the type of pemphigus was not specified (33). Desmosomes are of importance in interepidermal cell adhesion; hence, the finding of reactivity in some foliaceous antibodies for a desmosomal component is most intriguing. In an electron microscopic study of pemphigus foliaceous lesions (76), the earliest change noted was separation of tonofilaments from the desmosomes.

The finding that foliaceous and vulgaris antibodies recognize different molecules is an important step in understanding why the diseases are clinically and histologically different. It has been found that calcium ion concentration (65) and retinoic acid (70) can alter, in a complex way, the expression of pemphigus vulgaris antigen in cultured keratinocytes. This suggests that the levels of expression of the antigens *in vivo* may be modulated by the process of epidermal differentiation. However, only in limited cases have immunofluorescent studies revealed any variation in staining intensity with pemphigus antibodies at

different levels of differentiation of the epidermis. Some foliaceous antisera did preferentially bind to the upper, more differentiated layers of epidermis, precisely where the acantholytic split occurred (9,10). However, most pemphigus sera, whether vulgaris or foliaceous, bound to all layers of epidermis (9,10). It is possible that immunofluorescence is not, in general, sensitive enough to detect subtle differences in the concentrations of pemphigus antigens at different levels of the epidermis. Although it has been clearly shown that the foliaceous and vulgaris antigens are different, further work will be required to understand how this biochemical difference results in the distinct histological and clinical patterns of the two diseases.

Pathogenicity

Several lines of evidence have proved conclusively that pemphigus autoantibodies are pathogenic and directly responsible for the cutaneous lesions observed in the diseases.

The first series of observations came from studies using fragments of whole, normal human skin, which can be maintained in explant culture, without significant degeneration, for approximately 2 days. Early experiments showed that the addition of pemphigus serum to such organ cultures led to the development of acantholytic changes that mimicked the abnormalities characteristic of pemphigus lesions (4,43). The immunoglobulin fraction, specifically IgG, was responsible for the development of the epidermal abnormality (60); importantly, complement was not required and was not detected in the explants (43,60). In explant culture, the location of the intraepidermal split was low in the epidermis when pemphigus vulgaris IgG was added, and high when pemphigus foliaceous IgG was added (25,78), mimicking the pattern observed in patient lesions. Ultrastructurally, the lesions induced in explant culture resembled the patient lesions. The first pathological changes observed were widening of the intercellular spaces and dissolution of the intercellular substance; in the early *in vitro* lesions, many basal cells retained their desmosomal plaques with inserted tonofilaments (2).

Investigations with an animal model also have provided clear evidence for the pathogenicity of pemphigus antibody. When injected with pemphigus vulgaris IgG (1.5–16 mg per gram of body weight per day), neonatal mice developed pemphigus-like lesions within 18 to 72 hr of the first injection (1). Immunofluorescence revealed binding of IgG to lesional and perilesional epidermis. Discrete vesicles, extensive sloughing of the epidermis, and a positive Nikolsky sign were all noted on the animals. Histologically, intraepidermal lesions were observed either immediately above the basal cells or, in animals given very high doses of IgG, immediately below the granular cell layer. Dramatic widening of the intercellular spaces was noted at the electron micrograph level. Interestingly, both noninflammatory and inflammatory lesions (containing many polymorphonuclear leukocytes) were observed, frequently at the same time in the same animal.

Acantholytic lesions were also induced in neonatal mice by injection of IgG (40 mg per gram body weight) from patients with Brazilian pemphigus foliaceous. In contrast to the results with pemphigus vulgaris IgG, intraepidermal clefts developed in the upper, granular layer. Widening of the intercellular spaces between desmosomes was the first ultrastructural change detected, followed by separation and then disappearance of desmosomes. The lower layers of epidermis did not show any alterations (56). Thus, injection of neonatal mice with large doses of pemphigus IgG led to cutaneous alterations that clinically, histologically, and ultrastructurally resembled the human disease.

This model was further exploited in conjunction with studies on purified pemphigus antigen. A molecule that reacted with pemphigus vulgaris antisera was purified from normal human epidermis and injected into a rabbit in order to make a specific antiserum. When large amounts of this rabbit anti-pemphigus-antigen antiserum were injected into neonatal mice, the mice developed lesions that clinically and histologically resembled human pemphigus (52).

The experiments summarized in this section, utilizing both *in vivo* and *in vitro* models, prove the central role of pemphigus autoantibody in the induction of pemphigus lesions. As demonstrated by the *in vitro* studies, complement clearly is not required for initial development of the lesions, although a secondary role for complement should be considered (*vide infra*).

MECHANISM OF LESION INDUCTION

Involvement of a Proteinase

Early experiments by several groups suggested the possibility that pemphigus autoantibody might function by activation of proteinase activity (20,61,62). The general hypothesis suggests that localized increases in activity or concentration of a proteinase lead to cleavage of cell-cell adhesion molecules and hence produce a fragile and disrupted epidermis.

Murine epidermal cells in culture bound pemphigus antibody at their cell surfaces, and the antibody induced detachment of the epidermal cells from their culture plates (20). Most interestingly, the pemphigus-antibody-induced detachment was blocked by addition of a serine proteinase

inhibitor, soybean trypsin inhibitor, or by addition of a general proteinase inhibitor, α_2-macroglobulin. Control experiments demonstrated that complement was not required for detachment, that detachment was not a consequence of cell death, and that the binding of pemphigus IgG to the cell surface was not decreased by soybean trypsin inhibitor (20). These experiments demonstrate that pemphigus IgG can induce dyshesion in tissue culture, and they suggest that a proteolytic enzyme, specifically of the serine proteinase class, may mediate the effect. This view is supported by data obtained from explant culture experiments.

Enhanced proteolytic enzyme activity was observed in the conditioned medium of normal human explant cultures that were incubated with pemphigus IgG. Furthermore, the conditioned medium was able to induce acantholysis in fresh explants, even when totally depleted of remaining IgG (61). Pepstatin A, an inhibitor of carboxyl-type proteinases, or high concentrations of soybean trypsin inhibitor, an inhibitor of serine-type proteinases, were able to prevent pemphigus-IgG-induced acantholysis in organ culture. These reagents did not block binding of pemphigus IgG to the epidermal cells (45).

Plasminogen Activator Involvement in Acantholysis

The concept that pemphigus IgG may exert its pathogenicity through one or more proteolytic enzymes, without the involvement of complement, represents a rather unconventional mode of action for an antibody. However, recent work has suggested a hypothesis that accommodates both the clear pathogenetic role of pemphigus antibody and the involvement of a proteinase in pemphigus. The addition of pemphigus IgG to human epidermal cells in culture induced increased activity of the proteinase plasminogen activator (PA) both in the conditioned medium and in the cell lysate (25). Cycloheximide, at concentrations that blocked protein synthesis by 80%, prevented the pemphigus-IgG-induced PA activation, suggesting that the antibody induced synthesis of PA. The induction of PA by pemphigus IgG was rather specific; neither the lysosomal enzyme cathepsin D nor general protein synthesis was enhanced by addition of pemphigus antibody to epidermal cells.

The mechanism by which pemphigus IgG increases PA in epidermal cells is unclear, but it is intriguing to note that the enzyme induction is not limited to pemphigus antibody nor epidermis. Cell surface antibodies directed against kidney cells (3) and against melanoma (63) cells were also shown to induce enhanced PA activity on binding to their target tissues.

PA is a serine-type proteinase that converts the inactive proenzyme plasminogen into the broad-specificity proteinase plasmin by cleaving a single peptide bond, as reviewed elsewhere (16,53). Because of the high circulating levels of plasminogen and the nonselectivity of plasmin action, the PA/plasmin system represents a supply of proteolytic activity available and adaptable to a wide range of physiological and pathological functions. Historically, the PA/plasmin system has been most extensively studied for its role in fibrinolysis. However, more recent work has demonstrated the rather ubiquitous nature of the enzyme system and suggested many diverse areas of its involvement (16,58).

There are two types of PAs that are products of different genes (18,21,47,51,54) and immunologically are non-cross-reactive (5,55,75). The tissue-type PA plays a critical role in fibrinolysis (13,77) and hence in maintenance of plasma fluidity. This function is reflected by the biochemical finding that tissue PA binds to fibrin (55) and is fully active only in the presence of fibrin (11,28). It is likely that tissue-type PA has physiological roles other than fibrinolysis; recent studies have shown that tissue PA is made by a number of cell types (74,75), including melanoma cells in culture (55), granulosa cells (12), oocytes (29), and endothelial cells (42).

Urokinase-type PA has a very wide distribution and appears to initiate localized extracellular proteolysis for diverse physiological and pathological functions, including mammary gland involution (49), blastocyst implantation (68,69), ovulation (12,67), macrophage migration (73), and metastasis (50). In each of these cases, localized extracellular proteolysis is required during tissue degradation and remodeling and/or migration. A complex regulation system for urokinase yields active enzyme in the appropriate tissue at the required time for each physiological function listed earlier. Regulation of urokinase occurs at many levels: (a) synthesis is hormonally controlled, (b) inactive proenzyme must be converted to active enzyme by proteolytic cleavage, and (c) inhibitors of several types are present in serum and tissues.

Urokinase-type PA is made by a great many cell types (16); it is of particular interest that some cells appear to make both urokinase- and tissue-type PA (42,57,74,75).

The components of the PA/plasmin system are present in human skin. Human epidermal cells in culture, under both control and pemphigus-IgG-stimulated conditions, synthesized urokinase-type PA (25,46). In extracts of normal epidermis, the great majority of the PA activity was also the urokinase type (P. Jensen, *unpublished observations*). Plasminogen was immunocytochemically detectable in the epidermis, with the highest concentration in the basal layers (30). Inhibitors of PA were found in conditioned medium of keratinocyte cultures (8,26) and in low-salt extracts of normal human epidermis (S. Morioka and P. Jensen, *unpublished observations*). The physiological role of epidermal PA is not understood at present,

nor is its regulation defined. The highest level of PA was associated with the more differentiated epidermal cells (31,46). Compatible with this localization is evidence (23) to implicate a role for plasmin in the nuclear dissolution that occurs during terminal differentiation of epidermal cells. In addition, urokinase was immunocytochemically detected in migrating epidermal cells, suggesting a role for the enzyme in the migration of keratinocytes that occurs in the early stages of cutaneous wound healing (46).

The hypothesis that links PA with acantholysis in pemphigus is summarized in Fig. 2. Binding of pemphigus IgG to the surfaces of epidermal cells leads to increased PA; enhanced PA produces localized increases in epidermal plasmin levels. Plasmin cleaves one or more cell-cell adhesion molecules, producing a fragile epidermis that is easily induced to blister.

In testing this hypothesis, experiments in skin explant culture have been informative. As described earlier (45), an inhibitor of serine proteinases, soybean trypsin inhibitor, was able to prevent pemphigus-IgG-induced acantholysis in organ culture. Because soybean trypsin inhibitor blocks many serine proteinases, this finding did not conclusively demonstrate that the PA/plasmin system was involved in acantholysis. An inhibitor that is specific for urokinase, i.e., that does not affect other proteinases, is provided by antiserum made against purified urokinase. Addition of purified antiurokinase IgG along with pemphigus IgG to explant cultures prevented the development of acantholysis (78). Because of the specificity of the antiurokinase IgG, this experiment provides strong evidence for the involvement of PA in pemphigus acantholysis.

Addition of exogenous plasminogen to explant culture was not generally required for pemphigus-IgG-induced acantholysis; however, addition of plasminogen dramat-

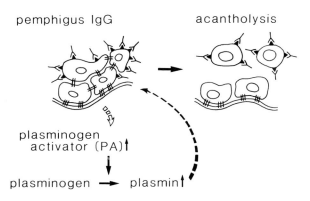

FIG. 2. A model of pemphigus lesion formation. Pemphigus IgG binds to the surfaces of epidermal cells, inducing plasminogen activator. Local high concentrations of plasminogen activator convert plasminogen into plasmin, which cleaves one or more cell surface molecules required for cell-cell adhesion. A fragile and easily disrupted epidermis results.

ically decreased the time of onset and increased the extent of acantholytic damage (25,78). The endogenous stores of plasminogen present in skin may be sufficient to support acantholysis in the absence of additional exogenous plasminogen. High concentrations (200–300 μg/ml) of plasminogen alone, in the absence of any pemphigus IgG, were able to induce foliaceous-like acantholysis in explant culture (78).

Inappropriate, localized activation of the PA/plasmin system thus appears to be pivotal early in the development of the pathological changes characteristic of pemphigus vulgaris and foliaceous.

CUTANEOUS INFLAMMATION IN PEMPHIGUS

In their early stages, pemphigus lesions are most commonly observed with minimal or no accompanying inflammatory response (17,41). Although inflammatory cells are typically sparse in new lesions, a small group of patients was reported in whom a dense eosinophilic infiltrate and intercellular edema preceded obvious acantholytic changes (19). More typically, older acantholytic lesions showed an infiltrate of neutrophils, eosinophils, and lymphocytes.

The role of complement in the development of pemphigus lesions has been controversial. Complement deposition was generally observed in acantholytic areas (14,37,72); however, biopsies from lesions that appeared in patients who were undergoing corticosteroid therapy showed reduced or no detectable complement deposition (15,35). In biopsies taken from clinically normal-appearing skin adjacent to pemphigus lesions, IgG deposits were present, but complement components (C1q, C3, C3 proactivator) could not be detected (37). An important characteristic of pemphigus is that blisters frequently can be elicited on such normal-appearing areas with gentle pressure (Nikolsky sign) (22). These clinical observations are consistent with experimental data showing that pemphigus IgG can induce acantholysis in the absence of complement, and they suggest that acantholytic lesions develop *in vivo* as well without the intervention of complement.

In spite of the fact that pemphigus antibody activity has been found in all four subclasses of IgG (59), the ability of pemphigus antibody to fix complement has been the subject of conflicting reports. Although early findings suggested the contrary (35,59), several groups have now clearly shown that pemphigus IgG can indeed fix complement (27,38,48). Pemphigus sera were found to fix complement components C1q and C4 as well as C3 to epidermis *in vitro,* suggesting classical activation of com-

plement following immune complex formation between pemphigus antibodies and epidermal antigens (27). In addition, purified pemphigus IgG was found to fix complement components C1q, C3, and C4 both in murine epidermal cell monolayer cultures and in human skin organ culture (38).

There is further evidence for activation of complement in pemphigus lesions. Total hemolytic complement was reduced in pemphigus blister fluids when compared with complement levels either in sera from the same patients or in other types of blister fluids (36). Cryoproteins were observed in sera of pemphigus patients with clinically active disease; these abnormal complexes contained complement components C3 and C4 as well as IgG that had pemphigus antibody activity (44). Thus, complement appears to be activated once acantholytic changes begin, and hence is likely to play a role in exacerbation of the primary cutaneous damage in pemphigus.

Complement activation may be responsible for the influx of inflammatory cells that occurs in developing lesions. In the presence of complement, pemphigus antibodies were shown to mediate attachment of polymorphonuclear leukocytes to epidermis *in vitro* (32). Furthermore, a proteinase obtained from human epidermis has been shown to induce polymorphonuclear leukocyte chemotaxis via a complement-mediated mechanism (71). The presence of activated infiltrating cells in the epidermis and dermis of acantholytic lesions may lead to further cutaneous damage.

CONCLUSION

Pemphigus is an autoimmune dermatosis in which autoantibody appears able to induce cutaneous lesions independent of mediators of inflammation such as complement or infiltrating cells. *In vitro* and *in vivo* experiments, as well as clinical and histological observations, support the primary and independent role of antibody in this disease. In epidermal cell culture, pemphigus antibody is able to induce PA, which converts plasminogen into the broad-specificity proteinase plasmin. Experiments in skin explant culture provide strong evidence that PA, through plasmin, mediates the interepidermal cell dyshesion characteristic of pemphigus lesions. Complement components and inflammatory cells are generally present in pemphigus lesions, except at their earliest stages, and hence are likely to play a role in exacerbation of the cutaneous damage.

REFERENCES

1. Anhalt, G. J., Labib, R. S., Voorhees, J. J., Beald, T. F., and Diaz, L. A. (1982): Induction of pemphigus in neonatal mice by passive

transfer of IgG from patients with the disease. *N. Engl. J. Med.,* 306:1189–1196.

2. Barnett, M. L., Buetner, E. H., and Chorzelski, T. P. (1977): Organ culture studies of pemphigus antibodies. II. Ultrastructural comparison between acantholytic changes in vitro and human pemphigus lesions. *J. Invest. Dermatol.,* 68:265–271.

3. Becker, D., Ossowski, L., and Reich, E. (1981): Induction of plasminogen activator synthesis by antibodies. *J. Exp. Med.,* 154:385–396.

4. Bellone, A. G., and Leone, V. (1956): Richerche sull influenza esercitata da sieri di soggetti san o affetti da pemfigo su pelle umana normale a pemfigosa coltivata in vitro. *G. Ital. Dermatol. Sifilol.,* 2:97–109.

5. Bernik, M. B., Wijngaards, G., and Rijken, D. C. (1981): Production by human tissues in culture of immunologically distinct, multiple molecular weight forms of plasminogen activators. *Ann. N.Y. Acad. Sci.,* 370:529–608.

6. Beutner, E. H., and Jordon, R. E. (1964): Demonstration of skin antibodies in sera of pemphigus vulgaris patients by indirect immunofluorescent staining. *Proc. Soc. Exp. Biol. Med.,* 117:505–510.

7. Beutner, E. H., Lever, W. F., Witebsky, E., Jordon, R., and Chertock, B. (1965): Autoantibodies in pemphigus vulgaris. *J.A.M.A.,* 192:682–688.

8. Birkedah-Hansen, H., and Taylor, R. E. (1983): Production of three plasminogen activators and an inhibitor in keratinocyte cultures. *Biochim. Biophys. Acta,* 756:308–318.

9. Bystryn, J. C., Abel, E., and deFeo, C. (1974): Pemphigus foliaceus: Subcorneal intercellular antibodies of unique specificity. *Arch. Dermatol.,* 110:857–861.

10. Bystryn, J. C., and Rodriguez, J. (1978): Absence of intercellular antigens in the deep layers of the epidermis in pemphigus foliaceus. *J. Clin. Invest.,* 61:339–348.

11. Camiolo, S. M., Thorsen, S., and Astrup, T. (1971): Fibrinogenolysis and fibrinolysis with tissue plasminogen activator, urokinase, streptokinase-activated human globulin, and plasmin. *Proc. Soc. Exp. Biol. Med.,* 138:277–280.

12. Canipari, R., and Strickland, S. (1985): Plasminogen activator in the rat ovary. *J. Biol. Chem.,* 260:5121–5125.

13. Collen, D. (1980): On the regulation and control of fibrinolysis. *Thromb. Haemosta.,* 43:77–89.

14. Cormane, R. H., and Chorzelski, T. P. (1967): "Bound" complement in the epidermis of patients with pemphigus vulgaris. *Dermatologica,* 134:463–466.

15. Cram, D. L., and Fukuyama, K. (1972): Immunohistochemistry of ultraviolet-induced pemphigus and pemphigoid lesions. *Arch. Dermatol.,* 106:819–824.

16. Dano, K., Andreasen, P. A., Grondahl-Hansen, J., Kristen, P., Nielsen, L. S., and Skriver, L. (1985): Plasminogen activators, tissue degradation, and cancer. *Adv. Cancer Res.,* 44:139–266.

17. Director, W. (1952): Pemphigus vulgaris: a clinicopathological study. *Arch. Dermatol. Syphilol.,* 65:155–169.

18. Edlund, T., Ny, T., Ranby, M., Heden, L., Palm, G., Holmgren, E., and Josephson, S. (1983): Isolation of cDNA sequences coding for a part of human tissue plasminogen activator. *Proc. Natl. Acad. Sci. USA,* 80:349–352.

19. Emmerson, R. W., and Wilson-Jones, E. (1968): Eosinophilic spongiosis in pemphigus. *Arch. Dermatol.,* 97:252–257.

20. Farb, R. M., Dykes, R., and Lazarus, G. S. (1978): Anti-epidermal-cell-surface pemphigus antibody detaches viable epidermal cells from culture plates by activation of proteinase. *Proc. Natl. Acad. Sci. USA,* 75:459–463.

21. Fisher, R., Waller, E. K., Grossi, G., Thompson, D., Tizard, R., and Schleuning, W.-D. (1985): Isolation and characterization of the human tissue-type plasminogen activator structural gene including its 5' flanking region. *J. Biol. Chem.,* 260:11223–11230.

22. Goodman, H. (1953): Nikolsky sign. *Arch. Dermatol. Syphilol.,* 68:334–335.

23. Green, H. (1977): Terminal differentiation of cultured human epidermal cells. *Cell,* 11:405–416.

24. Hashimoto, K., and Lever, W. F. (1967): An electronmicroscopic study on pemphigus vulgaris of the mouth and the skin with special reference to the intercellular cement. *J. Invest. Dermatol.,* 48:540–552.

25. Hashimoto, K., Shafran, K. M., Webber, P. S., Lazarus, G. S., and Singer, K. H. (1983): Anti-cell surface pemphigus autoantibody stimulates plasminogen activator activity of human epidermal cells. *J. Exp. Med.,* 157:259–272.

26. Hashimoto, K., Katayama, I., and Nishioka, K. (1985): Tissue plasminogen activator inhibitor in the epidermis. *Br. J. Dermatol.,* 113:523–527.

27. Hashimoto, T., Sugiura, M., Kurihara, S., and Nishikawa, T. (1982): In vitro complement activation by intercellular antibodies. *J. Invest. Dermatol.,* 78:316–318.

28. Hoylaerts, M., Rijken, D. S., Lijnen, H. R., and Collen, D. (1982): Kinetics of the activation of plasminogen by human tissue plasminogen activator. *J. Biol. Chem.,* 257:2912–2919.

29. Huarte, J., Belin, D., and Vassalli, J. D. (1985): Plasminogen activator in mouse and rat oocytes: Induction during meiotic maturation. *Cell,* 43:551–558.

30. Isseroff, R. R., and Rifkin, D. B. (1983): Plasminogen is present in the basal layer of the epidermis. *J. Invest. Dermatol.,* 80:297–299.

31. Isseroff, R. R., Fusenig, N. E., and Rifkin, D. B. (1983): Plasminogen activator in differentiating mouse keratinocytes. *J. Invest. Dermatol.,* 80:217–222.

32. Iwatsuki, K., Tagami, H., and Yamada, M. (1983): Pemphigus antibodies mediate the development of an inflammatory change in the epidermis. *Acta Derm. Venereol. (Stockh.),* 63:495–500.

33. Jones, J. C. R., Arnn, J., Staehelin, L. A., and Goldman, R. D. (1984): Human autoantibodies against desmosomes: Possible causative factors in pemphigus. *Proc. Natl. Acad. Sci. USA,* 81:2781–2785.

34. Jordon, R. E. (1971): Direct immunofluorescent studies of pemphigus and bullous pemphigoid. *Arch. Dermatol.,* 103:486–491.

35. Jordon, R. E., Sams, W. M., Jr., Diaz, G., and Beutner, E. H. (1971): Negative complement immunofluorescence in pemphigus. *J. Invest. Dermatol.,* 57:407–410.

36. Jordon, R. E., Day, N. K., Luckasen, J. R., and Good, R. A. (1973): Complement activation in pemphigus vulgaris blister fluid. *Clin. Exp. Immunol.,* 15:53–63.

37. Jordon, R. E., Schroeter, A. L., Rogers, R. S., III, and Perry, H. O. (1974): Classical and alternate pathway activation of complement in pemphigus vulgaris lesions. *J. Invest. Dermatol.,* 63:256–259.

38. Kawana, S., Janson, M., and Jordon, R. E. (1984): Complement fixation by pemphigus antibody. I. In vitro fixation to organ and tissue culture skin. *J. Invest. Dermatol.,* 82:506–510.

39. Koulu, L., Kusumi, A., Steinberg, M. S., Klaus-Kovtun, V., and Stanley, J. R. (1984): Human autoantibodies against a desmosomal core protein in pemphigus foliaceous. *J. Exp. Med.,* 160:1509–1518.

40. Lever, W. F. (1979): Pemphigus and pemphigoid: A review of the advances made since 1964. *J. Am. Acad. Dermatol.,* 1:2–31.

41. Lever, W. F. (1965): *Pemphigus and Pemphigoid.* Charles C Thomas, Springfield, Ill.

42. Levin, E. G., and Loskutoff, D. J. (1982): Cultured bovine endothelial cells produce both urokinase and tissue-type plasminogen activators. *J. Cell Biol.,* 94:631–636.

43. Michel, B., and Ko, C. S. (1977): An organ culture model for the study of pemphigus acantholysis. *Br. J. Dermatol.,* 96:295–302.

44. Miyagawa, S., and Sakamoto, L. (1977): Characterization of cryoprecipitates in pemphigus: Demonstration of pemphigus antibody activity in cryoprecipitates using the immunofluorescent technique. *J. Invest. Dermatol.,* 69:373–375.

45. Morioka, S., Naito, K., and Ogawa, H. (1981): The pathogenic role of pemphigus antibodies and proteinase in epidermal acantholysis. *J. Invest. Dermatol.,* 76:337–341.

46. Morioka, S., Jensen, P. J., and Lazarus, G. S. (1985): Human epidermal plasminogen activator: Characterization, localization, and modulation. *Exp. Cell Res.,* 161:364–372.

47. Nagamine, Y., Pearson, D., Altos, M. S., and Reich, E. (1984): cDNA and gene nucleotide sequence of porcine plasminogen activator. *Nucleic Acids Res.,* 12:9525–9541.

48. Nishikawa, T., Kurihara, S., Harrada, T., Sugawara, M., and Hatano, H. (1977): Capability of fixation of pemphigus antibodies in vitro. *Arch. Dermatol. Res.,* 260:1–6.

49. Ossowski, L., Biegel, D., and Reich, E. (1979): Mammary plasminogen activator: Correlation with involution, hormonal modulation and comparison between normal and neoplastic tissue. *Cell*, 16: 929–940.

50. Ossowski, L., and Reich, E. (1983): Antibodies to plasminogen activator inhibit human tumor metastasis. *Cell*, 35:611–619.

51. Pennica, D., Holmes, W. E., Kohr, W. J., Harkins, R. N., Vehar, G. A., Ward, C. A., Bennett, W. F., Yelverton, E., Seeburg, P. H., Heyneker, H. L., Goeddel, D. V., and Collen, D. (1983): Cloning and expression of human tissue-type plasminogen activator cDNA in *E. coli*. *Nature*, 301:214–221.

52. Peterson, L. L., and Wuepper, K. D. (1984): Isolation and purification of a pemphigus vulgaris antigen from human epidermis. *J. Clin. Invest.*, 73:1113–1120.

53. Reich, E. (1978): Activation of plasminogen: A widespread mechanism for generating localized extracellular proteolysis. In: *Biological Markers of Neoplasia: Basic and Applied Aspects,* edited by R. W. Ruddon. pp. 491–498. Elsevier/North Holland, Amsterdam.

54. Riccio, A., Gormaldi, G., Verde, P., Sebastio, G., Boast, S., and Blasi, F. (1985): The human urokinase-plasminogen activator gene and its promoter. *Nucleic Acids Res.*, 13:2759–2771.

55. Rijken, D. C., and Collen, D. (1981): Purification and characterization of the plasminogen activator secreted by human melanoma cells in culture. *J. Biol. Chem.*, 256:7035–7041.

56. Roscoe, J. T., Diaz, L., Sampaio, S. A. P., Castro, R. M., Labb, R. S., Takahashi, Y., Patel, H., and Anhalt, G. J. (1985): Brazilian pemphigus foliaceous antibodies are pathogenic to BALB/c mice by passive transfer. *J. Invest. Dermatol.*, 85:538–541.

57. Ryan, T. J., Seeger, J. I., Kumar, A., and Dickerman, H. W. (1984): Estradiol preferentially enhances extracellular tissue plasminogen activators of MCF-7 breast cancer cells. *J. Biol. Chem.*, 259:14324–14327.

58. Saksela, O. (1985): Plasminogen activation and regulation of pericellular proteolysis. *Biochim. Biophys. Acta*, 823:35–65.

59. Sams, W. M., and Schur, P. H. (1973): Studies of the antibodies in pemphigoid and pemphigus. *J. Lab. Clin. Med.*, 82:249–254.

60. Schiltz, J. R., and Michel, B. (1976): Production of epidermal acantholysis in normal human skin in vitro by the IgG fraction from pemphigus serum. *J. Invest. Dermatol.*, 67:254–260.

61. Schiltz, J., Michel, B., and Papay, R. (1979): Appearance of "pemphigus acantholysis factor" in human skin cultured with pemphigus antibody. *J. Invest. Dermatol.*, 73:575–581.

62. Singer, K. H., Sawka, N. J., Samowitz, H. R., and Lazarus, G. S. (1980): Proteinase activation: A mechanism for cellular dyshesion in pemphigus. *J. Invest. Dermatol.*, 74:363–367.

63. Singer, K. H., Robertson, A., and Stuhlmiller, G. (1983): Binding of anti-cell surface antibody to human melanoma cells stimulates plasminogen activator. *Clin. Res.*, 31:601A.

64. Singer, K. H., Hashimoto, K., Jensen, P. J., Morioka, S., and Lazarus, G. S. (1985): Pathogenesis of autoimmunity in pemphigus. *Annu. Rev. Immunol.*, 3:87–108.

65. Stanley, J. R., and Yuspa, S. H. (1983): Specific epidermal protein markers are modulated during calcium-induced terminal differentiation. *J. Cell Biol.*, 96:1809–1814.

66. Stanley, J. R., Koulu, L., and Thivolet, C. (1984): Distinction between epidermal antigens binding pemphigus vulgaris and pemphigus foliaceous autoantibodies. *J. Clin. Invest.*, 74:313–320.

67. Strickland, S., and Beers, W. H. (1976): Studies on the role of plasminogen activator in ovulation. *J. Biol. Chem.*, 251:5694–5702.

68. Strickland, S., Reich, E., and Sherman, M. I. (1976): Plasminogen activator in early embryogenesis: Enzyme production by trophoblast and parictal endoderm. *Cell*, 9:231–240.

69. Strickland, S., and Mahdavi, V. (1978): The induction of differentiation in teratocarcinoma stem cells by retinoic acid. *Cell*, 15:393–403.

70. Thivolet, C. H., Hintner, H. H., and Stanley, J. R. (1984): The effect of retinoic acid on the expression of pemphigus and pemphigoid antigens in cultured human keratinocytes. *J. Invest. Dermatol.*, 82: 329–334.

71. Thomas, C. A., Yost, F. J., Jr., Snyderman, R., Hather, V. B., and Lazarus, G. S. (1977): Cellular serine proteinase induces chemotaxis by complement activation. *Nature*, 269:521–522.

72. Van Joost, T. H., Cormane, R. H., and Pondman, K. W. (1972): Direct immunofluorescent study of the skin on occurrence of complement in pemphigus. *Br. J. Dermatol.*, 87:466–474.

73. Vassalli, J. D., Baccino, D., and Belin, D. (1985): A cellular binding site for the M_r 55,000 form of the human plasminogen activator, urokinase. *J. Cell Biol.*, 100:86–92.

74. Vetterlein, D., Young, P. L., Bell, T. E., and Roblin, R. (1979): Immunological characterization of multiple molecular weight forms of human cell plasminogen activators. *J. Biol. Chem.*, 254:575–578.

75. Vetterlein, D., Bell, T. E., Young, P. L., and Roblin, R. (1980): Immunological quantitation and immunoadsorption of urokinase-like plasminogen activators secreted by human cells. *J. Biol. Chem.*, 255:3665–3672.

76. Wilgram, G. F., Caulfield, J. B., and Modaic, E. B. (1964): An electron microscopic study of acantholysis and dyskeratosis in pemphigus foliaceous. *J. Invest. Dermatol.*, 43:287–299.

77. Wiman, B., and Collen, D. (1978): Molecular mechanism of physiological fibrinolysis. *Nature*, 272:549–550.

78. Morioka, S., Lazarus, G. S., and Jensen, P. J. (1987): Involvement of urokinase-type plasminogen activator in acantholysis induced by pemphigus IgG. *J. Invest. Dermatol. (in press)*.

Inflammation: Basic Principles and Clinical Correlates.
Edited by J. I. Gallin, I. M. Goldstein, and R. Snyderman.
Raven Press, Ltd., New York © 1988.

CHAPTER 38

Vasculitis: Mechanisms of Vessel Damage

Paula Kadison and Barton F. Haynes

Pathogenic Immune Complex Formation
Evidence for Pathogenic Immune Complex Formation in
  Specific Human Vasculitis Syndromes
Immediate Hypersensitivity Reactions Mediated by IgE
Direct Antibody-Mediated Vessel and Tissue Damage
Cellular Immune Responses and Granuloma Formation

Vessel Damage or Altered Vessel Function Mediated Directly by Infectious Agents
Tumor-Cell-Mediated Vascular Damage
Disordered Immunoregulation Associated with Vasculitis
  Syndromes
Summary
References

The necrotizing vasculitides are diseases characterized by inflammation and necrosis of blood vessels, resulting in vessel occlusion and ischemic changes in tissues supplied by involved vessels (34,36,48,49,88,131). The clinical spectrum of vasculitis ranges from diseases thought to be primary vasculitis syndromes to diseases associated with underlying conditions such as collagen vascular diseases, infections, or malignancies. Although no single classification system has been able to appropriately categorize every vasculitis syndrome, it is useful to attempt to properly categorize types of vasculitis in order to institute appropriate treatment (Table 1) (49). In general, vasculitis syndromes are thought to be mediated by immunologic mechanisms (29). That immune mechanisms are operative in vasculitis has been suggested from observations in animal models of immune-complex-mediated disease, from immunologic studies in patients with vasculitis, and from the responses of vasculitis patients to various modes of antiinflammatory and immunosuppressive therapy (34).

The goal of this chapter is to provide a survey of mechanisms potentially operative in the pathogenesis of primary vasculitis syndromes (Table 2). Mediators of inflammation necessary for the full expression of immune-mediated vasculitis syndromes, such as activated complement components, prostaglandins, and other soluble factors,

will be alluded to here, but are discussed in depth elsewhere in this volume.

PATHOGENIC IMMUNE COMPLEX FORMATION

The deposition of immune complexes in and around vessel walls is thought to be an important event in the genesis of vasculitis lesions in many of the syndromes listed in Table 1. Studies in animal models of acute serum sickness have demonstrated a series of events that lead to immune-complex-mediated vascular damage (reviewed in ref. 106). Rabbits given a single intravenous injection of bovine serum albumin (BSA) developed necrotizing arteritis and glomerulonephritis, similar to the lesions seen in humans with polyarteritis nodosa (PAN) (64,76). These lesions appeared at 10 to 14 days, the period when circulating immune complexes were being formed in slight antigen excess. Immunofluorescence studies of the affected vessel walls and glomeruli showed the presence of immunoglobulins, BSA, and complement (40). In this model, antigen equilibrated extravascularly during the preimmune phase of antigen elimination (19). When antibodies formed, they reacted with antigen in both the intravascular and extravascular spaces. Intravascular im-

TABLE 1. *Diseases within the spectrum of vasculitis*[a]

Polyarteritis nodosa group of systemic necrotizing vasculitis
    Classic polyarteritis nodosa
    Allergic granulomatosis
    Systemic necrotizing vasculitis "overlap syndrome"

Hypersensitivity vasculitis
    Serum sickness and serum-sickness-like reactions
    Henoch-Schönlein purpura
    Essential mixed cryoglobulinemia with vasculitis
    Vasculitis associated with malignancies
    Vasculitis associated with other primary disorders

Wegener's granulomatosis

Lymphomatoid granulomatosis

Giant cell arteritides
    Temporal arteritis
    Takayasu's arteritis

Thromboangiitis obliterans (Buerger's disease)

Mucocutaneous lymph node syndrome (Kawasaki's syndrome)

Miscellaneous vasculitides (Cogan's syndrome, Behçet's disease, erythema elevatum diutinum)

    [a] Adapted from Fauci et al. (49).

mune complexes were rapidly cleared, whereas extravascular sites of immune complex formation (perivascular spaces) remained targets of immune attack, giving rise to vascular lesions (19). Complement fixation, histamine release, and the presence of neutrophils were important for vascular damage in this model, because depletion of complement or neutrophils, as well as administration of antihistamines, prevented the development of arteritis (26).

In the chronic serum sickness model (antigen injected in daily small doses over weeks to months), the host response was variable (39). Some animals were tolerant to the antigen and made no immune response, whereas others cleared antigen rapidly, and the remainder developed chronic glomerulonephritis without generalized arteritis. In this animal model, antigen was given after antibodies appeared; immune complexes were limited to intravascular spaces, and tissue damage was limited to renal glomeruli (39).

A third animal model of serum sickness was produced by intermittent intravenous injections of protein and was characterized by the development of severe arteritis without glomerulonephritis (65).

Finally, the Arthus reaction is a fourth model of immune-complex-mediated vasculitis (reviewed in ref. 28). In this model, necrotizing vasculitis was seen at the site of locally injected antigen in animals preimmunized with the same antigen. Vessel damage occurred due to reaction of preformed antibody with locally injected antigen in vessel walls (28).

In 1982, Lawley et al. (105) documented the clinical and immunologic features of human serum sickness in patients with aplastic anemia who had received horse antithymocyte globulin. These patients developed fever, skin lesions, arthralgias, gastrointestinal symptoms, and proteinuria 8 to 13 days after initiation of therapy. Similar to observations in animal models, the development of clinical manifestations of serum sickness in humans was related to the formation of immune complexes. Increased levels of serum immune complexes were accompanied by decreases in serum levels of C3 and C4 and increases in serum levels of C3a/C3a-Des-Arg. In indirect immunofluorescence assays, three of five skin biopsies showed immunoglobulin and/or complement deposition in small dermal blood vessels (105).

Both the quantity and quality of the host immune response have been thought to be responsible for the variable vasculitic manifestations of immune complex disease in animal models and humans (19). Specific factors that govern the deposition of immune complexes in vessel walls include (a) physical properties of the immune complex (26), (b) the ability of the immune complex to activate complement (98), and (c) local vasoactive factors that influence vascular permeability (24,25).

Critical factors that determine immune complex size and composition are antigen and antibody valences and the relative and absolute concentrations of antigen and antibody (96). Monovalent and oligovalent antigens bind only one or few antibody molecules and therefore form small immune complexes. In contrast, multivalent antigens bind and cross-link many antibody molecules, forming large lattice-like structures (9). The antigen-antibody combining ratio of immune complexes can vary from antigen excess through equivalence to antibody excess. Immune complexes formed at slight antigen or antibody excess are most pathogenic because of their longevity in the circulation and appropriate size for efficient complement fixation (171).

Antibody affinity, class, and subclass also influence immune complex pathogenicity. IgG1, IgG2, IgG3, and IgM all activate the classic complement pathway efficiently. In contrast, IgG4, IgA, and aggregates of IgE interact with

TABLE 2. *Possible mechanisms of vascular damage in vasculitis syndromes*

1. Pathogenic immune complex formation
2. Immediate hypersensitivity reactions mediated by IgE
3. Direct antibody-mediated vessel or tissue damage
4. Cellular immune responses and granuloma formation
5. Vessel damage or altered vessel function mediated directly by infectious agents
6. Tumor-cell-mediated vessel damage
7. Disordered immunoregulation associated with vasculitis syndromes

the complement system via the alternative pathway (79). The Fc portion of immunoglobulin is important for binding to cellular receptors, as well as for binding complement components. Moreover, immune complex networks can be held together not only by immunoglobulin Fab-region interactions with antigen but also by Fc-Fc immunoglobulin interactions (127).

Interaction of complement components with immune complexes serves two major biologic functions in the clearance of these molecules. First, classic- and alternative-pathway activation normally results in the deposition of many C3b molecules in the complex. Binding of C3b to both antigen and antibody leads to reductions in the antigen-antibody bonds and in Fc-Fc interactions holding the complex together (125). This effect of C3b can in certain circumstances promote immune complex solubilization and diffusion away from the site of formation, thus inhibiting the initiation of a local immune response (157). Second, coating of antigen-antibody complexes with large amounts of C3 fragmentation products (opsonization) facilitates clearance of immune complexes by the mononuclear phagocyte system (168).

Once coated with C3b, immune complexes are normally removed from the circulation in two steps. First, C3b-coated immune complexes bind to specific receptors for C3b (complement receptor type 1, CR-1) on the surfaces of various cell types. Erythrocytes, polymorphonuclear leukocytes, macrophages, B cells, dendritic reticular cells in germinal centers, and glomerular podocytes all express CR-1 in humans (52,151). However, the primary cell type expressing CR-1 intravascularly is the erythrocyte, which normally provides a pool of cells capable of binding large quantities of immune complexes. Binding of C3b-coated immune complexes serves to prevent immune complex interactions with vascular endothelium and also functions to deliver immune complexes to spleen and liver macrophages (30). The CR-1 molecule itself normally can function as an inhibitor of complement activation by serving as a cofactor in the cleavage, and thus inactivation, of C3b (122).

In liver and spleen, macrophages bind immune complexes via CR-1 and Fc receptors, removing the complex from erythrocytes, thereby effecting release of normal red cells back into the circulation. Thus, complement is a major component of an efficient physiologic system that is capable of promoting immune complex elimination via tissue macrophages (157). Failure of this normal complement-dependent system for elimination of immune complexes can occur for several reasons: (a) depletion or deficiency of complement components, (b) failure of various antibody classes within immune complexes to bind complement, (c) depletion or blockade of CR-1, and (d) impairment of tissue macrophage function (157).

The association of various forms of immune complex disease with genetic complement deficiencies has provided the clearest suggestion for the importance of this system. Glomerulonephritis, systemic lupus erythematosus (SLE), and other connective-tissue diseases, some associated with vasculitis, all appear to occur with increased frequency in individuals with inherited complement deficiencies (153).

A defect in CR-1 expression is another possible mechanism of abnormal immune complex clearance. In dermatitis herpetiformis, a genetically associated defect in clearance of opsonized red cells associated with HLA-B8 DRw3 occurs and may predispose toward the development of autoimmune disease (104).

A major factor influencing vascular permeability and enhanced susceptibility to immune-complex-mediated damage is the release of vasoactive soluble mediators. Cochrane and Hawkins demonstrated that immune aggregates injected into animals did not localize subendothelially until histamine was given (27). Mediators derived from mast cells or platelets that increase vascular permeability (directly or indirectly) include histamine, bradykinin, serotonin, leukotrienes, prostaglandins, angiotensin, and platelet-activating factors (45). Both histamine and bradykinins have been shown to induce contraction of vascular endothelial cells, disrupting their close apposition and producing interendothelial gaps through which immune complexes, platelets, and lipoproteins can travel and be trapped against vascular basement membranes (6,118). Leukocyte-produced leukotrienes, as well as histamine, have been shown to be potent inducers of increased vascular permeability in postcapillary venules (72). Local characteristics of vessels themselves also influence immune complex deposition. The focal distribution of vasculitis lesions in animals and humans can be explained partially by structural and hemodynamic differences among various blood vessels and by the tendency of immune complexes to deposit at the branch point of the vessels (66,91).

Fauci et al. (49) and Van Es et al. (176) have outlined the scenario for vascular damage when immune complexes are not cleared by normal mechanisms (Fig. 1). Pathogenic immune complexes can activate complement components that participate in the amplification phases of the inflammatory response via generation of chemotactic factors for polymorphonuclear cells and monocytes (e.g., C3a, C5a). Further activation of complement can lead to assembly of the membrane attack complex (C5–C9), thus effecting cellular damage. Polymorphonuclear cells and monocytes are activated and adhere to endothelium, then extravasate and migrate toward the site of immune complex deposition. Immune complexes associated with vasculitis generally become enmeshed in the basement membranes of affected blood vessels. Such complexes cannot be ingested by leukocytes; yet they stimulate the secretory and respiratory burst activity of

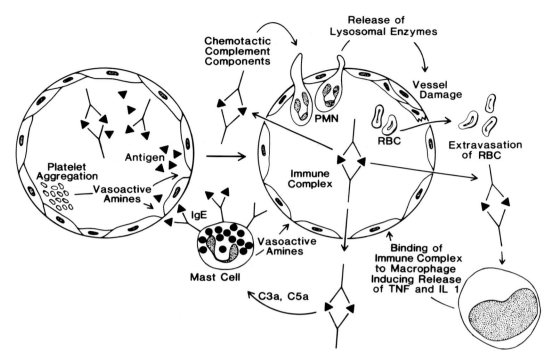

FIG. 1. Mechanisms of immune-complex-mediated vessel damage. Soluble immune complexes formed in antigen excess circulate and are ultimately deposited in blood vessel walls, related to increased vascular permeability at the site of deposition. The increased vascular permeability results from the action of vasoactive amines derived from platelets and IgE-triggered reactions. Immune complexes become trapped, and complement components are activated, some of which are chemotactic for polymorphonuclear leukocytes (PMNs) that migrate in and around the vessel wall. PMNs release their lysosomal enzymes, which damage the blood vessel wall, leading to extravasation of red blood cells and eventual vessel occlusion. Immune complexes also bind to activated macrophages and induce interleukin-1 (IL-1) and tumor necrosis factor (TNF), both factors capable of effecting changes in endothelial cells that may lead to vessel damage. (Adapted from refs. 49 and 176.)

the cells. Further phagocyte activation effects release of proteolytic enzymes, reactive oxygen metabolites, and proinflammatory substances such as platelet-activating factor, leukotrienes, and prostaglandins. Platelets may adhere to locally damaged endothelium and aggregate, obstruct blood vessels, and release more inflammatory mediators, augmenting vessel and tissue necrosis. Thus, the reaction spirals into an amplification cascade, causing damage to vessel walls and other surrounding tissues (49,176).

EVIDENCE FOR PATHOGENIC IMMUNE COMPLEX FORMATION IN SPECIFIC HUMAN VASCULITIS SYNDROMES

In the early 1970s, an association between persistent hepatitis B infection and a systemic necrotizing vasculitis syndrome indistinguishable from classic PAN was noted (69,174). In 1977, the association of essential mixed cryoglobulinemia and vasculitis with hepatitis B was described (111). In hepatitis-B-associated vasculitis, hepatitis B sur-

face antigen is present in circulating and tissue-bound immune complexes (69), strongly suggesting that hepatitis B antigen-antibody immune complexes are causally related to the development of vasculitis. A spectrum of vasculitis syndromes ranging from urticarial vasculitis to systemic necrotizing vasculitis have been associated with hepatitis B infection (37). In addition, tumor antigens (i.e., as seen in hairy cell leukemia) (87), drugs (amphetamines) (23), and infectious serous otitis media have all been associated with PAN syndromes (93,162). In PAN not associated with hepatitis B or other defined antigens, immunoglobulin deposits in vascular lesions have been seen in some, but not all, cases (15,58,107,123,132,138,181). In a recent retrospective study of PAN, immunoglobulin deposition was found in glomeruli and arteries in only a small percentage of cases (150). However, elevated serum immune complexes produced by C1q binding were present in 90% of patients, with serum cryoglobulins being present in 20% and elevated serum rheumatoid factor in 30% (150).

Churg-Strauss syndrome, or allergic angiitis and granulomatosis, was first described in 1950 and can be considered as a clinical subset of systemic necrotizing vasculitis (20,49). This syndrome occurs in patients with a prior history of asthma or other atopic diseases and is characterized by eosinophilia, eosinophilic tissue infiltration of various organs (particularly lung), extravascular granulomas, and necrotizing vasculitis of small arteries and veins (20). Elevated serum IgE levels during the vasculitic phase of the illness are typical (29), and elevated serum levels of IgE-containing immune complexes have been reported (120). In a recent review of this syndrome, 2 of 14 sera contained elevated levels of immune complexes, and study of renal biopsies showed IgM deposits in 4 patients, with C3 deposition in 3 patients and IgA in 1 patient (103).

Circulating and deposited immune complexes frequently have been reported in Wegener's granulomatosis, another form of systemic necrotizing vasculitis (49,84,85,149). Pinching et al. (141) showed that C3, IgM, or IgG was present in a granular pattern in most renal biopsies, with C3 detected in vessel walls. In addition, 16 of 18 patients had elevated serum levels of either or both immune complex and rheumatoid factor. Others have demonstrated IgG, IgA, or IgM in glomeruli in 4 of 11 renal biopsies, with C3 present in 55% of cases (150). In this series, 86% of patients with Wegener's granulomatosis had elevated serum immune complex levels that decreased with immunosuppressive therapy (150). Immunofluorescence studies on lung tissues from patients with Wegener's granulomatosis have demonstrated C3 and IgG deposition in a granular pattern in alveoli, as well as within medium-size pulmonary vessels (163).

Two connective-tissue diseases frequently associated with formation of immune complexes and vasculitis are rheumatoid arthritis (RA) and SLE. The spectrum of rheumatoid vasculitis ranges from a hypersensitivity vasculitis affecting small vessels, resulting in skin and nerve involvement, to a severe systemic necrotizing vasculitis syndrome similar to that seen in classic PAN (2). Patients with RA and vasculitis are more likely to have severe erosive joint disease, hypocomplementemia, circulating cryoglobulins, and low-molecular-weight IgM and IgG rheumatoid factors (146). In RA, elevated serum immune complexes are common, and immunoglobulin and complement deposition have been found in vessels of perineural tissue, rheumatoid nodules, synovium, and skin. Immune deposits have also been found in normal skin of patients with rheumatoid vasculitis (147).

Jorizzo et al. (94) injected histamine into 4 seropositive and 4 seronegative RA patients and performed preinjection and postinjection skin biopsies to study the development of vasculitis. Four hours after histamine injection, all seropositive patients had IgM and complement components present in dermal vessels, and by 24 hr a leukocytoclastic vasculitis was noted. All patients studied had increased circulating immune complexes detected by Raji cell or C1q binding assays prior to histamine injection. In contrast, none of the seronegative RA patients developed cutaneous vasculitis after histamine injection. These studies suggested that potentially pathogenic immune complexes may circulate in seropositive RA patients and that vasoactive amines such as histamine can trigger their deposition in vessels, causing a small-vessel vasculitis (94).

IgM rheumatoid factors have been demonstrated in cryoglobulins in rheumatoid vasculitis, and their levels have been correlated with disease activity (179). Stage and Mannik found that the presence of low-molecular-weight (7S) serum IgM in RA was associated with severe articular disease, rheumatoid nodules, high erythrocyte sedimentation rate, antinuclear antibodies, and rheumatoid vasculitis (166). IgG rheumatoid factors have been shown to occur more frequently and in higher titer in patients with rheumatoid vasculitis and in patients with RA and active extraarticular disease (3). Studies of serum IgG rheumatoid factor (RF) and C4 levels showed that IgG RF levels and anticomplement activity rose, whereas C4 levels fell with clinical relapse and returned to normal during remission (160). In addition, immune complexes containing complement-activating RFs have been found in sera of rheumatoid vasculitis patients (44). Some IgG RFs can form unique immune complexes (cyclic homodimers) with themselves, as well with as with normal IgG, and in doing so activate complement via the classic pathway (121).

Other studies have shown reductions of monocyte CR-1, but not Fc-receptor-mediated phagocytosis, in rheumatoid vasculitis patients, as compared with RA patients without vasculitis (89). Abnormal C3-mediated immune complex clearance in these patients has been correlated with low serum C3 concentrations. Cunningham et al. (33) used C3b-coated autologous erythrocytes to measure CR-1 function *in vivo* in patients with RA with and without vasculitis and found that C3b-mediated clearance was decreased only in rheumatoid vasculitis patients.

In SLE, elevated levels of circulating immune complexes are common, and immune complex deposition can be easily demonstrated in vessels in multiple organs (170). Coronary artery immune complex deposition has recently been described in 2 SLE patients with vasculitis who died of myocardial infarction (99).

In SLE, IgG anti-DNA antibodies have been associated with more severe disease than IgM anti-DNA antibodies (170). SLE vasculitis is more likely to be seen with large immune complexes, whereas smaller immune complexes are found in patients with SLE glomerulonephritis (170). The relevance of elevated serum immune complexes in SLE is strongly suggested by the common occurrence of hypocomplementemia associated with disease activity (170). Patients with SLE have abnormally long clearance times for IgG-coated erythrocytes; patients with higher immune complex levels have greater defects in CR-1 and Fc-receptor-mediated clearance (55,56). There is also a significant correlation between SLE disease activity and the magnitude of immune complex clearance defects (73), although some decrease in CR-1-mediated clearance in SLE may be inherited (182).

Giant cell arteritis (GCA) is another vasculitis syndrome in which immune complex deposition has been implicated in disease pathogenesis (119). Elevated serum IgG, IgA, and IgM have been noted in patients with GCA, and immunofluorescence studies of involved arterial walls have demonstrated deposition of both immunoglobulin and complement (113,136). Using a variety of assays, Espinoza et al. (46) and Park et al. (137) found elevated serum immune complex levels in patients with GCA and/or polymyalgia rheumatica.

Hypersensitivity vasculitis syndromes compose a broad category of diseases whose clinical hallmark is necrotizing arteritis of the skin manifested clinically as palpable purpura or recurrent urticaria (Table 1). Forms of hypersensitivity vasculitis have been associated with connective-tissue diseases, certain medications, malignancies, and infections (165). In hypersensitivity vasculitis, the vascular lesions may remain localized to skin or may involve various organ systems (165). In most forms of hypersensitivity vasculitis, immune complexes have been demonstrated in cutaneous vessels by immunofluorescence and electron microscopic analysis (13,159).

Henoch-Schönlein purpura (HSP) is a form of hypersensitivity vasculitis in which cutaneous palpable purpura is accompanied by arthralgias, nephritis, gastrointestinal bleeding, and abdominal pain (156). In HSP, biopsy of affected skin shows small-vessel vasculitis (60). Immunofluorescence of these lesions reveals granular IgA deposition in vessel walls, with C3, fibrin, and fibrinogen present (67). Immune deposits may be present in uninvolved skin as well (7). Gastrointestinal symptoms result from bowel-wall edema and hemorrhage due to vasculitis, with IgA deposits found in bowel-wall small vessels (167). Characteristic findings in the kidney range from minimal change to diffuse mesangial proliferation, with mesangial deposits of IgA1 predominating (7,100,167). C3, IgG, properdin, and factor B glomerular deposits have also been reported in HSP (45). Approximately 60% of patients with HSP have elevated serum IgA levels. Elevated serum immune complexes containing IgA have been documented in HSP, as have increased numbers of IgA-producing lymphocytes (95,101,175). Finally, many patients with HSP have low total hemolytic complement levels, with decreased alternative-pathway components (62). Both inability of IgA to activate the classic complement pathway and inefficient C3 binding by IgA immune complexes can result in pathogenic immune complex formation and defective C3b-mediated immune complex clearance (157).

Cryoglobulins are immunoglobulins that precipitate from blood at low temperatures. Elevated serum levels of cryoglobulins are found in a wide variety of diseases, in addition to occurring as a primary disorder (14). Type I cryoglobulins are monoclonal immunoglobulins that aggregate to form cryoprecipitates. Type II cryoglobulins consist of monoclonal immunoglobulins that bind to polyclonal IgG, and type III cryoglobulins generally are polyclonal RFs that activate complement via the classic pathway (115). In general, type I cryoprecipitates aggregate on a nonimmune basis and mediate vessel damage by complement activation via the alternative pathway (115). The clinical syndromes produced by type I cryoprecipitates usually are hyperviscosity syndromes, or less commonly a hypersensitivity vasculitis (115). The most common type of cryoglobulinemia associated with systemic vasculitis is the mixed (type III) variety that produces the distinctive mixed cryoglobulin-purpura-nephritis-vasculitis syndrome (70,124). Cryoglobulins can also directly stimulate the release of polymorphonuclear leukocyte lysosomal enzymes. Cold-induced cutaneous PAN has been described with a mixed cryoglobulin complex containing hepatitis B surface antigen and IgG, IgA, IgM, and C3. *In vitro* studies demonstrated that these immune complexes could be phagocytized by polymorphonuclear cells, resulting in release of lysosomal enzymes (139).

IMMEDIATE HYPERSENSITIVITY REACTIONS MEDIATED BY IgE

Immediate-hypersensitivity-type immune reactions may also be important in the pathogenesis of some of the vasculitis syndromes. In addition to playing a role in IgM, IgG, and IgA immune-complex-mediated vasculitic lesions via triggering release of soluble mediators from mast cells and basophils (*vide supra*), IgE in immune complexes has been postulated to directly mediate vascular damage. Frayha and associates have described 2 patients with trichinosis who developed a systemic necrotizing vasculitis similar to PAN and had elevated serum IgE and serum immune complex levels (57). Phanuphak and Kohler reported 6 patients who developed PAN after a course of allergic hyposensitization (140). In these patients, elevated serum immune complexes and hypocomplementemia were commonly present. These authors postulated that a combination of heightened reactivity to protein antigens with IgE-mediated release of vasoactive amines may have triggered the PAN syndrome (140). Finally, 5 patients with Churg-Strauss syndrome have been reported who had IgE-containing serum immune complexes (120). Although serum C3d levels were increased, C1q binding was negative, suggesting that complement activation by IgE immune complexes occurred in these patients via the alternative pathway (120).

DIRECT ANTIBODY-MEDIATED VESSEL AND TISSUE DAMAGE

Cytotoxic antibody reactions are important clinically in the syndromes of hemolytic transfusion reactions, juvenile-onset diabetes mellitus, and Goodpasture's syndrome (79). That direct antibody-mediated vascular damage occurs in vasculitis syndromes is only speculative; however, endothelial cells possess characteristics that make them participants in, and potential targets of, immune injury (8). Endothelial cells can replace macrophages as antigen-presenting cells (82) and are capable of stimulating allogeneic T-cell activation (81). Endothelial cells express ABO, HLA class I, HLA class II, and endothelial-cell-specific antigens, with the quantity of HLA class II antigens expressed varying according to vessel location and the degree of local inflammatory response (83,161).

Tissue injury itself may modify the expression of endothelial antigens, making vascular endothelial cells more susceptible to immune-mediated damage (8). Gamma-interferon induces endothelial cell major histocompatibility complex (MHC) class II molecule expression during viral infections, and transferrin receptors [recognized on target cells by natural killer (NK) cells] can be expressed during endothelial cell growth or after vessel injury (8).

Cines et al. (22) have reported complement-fixing antiendothelial cell antibodies in patients with active SLE (22). Furthermore, endothelial cells in culture with IgG from SLE sera separated and assumed a rounded appearance, indicating endothelial cell injury. Cells treated in this manner also exhibited increased prostaglandin I_2 secretion and abnormally bound platelets in vitro (22).

In addition, IgM serum antibodies that are cytotoxic for gamma-interferon-treated vascular endothelial cells have been described in the acute phase of mucocutaneous lymph node syndrome (110).

A recently described marker for vasculitic disease activity is the presence of serum cold-reacting lymphocytotoxic antibodies (145). Serum from patients with Wegener's granulomatosis, PAN, GCA, Churg-Strauss syndrome, and forms of cutaneous vasculitis have been found to contain IgM antibodies that are cytotoxic for B and T cells. Moreover, the presence of these antibodies has correlated with vasculitic disease activity (145). Whether or not these antibodies play a pathogenic role in vessel damage in these syndromes is unknown.

Autoantibodies against neutrophils (184), as well as anti-Ro and anti-La antibodies (5) in Wegener's granulomatosis, have recently generated interest as diagnostic tools and as markers of disease activity. The relationship of these antibodies to disease pathogenesis is unclear. However, intravascular lysis of polymorphonuclear cells in Wegener's granulomatosis vasculitic lesions has been described (42).

CELLULAR IMMUNE RESPONSES AND GRANULOMA FORMATION

It is clear that immune complexes can mediate vascular injury. However, cellular immune mechanisms may also initiate and/or perpetuate the formation of vasculitic lesions (reviewed in refs. 34, 48, and 49). Cell-mediated immunity may occur via antigen interaction with sensitized T lymphocytes, followed by amplification of the immune response by soluble mediators such as interleukin-1 (IL-1) and macrophage inhibitory factor (MIF). Recruitment and activation of other T cells and macrophages, with T-cell production of gamma-interferon (178), can lead to granuloma formation. These mechanisms may be responsible for the mononuclear infiltration seen in some types of cutaneous vasculitis (165) and may explain the presence of granulomata in diseases also associated with circulating and deposited immune complexes (Fig. 2) (34,49).

Several animal models have recently been developed for investigation of cell-mediated mechanisms of vascular damage. Of interest are studies in mice in which systemic vasculitis was produced by injection of animals with syngeneic T cells sensitized in vitro to cultured vascular smooth-muscle cells (74); 20% of animals developed granulomatous inflammation of the pulmonary arterioles, with both Lyt-1$^+$ (helper) and Lyt-2,3$^+$ (suppressor, cytotoxic) cells present (74). Moyer and Reinisch studied immune-complex-mediated vasculitis in MRL/lpr mice and found evidence for T-cell-mediated vascular damage in this model as well (129).

Winkleman et al. (183) examined skin biopsy specimens from 4 patients with forms of cutaneous granulomatous vasculitis and found that CD4 (T4$^+$) T lymphocytes were consistently found around inflamed vessel walls. Gephardt et al. (63) performed phenotypic analysis of pulmonary infiltrates in a patient with Wegener's granulomatosis. Monocytes and T lymphocytes composed the majority of cells in the vascular infiltrates, with both CD4 (T4$^+$) and CD8 (T8$^+$) T cells present. Ten Berge et al. (169) found normal circulating T-cell subsets and functional lymphocyte reactivity in vitro in 12 patients with Wegener's granulomatosis. Renal biopsy specimens from these patients obtained prior to initiation of therapy revealed cellular infiltrates consisting predominantly of T cells, with a CD4(T4)-to-CD8(T8) ratio of 5:1. Ten to 40% of infiltrating mononuclear cells were monocytes (169). A similar distribution of T-lymphocyte subtypes has been seen in cutaneous mononuclear cell infiltrates in classic delayed-type hypersensitivity lesions (180), in RA synovial lesions (102), and in drug-induced lupus nephritis (31).

Efforts to elucidate the nature of the immunologic disorder in GCA or temporal arteritis have included study of the cellular immune response to arterial-wall components (92,134). Studies of temporal artery biopsies have

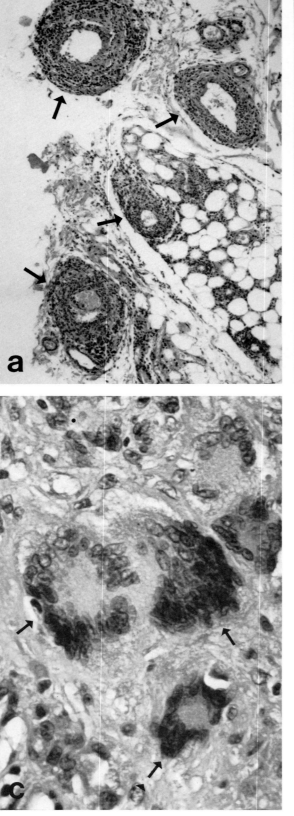

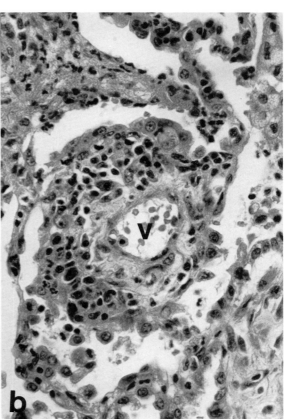

FIG. 2. Granulomatous vasculitis in Wegener's granulomatosis. Panel **a** shows local granulomatous vasculitis (*arrows*) of medium-size muscular arteries from biopsy of an orbital mass. ×70. Panel **b** shows vasculitis of a pulmonary artery (v). ×100. Panel **c** shows multinucleated giant cells within a Wegener's granulomatosis lung biopsy (*arrows*). ×700.

demonstrated few B lymphocytes and approximately equal numbers of CD4 (T4$^+$) and CD8 (T8$^+$) lymphocytes (18). Only 25% of temporal artery biopsies have shown IgM or IgG in endothelial or intimal vessel layers by immunofluorescence assay (18).

Finally, macrophages may be directly involved in inducing vascular damage, either via direct cell cytotoxicity or via the production of IL-1 (38) and tumor necrosis factor (TNF) (17). IL-1 and TNF have been shown to cause normally "anticoagulant" endothelial cells to become "procoagulant" via induction of expression of endothelial cell activation antigens (11). Induction of expression of these endothelial antigens by TNF and IL-1 is associated with increased platelet, mononuclear cell, and PMN adherence to endothelial cells, an important event that could lead to vessel inflammation and occlusion (12,16,61,128,142,143).

VESSEL DAMAGE OR ALTERED VESSEL FUNCTION MEDIATED DIRECTLY BY INFECTIOUS AGENTS

In theory, any infectious agent (or antigen) that induces an immune response could cause vasculitis. Possible mechanisms of vascular damage caused by infections are (a) the presence of the organism in the vessel by direct invasion or embolization, with resultant inflammatory response, (b) immune complex formation and deposition, (c) induction of cytotoxic antiendothelial cell antibodies, (d) induction of aberrant-cell-mediated immune reactions, and (e) toxin-induced vascular damage.

For instance, herpesvirus infections, including varicella zoster, herpes simplex (HSV), and cytomegalovirus, have been described associated with arteritis in the presence or absence of lymphoproliferative disease (34,41,75,97). Viral inclusion bodies in or near vessels have been described in many of these cases (148). Cines et al. (21) showed that HSV-1 infection of human endothelial cells resulted in expression of C3b and Fc receptors by those cells. Glycoproteins of HSV-1 can function as Fc receptors for immunoglobulin and receptors for C3b on the surfaces of HSV-1-infected cells (59,135), possibly promoting the binding of immune complexes to endothelial cells.

Mycoplasma pneumoniae infections in humans can cause disease in sites distant from the lungs, and cases of meningoencephalitis with vasculitis have been reported (43,53,54). Two animal models of *Mycoplasma* infection, *Mycoplasma neurolyticum* in mice and *Mycoplasma gallisepticum* in turkeys, have been reported that are associated with forms of vasculitis (172,173). In both of these animal models, vascular inflammation was caused by *Mycoplasma* production of substances toxic for vascular endothelium (172,173).

Vasculitis involving small arterioles is characteristic of rickettsial infections such as Rocky Mountain spotted fever. Endothelial cells are the primary targets of rickettsial infection, leading to mural thrombus formation, vessel occlusion, and mononuclear cell perivascular infiltrations (177).

Finally, the human retrovirus HTLV-1 has been shown to infect human endothelial cells *in vitro* (86) and likely explains the clinical syndrome of cutaneous lymphomatous vasculitis seen associated with HTLV-1-induced T-cell leukemia (Fig. 3) (77).

TUMOR-CELL-MEDIATED VASCULAR DAMAGE

Many vasculitis syndromes have been described in association with various malignant diseases (reviewed in ref. 34). These include the association of PAN with hairy cell leukemia (87), granulomatous vasculitis associated with Hodgkin's disease (34), and various forms of hypersensitivity vasculitis associated with a wide spectum of malignant disease types (155). The pathophysiology of most vasculitis syndromes associated with malignancies has been related to the formation of immune complexes containing tumor-associated antigens (4,80). However, in some malignant diseases associated with vasculitis, tumor cells have a predilection for direct invasion of vessel walls, thereby causing vessel damage. This type of vascular damage occurs in mycosis fungoides (71), HTLV-1-associated T-cell leukemia (77), and the premalignant syndrome of lymphomatoid granulomatosis (LyG) (51). The latter is a disease characterized by infiltration of various organs with a polymorphic cellular infiltrate of lymphoid and plasmacytoid cells, together with an angiocentric, angiodestructive pattern of inflammation (51,114). The disease has characteristics of both a primary vasculitis and a lymphoproliferative disease and evolves into a T-cell lymphoma in approximately 50% of cases (Fig. 4) (51).

Finally, a systemic vasculitis syndrome can occur associated with a cardiac left atrial myxoma, with embolization of tumor from the primary source to distal arteries and subsequent invasion of vessels by the malignant myxoma cells (90).

DISORDERED IMMUNOREGULATION ASSOCIATED WITH VASCULITIS SYNDROMES

Although vessel inflammation leading to vasculitis syndromes most often occurs via immune mechanisms, the precise immunoregulatory abnormalities that lead to B- and T-cell hypersensitivity are poorly understood in humans. Although it is clear that immune abnormalities

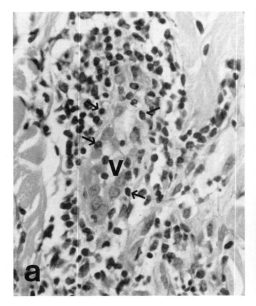

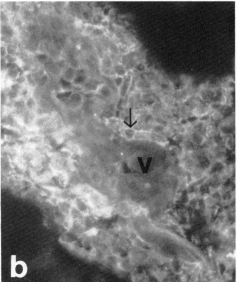

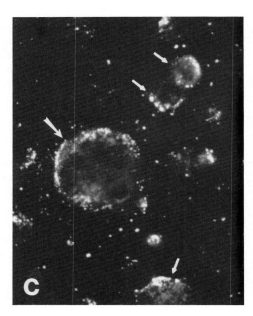

FIG. 3. HTLV-I-associated adult T-cell lymphoma/leukemia (ATL). **a:** Dermal infiltrating malignant T cells in a skin biopsy from patient with HTLV-I-associated ATL, with a vessel shown (v) with invading ATL cells (*arrows*). ×280. **b:** Indirect immunofluorescence of the skin lesion shown in panel a demonstrating reactivity of the malignant cells with an antibody against the T-cell-receptor-associated CD3(T3) antigens (v shows a vessel, and *arrow* points to malignant ATL cells in and around vessel wall). ×280. Panel **c** demonstrates identification of HTLV-I-infected T cells grown *in vitro* using an anti-HTLV-I p19 gag protein monoclonal antibody in indirect immunofluorescence assay. Arrows show HTLV-I+ small T cells and a large HTLV-I-infected multinucleated giant cell. ×280. Panels A and B from Haynes, B. F., Miller, S. E., Palker, T. J., et al. (1983). Identification of human T cell leukemia virus in a Japanese patient with adult T cell leukemia and cutaneous lymphomatous vasculitis. *Proc. Natl. Acad. Sci. (USA)*, 80:2054–2058.

can be identified in autoimmune diseases associated with vasculitis, it is not known if these abnormalities are primary and lead to immune-system hyperreactivity or are secondary and result from normal immune-system triggering by infectious or other unknown stimuli.

For example, in HSP (10), SLE (50), and rheumatoid vasculitis (1), mitogen-activated suppressor T-cell function has been found to be reduced or absent. In some studies, reduction in the number of suppressor T cells correlated with the presence of circulating anti-T-cell antibodies (154). In mucocutaneous lymph node syndrome, there is a relative decrease in circulating CD8 (T8$^+$) (suppressor) cells and an increase in CD4 (T4$^+$) (helper) cells that are associated with an increase in circulating immunoglobulin-secreting B cells (108,109). Similar observations have been made in human SLE and RA and in extensive studies of SLE-like syndromes in NZB mice (reviewed in ref. 185).

Current models of the genesis of autoimmune diseases suggest that genetically susceptible individuals prone to hyperreactive B- and T-cell responses develop clinical autoimmune disease when the immune system is stimulated by a variety of precipitating factors that could be infectious agents, drugs, tumor antigens, or environmental antigens (158). Even if disordered immunoregulatory events are

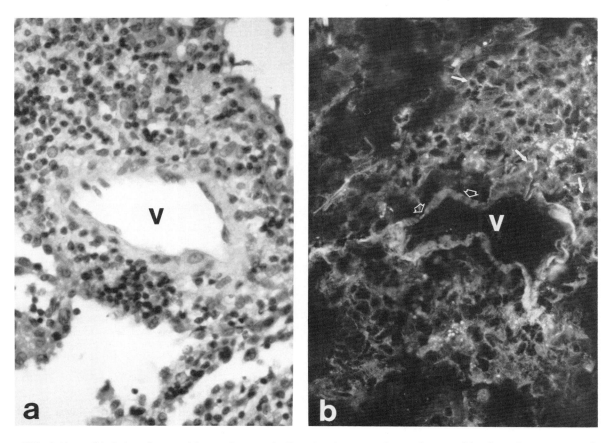

FIG. 4. Vasculitis in lymphomatoid granulomatosis. Panel **a** shows angiocentric vasculitis of a pulmonary vessel (v), with a lymphoid infiltrate. Panel **b** shows the cells to be primarily CD3(T3)+ T cells (*arrows*) in indirect immunofluorescence assay (v identifies vessel lumen; *open arrows* point out autofluorescent elastic lamina of vessel). ×280.

not primarily associated with the development of immune-mediated vascular lesions, they may well be important in maintaining ongoing pathologic immune responses. Thus, the development of ways to specifically abrogate pathologic immune responses would be of enormous importance for the development of safer and more effective therapies for vasculitis syndromes.

SUMMARY

Although a number of discrete mechanisms of vascular damage have been reviewed in this chapter, it is clear that in most clinical forms of vasculitis, multiple pathogenic mechanisms can occur simultaneously. Recognition of the types of pathogenic mechanisms present in a given clinical syndrome is important and can lead to the institution of appropriate therapy. Categorization of patients into one of the disease categories listed in Table 1 is likewise important. However, in many vasculitis syndromes, there is considerable overlap in clinical manifestations,

thus preventing precise disease categorization. In these cases, delineation of the extent of disease and determination of pathogenic mechanisms involved are critical steps toward determining appropriate therapeutic strategies (reviewed in ref. 78). Further clarification at the cellular and molecular levels of the events that can lead to vascular damage should allow for future development of specific treatments for each of these clinical syndromes.

REFERENCES

1. Abe, T., Takeuchi, I., Koide, J., Hosono, O., Homm, M., Morimoto, C., and Yokohari, R. (1984): Suppressor T cell function in patients with rheumatoid arthritis complicated by vasculitis. *Arthritis Rheum.*, 27:752–759.
2. Abel, T., Andrews, B., Cunningham, P., Brunner, C., Davis, J., and Horwitz, D. (1980): Rheumatoid vasculitis: Effect of cyclophosphamide on the clinical course and levels of circulating immune complexes. *Ann. Rheum. Dis.*, 93:407–413.
3. Allen, C., Elson, C., Scott, D. G. I., Bacon, P. A., and Bucknall, R. C. (1981): IgG antiglobulins in rheumatoid arthritis and other arthritides: Relationship with clinical features and other parameters. *Ann. Rheum. Dis.*, 93:127–131.

4. Ambrose, K. R., Anderson, N., and Coggin, J. (1971): Cytostatic antibody and SV40 tumor immunity in hamsters. *Nature,* 233:321–324.

5. Andrassy, K., Darai, G., Koderisch, J., and Riza, E. (1983): Anti-Ro antibodies in Wegener's granulomatosis. *Klin. Wochenschr.,* 61:873–875.

6. Arfors, K., Rutili, G., and Svensjo, E. (1979): Microvascular transport of macromolecules in normal and inflammatory conditions. *Acta Physiol. Scand.,* 463:93–103.

7. Baart de la Faille-Kuyser, E., Kater, L., and Kuitjten, R. (1976): Occurrence of IgA deposits in clinically normal skin of patients with renal disease. *Kidney Int.,* 9:424–429.

8. Bacon, P. A. (1985): Evolving concepts in vasculitis. *Q. J. Med.,* 57:609–610.

9. Barnett, E., Knutsen, D., Abrass, C., Chia, D., Young, L., and Liebling, M. (1979): Circulating immune complexes: Their immunochemistry, detection and importance. *Ann. Intern. Med.,* 91:430–440.

10. Beale, M., Nash, G., Bertovich, J., and MacDermott, R. (1982): Similar disturbances in B cell activity and regulatory T cell function on Henoch-Schönlein purpura and systemic lupus erythematosus. *J. Immunol.,* 128:486–491.

11. Bevilacqua, M., Pober, J., Majeau, G., Cotran, R., and Gimbrone, M. (1984): Interleukin-1 induces biosynthesis and cell surface expression of procoagulant activity in human vascular endothelial cells. *J. Exp. Med.,* 160:618–623.

12. Bevilacqua, M., Pober, J., Wheeler, M., Cotran, R., and Gimbrone, M. (1985): Interleukin-1 acts on cultured human vascular endothelium to increase the adhesion of polymorphonuclear leukocytes, monocytes, and related leukocyte cell lines. *J. Clin. Invest.,* 76:2003–2011.

13. Braverman, I., and Yen, A. (1975): Demonstration of complexes in spontaneous and histamine induced lesions and in normal skin of patients with leukocytoclastic angiitis. *J. Invest. Dermatol.,* 64:105–112.

14. Brouet, J., Clauvel, J., Damon, F., Klein, M., and Seligmann, M. (1974): Biological and clinical significance of cryoglobulins: A report of 86 cases. *Am. J. Med.,* 57:775–787.

15. Burkholder, P. (1968): Immunology and immunohistopathology of renal diseases. In: *The Structural Basis of Renal Disease,* edited by E. L. Becker, p. 211. Harper & Row, New York.

16. Cavender, D., Haskard, D., Joseph, B., and Ziff, M. (1986): Interleukin-1 increases the binding of human B and T lymphocytes to endothelial cell monolayers. *J. Immunol.,* 136:203–207.

17. Cerami, A., and Beutler, B. (1986): Cachectin and tumor necrosis factor as two sides of the same biological coin. *Nature,* 320:582–588.

18. Chess, J., Daniel, M., Bhan, A., Paluk, E., Robinson, N., Collins, B., and Kaynor, B. (1983): Serologic and immunopathologic findings in temporal arteritis. *Am. J. Ophthalmol.,* 96:283–289.

19. Christian, C., and Sargent, J. (1976): Vasculitis syndromes: Clinical and experimental models. *Am. J. Med.,* 61:385–392.

20. Churg, J., and Strauss, L. (1951): Allergic granulomatosis, allergic angiitis and periarteritis nodosa. *Am. J. Pathol.,* 27:277–301.

21. Cines, D. B., Lyss, A., Mahin, B., Corkey, R., Kefalides, N., and Friedman, H. (1983): Fc and C3 receptors induced by herpes simplex virus on cultured human endothelial cells. *J. Clin. Immunol.,* 63:123–128.

22. Cines, D., Lyss, A., Reeber, M., Bina, M., and DeHoratius, R. (1984): Presence of complement fixing anti-endothelial cell antibodies in systemic lupus erythematosus. *J. Clin. Immunol.,* 73:611–625.

23. Citron, B., Halpern, M., McCarron, M., Lundberg, G., McCormick, R., Pincus, I., Tatter, D., and Haverback, B. (1970): Necrotizing angiitis associated with drug abuse. *N. Engl. J. Med.,* 283:1003–1011.

24. Cochrane, C. G. (1963): Studies on the localization of circulating antigen-antibody complexes and other macromolecules in vessels. I. Structural studies. *J. Exp. Med.,* 118:489–502.

25. Cochrane, C. G. (1963): Studies on the localization of circulating antigen-antibody complexes and other macromolecules in vessels.

II. Pathogenic and pharmacodynamic studies. *J. Exp. Med.,* 118:503–515.

26. Cochrane, C. G. (1971): Mechanisms involved in the deposition of immune complexes in tissue. *J. Exp. Med.,* 134:75s–89s.

27. Cochrane, C., and Hawkins, D. (1968): Studies on circulating immune complexes. III. Factors governing the ability of circulating complexes to localize in blood vessels. *J. Exp. Med.,* 127:137–154.

28. Cochrane, C., and Janoff, A. (1974): The Arthus reaction: A model of neutrophil and complement mediated injury. In *The Inflammatory Process, Vol. 3,* ed. 2, edited by B. Zweifach, L. Grant, and R. McCluskey, pp. 85–162. Academic Press, New York.

29. Conn, D., McDuffie, F., Holley, K., and Schroeter, A. (1976): Immunologic mechanisms in systemic vasculitis. *Mayo Clin. Proc.,* 51:511–518.

30. Cornacoff, J., Hebert, L., Smead, W., Van Aman, M., Birmingham, D., and Waxman, F. (1983): Primate erythrocyte-immune-complex-clearance mechanisms. *J. Clin. Immunol.,* 71:236–247.

31. Couser, W., and Salant, K. (1980): In situ immune complex formation and glomerular injury. *Kidney Int.,* 17:1–13.

32. Culbertson, J. T. (1935): The relationship of circulating antibody to the local inflammatory reaction to antigen (the Arthus phenomenon). *J. Immunol.,* 29:29–45.

33. Cunningham, T., Nicholls, K., and Chen, S. (1985): Defective reticuloendothelial system C3b clearance in rheumatoid arthritis and vasculitis. *J. Rheum.,* 12:675–679.

34. Cupps, T., and Fauci, A. (1981): *Major Problems in Internal Medicine. Vol. 21: The Vasculitides.* W. B. Saunders, Philadelphia.

35. Cupps, T., and Fauci, A. (1982): Neoplasia and systemic vasculitis: A case report. *Arthritis Rheum.,* 25:475–477.

36. Cupps, T., and Fauci, A. (1982): The vasculitic syndromes. *Adv. Intern. Med.,* 27:315–344.

37. Dienstag, J. L. (1981): Hepatitis B as an immune complex disease. *Semin. Liver Disease,* 1:45–57.

38. Dinarello, C. A. (1985): An update on human IL-1: From molecular biology to clinical significance. *J. Clin. Immunol.,* 5:287–297.

39. Dixon, F., Feldman, J., and Vazquez, J. (1961): Experimental glomerulonephritis. *J. Exp. Med.,* 113:899–917.

40. Dixon, F., Vazquez, J., Weigle, W., and Cochrane, C. (1958): Pathogenesis of serum sickness. *Arch. Pathol.,* 65:18–28.

41. Doherty, A., and Bradfield, J. (1981): Polyarteritis nodosa associated with acute cytomegalovirus infection. *Ann. Rheum. Dis.,* 8:49–51.

42. Donald, K., Edwards, R., and McEvoy, J. (1976): An ultrastructural study of the pathogenesis of tissue injury in limited Wegener's granulomatosis. *Pathology,* 8:161–169.

43. Dorff, B., and Lind, K. (1976): Two fatal cases of meningoencephalitis associated with *Mycoplasma pneumoniae* infection. *Scand. J. Infect. Dis.,* 8:49–51.

44. Elson, C., Scott, D., Blake, D., Bacon, P., and Holt, P. (1983): Complement activating rheumatoid-factor-containing complexes in patients with rheumatoid vasculitis. *Ann. Rheum. Dis.,* 42:147–150.

45. Es, L. van, Daha, M., Valentijn, R., and Kauffman, R. (1984): The pathogenetic significance of circulating immune complexes. *Neth. J. Med.,* 27:350–358.

46. Espinoza, L., Bridgeford, P., Lowenstein, M., Bocanegra, T., Basey, F., and Germain, B. (1982): Polymyalgia rheumatica and giant cell arteritis: Circulating immune complexes. *J. Rheum.,* 9:556–560.

47. Evans, D., Williams, D., and Peters, D. (1973): Glomerular deposition of properdin in Henoch-Schönlein syndrome and idiopathic focal nephritis. *Br. Med. J.,* 3:326–328.

48. Fauci, A. S. (1983): Vasculitis. *J. Allergy Clin. Immunol.,* 72:211–223.

49. Fauci, A., Haynes, B., and Katz, P. (1978): The spectrum of vasculitis: Clinical, pathological, immunologic, and therapeutic considerations. *Ann. Intern. Med.,* 89:660–676.

50. Fauci, A., Steinberg, A., Haynes, B., and Whalen, G. (1978): Immunoregulatory aberrations in systemic lupus erythematosus. *J. Immunol.,* 121:1473–1479.

51. Fauci, A., Haynes, B., Costa, J., Katz, P., and Wolff, S. (1982): Lymphomatoid granulomatosis, prospective clinical and therapeutic experience over ten years. *N. Engl. J. Med.,* 306:68–74.

52. Fearon, D. T. (1984): Cellular receptors for fragments of the third component of complement. *Immunol. Today,* 5:105–110.
53. Feder, H., Watkin, T., Cole, S., and Quinfiliare, R. (1981): Severe meningoencephalitis complicating *Mycoplasma* pneumonia infection in a child. *Arch. Pathol. Lab. Med.,* 105:619–621.
54. Fernald, G. W. (1982): Immunologic interactions between host cells and mycoplasmas. *Rev. Infect. Dis.,* 4:S201–S204.
55. Frank, M., Hamburger, M., Lawley, T., Kimberly, R., and Plotz, P. (1979): Defective reticuloendothelial system Fc receptor function in systemic lupus erythematosus. *N. Engl. J. Med.,* 300:518–523.
56. Frank, M., Lawley, T., Hamburger, M., and Brown, E. (1983): Immunoglobulin G Fc receptor mediated clearance in autoimmune diseases. *Ann. Intern. Med.,* 98:206–218.
57. Frayha, R. A. (1981): Trichinosis related polyarteritis nodosa. *Am. J. Med.,* 71:307–312.
58. Freedman, P., Peters, J., and Kark, R. (1960): Localization of gammaglobulin in the diseased kidney. *Arch. Intern. Med.,* 105:524–535.
59. Friedman, H., Cohen, G., Eisenberg, R., Seidel, C., and Cines, D. (1984): Glycoprotein C of herpes simplex virus I acts as a receptor for C3b complement component in infected cells. *Nature,* 309:633–635.
60. Gairdner, D. (1947): The Schönlein-Henoch syndrome. *Q. J. Med.,* 17:95–122.
61. Gamble, J. R., Harlan, J., Klebanoff, S., and Vadas, M. (1985): Stimulation of the adherance of neutrophils to umbilical vein endothelium by human recombinant tumor necrosis factor. *Proc. Natl. Acad. Sci. USA,* 82:8667–8671.
62. Garcia-Fuentes, M., Martin, A., Chantler, C., and Williams, D. (1978): Serum complement components in Henoch-Schönlein purpura. *Arch. Dis. Child.,* 53:417–419.
63. Gephardt, G., Ahmad, M., and Tubbs, R. (1983): Pulmonary vasculitis (Wegener's granulomatosis): Immunohistochemical studies of T and B cell markers. *Am. J. Med.,* 74:700–703.
64. Germuth, F. G. (1953): A comparative histologic and immunologic study in rabbits of induced hypersensitivity of the serum sickness type. *J. Exp. Med.,* 97:257–281.
65. Germuth, F., and Heptinstall, R. (1957): The development of arterial lesions following prolonged sensitization of bovine gammaglobulin. *Bull. Johns Hopkins Hosp.,* 100:58–98.
66. Giacomelli, F., and Wiener, J. (1974): Regional variation in the permeability of rat thoracic aorta. *Am. J. Pathol.,* 75:513–528.
67. Giangiocomo, J., and Tisai, C. (1977): Dermal and glomerular deposition of IgA in anaphylactoid purpura. *Am. J. Dis. Child.,* 131:981–983.
68. Gilbert, G. J. (1977): Evidence of viral cause in granulomatous angiitis. *Neurology (Minneap.),* 27:100–101.
69. Gocke, D., Hsu, K., Morgan, C., Bombarieri, S., Lochshin, M., and Christain, C. (1970): Association between polyarteritis and Australia antigen. *Lancet,* 2:1149–1153.
70. Gorevic, P., Kassab, J., Levo, V., Kuhn, R., Meltzer, M., Prouse, P., and Franklin, E. (1980): Mixed cryoglobulins: Clinical aspects and long-term follow-up of 40 patients. *Am. J. Med.,* 9:128–133.
71. Granstein, R., Soter, N., and Haynes, H. (1981): Necrotizing vasculitis within cutaneous lesions of mycosis fungoides. *J. Am. Acad. Dermatol.,* 9:128–133.
72. Granstrom, E., and Hedqvist, P. (1982): Prostaglandins, thromboxanes, and leukotrienes. In: *Pathobiology of Endothelial Cells,* edited by H. Nossel and H. Vogel, pp. 287–300. Academic Press, New York.
73. Hamburger, M., Lawley, T., Kimberly, R., Plotz, P., and Frank, M. (1982): A serial study of splenic macrophage reticuloendothelial system Fc function in systemic lupus erythematosus. *Arthritis Rheum.,* 25:48–54.
74. Hart, M., Tassell, S., Sadenwasser, K., Schelper, R., and Moore, S. (1985): Autoimmune vasculitis resulting from *in vitro* immunity of lymphocytes to smooth muscle. *Am. J. Pathol.,* 119:448–455.
75. Hawley, D., Schaefer, J., Schulz, D., and Mulle, R. (1983): Cytomegalovirus encephalitis in acquired immunodeficiency syndrome. *Am. J. Clin. Pathol.,* 80:874–877.
76. Hawn, C., and Janeway, C. (1947): Histological and serological sequences in experimental hypersensitivity. *J. Exp. Med.,* 85:571–589.
77. Haynes, B., Miller, S., Moore, J., Dunn, P., Bolognesi, D., and Metzgar, R. (1983): Identification of human T cell leukemia virus in a Japanese patient with adult T cell leukemia and cutaneous lymphomatous vasculitis. *Proc. Natl Acad. Sci. USA,* 80:2054–2058.
78. Haynes, B., Allen, N., and Fauci, A. (1986): Diagnostic and therapeutic approach to the patient with vasculitis. *Med. Clin. North Am.,* 78:355–368.
79. Haynes, B., and Fauci, A. (1987): Introduction to clinical immunology. In: *Harrison's Principles of Internal Medicine,* ed. 11, edited by E. Braunwald, K. Isselbacher, R. Petersdorf, J. Wilson, J. Martin, and A. Fauci, pp. 328–336. McGraw-Hill, New York.
80. Hellstrom, I., Hellstrom, K., Sjogren, H., and Warner, G. (1971): Serum factors in tumor free patients cancelling the blocking of cell mediated tumor immunity. *Int. J. Cancer.,* 8:185–191.
81. Hirschberg, H., Evensen, S., Henriksen, T., and Thorsby, E. (1975): The human mixed lymphocyte-endothelium culture interaction. *Transplantation,* 19:495–501.
82. Hirschberg, H., Bergh, O., and Thorsby, E. (1980): Antigen presenting properties of vascular endothelial cells. *J. Exp. Med.,* 152:249s–255s.
83. Hirschberg, H., Braathen, L., and Thorsby, E. (1982): Antigen presentation by vascular endothelial cells and epidermal Langerhans cells: The role of HLA-DR. *Immunol. Rev.,* 66:57–77.
84. Horn, R., Fauci, A., Rosenthal, A., and Wolff, S. (1974): Renal biopsy pathology in Wegener's granulomatosis. *Am. J. Pathol.,* 74:423–433.
85. Howell, S., and Epstein, W. (1976): Circulating immune complexes in Wegener's granulomatosis. *Am. J. Med.,* 60:259–268.
86. Hoxie, J., Matthews, D., and Cines, D. (1984): Infection of human endothelial cells by human T cell leukemia virus type I. *Proc. Natl. Acad. Sci. USA,* 81:7591–7595.
87. Hughes, G., Elkon, K., Spiller, R., Catovsky, D., and Jamieson, I. (1979): Polyarteritis nodosa and hairy cell leukemia. *Lancet,* 1:678.
88. Hunder, G., and Lie, J. (1983): The vasculitides. *Cardiovasc. Clin.,* 13:261–291.
89. Hurst, N., and Nuki, G. (1981): Evidence for defect of complement mediated phagocytosis by monocytes from patients with rheumatoid arthritis and cutaneous vasculitis. *Br. Med. J.,* 282:2081–2083.
90. Huston, K., Combs, J., Lie, J., and Giuliani, E. (1978): Left atrial myxoma simulating peripheral vasculitis. *Mayo Clin. Proc.,* 53:752–756.
91. Huttner, I., More, R., and Rona, G. (1970): Fine structural evidence of specific mechanism for increased endothelial permeability in experimental hypertension. *Am. J. Pathol.,* 61:395–404.
92. Jones, J., Park, J., Hazleman, B., Ward, M., and Bulgen, D. (1980): Lack of consistent peripheral blood lymphocyte transformation responses in polymyalgia rheumatica and giant cell arteritis. *J. Rheum.,* 7:891–894.
93. Jonkers, G., Kwaduk, E., and Tio, L. (1975): Necrotizing polyarteritis nodosa and serous otitis media. *Neth. J. Med.,* 18:142–144.
94. Jorizzo, J., Daniels, J., Apisarnthanaraz, P., Gonzalez, B., and Cavallo, D. (1983): Histamine triggered localized cutaneous vasculitis in patients with seropositive rheumatoid arthritis. *J. Am. Acad. Dermatol.,* 9:845–851.
95. Kauffman, R., Herrman, N., Meyer, C., Daha, M., and Van Es, L. (1978): Circulating IgA immune complexes in Henoch-Schönlein purpura. *Am. J. Med.,* 69:859–866.
96. Knutsen, D., Van Es, L., Kayser, B., and Glassock, R. (1979): Soluble oligovalent antigen-antibody complexes. II. The effect of various selective forces upon relative stability of isolated complexes. *Immunology,* 37:495–503.
97. Koeppen, A., Lansing, L., Peng, S., and Smith, R. (1981): Central nervous system vasculitis in cytomegalovirus infection. *J. Neurol. Sci.,* 51:395–410.
98. Kohler, P. F. (1973): Clinical immune complex disease. *Medicine (Baltimore),* 52:419–428.
99. Korbet, S., Schwartz, M., and Lewis, E. (1984): Immune complex

deposition and coronary vasculitis in systemic lupus erythematosus. *Am. J. Med.,* 77:141–146.

100. Koskimies, O., Rapola, J., Savilahti, E., and Vilska, J. (1974): Renal involvement in Schönlein-Henoch purpura. *Acta Paediatr. Scand.,* 63:357–363.

101. Kuno-Sakai, H., Sakai, H., Nomoto, V., Takakura, I., and Kimura, M. (1979): Increase of IgA-bearing peripheral blood lymphocytes in children with Henoch-Schönlein purpura. *Pediatrics,* 64:918–922.

102. Kurosaka, M., and Ziff, M. (1983): Immunoelectron microscopic study of the distribution of T cell subsets in rheumatoid synovium. *J. Exp. Med.,* 158:1191–1210.

103. Lanham, J., Elkon, K., Pusey, C., and Hughes, G. (1984): Systemic vasculitis with asthma and eosinophilia: A clinical approach to the Churg-Strauss syndrome. *Medicine (Baltimore),* 63:65–81.

104. Lawley, T., Hall, R., Fauci, A., Katz, S., Hamburger, M., and Frank, M. (1981): Defective Fc receptor functions associated with HLA-B8 DRw3 haplotype. *N. Engl. J. Med.,* 314:185–192.

105. Lawley, T., Bielory, L., Gascon, P., Yancey, K., Young, N., and Frank, M. (1982): A prospective clinical and immunological analysis of patients with serum sickness. *N. Engl. J. Med.,* 311:1407–1413.

106. Leber, P., and McCluskey, R. (1974): Immune complex disease. In: *The Inflammatory Process, Vol. 3,* ed. 2, edited by B. Zweifach, L. Grant, and R. McCluskey, pp. 401–438. Academic Press, New York.

107. Leib, E., Chia, D., and Bernett, E. (1979): Immune complexes in polyarteritis nodosa. *Clin. Res.,* 27:87.

108. Leung, D., Siegal, R., Grady, A., Krensky, A., Meade, R., Reinherz, E., and Geha, R. (1982): Immunoregulatory abnormalities in mucocutaneous lymph node syndrome. *Clin. Immunol. Immunopathol.,* 23:100–112.

109. Leung, D., Chu, E., Wood, N., Grady, S., Meade, R., and Geha, R. (1983): Immunoregulatory T cell abnormalities in mucocutaneous lymph node syndrome. *J. Immunol.,* 130:2002–2004.

110. Leung, D., Collins, T., LaPierre, L., Geha, R., and Pober, J. (1986): Immunoglobulin M antibodies present in the acute phase of Kawasaki syndrome lyse cultured vascular endothelial cells stimulated by gamma interferon. *J. Clin. Immunol.,* 77:1428–1435.

111. Levo, Y., Gorevic, P., Kassab, H., Zucker, T., Franklin, D., and Franklin, E. (1977): Association between hepatitis B virus and essential mixed cryoglobulinemia. *N. Engl. J. Med.,* 296:1501–1503.

112. Levy, M., Broyer, M., Arsan, A., Levy-Bentolila, D., and Habib, R. (1976): Anaphylactoid purpura nephritis in childhood; nature history and immunopathology. *Adv. Nephrol.,* 6:183–228.

113. Liang, G., Simpkin, P., and Mannik, M. (1974): Immunoglobulins in temporal arteritis. *Ann. Intern. Med.,* 81:19–24.

114. Liebow, A., Carrington, C., and Friedman, P. (1972): Lymphomatoid granulomatosis. *Hum. Pathol.,* 3:457–558.

115. Lightfoot, R. W., Jr. (1985): Cryoglobulinemias and other dysproteinemias. In: *Textbook of Rheumatology, Vol. 2,* ed. 2, edited by W. Kelley, E. Harris, S. Ruddy, and C. Sledge, pp. 1337–1350. W. B. Saunders, Philadelphia.

116. Linneman, C., and Alvira, M. (1980): Pathogenesis of varicella zoster angiitis in the CNS. *Arch. Neurol.,* 37:239–240.

117. London, W. T. (1977): Hepatitis B virus and antigen-antibody complex disease. *N. Engl. J. Med.,* 296:1528–1529.

118. Majno, G., Shea, S., and Leventhal, M. (1969): Endothelial contraction induced by histamine-type mediators. *J. Cell Biol.,* 42:647–672.

119. Malmvall, B., Bengtsson, B., Kaijser, B., Nilsson, L., and Alestig, K. (1976): Serum levels of immunoglobulin and complement in giant cell arteritis. *J.A.M.A.,* 236:1876–1878.

120. Manger, B., Krapf, F., Granatzki, M., Nusslein, H., Burmester, G., Kaldene, J., and Krailedat, P. (1985): IgE containing circulating immune complexes in Churg-Strauss vasculitis. *Scand. J. Immunol.,* 21:369–370.

121. Mannik, M., and Nardella, F. (1985): IgG rheumatoid factors and self-association of these antibodies. *Clin. Rheum. Dis.,* 11:551–572.

122. Medof, M., Iida, K., Mold, C., and Nussenzweig, V. (1982): Unique role of the complement receptor CR in the degradation of C3b associated immune complexes. *J. Exp. Med.,* 156:1739–1754.

123. Mellors, R., and Ortega, L. (1956): Analytical pathology. III. New observations on pathogenesis of glomerulonephritis, lipid nephrosis, polyarteritis nodosa and secondary amyloid. *Am. J. Pathol.,* 32:455–499.

124. Meltzer, M., and Franklin, E. (1966): Cryoglobulinemia—a study of twenty-nine patients. *Am. J. Med.,* 40:828–836.

125. Miller, G., and Nussenzweig, V. (1975): A new complement function: Solubilization of antigen-antibody aggregates. *Proc. Natl. Acad. Sci. USA,* 72:418–422.

126. Mittal, K., Rossen, R., and Sharp, J. (1970): Lymphocyte cytotoxic antibodies in systemic lupus erythematosus. *Nature,* 225:1255–1256.

127. Moller, N. P. H. (1979): Fc mediated immune precipitation. I. A new role of the Fc portion of immunoglobulin G. *Immunology,* 38:631–640.

128. Montesano, R., Orci, L., and Vassalli, P. (1985): Human endothelial cell cultures: Phenotypic modulation by leukocyte interleukins. *J. Cell Physiol.,* 122:424–434.

129. Moyer, C., and Reinisch, C. (1984): The role of vascular smooth muscle cells in experimental autoimmune vasculitis. *Am. J. Pathol.,* 117:380–390.

130. McCluskey, R., and Bhan, A. (1982): Cell mediated mechanisms in renal diseases. *Kidney Int. (Suppl. 11),* 21:6–12.

131. McCluskey, R., and Fienberg, R. (1983): Vasculitis in primary vasculitides, granulomatoses and connective tissue diseases. *Hum. Pathol.,* 14:305–315.

132. McIntosh, R., Tinglof, B., and Kaufman, D. (1971): Immunohistology of renal disease. *Q. J. Med.,* 40:385–390.

133. Opie, E. L. (1924): Inflammatory reaction of the immune animal to antigen (Arthus phenomenon) and its relation to antibodies. *J. Immunol.,* 9:231–246.

134. Papaioannou, C., Hunder, G., and McDuffie, F. (1979): Cellular immunity in polymyalgia rheumatica and giant cell arteritis. *Arthritis Rheum.,* 22:740–745.

135. Para, M., Baucke, R., and Spear, P. (1982): Glycoprotein IgE of herpes simplex virus type. I: Effects of anti-IgE on virion infectivity and on virus induced Fc binding receptors. *J. Virol.,* 41:129–136.

136. Park, J., and Hazleman, B. (1978): Immunological and histological study of temporal arteries. *Ann. Rheum. Dis.,* 37:238–243.

137. Park, J., Jones, J., Harkiss, G., and Hazleman, B. (1981): Circulating immune complexes in polymyalgia rheumatica and giant cell arteritis. *Ann. Rheum. Dis.,* 40:360–365.

138. Paronetto, F., and Strauss, L. (1962): Immunocytochemical observations on polyarteritis nodosa. *AIM,* 56:289–296.

139. Pette, J. van de, Jarvis, J., Wilton, J., and MacDonald, D. (1984): Cutaneous periarteritis nodosa. *Arch. Dermatol.,* 120:109–111.

140. Phanuphak, P., and Kohler, P. (1980): Onset of polyarteritis nodosa during allergic hyposensitization treatment. *Am. J. Med.,* 68:479–485.

141. Pinching, A., Lockwood, C., Pussell, B., Rees, A., Swaney, P., Evans, D., Bowley, N., and Peters, D. (1983): Wegener's granulomatosis: Observations on 18 patients with severe renal disease. *Q. J. Med.,* 208:435–460.

142. Pober, J., Gimbrone, M., Contran, R., Reiss, C., Burakoff, S., Fiers, W., and Ault, K. (1983): Ia expression by vascular endothelium is inducible by activated T cells and by human gamma-interferon. *J. Exp. Med.,* 157:1339–1353.

143. Pober, J., Bevilaqua, M., Mendrich, K., LaPierre, L., Fiers, W., and Gimbrone, M. (1986): Two distinct monokines, interleukin-1 and tumor necrosis factor each independently induce biosynthesis and transient expression of the same antigen on the surface of cultured human vascular endothelial cells. *J. Immunol.,* 136:1680–1687.

144. Pober, J., Gimbrone, M., LaPierre, L., Mendrich, D., Fiers, W., Rothlein, R., and Springer, T. (1986): Overlapping patterns of activation of human endothelial cells by interleukin-1, tumor necrosis factor, and immune interferon. *J. Immunol.,* 137:1893–1896.

145. Pruzanski, W., Sarraf, D., Klein, M., Lau, C., Richardson, J., and Keystone, E., (1986): Lymphocytotoxins in vasculitis: Correlation with clinical manifestations and laboratory variables. *J. Rheum.,* 13:1066–1071.

146. Quismorio, F., Beardmore, T., Kaufman, R., and Mongan, P.

(1983): IgG rheumatoid factors and antinuclear antibodies in rheumatoid vasculitis. *Clin. Exp. Immunol.,* 52:333–340.

147. Rapoport, R., Kozin, F., Mackel, S., and Jordon, R. (1980): Cutaneous vascular immunofluorescence in rheumatoid arthritis. *Am. J. Med.,* 68:325–331.

148. Reyes, M., Fresco, R., Chokroverty, S., and Salud, E. (1976): Virus-like particles in granulomatous angiitis of the central nervous system. *Neurology (Minneap.),* 26:797–799.

149. Roback, S., Herdman, R., Hoyer, J., and Good, R. (1969): Wegener's granulomatosis in a child: Observations on pathogenesis and treatment. *Am. J. Dis. Child.,* 118:608–614.

150. Ronco, P., Verrous, T., Mignon, F., Kourilsky, D., Van Hille, P., Meyrier, A., Mery, J., and Morel-Maroger, L. (1983): Immuno-pathological studies of polyarteritis nodosa and Wegener's granulomatosis: A report of 43 patients with renal biopsies. *Q. J. Med.,* 52:121–123.

151. Ross, G., and Medof, M. (1985): Membrane complement receptors specific for bound fragments of C3. *Adv. Immunol.,* 37:217–267.

152. Rothstein, T., and Kenney, G. (1979): Cranial neuropathy, myeloradiculopathy and myositis: Complications of *Mycoplasma pneumoniae* infection. *Arch. Neurol.,* 36:476.

153. Ruddy, S. (1985): Complement deficiencies and rheumatic disease. In: *Textbook of Rheumatology, Vol. 1,* ed. 2, edited by W. Kelley, E. Harris, S. Ruddy, and C. Sledge, p. 1354. W. B. Saunders, Philadelphia.

154. Sakane, T., Steinberg, A., and Green, I. (1978): Studies of immune function of patients with systemic lupus erythematosus; dysfunction of suppressor T cell activation related to impaired generation rather than response of suppressor cells. *Arthritis Rheum.,* 21:657–664.

155. Sams, W., Claman, H., and Kohler, P. (1975): Human necrotizing vasculitis: Immunoglobulins and complement in vessel walls of lesions and normal skin. *J. Invest. Dermatol.,* 64:441–445.

156. Saulsbury, F. T. (1984): Henoch-Schönlein purpura. *Pediatr. Dermatol.,* 1:195–201.

157. Schifferli, J., Yin, C., and Peters, D. (1986): The role of complement and its receptor in the elimination of immune complexes. *N. Engl. J. Med.,* 315:488–495.

158. Schoenfeld, Y., and Schwartz, R. (1984): Immunologic and genetic factors in autoimmune disease. *N. Engl. J. Med.,* 311:1019–1029.

159. Schroeter, A., Copeman, P., Jordon, R., Sams, W., and Winkelman, R. (1971): Immunofluorescence of cutaneous vasculitis associated with systemic disease. *Arch. Dermatol.,* 104:254–259.

160. Scott, D., Bacon, P., Allen, C., Elson, C., and Wallington, T. (1981): IgG rheumatoid factor, complement and immune complexes in rheumatoid synovitis and vasculitis: Comparative and serial studies during cytotoxic therapy. *Clin. Exp. Immunol.,* 104:254–259.

161. Scott, H., Bradtzaeg, P., Hirschberg, H., Solheim, G., and Thorsby, E. (1981): Vascular and renal distribution of HLA-DR like antigens. *Tissue Antigens,* 18:195–202.

162. Sergent, J., and Christian, C. (1974): Necrotizing vasculitis after acute serous otitis media. *AIM,* 81:195–199.

163. Shasby, D., Schwarz, M., and Forstot, J. (1982): Pulmonary immune complex deposition in Wegener's granulomatosis. *Chest,* 81:338–340.

164. Siegal, I., Liu, T., and Gleicher, N. (1981): The red cell immune system. *Lancet,* 2:556–559.

165. Soter, N. A. (1976): Clinical presentations and mechanisms of necrotizing angiitis of the skin. *J. Invest. Dermatol.,* 67:354–359.

166. Stage, D., and Mannik, M. (1971): IgM-globulin in rheumatoid arthritis: Evaluation of its clinical significance. *Arthritis Rheum.,* 14:440–450.

167. Stevenson, J., Leong, L., Cohen, A., and Border, W. (1982): Henoch-Schönlein purpura: Simultaneous demonstration of IgA deposition in involved skin, intestine and kidney. *Arch. Pathol. Lab. Med.,* 106:192–195.

168. Takahashi, M., Czop, J., Ferreira, A., and Nussenzweig, W. (1976): Mechanism of solubility of immune aggregates by complement: Implications for immunopathology. *Transplant. Rev.,* 32:121–129.

169. Ten Berge, I., Wilmink, J., Meyer, C., Surachno, J., Ten Veen, K., Balk, T., and Schellekens, P. (1985): Clinical and immunologic follow-up of patients with severe renal disease in Wegener's granulomatosis. *Am. J. Nephrol.,* 5:21–29.

170. Theofilopoulos, A. (1980): Evaluation and clinical significance of circulating immune complexes. *Prog. Clin. Immunol.,* 4:63–92.

171. Theofilopoulos, A., and Dixon, F. (1979): The biology and detection of immune complexes. *Adv. Immunol.,* 28:89–220.

172. Thomas, L., Davidson, M., and McCluskey, R. (1966): Studies of PPLO infection. I. The production of cerebral polyarteritis by *Mycoplasma gallisepticum* in turkeys. The neurotoxic property of the *Mycoplasma. J. Exp. Med.,* 123:897–911.

173. Thomas, L., Aleu, F., Bitensky, M., Davidson, M., and Gesner, B. (1966): Studies of PPLO infection. II. The neurotoxin of *Mycoplasma neurolyticum. J. Exp. Med.,* 124:1067–1081.

174. Trepo, C., and Thivolet, J. (1970): Hepatitis associated antigen and periarteritis nodosa. *Vox Sang.,* 19:410–411.

175. Trygstad, C. W. (1971): Elevated serum IgA globulin in anaphylactoid purpura. *Pediatrics,* 47:1023–1028.

176. Van Es, L. A., Dana, M. R., Valentijn, R. M., and Kaufman, R. H. (1984): The pathogenic significance of circulating immune complexes. *Neth. J. Med.,* 27:350–358.

177. Walker, D., and Mattern, W. (1980): Rickettsial vasculitis. *Am. Heart J.,* 6:896–906.

178. Weinberg, B., Hobbs, M., and Misukonis, M. (1984): Recombinant human gamma-interferon induces human monocyte polykaryon formation. *Proc. Natl. Acad. Sci. USA,* 81:4554–4557.

179. Weisman, M., and Zvaifler, N. (1975): cryoimmunoglobulinemia in rheumatoid arthritis. *J. Clin. Immunol.,* 56:725–739.

180. Willemze, R., Graafereitsma, C. de, Cnossen, J., Vloten, W. Van, and Meyer, C. (1983): Characterization of T cell subpopulations in skin and peripheral blood of patients with cutaneous T cell lymphomas and benign inflammatory dermatoses. *J. Invest. Dermatol.,* 80:60–66.

181. Williams, R. C. (1980): *Immune Complexes in Clinical and Experimental Medicine.* Harvard University Press, Cambridge, Mass.

182. Wilson, J. G., Wong, W. W., Schur, P. H., and Fearon, D. T. (1982): Mode of inheritance of decreased C3b receptors on erythrocytes of patients with systemic lupus erythematous. *N. Engl. J. Med.,* 307:981–986.

183. Winkleman, R., Buechner, S., Powell, F., and Banks, P. (1983): The T lymphocyte and cutaneous Churg-Strauss granuloma. *Acta Dermatol. Venerol.,* 63:199–204.

184. Woude, F. Van der, Rasmussen, N., Lobatto, S., Wiik, A., Permin, H., Es, L. Van, Giessen, M. Vander, Hem, G. Vander, and The, T. (1985): Auto-antibodies to neutrophils and monocytes: A new tool for diagnosis and a marker of disease activity in Wegener's granulomatosis. *Lancet,* 1:425–429.

185. Zvaifler, N., and Woods, V. (1985): Etiology and pathogenesis of systemic lupus erythematosus. In: *Textbook of Rheumatology, Vol. 1,* ed. 2, edited by W. Kelley, E. Harris, S. Ruddy, and C. Sledge, pp. 1042–1070. W. B. Saunders, Philadelphia.

Inflammation: Basic Principles and Clinical Correlates.
Edited by J. I. Gallin, I. M. Goldstein, and R. Snyderman.
Raven Press, Ltd., New York © 1988.

CHAPTER 39

Graft-Versus-Host Disease

Julio C. Voltarelli and Marvin R. Garovoy

Graft-versus-host (GVH) reactions are immunological responses of donor lymphoid cells to disparate histocompatibility antigens expressed on cells of an immunodeficient host. The effects of GVH reactions in different organs, combined with other factors, such as secondary infections, result in the complex clinical syndrome of GVH disease (27,105). With the progressive use of allogeneic bone marrow transplantation to treat a variety of human diseases, GVH reactions have been recognized as a major clinical problem.

Several excellent reviews have been published on the experimental (13,27,34,43,88,92) and clinical (23,30, 89,100,104,105,111) aspects of GVH reactions. Consequently, these aspects will not be discussed in detail. Instead, this review will focus on basic mechanisms of GVH disease in humans.

CLINICAL FEATURES

Clinical GVH disease in humans is most frequently observed after allogeneic bone marrow transplantation. In fact, a recent study showed that all recipients of HLA-identical bone marrow developed severe acute GVH disease if they did not receive posttransplantation immunosuppression (106). With the use of prophylactic immunosuppression, about one-half of HLA-identical recipients and 70 to 80% of HLA-incompatible recipients develop acute GVH disease. Approximately 20% of all allogeneic marrow recipients die from complications of this disease.

Acute GVH disease appears during the first 100 days (usually 3–4 weeks) of the posttransplantation period and is manifested by dermatitis, enteritis, and hepatitis of variable severity (67,68). The onset of acute GVH disease usually is marked by a maculopapular rash involving the palms and soles that may spread to the entire body, leading to toxic epidermal necrosis. Intestinal and hepatic manifestations usually follow skin involvement. Symptoms of enteric GVH disease include watery diarrhea, along with abdominal pain, nausea, anorexia, vomiting, and, in severe cases, ileus. The hepatic manifestations of acute GVH disease include cholestatic jaundice, with striking elevations of bilirubin and liver enzymes, but usually without progression to hepatic failure or encephalopathy. Ascites and hepatorenal syndrome may occur in severe cases. A histological diagnosis of acute GVH disease should be established whenever possible, because many of the manifestations of this disease are nonspecific and may be confused with other disorders, particularly drug and radiation toxicity, as well as infections. The clinical stage of acute GVH disease is determined by the degree of damage to skin, liver, and gut. Thus, grade I GVH disease is mild and limited to the skin; grade II is moderate disease in multiple organs, with a mild decrease in clinical performance; grade III is severe disease, with a marked decrease in clinical performance; grade IV is life-threatening GVH disease. Acute GVH disease may be transient or sustained; 30 to 60% of patients with severe (grades II–IV) GVH disease die from complications of the disease or its therapy. Likewise, acute GVH disease seems to increase the incidence of, and mortality from, interstitial pneumonia, another major complication of bone marrow transplantation (118).

With the increased numbers of long-term survivors of bone marrow transplantation, a chronic relapsing pattern of GVH disease has emerged, developing 100 to 400 days after the transplantation and affecting one-third of patients. Most patients with chronic GVH disease have antecedent acute GVH disease, but 20 to 30% of patients do not.

The manifestations of chronic GVH disease frequently include a lichen-planus-like eruption, scleroderma, chronic hepatitis, Sjögren's syndrome, esophagitis, interstitial pneumonitis, and, more rarely, polyserositis, enteritis, and polymyositis (42,68,95,105). The manifestations of chronic GVH disease resemble those of collagen vascular diseases, but in contrast to several of these disorders, renal and central nervous system involvements are rare. The skin is involved in almost all patients, exhibiting dryness, hyperpigmentation and hypopigmentation, alopecia, lichen-planus-like lesions, and photosensitivity. Without treatment, progressive scleroderma with joint contractures may develop. The oral mucosa may show lichenoid lesions, and a sicca syndrome involving lacrimal and salivary glands may develop. Esophageal symptoms include dysphagia, retrosternal pain, and weight loss. Mucosal desquamation, strictures, and submucosal fibrosis are observed, but the characteristic muscle and neuronal abnormalities of scleroderma are not seen. Chronic liver disease is observed in 90% of patients with chronic GVH disease, with manifestations of cholestasis, but without progression to cirrhosis or hepatic failure. About 5 to 10% of long-term survivors develop obstructive lung disease, with histologic lesions of obliterative bronchiolitis. The prognosis is favorable for patients with chronic GVH disease limited to the skin and liver, but it is poor for patients with disseminated disease. In contrast to acute GVH disease, mortality is not high for chronic GVH disease, but long-lasting morbidity is common and includes dermal pain and joint contractures from skin lesions, wasting from esophagitis and malabsorption, pulmonary insufficiency, and growth retardation (91). Systemic infection due to protracted immunodeficiency is the most frequent cause of death.

In addition to being caused by bone marrow transplantation, GVH disease can be caused by whole-blood or leukocyte transfusions to patients with congenital or acquired immunodeficiencies (16,117). Transfusion-associated GVH disease is more acute, more severe, and more often associated with pancytopenia, but is associated with fewer constitutional symptoms than is posttransplantation GVH disease (16). GVH reactions can also be caused by engrafted maternal cells in immunodeficient children (110), by transplantation of small bowel (25),

pancreas-spleen (24), or fetal liver cells (65), or by chemical agents (50) (Table 1).

EXPERIMENTAL MODELS OF GVH DISEASE

Deliberate induction of a GVH reaction in animals provides an experimental model for assessing immunocompetence of lymphoid cells from different sources *in vivo* (reviewed in refs. 13,27,28,43,88). The requirements for inducing a GVH reaction include immunologically competent cells in the graft, histoincompatibility between donor and recipient, and immunologic incompetence of the host. In this regard, suitable hosts for GVH reactions include embryonic and neonatal animals ("runt disease"), F₁ hybrids injected with parental cells ("allogeneic disease"), genetically disparate animals sharing blood circulation ("parabiosis intoxication"), animals immunosuppressed by total-body irradiation ("secondary disease"), and animals suffering from congenital immunodeficiencies (e.g., nude mice).

The kinetics and severity of GVH reactions largely depend on the degree of histocompatibility differences and on the number of mature T cells present in the graft. Human bone marrow contains high proportions of T cells that frequently cause a fatal form of acute GVH disease. In contrast, mouse bone marrow contains few mature T cells, which cause a mild and delayed form of chronic GVH disease in some strain combinations disparate for the major histocompatibility complex (MHC). Thus, induction of acute fatal GVH disease in mice requires addition to the bone marrow inoculum of T cells from the spleen, lymph nodes, or thoracic duct. Finally, dog bone marrow appears to contain intermediate numbers of T cells (13,54,112).

Animal models of chronic GVH disease have been developed in rats (8), mice (82), and dogs (88). F₁ hybrid

TABLE 1. *Causes of GVH disease in humans*

HLA-matched bone marrow transplantation
HLA-mismatched bone marrow transplantation
Syngeneic bone marrow transplantation
Autologous bone marrow transplantation
Fetal liver transplantation
Transplantation of small bowel
Transplantation of pancreas-spleen
Maternal-fetal engraftment
Toxic-oil syndrome
Transfusion of whole blood, blood products, or leukocytes
    to patients with:
    Severe combined immunodeficiency
    Wiskott-Aldrich syndrome
    Hemolytic anemia of the newborn
    Hematological malignancies
    Neuroblastoma
    Immunosuppression due to chemotherapy

mice injected with parental cells may develop chronic GVH disease with or without a preceding phase of acute GVH disease (34). This syndrome resembles human autoimmune diseases such as systemic lupus erythematosus or overlap syndrome. In addition, chronic GVH disease that develops spontaneously in the rat radiation chimera has many immunopathological similarities with human chronic GVH disease (8). Moreover, chronic GVH disease also can be induced in the rat radiation chimera by adoptive transfer of immunocompetent cells (9).

Experimental GVH reactions may be systemic (due to dissemination of immunoreactive cells to several organs), local (induced by administering reactive cells into a site such as the skin from which they do not migrate), or regional (due to limited dissemination of reactive cells to draining lymph nodes).

Genetic Requirements

In a variety of animal species, including the mouse, rat, dog, monkey, and chicken, most severe GVH reactions occur when donor and recipient differ at the genes of the MHC (13). Most studies have been performed in mice, in which the organization of the MHC is known best. The MHC in the mouse (H-2 complex) is located on chromosome 17 and is composed of three classes of genes: class I genes in the K and D regions, class II genes in the I region, and class III genes in the S region.

The contributions of different MHC gene products to the development of GVH reactions vary according to whether the induction or the effector phase is measured with a particular assay. Thus, class II MHC differences cause strong proliferative responses, as measured by the splenomegaly assay, by delayed-type hypersensitivity reactions, and by mixed leukocyte cultures. In contrast, in assays measuring the effector phase of GVH reactions, e.g., mortality, an entire MHC difference appears to be required (52).

Proliferative responses, delayed-type hypersensitivity reactions, and GVH reactions also can be elicited by antigens outside of the MHC. These so-called minor histocompatibility antigens frequently cause severe or fatal GVH disease (64). Experimental GVH reactions produced by minor histocompatibility antigen differences have important implications for human GVH disease, which most commonly is observed after MHC-compatible bone marrow transplantation. In the mouse, well-characterized minor histocompatibility antigens are encoded at the Mls locus, which is located on chromosome 1. These antigens appear late in neonatal life and are present on B cells, macrophages, and bone marrow stem cells, but not on T cells. Differences in Mls antigens induce strong proliferative and delayed-type hypersensitivity reactions in models of GVH disease. However, Mls antigens do not seem to influence mortality from GVH disease, suggesting that other minor histocompatibility antigens are important for the effector phase of the reaction (54).

Finally, histocompatibility differences do not seem to be an absolute requirement for the development of GVH reactions, because acute GVH disease can be induced by cyclosporin treatment in syngeneic mice (18) and rats (48), chronic GVH disease develops in cyclophosphamide-treated syngeneic rats (73), and D-penicillamine can induce *in vitro* GVH reactions in syngeneic mice (72).

Cellular Mechanisms

Several studies have shown that mature T cells present in bone marrow grafts are the main cause of GVH disease and that other cells, such as macrophages, B cells, and natural killer (NK) cells, are not necessary for the development of the disease. However, these non-T cells can contribute to the pathogenesis of GVH disease and certainly are involved in related phenomena such as immunodeficiency, autoimmunity, suppressor cell dysfunction, or graft-versus-leukemia effects.

Studies of the phenotypes of cells involved in producing GVH disease in adoptive-transfer experiments indicate that effector cells of GVH reactions are mature T cells. Donor NK cells do not seem to be effectors of GVH reactions in mice (55,114). However, recipient NK cells seem to contribute to the intensity of GVH reactions, because treatment of recipients with anti-asialo-GM1 reduces the intensity of GVH disease (17). Furthermore, NK cells are the predominant mononuclear cells infiltrating the skin of mice with minor-histocompatibility-antigen-incompatible acute GVH disease (26). These findings suggest that NK cells may participate in acute GVH disease either as minor-histocompatibility-antigen-presenting cells (17) or as effector cells after being recruited and activated by lymphokines released during classic delayed-type hypersensitivity reactions (70).

Experimental Acute GVH Disease

Acute lethal GVH reactions directed against class I H-2 and minor histocompatibility antigen disparities are mediated by cytotoxic T cells, whereas GVH reactions directed to whole H-2 or class II differences are predominantly caused by T helper cells (55,99). Recognition of minor histocompatibility antigens by cytotoxic T cells (Lyt-2$^+$) is restricted by class I MHC molecules. Thus, minor histocompatibility antigens are stimulatory only when seen together with K/D antigens common to the effector cells (54,75). In addition, acute GVH disease developing in syngeneic transplanted rats after withdrawal of cyclosporin is mediated by cytotoxic T cells against Ia autoantigens (48).

In GVH reactions directed both to MHC and minor histocompatibility antigen differences, it is probable that T helper cells (L3T4$^+$) contribute to the maturation of an Lyt-1$^+$2$^+$ precursor cell into an Lyt-1$^+$ cytotoxic cell (74) or that T helper cells participate as mediators of delayed-type hypersensitivity reactions (75). Delayed-type hypersensitivity as a mechanism of tissue injury was best studied in the mouse model of acute intestinal GVH disease (44,70). The proposed sequence of events leading to mucosal damage in this model is as follows:

1. L3T4$^+$ T helper cells are activated by the recognition of foreign Ia antigens (in class II MHC-unmatched transplants) or by minor histocompatibility antigens presented in connection with self Ia (in MHC-matched transplants). These antigens are found on dendritic cells in Peyer's patches and on enterocytes.

2. Activated T helper cells secrete several lymphokines, including interleukin-2 (IL-2), IL-3, and gamma-interferon, that act on different cells and contribute to the inflammatory lesions. Thus, IL-2 causes proliferation of T helper cells that recirculate through the thoracic duct and migrate back to the gut mucosa. In addition, IL-2 could stimulate cytotoxic activity of NK cells. IL-3 stimulates production and release of various hematopoietic cells, especially mast cells that infiltrate the intestinal mucosa in GVH reactions. The temporal relation between mast cell infiltration and gut injury suggests, but does not prove, that these cells are involved in producing tissue damage (58). Finally, helper T cells produce gamma-interferon, which induces Ia expression on epithelial cells, amplifying the stimulation of T helper cells. Gamma-interferon also activates NK cells and macrophages. Activated NK cells (71) and macrophages (37) may also act as effector cells in mucosal damage. Some of the lymphokines produced by activated T helper cells also may stimulate the proliferation of epithelial cells of the intestinal mucosa.

3. Mucosal damage may increase the absorption of bacterial products through the intestine that produce additional lesions (71). There is only indirect evidence that delayed-type hypersensitivity inflammatory events occur in other target organs, such as the skin, during acute GVH disease in mice (89) or in humans (85).

Experimental Chronic GVH Disease

Chronic GVH disease is caused by Lyt-2$^-$/L3T4$^+$ cells that recognize class II H-2 autoantigens or alloantigens (34,75). These cells provide help to autoreactive B-cell clones that produce IgG and IgM complement-fixing antibodies that induce widespread inflammatory reactions.

Helper T cells also secrete lymphokines that stimulate fibroblast proliferation and collagen production (22,75).

Clonal analysis of MHC-identical mouse GVH disease revealed the presence of two types of T helper cells in the early phases of the disease: T cells that react to minor histocompatibility antigens and that can stimulate fibroblast proliferation (primarily responsible for acute GVH disease) and T cells that react to autologous Ia antigens and that stimulate collagen secretion, but not fibroblast proliferation. These findings may explain the collagen deposition that characterizes tissue lesions of chronic GVH disease and also may clarify the relationship between acute and chronic GVH disease. Thus, recipient-specific acute GVH disease clones may release lymphokines that stimulate fibroblast proliferation, as well as gamma-interferon that stimulates Ia expression on epithelial cells.

If the recipient does not die from acute GVH disease, Ia+ epithelial cells become targets for autoreactive T-cell clones. These cells secrete lymphokines that increase collagen production by fibroblasts. The synergistic effect of increasing fibroblast number and collagen production results in sclerosis of organs previously damaged by cytotoxic attack during acute GVH disease (skin, liver, gut) or of organs damaged by autoantibodies (lacrimal and salivary glands). It has been shown that T-cell clones that cause chronic GVH disease are present early after transplantation (75), indicating that the immunological events that ultimately lead to chronic GVH disease occur in the early posttransplantation period.

The mechanisms by which T-cell subpopulations cause acute and chronic GVH disease are probably different (34,99). Symptoms of acute GVH disease result from direct attack on host tissues by cytotoxic T cells, causing hypoplasia of the lymphohematopoietic system, manifested by hypogammaglobulinemia, thymic hypoplasia, and aplastic anemia. On the other hand, the symptoms of chronic GVH disease resemble those of disseminated autoimmune disease and are caused by activation of autoreactive B cells by allogeneic T helper cells (34) (Fig. 1). Autoreactive B-cell clones produce a variety of IgG autoantibodies that induce widespread inflammatory reactions, whereas T helper cells secrete factors that stimulate fibroblast proliferation and collagen secretion (22). Moreover, in some strain combinations, F$_1$ mice with GVH disease develop a B-cell lymphoproliferative disease that may culminate in malignant lymphoma (34).

GVH DISEASE IN HUMANS

Genetic Requirements

Until very recently, the great majority of bone marrow transplants in humans were performed between HLA genotypically identical siblings, with significant acute

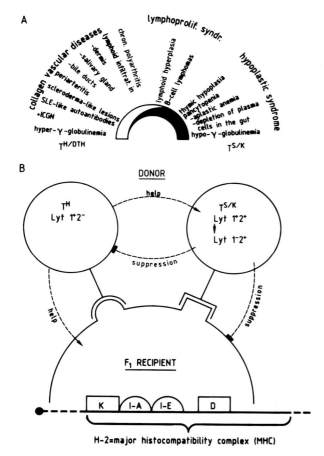

FIG. 1. Cellular pathogenesis of GVH reactions. **A:** Spectrum of stimulatory (**left**) and suppressive (**right**) pathological lesions that may develop during GVH reactions in F_1 mice. Suppressive effects are common in acute GVH disease, and stimulatory effects are common in chronic GVH disease. **B:** Cellular and genetic requirements for induction of stimulatory (**left**) and suppressive (**right**) GVH reactions. The F_1 cell depicted at the bottom of the figure with class I (*square*) and class II (*round*) MHC antigens represents stimulator and target cells located in lymphohematopoietic tissues and on epithelial surfaces. This basic concept was confirmed recently using cloned cell lines and a monoclonal antibody to L3T4 as a marker for mouse T helper cells (75,99). (From ref. 34.)

GVH disease developing in about one-third to one-half of recipients. The probable cause of GVH disease following HLA-identical transplants is sensitization to minor histocompatibility antigens. A series of six minor histocompatibility antigens was identified by the cytotoxic activity of donor lymphocytes repopulating HLA-identical marrow recipients against pretransplantation host cells (38). Recognition of minor histocompatibility antigens was restricted by class I HLA antigens, and mismatching for these antigens was strongly associated with the occurrence of chronic GVH disease. Another cause of GVH disease in HLA-matched transplants is HLA-DP incom-

patibility due to the relatively high rate of recombination between HLA-DQ and -DP (46).

In an attempt to extend the benefits of bone marrow transplantation to patients without HLA-matched donors, marrow transplants have recently been attempted between HLA partially identical relatives or between HLA phenotypically identical, unrelated individuals. In one study, patients with one to three HLA-incompatible loci had more and earlier GVH disease than did patients who were either genotypically or phenotypically HLA-identical. The nature of the locus mismatched, i.e., HLA-A, -B, or -DR, did not influence the outcome of GVH disease (Fig. 2). Thus, HLA matching clearly is relevant for the development of GVH disease, but there probably is no difference between class I or class II antigen disparity either genotypically or phenotypically (6). On the other hand, another study suggested that class II HLA mismatch conferred a higher risk for acute GVH disease than did class I mismatch (33).

Associations between particular HLA antigens and GVH disease also have been reported. Thus, the presence in the recipient of HLA-B18, -Bw21, -B49, and -B50 correlated with increased risk for acute GVH disease, whereas the presence of HLA-B8, -Bw35, or -Aw19 was associated with decreased risk (15,102). On the other hand, no association was found between HLA-A or -B antigens and the incidence of chronic GVH disease (103). The mechanism of the association between HLA-B antigens and acute GVH disease is unknown, but probably involves genes linked to particular HLA-B loci that control the intensity of allogeneic immune responses.

Genetic factors other than MHC antigens have been analyzed in relation to GVH disease. Incompatibility in the ABO system or in the antigens of the leukocyte group 5 system appears not to increase the risk of GVH disease (46). In contrast, disparity in the MNSs blood group may be an important factor (98). The effect of sex matching on the incidence of acute GVH disease is controversial (30,46). The International Bone Marrow Transplant Registry reported an increased risk for acute GVH disease in female-to-male transplants and suggested that the mechanism could involve an immune response to the H-Y antigen (11). In fact, the H-Y antigen can be a target of HLA class I restricted killing by cytotoxic cells from transfusion-sensitized patients (113). However, more recent data show an association between increased donor parity and augmented risk of acute GVH disease that may be due to presensitization to recipient male cells (2). No relationship was found between sex matching and the development of chronic GVH disease (87,103).

Finally, reports of GVH disease occurring in a few recipients of syngeneic or autologous bone marrow (35,83,107) argue against the need for genetic incompatibility in the development of GVH disease. However, there

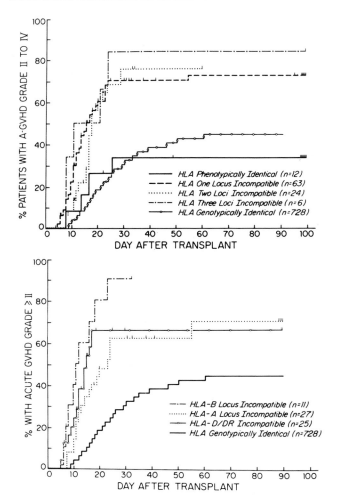

FIG. 2. Risk of acute GVH disease in relation to the number of disparate HLA loci (**top**) or in relation to the particular locus of HLA incompatibility (**bottom**). (From ref. 6.)

is always the question whether or not these cases constitute true GVH disease, as well as whether or not donors and recipients were truly syngeneic pairs (30). If this is the case, GVH disease could result from an autoimmune reaction triggered by virally modified autoantigens or by immunoregulatory disturbances of T-cell subsets in the host (54,84).

Nongenetic Factors

Many other factors besides genetic disparity have been investigated as contributing or aggravating causes of GVH disease in humans (10). The most striking predisposing factor for both acute and chronic GVH disease is increased age, either of the recipients (10,104) or of the donors (87). Older patients also tolerate the complications of GVH disease less well than do younger patients. An attractive

explanation for the adverse effect of age on the incidence of GVH disease is that decreased thymic function in older bone marrow recipients leads to impaired maturation of T cells generated by the transplanted marrow. Defective T-cell maturation would result in increased susceptibility to infections and immunoregulatory changes in T suppressor cells supposedly involved in the maintenance of GVH tolerance. In fact, patients older than 30 years have both a high incidence of GVH disease and low levels of the thymic hormone "facteur thymique serique" (1). Based on these findings, thymic transplantation and administration of thymic hormones have been attempted to prevent the development of chronic GVH disease, but with no success (1). In addition, a recent immunohistological study failed to provide evidence of a role for the thymus in the maturation of donor-derived T cells during the early posttransplantation period (109). Thus, the cause of the increased incidence of GVH disease in elderly patients is not known.

Bacterial decontamination in a protective environment significantly reduced the incidence and delayed the onset of acute GVH disease in patients who underwent transplantation because of aplastic anemia (101). Based on a similar effect seen in animals, it was hypothesized that enteric and skin bacteria sharing antigenic determinants with host epithelium activate lymphocyte clones to react against recipient tissues (112). However, there is no direct evidence for this mechanism in humans.

The association between GVH disease and viral infections has also been intensively investigated. The peak period for the occurrence of GVH disease coincides with the time during which cytomegalovirus (CMV) infection appears, and GVH disease is an important factor influencing the outcome of CMV infection (29). Thus, GVH disease could lead to reactivation of CMV infection or could interfere with the recovery of the immune system, thereby facilitating acquisition of infection (104). The idea that GVH disease leads to CMV infection is supported by the recent finding that acute GVH disease precedes CMV infection in a significant number of patients following marrow transplantation (69). However, the alternative view that CMV infection predisposes to GVH disease is supported by the observations that CMV infections precede the development of chronic GVH disease (60) and that prevention of CMV infections decreases the incidence of GVH disease (20). In addition, a correlation was observed between donor anti-CMV immunity and the development of chronic GVH disease (49), implying that chronic GVH disease might be mediated by a reaction of donor lymphocytes against cells of CMV-infected recipients. Indeed, because acute GVH disease usually is followed by chronic GVH disease (104), it is tempting to speculate that acute GVH disease predisposes to CMV infection, which in turn causes chronic GVH disease.

The risk for developing acute GVH disease is higher in patients with acute lymphoblastic leukemia (15) than in patients with aplastic anemia. Addition of total-body irradiation to the conditioning regimen for patients with aplastic anemia increased the incidence of GVH disease in some studies (11,36), but not in others (2,15). Refractoriness to random-donor platelet transfusions is associated with increased risk for severe GVH disease and poor survival among aplastic anemia patients (101), probably because these patients are hyperresponsive to minor histocompatibility antigens.

Finally, although the presence of GVH disease usually influences significantly the overall survival of transplant recipients (36,101), the presence of a particular factor associated with GVH disease may not affect the survival rate. For example, the addition of total-body irradiation to the preparative regimen increases the risk of GVH disease, but reduces the incidence of graft rejection, so that total-body irradiation has no net effect on survival (36). Likewise, several procedures that decrease the incidence of GVH disease, such as marrow T-cell depletion, may increase the risk for leukemia relapse and probably for graft failure, producing no significant effect on survival. These facts illustrate the complex and poorly understood interrelationship among GVH disease, graft failure, and allogeneic responses to leukemia (31).

Target Antigens

Dendritic cells (Langerhans cells), mature keratinocytes, and rete ridge stem cells are probable targets in skin GVH disease. Langerhans cells are the only cells in the normal epidermis that express class II MHC antigens and presumably are the most important cells involved in antigen presentation in the skin. The proposed role for DR antigens in triggering GVH disease is based on the fact that Langerhans cells are significantly reduced during episodes of clinical GVH disease (12,78) and are seen interacting with lymphocytes (32). Moreover, Langerhans cells of host origin persist for several months after transplantation and may express relevant antigens for the induction of GVH disease (77). However, a decrease in DR$^+$ dendritic cells was also observed after autologous bone marrow transplantation (45) and thus might be a consequence of pretransplantation irradiation (12). One recent study showed that reduction of Langerhans cells in the skin was specifically related to chronic, but not to acute, GVH disease (3).

Epidermal keratinocytes do not express class II MHC antigens in normal skin, but they exhibit these antigens in GVH disease and in other lymphocyte-mediated skin diseases (3,12). DR antigens in these conditions are synthesized by the keratinocytes themselves, probably stim-

ulated by gamma-interferon secreted by activated T cells. These antigens may contain polymorphic moieties not expressed on lymphoid cells, thus behaving as minor histocompatibility antigens and triggering strong immune responses by T lymphocytes (89). In addition, epidermal keratinocytes conserve the host HLA type after marrow transplantation (108); so they may be important targets for immune responses in skin. Thus, DR$^+$ host-derived keratinocytes that secrete IL-1 in the marrow recipient may be able to present antigen to allogeneic T helper cells, leading to the development of delayed-type hypersensitivity reactions. Alternatively, keratinocytes harboring both class I and class II HLA determinants may be targets for attack by allogeneic T cytotoxic cells in cooperation with helper T cells (12).

A recent morphological study suggested that the main targets for cutaneous GVH disease are the stem cell keratinocytes concentrated in the basal layer of the rete ridges (90). These primitive keratinocytes would be more susceptible to immune attack by donor T cells because of their osmotic fragility and their expression of unique differentiation antigens, like polymorphic DR. This hypothesis remains to be examined.

In chronic GVH disease, an ultrastructural study documented damage directed to keratinocytes, melanocytes, and Langerhans cells (32), and immunofluorescence studies suggested that targets are differentiation antigens present on keratinocytes of the basal layer of the skin (93).

Few studies have investigated the nature of target antigens in extracutaneous GVH disease, but it seems that DR$^+$ enterocytes (89) and bile duct cells (26) are the preferred targets for intestinal and hepatic GVH disease, respectively.

Besides the direct attack on tissues by immune cells, lesions of GVH disease could also result from donor immune reactions directed against host antigens on passenger leukocytes, leading to the release of lymphokines and development of delayed-type inflammatory reactions.

Cellular Mechanisms

T Cells

Evidence for T-cell involvement in human GVH disease has only recently begun to emerge and includes pathological as well as immunohistological data on target tissues, effects of depleting T cells from the marrow and of different forms of immunosuppression, and *in vitro* studies of T-lymphocyte markers and functions in patients (111,116).

Peripheral E-rosetting T cells are depressed during the first months after transplantation, regardless of the presence of GVH disease (111). Suppressor T cells, identified by the heteroantiserum TH2, were very low in 3 patients with acute GVH disease studied by Reinherz et al. (84). Interestingly, one of these patients received marrow from an identical twin and developed acute GVH disease indistinguishable from that observed in recipients of allogeneic transplants. The findings in chronic GVH disease were more heterogeneous, because in 2 patients suppressor cells were also lacking, but they were increased in 4 patients. This study suggests that immunoregulatory abnormalities are different in acute and chronic GVH disease and that these abnormalities may contribute to GVH disease.

More recently, the production of monoclonal antibodies to T-cell subpopulations has permitted extensive investigation of the dynamics of these subpopulations in human GVH disease. Earlier studies showed that T-helper/T-suppressor (CD4/CD8) cell ratios were reversed when measured 1 month or more after transplantation (reviewed in ref. 111). The use of flow cytometry permitted the evaluation of lymphocyte subsets in small amounts of peripheral blood as early as 4 days after transplantation. In these studies, a decrease in the T-helper/T-suppressor cell ratio to less than 2.5 at day 19 posttransplantation predicted the outcome of GVH disease in 9 of 10 patients, whereas only 2 of 14 patients with a ratio greater than 2.5 developed GVH disease (39). When these alterations are present, the T-cell compartment of the peripheral blood is composed of a mixture of donor and recipient cells. All patients in this study were receiving methotrexate as prophylaxis against GVH disease. In contrast, these changes in T-cell subsets were not observed in patients receiving cyclosporin in the posttransplantation period. It seems that cyclosporin A, but not methotrexate, is able to block the selective proliferation of T8$^+$ cells that occurs in peripheral blood during the early stages of acute GVH disease (41). In a separate study, the presence of GVH disease was not associated with any particular lymphocyte surface marker, but with the cytoplasmic content of several hydrolytic enzymes in lymphocytes and monocytes. There was a negative correlation between the outcome of GVH disease and the percentage of T cells displaying these hydrolases, and a positive correlation with the amount of the hydrolases in non-T cells and monocytes (86). These results can be explained by the loss of cytoplasmic enzymes from activated T cells during episodes of GVH disease.

Analysis of T-cell phenotypes in target tissues of GVH disease, rather than in peripheral blood, may help to elucidate the role of T cells in the pathogenesis of the disease. Some studies have shown an increase of T8$^+$ cells infiltrating the skin of patients with GVH disease and a correlation between the magnitude of the infiltrate and the severity of disease (56,57). These observations suggest that

T8$^+$ cells, probably with cytotoxic function, play a central role in producing the skin lesions of GVH disease. However, other studies failed to show any correlation between phenotypic abnormalities of lymphoid cells in the skin and the occurrence or grade of acute GVH disease (3,45,108). In one of these studies, few T cells of donor origin were seen infiltrating eczematous and normal skin after bone marrow transplantation (108). In another study, the scantiness of the cellular infiltrate suggested that soluble mediators rather than cytotoxic cells were responsible for the lesions of acute GVH disease, whereas in chronic GVH disease there was a predominance of T8$^+$ cells (3). Some studies also failed to demonstrate the presence of activation markers (DR, T10, IL-2 receptor) on lymphoid cells infiltrating cutaneous lesions (3,56), although this abnormality was reported in other studies (26,51).

Phenotypic abnormalities in the inflammatory cell infiltrate were also reported in target organs of GVH disease other than skin. In hepatic lesions, there are increases in T8$^+$ and Leu-7$^+$ cells and monocytes, as compared with transplantation patients without acute GVH disease. These cells are seen in the portal tracts and in the bile duct epithelium and do not express activation markers (26). Based on these findings, cytotoxic T cells, NK cells, or macrophages, acting alone or synergistically, could be implicated in the pathogenesis of hepatic GVH disease. Caution, however, must be exercised in interpreting increases in T8$^+$ and DR$^+$ cells in the gut during GVH disease (26), because T8$^+$ cells are numerous in normal intestinal mucosa, and there is little apparent association of lymphocytes with crypt necrosis (7). Likewise, interpretation of the increase in T8$^+$ lymphocytes in lung biopsies of patients with chronic GVH disease and lymphoid interstitial pneumonia requires more information about lung lymphocyte subsets in patients without GVH disease (79).

The most direct evidence for the involvement of T cells in the pathogenesis of GVH disease is derived from demonstrations in vitro of proliferation and cytotoxicity of donor T lymphocytes against recipient cells. In HLA-identical pairs, this reactivity is directed against minor histocompatibility antigens on host cells. In one study, circulating lymphocytes from approximately one-third of patients with chronic GVH disease showed unidirectional positive proliferative responses to cryopreserved recipient cells obtained prior to transplantation (111). Antihost proliferative responses have also been associated with acute GVH disease when skin cells have been used in the test either as a primary or secondary stimulus. In one study, T cells recovered from skin biopsies of 5 of 6 patients with acute GVH disease following HLA-matched transplantation showed proliferation in response to recipient and allogeneic cells in a primed lymphocyte test. This proliferative response against minor histocompatibility antigens was restricted by class II HLA antigens, and a cytotoxic response was observed in only 1 of 6 patients. These findings suggest that the predominant cell type present in skin during GVH disease is a noncytotoxic T helper cell that mediates a local delayed-type hypersensitivity reaction (85). Another recent study showed that proliferation of donor lymphocytes in response to recipient epidermal cells is associated with the further development of acute GVH disease (5).

Using another approach, donor lymphocytes sensitized to recipient cells in a mixed leukocyte culture were shown to cause the histologic picture of severe GVH disease involving skin *in vitro*. Reactivity was not demonstrated either by a proliferation or by a cytotoxicity assay. Interestingly, the target minor histocompatibility antigens were expressed either on the recipient or donor skin cells and lymphocytes from 10% of the patients, but from none of the donors showing autoreactivity against autologous skin (115).

Cytotoxic lymphocytes against host fibroblasts are found in about one-half of patients during the first 2 months after bone marrow transplantation, with an apparent correlation between a positive test and acute GVH disease (111). These results were confirmed using a more sensitive chromium-labeling assay, because 64% of the patients with acute GVH disease had cytotoxic cells directed against host fibroblasts. T cells were identified as responsible for the cytotoxicity against host fibroblasts in acute GVH disease, and no serum factors blocking cytotoxicity in patients without GVH disease were found. In another study, *in vitro* stimulation of peripheral blood lymphocytes with host cells from 2 patients with acute GVH disease generated cytotoxic cells that reacted against the recipients' normal and blast cells (80).

When expanded and tested against pretransplantation host lymphocytes, cytotoxic T-cell lines obtained 6 days after HLA-identical transplantation showed reactivity in acute and, particularly, in chronic GVH disease (38). This reactivity against minor histocompatibility antigens is supposed to be the primary cellular event in the induction and effector phases of GVH disease and was found to be restricted by class I HLA antigens. Interestingly, this cytotoxic reaction provided a cellular typing test for minor histocompatibility antigens that may permit the selection of donor-recipient pairs with less risk for GVH disease in the near future.

Immunoregulatory disturbances, particularly of suppressor cell activity, are observed in a large number of patients with GVH disease and may also play a role in the pathogenesis of the disease. Nonspecific suppressor cells inhibiting mixed leukocyte culture responses, proliferative responses to mitogens, and immunoglobulin synthesis are found in chronic GVH disease and correlate with the active stage of the disease (111). In most cases,

the cells responsible for suppression in chronic GVH disease are nonadherent, radioresistant $T8^+DR^-$ lymphocytes. The suppressive effect can be overcome by helper factors containing IL-2, suggesting that the target or the mechanism of the suppression is related to T helper cells. More recently, prostaglandin E_2 also was shown to be involved in the induction of suppressor cell activity in chronic GVH disease (53). In addition, patients with chronic GVH disease lack cells that specifically suppress proliferative responses to host antigens. These cells are also radiosensitive $T8^+$ lymphocytes that are present in healthy long-term chimeras, where conceivably they may be necessary to maintain the tolerance state between host and donor cells (111). Lack of appropriate suppressor cells is also postulated as being the cause of acute GVH disease, which would then result from an attack on host tissues by autocytotoxic null cells (76). However, neither the autocytotoxic effector cells nor the regulatory suppressor cells involved in GVH disease have been characterized.

B Cells

Hyperactive B-cell function has been detected by several tests in GVH disease, but it is unclear whether B cells contribute to the pathogenesis of the disease or simply are epiphenomena (111,116). Thus, lymphocytotoxic antibodies have been observed after bone marrow transplantation, but in most cases they are not related to GVH disease. Skin-reactive antibodies also have been found in patients with GVH disease (111). A pathogenic role of autoantibodies in chronic GVH disease was suggested by the findings of anti-acetylcholine-receptor antibodies in cases of myasthenia gravis associated with chronic GVH disease (97). The importance of other autoantibodies that have been detected in chronic GVH disease, such as antinuclear, antimitochondrial, and antierythrocyte antibodies, is questionable, because they are not regularly associated with clinical syndromes.

Circulating immune complexes also have been found after marrow transplantation, especially in patients with GVH disease. In one study, the immunoenzymatic conglutinin-binding assay detected elevated levels of immune complexes in patients with acute GVH disease, whereas the C1q-binding assay revealed the presence of immune complexes in long-term healthy survivors, but not in patients with chronic GVH disease. The significance of these observations is unclear, but it may be related to the ability of different methods to detect qualitatively distinct immune complexes (66). More recently, immune complexes containing casein and anticasein antibodies were observed in patients with acute and chronic GVH disease. These may be associated with increased absorption of milk proteins through the damaged intestinal tract. Although these complexes fix complement, and there was a tendency for an association between high antibody titers and more severe GVH disease, their inflammatory potential remains undetermined (21).

Monocytes and Macrophages

In light of the profound influence of macrophages on immunological interactions and function, it is surprising that few studies have addressed the roles of monocytes and macrophages as inducers or effectors of human GVH disease. Host macrophages survive the chemoirradiation pretransplantation regimen, but after the first month following grafting, they are replaced by donor cells. Thus, donor T helper cells in the recipient of a marrow transplant could interact with monocytes of either recipient or donor origin to proliferate in response to soluble antigens (19). In fact, accessory functions of blood monocytes for T-cell proliferation and IL-1 production are normal in patients with GVH disease (14,111). In addition, in the skin of patients with GVH disease, numerous OKM1[+] macrophages are present (51), and they can act as antigen-presenting cells or possibly as effector cells. Furthermore, persisting host Langerhans cells may also present minor histocompatibility antigens to donor T cells in the process of triggering GVH reactions (77). Finally, in a small number of patients with chronic GVH disease, monocytes capable of suppressing nonspecific and specific immunoglobulin synthesis were found, but their importance in the events leading to the development or termination of GVH disease is unclear (81,94).

Natural Killer Cells

Contradictory evidence exists for the role of natural killer (NK) cells in causing acute GVH disease (116). The most compelling support for this role comes from the observation that pretransplantation and posttransplantation levels of NK activity against fibroblasts infected with herpes simplex virus 1 (HSV-1) strongly correlate with the outcome of acute GVH disease (61,63). Thus, 7 of 13 patients with normal NK activity before transplantation acquired GVH disease, whereas 6 with low NK activity did not. Because there was no correlation between the degree of NK activity and the severity of GVH disease, NK cells from the host might provide the allogeneic stimulus required for the induction of GVH disease. This explanation is supported by the occurrence of GVH disease in severe combined immunodeficiency patients having normal or elevated NK activity (61) and by the prompt regression of GVH disease in one such patient when NK activity declined (96).

However, there is also evidence against the participation of host NK cells in the induction of GVH disease. First, NK activity is very low following transplantation and recovers gradually, suggesting a donor origin for NK cells even in the early posttransplantation period. In fact, a donor origin for NK cells was found in a small number of cases by DNA polymorphism analysis (4). Second, several other studies failed to confirm the relationship between low levels of NK activity against K-562 cells before or after transplantation and the development of GVH disease (40,47,59). One can argue about the different natures of effector NK cells that kill herpesvirus-infected fibroblasts versus those that kill K-562 cells. Only NK cells that are cytotoxic to herpesvirus-infected cells would be targets in GVH disease (62). In addition, cells with an NK phenotype have been identified in the skin and rectal epithelium of patients with acute GVH disease (71,119), suggesting that NK cells may be involved in producing tissue damage. However, until the association between NK activity and GVH disease is confirmed in a larger number of patients and more direct evidence from experimental and *in vitro* studies is obtained, a stimulatory or effector role for NK cells in GVH disease is uncertain.

REFERENCES

1. Atkinson, K., Incefy, G. S., Storb, R., Sullivan, K. M., Iwata, T., Dardenne, M., Ochs, H. D., Good, R. A., and Thomas, E. D. (1982): Low serum thymic hormone levels in patients with chronic graft-versus-host disease. *Blood*, 59:1073–1077.
2. Atkinson, K., Farrell, C., Chapman, G., Penny, R., and Biggs, J. (1986): Female marrow donors increase the risk of acute graft-versus-host disease: Effect of donor age and parity and analysis of cell populations in the donor marrow inoculum. *Br. J. Haematol.*, 63:231–239.
3. Atkinson, K., Munro, V., Vasak, E., and Biggs, E. (1986): Mononuclear cell subpopulations in the skin defined by monoclonal antibodies after HLA-identical sibling marrow transplantation. *Br. J. Dermatol.*, 114:145–160.
4. Ault, K. A., Autin, J. H., Ginsburg, D., Oakin, S. H., Rappeport, J. M., Keohan, M. L., Martin, P., and Smith, B. R. (1985): Phenotype of recovering lymphoid cell populations after marrow transplantation. *J. Exp. Med.*, 161:1483–1502.
5. Bagot, M., Cordonnier, C., Tilkin, A. F., Heslan, M., Vernant, J. P., Dubertret, L., and Levy, J. P. (1986): A possible predictive test for graft-versus-host disease in bone marrow graft recipients: The mixed epidermal cell–lymphocyte reaction. *Transplantation*, 41:316–319.
6. Beatty, P. G., Clift, R. A., Mickelson, E. M., Nisperos, B. B., Flournoy, N., Martin, P. J., Sanders, J., Stewart, P., Buckner, C. D., Storb, R., Thomas, E. D., and Hansen, J. A. (1985): Marrow transplantation from related donors other than HLA-identical siblings. *N. Engl. J. Med.*, 313:765–771.
7. Beschorner, W. E. (1984): Destruction of the intestinal mucosa after bone marrow transplantation and graft-versus-host disease. *Surv. Synth. Pathol. Res.*, 3:264–274.
8. Beschorner, W. E., Tutschka, P. J., and Santos, G. W. (1982): Chronic graft-versus-host disease in the rat radiation chimera. I. Clinical features, hematology, histology, and immunopathology in long-term chimeras. *Transplantation*, 33:393–399.
9. Beschorner, W. E., Tutschka, P. J., and Santos, G. W. (1983): Chronic graft-versus-host disease in the rat radiation chimera. III.

Immunology and immunopathology in rapidly induced models. *Transplantation*, 35:224–230.

10. Bortin, M. M. (1986): Risk factors for acute graft-vs.-host disease in humans. In: *Experimental Hematology Today*, edited by S. J. Baum, D. H. Pluznik, and L. A. Rozenszajin, pp. 114–121, Springer-Verlag, New York.

11. Bortin, M. M., Gale, R. P., and Rimm, A. A. (1981): Allogeneic bone marrow transplantation for 144 patients with severe aplastic anemia. *J.A.M.A.*, 245:1132–1139.

12. Breathnach, S. M. (1986): Current understanding of the aetiology and clinical implications of cutaneous graft-versus-host disease. *Br. J. Dermatol.*, 114:139–143.

13. Bril, H., and Benner, R. (1985): Graft-versus-host reactions: Mechanisms and contemporary theories. *CRC Crit. Rev. Clin. Lab. Sci.*, 22:43–95.

14. Brkic, S., Tsoi, M. S., Mori, T., Lachman, L., Gillis, S., Thomas, E. D., and Storb, R. (1985): Cellular interactions in marrow grafted patients. III. Normal interleukin-1 and defective interleukin-2 production in short-term patients and in those with chronic graft-versus-host disease. *Transplantation*, 39:30–35.

15. Bross, D. S., Tutschka, P. J., Farmer, E. R., Beschorner, W. E., Braine, H. G., Mellits, E. D., Bias, W. B., and Santos, G. W. (1984): Predictive factors for acute graft-versus-host disease in patients transplanted with HLA-identical bone marrow. *Blood*, 63:1265–1270.

16. Brubaker, D. B. (1986): Transfusion associated graft-versus-host disease. *Hum. Pathol.*, 17:1085–1088.

17. Charley, M. R., Mikhael, A., Hoot, G., Hackett, M. D., and Bennett, M. (1985): Studies addressing the mechanism of anti-asialo GM1 prevention of graft-versus-host disease due to minor histocompatibility antigenic differences. *J. Invest. Dermatol.*, 85:121s–123s.

18. Cheney, R. T., and Sprent, J. (1985): Capacity of cyclosporine to induce auto-graft-versus-host disease and impair intrathymic T cell differentiation. *Transplant. Proc.*, 17:528–530.

19. Chu, E., Umetsu, D., Rosen, F., and Geha, R. S. (1983): Major histocompatibility restriction of antigen recognition by T cells in a recipient of haplotype mismatched human bone marrow transplantation. *J. Clin. Invest.*, 72:1124–1129.

20. Condie, R. M., and O'Reilly, R. J. (1984): Prevention of cytomegalovirus infection by prophylaxis with intravenous, hyperimmune, native, unmodified cytomegalovirus globulin. Randomized trial in bone marrow transplant recipients. *Am. J. Med.*, 76:134.

21. Cunningham-Rundles, C., and O'Reilly, R. (1986): Association of circulating immune complexes containing bovine proteins and graft-versus-host disease. *Clin. Exp. Immunol.*, 64:323–329.

22. De Clerck, Y., Draper, V., and Parkman, R. (1986): Clonal analysis of murine graft-versus-host disease. II. Leukokines that stimulate fibroblast proliferation and collagen synthesis in graft-versus-host disease. *J. Immunol.*, 136:3549–3552.

23. Deeg, H., and Storb, R. (1986): Acute and chronic graft-versus-host disease: Clinical manifestations, prophylaxis and treatment. *J. Natl. Cancer Inst.*, 76:1325–1328.

24. Deierhoi, M. H., Sollinger, H. W., Bozdech, M. J., and Belzer, F. O. (1986): Lethal graft-versus-host disease in a recipient of pancreas-spleen transplant. *Transplantation*, 41:544–545.

25. Deltz, E., Ulrichs, K., Shack, T., Friedrichs, B., Muller-Ruchholtz, W., Muller-Hermelink, H. K., and Thiede, A. (1986): Graft-versus-host reaction in small bowel transplantation and possibilities for its circumvention. *Am. J. Surg.*, 151:379–386.

26. Dilly, S. A., and Sloane, J. P. (1985): An immunohistological study of human hepatic graft-versus-host disease. *Clin. Exp. Immunol.*, 62:545–553.

27. Elkins, W. L. (1971): Cellular immunology and the pathogenesis of graft-versus-host reactions. *Prog. Allergy*, 15:78–187.

28. Ford, W. L. (1978): Measurement of graft-versus-host activity. In: *Handbook of Experimental Immunology*, edited by D. M. Weir, pp. 30.1–30.12. Blackwell Scientific, Oxford, U.K.

29. Forman, S. J., and Gallagher, M. T. (1983): Reconstitution of the immune system. In: *Clinical Bone Marrow Transplantation*, edited by K. G. Blume and L. D. Petz, pp. 65–90. Churchill Livingstone, New York.

30. Gale, R. P. (1985): Graft-versus-host disease. *Immunol. Rev.*, 88:193–214.

31. Gale, R. P., and Reisner, Y. (1986): Graft rejection and graft-versus-host disease: Mirror images. *Lancet*, 1:1468–1470.

32. Gallucci, B. B., Shulman, H. M., Sale, G. E., Lerner, K. G., Caldwell, L. E., and Thomas, E. D. (1979): The ultrastructure of the human epidermis in chronic graft-versus-host disease. *Am. J. Pathol.*, 95:643–662.

33. Gingrich, R., Howe, C., Goeken, N., Ginder, G., and Fye, M. (1985): Successful bone marrow transplantation with partially matched unrelated donors. *Transplant. Proc.*, 17:450–452.

34. Gleichmann, E., Pals, S. T., Rolink, A. G., Radaskiewicz, T., and Gleichmann, H. (1984): Graft-versus-host reactions: Clues to the etiopathology of a spectrum of immunologic diseases. *Immunol. Today*, 5:324–332.

35. Gluckman, E., Devergie, A., Schier, J., and Saurat, J. H. (1980): Graft-versus-host disease in recipients of syngeneic bone marrow. *Lancet*, 1:253–254.

36. Gluckman, E., Barrett, A. J., Arcese, W., Devergie, A., and Degoulet, P. (1981): Bone marrow transplantation in severe aplastic anemia: A survey of the European Group for Bone Marrow Transplantation (EGBMT). *Br. J. Haematol.*, 49:165–173.

37. Goldin, H., and Keisari, Y. (1986): Increased oxidative burst potential exhibited by macrophages during graft-versus-host reactions. *Transplantation*, 41:755–758.

38. Goulmy, E., Bokland, E., Gratama, J. W., Zwaan, F. E., and van Rood, J. J. (1984): Detection of minor histocompatibility antigens by MHC restricted cytotoxic T lymphocytes generated during graft-versus-host disease. *Exp. Hematol. (Suppl. 15)*, 12:77–78.

39. Gratama, J. W., Naipal, A., Oljans, P., Zwaan, F. E., Verdonck, L. F., De Witte, T., Vossen, M. J. J., Bolhuis, R. L. H., De Gast, G. C., and Jansen, J. (1984): T lymphocyte repopulation and differentiation after bone marrow transplantation. Early shifts in the ratio between T4+ and T8+ T lymphocytes correlate with the occurrence of acute graft-versus-host disease. *Blood*, 63:1416–1423.

40. Gratama, J. W., Lipovich-Oosterveer, M. A., Ronteltap, C., Sinnige, L. G. F., Jansen, J., van der Griend, R. J., and Bolhuis, R. L. H. (1985): Natural immunity and graft-versus-host disease. *Transplantation*, 40:256–260.

41. Gratama, J. W., Wursch, A. M., Nissen, C., Gratwohl, A., D'Amaro, J., De Gast, G. C., and Speck, B. (1986): Influence of graft-versus-host disease prophylaxis on early T-lymphocyte regeneration following allogeneic bone marrow transplantation. *Br. J. Haematol.*, 62:355–365.

42. Graze, P. R., and Gale, R. P. (1979): Chronic graft-versus-host disease: A syndrome of disordered immunity. *Am. J. Med.*, 66:611–620.

43. Grebe, S. C., and Streilein, J. W. (1976): Graft-versus-host reactions: A review. *Adv. Immunol.*, 22:119–221.

44. Guy-Grand, D., and Vassali, P. (1986): Gut injury in mouse graft-versus-host reaction. Study of its occurrence and mechanism. *J. Clin. Invest.*, 77:1584–1595.

45. Guyotat, D., Mauduit, G., Chouvet, B., Kanitatkis, J., Van, H. V., Fierce, D., and Thivolet, J. (1986): A sequential study of histological and immunological changes in the skin after allogeneic bone marrow transplantation. *Transplantation*, 41:340–342.

46. Hansen, J. A., Mickelson, E. M., Beatty, P. G., and Thomas, E. D. (1986): Clinical bone marrow transplantation: Donor selection and recipient monitoring. In: *Manual of Clinical Laboratory Immunology*, edited by N. R. Rose, H. Friedman, and J. L. Fahey, pp. 892–901. American Society for Microbiology, Washington, D.C.

47. Heidemann, E., Schmidt, H., Schuch, K., Ostendorf, P., and Waller, H. D. (1986): Natural killer cell activity against a thymoma cell line Thy 121 in bone marrow transplant recipients. *Klin. Wochenschr.*, 64:125–130.

48. Hess, A. D., Horwitz, L., Beschorner, W. E., and Santos, G. W. (1985): Development of graft-versus-host disease-like syndrome in cyclosporine-treated rats after syngeneic bone marrow transplantation. I. Development of cytotoxic T lymphocytes with apparent polyclonal anti-Ia specificity, including autoreactivity. *J. Exp. Med.*, 161:718–730.

49. Jacobsen, N., Andersen, H. K., Akinhoj, P., Ryder, L. P., Platz,

P., Jerne, D., and Faber, V. (1986): Correlation between donor cytomegalovirus immunity and chronic graft-versus-host disease after allogeneic bone marrow transplantation. *Scand. J. Haematol.,* 36:499–506.

50. Kammuller, M. E., Penninks, A. H., and Seinen, W. (1984): Spanish toxic oil syndrome is a chemically induced GVHD-like epidemic. *Lancet,* 1:1174–1175.

51. Kaye, V. N., Neumann, P. M., Kersey, J., Goltz, R. W., Baldridge, B. D., Michael, A. F., and Platt, J. L. (1986): Identity of immune cells in graft-versus-host disease of the skin. Analysis using monoclonal antibodies by indirect immunofluorescence. *Am. J. Pathol.,* 116:436–440.

52. Klein, J., and Chang, C. J. (1976): Ability of H-2 regions to induce graft-versus-host disease. *J. Immunol.,* 117:736–740.

53. Klingemann, H. G., Tsoi, M. S., and Storb, R. (1986): Inhibition of prostaglandin E$_2$ restores effective lymphocyte proliferation and cell-mediated lympholysis in recipients after allogeneic marrow grafting. *Blood,* 68:102–107.

54. Korngold, R., and Sprent, J. (1983): Lethal GVHD across minor histocompatibility barriers: Nature of the effector cells and role of the H-2 complex. *Immunol. Rev.,* 71:5–29.

55. Korngold, R., and Sprent, J. (1985): Surface markers of T cells causing lethal graft-versus-host disease to class I vs. class II H-2 differences. *J. Immunol.,* 135:3004–3009.

56. Lampert, I. A., Janossy, G., Suitters, A. J., Bofill, M., Palmer, S., Gordon-Smith, E., Prentice, H. G., and Thomas, J. A. (1982): Immunological analysis of the skin in graft-versus-host disease. *Clin. Exp. Immunol.,* 50:123–131.

57. Lever, R., Turbitt, M., Mackie, R., Hann, I., Gibson, B., Burnett, J. N., and Willoughby, M. (1986): A prospective study of the histological changes in the skin in patients receiving bone marrow transplants. *Br. J. Dermatol.,* 114:161–170.

58. Levy, D. A., and Wefald, A. (1986): Gut mucosal mast cells and goblet cells during acute graft-versus-host disease in rats. *Ann. Inst. Pasteur Immunol.,* 137D:281–288.

59. Livnat, S., Seigneuret, M., Storb, R., and Prentice, R. L. (1980): Analysis of cytotoxic effector cell function in patients with leukemia or aplastic leukemia before and after bone marrow transplantation. *J. Immunol.,* 124:481–490.

60. Lonnqvist, B., Ringden, O., Walnen, B., Gahrton, G., and Lundgren, G. (1984): Cytomegalovirus infection associated with and predeeding chronic graft-versus-host disease. *Transplantation,* 38:465–468.

61. Lopez, C., Kirkpatrick, D., Sorell, M., O'Reilly, R. J., and Ching, C. (1979): Association between pre-transplant natural killing and graft-versus-host disease after stem cell transplantation. *Lancet,* 2:1103–1106.

62. Lopez, C., Kirkpatrick, D., Livnat, S., and Storb, R. (1980): Natural killer cells in bone marrow transplantation. *Lancet,* 1:1025.

63. Lopez, C., Schindler, B., Fitzgerald, P. A., and Kirkpatrick, D. (1984): The importance of natural killer cells in natural defense against severe viral infections and in graft-versus-host disease. In: *Natural Killer Activity and Its Regulation,* edited by T. Hoshino, H. S. Koren, and A. Uchida, pp. 395–399. Excerpta Medica, Amsterdam.

64. Loveland, B., and Simpson, E. (1986): The non-MHC transplantation antigens: Neither weak nor minor. *Immunol. Today,* 7:223–229.

65. Lowenberg, B., Vossen, J. M. J. J., and Doren, L. J. (1977): Transplantation of fetal liver cells in the treatment of severe combined immunodeficiency disease. *Blut,* 34:181–195.

66. Manca, F., Bacigalupo, A., van Lint, M. T., Trovatello, G., Cantarella, S., Frassoni, F., Marmont, A., and Celada, F. (1984): Circulating immune complexes in allogeneic marrow graft recipients. *Transplantation,* 38:428–430.

67. McDonald, G. B., Shulman, H. M., Sullivan, K. M., and Spencer, G. D. (1986): Intestinal and hepatic complications of human bone marrow transplantation. Part I. *Gastroenterology,* 90:460–477.

68. McDonald, G. B., Shulman, H. M., Sullivan, K. M., and Spencer, G. D. (1986): Intestinal and hepatic complications of human bone marrow transplantation. Part II. *Gastroenterology,* 90:770–784.

69. Miller, W., Flynn, P., McCullough, J., Balfour, H. H., Jr., Goldman,

A., Haake, J., McGlave, P., Ramsay, N., and Kersey, J. (1986): Cytomegalovirus infection after bone marrow transplantation: An association with acute graft-versus-host disease. *Blood,* 67:1162–1167.

70. Mowat, A. M., Borland, A., and Parrott, D. M. V. (1985): Augmentation of natural killer cell activity by anti-host delayed-type hypersensitivity during the graft-versus-host reaction in mice. *Scand. J. Immunol.,* 22:389–399.

71. Muller, C., Schuch, K., Pawelec, G., Wilms, K., and Wernet, P. (1982): Immunohistology of graft-versus-host disease mediated skin lesions and its correlation to a large-granular lymphocyte surface phenotype and function. *Blut,* 44:89–94.

72. Nagata, N., Hurteubach, V., and Gleichmann, E. (1986): Specific sensitization by Lyt1+2- T cells to spleen cells modified by the drug D-penicillamine or a stereoisomer. *J. Immunol.,* 136:136–142.

73. Oaks, M. K., and Cramer, D. V. (1985): Chronic graft-versus-host disease in rats after syngeneic bone marrow transplantation. *Transplantation,* 39:504–510.

74. Okunewick, J. P. (1985): Review of the effects of anti-T cell monoclonal antibodies on major and minor GVHR in mouse. In: *Experimental Hematology Today,* edited by S. G. Baum, D. H. Pluznik, and G. Ledney, pp. 133–143. Springer-Verlag, New York.

75. Parkman, R. (1986): Clonal analysis of murine graft-versus-host disease. I. Phenotypic and functional analysis of T lymphocyte clones. *J. Immunol.,* 136:3543–3552.

76. Parkman, R., Rappeport, J., and Rosen, R. (1980): Human graft-versus-host disease. *J. Invest. Dermatol.,* 74:276–279.

77. Perreault, C., Pelletier, M., Belanger, R., Montplaisir, S., Boileau, J., Bonny, Y., David, M., and Lacombe, M. (1984): Persistence of host Langerhans cells (LC) following allogeneic bone marrow transplantation (BMT). *Blood,* 64:219a.

78. Perreault, C., Pelletier, M., Landry, D., and Gyger, M. (1984): Study of Langerhans cells after allogeneic bone marrow transplantation. *Blood,* 63:807–811.

79. Perreault, C., Cousineau, S., D'Angleo, G., Gyger, M., Nepveu, F., Boileau, J., Bonny, Y., Lacombe, M., and Lavallee, R. (1985): Lymphoid interstitial pneumonia after allogeneic bone marrow transplantation. A possible manifestation of chronic graft-versus-host disease. *Cancer,* 55:1–9.

80. Pierson, G. R., and Elkins, W. L. (1983): In vitro generation of cytotoxic cells with graft vs host specificity from the blood of patients with graft vs. host disease. These effectors may detect minor alloantigens on leukemic targets from the host. In: *Recent Advances in Bone Marrow Transplantation,* edited by R. P. Gale, pp. 223–226. Alan R. Liss, New York.

81. Pollack, S., O'Reilly, R., Koziner, B., Good, R. A., and Hoffman, M. K. (1986): Reconstitution of *in vitro* humoral immune function in bone marrow transplant recipients. *Immunobiology,* 171:93–111.

82. Rappaport, H., Khalil, A., Halle-Pannenko, O., Pritchard, L., Dantchev, D., and Mathe, G. (1979): Histopathologic sequence of events in adult mice undergoing lethal graft-versus-host reaction developed across H-2 and/or non-H-2 histocompatibility barriers. *Am. J. Pathol.,* 96:121–142.

83. Rappeport, J., Mihm, M., Reinherz, E., Lopanski, S., and Parkman, R. (1979): Acute graft-versus-host disease in recipients of bone marrow transplants from identical twin donors. *Lancet,* 2:717–720.

84. Reinherz, E. L., Parkman, R., Rappeport, J., Rosen, F. S., and Schlossman, S. F. (1979): Aberrations of suppressor T cells in human graft-versus-host disease. *N. Engl. J. Med.,* 300:1061–1068.

85. Reinsmoen, N. L., Kersey, J. H., and Bach, F. H. (1984): Detection of HLA-restricted anti-minor histocompatibility antigen(s) reactive cells from skin GVHD lesions. *Human Immunol.,* 11:249–257.

86. Repetto, M., Bacigalupo, A., Viale, M., Gandini, M., Frassoni, F., Marmont, A. M., and Van Lint, M. T. (1985): Cytochemical analysis of peripheral blood mononuclear cells following allogeneic bone marrow transplantation: Correlation of hydrolase expression with graft-versus-host disease. *Blood,* 66:1011–1016.

87. Ringden, O., Paulin, T., Lonnqvist, B., and Nilsson, B. (1985): An

analysis of factors predisposing to chronic graft-versus-host disease. *Exp. Hematol.,* 13:1062–1067.

88. Sale, G. E. (1984): In vitro and in vivo animal models of GVHR and GVHD. In: *The Pathology of Bone Marrow Transplantation,* edited by G. E. Sale and H. M. Shulman, pp. 19–30. Year Book, Chicago.

89. Sale, G. E. (1984): Pathology and recent pathogenic studies in human graft-versus-host disease. *Surv. Synth. Pathol. Res.,* 3:235–253.

90. Sale, G. E., Shulman, H. M., Galucci, B. B., and Thomas, E. D. (1985): Young rete ridge keratinocytes are preferred targets in cutaneous graft-versus-host disease. *Am. J. Pathol.,* 118:278–287.

91. Sanders, J. E., Pitchard, S., Mahoney, P., Amos, D., Buckner, C. D., Witherspoon, R. P., Deeg, H. J., Doney, K. C., Sullivan, K. M., Appelbaum, F. R., Storb, R., and Thomas, E. D. (1986): Growth and development following marrow transplantation for leukemia. *Blood,* 68:1129–1135.

92. Santos, G. W., Hess, A. D., and Vogelsang, G. B. (1985): Graft-versus-host reactions and disease. *Immunol. Rev.,* 88:169–192.

93. Saurat, J. H., Didijean, L., Beucher, F., and Gluckman, E. (1978): Immunofluorescent tracing of cytoplasmic components involved in keratinocyte differentiation. *Br. J. Dermatol.,* 98:155–163.

94. Shiobara, S., Witherspoon, R. P., Lum, L. G., and Storb, R. (1984): Immunoglobulin synthesis after HLA identical marrow grafting. V. The role of peripheral blood monocytes in the regulation of in vitro immunoglobulin secretion stimulated by pokeweed mitogen. *J. Immunol.,* 132:2850–2856.

95. Shulman, H. M., Sullivan, K. M., Weiden, P. L., McDonald, G. B., Stricker, G. E., Sale, G. E., Hackman, R., Tsoi, M. S., Storb, R., and Thomas, E. D. (1980): Chronic graft-versus-host syndrome in man. A long-term clinicopathologic study of 20 Seattle patients. *Am. J. Med.,* 69:204–217.

96. Sindel, L. J., Buckley, R. H., Schiff, S. E., Ward, F. E., Mickey, G. H., Huand, A. T., Naspitz, C., and Koren H. (1984): Severe combined immunodeficiency with natural killer predominance: Abrogation of graft-versus-host disease and immunological reconstitution with HLA-identical bone marrow cells. *J. Allergy Clin. Immunol.,* 73:829–836.

97. Smith, C. I. E., Aarli, J. A., Biberfield, P., Bolme, P., Christensson, B., Gahurton, G., Hammarstrom, L., Lefvert, A. K., Lonnqvist, B., Mattel, G., Pirskanen, R., Ringden, O., and Svanborg, E. (1983): Myasthenia gravis after bone marrow transplantation: Evidence for a donor origin. *N. Engl. J. Med.,* 309:1565–1568.

98. Sparkes, R. S., Sparkes, M. C., Crist, M., Yale, C., Mickey, M. R., and Gale, R. P. (1980): MNSs antigens and graft versus host disease following bone marrow transplantation. *Tissue Antigens,* 15:212–215.

99. Sprent, J., Schaefer, M., Lo, D., and Korngold, R. (1986): Functions of purified L3T4+ and Lyt-2+ cells in vitro and in vivo. *Immunol. Rev.,* 91:195–218.

100. Storb, R. (1984): Pathophysiology and prevention of graft-versus host disease. In: *Advances in Immunology: Blood Cell Antigens and Bone Marrow Transplantation,* edited by J. McCullough and S. G. Sandler, pp. 337–366. Alan R. Liss, New York.

101. Storb, R., Prentice, R. L., Buckner, C. D., Clift, R. A., Appelbaum, F., Deeg, J., Doney, K., Hansen, J. A., Mason, M., Sanders, J. E., Singer, J., Sullivan, K. M., Witherspoon, R. P., and Thomas, E. D. (1983): Graft-versus-host disease and survival in patients with aplastic anemia treated by marrow grafts from HLA-identical siblings. Beneficial effect of a protective environment. *N. Engl. J. Med.,* 308:302–307.

102. Storb, R., Prentice, R. L., Hansen, J. A., and Thomas, E. D. (1983): Association between HLA-B antigens and acute graft-versus host disease. *Lancet,* 2:816–819.

103. Storb, R., Prentice, R. L., Sullivan, K. M., Shulman, H. M., Deeg, H. J., Doney, K. C., Buckner, C. D., Clift, R. A., Witherspoon, R. P., Appelbaum, F. A., Sanders, J. E., Stewart, P., and Thomas, E. D. (1983): Predictive factors in chronic graft-versus-host disease in patients with aplastic anemia treated by marrow transplantation from HLA-identical siblings. *Ann. Intern. Med.,* 98:461–466.

104. Storb, R., and Thomas, E. D. (1985): Graft-versus-host disease in dog and man: The Seattle experience. *Immunol. Rev.,* 88:215–238.

105. Sullivan, K. M. (1986): Acute and chronic graft-versus-host disease in man. *Int. J. Cell. Cloning (Suppl. 1),* 4:29–93.

106. Sullivan, K. M., Deeg, H. J., Sanders, J., Klosterman, A., Amos, D., Shulman, H., Sale, G., Martin, P., Witherspoon, R., Appelbaum, F., Doney, K., Stewart, P., Meyers, J., McDonald, G. B., Weiden, P., Fefer, A., Buckner, C. D., and Thomas, E. D. (1986): Hyperacute graft-versus-host disease in patients not given immunosuppression after allogeneic marrow transplantation. *Blood,* 67:1172–1175.

107. Thein, S. L., Goldman, J. M., and Galton, D. A. G. (1981): Acute "graft-versus-host disease" after autografting for chronic granulocytic leukemia in transformation. *Ann. Intern. Med.,* 94:210–211.

108. Thomas, J. A., Wakeling, W. F., Imrie, S. F., Sloane, J. P., Powles, R. P., and Lawler, S. D. (1984): Chimerism in the skin of bone marrow transplant recipients. *Transplantation,* 38:475–478.

109. Thomas, J. A., Sloane, J. A., Imrie, S. F., Ritter, M. A., Schuurman, H. J., and Huber, J. (1986): Immunohistology of the thymus in bone marrow transplant recipients. *Am. J. Pathol.,* 122:531–540.

110. Thompson, L. F., O'Connor, R. D., and Bastian, J. F. (1984): Phenotype and function of engrafted maternal T cells in patients with severe combined immunodeficiency. *J. Immunol.,* 133:2513–2517.

111. Tsoi, M. S. (1984): Immunologic studies of human GVHD. In: *The Pathology of Bone Marrow Transplantation,* edited by G. E. Sale and H. M. Shulman, pp. 11–18. Year Book, Chicago.

112. Van Bekkum, D. W. (1980): Immunological basis of graft-versus-host disease. In: *Biology of Bone Marrow Transplantation,* edited by R. P. Gale and C. F. Fox, pp. 175–193. Academic Press, New York.

113. Van Rood, J. J., Jongh, B., Claas, F. H. J., Goulmy, E., Gratama, J. M., and Gihpart, M. J. (1984): New facts on HLA genetics: Are they relevant in bone marrow transplantation? *Semin. Hematol.,* 21:65–80.

114. Varkila, K., and Hurme, M. (1985): Natural killer cells and graft-versus-host disease (GVHD): No correlation between the NK levels and GVHD in the murine P to F_1 model. *Immunology,* 54:121–126.

115. Vogelsang, G. B., Hess, A. D., Berkman, A. W., Tutschka, P. J., Farmer, E. R., Converse, P. J., and Santos, G. W. (1985): An in vitro predictive test for graft versus host disease in patients with genotypic HLA-identical bone marrow transplants. *N. Engl. J. Med.,* 313:645–650.

116. Voltarelli, J. C., and Stites, D. P. (1986): Immunological monitoring of bone marrow transplantation. *Diagn. Immunol.,* 4:171–193.

117. Von Fliedner, V., Higby, D. J., and Kim, U. (1982): Graft-versus-host reaction following blood product transfusion. *Am. J. Med.,* 72:951–961.

118. Weiner, R. S., Bortin, M. M., Gale, R. P., Gluckman, E., Kay, H. E. M., Kolb, H. J., Hartz, A. J., and Rimm, A. A. (1986): Interstitial pneumonitis after bone marrow transplantation. Assessment of risk factors. *Ann. Intern. Med.,* 104:168–175.

119. Weisdorf, S. A., Platt, J. L., Snover, D. C., Kernet, J. H., and Sharp, H. L. (1983): In situ analysis of T and killer lymphocyte subpopulations in rectal biopsies from bone marrow transplant recipients. *Gastroenterology,* 84:1348.

Inflammation: Basic Principles and Clinical Correlates.
Edited by J. I. Gallin, I. M. Goldstein, and R. Snyderman.
Raven Press, Ltd., New York © 1988.

CHAPTER 40

Histoplasmosis: A Granulomatous Inflammatory Response

George S. Deepe, Jr. and Ward E. Bullock

Until the mid-1940s, physicians generally presumed
that the presence of intrathoracic calcifications revealed
by X-rays signified prior tuberculosis, the classic paradigm
of infection-mediated, delayed-type hypersensitivity
(DTH). In the midwestern United States, however, the
low frequency of positive tuberculin skin tests in individuals with pulmonary calcifications raised increasing
doubts about that assumption. Although such failure to
mount a tuberculin skin test could be attributable to mal-
nourishment, overwhelming infection with *Mycobacterium tuberculosis,* or injection of insufficient antigen, it
was found that this could be verified in only a minority
of cases and did not explain the frequency of negative
reactions to tuberculin. It was not until 1945 that Christie
and Peterson (19) demonstrated the high incidence of
positive skin-test reactions to histoplasmin in many mid-
dle-Tennessee children with intrathoracic calcifications.
This landmark finding was confirmed by others (39,67),
and it was established unequivocally that histoplasmosis,
like tuberculosis, could effect a DTH response as manifested by a positive skin test and a healed primary complex
consisting of a pulmonary focus and satellite lymph nodes.
Cases of histoplasmosis have been reported from every

continent except Antarctica (81). In the United States,
histoplasmosis is endemic to the Ohio and Mississippi
river valleys, and it is estimated that 500,000 new infections occur in the United States each year (1). Although
many new infections are acquired sporadically, more than
40 epidemics have been reported. From 1978 to 1982,
more than 150,000 individuals were infected with *Histoplasma capsulatum* during a massive outbreak in Indianapolis, Indiana (103,106).

Infection with the dimorphic fungus *H. capsulatum* is
acquired by incidental inhalation of microconidia (5–8
µm) or small mycelial fragments that are deposited within
terminal bronchioles and alveoli, where they undergo
transformation to the pathogenic yeast phase within a period of hours to days. The morphological transition from
mycelial phase to yeast phase is accompanied by an orderly progression of biochemical events. Three distinct
stages have been described (75). Initially there is a decline
in intracellular adenosine triphosphate and a progressive
reduction in the respiration rate of organisms (stage 1).
The cells then enter a dormant phase for 4 to 6 days (stage
2). Finally, the respiratory rate returns to normal, and
there is an induction of yeast-phase-specific cysteine ox-

idase. At this point, the morphological transformation to yeast cells is completed (stage 3). Virtually all clinical manifestations of histoplasmosis are caused by yeast-phase organisms that evoke a characteristic inflammatory response of caseating or noncaseating granuloma formation.

Like leprosy and tuberculosis, histoplasmosis can be considered in the context of a spectrum of disease presentations regarding both its clinicopathological and immunological manifestations (Table 1). Clinically, infection with *H. capsulatum* produces a diversity of illnesses ranging from acute pulmonary disease to a chronic pulmonary infection to a progressive disseminated form. Among exposed individuals, it is estimated that acute pulmonary disease develops in more than 95%, whereas less than 1% progress to either chronic pulmonary disease or disseminated infection. Both acute pulmonary histoplasmosis and chronic pulmonary histoplasmosis are characterized by discrete granuloma formation, whereas in acute disseminated disease, granulomas generally are formed poorly, if at all. Instead, infected tissues are massively infiltrated by mononuclear phagocytes engorged with yeasts. Correspondingly, there are pronounced differences in the immunological manifestations of histoplasmosis among the various clinical groups. The *in vivo* and *in vitro* cellular immune responses of those with acute and chronic pulmonary diseases are generally intact; conversely, skin-test anergy and impaired blastogenic responses to mitogens and *Histoplasma* antigens are observed frequently among those with disseminated infection (58,64,71,85). In this chapter we shall examine the interrelationship between the inflammatory response and cell-mediated immunity in the various forms of histoplasmosis.

PATHOGENESIS OF ACUTE PULMONARY DISEASE

Immunopathology in Experimental Models

Inflammatory Response to Histoplasma *Conidia*

In the vast majority of individuals who inhale conidia and mycelial fragments of *H. capsulatum,* the infection is inapparent clinically or presents as a mild influenza-like illness. Although the early inflammatory response to *H. capsulatum* yeast in the lungs is of critical importance to both host and parasite, it is poorly understood in humans because acute pulmonary histoplasmosis is rarely fatal. However, animal models of pulmonary histoplasmosis have proved helpful in this regard. Three to 6 hr after intranasal inoculation of 5,000 to 20,000 conidia of *H. capsulatum,* Procknow et al. (70) observed conidial forms in the bronchioles and alveoli of outbred mice, but there was little or no surrounding cellular reaction. Small numbers of spores were ringed by a few polymorphonuclear leukocytes (PMNs, or neutrophils). Subsequently,

TABLE 1. *The spectrum of* H. capsulatum (Hc)-*induced disease*

Manifestations	Acute pulmonary disease	Chronic pulmonary disease	Acute disseminated disease
Clinical	Often asymptomatic	Fever, productive cough, pleuritic pain	Fever, weight loss, hepatosplenomegaly, hematologic disturbances[a]
Immunological			
Positive *Hc* skin test (≥5 mm)	>90%	70–90%	30–55%
Lymphocyte transformation to antigen or mitogen	+++[b]	+ to +++	±
Anti-*Hc* antibody[c]	25–85%[d]	75–95%	70–90%
Hc antigenuria[e]	20–50%	5–10%	60–90%
Pathological			
Positive sputum culture	<25%	50–70%	50–70%
Histology	Aggregates of lymphocytes and macrophages in alveolar walls; caseating and noncaseating granulomas; few yeasts; giant cells	Noncaseating granulomas; interstitial fibrosis; bullae; necrosis; thick-walled cavities; few to moderate yeasts	Diffuse macrophage proliferation and abundant yeasts in lymphoreticular system; few lymphocytes and giant cells

[a] Hematologic disturbances include anemia, leukopenia, and thrombocytopenia.

[b] + indicates proliferative response to antigen or mitogen that is 3–5-fold higher than background; ++ indicates 5–10-fold higher, and +++ indicates >10-fold higher.

[c] Complement-fixation titer ≥1:8.

[d] Higher incidence in those with symptomatic primary infection.

[e] Antigenuria measured by radioimmunoassay; ranges of percentages obtained from L. J. Wheat (*personal communication* and ref. 102).

large numbers of neutrophils entered lung parenchyma and surrounded conidia to form exudative lesions. From the outset until 36 hr, neutrophils were the predominant inflammatory cell type present. Infiltrating macrophages were detected first at the peripheries of inflammatory lesions at 9 hr after inoculation and became increasingly prominent thereafter. Despite the massive influx of PMNs in response to fungal elements, they did not appear to exert significant fungicidal activity *in vivo*. By light microscopy, conidia seemed relatively resistant to ingestion by neutrophils, although fragments of disrupted conidia were phagocytized. Ingestion of conidia by lung macrophages was not observed.

Why conidia used in the preceding experiments were not phagocytized is unknown. These results differ from the *in vitro* findings of other investigators. Both human and guinea pig PMNs and murine alveolar macrophages are capable of ingesting *H. capsulatum* conidia (47,54,77). Moreover, conidia can be killed efficiently by human neutrophils and are susceptible to the combination of hydrogen peroxide, halides, and myeloperoxidase (48). The most likely explanation for the discrepant findings is that Procknow used a strain of *Histoplasma* that was productive of a large number of macroconidia that are 8 to 16 μm in diameter. The large physical dimensions of these conidia alone could have inhibited phagocytosis by neutrophils and macrophages. That this property of an organism prevents ingestion by professional phagocytes has been demonstrated for the large yeast cells of *Blastomyces dermatitidis* (34), hyphae from *Candida albicans* (32), and spherules of *Coccidioides immitis* (36).

These *in vitro* studies strongly suggest that PMNs and alveolar macrophages are important mediators of natural resistance to *H. capsulatum* conidia; yet the *in vivo* role of these cells is not understood clearly. Because the incidence of histoplasmosis is high in endemic regions (up to 90% in some areas), this finding suggests that PMNs and alveolar macrophages frequently fail to eliminate all conidia. If these constituents of host defense were as efficient *in vivo* as they appear to be *in vitro*, it is doubtful that the incidence of histoplasmosis could have reached the level that it has. Moreover, it is unlikely that the failure of phagocytes to eliminate conidia is a consequence of exposure to large numbers of conidia that overwhelm host defenses, because most asymptomatic infections are thought to occur by inhalation of small numbers of conidia. For example, intranasal inoculation of mice with as little as one conidium can induce infection in 100% of animals (2).

Inflammatory Response to Histoplasma *Yeasts*

Small numbers of *Histoplasma* yeasts can be detected in infected areas of lung within 36 hr after inhalation of conidia (70). The yeasts are present almost exclusively in macrophages, within which they multiply, with a generation time of 9 to 11 hr (46). Indeed, it is quite uncommon to observe extracellular yeasts in tissue except in cases of overwhelming histoplasmosis. Subsequent to the initial appearance of yeasts, macrophages and lymphocytes become the predominant cells infiltrating lungs. In several models of acute pulmonary histoplasmosis, aggregates of macrophages and lymphocytes are found uniformly in alveoli and small bronchioles during the first week of infection (9,70,78). By the second week, discrete granulomas are present. These are composed of compact aggregates of macrophages, epithelioid cells, and lymphocytes. In rodents with experimental histoplasmosis, giant cells are notably absent in lungs. Resolution of the inflammatory response generally begins during the fourth week of infection. Moreover, infection in rodents does not lead to cavity formation or progressive fibrosis (9,70,78).

In pulmonary infection of inbred mice induced by intranasal inoculation of *H. capsulatum*, Baughman et al. (9) have correlated the histopathological changes in lungs with the alterations in cellular composition of bronchoalveolar lavage (BAL) fluid (Fig. 1). During the first week

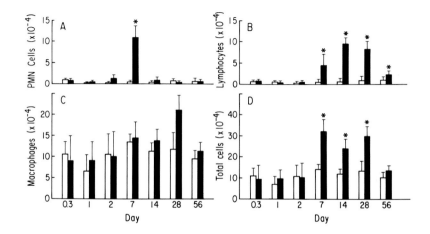

FIG. 1. Analysis of various cell populations retrieved from BAL fluid of mice with experimental pulmonary histoplasmosis (*black bars*) and age-matched control mice (*white bars*) at increasing time intervals after intranasal inoculation of 1 × 10⁵ *H. capsulatum* yeast cells. Asterisks indicate significant elevation (*p* < 0.02) above normal. (Reproduced with permission from authors and publisher).

of infection, there is a large influx of PMNs, with a rapid return to the normal range by the second week. At this time, when granulomas are evident in tissue sections of lungs, there is a 10-fold increase in the proportion of lymphocytes within the BAL fluid and a ninefold increase in absolute numbers of these cells. The lymphocytosis in BAL fluid persists through week 8 of infection, although it is considerably diminished. The number of macrophages in BAL fluid from infected mice is increased at day 28. Thus, analysis of cells within BAL fluid appears to reflect accurately the changes observed in the histology of lungs.

Human Pathology

The very limited information available concerning the early pathogenesis of acute pulmonary histoplasmosis in humans indicates that the initial inflammatory response is a bronchopneumonia in which alveoli are filled with macrophages containing yeast cells. Only small numbers of neutrophils have been observed in these lesions. In the pulmonary parenchyma, yeasts multiply within macrophages; concomitantly, there is spread of infection via the lymphatics and bloodstream to the regional lymph nodes and to the lymphoreticular system, especially the liver and spleen. Because yeasts rarely are found extracellularly, it is presumed that organisms disseminate within macrophages to other organs.

In humans, the specific cellular immune responses are thought to be activated in lymphoid organs and other tissues from 7 to 18 days after inhalation of large inocula of conidia, and somewhat later after inhalation of small to moderate numbers of organisms (41). With the generation of a specific immune response, lesions begin to heal. Giant cells are formed. Necrosis develops within the central areas of granulomas, and, often, numerous yeasts can be found in the caseous center. Draining regional lymph nodes become enlarged, sometimes massively. Eventually the lesions resolve by encapsulation with fibrous tissue, after which they frequently calcify.

Macrophage Attachment and Ingestion of *H. capsulatum* Yeasts

Crucial events that are required for establishment of *Histoplasma* infection are the recognition, binding, and phagocytosis of *H. capsulatum* yeasts by macrophages, thereby providing a permissive intracellular environment within which the organism multiplies. Thus, successful parasitization of the host is ensured prior to maturation of a specific cell-mediated immune response that renders macrophages capable of inhibiting or killing ingested yeasts.

Recently, the major receptor mechanism has been identified that mediates attachment of unopsonized *H. capsulatum* to human monocyte-derived macrophages from peripheral blood (15). Binding of *H. capsulatum* yeasts by macrophages is rapid and temperature-dependent and requires both Ca^{2+} and Mg^{2+} ions for optimum activity. Recognition of *H. capsulatum* yeasts does not require Fc receptors, mannosyl-fucosyl receptors, β-glucan receptors, or secretion of C3 by macrophages. Thus, the binding of unopsonized yeasts is quite different from that of other yeasts, such as *Candida glabrata*, *Candida krusei*, and *Saccharomyces cerevisiae*, which are bound via the mannosyl-fucosyl receptors of phagocytic cells (15,89,96).

To assess the role of the complement receptor 3 (CR3)/LFA-1/p150,95 family of adherence-promoting glycoproteins, macrophages can be plated on surfaces coated with monoclonal antireceptor antibodies. Such antibody-coated surfaces cause specific down-modulation of their target antigen from the apical portions of the macrophages (108). Each molecule of the CR3/LFA-1/p150,95 family contains a different α subunit that is associated noncovalently with a common β subunit ($M_r = 95,000$) in an $\alpha_1\beta_1$ configuration. Both the α chains and the common β chain are surface-exposed. Anti-β-chain monoclonal antibodies that recognize all three of the intact adhesion proteins block binding of the yeasts, as shown in Fig. 2. However, removal of individual receptors with antibody against α-chain polypeptides causes negligible depression of binding, and removal of any pair causes only modest depression. Thus, each of the members of the CR3/LFA-1/p150,95 family is independently capable of binding *H. capsulatum*. (The reader is referred to chapter by Gallin for more information on the CR3/LFA-1/p150,95 proteins.)

The structural basis for the finding that all three members of the CR3/LFA-1/p150,95 family share the ability to recognize *H. capsulatum* is not clear. One possibility is that the recognition site for *H. capsulatum* is located on the shared β chain. This assertion is supported by two observations. First, all three family members must be removed from macrophages to fully inhibit binding of *H. capsulatum*. Second, soluble anti-β antibodies inhibit binding of *H. capsulatum*. The binding site for C3bi, on the other hand, appears to be on the α chain of CR3, because LFA-1 and p150,95 do not recognize C3bi, and the anti-α monoclonal antibody OKM10 directly blocks the binding of C3bi to CR3 (109). Thus, CR3 may express two distinct binding sites, one for C3bi on the α chain, and the other for *Histoplasma* on the β chain. Such a view is consistent with experiments of Ross et al. (73) suggesting that CR3 expresses a lectin-like binding site that is distinct from the C3bi binding site. An alternative explanation for the data is that *H. capsulatum* expresses a variety of surface structures, some of which are recog-

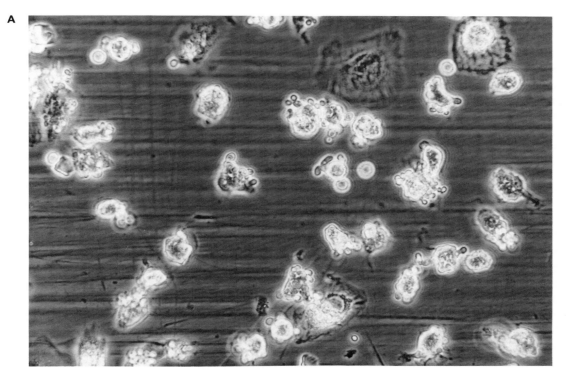

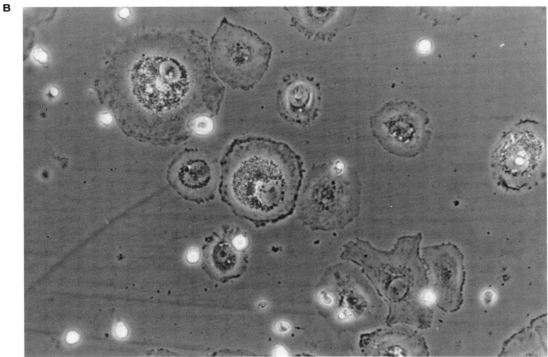

FIG. 2. A: In control monolayers of 7-day-cultured macrophages there is extensive binding of unopsonized *H. capsulatum* yeast cells by macrophages at 45 min at 37°C. **B:** In the presence of monoclonal antibody 1B4 (anti-β-chain-specific) at 25 μg/ml, binding of *H. capsulatum* is reduced greatly. Two yeasts bound to a macrophage are visible in the right lower portion of the field. ×234.

nized by CR3, others by LFA-1, and still others by p150,95.

Additional observations indicate that attachment and ingestion of *H. capsulatum* yeasts effectively induce generation of superoxide anion by human monocyte-derived macrophages, as measured by nitroblue tetrazolium reduction, and also promote the release of hydrogen peroxide (15). The time course and extent of hydrogen peroxide release is comparable to that induced by IgG-coated particles. This finding is of interest in light of the observation that ligation of CR3 by C3bi does not trigger the release of peroxide (109). However, since *H. capsulatum* also is recognized by LFA-1 and p150,95, it is possible that these receptors differ from CR3 in their capacity to trigger peroxide secretion or that they synergize with CR3 to induce peroxide release. Alternatively, CR3 may contain two binding sites, one for C3bi that does not initiate an oxidative burst and a second site that does. Moreover, it is possible that this fungus bears ligands recognized by other types of receptors, and these may initiate peroxide release after yeasts bind to CR3, LFA-1, or p150,95 on the macrophage surface. The actual role of toxic oxygen metabolites in the inhibition of killing of *H. capsulatum* yeasts intracellularly is unclear at present, because many ingested *Histoplasma* yeasts of strain 217B appear to remain viable within human macrophages for at least 2 hr after uptake, as determined by electron microscopy (P. A. Detmers and W. E. Bullock, *unpublished observations*).

Dynamics of Lymphocyte Populations in Pulmonary Histoplasmosis

Experimental Acute Pulmonary Histoplasmosis

Previous studies of the inflammatory response in lungs of humans or experimental animals with pulmonary histoplasmosis have described the organization of the cells infiltrating the lung tissues. Although these studies have detailed the serial changes in the inflammatory response to *H. capsulatum,* no information has been available regarding the dynamics of immunocompetent cells within lungs and other organs during the course of infection. Recently, however, flow microfluorometry has been employed to examine the flux of lymphocyte populations in the lungs of mice with acute pulmonary histoplasmosis (14). At weeks 2 and 4 after intranasal inoculation of *H. capsulatum* yeasts, the percentages of Thy-1.2$^+$ and Lyt-1$^+$ cells were significantly greater in infected lung homogenates than in homogenates from control animals. Similarly, the percentage of L3T4$^+$ cells was increased at week 2. By week 8, these differences were no longer discernible. Therefore, the influx of helper/inducer cells correlated with the period of peak inflammation within lungs.

Conversely, in infected lungs, the percentage of surface immunoglobulin-positive (sIg$^+$) cells was decreased relative to controls at weeks 2 and 4, but was increased at week 8.

Concomitant with the elevations in the helper/inducer T cells in lungs, there are reductions in the percentages of Thy-1.2$^+$, Lyt-1$^+$, and L3T4$^+$ cells in the spleens of infected mice at weeks 2, 4, and 8. No alterations in T-cell subpopulations are detectable in the thymuses of infected animals. These results indicate that acute pulmonary histoplasmosis induces an influx of cells of the helper/inducer phenotype into lung tissue. Because expansion of the helper/inducer cells in lungs is associated with a reduction of these cells in the spleen, it is possible that these cells may have migrated selectively into infected lung from the recirculating pool of T cells. It is also conceivable that the increased number of helper/inducer T cells could be accounted for by *in situ* proliferation in response to *H. capsulatum*. This seems unlikely, however, because more than 90% of the nonadherent cells are in the G_0/G_1 phase of the cell cycle (14).

Reinfection Histoplasmosis

In highly endemic areas, exogenous reinfections of the lung by *H. capsulatum* probably are common, although most of these episodes are unrecognized clinically. In some cases, reinfection of persons with acquired immunity may cause an acute, exuberant reaction in the lung, as typified by the presence of diffuse nodular infiltrates or miliary changes on chest roentgenograms (41). In mice challenged with three successive intranasal injections of yeast-phase *H. capsulatum* at 6-week intervals, there are marked elevations in the percentages of Thy-1.2$^+$ and L3T4$^+$ helper cells within the lungs shortly after each inoculation. Thus, 1 week after a second injection of yeast cells (week 7 after primary infection), the percentages of Thy-1.2$^+$ and L3T4$^+$ cells are increased by approximately 25% over the percentages of these T-cell subsets in age-matched control animals (W. E. Bullock, *unpublished observations*). By the second week after reexposure to yeast cells, the difference in percentage of this T-cell subset between infected and control animals diminishes considerably. With a third rechallenge, 12 weeks after the primary infection, there again are substantial elevations in the percentages of Thy-1.2$^+$ and L3T4$^+$ cells in lung at 1 week after inoculation, with rapid normalization thereafter. Of note is that repeated infections of the lung by *H. capsulatum* in this model system are not associated with development of cavity formation or fibrosis in areas of granulomatous inflammation. These findings are of interest relative to the putative immunologic events that may occur in the lungs of normal individuals who, because of occupation

Lymphocyte Populations in Lungs and Peripheral Blood of Humans with Acute Pulmonary Histoplasmosis

In a single study of 7 humans who were convalescing from acute pulmonary histoplasmosis, T-cell subsets were measured in BAL fluid and peripheral blood at one time point approximately 8 weeks after environmental exposure to *H. capsulatum*. The percentage of CD3+ cells in the lavage fluid of these individuals was significantly greater than for normal controls. Conversely, the percentage of CD3+ in the peripheral blood was equal to that in controls. The CD4/CD8 ratios in lavage fluid and peripheral blood of the patients were highly variable, but did not differ from those for controls. Nonetheless, an inverse correlation did exist between the CD4/CD8 ratios in BAL fluid and peripheral blood in patients (57). In another study of patients with acute pulmonary histoplasmosis following an epidemic, a significant reduction in the percentage of CD4+ cells in peripheral blood was demonstrated, and this decrement resolved after recovery from disease (68). Taken together, these studies suggest that there is a compartmentalization of immune T cells in lungs of humans with acute pulmonary histoplasmosis similar to that observed in experimental pulmonary infections.

Although the signal(s) that trigger lymphocyte influx into lungs and the function of the immunoregulatory cells within this organ are not yet understood, an analogy may be drawn to sarcoidosis, a granulomatous disease of unknown cause that principally involves lungs. Lavage fluid from patients with sarcoidal alveolitis contains significantly greater numbers of CD4+ cells than lavage fluid from normal controls. Concurrently, the number of CD4+ cells in peripheral blood is reduced markedly in sarcoid patients (49). Thus, there is a compartmentalization of the helper/inducer T cells within the lungs of patients with sarcoidosis that is similar to the influx of L3T4+ cells observed in experimental histoplasmosis. However, in acute pulmonary histoplasmosis, the influx of helper/inducer T lymphocytes is transient, and the number of these cells in lung tissue declines as the infection wanes. In sarcoidosis, on the other hand, the unknown stimulus to expansion of the helper/inducer T-cell population in lungs often persists for a prolonged period of time.

Clinical Manifestations of DTH in Histoplasmosis

Temporal Appearance of DTH

It is estimated that nearly 100% of individuals with acute pulmonary histoplasmosis show positive skin tests to histoplasmin (41,81). In humans, it has been difficult to determine the time interval between infection and the appearance of specific immunity because many infections are asymptomatic and the time of exposure cannot be ascertained precisely. Clinical studies of epidemics of histoplasmosis have suggested that 4 weeks after exposure to the fungus may be the earliest time in which delayed hypersensitivity may be detected, but the time frame is highly variable (61,63). In addition, it should be pointed out that in primary histoplasmosis, granuloma formation within the lungs and lymphoid tissues seems to precede by 1 or 2 weeks the appearance of cutaneous DTH. The reasons for this discrepancy have not been explored.

Under controlled experimental conditions, antigen-specific DTH measured *in vivo* can be detected approximately 2 to 4 weeks after animals have been challenged with *H. capsulatum* via the respiratory tract (9,78). The differences in onset of DTH among the various studies may be attributed to experimental variables, including the strain of organism, the phase of the organism, the experimental animal employed, and the size of the inoculum. In experimental pulmonary histoplasmosis, little is known concerning the temporal development of *in vitro* correlates of DTH either in the lung or in the extrapulmonary lymphoid tissue. In a single study of mice inoculated intratracheally with *Histoplasma* yeasts, spleen cells from infected mice proliferated in response to heat-killed *Histoplasma* yeasts as early as 1 week post-inoculation; the antigen-specific response peaked at week 2 and persisted for the duration (5 weeks) of the study (65).

Cells That Confer DTH and Protective Immunity to H. capsulatum

There have been few studies on the identity of cells conferring DTH and protective immunity to *H. capsulatum*. Thy-1.2+ spleen cells from mice immunized with viable *Histoplasma* yeasts can transfer DTH adoptively, as well as provide protective immunity to naive recipients, whereas B cells or immune sera fail to do so (53). More recent studies employing *H. capsulatum*-reactive murine T-cell clones have characterized the cell conferring DTH as Thy-1.2+, L3T4+ (25). Whether or not these antigen-specific L3T4+ T cells also can transfer protective immunity, as do splenic T cells harvested from immunized mice, is unknown. However, two lines of evidence suggest that this is the case. First, *Histoplasma*-specific T-cell clones (L3T4+) release a factor, closely resembling gamma-interferon, that causes inhibition of intracellular growth of *Histoplasma* yeasts *in vitro* (25). Second, *in vivo* administration of anti-L3T4 monoclonal antibody GK-1.5 to mice with systemic histoplasmosis reduces by 80% the number of L3T4+ T cells in spleens and lymph nodes. The loss of L3T4+ cells is associated with a threefold increase in the number of *Histoplasma* colony-forming units in spleens, as compared with infected control animals (A. E. Gomez, *unpublished observations*). It is reasonable to conclude, therefore, that *Histoplasma*-specific L3T4⁺ T cells also may be involved in protective immunity. That the same subpopulation of T cells can mediate DTH and protective immunity is supported by the finding that *Listeria monocytogenes*-specific T-cell clones can adoptively transfer both DTH and protective immunity (52).

Duration of Skin-Test Sensitivity

Conflicting data exist as to the duration of skin-test sensitivity to histoplasmin. One of the major difficulties regarding these data is the lack of standardization among various lots of histoplasmin. Nevertheless, it has been found that the skin tests of individuals who moved from the Midwest to reside in California remained positive 10 to 20 years later (84). In endemic areas, skin tests have been shown to be positive for at least 9 years after an epidemic (38). On the other hand, Zeidberg et al. (111) observed that 15.8% of 506 people reactive to histoplasmin who lived in a rural Tennessee county had become skin-test-negative when retested at an average of 25 months later. Reversion to negativity was most prevalent among those who were less than 1 year of age or greater than 40 years of age when the first skin test was performed. On retesting, skin reactions were negative in 23% of those less than 1 year of age and 29% of those older than 40. A criticism of this study is that definition of a positive skin test was not provided. Small changes (1–2 mm) in the size of induration may have accounted for the majority of negative skin tests on rechallenge, and these differences easily could have been caused by errors in antigen inoculation or errors in reading. Zeidberg's data require further confirmation; however, should the cutaneous DTH reactivity to histoplasmin prove to be of a more ephemeral nature, it would stand in contrast to the life-long duration of skin-test reactivity to tuberculin that follows infection with *M. tuberculosis*. Indeed, the putatively shorter duration (<2 years) of skin-test sensitivity to histoplasmin is all the more remarkable given the fact that *H. capsulatum*, like *M. tuberculosis*, persists for years in tissues of many individuals after primary infection (81). Thus, the apparent decline of skin-test reactivity observed by Zeidberg probably did not result from complete elimination of antigen from tissues. Moreover, because sensitized T lymphocytes that mediate DTH are believed to be long-lived, Zeidberg's study raises intriguing questions about the nature of *Histoplasma*-sensitized T cells.

Clinical Manifestations of DTH

Acute histoplasmosis in humans is associated with a number of extrapulmonary symptoms that presumably develop as a result of DTH reactions in tissues. The scope of these manifestations has best been determined from epidemics, because in such outbreaks the incidence of infection can be calculated with fair accuracy. Rheumatologic sequelae appear to be most common among the various clinical manifestations. Acute arthritis, arthralgias, erythema multiforme, and erythema nodosum develop in approximately 5 to 30% of individuals following exposure to *H. capsulatum* (72). The incidence of erythema nodosum associated with acute histoplasmosis is estimated to be 0.5% (82). In patients with acute arthritis, organisms rarely are recovered from joint fluid, and joint effusions contain little cellular reaction (10). Other unusual and infrequent manifestations that presumably are related to the inflammatory response include parotitis, interstitial nephritis, uveitis, and fibrosing mediastinitis. The latter is a rare and life-threatening sequela of histoplasmosis and arises from an exuberant host response to antigen. In this disorder, the involved tissues contain only a few organisms; yet there is massive proliferation of fibrous tissue outside the lymph nodes, leading to constriction of vital organs within the mediastinum. It appears, therefore, that the amount of fibrosis is excessive in relation to the small quantity of detectable antigen (42). Although no information exists as to what prompts this response in histoplasmosis or in tuberculosis, it is possible that products of macrophages or of antigen-specific lymphocytes (e.g., interleukin-1 and fibroblast-activating factor, respectively) initiate and sustain the process of fibrosis (56,79).

Nature of the Antigen Recognized in DTH Reactions

Most commonly, the antigenic preparation employed for immunological studies is a culture filtrate of either mycelial or yeast-phase organisms that is a mixture of crude antigens. Unfortunately, diverse strains of *H. capsulatum* have been employed to produce histoplasmin, and these preparations have not been standardized. Not surprisingly, several substances from mycelial or yeast-phase organisms have been proposed as antigens. These include galactomannan (7), a polysaccharide-protein complex or a polysaccharide (86,91), a protein, termed M-protein (12), ribosomal protein (93), and a sphingolipid (8). In those studies that have examined the antigen responsible for an *in vivo* DTH reaction, polysaccharides or glycoproteins have been identified most frequently as the antigenic component of the culture filtrate (81).

PATHOLOGY OF CHRONIC PULMONARY HISTOPLASMOSIS

Pathogenesis

Much less is known about the pathogenesis of chronic pulmonary histoplasmosis than of acute pulmonary disease, largely because a suitable animal model is lacking. The radiographic and anatomical manifestations of this form of histoplasmosis include either a pneumonic process or cavity formation. Some have proposed that chronic pulmonary histoplasmosis occurs predominantly, if not exclusively, in structurally damaged lungs (43). This assertion is supported by clinical and autopsy data showing that many individuals suffering from chronic pulmonary histoplasmosis have underlying lung disease, such as chronic obstructive lung disease. Thus, in some cases it is probable that cavitary histoplasmosis is caused by proliferation of yeasts within preexisting bullae, not as a consequence of DTH reaction in lung tissue.

In chronic pulmonary histoplasmosis, the earliest lesions that have been recognized in humans are characterized by an interstitial collection of lymphocytes, macrophages, occasional plasma cells, and intracellular yeasts (43). The alveoli in affected areas are thickened markedly. Within the central portion of the interstitial pneumonitis, there are scattered areas of necrosis. Because many small and medium-size arteries have narrowed lumina in the involved interstitial areas, it has been argued that the process of necrosis is a consequence of vascular compromise (43). In addition to the pneumonitis, granulomas may be observed within the interstitium. Eventually, fibrosis develops in the inflamed areas.

DTH in Chronic Pulmonary Histoplasmosis

In large series, cutaneous DTH responses to histoplasmin are absent from approximately 20% of individuals with chronic pulmonary histoplasmosis (3,37,43,64,106). In one smaller series, 6 of 10 individuals with chronic pulmonary histoplasmosis did not react to histoplasmin (20). Despite the findings in the latter study, anergy appears to be relatively infrequent in this form of the disease.

Studies of *in vitro* cellular immune responses have shown that, in general, lymphocytes from individuals with chronic pulmonary histoplasmosis are reactive to histoplasmin, as measured by ^{3}H-thymidine incorporation. *In vitro*, antigen reactivity has correlated with skin testing; thus, those individuals who manifest positive skin tests are also those whose lymphocytes proliferate in response to histoplasmin. Lymphocytes from those who are anergic by skin testing often fail to be stimulated by histoplasmin (3,20,64). In one study, hyporesponsiveness *in vitro* was observed when lymphocytes from anergic individuals were cultured with autologous serum (20). However, incubation of the same lymphocytes in serum from healthy humans reversed the poor responses. Of importance is the fact that serum from patients did not alter responsiveness to an irrelevant antigen prepared from *Candida albicans*. Because the capacity of autologous serum to depress antigen-specific responses was correlated with elevated levels

of complement-fixing antibody, it has been proposed that specific antibody or immune complexes may cause the serum-mediated suppression (20). This argument is supported by some work indicating that addition of serum from patients with high levels of anti-*Histoplasma* antibody can reduce proliferative responses to histoplasmin (64).

IMMUNOPATHOGENESIS OF DISSEMINATED HISTOPLASMOSIS

Yeast-phase organisms commonly disseminate by the lymphohematogenous route to involve the spleen and liver during the primary infection; however, this spread of organisms usually is self-limited and is undetected. Only later does the incidental finding of splenic or liver calcifications on X-ray indicate that "benign" dissemination of *H. capsulatum* has transpired. Infrequently, the organism may spread to the mononuclear phagocyte system and cause a life-threatening illness. It is often difficult to ascertain whether progressive disseminated histoplasmosis results from reactivation of a primary focus or from a reinfection. This is especially true in cases that develop in endemic areas. Nevertheless, reactivation disease has been well documented (21). Risk factors include age (elderly or infants) or immunosuppression that is caused by either an underlying illness or administration of immunosuppressive drugs (44,104). The latter risk factor is of importance for two reasons. First, major advances in the development and use of immunosuppressive therapy as adjuncts for transplantation or for treatment of various malignancies or immunological diseases have served to increase the number of individuals who will receive such therapy. In this group of patients, *Histoplasma* infection is disseminated in up to 88% of cases (33,51,76). Second, the epidemic of the acquired immune-deficiency syndrome (AIDS) is creating a large new population that is at risk for disseminated disease. In fact, nearly all AIDS patients with histoplasmosis manifest the disseminated form (11,92,105). The extremely high incidence of disseminated disease in high-risk groups can be contrasted with the incidence in the general population of 1 case in every 2,000 infected individuals (104).

Inflammatory Response in Disseminated Histoplasmosis

The spectrum of histopathology in disseminated histoplasmosis is broad. Most workers have attempted to categorize this form of disease on the basis of clinical manifestations, pathology, and degree of macrophage parasitization by yeast cells. Three forms have been established (infantile or acute disseminated, subacute, and chronic disseminated) (40,44), with the severity of clinical illness, as well as outcome, correlating well for each form. Thus, acute disseminated histoplasmosis is associated with the greatest degree of illness, whereas the illness is mild in the chronic form (22).

Acute Disseminated Histoplasmosis

In the infantile or acute disseminated form, unrelenting fevers, wasting, and hematologic abnormalities are common. Mononuclear phagocytes engorged with yeasts are scattered diffusely throughout lymphoreticular organs. In the most advanced cases, extracellular yeasts may be observed. Only a few lymphocytes, plasma cells, and neutrophils are present. Giant cells, granulomas, and epithelioid cells are absent. In less severe cases, focal collections of mononuclear phagocytes containing yeasts are found within tissues; lymphocytes are uncommon. Epithelioid cells and giant cells, if present, are rare (22,44). Thus, in this form of disseminated histoplasmosis, the only significant inflammatory response appears to be a massive collection of mononuclear phagocytes.

More than 80% of individuals with acute disseminated histoplasmosis manifest hematologic abnormalities, including leukopenia, anemia, and thrombocytopenia. In some cases these disturbances may result from hypersplenism, although this is unlikely to be the sole mechanism. For example, prostaglandins of the E series regulate, in part, the growth of a population of hematopoietic precursors, termed CFU-C, that have the potential to differentiate into macrophages or granulocytes (69). The possibility that prostaglandins contribute to the hematologic disturbances evident in disseminated histoplasmosis has been explored in a murine model. Adherent splenocytes from infected mice release high levels of prostaglandin E that are 100-fold greater than those in supernatants from normal adherent splenocytes and 50-fold greater than those found in supernatants of adherent cells from mice injected with heat-killed yeasts. These same culture supernatants of adherent splenocytes from infected mice sharply reduce the number of human CFU-C, and generation of granulocyte and macrophage colonies is suppressed equally. Treatment of actively infected mice with indomethacin, an inhibitor of prostaglandin synthesis, partially reverses the inhibitory effect of the culture supernatants from infected mice. Prostaglandins, therefore, may contribute to the alterations in myelopoiesis associated with disseminated histoplasmosis (16).

Thrombocytopenia is observed in a very high percentage of individuals with acute disseminated histoplasmosis (44). The mechanism of this disorder is speculative. However, it has been shown that *Histoplasma* yeasts can cause platelet aggregation *in vitro* when complexed with IgG and fibrinogen and thus may increase platelet elimination

(31). Whether or not intracellular yeasts can trigger identical events is unknown. Others have proposed that platelet destruction is mediated by immune mechanisms, based on the observation that an elevated platelet-associated IgG level has been detected in a patient with histoplasmosis (55).

Subacute and Chronic Disseminated Histoplasmosis

Acute disseminated histoplasmosis is life-threatening, whereas subacute and chronic disseminated diseases are associated with moderate to mild clinical symptoms. The liver and spleen frequently are enlarged. The pathology of subacute disseminated histoplasmosis is characterized by focal aggregates of mononuclear phagocytes containing yeasts. Often there is a paucity of lymphocytes, giant cells, and epithelioid cells, and granulomas are not present. Only in the chronic form of disseminated histoplasmosis are noncaseating granulomas commonly present. In both of these disease states, parasitization of macrophages by yeasts is considerably less extensive than in the acute form (44). In some cases of disseminated histoplasmosis, the principal manifestations of disease may arise from immunopathology that appears to be unrelated to granulomatous inflammation. For example, immune complex glomerulonephritis has been observed as an outstanding clinical feature in a case of disseminated histoplasmosis (13).

Disseminated Histoplasmosis in Immunosuppressed Patients

The histology of disseminated histoplasmosis in the immunosuppressed patient most often resembles that of the acute disseminated form. It is presumed that immunosuppression, whether induced by pharmacological agents or by an underlying disease, inhibits the normal immunoregulatory mechanisms and provides a safe "haven" for yeast cell replication. Of recent concern is infection with human immunodeficiency virus (HIV), which produces profound alterations in cellular and humoral immunity. Indeed, disseminated histoplasmosis has become a major opportunistic pathogen in AIDS patients of Midwestern or Caribbean origin or residence, and this disease constitutes one of the criteria for the definition of AIDS. Despite the considerable loss of CD4[+] lymphocytes in AIDS patients, those with disseminated histoplasmosis often have granulomas found in tissues (11,50,92,105). One issue that has not been addressed in these reports is whether the granulomas are "old" or whether they are of more recent origin. Nonetheless, this histopathological picture differs from that caused by another intracellular pathogen, *Mycobacterium avium-intracellulare*, in which sheets of acid-fast organisms are associated with a little inflammatory response or no response.

The finding of granulomas in AIDS patients with histoplasmosis raises important questions about the role of CD4$^+$ T cells in the formation of granulomas. Studies of other granulomatous diseases have suggested that the number of T-lymphocyte subpopulations within the granulomatous inflammatory response correlates with the efficacy of the host response. Thus, in diseases associated with the presence of discrete granulomas, including tuberculoid leprosy, sarcoidosis, and localized coccidioidomycosis, CD4$^+$ T cells compose a majority of the T cells within the granulomas. On the other hand, skin lesions from patients with lepromatous leprosy and disseminated coccidioidomycosis, in which discrete granulomas are absent, contain fewer CD4$^+$ cells (49,62,95). By contrast, experimental studies using athymic mice indicate that functional, mature helper T cells may not be required for granuloma formation. Granulomas do form in athymic mice infected with *Schistosoma mansoni* (35) and in nude rats inoculated with muramyl dipeptide (90). However, in both the *Schistosoma*-infected mice and the nude rats, the granulomas are smaller and more loosely formed than those seen in euthymic animals.

Immunoregulation in Disseminated Histoplasmosis

Forty-five to 70% of individuals with untreated disseminated histoplasmosis are anergic to skin testing with histoplasmin (37,71,85). Because these same individuals often have not been tested with other recall antigens, it is not known if cutaneous anergy in these individuals is exclusively antigen-specific. Peripheral blood mononuclear cells from approximately 70% of patients with disseminated infection display impaired blastogenic responses to

mitogens or to specific antigen (6,58,64,88). The basis for these disturbances in disseminated histoplasmosis has been examined both in experimental animals and in the human disease state.

Immunoregulatory Pathways

Disseminated infection by *H. capsulatum* in mice induces the generation of potent suppressor cells in the spleen and lymph nodes; concomitantly, there is severe depression of the *in vitro* cellular immune responses and DTH responses of infected mice (4,5) (Fig. 3). Two populations of cells exert nonspecific suppressor activity. One population is characterized as a cyclophosphamide-sensitive, Thy-1.2$^+$, Lyt-2$^+$, I-J$^+$ T cell; the other is a macrophage-like cell that is poorly adherent to glass or plastic surfaces, but adherent to nylon wool (24,69,102).

Because macrophage-like cells exert potent suppressor activity in experimental disseminated histoplasmosis, Deepe et al. (24) examined whether or not prostaglandins of the E series, which are products of macrophages, could mediate immunosuppression. Blockade of prostaglandin synthesis by indomethacin does not modify the *in vitro* suppressor capacity of whole spleen cells or of macrophage-like cells. The failure of indomethacin to reverse suppressor cell activity strongly suggests that prostaglandins are not a cause of immunosuppression in *Histoplasma* infection.

Additional studies have demonstrated the presence of complex immunoregulatory circuits in mice with disseminated histoplasmosis. Although spleen cells from infected C57BL/6 and C3H/HeJ mice mediate immunosuppression *in vitro,* spleen cells from these strains spontaneously release soluble mediators with disparate regulatory functions and biologic properties. Thus, spleen cells from in-

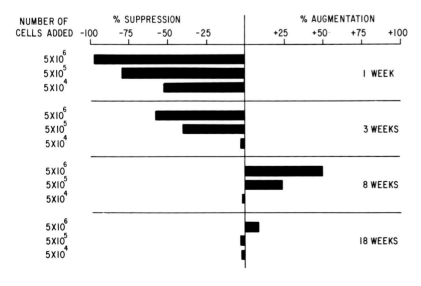

FIG. 3. Effects of decreasing numbers of spleen cells from C3H/Anf mice infected with 6 × 10^5 *H. capsulatum* yeast cells on the primary antibody response to sheep erythrocytes by 1 × 10^7 syngeneic spleen cells from age-matched normal mice. (Reproduced with permission from authors and publisher).

fected C3H/HeJ mice secrete a nonspecific suppressor factor; splenocytes from infected C57BL/6 mice release a nonspecific helper factor. Both factors have been characterized as proteins or glycoproteins that differ in regard to heat sensitivity, acid lability, and molecular weight. Neither the helper nor the suppressor factor exerts effector function; rather, they act only during the inductive phase of the immune response *in vitro* (28).

The operative helper and suppressor pathways have been analyzed to delineate the cellular interactions required for production of these factors and to identify the target cells on which the factors act (Fig. 4). Suppressor factor from C3H/HeJ mice is secreted by a Thy-1.2$^+$, Lyt-2$^+$, I-J$^+$ T cell, and its target is a Thy-1.2$^+$, Lyt-1$^+$2$^+$, I-J$^+$ T cell. In contrast, helper factor is produced by a Thy-1.2$^+$, Lyt-1$^+$ T cell, and its target is a Thy-1.2$^+$, Lyt-1$^+$ T cell. Optimal production of both factors requires the presence of accessory cells (29). Elucidation of these pathways has important implications for potential development of immunotherapeutic agents for treatment of disseminated histoplasmosis. Thus, as further definition of the immunoregulatory circuits is achieved, it should be possible to test the effect of immunomodulatory drugs on the natural course of this disease.

In comparison with murine studies, our knowledge of immunoregulatory pathways in humans with disseminated histoplasmosis is very limited. One group has isolated a population of short-lived T cells from peripheral blood of some patients with disseminated histoplasmosis that exert suppressor activity. The generation of these regulatory cells appears to be dependent on a factor released by macrophages (87,88). Others have demonstrated that there is a defect in the activation of concanavalin-A-inducible suppressor T cells from peripheral blood of anergic individuals with disseminated histoplasmosis (6). Thus, subjects' cells pretreated with concanavalin A are substantially less effective in suppressing the responses of normal peripheral blood mononuclear cells than are similarly treated cells from healthy controls. To date, the defective induction of suppressor T cells is a phenomenon observed only in subjects with disseminated disease; concanavalin-A-induced suppressor T-cell activity in those with localized histoplasmosis does not differ from that in healthy controls. Although the data are limited, the aforementioned results indicate that disseminated infection with *H. capsulatum* produces complex disturbances of immunoregulation in humans. Moreover, the results of the two studies cited earlier indicate that functional impairment of one suppressor population does not preclude the existence of another regulatory subpopulation that is suppressive.

Interleukins

There is increasing evidence that poor cell-mediated immune responses in histoplasmosis may, in part, be sec-

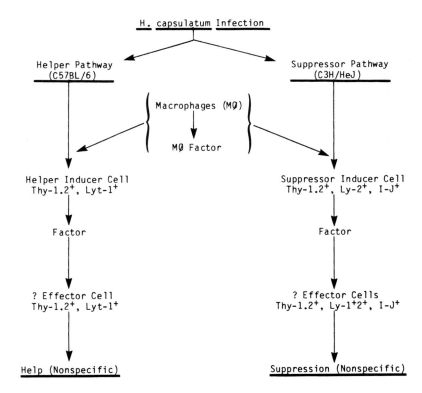

FIG. 4. Immunoregulatory pathways in C57BL/6 and C3H/HeJ mice with disseminated histoplasmosis. Thy-1.2$^+$, Lyt-1$^+$ T cells from C57BL/6 mice infected with *H. capsulatum* for 1 week release a factor that enhances the plaque-forming-cell response to sheep erythrocytes by normal syngeneic splenocytes. Conversely, Thy-1.2$^+$, Lyt-2$^+$, I-J$^+$ T cells from infected C3H/HeJ mice release a factor that suppresses the plaque-forming-cell response to sheep erythrocytes by normal syngeneic splenocytes. Optimal production of either factor requires macrophages or a factor secreted by macrophages. The helper mediates its regulatory effect by inducing a Thy-1.2$^+$, Lyt-1$^+$ T cell to exert nonspecific help, whereas the suppressor factor induces a Thy-1.2$^+$, Lyt-1$^+$2$^+$, I-J$^+$ T-cell population to function in the suppressor mode.

ondary to impaired production of cytokines necessary for amplification of the immune response. In this regard, Watson et al. (99) have examined the production of interleukins-1 and -2 (IL-1 and IL-2), two cytokines that are critical to T-cell growth, by splenocytes from mice with disseminated histoplasmosis. Generation of both IL-1 and IL-2 is depressed profoundly during the period of immunoregulatory disturbances at 2 to 4 weeks after inoculation. With resolution of the infection, the release of these cytokines returns to normal by week 8. It was found that impaired secretion of IL-1 could not be attributed either to differences in the numbers of adherent macrophages present in cultures of splenocytes from infected and normal mice or to the inhibitory influences of hydrogen peroxide or prostaglandins. Defective IL-2 secretion cannot be restored by exogenous IL-1 or by passage of splenocytes through nylon wool. In addition, a factor partially suppressive of IL-2 activity was detected in culture supernatants of concanavalin-A-stimulated splenocytes from infected animals. Therefore, the diminished IL-2 activity in supernatants of splenocyte cultures may be a consequence of both the suppressor factor and impaired production. Because disseminated histoplasmosis in mice is associated with marked perturbations of cellular immunity, it may well be that these two cytokines are responsible, partially, for the observed alterations in immunity.

The profound reduction in IL-2 production has prompted further studies to determine if exogenous recombinant IL-2 can restore immune responses and alter the severity of infection. Although it augments considerably the *in vitro* immune responses, *in vivo* administration of recombinant IL-2 fails to modify the severity of infection (26). On the other hand, recombinant IL-2 has been shown to be beneficial in several other experimental infections. Administration of recombinant IL-2 enhances survival of mice injected with *Toxoplasma gondii* (83), protects guinea pigs against a challenge with herpes simplex virus (100), and reduces the number of circulating *Trypanosoma cruzi* organisms in the blood of mice and prolongs survival (18). Why this lymphokine lacks therapeutic efficacy in murine histoplasmosis is not clear. However, it is possible that the effect of this lymphokine is compromised by its short half-life *in vivo* (17), by a serum inhibitor of IL-2 activity (45), or by a factor produced by splenocytes of infected mice that inhibits IL-2 activity (99).

Angiotensin-Converting Enzyme

Angiotensin-converting enzyme is an exopeptidase that converts angiotensin I to angiotensin II and inactivates bradykinin. Earlier studies of this enzyme have focused principally on its involvement in the regulation of peripheral vascular resistance. However, angiotensin-converting enzyme activity is elevated in the sera of some individuals with granulomatous disease, including sarcoidosis (30,59), berylliosis (60), and leprosy (60). Furthermore, serum levels of this enzyme are increased in up to 25% of individuals with histoplasmosis (23,74). Although the biological significance of elevated angiotensin-converting enzyme activity in granulomatous disease is unknown, recent studies have suggested that this enzyme may be involved in the regulation of granulomatous inflammation. Thus, treatment of mice infected with *Schistosoma mansoni* (101) or mice injected with nonviable *Mycobacterium bovis* BCG (80) with inhibitors of angiotensin-converting enzyme produces a striking reduction in granulomatous inflammation.

The foregoing studies employed model systems of inert antigens rather than actively replicating organisms. In murine disseminated histoplasmosis, angiotensin-converting enzyme activity is elevated during the height of infection. However, in sharp contrast to the beneficial effects observed in other models, administration of inhibitors of angiotensin-converting enzyme to mice injected with *H. capsulatum* produces unequivocal worsening of the clinical severity of infection, as well as increases of sixfold to sevenfold in the number of *Histoplasma* colony-forming units in spleens and livers of infected mice. The histopathologic changes in spleens of mice treated with these inhibitors were more severe than those in infected controls given saline and were characterized by massive proliferation of macrophages, with large aggregates of yeasts scattered throughout the red and white pulp. The mechanism by which these drugs alter susceptibility to infection is not understood. They do not appear to be cytotoxic to leukocytes, and they do not impair *in vitro* blastogenic responses to mitogens or DTH responses to nonspecific antigens. Thus, as measured by these assays, angiotensin-converting enzyme inhibitors are not immunosuppressive (27). It may well be that they alter the capacity of macrophages to become "activated." The process of macrophage activation that occurs during systemic histoplasmosis is a critical step in the capacity of the host to control the infection (94). Thus, it is conceivable that in compensation for an ineffectual resistance mechanism (suppression of macrophage activation) there is a massive influx of effector cells (macrophages) into infected areas in a futile attempt to limit replication of organisms.

Flux of T Lymphocytes in Disseminated Histoplasmosis

Although much is known of the histopathologic features of disseminated histoplasmosis, relatively little information is available concerning the changes in immunoregulatory cell populations that are associated with this disease state. During the acute phase of infection (days 0–21), splenomegaly and increased splenic cellularity are coincident with severe thymic involution and loss of cellularity. With convalescence, the spleen size decreases, and the thymic cellularity returns to normal by week 8 after intravenous inoculation with yeast-phase *H. capsulatum.* The thymic events are not explained by elevation of corticosterone levels secondary to the stress of infection, as similar changes are observed in adrenalectomized animals (98). Thus, the decreased cellularity of thymuses in infected mice may result from trafficking of thymocytes predominantly to the spleen. Evidence for this hypothesis has been provided by flow microfluorometry studies in which the flux of T cells and T-cell subsets was analyzed in the lymphoid organs and peripheral blood of infected animals (98). Involution of the thymus was associated with considerable loss of lymphocytes bearing a low density of Thy-1.2 surface antigen; a low surface density of Thy-1.2 is a property of mature T cells, whereas immature T cells bear greater amounts of this surface antigen. There also were reductions of mature T cells in the peripheral blood and bone marrow compartments. Conversely, however, mature T cells were increased within the spleen and to a lesser extent within mesenteric lymph nodes. These results suggest that systemic infection with *H. capsulatum* involves massive trafficking of mature T cells from the thymus to the spleen and, to a lesser degree, to central lymph nodes, both of which are infected extensively by *Histoplasma* yeasts.

In humans with disseminated histoplasmosis, shifts of immunoregulatory cell populations have been detected in peripheral blood. Analysis of the T-cell subsets in 7 patients revealed low CD4/CD8 ratios in all cases. In 3 of 7 patients, the low CD4/CD8 ratio could be accounted for by a reduction in the percentage of CD4$^+$ cells and an increase in CD8$^+$ cells (68). Recovery was associated with normalization of the percentages of CD4$^+$ and CD8$^+$ and the CD4/CD8 ratio in 2 of 3 patients studied. Thus, the reduction in CD4$^+$ cells in peripheral blood raises the possibility that these cells may have migrated to or become trapped within another organ system or systems involved by granulomatous abnormalities.

SUMMARY

The observations reviewed in this chapter delineate the spectrum of the clinical, pathological, and immunological manifestations associated with *H. capsulatum* infection. In addition, the many studies illustrate the complexities of the host response to *Histoplasma.* Indeed, it appears that an effective response to this fungus requires an interaction between antigen-specific T cells and macrophages, with the subsequent development of a granulomatous inflammatory response. When the communication between these cells is disrupted, for whatever reason, it is likely that the host will fail to control the replication of the organism and that eventually the organism will spread to involve many organs of the mononuclear phagocyte system. Consequently, in disseminated disease, there is not only a discrete lack of granuloma formation but also perturbations of immunoregulation. As we gain a better understanding of the signals that either trigger a successful outcome or are inimical to host resistance, we hope that it will be possible to manipulate those signals by the use of selective immunotherapy and thus greatly improve therapy for this fungal pathogen.

ACKNOWLEDGMENTS

This work was supported by grants AI-17339 and AI-23017 from the National Institutes of Health. The authors acknowledge the excellent secretarial assistance of Mrs. Angela Birch Smith.

REFERENCES

1. Ajello, L. (1971): Distribution of *Histoplasma capsulatum* in the United States. In: *Histoplasmosis,* edited by L. Ajello, E. W. Chick, and M. F. Furculow, pp. 103–122. Charles C Thomas, Springfield, Ill.
2. Ajello, L., and Runyon, L. C. (1953): Infection of mice with single spores of *Histoplasma capsulatum. J. Bacteriol.,* 66:34–40.
3. Alford, R. H., and Goodwin, R. A. (1972): Patterns of immune response in chronic pulmonary histoplasmosis. *J. Infect. Dis.,* 125:269–275.
4. Artz, R. P., and Bullock, W. E. (1979): Immunoregulatory responses in experimental disseminated histoplasmosis: Lymphoid organ histopathology and serological studies. *Infect. Immun.,* 23:884–892.
5. Artz, R. P., and Bullock, W. E. (1979): Immunoregulatory responses in experimental disseminated histoplasmosis: Depression of T-cell-dependent and T-effector responses by activation of splenic suppressor cells. *Infect. Immun.,* 23:893–902.
6. Artz, R. P., Jacobson, R. R., and Bullock, W. E. (1980): Decreased suppressor cell activity in disseminated granulomatous infections. *Clin. Exp. Immunol.,* 41:343–352.
7. Azuma, I., Kanetsuna, F., Tanaka, Y., Yamamura, Y., and Carbonell, L. M. (1974): Chemical and immunological properties of galactomannan obtained from *Histoplasma dubosii, Histoplasma capsulatum, Paracoccidioides brasiliensis,* and *Blastomyces dermatitidis. Mycopathol. Mycol. Appl.,* 54:111–126.
8. Barr, K. L., Laine, R. A., and Lester, R. L. (1984): Carbohydrate structures of three novel phosphoinositol-containing sphingolipids from the yeast *Histoplasma capsulatum. Biochemistry,* 23:5589–5596.
9. Baughman, R. B., Kim, K. C., Vinegar, A., Hendricks, D. E., Phillips, D., and Bullock, W. E. (1986): The pathogenesis of experimental pulmonary histoplasmosis: Correlative studies of histopathology, bronchoalveolar lavage cytology and respiratory function. *Am. Rev. Respir. Dis.,* 134:771–776.
10. Bayer, A. S., Choi, C., Tillman, D. B., and Guze, L. B. (1980): Fungal arthritis. V. Cryptococcal and histoplasmal arthritis. *Semin. Arthritis Rheum.,* 9:218–227.
11. Bonner, J. R., Alexander, W. J., Dismukes, W. E., App, W., Griffin, F. M., Little, R., and Shin, M. S. (1984): Disseminated histoplas-

mosis in patients with the acquired immune deficiency syndrome. *Arch. Intern. Med.,* 144:2178–2181.

12. Brock, E. G., Reiss, E., Pine, L., and Kaufman, L. (1984): Effect of periodate oxidation on the detection of antibodies against the M-antigen of histoplasmin by enzyme immunoassay (EIA) inhibition. *Curr. Microbiol.,* 10:177–184.

13. Bullock, W. E., Artz, R. P., Bhathena, D., and Tung, K. S. K. (1979): Histoplasmosis. Association with circulating immune complexes, eosinophilia, and mesangiopathic glomerulonephritis. *Arch. Intern. Med.,* 139:700–702.

14. Bullock, W. E., Hendricks, D. E., Baughman, R. B., and Townsend, W. (1987): The flux of lung lymphocyte populations during experimental pulmonary infection by *Histoplasma capsulatum:* Serial analysis by flow microfluorometry. (in press).

15. Bullock, W. E., and Wright, S. D. (1987): The role of the adherence-promoting receptors, CR3, LFA-1, and p150,95 in binding of *Histoplasma capsulatum* by human macrophages. *J. Exp. Med.,* 165: 195–210.

16. Caldwell, C. W., Yesus, Y. W., and Sprouse, R. F. (1983): In vitro suppression of myelopoiesis by adherent murine splenocytes in experimental disseminated histoplasmosis. *Am. J. Pathol.,* 110:247–253.

17. Cheever, M. A., Thompson, J. A., Kern, D. E., and Greenberg, P. D. (1985): Interleukin 2 (IL-2) administered in vivo: Influence of IL-2 route and timing on T cell growth. *J. Immunol.,* 134:3895–3990.

18. Choromanski, L., and Kuhn, R. E. (1985): Interleukin 2 enhances specific and nonspecific immune responses in experimental Chagas' disease. *Infect. Immun.,* 50:354–357.

19. Christie, A., and Peterson, J. C. (1945): Pulmonary calcification in negative reactors to tuberculin. *Am. J. Public Health,* 35:1131–1147.

20. Cox, R. A. (1979): Immunologic studies of patients with histoplasmosis. *Am. Rev. Respir. Dis.,* 120:143–149.

21. Davies, S. F., Khan, M., and Sarosi, G. A. (1978): Disseminated histoplasmosis in immunologically suppressed patients. Occurrence in a nonendemic area. *Am. J. Med.,* 64:94–100.

22. Davies, S. F., McKenna, R. W., and Sarosi, G. W. (1979): Trephine biopsy of the bone marrow in disseminated histoplasmosis. *Am. J. Med.,* 67:617–622.

23. Davies, S., Rohrbach, M. S., Thelen, V., Kuritsky, J., Gruninger, R., Simpson, M. L., and DeRemee, R. A. (1984): Elevated serum angiotensin-converting enzyme (SACE) activity in acute pulmonary histoplasmosis. *Chest,* 85:307–310.

24. Deepe, G. S., Jr., Kravitz, G. K., and Bullock, W. E. (1983): Pharmacological modulation of suppressor cell activity in mice with disseminated histoplasmosis. *Infect. Immun.,* 41:114–120.

25. Deepe, G. S., Jr., Smith, J. G., Sonnenfeld, G., Denman, D., and Bullock, W. E. (1986): Development and characterization of *Histoplasma capsulatum*-reactive murine T cell lines and clones. *Infect. Immun.,* 54:714–722.

26. Deepe, G. S., Jr., Taylor, C. L., Harris, J. E., and Bullock, W. E. (1986): Modulation of the cellular immune responses in mice with disseminated histoplasmosis by recombinant interleukin-2. *Infect. Immun.,* 53:6–12.

27. Deepe, G. S., Jr., Taylor, C. L., Srivastava, L., and Bullock, W. E. (1985): Impairment of granulomatous inflammatory response to *Histoplasma capsulatum* by inhibitors of angiotensin-converting enzyme. *Infect. Immun.,* 48:395–401.

28. Deepe, G. S., Jr., Watson, S. R., and Bullock, W. E. (1982): Generation of disparate immunoregulatory factors in two inbred strains of mice with disseminated histoplasmosis. *J. Immunol.,* 129:2186–2191.

29. Deepe, G. S., Jr., Watson, S. R., and Bullock, W. E. (1984): Cellular origins and target cells of immunoregulatory factors in mice with disseminated histoplasmosis. *J. Immunol.,* 132:2064–2071.

30. DeRemee, R. A., and Rohrbach, M. S. (1980): Serum angiotensin-converting enzyme in evaluating the clinical course of sarcoidosis. *Ann. Intern. Med.,* 92:361–365.

31. Des Prez, R. M., Steckley, S., Stroud, R. M., and Hawiger, J. (1980): Interaction of *Histoplasma capsulatum* with human platelets. *J. Infect. Dis.,* 142:32–39.

32. Diamond, R. D., Krzesicki, R., and Jao, W. (1978): Damage to pseudohyphal forms of *Candida albicans* by neutrophils in the absence of serum in vitro. *J. Clin. Invest.,* 61:349–359.

33. Dismukes, W. E., Royal, S. A., and Tynes, B. S. (1978): Disseminated histoplasmosis in corticosteroid-treated patients. *J.A.M.A.,* 240:1495–1498.

34. Drutz, D. J., and Frey, C. L. (1985): Intracellular and extracellular defenses of human phagocytes against *Blastomyces dermatitidis* conidia and yeasts. *J. Lab. Clin. Med.,* 105:737–750.

35. Epstein, W. L., Fukuyama, K., Danno, K., and Kwan-Wong, E. (1979): Granulomatous inflammation in normal and athymic mice infected with *Schistosoma mansoni:* An ultrastructural study. *J. Pathol.,* 127:207–219.

36. Frey, C. L., and Drutz, D. J. (1986): Influence of fungal surface components on the interaction of *Coccidioides immitis* with polymorphonuclear neutrophils. *J. Infect. Dis.,* 153:933–942.

37. Furculow, M. L. (1963): Comparison of treated and untreated severe histoplasmosis. *J.A.M.A.,* 183:823–829.

38. Furculow, M. L., and Grayston, J. T. (1955): Occurrence of histoplasmosis in epidemics: Etiologic studies. *Am. Rev. Tuberc.,* 68:307–320.

39. Goddard, J. C., Edwards, L. B., and Palmer, C. E. (1949): Relationship of pulmonary calcification with sensitivity to tuberculin and histoplasmin. *Public Health Rep.,* 64:820–844.

40. Goodwin, R. A., and Des Prez, R. M. (1978): Histoplasmosis. *Am. Rev. Respir. Dis.,* 117:929–956.

41. Goodwin, R. A., Loyd, J. E., and Des Prez, R. M. (1981): Histoplasmosis in normal hosts. *Medicine (Baltimore),* 60:231–266.

42. Goodwin, R. A., Nickell, J. A., and Des Prez, R. M. (1972): Mediastinal fibrosis complicating healed primary histoplasmosis and tuberculosis. *Medicine (Baltimore),* 51:227–246.

43. Goodwin, R. A., Jr., Owens, F. T., Snell, J. D., Hubbard, W. W., Buchanan, R. D., Terry, R. T., and Des Prez, R. M. (1976): Chronic pulmonary histoplasmosis. *Medicine (Baltimore),* 55:413–451.

44. Goodwin, R. A., Shapiro, J. L., Thurman, G. H., Thurman, S. S., and Des Prez, R. M. (1980): Disseminated histoplasmosis: Clinical and pathologic correlations. *Medicine (Baltimore),* 59:1–31.

45. Hardt, C., Rollinghoff, M., Pfizenmaier, M., Mosmann, M., and Wagner, H. (1981): Lyt-23⁺ cyclophosphamide-sensitive T cells regulate the activity of an interleukin 2 inhibitor in vivo. *J. Exp. Med.,* 154:262–274.

46. Howard, D. H. (1965): Intracellular growth of *Histoplasma capsulatum. J. Bacteriol.,* 89:518–523.

47. Howard, D. H. (1973): Fate of *Histoplasma capsulatum* in guinea pig polymorphonuclear leukocytes. *Infect. Immun.,* 8:412–419.

48. Howard, D. H. (1981): Comparative sensitivity of *Histoplasma capsulatum* conidiospores and blastospores to oxidative antifungal systems. *Infect. Immun.,* 32:381–387.

49. Hunninghake, G. W., and Crystal, R. G. (1981): Pulmonary sarcoidosis. A disorder mediated by excess helper T-lymphocyte activity at sites of disease activity. *N. Engl. J. Med.,* 305:429–434.

50. Jagadha, V., Andavolu, R. H., and Huang, C. T. (1985): Granulomatous inflammation in the acquired immune deficiency syndrome. *Am. J. Clin. Pathol.,* 84:598–602.

51. Kauffman, C. A., Israel, K. S., Smith, J. W., White, A. C., Schwarz, J., and Brooks, G. F. (1978): Histoplasmosis in immunosuppressed patients. *Am. J. Med.,* 64:923–932.

52. Kaufmann, S. H. E., and Hahn, H. (1982): Biological functions of T cell lines with specificity for the intracellular bacterium *Listeria monocytogenes* in vitro and in vivo. *J. Exp. Med.,* 155:1754–1765.

53. Khardori, N., Chaudhary, S., McConnachie, P., and Tewari, R. P. (1983): Characterization of lymphocytes responsible for protective immunity to histoplasmosis in mice. *Mykosen,* 26:523–532.

54. Kimberlin, C. L., Hariri, A. R., Hempel, H. O., and Goodman, N. L. (1981): Interactions between *Histoplasma capsulatum* and macrophages from normal and treated mice: Comparison of the mycelial and yeast phases in alveolar and peritoneal macrophages. *Infect. Immun.,* 34:6–10.

55. Kucera, J. C., and Davis, R. B. (1983): Thrombocytopenia associated with histoplasmosis and an elevated platelet IgG. *Am. J. Clin. Pathol.,* 79:644–646.

56. Lammie, P. J., Michael, A. I., Prystowsky, M. B., Linette, G. P.,

and Phillips, S. M. (1986): Production of a fibroblast-stimulating factor by *Schistosoma mansoni* antigen-reactive T cell clones. *J. Immunol.,* 136:1100–1106.

57. Leatherman, J. W., Michael, A. F., Simpson, M., and Hoidal, J. (1983): Characterization of cell-mediated immunity in the lung in histoplasmosis by monoclonal antibodies. *Am. Rev. Respir. Dis.,* 127:S195.

58. Lehmann, P. F., Gibbons, J., Senitzer, D., Ribner, B., and Freimer, E. H. (1983): T lymphocyte abnormalities in disseminated histoplasmosis. *Am. J. Med.,* 75:790–794.

59. Lieberman, J., Nosal, A., Schlesser, L. A., and Sastre-Foken, A. (1979): Serum angiotensin-converting enzyme for diagnosis and therapeutic evaluation of sarcoidosis. *Am. Rev. Respir. Dis.,* 120:329–335.

60. Lieberman, J., and Rea, T. H. (1977): Serum angiotensin-converting enzyme in leprosy and coccidioidomycosis. *Ann. Intern. Med.,* 87:422–425.

61. Loosli, C. G., Grayston, J. T., Alexander, E. R., and Tanzi, F. (1952): Epidemiological studies of pulmonary histoplasmosis in a farm family. *Am. J. Hyg.,* 55:392–401.

62. Modlin, R. L., Segal, G. P., Hofman, F. M., Walley, M. S., Johnson, R. H., Taylor, C. R., and Rea, T. H. (1985): In situ localization of T lymphocytes in disseminated coccidioidomycosis. *J. Infect. Dis.,* 151:314–319.

63. Murray, J. F., Lurie, H. I., Kaye, J., Komins, C., Borok, R., and Way, M. (1957): Benign pulmonary histoplasmosis (cave disease) in South Africa. *S. Afr. Med. J.,* 31:245–253.

64. Newberry, W. M., Jr., Chandler, J. W., Jr., Chin, T. D. Y., and Kirkpatrick, C. H. (1968): Immunology of the mycoses. I. Depressed lymphocyte transformation in chronic histoplasmosis. *J. Immunol.,* 100:436–443.

65. Nickerson, D. A., and Fairclough, P. (1984): Immune responsiveness following intratracheal inoculation with *Histoplasma capsulatum* yeast cells. *Clin. Exp. Immunol.,* 56:337–344.

66. Nickerson, D. A., Havens, R. A., and Bullock, W. E. (1981): Immunoregulation in disseminated histoplasmosis: Characterization of splenic suppressor cells. *Cell. Immunol.,* 60:287–297.

67. Palmer, C. E. (1945): Nontuberculous pulmonary calcification and sensitivity to histoplasmin. *Public Health Rep.,* 60:513–520.

68. Payan, D. G., Wheat, L. J., Brahmi, Z., Ip, S., Hansen, W. P., Hoffman, R. A., Healey, K., and Rubin, R. H. (1984): Changes in immunoregulatory lymphocyte populations in patients with histoplasmosis. *J. Clin. Immunol.,* 4:98:107.

69. Pelus, L. M., Broxmeyer, H. W., Kurland, J. I., and Moore, M. A. S. (1979): Regulation of macrophage and granulocyte proliferation. Specificities of prostaglandin E and lactoferrin. *J. Exp. Med.,* 150:277–292.

70. Procknow, J. J., Page, M. I., and Loosli, C. G. (1960): Early pathogenesis of experimental histoplasmosis. *Arch. Pathol.,* 69:413–426.

71. Reddy, P., Gorelick, D. F., Brasher, C. A., and Larsh, H. (1970): Progressive disseminated histoplasmosis as seen in adults. *Am. J. Med.,* 48:629–636.

72. Rosenthal, J., Brandt, K. K., Wheat, L. J., and Slama, T. G. (1983): Rheumatologic manifestations of histoplasmosis in the recent Indianapolis epidemic. *Arthritis Rheum.,* 26:1065–1070.

73. Ross, G. D., Cain, J. A., and Lachmann, P. J. (1985): Membrane complement receptor type three (CR_3) has lectin-like properties analogous to bovine conglutinin and functions as a receptor for zymosan and rabbit erythrocytes as well as a receptor for iC3b. *J. Immunol.,* 134:3307–3315.

74. Ryder, K. W., Jay, S. J., Kiblawi, S. O., and Hull, M. T. (1983): Serum angiotensin converting enzyme activity in patients with histoplasmosis. *J.A.M.A.,* 249:1888–1889.

75. Sacco, M., Medoff, G., Lambowitz, A. M., Kumar, B. V., Kobayashi, G. S., and Painter, A. (1983): Sulfhydryl induced respiratory "shunt" pathways and their role in morphogenesis in the fungus, *Histoplasma capsulatum. J. Biol. Chem.,* 258:8223–8230.

76. Sarosi, G. A., Voth, D. W., Dahl, B. A., Doto, I. L., and Tosh, F. E. (1971): Disseminated histoplasmosis: Results of long-term follow-up. *Ann. Intern. Med.,* 75:511–516.

77. Schaffner, A., Davis, C. E., Schaffner, T., Markert, M., Douglas, H., and Braude, A. I. (1986): In vitro susceptibility of fungi to killing by neutrophil granulocytes discriminates between primary pathogenicity and opportunism. *J. Clin. Invest.,* 78:511–524.

78. Schlitzer, R. L., Chandler, F. W., and Larsh, H. W. (1981): Primary acute histoplasmosis in guinea pigs exposed to aerosolized *Histoplasma capsulatum. Infect. Immun.,* 33:575–582.

79. Schmidt, J. A., Mizel, S. B., Cohen, D., and Green, I. (1982): Interleukin 1, a potential regulator of fibroblast proliferation. *J. Immunol.,* 128:2177–2182.

80. Schrier, D. J., Ripani, L. M., Katzenstein, A., and Moore, V. L. (1982): Role of angiotensin-converting enzyme in bacille Calmette-Guérin-induced granulomatous inflammation. *J. Clin. Invest.,* 65:1257–1264.

81. Schwarz, J. (1981): *Histoplasmosis.* Praeger, New York.

82. Sellers, T. F., Price, W. N., and Newberry, W. M. (1965): An epidemic of erythema multiforme and erythema nodosum caused by histoplasmosis. *Ann. Intern. Med.,* 62:1244–1262.

83. Sharma, S. D., Hofflin, J. M., and Remington, J. S. (1985): In vivo recombinant interleukin-2 administration enhances survival against a lethal challenge with *Toxoplasma gondii. J. Immunol.,* 135:4160–4163.

84. Smith, C. E. (1956): Analogy of coccidioidin and histoplasmin sensitivity. In: *Proceedings of a Conference on Histoplasmosis,* Public Health Service publication no. 465, pp. 173–177. U.S. Government Printing Office, Washington, D.C.

85. Smith, J. W., and Utz, J. P. (1972): Progressive disseminated histoplasmosis. A prospective study of 26 patients. *Ann. Intern. Med.,* 76:557–565.

86. Sprouse, R. F. (1977): Determination of molecular weight, isoelectric point, and glycoprotein moiety for the principal skin test-reactive component of histoplasmin. *Infect. Immun.,* 15:263–271.

87. Stobo, J. D. (1977): Immunosuppression in man: Suppression by macrophages can be mediated by interactions with regulatory T cells. *J. Immunol.,* 119:918–924.

88. Stobo, J. D., Paul, S., Van Scoy, R. E., and Hermans, P. E. (1976): Suppressor thymus-derived lymphocytes in fungal infection. *J. Clin. Invest.,* 57:319–328.

89. Sung, S. J., Nelson, R. S., and Silverstein, S. C. (1983): Yeast mannan inhibit binding and phagocytosis of zymosan by mouse peritoneal macrophages. *J. Cell Biol.,* 96:160–166.

90. Tanaka, A., Emori, K., Nago, S., Kushima, K., Kohashi, O., Saitoh, M., and Kataoka, T. (1982): Epithelioid granuloma formation requiring no T-cell function. *Am. J. Pathol.,* 106:165–170.

91. Taylor, M. L., Reyes Montes, M. R., Lanchica, A., Eslava Campos, C., Olvera, J., and Maxwell, R. (1980): Immunology of histoplasmosis: Humoral and cellular activity from a polysaccharide-protein complex and its deproteinized fraction in experimentally immunized mice. *Mycopathologia,* 71:159–166.

92. Taylor, M. N., Baddour, L. M., and Alexander, J. M. (1984): Disseminated histoplasmosis associated with the acquired immune deficiency syndrome. *Am. J. Med.,* 77:579–580.

93. Tewari, R. P., Khardori, N., McConnachie, P., von Behren, L. A., and Yamada, T. (1982): Blastogenic responses of lymphocytes from mice immunized by sublethal infection with yeast cells of *Histoplasma capsulatum. Infect. Immun.,* 36:1013–1018.

94. Tiku, M. L., McNabb, P. C., and Tomasi, T. B., Jr. (1985): Macrophage-related fibrinolysis in experimental disseminated histoplasmosis. *Infect. Immun.,* 49:641–646.

95. Van Voorhis, W. C., Kaplan, G., Nunes Sarno, E., Horwitz, M. A., Steinman, R. M., Levis, W. R., Nogueira, N., Hair, L. S., Rocha Gattass, C., Arrick, B. A., and Cohn, Z. A. (1982): The cutaneous infiltrates of leprosy. Cellular characteristics and the predominant T-cell phenotype. *N. Engl. J. Med.,* 307:1593–1597.

96. Warr, G. A. (1980): A macrophage receptor for (mannose/glucosamine)-glycoproteins of potential importance in phagocytic activity. *Biochem. Biophys. Res. Commun.,* 93:737–745.

97. Watson, S. R., and Bullock, W. E. (1982): Immunoregulation in disseminated histoplasmosis: Characterization of the surface phenotype of splenic suppressor T lymphocytes. *Infect. Immun.,* 37:940–945.

98. Watson, S. R., Miller, T. B., Redington, T. J., and Bullock, W. E. (1983): Immunoregulation in experimental disseminated histoplasmosis: Flow microfluorometry (FMF) studies of the Thy and

Lyt phenotypes of T lymphocytes from infected mice. *J. Immunol.,* 131:984–990.

99. Watson, S. R., Schmitt, S. K., Hendricks, D. E., and Bullock, W. E. (1985): Immunoregulation in disseminated murine histoplasmosis: Disturbances in the production of interleukins 1 and 2. *J. Immunol.,* 135:3487–3493.

100. Weinberg, A., Rasmussen, L., and Merigan, T. C. (1986): Acute genital infection in guinea pigs: Effect of recombinant interleukin-2 on herpes simplex virus type 2. *J. Infect. Dis.,* 154:134–140.

101. Weinstock, J. V., Ehrinpreis, M. N., Boros, D. L., and Gee, J. B. (1981): Effect of SQ 14225, an inhibitor of angiotensin I-converting enzyme on the granulomatous response to *Schistosoma mansoni* eggs in mice. *J. Clin. Invest.,* 67:931–936.

102. Wheat, L. J., Kohler, R. B., and Tewari, R. P. (1986): Diagnosis of disseminated histoplasmosis by detection of *Histoplasma capsulatum* antigen in serum and urine specimens. *N. Engl. J. Med.,* 314:83–88.

103. Wheat, L. J., Slama, T. G., Eitzen, H. E., Kohler, R. B., French, M. L. V., and Biesecker, J. L. (1981): A large urban outbreak of histoplasmosis: Clinical features. *Ann. Intern. Med.,* 94:331–337.

104. Wheat, L. J., Slama, T. G., Norton, J. A., Kohler, R. B., Eitzen, H. E., French, M. L. V., and Sathapatayavongs, B. (1982): Risk factors for disseminated or fatal histoplasmosis. Analysis of a large urban outbreak. *Ann. Intern. Med.,* 96:159–163.

105. Wheat, L. J., Slama, T. G., and Zeckel, M. L. (1985): Histoplasmosis in the acquired immune deficiency syndrome. *Am. J. Med.,* 78:203–210.

106. Wheat, L. J., Wass, J., Norton, J., Kohler, R. B., and French, M. L. V. (1984): Cavitary histoplasmosis occurring during two large urban outbreaks. Analysis of clinical, epidemiologic, roetgenographic, and laboratory features. *Medicine (Baltimore),* 63:201–209.

107. Wright, S. D., and Jong, M. T. C. (1987): Adhesion-promoting receptors on human macrophages recognize *E. coli* by binding to lipopolysaccharide. (in press).

108. Wright, S. D., Rao, P. E., Van Voorhis, W. C., Craigmyle, L. S., Iida, K., Talle, M. A., Westberg, E. F., Goldstein, G., and Silverstein, S. C. (1983): Identification of the C3bi receptor of human monocytes and macrophages by using monoclonal antibodies. *Proc. Natl. Acad. Sci. USA,* 80:5699–5703.

109. Wright, S. D., and Silverstein, S. C. (1983): Receptors for C3b and C3bi promote phagocytosis but not the release of toxic oxygen from human phagocytes. *J. Exp. Med.,* 158:2016–2023.

110. Wu-Hsieh, B., and Howard, D. H. (1984): Inhibition of growth of *Histoplasma capsulatum* by lymphokine-stimulated macrophages. *J. Immunol.,* 132:2593–2597.

111. Zeidberg, L. D., Dillon, A., and Gass, R. S. (1951): Some factors in the epidemiology of histoplasmin sensitivity in Williamson County, Tennessee. *Am. J. Public Health,* 41:80–89.

Inflammation: Basic Principles and Clinical Correlates.
Edited by J. I. Gallin, I. M. Goldstein, and R. Snyderman.
Raven Press, Ltd., New York © 1988.

CHAPTER 41

Pathogenesis of Rheumatoid Arthritis: A Disorder Associated with Dysfunctional Immunoregulation

Edward D. Harris, Jr.

Several general principles have evolved from study of the pathogenesis and clinical syndromes of rheumatoid arthritis (RA). One is that there are frequent interactions among different types of cells in this disease. A second is that the cytokines that control cellular interactions amplify the inflammatory cycles at many points in the evolution of the disease. A third, which follows logically from the first two, is that varied and plentiful inhibitor pathways are activated by inflammation. A fourth principle has been generated from evidence that spontaneous remissions are not infrequent in RA. This may mean that small adjustments in the regulatory factors that activate or suppress the rheumatoid process are sufficient to dampen the entire process, resulting in control of the immune response and suppression of inflammation and the proliferative response of mesenchymal cells. Parenthetically, it can be stated that for the future, a truly effective "remission-inducing" therapy for RA probably will not involve a cytotoxic drug nor a potent immune suppressant but rather one or more defined polypeptides that, introduced in the right manner to the patient, can trigger a healing process.

Adequate representation of the interactions and complexity of pathogenic mechanisms in RA could best be presented by a three-dimensional model; however, such a model would be too complex to understand. Given the space limitations of a text chapter, the compromise must be to present the inflammatory sequences in series, one after the other. The reader must remember that most are activated simultaneously.

PREDISPOSING FACTORS

Environment

RA exhibits approximately the same incidence in most populations throughout the world: about 1% of adult females and 0.5% of men. Rare pockets of higher incidence have not been explained when other infectious causes of polyarticular synovitis have been ruled out, but, in general, no environmental cause has been supported by good data. Stress, physical or mental, is mentioned as a process related to the onset of RA, but there are only anecdotal data to support the association.

Sex

The role of sex appears to be stronger than any geographic or racial factors as a determinant of the disease. It was not unreasonable, therefore, to examine the possible role of sex hormones in altering the incidence of new cases. Linos et al. (118) studied the incidence of RA and mortality from RA in Rochester, Minnesota, during the period 1950 through 1974. Whereas age-specific incidence rates for males remained relatively stable throughout the entire 25-year period, rates for females declined dramatically from 1964 to 1974. It was inferred that the introduction of oral contraceptives and estrogens for postmenopausal women could be the cause of the decline in incidence among females. Two additional studies have supported this hypothesis (191,211); however, two subsequent studies from the Rochester group have failed to confirm this association (47,117). In the most recent study (47), comparing any prior use of oral contraceptives with never having used them, the relative risk for RA estimated from 82 cases and 182 matched controls was 1:1, and the lack of a protective effect was independent of age, disease severity, and the date of confirmed diagnosis or symptom onset. A rebuttal to this has come from Dutch investigators (192), who compared 490 women with RA and a control group of 659 women. A negative association was found between the onset of RA and previous use of noncontraceptive hormones, confirming their earlier evidence for a protective effect. What can explain the discrepancy? Differences in methods and patient populations seem too minor to explain the difference, and thus further epidemiologic studies will be necessary, with special attention paid to a precise description of composition, as well as dose and duration of hormone therapy.

In experimental animals and humans, autoimmune disease is more common in females. Some diseases have a much greater female:male susceptibility ratio; for Hashimoto's thyroiditis, it is 25:1 to 50:1. The basis for the sex difference in this disease, as well as others, including RA, may be in the reactivity of lymphocytes in females as compared with males. Pregnancy is associated with decreased numbers of T lymphocytes (18,177). Sex hormones also affect stem cells, pre-B cells, and macrophages (4). Hench recognized long ago the ameliorative effects of pregnancy on RA (81). However, the complexity of the effects of sex on such diseases is illustrated by the fact

that pregnancy does not ameliorate all autoimmune diseases, and may indeed exacerbate systemic lupus erythematosus (SLE) (79). There is a negative correlation between serum α_2-glycoprotein concentration and RA disease activity during pregnancy (189). Another possibility for the "female effect" is the suppression of neutrophil responsiveness demonstrated *in vitro* by female sex hormones (26).

Genetics of the Immune Response

The propensity to develop RA appears to be associated with class II antigens of the major histocompatibility complex (MHC). The class II glycoproteins (often referred to as Ia) are formed of two transmembrane glycoproteins, an α chain and a β chain. Genes for both α and β chains are contained in contiguous regions of the sixth chromosome. Subregions code for DP, DQ, and DR. DR, the subregion with apparent relevance for RA, has two β chains (β_1 and β_2) and one α chain. More than 10 alleles of DR β genes have been demonstrated. Similar to the situation for immunoglobulins, there are variable, constant, and hypervariable regions of amino acid sequences. It appears that hypervariable areas are located at bends on the outside of the molecule as it is folded in space at locations where a small difference in amino acid composition can affect the fit among antigen, the MHC, and the T-cell receptor.

In early studies, DR haplotypes were determined using banks of alloantisera, much as were class I antigens such as HLA-B27. Using these techniques, Stastny (171) demonstrated that HLA-DR4 was associated with an approximately fourfold relative risk for RA in North American populations. However, several lines of data have indicated that more specific association of the MHC with RA is not measured by conventional typing for DR specificities. One is that DR4 determinants are not shared significantly by RA patients in the same family (209). Another is that in certain subpopulations (e.g., Israeli Jews), RA is more often associated with DR1 than DR4 (222). To investigate this problem by comparing epitopes rather than haplotypes, Lee et al. (113) used monoclonal antibodies against polymorphic Ia epitopes on cells of DR4-homozygous individuals. One of these epitopes, 109d6, identified by a monoclonal antibody, is more closely associated with disease susceptibility in some subgroups of the population (relative risk > 10) than are the allelic forms of Ia molecules typed by conventional DR4 alloantisera. The 109d6 epitope has been found to be present on more than one haplotype.

Recombinant DNA technology is providing base sequences for class II glycoproteins; rigorous comparison of clinical data with derived amino acid sequences for these surface markers may enable investigators to identify primary sequences of these DR chains that are linked tightly to susceptibility or expression of RA. The use of gene structure as a primary tool may provide similar associations; this involves the tools of restriction fragment length polymorphism (RFLP). DNA prepared from RA patients or controls is digested by endonucleases that cleave DNA at very specific base sequences. The digested DNA is then electrophoresed on gels. By use of radiolabeled complementary DNA (cDNA) probes complementary to β chains of class II antigens, autoradiographs of the gels can be developed that have patterns corresponding to the relative sizes of DNA fragments produced by the endonuclease. Using this technology, investigators from the University of Alabama (122) were able to detect one fragment of β-chain DNA produced by one endonuclease that appears to carry with it a 50-fold increased susceptibility for RA. It should follow that data using monoclonal antibodies and RFLP should converge on the same primary sequence or sequences of protein. The power of this association will reveal whether there are one, several, or many genetic determinants of susceptibility for RA.

POSSIBLE ETIOLOGIC FACTORS

That genetic determinants of the MHC are closely related to RA rests on better data than does any evidence for a specific cause of the disease. There are several broad hypotheses currently in favor for "the cause." One is that a foreign antigen such as a persistent but only weakly cytotoxic virus generates an immune reaction that becomes self-sustaining. A second is that certain individuals who express class II antigens associated with enhanced susceptibility to develop RA also have abnormal lymphocytes (determined by genes different from those controlling MHC expression) that allow a chronic persistent arthritis to develop in response to one or many different stimuli, including connective-tissue components such as type II collagen. An example of this exists in animals: the MRL/1 mouse has hyperactive T helper cells that lead to uncontrolled B-lymphocyte activation and polyclonal antibody production. This lymphocyte abnormality is controlled by a single recessive gene (182). A third possibility involves components of the two theories mentioned earlier: An infection in a susceptible person could result in production of antibodies that cross-react with tissue antigens in and around the joint, or (as can be the case with viral infections) the infected host cell could be programmed to produce abnormal proteins or glycoproteins that could then serve as antigens. If these infected cells were lymphocytes, a sustained inflammation could follow clonal expansion of cells, producing antibodies against the abnormal surface or transmembrane proteins.

Studies in recent years have generated interest in many potential etiologic factors. Two viruses (Epstein-Barr virus and parvovirus) and one host protein (collagen) will be discussed for the broad range of possibilities they present.

Epstein-Barr Virus

Large numbers of patients with seropositive RA (i.e., RA with circulating rheumatoid factor) have circulating antibody in high titers directed against an Epstein-Barr (EB) viral nuclear antigen (7). The EB virus receptor on the B lymphocyte, the target cell, is identical with a single membrane protein, the complement receptor type 2 (CR2) (60), that binds C3d, iC3b (the first product of factor I cleavage), and, with less affinity, C3b. EB virus infection of B cells results in polyclonal activation and production of as many antibodies as there are clones activated. B cells from patients with RA have a fivefold greater spontaneous infection rate with EB virus than do normal cells (166). B cells infected with EB virus have been demonstrated in rheumatoid synovium, but not in nonrheumatoid tissues (195). Why are more rheumatoid cells infected with EB virus? It appears that rheumatoid T lymphocytes carry an inherent defect that prevents them from adequately suppressing EB-virus-induced polyclonal B-cell proliferation (48,186). This defect in T cells is complex, culminating in insufficient gamma-interferon (IFNγ) being produced by the T cells to suppress EB virus proliferation. The deficient IFNγ production results from insufficient interleukin-2 (IL-2) biosynthesis by the rheumatoid T cells, a defect that in turn may be caused by insufficient interleukin-1 (IL-1) production by the rheumatoid monocyte/macrophage populations or by an excess of IL-1 inhibitor produced. IFNγ and IL-2 also combine to activate natural killer (NK) cells. A deficiency of these autacoids could lead to inadequate NK cell function. Because increased antibody titers against EB virus are not found in early RA (166), there is no way to relate the virus and disease as cause and effect. However, it could easily follow that once the initial rheumatoid inflammation has been initiated, EB viral infection of B cells in these hosts incapable of suppressing it can markedly amplify the immune response and perhaps even guarantee persistence and autonomy of the disease process.

Parvovirus

Parvoviruses are small, ubiquitous DNA viruses that produce several diseases in humans and in animals, including Aleutian mink disease. An arthropathy in adults, usually self-limited, is the most relevant of these (149,207). It can occur without viral prodromata or skin rash and has presented as a symmetrical polyarthropathy of sudden onset and moderate severity affecting, as does RA, the small joints of the hands, wrists, and knees. Some patients (up to 50%) have a typical erythematous "slapped-cheek" appearance to the face, a manifestation much more common when it affects children as erythema infectiosum or "fifth disease." It is more common in women than in men. Rheumatoid factor is not present. Joint destruction has not been described. The appearance of significant titers of antihuman parvovirus (anti-HPV) IgM closely follows the onset of symptoms; these fall to normal in 3 months as anti-HPV IgG rises.

These observations are particularly interesting in light of data from Simpson et al. (167), who isolated a parvovirus from rheumatoid synovium after maintaining it by inoculation into brains of newborn mice. Called RA-1, this virus is different from other HPVs, such as B19, which is the putative cause of the transient arthritis mentioned earlier (149,207). Using antibody to RA-1, antigen was found in synovium in 13 of 14 rheumatoid patients, but in none with osteoarthritis. Again, there is no proof that RA-1 caused RA in the patient from whom it was isolated, or in any other patient. However, the nature of RA-1 and other HPVs makes it essential to extend and expand these studies.

Parvovirus can integrate its own DNA into human chromosomes, perhaps leading to expression of antigens that generate an immune response. Infection of lymphoid cells by HPV or a similar virus may cripple them by permitting unbridled EB viral infection, and a polyclonal B-cell proliferation could become self-sustaining. Thus, although the ideal single viral pathogen that could cause RA should be ubiquitous, persistent, and arthrotropic and have the capability to alter immune responses, it is possible that these qualities might be distributed among two or more viruses that would work in series or parallel to produce RA in the genetically susceptible host. Other viruses, such as rubella (35,66), have been implicated as causative agents, but the same rigorous criteria for proof of causation must be applied to these as to EB virus and HPV.

Collagen as an Autoimmunogen

The discovery that type II collagen can cause arthritis in rats and mice and that the disease and/or some of its manifestations can be passively transferred by IgG fractions containing anticollagen antibodies (174) or by transfer of lymphocytes from affected animals (188) has generated much interest in autoimmunity to collagen as a cause of RA. Type II collagen is found almost exclusively in articular cartilage. A number of the findings in these rats and mice have been particularly provocative:

1. In both rats and mice, the immune response toward type II collagen is under strict MHC (Ia) gene control (219).

2. Athymic, nude rats do not develop arthritis in response to type II collagen injection, emphasizing the necessity for functional T cells to initiate collagen-induced arthritis (103).
3. A T-cell-derived arthritogenic lymphokine that produces synovitis and binds to type II collagen has been isolated from T cells obtained from animals after type II collagen immunization (80).
4. Type-II-collagen-reactive T-cell clones have been isolated from mice with collagen-induced arthritis (43,88).
5. Homologous (rather than heterologous) type-II-collagen-induced arthritis in male, but not in female, DBA/1 mice and was associated with clinical features (e.g., late onset, progressive development, exacerbations/remissions) resembling RA not previously reported in other experimental models of arthritis (87). Hybridization of spleen cells from DBA/1 mice immunized with immune complexes containing native type II collagen and a monoclonal anti-collagen-II antibody resulted in lymphocyte clones that produced two monoclonal IgG rheumatoid factors, one of which appeared to be an antiidiotype of anti-collagen-II antibodies (89).
6. A major immunogenic and arthritogenic epitope on type II collagen has been shown to reside in one (CB-11) of 12 polypeptides of type II α chains produced by cyanogen bromide cleavage (180).

In the aggregate, these data have shown that specific epitopes on homologous or heterologous type II collagen induce an MHC-restricted immune response dependent on T-cell help, resulting in activation of both a cellular immune response and a humoral immune response and destructive synovitis within the joints.

Collagen-induced arthritis is, of course, not a spontaneous disease. In an animal model of arthritis that is genetically mediated (i.e., that appearing in MRL/1 mice), the patterns of autoreactivity to type II collagen are different from those in collagen-induced forms (178). Severe synovitis and polyclonal B-cell activation precede the humoral immune response to collagen. Spontaneous collagen-II-specific antibody production is unaffected by collagen II immunization, suggesting that the antibody response against type II collagen is independent of MHC-restricted T-cell help in these rodents.

How do the data from rodents apply to RA? Although arthritis has been induced in mice by anticollagen antibodies from a patient with RA (218) and in monkeys by immunization with type II collagen (34), there is no answer yet to the question whether autoimmunity to collagen is related to the genesis of RA or is a reaction to excessive collagen turnover as joints are progressively destroyed and soluble type II denatured collagen fragments become abundant in extracellular spaces (175). If production of IL-1 by synovial tissue can be used as a measure of a "rheumatoid-like" synovitis, then type-II-collagen-induced arthritis appears to be more similar to the human disease than adjuvant arthritis or the spontaneous arthritis in MRL/1 mice.

Monoclonal antibodies to native type II collagen have been shown by immunofluorescence to react with cells within the invasive synovium at the pannus/cartilage junction in material taken from rheumatoid joints (105). Most interesting, however, are data from the same experiments showing no collagen antigenic determinants in normal cartilage; hyaluronidase treatment unmasked binding sites blocked in normal cartilage. In contrast, abundant staining of the cartilage around the pannus/cartilage junction in RA was found.

In RA, anticollagen antibodies are present in synovial fluid as well as in serum (10). However, only recently have investigators been careful to precisely differentiate antibodies to native and denatured collagens in RA. In one such study (155) using a solid-phase radioimmunoassay, sera from patients with RA contained antibody titers significantly higher to denatured bovine type II collagen than did control sera, whereas there was no difference in antibody titers to native collagen.

It seems reasonable to conclude from the data now available that autoantibody formation to collagen is not a primary event in the disease, but that the activated immune system in RA readily develops clonal proliferation of B cells expressing antibody against epitopes of type II collagen normally masked by the native helical conformation of collagen and its coating with proteoglycan and other noncollagen glycoproteins. Whether or not the antibodies appearing that are directed against the degraded, fragmented type II collagen can then participate in amplifying the immune response is unknown.

THE EARLY IMMUNE RESPONSE IN SYNOVIUM

Studies of early events in RA must focus on the synovial lining. It seems probable that the antigen that triggers the disease must be arthrotropic; that is, it (they) must somehow migrate to and localize in the synovium. Synovial lining cells that can be obtained by postmortem trypsin injection into intact joints from patients with arthritis are macrophage-like, with positive staining for esterases and Fc receptors. Most express HLA-DR antigens and can be shown to present antigen to T lymphocytes (101), resulting in their activation. Lymphocytes are recruited to the synovium from peripheral lymph nodes and traverse the synovial endothelial lining to the lining sublayers. It is known that the exit of lymphocytes from the circulation into lymph nodes or Peyer's patches occurs specifically at "high endothelial venules" characterized by tall endothelial cells. Specific membrane molecules (148) on mature T and B lymphocytes that are missing from thymus- or

bone-marrow-derived cells mediate adhesion to the endothelial cells. IL-1 (17) may facilitate lymphocyte adherence and/or migration through the venules. Rheumatoid synovial tissue has been examined for the relationship between the endothelium and the cellular infiltrate. Tall capillary endothelial cells were found in areas where there were dense collections of lymphocytes (91) in the surrounding tissue. Normal human mononuclear cells have been shown to bind to these endothelial cells in the rheumatoid synovium.

Thus, the synovial lining becomes a peripheral lymphoid organ manifesting a delayed-type hypersensitivity reaction. The rheumatoid synovial cells stain brightly for HLA-DR antigens (94). Functionally, the rheumatoid synovial macrophage-like dendritic cells are extremely efficient T-cell activators (101). The synovial lymphocytes express HLA-DR antigens, a manifestation of their activated state (102). The activated T lymphocytes, most of which express T4 (helper) antigens (146,147), surround the interdigitating dendritic macrophage-like HLA-DR$^+$ cells.

Activation of T Lymphocytes

Activation of T cells is an important amplification step in RA (Fig. 1). At the molecular level, the T-cell receptor (Ti/T3), antigen, and MHC form a trimolecular complex that results in activation of the T lymphocytes by specific antigen. Once activated by a specific foreign antigen/MHC combination, T cells react to the same antigen only in combination with the same MHC molecule. There is evidence that the antigen is presented, but not further "processed" (198), by the antigen-presenting cell.

Functional and structural studies indicate that the T-cell antigen-receptor complex consists of at least five polypeptide chains: the polymorphic α and β subunits of the Ti molecule, two glycosylated T3 subunits, and one nonglycosylated subunit (2,202). The Ti molecule is clonally specific and presumably serves as the antigen-binding site. The T3 molecules probably serve in transduction of signals from the surface into the cytosol following the ligand/Ti binding that results in T-cell activation. T4 and T8 are separate membrane antigens that are markers for the functional state of cells as helper (T4) or suppressor (T8) cells.

Although the combined presentation of antigen and MHC to the T-cell antigen receptor is *necessary* for T-cell activation, it appears that it is not *sufficient*. Another stimulus is needed, probably IL-1 provided by monocyte/macrophages (127) (see Chapters 13 and 33).

Similar to activation pathways in polymorphonuclear leukocytes and B lymphocytes, T-cell activation is related to an increase in the concentration of cytoplasmic free calcium (Ca^{2+}). The calcium is mobilized from intracel-

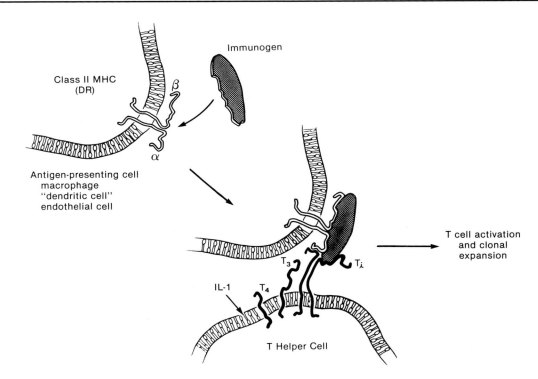

FIG. 1. The antigen/MHC/T-cell-receptor complex leads to activation of T lymphocytes. This process is facilitated by IL-1.

lular stores by inositol triphosphate (IP$_3$) that is generated in turn from phosphatidylinositol as a result of perturbation of the Ti/T3 antigen receptor in response to MHC-restricted presentation of antigen (54). A product of hydrolysis of phosphatidylinositol diphosphate (PIP$_2$) to IP$_3$ is diacylglycerol (DAG). DAG is the putative physiologic activator of protein kinase C, the intracellular enzyme that phosphorylates many different proteins and triggers new gene expression.

Lymphokines: Principal Regulators of the Proliferative Immune Response

Many soluble products of activated lymphocytes have been identified. These are described in detail in Chapters 14 to 16. Most studies of RA have focused on two lymphokines (IL-2 and IFNγ), although interest in tumor necrosis factor (TNF) has been increasing. There is growing evidence that in RA, the production of and cellular responses to these lymphokines may be abnormal.

IL-2

Formation of the heterotrimer (the aggregate of MHC/antigen with Ti/T3) on a helper T-cell membrane results in activation of the T cell. IL-2 receptors appear on the cell surface, and IL-2 synthesis and secretion are generated. The IL-2 receptor is a glycoprotein of 55 kd and has been

cloned and sequenced (190). The gene encoding for the human IL-2 receptor is on the short arm of chromosome 10 (115), whereas the genes for Ti/T3 are on chromosome 7, and the gene for IL-2 itself is on chromosome 4 (152). Mature T cells from all three subsets (helper, suppressor, killer) express IL-2 receptors and proliferate in the presence of IL-2. *In vitro,* if T cells are cultured for 2 weeks or more and are given frequent exposure to IL-2, T8 cells proliferate, but T4 cells diminish. So long as specific antigen remains available in the microenvironment, IL-2 receptors will be present on the activated cell surface, and proliferation of this clone will occur. When specific antigen is removed from the microenvironment, the IL-2 receptors disappear, and the Ti/T3 receptor is again expressed again on the cell surface. A new steady state is reached marked by an IL-2-induced clonal expansion. This gives a molecular explanation for immunologic memory (3); when specific antigen is reinserted into the system, there are many more cells with Ti/T3 receptors for that specific antigen available. IL-2 receptors have been identified on cells other than T lymphocytes, but a function mediated by IL-2 in these non-T cells is not known (Fig. 2).

Interferon

IFNγ, or immune interferon, is produced by antigen-activated T lymphocytes or by large granular lymphocytes that have natural killer activity. Receptors for IFNγ are

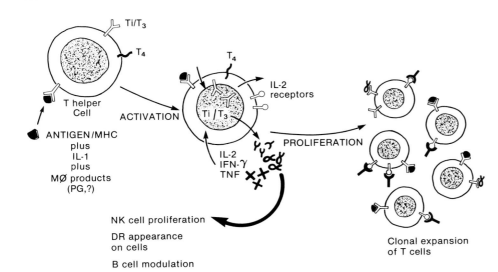

FIG. 2. The consequences of T4 cell activation. The Ti/T3 receptors disappear from the cell surface, and IL-2 receptors are expressed on the cell surface. IL-2, IFNγ, and TNFβ are expressed by the cells, resulting in clonal expansion of these cells, as well as changes toward activation and differentiation in other cells. This gives a molecular basis for immunologic memory. When the antigen is gone from the microenvironment, Ti/T3 are expressed again, and IL-2 receptors disappear. In the new steady state there are more cells with Ti/T3 specific for the initial antigen/MHC that activated the first T cells. Clonal expansion already has occurred, and these T cells are primed for activation.

present on many different types of cells, initiating many effects on these cells. Because of these broad actions, its role as autacoid in the heterogeneous cell population in rheumatoid synovial tissue is amplified. A short précis of its effects could be that it slows growth and leads to specialized and differentiated functions of cells. IFNγ contains 146 amino acids (molecular mass 17 kd) and is variably glycosylated (196). Similar to IL-2, its gene is expressed when the resting T cell is stimulated by antigen in conjunction with the MHC gene products at the Ti/T3 receptor in the presence of IL-1 (72). IFNγ inhibits the proliferation of a wide variety of cells, perhaps by reducing the expression of receptors such as that for insulin (57). Synthesis of types I and III collagen by rheumatoid synovial cells in culture is inhibited by IFNγ; this is associated with decreases in types I and III procollagen in messenger RNAs (mRNAs) in these cells (172). An important exception to this antiproliferative effect may be the apparent stimulation of mitogenesis in synovial fibroblasts by recombinant IFNγ (19).

The modulation/maturation effects of IFNγ are illustrated by its effects on macrophages. It increases accessory cell functions and decreases immunosuppressive functions; IFNγ reduces phospholipase A_2 activity, cutting down on the supply of arachidonic acid, the precursor of prostaglandins and leukotrienes (136). Fc receptors are increased on the macrophages. A major function of IFNγ in many cell types is induction of expression of class I and II MHC antigens on the cell surface. In the presence of IFNγ, many cells found in the rheumatoid synovium, including endothelial cells, fibroblasts, mast cells, and perhaps even B cells, can express accessory cell capability (136).

Most intriguing of the effects of IFNγ are its actions in collaboration with other autacoids. For example, IFNγ from lymphocytes and IFNβ from macrophages inhibit growth of and collagen production by human dermal fi-

broblasts (54). IL-2 and IFNγ in collaboration have important effects on generation and activity of natural killer (NK) cells. IL-2 stimulates T cells to produce IFNγ, which in turn acts as a differentiation signal that appears to be involved in the IL-2-initiated activation of NK cells (93).

NK cells can be defined operationally as a population of cells capable of mediating direct cytotoxicity against various types of target cells without any specific antigenic stimulus. In peripheral blood they appear as a morphologically homogeneous population of large granular lymphocytes. NK cells express T11 surface proteins and variably express Ti protein (151). It appears, therefore, that they are derived from T-lineage precursors and that the T11 molecule may be important in the activation of NK cells (151).

In RA, the production and/or cellular receptors of IL-2 and IFNγ may be abnormal. For example, using the autologous mixed leukocyte reaction with added IL-2 to generate cytotoxic cells, Goto and Zvaifler (65) demonstrated that cytotoxic cells from patients with active RA could not proliferate and had poor cytotoxic capabilities. This could be related to the reduced production of IL-2 by T lymphocytes in RA in response to activation stimuli (38) or to impaired production of IFNγ by these cells. In RA, the macrophage may be at fault. The inability of rheumatoid T lymphocytes to down-regulate EB-virus-induced B-cell proliferation (48,186) is probably related in part to an excessive sensitivity of the T cells to the suppressive influence of prostaglandins on IL-2 production (65) and/or insufficient IL-1 production of these cells. An additional mechanism could be production of IL-1 inhibitor(s) within the joint.

Other Lymphokines and Their Significance in RA

Another abnormality in lymphocyte function reported in RA is impaired suppressor cell function. It remains to be determined whether or not suppressor-activating factor (SAF) is a discrete protein (111) not related to others already cloned and sequenced. SAF-treated T lymphocytes release a T-cell-specific suppressor activity (TRSA) into culture medium. Patients with RA whose T cells demonstrated impaired TRSA release in response to SAF exhibited evidence for more active clinical disease than did RA patients with normal TRSA release (111). These factors must be purified, cloned, and expressed before their significance can be evaluated.

Tumor necrosis factor (TNFβ) is secreted by activated lymphocytes (176). This factor, formally called lymphotoxin, has structural homology with TNFα produced by stimulated macrophages. The potential role of TNFβ in RA has not been defined, but its potential for interaction with other autacoids in the disease is large. TNFβ may be synergistic with IL-1 in many actions on cells, with the exception of T-cell activation.

IL-2 binding to IL-2 receptors on activated T cells induces synthesis and secretion of IL-3, a hematopoietic growth and differentiation factor (221). It is interesting to speculate that insufficient production of IL-3 or other colony-stimulating factors (124) may be at the root of the red cell aplasia that occasionally is seen in RA (49).

Appreciation of the complexity of T-cell regulation makes it probable that additional factors, some known and others unknown, will be found that affect these cells. It may evolve that therapeutic use of one or another of these will be sufficient to begin a cycle of regulation that can gear down the inflammatory response and induce remission in this disease. For example, calcitriol [1,25(OH)$_2$D$_3$] has been shown to affect activation and proliferation of human T lymphocytes. Calcitriol blocks the transition of lymphocytes through the G$_1$ phase of the cell cycle, effectively inhibiting IL-2 production. It also inhibits the expression of transferrin receptors needed for cell growth (150), but does not affect expression of IL-2 receptors (150). Thus, calcitriol appears to act on lymphocytes by mechanisms similar to those of dexamethasone and PGE$_2$ (16,199).

Clinical Manifestations of Immunocyte Activation

Measurement of circulating lymphocyte subsets in RA has not been useful. It is generally agreed that these do not reflect activity in the synovium, the seat of the response. The one consistent finding has been an increase in the numbers of circulating lymphocytes that are expressing HLA-DR antigens on cell membranes (30,222). Similarly, increased expression of Fc receptors on peripheral-blood monocytes in RA has been measured and gives a measure of activation of these cells (31).

Assessment of cellular immunity in RA, as measured

by the state of responsiveness *in vitro* of lymphocytes after stimulation by soluble antigens, has produced interesting results (46,208). Some rheumatoid patients have anergic circulating lymphocytes; these people have increased T8$^+$ and DR$^+$ cells in peripheral blood, increased T4$^+$ and DR$^+$ cells in synovium, and weakly reactive or negative skin tests to PPD antigen. In contrast, patients with normally reactive lymphocytes *in vitro* have normal T8$^+$:T4$^+$ ratios in peripheral blood and little evidence for intense immunological activity in synovial biopsies. Both cellular anergy and dermal anergy in the first group disappeared immediately after leukapheresis, a phenomenon that paralleled a short-lived beneficial clinical response. Leukapheresis presumably removed a large quantity of the committed, already activated T cells in the circulation. Naive cells then entered the circulation from the marrow, and these cells were capable of responding to mitogens *in vitro*.

MULTIPLE CAPABILITIES OF ENDOTHELIAL CELLS

Proliferation of endothelial cells in the rheumatoid synovium is one of the most important components of the inflammation and proliferation in this disease. Angiogenesis provides the scaffold of new capillaries on which all new synovial cell and immunocyte proliferation is based. Angiogenesis factors can be provided by activated macrophages within the synovium (106,144). Major subpopulations of macrophages from rheumatoid synovium that are Fc- and C3-receptor-positive, esterase-positive, and peroxidase-negative and that stain positively with anti-DR and other antibodies against macrophage surface markers are particularly potent inducers of neovascularization (106). In addition, it has been determined that class II MHC (DR, Ia) antigens can be induced to appear on the surface membranes of vascular endothelium by human IFNγ (143). This could present a specific MHC/antigen complex to the circulation and possibly serve to recruit antigen-specific T helper cells into the site of an immune response. Indeed, it has been demonstrated that lymphocyte-rich areas in synovium from patients with RA contain blood vessels adhesive *in vitro* for mononuclear cells (137). These reactive vessels showed morphologic similarity to the high endothelial venules of lymph nodes where normal lymphocyte adhesion and emigration into surrounding tissue occurs. In experimental studies using dogs, it has been shown that cyclosporin A can prevent class II MHC antigen expression on endothelial cells (67), presumably by suppressing IFNγ production by T cells. It also has been documented that *in vitro* IL-1 increases the adhesion to endothelium of polymorphonuclear leukocytes and monocytes (17). During the early synovial inflammation in RA, the presence of IL-1 and IFNγ around synovial capillaries could result in recruitment of cells for the developing synovial lymphoid organ as well as for the inflammatory "sink" in synovial fluid. Regulation, modulation, and suppression of angiogenesis in the future may be possible by using a class of "angiostatic" steroids that lack glucocorticoid or mineralocorticoid activity. In the presence of specific heparin fragments not associated with anticoagulant function, these steroids are effective inhibitors of angiogenesis (42).

B-CELL PROLIFERATION IN RHEUMATOID SYNOVIUM

B-lymphocyte activation is the final immunological event in early rheumatoid synovitis. B lymphocytes, similar to T lymphocytes, are in the resting or G_0 phase of the cell cycle before activation. There are several ways that activation is initiated. If the currently unknown initiating antigen in RA has multiple repeating copies of an epitope, this antigen alone could bind to surface Ig and lead to receptor cross-linking and to an excited state susceptible to proliferative factors (140). This is a T-cell-independent process resulting in polyclonal activation. A second principal pathway of B-cell activation depends on interaction of T4 (helper) cells with a B cell in an antigen-specific, histocompatibility-restricted manner (27,90). The transmembrane signaling mechanisms involving phosphatidylinositol metabolism, diacylglycerol formation, an increase in cytoplasmic calcium, and protein kinase C activation are basically the same for B cells as for T cells (27). After initial excitation (or activation), receptors for B-cell growth and differentiation factors appear on the B-cell surface membrane (90). IL-1 (56) and IL-2 (91) both appear to have roles as cofactors (costimulant) in the activation process, and a 60-kd human protein, B-cell growth factor (BCGF, distinct from IL-2), has been purified. BCGF binds to receptors on activated B cells and drives them into a proliferative state (8). This clonal expansion is critical for physiological immune responses, but B-cell differentiation factors are needed to lift the cells into an antibody-secreting state (140,159). It is probable that T lymphocytes produce both B-cell growth and differentiation factors.

RHEUMATOID FACTORS AND PATHOGENESIS

Rheumatoid factors (RFs) and RA have always been linked, but the significance and specificity of that linkage are under continuing investigation. RFs are autoantibodies directed against epitopes on the Fc fragment of IgG. They are not specific for RA and appear to be associated with inflammatory states in which the immunologic stimulus persists in the body, and when polyclonal B-lymphocyte activation is present. Many mechanisms to explain why IgG becomes antigenic have been postulated (29). One of the most recent suggests that autoantigenic reactivity of IgG in RA is related to changes in the relative extent of asparagine-linked galactosylation of the proteins (139). The following are some reasons for linking RA and RFs in schemes of pathogenesis:

1. RA patients with positive tests for RFs have more severe disease and extraarticular manifestations than do patients with "seronegative" RA (33).
2. IgM RFs fix complement (158).
3. Levels of RFs correlate positively with *in vivo* complement turnover rates in patients with RA (99).
4. Immune complexes from rheumatoid synovial fluid and tissue contain RFs, IgG, and no other detectable antigen (210).
5. Appearance of anti-IgG plaque-forming cells in bone marrow and synovial fluid correlates positively with clinical activity of RA (194).
6. RFs are associated with a high frequency of subcutaneous nodules and vasculitis (181).

Recent studies of RF synthesis in synovial membrane cell cultures have indicated that only cells from patients with seropositive RA make RFs spontaneously (206). IgM RF represented $7.3 \pm 0.7\%$ of total IgM produced by cells from 12 patients, and IgG RF represented $2.6 \pm 1.1\%$ of IgG synthesized in those cultures with detectable IgG RF. These values are lower than those reported previously using less specific methods, but the specificity accentuates even more the growing appreciation that seronegative RA is, more often than not, a disease of different cause and pathogenesis than is seropositive RA. It is interesting that although the synovium is the focus for clinical inflammation in RA, production of RFs is not limited to synovium in either rheumatoid patients or normals. A marked EB virus inducibility of RF production by human marrow cells from aged subjects substantiates the belief that polyclonal B-cell activation in and of itself is associated with RF synthesis (62).

An interesting property of IgG RF is the capability of these molecules, which each express two antigen-binding sites, to self-associate to form dimers or larger polymers (145). Although less efficient in fixing complement than are aggregated IgG and large-lattice immune complexes, it is possible that self-associating IgG can have a role in immune pathogenesis in RA.

As many as 60% of human monoclonal anti-IgG antibodies from unrelated individuals share cross-reactive idiotypes (CRIs). Use of synthetic hyper-variable-region peptides and immunoblotting techniques has enabled investigators to identify these common regions (36). The majority of human monoclonal IgM RFs share one or two primary-sequence-dependent CRIs, both on the κ light chain (37). The data suggest that one gene or very few genes for the variable region of light chains, but large numbers of genes for the variable region of heavy chains, are used to code for IgM RF antoantibodies. Studies of affinity-purified RFs from rheumatoid patients, patients with Sjögren's syndrome, and normal elderly patients were screened with a panel of three antibodies, each directed against a different determinant on CRIs (61). The pattern of reaction against the three antibodies was different for each group.

It is conceivable that these anti-CRIs could bind to and inactivate RF-bearing B lymphocytes or that CRIs could be used as immunogens to induce clonal proliferation of the suppressor T cells against cells producing RF auto-antibodies (36). Such experiments will focus on the growing awareness that in the future the most effective therapy for the most complex diseases, including RA, will be built around the primary structures of human peptides and proteins.

As noted earlier, 90% or more of immunoglobulins produced by rheumatoid synovial B lymphocytes and plasma cells are *not* RFs. Data are variable regarding the expression of IgG subtypes by cells in rheumatoid synovium; if one subtype were produced in much greater quantity than others, it would be evidence for committed clones directed, perhaps, at the causative antigen. IgG produced by synovial explants *in vitro* has been typed. In early studies, IgG3 represented 41% of IgG, compared with a serum IgG3 concentration of 12% of IgG in the same patients (84). In contrast, in more recent studies, examination by immunofluorescence of the plasma cells in rheumatoid synovial samples showed only a slight increase in IgG3-containing cells (69).

IMMUNE COMPLEXES IN RA

A constant finding in RA is the centripetal orientation of the invasive, proliferating synovial tissue. It moves in toward the center of the joint, with an apparent special avidity for articular cartilage, despite the proteinase and angiogenesis inhibitors normally present in this tissue. As a corollary to this, it has been observed by many orthopedic surgeons and rheumatologists that when residual cartilage is completely removed from a joint during total joint replacement, that particular joint is less likely to be involved in a subsequent attack of rheumatoid synovitis, even if most of the synovium is not removed from the joint at time of surgery.

A major hypothesis that would link the immune lesion of RA more tightly to the proliferative/destructive lesion is that immune complexes produced in the synovium and deposited in the superficial regions of the articular cartilage serve as a fixed source of chemoattractant for the cellular pannus (Fig. 3). Some connections to support this hypothesis have been made:

1. Immunoglobulins and complement have been identified by immunofluorescence in the superficial layers of articular cartilage in RA (39). They can also be identified by electron microscopy (134).
2. In experimental animals it has been established that antigen and antibody, or soluble complexes of both, can diffuse into cartilage and be trapped there (95).
3. Immune complexes are absent from the cartilage that lies directly under invasive pannus tissue, implying that the deposits there were phagocytosed or otherwise freed into the synovial fluid by the pannus (165). If the former were true, immune complexes could have a dual role, first to serve as a chemoattractant, and then to induce synovial cells that have phagocytosed them to produce matrix proteinases (28,45).

To examine the antibody specificity of immune complexes sequestered in articular cartilage, Jasin (96) has extracted articular cartilage from patients with RA, osteoarthritis (OA), and traumatic injury. Rheumatoid cartilage contained 37 times more IgM and 14 times more IgG than did normal cartilage. IgM RF was found in 13 of 16 RA cartilage extracts, but in none from patients with OA or traumatic arthritis. Consistent with a possible role for autoimmunity to collagen in the pathophysiology of RA, more than 60% of rheumatoid cartilage extracts were positive for antibodies to native and denatured type II collagen (96). Blunting the significance of this, however, was the finding that OA cartilage extracts also contained anticollagen antibodies. That the presence of anticollagen antibodies can accentuate and amplify experimental arthritis is provided by evidence that prior injection of anticollagen antibodies into rats leads to more severe adjuvant arthritis transferred by immune spleen cells (179).

Applications of modern techniques to the search for specific antigens in RA have, appropriately, focused on immune complexes (ICs). Among the techniques used is immunoblotting after sodium dodecylsulfate/polyacrylamide-gel electrophoresis (SDS-PAGE) with antisera raised to ICs isolated from rheumatoid tissues (92). Although IgG is the principal immunoglobulin, and also the principal constituent of immune complexes, IgM, IgA, and C1q also are constituents of ICs from RA synovial fluid. Although "unidentified" constituents of ICs have been characterized on the basis of apparent molecular size, no further information about them is available. Data are sparse that would suggest that routine measurement of ICs in venous or arterial blood can be useful in monitoring disease activity in RA (138).

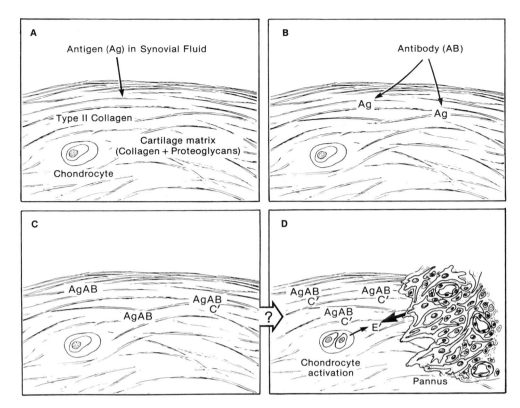

FIG. 3. A hypothesis to explain pannus invasion of articular cartilage. Antigen in synovial fluid may diffuse into superficial layers of cartilage (**A**), and antibody may joint it (**B**), forming antigen/antibody complexes (**C**) that—perhaps after fixing complement—may serve as chemoattractants for the proliferating pannus (**D**).

SYNOVIAL FLUID AND ACTIVATED POLYMORPHONUCLEAR LEUKOCYTES IN RA

Synovial fluid accumulation in inflamed joints is one of the first manifestations of disease activity in RA. In normal joints, this fluid is an ultrafiltrate of plasma that passes through the fenestrations along capillary endothelium in fine capillaries that lie in the matrix below synovial lining cells. Once in the extracellular space, there is no barrier to collection of fluid in the joint cavity, because pressure in the normal joint cavity is negative, compared even with that within postcapillary venules (131). As synovial fluid accumulates in a joint, the intraarticular pressure increases even to the point that synovial blood flow is compromised (97). This increase in pressure, combined with a capillary network that appears inadequate to provide sufficient O_2 to the enormous mass of proliferating cells, leads to low PO_2 and acidosis in joints of the most severely affected patients (55). Whereas intraarticular temperature in acutely inflamed joints is higher than that found in normal joints, joint temperature in severe proliferative chronic RA may be lower than normal (200), implying that blood flow in these most affected joints is insufficient to provide adequate perfusion.

From the standpoint of both diagnosis and importance in pathophysiology, it is the large numbers of polymorphonuclear (PMN) leukocytes that accumulate in rheumatoid synovial fluid that deserve our attention (Fig. 4). More than 1 billion PMN leukocytes may be drawn into the joint cavity of the knee each day in a rheumatoid patient with moderately active disease (86). This occurs by directed migration (chemotaxis) of PMN leukocytes to chemoattractants produced and released in the joint space (170). The most important of these in RA are as follows:

Chemotactic factor	Cell or cascade source
Leukotriene B_4	PMN membrane phospholipids
Platelet-activating factor	Cell membrane phospholipids (PMN, other cells)
C5a	From activation of complement
Thrombin	From activation of clotting
Lymphocyte-derived chemotactic factor	Lymphocytes

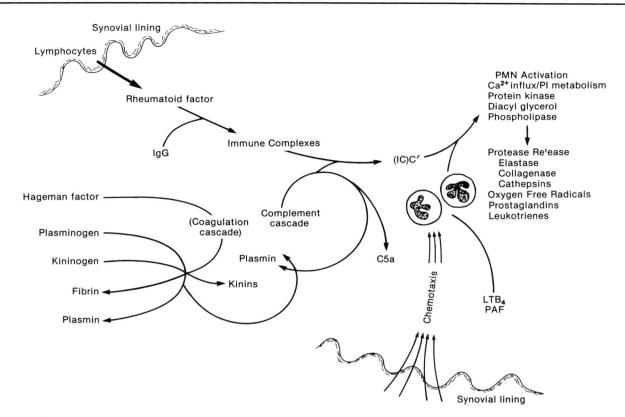

FIG. 4. Inflammatory events in the rheumatoid joint space. Lymphocytes in the synovium (**upper left**) produce RF; RF/IgG complexes can fix complement [(IC)C'] and as such are phagocytosed by PMN leukocytes. These are activated and release proteinases, oxygen-derived free radicals, prostaglandins, and leukotrienes. LTB_4 and platelet-activating factor are potent chemoattractants that attract more PMN leukocytes, amplifying the inflammation. In the fluid phase (**left**), the clotting, kinin, fibrinolytic, and complement cascades all interact, contributing also to the inflammation.

These substances bind to specific receptors on the PMN leukocyte membrane and are necessary and sufficient to activate these cells as they enter the joint space. Activation of the PMN leukocyte involves transmembrane signal transduction that utilizes a guanine nucleotide regulatory protein (169) (see Chapter 20), leading to phosphatidyl-inositol 4,5-diphosphate (PIP_2) hydrolysis by a specific phospholipase C to myoinositol 1,4,5-triphosphate (IP_3) and diacylglycerol (168). Similar to the activation of lymphocytes, these two substances act as second messengers; IP_3 stimulates release of Ca^{2+} from endoplasmic reticular stores, and diacylglycerol activates protein kinase C. Because the increase in intracellular Ca^{2+} leads to rapid increases in cAMP levels that can inhibit PIP_2 hydrolysis and Ca^{2+} mobilization, the regulation of intracellular Ca^{2+} concentrations appears to be crucial for controlling PMN leukocyte responses to chemoattractants.

The immediate result of this receptor/ligand binding on the PMN leukocyte surface and activation of the pathways described earlier is activation of the PMN leukocytes, a process that enables them to aggregate and adhere to other cell membranes, to generate oxygen-derived free radicals, to degranulate and release multiple enzymes, and to generate biologically active products of arachidonic acid by activating cyclooxygenase and lipoxygenase.

Of the leukotrienes, the PMN leukocyte makes only leukotriene B_4 (LTB_4). Peroxidation of arachidonic acid to 5-HPETE, and subsequent conversion of 5-HPETE to LTB_4, is catalyzed by a single protein (154). In addition to being a very potent chemoattractant for other PMN leukocytes, eosinophils, and macrophages, LTB_4 has these other actions (153).

1. promotion of neutrophil aggregation
2. enhancement of neutrophil adherence to endothelium
3. enhancement of proliferation of suppressor T cells and inhibition of proliferation of helper T cells in the presence of macrophages
4. enhancement of NK cytotoxic activity

The inflammatory prostaglandins (e.g., PGE_2) generated by PMN leukocytes have the following capabilities in and around the rheumatoid joint (129).

1. vasodilation, resulting in increased capillary permeability in concert with LTB$_4$
2. fever promotion (additive to IL-1)
3. sensitization of receptors to painful stimuli
4. increases in bone resorption by osteoclasts
5. modulation of immune reactions (e.g., mild inhibition of antigen-induced IL-2 production)

Neutral proteinases also are secreted from the activated PMN leukocyte. There are three principal activities: a gelatinase, an interstitial collagenase, and elastase. These proteases are released within 30 min of binding of various ligands to receptors on the PMN leukocyte membrane (83).

Substances produced by activated T lymphocytes can affect PMN leukocyte function. For instance, recombinant human IFNγ and human TNFβ (previously called lymphotoxin) enhance the phagocytic and antibody-dependent cellular cytotoxicity (ADCC) activities of PMN leukocytes (164). The mechanism of ADCC may be related to the capacity of the PMN leukocyte to produce active oxygen species (201).

It is only when biochemical pathways and cellular mechanisms are well worked out that ways of inhibiting them can be studied. This certainly is true for PMN leukocyte activation. Recent studies by Abramson and colleagues have indicated that the inhibitory effects of non-steroidal antiinflammatory drugs on PMN leukocyte function are not caused principally by inhibition of cyclooxygenase, but rather by inhibiting early steps in activation of the cells after stimuli have coupled with membrane receptors (1). Comprehension of the pathways involved in arachidonic acid metabolism has led even to modulation by diet. It has been determined that the marine fatty acids eicosapentaenoic acid and docosahexaenoic acid competitively inhibit the utilization of arachidonic acid by cyclooxygenase. Normal subjects who supplemented their usual diet with daily doses of these fish oils manifested a 37% decrease in release of arachidonic acid after activation of their PMN leukocytes, a 48% reduction of leukotriene production, and decreased chemotactic responses and adherence capabilities (114). Early reports from studies of fish oil supplementation in diets of rheumatoid patients have been encouraging (110).

SOLUBLE-PHASE INFLAMMATORY PATHWAYS IN SYNOVIAL FLUID

In addition to the activated PMN leukocytes in rheumatoid synovial fluid and the products of synovial lining cells that diffuse into the joint space, there are manifestations of activation of the kinin, clotting, fibrinolytic, and complement pathways in rheumatoid synovial fluid.

RF complexed with IgG can activate kallikrein (123), the versatile proteinase that can produce plasmin from plasminogen and convert latent metalloproteinases to their active forms. Through activation of the clotting system there is accumulation of fibrin within the rheumatoid joint. The coagulation cascade can be activated by tissue injury, as when hemorrhage occurs within or on the surfaces of villous fronds of rheumatoid synovial tissue, or by direct activation of Hageman factor by one of many proteases activated in the rheumatoid joint. Whether fibrinolysis proceeds at a normal or reduced rate in rheumatoid joints has not been settled (193).

In part because all of its component parts are available in plasma or serum, detailed chemical analysis of complement has been possible. This system exemplifies well the principle that following a thorough understanding of activation of a complicated biochemical pathway comes awareness that there are equally complex mechanisms of inhibition set in place for all the activation steps. The details of the complement system and the biologic consequences of complement activation have been covered in Chapters 4 and 5.

In RA, serum complement levels usually are elevated, except in patients with systemic rheumatoid vasculitis. Synovial fluid complement levels are often depressed, reflecting the activation of complement within the joint space (156). Levels of C3 or total hemolytic complement in synovial fluid are rarely useful in assessing disease activity.

In summary, synovial fluid in RA reflects the inflammatory events within the joint. The total leukocyte count is the best quantitative test that correlates with disease activity. The joint space is a "sink" for PMN leukocytes as well as for soluble products of inflammation. In rough proportion to the number of leukocytes are neutral proteinase, collagenase, and elastase (5) activities in the synovial fluid, as well as IgG, proteinases, and proteinase inhibitor complexes (68), the spent products of complement activation, and cytokines such as IL-1 (213) and IL-2 (133). While reflecting inflammation, however, the synovial fluid gives only a hint of the proliferative, destructive synovitis surrounding it.

THE RHEUMATOID SYNOVIUM AND DESTRUCTION OF TENDONS, LIGAMENTS, CARTILAGE, AND BONE

Shortly after the first lymphocytes appear in the edematous tissue below the lining cells of the synovium and around the newly proliferating small blood vessels, a generalized proliferation of synovial cells begins that leads to an enormous increase in cell numbers. The normal synovium, only a few cell layers in thickness, is replaced by thick tissue with a 10-fold to 100-fold increase in cell numbers.

Unlike a malignant proliferation of cells, however, the rheumatoid synovium is markedly heterogeneous. The following are some of the cells that can be identified by light and immunofluorescence microscopy:

1. endothelial cells
2. synovial cells (fibroblast-like, macrophage-like)
3. lymphocytes
4. plasma cells
5. multinucleate cells
6. mast cells
7. PMN leukocytes (rare)

In addition to being increased in number, virtually every cell type shows evidence for activation. As mentioned earlier, most cells manifest HLA-DR class II MHC antigens on their membranes, possibly induced by IFNγ. Cells at the border between the invasive pannus and cartilage also express the transferrin receptor (104) that is found on activated and proliferating cells. Even chondrocytes manifest surface class II MHC antigens (25) and can present antigen to T cells (183). Using immunoperoxidase staining of rheumatoid synovial tissue, it has been shown that a majority of nonlymphoid cells stain with monoclonal antibodies directed against membrane markers of the mononuclear phagocyte (monocyte) lineage (85): In synovium that is minimally inflamed, most cells bear markers for mature macrophage epitopes, whereas in sections of active synovitis, synovial cells bear epitopes that are largely restricted to blood monocytes. It has been inferred from these findings that much of the increase in cell number reflects recruitment of cells from the circulation, not hyperplasia of resident cells.

If rheumatoid synovial tissue is enzymatically dissociated and the suspended cells are washed and placed into monolayer cultures, up to 40% of the cells have a stellate appearance and lack monocyte antigens and Fc receptors (24). Substances such as IL-1 that induce collagenase biosynthesis in synovial cell cultures also lead to a stellate appearance of many cells in culture (12). Immunolocalization studies with a monospecific antibody to human rheumatoid synovial collagenase have shown that these cells contain large amounts of collagenase (compared with other adherent cells) and release enzymes into culture medium. If the cells are cultured on a substratum of collagen, collagenase protein released by the dendritic extensions of the cells binds to the collagen, leaving an exact "footprint" of the dendritic process if the cell is removed from the culture plate (216).

If the assumption is made that many mononuclear phagocytes (macrophages) are recruited to the sites of synovial inflammation in RA, another assumption must be that there is active differentiation of these cells from he-matopoietic progenitor cells. Human-macrophage-specific colony-stimulating factor (CSF-1) has been well defined, and molecular cloning of a complementary DNA that encodes it has been performed (100). Human urine was used as the source of CSF-1. The complementary DNA has been used to induce biosynthesis of biologically active CSF-1 in *Xenopus* oocytes. It will be important to determine whether or not CSF-1 is the initiator of monocyte proliferation in this disease.

Growth and Activation Factors for Synovial Cells

Unlike stem cells in marrow that may respond to a pluripotent proliferation factor similar to murine IL-3 (204) (and subsequent expansion of specific populations by factors such as CSF-1), synovial cells are washed in a milieu containing many types of factors that influence cell growth and maturation, including some that have opposing effects. Some of these are as follows:

Synovial fibroblast-activating factor (SFAF)

This activity (197), produced by lymphocytes and/or macrophages isolated from rheumatoid synovium, is not produced by similar numbers of peripheral blood mononuclear cells. It is found in cultures of mononuclear cells from rheumatoid synovial fluid, but not in cultures of synovial cells from noninflammatory synovitis.

Platelet-derived growth factor (PDGF)

There has been great interest in this substance, described first more than a decade ago (157) and recently purified (50). PDGF has a primary sequence homologous with the products of a major oncogene (53) from cells transformed with simian sarcoma virus (SSV). The SSV-transforming gene product is capable of binding specifically to cell membrane receptors for PDGF (112). Thus, some of the effector mechanisms for cellular proliferation are shared by malignant and nonmalignant proliferative states. PDGF, or a protein highly homologous with it, may be expressed by other cells, such as mononuclear cells. It is a potent stimulus to cell growth and very likely plays a major role in synovial cell proliferation in RA because of the many situations within synovial fronds in which clots form or hemorrhage develops. It should be noted that in addition to being a mitogen for synovial cells, PDGF stimulates collagenase expression by skin fibroblasts (14).

Connective-tissue-activating peptide III (CTAP-III)

This interesting peptide, also isolated from platelets, has a molecular mass of approximately 9.3 kD and similar amino-terminal sequences as β-thromboglobulin (β-TG) and platelet factor 4 (PF-4) (32). Biologic activities in cultured synovial cells demonstrated for CTAP-III include stimulation of DNA synthesis, hyaluronic acid and glycosaminoglycan synthesis, glycolysis, and PGE_2 secretion. Despite the sequence homologies, neither β-TG nor PF-4 has these stimulatory qualities, a fact perhaps related to small differences in NH_2-terminal amino acids.

Fibroblast chemotactic agents

In addition to mitogenic agents, synovial cell populations may be influenced by chemoattractants for mesenchymal cells. These have been described often (6). Chemotactic properties for fibroblasts appear to reside in many types of molecules, including structural and matrix proteins (e.g., fibronectin, collagen, elastin), as well as "factors" produced by lymphocytes and factors (e.g., PDGF, TGFβ) that were characterized first as mitogens.

IL-1.

This substance, present in humans as four biochemically distinct species that all exhibit similar biologic activities (212), is a prototype for autacoids (i.e., small polypeptides released by one cell and having receptors on a neighboring but different cell type) and proinflammatory hormones. In its most fundamental expression, IL-1 induces both laboratory and clinical aspects of an acute-phase response and continues its effects on cells with involvement in chronic immune and proliferative responses (52). In RA, IL-1 is involved in lymphocyte activation in the presence of antigen. It may be capable of stimulating lymphocyte adherence to endothelial cells. If local inflammation is sufficient, IL-1 will diffuse into the circulation and cause systemic effects, including fever and neutrophilia (98). IL-1 affects synovial cells and other mesenchymal cells such as chondrocytes, inducing them to produce prostaglandins and metalloproteinases in large quantity (108). Whereas the latter enzymes are primarily responsible for destruction of joint tissues in RA, the prostaglandins are involved in a complex series of effects—some antiinflammatory and others phlogistic—on many types of cells. IL-1 is found in human synovial tissue (215) and in synovial fluid of patients with RA (126,214), where it may serve a role as a chemoattractant for PMN leukocytes (126). Recent data suggest that PMN leukocytes release and probably synthesize IL-1 (185), a phenomenon that could contribute to the chronic stimulation to proliferation that rheumatoid synovial cells appear to manifest.

The synthesis of IL-1 is under complex control mechanisms. It has been shown, for example, that a soluble product from cloned human T lymphocytes is capable of stimulating a human monocyte line (U937) to produce IL-1 (9). This lymphokine is different from IFNγ, even though IFNγ also stimulates IL-1 biosynthesis by these cells. 1,25-Dihydroxyvitamin D suppresses IL-2 production by T cells, but stimulates IL-1 production by mononuclear phagocytes. In a twisting feedback, IL-1 stimulates prostaglandin (PG) biosynthesis; PGs inhibit collagen synthesis by the same fibroblast cell population that produces PGs. IL-1 and indomethacin together, *in vitro,* cause a striking increase in collagen biosynthesis (9). In the presence of IFNγ, IL-1 decreases collagen biosynthesis by synovial fibroblasts.

Studies in the past 5 years have shown that many "factors" isolated because of their biologic behavior in a certain assay system are in fact closely related to, if not identical with, IL-1. "Catabolin," for example, the substance that is produced by synovium and activates chondrocytes, is IL-1 (161,160). Human osteoclast-activating factor has been shown to have a primary sequence identical with that of one form of human IL-1 (51). Brain-derived acidic fibroblast growth factor—a substance that is an angiogenic substance *in vivo*—has homology with human IL-1 (63). Fibroblast proliferation factor is probably part of the IL-1 family (121). Various factors thought to be distinct from others, for instance, those that are derived from peripheral blood mononuclear cells and stimulate plasminogen activator production (71), may well turn out to be related to IL-1 when they are purified and sequenced. It is known that human monocyte IL-1 increases production of plasminogen activator activity 30-fold to 40-fold by cultured human synovial cells (129).

Inhibition of "Activating" Factors

An inhibitor for any cytokine cannot even be searched for until the active cytokine has been isolated and characterized. Thus, it is not surprising that information about natural, biologic compounds that inhibit the actions of activating factors has only recently been published. Again, inhibition of IL-1 is a useful prototype for other systems in which it is highly probable that physiologic mechanisms exist and can be induced that will specifically counteract the activating effects of cytokines.

One IL-1 inhibitor (IL-1 INH) has been partially purified from human urine (116). It is found in increased amounts during fever, indicating that situations generated by IL-1 simultaneously induce expression of IL-1 INH. This IL-1 INH can be precipitated by antibodies to low-molecular-mass (50 kD) trypsin inhibitors. An interesting report, in light of the potential role for EB virus in RA, is the evidence that B lymphocytes transformed by EB virus produce a polypeptide that inhibits IL-1 (162). Normal human neutrophils also are sources of a specific IL-1 inhibitor (184). The PMN leukocyte IL-1 INH is found in lysates of fresh cells, as well as in culture media from stimulated and unstimulated cells.

All of the IL-1 inhibitors mentioned earlier are detected by gel-filtration chromatography as multiple forms of differing molecular weights, a probable function of subunit aggregation. Whether or not these factors are related will be determined initially by their derived sequences from cDNA clones. These IL-1 INH are specific for inhibiting IL-1-induced thymocyte proliferation; they do not inhibit the effect on thymocytes of IL-2. Therefore, we can only speculate whether or not such IL-1 INHs will be capable of modulating immune responses once clonal expansion and activation of T cells have occurred.

DESTRUCTION OF JOINTS

Histopathologic examination at the interfaces among cartilage, tendon or bone, and synovial tissue in RA reveals several important general principles and allows certain inferences to be made from them:

1. There is marked cellular heterogeneity both in single areas and in different areas of synovium from a given patient compared with each other. For instance, there is little doubt that small foci of PMN leukocytes are seen at the pannus/cartilage junction (130), but these foci are rare, and there is little evidence that PMN leukocytes have a major involvement in destruction of cartilage by pannus (Fig. 5).

2. Although the cellular element of pannus is in direct contact with cartilage matrix, there is variability in the tightness of this bond. In some cases the leading edge of a synovial lining cell may extend into cartilage and actively phagocytose fibrillar collagen (77). In other cases a distinct

area bordered by cartilage, with virtually no matrix, may surround invasive cell processes; the inference from the latter, more commonly found abnormality is that extracellular proteinases are being released from the activated synovial cells.

3. Regardless of the nature of the cell/cartilage interface, proteoglycans become depleted from cartilage early in the inflammatory process, before there has been significant loss of cartilage. Specific stains for proteoglycans show the same changes *in vitro* when cartilage slices are incubated with rheumatoid synovial cells (70). Further, it has been demonstrated that cartilage depleted of proteoglycans has lost its capacity to rebound from a deforming load, a quality that predisposes it to permanent damage from weight bearing (78). It can be inferred that IL-1 and other "activating" polypeptides produced by the inflammatory synovitis diffuse into cartilage and induce proteinase synthesis by chondrocytes that leads to breakdown of proteoglycans.

Combining histopathologic and biochemical data, the following sequence can be structured that leads from the inflammatory process through to joint destruction:

1. Mononuclear phagocytes are drawn into the rheumatoid synovial tissue and release IL-1 in response to the early inflammatory response to activation of the immune system (109,141) (Fig. 6).

2. IL-1 and other growth/activation factors, including TNF/cachectin (44), stimulate proliferation of the synovial cells and induce biosynthesis of prostaglandins and proteinases by the synovial cells (128). Adherent synovial cells respond by mitogenesis to factors that do not stim-

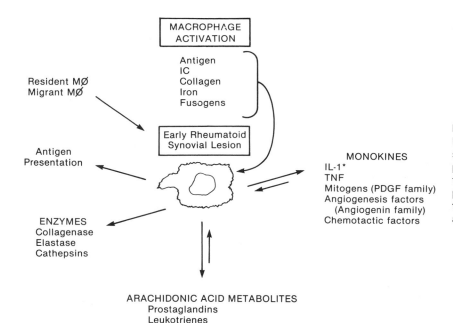

FIG. 5. The multipotential macrophage in RA. Many macrophages are not resident, but respond to synovial inflammation and become a part of the heterogeneous cellular infiltrate of the synovium. In the activated state they can present antigen and produce and release proteolytic enzymes, prostaglandins, leukotrienes, and monokines.

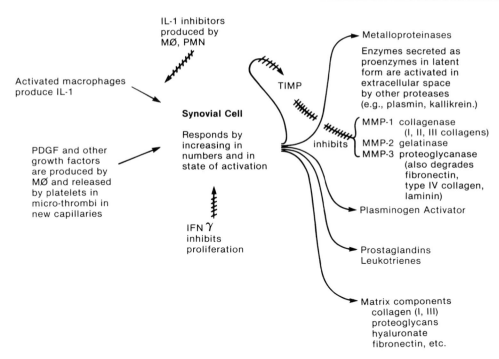

FIG. 6. Synovial cell activation and phenotypic expression in RA. Driven by proliferative factors, the synovial cells are induced to produce metalloproteinases, plasminogen activator, and arachidonic acid metabolites, as well as matrix components. TIMP is the principal inhibitor of these enzymes in tissues.

ulate production of prostaglandins and/or proteinases, i.e., products from lymphocyte-enriched cultures (11) and recombinant immune interferon (19). Other substances, such as substance P, are not mitogenic, but do induce prostaglandin and/or proteinase production by adherent rheumatoid synoviocytes (119).

3. In culture, synovial cells exposed to IL-1, perhaps in combination with prostaglandins and/or other substances that affect metabolism of cyclic nucleotides within cells (114), synthesize large amounts of prostaglandins and collagenase (Fig. 6). By immunohistochemistry it can be shown that the collagenase is concentrated around the thin tendrils of cellular extensions of stellate cells, whereas there is little evidence for enzyme production by cells with more characteristic fibroblast or macrophage appearances (217).

4. The advancing front of synovial cells releases at least three neutral matrix metalloproteinases (MMP) that, in active form, can degrade virtually all proteins within the extracellular matrix. They include: (a) MMP-1 (collagenase), (b) MMP-2 (gelatinase), and (c) MMP-3 (a proteinase with capability of degrading proteoglycans, fibronectin, laminin, and type IV collagen) (135). All three enzymes are active at neutral pH, depend for activity on the presence of calcium ions in their local environment, and are released from cells as proenzymes. The mechanism of activation of these proenzymes to their active

forms *in vivo* is not known, but may involve proteinases found in the inflammatory lesion itself, such as plasmin generated by plasminogen activator produced by rheumatoid synovial cells (205).

An interstitial collagenase purified from human skin (most assuredly identical with MMP-1) has been cloned, and the complete primary sequence of the proenzyme has been determined (64). MMP-2, the gelatinase of rheumatoid synovium, has not been characterized completely. MMP-3, a multisubstrate protease with no collagenase activity, has been purified and characterized (135). This proteinase is synthesized as a 55-kd proenzyme. It is activated to two active forms of 45 kd and 28 kd by proteinases, and both active forms degrade proteoglycans, type IV collagen, fibronectin, and laminin.

5. PMN leukocytes in the synovial fluid may bind to the surface of articular cartilage, discharge proteases in an act of "frustrated phagocytosis," and contribute in this fashion to joint destruction (107). The major PMN leukocyte granule enzyme is elastase, a multisubstrate neutral serine protease that can degrade proteoglycans and type IV collagen as well as elastin (see Chapter 32). The PMN enzymes can degrade the surface of cartilage, but probably have only a minor role at the pannus/cartilage junction.

6. Just as inhibitors are produced that have potential for regulating the activity of IL-1 and other cytokines, there are abundant natural inhibitors of MMP. The most

prevalent of these in many diverse tissues is a protein (or family of proteins) with M_r values about 30 kd that is found in all connective tissue and is called tissue inhibitor of metalloproteinases (TIMP) (173). In many instances, the same population of cells that produce the proenzymes also produce TIMP. For example, stimulated capillary endothelial cells produce procollagenase, proteoglycanase (stromelysin), and TIMP (82,203). If the proteinases are activated *in vitro,* the TIMP immediately complexes and inactivates them. This coordinate release of proenzymes and specific inhibitors may be a recurrent theme in mesenchymal inflammation. Fibroblasts also release a serine protease inhibitor named protease nexin (163). This protease is capable of inactivating trypsin, thrombin, and plasmin, but does not inhibit chymotrypsin-like proteases such as elastase.

7. Mast cells have been appreciated recently to make up a significant portion of cells at some areas of the invasive pannus/cartilage junction in RA (21,40). The role of these pluripotent cells in destruction of joint structures is not determined. However, it has been reported that mast cells added to cultures of adherent rheumatoid synovial cells *in vitro* generate a 50- to 400-fold increase in prostaglandin synthesis and a 10- to 50-fold stimulation of collagenase production (220). Mast cell heparin could potentiate capillary invasion of previously avascular tissue and/or, as a "second messenger," amplify the effects of hormones such as parathyroid hormone on bone cells (41). Occasionally, mast cells can be found in rheumatoid synovial fluid (120).

8. In studies of bone/cartilage junctions in RA, multinucleated cells staining positively for esterase activity are often found (23). Their role in destruction of subchondral bone may be important, particularly when one considers that multinucleated cells probably are very much activated to produce proteases and prostaglandins, as compared with populations of mononucleated cells (20).

9. Bone resorption in RA may be mediated by osteoclast action, stimulated to form and resorb bone by IL-1. In addition, it has been shown that both forms of human TNF (TNFα and TNFβ) cause osteoclastic bone resorption and inhibit bone collagen biosynthesis (15).

In review, there are many different species of cells at the synovial cartilage/bone junction (22). The "pannus" is of synovial origin, and it aggressively invades the cartilage and tendons, much as does a locally invasive tumor. The proliferative rheumatoid tissue does not simply replace dead cartilage; the cartilage cells, if anything, are in a stimulated, activated state and contribute their own proteinases to the degradative processes. The tumor-like quality of the synovial tissue was first emphasized by Harris et al. (73–76) in the 1970s and has been reiterated by

Fassbender (58,59) in the 1980s. The destructive power of the lesion is related to multiple cell-cell interactions, with one group of cells inducing potent proteinase production by others. Inexorably, unless an intervention by drugs or spontaneous remission occurs, there is destruction of the joint.

REFERENCES

1. Abramson, S., Korchak, H., Ludewig, R., and Weissmann, G. (1985): The modes of action of aspirin-like drugs. *Proc. Natl. Acad. Sci. USA,* 82:7227–7231.
2. Acuto, O., Fabbi, M., Bensussan, A., Milanese, C., Campen, T. J., Royer, H. D., and Reinherz, E. L. (1985): The human T-cell receptor. *J. Clin. Immunol.,* 5:141–157.
3. Acuto, O., and Reinherz, E. L. (1985): The human T-cell receptor: Structure and function. *N. Engl. J. Med.,* 312:1100–1111.
4. Ahmed, S. A., Penhale, W. J., and Talal, N. (1985): Sex hormones, immune responses, and autoimmune diseases: Mechanisms of sex hormone action. *Am. J. Pathol.,* 121:531–551.
5. Al-Haik, N., Lewis, D. A., and Struthers, G. (1984): Neutral protease, collagenase and elastase activities in synovial fluids from arthritic patients. *Agents Actions,* 15:436–442.
6. Albini, A., Adelmann-Grill, A. C., and Miller, P. K. (1985): Fibroblast chemotaxis. *Collagen Rel. Res.,* 5:283–296.
7. Alspaugh, M. A., and Tan, E. M. (1976): Serum antibody in rheumatoid arthritis reactive with a cell-associated antigen: Demonstration by precipitation and immunofluorescence. *Arthritis Rheum.,* 19:711.
8. Ambrus, J. L., Jr., Jurgensen, C. H., Brown, E. J., and Fauci, A. S. (1985): Purification to homogeneity of a high molecular weight human B cell growth factor; demonstration of specific binding to activated B cells; and development of a monoclonal antibody to the factor. *J. Exp. Med.,* 162:1319–1335.
9. Amento, E. P., Kurnick, J. T., and Krane, S. M. (1985): Interleukin 1 production by the human monocyte cell line U937 requires a lymphokine induction signal distinct from interleukin 2 or interferons. *J. Immunol.,* 134:350–357.
10. Andriopoulos, N. H., Mestecky, J., Miller, E. J., and Bennett, J. C. (1976): Antibodies to human native and denatured collagens in synovial fluids of patients with RA. *Clin. Immunol. Immunopathol.,* 6:209–212.
11. Baker, D. G., Baumgarten, D. F., and Chen, T.-S. (1986): Mediator and target cell variability in proliferation response of human adherent synovial cells in culture. *J. Rheumatol.,* 13:505–511.
12. Baker, D. G., Dayer, J.-M., Roelke, M., Schumacher, H. R., and Krane, S. M. (1983): Rheumatoid synovial cell morphologic changes induced by a mononuclear cell factor in culture. *Arthritis Rheum.,* 26:8–14.
13. Baker, D. G., Dayer, J.-M., Roelke, M., Schumacher, H. R., and Krane, S. M. (1983): Rheumatoid synovial morphologic changes induced by a mononuclear cell factor in culture. *Arthritis Rheum.,* 26:8–14.
14. Bauer, E. A., Cooper, T. W., Huang, J. S., Altman, J., and Deuel, T. F. (1985): Stimulation of in vitro human skin collagenase expression by platelet-derived growth factor. *Proc. Natl. Acad. Sci. USA,* 82:4132–4136.
15. Bertolini, D. R., Nedwin, G. E., Bringman, T. S., Smith, D. D., and Mundy, G. R. (1986): Stimulation of bone resorption and inhibition of bone formation *in vitro* by human tumour necrosis factors. *Nature,* 319:516–519.
16. Bettens, F., Kristensen, F., Walker, C., Schwalera, U., Bonnard, G. D., and de Weck, A. L. (1984): Lymphokine regulation of activated (G_1) lymphocytes. II. Glucocorticoid and anti-Tac-induced inhibition of human T lymphocytes. *J. Immunol.,* 132:261.
17. Bevilacqua, M. P., Pober, J. S., Wheeler, M. E., Cotran, R. S., and Gimbrone, M. A., Jr. (1985): Interleukin 1 acts on cultured human vascular endothelium to increase the adhesion of polymorpho-

nuclear leukocytes, monocytes, and related leukocyte cell lines. *J. Clin. Invest.*, 76:2003–2011.

18. Birkeland, S. A., and Kristofferson, K. (1977): Cellular immunity in pregnancy. *Clin. Exp. Immunol.*, 30:408–412.

19. Brinckerhoff, C. E., and Guyre, P. M. (1985): Increased proliferation of human synovial fibroblasts treated with recombinant immune interferon. *J. Immunol.*, 134:3142–3146.

20. Brinckerhoff, C. E., and Harris, E. D., Jr. (1978): Collagenase production by cultures containing multinucleated cells derived from synovial fibroblasts. *Arthritis Rheum.*, 21:745–754.

21. Bromley, M., Fisher, W. D., and Wooley, D. E. (1984): Mast cells at sites of cartilage erosion in the rheumatoid joint. *Ann. Rheum. Dis.*, 43:76–79.

22. Bromley, M., and Wooley, D. E. (1984): Histopathology of the rheumatoid lesion. *Arthritis Rheum.*, 27:857–863.

23. Bromley, M., and Wooley, D. E. (1984): Chondroclasts and osteoclasts at subchondral sites of erosion in the rheumatoid joint. *Arthritis Rheum.*, 27:968–975.

24. Burmester, G. R., Dimitriu-Bona, A., Waters, S. J., and Winchester, R. J. (1983): Identification of three major synovial lining cell populations by monoclonal antibodies directed to Ia antigens and antigens associated with monocyte/macrophages and fibroblasts. *Scand. J. Immunol.*, 17:69.

25. Burmester, G. R., Menche, O., Merryman, P., Klein, M., and Winchester, R. (1983): Application of monoclonal antibodies to the characterization of cells eluted from human articular cartilage. *Arthritis Rheum.*, 26:1187–1195.

26. Buyon, J. P., Korchak, H. M., Rutherford, L. E., et al. (1984): Female hormones reduce neutrophil responsiveness *in vitro*. *Arthritis Rheum.*, 27:623–630.

27. Cambier, J. C., Monroe, J. G., Coggeshall, K. M., and Ransom, J. T. (1985): The biochemical basis of transmembrane signalling by B lymphocyte surface immunoglobulin. *Immunol. Today*, 6: 218–222.

28. Cardella, C. J., Davies, P., and Allison, A. C. (1974): Immune complexes induce selective release of lysosomal hydrolases from macrophages. *Nature*, 274:46.

29. Carson, D. (1985): Rheumatoid factor. In: *Textbook of Rheumatology, ed. 2*, edited by W. N. Kelley, E. D. Harris, Jr., S. Ruddy, and C. B. Sledge, pp. 664–679. W. B. Saunders, Philadelphia.

30. Carter, S. D., Bacon, P. A., and Hall, N. D. (1981): Characterization of activated lymphocytes in the peripheral blood of patients with rheumatoid arthritis. *Ann. Rheum. Dis.*, 40:293–298.

31. Carter, S. D., Bourne, J. T., Elson, C. J., Hutton, C. W., Czudek, R., and Dieppe, P. A. (1984): Mononuclear phagocytes in rheumatoid arthritis: Fc-receptor expression by peripheral blood monocytes. *Ann. Rheum. Dis.*, 43:424–429.

32. Castor, C. W., Miller, J. W., and Walz, D. A. (1983): Structural and biological characteristics of connective tissue activating peptide (CTAP-III), a major human platelet-derived growth factor. *Proc. Natl. Acad. Sci. USA*, 80:765–769.

33. Cats, A., and Hazevoet, H. M. (1970): Significance of positive tests for rheumatoid factor in the prognosis of rheumatoid arthritis. *Ann. Rheum. Dis.*, 29:254.

34. Cathcart, E. S., Hayes, K. C., Gonnerman, W. A., Lazzari, A. A., and Franzblau, C. (1986): Experimental arthritis in a non-human primate. I. Induction by bovine type II collagen. *Lab. Invest.*, 54: 26–31.

35. Chantler, J. K., Tingle, A. J., and Petty, R. E. (1985): Persistent rubella virus infection associated with chronic arthritis in children. *N. Engl. J. Med.*, 313:1117–1123.

36. Chen, P. P., Goni, F., Fong, S., Jirik, F., Vaughan, J. H., Frangione, B., and Carson, D. A. (1985): The majority of human monoclonal IgM rheumatoid factors express a "primary structure-dependent" cross-reactive idiotype. *J. Immunol.*, 134:3281–3285.

37. Chen, P. P., Goni, F., Houghten, R. A., Fong, S., Goldfien, R., Vaughan, J. H., Frangione, B., and Carson, D. A. (1985): Characterization of human rheumatoid factors with seven antiidiotypes induced by synthetic hypervariable region peptides. *J. Exp. Med.*, 162:487–500.

38. Combe, B., Pope, R. M., Fischback, M., Darnell, B., Baron, S., and Talal, N. (1985): Interleukin 2 in rheumatoid arthritis: Production of and response to interleukin 2 in rheumatoid synovial fluid, synovial tissue, and peripheral blood. *Clin. Exp. Immunol.*, 59:520–528.

39. Cooke, T. D., Hurd, E. R., and Jasin, H. E. (1975): Identification of immunoglobulins and complement in rheumatoid articular collagenous tissues. *Arthritis Rheum.*, 18:563–576.

40. Crisp, A. J., Chapman, C. M., Kirkham, S. E., Schiller, A. L., and Krane, S. M. (1984): Articular mastocytosis in rheumatoid arthritis. *Arthritis Rheum.*, 27:845–851.

41. Crisp, A. J., Roelke, M. S., Goldring, S. R., and Krane, S. M. (1984): Heparin modulates intracellular cyclic AMP in human trabecular bone cells and adherent rheumatoid synovial cells. *Ann. Rheum. Dis.*, 43:628–634.

42. Crum, R., Szabo, S., and Folkman, J. (1985): A new class of steroids inhibits angiogenesis in the presence of heparin or a heparin fragment. *Science*, 230:1375–1378.

43. Dallman, M., and Fathman, C. G. (1985): Type II collagen-reactive T cell clones from mice with collagen-induced arthritis. *J. Immunol.*, 135:1113–1118.

44. Dayer, J.-M., Beutler, B., and Cerami, A. (1985): Cachectin/tumor necrosis factor stimulates collagenase and PGE_2 production by human synovial cells and dermal fibroblasts. *J. Exp. Med.*, 162:2163–2168.

45. Dayer, J.-M., Parswell, J. H., Schnaeberger, E. E., and Krane, S. M. (1980): Interactions among rheumatoid synovial cells and monocyte-macrophages: Production of collagenase-stimulating factor by human monocytes exposed to concanavalin A or immunoglobulin Fc fragments. *J. Immunol.*, 124:1712–1720.

46. Decker, J. L. (1984): Rheumatoid arthritis: Evolving concepts of pathogenesis and treatment. *Ann. Intern. Med.*, 101:810–824.

47. del Junco, D. J., Annegers, J. F., Luthra, H. S., Coulam, C. B., and Kurland, L. T. (1985): Do oral contraceptives prevent rheumatoid arthritis? *J.A.M.A.*, 254:1938–1941.

48. Depper, J. M., Bluestein, H. G., and Zvaifler, N. J. (1981): Impaired regulation of Epstein-Barr virus-induced lymphocyte proliferation in rheumatoid arthritis is due to a T cell deficit. *J. Immunol.*, 127: 1899.

49. Dessypris, E. N., Baer, M. R., Sergent, J. S., and Krantz, S. B. (1984): Rheumatoid arthritis and pure red cell aplasia. *Ann. Intern. Med.*, 100:202–206.

50. Deuel, T. F., and Hvang, J. S. (1984): Platelet-derived growth factor. Structure, function, and roles in normal and transformed cells. *J. Clin. Invest.*, 74:669–676.

51. Dewhirst, F. E., Stashenko, P. P., Mole, J. E., and Tsurumachi, T. (1985): Purification and partial sequence of human osteoclast-activating factor: Identity with interleukin 1. *J. Immunol.*, 135:2562–2568.

52. Dinarello, C. A. (1985): An update on human interleukin-1: From molecular biology to clinical relevance. *J. Clin. Immunol.*, 5:287–297.

53. Doolittle, R. F., Hunkapiller, M. W., Hood, L. E., et al. (1983): Simian sarcoma virus onc gene, v-sis, is derived from the gene (or genes) encoding a platelet-derived growth factor. *Science*, 221:275–277.

54. Duncan, M. R., and Berman, B. (1985): γ-interferon is the lymphokine and β-interferon the monokine responsible for inhibition of fibroblast collagen production and late but not early fibroblast proliferation. *J. Exper. Med.*, 162:516–527.

55. Falchuk, K. H., Goetzl, E. J., and Kulka, J. P. (1970): Respiratory gases of synovial fluids. An approach to synovial tissue circulatory-metabolic imbalance in rheumatoid arthritis. *Am. J. Med.*, 49:223.

56. Falkoff, R. J. M., Muraguchi, A., Hong, J.-X., Butler, J. L., Dinarello, C. A., and Fauci, A. S. (1983): The effects of interleukin 1 on human B cell activation and proliferation. *J. Immunol.*, 131: 801–805.

57. Faltynek, C. R., McCandless, S., and Baglioni, C. (1984): Treatment of lymphoblastoid cells with interferon decreases insulin binding. *J. Cell. Physiol.*, 121:437–441.

58. Fassbender, H.-G. (1983): Structural basis of articular cartilage destruction in rheumatoid arthritis. *Collagen Rel. Res.*, 3:141–155.

59. Fassbender, H.-G. (1984): Is pannus a residue of inflammation? *Arthritis Rheum.*, 27:956–957 (letter).

60. Fingeroth, J. D., Weis, J. J., Tedder, T. F., Strominger, J. L., Biro, P. A., and Fearon, D. T. (1984): Epstein-Barr virus receptor of human B lymphocytes is the C3d receptor CR2. *Proc. Natl. Acad. Sci. USA*, 81:4510–4514.

61. Fong, S., Chen, P. P., Gilbertson, T. A., Weber, J. R., Fox, R. I., and Carson, D. A. (1986): Expression of three cross-reactive idiotypes on rheumatoid factor autoantibodies from patients with autoimmune diseases and seropositive adults. *J. Immunol.*, 137:122–128.

62. Fong, S., Gilbertson, T. A., Hueniken, R. J., Singhal, S. K., Vaughan, J. H., and Carson, D. A. (1985): IgM rheumatoid factor autoantibody and immunoglobulin-producing precursor cells in the bone marrow of humans. *Cell. Immunol.*, 95:157–172.

63. Gimenez-Gallego, G., Rodkey, J., Bennett, C., Rios-Candelore, M., DiSalvo, J., and Thomas, K. (1985): Brain-derived acidic fibroblast growth factor: Complete amino acid sequence and homologies. *Science*, 230:1385–1388.

64. Goldberg, G. I., Wilhelm, S. M., Kronberger, A., Bauer, E. A., Grant, G. A., and Eisen, A. Z. (1986): Human fibroblast collagenase. *J. Biol. Chem.*, 261:6600–6605.

65. Goto, M., and Zvaifler, N. J. (1985): Impaired killer cell generation in the autologous mixed leukocyte reaction by rheumatoid arthritis lymphocytes. *Arthritis Rheum.*, 28:731–741.

66. Grahame, R., Armstrong, R., Simmons, N., Wilton, J. M. A., Laurent, R., Millis, R., and Mims, C. A. (1983): Chronic arthritis associated with the presence of intrasynovial rubella virus. *Ann. Rheum. Dis.*, 42:2–13.

67. Groenewegen, G., Buurman, W. A., and van der Linden, C. J. (1985): Lymphokine dependence of *in vivo* expression of MHC class II antigens by endothelium. *Nature*, 316:361–366.

68. Gysen, P., Malaise, M., Gaspar, S., and Franchimont, P. (1985): Measurement of proteoglycans, elastase, collagenase and protein in synovial fluid in inflammatory and degenerative arthropathies. *Clin. Rheum.*, 4:39–50.

69. Haber, P. L., Kubagawa, H., and Koopman, W. J. (1985): Immunoglobulin subclass distribution of synovial plasma cells in rheumatoid arthritis determined by use of monoclonal anti-subclass antibodies. *Clin. Immunol. Immunopathol.*, 35:346–351.

70. Hamerman, D., Janis, R., and Smith, C. (1967): Cartilage matrix depletion by rheumatoid synovial cells in tissue culture. *J. Exp. Med.*, 126:1005.

71. Hamilton, J. A., Fabriskie, J. B., Lachman, L. B., et al. (1982): Streptococcal cell walls and synovial activation. *J. Exp. Med.*, 155:1702–1718.

72. Hardy, K. J., Peterlin, B. M., Atchison, R. E., and Stobo, J. D. (1985): Regulation of expression of the human interferon gene. *Proc. Natl. Acad. Sci. USA*, 82:8173–8177.

73. Harris, E. D., Jr. (1976): Recent insights into the pathogenesis of the proliferative lesion in rheumatoid arthritis. *Arthritis Rheum.*, 19:68–72.

74. Harris, E. D., Jr., DiBona, D. R., and Krane, S. M. (1970): A mechanism for cartilage destruction in rheumatoid arthritis. *Trans. Assoc. Am. Physicians*, 83:267–274.

75. Harris, E. D., Jr., DiBona, D. R., and Krane, S. M. (1971): Mechanisms of destruction of articular structures in rheumatoid arthritis. In: *Proceedings of the 3rd International Symposium on Inflammation* (International Congress Series no. 229), edited by B. Forscher, pp. 243–253. Excerpta Medica, Amsterdam.

76. Harris, E. D., Jr., Faulkner, C. S., II, and Brown, F. E. (1975): Collagenolytic systems in rheumatoid arthritis. *Clin. Orthop.*, 110:303–316.

77. Harris, E. D., Jr., Glauert, A. M., and Murley, A. H. G. (1977): Intracellular collagen fibrils at the pannus/cartilage junction in rheumatoid arthritis. *Arthritis Rheum.*, 20:657–665.

78. Harris, E. D., Jr., Parker, H. D., Radin, E. L., and Krane, S. M. (1972): Effects of proteolytic enzymes on structural and mechanical properties of cartilage. *Arthritis Rheum.*, 15:497–503.

79. Hayslett, J. P., and Lynn, R. (1980): Effect of pregnancy in patients with lupus nephropathy. *Kidney Int.*, 18:207–220.

80. Helfgott, S. M., Dynesius-Trentham, R., Brahn, E., and Trentham, D. E. (1985): An arthritogenic lymphokine in the rat. *J. Exp. Med.*, 162:1531–1545.

81. Hench, P. A. (1949): The potential reversibility of rheumatoid arthritis. *Mayo Clin. Proc.*, 24:167–178.

82. Herron, G. S., Banda, M. J., Clark, E. J., Gavrilovic, J., and Werb, Z. (1986): Secretion of metalloproteinases by stimulated capillary endothelial cells. *J. Biol. Chem.*, 261:2814–2818.

83. Hibbs, M. S., Hasty, K. A., Kang, A. H., and Mainardi, C. A. (1984): Secretion of collagenolytic enzymes by human polymorphonuclear leukocytes. *Collagen Rel. Res.*, 4:467–477.

84. Hoffman, W. L., Goldberg, M. S., and Smiley, J. D. (1982): Immunoglobulin G3 subclass production by rheumatoid synovial tissue cultures. *J. Clin. Invest.*, 69:136–144.

85. Hogg, N., Palmer, D. G., and Revell, P. A. (1985): Mononuclear phagocytes of normal and rheumatoid synovial membrane identified by monoclonal antibodies. *Immunology*, 56:673–681.

86. Hollingsworth, J. W., Siege, E. R., and Creasey, W. A. (1967): Granulocyte survival in synovial exudate of patients with rheumatoid arthritis and other inflammatory joint diseases. *Yale J. Biol. Med.*, 39:289–296.

87. Holmdahl, R., Jansson, L., Larsson, E., Rubin, K., and Klareskog, L. (1986): Homologous collagen type II induces chronic and progressive arthritis in mice. *Arthritis Rheum.*, 29:106–113.

88. Holmdahl, R., Klareskog, L., Rubin, K., Larsson, E., and Wigzell, H. (1985): T lymphocytes in collagen II-induced arthritis in mice. *Scand. J. Immunol.*, 22:295–306.

89. Holmdahl, R., Nordling, C., Rubin, K., Tarkowski, A., and Klareskog, L. (1986): Generation of monoclonal rheumatoid factors after immunization with collagen II–anti-collagen II immune complexes: An anti-idiotype antibody to anti-collagen II is also a rheumatoid factor. *Scand. J. Immunol.*, (in press).

90. Howard, M., and Paul, W. E. (1983): Regulation of B-cell growth and differentiation by soluble factors. *Annu. Rev. Immunol.*, 307–333.

91. Iguchi, T., and Ziff, M. (1986): Electron microscopic study of rheumatoid synovial vasculature: Intimate relationship between tall endothelium and lymphoid aggregates. *J. Clin. Invest.*, 77:355–361.

92. Inman, R. D., Hamilton, N. C., Redecha, P. B., and Hochhauser, D. M. (1986): Electrophoretic transfer blotting analysis of immune complexes in rheumatoid arthritis. *Clin. Exp. Immunol.*, 63:32–40.

93. Itoh, K., Shiiba, K., Shimizu, Y., Suzuki, R., and Kumagai, K. (1985): Generation of activated killer (AK) cells by recombinant interleukin 2 (rIL-2) in collaboration with interferon γ (IFNγ). *J. Immunol.*, 134:3124–3129.

94. Janossy, G., Panayi, G., Duke, O., Poulter, L. W., Bafill, M., and Goldstein, G. (1981): Rheumatoid arthritis: A disease of T-lymphocyte/macrophage immunoregulation. *Lancet*, 2:839–842.

95. Jasin, H. E. (1975): Mechanism of trapping of immune complexes in joint collagenous tissues. *Clin. Exp. Immunol.*, 22:473.

96. Jasin, H. E. (1985): Autoantibody specificities of immune complexes sequestered in articular cartilage of patients with rheumatoid arthritis and osteoarthritis. *Arthritis Rheum.*, 28:241–248.

97. Jayson, M. I. V., and Dixon, A. S. J. (1970): Intra-articular pressure in rheumatoid arthritis of the knee. II. Effect of intra-articular pressure on blood circulation to the synovium. *Ann. Rheum. Dis.*, 29:266–268.

98. Kampschmidt, R. F. (1984): Infection, inflammation and interleukin 1. *Lymphokine Res.*, 2:97–110.

99. Kaplan, R. A., DeHeer, D. H., Carson, D. A., Pangburn, M. K., Muller-Eberhard, H. J., and Vaughan, J. H. (1980): Metabolism of C4 and factor B in rheumatoid arthritis: Relation to rheumatoid factor. *Arthritis Rheum.*, 23:911–920.

100. Kawasaki, E. S., Ladner, M., Wang, A. M., Van Arsdell, J., Warren, M. K., Coyne, M. Y., Schweickart, V. L., Lee, M.-T., Wilson, K. J., Boosman, A., Stanley, E. R., Ralph, P., and Mark, D. F. (1985): Molecular cloning of a complementary DNA encoding human macrophage-specific colony-stimulating factor (CSF-1). *Science*, 230:291–296.

101. Klareskog, L., Forsum, U., Scheynius, A., Kabelitz, D., and Wigzell, H. (1982): Evidence in support of a self-perpetuating HLA-DR-dependent delayed-type cell reaction in rheumatoid arthritis. *Proc. Natl. Acad. Sci. USA*, 79:3632–3636.

102. Klareskog, L., Forsum, U., Tjernlund, U. M., Kabelitz, D., and

Wigren, A. (1981): Appearance of anti-HLA-DR-reactive cells in normal and rheumatoid synovial tissue. *Scand. J. Immunol.,* 14: 183–192.

103. Klareskog, L., Holmdahl, R., Larsson, E., and Wigzell, H. (1983): Role of T lymphocytes in collagen II induced arthritis in rats. *Clin. Exp. Immunol.,* 51:117–125.

104. Klareskog, L., Johnell, O., and Hulth, A. (1984): Expression of HLA-DR and HLA-DQ antigens on cells within the cartilage-pannus junction in rheumatoid arthritis. *Rheumatol. Int.,* 4:11–15.

105. Klareskog, L., Johnell, O., Hulth, A., Holmdahl, R., and Rubin, K. (1986): Reactivity of monoclonal anti-type II collagen antibodies with cartilage and synovial tissue in rheumatoid arthritis and osteoarthritis. *Arthritis Rheum.,* 29:1–9.

106. Koch, A. E., Polverini, P. J., and Leibovich, S. J. (1986): Stimulation of neovascularization by human rheumatoid synovial tissue macrophages. *Arthritis Rheum.,* 29:471–478.

107. Korchak, H. M., Vienne, K., Rutherford, L. E., and Weissmann, G. (1984): Neutrophil stimulation, receptor, membrane, and metabolic events. *Fed. Proc.,* 43:2749–2754.

108. Krane, S. M., Goldring, S. R., and Dayer, J.-M. (1982): Interactions among lymphocytes, monocytes and other synovial cells in the rheumatoid synovium. In: *Lymphokines,* edited by E. Pick and M. Landy, pp. 75–95. Academic Press, New York.

109. Krane, S. M., Goldring, S. R., and Dayer, J.-M. (1982): Interactions among lymphocytes, monocytes and other synovial cells in the rheumatoid synovium. *Lymphokines,* 7:75–136.

110. Kremer, J. M., Rynes, R. I., Bartholomew, L. E., Michalek, A., and Jubiz, W. (1986): A double-blinded placebo controlled crossover study of eicosapentaenoic acid (EPA) supplementation in active rheumatoid arthritis (RA). *Arthritis Rheum.,* 29:511.

111. Lau, C., Budz-Tymkewycz, S., Ramsden, M., Lee, P., and Keystone, E. C. (1985): Impaired release of a T-cell specific suppressor factor in rheumatoid arthritis. *Clin. Exp. Immunol.,* 61:489–495.

112. Leal, F., Williams, L. T., Robbins, K. C., and Aaronson, S. A. (1985): Evidence that the v-sis gene product transforms by interaction with the receptor for platelet-derived growth factor. *Science,* 230:327–328.

113. Lee, S. H., Gregersen, P. K., Shen, H. H., Silver, J., and Winchester, R. J. (1984): Strong association of rheumatoid arthritis with the presence of a polymorphic Ia epitope defined by a monoclonal antibody: Comparison with the allodeterminant DR$_4$. *Rheumatol. Int.,* 4:17–23.

114. Lee, T. H., Hoover, R. L., Williams, J. D., Sperling, R. I., Ravalese, J., III, Spur, B. W., Robinson, D. R., Corey, E. J., Lewis, R. A., and Austen, K. F. (1985): Effect of dietary enrichment with eicosapentaenoic and docosahexaenoic acids on in vitro neutrophil and monocyte leukotriene generation and neutrophil function. *N. Engl. J. Med.,* 312:1217–1224.

115. Leonard, W. J., Donlon, T. A., Lebo, R. V., and Greene, W. C. (1985): Localization of the gene encoding the human interleukin-2 receptor on chromosome 10. *Science,* 228:1547–1549.

116. Liao, Z., Haimovitz, A., Chen, Y., Chan, J., and Rosenstreich, D. L. (1985): Characterization of a human interleukin 1 inhibitor. *J. Immunol.,* 134:3882–3886.

117. Linos, A., O'Fallon, W. M., Worthington, J. W., and Kurland, L. T. (1983): Case-control study of rheumatoid arthritis and prior use of oral contraceptives. *Lancet,* 2:1299–1300.

118. Linos, A., Worthington, J. W., O'Fallon, W. M., and Kurland, L. T. (1980): The epidemiology of rheumatoid arthritis in Rochester, Minnesota: A study of incidence, prevalence, and mortality. *Am. J. Epidemiol.,* 111:87–98.

119. Lotz, M., and Vaughan, J. H. (1986): Effects of the neuropeptide substance P on rheumatoid synoviocytes. *Arthritis Rheum.,* 29: S41.

120. Malone, D. G., Inani, A.-M., Schwartz, L. B., Barrett, K. E., and Metcalfe, D. D. (1986): Mast cell numbers and histamine levels in synovial fluids from patients with diverse arthritides. *Arthritis Rheum.,* 29:956–963.

121. Matsushima, K., Durum, S. K., Kimball, E. S., and Oppenheim, J. J. (1985): Purification of human interleukin 1 from human monocyte culture supernatants and identity of thymocyte comitogenic factor, fibroblast-proliferation factor, acute-phase protein-inducing factor, and endogenous pyrogen. *Cell. Immunol.,* 92:290–301.

122. McDaniel, D. O., Barger, B. O., Koopman, W. J., Acton, R. T., and Alarcon, G. (1980): Class II MHC restriction fragment length polymorphisms (RFLP) and HLA-DR4 in rheumatoid arthritis. *Arthritis Rheum.,* 29:511.

123. Melmon, K. L., and Cline, M. J. (1967): Kallikrein activator and kinase in human granulocytes: A model of inflammation. In: *Symposium on Vasoactive Polypeptides: Bradykin and Related Kinins,* edited by E. Rocha and M. Silva, Pergamon Press, Oxford.

124. Metcalf, D. (1985): The granulocyte-macrophage colony-stimulating factors. *Science,* 229:16–22.

125. Milanese, C., Richardson, N. E., and Reinherz, E. L. (1986): Identification of a T helper cell-derived lymphokine that activates resting T lymphocytes. *Science,* 231:1118–1122.

126. Miossec, P., Dinarello, C. A., and Ziff, M. (1986): Interleukin-1 lymphocyte chemotactic activity in RA synovial fluid. *Arthritis Rheum.,* 29:461–470.

127. Mizel, S. B. (1982): Interleukin 1 and T cell activation. *Immunol. Rev.,* 63:51.

128. Mizel, S. B., Dayer, J.-M., Krane, S. M., and Mergenhagen, S. E. (1981): Stimulation of rheumatoid synovial cell collagenase and prostaglandin production by partially purified lymphocyte-activating factor (IL-1). *Proc. Natl. Acad. Sci. USA,* 78:2474–2477.

129. Mochan, E., Uhl, J., and Newton, R. (1986): Interleukin 1 stimulation of synovial cell plasminogen activator production. *J. Rheumatol.,* 13:15–19.

130. Mohr, W., and Wessinghage, D. (1978): The relationship between polymorphonuclear granulocytes and cartilage destruction in rheumatoid arthritis. *J. Rheumatol.,* 37:81–86.

131. Mueller, W. (1929): Ueber den negativen Luftdruck im Gelenkram. *Dtsch. Z. Chirurgie,* 218:395.

132. Muraguchi, A., Kehrl, J. H., Longo, D. L., Volkman, D. J., Smith, K. A., and Fauci, A. S. (1985): Interleukin 2 receptors on human B cells. Implications for the role of interleukin 2 in human B cell function. *J. Exp. Med.,* 161:181–197.

133. Nouri, A. M. E., Panayi, G. S., and Goodman, S. M. (1984): Cytokines and the chronic inflammation of rheumatic disease. II. The presence of interleukin-2 in synovial fluids. *Clin. Exp. Immunol.,* 58:402–409.

134. Ohno, O., and Cooke, T. D. (1978): Electronmicroscopic morphology of immunoglobulin aggregates and their interactions in rheumatoid articular collagenous tissues. *Arthritis Rheum.,* 21:516–527.

135. Okada, Y., Nagase, H., and Harris, E. D., Jr. (1986): A metalloproteinase from human rheumatoid synovial fibroblasts that digest connective tissue matrix components. Purification and characterization. *J. Biol. Chem.,* 261:14,245–14,255.

136. Oppenheim, J. J. (1986): *Interleukins and Interferons in Inflammation.* Upjohn, Kalamazoo, Mich.

137. Oppenheimer-Marks, N., and Ziff, M. (1986): Binding of normal human mononuclear cells to blood vessels in rheumatoid arthritis synovial membrane. *Arthritis Rheum.,* 29:789–792.

138. Panush, R. S., Katz, P., Longley, S., and Yonker, R. A. (1985): Detection and quantitation of circulating immune complexes in arterial blood of patients with rheumatic disease. *Clin. Immunol. Immunopathol.,* 36:217–226.

139. Parekh, R. B., Dwek, R. A., Sutton, B. J., Fernandes, D. L., Leung, A., Stanworth, D., and Rademacher, T. W. (1985): Association of rheumatoid arthritis and primary osteoarthritis with changes in the glycosylation pattern of total serum IgG. *Nature,* 316:452–457.

140. Paul, W. E. (1983): Regulation of B-cell response: Activation and differentiation: A personal synthesis. In: *Fifth International Conference of Immunology,* edited by Y. Yamamora and T. Tada, pp. 727–731. Academic Press, Tokyo.

141. Penbelle, P., Damon, M., Blotman, F., and Dayer, J.-M. (1985): Production of MCF by mononuclear phagocytes from rheumatoid synovial fluid. *J. Rheumatol.,* 12:412–417.

142. Phadke, K., Carlson, D. G., Gitter, B. D., and Butler, L. D. (1986): Role of interleukin 1 and interleukin 2 in rat and mouse arthritis models. *J. Immunol.,* 136:4085–4091.

143. Pober, J. S., Gimbrone, M. A., Jr., Cotran, R. S., Reiss, C. S.,

Burakoff, S. J., Fiers, W., and Ault, K. A. (1983): Ia expression by vascular endothelium is inducible by activated T cells and by human γ-interferon. *J. Exp. Med.,* 157:1339–1353.

144. Polverini, P. J., Cotran, R. S., Gimbrone, M. A., Jr., and Unanue, E. R. (1977): Activated macrophages induce vascular proliferation. *Nature,* 269:804–806.

145. Pope, R. M., Teller, D. C., and Mannik, M. (1974): The molecular basis of self-association of antibodies to IgG (rheumatoid factor) in rheumatoid arthritis. *Proc. Natl. Acad. Sci. USA,* 71:517–521.

146. Poulter, L. W., Duke, O., Panayi, G. S., Hobbs, S., Raftery, M. J., and Janossy, G. (1985): Activated T lymphocytes of the synovial membrane in rheumatoid arthritis and other arthropathies. *Scand. J. Immunol.,* 22:683–690.

147. Poulter, L. W., and Janossy, G. (1985): The involvement of dendritic cells in chronic inflammatory disease. *Scand. J. Immunol.,* 21:401–407.

148. Rasmussen, R. A., Chin, Y., Woodruff, J. J., and Easton, T. G. (1985): Lymphocyte recognition of lymph node high endothelium: II. Cell surface proteins involved in adhesion defined by monoclonal anti-HEBF$_{LN}$ (A.11) antibody. *J. Immunol.,* 135:19–24.

149. Reid, D. M., Brown, T., Reid, T. M. S., Rennie, J. A. N., and Eastmond, C. J. (1985): Human parvovirus-associated arthritis: A clinical and laboratory description. *Lancet,* 1:422–425.

150. Rigby, W. F. C., Noelle, R. J., Krause, K., and Fanger, M. W. (1985): The effects of 1,25-dihydroxyvitamin D$_3$ on human T lymphocyte activation and proliferation: A cell cycle analysis. *J. Immunol.,* 135:2279–2285.

151. Ritz, J., Campen, T. J., Schmidt, R. E., Royer, H. D., Hercend, T., Hussey, R. E., and Reinherz, E. L. (1985): *Science,* 228:1540–1543.

152. Robb, R. J. (1984): Interleukin 2: The molecule and its function. *Immunol. Today,* 5:203–209.

153. Robinson, D. R. (1985): Low molecular weight mediators of inflammation. In: *Textbook of Rheumatology,* edited by W. N. Kelley, E. D. Harris, Jr., S. Ruddy, and C. S. Sledge, pp. 71–83. W. B. Saunders, Philadelphia.

154. Rouzer, C. A., Matsumoto, T., and Samuelsson, B. (1986): Single protein from human leukocytes possesses 5-lipoxygenase and leukotriene A$_4$ synthase activities. *Proc. Natl. Acad. Sci. USA,* 83:857–861.

155. Rowley, M., Tait, B., Mackey, I. R., Cunningham, T., and Phillips, B. (1986): Collagen antibodies in rheumatoid arthritis. *Arthritis Rheum.,* 29:174–184.

156. Ruddy, S., and Austen, K. F. (1973): Activation of the complement system in rheumatoid arthritis. *Fed. Proc.,* 32:134–137.

157. Rutherford, R. B., and Ross, R. (1976): Platelet factors stimulate fibroblasts and smooth muscle cells quiescent in plasma-serum to proliferate. *J. Cell Biol.,* 69:196.

158. Sabharwal, U. K., Vaughan, J. H., Fong, S., Bennett, P. H., Carson, D. A., and Curd, J. G. (1982): Activation of the classical pathway of complement by rheumatoid factors: Assessment by radioimmunoassay for C4. *Arthritis Rheum.,* 25:161–167.

159. Sakane, T., Ueda, Y., Suzuki, N., Niwa, Y., Hoshino, T., and Tsunematsu, T. (1985): OKT4$^+$ and OKT8$^+$ T lymphocytes produce soluble factors that can modulate growth and differentiation of human B cells. *Clin. Immunol.,* 62:112–120.

160. Saklatvala, J., Pilsworth, L. M. C., Sarsfield, S. J., Gavrilovic, J., and Heath, J. K. (1984): Pig catabolin is a form of interleukin 1. *Biochem. J.,* 224:461–466.

161. Saklatvala, J., Sarsfield, S. J., and Townsend, Y. (1985): Pig interleukin 1. *J. Exp. Med.,* 162:1208–1222.

162. Scala, O., Kuang, Y. D., Hall, R. E., Muchmore, A. V., and Oppenheim, J. J. (1984): Accessory cell function of human B-cells. *J. Exp. Med.,* 159:1637–1652.

163. Scott, R. W., Bergman, B. L., Bajpai, A., Hersh, R. T., Rodriguez, H., Jones, B. N., Barreda, C., Watts, S., and Baker, J. B. (1985): Protease nexin: Properties and a modified purification procedure. *J. Biol. Chem.,* 260:7029–7035.

164. Shalaby, M. R., Aggarwal, B. B., Rinderknecht, E., Svedersky, L. P., Finkle, B. S., and Palladino, M. A., Jr. (1985): Activation of human polymorphonuclear neutrophil functions by interferon-γ and tumor necrosis factors. *J. Immunol.,* 135:2069–2073.

165. Shiozawa, S., Jasin, H. E., and Ziff, M. (1980): An absence of immunoglobulins in rheumatoid cartilage-pannus junctions. *Arthritis Rheum.,* 23:816–821.

166. Silverman, S. L., and Schumacher, H. R. (1981): Antibodies to Epstein-Barr viral antigens in early rheumatoid arthritis. *Arthritis Rheum.,* 24:5115.

167. Simpson, R. W., McGurty, L., Simon, L., Smith, C. A., Godzeski, C. W., and Boyd, R. J. (1984): Association of parvoviruses with rheumatoid arthritis of human. *Science,* 223:1425–1428.

168. Smith, C. D., Cox, C. C., and Snyderman, R. (1986): Receptor-coupled activation of phosphoinositide-specific phospholipase C by an N protein. *Science,* 232:97–100.

169. Smith, C. D., Verghese, M. W., and Snyderman, R. (1985): Chemoattractant receptor-induced leukocyte activation and polyphosphoinositide degradation is mediated by a guanine nucleotide regulatory protein. In: *Sensing and Response in Microorganisms,* edited by M. Eisenbach and M. Balaban, pp. 215–233. Elsevier Science, Philadelphia.

170. Snyderman, R., and Lane, B. C. (1985): Inflammation and chemotaxis. In: *Endocrinology,* ed. 2, edited by L. J. DeGroot, Grune & Stratton, Orlando.

171. Stastny, P. (1978): Association of the B-cell alloantigen DR4 with rheumatoid arthritis. *N. Engl. J. Med.,* 298:869.

172. Stephenson, M. L., Krane, S. M., Amento, E. P., McCroskery, P. A., and Byrne, M. (1985): Immune interferon inhibits collagen synthesis by rheumatoid synovial cells associated with decreased levels of the procollagen mRNAs. *FEBS Lett.,* 180:43–50.

173. Stricklin, G. P., and Welgus, H. G. (1983): Human skin fibroblast collagenase inhibitor. *J. Biol. Chem.,* 258:12252–12258.

174. Stuart, J. M., Cremer, M. A., Townes, A. S., and Kang, A. H. (1982): Type II collagen-induced arthritis in rats: Passive transfer with serum. *J. Exp. Med.,* 155:1.

175. Stuart, J. M., and Kang, A. H. (1986): Monkeying around with collagen autoimmunity and arthritis. *Lab. Invest.,* 54:1–3.

176. Sugarman, B. J., Aggarwal, B. B., Hass, P. E., Figari, I. S., Palladino, M. A., Jr., and Shepard, H. M. (1985): Recombinant human tumor necrosis factor-β: Effects on proliferation of normal and transformed cells in vitro. *Science,* 230:943–945.

177. Tallon, D. F., Corcoran, D. J. D., O'Dwyer, E. M., and Greally, J. F. (1984): Circulating lymphocyte subpopulations in pregnancy. *J. Immunol.,* 132:1784–1787.

178. Tarkowski, A., Holmdahl, R., Rubin, K., Klareskog, L., Nilsson, L. A., and Gunnarsson, E. (1986): Patterns of autoreactivity to collagen type II in autoimmune MRL/1 mice. *Clin. Exp. Immunol.,* 63:441–449.

179. Taurog, J. D., Kerwar, S. S., McReynolds, R. A., Sandberg, G. P., Leary, S. L., and Makowald, M. L. (1985): Synergy between collagen-induced and adjuvant arthritis in rats. *J. Exp. Med.,* 162:962–978.

180. Terato, K., Hasty, K. A., Cremer, M. A., Stuart, J. M., Townes, A. S., and Kang, A. H. (1985): Collagen-induced arthritis in mice: Localization of an arthritogenic determinant to a fragment of the type II collagen molecule. *J. Exp. Med.,* 162:637–646.

181. Theofilopoulos, A. N., Burtonboy, G., LoSpalluto, J. J., and Ziff, M. (1974): IgM rheumatoid factor and low molecular weight IgM: An association with vasculitis. *Arthritis Rheum.,* 17:272–284.

182. Theofilopoulos, A. N., and Dixon, F. J. (1982): A spontaneous rheumatoid arthritis-like disease in MRL/1 mice. *J. Exp. Med.,* 155:1690–1701.

183. Tiku, M. L., Liu, S., Weaver, C. W., Teodorescu, M., and Skosey, J. L. (1985): Class II histocompatibility antigen-mediated immunologic function of normal articular chondrocytes. *J. Immunol.,* 135:2923–2928.

184. Tiku, K., Tiku, M. L., Liu, S., and Skosey, J. L. (1986): Normal human neutrophils are a source of a specific interleukin 1 inhibitor. *J. Immunol.,* 136:3686–3692.

185. Tiku, K., Tiku, M. L., and Skosey, J. L. (1986): Interleukin 1 production by human polymorphonuclear neutrophils. *J. Immunol.,* 136:3677–3685.

186. Tosato, G., Steinberg, A. D., and Blaese, R. M. (1981): Defective EBV-specific suppressor T cell function in rheumatoid arthritis. *N. Engl. J. Med.,* 305:1238.

187. Tosato, G., Steinberg, A. D., Yarchoan, R., Hedman, C. A., Pike, S. E., DeSean, V., and Blaese, R. M. (1984): Abnormally elevated frequency of Epstein-Barr virus-infested B cells in the blood of patients with rheumatoid arthritis. *J. Clin. Invest.*, 73:1789–1796.

188. Trentham, D. E., Dynesius, R. A., and David, J. R. (1978): Passive transfer by cells of type II collagen-induced arthritis in rats. *J. Clin. Invest.*, 62:359–366.

189. Unger, A., Kay, A., Griffin, A. J., et al. (1983): Disease activity and pregnancy associated $_2$-glycoprotein in rheumatoid arthritis during pregnancy. *Br. Med. J.*, 286:750–792.

190. Urdal, D. L., March, C. J., Gillis, S., et al. (1984): Purification and chemical characterization of the receptor for interleukin 2 from activated human T lymphocytes and from a human T-cell lymphoma cell line. *Proc. Natl. Acad. Sci. USA*, 81:6481–6485.

191. Vandenbroucke, J. P., Valkenburg, H. A., Boersma, J. W., et al. (1982): Oral contraceptives and rheumatoid arthritis: Further evidence for a preventive effect. *Lancet*, 1:839–842.

192. Vandenbroucke, J. P., Witteman, J. C. M., Valkenburg, H. A., Boersma, J. W., Cats, A., Festen, J. J. M., Hartman, A. P., Huber-Bruning, O., Rasker, J. J., and Weber, J. (1986): Noncontraceptive hormones and rheumatoid arthritis in perimenopausal and postmenopausal women. *J.A.M.A.*, 255:1299–1303.

193. Van de Putte, L. B. A., Hegt, V. N., and Overbeck, T. E. (1977): Activators and inhibitors of fibrinolysis in rheumatoid and nonrheumatoid synovial membranes. *Arthritis Rheum.*, 20:671–678.

194. Vaughan, J. H. (1975): Lymphocyte function in rheumatoid disorders. *Arch. Intern. Med.*, 135:1324–1328.

195. Vaughan, J. H., Carson, D. A., and Fox, R. I. (1983): The Epstein-Barr virus and rheumatoid arthritis. *Clin. Exp. Rheum.*, 1:265–272.

196. Velcek, J. (editor) (1984): *Interferons and the Immune System.* Elsevier/North Holland, Amsterdam.

197. Wahl, S. M., Malone, D. G., and Wilder, R. I. (1985): Spontaneous production of fibroblast-activating factor(s) by synovial inflammatory cells. *J. Exp. Med.*, 161:210–222.

198. Walden, P., Nagy, Z. A., and Klein, J. (1985): Induction of regulatory T-lymphocyte responses by liposomes carrying major histocompatibility complex molecules and foreign antigen. *Nature*, 315:327–329.

199. Walker, C., Kristensen, F., Bettens, F., and de Weck, A. L. (1983): Lymphokine regulation of activated (G_1) lymphocytes. I. Prostaglandin E_2-induced inhibition of interleukin 2 production. *J. Immunol.*, 130:1770.

200. Wallis, W. J., Simkin, P. A., and Nelp, W. B. (1985): Low synovial clearance of iodide provides evidence of hypoperfusion in chronic rheumatoid arthritis. *Arthritis Rheum.*, 28:1096–1104.

201. Weiss, S. J. (1980): The role of superoxide in the destruction of erythrocyte targets by human neutrophils. *J. Biol. Chem.*, 255:9912.

202. Weiss, A., Imboden, J., Hardy, K., Manger, B., Terhorst, C., and Stobo, J. (1986): The role of the T3/antigen receptor complex in T-cell activation. *Annu. Rev. Immunol.*, 4:593–619.

203. Welgus, H. G., and Stricklin, G. P. (1983): Human skin fibroblast collagenase inhibitor. *J. Biol. Chem.*, 258:12259–12264.

204. Welte, K., Platzer, E., Lu, L., Gabrilove, J. L., Levi, E., Mertelsmann, R., and Moore, M. A. S. (1985): Purification and biochemical characterization of human pluripotent hematopoietic colony-stimulating factor. *Proc. Natl. Acad. Sci. USA*, 82:1526–1530.

205. Werb, Z., Mainardi, C. L., Vater, C. A., and Harris, E. D., Jr. (1977): Endogenous activation of collagenase secreted by rheumatoid synovial cells: Evidence for the role of plasminogen activator. *N. Engl. J. Med.*, 296:1017–1023.

206. Wernick, R. M., Lipsky, P. E., Marban-Arcos, E., Maliakkal, J. J., Edelbaum, D., and Ziff, M. (1985): IgG and IgM rheumatoid factor synthesis in rheumatoid synovial membrane cell cultures. *Arthritis Rheum.*, 28:742–752.

207. White, D. G., Mortimer, P. P., Blake, D. R., Woolf, A. D., Cohen, B. J., and Bacon, P. A. (1985): Human parvovirus arthropathy. *Lancet*, 1:419–421.

208. Wilder, S. M., Wilder, R. L., Katona, I. M., et al. (1983): Leukapheresis in rheumatoid arthritis: Association of clinical improvement with reversal of anergy. *Arthritis Rheum.*, 26:1076–1084.

209. Winchester, R. J. (1981): Genetic aspects of rheumatoid arthritis. *Semin. Immunopathol.*, 4:89–102.

210. Winchester, R. J., Agnello, V., and Kunkel, H. G. (1970): Gamma globulin complexes in synovial fluids of patients with rheumatoid arthritis. Partial characterization and relationship to lowered complement levels. *Clin. Exp. Immunol.*, 6:689.

211. Wingrove, S., and Kay, C. R. (1978): Reduction in incidence of rheumatoid arthritis associated with oral contraceptives. *Lancet*, 1:569–571.

212. Wood, D. D., Bayne, E. K., Goldring, M. B., Gowen, M., Hamerman, D., Humes, J. L., Ihrie, E. J., Lipsky, P. E., and Staruch, M.-J. (1985): The four biochemically distinct species of human interleukin 1 all exhibit similar biologic activities. *J. Immunol.*, 134:895–903.

213. Wood, D. D., Ihrie, E. J., Dinarello, C. A., and Cohen, P. L. (1983): Isolation of an interleukin-1-like factor from human joint effusion. *Arthritis Rheum.*, 26:975–983.

214. Wood, D. D., Ihrie, E. J., Dinarello, C. A., and Cohen, P. L. (1983): Isolation of an interleukin 1-like factor from human joint effusions. *Arthritis Rheum.*, 26:975–983.

215. Wood, D. D., Ihrie, E. J., and Hamerman, D. (1985): Release of interleukin-1 from human synovial tissue *in vitro*. *Arthritis Rheum.*, 28:853–862.

216. Wooley, D. E., Brinckerhoff, C. E., Mainardi, C. L., Vater, C. A., Evanson, J. M., and Harris, E. D., Jr. (1979): Collagenase production by rheumatoid synovial cells: Morphological and immunohistochemical studies of the dendritic cell. *Ann. Rheum. Dis.*, 38:262–270.

217. Wooley, D. E., Harris, E. D., Jr., Mainardi, C. L., and Brinckerhoff, C. E. (1978): Collagenase immunolocalization in cultures of rheumatoid synovial cells. *Science*, 200:773–775.

218. Wooley, P. H., Luthra, M. S., Singh, S., Huse, A., Stuart, J. M., and David, C. S. (1984): Passive transfer of arthritis in mice by human anti-type II collagen antibody. *Mayo Clin. Proc.*, 59:737–743.

219. Wooley, P. H., Luthra, M. S., Stuart, J. M., and David, C. S. (1981): Type II collagen-induced arthritis in mice. I. Major histocompatibility complex linkage and antibody correlates. *J. Exp. Med.*, 154:688.

220. Yoffe, J. R., Taylor, D. J., and Wooley, D. E. (1984): Mast cell products stimulate collagenase and prostaglandin E production by cultures of adherent rheumatoid synovial cells. *Biochem. Biophys. Res. Commun.*, 122:270–276.

221. Ythier, A. A., Abbud-Filho, M., Williams, J. M., Loertscher, R., Schuster, M. W., Nowill, A., Hansen, J. A., Maltezos, D., and Strom, T. B. (1985): Interleukin 2-dependent release of interleukin 3 activity by $T4^+$ human T-cell clones. *Proc. Natl. Acad. Sci. USA*, 82:7020–7024.

222. Yu, D. T., Winchester, R. J., Fu, S. M., Gwofsky, A., Ko, H. S., and Kunkel, H. G. (1980): Peripheral blood Ia-positive T cells: Increases in certain diseases and after immunization. *J. Exp. Med.*, 151:91–100.

Inflammation: Basic Principles and Clinical Correlates.
Edited by J. I. Gallin, I. M. Goldstein, and R. Snyderman.
Raven Press, Ltd., New York © 1988.

CHAPTER 42

Gout: Crystal-Induced Inflammation

Thomas P. Gordon, Robert Terkeltaub,
and Mark H. Ginsberg

Over the past two decades, several distinct microcrystals have been implicated in the pathogenesis of acute and chronic articular syndromes. These disorders have been grouped under the term "crystal-deposition diseases," based on the concepts that a local or systemic metabolic disturbance leads to supersaturated body fluids, with consequent crystal formation, that the crystals then induce acute or chronic tissue inflammation, and that a chemically defined crystal is specific for the disease (52). Crystals believed to be involved in the pathogenesis of joint disease include monosodium urate monohydrate (53,75), calcium pyrophosphate dihydrate (54), hydroxyapatite and related basic calcium phosphates (11,74), brushite (14), and calcium oxalate (32).

This chapter discusses the pathogenesis and modulation of acute gouty arthritis, which has been recognized for centuries as one of the most severe, painful forms of acute inflammation occurring in humans, and which serves as the prototype of these arthritic diseases caused by crystal deposition.

PATHOGENESIS OF URATE-CRYSTAL-INDUCED INFLAMMATION

Activation of Humoral and Cellular Mediators of Inflammation

The virtually constant finding of monosodium urate crystals in joint fluid from patients with acute gouty arthritis (53), and reproduction of the syndrome by injection of synthetic crystals (13,75), established the urate crystal as the causative agent of human gout. Studies during the last 25 years have suggested that the severity of many cases of gouty arthritis may arise from the ability of urate crystals to activate a remarkable variety of humoral and cellular inflammatory mediator systems (Table 1).

Direct activation of the classic complement pathway by urate crystals occurs *in vitro* (16,59), and there is evidence of complement activation in many gouty synovial fluids (28,38). Urate crystals bind and activate purified macromolecular C1 in the absence of immunoglobulin

TABLE 1. *Mediators involved in urate-crystal-induced inflammation*

Source	Products
Neutrophils	Lysosomal proteases
	Leukotriene B$_4$
	HETEs (hydroxyeicosatetraenoic acids)
	Crystal-induced chemotactic factor
	Oxygen-derived free radicals
Synovial fibroblasts	Prostaglandins
	Lysosomal proteases
Mononuclear phagocytes	Prostaglandins
	Lysosomal proteases
	Interleukin 1
	Oxygen-derived free radicals
Platelets	Arachidonic acid metabolites
	Lysosomal proteases
	Biogenic amines
Complement system	C3a, C5a
Contact system	Kallikrein
	Bradykinin
	Plasmin

(16), and the activation products, $\overline{C1r}$ and $\overline{C1s}$, have been detected on the surfaces of monosodium urate crystals exposed to plasma (87). Classic complement pathway activation may also be amplified by IgG (29) and by C-reactive protein (68). Alternative complement pathway activation occurs *in vitro* at higher concentrations of crystals (15). Cleavage of C5 to C5b and C5a via a stable C5 convertase formed on the crystal surface was demonstrated by Russell et al. (67). Despite the possibility that the potent chemoattractant C5a and the anaphylatoxins C3a and C5a could play a role in the pathogenesis of gouty synovitis, the degree of urate-crystal-induced inflammation has only slightly, if at all, been reduced in complement-depleted animals (62,82,93). This reinforces the concept of the redundancy of the inflammatory response to urate crystals (Table 1) and suggests that complement is not required as a mediator in acute gout.

Joint fluids from patients with gouty arthritis and from experimental animals with synthetic urate-crystal-induced inflammation contain elevated levels of kinins that could contribute to the pain and vascular changes of gout (37,57). Monosodium urate crystals activate Hageman factor and the contact system of coagulation *in vitro* to generate kallikrein, bradykinin, plasmin, and other mediators (21). However, the contact system, like the complement system, does not appear necessary for acute gouty arthritis. Acute gout occurs in patients with Hageman factor deficiency (27,44), and an acute inflammatory response to injected urate crystals is seen in chickens, which lack Hageman factor (81).

In contrast to the fluid-phase mediators of inflammation, there is considerable evidence supporting a central role for neutrophils in gouty inflammation. There is a striking accumulation of these cells in both the joint fluid and synovial membrane in natural gout (3,53) and in acute crystal-induced experimental synovitis (13,75), together with active phagocytosis of urate crystals. Experimental urate-induced synovitis is diminished when neutrophils are depleted with cytotoxic drugs (61) or with antipolymorphonuclear leukocyte serum (9). Results of crystal-neutrophil interactions include release of lysosomal proteases (96) and generation of oxygen-derived free radicals (1,77), lipoxygenase products of arachidonic acid (leukotriene B$_4$, hydroxyeicosatetraenoic acids) (64,76), and a chemotactic, low-molecular-weight glycoprotein known as crystal-induced chemotactic factor (60). Injection of purified crystal-induced chemotactic factor induces a marked polymorphonuclear leukocyte response in rabbit joints without altering vascular permeability (84). Crystal-induced chemotactic factor has also been identified in human gouty synovial fluid (63). These and other properties of crystal-induced chemotactic factor have been reviewed recently (86).

Cells other than neutrophils are involved in the pathogenesis of gouty inflammation. Although outnumbered by neutrophils during the acute phase, synovial fluid mononuclear phagocytes become proportionately greater with time and often are seen to ingest urate crystals (70). Monosodium urate crystals stimulate synthesis of prostaglandin E$_2$ and release of lysosomal enzymes from these cells *in vitro* (56).

Interactions of urate crystals with resident macrophages in the synovial lining (type A synoviocytes) and synovial fibroblasts (type B synoviocytes) are likely to play a role in the development of gouty arthritis, because phagocytosis of crystals by synoviocytes occurs soon after their injection into canine joints (72), and urate crystals stimulate the synthesis of vasodilator prostaglandins (prostaglandin I$_2$, prostaglandin E$_2$) from synovial fibroblasts in tissue culture (97). Monosodium urate crystals have recently been shown to stimulate the production of endogenous pyrogen, or interleukin 1 (IL-1), from mononuclear phagocytes *in vitro,* a property shared by silica, but not by calcium pyrophosphate dihydrate or apatite crystals (49). In addition to mediating the fever of gout, it has been proposed that IL-1 may be involved in the initiation of acute gouty arthritis by stimulating synovial influx of neutrophils (49).

Monosodium urate crystals also interact with platelets and trigger rapid secretion of adenosine diphosphate, adenosine triphosphate, and serotonin, followed by a cytolytic phase. Electron microscopic studies reveal morphological evidence of platelet secretion and crystal internalization (18). Although the uncoated crystal surface is sufficient to trigger the secretory response, stimulation is also mediated by interaction of the Fc regions of adsorbed IgG with Fc receptors on the platelet membrane (19,20).

Further evidence for the importance of cells in the pathogenesis of gouty inflammation comes from studies indicating that most of the agents used to manage crystal-induced inflammation act on cells rather than on soluble mediator systems. Colchicine, a drug with little general antiinflammatory effects, inhibits (albeit modestly) many leukocyte functions, including neutrophil random motility, chemotaxis, margination, and phagocytosis (46). In addition, colchicine inhibits the synthesis of crystal-induced chemotactic factor (85) and leukotriene B$_4$ (76) by neutrophils exposed to urate crystals. Indomethacin and phenylbutazone, drugs often used in the treatment of gout, inhibit crystal phagocytosis (83) in addition to prostaglandin synthetase. It is unclear, however, whether or not any effects on cells account for the ability of these drugs to inhibit gouty inflammation.

Mechanisms of Cellular Interactions with and Stimulation by Urate Crystals

Using X-ray crystallography, Mandel (50) has determined the three-dimensional crystal structure of monosodium urate monohydrate. In brief, the crystal contains parallel stacks of purine rings interspersed with sodium ions that bond to the oxygen atoms of the urate anions. The water molecules of crystallization form hydrogen bonds to the purine rings and lie in channels between the rings. Heating monosodium urate crystals at high temperatures drives off the water of crystallization and alters the internal structure and surface structure of the crystals (51). This alteration in the crystal lattice is the likely reason for the diminished capacity of heated crystals to activate complement (59). The crystals possess a net negative charge, in keeping with the negatively charged oxygen atoms prominent on the crystal surfaces, and are capable of binding to membranes either through hydrogen bonding (where the crystals would contain the receptor) or by electrostatic interactions with positively charged phospholipid head groups. Surface roughness on an atomic scale appears to be an important structural requirement for biological activity, because the crystal faces of phlogistic crystals (monosodium urate, calcium pyrophosphate dihydrate) are irregular, whereas the surfaces of nonphlogistic crystals are smooth (50).

Following phagocytosis of urate crystals by neutrophils, rapid dissolution of the phagolysosomal membrane is observed, with internal release of lysosomal contents and cellular swelling and death (33,71,95). These observations have led to the "suicide-sac" or "perforation-from-within" hypothesis. When protein-coated crystals are phagocytosed and come to lie within phagolysosomes, it is proposed that enzymes digest the adsorbed proteins, allowing lysis of phagolysosomes to proceed with cell death and release to the exterior of neutrophil contents, which amplify tissue injury and inflammation. The apparent lack of direct injury to the plasma membrane by the crystals has been thought to be due to the inhibitory effect of proteins coating the crystal surface (92,94,96).

In addition, the interaction of crystals with the external plasma membrane provokes extracellular release of lysosomal enzymes (17,33) and superoxide anion radicals (1) by noncytolytic mechanisms. To test whether or not cellular stimulation was mediated by crystal–membrane protein interactions, we studied the interaction between platelets and monosodium urate crystals (36). Urate crystals bound the platelet membrane glycoproteins GPIIb/IIIa and GPIb. Moreover, proteolytic removal of these proteins from the cell surface, or antibodies directed against these proteins, inhibited urate-induced platelet secretion, indicating that crystal–membrane protein interactions mediated platelet stimulation by the crystals. Because clustering of membrane proteins, such as might be induced by multivalent ligands, is a stimulus for secretion (31), we hypothesize that these crystals stimulate cells by binding to membrane proteins, leading to their clustering in the plane of the membrane. Because a membrane protein bound to the surface of a rigid crystal is probably immobile, it is likely that such clustering events occur at the junction between crystal-contacted and noncontacted plasma membrane. Freely diffusing membrane proteins could enter this zone and be immobilized by binding to the crystal (Fig. 1). Cellular stimulation may also be mediated by interactions between exposed Fc regions of IgG adsorbed to the crystal surface and cellular Fc receptors (see following).

Temporal Events in Urate-Crystal-Induced Synovitis

The sequence of events leading to the initial synovial influx of neutrophils and the onset of pain and vascular changes of gout remains uncertain. A simplified scheme of the possible events leading to the development of acute gouty arthritis is presented in Fig. 2. Crystals deposited in cartilage or synovium may be released into the joint fluid following mechanical disruption or partial crystal dissolution and loosening (79). Alternatively, *de novo* precipitation of crystals in synovial fluid may follow a fall in temperature (43) or a transient rise in synovial urate concentration (78). Once present in the joint fluid, the

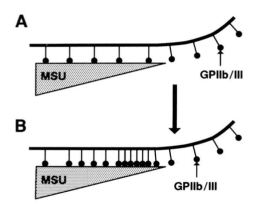

FIG. 1. Hypothesis for the clustering of plasma membrane urate-crystal-binding proteins (e.g., GPIIb/IIIa) at the junctional zone between crystal-contacted and noncontacted plasma membrane. **A:** GPIIb/IIIa is initially homogeneously distributed in the membrane. GPIIb/IIIa in close proximity to the rigid crystal surface binds to it, thereby immobilizing the glycoprotein in the plane of the membrane. Continued lateral diffusion of the unbound GPIIb/IIIa brings it to the junctional zone, where it becomes immobilized by binding to the crystal surface (**B**). Thus, initial clustering will be in this junctional zone and may be limited by (a) local saturation of crystal binding sites with GPIIb/IIIa, (b) steric hindrance between GPIIb/IIIa molecules, and/or (c) hindrance by another large entity bound to the crystal surface, e.g., low-density lipoprotein.

crystals presumably would be free to activate mediators of inflammation.

Neutrophils probably are not involved in the initial stages of inflammation, because neutrophil infiltration lags behind rises in intraarticular pressure (55) and phagocytosis of crystals by synoviocytes (72) during urate-crystal-induced synovitis in dogs. In monosodium-urate-crystal-induced air-pouch inflammation in the rat, prostaglandin synthesis and ingestion of crystals by lining cells with the characteristics of type A and type B synoviocytes occurred before the appearance of neutrophils (24). Thus, the triggering event in gouty inflammation may be phagocytosis of urate crystals by type B synoviocytes, with synthesis of prostaglandins (97), release of lysosomal enzymes, and production of IL-1 by type A synoviocytes (49). Prostaglandin E_2 and prostaglandin I_2 (prostacyclin) would produce vasodilatation, enhance vascular leakage, and contribute to the pain of gout. Activation by the crystal surface of the complement pathways and contact system would also contribute to the early stages of urate-induced synovitis.

Once sufficient neutrophils had migrated into the joint space under the influence of C5a, and perhaps synoviocyte-derived chemotactic factors, extracellular release of mediators such as crystal-induced chemotactic factor and

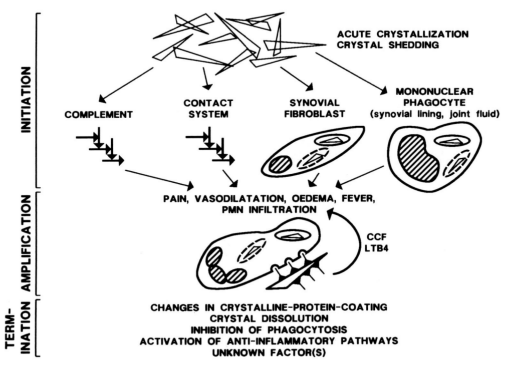

FIG. 2. Schematic outline of possible events leading to the development and termination of acute urate-crystal-induced synovitis: CCF, crystal-induced chemotactic factor; LTB_4, leukotriene B_4.

leukotriene B_4 from crystal-neutrophil interactions would establish a vicious cycle of leukocyte infiltration and would amplify as well as propagate acute gouty inflammation (47,49).

Possible mechanisms contributing to the spontaneous termination of acute gouty attacks include crystal dissolution by lysosomal myeloperoxidase (35,65), ingress of apoprotein B (apo-B) lipoproteins into the joint space (see following), enzymic digestion of IgG attached to the crystal surface (10), production of inhibitors of phagocytosis, including crystal-induced chemotactic factor (4,86), and generation of endogenous antiinflammatory factors such as adrenal cortical hormones.

Variable Inflammatory Responses to Urate Crystals

Despite the ability of monosodium urate crystals to activate numerous inflammatory mediators, clinical observations suggest that there is no direct relationship between urate crystal deposition and the inflammatory reactions seen in gouty patients. Large quantities of crystals ("joint milk") may be aspirated from joints that show little or no signs of inflammation; yet in other patients, few crystals may be detected, despite full-blown acute gouty arthritis. Patients with gout often have a striking lack of inflammation around subcutaneous deposits of urate crystals (so-called quiescent crystals) (1), and some patients with tophaceous gout give no history of acute attacks of arthritis (34). Thus, factors must be present that either trigger or inhibit the development of an acute inflammatory response to urate crystals. Additional observations suggesting that the biological activity of urate crystals and expression of gouty arthritis are modulated by multiple factors include the following: the sporadic nature and spontaneous termination of the gouty attack, with crystals commonly identified in joint fluids after inflammation has resolved; the variation in the inflammatory response to synthetic crystals injected into knee joints of gouty volunteers (75); the finding of monosodium urate crystals in asymptomatic first metatarsophalangeal joints (2,66) and knee joints (22); and the rarity of acute gout in patients with rheumatoid arthritis (91).

FACTORS THAT MODULATE THE INFLAMMATORY POTENTIAL OF URATE CRYSTALS

As noted earlier, striking variability of the inflammatory response in gouty patients challenges the assumption that the presence of urate crystals in joints is a sufficient precondition for acute gout. Several factors have been identified that may modulate the inflammatory activity of urate crystals and account for such observations as the higher incidence of gout in men, the short duration of acute gout, and the puzzle of finding crystals without inflammation.

Sex Hormones

A role for sex steroids in the pathogenesis of gout is suggested by the higher serum urate levels and young-age incidence of gout in males (98), as well as by a deficiency in production of β-estradiol in patients with gout (58). Evidence from *in vitro* systems suggests that estrogens may protect plasma membranes from membranolysis, because incorporation of estradiol into liposomes inhibited monosodium-urate-crystal-induced lysis. Enhanced lysis was observed in liposomes containing androgens (96).

Crystal Size and Morphology

Crystal size may be important, because smaller crystals are phagocytosed more avidly by human neutrophils than are larger ones and yield higher leukocyte counts and phagocytic indices when injected into canine joints (73). Furthermore, "small" crystals (about 5 μm in length) were found to be more inflammatory than "large" crystals (greater than 20 μm in length) after injection into a rat's paw (12). It appears that very small "amorphous" urate particles (less than 0.1 μm long) produce little or no inflammation (12,75). In studies with natural crystals aspirated from patients with gout, however, Antommattei et al. (6) could find no correlation between crystal size or shape and severity of inflammation. Other reports concerning the role of crystal shape are conflicting, with both blunt (66) and needle-shaped (22) crystals being found in asymptomatic joints or in joints with subacute gouty arthritis.

Hyaluronic Acid Concentration

Large polymeric hyaluronic acid has been shown to inhibit phagocytosis of monosodium urate crystals in a concentration-dependent manner (8). The hyaluronate content is relatively constant in a joint, but a fall in hyaluronic acid concentration in a joint effusion, for example, following trauma, might remove its inhibitory effect on crystal-cell interactions and render the crystals more inflammatory.

Urate in Solution

Clinical observations suggest a possible effect of urate in solution on gouty inflammation, because changes in serum uric acid concentrations may precipitate attacks of gout. Malawista et al. (48) have demonstrated a suppressive effect of physiologic concentrations of urate on protein adsorption by neutrophil membranes; this could result in a loss of membrane protective effect and enhanced membranolysis by monosodium urate crystals. This was supported by experiments with silica crystals, which showed increased cell lysis in the presence of dissolved urate (48). Other studies suggest that urate in solution may have an antiinflammatory or immunosuppressive effect. Uric acid is known to be a potent antioxidant (5) and inhibits adjuvant-induced arthritis in the rat (45).

With the realization that crystal size, morphology, and number may not be important in modifying natural gouty arthritis (6), attention has focused on the crystal surface as a possible critical determinant of phlogistic activity.

Binding of Proteins to Urate Crystals

Kozin and McCarty (39,40) were the first workers to investigate the adsorptive properties of urate crystals. The binding isotherm for IgG showed a plateau above IgG concentrations of 5 mg/ml and a second rise above about 20 mg/ml. It has been postulated that the plateau phase corresponds to monolayer formation and that the secondary rise reflects molecular aggregation (42,80). Thus, at concentrations found in joint fluid, IgG is likely to be adsorbed on the crystal surface as a monolayer. Studies have suggested that the Fc fragments of adsorbed IgG molecules are fully exposed (41), and Bardin et al. (7) have confirmed the functional availability of Fc fragments by immunoelectron microscopy. A number of biologically significant proteins were observed to bind to urate crystals *in vivo,* including fibrin and C1q (reviewed in ref. 30).

The plasma protein coat of urate crystals has been assessed by two-dimensional polyacrylamide-gel electrophoresis (87). More than 30 crystal-associated polypeptides of both anionic and cationic species were detected in gels of proteins eluted from plasma-exposed crystals. Proteins more abundant in the crystal pellet than in starting plasma included C1q, C1r, C1s, fibronectin, fibrinogen, and kininogen. Apo-B-containing lipoproteins were also well represented in the plasma coat (88). In contrast, a number of polypeptides abundant in starting plasma (e.g., albumin, IgG) were relatively impoverished in the crystal pellet. These studies highlighted the complexity of crystal-protein interactions and showed that overall protein charge was not necessarily a critical factor.

Modulating Effect of Crystalline Protein Coating on Crystal-Cell Interactions

The interaction of monosodium urate crystals with neutrophils is a critical feature in the pathogenesis of acute gout (61), but the factors modulating this interaction are still uncertain. One modulator likely to be important is crystalline protein coating. It was found that binding of IgG alone resulted in enhanced platelet secretion (19) and increases in superoxide generation and lysosomal enzyme release from neutrophils (1,92), apparently mediated by interactions of exposed Fc fragments with cellular Fc receptors (19). An IgM monoclonal rheumatoid factor bound preferentially to monosodium urate crystals coated with a monolayer of IgG and inhibited the neutrophil chemiluminescence response (a marker of crystal-membrane perturbation) by blocking the interaction of crystal-bound IgG with Fc receptors (23). The coating of urate crystals by rheumatoid factor might explain the rarity of acute gouty arthritis in patients with rheumatoid arthritis (91).

Although coating of urate crystals with purified IgG enhances cellular stimulation, adsorption of whole plasma or serum to the crystal surface was shown to markedly inhibit membranolysis (92), platelet secretion (18), and neutrophil superoxide generation (1). Using measurements of luminol-dependent chemiluminescence and selective protein depletion and reconstitution, we identified apo-B-containing low-density lipoproteins and very-low-density lipoproteins as the major inhibitory proteins of crystal-neutrophil interactions (88). Recent work has shown that low-density lipoproteins abrogate a range of cellular responses to urate and other crystals by inhibiting the physical interactions between crystals and cells (90) and that apo-B is the component responsible (89). Because apo-B lipoproteins are normally excluded from uninflamed joints (69), it has been proposed that ingress of lipoproteins into the joint space during urate-crystal-induced synovitis may be responsible for terminating acute attacks of gout (88). The inhibitory effect of low-density lipoproteins on crystal-cell interactions *in vitro* has been confirmed, but human low-density lipoproteins did not appear inhibitory in the rat in either urate-crystal-induced air-pouch inflammation (25) or urate-crystal-induced footpad swelling and pleurisy (P. Dieppe, *personal communication*). Further clinical and animal studies will be required to clarify the role of apo-B lipoproteins in the pathogenesis of gouty arthritis. For example, it would be interesting to study the effects of low-density lipoproteins in the neutrophil-dependent canine and primate models of urate-induced synovitis, which may be closer analogues of human gout. Preliminary studies have indicated the presence of inhibitory coating material on natural urate crystals, but the nature of this *in vivo* inhibitor has yet to be determined (26).

CONCLUSION

The dramatic clinical picture of acute gouty arthritis, together with unexplained observations such as the short duration of attacks and asymptomatic crystal deposition, continues to stimulate investigation into this venerable disease. The association of gouty arthritis with a chemically defined crystal has been an advantageous feature of the disease for investigators and has facilitated new insights into the pathogenesis of tissue damage caused by negatively charged particles (i.e., urate, silica, and calcium pyrophosphate dihydrate crystals). Further investigation into the mechanisms by which crystal-cell interactions are modulated would appear worthwhile, because interactions of cells with surfaces are important in a broad range of medical conditions. Finally, the credibility of any hypothesis concerning the pathogenic mechanisms of human gout must be judged by its ability to predict the unique clinical features of this disease.

ACKNOWLEDGMENTS

Supported by NIH grants AM-36702 and AM-27214, an NH and MRC Neil Hamilton Fairley Fellowship, the Veterans Administration Research Service, and the D. E. V. Starr Research Fellowship in Rheumatology. This is manuscript 4478 from the Department of Immunology of the Research Institute of Scripps Clinic.

REFERENCES

1. Abramson, S., Hoffstein, S. T., and Weissmann, G. (1982): Superoxide anion generation by human neutrophils exposed to monosodium urate. Effect of protein adsorption and complement activation. *Arthritis Rheum.*, 25:174–180.
2. Agudelo, C. A., Schumacher, H. R., and Phelps, P. (1972): Effect of exercise on urate crystal-induced inflammation in canine joints. *Arthritis Rheum.*, 15:609–616.
3. Agudelo, C., and Schumacher, H. R. (1973): The synovitis of acute gouty arthritis. A light and electron microscopic study. *Hum. Pathol.*, 4:265–279.
4. Alvarellos, A., and Spilberg, I. (1985): An inhibitor of superoxide generation and phagocytosis in synovial fluid of gout and pseudogout patients. *Arthritis Rheum. (Suppl.)*, 28:48 (abstract).
5. Ames, B. N., Cathcart, R., Schwiers, E., and Hochstein, P. (1981): Uric acid provides an antioxidant defense in humans against oxidant- and radical-caused aging and cancer: A hypothesis. *Proc. Natl. Acad. Sci. USA*, 78:6858–6862.
6. Antommattei, O., Schumacher, H. R., Reginato, A. J., and Clayburne, G. (1984): Prospective study of morphology and phagocytosis of synovial fluid monosodium urate crystals in gouty arthritis. *J. Rheumatol.*, 11:741–744.
7. Bardin, T., Cherian, P. V., and Schumacher, H. R. (1984): Immunoglobulins on the surface of monosodium urate crystals: An immunoelectron microscopic study. *J. Rheumatol.*, 11:339–341.
8. Brandt, K. D. (1974): The effect of synovial hyaluronate on the ingestion of monosodium urate crystals by leukocytes. *Clin. Chim. Acta*, 55:307–315.
9. Chang, Y. H., and Gralla, E. J. (1968): Suppression of urate crystal-induced canine joint inflammation by heterologous anti-polymorphonuclear leukocyte serum. *Arthritis Rheum.*, 11:145–150.
10. Dieppe, P. A. (1984): Crystal deposition and inflammation. *Q. J. Med.*, 53:309–316.
11. Dieppe, P. A., Huskisson, E. C., Crocker, P., and Willoughby, D. A. (1976): Apatite deposition disease. *Lancet*, 1:266–269.
12. Dieppe, P. A., and Calvert, P. (1983): *Crystals and Joint Disease.* Chapman & Hall, London.
13. Faires, J. S., and McCarty, D. J. (1962): Acute arthritis in man and dog after intrasynovial injection of sodium urate crystals. *Lancet*, 2: 682–684.
14. Faure, G., Netter, P., Malanan, B., and Steinmetz, J. (1977): Monocrystalline calcium hydrogen phosphate dihydrate in destructive arthropathy of chondrocalcinosis. *Lancet*, 2:142–143.
15. Fields, T. R., Abramson, S. B., Weissmann, G., Kaplan, A. P., and Ghebrehiwet, B. (1983): Activation of the alternate pathway of complement by monosodium urate crystals. *Clin. Immunol. Immunopathol.*, 26:249–257.
16. Giclas, P. C., Ginsberg, M. H., and Cooper, N. R. (1979): Immunoglobulin G independent activation of the classical complement pathway by monosodium urate crystals. *J. Clin. Invest.*, 63:759–764.
17. Ginsberg, M. H., Kozin, F., Chow, D., May, J., and Skosey, J. L. (1977): Adsorption of polymorphonuclear leukocyte lysosomal enzymes to monosodium urate crystals. *Arthritis Rheum.*, 20:1538–1542.
18. Ginsberg, M. H., Kozin, F., O'Malley, M., and McCarty, D. J. (1977): Release of platelet constituents by monosodium urate crystals. *J. Clin. Invest.*, 60:999–1007.
19. Ginsberg, M. H., and Kozin, F. (1978): Mechanisms of cellular interaction with monosodium urate crystals: IgG-dependent and IgG-independent platelet stimulation by urate crystals. *Arthritis Rheum.*, 21:896–903.
20. Ginsberg, M. H., Henson, P. M., Henson, J., and Kozin, F. (1979): Mechanisms of platelet response to monosodium urate crystals. *Am. J. Pathol.*, 94:549–557.
21. Ginsberg, M. H., Jaques, B., Cochrane, C. G., and Griffin, J. H. (1980): Urate crystal-dependent cleavage of Hageman factor in human plasma and synovial fluid. *J. Lab. Clin. Med.*, 95:497–506.
22. Gordon, T. P., Bertouch, J., Walsh, B., and Brooks, P. M. (1982): Monosodium urate crystals in asymptomatic knee joints. *J. Rheumatol.*, 9:967–969.
23. Gordon, T. P., Ahern, M. J., Reid, C., and Roberts-Thomson, P. J. (1985): Studies on the interaction of rheumatoid factor with monosodium urate crystals and case report of coexistent tophaceous gout and rheumatoid arthritis. *Ann. Rheum. Dis.*, 44:384–389.
24. Gordon, T. P., Kowanko, I. C., James, M., and Roberts-Thomson, P. J. (1985): Monosodium urate crystal-induced prostaglandin synthesis in the rat subcutaneous air pouch. *Clin. Exp. Rheumatol.*, 3: 291–296.
25. Gordon, T. P., Clifton, P., James, M. J., and Roberts-Thomson, P. J. (1986): Lack of correlation between in vitro and in vivo effects of low density lipoprotein on the inflammatory activity of monosodium urate crystals. *Ann. Rheum. Dis.*, 45:673–676.
26. Gordon, T. P., and Roberts-Thomson, P. J. (1986): Preliminary evidence for the presence of an inhibitor on the surface of natural monosodium urate crystals. *Arthritis Rheum.*, 29:1172 (letter).
27. Green, D., Arsever, C. L., Grumet, K. A., and Ratnoff, O. D. (1982): Classic gout in Hageman factor (factor XII) deficiency. *Arch. Intern. Med.*, 142:1556–1557.
28. Hasselbacher, P. (1979): Immunoelectrophoretic assay for synovial fluid C3 with correction for synovial fluid globulin. *Arthritis Rheum.*, 22:243–250.
29. Hasselbacher, P. (1979): C3 activation by monosodium urate monohydrate is enhanced by surface IgG. *Arthritis Rheum.*, 22:620 (abstract).
30. Hasselbacher, P. (1982): Crystal-protein interactions in crystal-induced arthritis. In: *Advances in Inflammation Research,* edited by G. Weissmann, pp. 25–44. Raven Press, New York.
31. Henson, P. M., Ginsberg, M. H., and Morrison, D. C. (1978): Mechanisms of mediator release from inflammatory cells. In: *Cell Surface Reviews, Vol. V,* edited by G. Poste and G. L. Nicholson, pp. 407–481. Elsevier, New York.
32. Hoffman, G. S., Schumacher, H. R., Paul, H., Cherian, V., Reed, R., Ramsay, A. G., and Franck, W. A. (1982): Calcium oxalate microcrystalline associated arthritis in end stage renal disease. *Ann. Intern. Med.*, 97:36–42.
33. Hoffstein, S., and Weissmann, G. (1975): Mechanisms of lysosomal

enzyme release from leukocytes. IV. Interaction of monosodium urate crystals with dogfish and human leukocytes. *Arthritis Rheum.,* 18:153–165.

34. Hollingworth, P., Scott, J. T., and Burry, H. C. (1983): Nonarticular gout: Hyperuricaemia and tophus formation without gouty arthritis. *Arthritis Rheum.,* 26:98–101.

35. Howell, R. R., and Seegmiller, J. E. (1962): Uricolysis by human leukocytes. *Nature (Lond.),* 196:482–483.

36. Jaques, B. C., and Ginsberg, M. H. (1982): The role of cell surface proteins in platelet stimulation by monosodium urate crystals. *Arthritis Rheum.,* 25:508–521.

37. Kellermeyer, R. W., and Breckenridge, R. T. (1966): The inflammatory process in acute gouty arthritis. II. The presence of Hageman factor and plasma thromboplastin antecedent in synovial fluid. *J. Lab. Clin. Med.,* 67:455–460.

38. Kim, H. J., McCarty, D. J., Kozin, F., and Koethe, S. (1980): Clinical significance of synovial fluid total hemolytic complement activity. *J. Rheumatol.,* 7:143–152.

39. Kozin, F., and McCarty, D. J. (1976): Protein adsorption to monosodium urate, calcium pyrophosphate dihydrate, and silica crystals. *Arthritis Rheum.,* 19:433–438.

40. Kozin, F., and McCarty, D. J. (1977): Protein binding to monosodium urate monohydrate, calcium pyrophosphate dihydrate, and silicon dioxide crystals. I. Physical characteristics. *J. Lab. Clin. Med.,* 89:1314–1325.

41. Kozin, F., and McCarty, D. J. (1980): Molecular orientation of immunoglobulin G adsorbed to microcrystalline monosodium urate monohydrate. *J. Lab. Clin. Med.,* 95:49–58.

42. Levine, S. N. (1969): Thermodynamics of adsorbed protein films. *J. Biomed. Mater. Res.,* 3:83–94.

43. Loeb, J. N. (1972): The influence of temperature on the solubility of monosodium urate. *Arthritis Rheum.,* 15:189–192.

44. Londino, A. V., and Luparello, F. J. (1984): Factor XII deficiency in a man with gout and angioimmunoblastic lymphadenopathy. *Arch. Intern. Med.,* 144:1497–1498.

45. Lussier, A., and DeMedicis, R. (1978): Inhibition of adjuvant-induced arthritis in the hyperuricaemic rat. *Agents Actions,* 8:536–542.

46. Malawista, S. E. (1975): The action of colchicine in acute gouty arthritis. *Arthritis Rheum. (Suppl.),* 18:835–846.

47. Malawista, S. E. (1977): Gouty inflammation. *Arthritis Rheum. (Suppl.),* 20:241–248.

48. Malawista, S. E., Van Blaricom, G. V., Cretella, S. B., and Schwartz, M. L. (1979): The phlogistic potential of urate in solution. Studies on the phagocytic process in human leukocytes. *Arthritis Rheum.,* 22:728–736.

49. Malawista, S. E., Duff, G. W., Atkins, E., Cheung, H. S., and McCarty, D. J. (1985): Crystal-induced endogenous pyrogen production. A further look at gouty inflammation. *Arthritis Rheum.,* 28:1039–1046.

50. Mandel, N. S. (1976): The structural basis of crystal-induced membranolysis. *Arthritis Rheum.,* 19:439–445.

51. Mandel, N. S. (1980): Structural changes in sodium urate crystals on heating. *Arthritis Rheum.,* 23:772–776.

52. McCarty, D. J. (1974): Crystal deposition joint disease. *Annu. Rev. Med.,* 25:279–288.

53. McCarty, D. J., and Hollander, J. L. (1962): Identification of urate crystals in gouty synovial fluid. *Ann. Intern. Med.,* 54:452–460.

54. McCarty, D. J., Kohn, N. N., and Faires, J. S. (1962): The significance of calcium phosphate crystals in the synovial fluid of arthritis patients: The "pseudogout syndrome." I. Clinical aspects. *Ann. Intern. Med.,* 56:711–737.

55. McCarty, D. J., Phelps, P., and Pyensen, J. (1966): Crystal-induced inflammation in canine joints. I. An experimental model with quantification of the host response. *J. Exp. Med.,* 124:99–114.

56. McMillan, R. M., Hasselbacher, P., Hahn, J. L., and Harris, E. D. (1981): Interactions of murine macrophages with monosodium urate crystals: Stimulation of lysosomal enzyme release and prostaglandin synthesis. *J. Rheumatol.,* 8:555–562.

57. Melmon, K. L., Webster, M. E., Goldfinger, S. E., and Seegmiller, J. E. (1967): The presence of a kinin in inflammatory synovial effusions from arthritides of varying etiologies. *Arthritis Rheum.,* 10:13–20.

58. Merinello, E., Riario-Sforza, G., and Marcolongo, R. (1985): Plasma follicle-stimulating hormone, luteinizing hormone, and sex hormones in patients with gout. *Arthritis Rheum.,* 28:127–131.

59. Naff, G. B., and Byers, P. H. (1973): Complement as a mediator of inflammation in acute gouty arthritis. I. Studies on the reaction between human serum complement and sodium urate crystals. *J. Lab. Clin. Med.,* 81:747–760.

60. Phelps, P. (1969): Polymorphonuclear leukocyte motility *in vitro.* III. Possible release of a chemotactic substance after phagocytosis of urate crystals by polymorphonuclear leukocytes. *Arthritis Rheum.,* 12:197–203.

61. Phelps, P., and McCarty, D. J. (1966): Crystal-induced inflammation in canine joints. II. Importance of polymorphonuclear leukocytes. *J. Exp. Med.,* 124:115–125.

62. Phelps, P., and McCarty, D. J. (1969): Crystal-induced arthritis. *Postgrad. Med.,* 45:87–93.

63. Phelps, P., Andrews, R., and Rosenbloom, J. (1981): Demonstration of chemotactic factor in human gout. *J. Rheumatol.,* 8:889–894.

64. Rae, S. A., Davidson, E. M., and Smith, M. J. H. (1982): Leukotriene B₄, an inflammatory mediator in gout. *Lancet,* 2:1122–1123.

65. Reardon, J. A., and Scott, J. T. (1980): Resolution of acute gout attacks: A possible mechanism. *Ann. Rheum. Dis.,* 39:189 (abstract).

66. Roualt, T., Caldwell, D. S., and Holmes, E. W. (1982): Aspiration of the asymptomatic metatarsophalangeal joint in gout patients and asymptomatic controls. *Arthritis Rheum.,* 25:209–212.

67. Russell, I. J., Mansen, C., Kolb, L. M., and Kolb, W. P. (1982): Activation of the fifth component of human complement (C5) induced by monosodium urate crystals: C5 convertase assembly on the crystal surface. *Clin. Immunol. Immunopathol.,* 24:239–250.

68. Russell, I. J., Papaioannou, C., McDuffie, F. C., Macintyre, S., and Kushner, I. (1983): Effect of IgG and C-reactive protein on complement depletion by monosodium urate crystals. *J. Rheumatol.,* 10:425–433.

69. Schmid, M., and Macnair, M. (1956): Characterization of the proteins of certain post-mortem human synovial fluids in certain disease states. *J. Clin. Invest.,* 35:708–718.

70. Schumacher, H. R. (1977): Pathogenesis of crystal-induced synovitis. *Clin. Rheum. Dis.,* 3:105–131.

71. Schumacher, H. R., and Phelps, P. (1971): Sequential changes in human polymorphonuclear leukocytes after urate crystal phagocytosis. An electron microscopic study. *Arthritis Rheum.,* 14:513–526.

72. Schumacher, H. R., Phelps, P., and Agudelo, C. A. (1974): Urate crystal induced inflammation in dog joints: Sequence of synovial changes. *J. Rheumatol.,* 1:102–113.

73. Schumacher, H. R., Fishbein, P., Phelps, P., Tse, R., and Krauser, R. (1975): Comparison of sodium urate and calcium pyrophosphate crystal phagocytosis by polymorphonuclear leukocytes. Effects of crystal size and other factors. *Arthritis Rheum. (Suppl.),* 18:783–792.

74. Schumacher, H. R., Sorylo, A. P., and Tse, R. L. (1977): Arthritis associated with apatite crystals. *Ann. Intern. Med.,* 87:411–416.

75. Seegmiller, J. E., Howell, R. R., and Malawista, S. E. (1962): The inflammatory reaction to sodium urate. *J.A.M.A.,* 180:125–131.

76. Serhan, C. N., Lundberg, S., Abramson, S., Samuelsson, B., and Weissmann, G. (1984): Formation of leukotrienes and hydroxy acids by human neutrophils and platelets exposed to monosodium urate. *Prostaglandins,* 27:563–581.

77. Simchowitz, L., Atkinson, J. P., and Spilberg, I. (1982): Stimulation of the respiratory burst in human neutrophils by crystal phagocytosis. *Arthritis Rheum.,* 25:181–188.

78. Simkin, P. A. (1977): The pathogenesis of podagra. *Ann. Intern. Med.,* 86:230–233.

79. Simkin, P. (1978): Role of local factors in the precipitation of urate crystals. In: *Uric Acid,* edited by W. N. Kelley and I. M. Weiner, pp. 379–395. Springer-Verlag, Berlin.

80. Soderquist, M. E., and Walton, A. G. (1980): Structural changes in proteins adsorbed on polymer surfaces. *J. Colloid Interface Sci.,* 75:386–396.

81. Spilberg, I. (1974): Urate crystal arthritis in animals lacking Hageman factor. *Arthritis Rheum.,* 17:143–148.

82. Spilberg, I., and Osterland, C. K. (1970): Anti-inflammatory effect

of the trypsin-kallikrein inhibitor in acute arthritis induced by urate crystals in rabbits. *J. Lab. Clin. Med.,* 76:472–479.

83. Spilberg, I., Gallacher, A., Mandell, B., and Rosenberg, D. (1977): A mechanism of action for non-steroidal anti-inflammatory agents in calcium pyrophosphate dihydrate (CPPD) crystal induced arthritis. *Agents Actions,* 7:153–155.

84. Spilberg, I., Rosenberg, D., and Mandell, B. (1977): Induction of arthritis by purified cell-derived chemotactic factor. Role of chemotaxis and vascular permeability. *J. Clin. Invest.,* 59:582–585.

85. Spilberg, I., Mandell, B., Mehta, J., Simchowitz, L., and Rosenberg, D. (1979): Mechanism of action of colchicine in acute urate crystal-induced arthritis. *J. Clin. Invest.,* 64:775–780.

86. Spilberg, I., and Mandell, B. (1982): Crystal-induced chemotactic factor. In: *Advances in Inflammation Research,* edited by G. Weissmann, pp. 57–65. Raven Press, New York.

87. Terkeltaub, R., Tenner, A. J., Kozin, F., and Ginsberg, M. H. (1983): Plasma protein binding by monosodium urate crystals. Analysis by two-dimensional gel electrophoresis. *Arthritis Rheum.,* 26:775–783.

88. Terkeltaub, R., Curtiss, L. K., Tenner, A. J., and Ginsberg, M. H. (1984): Lipoproteins containing apoprotein B are a major regulator of neutrophil responses to monosodium urate crystals. *J. Clin. Invest.,* 73:1719–1730.

89. Terkeltaub, R., Martin, J., Curtiss, L. K., and Ginsberg, M. H. (1986): Apoprotein B is the constituent of low density lipoprotein (LDL) responsible for specific inhibition of neutrophil (PMN)–urate crystal (UC) interaction. *Arthritis Rheum. (Suppl.),* 29:36 (abstract).

90. Terkeltaub, R., Smeltzer, D., Curtiss, L. K., and Ginsberg, M. H. (1986): Low density lipoprotein inhibits the physical interaction of phlogistic crystals and inflammatory cells. *Arthritis Rheum.,* 29:363–370.

91. Wallace, D. J., Klinenberg, J. R., Morhaim, D., Berlanstein, B., Biren, P. C., and Callis, G. (1979): Coexistent gout and rheumatoid arthritis. Case report and literature review. *Arthritis Rheum.,* 22:81–86.

92. Wallingford, W. R., and McCarty, D. J. (1971): Differential membranolytic effects of microcrystalline sodium urate and calcium pyrophosphate dihydrate. *J. Exp. Med.,* 133:100–112.

93. Webster, M. E., Maling, H. M., Zweig, M. H., Williams, M. A., and Anderson, W. (1973): Urate crystal induced inflammation in the rat: Evidence for the combined actions of kinins, histamine and components of complement. *Immunol. Commun.,* 1:185–198.

94. Weissmann, G. (1974): Crystals, lysosomes and gout. *Adv. Intern. Med.,* 19:239–257.

95. Weissmann, G., Zurier, R. B., Spieler, P. J., and Goldstein, I. M. (1971): Mechanisms of lysosomal enzyme release from leukocytes exposed to immune complexes and other particles. *J. Exp. Med. (Suppl.),* 134:149s–165s.

96. Weissmann, G., and Rita, G. A. (1972): Molecular basis of gouty inflammation: Interaction of monosodium urate crystals with lysosomes and liposomes. *Nature (New Biol.),* 240:167–172.

97. Wigley, F. M., Fine, I. T., and Newcombe, D. S. (1983): The role of the human synovial fibroblast in monosodium urate crystal-induced synovitis. *J. Rheumatol.,* 10:602–611.

98. Wyngaarden, J. B., and Kelley, W. N. (1976): *Gout and Hyperuricemia.* Grune & Stratton, New York.

Inflammation: Basic Principles and Clinical Correlates.
Edited by J. I. Gallin, I. M. Goldstein, and R. Snyderman.
Raven Press, Ltd., New York © 1988.

CHAPTER **43**

Neutrophilic Dermatoses: Sweet's Syndrome and Pyoderma Gangrenosum

Joseph L. Jorizzo

The primary emphasis of this review will be to discuss the vessel-based neutrophilic dermatoses as models of immune-complex-mediated, neutrophil-induced dermal vessel damage. Basic aspects of neutrophil biology have been reviewed elsewhere, and some issues of relevance to this review have been published (17,80,145,153). Non-infectious dermatoses in which neutrophils play a prominent role in pathogenesis are summarized in Table 1. These dermatoses include psoriasiform dermatoses, autoimmune bullous dermatoses, and the vessel-based neutrophilic dermatoses, as well as pyoderma gangrenosum. Pyoderma gangrenosum is a partially vessel-based cutaneous disease whose pathogenesis remains more obscure than those of the vessel-based neutrophilic dermatoses. Neutrophils are a prominent feature of the histopathology of pyoderma gangrenosum. A variant of pyoderma gangrenosum (i.e., bullous pyoderma gangrenosum) appears to be closely related to Sweet's syndrome (a vessel-based neutrophilic dermatosis).

PSORIASIFORM DERMATOSES

Psoriasis vulgaris is a chronic proliferative dermatosis that affects approximately 2% of the world's population. Clinically the disease is characterized by scaling plaques of proliferative epithelium (140). One of the earliest histopathologic features is an exocytosis (i.e., emigration) of neutrophils from dermal papillary capillaries into the epidermis (190). Cells of the stratum corneum that retain their nuclei in the rapidly proliferating epidermis of psoriasis are called parakeratotic cells. Admixtures of the parakeratotic mounds with neutrophils are called Monro microabscesses, a diagnostic feature of psoriasis (112). Collections of neutrophils to form micropustules below the stratum corneum, but still in the epidermis, are called spongiform pustules of Kogoj. These microabscesses are also a hallmark of histopathologic diagnosis of psoriasis (48).

Even an overview of the multitude of theories regarding the pathogenesis of psoriasis is beyond the scope of this review (25). Revelant to the current review are early studies that attempted to explain the diagnostic early exocytosis of neutrophils into psoriatic epidermis. Crude extracts of psoriatic epidermal scale, investigated using modified Boyden chamber techniques, have been shown to have highly potent chemotactic properties for peripheral blood neutrophils (133). Over the past 10 years, several theories have been advanced to account for neutrophil

TABLE 1. *Noninfectious neutrophilic dermatoses*

I. Psoriasiform dermatoses
   A. Psoriasis
   B. Reiter's syndrome
   C. Variants
II. Autoimmune bullous dermatoses
III. Vessel-based neutrophilic dermatoses
   A. Leukocytoclastic vasculitis
      1. Small-vessel variants
      2. Large-vessel variants
   B. Sweet's syndrome
   C. Pustular vasculitis
      1. Behçet's disease
      2. Bowel-associated dermatosis-arthritis syndrome
   D. Erythema nodosum
   E. Familial Mediterranean fever
IV. Pyoderma gangrenosum

chemotactic activity in psoriatic epidermis. An immunopathologic theory proposes anti-stratum-corneum and/or anti-basal-epithelial-cell antibody deposition in psoriatic epidermis, with resultant activation of the complement cascade, with subsequent neutrophil chemotaxis directed toward immune-complex-activated complement components (24). Another hypothesis proposes abnormal production of leukotriene B_4 and other lipoxygenase pathway products in psoriatic epidermis. Both leukotriene B_4 and 12-hydroxyeicosatetraenoic acid (12-HETE) have significant neutrophil chemoattractant properties. Once attracted into the psoriatic epidermis, neutrophils themselves might release additional leukotriene B_4, with further propagation of the disease process (141).

The generalized and localized pustular variants of psoriasis vulgaris are outlined in Table 2. These clinically distinct variants of psoriasis underscore the prominence of neutrophils in psoriasis. Whereas in psoriasis vulgaris the spongiform pustules of Kogoj are micropustules, in pustular psoriasis these neutrophil-containing pustules are macroscopic and are the most striking clinicopathologic feature of the disease (124).

Reiter's disease, with its classic triad of urethritis, axial arthritis (usually HLA-B27-positive), and conjunctivitis, is also characterized by typical cutaneous lesions such as circinate balanitis and keratoderma blennorrhagica (146). These cutaneous lesions are clinicopathologically indis-

TABLE 2. *Generalized and localized variants of psoriasis*

I. Generalized pustular psoriasis
   A. Pustular psoriasis of von Zumbusch
   B. Acral pustular psoriasis (Hallopeau)
   C. Impetigo herpetiformis
II. Localized pustular psoriasis
   A. Psoriasis with pustules
   B. Localized acrodermatitis continua (Hallopeau)
   C. Palmar-plantar pustulosis

tinguishable from psoriasis lesions, with both diseases having typical neutrophilic spongiform micropustules and occasionally macropustules (143). Lesions on the tongue and palate may be seen in generalized pustular psoriasis and in Reiter's disease. These lesions also are characterized by neutrophilic microabscesses (142).

Subcorneal pustular dermatosis (Sneddon-Wilkinson) is a disease considered by some to be a variant of pustular psoriasis and by others to be a distinct entity. The striking histopathologic feature is the occurrence of large neutrophilic pustules in a subcorneal location in the absence of spongiform micropustules of Kogoj (126). The phenomenon of extensive neutrophil exocytosis into epidermis is shared with the psoriasis group of dermatoses.

AUTOIMMUNE BULLOUS DERMATOSES

The autoimmune bullous dermatoses are reviewed in detail in the chapter by Lazarus. A role for the neutrophil has been reviewed for pemphigus vulgaris (60,61,125,134). Bullous pemphigoid is thought to represent a type II immunologic reaction. Circulating IgG antibody is directed against bullous pemphigoid antigen in the lamina lucida of the dermal-epidermal junction and results in complement-mediated neutrophilic infiltration, with production of a generalized bullous disorder characterized clinically by tense blisters. An *in vitro* model of bullous pemphigoid has been developed using rabbit cornea (3). Gammon and colleagues have demonstrated *in vitro* that directed migration of neutrophils occurs following the binding of bullous pemphigoid antibody and that this reaction is complement-dependent (42).

Dermatitis herpetiformis is an HLA-B8- and HLA-Dw3-associated autoimmune disease characterized by an intensely pruritic vesicular dermatosis and a gluten-sensitive enteropathy (76). A hypothesis for the pathogenesis of lesions in dermatitis herpetiformis is the following: An antigen (e.g., gluten) may be presented to a genetically susceptible host (HLA-B8 and HLA-Dw3) in the gastrointestinal tract, with IgA immune complex formation. IgA deposition in dermal papillae may lead to activation of the alternative complement pathway. Complement-derived chemotactic factors may lead to neutrophil-mediated damage to the dermal-epidermal junction above the dermal papillae, with resultant blister formation (76).

In summary, the autoimmune bullous dermatoses, despite clinicopathologic similarities, are quite distinct in terms of mechanisms of neutrophil-induced inflammation. In pemphigus, the complement cascade and neutrophils appear to be bystanders or at best secondary role players in an antibody-induced reaction in which direct enzyme activation may occur. Bullous pemphigoid seems to represent a situation in which specific IgG antibody circulates and activates the classic complement cascade at the peripheral site of antigen binding, with subsequent neutrophil-induced tissue damage. Dermatitis herpetiformis may represent a disease with circulating IgA-antigen immune complexes in which complement-derived chemotactic factors result from activation of the alternative complement pathway. Again, neutrophils may mediate the ultimate tissue injury.

VESSEL-BASED NEUTROPHILIC DERMATOSES AND PYODERMA GANGRENOSUM

The remainder of this review will deal with dermatoses whose unifying feature is the histopathologic presence of an angiocentric (i.e., vessel-based), primarily neutrophilic infiltrate. Leukocytoclastic vasculitis will be reviewed as the dermatopathologic model of circulating-immune-complex-mediated (CIC-mediated), neutrophil-induced vessel damage. This will be followed by detailed reviews of Sweet's syndrome and pustular vasculitis (i.e., our unifying concept for other dermatoses characterized by a vessel-based histopathology similar to that seen in lesions of Sweet's syndrome) and a brief overview of erythema nodosum and cutaneous lesions of familial Mediterranean fever. Pyoderma gangrenosum, as it relates to these dermatoses, will also be reviewed.

LEUKOCYTOCLASTIC VASCULITIS: A MODEL OF CIC-MEDIATED, NEUTROPHIL-INDUCED VESSEL DAMAGE

"Leukocytoclastic vasculitis" is a histopathologic term referring to the following constellation of microscopic findings: endothelial swelling, frequently with occlusion of the blood vessel, infiltration of the blood vessel wall by neutrophils, with leukocytoclasis (i.e., karyorrhexis of nuclei of these neutrophils), fibrinoid necrosis of blood vessel walls, and extravasation of erythrocytes (47,150) (Fig. 1).

The categorization of clinical syndromes characterized by histopathologic leukocytoclastic vasculitis, or variants of this process, has been confused by the needless proliferation of eponymal designations and by jargon. We have published a classification of necrotizing vasculitis (which is basically a variation of many others) as a part of a classification of reactive inflammatory vascular dermatoses (Table 3) (68). We prefer Soter's designation "necrotizing venulitis" for small-vessel-based leukocytoclastic vasculitis involving postcapillary venules. Large-vessel-based leukocytoclastic vasculitis and variants can be classified as polyarteritis nodosa, granulomatous vasculitis, and giant-cell arteritis, each with subclassifications. Reviews of the clinicopathologic features of various forms of necrotizing vasculitis are available in recent publications (36,39,43,118,119,151).

Studies of the pathogenesis of leukocytoclastic vasculitis affecting small blood vessels (i.e., necrotizing venulitis) have been the basis for construction of a hypothetical model of CIC-mediated, neutrophil-induced damage to cutaneous blood vessels (117). Several electron and immunoelectron microscopic studies have clarified the morphologic features of early lesions of necrotizing venulitis, with the following conclusions: (a) postcapillary venules with a minimal smooth-muscle coat and numerous pericytes are affected; (b) endothelial swelling may lead to venular occlusion; (c) venular basement membrane is thickened, with layered intramural deposition of fibrin; (d) endothelial cells show large numbers of pinocytotic vesicles; (e) fibrin is also deposited in association with

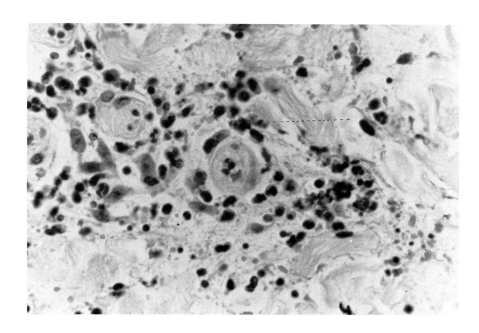

FIG. 1. Histopathologic finding of leukocytoclastic vasculitis. Note the endothelial swelling, fibrinoid necrosis of blood vessel walls, leukocytoclasia, infiltration of vessel walls by neutrophils, and extravasation of erythrocytes. ×280.

TABLE 3. Necrotizing vasculitis

I. Necrotizing venulitis
  A. Usual variety
  B. Henoch-Schönlein purpura
  C. Essential mixed cryoglobulinemia
  D. Waldenström's hypergammaglobulinemic purpura
  E. Associated with collagen vascular disease
  F. Urticarial vasculitis
  G. Erythema elevatum diutinum
  H. Nodular vasculitis
  I. Rheumatoid nodule
II. Polyarteritis nodosa
  A. Systemic form
  B. Cutaneous form
III. Granulomatous vasculitis
  A. Wegener's granulomatosis
  B. Allergic granulomatosis of Chung and Straus
  C. Lymphomatoid granulomatosis
IV. Giant-cell arteritis
  A. Temporal arteritis
  B. Takayasu's disease

collagen fibrils around affected venules; (f) fragmented neutrophils are present within and around blood vessels; (g) electron-dense, amorphous deposits lacking the periodicity of fibrin and suggestive of immune complexes are detectable on the luminal side of the basement membrane in the walls of postcapillary venules in early lesions; (h) similar immune-complex-like material is present in cytoplasmic vacuoles of perivenular neutrophils, suggesting their phagocytosis and removal (14,116,152).

Whereas older clinical lesions rarely demonstrate immunoreactants or fibrin in dermal blood vessels on direct immunofluorescence microscopic assessment, lesions less than 24 hr old often show these materials (Fig. 2). The most common finding is deposition of C3, IgM, IgA, IgG, and sometimes fibrin in upper dermal blood vessels (119). It is postulated that lesions older than 24 hr do not show these immunoreactants because of their phagocytosis by neutrophils, with subsequent lysosomal destruction.

Intradermal injection of small doses of histamine phosphate (e.g., 0.05 ml of a 1-mg/ml solution) has been used to induce lesions as a means of investigating the time sequence of the development of early lesions in necrotizing venulitis (14,152). This procedure has become known as Braverman's "histamine trap test." The postulate is that histamine produces gaps between endothelial cells, which then serve as a "trap" for CICs. The optimal time to biopsy histamine injection sites for the detection of immunoreactant deposition by direct immunofluorescence microscopy is from 1 to 4 hr after injection. Leukocytoclastic vasculitis is detectable on routine histology after 24 hr (49).

CICs are detectable by routine *in vitro* assays (e.g., C1q binding assay or Raji cell assay) in a high percentage of patients with necrotizing venulitis (29,136,151). Specific antigen, such as hepatitis B surface antigen, has been detected in association with immunoreactants in affected dermal blood vessels in some subgroups of patients (11). Other antigens, such as from streptococcus or herpesvirus, have also been reported (106).

Various animal models, including experimental serum sickness in rabbits, have provided support for a CIC-mediated pathogenesis of necrotizing venulitis. CICs are detectable in serum from affected rabbits, and immunoreactants are detectable in dermal blood vessels and in kidney. The routine histopathologic finding of leukocy-

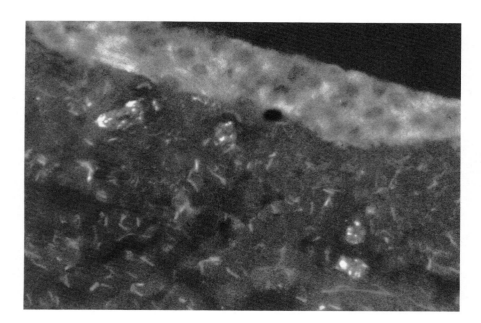

FIG. 2. Direct immunofluorescence photomicrograph of C3 deposition in upper dermal blood vessels. ×280.

toclastic vasculitis 24 hr after intradermal histamine injection is also a feature of lesions in this model (118).

The prevailing hypothesis based on the aforementioned data is that necrotizing venulitis results from the deposition of CICs in the walls of dermal venules. Subsequent activation of the classic complement cascade, with elaboration of C5a, leads to the attraction of neutrophils. Neutrophils then release lysosomal enzymes, such as collagenase and elastase, that result in the fibrinoid change seen in blood vessel walls. The trapping of CICs at specific sites may depend on local triggering factors such as vasoactive amines (14,65). Other factors, such as the amount of antibody formed, the size of CICs, the clearance of CICs, and the ratio of antigen and antibody, determine whether or not clinical necrotizing venulitis will develop in a given patient.

SWEET'S SYNDROME

Acute febrile neutrophilic dermatosis was first described by Sweet in 1964 (131). The condition that has come to be known as Sweet's syndrome is an uncommon reactive inflammatory dermatosis that occurs most commonly in women, but has been described in males and in children (84). The syndrome is best defined by its original non-eponymal designation. The cardinal features include acute inflammatory cutaneous plaques, fever and arthralgias, peripheral blood neutrophilia, and a vessel-based histopathology dominated by neutrophils, all occurring in the absence of infection. Complete recovery is the rule. Cutaneous lesions resolve completely, without scarring. Individual episodes last from weeks up to 2 months. Patients may experience several attacks of the disease (50,52,132).

Clinical Features

The cutaneous lesions of Sweet's syndrome are distinctive (Fig. 3). They are erythematous, raised, tender, inflammatory lesions that are sharply marginated. They may be geographic in outline and may reach diameters of several centimeters. The plaques may be composed of grouped, translucent-appearing papules that may mimic vesicles. Although pustulation has been described and mild desquamation may occur, epidermal changes usually are not prominent (132).

The upper body, including face, neck, trunk, and upper extremities, provides the favored sites; however, lesions may occur elsewhere. The process may be generalized, although solitary lesions have been reported. Lesions may recur at particular sites (132). Lesions often occur in crops over 1 to 2 weeks and resolve over 4 to 8 weeks. Lesions heal without scarring, although they may leave a transient brown staining of the skin.

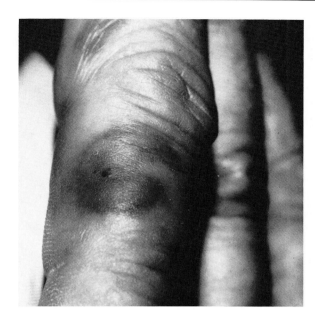

FIG. 3. Typical inflammatory plaques seen in Sweet's syndrome (acute febrile neutrophilic dermatosis).

Serum-sickness-like features of fever, arthralgias, and myalgias are typical. Other systemic signs and symptoms may include headache, malaise, vomiting, and prostration. Conjunctivitis and/or episcleritis may occur in up to 60% of patients (52). Oral manifestations are not frequent, but have been described (35). An individual patient may lack fever, any of the other systemic features, or even leukocytosis. White cell counts of 20,000/cm^3, with 80 to 90% neutrophils, are not uncommon. The erythrocyte sedimentation rate, platelet count, and other acute-phase reactants may be elevated. No specific laboratory abnormalities occur.

Cutaneous lesions usually are the presenting features of the syndrome. Systemic signs and symptoms and leukocytosis usually follow the appearance of cutaneous lesions by up to 1 week. The combination of the aforementioned clinical features with the diagnostic histopathology (*vide infra*) excludes other diagnoses such as erythema multiforme, erythema nodosum, or cutaneous infections.

Histopathology

The histopathologic hallmark of Sweet's syndrome is a dense, perivascular, predominantly neutrophilic dermal infiltrate (27). Mononuclear cells and rare eosinophils may also be seen. Leukocytoclasia (a breaking up of the nuclei of neutrophils) is a prominent feature. Endothelial swelling is prominent; however, the fibrinoid necrosis of blood vessel walls and the extravasation of erythrocytes that typify leukocytoclastic vasculitis are absent (Fig. 4). Whereas dermal edema may be so marked that dermal vesiculation may occur (38), intraepidermal vesiculation is not common (50). Extention of the inflammatory process into the subcutaneous tissue has been described recently (22), as has a septal granulomatous panniculitis (12).

Pathogenesis

The pathogenesis of Sweet's syndrome remains unknown. Investigators have been intrigued, from the earliest reports, by the variety of underlying conditions with which Sweet's syndrome has been associated. Leukemia has been identified in up to 10% of patients with Sweet's syndrome (13,23,50,130). Associations with metastatic adenocarcinoma (50), testicular carcinoma (122), lymphoma (78), multiple myeloma (5), and ovarian carcinoma (99) have also been described. Immunologically mediated diseases such as Sjögren's syndrome (111), bowel bypass syndrome (10), lupus erythematosus (subacute cutaneous) (44), ulcerative colitis (11), and rheumatoid arthritis (55) have also been anecdotally associated with Sweet's syndrome. Extensive investigation has failed to reveal any underlying infectious cause of Sweet's syndrome (130).

The association of Sweet's syndrome with underlying conditions that are often associated with CICs, and the vessel-based dermal neutrophilic histology with leukocytoclasia, naturally would lead to the postulate of a pathogenesis similar to that proposed for necrotizing venulitis (leukocytoclastic vasculitis). The evidence to support this hypothesis for the pathogenesis of cutaneous lesions

in Sweet's syndrome is meager. Detailed studies of CICs with *in vitro* assays (e.g., C1q binding or Raji cell assays) are lacking in Sweet's syndrome. Immunoreactants (e.g., IgM, C3) have been reported to be detectable microscopically in dermal blood vessels of early lesions in the rare patients in whom direct immunofluorescence microscopy was performed (89,101). Other investigators have reported negative direct immunofluorescence microscopic findings (111). One patient with both Sweet's syndrome and pustular psoriasis has been reported to have had cryoglobulin-bowel-flora-antigen complexes (104). Clearly, the possibility of CIC-mediated vessel damage has not yet been systematically assessed as a component in the pathogenesis of lesions in Sweet's syndrome. Complement component levels (e.g., C3) and total hemolytic complement levels are normal in patients with Sweet's syndrome (130), although assays for complement split products and other more sensitive assays of complement consumption have not been performed.

The dramatic neutrophilia that characterizes lesions of Sweet's syndrome histopathologically has led investigators to assess various parameters of neutrophil function, including phagocytosis, metabolic activation, and bacterial killing. These anecdotal reports have described findings that were within normal limits or have shown minimal elevations of these neutrophil functional parameters (75,101,130). Of interest is the recent report (in a solitary patient) of a heat-stable, nonlipid factor in serum from a patient with Sweet's syndrome that enhanced the migration of neutrophils as measured using a Boyder chamber assay (75). This is similar to our own reported findings in various forms of pustular vasculitis that will be reviewed. Confirmation of this finding and clarification of the exact

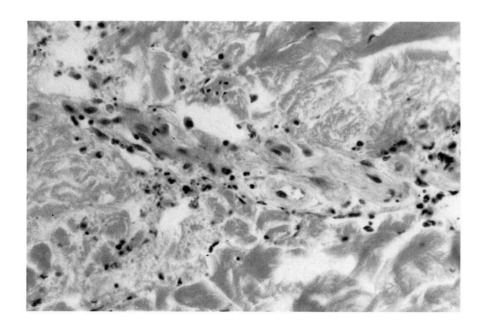

FIG. 4. Neutrophilic vascular reaction seen in Sweet's syndrome (and in pustular vasculitis lesions of Behçet's disease and bowel-associated dermatosis-arthritis syndrome). Note the absence of fibrinoid necrosis of blood vessel wall. ×280.

nature of this neutrophil migration enhancement factor in serum of patients with Sweet's syndrome are required. It is tempting to speculate that such enhancement of neutrophil migration might play a role in the pathogenesis of this "neutrophilic dermatosis."

Therapy

Systemic corticosteroid therapy is the most accepted therapy for Sweet's syndrome. Most reports of Sweet's syndrome have described treatment of only 1 or 2 patients. Prospective double-blind studies of experimental therapy are totally lacking. However, systemic corticosteroid therapy in the dose range of $\frac{1}{2}$ to 1 mg/kg/day tapered over several weeks seems to be the treatment of choice (52,130,132). It is unclear if indomethacin, aspirin, or other nonsteroidal antiinflammatory agents provide more than symptomatic relief (57,130). Other therapies with some reports of success in small groups of patients include oral potassium iodide (58), oral colchicine (108), oral dapsone (6), and oral isotretinoin (75). Direct or indirect effects on neutrophils were the postulated mechanisms of action for each of these agents; however, objective evidence concerning their possible mechanisms of action is lacking.

PUSTULAR VASCULITIS

Pustular cutaneous vasculitis results from a heterogeneous group of disorders characterized by pustules on purpuric bases. These lesions may occur in Behçet's syndrome, bowel-associated dermatosis-arthritis syndrome, gonococcemia, or a primary idiopathic cutaneous eruption (62,92). Although these conditions have previously been considered to be unrelated entities, clinicopathologic comparison reveals similarities among these conditions (63). The histopathology of pustular vasculitic lesions in each of the aforementioned conditions shows vessel changes similar to those seen in Sweet's syndrome or fully developed leukocytoclastic vasculitis, depending on the lesion sampled. The histopathology of cutaneous lesions seen in necrotizing venulitis (leukocytoclastic vasculitis) and in Sweet's syndrome was reviewed earlier. We had used the term "Sweet's-like vasculitis" to describe changes in the dermal vasculature that are histopathologically separable from those seen in leukocytoclastic vasculitis. Leukocytoclastic vasculitis, as we have discussed, is characterized by karyorrhexis of neutrophils, fibrinoid necrosis of the walls of small blood vessels, and extravasation of large numbers of erythrocytes into the dermis. "Sweet's-like vasculitis" derives its name from Sweet's syndrome (acute febrile neutrophilic dermatosis). In this disorder and in "Sweet's-like vasculitis" the dermal vessel damage

is not as severe as in true leukocytoclastic vasculitis. Leukocytoclasia is minimal or absent, and fibrinoid necrosis does not occur. Extravasated erythrocytes are also found in fewer numbers, and the main finding is the presence of neutrophils, lymphocytes and occasional eosinophils in and around the walls of small dermal vessels. We have recently substituted the designation "neutrophilic vascular reaction" for "Sweet's-like vasculitis" (72,91). In addition to the clinicopathologic similarities among diseases characterized by cutaneous pustular vasculitis, there is preliminary evidence that these diseases may all have a pathogenesis related to CIC-mediated vessel damage and serum enhancement of neutrophil migration. The dramatic accumulation of neutrophils might account for the pustulo-purpuric, rather than simply purpuric, nature of the cutaneous pustular vasculitic lesions.

Behçet's Disease

Clinical Features

Behçet's disease must be diagnosed using clinical criteria, because no pathognomonic laboratory parameters exist. Although several sets of diagnostic criteria have been published, we have found the O'Duffy criteria to be particularly useful. These are based on the presence of recurrent oral aphthae (canker sores) and at least two of the following five features: recurrent genital aphthae, uveitis, synovitis, cutaneous pustular vasculitis (pathergy), and meningoencephalitis (20,103). Inflammatory bowel disease is associated with an increased incidence of aphthosis (137) and may be associated with enteropathic arthritis (105). We agree with O'Duffy and Rogers that inflammatory bowel disease should be excluded before a diagnosis of Behçet's disease is made (115).

Oral aphthae are identical with the simple aphthae seen in recurrent aphthosis. They are very tender ulcers that begin as erythematous macules on the buccal mucosa, the tongue, the lips, the pharynx, and even the gastrointestinal tract after mild trauma (114). These simple aphthae rarely exceed 1 cm in size; they are self-limited (resolving over a maximum of 3–4 weeks) and usually heal without scarring. Patients at times develop major aphthous lesions that heal slowly, with scarring. Genital aphthae are lesions identical with simple oral aphthae; however, they occur on the genital mucosa. As 20% of normal individuals may have oral aphthosis, the concomitant occurrence of genital aphthosis is particularly relevant in the diagnosis of Behçet's disease.

Posterior uveitis (i.e., vasculitis of retinal vasculature) is not only a common ocular lesion of Behçet's disease but also a significant cause of blindness and the major cause of significant morbidity in this disease (21). Conjunctivitis and anterior uveitis occur, and secondary ocular changes include cataracts, glaucoma, and neovascularization of the iris and retina.

The characteristic arthritis of Behçet's disease is a non-erosive inflammatory polyarthritis affecting both large and small joints (20). Patients who have been described with HLA-B27-positive sacroileitis and axial arthritis are best classified as having the Reiter's syndrome spectrum or as having enteropathic arthritis, not as having Behçet's disease.

Neurologic manifestations of Behçet's disease may be mild and difficult to substantiate, often presenting as migraine-like headaches or psychiatric symptoms. Life-threatening manifestations may occur, as may motor paresis, brainstem dysfunction, intracranial hypertension, and multiple sclerosis-like signs (102).

Vascular manifestations occur in up to one-fourth of patients with Behçet's disease. These include superficial and deep thrombophlebitis, even of major veins such as the superior or inferior vena cava.

An additional major cutaneous feature of Behçet's disease is the pustular vasculitis that occurs either after trauma, such as from pinprick or intradermal injection, or spontaneously (Fig. 5). Similar clinicopathologic lesions occurring in subcutaneous tissue present as erythema-nodosum-like nodules. The clinical and pathologic features of these pustular vasculitis (pathergy) lesions and the deeper lesions have been elegantly investigated by Nazarro (97).

Significant cardiac or renal manifestations of Behçet's disease are rare. Pulmonary vasculitis may occur and may mimic pulmonary embolism or pulmonary tuberculosis clinically. Hemoptysis may be a presenting feature (51).

The relationship of Behçet's disease and inflammatory bowel disease is controversial. While some authors use the label Behçet's disease for patients with inflammatory bowel disease (154), we agree with O'Duffy that because patients with inflammatory bowel disease may have oral aphthae and enteropathic arthritis, these patients, many of whom are HLA-B27-positive, should be excluded when using clinical criteria for Behçet's disease (103,115).

Histopathology

Many published reports of the histopathologic features of Behçet's disease have been based on autopsy registry data (79). It is our contention that the study of late lesions with their almost exclusively mononuclear cell infiltrations has led to theories of pathogenesis that ignore the neutrophils that are present in early lesions. Recent interpretations of light, electron, and immunofluorescence microscopic data from the earliest mucosal or cutaneous lesions (i.e., the tissue most accessible for the study of early lesions) are compatible with an underlying neutrophilic vascular reaction that produces the aphthae, cutaneous pustular vasculitis, and possibly other lesions of Behçet's disease (41,66,85,96,97). Biopsies from the earliest pustular vasculitic lesions of Behçet's disease have revealed either leukocytoclastic vasculitis or at least a neutrophilic vascular reaction similar to the perivascular and vascular changes seen in the lesions of Sweet's syndrome (66,97). Histopathologic findings in the erythema-nodosum-like lesions are similar to those in the more superficial pustular vasculitic lesions (97).

Pathogenesis

A detailed review of the various theories regarding the pathogenesis of Behçet's disease is beyond the scope of

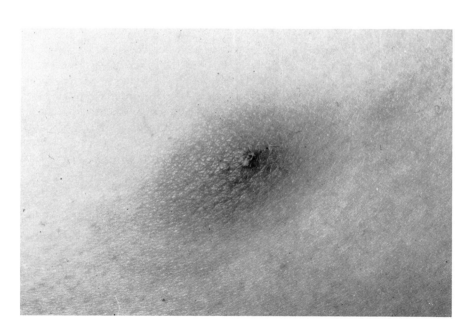

FIG. 5. Pustular vasculitis (pathergy) lesions occurring in a patient with Behçet's disease after cutaneous trauma.

this overview. IgG-containing CIC and reduced serum complement, correlating with disease activity, may be detected in sera from more than half of patients with Behçet's disease using a variety of *in vitro* assays (41,53,66,82,83,139,147).

Early histopathologic studies of mucocutaneous and systemic lesions from patients with Behçet's disease reported a lymphohistiocytic process that led investigators to postulate pathomechanisms relating to delayed hypersensitivity reactions. More recent interpretations of light, electron, and immunofluorescence microscopic data have focused on the presence of varying degrees of neutrophilic vascular reactions, including leukocytoclastic vasculitis, in biopsies taken from the earliest mucocutaneous lesions and pathergy lesions of patients with Behçet's disease (41,66,69,96,97,139). The discrepancy between neutrophilic versus lymphohistiocytic histopathology can probably be explained best by analogy to leukocytoclastic vasculitis, where the early diagnostic neutrophil-dominated histopathologic changes give way rapidly to nondiagnostic lymphocytic changes after 24 to 36 hr. The life-span of lesions must be considered when attempting to draw mechanistic conclusions from morphologic data.

Early studies in Japan, followed by confirmation from the Middle East and Europe, showed that neutrophils from patients with Behçet's disease demonstrate increased migration to standard chemoattractants (as assessed by either Boyden chamber or subagarose methods), when compared with neutrophils from a normal control population (33,95,127,135). This early work left in doubt whether the mechanism of increased neutrophil migration was related to serum or to the neutrophil itself. These investigators advocated systemic therapy with colchicine as a way to modify this increased migration, possibly via effects of colchicine on the microtubules of neutrophils (94,95). Colchicine is known to affect neutrophil adherence (88), locomotion (13,138), and phagocytosis (81), possibly via an effect on microtubules (91).

In a study comparing neutrophil migration in 6 patients with Behçet's disease to neutrophil migration in 7 control patients using a modified subagarose technique, we confirmed increased migration of the neutrophils from patients. The data indicated that without colchicine pretreatment, heat-inactivated serum (placed in the agar) from all of the patients with Behçet's disease increased the migration of neutrophils from the patients (5.07 ± 1.99, increased to 7.45 ± 2.56, $p \leq 0.01$) and of neutrophils from the controls (6.62 ± 1.99, increased to 8.85 ± 1.91, $p \leq 0.01$). Serum from the controls did not produce this effect (66). Therefore, in our experience, the enhancement of neutrophil migration seemed to result from a heat-stable serum factor. Interestingly, pretreating patients with oral colchicine (0.6 mg, by mouth, three times daily for 4 weeks, followed by 4 weeks "off" treatment, followed by 4 weeks "on" treatment) did not affect the migration

of normal neutrophils. However, the ability of serum from patients with Behçet's disease to enhance the migration of patients' cells or control cells was completely eliminated when comparing "on" colchicine data to "off" colchicine data (66). These results await confirmation in a larger series of patients.

In a subsequent small study, we assessed the effects of another experimental therapy, oral thalidomide, for Behçet's disease in a carefully monitored group of patients. Despite *in vitro* evidence from France that thalidomide might have an inhibitory effect on neutrophil migration, we found no effects on neutrophil migration in our small patient group (74). In that study we also qualitatively assessed the LFA-1/Mac-1/p150,95 family of glycoproteins, which have been associated with neutrophil adherence, by tritium labeling of neutrophil cell surfaces. Recent evidence has suggested that the LFA-1/Mac-1/p150,95 family of cell surface glycoproteins is necessary for optimal neutrophil adherence, chemotaxis, and phagocytosis (1,2,7,28,46). We found no qualitative abnormalities in this group of glycoproteins in patients with Behçet's disease and no effect on them as a result of oral thalidomide therapy (74). Preliminary results from our ongoing studies suggest that the enhancement of neutrophil migration seen when serum from Behçet's patients is mixed with agarose may not be seen with a more adherence-independent system such as collagen (F. C. Schmalstieg, and J. L. Jorizzo, *unpublished observations,* 1986). Our hypothesis remains that neutrophil-adherence-related phenomena may be relevant to the enhancement of neutrophil migration induced by serum from patients with Behçet's disease.

In addition to assessing neutrophil migration, our work in patients with Behçet's disease has also involved an attempt to address CIC-mediated vessel damage as a factor in the pathogenesis of Behçet's lesions. We have studied 10 patients with Behçet's disease using our modification of Braverman's histamine trap test (19,66,69,73,74,117). We believe this test to be particularly relevant in the assessment of patients with Behçet's disease because the pustular vasculitic (pathergy) cutaneous lesions may be induced by intradermal injection. Test sites are assessed by immunofluorescence microscopy (4 hr) and by routine microscopy (24 hr), using suitable controls, for the presence of immunoreactant deposition (4 hr) and neutrophilic vascular reactions (24 hr), respectively. All 10 patients tested during active disease had evidence of either neutrophilic vascular reactions (as in lesions of Sweet's syndromes) or leukocytoclastic vasculitis detected by routine microscopic assessment of histamine-induced lesions (69,74). Eight of these 10 patients also had immunoreactants (usually C1q, C2, or IgG) or fibrin detected in dermal blood vessels by immunofluorescence microscopy from biopsies taken 4 hr after histamine injection (69,74). Six patients were retested during disease remission. All 6 patients showed changes like those seen in normal controls (i.e., rare lymphocytes or eosinophils) on routine histology of histamine-injected skin during remission. Five of 6 patients converted to negative on immunofluorescence microscopic assessment of biopsied skin during remission (69). Our hypothesis is that a CIC-mediated neutrophilic vascular reaction localizes to sites of mucocutaneous trauma, possibly by endogenous histamine release from mast cells, producing endothelial gaps that trap CICs. A heat-stable serum factor that is not yet classified might facilitate the brisk accumulation of neutrophils producing the typical pustular vasculitic (rather than simple palpable purpuric lesions produced in CIC-induced leukocytoclastic vasculitis) mucocutaneous lesions of Behçet's disease. Systemic lesions might be produced by a similar mechanism.

A major diagnostic problem is the healthy patient with only recurrent oral and genital aphthosis or with almost constant, multiple (>3) oral aphthae. Heretofore, a laboratory approach to excluding Behçet's disease has not been available. We have labeled these patients as having complex aphthosis. In our laboratory study of 6 patients with this rare affliction, 5 patients were indistinguishable from control patients (e.g., normal neutrophil migration, no abnormalities on the Braverman histamine trap test, and negative C1q and Raji cell assays for CICs). One patient was identical with patients with Behçet's disease with respect to results of these tests and went on to develop florid Behçet's disease (70). All 6 patients have been followed for 3 years now, and the 5 patients with normal laboratory parameters show no signs of Behçet's disease (70).

These preliminary findings suggest that *in vitro* and *in vivo* evidence of CICs and the finding of enhanced neutrophil migration are associated with cutaneous pustular vasculitic and systemic disease in patients with Behçet's disease. Simple or complex aphthosis may occur without these findings. In fact, simple aphthosis may occur in 20% of the normal population (4,114). The etiology of simple aphthosis remains obscure.

Therapy

A brief summary of recent advances in therapy for patients with Behçet's disease, as discussed at the 1985 International Conference on Behçet's Disease held in London, England, has been published (73). The major morbidity in the disease is blindness from posterior uveitis. Patients with this problem usually are treated with a combination of systemic corticosteroids (e.g., prednisone at 1 mg/kg/day) and azathioprine (200 mg/day). Other systemic therapies include chlorambucil (0.1 mg/kg/day, with tapering to as low as 2 mg/day maintenance) and cyclosporin A. Chlorambucil is associated with the risks of in-

fertility and chromosomal damage. Cyclosporin A may affect the disease process via its known effects on T helper cells; however, there is a risk of renal interstitial fibrosis and arteriolar hyalinization, and the cost of treatment is very high. Mucocutaneous and, to a lesser degree, ocular lesions may be dramatically benefited by oral thalidomide therapy. There are well-known risks of teratogenicity and peripheral neuropathy associated with thalidomide therapy. These risks have caused the availability of this agent to be restricted to patients with erythema nodosum leprosum, and it has recently become unobtainable for use in treating patients with Behçet's disease, even under the strictest of protocols (71,74). Oral colchicine is far less effective than oral thalidomide; however, providing that complete blood counts are monitored to guard against neutropenia, this is a safe therapy for those individuals in whom it works (66,95).

Bowel-Associated Dermatosis-Arthritis Syndrome

Since the early 1970s, physicians have been aware of a syndrome consisting of typical cutaneous lesions, polyarthralgias and nonerosive polyarthritis, fever, and myalgias occurring in up to 20% of patients following jejunoileal bypass surgery for morbid obesity (18,34,123,148). In 1983, we expanded the concept of bowel bypass syndrome to include patients with an identical syndrome occurring without bowel bypass surgery, but associated with other bowel disease (64). The name bowel-associated dermatosis-arthritis syndrome was suggested, and others have now adopted this nomenclature (31).

Clinical Features

The typical cutaneous lesions of this syndrome provide the reason for inclusion of this condition in this review: a pustular vasculitis with a histopathologic appearance of a neutrophilic vascular reaction identical with that seen in pustular vasculitic lesions of Behçet's disease (i.e., with vessel changes and leukocytoclasia like those seen in lesions of Sweet's syndrome). Lesions begin as erythematous macules less than 1 cm in diameter. After an urticarial stage, the lesions become pustular, with purpuric bases over a 24- to 48-hr period (30,37,45,54,64) (Fig. 6). Lesions occur primarily in an upper truncal distribution, as distinguished from the palpable purpuric eruption on dependent sites characteristic of necrotizing venulitis. Cutaneous lesions last from 2 to 8 days and recur in bouts every 4 to 6 weeks (although this may be quite variable). As in patients with Behçet's disease, subcutaneous lesions very similar to erythema nodosum may occur (37).

The onset of the syndrome is heralded by fever, chills, and flu-like symptoms. The synovitis, myalgias, and cu-

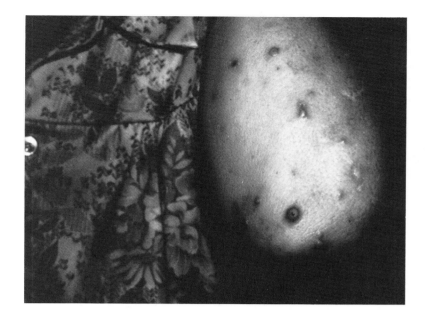

FIG. 6. Spontaneously appearing pustular vasculitis lesions in a patient with bowel-associated dermatosis-arthritis syndrome.

taneous eruption follow. The polyarticular arthralgias often affect the hands, wrists, and other peripheral (rather than axial) joints. A nonerosive polyarthritis may affect the same joints (18,24,123). Tendinitis and other systemic features may occur.

Histopathology

Early reports described the histopathologic features of cutaneous lesions of bowel bypass syndrome as showing leukocytoclastic vasculitis. More recent accounts agree that fibrinoid necrosis of blood vessel walls is not a feature of lesions and that the vessel changes are similar to those seen in Sweet's syndrome (37,64,77). As discussed earlier, we now prefer the designation "neutrophilic vascular reaction" to "Sweet's-like vasculitis" or other descriptions for this constellation of histopathologic features. We have been unable to distinguish cutaneous biopsies of pustular vasculitis lesions taken from patients with Behçet's disease from cutaneous biopsies taken from patients with bowel-associated dermatosis-arthritis syndrome (J. L. Jorizzo and A. R. Solomon, *unpublished data, 1985*).

Pathogenesis

The pathogenesis of lesions of bowel bypass syndrome, and, by extension, bowel-associated dermatosis-arthritis syndrome, may involve CICs, perhaps related to bacterial peptidoglycans from bowel flora (37). Indirect evidence to support a CIC-mediated pathogenesis includes positive results on *in vitro* assays (e.g., C1q binding and Raji cell assays), immunoreactant deposition in dermal blood vessels from biopsies of early cutaneous lesions, and evidence

on Braverman's histamine trap test for immunoreactant deposition (4 hr after histamine injection) and neutrophilic vascular reaction (24 hr after histamine injection) (30,37,67,77,129). Bacterial overgrowth in a blind loop of bowel or bowel diverticulum or increased access of bowel antigens to the circulation in inflammatory bowel disease could result in bowel antigen-containing CICs. These CICs could deposit in target tissues, such as the dermal vasculature and synovium. Obviously, specific studies such as isolation of bacterial peptidoglycans and other gut antigens in CICs by immunoblot techniques and the detection of these antigens in lesional tissue by immunoperoxidase or fluorescein labeling of specific antibody will be required to further support this hypothesis.

Preliminary evidence in a very small patient group also suggests that patients with bowel-associated dermatosis-arthritis syndrome have enhanced neutrophil migration. Serum from 3 patients appeared to act in a manner similar to serum from patients with Behçet's disease in its ability to enhance the migration of patient and control neutrophils (67). Obviously, confirmation in a larger patient population is required. It is possible that pustular vasculitis lesions in both Behçet's disease and bowel-associated dermatosis-arthritis syndrome may result from CIC-mediated vessel damage, with accumulation of neutrophils being promoted by a still unclassified heat-stable serum factor that enhances neutrophil migration.

Therapy

The cutaneous lesions and serum-sickness-like signs and symptoms of bowel-associated dermatosis-arthritis syndrome may be dramatically controlled by systemic corticosteroid therapy (e.g., prednisone at 1 mg/kg/day). However, the relapsing and non-life-threatening nature of the illness usually does not justify this approach. Systemic antibiotics such as tetracycline, metronidazole, or even erythromycin are beneficial (37,64). It is unclear whether these antibiotics are beneficial via reduction of overgrown bowel flora (e.g., in a blind loop) or whether there is a direct effect on neutrophil migration. Our preliminary observations did not support the latter hypothesis (67). By analogy with the pustular vasculitis of Behçet's disease, oral colchicine therapy might be beneficial. Oral thalidomide was beneficial in 1 patient whom we treated (74). In patients who have had jejunoileal bypass, restoration of normal bowel anatomy is curative (37).

OTHER NEUTROPHILIC VASCULAR DERMATOSES

Erythema Nodosum

Erythema nodosum is a distinct entity characterized by painful, inflammatory, bruise-like nodules, usually located on the anterior tibial surfaces. Serum-sickness-like signs and symptoms of fever, malaise, arthralgias, and arthritis often are associated.

The histopathology is dominated by findings in the septal panniculus (i.e., around blood vessels in the subcutaneous fat). Endothelial swelling, edema, and an angiocentric mixed infiltrate, which may be dominated by neutrophils in early lesions, are characteristic (149).

Although a pathogenesis involving CIC-mediated vessel damage has long been suspected because of the serum-sickness-like features and neutrophil-dominated histopathology, supporting evidence remains meager. Patients usually have late lesions biopsied because of the deep location and sometimes gradual evolution of lesions. The nonspecific finding of immunoreactant deposition in cutaneous blood vessels in lesions of erythema nodosum is an inconstant feature (100). Erythema nodosum may be associated with streptococcal infection, sarcoidosis, tuberculosis, and drug allergy (144). Its occurrence with inflammatory bowel disease, Behçet's disease, and bowel-associated dermatosis-arthritis syndrome is particularly relevant to this review (63,97).

Familial Mediterranean Fever

Familial Mediterranean fever is an autosomal recessive, uncommon condition. It consists of serum-sickness-like signs and symptoms (i.e., fever, polyserositis and/or polyarthritis or monoarthritis, abdominal crisis, pleurisy, and an associated inflammatory vascular dermatosis) occur-

ring in Mediterraneans as idiopathic, recurring, self-limited episodes (93,128). Amyloidosis may be associated (93).

Cutaneous manifestations may range from erysipelas-like erythemas to erythema-nodosum-like nodules to fully developed necrotizing venulitis or a polyarteritis-nodosa-like vasculitis (89). The histopathologic findings range from nonspecific perivascular inflammation to fully developed leukocytoclastic vasculitis.

Laboratory evaluation reveals that patients have peripheral blood neutrophilia and elevated erythrocyte sedimentation rates. Over half the patients tested have in vitro evidence of CICs and complement consumption (40,120). Interestingly, oral colchicine is a mainstay of treatment for patients with familial Mediterranean fever (32). The mechanism by which colchicine exerts its beneficial effect is unknown; however, it is tempting to speculate that effects on neutrophils may be important.

PYODERMA GANGRENOSUM

Pyoderma gangrenosum is an ulcerative skin disease characterized by ulcers with raised, undermined, purple borders and irregular bases. The clinical appearance is often quite characteristic, and the clinical course can be explosive. The title is a misnomer, as this is not a pyoderma. The diagnosis actually depends on the exclusion of underlying infection. Pyoderma gangrenosum has been reported to occur in association with a number of internal diseases.

Clinical Features

Lesions of pyoderma gangrenosum begin as small inflammatory pustules that may be tender. They may begin as solitary lesions, or they may occur in crops. The fully developed lesions have a characteristic appearance, with a dusky purple border that is undermined (Fig. 7). The ulcer base is irregular, with granulation material and purulent debris. Lesions heal spontaneously or with therapy to leave irregular cribriform scars. Any body site may be affected; however, lesions often demonstrate pathergy (the tendency to start or spread to sites of needle puncture or other trauma) (56). A superficial bullous variant appears to occur as a marker for myeloproliferative disorders and is also called atypical Sweet's syndrome (19,87,107).

The diagnosis of pyoderma gangrenosum is a clinical diagnosis of exclusion. Conditions to be excluded are infections (bacterial, fungal, mycobacterial, other infections), collagen vascular or vasculitic diseases (e.g., systemic lupus erythematosus, rheumatoid vasculitis, Behçet's disease, Wegener's granulomatosis), factitial dis-

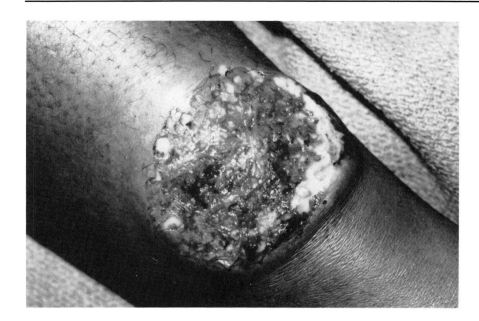

FIG. 7. A typical, fully developed, ulcerative lesion of pyoderma gangrenosum. Note the dusky, undermined border.

ease, iododerma, bromoderma, and malignancy (56). Pyoderma gangrenosum may occur with a host of internal diseases, including inflammatory bowel disease, chronic active hepatitis, polyarthritis, and myeloproliferative disorders (16). Over 50% of patients have no associated diseases (98).

Histopathology

The biopsy findings from lesions of pyoderma gangrenosum may be supportive of the diagnosis, but are nondiagnostic. Early lesions demonstrate epidermal necrosis, dermal edema, and a mixed perivascular infiltrate with prominent neutrophilia. Older lesions show more epidermal acanthosis and a more mononuclear cell infiltrate. There is controversy as to the degree of vessel damage present. Early lesions may resemble a neutrophilic vascular reaction with endothelial swelling (56). The lesions in bullous pyoderma gangrenosum are particularly likely to show this histology. The fully developed leukocytoclastic vasculitis seen in some lesions may be an epiphenomenon secondary to lesion ulceration or may be primary.

Pathogenesis

The pathogenesis of pyoderma gangrenosum remains unknown. The detection of a neutrophilic vascular reaction in early lesions, the nonspecific finding of immunoreactants in dermal blood vessels (12), the similarity of bullous pyoderma gangrenosum to Sweet's syndrome, and the association of pyoderma gangrenosum with diseases associated with CICs, such as inflammatory bowel disease and chronic active hepatitis, would prompt speculation that pyoderma gangrenosum might represent a localized CIC-mediated vasculopathy. Hard evidence, such as detection of CICs and specific antigen in serum and the demonstration of specific antigen associated with immunoreactant deposition in cutaneous vasculature or complement split products, is completely lacking. The disease process tends to be chronic, and patients are promptly treated with systemic corticosteroids, which are factors that have impeded the study of this disease. Investigations of cellular immunity, circulatory immunoglobulins, and CICs by *in vitro* assays have not yielded any consistent abnormalities (56).

Although neutrophil function has been studied in several small series of patients, results are contradictory. One patient demonstrated impaired neutrophil migration by Boyden chamber assessment (56); another patient showed decreased neutrophil phagocytosis, with normal killing; 2 brothers have been reported with deficient random motility and phagocytosis, but normal chemotaxis (56). It has been suggested that impaired neutrophil chemotaxis may be an epiphenomenon related to increased serum IgA in patients with long-standing neutrophilic dermatoses (56). It is interesting that one group reported a "streaking leukocyte factor" in serum from patients with pyoderma gangrenosum that enhanced neutrophil and monocyte migration *in vitro* (56). Although this last finding is similar to our findings in the pustular vasculitis of Behçet's disease and possibly bowel-associated dermatosis-arthritis syndrome and that seen in 1 patient with Sweet's syndrome, conclusions as to the pathogenic significance of this finding remain premature and speculative.

Therapy

Topical therapy is important in pyoderma gangrenosum as a means of limiting bacterial colonization. Bacterial overgrowth may, by a pathergy-related mechanism, cause the local lesions to expand. Intralesional corticosteroids may be of benefit in mild localized cases. Systemic therapy with corticosteroids (e.g., prednisone at 1 mg/kg/day) is required for control of rapidly expanding lesions. Higher doses may be required to achieve control in resistant cases (56). Rebound after tapering systemic therapy too rapidly is a very real concern. Megadose "steroid pulse" therapy may prove to have a role in patients with resistant disease, but its use is limited because of concern regarding cardiac arrhythmias (59). Adjunctive systemic therapies that appear to be efficacious in treating pyoderma gangrenosum include azathioprine (100–200 mg/day) (15), cyclophosphamide (100–200 mg/day) (26), dapsone (100–200 mg/day), and sulfapyridine (500–1,000 mg three times daily) (86).

SUMMARY

Four different models of neutrophilic dermatosis have been mentioned: psoriasiform dermatoses, autoimmune bullous dermatosis, vessel-based neutrophilic dermatoses, and pyoderma gangrenosum. Only the last two models were reviewed in detail. The diagnostic histopathologic feature of the psoriasiform dermatoses (e.g., psoriasis, Reiter's syndrome) is the exocytosis of neutrophils into the proliferating epidermis. Future investigations may focus on pharmacologic or immunologic mediators that may direct this migration. Also, factors relating to the neutrophils themselves that might predispose to this striking movement into the epidermis must be clarified.

The autoimmune bullous dermatoses (e.g., pemphigus group, bullous pemphigoid, dermatitis herpetiformis) have been well studied immunologically. The first two diseases may occur as modifications of a type II immunologic reaction. Pemphigus vulgaris may be produced in an animal model in the absence of complement. The role of the neutrophil and signals for accumulation of neutrophils without complement await clarification in this disease. Bullous pemphigoid may be a disease in which complement is activated by immunoglobulin binding to target antigen (i.e., bullous pemphigoid antigen in the lamina lucida of the dermal-epidermal junction), with complement activation leading to neutrophil chemotaxis to the site of target tissue injury. Dermatitis herpetiformis appears to be a disease in which IgA-containing CICs activate complement via the alternative pathway. Neutrophils are attracted to the dermal papillae, with subsequent tissue damage and blister formation at this site.

The model for CIC-mediated, neutrophil-induced, vessel-based disease is necrotizing venulitis (leukocytoclastic vasculitis). This disease appears to be a model for type III immune injury in the skin. Sweet's syndrome and the pustular vasculitis of Behçet's disease and bowel-associated dermatosis-arthritis syndrome are characterized by less severe vessel damage than is leukocytoclastic vasculitis (i.e., neutrophilic vascular reaction, with no fibrinoid necrosis of blood vessel walls). However, there may be more accumulation of neutrophils than in leukocytoclastic vasculitis, producing clinical pustular vasculitic lesions rather than simple palpable purpura. More research is needed to clearly establish a primary role for CICs in producing these vascular reactions. The preliminary finding of a heat-stable serum factor that enhances neutrophil migration in each of these reactions is provocative and may eventually help to clarify the pustular nature of these lesions. The nature of this factor and its mechanism of action are totally unknown, although there may be a relationship to neutrophil adherence.

Pyoderma gangrenosum remains a particularly enigmatic neutrophilic dermatosis. The overlap between the superficial bullous variant of pyoderma gangrenosum and atypical Sweet's syndrome in patients with myeloproliferative disease, the detection of a neutrophilic vascular reaction in early lesions, and the finding of a "neutrophil streaking factor" in 1 patient are very tentative but provocative suggestions that pyoderma gangrenosum might represent a chronic localized variant of the aforementioned neutrophilic vessel-based dermatoses.

REFERENCES

1. Abramson, J. S., Mills, E. L., Sawyer, M. K., Regalmann, W. R., Nelson, J. D., and Quie, P. G. (1981): Recurrent infections and delayed separation of the umbilical cord in an infant with abnormal phagocytic cell locomotion and oxidative response during partial phagocytosis. *J. Pediatr.*, 99:887–894.
2. Anderson, D. C., Schmalstieg, F. C., Kohl, S., Hughes, B. J., Tosi, M. F., Buffone, G. J., Dickey, W. D., Abramson, J. S., Boxer, L. A., Brinkley, B. R., Hollers, T. M., and Smith, C. W. (1984): Abnormalities of polymorphonuclear leukocyte function associated with a heritable deficiency of high molecular weight surface glycoprotein (GP138): Common relationships to diminished cell adherence. *J. Clin. Invest.*, 74:536–551.
3. Anhalt, G. J., Bahn, C. F., Labib, R. S., Voorhees, J. J., Sugar, A., and Diaz, L. A. (1981): Pathogenic effects of bullous pemphigoid autoantibodies on rabbit corneal epithelium. *J. Clin. Invest.*, 68:1097–1101.
4. Antoon, J. W., and Miller, R. L. (1980): Aphthous ulcers: A review of the literature on etiology, pathogenesis, diagnosis, and treatment. *J.A.D.A.*, 101:803–808.

5. Apted, J. H. (1984): Sweet's syndrome (acute febrile neutrophilic dermatosis) associated with multiple myeloma. *Australas. J. Dermatol.,* 25:15–17.

6. Aram, H. (1984): Acute febrile neutrophilic dermatosis (Sweet's syndrome): Response to dapsone. *Arch. Dermatol.,* 120:245–247.

7. Arnaout, M. A., Pitt, J., Cohen, H. J., Melamed, J., Rosen, F. S., and Colten, H. R. (1982): Deficiency of a granulocyte-membrane glycoprotein (gp-150) in a boy with recurrent bacterial infections. *N. Engl. J. Med.,* 306:693–699.

8. Azizi, E., and Fisher, B. K. (1976): Cutaneous manifestations of familial Mediterranean fever. *Arch. Dermatol.,* 112:364–366.

9. Baumal, A., and Kantor, I. (1961): Urticaria and dermographism with Mediterranean fever: Report of a case. *Arch. Dermatol.,* 84:630–632.

10. Bechtel, M. A., and Callen, J. P. (1981): Acute febrile neutrophilic dermatosis: Sweet's syndrome. *Arch. Dermatol.,* 117:664–666.

11. Benton, E. C., Rutherford, D., and Hunter, J. A. (1985): Sweet's syndrome and pyoderma gangrenosum associated with ulcerative colitis. *Acta. Derm. Venereol.,* 65:77–80.

12. Blaustein, A., Moreno, A., Noguera, J., and de Moragas, J. M. (1985): Septal granulomatous panniculitis in Sweet's syndrome. *Arch. Dermatol.,* 121:785–788.

13. Borel, J. F. (1973): Effect of some drugs on the chemotaxis of rabbit neutrophils *in vitro. Experimentia,* 27:676–678.

14. Braverman, I. M., and Yen, A. (1975): Demonstration of immune complexes in spontaneous and histamine-induced lesions and in normal skin of patients with leukocytoclastic angiitis. *J. Invest. Dermatol.,* 64:105–112.

15. Byrne, J. P. H., Hewitt, M., and Summerly, R. (1976): Pyoderma gangrenosum associated with active chronic hepatitis. *Arch. Dermatol.,* 112:1297–1301.

16. Callen, J. P., and Taylor, W. B. (1978): Pyoderma gangrenosum: A literature review. *Cutis,* 21:61–64.

17. Camp, R. D. R., Coutts, A. A., Greaves, M. W., Kay, A. B., and Walport, M. J. (1983): Responses of human skin to intradermal injection of leukotrienes C4, D4, and B4. *Br. J. Pharmacol.,* 80:497–502.

18. Campbell, J. M., Hunt, T. K., Karam, J. H., and Forsham, P. H. (1977): Jejunoilial bypass as a treatment of morbid obesity. *Arch. Intern. Med.,* 137:602–610.

19. Caughman, W., Stern, R., and Haynes, H. (1983): Neutrophilic dermatosis of myeloproliferative disorders: Atypical forms of pyoderma gangrenosum and Sweet's syndrome associated with myeloproliferative disorders. *J. Am. Acad. Dermatol.,* 9:751–758.

20. Chajek, T., and Fainaru, M. (1975): Behçet's disease: Report of 41 cases and review of the literature. *Medicine (Baltimore),* 54:179–196.

21. Colvard, D. M., Robertson, D. M., and O'Duffy, J. D. (1977): The ocular manifestations of Behçet's disease. *Arch. Ophthalmol.,* 95:1813–1817.

22. Cooper, P. H., Freierson, H. D., and Green, K. E. (1983): Subcutaneous neutrophilic infiltrates in acute febrile neutrophilic dermatosis. *Arch. Dermatol.,* 119:610–611.

23. Cooper, P. H., Innes, D. J., and Green, K. E. (1983): Acute febrile neutrophilic dermatosis and myeloproliferative disorders. *Cancer,* 51:1518–1526.

24. Cormane, R. H. (1981): Immunopathology of psoriasis. *Arch. Dermatol. Res.,* 270:201–215.

25. Cram, D. L. (1981): Psoriasis: Current advances in etiology and treatment. *J. Am. Acad. Dermatol.,* 4:1–14.

26. Crawford, S. E., Sherman, R., and Favara, B. (1957): Pyoderma gangrenosum with response to cyclophosphamide therapy. *J. Pediatr.,* 71:255–258.

27. Crow, K. D., Kerdel-Vegas, F., and Rook, A. (1969): Acute febrile neutrophilic dermatosis: Sweet's syndrome. *Dermatologica,* 139:123–134.

28. Crowley, C. A., Curnutte, J. T., Rosin, R. E., Andre-Schwarz, J., Gallin, J. I., Klempner, J. I., Synderman, R., Southwide, R. S., Stossel, T. P., and Babior, B. M. (1980): An inherited abnormality

of neutrophil adhesion: Its genetic transmission and its association with a missing protein. *N. Engl. J. Med.,* 302:1163–1168.

29. Dambuyant, C., and Thivolet, J. (1981): Antigenic similarities within circulating immune complexes in patients suffering from cutaneous vasculitis. *Dermatologica,* 162:429–437.

30. Dicken, C. H., and Sheehafer, J. R. (1979): Bowel bypass syndrome. *Arch. Dermatol.,* 115:837–839.

31. Dicken, C. H. (1984): Bowel-associated dermatosis-arthritis syndrome: Bowel bypass syndrome without bowel bypass. *Mayo Clin. Proc.,* 59:43–46.

32. Dinarello, C. A., Wolff, S. M., Goldfinger, S. E., Dale, D., and Arling, W. (1974): Colchicine therapy for familial Mediterranean fever: A double-blind trial. *N. Engl. J. Med.,* 291:934–937.

33. Djawari, D., Hornstein, O. P., and Schotiz, J. (1981): Enhancement of granulocyte chemotaxis in Behçet's disease. *Arch. Dermatol. Res.,* 270:81–88.

34. Drenick, E. J., Ament, M. R., Finegold, S. M., Corrodi, P., and Passaro, E. (1976): Bypass enteropathy: Intestinal and systemic manifestations following small bowel bypass. *J.A.M.A.,* 236:269–272.

35. Driban, N. E., and Alvarez, M. A. (1984): Oral manifestations of Sweet's syndrome. *Dermatologica,* 169:102–103.

36. Ekenstam, E. A., and Callen, J. P. (1984): Cutaneous leukocytoclastic vasculitis: Clinical and laboratory features of 82 patients seen in private practice. *Arch. Dermatol.,* 120:484–489.

37. Ely, P. H. (1980): The bowel bypass syndrome: A response to bacterial peptidoglycans. *J. Am. Head Dermatol.,* 2:473–487.

38. Evans, S., and Evans, C. C. (1971): Acute febrile neutrophilic dermatosis: Two cases. *Dermatologica,* 193:153–159.

39. Fauci, A. S., Haynes, B. F., and Katz, P. (1978): The spectrum of vasculitis: Clinical, pathologic, immunologic and therapeutic considerations. *Ann. Intern. Med.,* 89:660–676.

40. Flatau, E., Kohn, D., Schiller, D., Lurie, M., and Levy, E. (1982): Schönlein-Henoch syndrome in patients with familial Mediterranean fever. *Arthritis Rheum.,* 25:42–47.

41. Gamble, C. N., Wiesner, K. B., Shapiro, E. F., and Boyer, W. J. (1979): The immune complex pathogenesis of glomerulonephritis and pulmonary vasculitis in Behçet's disease. *Am. J. Med.,* 66:1031–1039.

42. Gammon, W., Lewis, D., Carol, J., Sams, W. M., Jr., and Wheeler, C. E. (1980): Pemphigoid antibody mediated attachment of peripheral blood leukocytes at the dermal-epidermal junction of human skin. *J. Invest. Dermatol.,* 75:334–339.

43. Gilliam, J. N., and Smiley, J. D. (1976): Cutaneous necrotizing vasculitis and related disorders. *Ann. Allergy,* 37:328–329.

44. Goette, D. K. (1985): Sweet's syndrome in subacute cutaneous lupus erythematosus. *Arch. Dermatol.,* 121:789–791.

45. Goldman, J. A., Casey, H. L., Davidson, E. D., Hersh, T., and Pirozzi, D. (1979): Vasculitis associated with intestinal bypass surgery. *Arch. Dermatol.,* 115:725–727.

46. Goldstein, I., Hoffstein, S., Gallin, J., and Weissman, G. (1973): Mechanisms of lysosomal enzyme release from human leukocytes: Microtubule assembly and membrane fusion induced by a component. *Proc. Natl. Acad. Sci. USA,* 70:2916–2920.

47. Goltz, R. W. (1962): Cutaneous manifestations of allergic angiitis. *Lancet,* 82:219–222.

48. Gordon, M., and Johnson, W. C. (1967): Histopathology and histochemistry of psoriasis. *Arch. Dermatol.,* 95:402–407.

49. Gower, R. G., Sams, W. M., Jr., Thorne, E. G., Kohler, P. F., and Claman, H. N. (1977): Leukocytoclastic vasculitis: Sequential appearance of immunoreactants and cellular changes in serial biopses. *J. Invest. Dermatol.,* 69:477–484.

50. Greer, K. W., Pruitt, J. L., and Bishop, G. F. (1975): Acute febrile neutrophilic dermatosis (Sweet's syndrome). *Arch. Dermatol.,* 111:1461–1463.

51. Grenier, P., Bletry, O., Gornud, F., Godeau, S., and Nahum, H. (1981): Pulmonary involvement in Behçet's disease. *A.J.K.,* 137:565–569.

52. Gunawardena, D. A., Gunawardena, K. A., Ratanayka, R. S., and

Vasantnanathan, N. S. (1975): The clinical spectrum of Sweet's syndrome (acute febrile neutrophilic dermatosis): A report of eighteen cases. *Br. J. Dermatol.*, 92:363–373.

53. Gupta, R. C., O'Duffy, J. D., McDuffie, F. C., Meurer, M., and Jordon, R. E. (1973): Circulatory immune complexes in active Behçet's disease. *Clin. Exp. Immunol.*, 34:213–218.

54. Hansen, D. D., Lopez, D. A., and Jenson, K. K. (1978): Pustulosis associated with bypass surgery for obesity: A dermato-arthritis syndrome. *J. Assoc. Milit. Dermatol.*, 4:32–37.

55. Harary, A. M. (1983): Sweet's syndrome associated with rheumatoid arthritis. *Arch. Intern. Med.*, 143:1993–1995.

56. Hickman, J. G. (1983): Pyoderma gangrenosum. *Clin. Dermatol.*, 1:102–113.

57. Hoffman, G. S. (1977): Treatment of Sweet's syndrome (acute febrile neutrophilic dermatosis) with indomethacin. *J. Rheumatol.*, 4:201–206.

58. Horio, T., Inamura, S., Danno, K., Furukawa, F., and Ofuji, S. (1980): Treatment of acute neutrophilic dermatosis (Sweet's syndrome) with potassium iodide. *Dermatologica*, 160:341–347.

59. Johnson, R. B., and Lazarus, G. S. (1982): Pulse therapy: Therapeutic efficacy in the treatment of pyoderma gangrenosum. *Arch. Dermatol.*, 118:76–84.

60. Jordon, R. E., Trifthauser, C. T., and Schroeter, A. L. (1971): Direct immunofluorescent studies of pemphigus and bullous pemphigoid. *Arch. Dermatol.*, 103:486–491.

61. Jordon, R. E., and McDuffie, F. C. (1976): Serum and blister fluid anticomplementary activity in pemphigus and bullous pemphigoid: Sucrose density gradient studies. *Proc. Soc. Exp. Biol. Med.*, 151:594–598.

62. Jorizzo, J. L. (1983): Pustular vasculitis: An emerging disease concept. *J. Am. Acad. Dermatol.*, 9:160–162.

63. Jorizzo, J. L. (1983): Pustular vasculitis: Common ground among Behçet's, bowel bypass, and disseminated gonorrhea syndromes. *Dermatol. Clin.*, 1:607–613.

64. Jorizzo, J. L., Apisarnthanarax, P., Subrt, P., Hebert, A. A., Henry, J. C., Raimer, S. S., Dinehart, S. M., and Reinarz, J. A. (1983): Bowel-bypass syndrome without bowel bypass: Bowel-associated dermatosis-arthritis syndrome. *Arch. Intern. Med.*, 143:457–461.

65. Jorizzo, J. L., Daniels, J. C., and Apisarnthanarax, P. (1983): Histamine-triggered localized vasculitis in patients with seropositive rheumatoid arthritis. *J. Am. Acad. Dermatol.*, 9:845–851.

66. Jorizzo, J. L., Hudson, R. D., Schmalstieg, F. C., Daniels, J. C., Apisarnthanarax, P., Henry, J. C., Gonzalez, E. B., Ichikawa, Y., and Cavallo, T. (1984): Behçet's syndrome: Immune regulation, circulating immune complexes, neutrophil migration, and colchicine therapy. *J. Am. Acad. Dermatol.*, 10:205–214.

67. Jorizzo, J. L., Schmalstieg, F. C., Dinehart, S. M., Daniels, J. C., Cavallo, T., Apisarnthanarax, P., Rudloff, H. B., and Gonzalez, E. B. (1984): Bowel-associated dermatosis-arthritis syndrome: Immune complex-mediated vessel damage and increased neutrophil migration. *Arch. Intern. Med.*, 144:738–740.

68. Jorizzo, J. L. (1985): Classification of urticaria and reactive inflammatory vascular dermatoses. *Dermatol. Clin.*, 3:3–11.

69. Jorizzo, J., Solomon, A. R., and Cavallo, T. (1985): Behçet's syndrome: Immunopathologic and histopathologic assessment of pathergy lesions is useful in diagnosis and follow-up. *Arch. Pathol. Lab. Med.*, 109:747–751.

70. Jorizzo, J. L., Taylor, R. S., Schmalstieg, F. C., Solomon, A. R., Daniels, J. C., Rudloff, H. E., and Cavallo, T. (1985): Complex aphthosis: A forme fruste of Behçet's syndrome? *J. Am. Acad. Dermatol.*, 13:80–84.

71. Jorizzo, J. L., Schmalstieg, F. C., Solomon, A. R., Cavallo, T., Taylor, R. S., Rudloff, H. B., Schmalstieg, E. J., and Daniels, J. C. (1986): Thalidomide effects in Behçet's syndrome and pustular vasculitis. *Arch. Intern. Med.*, 146:878–881.

72. Jorizzo, J. L., McNelly, M. C., Baughn, R. B., Solomon, A. R., Cavallo, T., and Smith, F. B. (1986): Circulatory immune complexes play a role in human secondary syphilis. *J. Infect. Dis.*, 153:1014–1022.

73. Jorizzo, J. L. (1986): Behçet's disease: An update based on the

1985 International Conference in London, England. *Arch. Dermatol.*, 122:556–558.

74. Jorizzo, J. L., Schmalstieg, F. C., Solomon, A. R., Taylor, R. S., and Cavallo, T. (1986): Studies of circulatory immune complexes, neutrophils, and effects of oral colchicine or thalidomide in Behçet's disease. In: *Recent Advances in Behçet's Disease*, edited by T. Lehner and C. G. Barnes, pp. 89–95. Royal Society of Medicine Press, London.

75. Kaplan, S. S., Wechsler, H. L., Basford, R. E., Zdziarski, U. E., and Kuhns, D. B. (1985): Increased plasma chemoattractant in Sweet's syndrome. *J. Am. Acad. Dermatol.*, 12:1013–1021.

76. Katz, S. I., Hall, R. P., Lawley, T. J., and Stober, W. (1980): Dermatitis herpetiformis: The skin and the gut. *Ann. Intern. Med.*, 93:857–874.

77. Kennedy, C. (1981): The spectrum of inflammatory skin disease following jejuno-ileal bypass for morbid obesity. *Br. J. Dermatol.*, 105:425–435.

78. Krolikowski, F. J., Reuter, K., and Shultis, E. W. (1985): Acute febrile neutrophilic dermatosis (Sweet's syndrome) associated with lymphoma. *Hum. Pathol.*, 16:520–522.

79. Lakhanpal, S., Tani, K., Lie, J. T., Katoh, K., Ishigatsubo, Y., and Ohokubo, T. (1985): Pathologic features of Behçet's syndrome: A review of Japanese autopsy registry data. *Hum. Pathol.*, 16:790–795.

80. Lazarus, G. S., Daniels, J. R., Lian, J., and Burleigh, M. C. (1972): Role of granulocyte collagenase in collagen degradation. *Am. J. Pathol.*, 68:565–578.

81. Lehrer, R. I. (1973): Effects of colchicine and chloramphenicol of the oxidative metabolism and phagocytic activity of human neutrophils. *J. Infect. Dis.*, 127:40–48.

82. Lehner, T., Almeida, J. D., and Levinsky, R. J. (1978): Damaged membrane fragments and immune complexes in the blood of patients with Behçet's syndrome. *Clin. Exp. Immunol.*, 34:206–212.

83. Lehner, T., Welshi, K., and Batchelor, J. R. (1981): Relationship of HLA phenotype to immunoglobulin class present in immune complexes from patients with Behçet's syndrome. *Tissue Antigens*, 17:357–361.

84. Levin, D. L., Esterly, M. B., Herman, J. J., and Boxall, L. B. H. (1981): The Sweet syndrome in children. *J. Pediatr.*, 99:73–78.

85. Levinsky, R. J., and Lehner, T. (1978): Circulating soluble immune complexes in recurrent oral ulceration and Behçet's syndrome. *Clin. Exp. Immunol.*, 32:192–198.

86. Lorincz, A. L., and Pearson, R. W. (1962): Sulfapyridine and sulfone type drugs in dermatology. *Arch. Dermatol.*, 85:42–56.

87. Lynch, P. J. (1982): Bullous pyoderma gangrenosum. *Cutis*, 30:496–497.

88. MacGregor, R. R. (1976): The effect of antiinflammatory agents and inflammation on granulocyte adherence: Evidence for regulatory plasma factors. *Am. J. Med.*, 61:597–607.

89. Maekawa, Y., Kageshita, T., and Nagata, T. (1984): A case of acute febrile neutrophilic dermatosis (Sweet's syndrome): A demonstration of IgM and C_3 deposits on the vessel walls in involved skin. *J. Dermatol.*, 11:560–564.

90. Malawista, S. E. (1968): Colchicine: A common mechanism for its anti-inflammatory and antimitotic effects. *Arthritis Rheum.*, 11:191–197.

91. McNeely, M. C., Jorizzo, J. L., Solomon, A. B., Smith, E. B., Cavallo, T., and Sanchez, R. L. (1986): Cutaneous secondary syphilis: Preliminary immunohistopathologic support for a role for immune complexes in lesion pathogenesis. *J. Am. Acad. Dermatol.*, 14:564–571.

92. McNeely, M. C., Jorizzo, J. L., Solomon, A. R., Schmalstieg, F. C., and Cavallo, T. (1986): Primary idiopathic cutaneous pustular vasculitis. *J. Am. Acad. Dermatol.*, 14:939–944.

93. Meyerhoff, J. (1980): Familial Mediterranean fever: Report of a large family, review of the literature, and discussion of the frequency of amyloidosis. *Medicine (Baltimore)*, 59:66–77.

94. Miyachi, Y., Taniguchi, S., Ozaki, M., and Horio, T. (1981): Colchicine in the treatment of the cutaneous manifestations of Behçet's disease. *Br. J. Dermatol.*, 104:67–69.

95. Mizushima, Y., Matsumura, N., and Mori, M. (1979): Chemotaxis of leukocytes and colchicine treatment in Behçet's disease. *J. Rheumatol.*, 6:108–110.

96. Muller, W., and Lehner, T. (1982): Quantitative electron microscopical analysis of leukocyte infiltration in oral ulcers of Behçet's syndrome. *Br. J. Dermatol.*, 106:535–544.

97. Nazarro, P. (1966): Cutaneous manifestations of Behçet's disease, In: *International Symposium on Behçet's Disease*, edited by M. Monacelli and P. Nazarro, pp. 15–41. S. Karger, Basel.

98. Newell, L. M., and Malkinson, F. D. (1982): Pyoderma gangrenosum. *Arch. Dermatol.*, 118:769–775.

99. Nguyen, K. Q., Hurst, C. G., Pierson, D. L., and Rodman, O. G. (1983): Sweet's syndrome and ovarian carcinoma. *Cutis*, 32:152–154.

100. Niemi, K. M., Forstrom, L., Hannuksela, M., Mustakallio, K. K., and Salo, O. P. (1977): Nodules on the legs. *Acta Derm. Venereol.*, 57:145–154.

101. Nunzi, E., Covato, F., Dallegri, F., Patrone, F., and Cormane, R. M. (1981): Immunopathological studies on a case of Sweet's syndrome. *Dermatologica*, 163:393–400.

102. O'Duffy, J. D., and Goldstein, N. P. (1976): Neurologic involvement in seven patients with Behçet's disease. *Am. J. Med.*, 61:170–178.

103. O'Duffy, J. D. (1981): Behçet's disease. In: *Textbook of Rheumatology, Vol. 2*, edited by W. N. Kelly, E. D. Harris, Jr., S. Ruddy, et al. W. B. Saunders, Philadelphia.

104. Oseroff, A. R., Adler, L., Malloy, K., Soltani, K., and Medenica, M. (1981): Neutrophil abnormalities in a patient with Sweet's syndrome. *J. Invest. Dermatol.*, 76:331.

105. Palumbo, P. J., Ward, L. E., Sauer, W. G., and Scudamore, H. H. (1973): Musculoskeletal manifestations of inflammatory bowel disease: Ulcerative and granulomatous colitis and ulcerative proctitis. *Mayo Clin. Proc.*, 48:411–416.

106. Parish, W. E. (1980): Microbial antigens in vasculitis. In: *Vasculitis*, edited by K. Wolff, and R. K. Winkelmann, pp. 129–150. W. B. Saunders Philadelphia.

107. Perry, H. O., and Winkelmann, R. K. (1972): Bullous pyoderma gangrenosum and leukemia. *Arch. Dermatol.*, 106:901–905.

108. Petrozzi, J. W., and Warthan, T. L. (1976): Sweet's syndrome: Unique local response to streptococcal antigen. *Cutis*, 17:267–272.

109. Pinkus, H., and Mehregan, A. H. (1966): The primary histologic lesions of seborrheic dermatitis and psoriasis. *J. Invest. Dermatol.*, 46:109–116.

110. Popp, J. W., Jr., Harrist, T. J., Dienstag, J. L., Bahan, A. K., Wands, J. R., Lamont, J. T., and Mihm, M. C. (1981): Cutaneous vasculitis associated with acute and chronic hepatitis. *Arch. Intern. Med.*, 141:623–629.

111. Prystowsky, S. D., Fye, K. H., Goette, K. D., and Daniels, T. E. (1978): Acute febrile neutrophilic dermatosis associated with Sjögren's syndrome. *Arch. Dermatol.*, 114:1234–1235.

112. Ragaz, A., and Ackerman, A. B. (1979): Evolution, maturation, and regression of lesions of psoriasis. *Am. J. Dermatopathol.*, 1:119–214.

113. Raimer, S. S., and Duncan, W. C. (1978): Febrile neutrophilic dermatosis in acute myelogenous leukemia. *Arch. Dermatol.*, 114:413–414.

114. Rogers, R. S., III (1977): Recurrent aphthous stomatitis: Clinical characteristics and evidence for an immunopathogenesis. *J. Invest. Dermatol.*, 69:499–509.

115. Rogers, R. S., III, and O'Duffy, J. D. (1981): Behçet's syndrome and treatment with colchicine. *J. Am. Acad. Dermatol.*, 4:483–484.

116. Ruiter, M., and Molenaar, I. (1970): Ultrastructural changes in arteriolitis (vasculitis) allergica cutis superficialis. *Br. J. Dermatol.*, 83:14–26.

117. Sams, W. M., Jr., Thorne, E. G., Small, P., Mass, M. F., McIntosh, R. M., and Stanford, R. E. (1976): Leukocytoclastic vasculitis. *Arch. Dermatol.*, 112:219–226.

118. Sams, W. M., Jr. (1980): Models of necrotizing vasculitis. In: *Vasculitis*, edited by K. Wolff and R. K. Winkelmann, pp. 108–116. W. B. Saunders, Philadelphia.

119. Sams, W. M., Jr. (1980): Necrotizing vasculitis. *J. Am. Acad. Dermatol.*, 3:1–13.

120. Savi, M., Asinari, G., Gaudiano, V., Olivetti, G., and Neri, T. M. (1978): Unusual immunologic findings in familial Mediterranean fever. *Arch. Intern. Med.*, 138:644–645.

121. Schroeter, A. L., and Su, W. P. D. (1980): The vasculitis of pyoderma gangrenosum: A dermatopathologic and immunopathologic study. *Arch. Dermatol.*, 116:1388.

122. Shapiro, L., Baraf, C. S., and Rickhermier, L. L. (1971): Sweet's syndrome (acute febrile neutrophilic dermatosis): Report of a case. *Arch. Dermatol.*, 103:81–84.

123. Shagrin, J. W., Frame, B., and Duncan, H. (1971): Polyarthritis in obese patients with intestinal bypass. *Ann. Intern. Med.*, 75:377–380.

124. Shelley, W. B., and Kirschbaum, J. (1961): Generalized pustular psoriasis. *Arch. Dermatol.*, 84:73–78.

125. Singer, K. H., Sawka, N. J., Samowitz, H. R., and Lazarus, G. S. (1980): Proteinase activation: Mechanism for cellular dyshesion in pemphigus. *J. Invest. Dermatol.*, 74:363–367.

126. Sneddon, J. B., and Wilkinson, D. S. (1979): Subcorneal pustular dermatosis. *Br. J. Dermatol.*, 100:61–68.

127. Sobel, J. D., Haim, S., Obedeanu, N., Meshulam, T., and Merzbach, D. (1977): Polymorphonuclear leukocyte function in Behçet's disease. *J. Clin. Pathol.*, 30:250–253.

128. Sohar, E., Gafni, J., Pras, M., and Hiller, H. (1967): Familial Mediterranean fever: A survey of 470 cases and review of the literature. *Am. J. Med.*, 43:227–253.

129. Stein, H. B., Schlappner, O. L. A., Boyko, W., Gourlay, R. H., and Neeve, L. E. (1982): The intestinal bypass arthritis-dermatitis syndrome. *Arthritis Rheum.*, 24:684–690.

130. Storer, J. S., Nesbitt, L. T., Galen, W. K., and DeLeo, V. A. (1983): Sweet's syndrome. *Int. J. Dermatol.*, 22:8–12.

131. Sweet, R. D. (1964): An acute febrile neutrophilic dermatosis. *Br. J. Dermatol.*, 76:349–356.

132. Sweet, R. D. (1979): Acute febrile neutrophilic dermatosis, 1978. *Br. J. Dermatol.*, 100:93–99.

133. Tagami, H., and Ofuji, S. (1976): Leukotactic properties of soluble substance in psoriatic scales. *Br. J. Dermatol.*, 95:1–8.

134. Takahashi, Y., Patel, H. P., Labib, R. S., Diaz, L. A., and Anhalt, G. J. (1985): Experimentally induced pemphigus vulgaris in neonatal BALB/c mice: A time-course study of clinical, immunologic, ultrastructural, and cytochemical changes. *J. Invest. Dermatol.*, 84:41–46.

135. Takeuchi, A., Kobayashi, K., Mori, M., and Mizushima, Y. (1981): The mechanism of hyperchemotaxis in Behçet's disease. *J. Rheumatol.*, 8:40–44.

136. Tappeimer, G., Jordon, R. E., and Wolff, K. (1980): Circulating immune complexes in necrotizing vasculitis. In: *Vasculitis*, edited by K. Wolff and R. K. Winkelmann, pp. 68–75. W. B. Saunders, Philadelphia.

137. Truelove, S. C., and Morris-Owen, R. M. (1958): Treatment of aphthous ulceration of the month. *Br. Med. J.*, 1:603–607.

138. Valerius, N. H. (1978): *In vitro* effects of colchicine in neutrophil granulocyte locomotion. *Acta Pathol. Microbiol. Scand.*, 86:149–154.

139. Valesini, G., Picardo, M., Pastore, R., and Pivetti, P. (1981): Circulating immune complexes in Behçet's syndrome: Purification, characterization and cross-reactivity studies. *Clin. Exp. Immunol.*, 44:522–527.

140. Van Scott, E. J., and Ekel, T. W. (1963): Kinetics of hyperplasia in psoriasis. *Arch. Dermatol.*, 88:373–381.

141. Voorhees, J. J. (1983): Leukotrienes and other lipoxygenesis products in the pathogenesis and therapy of psoriasis and other dermatosis. *Arch. Dermatol.*, 119:541–547.

142. Wagoner, G., Luckasen, J. R., and Goltz, R. W. (1976): Mucous membrane involvement in generalized pustular psoriasis. *Arch. Dermatol.*, 112:1010–1014.

143. Weinberger, H. W., Ropes, M. W., Kulka, J. P., and Bauer, W. (1962): Reiter's syndrome: Clinical and pathologic observations. *Medicine (Baltimore)*, 41:35–91.

144. White, J. W. (1985): Erythema nodosum. *Dermatol. Clin.,* 3:119–127.

145. Whited, S. C., and Gallin, J. I. (1980): Neutrophil chemotaxis. *Int. J. Dermatol.,* 19:130–138.

146. Wilkens, R. F., Arnett, F. C., Bitter, T., Calin, A., Fisher, L., Ford, D. I. C., Good, A. E., and Masi, A. J. (1981): Reiter's syndrome: Evaluation of preliminary criteria for definite disease. *Arthritis Rheum.,* 24:844–849.

147. Williams, B. D., and Lehner, T. (1977): Immune complexes in Behçet's syndrome and recurrent oral ulceration. *Br. Med. J.,* 1:1387–1389.

148. Wills, C. E., Jr. (1972): Small bowel bypass for obesity: A discussion of four different approaches. *J. Med. Assoc. Ga.,* 61:322–328.

149. Winkelmann, R. K., and Forstrom, L. (1975): New observations in the histopathology of erythema nodosum. *J. Invest. Dermatol.,* 65:441–446.

150. Winkelmann, R. K., and Ditto, W. B. (1964): Cutaneous and visceral syndromes of necrotizing or "allergic" angiitis: A study of 38 cases. *Medicine (Baltimore),* 43:59–89.

151. Wolf, K., and Winkelmann, R. K. (editors) (1980): *Vasculitis.* W. B. Saunders, Philadelphia.

152. Wolff, H. H., Maciejewski, W., Scherer, R., and Braun-Falco, O. (1978): Immunoelectron microscopic examination of early lesions in histamine induced immune complex vasculitis in man. *Br. J. Dermatol.,* 99:13–24.

153. Wong, E., Camp, R. D., and Greaves, M. W. (1985): The responses of normal and psoriatic skin to single and multiple topical applications of leukotriene B_4. *J. Invest. Dermatol.,* 84:421–423.

154. Yim, C. W., and White, R. H. (1985): Behçet's syndrome in a family with inflammatory bowel disease. *Arch. Intern. Med.,* 145:1047–1050.

Inflammation: Basic Principles and Clinical Correlates.
Edited by J. I. Gallin, I. M. Goldstein, and R. Snyderman.
Raven Press, Ltd., New York © 1988.

CHAPTER 44

Emphysema: Proteinase–Antiproteinase Imbalance

Aaron Janoff

HISTORICAL OVERVIEW OF THE PROTEINASE–ANTIPROTEINASE IMBALANCE HYPOTHESIS

Pulmonary emphysema is characterized anatomically by destruction of lung parenchyma (Fig. 1), often involving walls of respiratory bronchioles (centrilobular lesion), but extending to true alveoli in panlobular disease. Approximately two decades ago it was suggested that unrestrained proteolysis of lung connective tissue might be responsible. This condition can arise when elastinolytic proteases are released or locally activated and are ineffectively down-regulated by endogenous proteinase inhibitors in the lower respiratory tract. Marginated neutrophils, resident alveolar macrophages, and mononuclear leukocytes in transit between blood capillaries and alveolar air spaces have all been implicated as likely sources of these lung-damaging elastases. α_1-Proteinase inhibitor (α_1-PI, α_1-antitrypsin), present in alveolar secretions primarily as a transudated protein from the pulmonary circulation, and low-molecular-weight bronchial mucus inhibitors, products of local secretory cells of the pulmonary epithelium (see following), have been implicated as important regulators of the neutrophil and monocyte elastases.

The proposal that deranged homeostasis between the foregoing enzymes and inhibitors is responsible for alveolar effacement in emphysema came to be known as the proteinase–antiproteinase imbalance hypothesis. It was based on the signal observations of Laurell and Eriksson (60) and Gross et al. (33), which have now been reproduced in many laboratories. Laurell and Eriksson were the first to recognize that a heritable deficiency in α_1-PI was often associated with early-onset, familial panlobular emphysema. Gross et al. (33) showed that intrapulmonary instillation of the plant protease papain (which possesses elastinolytic activity when used in crude form) produced anatomic derangements in animals characteristic of human emphysema. Others have since produced experimental emphysema with purified bacterial and pancreatic elastases and, perhaps more significantly, with human neutrophil elastase (45,91,93) and have observed physiologic as well as anatomic stigmata of the disease in their models.

Thus, the proteinase–antiproteinase imbalance hypothesis grew largely out of circumstantial evidence derived either from animal models of the disease induced by elastinolytic proteases or from a relatively small proportion of patients with emphysema whose disease was

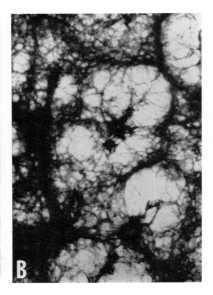

FIG. 1. Thick-section, low-power micrographs. **A:** Normal human lung. **B:** Emphysematous lung. Note the severe destruction of air-space walls and the relatively few, fine strands of remaining connective tissue in **B.** Magnification is the same in **A** and **B.** (Courtesy of Dr. Philip B. Kane, Department of Pathology, State University of New York at Stony Brook.)

genetically linked to a deficiency of antielastase. This pathogenetic schema has been extensively discussed in the recent literature (41,69,85,92,94).

Because pulmonary emphysema in the vast majority of affected individuals appears not to be due to genetic deficiency in circulating α_1-PI but rather to cigarette smoking, we shall address the question of proteinase–antiproteinase imbalance in the lungs of cigarette smokers in much of the following discussion.

INFLAMMATORY LEUKOCYTES AS POTENTIAL SOURCES OF ELASTINOLYTIC PROTEINASES IN LUNGS OF SMOKERS

Neutrophils appear in increased numbers in the lungs of cigarette smokers (37), and even more dramatic increases in pulmonary mononuclear phagocytes occur in such individuals (72,81). Neutrophils and monocytes both contain a well-described serine proteinase with potent elastinolytic activity. The chemical properties, endogenous substrates, and subcellular localization of this enzyme have been reviewed recently (8,40). These properties will be briefly summarized next.

The elastase of human neutrophil leukocytes is a serine proteinase; that is, a serine residue in position 195 of the enzyme's primary sequence contributes a nucleophilic hydroxyl group to attack carbonyl carbons of scissile peptide bonds. Valine or alanine residues are preferred in the P1 position of the target substrate (these are the amino acids whose α-carbonyl carbons undergo preferential attack). The enzyme is a single-chain polypeptide with a strongly basic isoelectric pH of 10 to 11. It has several isoenzyme forms, is active at neutral pH, has a molecular weight of 33,000, and contains 18 to 20% carbohydrate.

It is synthesized primarily in promyelocytes and stored in the cytoplasmic azurophil granules of maturing polymorphonuclear (PMN) leukocytes in amounts ranging up to 3 pg per cell. PMN elastase is discharged into tissues when the cell encounters objects to be phagocytized or undergoes postmortem autolysis.[1]

Monocytes contain small amounts of a serine protease closely resembling PMN elastase, both in physical-chemical properties and in antigenic behavior. In addition to its cytoplasmic granular distribution, the monocyte enzyme is also found on the cell membrane. In that location, it may attack extracellular substrates coming in contact with mononuclear phagocytes during their transit across endothelial barriers and through connective-tissue matrices. When observed in cell culture, monocytes gradually lose their serine protease as they differentiate into macrophages; they then develop a new elastase with properties of a metalloenzyme (that is, containing a coordinated zinc atom in its active site).

Little is known about the mechanisms responsible for attraction of inflammatory leukocytes into air spaces of the lung by tobacco smoke inhalation. Cigarette smoke can stimulate alveolar macrophages to produce and/or secrete chemoattractants and secretagogues for neutrophils. On the basis of their characterization to date, these macrophage-derived molecules may include bioactive lipids (38,68) such as leukotriene B_4, although newer evidence suggests that synthesis of this arachidonic acid metabolite by macrophages may actually be depressed in smokers (62). In addition, macrophage-derived peptides such as interleukin 1 (7,24,86) have been implicated in neutrophil recruitment. For more information about the chemotactic activity of lipid mediators, see Chapter 8. Interleukin 1 is discussed in Chapter 12.

Whatever the macrophage-derived factor may be, smokers' macrophages, cultured *in vitro,* release this activity, whereas macrophages recovered from nonsmokers do not. However, if the latter cells are exposed to cigarette smoke in culture, they then appear to liberate chemotactic factor(s) as well (38).

Recently it was reported (99) that nicotine itself is chemotactic at high concentrations, whereas at concentrations found in smokers, it enhances the chemotactic responsiveness of neutrophils to C5a. The latter is a chemotactically active peptide generated during activation of the complement cascade and is one of the most potent neutrophil and monocyte chemoattractants yet described.

We recently demonstrated that cigarette smoke components are capable of modifying C3 and activating the alternative pathway of complement *in vitro* (50). We also showed that the increase in chemotactic activity of rodent lung fluids immediately after acute cigarette smoke exposure is complement-dependent (51) and that pulmonary leukocytosis following long-term chronic exposure of mice to cigarette smoke is partly dependent on normal tissue levels of C5 (52).

Even if the foregoing mediators (leukotrienes, complement-independent peptides, complement-derived peptides, cytokines, and components of cigarette smoke itself) only initiate the ingress of small numbers of elastase-secreting leukocytes to the lung, connective-tissue breakdown accompanying this inflammatory response can then augment and perpetuate the pulmonary leukocyte accumulation. This occurs because among the peptides resulting from enzymatic breakdown of collagen (79) and elastin (90) are species with potent chemotactic activity for neutrophils and monocytes.

In addition, mast cells are capable of releasing chemoattractants for neutrophils (4) and eosinophils (30), and there is preliminary evidence suggesting that cigarette smoke may stimulate pulmonary mast cell secretory responses (100).[2]

RESIDENT LUNG CELLS AS POTENTIAL SOURCES OF ELASTINOLYTIC PROTEINASES IN SMOKERS

In addition to the large marginated pool of leukocytes in the lung, from which neutrophils and monocytes may enter pulmonary interstitium and air spaces when stimulated by the mechanisms discussed earlier, other cells possessing elastinolytic enzymes are normally found in this organ. These include fibroblasts, smooth-muscle cells, platelets, mast cells, and alveolar macrophages.

Smooth-muscle cells derived from porcine aorta have been shown to possess a serine type of elastase localized to their plasma membranes. Similar activity has been extracted from human aorta. The arterial enzyme can be distinguished from human neutrophil elastase by its amino acid composition and immunologic specificity. Aortic smooth-muscle cell elastase may participate in elastin turnover in normal arterial wall and in the pathologic elastinolysis of atherosclerosis. It is not known, however, if lung smooth-muscle cells also carry a cell-associated elastase or if such an enzyme plays any role in normal lung elastin turnover or in the pathogenesis of emphysema. Human skin fibroblasts also contain an elastase. On a per-cell basis, fibroblasts secrete about 2% of the enzyme activity extractable from neutrophils. Similarly, platelets have small amounts of elastase. Platelet elastase is clearly a different enzyme from that of the neutrophil on the basis of immunologic and other criteria (39). The platelet enzyme may also play a role in vascular injury, including perhaps injury to pulmonary endothelial cells during the adult respiratory distress syndrome. However, virtually nothing is known about the role of platelet elastase in pulmonary emphysema. On the other hand, platelet factor 4, a low-molecular-weight cationic protein that is released from platelets during clotting, has been reported to be a potent stimulator of neutrophil elastase. It has been suggested that this stimulation may be based on competition between platelet factor 4 and neutrophil elastase (which is also cationic, see above) for negatively charged domains on elastin that are unproductive cleavage sites for the protease. Thus, in an indirect way, platelets could be determinants of parenchymal destruction in emphysema by functioning synergistically with leukocytes. References to original articles describing the elastases of smooth-muscle cells, fibroblasts, and platelets can be found in Janoff (41).

Pulmonary mast cells are another potential source of elastinolytic proteinases that could be released into lung connective tissue as a result of smoking. Mast cells are found within pulmonary parenchyma, including alveolar walls. Their numbers have been reported to be as high as $350/mm^2$ of alveolar wall in uninflated lung (25), whereas another study (58) showed that, in smokers, 2% of all epithelial cells of terminal and respiratory bronchioles are mast cells. Human lung mast cells were recently reported to contain low levels of neutrophil-type serine-elastase (66). This enzyme is released in active form during mast cell degranulation triggered by immunological events and has been implicated as an inflammatory mediator in IgE-dependent reactions (67).

Interest in the possible role of mast cell elastase in the effacement of alveolar walls in emphysema has been heightened by reports that cigarette smoking causes degranulation of circulating basophils in humans (101) and of pulmonary mast cells in monkey lungs ventilated with tobacco smoke *ex situ* (100).[2] Mast cell degranulation can be induced by nonspecific stimuli, including amines and other basic molecules (44), and cigarette smoke contains such compounds (87). In addition to elastase, mast cell degranulation in alveolar septal connective tissue would release other mediators of injury. The mast cell degranulation process is associated with secretion of prostaglandin D_4, chemotactic factors for neutrophils (4) and eosinophils (30), and other proteinases (tryptase in humans, chymase in rats). The latter proteinases may produce injury directly or by acting synergistically with elastase. These hypothetical pathways of alveolar wall damage mediated by mast cell degranulation in response to smoking are summarized in Fig. 2. Should pulmonary parenchymal mast cells discharge their granule contents (including elastase and other mediators of inflammation) into the lung in response to cigarette smoking, then secretion of this proteinase and other enzymes and phlogistens in close proximity to alveolar interstitial elastic fibers could play an important role in the accelerated destruction of these critical connective-tissue elements in smokers' emphysema.

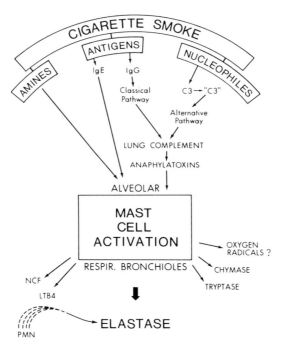

FIG. 2. Cigarette smoke may cause mast cell degranulation by several mechanisms: (a) direct stimulation of the mast cell release reaction by basic compounds in smoke; (b) IgE-mediated release reactions triggered by tobacco antigens in sensitized individuals; (c) anaphylatoxin-mediated release reactions after activation of the classic complement pathway by interaction of IgG with tobacco antigens, or after activation of the alternative complement pathway by tobacco-smoke-induced modification of C3, as described in the text. Degranulation of alveolar mast cells by any of these pathways might release: chemoattractants and secretagogues for neutrophils (and eosinophils), prostaglandins, leukotrienes, chymase (in rodents), tryptase, mast cell elastase, and perhaps toxic species of oxygen. All of these could play roles in alveolar wall damage. (From ref. 69.)

Alveolar macrophages may be yet another source of elastinolytic proteinases with the potential for causing lung damage. Murine alveolar macrophages synthesize and secrete a metalloendopeptidase with elastinolytic activity. Human alveolar macrophages display a surface-membrane-associated cysteinyl (thiol) proteinase with considerable activity against elastin. These cells are also capable of specific uptake, retention, and release of neutrophil elastase. To complicate matters further, degradation of matrix elastic fibers by macrophages involves the cooperative activity of still other proteolytic enzymes, especially plasminogen activator. The generated plasmin appears to be critical for hydrolyzing proteoglycans in the matrix and unmasking the embedded elastic fiber target. Some further discussion of these macrophage elastin-degrading enzyme systems now seems in order.

Murine macrophage elastase is a metal-dependent proteinase with a molecular weight of 22,000 (107). The enzyme prefers to cleave peptide bonds to which leucine[3] contributes the α-amino group (48). In a 24-hr culture period, approximately 200 mouse macrophages will secrete enzyme activity equivalent to that contained in one human neutrophil. However, the mouse macrophage enzyme is resistant to inhibition by α_1-PI and can actually digest this antiproteinase (5). For this reason, the possibility that a similar enzyme may be liberated by human alveolar macrophages has attracted widespread attention.

Human alveolar macrophages contain significant amounts of cathepsin B (73). This enzyme, or another[4] cell-associated cysteinyl proteinase (64), was recently implicated (18) as being responsible for 65 to 80% of human alveolar macrophage elastinolytic activity, rather than the metalloenzyme described in murine macrophages. The cysteinyl elastinolytic protease(s) is also displayed on the macrophage surface membrane (18) and partly for this reason is more resistant to the classic soluble proteinase inhibitors of serum and alveolar fluids.

In addition, macrophages also bind and internalize neutrophil elastase, by virtue of possessing a specific membrane receptor for this and other neutrophil glycoprotein enzymes (13). Macrophages can subsequently release the neutrophil enzyme in an active form, a process accelerated by macrophage cell injury (14). In this way, macrophages can serve as vectors for the harbored neutrophil protease, carrying it to tissue sites that it ordinarily might not reach and bringing it into closer proximity to its targets in the extracellular matrix than normally. Thus, macrophage-delivered neutrophil elastase might also partly escape the surveillance of soluble proteinase inhibitors.

Degradation of connective-tissue matrix macromolecules by macrophages appears to involve the cooperative interplay of several enzymes, primarily elastase and plasminogen activator (47,103,104). The latter not only is a secretory product of the cell but also is present on macrophage plasma membranes (19), and in that location it may help account for the extensive pericellular matrix dissolution characteristic of macrophages acting in close physical contact with matrix substrates. By converting plasminogen to plasmin in inflammatory exudative fluids, macrophage plasminogen activator can indirectly facilitate elastinolysis, plasmin being effective at stripping away proteoglycans and fibrin and thus unmasking target collagen and elastin fibers.

ANTIELASTASES IN THE LUNG

Table 1 lists some of the major inhibitors of leukocytic and macrophage elastases that probably play important roles in regulating the extracellular activity of these enzymes in lung connective tissue.

Bronchial mucus contains at least two of these antielastases that undoubtedly act to protect the mucous-lined airways against the potentially injurious effects of elastase released in the course of bronchial inflammation. The first (antileukoprotease or bronchial mucous inhibitor) inhibits trypsin, chymotrypsin, cathepsin G, and neutrophil elastase, but not other (e.g., pancreatic) elastases. Antileukoprotease is closely related to, if not identical with, low-molecular-weight inhibitors of neutrophil elastase found in other body secretions, e.g., cervical mucous inhibitor and human seminal plasma inhibitor. This agent has been purified recently, and its complete primary structure has been determined by protein sequencing (89,97), as well as by DNA sequencing (89). Antileukoprotease is a single-chain polypeptide containing 107 amino acid residues, including many cysteines. These, in turn, participate in the formation of 16 disulfide bridges. The latter undoubtedly help to stabilize the molecule. No carbohydrate has been detected in the purified inhibitor. Two reactive domains are present. One, containing an arginine-tyrosine center, inhibits trypsin; the second domain contains a leucine-methionine-reactive site and inhibits neutrophil elastase.

Using monoclonal antibodies and a two-step gold-labeling technique (56), antileukoprotease has been localized ultrastructurally to secretory granules of serous cells in bronchial mucous glands and to secretory granules of goblet cells and Clara cells in bronchiolar epithelium. The presence of this inhibitor in bronchioles suggests that it may function to protect peripheral lung, as well as central airways, against destruction mediated by neutrophil elastase and cathepsin G.

A second, low-molecular-weight, acid-stable protein present in bronchial mucus inhibits leukocyte elastase and pancreatic elastase, but not trypsin, chymotrypsin, or cathepsin G. This elastase-specific mucous inhibitor is currently undergoing intensive study (35).

Table 1 also lists a third antiproteinase that is locally produced in the lung, namely, the tissue inhibitor of metalloproteinases (TIMP). This uncharacterized agent is produced by human alveolar macrophages (3), and it can inactivate the metalloenzyme (elastase) secreted by rodent alveolar macrophages discussed earlier. Simultaneous secretion of TIMP by human alveolar macrophages may mask production of a comparable metalloelastase by these same cells. Human alveolar macrophage TIMP is functionally and immunologically identical with the TIMP released by human skin fibroblasts.

Also listed in the table are two major elastase inhibitors that are not produced locally in the lung, except for very small amounts synthesized and secreted by alveolar macrophages (105,106). These are the circulating plasmatic inhibitors, α_1-PI and α_2-macroglobulin, that are present in alveolar epithelial lining fluid, the former as a result of normal transudative processes, the latter because of increased permeability of the alveolar membranes in lung inflammation. α_1-PI is deemed to be a major regulator of neutrophil elastase in human alveolar secretions, and it will therefore be discussed in some detail in the following section.

α_1-PI

Is α_1-PI the Chief Regulator of Neutrophil Elastase in the Lower Respiratory Tract?

An important question, not yet fully resolved, is whether the low-molecular-weight mucous inhibitors discussed earlier contribute to the antiproteinase defense of the respiratory bronchioles and alveoli to a significant extent

TABLE 1. *Important elastase inhibitors in human lung*

Inhibitor	M_r (kd)	Source in the lung
Bronchial mucous inhibitor (antileukoprotease)	10	Serous cells of bronchial mucous glands, goblet cells, Clara cells
Elastase-specific mucous inhibitor	10	Mucous glands, non-ciliated-airway epithelial cells
TIMP	?	Macrophages (fibroblasts?)
α_1-PI	52	Plasma (liver), macrophages
α_2-Macroglobulin	725	Plasma (liver), macrophages

or whether their protective function is largely limited to mucus-lined airways, where they clearly predominate over the plasma transudated inhibitor, α_1-PI. This issue is especially important in the context of emphysema, in which the respiratory air spaces are the principal targets of proteolytic attack, rather than the bronchi. Immunocytochemical demonstration of antileukoprotease in secretory granules of Clara cells in small bronchioles (56) raises the distinct possibility that this low-molecular-weight inhibitor participates in the antielastase "screen" of the peripheral lung. On the other hand, in a number of α_1-PI-deficient subjects with the homozygous Z phenotype of the inhibitor, neutrophil elastase inhibitory activity of bronchoalveolar secretions recovered by lavage was reported as being less than 10% of normal (27). In one individual with the rare null-null phenotype for α_1-PI, in whom an α_1-PI gene-transcription defect was present, only 15% or less of the normal elastase inhibitory activity was detected in such secretions (R. Crystal, *personal communication*).[5]

Perhaps antileukoprotease and α_1-PI have independent and physiologically different functions. *In vitro, α_1-PI* can dissociate neutrophil elastase from its complex with the mucous inhibitor and then avidly bind the released proteinase. On the other hand, the low-molecular-weight elastase inhibitors appear to be more effective than α_1-PI when confronted with neutrophil elastase already bound to insoluble elastin. For these reasons it has been proposed that α_1-PI "inhibits free elastase and maintains bronchial inhibitor in a free state by continuously removing elastase bound to it, while bronchial inhibitor functions as an inhibitor of elastin-bound elastase" (28).

Deficiencies of α_1-PI and Susceptibility to Emphysema

Whether α_1-PI is or is not the chief regulator of neutrophil elastase in the lower respiratory tract in humans, it is clear that without a sufficient level of functional α_1-PI in the alveolar air spaces, risk of emphysema is greatly increased, especially in smokers (59). This follows whether α_1-PI is the only neutrophil elastase inhibitor shielding the alveolar structures or whether α_1-PI functions as the terminal inhibitor of this enzyme, as suggested earlier (28).

Genetic deficiency of α_1-PI has long been recognized as a major predisposing factor for emphysema (60). The molecular basis for the predominant form of heritable α_1-PI deficiency is now well understood and has been clearly described (6,9); it will not be reviewed here.

In the majority of emphysema victims, the foregoing genetic abnormality in α_1-PI is not apparent. To help explain their disease, investigators have suggested the presence of other, still unknown genetic polymorphisms of α_1-PI not affecting inhibitor levels but causing subtle genetic defects in inhibitor function. Alternatively, acquired derangements in the inhibitor resulting from environ-

mental influences have been proposed. Included in the second category is the concept of α_1-PI inactivation caused by smoking.

Acquired Deficiency of α_1-PI in the Lower Respiratory Tract in Smokers: The "Oxidation Hypothesis"

α_1-PI acts as a pseudosubstrate for its target proteinases, and the site in the inhibitor recognized and attacked by the proteinase represents the active site of the inhibitor. Structural studies have shown that the elastase-inhibitory active site of α_1-PI contains a methionine-serine peptide bond (46). When this methionine-serine bond is recognized by the proteolytic enzyme, a series of reactions begins that rapidly leads to formation of extremely stable complexes between 1 mol of protease and 1 mol of inhibitor. The high stability of this complex may be based on covalent or noncovalent bonding between the catalytic site of the proteinase and the active site of the inhibitor; the precise mechanism is not certain.

If the sulfur atom in the methionine side chain at position 358 (Met 358) in α_1-PI is converted to a sulfoxide (Met-O 358), the inhibitor becomes less effective in binding neutrophil elastase by at least three orders of magnitude (association rate constant of native α_1-PI for neutrophil elastase = 6.5×10^7 mole^{-1} sec^{-1}, versus 3.1×10^4 mole^{-1} sec^{-1} for the oxidized inhibitor) (65). This may result from steric effects of the bulkier sulfoxide moiety hindering the accommodation of Met-O 358 into the proteinase's substrate-binding pocket.

In vitro, both whole cigarette smoke (42) and oxidizing free radicals formed by interactions of NO, air, and organic constituents present in the gas phase of cigarette smoke (82) clearly inactivate α_1-PI. Recently, strong (albeit indirect) evidence was obtained showing that inactivation of human α_1-PI by gas-phase cigarette smoke is based on selective oxidation of the active-site (Met 358) residue, as is inactivation of this protein by chemical, enzymatic, and cellular oxidizing systems (43). On the other hand, mouse α_1-PI can also be oxidatively inactivated, even though in this species the plasma elastase inhibitor appears to contain a tyrosine residue rather than a methionine residue in the P1 position of its elastase-binding site (70).

In addition to oxidizing free radicals formed in smoke, alveolar macrophages present in smokers' lungs themselves generate increased amounts of activated oxygen species, especially hydrogen peroxide (36), and perhaps also hydroxyl radical. Human blood monocytes and alveolar macrophages, when stimulated with the membrane-perturbing agent phorbol myristate acetate, produce superoxide radical and other activated species of oxygen and partly inactivate the elastase inhibitory capacity of serum (15). In these experiments, serum elastase inhibitory capacity can be protected by superoxide dismutase (which scavenges the superoxide radical), catalase (which scavenges hydrogen peroxide), and sodium azide (which blocks myeloperoxidase activity). Moreover, serum elastase inhibitory capacity is not decreased if cells from a patient with chronic granulomatous disease are used (such cells cannot generate activated species of oxygen, even when stimulated with the phorbol ester).

Our laboratory found inactivated α_1-PI in lung secretions recovered from smokers by bronchoalveolar lavage and demonstrated the presence of methionine sulfoxide (4 moles/mol α_1-PI) in the inactivated inhibitor (16). However, it was not determined if the active-site methionine (Met 358) was one of the oxidized residues. Nonsmokers' α_1-PI was fully active and contained no methionine sulfoxide. Diminished α_1-PI function in human smokers' bronchoalveolar lavage had also been reported independently (26). On the other hand, two other laboratories found inactive α_1-PI in equal amounts in both smokers' and nonsmokers' lung fluids (11,95). In another investigation, the oxidized form of α_1-PI was detected equally in smokers and nonsmokers, although the latter were ex-smokers with chronic bronchitis (R. A. Stockley, *personal communication*).[6]

Abboud et al. (1) reported small (10%) but statistically significant decreases in functionally active α_1-PI in lung lavage fluid collected from subjects 1 hr after they smoked two cigarettes. Nearly fully active α_1-PI was found in the same subjects lavaged immediately before smoking (and after overnight abstinence). In other subjects, α_1-PI activity in lavage fluid collected 2 to 3 hr after smoking two cigarettes showed no change from presmoking base-line values. (These data suggest that for analysis of α_1-PI functional status, bronchopulmonary secretions should not be collected much later than 1 hr after acute smoking.) Abboud et al. (1) also found that at 30 to 60 min after smoking two cigarettes (the time at which detectable decreases in α_1-PI activity were observed), there is also maximal production of the superoxide radical (and presumably its derivative species of activated oxygen) by the macrophages recovered in the same lavage samples (2).

Small decreases, like those described earlier, in the functional activity of lung lavage α_1-PI caused by smoking could be physiologically meaningful, because lavage mixes the secretions from different regions of the acinus, whereas the distribution of inhaled smoke is uneven and tends to follow a centriacinar deposition pattern. Thus, severely inactivated α_1-PI washed up from centriacinar surfaces theoretically could be considerably diluted by undamaged inhibitor recovered from other portions of the lobule, leading to small observable decreases in overall inhibitor activity. Decreased inhibitor function could nevertheless be significant in the centriacinar zone, where the most common form of emphysema develops.[7] It may also be

worth noting that although ventilation is greater in basal portions of the lung during tidal breathing, inhalation of a bolus of cigarette smoke can increase the distribution of inhaled markers to apical lung zones (77). Developing lesions of emphysema in smokers typically are more severe in upper portions of the lung (98).

It may be, then, that episodes of acquired deficiency of lung α_1-PI occur in some smokers and lead, in turn, to "pulses" of lung connective-tissue proteolysis. Although this remains an attractive hypothesis, definitive proof of α_1-PI oxidation *in vivo* is lacking. In addition, we presently have no explanation for the apparent resistance of most smokers to emphysema (genetic variation in lung antioxidants?). Also, alternative mechanisms of α_1-PI inactivation (e.g., proteolytic degradation) (5,94) need to be more fully explored.

ASSESSMENT OF ELASTINOLYSIS IN SMOKERS

One reasonable prediction of the proteinase–antiproteinase hypothesis is that lung elastin turnover should be accelerated at some stage in the development of emphysema, and during this stage the concentration of elastin degradation peptides should be increased in plasma and/or urine. Several immunologic assays have been developed to test this prediction. Following acid hydrolysis of urine samples, excreted elastin peptides have been measured by radioimmunoassay of desmosine, the major cross-linking amino acid present in mature elastin (34,55). In one recent study involving over 150 subjects (23), urine desmosine levels were found to be unrelated to cigarette smoking or to spirometric function. The investigators concluded that "measurement of urine desmosine may not be useful as an indirect measurement of elastolysis in cigarette smokers." A second study involving persons with homozygous α_1-PI deficiency and severe emphysema failed to detect any increase in desmosine excretion in these patients over that in control subjects (78). However, greater success has been obtained using solid-phase radioimmunoassays (22) or enzyme-linked immunosorbent assays (ELISA) for elastin peptides in plasma. For example, one group (57) used an improved sensitive ELISA with a peroxidase-antiperoxidase complex as the "reporter group" and found that patients with chronic obstructive lung disease had plasma levels of elastin peptides two times higher than those found in normal nonsmokers, whereas normal smokers had values intermediate between those for the other two groups. Of interest, 20% of the normal smokers had elevated elastin peptide levels, similar to those in the emphysema group. This figure correlates closely to the percentage of smokers who are at risk for developing obstructive lung disease.

These same workers also used immunogold-staining methods to demonstrate neutrophil elastase bound to partly destroyed elastic fibers at sites of emphysematous change in smokers' lungs (53). Although immunological detection methods cannot differentiate between active and inactive enzyme, gold-particle counts indicating the presence of elastase showed a positive correlation with the mean linear intercept, a morphometric index of emphysema. Other evidence suggesting that active neutrophil elastase may be released in smokers can be found in the recent report of increased plasma levels of the neutrophil elastase-derived fibrinogen peptide ($A\alpha_{1-21}$) in smokers and especially in emphysema patients (102).

The observation of increased elastin peptides in smokers' plasma and the detection of elastin-bound, extracellular neutrophil elastase in smokers' lungs support the view that smoking enhances lung elastinolysis in susceptible individuals. In this connection, it is worth noting that augmentation of elastase-induced emphysema in experimental animals by cigarette smoke has also been observed in several laboratories (reviewed in ref. 54).

SOME OTHER VARIABLES THAT MAY AFFECT SUSCEPTIBILITY TO EMPHYSEMA IN SMOKERS

In addition to their actions on proteinase inhibitors, the oxidizing agents generated by leukocytes and macrophages, and perhaps those in cigarette smoke, can also damage the lung by acting directly on a variety of other molecules and cells. For example, gelation of collagen at 37°C can be inhibited if the collagen is first preincubated with xanthine oxidase and hypoxanthine (a superoxide-radical-generating system). The inhibitory effect on collagen is dependent on production of the superoxide radical during conversion of hypoxanthine to uric acid by xanthine oxidase and is completely blocked by addition of superoxide dismutase or catalase (31). Also, superoxide anion and other oxygen-derived free radicals (produced either by xanthine oxidase or from stimulated PMN) can depolymerize hyaluronic acid, as reflected in its decreased viscosity and the appearance of glycosaminoglycans of lower molecular weight. The depolymerized hyaluronic acid is then more susceptible to degradation by β-*N*-acetylglycosaminidase (32). Again, radical scavengers block all the foregoing changes. In addition to directly breaking covalent bonds in connective-tissue protein macromolecules such as collagen (see above), activated oxygen species may also induce subtle chemical modifications in proteins that in turn render them more susceptible to attack by proteases (see Chapter 23). Thus, in addition to their indirect contribution through inactivation of proteinase inhibitors, reactive oxygen species and oxidized halides may

well contribute to connective-tissue damage in emphysema by directly affecting collagen, proteoglycans, or even elastin (83).

Levels of antioxidants such as vitamin E are decreased in smokers' lung fluids, with corresponding increases in the content of oxidized vitamin E (76). Plasma levels of vitamin E are unaffected by smoking.

Relatively small doses of tobacco smoke have been reported to damage epithelial cell tight junctions in the respiratory tree (10). Resultant increases in mucosal permeability could facilitate penetration of enzymes (e.g., elastase) or other potentially injurious substances present in airway lumina into the underlying structures of the airway wall. In addition, proteinases themselves can stimulate alveolar epithelial transport processes (71), and this can be yet another mechanism by which proteinases residing within the alveolar spaces reach the interstitium.

In lungs of experimental animals, lysyl oxidase activity normally increases markedly after injury induced by elastase instillation (75). Lysyl oxidase is a copper-dependent enzyme involved in the formation of intermolecular cross-links between soluble collagen or tropoelastin monomers and would be expected to play an active role in tissue repair during healing. The rise in lung lysyl oxidase activity after elastase-induced injury is severely blunted by exposure of the animals to cigarette smoke inhalation during the repair phase (74). As a result, neosynthesis of cross-linked elastin and collagen is blunted, with consequent reduction in the capacity of the lung to repair itself. These results, together with the independent observation that aqueous solutions of cigarette smoke can inhibit the activity of lysyl oxidase on elastin and the formation of desmosine cross-links *in vitro* (61), suggest that in some human smokers, long-term interference with elastin synthesis may also contribute to the development of the connective-tissue abnormalities characteristic of emphysema.

Although no heritable diseases have as yet been shown to be caused by molecular defects of elastin, predisposition to emphysema in selected smokers might result from such defects. Application of the newer techniques of genetic analysis to elucidate possible polymorphisms of the elastin gene may, in the future, demonstrate relevant derangements at this level.

RATIONAL THERAPIES FOR EMPHYSEMA

α_1-PI Deficiency

Individuals at increased risk for emphysema because of a genetic deficiency in α_1-PI will have newer treatment modalities available to them in the near future based on inhibitor-replacement therapy. α_1-PI purified from human plasma has already undergone preliminary clinical trials in homozygous-deficient persons (21). The results show that weekly intravenous doses of 60 mg/kg of the purified protein are sufficient to maintain a concentration of the inhibitor in serum and bronchoalveolar lavage fluid significantly above that for the untreated patient, despite rapidly declining levels beginning 2 to 3 days after each α_1-PI injection. No circulating anti-α_1-PI antibodies, immediate hypersensitivity reactions, immune complex disease, hepatitis (A or non-A,B), or coagulation dysfunctions were noted over 26 weeks of α_1-PI replacement therapy. As encouraging as these biochemical and immunologic data are, physiological evidence of a decreased rate of decline in pulmonary function would also be required in order to consider replacement therapy beneficial.

Less expensive, recombinant forms of α_1-PI may also become available soon for replacement therapy programs (12). However, the proteins produced by microbial organisms bearing the cloned human α_1-PI gene lack the normal carbohydrate side chains of the endogenous mammalian inhibitor. As a result, clearance of the unglycosylated protein from the circulation is greatly accelerated (17). Still, pulmonary retention of the transudated recombinant inhibitor is not significantly less than that of the native plasma protein (17). The risk of immunological reactions may also be increased by the absence of carbohydrate side chains.

Ultimately, gene therapy (i.e., introduction of the normal α_1-PI gene into deficient individuals) may become feasible. Before this approach can be optimally utilized, we need to know how cells regulate α_1-PI gene expression under normal conditions and during acute-phase reactions.

The mutant α_1-PI allele (Z) most often associated with severe inhibitor deficiency is apparently transcribed and translated normally, but posttranslational modification of its protein product is abberant and leads to defective secretion of the protein from hepatocytes and macrophages (6,9). Understanding the mechanism of the secretory defect may provide alternative means of therapeutic intervention.

Emphysema in α_1-PI-Sufficient Persons

Current projections of treatment modalities to arrest the progression of emphysema in α_1-PI-sufficient persons are also geared toward supplementation of lung antiproteinase defense. Inhibitors that are under consideration include the following: genetically engineered, oxidation-resistant mutants of α_1-PI (20,29,84); recombinant forms of the low molecular-weight, stable antileukoprotease of bronchial mucus (see above); eglin c (88); various synthetic, low-molecular-weight elastase inhibitors (49,63,80). Antioxidant drugs, which can be administered by aerosol,

also deserve attention (96). However, in the long run, the most rational approach to decreasing the incidence of chronic destructive lung disease in the general population would be elimination of cigarette smoking, because antiproteinase therapy for individuals who may have an acquired form of α_1-PI deficiency (induced by cigarette smoking) is not likely to be as effective as smoking cessation itself. Also, it should be borne in mind that antiproteinase therapy, in any form, is a prophylactic measure designed to prevent further damage. It cannot be a curative measure designed to restore the damaged lung to some earlier state.

ACKNOWLEDGMENTS

This work was supported in part by USPHS grants HL-14262 and HL-32429 and by a contract from Cortech, Inc., Denver, Colorado.

REFERENCES

1. Abboud, R. T., Fera, T., Richter, A., Tabona, M. Z., and Johal, S. (1985): Acute effect of smoking on the functional activity of alpha$_1$-proteinase inhibitor in bronchoalveolar lavage fluid. *Am. Rev. Respir. Dis.,* 131:79–85.
2. Abboud, R. T., Richter, A., Fera, T., and Johal, S. (1984): Acute effect of smoking on superoxide production by pulmonary alveolar macrophages. *Am. Rev. Respir. Dis.,* 129(2):315 (abstract).
3. Albin, R. J., Senior, R. M., Welgus, H. G., and Campbell, E. J. (1986): Modulation of macrophage elastase activity: Identification and quantification of a metalloproteinase elastase inhibitor released by human alveolar macrophages. In: *Second International Symposium on Pulmonary Emphysema and Proteolysis,* edited by C. Mittman and J. C. Taylor. Academic Press, New York.
4. Atkins, P. C., Norman, M., Zweiman, B., and Rosenblum, F. (1979): Further characterization and biologic activity of ragweed antigen-induced neutrophil chemotactic activity in man. *J. Allergy Clin. Immunol.,* 64:251–258.
5. Banda, M. J., Clark, E. J., and Werb, Z. (1980): Limited proteolysis by macrophage elastase inactivates human alphal-proteinase inhibitor. *J. Exp. Med.,* 152:1563–1570.
6. Bathurst, I. C., Travis, J., George, P. M., and Carrell, R. W. (1984): Structural and functional characterization of the abnormal Z alpha$_1$-antitrypsin isolated from human liver. *FEBS Lett.,* 177:179–183.
7. Beck, G., Habicht, G. S., Benach, J. L., and Miller, F. (1986): Interleukin 1: A common endogenous mediator of inflammation and the local Shwartzman reaction. *J. Immunol.,* 136:3025–3031.
8. Bieth, J. G. (1986): Elastases: Catalytic and biological properties. In: *Biology of Extracellular Matrix,* edited by R. P. Mecham, (publisher), (city).
9. Boswell, D. R., and Bathurst, I. C. (1985): Molecular physiology and pathology of alpha$_1$-antitrypsin. *Biochem. Educ.,* 13:98–104.
10. Boucher, R. C., Johnston, J., Inoue, S., Hulbert, W., and Hogg, J. C. (1980): The effect of cigarette smoke on the permeability of guinea pig airways. *Lab. Invest.,* 43:94–100.
11. Boudier, C., Pelletier, A., Pauli, G., and Bieth, J. G. (1983): The functional activity of alpha$_1$-proteinase inhibitor in bronchoalveolar lavage fluids from healthy human smokers and nonsmokers. *Clin. Chim. Acta,* 132:309–315.
12. Cabezon, T., Dewilde, M., Herion, P., Loriau, R., and Bollen, A. (1984): Expression of human alpha$_1$-antitrypsin cDNA in the yeast *Saccharomyces cerevisiae. Proc. Natl. Acad. Sci. USA,* 81:6594–6598.
13. Campbell, E. J. (1982): Human leukocyte elastase, cathepsin G,

and lactoferrin: Family of neutrophil granule glycoproteins that bind to an alveolar macrophage receptor. *Proc. Natl. Acad. Sci. USA,* 79:6941–6945.

14. Campbell, E. J., and Wald, M. S. (1983): Hypoxic injury to human alveolar macrophages accelerates release of previously bound neutrophil elastase: Implications for lung connective tissue injury including pulmonary emphysema. *Am. Rev. Respir. Dis.,* 127:631–635.

15. Carp, H., and Janoff, A. (1980): Potential mediator of inflammation. Phagocyte-derived oxidants suppress the elastase inhibitory capacity of alpha₁-proteinase inhibitor in vitro. *J. Clin. Invest.,* 66:987–995.

16. Carp, H., Miller, F., Hoidal, J., and Janoff, A. (1982): Alpha₁-proteinase inhibitor purified from lungs of cigarette smokers contains oxidized methionine and has decreased elastase inhibitory capacity. *Proc. Natl. Acad. Sci. USA,* 779:2041–2045.

17. Casolaro, A., Fells, G., Wewers, M., Pierce, J., and Crystal, R. (1986): Evaluation of parenteral administration of recombinant DNA produced alpha₁-antitrypsin to primates. In: *Second International Symposium on Pulmonary Emphysema and Proteolysis,* edited by C. Mittman and J. C. Taylor, Academic Press, New York.

18. Chapman, H. A., and Stone, O. L. (1984): Comparison of live human neutrophil and alveolar macrophage elastolytic activity in vitro. Relative resistance of macrophage elastolytic activity to serum and alveolar proteinase inhibitors. *J. Clin. Invest.,* 74:1693–1700.

19. Chapman, H. A., Stone, O. L., and Vavrin, Z. (1984): Degradation of fibrin and elastin by intact human alveolar macrophages in vitro. Characterization of a plasminogen activator and its role in matrix degradation. *J. Clin. Invest.,* 73:806–815.

20. Courtney, M., Jallat, S., Tessier, L.-H., Benavente, A., Crystal, R. G., and Lecocq, J.-P. (1985): Synthesis in *E. coli* of alpha₁-antitrypsin variants of therapeutic potential for emphysema and thrombosis. *Nature,* 313:149–151.

21. Crystal, R. (1986): Results of clinical trial of alpha₁PI replacement therapy. In: *Second International Symposium on Pulmonary Emphysema and Proteolysis,* edited by C. Mittman and J. C. Taylor, Academic Press, New York.

22. Darnule, T. V., McKee, M., Darnule, A. T., Turino, G. M., and Mandl, I. (1982): Solid phase radioimmunoassay for estimation of elastin peptides in human sera. *Anal. Biochem.,* 122:302–307.

23. Davies, S. F., Offord, K. P., Brown, M. G., Campe, H., and Niewoehner, D. (1983): Urine desmosine is unrelated to cigarette smoking or to spirometric function. *Am. Rev. Respir. Dis.,* 128:473–475.

24. Elias, J. A., Schreiber, A. D., Gustilo, K., Chien, P., Rossman, M. D., Lammie, P. J., and Daniele, R. P. (1985): Differential interleukin 1 elaboration by unfractionated and density fractionated human alveolar macrophages and blood monocytes: Relationship to cell maturity. *J. Immunol.,* 135:3198–3204.

25. Fox, B., Bull, T. B., and Guz, A. (1981): Mast cells in the human alveolar wall: An electromicroscopic study. *J. Clin. Pathol.,* 34:1333–1342.

26. Gadek, J. E., Fells, G. A., and Crystal, R. G. (1979): Cigarette smoking induces functional antiprotease deficiency in the lower respiratory tract of humans. *Science,* 206:1315–1316.

27. Gadek, J. E., Fells, G. A., Zimmerman, R. L., Rennard, S. I., and Crystal, R. G. (1981): Anti-elastases of the human alveolar structures. Implications for the protease-antiprotease theory of emphysema. *J. Clin. Invest.,* 68:889–898.

28. Gauthier, F., Fryksmark, V., Ohlsson, K., and Bieth, J. G. (1982): Kinetics of the inhibition of leukocyte elastase by the bronchial inhibitor. *Biochim. Biophys. Acta,* 700:178–183.

29. George, P. M., Travis, J., Vissers, M. C. M., Winterbourn, C. C., and Carrell, R. W. (1984): A genetically-engineered mutant of alpha₁-antitrypsin protects connective tissue from neutrophil damage and may be useful in lung disease. *Lancet,* 2:1426–1428.

30. Goetzl, E. J., and Austen, K. F. (1975): Purification and synthesis of eosinophilotactic tetrapeptides of human lung tissue: Identification as eosinophil chemotactic factor of anaphylaxis. *Proc. Natl. Acad. Sci. USA,* 72:4123–4127.

31. Greenwald, R. A., and Moy, W. W. (1979): Inhibition of collagen gelation by action of the superoxide radical. *Arthritis Rheum.,* 22:251–259.

32. Greenwald, R. A., and Moy, W. W. (1980): Effect of oxygen-derived free radicals on hyaluronic acid. *Arthritis Rheum.,* 23:455–463.

33. Gross, P., Pfitzer, E. A., Toker, E., Babyak, M. A., and Kaschak, A. (1965): Experimental emphysema. Its production with papain in normal and silicotic rats. *Arch. Environ. Health,* 11:50–58.

34. Harel, S., Janoff, A., Yu, S. Y., Hurewitz, A., and Bergofsky, E. H. (1980): Desmosine radioimmunoassay for measuring elastin degradation *in vivo. Am. Rev. Respir. Dis.,* 122:769–773.

35. Hochstrasser, K., Albrecht, G. J., Schonberger, O. L., Rasche, B., and Lempart, K. (1981): An elastase-specific inhibitor from human bronchial mucus. Isolation and characterization. *Hoppe Seylers Z. Physiol. Chem.,* 362:1369–1375.

36. Hoidal, J., Fox, R., LeMarbe, P., Perri, R., and Repine, J. (1981): Altered oxidative metabolic responses of alveolar macrophages from asymptomatic cigarette smokers. *Am. Rev. Respir. Dis.,* 123:85–89.

37. Hunninghake, G. W., and Crystal, R. G. (1983): Cigarette smoking and lung destruction: Accumulation of neutrophils in the lungs of cigarette smokers. *Am. Rev. Respir. Dis.,* 128:833–838.

38. Hunninghake, G., Gadek, J., and Crystal, R. (1980): Human alveolar macrophage neutrophil chemotactic factor: Stimuli and partial characterization. *J. Clin. Invest.,* 66:473–483.

39. James, H. L., Wachtfogel, Y. T., James, P. L., Zimmerman, M., Coleman, R. W., and Cohen, A. B. (1985): A unique elastase in human blood platelets. *J. Clin. Invest.,* 76:2330–2337.

40. Janoff, A. (1985): Elastase in tissue injury. *Annu. Rev. Med.,* 36:207–216.

41. Janoff, A. (1985): Elastases and emphysema. Current assessment of the protease-antiprotease hypothesis. *Am. Rev. Respir. Dis.,* 132:417–433.

42. Janoff, A., and Carp, H. (1977): Possible mechanism of emphysema in cigarette smokers: Cigarette smoke condensate suppresses proteinase inhibitors in vitro. *Am. Rev. Respir. Dis.,* 116:65–72.

43. Janoff, A., George-Nascimento, C., and Rosenberg, S. (1986): A genetically-engineered, mutant human alpha₁-proteinase inhibitor is more resistant than the normal inhibitor to oxidative inactivation by chemicals, enzymes, cells and cigarette smoke. *Am. Rev. Respir. Dis.,* 133:353–356.

44. Janoff, A., and Schaefer, S. (1967): Mediators of acute inflammation in leukocyte lysosomes. *Nature,* 213:144–147.

45. Janoff, A., Sloan, B., Weinbaum, G., Damiano, V., Sandhaus, R. A., Elias, J., and Kimbel, P. (1977): Experimental emphysema induced with purified human neutrophil elastase: Tissue localization of the instilled protease. *Am. Rev. Respir. Dis.,* 115:461–478.

46. Johnson, D., and Travis, J. (1978): Structural evidence for methionine at the reactive site of human alpha₁-proteinase inhibitor. *J. Biol. Chem.,* 253:7142–7144.

47. Jones, P. A., and Werb, Z. (1980): Degradation of connective tissue matrices by macrophages. II. Influence of matrix composition on proteolysis of glycoproteins, elastin and collagen by macrophages in culture. *J. Exp. Med.,* 152:1527–1536.

48. Kettner, C., Shaw, E., White, R., and Janoff, A. (1981): The specificity of macrophage elastase on the insulin B-chain. *Biochem. J.,* 195:369–372.

49. Kettner, C., and Shenvi, A. (1986): Peptide boronic acid inhibitors of elastase. In: *Second International Symposium on Pulmonary Emphysema and Proteolysis,* edited by C. Mittman and J. C. Taylor, Academic Press, New York.

50. Kew, R. R., Ghebrehiwet, B., and Janoff, A. (1985): Cigarette smoke can activate the alternative pathway of complement *in vitro* by modifying C3. *J. Clin. Invest.,* 75:1000–1007.

51. Kew, R. R., Ghebrehiwet, B., and Janoff, A. (1986): The role of complement in cigarette smoke-induced chemotactic activity of lung fluids. *Am. Rev. Respir. Dis.,* 133:478–481.

52. Kew, R. R., Ghebrehiwet, B., and Janoff, A. (1987): The fifth component of complement (C5) is necessary for maximal pulmonary leukocytosis in mice chronically-exposed to cigarette smoke. *Clin. Immunol. Immunopathol.,* 43:73–81.

53. Kimbel, P., Weinbaum, G., and Damiano, V. V. (1986): Immunolocalization of elastase in human emphysematous lungs. In: *Second International Symposium on Pulmonary Emphysema and*

Proteolysis, edited by C. Mittman and J. C. Taylor, Academic Press, New York.

54. Kimmel, E. C., Winsett, D. W., and Diamond, L. (1985): Augmentation of elastase-induced emphysema by cigarette smoke. Description of a model and a review of possible mechanisms. *Am. Rev. Respir. Dis.,* 132:885–893.

55. King, G. S., Starcher, B. C., and Kuhn, C. (1980): The measurement of elastin turnover by the radioimmunoassay of urinary desmosine excretion. *Clin. Respir. Physiol. (Suppl.),* 16:61–64.

56. Kramps, J. A., de Water, R., Willems, L. N. A., Van Muijen, G. N. P., Fransen, J. A. M., Franken, C., and Dijkman, J. H. (1986): Ultrastructural localization of antileukoprotease in serous cells of bronchial glands and in non-ciliated bronchiolar epithelial cells of human lung. In: *Second International Symposium on Pulmonary Emphysema and Proteolysis,* edited by C. Mittman and J. C. Taylor, Academic Press, New York.

57. Kucich, U., Christner, P., Lippmann, M., Kimbel, P., Williams, G., Rosenbloom, J., and Weinbaum, G. (1985): Utilization of a peroxidase antiperoxidase complex in an enzyme-linked immunosorbent assay of elastin-derived peptides in human plasma. *Am. Rev. Respir. Dis.,* 131:709–713.

58. Lamb, D., and Lumsden, A. (1982): Intraepithelial mast cells in human distal airway epithelium: Evidence for smoking-induced changes in their frequency. *Thorax,* 37:334–342.

59. Larsson, C. (1978): Natural history and life expectancy in severe alpha$_1$-antitrypsin deficiency, PiZ. *Acta Med. Scand.,* 204:345–351.

60. Laurell, C. B., and Eriksson, S. (1963): The electrophoretic alpha$_1$-globulin pattern of serum in alpha$_1$-antitrypsin deficiency. *Scand. J. Clin. Invest.,* 15:132–140.

61. Laurent, P., Janoff, A., and Kagan, H. M. (1983): Cigarette smoke blocks cross-linking of elastin *in vitro. Am. Rev. Respir. Dis.,* 127:189–192.

62. Laviolette, M., Coulombe, R., Picard, S., Braquet, P., and Borgeat, P. (1986): Decreased leukotriene B$_4$ synthesis in smokers' alveolar macrophages *in vitro. J. Clin. Invest.,* 77:54–60.

63. Martorana, P. A., Lungarella, G., Share, N. N., Gardi, C., and Zimmerman, M. (1986): The effect of furoyl saccharin, a novel non-peptidic acylating protease inhibitor in various animal models of emphysema. In: *Second International Symposium on Pulmonary Emphysema and Proteolysis,* edited by C. Mittman and J. C. Taylor, Academic Press, New York.

64. Mason, R. W., Johnson, D. A., Barrett, A. J., and Chapman, H. A. (1986): Elastinolytic activity of human cathepsin L. *Biochem. J.,* 233:925–927.

65. Matheson, N. R., Janoff, A., and Travis, J. (1982): Enzymatic oxidation of alpha$_1$-proteinase inhibitor in abnormal tissue turnover. *Mol. Cell. Biochem.,* 45:65–71.

66. Meier, H. L., Heck, L. W., Schulman, E. S., and MacGlashen, D. W., Jr. (1985): Purified human mast cells and basophils release human elastase and cathepsin G by an IgE-mediated mechanism. *Int. Arch. Allergy Appl. Immunol.,* 77:179–183.

67. Meier, H. L., Heck, L. W., Schulman, E. S., MacGlashen, D. W., Jr., Kaplan, A., and Newball, H. H. (1987): Release of elastase from human mast cells and basophils and its identification as a Hageman factor cleaving enzyme (*in press*).

68. Merril, W. W., Naegel, G. P., Mathay, R. A., and Reynolds, H. Y. (1980): Alveolar macrophage-derived chemotactic factor. Kinetics of in vitro production and partial characterization. *J. Clin. Invest.,* 65:268–276.

69. Mittman, C., and Taylor, J. C. (editors) (1986): *Second International Symposium on Pulmonary Emphysema and Proteolysis.* Academic Press, New York.

70. Nathoo, S. A., and Finlay, T. H. (1986): Immunological and chemical properties of mouse alpha$_1$-protease inhibitors. *Arch. Biochem. Biophys.,* 246:162–174.

71. Niewoehner, D. E. (1986): The protective role of the alveolar epithelium in the pathogenesis of emphysema. In: *Second International Symposium on Pulmonary Emphysema and Proteolysis,* edited by C. Mittman and J. C. Taylor, Academic Press, New York.

72. Niewoehner, D. E., Kleimerman, J., and Rice, D. P. (1974): Pathologic changes in the peripheral airways of young cigarette smokers. *N. Engl. J. Med.,* 291:755–758.

73. Orlowski, M., Orlowski, J., Lesser, M., and Kilburn, K. H. (1981): Proteolytic enzymes in bronchopulmonary lavage fluids: Cathepsin B-like activity and prolylendopeptidase. *J. Lab. Clin. Med.,* 97:467–476.

74. Osman, M., Cantor, J. O., Roffman, S., Keller, S., Turino, G. M., and Mandl, I. (1985): Cigarette smoke impairs elastin resynthesis in lungs of hamsters with elastase-induced emphysema. *Am. Rev. Respir. Dis.,* 132:640–643.

75. Osman, M., Kaldany, R.-R. J., Cantor, J. O., Turino, G. M., and Mandl, I. (1985): Stimulation of lung lysyl oxidase activity in hamsters with elastase-induced emphysema. *Am. Rev. Respir. Dis.,* 131:169–170.

76. Pacht, E. R., Kaseki, H., Mohammed, J. R., Cornwell, D. G., and Davis, W. B. (1986): Deficiency of vitamin E in the alveolar fluid of cigarette smokers. Influence on alveolar macrophage cytotoxicity. *J. Clin. Invest.,* 77:789–796.

77. Pearson, M. G., Chamberlain, M. J., Morgan, W. K. C., and Vinitski, S. (1985): Regional deposition of particles in the lung during cigarette smoking in humans. *J. Appl. Physiol.,* 59:1828–1833.

78. Pelham, F., Wewers, M., Crystal, R., Buist, A. S., and Janoff, A. (1985): Urinary excretion of desmosine (elastin cross-links) in subjects with PiZZ alpha$_1$-antitrypsin deficiency, a phenotype associated with hereditary predisposition to pulmonary emphysema. *Am. Rev. Respir. Dis.,* 132:821–823.

79. Postlethwaite, A. E., and Kang, A. H. (1976): Collagen and collagen peptide-induced chemotaxis of human blood monocytes. *J. Exp. Med.,* 143:1299–1307.

80. Powers, J. (1986): Mechanism-based inhibitors of human leucocyte elastase. In: *Second International Symposium on Pulmonary Emphysema and Proteolysis,* edited by C. Mittman and J. C. Taylor, Academic Press, New York.

81. Pratt, S., Finley, T., Smith, M., and Ladman, A. (1969): A comparison of alveolar macrophages and pulmonary surfactant obtained from lungs of human smokers and non-smokers by endobronchial lavage. *Anat. Rec.,* 163:497–506.

82. Pryor, W. A., Dooley, M. M., and Church, D. F. (1985): Mechanisms of cigarette smoke toxicity: The inactivation of human alpha$_1$-proteinase inhibitor by nitric oxide/isoprene mixtures in air. *Chem. Biol. Interact.,* 54:171–183.

83. Rao, N. V., and Hoidal, J. R. (1986): Oxidized halogens degrade elastin: A potential mechanism for smoking-induced emphysema. In: *Second International Symposium on Pulmonary Emphysema and Proteolysis,* edited by C. Mittman and J. C. Taylor, Academic Press, New York.

84. Rosenberg, S., Barr, P. J., Najarian, R. C., and Hallewell, R. A. (1984): Synthesis in yeast of a functional oxidation-resistant mutant of human alpha$_1$-antitrypsin. *Nature,* 312:77–80.

85. Sandhaus, R. A. (1986): Genetic basis of chronic obstructive pulmonary disease. *Semin. Respir. Med.,* 7:353–357.

86. Sauder, D. N., Mounessa, N. L., Katz, S. I., Dinarello, C. A., and Gallin, J. I. (1984): Chemotactic cytokines: The role of leukocyte pyrogen and epidermal cell thymocyte-activating factor in neutrophil chemotaxis. *J. Immunol.,* 132:828–832.

87. Schmeltz, I., and Hoffmann, D. (1977): Nitrogen-containing compounds in tobacco and tobacco smoke. *Chem. Rev.,* 77:295–311.

88. Schnebli, H. P. (1986): Eglin c, an elastase/cathepsin G inhibitor with therapeutic potential in emphysema and ARDS: A review. In: *Second International Symposium on Pulmonary Emphysema and Proteolysis,* edited by C. Mittman and J. C. Taylor, Academic Press, New York.

89. Seemuller, U., Fritz, H., Wiedenmann, K., Machleidt, W., Heinzel, R., Appelhans, H., Gassen, H.-G., and Lottspeich, F. (1986): The acid-stable proteinase inhibitor of human mucous secretions (HUSI-I, antileukoprotease). Complete amino acid sequence as revealed by protein and cDNA sequencing and structural homology to whey proteins and red sea turtle proteinase inhibitor. *FEBS Lett., (in press).*

90. Senior, R. M., Griffen, G. L., and Mecham, R. P. (1980): Chemotactic activity of elastin-derived peptides. *J. Clin. Invest.,* 66:859–862.

91. Senior, R. M., Tegner, H., Kuhn, C., Ohlsson, K., Starcher, B. C.,

and Pierce, J. A. (1977): The induction of pulmonary emphysema with leukocyte elastase. *Am. Rev. Respir. Dis.,* 116:469–475.

92. Snider, G. L. (1984): Two decades of research in the pathogenesis of emphysema. *Schweiz. Med. Wochenschr.,* 114:898–906.

93. Snider, G. L., Lucey, E. C., Christensen, T. G., Stone, P. J., Calore, J. D., Catanese, A., and Franzblau, C. (1984): Emphysema and bronchial secretory cell metaplasia induced in hamsters by human neutrophil products. *Am. Rev. Respir. Dis.,* 129:155–160.

94. Stockley, R. A. (1983): Proteolytic enzymes, their inhibitors and lung disease. *Clin. Sci.,* 64:119–126.

95. Stone, P. J., Calore, J. D., McGowan, S. E., Bernado, J., Snider, G. L., and Franzblau, C. (1983): Functional alpha$_1$-protease inhibitor in the lower respiratory tract of cigarette smokers is not decreased. *Science,* 221:1187–1189.

96. Theron, A., and Anderson, R. (1985): Investigation of the protective effects of the antioxidants ascorbate, cysteine and dapsone on the phagocyte-mediated oxidative inactivation of human alpha$_1$-protease inhibitor *in vitro. Am. Rev. Respir. Dis.,* 132:1049–1054.

97. Thompson, R., and Ohlsson, K. (1986): The secretory leukocyte protease inhibitor: Biochemical and biomedical aspects. In: *Second International Symposium on Pulmonary Emphysema and Proteolysis,* edited by C. Mittman and J. C. Taylor, Academic Press, New York.

98. Thurlbeck, W. M. (1963): The incidence of pulmonary emphysema with observations on the relative incidence and spatial distribution of various types of emphysema. *Am. Rev. Respir. Dis.,* 87:206–215.

99. Totti, N., McCusker, K. T., Campbell, E. J., Griffen, G. L., and Senior, R. M. (1984): Nicotine is chemotactic for neutrophils and enhances neutrophil responsiveness to chemotactic peptides. *Science,* 233:169–171.

100. Walter, A., and Walter, S. (1982): Mast cell density in isolated monkey lungs on exposure to cigarette smoke. *Thorax,* 37:699–702.

101. Walter, S., and Walter, A. (1982): Basophil degranulation induced by cigarette smoking in man. *Thorax,* 37:756–759.

102. Weitz, J. I., Landman, S. L., Crowley, K. A., Birken, S., and Morgan, F. J. (1986): Development of an assay for *in vivo* human neutrophil elastase activity. *J. Clin. Invest.,* 78:155–162.

103. Werb, Z., Bainton, D. F., and Jones, P. A. (1980): Degradation of connective tissue matrices by macrophages. III. Morphological and biochemical studies on extracellular, pericellular and intracellular events in matrix proteolysis by macrophages in culture. *J. Exp. Med.,* 152:1537–1553.

104. Werb, Z., Banda, M. J., and Jones, P. A. (1980): Degradation of connective tissue matrices by macrophages. I. Proteolysis of elastin, glycoproteins and collagen by proteinases isolated from macrophages. *J. Exp. Med.,* 152:1340–1357.

105. White, R., Janoff, A., and Godfrey, H. P. (1980): Secretion of alpha$_2$-macroglobulin by human alveolar macrophages. *Lung,* 158:9–14.

106. White, R., Lee, D., Habicht, G. S., and Janoff, A. (1981): Secretion of alpha$_1$-proteinase inhibitor by cultured rat alveolar macrophages. *Am. Rev. Respir. Dis.,* 123:447–449.

107. White, R. R., Norby, D., Janoff, A., and Dearing, R. (1980): Partial purification and characterization of mouse peritoneal exudative macrophage elastase. *Biochim. Biophys. Acta,* 612:233–244.

RECENT UPDATE

[1] Since this chapter was submitted, the complete sequence of PMN elastase has been published [Sinha et al., *P.M.A.S.* (1987), 84:2228–2232].

[2] Additional evidence of pulmonary mast cell stimulation in human smokers has since been obtained [Kalenderian et al., *Am. Rev. Respir. Dis.* (1987), 135:A153].

[3] and/or methionine. See Banda et al., *J. Clin. Invest.* (1987), 79:1314–1317.

[4] e.g., cathepsin L.

[5] These data have since been published [Wewers et al., *Am. Rev. Resp. Dis.* (1987), 135:539–543].

[6] These results have since been published [Stockley et al., *Thorax* (1986), 41:442–447].

[7] The surface area of the terminal and respiratory bronchioles combined is only 0.1% of the total surface area of the lung [Whitcomb (1982), *The Lung—Normal and Diseased,* p. 4. C. V. Mosby Co., St. Louis]. Even complete inactivation of α_1-PI, limited to this centrilobular zone, would be nearly impossible to detect.

Inflammation: Basic Principles and Clinical Correlates.
Edited by J. I. Gallin, I. M. Goldstein, and R. Snyderman.
Raven Press, Ltd., New York © 1988.

CHAPTER 45

Adult Respiratory Distress Syndrome

Richard H. Simon and Peter A. Ward

For the lung to function as an effective gas-exchange organ, ambient air must come into close juxtaposition to blood contained within alveolar capillaries. This can be accomplished only if the alveolar spaces are filled with air, not with fluid, and if an adequately low surface tension is maintained in the alveolar compartment. The responsibility for limiting fluid accumulation within alveoli belongs to the complex structures of the alveolar-capillary wall. Loss of integrity of this membrane causes alveolar flooding and subsequent respiratory failure. In this chapter we shall discuss the pathophysiology and treatment of respiratory failure that develops secondarily to diffuse injury of the capillary-alveolar wall.

In 1967, Ashbaugh et al. (1) described a group of 12 critically ill patients who had a variety of underlying illnesses and who abruptly developed pulmonary edema and respiratory failure. Prior to that time, others had reported the occurrence of respiratory failure in patients with certain specific underlying conditions. However, Ashbaugh and colleagues noted that despite the diversity of diagnoses in their patients, striking clinical and pathological similarities were present in their pulmonary abnormalities. They also noted that the lungs of their patients shared many physiological and histological features with those of neonates having infant respiratory distress syndrome. These observations spawned the term "adult respiratory distress syndrome" (ARDS), which has been widely used to describe this pulmonary process. In its broadest use, ARDS is applied to the condition in which there is acute severe injury of pulmonary capillary-alveolar walls leading to alveolar flooding and respiratory failure.

DIAGNOSIS

At present, there is no single, readily available clinical test that can be used to define ARDS. As a result, the diagnosis continues to be based on fulfilling a set of criteria. Although a universally accepted set of criteria does not exist, most definitions encompass the following requirements:

1. Respiratory impairment must develop acutely and then rapidly progress to respiratory failure. Not included are those chronic pulmonary diseases that eventually cause pulmonary insufficiency. In general, the term ARDS has been restricted to those patients with severe abnormalities (i.e., patients requiring mechanical ventilation). If, in the future, more sensitive and specific diagnostic tests are developed, the designation "ARDS" may also be applied to patients with milder degrees of lung injury.

2. Bilateral, diffuse alveolar infiltrates must be evident on chest roentgenograms. The abnormality must not be limited to a distinct anatomic area, but be representative of a generalized pathological condition.

3. Hemodynamic abnormalities must not be the sole

causes of the pulmonary dysfunction. Pulmonary edema that occurs secondary to elevated pulmonary capillary hydrodynamic pressure is excluded from the diagnosis of ARDS. Thus, patients with left ventricular failure or mitral valve disease are not included in the ARDS category. There is general agreement that for the diagnosis of ARDS to be made, the pulmonary arterial wedge pressure must not be elevated (e.g., <16–18 mm Hg). Unfortunately, this criterion excludes patients who have *both* primary capillary-alveolar wall injury and elevated pulmonary arterial wedge pressure.

4. The lungs must be noncompliant (i.e., increased airway pressure must be required to overcome the elastic forces of the lung). In their original description of ARDS, Ashbaugh et al. (1) noted that their patients had "congestive atelectasis" and decreased lung compliance. Many investigators require the total static respiratory system compliance to be less than 50 ml/cm H_2O.

5. The patients must be hypoxemic and respond poorly to administration of high concentrations of inspired oxygen. One frequently used criterion stipulates that the ratio of arterial to alveolar oxygen tension must be less than 0.2.

PATHOLOGY

On gross examination, the lungs are heavy and airless. By light microscopy, the alveolar walls are edematous, and capillaries frequently contain clusters of neutrophils, platelets, and fibrin clots (41,72). The alveolar spaces contain edema fluid and often are lined by hyaline membranes that consist largely of fibrin and cellular debris. The cellular component of the alveolar compartment includes red blood cells, macrophages, and neutrophils. When studied early in the course of ARDS, electron microscopy has demonstrated varying degrees of endothelial cell blebbing and necrosis (3,66). The thin type I epithelial cells that line the alveolar air spaces frequently show evidence of injury. Endothelial and/or epithelial cells may be lifted off their basement membranes, leaving large denuded areas. With the passage of time, type II epithelial cells proliferate in an effort to cover the alveolar basement membrane. The numbers of fibroblasts and the amount of connective tissue within the alveolar septae also increase, especially in ARDS patients surviving the first week of illness.

PHYSIOLOGY

The accumulation of fluid within the air spaces leads to alveolar collapse, causing a reduction in functional re-

sidual capacity of the lung (1). As mentioned previously, lung compliance is reduced. Hemodynamic measurements demonstrate an increase in pulmonary arterial resistance, with concomitant pulmonary hypertension. The alveolar flooding extensively disrupts normal gas exchange. Severe hypoxemia occurs due to passage of blood through capillaries of nonventilated alveoli (19).

RISK FACTORS

ARDS has been noted to occur as a complication of a large number of acute illnesses. Several large prospective studies have measured the frequency with which ARDS occurs as a complication of various diseases. In one study, all hospitalized patients at a medical center were monitored for the development of ARDS (25). Concurrently, the investigators monitored all patients who carried specific diagnoses that were thought to predispose to ARDS. Based on these data, it was concluded that the highest risk factors for subsequent development of ARDS were pulmonary aspiration (36%), diffuse intravascular coagulation (22%), severe pneumonia in the intensive-care unit (12%), hypertransfusion (5%), long-bone or pelvic fracture (5%), bacteremia (4%), cutaneous burns (2%), and cardiopulmonary bypass surgery (2%). The appearance of multiple risk factors in a given patient greatly increased the risk for development of ARDS. Another study found similar results (70). One of the diagnostic categories in this latter study was "sepsis syndrome," defined as the clinical picture of serious bacterial infection, with a concurrent adverse systemic response, e.g., hypotension. Of 13 patients in the study with sepsis syndrome, 5 (38%) developed ARDS. Thus, the risk of ARDS in bacteremic patients is markedly increased if there are associated abnormalities such as hypotension.

TYPES OF LUNG INJURIES THAT LEAD TO ALVEOLAR EDEMA

Despite the wide diversity of illnesses that predispose to ARDS, the clinical and pathological characteristics of the lung disease are remarkably consistent. This has led many investigators to postulate that there is a final, common pathway that leads to ARDS, regardless of differences in initiating factors. However, at present, a unifying pathophysiologic mechanism has not been identified. Instead, there is reason to believe that a single pathway might not exist. The permeability barrier formed by the capillary-alveolar wall is a complex structure (100). Prevention of alveolar edema is dependent on proper functioning of many different components. Serious injury to any of the individual components will lead to alveolar flooding, and the criteria for ARDS will be fulfilled.

The capillary endothelium provides the first impediment to movement of fluid from capillary lumen to alveolar air space. However, the endothelial barrier is incomplete; the tight junctions between endothelial cells do not completely exclude plasma macromolecules from the interstitial space (92). Under normal circumstances, the plasma proteins and fluid that reach the interstitial space are cleared by the pulmonary lymphatic system (89).

Theoretically, a large variety of pathologic processes could increase the flux of fluid across the capillary endothelium. Any endothelial cell insult that loosens intercellular tight junctions, reduces the adherence of cells to their basement membranes, or reduces cell viability would be expected to cause increased transit of fluid into the interstitial space. If the increased flux of fluid across the endothelium exceeds the capacity of the lymphatic system to remove the fluid, the volume of the interstitial space will expand. Although the interstitial space is somewhat distensible, it can accommodate only a limited amount of fluid before interstitial pressure increases and fluid leaks into the alveolar air spaces.

The air side of the alveolar surface is lined by two types of epithelial cells (100). Type I cells are flat, squamous-like cells that extend thin cytoplasmic plates to cover approximately 95% of the alveolar basement membrane. Type II cells are compact, cuboidal cells that occupy the remaining surface area of the alveoli. Both types of epithelial cells are joined together by tight junctions that are less permeable to macromolecules than are the endothelial junctions (44,78). Thus, the epithelium forms a tighter barrier against fluid movement than does the endothelium (92). In addition to acting as a physical barrier, type II cells have several other known functions that can limit the flux of fluid into the alveoli. For example, type II cells actively transport solute molecules from the alveolar to the interstitial compartment (29,56). Type II cells also secrete into the alveolar space the surface-active, lipid-rich material surfactant (75). By decreasing the surface tension of the alveolar lining fluid, surfactant causes the hydrodynamic pressure in the alveolar fluid located below the air–liquid interface to be less negative (relative to the interstitium) than it otherwise would be (30). In this manner, surfactant causes less fluid to be drawn out of the interstitium and into the alveolar space. Thus, dysfunction of any of these epithelial cell properties would be expected to lead to fluid accumulation within the alveoli.

From these considerations, it is apparent that a large number of independent pathogenic mechanisms potentially could cause the types of lung injuries that lead to ARDS. Studies of humans with ARDS have revealed that several components of the alveolar wall are often damaged. In particular, histological and ultrastructural studies have shown that both endothelium and epithelium are frequently injured (3,66). In addition, analysis of bronchoalveolar lavage fluid from patients with ARDS has also revealed that surfactant is often abnormal (32).

AGENTS OF INJURY

Many different mechanisms have been suggested to explain the causes of lung injuries that occur in various types of ARDS. In special cases involving exogenous toxins, there is evidence to suggest that direct injury to components of the capillary-alveolar membrane is responsible for the initial damage. This mechanism has been suggested for agents such as paraquat (55), the sedative-hypnotic ethchlorvynol (23), and high tensions of oxygen (21). In most cases of ARDS, the agent responsible for the lung damage is not definitely known. Evidence accumulating over the last several years has strongly suggested that activation of inflammatory cascades may be involved in the series of pathological events that culminate in ARDS.

Neutrophils

Much emphasis has recently been placed on the role of neutrophils as being an important cause of injury. In human ARDS, the evidence implicating the neutrophil is indirect but substantial. More definitive data have been obtained from experiments using intact animals, isolated perfused animal lungs, or lung cells maintained in tissue culture. Based on these pieces of information, a schema for neutrophil-induced lung injury has evolved (Fig. 1).

Investigations have revealed that early in the course of ARDS, neutrophils are sequestered within lung capillaries (3), causing a transient decrease in the number of circulating white blood cells (93). Neutrophils harvested from peripheral blood of patients with ARDS show evidence of preexisting "activation" (106). These cells demonstrate enhanced chemotaxis and generate abnormally high levels of oxygen metabolites following *in vitro* stimulation. Elevated concentrations of neutrophil secretory products, such as lactoferrin, have been detected in the plasma of patients with ARDS (31). If patients with mild lung injury also have diseases that reduce the blood neutrophil count, lung impairment frequently worsens if circulating neutrophil counts recover to normal (73).

Some neutrophils that accumulate within lung capillaries leave the vascular space and migrate into the interstitium and alveolar air spaces (3,66). Normally, there are only a few neutrophils present within alveoli. Neutrophils constitute less than 3% of all cells obtained by bronchoalveolar lavage of healthy volunteers. In patients with ARDS, the percentage of neutrophils in the lavage is markedly increased to 76 to 85% (26,52,61).

Although the activities of neutrophils may be important in many cases of ARDS, they are not demonstrably in-

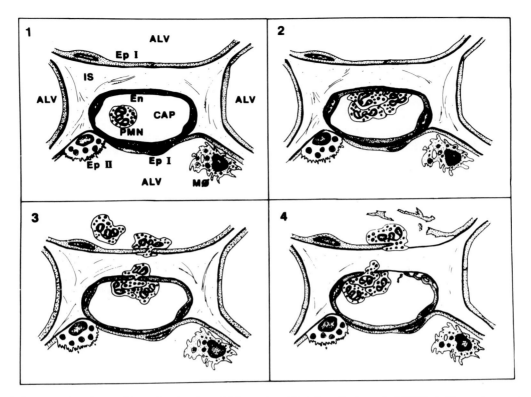

FIG. 1. Proposed pathogenic mechanism by which neutrophils injure the lung in ARDS. **1:** Normally, neutrophils (PMN) circulate through the pulmonary alveolar capillaries (CAP) without causing injury to capillary endothelial cells (En). The alveolar air spaces (ALV) are protected from flooding by endothelial cells, components of the interstitial space (IS), and alveolar epithelial cells. These latter cells consist of thin, type I epithelial cells (Ep I) and cuboidal, surfactant-producing type II cells (Ep II). An alveolar macrophage (Mϕ) is depicted within an alveolus. **2:** Secondary to a variety of pathological processes, inflammatory stimuli are introduced into the intravascular space, causing activation of various cascades, including complement. These products, such as complement fragment C5a, cause neutrophils to aggregate and become adherent to the endothelial surface. **3:** Neutrophils migrate through the endothelium into the interstitial space and then through the epithelium into the alveolar air space by passing through tight junctions. **4:** The activated neutrophils release agents that injure endothelial and epithelial cells, causing alveolar flooding and ARDS.

volved in all cases. ARDS has occasionally been reported to occur in patients who are severely neutropenic for days prior to the onset of lung injury (9,51,58). It is also possible that in some situations, lung injury may be initiated by certain toxic agents, and the damage is then amplified by the activities of neutrophils.

Although the evidence implicating neutrophils in the genesis of human ARDS is indirect, data demonstrating the importance of neutrophils in various animal models of acute lung injury are more definitive. The usual approach that is used to demonstrate neutrophil dependence is to deplete the animal of circulating neutrophils and measure any diminution in lung injury that occurs following administration of the stimulus. Although there have been several experimental models used to study neutrophil dependence of lung injury, only a few will be discussed in this chapter for illustrative purposes. One extensively studied model is administration of endotoxin to sheep (10). To monitor the various forces that govern

interstitial fluid accumulation, sheep were surgically instrumented, and hydrodynamic pressures, cardiac output, and lung lymph flow rate and content were measured. Using these measurements, any increase in extravascular fluid flux can be ascribed to changes in hydrodynamic pressures and/or capillary permeability. When endotoxin was infused into unanesthetized sheep, there was a brief period of pulmonary arterial hypertension with increased lymph flow that was not accompanied by increased capillary permeability. Several hours afterward, however, there was a second increase in lymph flow associated with a higher protein concentration indicating that an increase in permeability had occurred. Importantly, sheep previously depleted of neutrophils by administration of hydroxyurea had less of an increase in permeability following endotoxin infusion (40).

In another model system, lung injury occurred following intravenous infusion of cobra venom factor into rats (94). The cobra venom factor was found to induce systemic complement activation, neutrophil sequestration within the lungs, and an increase in extravascular leak of plasma macromolecules. Rats depleted of neutrophils prior to cobra venom factor infusion were totally resistant to lung injury. The ability of stimulated neutrophils to directly injure lung tissue has been demonstrated using perfused *ex vivo* animal lungs (63,82). When rabbit or rat lungs were perfused with solutions containing neutrophils that had been stimulated with phorbol myristate acetate, a brief period of increased pulmonary arterial resistance occurred, followed by an increase in vascular permeability. The injury was dependent on the presence of stimulated neutrophils, because perfusion with phorbol myristate acetate alone or resting neutrophils alone did not induce injury. Isolated endothelial cells and lung alveolar epithelial cells maintained in tissue culture are also susceptible to neutrophil-induced injury. Following exposure to stimulated neutrophils, endothelial (35) or epithelial (2) cells detach from the tissue culture plate. In many reports, clear evidence of cytotoxic events has been presented for both endothelial (76,96,104) and alveolar epithelial cells (86,90). If either result took place *in vivo,* increased lung permeability would occur.

Neutrophils possess many factors that potentially can injure lung tissue (Fig. 2). These armaments have been extensively studied in the context of neutrophil microbicidal functions. The cytotoxic agents include various degradative enzymes, lactoferrin, and cationic proteins that are contained within secretory granules. Another important group of toxic factors comprises oxygen metabolites.

Evidence exists to show that many neutrophil-derived products are detectable within the lungs of humans with ARDS. For example, bronchoalveolar lavage fluid obtained from patients with ARDS contains increased concentrations of the neutrophil secretory enzymes elastase (52,61) and collagenase (15). There are conflicting reports whether or not the elastase recovered in bronchoalveolar lavage fluid is catalytically active. In some studies, all elastase has been reported to be inactivated by being

bound to α_1-protease inhibitor that is also present within the lavage fluid (26,43). On the other hand, some investigators have found active elastase in bronchoalveolar lavage fluids retrieved from patients with ARDS (52,61). It remains to be determined whether these or other neutrophil degradative enzymes are responsible for injury in ARDS.

Neutrophil-derived oxygen metabolites represent another group of agents that have been incriminated as a cause of lung injury in humans with ARDS. Neutrophils contain a membrane-bound oxidase that, when activated, catalyzes the transfer of a single electron from NADPH to oxygen to form a free radical, superoxide anion. Superoxide is only the first of a chain of oxygen metabolites that are generated by this process. Superoxide interacts with itself in a dismutation reaction to form hydrogen peroxide. In the presence of chloride and myeloperoxidase (a neutrophil granule enzyme), hypochlorous acid is formed. If a transition metal is present and in the proper configuration, hydroxyl radical can be generated via the metal-catalyzed Haber-Weiss reaction. Once these oxygen metabolites are present, a large number of other toxic agents can be generated by free-radical reactions such as lipid peroxides.

With currently available methods, it is difficult to conclusively prove that neutrophil-generated oxygen metabolites cause human ARDS. However, it is known that oxygen metabolites are present within the lungs of patients who have the syndrome. For example, it was noted that some of the α_1-protease inhibitor that was present in bronchoalveolar lavage fluid of patients with ARDS was inactive (16). Analysis of the abnormal inhibitor molecules demonstrated that a critical sulfhydryl group had been oxidized to form a sulfoxide. Oxygen metabolites were shown to be able to induce this conversion and make the α_1-protease inhibitor inactive. More directly, analysis of condensates of expired breath from patients with ARDS revealed increased concentrations of hydrogen peroxide, when compared with other critically ill, intubated patients who did not have ARDS (6).

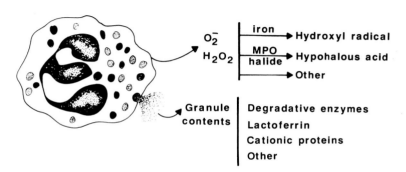

FIG. 2. Neutrophil products that are possible causes of lung injury in ARDS. Stimulated neutrophils release the free radical superoxide (O_2^-), which spontaneously dismutates to hydrogen peroxide (H_2O_2). The potential toxicities of superoxide and hydrogen peroxide are further enhanced in the presence of iron by forming the very reactive hydroxyl radical. In the presence of myeloperoxidase (MPO) and a halide, hydrogen peroxide is converted to hypohalous acid, with its own spectrum of reactivity. These agents and others can initiate free-radical chain reactions to produce additional toxic materials such as lipid peroxides. Neutrophils also contain within their granules other agents that may be responsible for lung injury. These include degradative enzymes (proteases, lipases, nucleases, and saccharidases), lactoferrin, cationic proteins, and possibly other agents.

There is strong evidence that neutrophil-derived products are able to cause lung injury in various animal models of ARDS. Rabbit lungs perfused *ex vivo* with xanthine and xanthine oxidase (produces superoxide and hydrogen peroxide) or with glucose and glucose oxidase (produces hydrogen peroxide) develop rapid vascular injury and pulmonary edema (91). These harmful effects are prevented by coinfusion of catalase (which converts H_2O_2 to oxygen and water), suggesting that H_2O_2 is a key product or intermediate. Recently it has been shown that xanthine/xanthine oxidase and leukocytic elastase may act synergistically in causing injury. Infusion of both agents together caused extensive damage, whereas each reagent alone produced no measurable lung injury (4). These studies suggest that lung microvascular injury might be the product of the combined effects of toxic oxygen products and proteases. This speculation has support from other studies in which it has been shown that (a) oxygen metabolites can alter substrates to increase their susceptibility to hydrolysis by proteases (24), (b) neutrophils exposed to proteases have substantial increases in their oxygen radical burst following addition of an appropriate agonist (45), and (c) oxygen metabolites can inactivate antiproteases, thus permitting increased proteolysis by neutrophil-derived proteases (16).

An *in vivo* model in which acute lung injury can be ascribed to neutrophil-derived oxygen metabolites is cobra venom factor infusion in the rat (94). Intravenous administration of cobra venom factor caused leukoaggregation and sequestration of neutrophils within the pulmonary microvasculature, leading to acute injury. Interstitial and intraalveolar edema with hemorrhage and fibrin deposition occurred. The development of lung injury was accompanied by the appearance of lipid peroxidation products in the lung and plasma (97). By the use of various interventions, the mediator pathways have been tentatively delineated. Neutrophil depletion is absolutely protective, as is infusion of catalase (a scavenger of hydrogen peroxide). Chelators of iron (deferoxamine and apolactoferrin) are highly protective, whereas infusion of iron salts accentuates the injury (98). Finally, hydroxyl-radical scavengers (dimethylthiourea and dimethylsulfoxide) are highly protective. These studies have suggested the following series of events (in order): complement activation, appearance in plasma of C5a, aggregation and activation of neutrophils, with production of superoxide and H_2O_2, iron-catalyzed conversion of H_2O_2 to hydroxyl radical, and finally focal destruction of endothelial cells within the lung microvasculature (Fig. 1). The infusion of venom factor causes abrupt and massive activation of complement. In other experimental models where the intensity of complement activation is probably less, it appears that an additional insult (such as anoxia, prostaglandin E_2, or sepsis with endotoxemia) probably is essential for the development of lung injury (99).

Other models in which oxygen metabolites mediate or participate in the development of acute lung injury include the following: IgG-immune-complex-induced injury of lung (in which neutrophils appear to be the source of the toxic oxygen products) (46); IgA-immune-complex-induced (49) and phorbol-ester-induced lung injury (in which lung macrophages may be the source of the oxygen metabolites) (47); and acute lung injury in sheep following infusion of bacterial endotoxin (in which blood neutrophils seem to be the source of toxic oxygen metabolites) (40). Finally, repetitive exposure of the rabbit airway to chemotactic peptides leads to acute lung injury that can be related to the combined effects of toxic oxygen radicals and released leukocytic proteases (81).

The ability of neutrophils to injure cells maintained in tissue culture has been demonstrated using a number of different types of cells. The identity of the agent responsible for the injury varies depending on the target cell used and the experimental protocol employed. In some circumstances, the injurious process appears to involve neutrophil granule enzymes. For example, neutrophil elastase has been implicated as a cause of endothelial cell detachment (35) and death (87). Similarly, neutrophil elastase was thought to be responsible for detachment of lung alveolar epithelial cells from their culture dish (2). In addition to the proteolytic enzymes contained within granules, plasma-membrane-associated neutral proteases have also been implicated in the cytotoxic activities of neutrophils (71). In another system, alveolar epithelial cells were killed by a process that required close neutrophil adherence to the alveolar cells but was independent of neutrophil-generated oxidants (86).

Various combinations of neutrophil-generated superoxide, hydrogen peroxide, hydroxyl radical, or hypochlorous acid have been identified as toxic agents in various *in vitro* cytotoxicity systems (103). Relevant to the lung, hydrogen peroxide was reported to be responsible for neutrophil-induced injury of isolated endothelial (76, 96,104) and alveolar epithelial cells (90). Using bovine pulmonary artery endothelial cells as a target, the iron chelator deferoxamine reduced the injury generated by stimulated neutrophils (96). This suggested a role for hydroxyl radical produced via the iron-catalyzed Haber-Weiss reaction. The neutrophil enzyme myeloperoxidase appeared not to be involved, because its inactivation by azide did not diminish (but actually increased) the cytotoxic effects of activated neutrophils on endothelial cells (96,104).

Macrophages

Other inflammatory cells may be involved in the development of human ARDS. Macrophages present within the pulmonary interstitium and alveolar air spaces possess many of the same potentially injurious agents as neutrophils. They contain a variety of enzymes and can release oxygen metabolites. In addition, they can take up enzymes released by other inflammatory cells, such as neutrophil elastase, and later release them at inflammatory sites (60). Whether or not macrophages are directly responsible for lung injury in human ARDS is speculative at the present time. When phorbol myristate acetate (an activator of neutrophils and macrophages) was instilled intratracheally into rats, the subsequent lung injury was found to be neutrophil-independent, but was inhibited by the addition of the hydrogen peroxide scavenger catalase (47). This led to the suggestion that oxidants released by lung macrophages were responsible for the damage. Similarly, acute lung injury in the rat caused by IgA immune complexes was found to be oxygen-metabolite-mediated; however, neutrophil depletion was not protective (49). It has therefore been suggested that stimulation of lung macrophages by IgA immune complexes and their subsequent generation of toxic oxygen products are central to the lung injury (48). In addition to directly causing lung injury, macrophages may be indirectly involved by their release of inflammatory mediators, including arachidonic acid metabolites, interleukin 1, tumor necrosis factor, and interferons.

Little information is available at present to evaluate the role of other inflammatory cells in ARDS, such as eosinophils, basophils, and lymphocytes.

MODULATORS OF LUNG INJURY

The signals that initiate and modulate the processes of lung injury are not well elucidated. In some circumstances, the stimulus may be introduced via the vascular system, and in other situations from the air-space side.

Endotoxin

Because septic shock is an important risk factor for ARDS, much interest has been directed toward the role of endotoxin as part of the initiating sequence. In humans, ARDS does not develop in all patients with bacteremia (25,70). Therefore, the presence of circulating endotoxin is not sufficient *per se* to cause ARDS. Because the incidence of ARDS is much higher when bacteremia is accompanied by shock, this suggests that endotoxin might work in concert with other factors to initiate the process of lung injury. In experimental systems using the rat (74) or sheep (10), endotoxin infusion induced lung injury, but the exact mechanism by which lung injury occurred has not been determined. As mentioned previously, the process is neutrophil-dependent, at least in the sheep. Endotoxin is known to influence inflammatory processes in several ways. It may participate indirectly by activating

complement via the alternative pathway (64). When present at low concentrations, endotoxin has been shown to greatly potentiate the ability of agonists to stimulate neutrophils to release toxic agents (36). For example, neutrophils preincubated with endotoxin and then stimulated with the chemotactic tripeptide formylmethionylleucylphenylalanine damaged endothelial cells, whereas neutrophils not preincubated with endotoxin did not (87). Endotoxin has also been shown to have direct toxicity for endothelial cells (34).

Complement

Activation of complement is another mechanism that has been suggested to be important in the genesis of ARDS. The ability of activated complement components to cause neutrophil sequestration within the lung was demonstrated in studies of patients undergoing hemodialysis (17) or cardiopulmonary bypass surgery (14). Exposure of plasma to the cellophane membranes caused the complement activation. Although extensive pulmonary neutrophil sequestration was shown to occur during hemodialysis, convincing evidence that clinically evident lung injury occurred is not available (68). In many patients with ARDS, complement activation has been detected by the presence of circulating complement fragments C3a and C5a (22,33,59,88,102). Of note, the presence of complement fragments is not sufficient to cause ARDS, because circulating complement fragments have also been detected in patients with risk factors for ARDS who do not develop the syndrome (22,59,88,102). Nevertheless, complement activation may still be an important step in the initiation of ARDS in many patients. In particular, complement may be critical by causing neutrophils to accumulate within the lungs, where they are stimulated by additional mediators to cause injury.

Arachidonic Acid Metabolites

Other suspected mediators of ARDS are the oxidative products of arachidonic acid. This suspicion is largely derived from knowledge that various arachidonate metabolites can induce many of the physiological alterations that occur in ARDS, such as vasoconstriction, increased microvascular permeability, aggregation of platelets, and chemotaxis of neutrophils. Reports of the results of direct measurements of arachidonic acid metabolites in human ARDS have been limited. In one study, the concentrations of arachidonic acid metabolites contained within respiratory secretions were measured in a group of 10 patients having ARDS and compared with those from a group of 5 patients with cardiogenic pulmonary edema (57). The ARDS patients had elevated concentrations of leukotriene

D_4, but not of leukotrienes B_4 and C_4, prostaglandin E_2, or thromboxane B_2.

Much of the interest in the role of arachidonic acid metabolites derives from animal studies. In a variety of animal models, elevations in arachidonic acid metabolites have been detected during the process of lung injury. In addition, inhibitors of various steps in the pathway of arachidonic acid metabolism were found to limit some of the changes associated with developing lung injury.

Products of the cyclooxygenase pathway of arachidonic acid metabolism have been detected in animal models of acute lung injury. Thromboxane B_2, the stable breakdown product of the active thromboxane A_2, has been found in lung lymph of sheep in which lung injury was induced by intravascular infusion of endotoxin (20) or thrombin (28). Thromboxane A_2 causes vasoconstriction, a prominent feature in ARDS. Other cyclooxygenase products have also been detected at increased concentrations in animal models of ARDS, including prostaglandin 6-keto-$F_{1\alpha}$ (the stable breakdown product of prostacyclin, a vasodilator and inhibitor of platelet aggregation), as well as more modest increases in prostaglandins $F_{2\alpha}$ and E_2 (20). In animal models, inhibitors of either cyclooxygenase or thromboxane synthetase reduced the pulmonary hypertension that occurred shortly after administration of endotoxin or thrombin (27). In some animal models, inhibition of these enzymes did not prevent the subsequent increase in microvascular permeability, suggesting that development of leaky lungs did not require thromboxane. However, in other animal models, nonsteroidal antiinflammatory drugs did reduce the severity of lung injury (7). Because ARDS occurs in some patients who take large amounts of aspirin (a potent cyclooxygenase inhibitor), it is apparent that products of the cyclooxygenase enzyme are not required for the development of human ARDS (38). This does not preclude their role in other types of ARDS.

Another important group of arachidonic metabolites includes those generated by the 5-lipoxygenase enzyme. Elevated levels of these molecules have been detected in various models of lung injury, including those utilizing intact animals and *ex vivo* perfused lung systems. Leukotrienes C_4, D_4, and E_4 constitute what was previously known as "slow-reacting substance of anaphylaxis." Depending on the species of animal tested, these agents generate varying degrees of increased microvascular permeability and airway constriction. As mentioned earlier, leukotriene D_4 has been detected in pulmonary secretions of humans with ARDS (57). Leukotriene B_4 is a potent neutrophil chemotactic agent, one source of which is stimulated alveolar macrophages. It has been hypothesized that macrophage-generated leukotriene B_4 is partially responsible for the neutrophil accumulation that occurs within the alveolar air spaces in ARDS. Another arachidonic acid metabolite with neutrophil chemotactic properties is 5-hydroxyeicosatetraenoic acid (5-HETE). Elevated levels of 5-HETE have been detected in the lung lymph of sheep infused with endotoxin (67). As opposed to the early appearance of thromboxane, 5-HETE was detected later and correlated temporally with the onset of increased permeability edema.

At the present time, no conclusive statements can be made regarding the role of arachidonic acid products in the acute lung injury of human ARDS. It appears likely that these products contribute to the full development of acute lung injury but that the arachidonate products are not essential mediators. It should also be pointed out that another unresolved question is the cellular origin of these products. Both platelets and neutrophils are rich sources of thromboxane A_2. Leukotriene C_4 is produced in large amounts by stimulated macrophages, mast cells, and basophils. From what source these arachidonate products emanate *in vivo* cannot presently be ascertained. With the continued development of arachidonic acid metabolite assays, analogues, and inhibitors, an improved understanding of the roles of these agents should be forthcoming.

Coagulation System

Indirect evidence of a role for coagulation products in ARDS is derived from several sources. Examination of lung tissue from patients with ARDS often reveals microthrombi and platelet aggregates within pulmonary vessels (95). Cross-linked fibrin is a major constituent of the hyaline membranes that are seen within the alveolar spaces. Diffuse intravascular coagulation is frequently associated with ARDS, occurring in 7 of 30 patients in one study (8). Based on other studies, however, it appears that diffuse intravascular coagulation may be secondary to the underlying disease process rather than the development of ARDS per se (62). Fibrinogen kinetics have been measured in critically ill patients, including those who have ARDS. Using intravenously administered ^{125}I-fibrinogen, patients with ARDS were found to have increased sequestration of radioactive label in their lungs, as compared with other critically ill patients who did not have ARDS (13). Using radiolabeled platelets, pulmonary accumulation of radiolabel has also been demonstrated in patients with ARDS (79). Plasma fibrinopeptide D, a product of fibrin degradation, has been detected in critically ill patients and has been shown to correlate with the development of ARDS (37). In one animal model, infusion of fibrinopeptide D initiated lung injury (53). When cultured confluent monolayers of endothelial cells were exposed to purified fragment D, the cells within the monolayer retracted (18). Whether activation of the coagulation system is the cause or merely the result of lung injury in human ARDS remains to be determined.

Other Mediators

Platelet-activating factor (acetylglyceryl ether phosphorylcholine) has properties that make it attractive as a mediator of ARDS. It induces pulmonary hypertension in sheep, possibly by causing thromboxane release (54). In some experimental systems, platelet-activating factor induces increased endothelial permeability (39). Its role in human ARDS remains speculative at the present time. Other agents that have been suggested to play a role in the development of ARDS are histamine (12) and serotonin (11).

Because there are extensive interactions between various components of the inflammatory system, it is difficult to discern which are initiating factors and which are merely secondary changes. As an example of the interdependence, it is known that Hageman factor can activate the coagulation cascade, the fibrinolytic system, the kinin pathway, and the complement system.

PREVENTION AND TREATMENT

Various approaches to prevent or treat ARDS have been suggested. Glucocorticoids have received the greatest interest. The results of glucocorticoid trials have been varied, possibly in part because of differences in the characteristics of the patient groups studied and the timing of drug administration. One study used the flux of ^{131}I-albumin from blood to lung secretions as an indirect measure of microvascular permeability. The investigators found that a high dose of glucocorticoid administered to patients with sepsis-related ARDS was temporally associated with a subsequent decrease in lung microvascular permeability (84). In this study, the patients with milder abnormalities of lung function responded to the glucocorticoid infusion, whereas those with more severe damage did not. In a double-blind, randomized study, methylprednisolone (7.5 mg/kg body weight every 6 hr for 12 doses) was administered to patients with trauma and fractures of major bones (80). The 21 patients receiving methylprednisolone had a reduced incidence of fat-emboli syndrome, as compared with the 43 receiving placebo. One of the hallmarks of fat-emboli syndrome is acute lung injury that has the features of ARDS. As opposed to the aforementioned studies, no benefit from glucocorticoids was reported for patients with gastric aspiration (105) or smoke inhalation (65), nor for a large group of critically ill patients at risk for ARDS (101). A few studies demonstrated a higher incidence of infection in the glucocorticoid-treated group (101,105). Importantly, preliminary results from a large, multicenter, randomized study do not support a beneficial effect of glucocorticoids in established human ARDS. Similar to the experience in humans, glucocorticoids in

animal models of lung injury have been shown to cause either beneficial (7) or deleterious (50) effects, possibly depending on animal species, type of injury, and timing of doses.

Prostaglandin E_1 has been reported to benefit patients with ARDS. Prostaglandin E_1 shares some properties with prostacyclin, e.g., it induces vasodilation. In a study of a small number of patients with ARDS, prostaglandin E_1 infusion was associated with a reduction in pulmonary arterial pressure and vascular resistance, an increase in cardiac output, and an increase in oxygen delivery to peripheral tissues (42,83). Before the use of prostaglandin E_1 can be advocated, a large-scale randomized study will be necessary.

In addition to the previously mentioned interventions, active research is being undertaken to develop and test agents that theoretically might limit ARDS. Based on their effectiveness in animal models, agents such as the oxygen metabolite scavengers superoxide dismutase and catalase, the iron chelators deferoxamine and dihydroxybenzoic acid (5), and various inhibitors of the arachidonic acid metabolic pathways might prove effective in some cases of ARDS.

Until generally effective pharmacologic agents become available, physicians will have to continue to use a number of supportive measures that lessen the physiological abnormalities of patients with ARDS. Over the last several years, important concepts of fluid management have been developed that are based on the Starling equation. This equation can be used to describe some of the forces that govern fluid flux across semipermeable membranes:

$$\text{fluid flux} = K_d[(\Delta P_{\text{hydro}}) - \sigma(\Delta P_{\text{oncot}})]$$

where K_d is the permeability constant of the membrane, ΔP_{hydro} and ΔP_{oncot} are the hydrodynamic and oncotic pressure gradients across the membrane, respectively, and σ is the reflection coefficient, which is a measure of how well the membrane limits the crossing of macromolecules.

Using this conceptual framework, studies in patients with ARDS have demonstrated that reduction of pulmonary capillary hydrostatic pressure reduces the main driving force that generates alveolar edema in ARDS (85). To reduce the hydrostatic pressure, fluid management is manipulated to maintain pulmonary arterial wedge pressure at the lowest level that still provides adequate cardiac output. In so doing, flux of fluid into the alveoli is minimized. However, the benefits to the lung have to be balanced against injury to other organs due to hypoperfusion.

As stated at the beginning of this chapter, the capillary-alveolar membrane in ARDS becomes permeable to macromolecules. This change can be expressed as a decrease in σ, the reflection coefficient of the Starling equation. With the loss of the permeability barrier, σ approaches zero, and plasma colloid osmotic pressure loses its effect on fluid flux across the damaged alveolar membrane. Therefore, the type of fluid (crystalloid or colloid) that is administered to patients with ARDS (in whom σ is close to zero) does not affect alveolar fluid flux (85).

In an effort to minimize the severe hypoxemia characteristic of ARDS, important concepts in ventilatory management have been developed. As mentioned previously, the hypoxemia of ARDS is secondary to the passage of blood through capillaries of alveoli that are collapsed or filled with fluid (19). It has been repeatedly demonstrated that reinflation of collapsed alveoli will reduce the shunt. This can be accomplished by adjusting the patient's ventilator to maintain an elevated airway pressure at the end of the expiratory cycle (positive end-expiratory pressure, or PEEP) (1). This manipulation increases lung volume at the end of exhalation and reduces the collapse of alveoli. With improved ventilation of alveoli, the shunt decreases, and arterial blood oxygen tension improves. The amount of positive end-expiratory pressure is chosen to provide adequate arterial oxygen tension at nontoxic inspired oxygen concentrations. However, it is also necessary to consider the adverse effects of positive end-expiratory pressure on cardiac output. At high levels of positive end-expiratory pressure, cardiac output is reduced by several mechanisms, including a reduction in venous return to the heart. Thus, to improve delivery of oxygen to peripheral tissues, a level of positive end-expiratory pressure must be selected that balances the beneficial increase in arterial oxygen tension against the decrease in cardiac output.

Because positive end-expiratory pressure improves arterial oxygen tension in ARDS, it has been suggested that it also reduces the extent of lung injury (77). Definitive studies that address this question are now available and have concluded that positive end-expiratory pressure does not alter the incidence or severity of lung injury, but only lessens the hypoxemia that develops when lung injury occurs (69).

PROGNOSIS AND FUTURE DIRECTIONS

Despite improved understanding of the pathophysiology of ARDS, the prognosis for patients with the syndrome remains poor. Mortality generally exceeds 50%, depending on the associated underlying conditions. It is unlikely that refinements in ventilator and fluid management will have a substantial impact on the survival of these severely ill patients. Only the development of agents that will block or limit the injury is likely to improve the outcome. To be effective, these interventions may have to be administered prophylactically or at least very early in the course of lung injury. Furthermore, there is increasing awareness that ARDS is a systemic condition

and that mortality is therefore also dependent on the extent of damage in other organ systems (e.g., heart, brain, and kidney). Any treatment regimen must then address the nonpulmonary manifestations of the syndrome. It has also become apparent that patients with ARDS who survive the first several days often succumb to subsequent infectious complications. Therefore, interventions that block parts of the inflammatory system (in an effort to prevent lung injury) must not cripple the body's ability to fight invading organisms. Only with a better understanding of the inflammatory processes that lead to ARDS can we expect to successfully develop such treatments.

ACKNOWLEDGMENTS

This work was supported in part by a grant from the National Heart, Lung and Blood Institute (HL-31963) and by a grant-in-aid from the American Heart Association, with funds contributed in part by the American Heart Association of Michigan (84-1058). The authors would like to thank Ms. Phyllis Green for secretarial assistance.

REFERENCES

1. Ashbaugh, D. G., Bigelow, D. B., Petty, T. L., and Levine, B. E. (1967): Acute respiratory distress in adults. *Lancet*, 2:319–323.
2. Ayars, G. H., Altman, L. C., Rosen, H., and Doyle, T. (1984): The injurious effect of neutrophils on pneumocytes *in vitro*. *Am. Rev. Respir. Dis.*, 130:964–973.
3. Bachofen, M., and Weibel, E. R. (1977): Alterations of the gas exchange apparatus in adult respiratory insufficiency associated with septicemia. *Am. Rev. Respir. Dis.*, 116:589–615.
4. Baird, B. R., Cheronis, J. C., Sandhaus, R. A., White, C. W., and Repine, J. E. (1986): Perfusion with hydrogen peroxide and neutrophil elastase synergistically causes acute edematous injury (ARDS) in isolated rat lungs which is inhibitable by non-oxidizable (Eglin) but not oxidizable (alpha-1-protease inhibitor) elastase inhibitors. *Clin. Res.*, 34:638A.
5. Baldwin, S. R., Simon, R. H., Boxer, L. A., Till, G. O., and Kunkel, R. G. (1985): Attenuation by 2,3-dihydroxybenzoic acid of cobra venom factor-induced acute lung injury in the rat. *Am. Rev. Respir. Dis.*, 132:1288–1293.
6. Baldwin, S. R., Simon, R. H., Grum, C. M., Ketai, L. H., Boxer, L. A., and Devall, L. J. (1986): Oxidant activity in expired breath of patients with adult respiratory distress syndrome. *Lancet*, 1:11–13.
7. Begley, C. J., Ogletree, J. L., Meyrick, B. O., and Brigham, K. L. (1984): Modification of pulmonary responses to endotoxemia in awake sheep by steroidal and nonsteroidal anti-inflammatory agents. *Am. Rev. Respir. Dis.*, 130:1140–1146.
8. Bone, R. C., Francis, P. B., and Pierce, A. K. (1976): Intravascular coagulation associated with adult respiratory distress syndrome. *Am. J. Med.*, 61:585–589.
9. Braude, S., Apperley, J., Krausz, T., Goldman, J. M., and Royston, D. (1985): Adult respiratory distress syndrome after allogeneic bone-marrow transplantation: Evidence for a neutrophil-independent mechanism. *Lancet*, 1:1239–1242.
10. Brigham, K. L., Bowers, R. E., and Haynes, J. (1979): Increased sheep lung vascular permeability caused by *Escherichia coli* endotoxin. *Circ. Res.*, 45:292–297.
11. Brigham, K. L., and Owen, P. J. (1975): Mechanism of the serotonin

effect on lung transvascular fluid and protein movement in awake sheep. *Circ. Res.*, 36:761–770.

12. Brigham, K. L., and Owen, P. J. (1975): Increased sheep lung vascular permeability caused by histamine. *Circ. Res.*, 37:647–657.

13. Busch, C., Dahlgren, S., Jakobson, S., Jung, B., Modig, J., and Saldeen, T. (1975): The use of ^{125}I-labelled fibrinogen for determination of fibrin trapping in the lungs in patients developing the microembolism syndrome. *Acta Anaesthesiol. Scand.* (*Suppl.*), 57: 45–54.

14. Chenoweth, D. E., Cooper, S. W., Hugli, T. E., Stewart, R. W., Blackstone, E. H., and Kirklin, J. W. (1981): Complement activation during cardiopulmonary bypass: Evidence for generation of C3a and C5a anaphylatoxins. *N. Engl. J. Med.*, 304:497–503.

15. Christner, P., Fein, A., Goldberg, S., Lippmann, M., Abrams, W., and Weinbaum, G. (1985): Collagenase in the lower respiratory tract of patients with adult respiratory distress syndrome. *Am. Rev. Respir. Dis.*, 131:690–695.

16. Cochrane, C. G., Spragg, R., and Revak, S. D. (1983): Pathogenesis of the adult respiratory distress syndrome. *J. Clin. Invest.*, 71:754–761.

17. Craddock, P. R., Fehr, J., Brigham, K. L., Kronenberg, R. S., and Jacob, H. S. (1977): Complement and leukocyte-mediated pulmonary dysfunction in hemodialysis. *N. Engl. J. Med.*, 296:769–774.

18. Dang, C. V., Bell, W. R., Kaiser, D., and Wang, A. (1985): Disorganization of cultured vascular endothelial cell monolayers by fibrinogen fragment D. *Science*, 227:1487–1490.

19. Dantzker, D. R., Brook, C. J., DeHart, P., Lynch, J. P., and Weg, J. G. (1979): Ventilation-perfusion distributions in the adult respiratory distress syndrome. *Am. Rev. Respir. Dis.*, 120:1039–1052.

20. Demling, R. J., Smith, M., Gunther, R., Flynn, J. T., and Gee, M. H. (1981): Pulmonary injury and prostaglandin production during endotoxemia in conscious sheep. *Am. J. Physiol.*, 240:H348–H353.

21. Deneke, S. M., and Fanburg, B. L. (1980): Normobaric oxygen toxicity of the lung. *N. Engl. J. Med.*, 303:76–86.

22. Duchateau, J., Haas, M., Schreyen, H., Radoux, L., Sprangers, L., Noel, F. X., Braun, M., and Lamy, M. (1984): Complement activation in patients at risk of developing the adult respiratory distress syndrome. *Am. Rev. Respir. Dis.*, 130:1058–1064.

23. Fairman, R. P., Glauser, F. L., and Falls, R. (1981): Increases in lung lymph and albumin clearance with ethchlorvynol. *J. Appl. Physiol.*, 50:1151–1155.

24. Fligiel, S. E. G., Lee, E. C., McCoy, J. P., Johnson, K. J., and Varani, J. (1984): Protein degradation following treatment with hydrogen peroxide. *Am. J. Pathol.*, 115:418–425.

25. Fowler, A. A., Hamman, R. F., Good, J. T., Benson, K. N., Baird, M., Eberle, D. J., Petty, T. L., and Hyers, T. M. (1983): Adult respiratory distress syndrome: Risk with common predispositions. *Ann. Intern. Med.*, 98:593–597.

26. Fowler, A. A., Walchak, S., Giclas, P. C., Henson, P. H., and Hyers, T. M. (1982): Characterization of antiproteinase activity in the adult respiratory distress syndrome. *Chest* (*Suppl.*), 81:50S–51S.

27. Frolich, J., Ogletree, M., and Brigham, K. L. (1980): Gram negative endotoxemia in sheep: Pulmonary hypertension correlated to pulmonary thromboxane synthesis. *Adv. Prostagland. Thrombox. Res.*, 7:745.

28. Garcia-Szabo, R. R., Peterson, M. B., Watkins, W. D., Bizios, R., Kong, D. L., and Malik, A. B. (1983): Thromboxane generation after thrombin. Protective effect of thromboxane synthetase inhibition on lung fluid balance. *Circ. Res.*, 53:214–222.

29. Goodman, B. E., and Crandall, E. D. (1982): Dome formation in primary cultured monolayers of alveolar epithelial cells. *Am. J. Physiol.*, 243:C96–C100.

30. Guyton, A. C., and Moffatt, D. S. (1981): Role of surface tension and surfactant in the transepithelial movement of fluid and in the development of pulmonary edema. *Prog. Respir. Res.*, 15:62–75.

31. Hallgren, R., Borg, T., Venge, P., and Modig, J. (1984): Signs of neutrophil and eosinophil activation in adult respiratory distress syndrome. *Crit. Care Med.*, 12:14–18.

32. Hallman, M., Spragg, R., Harrell, J. H., Moser, K. M., and Gluck,

L. (1982): Evidence of lung surfactant abnormality in respiratory failure. *J. Clin. Invest.*, 70:673–683.

33. Hammerschmidt, D. E., Weaver, L. J., Hudson, L. D., Craddock, P. R., and Jacob, H. S. (1980): Association of complement activation and elevated plasma-C5a with adult respiratory distress syndrome. *Lancet*, 1:947–949.

34. Harlan, J. M., Harker, L. A., Reidy, M. A., Gajdusek, C. M., Schwartz, S. M., and Striker, G. E. (1983): Lipopolysaccharide-mediated bovine endothelial cell injury *in vitro. Lab. Invest.*, 48:269–274.

35. Harlan, J. M., Killen, P. D., Harker, L. A., and Striker, G. E. (1981): Neutrophil-mediated endothelial injury *in vitro. J. Clin. Invest.*, 68:1394–1403.

36. Haslett, C., Guthrie, L. A., Kopaniak, M. M., Johnston, R. B., Jr., and Henson, P. M. (1985): Modulation of multiple neutrophil functions by preparative methods or trace concentrations of bacterial lipopolysaccharide. *Am. J. Pathol.*, 119:101–110.

37. Haynes, J. B., Hyers, T. M., Giclas, P. C., Franks, J. J., and Petty, T. L. (1980): Elevated fibrin(ogen) degradation products in the adult respiratory distress syndrome. *Am. Rev. Respir. Dis.*, 122:841–847.

38. Heffner, J. E., and Sahn, S. A. (1981): Salicylate-induced pulmonary edema. *Ann. Intern. Med.*, 95:405–409.

39. Heffner, J. E., Shoemaker, S. A., Canham, E. M., Patel, M., McMurtry, I. F., Morris, H. G., and Repine, J. E. (1983): Acetyl glyceryl ether phosphorylcholine-stimulated human platelets cause pulmonary hypertension and edema in isolated rabbit lungs. *J. Clin. Invest.*, 71:351–357.

40. Heflin, C., and Brigham, K. L. (1981): Prevention by granulocyte depletion of increased vascular permeability of sheep lung following endotoxemia. *J. Clin. Invest.*, 68:1253–1260.

41. Hill, J. D., Ratliff, J. L., Parrott, J. C. W., Lamy, M., Fallat, R. J., Koeniger, E., Yaeger, E. M., and Whitmer, G. (1982): Pulmonary pathology in acute respiratory insufficiency: Lung biopsy as a diagnostic tool. *J. Thorac. Cardiovasc. Surg.*, 71:64–71.

42. Holcroft, J. W., Vassar, M. J., and Weber, C. J. (1985): Prostaglandin E$_1$ and survival in patients with the adult respiratory distress syndrome. *Ann. Surg.*, 203:371–378.

43. Idell, S., Kucich, U., Fein, A., Kueppers, F., James, H. L., Walsh, P. N., Weinbaum, G., Colman, R. W., and Cohen, A. B. (1985): Neutrophil elastase-releasing factors in bronchoalveolar lavage from patients with adult respiratory distress syndrome. *Am. Rev. Respir. Dis.*, 132:1098–1105.

44. Inoue, S., Michel, R. P., and Hogg, J. C. (1976): Zonulae occludentes in alveolar epithelium and capillary endothelium of dog lungs studied with the freeze-fracture technique. *J. Ultrastruct. Res.*, 56:215–225.

45. Johnson, K. J., and Varani, J. (1981): Substrate hydrolysis by immune complex-activated neutrophils: Effects of physical presentation of complexes and protease inhibitors. *J. Immunol.*, 127:1875–1879.

46. Johnson, K. J., and Ward, P. A. (1981): Role of oxygen metabolites in immune complex injury of lung. *J. Immunol.*, 126:2365–2369.

47. Johnson, K. J., and Ward, P. A. (1982): Acute and progressive lung injury after contact with phorbol myristate acetate. *Am. J. Pathol.*, 107:29–35.

48. Johnson, K. J., Ward, P. A., Kunkel, R. G., and Wilson, B. S. (1986): Mediator of I$_g$A induced lung injury in the rat. Role of macrophages and reactive oxygen products. *Lab. Invest.*, 54:499–506.

49. Johnson, K. J., Wilson, B. S., Till, G. O., and Ward, P. A. (1984): Acute lung injury in rat caused by immunoglobulin A immune complexes. *J. Clin. Invest.*, 74:358–369.

50. Kehrer, J. P., Klein-Szanto, A. J. P., Sorensen, E. M. B., Pearlman, R., and Rosner, M. H. (1984): Enhanced acute lung damage following corticosteroid treatment. *Am. Rev. Respir. Dis.*, 130:256–261.

51. Laufe, M. D., Simon, R. H., Flint, A., and Keller, J. B. (1986): Adult respiratory distress syndrome in neutropenic patients. *Am. J. Med.*, 80:1022–1026.

52. Lee, C. T., Fein, A. M., Lippmann, M., Holtzman, H., Kimbel, P., and Weinbaum, G. (1981): Elastolytic activity in pulmonary

lavage fluid from patients with adult respiratory-distress syndrome. *N. Engl. J. Med.,* 304:192–196.

53. Luterman, A., Manwaring, D., and Curreri, P. W. (1977): The role of fibrinogen degradation products in the pathogenesis of the respiratory distress syndrome. *Surgery,* 82:703–709.

54. Malik, A. B., Selig, W. M., and Burhop, K. E. (1985): Cellular and humoral mediators of pulmonary edema. *Lung,* 163:193–219.

55. Martin, W. J., II, Gadek, J. E., Hunninghake, G. W., and Crystal, R. G. (1981): Oxidant injury of lung parenchymal cells. *J. Clin. Invest.,* 68:1277–1288.

56. Mason, R. J., Williams, M. C., Widdicombe, J. H., Sanders, M. J., Misfeldt, D. S., and Berry, L. C., Jr. (1982): Transepithelial transport by pulmonary alveolar type II cells in primary culture. *Proc. Natl. Acad. Sci. USA,* 79:6033–6037.

57. Matthay, M. A., Eschenbacher, W. L., and Goetzl, E. J. (1984): Elevated concentrations of leukotriene D_4 in pulmonary edema fluid of patients with the adult respiratory distress syndrome. *J. Clin. Immunol.,* 4:479–483.

58. Maunder, R. J., Hackman, R. C., Riff, E., Albert, R. K., and Springmeyer, S. C. (1986): Occurrence of the adult respiratory distress syndrome in neutropenic patients. *Am. Rev. Respir. Dis.,* 133:313–315.

59. Mayes, J. T., Schreiber, R. D., and Cooper, N. R. (1984): Development and application of an enzyme-linked immunosorbent assay for the quantitation of alternative complement pathway activation in human serum. *J. Clin. Invest.,* 73:160–170.

60. McGowan, S. E., Stone, P. J., Snider, G. L., and Franzblau, C. (1984): Alveolar macrophage modulation of proteolysis by neutrophil elastase in extracellular matrix. *Am. Rev. Respir. Dis.,* 130:734–739.

61. McGuire, W. W., Spragg, R. G., Cohen, A. B., and Cochrane, C. G. (1982): Studies on the pathogenesis of the adult respiratory distress syndrome. *J. Clin. Invest.,* 69:543–553.

62. Modig, J., Borg, T., Wegenius, G., Bagge, L., and Saldeen, T. (1983): The value of variables of disseminated intravascular coagulation in the diagnosis of adult respiratory distress syndrome. *Acta Anaesthesiol. Scand.,* 27:369–375.

63. Morganroth, M. L., Till, G. O., Kunkel, R. G., and Ward, P. A. (1986): Complement and neutrophil-mediated injury of perfused rat lungs. *Lab. Invest.,* 54:507–514.

64. Morrison, D. C., and Kline, L. F. (1977): Activation of the classical and properdin pathways of complement by bacterial lipopolysaccharides (LPS). *J. Immunol.,* 118:362–368.

65. Moylan, J. A., and Chan, C. K. (1978): Inhalation injury—an increasing problem. *Ann. Surg.,* 188:34–37.

66. Nash, G., Foley, F. D., and Langlinais, P. C. (1974): Pulmonary interstitial edema and hyaline membranes in adult burn patients. *Hum. Pathol.,* 5:149–161.

67. Ogletree, M. L., Oates, J. A., Brigham, K. L., and Hubbard, W. C. (1982): Evidence for pulmonary release of 5-hydroxyeicosatetraenoic acid (5-HETE) during endotoxemia in unanesthetized sheep. *Fed. Proc.,* 23:459–468.

68. Patterson, R. W., Nissenson, A. R., Miller, J., Smith, R. T., Narins, R. G., and Sullivan, S. F. (1981): Hypoxemia and pulmonary gas exchange during hemodialysis. *J. Appl. Physiol.,* 50:259–264.

69. Pepe, P. E., Hudson, L. D., and Carrico, C. J. (1984): Early application of positive end-expiratory pressure in patients at risk for the adult respiratory-distress syndrome. *N. Engl. J. Med.,* 311:281–286.

70. Pepe, P. E., Potkin, R. T., Reus, D. H., Hudson, L. D., and Carrico, C. J. (1982): Clinical predictors of the adult respiratory distress syndrome. *Am. J. Surg.,* 144:124–130.

71. Pontremoli, S., Melloni, E., Michetti, M., Sacco, O., Sparatore, B., Salamino, F., Damiani, G., and Horecker, B. L. (1986): Cytolytic effects of neutrophils: Role of a membrane-bound neutral protease. *Proc. Natl. Acad. Sci. USA,* 83:1685–1689.

72. Pratt, P. C. (1982): Pathology of adult respiratory distress syndrome: Implications regarding therapy. *Semin. Respir. Med.,* 4:79–85.

73. Rinaldo, J. E., and Borovetz, H. (1985): Deterioration of oxygenation and abnormal lung microvascular permeability during resolution of leukopenia in patients with diffuse lung injury. *Am. Rev. Respir. Dis.,* 131:579–583.

74. Rinaldo, J. E., Dauber, J. H., Christman, J., and Rogers, R. M. (1984): Neutrophil alveolitis following endotoxemia. *Am. Rev. Respir. Dis.,* 130:1065–1071.

75. Rooney, S. A. (1985): The surfactant system and lung phospholipid biochemistry. *Am. Rev. Respir. Dis.,* 131:439–460.

76. Sacks, T., Moldow, C. F., Craddock, P. R., Bowers, T. K., and Jacob, H. S. (1978): Oxygen radicals mediate endothelial cell damage by complement-stimulated granulocytes. *J. Clin. Invest.,* 61:1161–1167.

77. Schmidt, G. B., O'Neill, W. W., Kotb, K., Hwang, K. K., Bennett, E. J., and Bombeck, C. T. (1976): Continuous positive airway pressure in the prophylaxis of the adult respiratory distress syndrome. *Surg. Gynecol. Obstet.,* 143:613–618.

78. Schneeberger, E. E., and Karnovsky, M. J. (1976): Substructure of intercellular junctions in freeze-fractured alveolar-capillary membranes of mouse lung. *Circ. Res.,* 38:404–411.

79. Schneider, R. C., Zapol, W. M., and Carvalho, A. C. (1980): Platelet consumption and sequestration in severe acute respiratory failure. *Am. Rev. Respir. Dis.,* 122:445–451.

80. Schonfeld, S. A., Ploysongsang, Y., DiLisio, R., Crissman, J. D., Miller, E., Hammerschmidt, D. E., and Jacob, H. S. (1983): Fat embolism prophylaxis with corticosteroids. *Ann. Intern. Med.,* 99:438–443.

81. Schraufstatter, I. U., Revak, S. D., and Cochrane, C. G. (1984): Proteases and oxidants in experimental pulmonary inflammatory injury. *J. Clin. Invest.,* 73:1175–1184.

82. Shasby, D. M., Vanbenthuysen, K. M., Tate, R. M., Shasby, S. S., McMurtry, I., and Repine, J. E. (1982): Granulocytes mediate acute edematous lung injury in rabbits and in isolated rabbit lungs perfused with phorbol myristate acetate: Role of oxygen radicals. *Am. Rev. Respir. Dis.,* 125:443–447.

83. Shoemaker, W. C., and Appel, P. L. (1986): Effects of prostaglandin E_1 in adult respiratory distress syndrome. *Surgery,* 99:275–282.

84. Sibbald, W. J., Andersen, R. R., Reid, B., Holliday, R. L., and Driedger, A. A. (1981): Alveolar-capillary permeability in human septic ARDS. *Chest,* 79:133–142.

85. Sibbald, W. J., Driedger, A. A., Wells, G. A., Myers, M. L., and Lefcoe, M. (1983): The short-term effects of increasing plasma colloid osmotic pressure in patients with noncardiac pulmonary edema. *Surgery,* 93:620–633.

86. Simon, R. H., DeHart, P. D., Todd, R. F., and Curnutte, J. T. (1986): Neutrophil-induced injury of rat pulmonary alveolar epithelial cells. *J. Clin. Invest.,* 78:1375–1386.

87. Smedly, L. A., Tonnesen, M. G., Sandhaus, R. A., Haslett, C., Guthrie, L. A., Johnston, R. B., Jr., Henson, P. M., and Worthen, G. S. (1986): Neutrophil-mediated injury to endothelial cells. *J. Clin. Invest.,* 77:1233–1243.

88. Solomkin, J. S., Cotta, L. A., Satoh, P. S., Hurst, J. M., and Nelson, R. D. (1985): Complement activation and clearance in acute illness and injury: Evidence for C5a as a cell-directed mediator of the adult respiratory distress syndrome in man. *Surgery,* 97:668–678.

89. Staub, N. C. (1979): Pathways for fluid and solute fluxes in pulmonary edema. In: *Pulmonary Edema,* edited by A. P. Fishman and E. M. Renkin, pp. 113–124. American Physiological Society, Bethesda.

90. Suttorp, N., and Simon, L. M. (1982): Lung cell oxidant injury. *J. Clin. Invest.,* 70:342–350.

91. Tate, R. M., Van Benthuysen, K. M., Shasby, D. M., McMurtry, I. F., and Repine, J. E. (1982): Oxygen radical-mediated permeability edema and vasoconstriction in isolated perfused rabbit lungs. *Am. Rev. Respir. Dis.,* 126:802–806.

92. Taylor, A. E., and Gaar, K. A., Jr. (1970): Estimation of equivalent pore radii of pulmonary capillary and alveolar membranes. *Am. J. Physiol.,* 218:1133–1140.

93. Thommasen, H. V., Boyko, W. J., Russell, J. A., and Hogg, J. C. (1984): Transient leucopenia associated with adult respiratory distress syndrome. *Lancet,* 1:809–812.

94. Till, G. O., Johnson, K. J., Kunkel, R., and Ward, P. A. (1982): Intravascular activation of complement and acute lung injury. *J. Clin. Invest.,* 69:1126–1135.

95. Tomashefski, J. F., Davies, P., Boggis, C., Greene, R., Zapol, W. M., and Reid, L. M. (1983): The pulmonary vascular lesions

of the adult respiratory distress syndrome. *Am. J. Pathol.,* 112: 112–126.

96. Varani, J., Fligiel, S. E. G., Till, G. O., Kunkel, R. G., Ryan, U. S., and Ward, P. A. (1985): Pulmonary endothelial cell killing by human neutrophils: Possible involvement of hydroxyl radical. *Lab. Invest.,* 53:656–663.

97. Ward, P. A., Till, G. O., Hatherhill, J. R., Annesley, T. M., and Kunkel, R. G. (1985): Systemic complement activation, lung injury and products of lipid peroxidation. *J. Clin. Invest.,* 76:517–527.

98. Ward, P. A., Till, G. O., Kunkel, R., and Beauchamp, C. (1983): Evidence for role of hydroxyl radical in complement and neutrophil-dependent tissue injury. *J. Clin. Invest.,* 72:789–801.

99. Webster, R. O., Larsen, G. L., Mitchell, B. C., Goins, A. J., and Henson, P. M. (1982): Absence of inflammatory lung injury in rabbits challenged intravascularly with complement-derived chemotactic factors. *Am. Rev. Respir. Dis.,* 125:335–340.

100. Weibel, E. R., and Bachofen, H. (1979): Structural design of the alveolar septum and fluid exchange. In: *Pulmonary Edema,* edited by A. P. Fishman and E. M. Renkin, pp. 1–20. American Physiological Society, Bethesda.

101. Weigelt, J. A., Norcross, J. F., Borman, K. R., and Snyder, W. H., III (1985): Early steroid therapy for respiratory failure. *Arch. Surg.,* 120:536–540.

102. Weinberg, P. F., Matthay, M. A., Webster, R. O., Roskos, K. V., Goldstein, I. M., and Murray, J. F. (1984): Biologically active products of complement and acute lung injury in patients with the sepsis syndrome. *Am. Rev. Respir. Dis.,* 130:791–796.

103. Weiss, S. J., and LoBuglio, A. F. (1982): Biology of disease. Phagocyte-generated oxygen metabolites and cellular injury. *Lab. Invest.,* 47:5–18.

104. Weiss, S. J., Young, J., LoBuglio, A. F., Slivka, A., and Nimeh, N. F. (1981): Role of hydrogen peroxide in neutrophil-mediated destruction of cultured endothelial cells. *J. Clin. Invest.,* 68:714–721.

105. Wolfe, J. E., Bone, R. C., and Ruth, W. E. (1977): Effects of corticosteroids in the treatment of patients with gastric aspiration. *Am. J. Med.,* 63:719–722.

106. Zimmerman, G. A., Renzetti, A. D., and Hill, H. R. (1983): Functional and metabolic activity of granulocytes from patients with adult respiratory distress syndrome. *Am. Rev. Respir. Dis.,* 127: 290–300.

Inflammation: Basic Principles and Clinical Correlates.
Edited by J. I. Gallin, I. M. Goldstein, and R. Snyderman.
Raven Press, Ltd., New York © 1988.

CHAPTER 46

Inflammation Induced by
Staphylococcus aureus

John N. Sheagren

Inflammatory Components of *S. aureus*
  Cell Wall Components • The Staphylococcal Capsule
  and Slime Production • Toxins • Enzymes
**Clinical Manifestations of Inflammation Produced by
*S. aureus***
  Local Lesion Characteristics • Systemic Manifestations
Infections Caused by *S. aureus*

Toxin-Related Syndromes
  Staphylococcal Gastroenteritis • Toxic Shock Syn-
  drome • Staphylococcal Scalded-Skin Syndrome
Therapeutic Considerations
  Local Measures • Antibiotic Therapy • Anti-inflamma-
  tory Therapy for Staphylococcal Infections
Summary
References

Staphylococcus aureus continues to be a major cause of infectious morbidity and mortality both in the community and in the hospital setting (38,39). Especially within hospitals in this country, *S. aureus* is becoming more and more aggressive. *S. aureus* has now surpassed *Escherichia coli* as the leading cause of hospital-acquired bacteremia (20), with substantial resultant morbidity, mortality, and increases in the cost of hospitalization to those unfortunate enough to be so affected. This review will attempt to clarify mechanisms of inflammation generated by *S. aureus,* for, paradoxically, it is as much the inflammation generated by the organism as it is specific organism characteristics per se that lead to the types of tissue damage so characteristic of this accomplished pathogen.

INFLAMMATORY COMPONENTS OF
S. AUREUS

As microbes breach the barrier systems (primarily consisting of the skin and mucous membranes), proliferation occurs in subcutaneous tissues. Tissue damage is generated during *S. aureus* infection in two ways: First, the organism may directly injure the host by the production of toxic substances. Second, inflammation generated primarily through activation of the alternative complement pathway, the pathway triggered by a variety of high-molecular-weight, cell wall polysaccharides, also causes damage to host tissues. Of all bacterial high-molecular-weight, proinflammatory polysaccharide substances, endotoxin has been best studied, and it is a highly efficient activator of complement. Gram-positive microbes do not contain endotoxin (which consists of a lipid component, lipid A, along with polysaccharide, known together as the "core glycolipid"); however, they do generate inflammation as they proliferate through tissues, and it is important to realize that they, too, have highly inflammatory cell wall components, specifically able to activate complement via the alternative pathway (45). In addition, Gram-positive cocci, especially *S. aureus,* produce a variety of toxins and enzymes that can also generate inflammation; specifically, inflammation is produced both via complement activation and as the result of direct toxic or enzymatic damage to host cells and tissues, resulting secondarily in chemotactic fragment production and polymorphonuclear leukocyte accumulation in the area of the proliferating bacterium. The next several sections will describe how Gram-positive cocci generate inflammation through their cell wall components, toxins, or enzymes. This review depends heavily on data incorporated into a remarkable two-volume review of basic information concerning staphylococci and staphylococcal infections by Easmon and Adlam (12).

Cell Wall Components

The cell wall surface of *S. aureus* is composed of two structures: the external cell wall and the underlying cell membrane (15,33,48). The major components of the cell wall are peptidoglycan, teichoic acid, and protein A. The cell membrane is, like most microbial membranes, a lipid-protein bilayer. There are basic differences between Gram-positive and Gram-negative bacteria, most of which are discernible when one studies the ultrastructural and chemical composition of the cell surface components. Gram-positive organisms usually have a thick (up to 80 nm) homogeneous cell wall. In contrast, the Gram-negative microbial cell wall is thinner (20–30 nm) and characteristically has an outer membrane. As stated earlier, the polymers that make up the cell walls of Gram-negative and Gram-positive microbes are chemically quite different. Gram-positive bacteria contain peptidoglycan polysaccharides and/or teichoic acid or teichuronic acids with or without the presence of protein. The cell walls of Gram-negative bacteria are rich in lipophilic materials consisting of lipopolysaccharides, lipoproteins, phospholipids, proteins, and relatively little peptidoglycan (usually less than 10% of the cell wall components).

Staphylococci are typical of Gram-positive microbes in that the cell contents are surrounded by a unit membrane (known as the cytoplasmic or plasma membrane). The components of the microbe outside the plasma membrane consist of a thick, homogeneous, and only modestly electron-dense layer (the cell wall). The structure and characteristics of the cell envelope have recently been thoroughly reviewed (33). The walls of all staphylococci are composed of peptidoglycan and teichoic acid, the proportion of peptidoglycan being about 50 to 60% of the dry weight of cell wall preparations. Protein is also found in the cell walls of most staphylococci, with the best characterized cell wall protein being protein A, a protein found only in *S. aureus*.

The exact chemical composition of peptidoglycan, the main structural and shape-maintaining polymer in the staphylococcal cell wall, has been difficult to define. Peptidoglycan is a huge macromolecule, encasing the entire microbe in a semirigid container. It is best described as a heteropolymer consisting of glycan chains cross-linked through short peptides. The glycan component is fairly uniform and consists of alternating β-1,4-linked units of *N*-acetylglucosamine and *N*-acetylmuramic acid. In *S.*

aureus, about 50 to 70% of the muramic acid residues occur as *N*-6-*O*-diacetylmuramic acid, although some *O*-acetyl groups are also found in coagulase-negative staphylococci. The muramic acid phosphate may represent the attachment point between peptidoglycan and teichoic acid. The carboxyl group of muramic acid is substituted by an oligopeptide containing alternating L- and D-amino acids. Staphylococci almost always have a tetrapeptide as the oligopeptide, and adjacent oligopeptides are cross-linked either directly or by insertion of an interpeptide bridge. The end result of this chemistry is a semirigid structure that is rather resistant to degradation by a variety of tissue digestive enzymes and processes.

Cell wall teichoic acids are water-soluble polymers usually made up of glycerol or ribitol phosphate, sugar and/or *N*-acetylamino sugar, and sometimes D-alanine. Glycerol and ribitol residues are linked together through phosphodiester bridges. As stated earlier, the probable linkage between teichoic acid and peptidoglycan consists of a triglycerol phosphate that is attached through a phosphodiester linkage to the 4 position of the *N*-acetylglucosamine. Most strains of *S. aureus* contain a ribitol teichoic acid in their cell walls containing *N*-acetylglycosamine and D-alanine. Cell wall glycerol teichoic acids are widely distributed among coagulase-negative staphylococci, but may also be found among coagulase-positive microbes. All staphylococci contain a membrane glycerol teichoic acid. In fact, most Gram-positive bacteria contain a glycerol teichoic acid extractable from the ribosome-membrane fraction of disrupted cells. This material is known as lipoteichoic acid.

Staphylococcal peptidoglycans, when solubilized by ultrasonic treatment, have considerable biologic activities, the most important of which is that they are "endotoxin-like." Staphylococcal peptidoglycans are pyrogenic; they can cause gelation of amebocyte lysate (although requiring doses 1,000–400,000 times higher than endotoxin), can activate complement and thereby generate chemotactic factors, and can result in the aggregation and lysis of blood components, especially platelets. Intradermal injection of 10 to 100 μg of sonically solubilized peptidoglycan into a variety of experimental animals elicits a prompt inflammatory response. These responses have all the histologic and temporal characteristics of an "acute inflammatory reaction" beginning 4 to 6 hr after injection and peaking at about 24 hr. How peptidoglycan generates inflammation is not entirely clear, but it can activate complement both via the classic complement pathway and, in experiments in C2-deficient sera, via the alternative complement pathway (29). In that regard, studies by Peterson et al. (29), Wilkinson (48), and Verbrugh et al. (45) have shown that peptidoglycan is the major cell wall component involved in staphylococcal opsonization. Thus, the cell wall of *S. aureus* not only is important to structural integrity but also undoubtedly plays a major role in the generation of tissue inflammatory responses to the organism. Certainly a component of the "virulence" attributed to this aggressive organism is mediated by one or another cell wall constituent.

Protein A was first described among a variety of antigens in *S. aureus* in the late 1950s by Klaus Jensen (15). Protein A was found originally in about 75% of freshly isolated strains of *S. aureus,* and now it is believed that almost all pathogenic strains of the organism contain protein A. Protein A reacts with the Fc part of immunoglobulin molecules from a variety of different species. Protein A can elicit Arthus and anaphylactic types of reactions, histamine release from basophils, and activation of the complement system via the classic pathway. Protein A is also a valuable immunosorbent in affinity-chromatographic isolation of IgG from a wide variety of species. By using radioactively labeled myeloma γ-globulin, protein A is detected in the surface structures of over 90% of strains of *S. aureus* and is probably present in all coagulase-positive strains. Protein A itself has a number of interesting and probably pathogenetically important biologic effects, all recently reviewed in great detail by Forsgren et al. (15). These include complement activation, generation of both immediate and delayed hypersensitivity reactions, chemotactic activities and enhancement of phagocytosis, a variety of effects on lymphocytes and macrophages, including lymphocyte activation, and stimulation, as measured by the mitogenic response. Interestingly, cellular cytotoxicity is also dramatically enhanced by IgG–protein-A complexes, as determined by rosette-forming assays and cytotoxicity assays. Finally, as one might expect, protein A production is well correlated with pathogenicity, as measured by virulence in several experimental models of *S. aureus* infection.

The Staphylococcal Capsule and Slime Production

A complete and very well done review of the *S. aureus* capsule and a discussion of slime production have recently been published by Wilkinson (48). He points out that the phenomenon of encapsulation in staphylococci has been underappreciated by investigators, even though in recent years encapsulation of coagulase-negative staphylococci has been well described. The surface of *S. aureus,* as described in earlier sections, is, in fact, a mosaic in which all the major cell wall components and certain membrane components interact with both internal and external factors (29). The capsule is located external to the cell wall components and almost invariably comprises polysaccharides. Wilkinson defines the capsule as a covering layer outside the cell demonstrable by light microscopy and having a definite external surface. In addition to the clearly

defined capsule, another type of exopolysaccharide may be produced in some strains of *S. aureus* that is not attached to the bacterial surface. This material is termed "slime." Although it is known that the staphylococcal capsule consists of polysaccharide materials, biosynthetic studies of staphylococcal capsular polysaccharides continue to be a challenge. Also, the genetics and regulation of the biosynthesis of capsules and slime by staphylococci are as yet not well defined.

The relationship of encapsulation to virulence is an intriguing one. The major biologic differences between strain variants that do and do not possess capsules have been shown in mouse lethality studies: Encapsulated strains are highly resistant to phagocytosis and readily kill mice. In classic studies of encapsulated versus unencapsulated strains of staphylococci in 1965, Keonig and Melley, as summarized by Wilkinson (48), showed that in intraperitoneal infections in mice, relatively little phagocytosis of encapsulated strains occurred. Furthermore, intravenous immunization with the heat-killed vaccine made from the encapsulated strain subsequently protected mice from fatal infection. Encapsulated strains of *S. aureus* resist phagocytosis because the capsule acts as a physical barrier, preventing contact between cell-wall-associated C3 (the opsonic component of complement) and the membrane of the phagocyte, contact that is essential for engulfment and ultimately killing of the microbe.

Slime production is also likely to be associated with staphylococcal virulence, especially as regards infection around foreign bodies. Slime-producing organisms become completely surrounded by slime, a very amorphous material that is also a polysaccharide. Christensen et al. (7) noted that a high proportion of human *S. epidermidis* strains grew as a slimy film coating the culture flask. Such strains grew very well on intravascular catheters, and additional data have firmly linked slime-producing strains of *S. epidermidis* as more virulent in causing infections around foreign bodies, especially plastic catheters (7,9). No data are now available documenting whether or not slime-producing *S. aureus* strains are more virulent in foreign-body infections, which certainly seems to be a logical assumption.

Toxins

S. aureus produces a wide variety of extracellular toxins, and many earlier studies of the pathogenetic characteristics of *S. aureus* concentrated on establishing the identity of each toxin and its biologic activity. Seven toxins have emerged as being most important for understanding the pathogenesis of staphylococcal disease. These seven are the alpha, beta, gamma, and delta toxins, the so-called P.V. leukocidin, the epidermolytic toxin (responsible for the staphylococcal scalded-skin syndrome), and the enterotoxins, including enterotoxin F, now called "toxic shock syndrome toxin 1" (TSS toxin 1) and known to be the cause of the toxic shock syndrome (TSS) (5). A problem in studying the biologic effects of staphylococcal toxins is the fact that the highly purified toxins are very unstable, making especially difficult interpretation of negative biologic test results. Whereas early studies of staphylococcal toxins concentrated on their hemolytic effects, it is now known that those same properties are more broadly expressed against all types of cell membranes; thus, these toxins are in fact broadly cytolytic or cytotoxic. The next several sections will describe the individual effects of each toxin, drawing heavily on information contained in a recent review of the biologic effects of cell-damaging toxins by Wadstrom (47).

Alpha Toxin

Highly purified alpha toxins have been shown on repeated studies to be lethal for a variety of experimental animals. An experiment of nature in the 1930s, the so-called "Bundaberg disaster," strongly suggests that alpha toxogenic staphylococci are lethal for humans as well. In Bundaberg, Germany, several children died after having received a staphylococcal vaccine contaminated with alpha-toxin-producing microbes, an event that triggered a large number of *in vivo* studies in experimental animals strongly suggesting that alpha toxin is the major "lethal toxin" produced by *S. aureus*. The toxin seems to attack cell membranes relatively indiscriminately, damaging essentially every organ system that has been studied; however, alpha toxin has a particularly damaging action on the nervous system, producing a variety of dysfunctional effects on both the peripheral and central nervous systems. Alpha toxin also has a dramatic effect on vascular smooth muscle and/or endothelium, increasing the permeability of small vessels, a property inhibited by antihistamines. Alpha toxin also causes spastic contraction of large blood vessels and intestinal smooth muscle. Whether primarily or secondarily, blood pressure is elevated by alpha toxin injection, apparently because of catecholamine liberation. As stated earlier, alpha toxin is hemolytic and leukocidal and is able to lyse blood platelets. Other effects that have been attributed to alpha toxin include production of renal cortical and skin necrosis.

Beta, Gamma, and Delta Toxins

Each of these three toxins has been individually isolated and purified, so that at present there is no question that each is a unique entity. Not clear, however, is the exact degree to which each toxin produces damage to specific tissues and organs as has been demonstrated for alpha toxin. Further, how specific or different is each toxin's method of cytolysis also is not known. These substances probably act in a manner similar to alpha toxin.

Leukocidin

In addition to these four toxins, an entirely distinct toxin has been isolated that selectively damages phagocytes such as the neutrophil and the macrophage. Leukocidin, as it has been named, not only attacks individual leukocytes but also, when injected into experimental animals, dramatically stimulates phagocyte production, through mechanisms as yet unknown. Also, circulating granulocytes become activated by leukocidin, as measured by increased release of a variety of lysosomal enzymes and an increase in oxygen consumption.

Epidermolytic Toxins

Epidermolytic toxin (ET), the cause of staphylococcal scalded-skin syndrome (13,31), is made by a number of strains of staphylococci, most of which are typeable into phage group II. Several variants of ET have been identified, with molecular-weight estimates ranging from 24,000 to 32,000. It is clear now that at least two serotypes of ET exist that differ in terms of heat stability. Further, different toxin-producing strains of *S. aureus* may produce either or both of these serotypes. Despite some residual confusion, the two serotypes are now designated ET-A and ET-B. A complete summary of characteristics of the epidermolytic toxins has recently been published by Arbuthnott (1). ET seems to be produced by several genetic mechanisms still under investigation. The molecular basis of ET action remains unknown; however, both ET-A and ET-B produce the same histologic changes in the epidermis by causing separation of epidermal cells in the stratum granulosum, with resulting formation of intraepidermal clefts. Exactly how epidermal lysis occurs secondary to ET is not known. Also, whereas dramatic changes occur in the skin in both experimental animals and humans, little inflammation is evident. Polymorphonuclear leukocytes are absent, and minimal subcutaneous edema develops. In contrast to TSS, staphylococcal scalded-skin syndrome is benign, lacking any organ-system involvement other than the skin.

Enterotoxins

The enterotoxins (4) are a series of low-molecular-weight (25,000–30,000) proteins that are similar in activity and composition but are identifiable as separate proteins because of antigenic differences. Based on such differences, the enterotoxins have been termed enterotoxins A, B, C, etc. The clinical syndromes associated with enterotoxin production will be described later. The exact mechanism of action of the enterotoxins is not clear, but the presumption is that they have a direct toxic effect on cells, as do the other *S. aureus* protein toxins. The enterotoxins are the only biologically active substances produced by staphylococci whose toxic properties are resistant to proteolytic enzymes. Despite extensive studies trying to define the exact target substances of the enterotoxins that result in the dramatic clinical syndrome of gastroenteritis, no information is available at the present time that firmly defines their mode(s) of action.

Todd et al. (42) described TSS, a newly recognized disease associated with *S. aureus* infection. It is now known that the toxin responsible for this dramatic syndrome (see following) is an enterotoxin named "enterotoxin F" (5). The same toxin was called pyrogenic exotoxin C by Schlievert et al. (34). The toxin is now called TSS toxin 1, in case other forms of TSS should be identified in the future (5). Whereas TSS toxin 1 is the toxin that produces full-blown TSS, all other enterotoxins exhibit some similar toxic characteristics. For example, individual experiments

have shown other enterotoxins to affect organs other than the gastrointestinal tract; for example, some toxins affect circulating formed blood elements, especially the platelets, resulting in thrombocytopenia, and most enterotoxins produce hypotension. Thus, it appears that all enterotoxins express some of the biological characteristics of TSS toxin 1. The mechanism(s) by which staphylococcal enterotoxins produce inflammatory damage and the clinical syndrome will be addressed in a later section.

Enzymes

S. aureus strains produce large numbers of proteins that are released into their surrounding environments when grown either *in vitro* or *in vivo*. More than 25 different extracellular proteins have been identified. A complete review of extracellular enzymes from *S. aureus* was published by Arvidson in 1983 (2). Of the 25 extracellular proteins identified, 9 have been characterized as toxins, and the remaining are nontoxic enzymes or enzyme activators. Enzymes of importance that have been identified from *S. aureus* are listed in Table 1.

TABLE 1. *Important enzymes in* Staphylococcus aureus

Enzymes	Characteristics	References
Staphylocoagulase	Key marker of pathogenicity; causes polymerization of fibrinogen	21
Bacteriolytic enzymes ("lysozyme")	Probably an endo-β-N-acetylglucosaminidase	2
Hyaluronate lyase ("mucilase," "spreading factor," "hyaluronidase")	Polysaccharide-containing	2
Lipase	Associated with furunculosis-producing strains	2
Nuclease	A DNAase	2
Penicillinase	An inducible, extracellular β-lactamase; determined by plasmid DNA	2
Phosphatase	Both acid and alkaline varieties have been described	2
Proteinases	Three varieties produced: a serine protease, a metalloprotease, and a thiol protease	2
Staphylokinase	Activates plasminogen to plasmin; responsible for fibrinolytic activity by *S. aureus*	2

CLINICAL MANIFESTATIONS OF INFLAMMATION PRODUCED BY *S. AUREUS*

It is useful to divide the clinical manifestations of inflammation during *S. aureus* infections into those manifested locally versus systemically. Local lesion characteristics can, in turn, be due either to direct proliferation of the organism at the site of infection or to distant effects of toxins on the skin. Although systemic manifestations may be produced by toxins (e.g., staphylococcal scalded-skin syndrome and TSS), they are more commonly seen during bacteremia with *S. aureus,* which, not uncommonly, may result in septic shock and the syndrome of multiple-organ-system failure with or without the presence of disseminated intravascular coagulation.

Local Lesion Characteristics

Staphylococcal infections almost invariably are initiated by an endogenously carried organism (commonly colonized sites are the nose, throat, intertriginous areas, and the perineum) that enters a break in the dermal barriers. If such a break is associated with a foreign body (for example, a suture or an intravascular catheter), the inoculum of organisms required to produce an infection/lesion is dramatically reduced (38,39). Nonetheless, a localized staphylococcal lesion is quite characteristic: Initially, the site becomes painful, followed shortly thereafter by the presence of erythema and induration and, ultimately, the formation of an abscess containing thick, creamy pus. Histologically, the inflammatory reaction is typified by hyperemia, tissue edema, and a massive influx of polymorphonuclear leukocytes. Tissue necrosis is common, and fibrosis occurs during healing. In chronic, healing infections, mononuclear cells predominate, and giant cells are commonly seen. Special stains often will reveal that the organisms have moved through tissues more rapidly than the accumulation of polymorphonuclear leukocytes has contained them. The antiphagocytic properties of the capsule, combined with the microbe's ability to produce the variety of enzymes mentioned earlier, undoubtedly are related to their characteristic elusiveness.

Local lesions produced by toxins are quite different. The skin changes produced by the scalded-skin syndrome and TSS begin as dermal blotches that then progress to a diffuse erythroderma, reflecting increased vascularity of the skin. The mechanism underlying increased vascularity is not known; at biopsy, little, if any, inflammation is present in the skin in either syndrome. During staphylococcal scalded-skin syndrome, lysis of the intracellular connections within the epidermis itself produces the blistering skin lesions associated with the disease; however, we do not know what triggers the increased vascular flow to the skin, or whether or not other mediators of inflammation are involved (such as kinins, products of the arachidonic acid cascade, etc.). In TSS, the epidermal damage occurs in the deeper epidermal layers (22).

Systemic Manifestations

During bacteremia, *S. aureus* organisms can cause two different types of complications: microbiologic and metabolic. First, as regards microbiologic complications, the organism delights in seeding to multiple organs and tissues as well as to the heart valves (causing endocarditis) (38). How the organism seeds to peripheral sites is not clear, but increasing evidence implicates a variety of adhesins (11). Specifically, *S. aureus* has receptors on its cell surface for such subendothelial substances as fibronectin (43,46) and laminin (46). Further, fibronectin-induced agglutination of *S. aureus* correlates with invasiveness (30). Presumably, chronically inflamed or traumatized tissues will have had such subendothelial components exposed, so that during *S. aureus* bacteremia, organisms can easily adhere to the subendothelial and/or subcutaneous structures. Once having seeded to the area of inflammation, the organism can readily proliferate and invade into deeper tissues. Each metastatic lesion presumably will have the same inflammatory characteristics as the local lesion described earlier, namely, activation of all elements of tissue inflammation via complement, coagulation, and the kinin systems, accompanied by a dramatic subsequent influx of neutrophils to the area.

Other metabolic complications produced by *S. aureus* bacteremia/septicemia include the septic shock syndrome and the syndromes of multiple-organ-system failure and disseminated intravascular coagulation. The exact mechanism of systemic shock production by *S. aureus* is not clear, as recently reviewed in detail (38–40). One way *S. aureus* can produce shock is by severely damaging a variety of local organs responsible for hemodynamic stability; for example, myocardial abscess formation may lead to cardiogenic shock; rupture of vessels by mycotic aneurysm or extremely severe diarrhea may lead to hypovolemic shock. Yet, intravascular staphylococci can also trigger the classic syndrome of septic shock in exactly the same manner as Gram-negative organisms. The endotoxin-like substances in the staphylococcal cell wall (the peptidoglycan–teichoic acid complex) activate complement and a variety of other systemic inflammatory and endocrine systems, resulting in hemodynamic deterioration and septic shock, just as endotoxin in Gram-negative organisms mediates the same series of events (40). Inflammatory processes activated during bacteremia include the complement system, the coagulation system (whether directly by cell wall products or assisted by coagulase), the kinin system, and the ACTH-endorphin system.

Strains of *S. aureus* isolated from patients suffering from septic shock and disseminated intravascular coagulation (24,26) have been found to be highly efficient activators of complement (44).

Thus, pathologic manifestations of systemic infection with *S. aureus* consist of metastatic abscess formation in multiple organs and/or findings of multiple-organ-system failure such as adult respiratory-distress syndrome, renal failure, toxic hepatopathy, etc.

INFECTIONS CAUSED BY *S. AUREUS*

Clearly, the major reason why *S. aureus* is important as a human pathogen stems from its propensity to cause rapidly progressive infection in almost every tissue and organ system within the body (38). Skin and skin-structure infections are most commonly caused by *S. aureus*, and a general clinical rule is that one should initially consider *S. aureus* to be the responsible pathogen in *any* skin infection. Thus, initial treatment must appropriately cover *S. aureus*, even though a variety of other organisms may be involved (for example, the β-hemolytic streptococcus). In the community, *S. aureus* is the agent most commonly found to be responsible for a wide variety of skin infections such as recurrent boils, folliculitis, etc., as well as secondary infections of traumatic wounds produced in the skin and mucous membranes. Starting from a skin focus, the organism can work its way through tissues directly to involve deeper structures such as bones (osteomyelitis) and joints (septic arthritis). Involvement of muscle is a unique characteristic of debilitated, undernourished populations in tropical climates, and it results in the syndrome known as pyomyositis (32). *S. aureus* can directly produce overwhelming staphylococcal pneumonia (often complicating a viral pneumonia) as well as primary *S. aureus* urinary tract infection, although more commonly infections in the latter two organ systems result from seeding during bacteremia. Of course, *S. aureus* bacteremia can result in seeding of all the organ systems listed earlier, including skin, skin structures, muscles, bones, and joints. Central nervous system infections can result either from direct inoculation of the organism into the central nervous system (as following neurosurgery or trauma) or from systemic seeding to the central nervous system during an episode of staphylococcal bacteremia.

S. aureus bacteremia, as mentioned earlier, is extremely common, *S. aureus* being the single leading cause of hospital-acquired bacteremia (20). A 500-bed community or university hospital generally will record between three and five episodes of *S. aureus* bacteremia monthly. Such episodes usually are secondary to a peripheral site of infection that has seeded the bloodstream, intravascular catheters being the most common sources. Bacteremia may be asymptomatic, most commonly in debilitated patients; in otherwise healthy individuals, fever, chills, and other signs of systemic infection usually are present. Septicemia (self-perpetuating bacteremia associated with severe symptoms of systemic inflammation) may occur without endocarditis, but the more symptomatic an individual appears during an episode of *S. aureus* bacteremia, the more likely are multiple organs to have been seeded and endocarditis to have developed. Endocarditis is defined as *S. aureus* infection of cardiac valves. Any type of valvular abnormality, no matter how minor (as in the prolapsed-mitral-valve/click-murmur syndrome, minor aortic valve abnormalities such as a bicuspid aortic valve, fenestrated valve leaflets, etc.) will result in a very high likelihood of seeding and rapid progression of cardiac valve malfunction. Obviously, organically damaged valves (as from rheumatic fever) or congenital heart defects are at extremely high risk of involvement during an episode of staphylococcal bacteremia. There is also no question that neglected episodes of *S. aureus* bacteremia may, and not uncommonly do, seed to entirely normal valves, especially the aortic valve (39). Thus, the most devastating complication of *S. aureus* bacteremia in terms of the microbiologic complication is endocarditis. The epidemiology, clinical manifestations, diagnosis, and treatment of *S. aureus* endocarditis have recently been reviewed (38,39).

TOXIN-RELATED SYNDROMES

This section will review the syndromes of staphylococcal gastroenteritis, TSS, and the staphylococcal scalded-skin syndrome.

Staphylococcal Gastroenteritis

As stated earlier, the staphylococcal enterotoxins are the best-known causative agents of food-borne disease, and staphylococcal gastroenteritis is the leading cause of food-borne illness in the world (38). Of course, other causative agents such as salmonella, shigella, campylobacter, clostridia, and some species of vibrios may be more frequent causes of food poisoning in some countries.

The site of action of the enterotoxin in assumed to be the digestive tract, but, as evidenced most dramatically in TSS, enterotoxins may directly alter blood pressure, cause fever, and affect other organ systems as well. Preformed toxin is generated by enterotoxigenic strains of *S. aureus* when they are grown in high-carbohydrate-containing foodstuffs. High concentrations of carbohydrates apparently enhance the generation of toxin.

Evidence is strong that the preformed toxin is absorbed into the circulatory system: In experimental animals, more toxin in required intragastrically to duplicate the symptoms of staphylococcal food poisoning than when the toxin is given intravenously. The exact mechanism of how the staphylococcal enterotoxins produce the clinical syndrome of nausea, vomiting, and diarrhea, despite numerous studies in experimental animals and observations in humans, remains unclear. I assume that the toxin directly damages selected cells, producing the functional changes.

It is important to separate the syndrome of staphylococcal enteritis from staphylococcal food poisoning. Following the development of antibiotics in the early 1950s, patients occasionally developed an overwhelming gastrointestinal infection with pseudomembrane formation in which massive numbers of staphylococci were present in the stool. Such strains almost invariably were potent producers of enterotoxin (4), and it was concluded that the enterotoxins were the cause of the enteritis, as pseudomembrane formation is observed in some cases of staphylococcal gastroenteritis as well. Undoubtedly, some of the early cases of staphylococcal pseudomembranous enteritis or enterocolitis were caused by *Clostridium difficile,* which had not been discovered at that time. On the other hand, enterotoxigenic staphylococci produce a similar syndrome when present in extremely large numbers in the gastrointestinal tract.

Toxic Shock Syndrome

As stated earlier, Todd et al. (42) first described TSS. TSS is the result of *in vivo* production of a protein toxin (called TSS toxin 1) at the site of a localized and often relatively asymptomatic peripheral infection with a TSS-toxin-1-producing strain of *S. aureus.* Production of TSS toxin 1 has been shown by Schutzer et al. (37) to be the result of lysogeny, the presence of a temperate bacteriophage. The toxin has now been highly purified, and the syndrome has been reproduced in rabbits and primates. The exact mechanism of TSS toxin 1 tissue damage is not known. It is likely that, as with other enterotoxins, it directly attacks peripheral tissues. Alternatively, Schlievert (35) suggests that the toxin enhances the effect of Gram-negative bacterial cell wall endotoxins so that a very small, usually subtoxic, amount of endotoxin will cause extensive host damage. TSS toxin 1 slows clearance of endotoxin from the blood of rabbits (16). Newer studies have also shown that strains of *S. aureus* from patients with TSS are potent inducers of interleukin 1 (IL-1) when compared with non-TSS-associated strains (18,27). Interestingly, IL-1 induction was independent of the production of TSS toxin 1, raising a new question regarding the precise role of TSS toxin 1 in the pathogenesis of TSS.

Toxogenic strains of *S. aureus* exhibit enhanced TSS toxin 1 production when the concentration of magnesium in the culture medium is reduced (23), a condition produced *in vivo* by the chelation of magnesium by superabsorbent tampon material. When TSS was first recognized, most cases were related to menstruation; however, at present, approximately one-third of all cases are not menstrually associated. Of interest is the fact that superabsorbent tampon material in any site enhances toxin production, as has recently been illustrated by the association of TSS with nasal packing materials.

The clinical syndrome is dramatic. There is abrupt onset of high fever, chills, myalgias, nausea, vomiting, and profuse watery diarrhea, as would be expected with an enterotoxin. Within the first few days, however, a sunburn-like rash appears, along with conjunctival injection. On biopsy, the epidermis exhibits cleavage in the basal layers of the skin (22). Histologically, the site of epidermal cleavage differentiates it from the staphylococcal scalded-skin syndrome (described following) and from viral infections and drug eruptions. The patient becomes progressively hypotensive and begins to exhibit impairment of function in multiple organs: Most commonly seen are pulmonary failure, renal failure, altered mentation, a hepatopathy, a cardiomyopathy, and a myopathy (muscle enzymes are highly elevated in serum). Additional abnormalities are found in almost every other organ system studied. Unique to the syndrome is profound thrombocytopenia, usually without evidence of disseminated intravascular coagulation. The serum albumin drops dramatically, and levels of less than 2 g/dl are common. Out of proportion to the drop in albumin is the decline in serum calcium, and levels of calcitonin are highly elevated (6).

Therapy for TSS is supportive. It is important to identify the peripheral localized site of *S. aureus* infection in order to permit drainage. Antibiotics are indicated, as relapse is less frequent in patients with TSS associated with menstruation who are treated with antibiotics. Antibiotics do not, however, have much effect on the outcome of the initial clinical illness. TSS-toxin-1-producing strains of *S. aureus* usually are readily identified from the site of the peripheral infection; however, bacteremia is rare. It is conceivable that development of a monoclonal human antibody against TSS toxin 1 could shorten the course of the acute illness. Also, patients with TSS, in general, lack preexisting antibodies against TSS toxin 1 (38), suggesting that a vaccine might also be helpful.

Staphylococcal Scalded-Skin Syndrome

Staphylococcal scalded-skin syndrome (SSSS) is a benign, toxin-mediated disease produced by certain strains of *S. aureus,* usually of bacteriophage group II. These strains produce an exfoliative toxin. Whether epidermolytic toxin production is controlled by lysogeny, the presence of a plasmid, or some other mechanism is unknown. Again, staphylococci proliferate in a peripheral focus of infection, usually in an infant or young child, although adult cases have been described (25). Epidermolytic toxin is adsorbed systemically and circulates to the skin. There is cleavage of the middle layers of the epidermis, with bullae formation, and ultimately a slipping away of the superficial layer of the epithelium on gentle pressure (a positive Nikolsky sign). Histopathologically, there is cleavage of the epidermis, without any other visible signs of inflammation; no other organs are involved in this syndrome. The only morbidity due to SSSS is related to the site of initial infection: As with all staphylococcal infections, local progression of the infection and/or systemic spread of the organism may occur.

THERAPEUTIC CONSIDERATIONS

Prompt diagnosis of an *S. aureus* infection is the key to appropriate therapy. Standard microbiologic methods continue to be the primary methods of diagnosis: Gram stain of appropriately obtained specimens when a patient first appears with a peripheral focus suspected of being staphylococcal will almost always reveal the typical grape-like clusters of the staphylococci mixed with inflammatory debris. A high index of suspicion for staphylococcal infection should be maintained in patient groups known to have an increased rate of nasopharyngeal carriage of the organism. Those groups of patients have recently been thoroughly reviewed (38). All septic-appearing patients should be thoroughly evaluated with aspiration, Gram stain, and culture of all potentially septic foci. Whenever there is any possibility that *S. aureus* might be responsible (essentially *always* in hospital-acquired infections), initial empiric antibiotic regimens must be tailored effectively to cover *S. aureus.*

Local Measures

As with all other infections, but of special importance in infections due to *S. aureus,* drainage, debridement, and foreign-body removal are mandatory. Although one may suppress acute staphylococcal infections in and around foreign bodies, almost invariably it will be found that removal ultimately will be required to prevent relapses. Almost without exception, patients who fail to respond to an initial course of antibiotics for an organism found to be sensitive to the chosen antimicrobial agents will turn out to have an undrained collection of pus. Extensive efforts must be made to find and drain all deep, septic foci in patients with severe *S. aureus* sepsis.

Antibiotic Therapy

Whereas initially all strains of *S. aureus* were sensitive to penicillin and sulfa drugs, less than 5 to 10% are now sensitive to plain penicillin. The penicillinase-resistant penicillins (methicillin, nafcillin, and oxacillin) emerged as the treatments of choice in the late 1950s and throughout the 1960s, with the cephalosporins, erythromycin, and vancomycin being available as alternatives for penicillin-allergic patients. Throughout the 1960s, organisms resistant to all the β-lactam antibiotics (referred to commonly as methicillin-resistant staphylococci, a poor choice of terminology) began to appear (38). A present, β-lactam-antibiotic-resistant *S. aureus* are responsible for 10 to 30% of *S. aureus* infections, including bacteremia in large academic medical centers and community hospitals, and β-lactam-antibiotic-resistant *S. aureus* are increasing in frequency even in smaller hospitals and nursing homes. At present, the drug of choice for treatment of β-lactam-antibiotic-resistant *S. aureus* is vancomycin. An alternative drug is trimethoprim-sulfamethoxazole. The quinolone group of antibiotics, when clinically available, will offer several excellent alternatives for treatment of these multiresistant organisms. Quinolones presently under investigation that have shown excellent activity against β-lactam-antibiotic-resistant *S. aureus* are ciprofloxacin and norfloxacin. Other drugs under development that will be effective against β-lactam-antibiotic-resistant *S. aureus* include the teichoplanins and coumermycin.

Anti-inflammatory Therapy for Staphylococcal Infections

In overwhelming infection with bacteremia, various new approaches are being taken to tide the host through. Of course, antibiotics must be administered promptly, but antibiotics will do little to alter the metabolic deterioration generated by the endocrine and inflammatory sequelae of bacteremia that in the end may result in the syndrome of septic shock and multiple-organ-system failure. There are various therapeutic modalities that have a firm rationale for use in patients with septic shock, and such patients, when suffering from overwhelming infection with *S. aureus,* are no different from those in shock and/or multiple-organ-system failure secondary to Gram-negative bacteremia ("endotoxemia") or fungemia. Shock syndromes related to infection have recently been reviewed (40). As regards septic shock syndrome produced by infection with *S. aureus,* the following comments are relevant:

Antiserum Therapy for Septic Shock

In Gram-negative septicemia, an antiserum directed against the "core" glycolipid part of the endotoxin molecule has been found to be effective. These antibodies cross-react with endotoxins from many species of Gram-negative organisms. This antibody abrogates the development of septic shock in experimental animal models and has recently been shown to significantly reduce mortality among patients suffering from Gram-negative microbial bacteremia. As mentioned earlier, the "endotoxin" of staphylococci, in particular, and of Gram-positive microbes, in general, is the peptidoglycan–teichoic acid moiety in the cell wall that in the bloodstream can trigger all the sequelae of endotoxemia. Thus, although at present no studies have explored this possibility, an antiserum directed against peptidoglycan and/or teichoic acid probably will "neutralize" many of the shock symptoms caused by staphylococcal bacteremia. In the future, therefore, a "polyvalent" antiserum could be available to be administered to all patients who appear to be severely septic; that antiserum would contain antibodies to Gram-negative endotoxins, the Gram-positive peptidoglycan–teichoic acid complex, and the "endotoxin-like" yeast polysaccharides (e.g., zymosan).

Naloxone Therapy

During the stress of bacteremia, the ACTH/endorphin system is massively activated. Such events almost certainly occur during Gram-positive infections, just as they do in those caused by Gram-negative microbes. The rationale for the use of naloxone in bacteremic shock (naloxone being the opiate antagonist used to reverse opiate overdoses in clinical practice) is as follows: As stress causes the release of ACTH to provide metabolic and fluid and electrolyte support, endorphins are also released, providing anxiety relief and pain relief. The endorphins are very powerful opiate-like substances that provide both pain relief and anxiety relief during severe stress, especially as a result of trauma and bacteremia; however, the endorphins have the same side effects of hypotension and enhanced capillary leakage as do the synthetic opiates. In experimental Gram-negative infections, naloxone therapy can stabilize blood pressure (14) and, in some species, enhance survival (19). Survival in primates is not increased (17). Although septic patients experience a rise in blood pressure following naloxone administration (28), no clinical evidence has been generated to suggest enhancement of survival. Data on naloxone therapy in severe sepsis have been generated primarily in models using Gram-negative infections, and studies of the roles of endorphins in Gram-positive shock need to be carried out.

Anti-inflammatory Therapy

Glucocorticoids prevent shock in experimental animals following infusion either of endotoxin or of intact, live Gram-negative organisms (41). Extremely large doses of glucocorticoids are required in experimental animals to produce salutary effects. The doses of glucocorticoids that have been studied in humans (and, in some studies, found to be beneficial) are in the range of 30 mg/kg administered two or three consecutive times. The rationale for anti-inflammatory therapy in severe sepsis has recently been thoroughly reviewed (41). In at least one clinical study of bacteremic patients in whom glucocorticoids produced enhanced survival (36), patients suffering Gram-positive infections did as well as or better than those suffering Gram-negative infections. Recent data from two multi-center trials of steroids in severe sepsis have not, however, shown any clinical efficacy.

Nonsteroidal anti-inflammatory agents are also effective in reducing shock and mortality in experimental Gram-negative bacillary infections. The effects of nonsteroidals on Gram-positive infections need to be studied. Nonsteroidal agents may maximize the therapeutic index: Specifically, the ideal anti-inflammatory drug will maximize short-term anti-inflammatory effects, resulting in hemodynamic stabilization during bacteremia, while minimizing long-term immunosuppressive effects that will result in increased numbers of secondary infections.

SUMMARY

S. aureus is very effective at generating acute inflammation. The aggressiveness of the organism in invading host tissues results in rapid and extensive tissue destruction when compared with most other microbial pathogens. *S. aureus* produces inflammation through a variety of mechanisms: Its cell wall components are highly inflammatory, being "endotoxin-like" in their ability to activate complement, as well as the coagulation and kinin systems. The capsule of *S. aureus,* on the other hand, tends to reduce the generation of inflammation in tissues and in that regard is "antiphagocytic," permitting the organism to proliferate, escape phagocytosis, and move through tissue, avoiding the ensuing acute inflammatory response. Thus, the presence or absence of a capsule seems to be one of the keys as to how important a given strain of *S. aureus* is as either a tissue or bloodstream pathogen. Specifically, the presence of a capsule permits the organism to move rapidly through tissues and to reach the bloodstream more readily. Paradoxically, however, once in the bloodstream, the encapsulated organism is rather benign, not triggering as vigorously those endocrine and inflammatory systems that contribute to septic shock. Less well encapsulated organisms generate more tissue inflammation, are more readily phagocytized and killed locally, and therefore are less likely to reach the bloodstream; however, should such strains gain access to the bloodstream, as when causing an intravascular catheter infection, they can rapidly trigger the septic shock syndrome and multiple-organ-system failure.

Although cell wall components are very important to the generation of inflammation, the organism also produces a number of proteinaceous substances that are highly proinflammatory, i.e., a variety of protein toxins and extracellular enzymes. Those substances undoubtedly contribute to the pathogenicity of the organism, probably permitting tissue invasion to occur more readily and also enhancing inflammation and tissue destruction. Thus, the well-developed inflammatory capabilities of *S. aureus* undoubtedly contribute to its virulence as a pathogen and to its importance as the primary cause of serious localized and systemic infections in humans.

ACKNOWLEDGMENT

The assistance of Ms. Kathleen McCormick Schulz in the preparation of this manuscript is deeply appreciated.

REFERENCES

1. Arbuthnott, J. D. (1983): Epidermolytic toxins. In: *Staphylococci and Staphylococcal Infections,* edited by C. S. F. Easmon and C. Adlam, pp. 599–617. Academic Press, New York.
2. Arvidson, S. O. (1983): Extracellular enzymes from *Staphylococcus aureus.* In: *Staphylococci and Staphylococcal Infections,* edited by C. S. F. Easmon and C. Adlam, pp. 745–808. Academic Press, New York.
3. Bergdoll, M. S., Crass, B. A., Reiser, R. F., Robbins, R. N., and Davis, J. P. (1981): A new staphylococcal enterotoxin, enterotoxin F, associated with toxic shock syndrome *Staphylococcus aureus* isolates. *Lancet,* 1:1017–1020.
4. Bergdoll, M. S. (1983): Enterotoxins. In: *Staphylococci and Staphylococcal Infections,* edited by C. S. F. Easmon and C. Adlam, pp. 599–617. Academic Press, New York.
5. Bergdoll, M. S., and Schlievert, D. M. (1984): Toxic shock syndrome toxin. *Lancet,* 2:291–292.
6. Chesney, R. W., McCarron, D. M., Haddad, J. G., Hawker, C. D., DiBella, F. P., Chesney, P. J., and Davis, J. P. (1983): Pathogenic mechanisms of the hypocalcemia of the staphylococcal toxic-shock syndrome. *J. Lab. Clin. Med.,* 101:576–585.
7. Christensen, G. D., Simpson, W. A., Bisno, A. L., and Beachey, G. H. (1983): Experimental foreign body infections in mice challenged with slime-producing *Staphylococcus* epidermidis. *Infect. Immun.,* 40:407–410.
8. Crass, B. A., and Bergdoll, M. S. (1986): Toxin involvement in toxic shock syndrome. *J. Infect. Dis.,* 153:918–926.
9. Davenport, D. S., Massanari, R. M., Pfaller, M. A., Bale, M. J., Streed, S. A., and Hierholzer, W. J. (1986): Usefulness of a test for slime production as a marker for clinically significant infections with coagulase-negative staphylococci. *J. Infect. Dis.,* 153:332–339.
10. DeMaria, A., Heffernan, J. J., Grindlinger, G. A., Graven, D. E., McIntosh, T. K., and McCabe, W. R. (1985): Naloxone versus placebo in treatment of septic shock. *Lancet,* 1:1363–1365.
11. Dunkle, L. M., Blair, L. L., and Fortune, K. P. (1986): Transformation of a plasmid encoding an adhesin of *Staphylococcus aureus* into a nonadherent staphylococcal strain. *J. Infect. Dis.,* 153:670–675.
12. Easmon, C. S. F., and Adlam, C. (editors) (1983): *Staphylococci and Staphylococcal Infections.* Academic Press, New York.
13. Elias, P. M., Fritsch, P., and Epstein, E. H. (1977): Staphylococcal scalded skin syndrome: Clinical features, pathogenesis, and recent microbiological and biochemical developments. *Arch. Dermatol.,* 113:207–219.
14. Faden, A. I., and Holaday, J. W. (1980): Experimental endotoxic

15. shock: The pathophysiologic function of endorphin and treatment with opiate antagonists. *J. Infect. Dis.,* 142:229–238.
15. Forsgren, A., Ghetic, V., Lindmark, R., and Bjoquest, J. (1983): Protein A and its exploitation. In: *Staphylococci and Staphylococcal Infections,* edited by C. S. F. Easmon and C. Adlam, pp. 427–480. Academic Press, New York.
16. Fujikawa, H., Igarashi, H., Usami, H., Tanaka, S., and Tamura, H. (1986): Clearance of endotoxin from the blood of rabbits injected with staphylococcal toxic shock syndrome toxin-1. *Infect. Immun.,* 52:134–137.
17. Hinshaw, L. B., Beller, B. K., Chang, A. C. K., Flourney, D. J., Lahti, R. A., Passey, R. B., and Archer, L. T. (1984): Evaluation of naloxone for therapy of *E. coli* shock: Species differences. *Arch. Surg.,* 119:1410–1418.
18. Hirose, A., Ikejima, T., and Gill, D. M. (1985): Established macrophage-like cell lines synthesize interleukin-1 in response to toxic shock syndrome. *Infect. Immun.,* 50:765–770.
19. Holaday, J. W. (1985): Opioid antagonists in septic shock. In: *Septic Shock: Newer Concepts of Pathophysiology and Treatment,* edited by M. Sande and R. Root, pp. 201–218. Churchill Livingstone, New York.
20. Horan, T. C., White, J. W., Jarvis, W. R., Emori, T. G., Culber, D. H., Munn, V. P., Thornberry, C., Olson, D. R., and Hughes, J. M. (1986): Nosocomial infection surveillance, 1984. *Morbid. Mortal. Weekly Reports,* 35:17SS–29SS.
21. Jeljaszewicz, J., Switalski, L. M., and Adlam, C. (1983): Staphylocoagulase. In: *Staphylococci and Staphylococcal Infections,* edited by C. S. F. Easmon and C. Adlam, pp. 525–557. Academic Press, New York.
22. Kapral, F. A. (1982): Epidermal toxin production by *Staphylococcus aureus* strains from patients with toxic shock syndrome. *Ann. Intern. Med.,* 96:972–974.
23. Mills, J. T., Parsonnet, J., Tsai, Y., Kendrick, M., Hickman, R. K., and Kass, E. H. (1985): Control of production of toxic shock syndrome toxin-1 (Tsst-1) by magnesium ion. *J. Infect. Dis.,* 6:1158–1161.
24. Murray, H. W., Tuazon, C. U., and Sheagren, J. N. (1977): Staphylococcal septicemia and disseminated intravascular coagulation: *Staphylococcus aureus* endocarditis mimicking meningococcemia. *Arch. Intern. Med.,* 137:844–847.
25. Neefe, L. I., Tuazon, C. U., Cardella, T. A., and Sheagren, J. N. (1979): Staphylococcal scalded skin syndrome in adults: Case report and review of the literature. *Am. J. Med.,* 277:99–110.
26. O'Connor, D. T., Weisman, M. H., and Feirer, J. (1978): Activation of the alternate pathway in *Staph. aureus* infective endocarditis and its relationship to thrombocytopenia, coagulation abnormalities, and acute glomerulonephritis. *Clin. Exp. Immunol.,* 34:179–187.
27. Parsonnet, J., Gillis, Z. A., and Pier, G. B. (1986): Induction of interleukin-1 by strains of *Staphylococcus aureus* from patients with nonmenstrual toxic shock syndrome. *J. Infect. Dis.,* 154:55–65.
28. Peters, W. P., Friedman, P. A., Johnson, M. W., and Mitch, W. E. (1981): Pressor effect of naloxone in septic shock. *Lancet,* 1:529–532.
29. Peterson, P. K., Wilkinson, B. J., Kim, Y., Schmeling, D., and Quie, P. G. (1978): Influence of encapsulation on staphylococcal opsonization and phagocytosis by human polymorphonuclear leukocytes. *Infect. Immun.,* 19:943–949.
30. Proctor, R. A., Christman, G., and Mosher, D. F. (1984): Fibronectin-induced agglutination of *Staphylococcus aureus* correlates with invasiveness. *J. Lab. Clin. Med.,* 104:455–469.
31. Rogolsky, M. (1979): Nonenteric toxins of *Staphylococcus aureus. Microbiol. Rev.,* 43:320–360.
32. Schlech, W. F., III, Moulton, P., and Kaiser, A. B. (1981): Pyomyositis: Tropical disease in a temperate climate. *Am. J. Med.,* 71: 900–902.
33. Schleifer, K. H. (1983): The cell envelope. In: *Staphylococci and Staphylococcal Infections,* edited by C. S. F. Easmon and C. Adlam, pp. 385–428. Academic Press, New York.
34. Schlievert, P. M., Shands, K. N., Dan, B. B., Schmid, G. P., and Mishimura, R. D. (1981): Identification and characterization of an exotoxin from *Staphylococcus aureus* associated with toxic-shock syndrome. *J. Infect. Dis.,* 143:509–516.
35. Schlievert, P. M. (1983): Alteration of immune function by staph-

ylococcal pyogenic exotoxin type C: Possible role in toxic-shock syndrome. *J. Infect. Dis.,* 147:391–398.

36. Schumer, W. (1976): Steroids in the treatment of clinical septic shock. *Ann. Surg.,* 184:333–341.

37. Schutzer, S. E., Fischetti, V. A., and Zabriskie, J. B. (1983): Toxic shock syndrome and lysogeny in *Staphylococcus aureus. Science,* 220:316–318.

38. Sheagren, J. N. (1984): *Staphylococcus aureus:* The persistent pathogen. *N. Engl. J. Med.,* 310:1368–1373, 1437–1442.

39. Sheagren, J. N. (1984): Staphylococcal infections. In: *Cecil Textbook of Medicine,* ed. 17, edited by J. B. Wyngaarden and J. B. Smith, pp. 1543–1551. W. B. Saunders, Philadelphia.

40. Sheagren, J. N. (1985): Shock syndromes related to sepsis. In: *Cecil Textbook of Medicine,* ed. 17, edited by J. B. Wyngaarden and J. B. Smith, pp. 1473–1477. W. B. Saunders, Philadelphia.

41. Sheagren, J. N. (1985): Glucocorticoid therapy in the management of septic shock. In: *Septic Shock: Newer Concepts of Pathophysiology and Treatment,* edited by M. Sande and R. Root, pp. 201–218. Churchill Livingstone, New York.

42. Todd, J., Fishaut, M., Kapral, F., and Welch, T. (1978): Toxic-shock syndrome associated with phage group II staphylococci. *Lancet,* 2:1116–1118.

43. Toy, P. T. C. Y., Lai, L. L., Drake, T. A., and Sande, M. A. (1985): Effect of fibronectin on adherence of *Staphylococcus aureus* to fibrin thrombi *in vitro. Infect. Immun.,* 48:83–86.

44. Tuazon, C. U., Sheagren, J. N., and Quie, P. G. (1981): Variability in the degree of opsonization and phagocytosis of strains of *Staphylococcus aureus* isolated from patients with disseminated intravascular coagulation. *J. Lab. Clin. Med.,* 98:949–955.

45. Verbrugh, H. A., Van Dijk, W. C., Peters, R., Van Erne, M. E., Daha, M. R., Peterson, P. K., and Verhoef, J. (1980): Opsonic recognition of staphylococci mediated by cell wall peptidoglycan: Antibody-independent activation of human complement and opsonic activity of peptidoglycan antibodies. *J. Immunol.,* 124:1167–1173.

46. Vercellotti, G. M., Lussenhop, D., Peterson, P. K., Furcht, L. T., McCarthy, J. B., Jacob, H. S., and Moldow, C. F. (1984): Bacterial adherence to fibronectin and endothelial cells: A possible mechanism of bacterial tissue tropism. *J. Lab. Clin. Med.,* 103:34.

47. Wadstrom, T. (1983): Biological effects of cell damaging toxins. In: *Staphylococci and Staphylococcal Infections,* edited by C. S. F. Easmon and C. Adlam, pp. 671–704. Academic Press, New York.

48. Wilkinson, B. J. (1983): Staphylococcal capsules and slime. In: *Staphylococci and Staphylococcal Infections,* edited by C. S. F. Easmon and C. Adlam, pp. 481–523. Academic Press, New York.

Inflammation: Basic Principles and Clinical Correlates.
Edited by J. I. Gallin, I. M. Goldstein, and R. Snyderman.
Raven Press, Ltd., New York © 1988.

CHAPTER 47

Fibrosis: Bacterial-Cell-Wall-Induced Hepatic Granulomas

Sharon M. Wahl

Exudation and Cell Recruitment
    Acute Inflammation • Leukocyte Migration • Modulation of Leukocyte Recruitment • Genetic Susceptibility to SCW-Induced Inflammation
Chronic Inflammation
    Cellular Infiltrates • Cytokine Production

Angiogenesis
    Endothelial Cell Migration and Proliferation • Angiogenesis Factors
Fibroplasia and Repair
    Fibroblast Recruitment • Fibroblast Proliferation • Matrix Formation
Concluding Remarks
References

Tissue injury initiates an inflammatory response that results in removal of the causative stimulus and, ultimately, tissue repair. Without an inflammatory response, healing and restoration of structural and/or functional integrity of the injured tissue do not occur. However, in the absence of infection or a specific antigen, a wound can heal in an animal depleted of red blood cells (62,84), lymphocytes (146), neutrophils (141), or complement (167). Of the leukocyte population, only macrophages appear to be essential to resolution of this type of injury (82). In contrast to trauma-induced injury, infection or antigen deposition and the host's attempt to repair the resulting tissue injury are considerably more complex because of the involvement of additional cells, including T lymphocytes. This chapter will focus on an injury inflicted in the liver with a T-lymphocyte-dependent stimulus. Induction of hepatic granulomas by bacterial cell wall antigens provides a model of inflammation and repair that encompasses the entire cascade of events leading from injury to repair. Deposition of this poorly degradable, persistent bacterial cell wall antigen results in a prolonged attempt by the host to repair the tissue, culminating in fibroplasia and fibrogenesis. In this and in other fibrotic diseases, distinct immune inflammatory and vascular

events precede fibrosis and scarring and can be associated intimately, even causally, with the increased connective-tissue accumulation. The deposition of antigen (or other types of injury) leads to an exudation and cell recruitment phase, chronic inflammation, angiogenesis, and, finally, fibroblast accumulation and matrix synthesis and/or fibrosis. These events will be discussed sequentially, although the phases of inflammation are clearly interrelated and overlapping.

EXUDATION AND CELL RECRUITMENT

Acute Inflammation

Within 2 to 4 days following intraperitoneal injection of a group A streptococcal cell wall (SCW) preparation into genetically susceptible LEW/N rats, an acute reaction develops within the liver, characterized by edema, neutrophil accumulation, and deposition of fibrin. This initial phase develops coincident with the localization of SCW in the liver. The second, chronic phase of the response is characterized by a granulomatous-type inflammatory reaction that is dependent on persistence of the SCW in the tissue (172,173,182). The SCW peptidoglycan-polysaccharide complex, that portion of the bacterial cell wall that induces inflammation, contains repeating units of the disaccharide *N*-acetylglucosamine–muramic acid linked to a polysaccharide heteropolymer composed of a rhamnose backbone with rhamnose side chains terminating with *N*-acetylglucosamine residues (76). The group A polysaccharide renders the complex resistant to degradation by lysozyme (46), enabling it to persist in the tissue indefinitely.

In this model, the group A SCW are sequestered initially by components of the hepatic mononuclear phagocyte system. Thus, within hours after intraperitoneal injection, the SCW are widely disseminated throughout the sinusoidal Kupffer cells (5,172). Ultrastructurally, the SCW appear as an amorphous material within the cytoplasm of the Kupffer cells, which consequently become enlarged and project into the sinusoidal spaces (Fig. 1A). Furthermore, the liver sinusoidal spaces and microvessels in the SCW-injected animals become distended and filled with erythrocytes and leukocytes as the blood flow slows (Fig. 1A). This stasis within vessels at the site of inflammation is necessary for subsequent cell migration.

The initial observable event in the development of this SCW-induced inflammatory response is localized association of leukocytes with the endothelium. Localized adhesion of circulating leukocytes to the endothelial lining leads to their egress from the vasculature into the tissues. Because the peptidoglycan-polysaccharide complex of SCW activates the alternative complement pathway (131), this initial response may trigger the generation of vasopermeability, coagulation (190), and chemotactic factors (144) promoting leukocyte adherence (154) and emigration from the circulation into the extravascular parenchymal tissue. In support of a role for complement in the development of the SCW response, depletion of complement by cobra venom factor results in reduced acute inflammatory lesions (131). Moreover, the increased serum complement activity observed in SCW-injected rats may reflect SCW stimulation of macrophages to synthesize complement proteins (79).

In addition to complement activation, SCW also promote generation of arachidonic acid oxygenation products (189), an important source of chemical mediators that cause increased vascular permeability, vasodilation, migration, and chemoattraction (32,126). SCW dose-dependent production of prostaglandin E_2 (PGE_2) and leukotriene B_4 (LTB_4) measured in rat dermal air pouches peaks 3 days after SCW administration, concurrent with maximal neutrophil accumulation, and declines to lower levels that are maintained for an extended period (189). In this

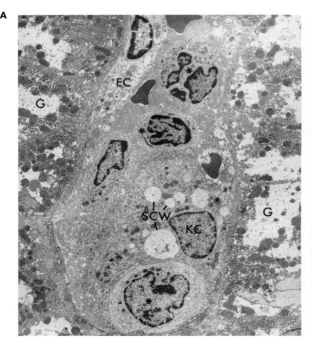 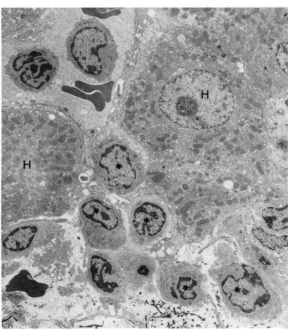

FIG. 1. A: Leukocyte accumulation in a hepatic sinusoid 3 days following intraperitoneal injection of SCW into a genetically susceptible LEW/N rat. Several leukocytes (*) and a Kupffer cell (KC) have nearly obliterated the lumen of the sinusoid. Phagocytic vacuoles containing SCW are present in the Kupffer cell. A damaged endothelial cell (EC) is present in the upper part of the micrograph. The adjacent hepatocytes contain abundant glycogen (G). ×3,200. **B:** Leukocyte migration from the hepatic sinusoids into the liver parenchyma. Several mononuclear cells (*) appear to be migrating through the hepatic parenchyma between the sinusoid (**top left**) and a granuloma (**bottom**). Hepatocytes (H) have a relatively normal appearance. ×3,700.

regard, lipoxygenase-dependent oxidation products of arachidonic acid metabolism recently were shown to promote the margination and sticking of neutrophils to the endothelium (45,61) via an endothelial-cell-dependent mechanism related to platelet-activating factor (PAF) synthesis (93). SCW-activated phagocytic Kupffer cells also may be a source of arachidonic acid metabolites, thereby increasing leukocyte adhesiveness to endothelial cells lining the liver sinusoids. Kupffer cells also produce interleukin 1 (IL-1) (123) and likely tumor necrosis factor (TNF), which act through specific binding sites on endothelial cells to promote activation of hemostatic mechanisms and to induce endothelial cell synthesis and release of IL-1 (99). In response to diverse stimuli, including neutrophil elastase and toxic O_2 species (142), the endothelial cells become procoagulant and phagocytic, express Fc and C3b receptors, and produce IL-1 (122,125,176,184). Thus, IL-1 derived from several sources may influence endothelial cell adherence and emigration of neutrophils, monocytes, and lymphocytes (17) and be an important regulator of leukocyte–vessel wall interactions at sites of inflammation. These events are crucial to accumulation of leukocytes at the inflammatory site.

Endothelial cells also appear to participate actively in the regulation of vascular permeability (reviewed in ref. 125). Development of edema in the liver is likely the consequence of several pathophysiological events, including activation, damage (Fig. 1A), and loss of endothelial cells, changes in vascular resistance, and degradation of vascular basement membranes (130). Neutrophils and stimulated endothelial cells produce PAF, a membrane lipid derivative that along with arachidonic acid metabolites (PGE_2, PGI_2, LTB_4), bradykinin, 5-hydroxytryptamine, and activated C3 and C5 enhances vascular permeability (130). Thus, endothelial cells, previously thought to be innocent bystanders in these events, now appear to be active and crucial participants (see Chapter 29).

In addition to altered vascular permeability and exudation of plasma components, SCW-induced activation of complement likely promotes activation of the coagulation and fibrinolytic cascades and aggregation of platelets. Aggregated platelets generate 12-hydroxyeicosatetraenoic acid (12-HETE), which enhances monocyte/macrophage-derived procoagulant activity (83). This enhancement of the coagulation cascade by monocytes culminates in conversion of soluble circulating fibrinogen into a network of fibrin at the site of injury (103). Fibrin, which is obvious in the early SCW liver lesions, may be an important forerunner of fibrotic events.

Leukocyte Migration

Localized adhesion of leukocytes to the vessel wall at sites of inflammation and their subsequent emigration

(Fig. 1B) are complex events that involve multiple humoral and cellular components. Recent *in vitro* studies reveal that a variety of ligands for which leukocytes have specific membrane receptors are associated with inflammatory lesions and induce directional movement of the cells in response to a diffusing concentration gradient (see Chapter 18). In this regard, products generated through activation of the clotting, kinin, and fibrinolytic systems (14,69,70) may regulate not only adherence but also leukocyte migration. In addition to these other acute inflammatory attractants, platelet aggregation results in the release of several chemotactically active products, including platelet factor 4 (34), platelet-derived growth factor (PDGF) (35), and transforming growth factor β (TGF-β) (174). Generation of arachidonic acid metabolites, especially LTB_4, also contributes to the attraction of leukocytes (156). SCW-induced complement activation produces C5a, which attracts polymorphonuclear leukocytes and monocytes (137), and its subsequent cleavage product, C5a-Des-Arg, which favors monocyte migration (86). In the event of an infection, bacterial products may also serve as potent inducers of leukocyte chemotaxis (85,127).

Following neutrophil accumulation, which peaks around 3 days after SCW injection, a noticeable increase in hepatic accumulation of mononuclear leukocytes occurs. The mechanisms responsible for this transition from neutrophil to mononuclear cell infiltrate and its maintenance are unknown, but are critical in the development and resolution of inflammation and in the healing process. Although accumulation of monocytes appears to occur in dermal wounds even in neutrophil-depleted animals (141), neutrophil depletion in other types of inflammation prevents monocyte recruitment (59). Neutrophil proteolytic activity identifiable as elastase can cleave Hageman factor, prekallikrein, kininogen, C4, C5, C3, and factor B of the complement system (130), and these events may provide important precursors for subsequent events at the inflammatory site. Once localized at the inflammatory site, activated monocytes apparently clear the neutrophil population by phagocytosis (59).

Additional chemotactic factors are elaborated by T lymphocytes in antigen-induced inflammation and injury. T lymphocytes attracted to the site adhere to the endothelium (20) and penetrate into the parenchyma (Fig. 1B), where they provide a source of recruitment factors for additional inflammatory cells. Granulomas from the livers of SCW-injected rats release significant amounts of chemotactic activity similar to lymphocyte-derived chemotactic factor (LDCF) produced by activated T cells (41). In addition to LDCF, lymphocytes generate TGF-β (71), recently shown to be an extremely potent chemoattractant for monocytes (174). TGF-β, a homodimer ($M_r = 25,000$) with two 112-amino-acid chains, induces monocyte migration at femtomolar concentrations and may play an important role in recruitment and activation of monocytes in chronic inflammatory lesions. These data suggest that release of chemotactic factor(s) by lymphocytes stimulated by the persistent SCW in the granulomatous lesion may provide a continual recruitment mechanism for mononuclear cells that accumulate for many weeks after the initial SCW injection (Fig. 1B).

As monocytes emigrate from the bloodstream through the basement membrane, one basement membrane glycoprotein, laminin, interacts with the monocytes to activate and enhance their phagocytic capacity (21). Laminin also serves as an attachment and attractant factor for neutrophils (153). After leaving the circulation, migration of the monocytes through the connective-tissue matrix into the parenchyma may involve secretion of proteolytic enzymes to facilitate a pathway to the inflammatory site. Whereas interaction of leukocyte receptors with chemotactic ligands initiates a series of intracellular events, including transmethylation reactions and activation of protein kinase C leading to cell motility, higher concentrations of these ligands induce leukocyte activation and increased oxidative metabolism, lysosomal enzyme release, and monokine production (144). Although these events provide bactericidal and/or cytotoxic host defense pathways, they also have the potential to inflict considerable tissue damage. Degradation and injury of the tissue matrix also release additional chemotactic fragments from collagen, fibronectin, and elastin (102,109,132). Thus, there appear to be mechanisms promoting leukocyte recruitment into the inflammatory site from the earliest onset of tissue injury into the later reparative phases.

Modulation of Leukocyte Recruitment

The previously described events are critical to evolution of the chronic inflammatory lesions, because interruption of exudation and cell recruitment inhibits granuloma formation. Site-specific inhibitors have provided valuable information concerning the mechanisms of cellular recruitment and their impact on evolution of granulomas. For example, antiinflammatory corticosteroids interrupt the earliest stages of inflammation and wound healing by inhibiting release of inflammatory mediators that regulate vascular permeability and recruitment of leukocytes (166). Production of LTB$_4$, a major arachidonic acid metabolite of leukocytes (22,48), may be blocked by corticosteroids (60), thereby reducing its early chemoattractant and other proinflammatory activities. Because the generation of other recruitment factors, including LDCF, also is inhibited by steroid administration (reviewed in ref. 166), a major action of corticosteroids may be to impair the accumulation of leukocytes at an inflammatory site by reducing the availability of chemoattractants. This reduced accumulation of both neutrophils and monocytes in the liver in SCW-treated animals appears to be the crucial

anti-inflammatory mechanism of corticosteroids in inhibiting granuloma development (7).

Another potential target for modulation of granuloma development is the T lymphocyte. In recent studies, we showed that treatment of LEW/N rats with cyclosporin A (CsA), the fungal metabolite that blocks T-lymphocyte proliferation and lymphokine production and that is commonly used as an immunosuppressive agent in organ transplantation, resulted in inability of the animals to develop hepatic granulomas (6,172). The SCW, identified by immunoperoxidase staining, localize within the Kupffer cells of the liver in both CsA-treated and placebo-treated animals to the same extent. However, following the initial uptake of the SCW antigens by the hepatic Kupffer cells and the acute neutrophil accumulation in the parenchyma, there was no subsequent mobilization of the mononuclear phagocytic cells containing the SCW into granulomas in the CsA-treated animals. Furthermore, the lymphoid cells from the CsA-treated animals did not generate a chemotactic factor(s) for monocytes when stimulated *in vitro*. These observations suggest that CsA exerts it inhibitory effect very early in the development of SCW-induced lesions, likely at the level of recruitment of monocytes/macrophages into the inflammatory site.

In related studies, congenitally athymic nude (rnu/rnu) rats, which also lack functional T lymphocytes, were shown to be incapable of generating a granulomatous response to SCW (5). Although an acute, primarily neutrophilic response occurs in the athymic animals, accumulation of mononuclear cells is clearly impaired. On reaching the inflammatory site, the neutrophils ingest SCW and debris, but apparently do not contribute to the subsequent granuloma and repair mechanisms. Small focal areas of loosely organized mononuclear cells were subsequently found in the periportal regions of the athymic rat, in contrast to the large organized aggregates of lymphocytes and mature macrophages present in the parenchyma and portal areas in the euthymic rats. There was a direct correlation between the tissue deposition of the SCW and the development of inflammation in the euthymic animals, which developed much more severe histologic evidence of disease than did the athymic rats. These studies indicate that functional T lymphocytes are required for the development of chronic hepatic granulomas, although they play a less significant or nonexistent role in the development of the acute, exudative hepatic inflammation.

Genetic Susceptibility to SCW-Induced Inflammation

The early development of the SCW-induced inflammatory lesion is controlled by multiple genes that are not associated with the major histocompatibility complex (9,181). Inbred rat strains that share the RTL.1 major histocompatibility complex haplotype are not universally susceptible to SCW-induced granulomatous lesions (181). However, susceptibility is strongly dependent on genetic background and is inherited as a dominant or codominant trait influenced by two or more genetic loci. Sex hormones also appear to modulate the incidence and severity of disease, with androgens enhancing and estrogens depressing clearance and sequestration of SCW by the mononuclear phagocyte system (4).

The mechanisms by which the genetic differences account for variation in susceptibility to SCW-induced chronic inflammation are unclear, but this may occur at the level of inflammatory mediator production (40). The differences are not due to failure to deposit and sequester bacterial cell walls, because there is no apparent difference in the distributions of SCW in resistant and susceptible animals. However, recent evidence suggests that there is a difference in the abilities of resistant and susceptible rat strains to elaborate PGE_2 and LTB_4 in response to the bacterial cell walls (189). Rat strains that develop chronic granulomatous lesions generate higher levels of these arachidonic acid metabolites than do strains that do not develop chronic disease. Consequently, the inability to provide sufficient initial levels of chemotactic and vasoactive mediators may contribute to the abbreviated response in the resistant animals. Furthermore, the resistant rat strains fail to demonstrate augmented class II major histocompatibility complex antigen (Ia) expression in the liver following SCW administration (8). The early differences in Ia expression and arachidonic acid metabolite synthesis following SCW administration suggested macrophage involvement in the regulation of susceptibility and resistance to the SCW. Based on these findings, studies

were initiated to define a role for monocytes/macrophages in the regulation of susceptibility. It appears that macrophages from the susceptible LEW/N rats generate higher levels of inflammatory mediators, including arachidonic acid metabolites and cytokines, in response to coculture with SCW than do macrophages from resistant F344/N rats (42). Thus, the macrophage may play a pivotal role in the development of susceptibility to SCW-induced chronic inflammation. Further identification of the genetically controlled differences in susceptibility will provide important information in defining critical pathogenic mechanisms in the disease process.

CHRONIC INFLAMMATION

Cellular Infiltrates

Evolution of SCW-induced liver lesions is characterized by chronic inflammation leading to parenchymal fibrosis and scarring. Mononuclear cells aggregate in the liver parenchyma and by 2 to 3 weeks after SCW administration organize into compact granulomatous lesions (Table 1). Identification of the cellular constituents of the granulomatous lesions using cell-specific monoclonal antibodies has revealed a predominance of T lymphocytes (W3/13$^+$) of the helper/inducer subset (W3/25$^+$), with fewer suppressor/cytotoxic (OX8$^+$) lymphocytes (172). This helper-T-cell/suppressor-T-cell imbalance may contribute to perpetuation of the highly inflammatory nature of the lesion. The prevalence of helper/inducer T lymphocytes (Fig. 2A) within the early granulomas is the consequence of lymphocyte emigration from the blood to the liver and

TABLE 1. *Cellular infiltrates in hepatic granulomas*

Cell	Localization	Products[a]	Functions
Neutrophils	Transient periportal, parenchymal	ROI, proteases, AA	Phagocytosis, acute inflammation
Mast cells	Dispersed in granuloma	Histamine, heparin	Angiogenesis, fibrosis (?)
Eosinophils	Dispersed in granuloma	Major basic protein, cationic protein	?
Monocytes/macrophages	Organized in center of granuloma; in peripheral fibroblast region	ROI, AA, PA, collagenase, IL-1, TNF, PDGF, TGF-β, FGF	Accessory cells, fibroplasia, angiogenesis
T lymphocytes			
Helper/inducer	Throughout granuloma and in peripheral fibroblast region	LDCF, IL-2, IL-3, GM-CSF, FAF, angiogenic factors	Proliferation, regulation
Suppressor/cytotoxic	Dispersed in granuloma	Suppressor factors (?)	Proliferation, regulation
B lymphocytes	Dispersed in granuloma	Lymphokines, antibodies	
Endothelial cells	Capillaries	AA, PAF, IL-1	Acute inflammation, angiogenesis
Fibroblasts	Periphery of granuloma	Collagen, fibronectin, proteoglycans, collagenase, AA, GM-CSF	Tissue repair

[a] ROI, reactive oxygen intermediates; AA, arachidonic acid metabolites; PA, plasminogen activator.

of local proliferation of T cells mediated by interleukin 2 (IL-2).

Monocytes/macrophages (Ia$^+$) are especially prominent at all stages of the granuloma evolution. The ability of these cells to phagocytize (Fig. 2A) is crucial to the clearance of debris, antigen, and/or microorganisms in the inflammatory site. After interaction of the SCW with the phagocytic cell membrane through Fc, C3b, or other receptors, ingestion occurs, with phagosome formation and lysosome-phagosome fusion. Granuloma macrophages contain an extensive phagolysosomal network containing debris, lipid, glycogen, and material identified as SCW (Fig. 2A). The ingested lysozyme-resistant and therefore poorly degradable SCW-complex persists and becomes concentrated within the macrophages, maintaining their heightened state of activation and thereby stimulating the generation of a spectrum of enzymes and monokines. In this regard, the SCW have been shown to persist within cultured macrophages as long as 40 days (143). Furthermore, multinucleated giant cells apparently formed by the fusion of macrophages under T-cell influence (113) are seen throughout the granuloma. Functional analysis of multinucleated giant cells indicates that these cells possess Ia antigens, are phagocytic, and kill microorganisms at least as effectively as macrophages (87,128). Less mature monocyte-like cells are also apparent throughout granuloma development because of continued mechanisms of recruitment of blood-borne cells to the lesion. In addition to recruitment of circulating monocytes, the expanded monocyte-macrophage population may be derived, in part, from a replicating population of cells in the liver and/or from recruited Kupffer cells (172).

In addition to the predominant T lymphocyte and monocyte-macrophage infiltrates, mast cells, eosinophils, and plasma cells can be identified throughout the granuloma (Fig. 2B–D).

Cytokine Production

Lymphocytes

Intact granulomas have been isolated from the livers of SCW-injected animals and enzymatically digested to free the cellular constituents of the granulomas from their matrix for in vitro culture and analysis (172,173). The W3/13$^+$ T-lymphocyte populations obtained from the granulomas spontaneously release lymphokines that recruit and activate mononuclear phagocytes, including LDCF, the lymphokine that recruits monocytes. T lymphocytes recovered from the liver granulomas also spontaneously release IL-2, the T-cell growth factor, in contrast to resting T cells obtained from other lymphoid organs, which require activation in order to release IL-2. These activated T cells and the IL-2 they generate may contribute to maintaining the persistent inflammation in response

to the nondegradable bacterial cell walls deposited in the liver. Interestingly, the recent observation that human monocytes transcribe and translate IL-2 receptors (175) suggests that IL-2 may also contribute to the regulation of mononuclear phagocyte function.

Colony-stimulating factors (CSF) that regulate the proliferation and differentiation of mononuclear phagocytes are also constitutively produced by the granuloma lymphocytes (172). Granulocyte-macrophage CSF (GM-CSF) is generated early in granuloma development, as is interleukin 3 (multi-CSF, IL-3). Not only does CSF stimulate proliferation and differentiation of granulocyte-macrophage precursors (106), but also it stimulates macrophages to produce diverse inflammatory mediators, including IL-1 (97), PGE$_2$ (78), interferon (97), and plasminogen activator (55). Macrophage function and Ia expression are likely also regulated by T-cell-derived γ-interferon (γ-IFN) (15,96). In addition to its colony-stimulating activity, IL-3 is a growth factor for mast cells (64) evident in the granulomas (Fig. 2C).

The contributions of these various cytokines have been investigated during the course of granuloma evolution (172). Cytokine production by early SCW-induced granulomas ($\leq$3 weeks), which are composed primarily of T helper/inducer lymphocytes and macrophages, was compared with that by later granulomas (>6 weeks). The 6-week granulomas are more organized and compact and contain mature macrophages, giant cells, and some fibroblasts. By comparison, granulomas of more than 12 weeks' duration are characterized by less intense inflammation, fewer T lymphocytes, more mature macrophage forms, and abundant fibroblast infiltration and matrix synthesis. Quantitation of IL-2 from these transitional forms of granulomas revealed highest levels of IL-2 in the earlier granulomas, when the numbers of T cells are maximal. Moreover, IL-2 activity declined over the ensuing 12 weeks, consistent with a decrease in T-lymphocyte numbers. Similarly, IL-3 produced by 3-week granulomas peaked at 6 weeks and subsequently declined. Whether or not the decreased inflammatory response to SCW that occurs in later granulomas and the attendant decline in cytokine production are related to a proportional increase in suppressor T cells, as occurs in Schistosoma mansoni liver granulomas (37,177), has not yet been determined. In contrast to IL-2 and IL-3, however, GM-CSF levels continued to increase even in the late-stage granulomas ($\geq$12 weeks), suggesting that cells other than the W3/13$^+$ T lymphocytes might be contributing to the production of this cytokine. Because fibroblasts have recently been shown to generate GM-CSF (191), and because these cells increasingly accumulate throughout granuloma development coincident with the presence of the lymphokine fibroblast-activating factor (FAF), the fibroblasts may contribute to the persistent GM-CSF levels. Together these mediators play an important role in the local aggregation,

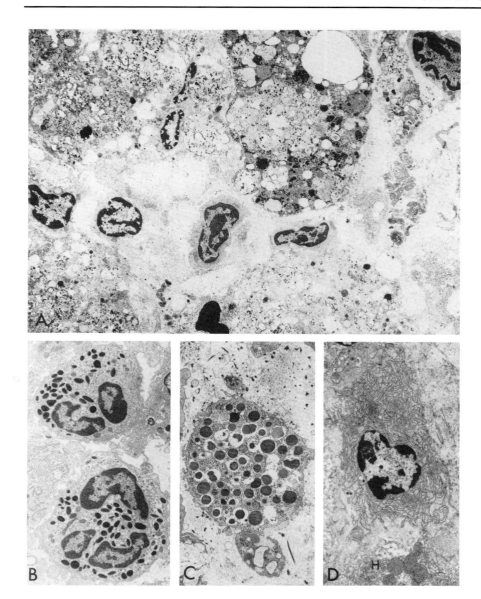

FIG. 2. Ultrastructural characterization of cellular components of SCW-induced granulomas. **A:** Lymphocytes and large macrophages engorged with phagocytized debris are evident. ×4,900. **B:** Limited numbers of eosinophils are seen throughout the granuloma. ×6,500. **C:** Mast cells are present in the granuloma. ×8,200. **D:** Plasma cell present at the periphery of a granuloma; (H) hepatocyte cytoplasm. ×7,200. (From ref. 172.)

division, and maturation of mononuclear phagocytes in the liver parenchyma and in the evolution of compact, organized granulomas.

The requirement for these T-cell cytokines in the evolution of SCW-induced granulomas is clear. Inhibition of T-cell lymphokine synthesis results in impaired or nonexistent granuloma formation. For example, CsA, which inhibits lymphokine production at the transcriptional level (77), blocks IL-2 synthesis and therefore the cascade of events dependent on IL-2. The inhibitory effects of CsA extend to the production of other lymphokines, including IL-3, γ-IFN, and FAF (173), although transcription and translation of GM-CSF appear to be resistant to CsA (18). Whereas the diminished recruitment of monocytes in the livers of rats treated with CsA beginning 24 hr prior to or on the day of injection of SCW (6,188) is likely due to decreased LDCF levels, CsA inhibits granuloma devel-

opment even when administered 12 days after SCW injection. Although macrophage function appears to remain intact in CsA-treated animals, activated macrophages cannot independently mediate SCW granuloma formation. Consequently, in the absence of functional T cells, presumably because of lack of macrophage recruitment (LDCF) and maturation factors (IL-2, CSF), the transition from monocytes to functionally active macrophages and maintenance of activation is incomplete, and granuloma development is abrogated. These observations indicate numerous T-cell-dependent events in the sequelae of granuloma development.

Monocytes/Macrophages

The presence of a granuloma indicates that the SCW have resisted destruction by the acute inflammatory response and are being sequestered by mature elements of the mononuclear leukocyte system (1,23). Ingestion of SCW by phagocytic mononuclear leukocytes initiates a complex series of events in which the macrophages undergo certain functional and metabolic changes. One such change, the respiratory burst, is characterized by an increase in O_2 consumption and increased glucose metabolism via the hexose monophosphate shunt, culminating in the generation of O_2^- and H_2O_2. These reactive metabolites of oxygen generated at or near the cell surface and within phagocytic vacuoles have antimicrobial and/or antitumor effects. Although the production of highly reactive oxygen species is central to the bactericidal process, these products are potent oxidizing agents that can contribute significantly to the tissue damage that accompanies inflammation. Regulation of the production of these and other secretory products can be enhanced by various receptor-ligand interactions, lymphokines, SCW, and other inflammatory factors (98).

As a major secretory cell, the activated macrophage produces a large number of mediators, including neutral proteases, hydrolytic enzymes, complement components, and coagulation factors (98). Macrophage-derived neutral proteases are elevated in inflammatory lesions and likely contribute to matrix destruction, clearance of the inflammatory site, and tissue remodeling and repair. One of these neutral proteases, plasminogen activator (PA) (55), activates plasminogen to plasmin, another neutral protease of broad specificity that can lyse fibrin, activate C1 and C3, and cleave activated Hageman factor. Regulation of PA activity may occur through production of an inhibitor of PA by monocytes (47,158), and a decrease in PA would favor fibrin deposition, which is apparent in SCW lesions (172). Other macrophage-derived neutral proteases include collagenase, which can be activated by plasmin (185) and is required for initiation of collagen degradation (56). Another macrophage enzyme that contributes to the destruction of connective-tissue matrix molecules, including elastin, collagen, and proteoglycans, is elastase. Elastase activity is regulated in part by an α_1-proteinase inhibitor produced by T-cell-stimulated macrophages (151). Thus, macrophages appear not only to generate tissue-degrading enzymes but also to produce inhibitors of some of the same enzymes. How the balance of these enzyme-inhibitor complexes contributes to tissue destruction is unclear, but excessive enzyme levels without corresponding inhibitors may promote the tissue breakdown that occurs in many chronic inflammatory lesions.

In addition to the plethora of enzymes, inflammatory macrophages secrete mediators that promote the local inflammatory response. One of these mediators, IL-1, is spontaneously elaborated by the granulomas and by the adherent macrophages recovered from the granulomas (172). IL-1, which represents a family of polypeptides, has multiple biologic activities in host responses to infection, injury, and other immunological reactions (36). Characterization of the IL-1 activity from the granulomas revealed a peptide similar to that produced by stimulated rat spleen (172) and peritoneal macrophages (68). IL-1 levels are highest in the earlier granulomas (3 weeks), concurrent with the presence of many newly recruited phagocytic cells. During the course of the subsequent 12 weeks, IL-1 levels attenuate in parallel with maturation of the granulomas and the constituent macrophages. These findings are consistent with recent observations that maturation of blood monocytes is associated with loss of ability to elaborate IL-1 (39,178) and point to the newly recruited cells as the primary cells producing IL-1.

Activated macrophages also generate bioactive lipids, including thromboxanes, leukotrienes, PAF, and PGE_2. PGE_2 levels increase with the maturation of the granulomas and may provide an immunoregulatory role in the later granulomas (172). As shown in other studies, PGE_2 acts as a feedback inhibitor of many cellular immune processes, including lymphocyte proliferation and lymphokine production (49), and in the maturing granulomas may contribute to the decreased IL-2 and IL-3 levels. Although proinflammatory in early inflammation, PGE_2 is antiinflammatory in the later stages of granuloma evolution. The increasing fibroblast population (see following) may also contribute to production of PGE_2 in the more mature granulomas.

Fibroblasts

Recent evidence suggests that IL-1 stimulates fibroblasts to synthesize and secrete PGE_2 and GM-CSF (191). GM-CSF, a family of glycoproteins that promote differentiation of hemopoietic progenitor cells to mature granulocytes and macrophages, is generally considered a product of activated T lymphocytes (31,124) and mononuclear phagocytes (28). However, when other T-cell products (IL-2, IL-3) and macrophage mediators (IL-1) decline in the later stages of the granulomatous response, levels of GM-CSF continue to rise substantially. During this phase of the granulomatous response, the accumulation of fibroblasts is pronounced, and these fibroblasts may generate substantial quantities of GM-CSF that regulate monocyte-macrophage differentiation. The production of PGE_2 by fibroblasts also provides a regulatory signal in modulating the intensity of the inflammation. Because the elevated PGE_2 levels in mature granulomas (12 weeks) are inversely proportional to the activities detected for the inflammatory mediators IL-1, IL-2, and IL-3, the expanding fibroblast population may contribute to this immunoregulatory circuit through elaboration of prostaglandins.

ANGIOGENESIS

Endothelial Cell Migration and Proliferation

Angiogenesis, the formation of a new capillary network, is essential to the formation of inflammatory granulation tissue, wound repair, and chronic inflammatory processes. The anastomosing capillary beds that bud from the vessels in the surrounding tissue allow delivery of nutrients necessary for fibroblast proliferation and protein synthesis. Because fibroplasia cannot proceed without this network of capillaries (Fig. 3), angiogenesis factors are of obvious importance in tissue repair and granuloma formation. Although the angiogenic stimuli may differ, the events that occur as new capillaries grow in granulation tissue are similar to the well-characterized, ordered sequence of capillary growth that occurs in association with tumors (reviewed in ref. 43). Initially, the basal lamina of the parent venule begins to fragment, possibly in response to endothelial-cell-derived proteases (117), such as types IV and V collagenases (67). Small villous processes of endothelial cells then protrude through the fragmented basal lamina as important precursors to angiogenic events.

TABLE 2. *Chemoattractants for endothelial cells and fibroblasts*

Source of chemoattractants	Responding cell populations	
	Endothelial cells	Fibroblasts
Complement		
C5 fragment		+
Platelets		
Platelet factor	+	
PDGF		+
TGF-β		+
Platelet factor 4		+
β-thromboglobulin		+
Inflammatory cells		
PDGF		+
LDCF-F		+
TGF-β		+
LTB$_4$		+
Heparin	+	
PGE$_2$	+	
Fibronectin	+	+
Connective tissue		
Collagen	+	+
Fibronectin	+	+

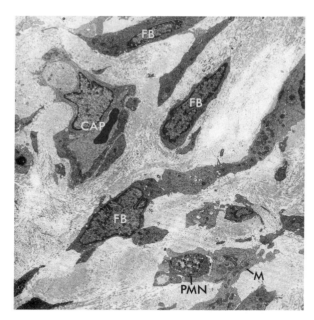

FIG. 3. Capillary formation in hepatic granulomas. Electron micrograph of peripheral region of hepatic granuloma 6 weeks after SCW injection. Abundant collagen and numerous fibroblasts (FB) are seen. A regenerating capillary (CAP) containing an erythrocyte (RBC) is present at the upper left. Portions of a PMN and a mononuclear cell (M) are visible. ×4,400. A new capillary sprout appears to be budding from the capillary into the perivascular connective tissue. The cylindrical vacuoles formed within the cytoplasm of the endothelial cells connect to similar vacuoles in adjacent endothelial cells to establish the lumen of a new vessel.

Following penetration of the basement membrane, the endothelial cells begin to migrate into the perivascular connective tissue. This migration appears to be a key component of neovascularization, because capillary buds develop at a distance from the parent vessel. Even when DNA synthesis is blocked, migration by the leading endothelial cells and capillary elongation continue, at least temporarily, indicating that chemotactic stimuli (Table 2) play an important role in neovascularization (138). Because fibronectin serves as an attractant for migrating endothelial cells (24), the production of this glycoprotein by endothelial cells (30) may provide an important directional signal. With the arrival of endothelial cells in the tissue, the first tube-like structures suggestive of vessels appear as cylindrical vacuoles that form within the cytoplasm of single endothelial cells (72) (Fig. 3). Contiguous cells also form vacuoles that connect to form the lumen of a new vessel. During the continued division of endothelial cells, additional bud-like structures form off nearby blood vessels that anastomose to form loops into which blood begins to flow. Although the generation of a hypoxic environment (72) and the local production of proteases (52) contribute to neovascularization, capillary endothelial cell migration and proliferation are largely dependent on diffusible angiogenic stimuli, as described later.

Angiogenesis Factors

Products of inflammatory cells that contribute to the regulation of proliferation and migration of endothelial cells are commonly identified functionally by their ability to induce angiogenesis in the embryonic chick chorioallantoic membrane or in the avascular rabbit cornea (43). Although these systems do not discriminate between mitotic and chemotactic agents, they provide information as to the involvement of cells and/or their products in neovascularization.

In an acute inflammatory response, aggregating platelets that contain 40 to 100 times as much TGF-β as other nonneoplastic tissues release this potent angiogenic stimulus (118). Interestingly, TGF-β may act as a bifunctional regulator of cell growth, inhibiting endothelial cell growth by delaying entry of G_1 cells into S phase and enhancing cell growth once the cells have passed the G_1/S border or are in G_2 (58). In addition to platelets, mast cells release angiogenic signals. One such mast cell factor, heparin, selectively stimulates endothelial cell migration (11). *In vivo,* heparin-enhanced angiogenesis is inhibitable by protamine, a specific inhibitor of heparin (152).

New capillary growth is also associated with mononuclear cell accumulation. Macrophages obtained from a wound spontaneously release a factor or factors that enhance endothelial cell proliferation and migration (13,73). Macrophage release of these factors is dependent on activation (107,135). Once activated, macrophages secrete proteases, macrophage angiogenesis factor (MAF) (135), and prostaglandins that are primarily chemotactic (44). In addition, macrophage-derived growth factor (MDGF) (89) and PDGF (136) have mitogenic activity for endothelial cells. Fibroblast growth factor (FGF), a potent endothelial cell mitogen (26), is also a product of stimulated macrophages (12). From these observations it is apparent that activation of macrophages triggers the release of numerous signals that regulate both endothelial cell recruitment and growth.

Angiogenesis that accompanies an immune response involves the release of additional angiogenesis factors (10,140), including T-cell-derived TGF-β (71). Although many pathways remain to be defined, inflammatory cells clearly participate in angiogenic events, likely through release of a network of cytokines. These cytokines influence the orderly sequence of events beginning with dissolution of vascular basal lamina, induction of cell migration, triggering of endothelial cell mitosis, formation of capillary sprouts, anastomosis, and, finally, reestablishment of blood flow. Within the SCW-induced liver granulomas, the capillary network is retained for months. When the angiogenic stimulus no longer persists, or if inhibitors of angiogenesis are produced, the capillaries undergo regression and deteriorate. Adherence of platelets to the deteriorating endothelial cells promotes vascular stasis and degeneration. Subsequently, phagocytic cells may ingest the degenerating capillary endothelial cells (43) during the formation of fibrous scar tissue.

FIBROPLASIA AND REPAIR

Fibroblast Recruitment

As the SCW are sequestered by phagocytes in the granulomas, an increased presence of fibroblasts around the peripheries of the granulomas becomes evident, and tissue repair is observed. Resting fibroblasts in the tissue divide, migrate toward the tissue injury, and produce collagen and other matrix components. Recruitment and expansion of the fibroblast population that synthesizes collagen are required for the normal postinflammatory repair phase of the fibrotic process. The signals that initiate, propagate, and terminate fibroblast recruitment, proliferation, and collagen synthesis have been investigated extensively in the past several years.

Fibroblast recruitment appears to occur in response to specific chemoattractants. Fibroblasts are motile *in vitro* and *in vivo* and migrate in response to a variety of inflammatory chemoattractants summarized in Table 2. Whether different subpopulations of fibroblasts are selectively recruited by these chemotactic ligands favoring the accumulation of a highly collagen synthetic or a highly proliferative phenotype is unknown. However, coordinated movement of the fibroblasts into the granuloma site is dependent on chemotaxis toward soluble stimuli and may also involve the process of haptotaxis along a substratum adhesion gradient and/or contact guidance in which the cells align along discontinuities in a three-dimensional substratum (reviewed in ref. 91). Such mechanisms of orientation may contribute to the highly oriented appearance of the fibroblasts around the granuloma.

Diffusible chemotactic stimuli for fibroblasts include both serum- and cell-derived molecules. Activation of serum complement by SCW or other agents releases a fragment from C5 that is distinct from C5a and uniquely chemotactic for fibroblasts (112). If tissue injury is associated with platelet aggregation, a plethora of fibroblast recruitment factors may be released. Likely candidates include LTB$_4$ (95), β-thromboglobulin (133), PDGF (53,134), and TGF-β (174). In addition to the platelets, recent demonstrations that activated macrophages produce PDGF (89,136) and TGF-β (174) indicate a continuing source of these recruitment signals for fibroblasts long after platelet involvement has ceased.

Continued serum-derived exudation of fibronectin into the tissue and macrophage- and/or fibroblast-derived fibronectin provide both chemotactic (155) and haptotactic (91) stimuli in the recruitment of fibroblasts. Fibronectin, a 440,000-dalton glycoprotein with multiple ligand-binding activities, is involved in regulating a number of important biological phenomena, including cell motility and adhesion. Fibronectin accumulates at sites of inflammation and wound healing (50,63), and enzymatic cleavage of the molecule appears to enhance its biologic activity. A 75,000-dalton tryptic fragment derived from the central portion of the molecule contains the recruitment activity (90). Although this fragment encompasses the minimum cell adhesion structure (57), consisting of the tetrapeptide arginyl-glycyl-aspartyl-serine (RGDS) (104), RGDS cannot independently induce cell motility (90).

Other matrix proteins, including types I, II, and III interstitial collagens (111), and their cleavage products influence fibroblast recruitment. Moreover, enzymatic disruption of these matrix proteins, accompanied by phagocytosis of the fragments, clears a pathway for fibroblast penetration through the extracellular matrix.

Additional mediators of fibroblast recruitment are

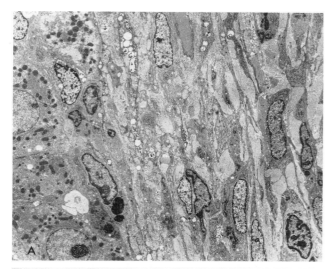

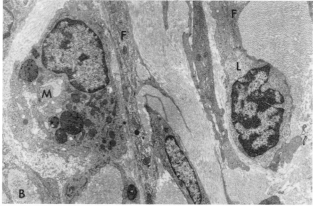

FIG. 4. Association of mononuclear cells and fibroblasts in hepatic granulomas. **A:** Section of the peripheral region of the granuloma adjacent to liver parenchyma **(left)** demonstrating mononuclear cells and numerous fibroblasts embedded in a collagenous matrix. ×2,900. **B:** A macrophage (M) and a lymphocyte (L) in direct contact with granuloma fibroblasts (F) and prominent collagen bundles. Banded collagen fibrils are seen in longitudinal section and in cross section. ×7,400. (From ref. 173.)

elaborated by inflammatory T cells. Antigen-activated lymphocytes produce a 22,000-dalton chemoattractant for fibroblasts (LDCF-F) (110) and also a factor that inhibits fibroblast migration (119). Accumulation and immobilization of the connective-tissue cells at the inflammatory site enable them to begin proliferating and generating matrix components for tissue repair. In the livers of SCW-injected animals, the fibroblasts localize around the periphery of the granuloma adjacent to the inflammatory cells (Fig. 4). With the appearance of fibroblasts, new capillaries, and granulation tissue, the reparative sequelae commence in the SCW-induced liver lesions, similar to those described in other injuries (121).

Fibroblast Proliferation

In addition to recruitment of fibroblasts to the site of tissue injury, expansion of the fibroblast population results from proliferation of local hepatic fibroblasts. This increase in fibroblast numbers is the critical step in the development of fibrosis and appears to be significantly influenced by inflammatory cell-derived products that enhance and/or inhibit fibroblast growth. The presence of such growth regulatory factors is commonly determined by *in vitro* fibroblast proliferation assays (165). Fibroblast growth factors are characterized by their ability to independently stimulate fibroblast growth or to function as comitogens in the induction of fibroblast growth. The complementation assay for cell growth requires a competence factor that renders the cells competent to replicate their DNA and a progression factor that enables the cells to progress from G_0/G_1 into S phase (150). If the factor being evaluated has competence or progression activity, it will, in combination with appropriate cofactors, provide an adequate stimulus for replication. Using these assays to monitor modulation of fibroblast growth, several inflammatory-cell-derived molecules have been identified that can alter the growth properties of primary fibroblast cultures. To understand the mechanisms of action of all these growth factors, it is important to realize that they probably act in sequence and/or in concert, with each peptide modulating the effects of additional peptides.

Once mononuclear leukocytes have infiltrated the granuloma, numerous polypeptide growth factors become available. Mast cells, also present throughout granuloma evolution (164,172), may contribute to the regulation of fibrotic events (29) through release of histamine and/or other mediators that regulate proliferation of fibroblasts (27). Because both T lymphocytes and macrophages produce cytokines capable of regulating fibroblast growth and function, these cytokines represent crucial molecular links between inflammation and repair and/or fibrosis. These mononuclear cell growth factors, by promoting fibroblast division, initiate resolution of the injury. Proliferation of fibroblasts and subsequent generation of connective-tissue matrix determine in large part the outcome of tissue injury in many inflammatory diseases. Cytokines that can enhance as well as inhibit fibroblast growth have been identified, indicating that a balance between these inflammatory cell products may lead to controlled tissue repair, or, alternatively, an imbalance might favor either fibrosis or loss of the matrix.

T-Lymphocyte-Derived Growth Factors

Many studies have demonstrated that T lymphocytes produce fibroblast growth factors both *in vitro* and *in vivo* (reviewed in ref. 165). Consistent with these observations, W3/13+ T lymphocytes obtained from SCW liver granulomas constitutively release a 40,000-dalton peptide that stimulates quiescent fibroblasts to proliferate (173). In view of the marked effect of this soluble T-lymphocyte product or products on fibroblast growth, further characterization of the FAF is relevant in understanding mechanisms of inflammatory-cell-mediated fibrosis. More extensive analysis of FAF, using human OKT3+ T lymphocytes as a source of FAF, has revealed that this cytokine has a major peak of activity around $M_r = 40,000$ and a primary isoelectric point of 5.0 to 5.5 and is protease-sensitive, heat-labile, and nondialyzable (169). The messenger RNA (mRNA) for this polypeptide, which is minimally detectable in resting T cells, but significantly elevated in mitogen-induced T cells, has been translated in the *Xenopus* oocyte system (2). This oocyte translation product is functionally and physicochemically similar to that generated by T cells, and therefore subsequent genetic cloning of this mediator will be possible. Because only activated T cells transcribe and translate FAF, this factor likely plays a regulatory role in connective-tissue growth *in vivo,* where it would be released only within the microenvironment of inflammation. Moreover, lymphoid cells isolated from inflammatory lesions constitutively release FAF activity (163,170,173), and the close proximity of lymphocytes and fibroblasts in fibrotic lesions (Fig. 4) favors exchange of such soluble regulatory molecules. Other T-cell-derived lymphokines such as IL-2 do not appear to play a major role in regulating mesenchymal cell growth. The role of γIFN is unclear, because it has been shown to enhance (25), to have no effect, or to inhibit (80,165) fibroblast replication. T lymphocytes also generate an inhibitor of fibroblast proliferation (100), providing a mechanism for down-regulating the repair process.

The importance of these T-cell lymphokines to fibrotic events has been defined in T-cell-deficient animals. Athymic (nude) rats do not develop fibrotic nodules when injected with SCW (5,173), consistent with the inability of the athymic animals to generate the 40,000-d peptide growth factor, FAF. Additionally, CsA, which inhibits FAF production, inhibits hepatic granuloma fibrosis in SCW-treated rats (6,173,189), even when CsA is administered after mononuclear cells have infiltrated into the liver. Thus, it appears that CsA directly inhibits lymphocyte production of the lymphokine or lymphokines that stimulate fibroblast proliferation, resulting in absence of fibrosis in the liver following SCW treatment.

Macrophage-Derived Growth Factors

In addition to the apparent direct regulation of fibroblast growth and function, T lymphocytes indirectly regulate fibrosis through their ability to recruit and activate macrophages that in turn influence connective-tissue metabolism. Recruitment via LDCF is instrumental in the accumulation of macrophages, as evidenced by the ability of CsA to inhibit LDCF production by activated T cells in SCW-treated rats and thereby interrupt macrophage chemotaxis and infiltration. Furthermore, T-lymphocyte products, including γIFN, CSF, and IL-2, are important in regulation of macrophage activation and presumably in promoting macrophage synthesis of fibroregulatory molecules. Thus, by inhibiting T-cell cytokine production, macrophage activation and the events dependent on that activation are also inhibited.

Macrophages are clearly associated with significant changes in connective-tissue cell proliferation and matrix deposition in SCW granulomas (Fig. 4). This was first demonstrated in experimentally wounded animals, in which depletion of macrophages resulted in delayed fibroblast infiltration and proliferation (82). Regulation of these fibroblast events was subsequently attributed to the release of soluble growth factors by activated macrophages (165,168). Recently, some of these factors were identified as PDGF (136), FGF (12), TNF (159), and IL-1 (129). In addition, macrophages isolated from inflammatory sites (19,186,187) spontaneously secrete fibroblast growth factors, reinforcing the concept that these molecules contribute to the regulation of fibroblast proliferation associated with inflammation. The availability of recombinant molecules and monoclonal antibodies will facilitate elucidation of the role each of these factors plays in regulating fibroblast proliferation.

With the additional production of a monocyte factor that inhibits fibroblast proliferation (74), potential elements for growth control are available. Monocyte regulation of fibroblast prostaglandin synthesis by IL-1 or TNF (33) may also inhibit growth. Recent evidence demonstrates that monocytes can chronically stimulate fibroblast PGE_2 synthesis by augmenting cyclooxygenase activity (179). Mesenchymal cell growth in the granuloma is ultimately held in check, the cells do not undergo transformation nor invade the liver, and fibroplasia is limited to the periphery of the granuloma. Considerably more research will be required to define the up- and down-regulation of fibroblast growth by these monocyte products.

Matrix Formation

Matrix Synthesis

As fibroblasts accumulate at an inflammatory site, they produce matrix components, including the collagen of connective-tissue fibers and the hyaluronic acid and proteoglycans of the ground substance, that are required for tissue repair. Under physiologic conditions of wound healing, a delicate balance of synthesis and degradation of collagen occurs. Disruption of this balance of synthesis and degradation can lead to pathologic manifestations. Within the granuloma, the connective-tissue cells generating matrix proteins frequently are found in close proximity to the mononuclear cells (Fig. 4) favoring a regulatory influence. Hyperplastic fibrous tissue with increased numbers of fibroblasts and small blood vessels becomes increasingly evident (Fig. 4A). Furthermore, because of the chronic nature of the SCW, prolonged stimulation of fibroblast matrix synthesis results in excessive connective-tissue formation, leading ultimately to scar tissue around the granuloma and hepatic fibrosis (173).

Although the cytokines produced by lymphocytes and macrophages that influence matrix synthesis are not as well defined as those that regulate fibroblast growth, considerable evidence indicates that mononuclear cell signals also modulate fibrogenesis (3,65,66,114,168). The activated fibroblasts transcribe collagen genes to precursor collagen mRNAs, which are processed to functional mRNA molecules coding for preprocollagen polypeptides (reviewed in refs. 101 and 157). The cytokine IL-1 enhances collagen gene expression (3), although levels of secreted collagen have been reported to be either increased (75) or decreased (180) following IL-1 administration. In contrast to IL-1, recombinant γIFN inhibits collagen synthesis at the transcriptional level (3,120,148). Although TGF-β increases collagen and glycosaminoglycan secretion by fibroblasts (118), the level of regulation is not known.

Following initiation of transcription, translation of the procollagen mRNA yields pro-α polypeptide chains that undergo extensive posttranslational modifications, including hydroxylation at proline and lysine residues, glycosylation of hydroxylysine residues, mannosylation of the extension peptides, and formation of the interchain disulfide bonds. Assembly of three pro-α polypeptide chains into a triple-helix conformation forms procollagen (115) ready for secretion (reviewed in ref. 81). The gran-

uloma fibroblasts possess prominent Golgi apparati and complex networks of dilated rough endoplasmic reticulum, consistent with active synthesis and secretion of collagen (Fig. 4B). Once secreted extracellularly, the triple-helix procollagen molecules are cleaved by specific proteases at the amino-terminal and carboxy-terminal ends, allowing alignment of the collagen molecules to form a fiber structure stabilized by lysine and hydroxylysine-derived cross-links (81) that is then deposited in the tissue. This entire multistep biosynthesis of the triple-helix collagen molecule provides numerous potential targets for inflammatory cell regulation of collagen production, including translation, posttranslational modifications, secretion, extracellular processing, and assembly to an ordered supramolecular structure.

Characterization of the interstitial collagens being generated by the activated granuloma fibroblasts identified both types I and III interstitial collagens in the periphery of the granuloma (173). Granuloma tissue also contains type V, without an apparent increase in type IV collagen. In dermal wounds and other fibrotic lesions, infiltration of fibroblasts and formation of granulation tissue normally coincide with initial increases in type III collagen fibers, hyaluronate, and fibronectin (50,116). Matrix assembly may be dependent on the availability of the newly secreted fibronectin, because antibodies directed against the collagen binding domain of fibronectin inhibit collagen fibril deposition (92). During the progression of fibrogenesis, production of type III declines, with type I collagen becoming the predominant matrix protein. The same fibroblasts that synthesize type I also synthesize type III collagen, although the mechanisms responsible for this switch are unclear. Recent data suggest that PGE$_2$ (147) and/or IL-1 promote type III over type I collagen synthesis, and the higher levels of IL-1 in the earlier granulomas may contribute to the early deposition of type III collagen (3).

In contrast to mononuclear cell regulation of collagen synthesis by fibroblasts, little is known regarding regulation of the synthesis of other matrix constituents, including proteoglycans, macromolecules composed of a protein core attached to long unbranched-polysaccharide-chain glycosaminoglycans. Activated mononuclear cell supernatants have been shown to increase glycosaminoglycan synthesis in fibroblast monolayers (180) and may likewise regulate fibroblast synthesis of other matrix components. The resulting connective-tissue matrix is a complex composite of different types of collagen, proteoglycans, and noncollagenous glycoproteins and proteins. In the later stages of granuloma evolution, the number of fibroblasts declines, the inflammatory infiltrate is reduced, and deposits of extracellular matrix remain as the major feature.

Deposition and accumulation of collagen can be modulated by antiinflammatory glucocorticoids that directly influence collagen synthesis (reviewed in refs. 38 and 166) and degradation (171). In this regard, recent evidence suggests selective inhibition of procollagen molecule synthesis, without an effect on certain other biosynthetic steps. Both procollagen types I and III syntheses are apparently inhibited by glucocorticoids (139). The glucocorticoid-mediated decrease in type I collagen may occur at the level of mRNA (149) and is reportedly due to stimulation of mRNA degradation, not to changes in transcriptional activity (54). Consequently, administration of steroids may provide an important mechanism for regulating the postinflammatory repair phase of tissue injury.

Matrix Turnover

Whereas normal healing is characterized by simple scar formation, chronic inflammatory lesions contain activated fibroblasts that continue to secrete matrix proteins, likely under the influence of mononuclear cell products. Furthermore, as fibroblasts synthesize collagen and other matrix proteins, these proteins are also being degraded. Collagenase produced by both macrophages (162) and fibroblasts (183) is the crucial enzyme in normal remodeling of collagen and scar tissue. Resting fibroblasts and/or monocytes/macrophages in culture rarely synthesize significant levels of collagenase, but, once activated, they undergo a shift in gene expression and enzyme translation. Although the intact collagen triple helix is largely stable against normal proteolytic enzymes, collagenase catalyzes the first and rate-limiting step in its proteolysis (51).

Collagenase synthesized by fibroblasts originates as a preproenzyme (183) that is secreted in two proenzyme forms (57,000 and 52,000 dalton). Cleavage of the latent procollagenase by plasmin, kallikrein, or cathepsin B yields active enzyme species (56). In addition to the enzyme, fibroblasts produce a metalloendoprotease inhibitor of collagenase, the synthesis of which does not correlate with collagenase production (183). After the initial collagenase cleavage of the collagen molecule, it then becomes susceptible to further attack by other proteolytic enzymes, both intracellularly and extracellularly. Intracellular collagen fibrils frequently are observed inside SCW-granuloma fibroblast vacuoles that appear to be secondary lysosomes (173). These observations suggest that fibroblast-dependent collagen degradation and tissue remodeling (94,105) are ongoing processes during granuloma development.

In addition to fibroblasts, macrophages are also sources of collagenolytic activity. Macrophages not only secrete collagenase when activated by lymphokines (160) and bacterial products (161) but also promote production of collagenase and PGE_2 by fibroblasts through secretion of TNF, IL-1, and PDGF (16,33). Activated macrophages also generate reactive oxygen intermediates that can attack

the α chains of collagen and hyaluronic acid (108). Over the course of several months, this remodeling of the fibrotic nodules associated with the SCW granulomas continues, with some resorption of the matrix. However, a thickened scar and a vascular supply surrounding the granuloma persist for months. The continual SCW activation of the cells, with residual inflammation, leads to a situation not dissimilar to hypertrophic scar formation. Macrophages containing ingested SCW can be found within the connective-tissue capsule as well as within the core of the granuloma months after the initial injection of SCW, providing an ongoing source of molecular signals to the fibroblasts.

CONCLUDING REMARKS

Although the association among inflammatory cells, wound healing, and fibrosis historically has been a subject of considerable investigation, only recently has the molecular basis of fibroplasia and fibrogenesis been partially characterized. From *in vitro* studies, the basic mechanisms of inflammatory cell regulation of connective-tissue metabolism have been defined. These observations have been extended with *in vivo* models of fibrosis, including the model of SCW-induced hepatic granuloma (Fig. 5). A variety of lymphocyte- and monocyte-derived peptide signaling molecules interact in a complex pattern to orchestrate the development and perpetuation of the SCW-induced inflammatory lesion that then influences the recruitment, growth, and matrix synthesis of connective-tissue cells. The repair essentially begins as soon as tissue injury occurs. However, because the inflammation is not resolved in the SCW-mediated granuloma, inflammation and repair continue concurrently. The SCW antigens become segregated within the core of the granuloma, and this walling off of the antigen provides a mechanism for the host to sequester the poorly biodegradable SCW. During the ensuing weeks there is a progressive fibroblast proliferative response, matrix generation, and formation of fibrotic nodules in association with the granuloma throughout the liver. Because of the persistence of the SCW antigen and the failure to completely resolve the inflammatory response, the tissue cannot heal, and continued efforts result in excessive scarring or fibrosis. The fibrotic response can result in replacement of the original tissue with collagen, impairing tissue and/or organ function. Continued definition of the events associated with this form of incomplete or altered resolution of the inflammatory response is of importance because it may lead to an understanding of the pathogenesis of a variety of diseases associated with unresolved or chronic inflammation.

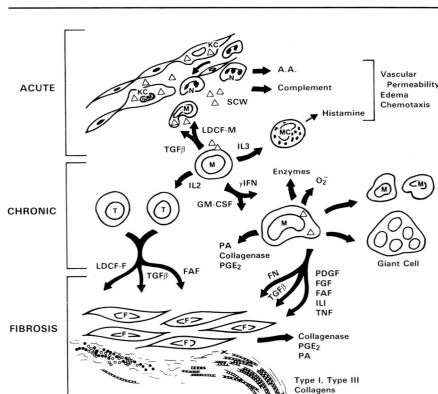

FIG. 5. Schematic summary of SCW-mediated inflammatory events leading to fibrosis. Injected SCW (△) that are phagocytized by Kupffer cells (KC) activate complement and arachidonic acid (A.A.) metabolism, leading to neutrophil (N) recruitment and acute inflammation. Recruitment of monocytes (M) and T lymphocytes (T) and persistence of the SCW result in a chronic inflammatory response. Activated T cells release lymphokines, including LDCF-M, TGF-β, IL-3, IL-2, γIFN, and CSF, that perpetuate and augment the inflammatory response. Macrophages are stimulated to secrete reactive oxygen intermediates (O$_2^-$), PA, PGE$_2$, hydrolytic enzymes, and neutral proteases. Both T cells and monocytes/macrophages release growth factors important in fibrosis and angiogenesis (PDGF, FGF, FAF, IL-1, TNF, and TGF-β). The expanded fibroblast population then secretes collagen and other matrix proteins to form the scar tissue associated with tissue repair.

Fibrotic sequelae to inflammation in lung (pulmonary fibrosis), liver (liver fibrosis and other cirrhoses), or other organs (scleroderma, rheumatoid arthritis, atherosclerosis) can be severe and life-threatening. Excessive accumulation of collagen and other extracellular matrix components in locations where they are not normally found is a frequent problem in a number of diseases. Although there are many circumstances of growth and wound healing in which increased synthesis and deposition of the extracellular matrix are required, these events can clearly become pathologic following a powerful inflammatory reaction. Thus, identification and characterization of the regulatory events during normal and aberrant wound repair should reveal approaches that can be used to modify or control the rate of repair. Because cell proliferation is essential in inflammation and repair, the key to controlling these events is most surely the peptide growth factors (145). The recent advances in purification procedures and recombinant DNA technology will enable further definition of the expression, functional relationships, and relevance of these products in inflammatory processes and in their fibrotic sequelae. The ability to therapeutically accelerate repair with growth-promoting substances could facilitate healing in disease or trauma. Alternatively, antagonists to growth factors may also be of benefit in certain circumstances to reduce scar formation. Specific antibodies, drugs, peptide inhibitors, and other antagonists to growth factors and/or their receptors are potential candidates for regulation of fibrosis. Future advances in this field likely will utilize many of these approaches to alter the course of wound healing and/or its potentially pathologic sequelae in connective-tissue disorders such as scleroderma, rheumatoid arthritis, and pulmonary fibrosis.

ACKNOWLEDGMENTS

The author is grateful to Dr. A. Hand for preparation of the electron micrographs, to Ms. D. A. Hunt for her expert assistance, to Ms. J. B. Allen, without whom these studies would not have been possible, and to Ms. P. Pace and Mrs. E. Walter for their patience in typing this manuscript.

REFERENCES

1. Adams, D. O. (1976): The granulomatous inflammatory response. A review. *Am. J. Pathol.*, 84:164–193.
2. Agelli, M., and Wahl, S. M. (1987): Synthesis of biologically active fibroblast activating factor (FAF) by *Xenopus* oocytes injected with T lymphocyte mRNA. *Cell. Immunol.*, (in press).

3. Agelli, M., Sobel, M. E., and Wahl, S. M. (1987): Cytokine modulation of fibroblast collagen production. *Fed. Proc.*, 46:924.

4. Allen, J. B., Blatter, D., Calandra, G. B., and Wilder, R. L. (1983): Sex hormonal effects on the severity of streptococcal cell wall-induced polyarthritis in the rat. *Arthritis Rheum.*, 26:560–563.

5. Allen, J. B., Malone, D. G., Wahl, S. M., Calandra, G. B., and Wilder, R. H. (1985): The role of the thymus in streptococcal cell wall-induced arthritis and hepatic granuloma formation: Comparative studies of pathology and cell wall distribution in athymic and euthymic rats. *J. Clin. Invest.*, 76:1042–1056.

6. Allen, J. B., Yocum, D. E., Wilder, R. L., and Wahl, S. M. (1986): Inhibition by cyclosporin A of streptococcal cell wall induced hepatic granulomas in LEW/N rats. *Ann. N.Y. Acad. Sci.*, 465:351–361.

7. Allen, J. B., Hunt, D. A., Feldman, G. M., Hand, A., Wahl, L., Ink, L., Swisher, J., and Wahl, S. (1987): Pharmacologic regulation of the development of streptococcal cell wall induced arthritis in rats. *Arthritis Rheum.*, (in press).

8. Allen, J. B., and Wilder, R. L. (1987): Variable severity and Ia antigen expression in streptococcal cell wall-induced hepatic granulomas in rats: dependence on rat strain and cell wall fragment size. *Infect. Immun.*, 55:674–679.

9. Anderle, S. K., Greenblatt, J. J., Cromartie, W. J., Clark, R., and Schwab, J. H. (1979): Modulation of the susceptibility of inbred and outbred rats to arthritis induced by cell walls of group A streptococci. *Infect. Immun.*, 25:484–490.

10. Auerbach, R. (1981): Angiogenesis-inducing factors: A review. *Lymphokines*, 4:69–88.

11. Azizkhan, R. G., Azizkhan, J. C., Zetter, B. R., and Folkman, J. (1980): Mast cell heparin stimulates migration of capillary endothelial cells *in vitro*. *J. Exp. Med.*, 152:931–944.

12. Baird, A., Mormede, P., and Bohlen, P. (1985): Immunoreactive fibroblast growth factor in cells of peritoneal exudate suggests its identity with macrophage-derived growth factor. *Biochem. Biophys. Res. Commun.*, 126:358–364.

13. Banda, M. J., Knighton, D. R., Hunt, T. K., and Werb, Z. (1982): Isolation of a nonmitogenic angiogenesis factor from wound fluid. *Proc. Natl. Acad. Sci. USA*, 79:7773–7777.

14. Bar-Shivat, R., Kahn, A., Fenton, J. W., and Wilner, G. D. (1983): Chemotactic response of monocytes to thrombin. *J. Cell Biol.*, 96:282–285.

15. Basham, T. Y., and Merigan, T. C. (1983): Recombinant interferon-γ increases HLA-DR synthesis and expression. *J. Immunol.*, 130:1492–1494.

16. Bauer, E. A., Cooper, T. W., Huang, J. S., Altman, J., and Deuel, T. F. (1985): Stimulation of *in vitro* human skin collagenase expression by platelet-derived growth factor. *Proc. Natl. Acad. Sci. USA*, 82:4132–4136.

17. Bevilacqua, M. P., Pober, J. S., Whellar, M. E., Cotran, R. S., and Gimbrone, M. A., Jr. (1985): Interleukin 1 acts on cultured human vascular endothelium to increase the adhesion of polymorphonuclear leukocytes, monocytes, and related leukocyte cell lines. *J. Clin. Invest.*, 76:2003–2011.

18. Bickel, M., Tsuda, H., Evequoz, V., Mergenhagen, S. E., Wahl, S. M., and Pluznik, D. H. (1987): Differential regulation of colony stimulating factors and interleukin 2 production by cyclosporin A. *Proc. Natl. Acad. Sci. USA*, 84:3274–3277.

19. Bitterman, P. B., Adelberg, S., and Crystal, R. G. (1983): Mechanisms of pulmonary fibrosis. Spontaneous release of the alveolar macrophage-derived growth factor in the interstitial lung disorders. *J. Clin. Invest.*, 72:1801–1813.

20. Bjerknes, M., Cheng, H., and Ottaway, C. (1986): Dynamics of lymphocyte-endothelial interactions in vivo. *Science*, 231:402–405.

21. Bohnsack, J. F., Kleinman, H. K., Takahashi, T., O'Shea, J. J., and Brown, E. J. (1985): Connective tissue proteins and phagocytic cell function. Laminin enhances complement and Fc-mediated phagocytosis by cultured human macrophages. *J. Exp. Med.*, 161:912–923.

22. Borgeat, P., and Samuelsson, B. (1979): Arachidonic acid metabolism in polymorphonuclear leukocytes: Effects of ionophore A23187. *Proc. Natl. Acad. Sci. USA*, 76:2148–2153.

23. Boros, D. L. (1978): Granulomatous inflammation. *Prog. Allergy*, 24:183–267.

24. Bowersox, J. C., and Sorgente, N. (1982): Chemotaxis of aortic endothelial cells in response to fibronectin. *Cancer Res.*, 42:2547–2551.

25. Brinckerhoff, C. E., and Guyre, P. M. (1985): Increased proliferation of human synovial fibroblasts treated with recombinant immune interferon. *J. Immunol.*, 134:3142–3146.

26. Burgess, W. H., Mehlman, T., Friesel, R., Johnson, W. V., and Maciag, T. (1985): Multiple forms of endothelial cell growth factor: Rapid isolation and biological and chemical characterization. *J. Biol. Chem.*, 260:11389–11392.

27. Castor, C. W. (1981): Autacoid regulation of wound healing. In: *Tissue Repair and Regeneration. Handbook of Inflammation, Vol. 3*, edited by L. E. Glynn, J. C. Houck, and G. Weissman, pp. 177–207. Elsevier/North Holland, Amsterdam.

28. Chervenick, P. A., and LoBuglio, A. F. (1972): Human blood monocytes: Stimulators of granulocyte and mononuclear cell colony formation *in vitro*. *Science*, 178:164–166.

29. Claman, H. N. (1985): Mast cells, T cells and abnormal fibrosis. *Immunol. Today*, 6:192–195.

30. Clark, R. A. F., Quinn, J. H., Winn, W. J., Lanigan, J. M., and Colvin, R. B. (1982): Fibronectin is produced by blood vessels in response to injury. *J. Exp. Med.*, 156:646–651.

31. Cline, M. J., and Golde, D. W. (1974): Production of colony stimulating activity by human lymphocytes. *Nature*, 248:703–704.

32. Davies, P., Bailey, P. J., Goldenberg, M. M., and Ford-Hutchinson, A. W. (1984): The role of arachidonic acid oxygenation products in pain and inflammation. *Annu. Rev. Immunol.*, 2:335–357.

33. Dayer, J. M., Beutler, B., and Cerami, A. (1985): Cachectin/tumor necrosis factor stimulates synovial cells and fibroblasts to produce collagenase and prostaglandin E₂. *J. Exp. Med.*, 162:2163–2167.

34. Deuel, T. F., Senior, R. M., Chang, D., Griffin, G. L., Heinrikson, R. L., and Kaiser, E. T. (1981): Platelet factor 4 is chemotactic for neutrophils and monocytes. *Proc. Natl. Acad. Sci. USA*, 78:4584–4587.

35. Deuel, T. F., Senior, R. M., Huang, J. S., and Griffin, G. L. (1982): Chemotaxis of monocytes and neutrophils to platelet-derived growth factor. *J. Clin. Invest.*, 69:1046–1049.

36. Dinarello, C. A. (1984): Interleukin 1. *Rev. Infect. Dis.*, 6:51–95.

37. Doughty, B. L., and Phillips, S. M. (1982): Delayed hypersensitivity granuloma formation and modulation around *Schistosoma mansoni* eggs *in vitro*. *J. Immunol.*, 128:37–42.

38. Durant, S., Duval, D., and Homo-Delarche, F. (1986): Factors involved in the control of fibroblast proliferation by glucocorticoids: A review. *Endocrine Reviews*, 7:254–269.

39. Elias, J. A., Schreiber, A. D., Gustilo, K., Chien, P., Rossman, M. D., Lammie, P. J., and Daniele, R. P. (1985): Differential interleukin 1 elaboration by unfractionated and density fractionated human alveolar macrophages and blood monocytes: Relationship to cell maturity. *J. Immunol.*, 135:3198–3204.

40. Esser, R. E., Anderle, S. K., Chetly, C., Stimpson, S. A., Cromartie, W. J., and Schwab, J. H. (1986): Comparison of inflammatory reactions induced by intraarticular injection of bacterial cell wall polymers. *Am. J. Pathol.*, 122:323–334.

41. Evequoz, V., Allen, J. B., Pluznik, D. H., Paglia, L., Yocum, D. E., Wilder, R. L., Malone, D. G., and Wahl, S. M. (1985): Streptococcal cell wall (SCW)-induced hepatic granuloma formation and fibrosis require T lymphocytes. *J. Leukocyte Biol.*, 38:118.

42. Feldman, G., Allen, J., Swisher, J., Pluznik, D., Wahl, L., and Wahl, S. (1987): Susceptibility to streptococcal cell wall (SCW)-induced polyarthritis is associated with differential macrophage activation. *J. Leukocyte Biol.*, (in press).

43. Folkman, J. (1983): Angiogenesis: Initiation and control. *Ann. N.Y. Acad. Sci.*, 401:212–227.

44. Form, D. M., and Auerbach, R. (1983): PGE₂ and angiogenesis. *Proc. Soc. Exp. Biol.*, 172:214–218.

45. Gimbrone, M. A., Jr., Brock, A. F., and Schafer, A. I. (1984): Leukotriene B₄ stimulates polymorphonuclear leukocyte adhesion to cultured vascular endothelial cells. *J. Clin. Invest.*, 74:1552–1555.

46. Glick, A. D., Ranhand, J. M., and Cole, R. M. (1972): Degradation

of group A streptococcal cell walls by egg-white lysozyme and human lysosomal enzymes. *Infect. Immun.*, 6:403–413.

47. Gold, M. R., Miller, C. L., and Mishell, R. I. (1985): Soluble non-cross-linked peptidoglycan polymers stimulate monocyte-macrophage inflammatory reactions. *Infect. Immun.*, 49:731–741.

48. Goldyne, M. E., Burrish, G. F., Poubelle, P., and Borgeat, P. (1984): Arachidonic acid metabolism among human mononuclear leukocytes: Lipoxygenase-related pathways. *J. Biol. Chem.*, 259:8815–8819.

49. Goodwin, J. S., and Webb, D. R. (1980): Regulation of immune responses by prostaglandins. *Clin. Immunol. Immunopathol.*, 15:106–122.

50. Grinnell, F. (1984): Fibronectin and wound healing. *J. Cell. Biochem.*, 26:107–116.

51. Gross, J., and Nagai, Y. (1965): Specific degradation of the collagen molecule by tadpole collagenolytic enzyme. *Proc. Natl. Acad. Sci. USA*, 54:1197–1204.

52. Gross, J. L., Moscatelli, D., and Rifkin, D. B. (1983): Increased capillary endothelial cell protease activity in response to angiogenic stimuli *in vitro*. *Proc. Natl. Acad. Sci. USA*, 80:2623–2627.

53. Grotendorst, G. R., Paglia, L., McIvor, C., Barsky, S., Martinet, Y., and Pencer, D. (1985): Chemoattractants in fibrotic disorders. In: *Fibrosis*, pp. 150–158. Pitman, London.

54. Hamalainen, L., Oikarinen, J., and Kivirikko, K. J. (1985): Synthesis and degradation of type I procollagen mRNAs in cultured human skin fibroblasts and the effect of cortisol. *J. Biol. Chem.*, 260:720–725.

55. Hamilton, J. A., Stanley, E. R., Burgess, A. W., and Shadduck, R. K. (1980): Stimulation of macrophage plasminogen activator activity by colony-stimulating factors. *J. Cell. Physiol.*, 103:435–445.

56. Harris, E. D., Jr. (1986): Regulation of collagenolysis in synovial cell systems. *Rheumatology*, 10:197–215.

57. Hayashi, M., and Yamada, K. M. (1983): Domain structure of the carboxy-terminal half of human plasma fibronectin. *J. Biol. Chem.*, 258:3332–3340.

58. Heimark, R. L., Twardzik, D. R., and Schwartz, S. M. (1986): Inhibition of endothelial regeneration by type-beta transforming growth factor from platelets. *Science*, 233:1078–1080.

59. Henson, P. M., Larsen, G. L., Henson, J. E., Newman, S. L., Musson, R. A., and Leslie, C. C. (1984): Resolution of pulmonary inflammation. *Fed. Proc.*, 43:2799–2806.

60. Hong, S. L., and Levine, L. (1976): Inhibition of arachidonic acid release from cells as the biochemical action of antiinflammatory corticosteroids. *Proc. Natl. Acad. Sci. USA*, 73:1730–1734.

61. Hoover, R. L., Karnovsky, M. J., Austen, K. F., Corey, E. J., and Lewis, R. A. (1984): LTB₄ modulates neutrophil-endothelial interactions. *Proc. Natl. Acad. Sci. USA*, 81:2192–2193.

62. Hugo, N. E., Thompson, L. W., Zook, E. G., et al. (1969): Effect of chronic anemia on the tensile strength of healing wounds. *Surgery*, 66:741–745.

63. Hynes, R. O., and Yamada, K. M. (1982): Fibronectins: Multifunctional modular glycoproteins. *J. Cell Biol.*, 95:369–377.

64. Ihle, J. N., Keller, J., Oroszlan, S., Henderson, L. E., Copeland, T. D., Fitch, F., Prystowsky, M. B., Goldwasser, E., Schrader, J. W., Palaszynski, E., Dy, M., and Lebel, B. (1983): Biologic properties of homogeneous interleukin 3. I. Demonstration of WEHI-3 growth factor activity, mast cell growth factor activity, P cell stimulating factor activity, colony stimulating factor activity, and histamine producing cell stimulating factor activity. *J. Immunol.*, 131:282–287.

65. Jimenez, S. A., Freundlich, B., and Rosenbloom, J. (1984): Selective inhibition of human diploid fibroblast collagen synthesis by interferons. *J. Clin. Invest.*, 74:1112–1116.

66. Johnson, R. L., and Ziff, M. (1976): Lymphokine stimulation of collagen accumulation. *J. Clin. Invest.*, 58:240–252.

67. Kalebic, T., Garbisa, S., Glaser, B., and Liotta, L. A. (1983): Basement membrane collagen: Degradation by migrating endothelial cells. *Science*, 221:281–283.

68. Kampschmidt, R. F., and Franks, T. (1985): The physical and biological properties of rat interleukin 1. *J. Leukocyte Biol.*, 37:715.

69. Kaplan, A. P., Kay, A. B., and Austen, K. F. (1972): A prealbumin activator of prekallikrein. III. Appearance of chemotactic activity for human neutrophils by the conversion of human prekallikrein to kallikrein. *J. Exp. Med.*, 135:81–97.

70. Kaplan, A. P., Goetzl, E. J., and Austen, K. F. (1973): The fibrinolytic pathway of human plasma. II. The generation of chemotactic activity by activation of plasminogen proactivator. *J. Clin. Invest.*, 52:2591–2595.

71. Kehrl, J. H., Wakefield, L. M., Roberts, A. B., Jakowlew, S., Alvarez-Mon, M., Derynk, R., Sporn, M. B., and Fauci, A. S. (1986): The production of TGF-β by human T lymphocytes and its potential role in the regulation of T cell growth. *J. Exp. Med.*, 163:1037–1050.

72. Knighton, D. R., Silver, I. A., and Hunt, T. K. (1981): Regulation of wound healing angiogenesis: Effect of oxygen gradients and inspired oxygen concentration. *Surgery*, 90:262–270.

73. Knighton, D. R., Silver, I. A., and Hunt, T. K. (1984): Studies on inflammation and wound healing: Angiogenesis and collagen synthesis stimulated *in vivo* by resident and activated wound macrophages. *Surgery*, 96:48–54.

74. Korn, J. H., Halushka, P. V., and LeRoy, E. C. (1980): Mononuclear cell modulation of connective tissue function. Suppression of fibroblast growth by stimulation of endogenous prostaglandin production. *J. Clin. Invest.*, 65:543–554.

75. Krane, S. M., Dayer, J. M., Simon, L. S., and Byrne, M. S. (1985): Mononuclear cell-conditioned medium containing mononuclear cell factor (MCF), homologous with interleukin 1, stimulates collagen and fibronectin synthesis by adherent rheumatoid synovial cells: Effects of prostaglandin E₂ and indomethacin. *Collagen Rel. Res.*, 5:99–117.

76. Krause, R. M. (1977): Cell wall antigens of gram-positive bacteria and their biological activities. In: *Microbiology—1977*, edited by D. Schlessinger, pp. 330–338. American Society for Microbiology, Washington, D.C.

77. Kronke, M., Leonard, W. J., Depper, J. M., Arya, S. K., Wong-Staal, F., Gallo, R. C., Waldmann, T. A., and Greene, W. C. (1984): Cyclosporin A inhibits T-cell growth factor gene expression at the level of mRNA transcription. *Proc. Natl. Acad. Sci. USA*, 81:5214–5218.

78. Kurland, J. I., Pelus, L. M., Ralph, P., Bockman, R. S., and Moore, M. A. S. (1979): Induction of prostaglandin E synthesis in normal and neoplastic macrophages: Role for colony-stimulating factor(s) distinct from effects on myeloid progenitor cell proliferation. *Proc. Natl. Acad. Sci. USA*, 76:2326–2330.

79. Lambris, J. D., Allen, J. B., and Schwab, J. H. (1982): *In vivo* changes in complement induced with peptidoglycan-polysaccharide polymers from streptococcal cell walls. *Infect. Immun.*, 35:377–380.

80. Lammie, P. J., Michael, A. I., Linette, G. P., and Phillips, S. M. (1986): Production of a fibroblast-stimulating factor by *Schistosoma mansoni* antigen-reactive T cell clones. *J. Immunol.*, 136:1100–1106.

81. Leblond, C. P., and Laurie, G. W. (1986): Morphological feature of connective tissues. *Rheumatology*, 10:1–28.

82. Leibovich, S. J., and Ross, R. (1975): The role of the macrophage in wound repair: A study with hydrocortisone and antimacrophage serum. *Am. J. Pathol.*, 78:71–91.

83. Lorenzet, R., Niemetz, J., Marcus, A. J., and Broekman, M. J. (1986): Enhancement of mononuclear procoagulant activity by platelet 12-hydroxyeicosatetraenoic acid. *J. Clin. Invest.*, 78:418–423.

84. Macon, W. L., and Pories, W. J. (1967): Effect of iron deficiency anemia on wound healing. *Surgery*, 69:792–796.

85. Marasco, W. A., Phan, S. H., Krutzsch, H., Showell, H. J., Feltner, D. E., Nairn, R., Becker, E. L., and Ward, P. A. (1984): Purification and indentification of formyl-methionyl-leucyl phenylalanine as the major peptide neutrophil chemotactic factor produced by *Escherichia coli*. *J. Biol. Chem.*, 259:5430–5439.

86. Marder, S. R., Chenoweth, D. E., Goldstein, I. M., and Perez, H. D. (1985): Chemotactic responses of human peripheral blood monocytes to the complement-derived peptides C5a and C5a des Arg. *J. Immunol.*, 134:3325–3331.

87. Mariano, M., Nikitin, T., and Malucelli, B. E. (1976): Immunological and nonimmunological phagocytosis by inflammatory macrophages, epithelioid cells and macrophage polykaryons from foreign body granulomata. *J. Pathol.*, 120:151–159.

88. Martin, B. M., Gimbrone, M. A., Unanue, E. R., and Cotran, R. S. (1981): Stimulation of nonlymphoid mesenchymal cell proliferation by a macrophage-derived growth factor. *J. Immunol.*, 126:1510–1515.

89. Martinet, Y., Bitterman, P. B., Mornex, J., Grotendorst, G. R., Martin, G. R., and Crystal, R. G. (1986): Activated human monocytes express the c-sis proto-oncogene and release a mediator showing PDGF-like activity. *Nature*, 319:158–160.

90. McCarthy, J. B., Hagen, S. T., and Furcht, L. T. (1986): Human plasma fibronectin contains multiple adhesive and motility promoting domains for metastatic melanoma cells. *J. Cell Biol.*, 102: 179–188.

91. McCarthy, J. B., Sas, D. B., and Furcht, L. T. (1987): Mechanisms of connective tissue migration into wounds. In: *Molecular and Cellular Biology of Wound Repair*, edited by R. A. F. Clark and P. Henson, Plenum Press, New York.

92. McDonald, J. A., Kelley, D. G., and Broekelmann, T. J. (1982): Role of fibronectin in collagen deposition: Fab' to the gelatin-binding domain of fibronectin inhibits both fibronectin and collagen organization in fibroblast extracellular matrix. *J. Cell Biol.*, 92:485–492.

93. McIntyre, T. M., Zimmerman, G. A., and Prescott, S. M. (1986): Leukotrienes C$_4$ and D$_4$ stimulate human endothelial cells to synthesize platelet-activating factor and bind neutrophils. *Proc. Natl. Acad. Sci. USA*, 83:2204–2208.

94. Melcher, A. H., and Chan, J. (1981): Phagocytosis and digestion of collagen by gingival fibroblasts *in vivo*: A study of serial sections. *J. Ultrastruct. Res.*, 77:1–36.

95. Mensing, H., and Czarnetzki, B. M. (1984): Leukotriene B$_4$ induces in vitro fibroblast chemotaxis. *J. Invest. Dermatol.*, 82:9–12.

96. Mokoena, T., and Gordon, S. (1985): Human macrophage activation. Modulation of mannosyl, fucosyl receptor activity *in vitro* by lymphokines, gamma and alpha interferons and dexamethasone. *J. Clin. Invest.*, 75:624–631.

97. Moore, R. N., Oppenheim, J. J., Farrar, J. J., Carter, C. S., Waheed, A., Jr., and Shadduck, R. K. (1980): Production of lymphocyte-activating factor (interleukin 1) by macrophages activated with colony stimulating factors. *J. Immunol.*, 1250–1302.

98. Nathan, C. F., Murray, H. W., and Cohn, Z. A. (1980): The macrophage as an effector cell. *N. Engl. J. Med.*, 303:622–625.

99. Nawroth, P. P., Bank, I., Handley, D., Cassimeris, J., Chess, L., and Stern, D. (1986): Tumor necrosis factor/cachectin interacts with endothelial cell receptors to induce release of interleukin 1. *J. Exp. Med.*, 163:1363–1375.

100. Neilson, E. G., Phillips, S. M., and Jimenez, S. (1982): Lymphokine modulation of fibroblast proliferation. *J. Immunol.*, 128:1484–1486.

101. Nerlich, A. G., Poschl, E., Voss, T., and Muller, P. K. (1986): Biosynthesis of collagen and its control. *Rheumatology*, 10:70–90.

102. Norris, D. A., Clark, R. A. F., and Swigart, L. M. (1982): Fibronectin fragments are chemotactic for human peripheral blood monocytes. *J. Immunol.*, 129:1612–1618.

103. Ogston, D., and Bennett, B. (1984): The blood coagulation cascade. In: *Recent Advances in Blood Coagulation, Vol. 4*, edited by L. Poller, pp. 1–10. Churchill Livingstone, New York.

104. Peirschbacher, M. D., and Ruoslahti, E. (1984): Cell attachment activity of fibronectin can be duplicated by a small synthetic fragment of the molecule. *Nature*, 309:30–33.

105. Perez-Tamayo, R. (1970): Collagen resorption in carrageenin granulomas. II. Ultrastructure of collagen resorption. *Lab. Invest.*, 22: 142–159.

106. Pluznik, D. H. (1985): CSF dependent proliferation is triggered in the early G$_1$ phase of the target cell cycle. In: *Cellular and Molecular Biology of Lymphokines*, edited by C. Sorg and A. Schimple, pp. 497–500. Academic Press, New York.

107. Polverini, P. J., Cotran, R. S., Gimbrone, M. A., and Unanue, E. R. (1977): Activated macrophages induce vascular proliferation. *Nature*, 269:804–806.

108. Poole, A. R. (1986): Changes in the collagen and proteoglycan of articular cartilage in arthritis. *Rheumatology*, 10:316–371.

109. Postlethwaite, A. E., and Kang, A. H. (1976): Collagen and collagen peptide-induced chemotaxis of human blood monocytes. *J. Exp. Med.*, 143:1299–1307.

110. Postlethwaite, A. E., Snyderman, R., and Kang, A. H. (1976): The chemotactic attraction of human fibroblasts to a lymphocyte derived factor. *J. Exp. Med.*, 144:1188–1203.

111. Postlethwaite, A. E., Seyer, J. M., and Kang, A. H. (1978): Chemotactic attraction of human fibroblasts to type I, II, and III collagens and collagen-derived peptides. *Proc. Natl. Acad. Sci. USA*, 75:871–875.

112. Postlethwaite, A. E., Snyderman, R., and Kang, A. H. (1979): Generation of a fibroblast chemotactic factor in serum by activation of complement. *J. Clin. Invest.*, 64:1379–1385.

113. Postlethwaite, A. E., Jackson, B. K., Beachey, E. H., and Kang, A. H. (1982): Formation of multinucleated giant cells from human monocyte precursors. Mediation by a soluble protein from antigen- and mitogen-stimulated lymphocytes. *J. Exp. Med.*, 155:168–178.

114. Postlethwaite, A. E., Smith, G. N., Mainardi, C. L., Seyer, J. M., and Kang, A. H. (1984): Lymphocyte modulation of fibroblast function *in vitro*: Stimulation and inhibition of collagen production by different effector molecules. *J. Immunol.*, 132:2470–2477.

115. Prockop, D. J., Berg, R. A., Kivirikko, K. I., and Uitto, J. (1976): Intracellular steps in the biosynthesis of collagen. In: *Biochemistry of Collagen, Vol. 163*, edited by G. N. Ramachandran and A. H. Reddi, pp. 273–287. Plenum, New York.

116. Repesh, L. A., Fitzgerald, T. J., and Furcht, L. T. (1982): Fibronectin involvement in granulation tissue and wound healing in rabbits. *J. Histochem. Cytochem.*, 30:351–358.

117. Rifkin, D. B., Gross, J. L., Moscatelli, D., and Jaffe, E. (1982): In: *Pathobiology of the Endothelial Cell*, edited by H. Nossel and H. J. Voge, pp. 191–197. Academic Press, New York.

118. Roberts, A. B., Sporn, M. B., Assoian, R. K., Smith, J. M., Roche, N. S., Wakefield, L. M., Heine, U. I., Liotta, L. A., Falanga, V., Kehrl, J. H., and Fauci, A. S. (1986): Transforming growth factor type β: Rapid induction of fibrosis and angiogenesis *in vivo* and stimulation of collagen formation *in vitro*. *Proc. Natl. Acad. Sci. USA*, 83:4167–4171.

119. Rola-Pleszcynski, M., Lieu, H., Hamel, J., and Lemaire, I. (1982): Stimulated human lymphocytes produce a soluble factor which inhibits fibroblast migration. *Cell. Immunol.*, 74:104–110.

120. Rosenbloom, J., Feldman, G., Freundlich, B., and Jimenez, S. A. (1984): Transcriptional control of human diploid fibroblast collagen synthesis by gamma-interferon. *Biochem. Biophys. Res. Commun.*, 123:365–372.

121. Ross, R. (1969): Wound healing. *Sci. Am.*, 220:40–55.

122. Rossi, V., Breviario, F., Ghezzi, P., Dejana, E., and Mantovani, A. (1985): Prostacyclin synthesis induced in vascular cells by interleukin 1. *Science*, 229:174–176.

123. Rubinstein, D., Roska, A. K., and Lipsky, P. E. (1986): Liver sinusoidal lining cells express class II major histocompatibility antigens but are poor stimulators of fresh allogeneic T lymphocytes. *J. Immunol.*, 137:1803–1810.

124. Ruscetti, F. W., and Chervenick, P. A. (1975): Release of colony stimulating activity from thymus-derived lymphocytes. *J. Clin. Invest.*, 55:520–527.

125. Ryan, U. S. (1986): The endothelial surface and responses to injury. *Fed. Proc.*, 45:101–108.

126. Samuelsson, B. (1983): Leukotrienes: Mediators of immediate hypersensitivity reactions and inflammation. *Science*, 220:568–578.

127. Schiffman, E., Corcoran, B. A., and Wahl, S. M. (1975): N-formylmethionylpeptides as chemoattractants for leucocytes. *Proc. Natl. Acad. Sci. USA*, 72:1059–1061.

128. Schlesinger, L., Musson, R. A., and Johnston, R. B., Jr. (1984): Functional and biochemical studies of multinucleated giant cells derived from the culture of human monocytes. *J. Exp. Med.*, 159: 1289–1294.

129. Schmidt, J. A., Mizel, S. B., Cohen, D., and Green, I. (1982): In-

terleukin 1, a potential regulator of fibroblast proliferation. *J. Immunol.*, 128:2177–2181.

130. Schraufstatter, I., Revak, S. D., and Cochrane, C. G. (1984): Biochemical factors in pulmonary inflammatory disease. *Fed. Proc.*, 43:2807–2810.

131. Schwab, J. H., Allen, J. B., Anderle, S. K., Dalldorf, F., Eisenberg, R., and Cromartie, W. J. (1982): Relationship of complement to experimental arthritis induced in rats with streptococcal cell walls. *Immunology*, 46:83–88.

132. Senior, R. M., Griffin, G. L., and Mecham, R. P. (1980): Chemotactic activity of elastin derived peptides. *J. Clin. Invest.*, 66:859–862.

133. Senior, R. M., Griffin, G. L., Huang, J. S., Walz, D. A., and Deuel, T. F. (1983): Chemotactic activity of platelet alpha granule proteins for fibroblasts. *J. Cell Biol.*, 96:382–385.

134. Seppa, H., Grotendorst, G., Seppa, S., Schiffmann, E., and Martin, G. (1982): Platelet-derived growth factor is chemotactic for fibroblasts. *J. Cell Biol.*, 92:584–588.

135. Shahabuddin, S., Kumar, S., West, D., and Arnold, F. (1985): A study of angiogenesis factors from five different sources using a radioimmunoassay. *Int. J. Cancer*, 35:87–91.

136. Shimokado, K., Raines, E. W., Madtes, D. K., Barrett, T. B., Benditt, E. P., and Ross, R. (1985): A significant part of macrophage-derived growth factor consists of at least two forms of PDGF. *Cell*, 43:277–286.

137. Shin, H. S., Snyderman, R., Friedman, E., Mellors, A., and Mayer, M. M. (1968): Chemotactic and anaphylatoxic fragment cleaved from the fifth component of guinea pig complement. *Science*, 162:361–363.

138. Sholley, M. M., Gimbrone, M. A., Jr., and Cotran, R. S. (1978): The effects of leukocyte depletion on corneal vascularization. *Lab. Invest.*, 38:32–40.

139. Shull, S., and Cutroneo, K. R. (1983): Glucocorticoids coordinately regulate procollagens type I and type III synthesis. *J. Biol. Chem.*, 258:3364–3369.

140. Sidky, Y. A., and Auerbach, R. (1975): Lymphocyte-induced angiogenesis (LIA): A quantitative and sensitive assay of the graft vs. host reaction. *J. Exp. Med.*, 141:1084–1108.

141. Simpson, D. M., and Ross, R. (1972): The neutrophilic leukocyte in wound repair. A study with antineutrophil serum. *J. Clin. Invest.*, 51:2009–2023.

142. Smedley, L. A., Tonnesen, M. G., Sandhaus, R. A., Haslett, C., Guthrie, L. A., Johnston, R. B., Jr., Henson, P. M., and Worthen, G. S. (1986): Neutrophil-mediated injury to endothelial cells. Enhancement by endotoxin and essential role of neutrophil elastase. *J. Clin. Invest.*, 77:1233–1243.

143. Smialowicz, R. J., and Schwab, J. H. (1977): Processing of streptococcal cell walls by rat macrophages and human monocytes *in vitro. Infect. Immun.*, 17:591–598.

144. Snyderman, R., and Pike, M. (1984): Chemoattractant receptors on phagocytic cells. *Annu. Rev. Immunol.*, 2:257–281.

145. Sporn, M. B., and Roberts, A. B. (1986): Peptide growth factors and inflammation, tissue repair and cancer. *J. Clin. Invest.*, 78:329–332.

146. Stein, J. M., and Levenson, S. M. (1966): Effect of the inflammatory reaction on subsequent wound healing. *Surg. Forum*, 17:484–485.

147. Steinman, B. U., Abe, S., and Martin, G. R. (1982): Modulation of type I and type II collagen production in normal and mutant human skin fibroblasts by cell density, prostaglandin E_2 and epidermal growth factor. *Collagen Rel. Res.*, 2:185–195.

148. Stephenson, M. L., Krane, S. M., Amento, E. P., McCroskery, P. A., and Byrne, M. (1985): Immune interferon inhibits collagen synthesis by rheumatoid synovial cells associated with decreased levels of the procollagen mRNAs. *FEBS Lett.*, 180:43–49.

149. Sterling, K. M., Harris, M. J., Mitchell, J. J., Petrillo, T. A., Delaney, L., and Cutroneo, K. R. (1983): Dexamethasone decreases the amounts of type I procollagen mRNAs *in vivo* and in fibroblast cultures. *J. Biol. Chem.*, 258:7644–7647.

150. Stiles, C. D., Capone, G. T., Scher, C. D., Antoniades, H. N., Van Wyk, J. J., and Pledger, W. J. (1979): Dual control of cell growth by somatomedins and platelet-derived growth factor. *Proc. Natl. Acad. Sci. USA*, 76:1279–1283.

151. Takemura, S., Rossing, T. H., and Perlmutter, D. H. (1986): A lymphokine regulates expression of alpha-1-proteinase inhibitor in human monocytes and macrophages. *J. Clin. Invest.*, 77:1207–1213.

152. Taylor, S., and Folkman, J. (1982): Protamine is an inhibitor of angiogenesis. *Nature*, 297:307–312.

153. Terranova, V. P., Diflorio, R., Hujanen, E., Lyall, R. M., Liotta, L. A., Thorgeirsson, U., Siegal, G. P., and Schiffmann, E. (1986): Laminin promotes rabbit neutrophil motility and attachment. *J. Clin. Invest.*, 77:1180–1186.

154. Tonnesen, M. G., Smedly, L. A., and Henson, P. M. (1984): Neutrophil endothelial cell interactions modulation of neutrophil adhesiveness induced by complement fragments C5a and C5a des arg and formyl-methionyl-leucyl-phenylalanine in vitro. *J. Clin. Invest.*, 74:1581–1592.

155. Tsukamoto, Y., Helsel, W. E., and Wahl, S. M. (1981): Macrophage production of fibronectin, a chemoattractant for fibroblasts. *J. Immunol.*, 127:673–678.

156. Turner, S. R., and Lynn, W. S. (1978): Lipid molecules as chemotactic factors. In: *Leukocyte Chemotaxis*, edited by J. I. Gallin and P. G. Quie, pp. 289–298. Raven Press, New York.

157. Uitto, J. L., Ryhanen, E. M., Tan, A., Oikarinen, I., and Zaragoza, E. J. (1984): Pharmacological inhibition of excessive collagen deposition in fibrotic disease. *Fed. Proc.*, 43:2815–2820.

158. Vassali, J. D., Dayer, J. M., Wohlwend, A., and Belin, D. (1984): Concomitant secretion of prourokinase and of a plasminogen activator-specific inhibitor by cultured human monocytes-macrophages. *J. Exp. Med.*, 159:1653–1668.

159. Vilcek, J., Palombella, V. J., Henriksen-DeStefano, D., Swenson, C., Feinman, R., Hirai, M., and Tsujimoto, M. (1986): Fibroblast growth enhancing activity of tumor necrosis factor and its relationship to other polypeptide growth factors. *J. Exp. Med.*, 163:632–643.

160. Wahl, L. M., Wahl, S. M., Mergenhagen, S. E., and Martin, G. R. (1975): Collagenase production by lymphokine activated macrophages. *Science*, 187:261–263.

161. Wahl, L. M., Wahl, S. M., Mergenhagen, S. E., and Martin, G. R. (1974): Collagenase production by endotoxin-activated macrophages. *Proc. Natl. Acad. Sci. USA*, 71:3598–3601.

162. Wahl, L. M., and Winter, C. C. (1984): Regulation of guinea pig macrophage collagenase production by dexamethasone and colchicine. *Arch. Biochem. Biophys.*, 230:661–667.

163. Wahl, S. M. (1986): Inflammatory cell regulation of connective tissue metabolism. In: *Rheumatology: Connective Tissue in Normal and Pathological States, Vol. 10*, pp. 404–429. Karger, Basel.

164. Wahl, S. M. (1987): Hepatic granulomas as a model of inflammation and repair. *Methods Enzymol., (in press).*

165. Wahl, S. M. (1987): Lymphocyte and macrophage derived growth factors. *Methods Enzymol., (in press).*

166. Wahl, S. M. (1987): Corticosteroids and wound healing. In: *Antiinflammatory Steroid Action: Basic and Clinical Aspects.* Academic Press, New York.

167. Wahl, S. M., Arend, W. P., and Ross, R. (1974): The effect of complement depletion on wound healing. *Am. J. Pathol.*, 74:73–83.

168. Wahl, S. M., Wahl, L. M., McCarthy, J. B., Chedid, L., and Mergenhagen, S. E. (1979): Macrophage activation by mycobacterial water soluble compounds and synthetic muramyl dipeptide. *J. Immunol.*, 122:2226–2231.

169. Wahl, S. M., and Gately, C. L. (1983): Modulation of fibroblast growth by a lymphokine of human T cell and T cell origin. *J. Immunol.*, 130:1226–1230.

170. Wahl, S. M., Malone, D. G., and Wilder, R. L. (1985): Spontaneous production of fibroblast activating factor(s) by synovial inflammatory cells. A potential mechanism for enhanced tissue destruction. *J. Exp. Med.*, 161:210–222.

171. Wahl, S. M., and Wahl, L. M. (1985): Regulation of macrophage collagenase, prostaglandin and fibroblast-activating factor production by anti-inflammatory agents: Different regulatory mechanisms for tissue injury and repair. *Cell. Immunol.*, 92:302–312.

172. Wahl, S. M., Allen, J. B., Dougherty, S., Evequoz, E., Pluznik, D. H., Wilder, R. L., Hand, A. R., and Wahl, L. M. (1986): T

lymphocyte dependent evolution of bacterial cell wall induced hepatic granulomas. *J. Immunol.,* 137:2199–2209.

173. Wahl, S. M., Hunt, D. A., Allen, J. B., Wilder, R. L., Paglia, L., and Hand, A. R. (1986): Bacterial cell wall induced hepatic granulomas. An *in vivo* model of T cell dependent fibrosis. *J. Exp. Med.,* 163:884–902.

174. Wahl, S., Hunt, D., Wakefield, L., McCartney-Francis, N., Wahl, L., Roberts, A., and Sporn, M. (1987): Transforming growth factor-beta (TGF-β) induces monocyte chemotaxis and growth factor production. *Proc. Natl. Acad. Sci. USA,* 84:5788–5792.

175. Wahl, S. M., McCartney-Francis, N., Hunt, D. A., Smith, P. D., Wahl, L. M., and Katona, I. M. (1987): Monocyte interleukin 2 receptor gene expression and IL2 augmentation of microbicidal activity. *J. Immunol.,* 139:1342–1347.

176. Warner, C. R., Vetto, R. M., and Burger, D. R. (1984): The mechanisms of antigen presentation by endothelial cells. *Immunobiology,* 168:453–469.

177. Wellman, S. R., Chensue, S. W., and Boros, D. L. (1980): Modulation of granulomatous hypersensitivity. Analysis by adoptive transfer of effector and suppressor T lymphocytes involved in granulomatous inflammation in murine schistosomiasis. In: *Basic and Clinical Aspects of Granulomatous Diseases,* edited by D. L. Boros and T. Yoshida, pp. 219–229. Elsevier/North Holland, Amsterdam.

178. Wewers, M. D., Rennard, S. I., Hance, A. J., Bitterman, P. B., and Crystal, R. G. (1984): Normal human alveolar macrophages obtained by bronchoalveolar lavage have a limited capacity to release interleukin 1. *J. Clin. Invest.,* 74:2208–2218.

179. Whiteley, P. J., and Needleman, P. (1984): Mechanism of enhanced fibroblast arachidonic acid metabolism by mononuclear cell factor. *J. Clin. Invest.,* 74:2249–2253.

180. Whiteside, T. L., Worrall, J. G., Prince, R. K., Buckingham, R. B., and Rodnan, G. P. (1985): Soluble mediators from mononuclear cells increase the synthesis of glycosaminoglycan by dermal fibroblast cultures derived from normal subjects and progressive systemic sclerosis patients. *Arthritis Rheum.,* 28:188–197.

181. Wilder, R. L., Calandra, G. B., Garvin, A. J., Wright, K. D., and Hansen, C. T. (1982): Strain and sex variation in the susceptibility to streptococcal cell wall-induced polyarthritis in the rat. *Arthritis Rheum.,* 25:1064–1072.

182. Wilder, R. L., Allen, J. B., Wahl, L. M., Calandra, G. B., and Wahl, S. M. (1983): The pathogenesis of group A streptococcal cell wall induced polyarthritis in the rat: Comparative studies in arthritis resistant and susceptible inbred rat strains. *Arthritis Rheum.,* 26:1442–1451.

183. Wilhelm, S. M., Eisen, A. Z., Teter, M., Clark, S. D., Kronberger, A., and Goldberg, G. (1986): Human fibroblast collagenase: Glycosylation and tissue specific levels of enzyme synthesis. *Proc. Natl. Acad. Sci. USA,* 83:3756–3760.

184. Windt, M. R., and Rossenwasser, L. J. (1984): Human vascular endothelial cells produce interleukin 1. *Lymphokine Res.,* 3:281a.

185. Woolley, D. E. (1984): Mammalian collagenase. In: *Extracellular Matrix Biochemistry,* edited by C. Piez and H. Reddi, p. 119. Elsevier, New York.

186. Wyler, D. J., Wahl, S. M., and Wahl, L. M. (1978): Hepatic fibrosis in schistosomiasis: Egg granulomas secrete fibroblast stimulating factor *in vitro. Science,* 207:438–440.

187. Wyler, D. J., Stadecker, M. J., Dinarello, C. A., and O'Dea, J. F. (1984): Fibroblast stimulation in shistosomiasis. V. Egg granuloma macrophages spontaneously secrete a fibroblast-stimulating factor. *J. Immunol.,* 132:3142–3148.

188. Yocum, D. E., Allen, J. B., Wahl, S. M., Calandra, G. B., and Wilder, R. L. (1986): Inhibition by cyclosporin A of streptococcal cell wall induced arthritis and hepatic granulomas in rats. *Arthritis Rheum.,* 29:262–273.

189. Yoshino, S., Cromartie, W. J., and Schwab, J. H. (1985): Inflammation induced by bacterial cell wall fragments in the rat air pouch. Comparison of rat strains and measurement of arachidonic acid metabolites. *Am. J. Pathol.,* 121:327–336.

190. Zimmerman, T. S., and Muller-Eberhard, H. J. (1971): Initiation of coagulation by complement activation: Generation of platelet associated clot promoting activity. *Blood,* 38:791.

191. Zucali, J. R., Dinarello, J. A., Oblon, D. J., Gross, M. A., Anderson, L., and Weiner, R. S. (1986): Interleukin 1 stimulates fibroblasts to produce granulocyte-macrophage colony stimulating activity and prostaglandin E$_2$. *J. Clin. Invest.,* 77:1857–1863.

Inflammation: Basic Principles and Clinical Correlates.
Edited by J. I. Gallin, I. M. Goldstein, and R. Snyderman.
Raven Press, Ltd., New York © 1988.

CHAPTER 48

Anti-Inflammatory Effects of Neoplasia

George J. Cianciolo

<table>
<tr>
<td>

Defects of Inflammatory Cell Accumulation Associated
  with Human Cancer
Defects of Inflammatory Cell Accumulation in Tumor-
  Bearing Animals
Defects of Inflammatory Cells Associated with Retrovirus
  Infections

</td>
<td>

Mechanisms of Anti-Inflammatory Defects in Neoplasia
  Chemotactic Factor Inactivators • Anti-Inflammatory
  Factors Produced by Neoplasms
Summary
References

</td>
</tr>
</table>

Phagocytic cells are important in host defenses against not only microbial and viral infections but also neoplastic disease. Macrophages have been extensively studied and shown to be capable of infiltrating tumors *in vivo* and destroying tumors both *in vitro* and *in vivo*. The role of host immune surveillance in providing resistance against neoplastic disease has been a subject of some debate (59,60,73–75,97). Nevertheless, numerous studies support the concept that phagocytic cells play an important role in immune surveillance against cancer. This chapter will report on those studies and studies by various investigators that indicate defects in inflammatory cell accumulation and migratory capability in humans and animals with neoplastic disease or retrovirus infections. Recent investigations on the mechanisms involved in such defects of inflammatory cells will be reported and discussed.

Many arguments against a role for immune surveillance in control of neoplastic disease were based on data using immunodeficient or immunosuppressed mice. For instance, Stutman (96) showed that nude mice showed no differences in either latent period or incidence of sarcomas or lung adenocarcinomas after administration of 3-methylcholanthrene at birth. He reported that these athymic mice, which congenitally lacked T-cell lymphocyte function, were also unable to reject allogeneic skin grafts at the same time. A more comprehensive study involving nude mice was that of Rygaard and Poolsen (80), who reported that no spontaneous tumors occurred in over 15,000 mice observed over a 6-year period. The use of

studies such as these to refute a role for immune surveillance in the control of cancer requires that one accept the assumption that T lymphocytes play the critical role in such surveillance, because the nude mouse still retains normal macrophage function. Much information has been accumulated to suggest that macrophages are capable not only of infiltrating tumors but also of destroying them.

In 1970, Evans and Alexander (31) reported that peritoneal macrophages from mice that had previously been immunized with a single injection of irradiated lymphoma cells were capable of killing those lymphoma cells in an *in vitro* cytotoxicity assay. They also showed that macrophages could be activated to become cytotoxic for tumor cells both *in vivo* and *in vitro* by either endotoxin or double-stranded RNA. Along a similar line, Droller and Remington (27) reported that *Toxoplasma*-infected mice were more resistant to *in vivo* tumor growth. Such mice had previously been shown to contain activated macrophages that were capable of *in vitro* inhibition of [^{3}H]thymidine incorporation by tumor cells.

Evidence to support the concept that macrophages play an important role in the control of tumor growth began to accumulate in the early 1970s. Eccles and Alexander (28,29) investigated the macrophage content of a group of chemically induced rat fibrosarcomas and demonstrated that the macrophage content in each of six different rat sarcomas was directly related to the immunogenicity of the sarcoma and inversely correlated with its capacity to metastasize in syngeneic recipients. In 1975, Gauci and

Alexander (36) reported studies designed to measure the numbers of macrophages in 27 human breast tumors and 17 melanomas. In patients who later developed metastatic disease, tumors contained 9% macrophages or less, whereas tumors from patients who did not develop metastases had up to 30% macrophages.

The defensive function that macrophages might exert within tumors was illustrated by studies such as those of Wood and Gillespie (107), in which they depleted macrophages from murine tumor cell suspensions and showed that such depletion increased the potential of transplanted tumor cells to metastasize and decreased the survival times of the recipient mice, as compared with inocula that still contained macrophages. In that same year, Haskill et al. (41) showed that two different rat sarcomas contained a large proportion of host cells that morphologically resembled macrophages and adhered to plastic. They showed that the proportion of host cells was greater in younger (10–12 days) than in older (35 days) tumors. The macrophage-like host cells that they isolated from tumors could inhibit tumor cell growth (colony formation) in vitro, in much the same manner as described for activated macrophages. They were also able to isolate and grow in vitro macrophage precursors from these tumors, but the in vitro growth of these precursors was inhibited by coculture with the tumor cells. This finding suggested that the macrophages and tumors might have mutual growth-inhibiting effects within the tumor microenvironment.

Further evidence that macrophages play an important role in immune defense against tumors came from studies in which administration of agents toxic to macrophages in vitro decreased host resistance to tumors in vivo. McBride et al. (56) reported that the numbers of lung tumor nodules following intravenous injection of tumor cells increased in mice that had previously been injected with gold salts, which are thought to exert their antiinflammatory effect on macrophages. In addition, it was found that the in vitro cytotoxicity toward tumor cells of macrophages from Corynebacterium parvum-treated mice could be significantly decreased if the mice were treated with gold salts (37). Enhanced growth of subcutaneously injected tumors was seen in mice that also received a single intravenous injection of silica or carageenan on the same day (49). The antitumor effects of macrophage-activating agents such as C. parvum and bacille Calmette-Guérin (BCG) can also be abrogated by such agents (50). Additional studies by Thomson and Fowler (102) demonstrated enhancement of tumor growth in mice receiving intraperitoneal injections of carageenan.

In a 1976 report, Russell et al. (78) showed that regressing Moloney sarcomas contained as many as five times the numbers of macrophages per gram of tumor as did progressively growing sarcomas. Whenever mononuclear cells were present, whether in progressively growing or regressively growing tumors, mitotic activity was negligible, suggesting that mononuclear phagocytes might be capable of interfering with in vivo tumor growth. Russell et al. (79) also demonstrated that macrophages isolated from regressing tumors were cytolytic for tumor cells in vitro, whereas those isolated from progressing tumors showed no such activity.

Thus, considerable evidence has been accumulated to support the concept that mononuclear phagocytes are capable of infiltrating tumors and that their presence correlates with decreased progression or metastasis. Furthermore, tumor-associated macrophages are capable of directly killing or inhibiting in vitro tumor growth. Finally, agents that cause decreased macrophage function in vivo also enhance the in vivo growth of transplanted syngeneic tumors.

DEFECTS OF INFLAMMATORY CELL ACCUMULATION ASSOCIATED WITH HUMAN CANCER

If, as described earlier, mononuclear phagocytes are capable of infiltrating tumors and restricting their growth or participating in their destruction, the question arises as to why this fails to occur under many circumstances. One possibility is that mononuclear phagocytes may be unable to migrate to the tumor site in sufficient numbers, or, once there, they may be unable to mount a successful cytolytic or cytostatic attack on the tumor cells. One of the earliest studies demonstrating tumor-associated mononuclear phagocyte dysfunction in its host was that of Berg (8). He examined the histological patterns of breast cancer biopsies and found that 73% of patients who survived 10 years or longer showed an inflammatory infiltrate, whereas only 23% of the patients who survived less than 10 years showed such a reaction. These results suggested that tumors might be capable of suppressing a normal inflammatory response and promoting their own growth. Several years later, Dizon and Southam (26) used a modification of the Rebuck skin-window assay to examine 101 breast cancer patients for their ability to mobilize tissue macrophages. Quantitating the number of macrophages that adhered to a glass coverslip placed over a light skin abrasion, they found that the numbers of accumulated macrophages were significantly depressed in cancer patients, as compared with patients with noncancerous diseases. Eighteen of the 101 cancer patients were classified as having early cancer, with no signs of disseminated disease. Of these 18 patients, 13 had responses similar to those of healthy controls, suggesting that the depressed mononuclear phagocyte responses were related to the severity of disease. Goldsmith et al. (38), using this same modified Rebuck assay, demonstrated that in addition to a decrease in the percentage of mononuclear phagocytes responding to skin abrasion in cancer patients, there was a decrease in the absolute number of monocytes responding. Johnson et al. (47) demonstrated that inflammation due to agents such as croton oil was depressed in cancer patients, as were reactions to the contact sensitizing agent 2,5-dinitrochlorobenzene.

The development by Snyderman et al. (85) of a quantitative assay for *in vitro* measurement of chemotactic responsiveness of human peripheral blood monocytes allowed examination of the nature of defects in inflammatory cell accumulation in cancer patients. Preliminary reports by Hausman et al. (42) and Snyderman et al. (87) indicated that *in vitro* chemotactic responses of blood monocytes from patients with a number of different types of malignancies were defective and that, in many instances, the responses returned to normal after BCG immunotherapy or surgical removal of the tumor. Boetcher and Leonard (11) studied *in vitro* monocyte chemotaxis in 44 cancer patients. Twenty-four of the 44 patients had decreased monocyte chemotactic responsiveness, whereas only 3 of 22 normal individuals and 2 of 24 control (noncancer) patients had defective responses. Abnormal monocyte chemotactic responsiveness was rarely seen in patients with minimal disease, but was detected in all other stages. Data from Boetcher and Leonard's studies showed that the appearance of nodal metastases was delayed in those melanoma patients who had normal monocyte chemotactic responsiveness. Hausman et al. (43) studied monocyte chemotaxis in patients with neoplasms of the urinary tract. They reported that 24 patients with various stages of renal carcinoma exhibited a mean defect of 34% when compared with healthy individuals or patients hospitalized with noncancerous disease. They also studied 12 persons who had transitional cell carcinoma of the bladder and found an average chemotactic defect of 29.8% compared with controls.

In one of the most comprehensive studies of monocyte chemotaxis in patients with neoplastic disease, Snyderman and Pike (89) reported that 38% (32/84) of patients with malignant melanoma, 59% (29/49) of patients with cancer of the breast, and 47% (35/74) of patients with a variety of other neoplasms had depressed *in vitro* monocyte chemotactic responsiveness. Nearly half (46%) of the 208 patients studied had depressed monocyte chemotactic responses. In the same study, Snyderman and Pike found that the polymorphonuclear leukocyte (PMN) chemotactic responses of these patients were normal. Rubin et al. (77) also reported depressed monocyte chemotaxis in patients with malignant melanoma. They suggested that an inverse relationship existed between *in vitro* monocyte chemotaxis and the clinical course of disease in patients in stages II and III. They postulated that such patients might develop lymphocyte-mediated reactivity to residual

tumor and elaborate high concentrations of lymphokines, which then might deactivate the monocytes *in vivo*. The inverse correlation observed by Rubin et al. (77) differed from the findings of Snyderman et al. (92) in a longitudinal study of 56 patients with malignant melanoma who were initially tested and then followed through immunotherapy and, in some cases, surgery. Of the 56 patients, 44% had initially depressed monocyte chemotactic responsiveness, but after two injections of BCG immunotherapy, only 8% had depressed responses. However, enhancement of chemotactic responses in patients undergoing BCG immunotherapy was not necessarily indicative of a good prognosis, because of the 19 patients who showed enhanced monocyte chemotactic responsiveness after BCG administration, 11 had recurrence or progression of the cancer. One of the most noteworthy findings that emerged from this study was that detected abnormalities (either enhanced or depressed) of chemotaxis were associated with a poor prognosis and frequently with extent of malignancy. On the other hand, normal chemotaxis was associated with a more favorable prognosis and usually with absence of clinically detectable disease.

Kay and McVie (48) measured monocyte chemotaxis in 31 patients with bronchial carcinoma and found that 13 patients with metastatic disease had significantly depressed responses, whereas those patients with disease confined to the chest, or with recurrent or operable bronchial carcinoma, had no significant depression of their responses. In 1978, Snyderman et al. (88) studied monocyte chemotactic responsiveness in patients with breast cancer. In 42 patients with benign breast masses and 17 patients with a history of breast cancer, but clinically free of disease after surgery, monocyte chemotaxis was not significantly different from that in 98 normal controls. However, in patients with active breast cancer, monocyte chemotaxis was significantly depressed. Of the 37 patients in this group, 57% had monocyte responses below the 90% confidence limit for the normal controls. Thirty-two patients suspected of having neoplasms were studied before and approximately 25 days after surgical removal of the tumor or mass. The histopathologic diagnosis for each patient was determined at the end of the study. Of 20 patients with malignant disease, 12 had depressed responses. Ten of the 12 patients with depressed responses had normal or above-normal responses after surgery. None of the 12 patients with benign disease had depressed monocyte chemotactic responsiveness prior to surgery.

Kjeldsberg and Pay (51) studied peripheral blood monocyte chemotaxis in 21 patients with cancer of the lung or prostate prior to treatment and found chemotaxis defective in 45% of the patients. They found chemotactic factor inactivators in the sera of 19 of the 21 patients, but no apparent correlation was seen between the level of chemotactic factor inactivators and the level of monocyte chemotactic responsiveness. In 2 of 4 patients, the chemotactic factor inactivators disappeared after surgery, but monocyte chemotaxis remained the same. Norris et al. (70) studied monocyte chemotaxis in 35 patients with acute lymphoblastic leukemia (ALL), 6 with chronic lymphocytic leukemia (CLL), 6 with acute myelogenous leukemia (AML), and 10 with chronic myelogenous leukemia (CML), all before beginning chemotherapy. Function was compared to that in age-matched control groups. Significant inhibition of chemotaxis was seen in patients with ALL and CLL, but there was no significant defect in CML and AML. The deficient monocyte chemotaxis was not due merely to decreased percentages of peripheral blood monocytes.

In a 1982 report, Israel et al. (45) used a modified Rebuck window technique to study macrophage migration in cancer patients in different clinical situations. Their data showed that macrophage migration was virtually abolished in patients with metastatic cancer as compared with healthy controls. In patients with resectable breast and lung tumors, the test performed preoperatively correlated closely with lymph node status as determined by pathological examination after surgery. Patients without lymph node involvement showed significantly stronger responses than did controls, whereas those with lymph node involvement had diminished responses or even no responses.

Nielsen et al. (65) studied monocyte chemotaxis in 14 patients with small cell bronchogenic carcinoma before and during combination chemotherapy. Monocyte chemotactic responsiveness was significantly depressed in all 14 patients before chemotherapy and returned to normal or near-normal values in 11 patients after therapy. They found that chemotactic factor inactivators in patients' plasma decreased following therapy and that improvement was significantly more pronounced in patients in complete remission. Dammacco et al. (24) evaluated chemotactic responsiveness of peripheral blood monocytes in three groups of subjects: 32 patients with multiple myeloma, 27 subjects with benign monoclonal gammapathy, and 64 normal controls. Monocyte chemotaxis was significantly depressed in multiple myeloma patients and in subjects with benign monoclonal gammapathy, although 75% of the multiple myeloma patients had monocyte chemotaxis values below the 95% confidence limits for the normal controls, whereas only 33% of the benign monoclonal gammapathy subjects had values below this limit.

Daunter et al. (25) observed a significant reduction in monocyte chemotactic responsiveness in cervical cancer patients, relative to healthy subjects, but no significant difference between ovarian cancer patients and controls. Mononuclear phagocyte function in patients with head and neck cancer was studied by Balm et al. (3). The numbers of blood monocytes, their ability to mature into macrophages, their nitroblue tetrazolium (NBT) reduction capacity, and their migration toward casein were studied in 29 patients with squamous cell carcinoma of the larynx and 12 patients with squamous cell carcinoma at other sites within the head and neck. A clear impairment of migration toward casein was found in the two groups of carcinoma patients, whereas the numbers of monocytes were only marginally affected, and maturation was found to be enhanced. Balm et al. (4) subsequently reported studies of 40 patients with squamous cell carcinoma of the head and neck. They found that chemotactic responsiveness was decreased in carcinoma patients and that this value appeared to be positively correlated in individual patients with the number of tumor-infiltrating macrophages as well as with the histologic grade of the tumor. Patients with poorly differentiated malignancies showed impaired monocyte chemotaxis and low numbers of tumor-infiltrating macrophages. Alveolar macrophage chemotaxis was studied by Lemare et al. (54) in 48 individuals with primary bronchial carcinoma and 14 patients with pulmonary metastases from various origins. Alveolar macrophage chemotaxis was significantly less in patients with bronchial carcinoma than in healthy volunteers. Chemotaxis was significantly more depressed in cells obtained from the neighborhood of the tumor than in cells from the opposite lung. In contrast, the presence of lung metastases did not affect alveolar macrophage chemotaxis.

Although no defect had been observed in monocyte chemotaxis in CML patients (70), Anklesara et al. (2) reported that chemotaxis of granulocytes from CML patients was defective. Whereas 84% of normal granulocytes were motile, only 30% of granulocytes from untreated patients, 34% of granulocytes from relapse patients, and 36% from patients in acute blast crisis were found to be motile. Nielsen et al. (66) studied the chemotactic responsiveness of blood monocytes in 16 patients with nonseminomatous testicular carcinoma before, during, and after chemotherapy. Their study showed normal monocyte chemotaxis in patients with testicular carcinoma, which is in contrast to the responses observed in the other solid tumors studied.

In a 1986 study, Tan et al. (100) used the monocyte polarization assay developed by Cianciolo and Snyderman (21) to test monocyte chemotactic responsiveness in 24 patients with head and neck cancer and reported that the results correlated well with those obtained using the traditional Boyden chamber assay (85). All patients tested had depressed responses as determined by the polarization assay. Nine of the patients were reexamined 2 to 6 weeks after surgery, and 7 of the 9 patients reexamined showed improvement after surgery, with the responses of 4 patients returning to within normal limits, further supporting the concept that depressed monocyte chemotactic responses were tumor-mediated.

In summary, defective *in vivo* accumulation of macrophages to an inflammatory event such as skin abrasion has been demonstrated for several types of neoplastic disease. Furthermore, defective *in vitro* monocyte chemotactic responsiveness has been demonstrated in patients with a large variety of tumors or leukemias. The variety of neoplasias in which defects in monocyte/macrophage migration have been observed are listed in Table 1. In many of the patients studied, defective *in vitro* monocyte chemotaxis improved during and after therapy or surgical intervention, suggesting that the tumor might mediate the defect by release of soluble factors.

DEFECTS OF INFLAMMATORY CELL ACCUMULATION IN TUMOR-BEARING ANIMALS

Although numerous investigators have presented extensive evidence documenting a defect in inflammatory cell accumulation in patients with cancer, the development of animal models has been an invaluable aid in understanding the potential mechanisms involved. One of the earliest demonstrations of depressed inflammatory responses in tumor-bearing animals was by Mahoney and Leighton (55), describing studies in which they implanted lengths of cotton thread in several transplantable mouse and rat tumors or in normal tissues such as liver, spleen, kidney, and subcutaneous connective tissue. After 1 week, tissue samples containing the implanted thread were removed and examined histologically. All normal tissues

TABLE 1. *Defects of mononuclear phagocyte function in human neoplasia*

Type of cancer	Defect	References
ALL	*In vitro* chemotaxis	69
Bladder	*In vitro* chemotaxis	43
Breast	*In vivo* inflammation	8,26,38,44
	In vitro chemotaxis	87,88
Bronchial	*In vitro* chemotaxis	47,53,64
Cervical	*In vitro* chemotaxis	25
CLL	*In vitro* chemotaxis	69
Head and neck	*In vitro* chemotaxis	3,4
	In vitro polarization	99
Larynx	*In vitro* chemotaxis	3
Lung	*In vivo* inflammation	44
	In vitro chemotaxis	50
Melanoma	*In vitro* chemotaxis	11,76,88,91
Myeloma	*in vitro* chemotaxis	24
Prostate	*In vitro* chemotaxis	50
Renal	*In vitro* chemotaxis	43

showed similar and very strong inflammatory responses, whereas the neoplastic tissues displayed only minimal inflammatory responses. One mouse tumor, studied for up to 23 days, had minimal inflammation at all times studied. The inflammatory response to implanted thread was normal in a regenerating liver, ruling out the possibility that the depressed inflammation was simply characteristic of the fact that the tumor site contained large numbers of rapidly dividing cells.

Bernstein et al. (9) reported that guinea pigs bearing large intramuscular tumors had impaired delayed cutaneous hypersensitivity to specific antigens and decreased cutaneous inflammatory reactivity to nonspecific agents. Furthermore, induced peritoneal exudates from tumor-bearing animals contained fewer cells than those from tumor-free animals, suggesting that the defect might be representative of a generalized inability to accumulate cells to inflammatory foci. Eccles and Alexander (29) reported that as tumors grew in size, there was a sharp decrease in the ability of tumor-bearing rats to produce inflammatory exudates in response to intraperitoneal oyster glycogen or cutaneous delayed hypersensitivity responses to PPD or sheep red blood cells. Suppression of the delayed hypersensitivity response was reversed by local injection of normal peritoneal macrophages, with the eliciting antigen suggesting that the defect was macrophage-related. In some instances, accumulation of macrophages in the peritoneal cavity after glycogen injection was totally inhibited. Fauve et al. (33) found that teratocarcinoma cells impaired local inflammation when injected in mice and that the tumor cells were capable of "repulsing" macrophages *in vitro*, suggesting that such tumor cells might possess a mechanism for preventing macrophages from accumulating in their vicinity.

In 1976, Snyderman et al. (91) developed an assay that allowed quantitative measurements of the effects of neoplasms and their products on *in vivo* accumulation of macrophages to inflammatory stimuli in inbred mice. This assay is based on the observation that intraperitoneal injection of purified phytohemagglutinin (PHA), concanavalin A (con-A), or protease peptone results in an inflammatory exudate that by 48 hr after injection consists largely of macrophages. The macrophages in the peritoneal cavity are quantitated by peritoneal lavage, followed by cell counts and differentials, allowing the effects of implanted tumors on the accumulation of macrophages to an inflammatory stimulus to be monitored. Snyderman et al. (91) showed that subcutaneous implantation of 2.5×10^6 sarcoma cells into the thigh resulted in a significant depression, 7 days later, of macrophage accumulation in response to intraperitoneal PHA, whereas injection of normal spleen cells had no effect. In a subsequent report, Snyderman and Pike (90) showed that inflammatory accumulation of macrophages could be inhibited not only by intact cells of four different tumor lines but also by cell-free extracts of the tumors and dialysates of such extracts.

Stevenson and Meltzer (95) demonstrated that the *in vitro* chemotactic responses of peritoneal macrophages from mice bearing transplantable syngeneic 3-methylcholanthrene-induced tumors in their footpads were depressed to about 50% of normal levels. This chemotactic defect was to both lymphocyte and complement-derived chemotactic stimuli and was evident even before the appearance of palpable tumors and persisted until the death of the animal 6 to 8 weeks later.

A number of additional investigators reported inhibition of inflammatory responses in normal mice by injections of tumor cells or tumor cell products. Lau et al. (53) inhibited the *in vivo* inflammatory reaction to 10^8 subcutaneously injected *Candida albicans* by coinjection with 5×10^4 L1210 leukemia cells. Meltzer and Stevenson (57) reported that the numbers of peritoneal exudate cells elicited in tumor-bearing mice 8 to 14 days after intraperitoneal infection with BCG were depressed. This inflammatory defect was detected 1 week after tumor implantation and persisted for more than 5 weeks. However, in contrast to resident peritoneal macrophages, peritoneal exudate macrophages induced by BCG in tumor-bearing mice were as responsive to chemotactic stimuli as BCG-activated macrophages from control mice. No differences in tumoricidal responses of BCG-activated macrophages obtained from tumor-bearing mice and control mice were noted.

Normann and Sorkin (69) showed a generalized impairment of monocyte migratory function in rats bearing dimethylbenzanthracene-induced tumors. The accumulation of peritoneal macrophages to an inflammatory stimulus was impaired, and the chemotactic responses of both resident and elicited peritoneal macrophages were depressed. Like Snyderman and co-workers, they found PMN function to be unaffected.

In contrast to earlier studies in rodents that used transplanted syngeneic tumors, Normann et al. (68) reported that SJL/J mice that developed spontaneous histiocytic lymphomas accumulated significantly fewer macrophages than did age-matched animals without tumors. Macrophage accumulation was depressed whether measured as cells adhering to subcutaneously implanted nitrocellulose filters or as peritoneal exudates in response to PHA. They also found no corresponding defect in neutrophil function. This was the first demonstration in an animal model system of an inflammatory defect associated with a spontaneously arising tumor. Using a different strain of mice, C3H/HEN, Cianciolo et al. (15) also found depressed accumulation of peritoneal macrophages in response to PHA in mice bearing spontaneous mammary adenocarcinomas. Cianciolo et al. (15) also showed that the de-

pressed inflammatory activity could be transferred to normal mice by submicroliter quantities of plasma or urine from the tumor-bearing mice, supporting the concept that a circulating mediator is involved in the inhibition of macrophage accumulation.

A different animal model system, but one that nevertheless depended on macrophage accumulation, was used by Nelson and Nelson (62). They reported that the mixing of fibrosarcoma cells with sheep red blood cells (SRBC) prior to injection into SRBC-sensitized mice resulted in inhibition of the subsequent delayed hypersensitivity reaction and that this inhibition was directly proportional to the number of tumor cells present in the injection mixture. They also showed that delayed hypersensitivity reactions could be inhibited equally well by supernatants of cultured tumor cells, whereas supernatants of normal mouse fibroblasts or macrophages were inactive. Activity was found in the supernatants of all human and rat tumor cell lines tested, indicating a broad spectrum of species reactivity. Nelson and Nelson found that the inhibitory activity present in the tumor cell culture supernatants was less potent for inhibiting *in vitro* macrophage migration than for inhibiting the *in vivo* delayed hypersensitivity responses, a result very similar to that observed by Snyderman and Pike (89,90), who found that inhibition of *in vitro* macrophage chemotaxis required extracts prepared from a substantially larger number of cells than required for inhibition of *in vivo* macrophage accumulation.

Thus, animal model systems employing rodents reproduce the *in vivo* inhibition of macrophage accumulation or delayed hypersensitivity reactions in tumor-bearing hosts that has been observed in humans with cancer. Furthermore, *in vitro* macrophage migration is inhibited in cells from animals bearing tumors, a result also observed in cancer patients. The fact that such results are observed in animals bearing spontaneous carcinomas lends support to their value in studying the underlying mechanisms of depressed inflammatory responses in neoplastic disease.

DEFECTS OF INFLAMMATORY CELLS ASSOCIATED WITH RETROVIRUS INFECTIONS

Until recently, there had been no direct connection of retroviruses to human neoplasia. However, the discovery of the human T-lymphotrophic viruses, such as HTLV-I (71), HTLV-II, and HIV (HTLV-III) (5,34), resulted in the observation that such retroviruses might be directly involved in human neoplasias, such as adult T-cell leukemia (ATL) (71), or that they might be indirectly involved through the induction of an immunosuppressed condition, such as frequently occurs in patients infected with HTLV-I or those infected with HTLV-III/LAV/HIV who suffer from the acquired immunodeficiency syndrome (AIDS) (30,32).

Previous studies in mice had suggested that retrovirus infection could result in impaired macrophage function. Bendinelli et al. (6) had shown that proteose-peptone-elicited peritoneal macrophages could restore the depressed plaque-forming-cell responsiveness of splenocytes from mice infected with Rowson-Parr retrovirus. Furthermore, Specter et al. (94) used isolated B lymphocytes, thymus-derived T lymphocytes, and sheep-erythrocyte-educated T cells plus whole spleen cell populations (devoid of macrophages) and found that none of these populations restored the antibody response of the Rowson-Parr-virus-infected spleen cells. These observations further support the possibility that macrophages are the cell type responsible for restoration of plaque-forming-cell responses.

Cianciolo et al. (19) reported that injection of subnanogram quantities of low-molecular-weight extracts prepared from certain oncogenic murine retroviruses could inhibit *in vivo* macrophage accumulation in normal mice. Why only certain retroviruses possessed this activity was not determined, but it is interesting that the active viruses all belonged to the FMR (Friend, Moloney, Rauscher) subgroup of murine leukemia viruses and that the Rowson-Parr virus used by Bendinelli et al. (6) and Specter et al. (94) is a component of the Friend complex.

Because human retroviruses have only recently been identified, there have been few studies of inflammatory cell function in patients infected exogenously with these viruses. However, Smith et al. (84) investigated *in vitro* monocyte chemotaxis in patients with AIDS. Using three different chemotactic stimuli, *N*-formyl-methionyl-leucyl-phenylalanine (FMLP), lymphocyte-derived chemotactic factor, and C5a-Des-Arg, they found that monocytes from AIDS patients with Kaposi's sarcoma and/or opportunistic infection exhibited a marked reduction in chemotaxis to all stimuli, as compared with those from healthy control subjects. The reduced chemotactic responses were observed over a wide range of concentrations for each stimulus. Monocytes from AIDS patients with opportunistic infections exhibited greater inhibition of monocyte chemotactic responsiveness than did monocytes from AIDS patients who had only Kaposi's sarcoma. Monocytes from three homosexuals who had lymphadenopathy and abnormal immunological profiles had monocyte chemotactic responses that were intermediate between those of the AIDS patients and those of healthy heterosexual controls. Monocytes from healthy homosexuals had normal chemotactic responsiveness to the same stimuli.

Further support for depressed mononuclear phagocyte function in AIDS patients comes from studies reported by Lane et al. (52). They found that although the proliferative responses of the unseparated total mononuclear cell populations from AIDS patients were depressed, when the lymphocyte subpopulations were isolated and stimulated separately they appeared to have normal responses. A potential mechanism for the depressed proliferative responses in AIDS, other than the obvious decrease in T4+ lymphocytes, could be a defect in antigen-presenting function by the monocytes of HIV-infected individuals.

The link between such viruses and cancer is only now beginning to be explored, but, as will be described later, there is already substantial evidence to suggest that anti-inflammatory proteins associated with neoplasia may be related to certain retrovirus gene products.

MECHANISMS OF ANTI-INFLAMMATORY DEFECTS IN NEOPLASIA

There is no evidence as yet to suggest that neoplasia causes a defect in the production of inflammatory cells. Much of the evidence to date has suggested modulation of inflammatory cell function by humoral factors, and such factors will be the focus of the following discussion. However, one system in which an intrinsic cell defect appears to play a role involves the migratory capacity of lymphocytes in patients with neoplasia. In studies reported in 1984, Hesse et al. (44) showed that patients with established malignancy showed depressed T-lymphocyte migration and that their lymphocytes failed to respond to both lymphocyte chemotactic factor and chemokinetic factors (casein). These authors attributed the depressed migration of patients' T cells to a direct inhibitory action of an E-rosetting suppressor cell. More recently, Cole et al. (23) reported that 15 of 22 patients with established malignancy produced lymphocyte chemotactic factor at levels that were more than two standard deviations below the mean for control cells. A significant correlation was observed between the response of T cells to a migration stimulus and the production of lymphocyte chemotactic factor by these same patients. The addition of patient mononuclear cells or T cells to normal mononuclear cells resulted in inhibition of lymphocyte chemotactic factor production by the normal cells. Separation of patient T cells showed that the inhibitory activity was associated with the Leu-2 T-cell subset.

Chemotactic Factor Inactivators

Circulating factors that suppress accumulation of inflammatory cells could act by affecting the responding cell or the inflammatory agent. This latter class of circulating factors has been termed chemotactic factor inactivators (CFIs), and these have been found in association with a variety of different neoplasms, as well as in normal serum. A CFI in normal human serum was first described by Berenberg and Ward (7) in 1973. In the following year, they reported (106) that elevated levels of CFIs could be found in the sera of 9 patients with Hodgkin's disease and that the inactivators from Hodgkin's sera were qualitatively similar to those found in normal sera and were capable of inactivating both C5 and bacterially derived chemotactic factors, but not those derived from the C3 component of complement. Till and Ward (103) determined that human CFIs consist of two inactivators: a β-globulin with a sedimentation velocity of approximately 7S and an α-globulin with a sedimentation velocity of approximately 4S. In addition to being found in human serum, CFIs have also been found in various cell extracts and ascites fluids of rats (12). Extracts prepared from either Walker sarcoma cells or Novikoff hepatoma cells inactivated bacterial chemotactic factor and chemotactic activity associated with either C3 or C5 fragments or lymphocyte-derived chemotactic factor. CFI activity was also identified in rat neutrophils, in alveolar macrophages, and in extracts of liver, spleen, and kidney from normal rats, suggesting that proteases could be responsible. Blumenfeld and Territo (10) reported a CFI found in the serum of a patient with ALL. The factor was characterized as heat-labile and blocked the activity of complement-dependent chemotactic factors, as well as the chemotactic activity produced by *Escherichia coli*. Supernatants from cultured lymphoblasts of the patient were also found to have CFI activity similar in nature to that found in the patient's serum.

Cohen et al. (22) reported that the ascites fluid or peritoneal washings from DBA/2 mice bearing the P-815 mastocytoma contained CFIs that inactivated not only bacterial chemotactic factor but also the chemotactic activity generated from C3 or C5 components of complement. They found that the amount of CFI was proportional to the number of tumor cells in the exudate and that activity could also be found in tumor cell homogenates as well as in the supernatants of tumor cells grown in culture. They reported that the CFI activity was heat-labile, but unaffected by protease inhibitors, and that its molecular mass was greater than 50,000 daltons. Furthermore, Cohen et al. (22) also reported that in C57BL/6 mice, which reject the mastocytoma, the level of CFIs decreased in proportion to the decreasing numbers of tumor cells.

Although a number of investigators have identified tumor-associated CFIs, their presence cannot explain why in many patients or tumor-bearing animals monocyte/macrophage migratory function has been found to be inhibited, whereas PMN migration has been unaffected. The presence of monocyte-directed anti-inflammatory factors might offer one explanation and are discussed in the following sections. Moreover, no definitive identification of such substances has been forthcoming.

Anti-Inflammatory Factors Produced by Neoplasms

Factors that Inhibit Production of Reactive Oxygen Intermediates

Among products secreted by macrophages that have potential for killing tumor cells are the reactive oxygen intermediates, which include superoxide anion (O_2^-) and hydrogen peroxide (H_2O_2). The ability of supernatants from cultured tumor cells to inhibit the production of H_2O_2 by macrophages was first reported by Nelson et al. (61), although the inhibition observed was somewhat variable, perhaps because of the relatively short incubation times used. In the same year, Szuro-Sudol and Nathan (99) reported that each of 11 murine tumors tested produced a factor that markedly suppressed the ability of caseinate-elicited peritoneal macrophages to release H_2O_2 or O_2^- in response to phorbol myristate acetate (PMA) or zymosan. They also found that four of seven normal cell types produced a similar inhibitory activity, although the activity associated with normal cells was 3.5 to 7 times lower in titer than that found in tumor-cell-conditioned medium. The inhibitory effects of tumor-cell-conditioned medium on H_2O_2 release were reversible, and the H_2O_2-releasing capacity of cells treated with tumor-cell-conditioned medium returned to normal by 6 days after its removal. Furthermore, tumor-cell-conditioned medium was found to inhibit the augmentation of H_2O_2 release in macrophages stimulated with lymphokine-rich supernatants of con-A-stimulated lymphocyte cultures. Suppression of the release of H_2O_2 or O_2^- by tumor-cell-conditioned medium appeared to be relatively specific, because it increased macrophage spreading and adherence to glass, whereas it had little effect on rates of phagocytosis, protein synthesis, or secretion of lysozyme, plasminogen activator, arachidonic acid, or its metabolites.

Szuro-Sudol et al. (98) found that after 24 hr of culture of mouse peritoneal macrophages with tumor-cell-conditioned medium, both *in vivo* and *in vitro* activated macrophages could no longer kill toxoplasma or inhibit their replication. Furthermore, they found that *in vivo* administration of tumor-cell-conditioned medium resulted in similar impairment. The ability of resident and activated macrophages to kill *Leishmania donovani* was also markedly suppressed by *in vitro* incubation with tumor-cell-conditioned medium, but exogenous H_2O_2 restored killing activity, suggesting that tumor-cell-conditioned medium suppressed both macrophage oxidative metabolism and antiparasitic activities.

Tsunawaki and Nathan (104) examined the mechanism of suppression by the macrophage deactivation factor present in tumor-cell-conditioned medium. They showed that inhibition of H_2O_2 release could not be overcome by increasing the concentration of phorbol esters used to trigger the respiratory burst and that deactivated macrophages consumed H_2O_2 at the same rate as normally activated cells. Furthermore, cells treated with macrophage deactivation factor transported glucose with the same kinetics and maintained similar intracellular concentrations of NADPH and NADP as untreated cells. Incubation of activated macrophages in macrophage deactivation factor resulted in an increase in the K_m of its oxidase for NADPH from 0.06 mM to 0.67 mM, and V_{max} fell approximately 1.7-fold. The kinetic changes, together with the measured intracellular concentration of NADPH, could account quantitatively for the suppression of H_2O_2 release by deactivated macrophages.

Factors that Inhibit Migratory Function

One of the first reports to show direct inhibition of migratory function by tumor-derived products was that of Fauve et al. (33). They showed that teratocarcinoma cells produced an antiinflammatory factor of molecular mass between 1,000 and 10,000 daltons. Snyderman and Pike (90) demonstrated *in vivo* inhibition of peritoneal macrophage accumulation to inflammatory agents such as PHA, con-A, and proteose-peptone by prior subcutaneous injection of tumor cells or cell-free extracts of sonicated tumor cells. They also showed that the inhibitory activity in sonicated tumor cell supernatants was dialyzable, indicating a molecular mass of approximately 15,000 daltons or less.

Nelson and Nelson (62,63) found that tumors contained both low-molecular-mass (<10,000 daltons) and high-molecular-mass (>10,000 daltons) inhibitors of inflammation and delayed-type hypersensitivity (DTH) responses. They demonstrated that the two fractions exhibited different kinetics of activity: The high fraction inhibited later (35–70 hr) delayed hypersensitivity responses, and the low fraction inhibited early (18–35 hr) delayed hypersensitivity responses. Furthermore, they demonstrated that older mice were more sensitive to the inhibitory effects of the tumor-related antiinflammatory factors.

Normann and Cornelius (67) also identified two different-size anti-inflammatory factors produced by murine neoplasms. P-815 mastocytoma cells from DBA/2 mice and a 3-methylcholanthrene-induced fibrosarcoma from C57BL/6 mice produced in culture at least two soluble factors that inhibited macrophage accumulation *in vivo* when injected subcutaneously into syngeneic recipients. One factor was a low-molecular-mass (<1,000 daltons) peptide, as judged by ultrafiltration, and the second factor had a molecular mass between 30,000 and 100,000 daltons. These anti-inflammatory factors depressed both granulocyte and macrophage responses.

Cianciolo et al. (19) reported that oncogenic murine retroviruses of the Friend-Moloney-Rauscher subgroup were capable of inhibiting macrophage accumulation in mice and that the purified transmembrane envelope protein of these viruses, p15E, could also inhibit macrophage accumulation. The low-molecular-weight inhibitory factors from murine tumor cells (89,90) and the retrovirus extracts (19) shared many physicochemical properties. Cianciolo and colleagues therefore examined a series of murine tumor cell lines to determine if retroviral p15E was routinely expressed by such cells, perhaps from endogenous loci. Using metabolic labeling with ^{35}S-methionine and immunoprecipitation with monoclonal anti-p15E antibodies, they showed that all six murine tumor cell lines examined expressed p15E (18). Although primary tumors could not be examined using these techniques, they developed a competition enzyme-linked immunoassay (ELISA) for p15E using a high-titer polyclonal rabbit antiserum. Using this assay, they demonstrated that p15E-related proteins were also present in extracts prepared from spontaneous murine mammary adenocarcinomas or primary fibrosarcomas induced with 3-methylcholanthrene (MCA). They also found p15E in the ascites fluid of mice injected intraperitoneally with several different murine tumor cell lines. Most significant was the demonstration that the anti-inflammatory activity in extracts prepared from MCA-induced primary tumors could be absorbed by anti-p15E monoclonal antibodies.

Further evidence that p15E-related proteins play a significant role in the antiinflammatory effects of murine neoplasms comes from studies by Nelson et al. (64). They demonstrated that murine tumor cell culture supernatants contained two factors (one of 1,000–10,000 daltons and one >10,000 daltons) that inhibited the early and late phases of DTH reactions, respectively. Inhibition of the late phase of DTH reactions by murine tumor cell supernatants was prevented by prior passive immunization of the recipient mice with monoclonal anti-p15E antibodies. Immunization with control antibodies of the same isotypes was ineffective in preventing inhibition of DTH reactions. In addition, they reported that an extract prepared from bovine ocular squamous cell carcinoma inhibited murine DTH reactions, and this inhibition could also be blocked by passive immunization with anti-p15E antibodies. Their findings supported the idea that p15E-related proteins might play an important role in the anti-inflammatory effects of not only murine tumors but also those originating in other species.

Warabi et al. (105) described the partial characterization of a low-molecular-weight inhibitor of chemotaxis from T-241 murine fibrosarcoma cells. This factor (<1,000 daltons) had antichemotactic activity for both macrophages and PMNs, properties that suggested that it was different from that described by Snyderman and Pike (89,90) or Cianciolo et al. (18,19). However, it is possible that it may be related to the low-molecular-weight factor that Nelson et al. (62–64) described as being responsible for inhibition of the early phase of DTH reactions. Studies by Cheung et al. (13) also identified a factor of approximately 500 daltons derived from murine lung carcinoma that was capable of inhibiting macrophage migration, and this factor had characteristics of a prostaglandin. Thus non-p15E-related anti-inflammatory factors are associated with neoplasms.

The monocyte polarization assay measures the morphological shape change of monocytes in suspension to chemotactic stimuli (21), and its development allowed accurate quantification of monocyte responses to chemoattractants in the presence of factors that could nonspecifically affect cellular adherence. Using this assay, Cianciolo et al. (16) demonstrated that fluids (pleural effusions, ascites) from patients with neoplastic diseases blocked the polarization responses of monocytes to a variety of chemotactic stimuli such as FMLP, C5a, and lymphocyte-derived chemotactic factor. No activity was found in the fluids from patients with noncancerous diseases. The inhibitory activity was specific for monocytes in that neutrophil polarization responses were unaffected. The inhibitory activity was heat-stable (56°C, 30 min) and trypsin-sensitive, suggesting that it was protein in nature. Fractionation of inhibitory fluids by high-performance liquid chromatography (HPLC) revealed three peaks of activity (>200,000, ca. 46,000, and ca. 21,000 daltons). Perhaps the most surprising observation was that the inhibitory activity in human malignant fluids could be absorbed by any of three different monoclonal antibodies to murine retroviral p15E. Furthermore, any of the three peaks of inhibitory activity obtained by HPLC could be absorbed by anti-p15E monoclonal antibodies. In addition, Cianciolo et al. (16) demonstrated that low-molecular-mass (<25,000 daltons) ultrafiltrates of Rauscher leukemia virus (RLV) were capable of inhibiting the polarization responses of human peripheral blood monocytes and that the inhibitory activity present in the RLV ultrafiltrates could also be absorbed by anti-p15E antibodies.

In a subsequent study, Cianciolo et al. (20) reported that cells from a variety of human tumor lines, but not normal peripheral blood cells, contained p15E-related antigens, as determined by fluorescence-activated cell sorting (FACS) of fixed cells stained with anti-p15E monoclonal antibodies and a fluorescence-labeled second antibody. Although normal human peripheral blood cells did not contain detectable levels of a p15E-related antigen, once such cells were mitogen-transformed with various lectins such as PHA, con-A, or pokeweed mitogen (PWM), the cells became reactive with anti-p15E. These findings led Snyderman and Cianciolo (86) to propose a two-stage model of tumorigenesis (Fig. 1) in which the first stage involves neoplastic transformation of a normal cell. They suggested that such transformation might involve activation of genes such as oncogenes, but that acquisition of a transformed phenotype would not in itself be sufficient for the transformed cell to grow as a tumor in a normal, immune-competent host. They suggested that the activation of a second gene or set of genes coding for an immunosuppressive or antiinflammatory protein(s) such as p15E would allow the transformed cell to escape immune surveillance and grow as a tumor. This model predicted that the human genome would contain genes coding for anti-inflammatory proteins that might normally be repressed or expressed at very low levels, but that could be activated under various conditions, including, but not restricted to, neoplastic transformation. Such endogenous genes might be, but would not have to be, related to p15E.

A 1986 study by Ji-Ming et al. (46) was designed to explore the relationship between chemotactic and antichemotactic products released by tumor cells. Culture supernatants of the human 8387 sarcoma and SW626 ovarian carcinoma cell lines were depleted of p15E-related antigens using immobilized anti-p15E monoclonal anti-

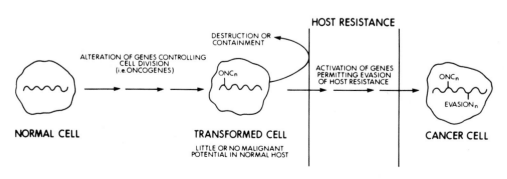

FIG. 1. A two-stage model for development of clinically apparent neoplasms. One stage relates to neoplastic transformation in regard to cell replication. To overcome natural host resistance, transformed cells must acquire additional alterations, such as the means to resist immune surveillance. These might include release of factors such as chemotactic factor inactivators, macrophage deactivation factors, or p15E-related inhibitors of monocyte/macrophage accumulation or migration. (From ref. 86.)

bodies. This treatment produced a consistent and significant increase in the polarizing and chemotactic activities of the tumor cell supernatants. Material that was eluted from the Sepharose-bound anti-p15E antibodies did not contain any polarizing or chemotactic activity, but was capable of suppressing the responses of normal monocytes to various chemoattractants. Thus, these studies demonstrated the coexistence in culture supernatants of two human tumor cell lines of factors with opposite influences on monocyte chemotaxis. Their data suggested that migration of monocytes into neoplastic tissue might be regulated by a balance between chemotactic factors and anti-inflammatory, p15E-related proteins produced by tumor cells.

Recently, Tan et al. (101) reported demonstration of anti-inflammatory p15E-related proteins in primary human neoplastic tissue. They isolated low-molecular-weight factors from 14 different head and neck carcinomas and tested them for their effects on chemotactic responsiveness, as measured by polarization of healthy donor monocytes. The factors inhibited polarization by 62 to 94%, whereas extracts derived from healthy mucosa inhibited polarization by only 12 to 29%. The inhibitory activity contained within the extracts of neoplastic tissues was specifically absorbed by either monoclonal or polyclonal antibodies to retroviral envelope protein p15E, suggesting that the previously described defects of monocyte chemotactic responsiveness observed in patients with head and neck cancers might be results of the release of p15E-related proteins from growing neoplasms.

Siegbahn et al. (81–83) have published a series of reports on a cell-directed inhibitory activity for PMN chemokinetic migration found in the sera of patients with CLL. This activity was heat-labile (56°C, 30 min) and could be detected in the supernatants of cultured tumor cells, but not in the supernatants of lymphoblastoid cell lines established from CLL patients, suggesting that the primary CLL cell was the origin of the activity. Further characterization of the chemokinetic inhibitory factor demonstrated it to be a glycoprotein of approximately 30,000 daltons. It was found in the sera of 64 of 89 CLL patients examined and gave significant inhibition of chemokinesis at a concentration of 0.02%. Furthermore, Siegbahn and associates reported that 31 of 89 patients had an increased propensity for infections and that more patients with chemokinetic inhibitory factor in their sera had infections than did a control group with normal susceptibility to infections. They concluded that chemokinetic inhibitory factor probably contributed to the increased susceptibility to infections seen in CLL patients.

Synthetic Peptides Based on P15E

Although recent evidence suggests a role for p15E-related proteins in the inflammatory dysfunction associated with neoplasia, little is known about how such proteins work. Cianciolo et al. (17) made the observation that within retroviral p15E there exists a 26-amino-acid region that has been extremely well conserved not only among the murine type C retroviruses (14,17) but also among feline, bovine, and avian type C viruses and among the simian type D retroviruses (72,93) (Fig. 2). A synthetic peptide (CKS-17) corresponding to the first 16 amino acids of this conserved region of p15E mimics many of the *in vitro* immunosuppressive activities of purified p15E, including inhibition of lymphocyte proliferation, monocyte respiratory-burst activity, natural killer (NK) cell activity, and inhibition of immunoglobulin synthesis by B cells (14,39,40,58). CKS-17, however, was incapable of inhibiting monocyte migration, and it was suggested that

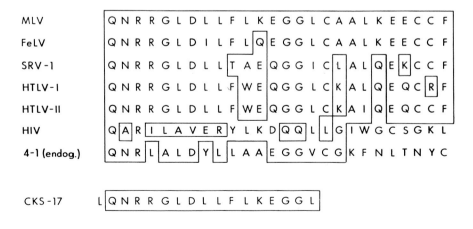

FIG. 2. Comparison of amino acid sequences from highly conserved regions of retrovirus transmembrane envelope proteins. Viruses represented are murine leukemia viruses (MLV), feline leukemia virus (FeLV), a simian acquired immune-deficiency syndrome virus (SRV-1), human T-lymphotropic viruses (HTLV-I and HTLV-II), human immune-deficiency virus (HIV), and an endogenous human retrovirus isolate (4-1). Also shown is the sequence for the immunosuppressive synthetic peptide CKS-17. Amino acids that are identical or that represent favored substitutions are contained within the large boxed area. Favored substitutions shown are G → A (4-1), L → I (FeLV, SRV-1, HTLV-II), F → Y (HIV), E → Q (SRV-1, HTLV-I, HTLV-II), E → D (HIV), L → V (4-1), A → G (HIV, 4-1).

other regions of p15E were involved in its antimigratory activity or that a longer peptide encompassing the whole conserved region might be required.

Cianciolo et al. (14) reported that this same conserved region occurs in the envelope proteins of the human retroviruses HTLV-I and -II and, to a lesser extent, HTLV-III/LAV (human immunodeficiency virus, HIV) (Fig. 2). More recently, Repaske et al. (76) identified an endogenous human retrovirus sequence (4-1) isolated from genomic DNA. The envelope region of this human endogenous virus also contains a region homologous to the highly conserved, immunosuppressive region of p15E (Fig. 2). Furthermore, Repaske and colleagues reported that the envelope sequence of this replication-defective endogenous human virus is expressed in human malignant tissues and placenta, but not in normal tissues. In addition, Gattoni-Celli et al. (35) have documented the expression of this envelope gene, as detected by Northern blot analysis, in primary human colon carcinomas and colon carcinoma cell lines. Whether or not this endogenous human retrovirus envelope protein is the p15E-related protein associated with anti-inflammatory activity in human neoplasia is a subject of extensive investigation.

SUMMARY

Defects in inflammatory cell accumulation *in vivo* and monocyte chemotactic responsiveness *in vitro* have been well documented in humans with cancer and in tumor-bearing animals. Furthermore, there appears to be an inverse correlation between the number of tumor-associated macrophages or the cytolytic activity of such macrophages and the progression of neoplastic disease. The preponderance of evidence has suggested that defects in monocyte function associated with neoplasia are mediated by soluble mediators. Such mediators include inhibitors of respiratory-burst function, such as macrophage deactivation factor, and inhibitors of chemotactic function, such as chemotactic factor inhibitors or monocyte/macrophage chemotaxis inhibitors. At least portions of the anti-inflammatory proteins associated with human and animal neoplasms appear to be antigenically related to the anti-inflammatory, immunosuppressive retroviral envelope protein p15E. Whether or not anti-inflammatory proteins produced by human neoplasms are encoded by endogenous retrovirus envelope loci has not yet been determined, although such loci have been shown to be activated in regard to mRNA expression in malignant tissues.

REFERENCES

1. Alexander, P., and Evans, R. (1972): Endotoxins and double-stranded RNA render macrophages cytotoxic. *Nature (New Biol.)*, 232:76–78.
2. Anklesara, P. N., Advani, S. H., and Bhisey, A. N. (1985): Defective chemotaxis and adherence in granulocytes from chronic myeloid leukemia (CML) patients. *Leuk. Res.*, 9:64–68.
3. Balm, T. A. J. M., Drexhage, H. A., von Blomberg, M. E., and Snow, G. B. (1982): Mononuclear phagocyte function in head and neck cancer: NTB-dye reduction maturation and migration of peripheral blood monocytes. *Laryngoscope*, 92:810–814.
4. Balm, T. A. J. M., Drexhage, H. A., von Blomberg, M., Weltevreden, E. T., Veldhuizen, R. W., Mullink, R., and Snow, G. B. (1984): Mononuclear phagocyte function in head and neck cancer: Chemotactic responsiveness of blood monocytes in correlation between histologic grade of the tumor and infiltration of these cells into the tumor area. *Cancer*, 54:1010–1015.
5. Barre-Sinoussi, F., Cherman, J. C., Rey, F., Nugeyre, M. T., et al. (1983): Isolation of a T-lymphotrophic retrovirus from a patient at risk for acquired immune deficiency syndrome (AIDS). *Science*, 220:868.
6. Bendinelli, M., Kaplan, G., and Friedman, H. (1975): Reversal of leukemia virus-induced immunosuppression in vitro by peritoneal macrophages. *J. Natl. Cancer Inst.*, 55:1425.
7. Berenberg, J. L., and Ward, P. A. (1973): Chemotactic factor inactivator in normal human serum. *J. Clin. Invest.*, 52:1200.
8. Berg, J. W. (1959): Inflammation and prognosis in breast cancer. *Cancer*, 12:714.
9. Bernstein, I. D., Zbar, B., and Rapp, H. J. (1972): Impaired inflammatory response in tumor-bearing guinea pigs. *J. Natl. Cancer Inst.*, 49:1641–1647.
10. Blumenfeld, W., and Territo, M. (1979): A chemotactic inhibitor produced in blast cells and present in the serum of a patient with acute lymphoblastic leukemia. *Blood*, 54:412–420.
11. Boetcher, D. A., and Leonard, E. J. (1974): Abnormal monocyte chemotactic response in cancer patients. *J. Natl. Cancer Inst.*, 52:1091–1099.
12. Brozna, J. P., and Ward, P. A. (1975): Antileukotactic properties of tumor cells. *J. Clin. Invest.*, 56:616.
13. Cheung, H. T., Cantarow, W. D., and Sundharadas, G. (1979): Characteristics of a low molecular weight factor from mouse tumors that affects in vitro properties of macrophages. *Int. J. Cancer*, 23:344–352.
14. Cianciolo, G. J., Copeland, T. D., Oroszlan, S., and Snyderman, R. (1985): Inhibition of lymphocyte proliferation by a synthetic peptide homologous to retroviral envelope proteins. *Science*, 230:453–455.
15. Cianciolo, G. J., Herberman, R. B., and Snyderman, R. (1980): Depression of murine macrophage accumulation by low molecular weight factors derived from spontaneous mammary carcinomas. *J. Natl. Cancer Inst.*, 65:829–834.
16. Cianciolo, G. J., Hunter, J., Silva, J., Haskill, J. S., and Snyderman, R. (1981): Inhibitors of monocyte responses to chemotaxins are present in human cancerous effusions and react with monoclonal antibodies to the P15(E) structural protein of retroviruses. *J. Clin. Invest.*, 68:831–844.
17. Cianciolo, G. J., Kipnis, R. J., and Snyderman, R. (1984): Similarity between p15E of murine and feline leukemia viruses and p21 of HTLV. *Nature*, 311(5986):515.
18. Cianciolo, G. J., Lostrom, M. E., Tam, M., and Snyderman, R. (1983): Murine malignant cells synthesize a 19,000 dalton protein which is physicochemically and antigenically related to the immunosuppressive retroviral protein, p15E. *J. Exp. Med.*, 158:885–900.
19. Cianciolo, G. J., Matthews, T. J., Bolognesi, D. P., and Snyderman, R. (1980): Macrophage accumulation in mice is inhibited by low molecular weight products from murine leukemia viruses. *J. Immunol.*, 124:2900–2905.
20. Cianciolo, G. J., Phipps, D., and Snyderman, R. (1984): Human malignant and mitogen transformed cells contain retroviral p15E-related antigen. *J. Exp. Med.*, 159:964–969.
21. Cianciolo, G. J., and Snyderman, R. (1981): Monocyte responsiveness to chemoattractants is a property of a subpopulation of cells that can respond to multiple chemoattractants. *J. Clin. Invest.*, 67:60–68.
22. Cohen, M. C., Brozna, J. P., and Ward, P. A. (1979): In vitro and

in vivo production of chemotactic inhibitors by tumor cells. *Am. J. Pathol.,* 94:603–614.

23. Cole, D., Van Epps, D. E., and Williams, R. C., Jr. (1986): Defective T-lymphocyte chemotactic factor production in patients with established malignancy. *Clin. Immunol. Immunopathol.,* 38:209–221.

24. Dammacco, F., Miglietta, A., Ventura, M. T., and Bonomo, L. (1982): Defective monocyte chemotactic responsiveness in patients with multiple myeloma and benign monoclonal gammapathy. *Clin. Exp. Immunol.,* 47:481–486.

25. Daunter, B., Khoo, S. K., and Mackay, E. V. (1982): Monocyte chemotaxis in patients with cervical or ovarian cancer. *Gynecologic Oncology,* 13:152–157.

26. Dizon, Q., and Southam, C. M. (1963): Abnormal cellular response to skin abrasion in cancer patients. *Cancer,* 16:1288–1292.

27. Droller, M. J., and Remington, J. S. (1975): A role for the macrophage in in vitro and in vivo resistance to murine bladder tumor cell growth. *Cancer Res.,* 35:49–53.

28. Eccles, S. A., and Alexander, P. (1974): Macrophage content of tumors in relation to metastatic spread and host immune reaction. *Nature (London),* 250:667–669.

29. Eccles, S. A., and Alexander, P. (1974): Sequestration of macrophages in growing tumors and its effect on the immunological capacity of the host. *Br. J. Cancer,* 30:42–49.

30. Essex, M. D., et al. (1984): Seroepidemiology of human T-cell leukemia virus in relation to immunosuppression and the acquired immunodeficiency syndrome. In: *Human T-Cell Leukemia/Lymphoma Virus,* edited by R. C. Gallo, M. E. Essex, and L. Gross, pp. 355–362. Cold Spring Harbor Press, Cold Spring Harbor, N.Y.

31. Evans, R., and Alexander, P. (1970): Cooperation of immune lymphoid cells with macrophages in tumor immunity. *Nature (London),* 228:620–622.

32. Fauci, A. S., and Lane, H. C. (1985): The acquired immunodeficiency syndrome (AIDS): An update. *Int. Arch. Allergy Appl. Immunol.,* 77:81.

33. Fauve, R. M., Hevin, B., Jacob, H., Gaillard, J. A., and Jacob, F. (1974): Antiinflammatory effects of murine malignant cells. *Proc. Natl. Acad. Sci. USA,* 71:4052.

34. Gallo, R. C., Salahuddin, S. Z., Popovic, M., Shearer, G. M., Kaplan, M., Haynes, B. F., Palker, T. J., Redfield, R., Oleske, J., Safai, B., White, G., Foster, P., and Markham, P. D. (1984): Frequent detection and isolation of cytopathic retroviruses (HTLV-III) from patients with AIDS and at risk for AIDS. *Science,* 224:501–503.

35. Gattoni-Celli, S., Kirsch, K., Kalled, S., and Isselbacher, K. J. (1986): Expression of type C-related endogenous retroviral sequences in human colon tumors and colon cancer cell lines. *Proc. Natl. Acad. Sci. USA,* 83:6127.

36. Gauci, C. L., and Alexander, P. (1975): The macrophage content of some human tumors. *Cancer Lett.,* 1:29.

37. Ghaffar, A., McBride, W. H., and Cullen, R. T. (1976): Interaction of tumor cells and activated macrophages in vitro: Modulation by *Corynebacterium parvum* and gold salts. *J. Reticuloendothel. Soc.,* 20:283–289.

38. Goldsmith, H. S., Levin, A. G., and Southam, C. M. (1965): A study of cellular responses in cancer patients by qualitative and quantitative Rebuck tests. *Surg. Forum,* 16:102.

39. Harrell, R. A., Cianciolo, G. J., Copeland, T. D., Oroszlan, S., and Snyderman, R. (1986): Suppression of the respiratory burst of human monocytes by a synthetic peptide homologous to envelope proteins of human and animal retroviruses. *J. Immunol.,* 136:3517–3520.

40. Harris, D. T., Cianciolo, G. J., Snyderman, R., Argov, S., and Koren, H. S. (1986): Inhibition of human natural killer cell activity by a synthetic peptide homologous to a conserved region in the retroviral protein p15E. *J. Immunol.,* 138:889.

41. Haskill, J. S., Proctor, J. W., and Yamamura, Y. (1975): Host responses within solid tumor. I. Monocytic effector cells within rat sarcomas. *J. Natl. Cancer Inst.,* 54:387.

42. Hausman, M., Brosman, S., Fahey, J. L., and Snyderman, R. (1973): Defective mononuclear leukocyte chemotactic activity in patients with genitourinary carcinoma. *Clin. Res.,* 21:646A.

43. Hausman, M. S., Brosman, S., Snyderman, R., Mickey, M. R., and Fahey, J. (1975): Defective monocyte function in patients with genitourinary carcinoma. *J. Natl. Cancer Inst.,* 55:1047–1054.

44. Hesse, D. G., Cole, D. J., Van Epps, D. E., and Williams, R. C., Jr. (1984): Decreased T lymphocyte migration in patients with malignancy mediated by a suppressor cell population. *J. Clin. Invest.,* 73:1078–1085.

45. Israel, L., Samak, R., Edelstein, R., Amouroux, J., Battesti, J.-P. and de Saint Florent, G. (1982): In vivo nonspecific macrophage chemotaxis in cancer patients and its correlation with extent of disease, regional lymph node status, and disease-free survival. *Cancer Res.,* 42:2489–2494.

46. Ji-Ming, W., Cianciolo, G. J., Snyderman, R., and Mantovani, A. (1986): Coexistence of a chemotactic factor and a retroviral p15E-related chemotaxis inhibitor in human tumor cell culture supernatants. *J. Immunol.,* 137:2726–2732.

47. Johnson, M. W., Maibach, H. I., and Salmon, S. E. (1971): Skin reactivity in patients with cancer. Impaired delayed hypersensitivity or faulty inflammatory response? *N. Engl. J. Med.,* 284:1255–1257.

48. Kay, A. B., and McVie, J. G. (1977): Monocyte chemotaxis in bronchial carcinoma and cigarette smokers. *Br. J. Cancer,* 36:461–465.

49. Keller, R. (1976): Promotion of tumor growth in vivo by anti-macrophage agents. *J. Natl. Cancer Inst.,* 57:1355–1361.

50. Keller, R. (1977): Abrogation of antitumor effects of *Corynebacterium parvum* and BCG by antimacrophage agents. *J. Natl. Cancer Inst.,* 59:1751–1753.

51. Kjeldsberg, C. R., and Pay, G. D. (1978): A qualitative and quantitative study of monocytes in patients with malignant solid tumors. *Cancer,* 41:2236–2241.

52. Lane, H. C., Depper, J. M., Greene, W. C., and Whalen, G. (1985): Qualitative analysis of immune function in patients with the acquired immunodeficiency syndrome. *N. Engl. J. Med.,* 313:79.

53. Lau, B. H. S., Masek, T. D., Chu, W. T., and Slater, J. M. (1976): Antiinflammatory reaction associated with murine L1210 leukemia. *Experimentia,* 15:1598.

54. Lemare, E., Carre, P., Legrand, M. F., Lavander, M., Boissinot, E., Renoux, M., and Renous, G. (1984): Alveolar macrophage dysfunction in malignant lung tumors. *Thorax,* 39:448–452.

55. Mahoney, M. J., and Leighton, J. (1961): The inflammatory response to a foreign body within transplantable tumors. *Cancer Res.,* 22:334–338.

56. McBride, W. H., Tuach, W., and Marmion, B. P. (1975): The effects of gold salts on tumor immunity and its stimulation by *Corynebacterium parvum. Br. J. Cancer,* 32:558–567.

57. Meltzer, M. S., and Stevenson, M. M. (1977): Macrophage function in tumor-bearing mice: Tumoricidal and chemotactic responses of macrophages activated by infection with *Mycobacterium bovis,* strain BCG. *J. Immunol.,* 118:2176–2181.

58. Mitani, M., Cianciolo, G. J., Snyderman, R., Yasuda, M., Good, R. A., and Day, N. K. (1987): Suppressive effect on polyclonal B-cell activation of a synthetic peptide homologous to a transmembrane component of oncogenic retroviruses. *Proc. Natl. Acad. Sci. USA,* 84:237–240.

59. Moller, G., and Moller, E. (1976): The concept of immunological surveillance against neoplasia. *Transplant. Rev.,* 28:3–16.

60. Moller, G., and Moller, E. (1978): Immunological surveillance against neoplasia. In: *Immunological Aspects of Cancer,* edited by J. E. Castro, pp. 205–217. University Park Press, Baltimore.

61. Nelson, M., Booth, M. L., and Nelson, D. S. (1982): Effects of tumor cell culture supernatants on some biochemical activities of macrophages. *Aust. J. Exp. Biol. Med. Sci.,* 59:229–237.

62. Nelson, M., and Nelson, D. S. (1978): Macrophages and resistance to tumors. I. Inhibition of delayed type hypersensitivity reactions by tumor cells and by soluble products affecting macrophages. *Immunology,* 34:277.

63. Nelson, M., and Nelson, D. S. (1980): Macrophages and resistance to tumors. IV. The influence of age on the susceptibility of mice to the antiinflammatory and antimacrophage effects of tumor cell products. *J. Natl. Cancer Inst.,* 65:781–789.

64. Nelson, M., Nelson, D. S., Spradbow, P. B., Kuchroo, V. K., Jennings, P. A., Cianciolo, G. J., and Snyderman, R. (1985): Successful tumor immunotherapy: Possible role of antibodies to anti-inflam-

matory factors produced by neoplasms. *Clin. Exp. Immunol.,* 61: 109–117.

65. Nielsen, H., Bennedsen, J., and Dombernowsky, P. (1982): Normalization of defective monocyte chemotaxis during chemotherapy in patients with small cell anaplastic carcinoma of the lung. *Cancer Immunol. Immunother.,* 14:13–15.

66. Nielsen, H., Rorth, M., and Bennedsen, J. (1985): Monocyte chemotaxis in patients with nonseminomatous testicular carcinoma. *Cancer Immunol. Immunother.,* 19:68–71.

67. Normann, S. J., and Cornelius, J. (1982): Characterization of antiinflammatory factors produced by murine tumor cells in culture. *J. Natl. Cancer Inst.,* 69:1321–1327.

68. Normann, S. J., Schardt, M., and Sorkin, E. (1979): Antiinflammatory effect of spontaneous lymphoma in SJL/J mice. *J. Natl. Cancer Inst.,* 63:825–833.

69. Normann, S. J., and Sorkin, E. (1976): Cell specific defect in monocyte function during tumor growth. *J. Natl. Cancer Inst.,* 57: 135–140.

70. Norris, D. A., Weston, W. L., Tubergen, D. G., Rose, B., and Odom, L. F. (1980): Monocyte chemotaxis in leukemia patients. *J. Lab. Clin. Med.,* 95:609–615.

71. Poiesz, B. J., Ruscetti, F. W., Reitz, M. S., Kalyanaraman, V. S., and Gallo, R. C. (1981): Isolation of a new type C retrovirus (HTLV) in primary uncultured cells of a patient with Sezary T-cell leukemia. *Nature,* 294:268–271.

72. Power, M. D., Marx, P. A., Bryant, M. L., Gardner, M. B., et al. (1986): Nucleotide sequence of SRV-1, a type D simian acquired immune deficiency syndrome retrovirus. *Science,* 231:1567.

73. Prehn, R. T. (1972): The immune reaction as a stimulator of tumor growth. *Science,* 175:170.

74. Prehn, R. T. (1976): Do tumors grow because of the immune response of the host? *Transplant. Rev.,* 28:34–42.

75. Prehn, R. T., and Lappe, M. A. (1971): An immunostimulation theory of tumor development. *Transplant. Rev.,* 7:26.

76. Repaske, R., Steel, P. E., O'Neill, R. R., Rabson, A. B., and Martin, M. A. (1985): Nucleotide sequence of a full-length human endogenous retroviral segment. *J. Virol.,* 54:764.

77. Rubin, R. H., Cosini, A. B., and Goetzl, E. J. (1976): Defective human mononuclear leukocyte chemotaxis as an index of host resistance to malignant melanoma. *Clin. Immunol. Immunopathol.,* 6:376–388.

78. Russell, S. W., Doe, S. F., and Cochrane, C. G. (1976): Number of macrophages and distribution of mitotic activity in regressing and progressing Moloney sarcomas. *J. Immunol.,* 116:164–166.

79. Russell, S. W., Doe, W. F., and McIntosh, A. T. (1977): Functional characterization of a stable, non-cytolytic stage of macrophage activation in tumors. *J. Exp. Med.,* 146:1511–1520.

80. Rygaard, J., and Poolsen, C. O. (1976): The nude mouse in the hypothesis of immunological surveillance. *Transplant. Rev.,* 28: 43–61.

81. Siegbahn, A., Simonsson, B., and Venge, P. (1984): The chemokinetic inhibitory factor (CIF) in serum of CLL patients: Correlation with infection propensity and disease activity.

82. Siegbahn, A., Venge, P., and Nilsson, K. (1983): Cellular origin of the chemokinetic inhibitor of polymorphonuclear leukocytes found in sera from patients with chronic lymphocytic leukemia. *Scand. J. Haematol.,* 31:184–192.

83. Siegbahn, A., Venge, P., Nilsson, K., and Simonsson, B. (1982): Identification of a chemokinetic inhibitor in serum from patients with chronic lymphocytic leukemia. *Scand. J. Haematol.,* 28:122–131.

84. Smith, P. D., Ohura, K., Masur, H., Lane, H. C., Fauci, A. S., and Wahl, S. M. (1984): Monocyte function in the acquired immunodeficiency syndrome. Defective chemotaxis. *J. Clin. Invest.,* 76: 2121–2128.

85. Snyderman, R., Altman, L. C., Hausman, M. S., and Mergenhagen, S. E. (1972): Human mononuclear leukocyte chemotaxis: A quantitative assay for humoral and cellular factors. *J. Immunol.,* 108: 857–860.

86. Snyderman, R., and Cianciolo, G. J. (1984): Immunosuppressive activity of the retroviral envelope protein p15E and its possible

relationship to neoplasia. In: *Immunology Today,* edited by J. Inglis, pp. 240–244. Elsevier, Amsterdam.

87. Snyderman, R., Dickson, J., Meadows, L., and Pike, M. (1974): Deficient monocyte chemotactic responsiveness in humans with cancer. *Clin. Res.,* 22:430A.

88. Snyderman, R., Meadows, L., Holder, W., and Wells, S., Jr. (1978): Abnormal monocyte chemotaxis in patients with breast cancer: Evidence for a tumor-mediated effect. *J. Natl. Cancer Inst.,* 60: 737–740.

89. Snyderman, R., and Pike, M. C. (1976): Defective macrophage migration produced by neoplasms: Identification of an inhibitor of macrophage chemotaxis. In: *The Macrophage in Neoplasia,* edited by M. A. Fink, Academic Press, New York.

90. Snyderman, R., and Pike, M. C. (1976): An inhibitor of macrophage chemotaxis produced by neoplasms. *Science,* 192:370–372.

91. Snyderman, R., Pike, M. C., Blaylock, B. L., and Weinstein, P. (1976): Effects of neoplasms on inflammation: Depression of macrophage accumulation after tumor implantation. *J. Immunol.,* 116: 585–589.

92. Snyderman, R., Seigler, H. F., and Meadows, L. (1977): Abnormalities of monocyte chemotaxis in patients with melanoma: Effects of immunotherapy and tumor removal. *J. Natl. Cancer Inst.,* 58: 37–41.

93. Sonigo, P., Barker, C., Hunter, E., and Wain-Hobson, S. (1986): Nucleotide sequence of Mason-Pfizer monkey virus: An immunosuppressive D-type retrovirus.

94. Specter, S. C., Bendinelli, M., Ceglowski, W. S., and Friedman, H. (1978): Macrophage-induced reversal of immunosuppression by leukemia viruses. *Fed. Proc.,* 37:97–101.

95. Stevenson, M. M., and Meltzer, M. S. (1976): Depressed chemotactic responses in vitro of peritoneal macrophages from tumor-bearing mice. *J. Natl. Cancer Inst.,* 57:847–852.

96. Stutman, O. (1974): Tumor development after 3-methylcholanthrene in immunologically deficient athymic nude mice. *Science,* 183:534–536.

97. Stutman, O. (1975): Immunodepression and malignancy. *Adv. Cancer Res.,* 22:261–422.

98. Szuro-Sudol, A., Murray, H. W., and Nathan, C. F. (1983): Suppression of macrophage antimicrobial activity by a tumor cell product. *J. Immunol.,* 131:384–387.

99. Szuro-Sudol, A., and Nathan, C. F. (1982): Suppression of macrophage oxidative metabolism by products of malignant and non-malignant cells. *J. Exp. Med.,* 156:945–961.

100. Tan, I. B., Drexhage, H. A., Scheper, R. J., von Blomberg, B. M. E., de Haan-Meulman, M., Snow, G. B., and Balm, A. J. M. (1986): Defective monocyte chemotaxis in patients with head and neck cancer: Restoration after treatment. *Arch. Otolaryngol. Head Neck Surg.,* 112:541–544.

101. Tan, I. B., Drexhage, H. A., Scheper, R. J., von Blomberg, B. M. E., van de Flier, M., de Haan-Meulman, M., Snow, G. B., and Balm, T. J. M. (1986): Immunosuppressive retroviral p15E-related factors in head and neck carcinomas. *Arch. Otolaryngol. Head Neck Surg.,* 112:942–945.

102. Thomson, A. W., and Fowler, E. J. (1977): Potentiation of tumor growth by carageenan. *Transplantation,* 24:397–400.

103. Till, G., and Ward, P. A. (1975): Two distinct chemotactic factor inactivators in human serum. *J. Immunol.,* 114:843.

104. Tsunawaki, S., and Nathan, C. F. (1986): Macrophage deactivation. Altered kinetic properties of superoxide-producing enzyme after exposure to tumor-cell conditioned medium. *J. Exp. Med.,* 164: 1319–1331.

105. Warabi, H., Venkat, K., Geetha, V., Kiotta, L. A., Brownstein, M., and Schiffman, E. (1984): Identification and partial characterization of a low-molecular-weight inhibitor of leukotaxis from fibrosarcoma cells. *Cancer Res.,* 44:915–922.

106. Ward, P. A., and Berenberg, J. L. (1974): Defective regulation of inflammatory mediators in Hodgkin's disease. *N. Engl. J. Med.,* 290:76.

107. Wood, B. W., and Gillespie, G. Y. (1975): Studies on the role of macrophages in regulation of growth and metastasis of murine chemically induced fibrosarcomas. *Int. J. Cancer,* 16:1022–1029.

Pharmacologic Modulation
of Inflammation

Inflammation: Basic Principles and Clinical Correlates.
Edited by J. I. Gallin, I. M. Goldstein, and R. Snyderman.
Raven Press, Ltd., New York © 1988.

CHAPTER 49

Adrenal Corticosteroids

Debra L. Bowen and Anthony S. Fauci

<table>
<tr><td>

Biochemistry/Pharmacology
Mechanisms of Action
Effects of GCC on Inflammatory and Immunologic Mediators
   Production and Function of Immunoglobulins • Production and Function of Soluble Factors

</td><td>

Effects of GCC on Cellular Components of Inflammation and Immunity
   Phagocytic Cells • Neutrophils • Monocytes and Macrophages • Eosinophils • Basophils • Mast Cells • Platelets • Fibroblasts • Lymphocytes
Summary
References

</td></tr>
</table>

Glucocorticoids (GCC) exert profound effects on the inflammatory and immune responses of mammals. Since clinical improvement was first reported in patients with rheumatoid arthritis who were treated with cortisone in 1949 (86), physicians have used GCC in the clinical management of inflammatory and immunologic diseases.

Many original observations regarding the regulatory effects of GCC on immune and inflammatory responses were made in other species, and generalization of many of those findings to humans has been limited by recognition of the unique lytic effects of GCC on immunoregulatory cells in some species, such as the rabbit, mouse, and rat, whereas lymphocytes from other species, such as the guinea pig and human, are resistant to such lytic effects. In this chapter we shall focus on the accumulated body of human research describing the effects of GCC on inflammation and immunity. However, in some instances important observations have been made in other species that may be relevant to the mechanisms of GCC regulation of human immune responses. Therefore, we identify and present this information, acknowledging that differences between species exist and that these differences may ultimately prevent generalization of certain animal studies to humans.

Inflammation is the result of a process that involves vasodilation, increased vascular permeability, initial cellular infiltrates with neutrophils, and subsequently infiltrates with mononuclear cells, with concomitant lysosomal enzyme release and tissue destruction. Much of the time, this process is salutary, as in host defenses against infection; sometimes, however, acute or chronic destructive inflammatory processes occur. GCC affect each of these inflammatory events and alter the production and release of many specific mediators of inflammation, as well as the function of cells responsible for an adequate inflammatory response.

BIOCHEMISTRY/PHARMACOLOGY

The adrenal cortex synthesizes and releases three classes of steroids: GCC, mineralocorticoids, and the sex hormones (102). GCC are endogenously synthesized through reactions that result in conversion of cholesterol to cortisol. Adults secrete approximately 20 mg of cortisol per day. Of the 5 to 25 μg of cortisol per 100 ml in plasma, 95% is bound to plasma proteins, an α-globulin transcortin, and albumin. About 5% of endogenous GCC and about 35% of exogenous synthetic GCC circulate in an unbound and active state. Cortisol is rapidly removed from the circulation and metabolized, with a plasma half-life of only 90 min; less than 2% is excreted in the urine unchanged. The 11β-hydroxyl group is the active GCC group; 11-ketosteroids such as prednisone lack activity until they are converted in the liver into their respective 11β-hydroxyl compounds, such as prednisolone. Some

GCC-responsive cells have 6,000 to 12,000 receptors that bind GCC with a dissociation constant of 10^{-9} M (102). For some of these cells it has been demonstrated that a steroid-receptor complex is translocated into the nucleus and associates with nuclear chromatin or DNA, and messenger RNA (mRNA) synthesis increases up to 10,000-fold over the following 2 to 24 hr (102).

MECHANISMS OF ACTION

Several mechanisms of action for GCC have been proposed. Classic theory has attributed GCC cellular effects to specific binding of GCC to intracellular GCC receptors, with subsequent initiation of a series of cellular events involving synthesis of new proteins (30). There is considerable experimental evidence in support of this theory, and it constitutes the current dogma of steroid hormone action. Over the past few years it has been proposed that some effects of GCC are mediated through synthesis of new phospholipid inhibitory proteins (PLIPs) or lipocortins that can affect the inflammatory and the teratogenic responses of certain cells exposed to GCC (12,77,78,88). However, other described mechanisms of GCC action include GCC-induced changes in cyclic nucleotide ratios, changes in membrane fluidity, and alterations in ion channels that occur too early for new protein synthesis and that may directly affect a subsequent cellular response (17,70,71,95). Data accumulated from these recent studies suggest that direct membrane changes may alter the number or function of nonsteroid membrane-level receptors that are involved in a usual cellular response. Each of these possible mechanisms of GCC action will be examined.

Classically, GCC responses have been attributed to the cascade of cellular events initiated by GCC binding to a specific intracellular GCC receptor. These receptors are widely distributed in mammalian tissue. *In vitro* studies have demonstrated that following binding to specific surface membrane receptors, GCC are internalized and can bind reversibly with high affinity to intracellular receptor proteins. This hormone-receptor complex can then migrate into the cell nucleus and can bind to nuclear chromatin or DNA. This steroid-receptor complex associates with nuclear DNA and modulates gene expression. Specific, newly synthesized mRNA then codes for proteins that are thought to regulate some functional expression of the GCC effects (29). This scheme is widely accepted as the primary mode of action of all steroid hormones.

The details of the mechanisms of GCC effects subsequent to receptor binding are complex and incompletely defined. Furthermore, this theoretical model, although resulting from a large body of experimental data, probably is not the sole mechanism of GCC effects on either the inflammatory response or the immune response. It is well known that the presence of specific intracytoplasmic GCC receptors does not predict GCC responsiveness in all malignancies (65,113). In fact, there is a definite lack of correlation between GCC receptor density and the *in vitro* growth-inhibitory effect of dexamethasone in human leukemia cell lines (125). However, it should be noted that cell-cycle phase parameters for these studies have never been reported concomitantly.

Nevertheless, specific intracytoplasmic GCC receptors are present widely in cells of the normal immune system: in human lymphocytes (112), monocytes (165), neutrophils, and eosinophils (132). The numbers of these specific intracytoplasmic receptors in mitogenically stimulated lymphocytes have been shown to vary in different stages of the cell cycle (35). In addition, selective T-lymphocyte populations vary in receptor parameters such as density, affinity, and binding constants (46,137). However, measurements of GCC functional responsiveness in immunoreactive cells have not directly correlated with specific intracytoplasmic receptor measurements (59,82,137,156).

Recently, some of the antiinflammatory effects of GCC have been attributed to synthesis of lipocortins. Lipocortins are a family of GCC-induced proteins with antiphospholipase activity that control the biosynthesis of the potent mediators of inflammation: prostaglandins and leukotrienes. Lipocortins have been hypothesized to prevent mobilization of arachidonic acid from membrane phospholipids by inhibiting hydrolysis of these phospholipids by phospholipase A_2 (Fig. 1).

The first lipocortins identified were isolated from immunologic cells and were named "macrocortin," which was derived from rat macrophages (12), and "lipomodulin," which was isolated from rabbit neutrophils (88). Subsequently, lipocortins were isolated from a wide variety of cells and tissues. Renocortins were isolated from rat renomedullary interstitial cells (33,144). Lipocortins were purified from human placenta (93), human endometrium (79), and human embryonic skin fibroblasts (52). These proteins are collectively known as lipocortins (45), with molecular weights ranging from 15,000 to 200,000 daltons (44). In immunologic studies, monoclonal antibodies raised to one lipocortin showed immunologic cross-reactivity to others (44,61), suggesting a functional identity and a structural heterogeneity in molecular weight brought about by proteolysis from the higher-molecular-weight species.

Functionally, lipocortins have been demonstrated to inhibit rat paw edema induced by carrageenin (44), to promote cellular differentiation in a human histiocytic lymphoma cell line (44), and to induce T cells to produce a glycosylation inhibitory factor that inhibits the IgE response (97). Similar lipocortins, called PLIPs by the authors, have been demonstrated to result in teratogenic effects in the mouse palate model (77,78). These are functions that support roles for these proteins in antiinflammatory and immunologic effects.

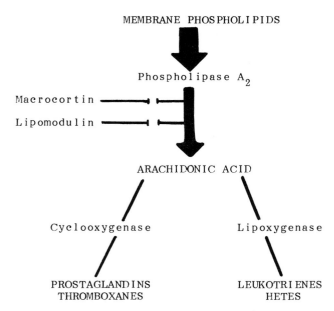

MEMBRANE PHOSPHOLIPIDS

Phospholipase A₂

Macrocortin ⟶

Lipomodulin ⟶

ARACHIDONIC ACID

Cyclooxygenase   Lipoxygenase

PROSTAGLANDINS   LEUKOTRIENES
THROMBOXANES   HETES

FIG. 1. Brief scheme for generation of lipid mediators from the phospholipase A₂ action on membrane phospholipids. GCC presumably stimulates synthesis of proteins (e.g., macrocortin and lipomodulin) that affect the early step in this process by inhibiting phospholipase A₂ activity.

Using amino acid sequence information obtained from the 40,000-dalton purified rat lipocortin, human lipocortin has been cloned from complementary DNA and expressed in *E. coli* (163). Most recently, the major cellular p35/36 substrates of tyrosine kinases (18,93,107) were demonstrated to share homology with the human lipocortins I and II (93,107) and also to inhibit phospholipase A₂ (18). Human lipocortin I appears to be the same protein as the epidermal growth factor receptor kinase substrate, and lipocortin II is the apparent human analogue of pp36, a major substrate for the retroviral protein tyrosine receptor kinase (93,107).

These recent findings have major implications for the theory suggesting that the lipocortins are the specific second-messenger protein(s) inducible by the GCC hormones. The specificity of GCC in inducing these cellular substrates for the ECF receptor kinase and retroviral receptor kinase may now be examined. At this time, the relationship between any lipocortin effect and specific or a net GCC effects on the inflammatory and immunologic responses remains unclear.

Thus, lipocortins are produced by a wide variety of cells and probably are best characterized as GCC-inducible proteins that may result in regulation of some cellular functions. Again, it is not yet clear whether or not GCC are the sole inducers of these proteins, although evidence to date would make this supposition appear unlikely.

Although new synthesis of some proteins may occur in response to GCC, GCC generally inhibit amino acid incorporation into protein. In splenic lymphocytes, GCC stimulate protein degradation and expand intracellular amino acid pools (116), inhibiting amino acid precursor incorporation into protein. Furthermore, this protein degradation in lymphocytes has been documented and quantitated by sodium dodecylsulfate gel electrophoresis (115,117).

In a similar fashion, GCC also inhibit total RNA synthesis. We have shown that in human B lymphocytes, tritiated-uridine incorporation is markedly diminished and total new RNA synthesis is decreased in the presence of hydrocortisone (HC) over a wide range of concentrations (15).

Additional intracellular mechanisms have been shown to be important in the direct immunoregulatory effect of GCC. Cyclic adenosine monophosphate (cAMP) levels are elevated within minutes following addition of GCC to human lymphocytes, too early for new protein synthesis. Furthermore, this accumulation of cAMP in lymphocytes has been demonstrated to increase cellular sensitivity to catecholamines *in vitro* (126). Other GCC-induced cell membrane changes have been demonstrated after brief incubations with immunoregulatory cells. Human macrophages have been demonstrated to up-regulate HLA-DR (72) and insulin receptor (6) expression in response to brief *in vitro* culture with GCC. At the same time, these monocytes exhibit a diminished functional response in antigen processing and presentation (71). Peripheral human lymphocytes, on the other hand, have been demonstrated to exhibit a 15% reduction in histocompatibility antigen expression, without a clear-cut demonstration that this effect is causally related to a functional change in the lymphocytes examined (91). However, phytohemagglutinin-induced Ia antigen expression in human T cells and proliferation of T cells stimulated with autologous phytohemagglutinin have been correlated, and both parameters have been shown to be inhibited by low-dose prednisone (96). A more significant reduction in HLA expression has been shown in purified human B-cell populations from tonsils using HC *in vitro* (D. L. Bowen and A. S. Fauci, *unpublished data*) and from peripheral blood using dexamethasone *in vivo* (119). This reduction in HLA expression is selective and dependent on cell-cycle phase and cell maturation in B cells (D. L. Bowen and A. S. Fauci, *unpublished data*). Furthermore, there is evidence that these GCC-induced alterations in Ia expression in B lymphocytes are T-cell- and accessory-cell-independent. In the mouse, GCC-induced suppression of B-cell immune response antigens has been demonstrated after intravenous administration of dexamethasone. A 75% reduction in the expression of Ia occurred within 6 hr, with return to base line by 12 hr, following GCC injection. This effect was dose-dependent and was observed after dexamethasone injection into athymic nude mice, suggesting that the alteration in B-cell Ia expression caused by GCC is a T-cell-independent process (43). These findings are of interest because the mechanisms by which T and B cells collaborate in the linked recognition of hapten and carrier suggest that antigen serves as a bridge between helper T cells and B cells and that B cells may process antigen independently for recognition in initial steps. Helper T cells cannot recognize free antigen, but must recognize antigen in conjunction with Ia on the surfaces of antigen-presenting cells. Resting B cells have been found to be incapable of presenting antigen, whereas activated B cells can both process and present antigen. It is likely that B cells bind, internalize, and process antigen (8). Activated B cells efficiently present antigen that has been bound specifically to surface membrane immunoglobulin (sIg) receptors, rather than antigen that has been taken up nonspecifically (26,28,101). Antigen is then complexed with membrane Ia and expressed on the B-cell surface and serves to focus antigen-specific T-cell help. Thus, if GCC suppress Ia expression in cells given an activating sIg mitogenic or antigenic signal, subsequent T-B interaction cannot occur, and cooperative amplication of an immune response will not result.

Other membrane-associated events in human leukocytes are altered by GCC after only brief incubations. Cholesterol-like molecules change the ratio of phospholipids in the cell membrane and inhibit cell membrane fluidity (92). Relatively high concentrations of HC have been shown to prevent capping in B lymphocytes (4), although these concentrations do not prevent an earlier membrane-associated event in sIg-mediated signaling, sIg cross-linkage, and attachment to the cytoskeleton (D. L. Bowen and A. S. Fauci, *unpublished data*).

Transient decreases in phospholipid methylation in lymphoid cells can be induced by dexamethasone (136). The functional effect of this finding is not yet clear, but phospholipid methylation was reported to be involved in early membrane activation events in many cells (87). To summarize, it is clear that membrane-related changes in immunoregulatory cells that are induced by GCC are cell-type- and cycle-selective and that many of these GCC-induced changes have not been shown to be mediated through the classic steroid-receptor cascade.

Whatever the mechanism of action, diverse effects of GCC have been described for all cellular components of the immune system and for many humoral events that relate to the normal human inflammatory and immune responses.

EFFECTS OF GCC ON INFLAMMATORY AND IMMUNOLOGIC MEDIATORS

GCC have multiple effects on the production and function of many inflammatory and immunologic mediators. Generally, GCC suppress production of these mediators,

but may also alter the function of normally produced mediators. The overall balance of these effects *in vivo* is to suppress the production and function of inflammatory mediators and to suppress the *in vivo* response. *In vitro* effects of GCC vary depending on culture conditions and the presence or absence of other factors in the *in vitro* conditions.

Production and Function of Immunoglobulins

Perhaps the greatest diversity can be seen in GCC effects on the production and function of Ig. It is quite clear that *in vivo* GCC suppress the production of total Ig (22). On the other hand, *in vitro* GCC may suppress, enhance, or have no discernible effect on the production of Ig by immunologic cells in culture (34,37,57). It is clear that multiple factors and cell types are important in the production and function of Ig *in vivo* and that only some of these factors and cells are affected by GCC *in vitro*. These effects will be outlined later.

In vivo administered GCC result in suppression of total Ig production, particularly IgG and IgA subtypes. Maximal suppression with a split-dose GCC regimen occurs at 2 to 4 weeks after institution of therapy. Initially the reduction in serum Ig is partially accounted for by an increased rate of Ig catabolism, although decreased serum levels several weeks later reflect a decreased rate of production (22). Daily doses of GCC may also reduce IgE levels. The first demonstration of altered IgE levels subsequent to GCC therapy was in 1971 with asthmatic children. GCC-treated children had IgE levels remarkably lower than those of untreated children. After GCC was discontinued, IgE levels rose and became higher after an increasing interval following GCC therapy (108). IgE production is also decreased following GCC therapy in other illnesses such as the idiopathic hypereosinophilic syndrome (21) and allergic bronchopulmonary aspergillosis (139).

The effects of *in vitro* GCC on Ig production vary with different culture and assay systems. Potentiation of total Ig production stimulated by pokeweed mitogen (PWM) has been demonstrated by measurement of plaque-forming cell responses (60) and of supernatant Ig (35). This GCC-induced enhancement of Ig production in response to mitogens or to a mixed leukocyte reaction may be seen with culture medium containing fetal calf serum or with serum-free medium containing defined nutrients to support cell growth (D. L. Bowen and A. S. Fauci, *unpublished observations*), although it is apparently absent when using a human source for serum in culture (37). Investigators have emphasized the need to determine the bioavailability of GCC in cultures that contain different GCC-binding proteins, because the same molar concentration of GCC may not result in the same effective concentration using different sources of supplemented medium.

In vivo GCC effects on *in vitro* B-cell function have also been described in humans. Spontaneous Ig production by B cells was enhanced by *in vivo* GCC when measured in an *in vitro* plaque-forming cell assay. The same increased response was also observed with a brief *in vitro* exposure of the B cells to GCC. The mitogen-induced B-cell differentiation response, however, varied with total course of *in vivo* GCC: A single *in vivo* pulse of a pharmacologic concentration of GCC reduced PWM-induced plaque-forming cell responses at 4 to 5 hr, with complete recovery by 24 hr; however, after a 5-day *in vivo* course of GCC, recovery of suppressed PWM-induced response was delayed to 60 hr. The mechanism of suppression of the PWM B-cell response appears multifactorial; it is not due simply to an enriched circulating OKT8 suppressor population. OKT8 suppressor/cytotoxic cells were enriched in the circulation 10 hr after the last GCC dose, with a return to normal numbers after 36 hr, even though the PWM response remained suppressed at that time (38).

Thus, GCC may suppress *in vivo* Ig production, enhance or suppress *in vitro* production after *in vivo* administration, and enhance *in vitro* Ig production when directly added to cell culture. These diverse effects of GCC on Ig production suggest that GCC interact with the system used to measure Ig production and function. Factors or cells present *in vivo* with GCC result in overall suppression of Ig production. More highly purified and processed *in vitro* culture systems, however, usually respond to GCC with enhanced Ig production. This diversity of GCC effects on Ig production emphasizes the complexity of the immune interactions required to stimulate or suppress Ig production.

Production and Function of Soluble Factors

Release of non-Ig soluble factors by immunoreactive cells is also affected by GCC. These factors represent all humoral components that mediate the inflammatory and immune responses in humans: complement components, kinins, products of the lipooxygenase and cyclooxygenase pathways, histamine, and numerous cytokines. Some of these mediators are more significantly affected than others by GCC, as discussed later.

Complement Components

Complement production and metabolism in humans appear to be resistant to GCC. Although suppression of serum complement components can be observed in guinea pigs with high-dose GCC administration (5),

there is little evidence that this is clinically relevant in humans (29).

Lipid Mediators

Eicosanoid release is important in the development of an adequate inflammatory response. GCC modulate this event. Initially, eicosanoid generation occurs by cleavage of arachidonic acid from precursor phospholipids by phospholipase A_2. The lipocortins, which are inducible by GCC, may inhibit this initial step, preventing all eicosanoid formation by either the cyclooxygenase or lipooxygenase pathway (102).

Eicosanoids have been demonstrated to affect pyrogenesis, vasodilation, vascular permeability, pain thresholds, neutrophil chemotaxis, and smooth-muscle contraction. Because of the diverse actions of the eicosanoids and their effectiveness at low concentrations, modulation of eicosanoid production and release is one mechanism by which GCC can affect the inflammatory response.

The eicosanoid leukotriene B_4 (LTB_4) is a potent chemotactic molecule for polymorphonuclear cells (102). Generation and release of LTB_4 at inflammatory sites have been shown to be inhibited by GCC and to correlate with diminished neutrophil accumulation at the site (161).

Leukotrienes C_4, D_4, and E_4 compose the slow-reacting substance of anaphylaxis (SRS-A). GCC inhibits leukotriene release *in vivo* in experimental animals (20) and in human lung tissue (81). Isolated human lung mast cells apparently do not respond to GCC (148).

GCC inhibit prostaglandin synthesis by interfering with phospholipase A_2 activity. This action appears to be mediated through inhibition of arachidonate release and to depend on new protein synthesis, because it can be prevented by inhibitors of protein synthesis such as cycloheximide (62).

Thus, GCC modulation of lipid mediator production and release is one mechanism by which GCC suppress the inflammatory response. This modulation may occur, at least partially, through GCC suppression of phospholipase A_2 activity.

Histamine

GCC are useful in treating urticaria and angioedema because they inhibit the vascular permeability caused by mediators such as histamine, prostaglandins, and leukotrienes. The mechanism of histamine depletion in tissue that is accompanied by a decrease in tissue mass after prolonged GCC therapy is undefined, although it has been observed since 1941 (143). However, IgE-mediated release of histamine from basophils has been shown to be inhibited by dexamethasone at a concentration of $10^{-7} M$ (147).

This time-dependent effect on histamine release occurs only after prolonged incubation and reaches 80% inhibition at 24 hr. The GCC effect was not demonstrated for histamine release induced by f-met-leu-phe (122), suggesting that GCC suppression of basophil histamine release was not the result of phospholipase A_2 inhibition (147). Although histamine release by human lung mast cells does not appear to be affected by GCC, mouse peritoneal mast cells are inhibited by low concentrations of dexamethasone (39). Again, histamine release induced by the ionophore A23187 was not affected by dexamethasone, suggesting that GCC affect early processes in cell activation.

Cytokines

Numerous cytokines have recently been described and differentiated from one another by physiochemical and functional studies. These factors are intricately involved in human inflammatory and immune responses. GCC generally inhibit the production and/or release of these cytokines. Effects of GCC on several of these mediators are outlined next.

Interleukin 1 (IL-1) is a known pyrogen and serves a permissive role in T-cell production of IL-2, which is also known as T-cell growth factor. IL-1 production by monocytes is suppressed by GCC (166).

Furthermore, GCC can inhibit *in vitro* production of IL-2 (73). It has previously been demonstrated that mitogen-induced T-cell proliferation may be restored in the presence of HC with the addition of exogenous IL-2 (73). GCC-induced inhibition of IL-2 and γ-interferon synthesis occur at the mRNA level in human T-cell clones (3). This GCC-induced inhibition of factor production is selective, because the production of HLA-specific message is not suppressed in the presence of dexamethasone in the same T-cell clones.

Inhibition of the synthesis of other soluble mediators such as lymphotoxin (167) and a monocyte chemotactic factor (145) has been reported with *in vitro* GCC.

The mechanisms of the GCC effects on cytokine production are not completely defined. However, one mechanism of GCC effect on the production of a recently described cytokine, IL-3, in the murine system may provide some insight. In the mouse, this GCC-induced effect appears to occur by direct inhibition of specific genomic transcription. Production of IL-3 in a concanavalin-A-stimulated murine helper T-cell clone was inhibited by dexamethasone. Furthermore, this effect was demonstrated for the supernatant IL-3 activity as well as for the accumulation of IL-3 mRNA in the cells. Similar to the finding reported earlier in human T-cell clones, this inhibition of IL-3 production was selective. The constitutive

synthesis of Thy-1 mRNA was not altered by dexamethasone. Because of the rapid action on IL-3 mRNA, the stability of IL-3 mRNA in the presence of dexamethasone, and the lack of dexamethasone inhibition of either mRNA processing or transport from the nucleus, this effect appeared to occur by direct inhibition of transcription of the IL-3 gene. Thus, GCC can regulate a set of mitogen-inducible genes in murine helper T cells (36).

Cytokine production is inhibited by GCC, and this effect of GCC can be separated from effects on cellular proliferation, at least in T-cell clones. Dexamethasone, even at physiologic concentrations, inhibits production of IL-2, macrophage-activating factor (MAF), colony-stimulating factor (CSF), and γ-interferon in long-term alloreactive T-cell clones (106). Furthermore, dexamethasone and an IL-2-containing supernatant exert opposing effects on clonal MAF production. GCC reduced the rate of secretion without causing a compensatory increase in the duration of secretion, whereas the IL-2 supernatant increased both the rate and the total amount of MAF secreted. Furthermore, in the presence of dexamethasone, the effect of IL-2 was abrogated. Effects of dexamethasone were seen within 4 hr after stimulation, and they increased with longer exposure, until MAF production ceased at 12 to 24 hr. Preexposure and removal of dexamethasone before concanavalin A stimulation also inhibited MAF release. Factor production by all 16 clones tested was inhibited by dexamethasone, but proliferation of two cytolytic clones was unaffected by dexamethasone (106).

However, GCC usually block both IL-2 production and DNA synthesis in bulk T-cell cultures. In another study, endogenous IL-2 production was blocked *in situ* by pharmacologic concentrations of dexamethasone, with a concomitant 80 to 90% reduction of T-cell tritiated-thymidine uptake (10). These cells remained in the G_{1a} phase because of insufficient RNA synthesis for proliferation. IL-2 addition allowed cells to synthesize more RNA so that they could enter S phase and proliferate. A monoclonal antibody, anti-Tac, inhibited exogenous IL-2-induced RNA synthesis in dexamethasone-treated phytohemagglutinin-stimulated T cells. However, anti-Tac did not diminish the endogenous response to IL-2 in phytohemagglutinin-stimulated cells, although anti-Tac bound just as well to these cells (10).

Nevertheless, GCC-induced suppression of factor production is not uniform, and the effect of GCC may depend on the lymphocyte subset involved. *In vitro*, GCC can augment Sendai-virus-induced interferon production in human tumor lines (1); it may enhance B-cell growth factor (BCGF) production in certain human tumor lines that have been mitogenically stimulated (D. L. Bowen and A. S. Fauci, *unpublished observations*) and enhance B-cell differentiation factor (BCDF) activity in the harvested supernatants of MLR and mitogenically stimulated human lymphocyte cultures (16).

EFFECTS OF GCC ON CELLULAR COMPONENTS OF INFLAMMATION AND IMMUNITY

Although the effects of GCC in regulating numerous humoral components of inflammation and immunity might alone account for significant suppression of these functions, GCC also exert marked effects on the cellular components that ensure modulation of the inflammatory and immunity cascades. In fact, the major antiinflammatory actions of GCC have been attributed to their effects on the polymorphonuclear leukocyte (neutrophil).

Phagocytic Cells

GCC alter the maturation, distribution, and function of phagocytic cells. GCC have primary effects on neutrophil and monocyte production and function. GCC modulate the ratio of neutrophils to monocytes in the bone marrow. GCC redistribute neutrophils, causing a peripheral blood neutrophilia and preventing ingress of neutrophils into inflammatory sites. GCC affect both phagocytic cell types by inhibiting chemotaxis directly and through suppression of LTB_4 production or release (110,161), by preventing production and release of other cellular products, by altering endocytosis (both phagocytosis and pinocytosis) (7,89,152), by suppressing oxidative antimicrobial function (superoxide generation by neutrophils) (33,123), and by decreasing cytotoxic function (141).

Neutrophils

Unlike the effects of GCC on other inflammatory and immunoregulatory cells in which there is a depletion of cells from the circulation, there is a moderate neutrophilia following *in vivo* administration of GCC that occurs within 4 to 6 hr. Within 24 hr, circulating neutrophils return to pretreatment levels (41,42). Granulocyte adherence is inhibited by GCC (118). Increased bone marrow release and delayed migration from the intravascular space are two important mechanisms of the GCC-induced neutrophilia observed in the peripheral blood (41,58).

GCC may also modulate granulocytosis by shifting production to the granulocyte line at a progenitor cell level. Dexamethasone has been shown to modulate CSF-dependent clonal growth of myeloid progenitor cells in semisolid agar cultures, enhancing the formation of granulocyte colonies (by 50–100%) and suppressing the formation of macrophage colonies (by 75–97%). This mod-

ulation occurs *in vitro* if GCC are added at the time of culture initiation and up to 72 hr later. The results suggest that GCC shift the balance of granulocyte formation versus macrophage formation at the earliest stages of precursor cell differentiation (153).

Nevertheless, there is circumstantial evidence that altered maturation of granulocytes also occurs in the presence of GCC. *In vivo*, GCC cause nuclear hypersegmentation of circulating granulocytes in normal humans. The nuclear lobe count is noted to increase by the third day of treatment, and nuclear segmentation increases even further with continued therapy during a week of observation. The mechanism of this effect is not known, but it is likely due to altered cellular maturation, which is the case with folate and vitamin B_{12} deficiencies (51).

In addition to the peripheral blood neutrophilia resulting from the aforementioned mechanism, there is inhibition of neutrophil influx to sites of an inflammatory response. The inhibition of neutrophil influx by GCC results from reduced margination, reduced sticking of the neutrophil to blood vessel walls, and inhibition of chemotaxis. In fact, it has been observed that GCC at pharmacologic concentrations are able to totally suppress neutrophil chemotaxis toward complement-derived anaphylatoxins (164).

Two possible mechanisms of GCC-induced inhibition of neutrophil chemotaxis have been proposed: a direct inhibitory effect on chemotaxis and an effect mediated through the reduced generation of LTB_4, one of the most potent chemotactic molecules discovered at inflammatory sites.

Pretreatment of human neutrophils with dexamethasone, at low concentrations, directly inhibits their chemotaxis, as determined by the modified Boyden chamber method (68). This effect was demonstrated to be independent of any factor released within the sample (110). On the other hand, rat neutrophils exposed to opsonized zymosan particles *in vitro* instantaneously and continuously released a chemotactic factor into the medium. This activity was attributed to LTB_4 based on the data obtained from high-performance liquid chromatography (HPLC). Dexamethasone at 0.25 μg/ml caused suppression of generation of LTB_4 from leukocytes in a time-dependent manner (110). Human studies also support a modulation of neutrophil chemotaxis by LTB_4 and its inhibition in the presence of dexamethasone (149). LTB_4 generated in inflammatory sites was identified by reverse-phase HPLC. Local application of dexamethasone in these inflammatory sites suppressed chemotactic activity of the lipophilic fraction containing LTB_4 activity, in parallel with inhibition of neutrophil infiltration.

After neutrophils arrive at sites of inflammation, lysosomal constituents are released either during phagocytosis or as a consequence of cytolysis. Among the lysosomal constituents released are several enzymes and proteins that support the inflammatory process. GCC inhibit macrophage, neutrophil, and lymphocyte secretory responses (102).

Inhibition of the release of mediators is somewhat selective and is most often described for those mediators dependent on phospholipase A_2 activity. For GCC-induced mediator release, phospholipase A_2 activity is diminished, and prostaglandin E_2 release in neutrophils is decreased, even though the activity of other membrane phosphotransferases is not altered by GCC (14).

The secretion of plasminogen activator has been correlated with cell migration into inflammatory loci. GCC block the production of plasminogen activator by human neutrophils (76).

The effect of GCC on enhancement of the neutrophil response to β-adrenergic stimulation has been described. Only 4 hr after in vivo administration of 100 mg hydrocortisone, granulocyte adenylate cyclase activity in response to prostaglandin E or isoproterenol is increased significantly (42). There is an increase in granulocyte β-adrenergic receptor number of 40% and an equivalent decrease in lymphocyte β-adrenergic receptor number of 40% only 4 hr after administration of 100 mg of cortisone acetate to normal subjects. After 24 hr, both types of leukocytes show increased numbers of β-adrenergic receptors. Thus, GCC facilitate β-adrenergic receptor responsiveness by increasing both leukocyte receptor number and their coupling to adenylate cyclase.

In addition, GCC may influence cAMP-dependent protein kinases and affect β-adrenergic responsiveness, with a rise in cAMP levels through this mechanism. There is a specific and marked reduction by GCC of ^{32}P incorporation into a protein of 54,000 d. Phosphorylation of this protein is also regulated by cAMP, and it is the regulatory subunit of type II cAMP-dependent protein kinase. GCC may affect not only the autophosphorylation of this protein kinase but also its cellular concentration and isoenzyme pattern (114).

It has been suggested by some investigators that the increase in β-receptor responsivenesses is affected by inhibition of extraneuronal uptake of β agonists (69).

In addition, there is evidence that superoxide generation, which is critical to effective neutrophil antimicrobial function, is altered with GCC treatment. Superoxide production and release of lactoferrin and lysozyme from human peripheral-blood polymorphonuclear leukocytes were inhibited in a dose-dependent manner by dexamethasone incubation for 20 min at 37°C (33). In another study, a change in the characteristics of membrane phospholipids was noted in human neutrophils after incubation with dexamethasone at low concentrations (123). Concomitantly, these cells were found to be deficient in

superoxide production. These results supported an effect of GCC-induced lipid changes on the subsequent activity of the oxidase responsible for superoxide anion production.

Selective peptide synthesis in human peripheral-blood neutrophils is also affected by GCC. The rate of incorporation of L-[^{35}S]methionine into nine polypeptides, as determined by two-dimensional gel electrophoresis, was consistently influenced by dexamethasone in a dose-dependent manner. Functional correlations with these observations have not yet been made (14).

Finally, malakoplakia is a chronic granulomatous inflammatory disorder in which leukocytes fail to kill *Staphylococcus aureus* and *E. coli* normally *in vitro*. Malakoplakia occurs most frequently in patients on chronic immunosuppression with prednisone. Recent reports cite *E. coli* as the most frequent infecting agent. The clinical features demonstrate evidence of redistributed cells and diminished cellular function *in vivo*. Thus, it has been suggested that this illness may represent a clinical correlate of the long-term overall GCC effect on inflammatory surveillance by the neutrophil (11).

Thus, GCC affect the function of polymorphonuclear leukocytes by inhibiting chemotaxis, preventing production and release of some cellular products, suppressing endocytosis, and preventing oxidative function through modulation of superoxide generation. As detailed earlier, these major GCC-induced effects on polymorphonuclear leukocytes result in some antiinflammatory actions of the hormone.

Monocytes and Macrophages

Monocytes are more susceptible to GCC-induced depletion from peripheral blood than are lymphocytes (80). Similar to the redistribution occurring with lymphocytes, however, the peak effect occurs 4 to 6 hr following GCC administration and lasts for 24 hr (55).

GCC inhibits the clearance of antibody-coated red cells by the mononuclear phagocyte system, probably by interfering with binding of antibody-coated cells to Fc receptors on macrophages (4). Monocyte IgG and C3 receptor functions are suppressed by pharmacologic doses of GCC (149). This observation serves as a rationale for the use of GCC in autoimmune hemolytic anemia and other hemolytic states in which receptors for the Fc portion of IgG are increased in number (63).

Monocyte chemotaxis is inhibited *in vitro* by GCC in pharmacologic concentrations (140). In fact, skin-window studies have demonstrated a much more sensitive response to GCC for monocytes than for neutrophils (41). However, when monocytes are harvested from patients receiving GCC therapy, suppression of chemotaxis cannot be induced by *in vitro* GCC (161).

Monocytes and macrophages are very important components of the pathologic process in illnesses such as giant cell arteritis, and GCC constitute a mainstay of chemotherapy for this illness (58). The modulation of lymphokine-induced giant cell formation by GCC has been examined in rabbits. Low concentrations of GCC consistently inhibited giant cell formation elicited by macrophage fusion factor (MFF) without affecting macrophage viability (67). GCC at pharmacologic concentrations affected the migration inhibition of alveolar macrophages induced by macrophage inhibition factor (MIF). MFF and MIF are released into the culture medium after 24 hr of incubation of rabbit lymph node lymphocytes with heat-killed Calmette-Guérin bacillus (BCG). Cell-free supernatants from these cultures induce giant cell formation and migration inhibition of homologous normal alveolar macrophages (67). Thus, lymphokine-induced giant cell formation was suppressed by GCC. GCC suppress production of plasminogen activator and of IL-1 by human monocytes (165). Thus, two primary monocyte regulatory cytokine functions are altered with GCC therapy.

GCC inhibit phagocytosis and cell spreading in cultures of murine peritoneal macrophages (7). This inhibition appears to be mediated through a dexamethasone-induced substance in supernatants from macrophage cultures and is not reversed by addition of arachidonic acid or inhibitors of prostaglandin and leukotriene biosynthesis. Thus, these important macrophage functions appear to be inhibited by GCC independent of any GCC effect on prostaglandin or leukotriene release (7).

There is evidence that changes in receptor numbers may alter lysosomal function and pinocytosis in macrophages. Dexamethasone increases expression of mannose receptors and decreases extracellular lysosomal enzyme accumulation in macrophages (152). Macrophages express a mannose-specific pinocytosis receptor that binds and internalizes lysosomal hydrolases. Treatment of rat bone-marrow-derived macrophages with dexamethasone results in a concentration- and time-dependent increase in mannose receptor activity. Half-maximal effects were observed at a dexamethasone concentration of 10^{-9} M. Cell surface binding was elevated 2.6-fold, and ^{125}I-β-glucuronidase uptake was increased 2.5-fold after dexamethasone treatment. Increased binding appeared to be due to an increase in receptor number without a change in affinity. Extracellular levels of hexosaminidase were sharply reduced by dexamethasone treatment and corresponded with the rise in mannose-receptor activity (152). Thus, pinocytosis and lysosome function may be altered by GCC at the receptor level.

Macrophage endocytic receptors are regulated by GCC. Dexamethasone modulates lipoprotein metabolism in cultured human-monocyte-derived macrophages (91).

These cells have receptors for native low-density lipoprotein (LDL) and acetylated LDL (ALDL). ALDL uptake can promote cellular cholesteryl ester accumulation, which results in the formation of foam cells that are involved in the development of atherosclerotic disease. GCC preincubation inhibited LDL degradation to 50% of control, but doubled ALDL degradation. These effects occurred maximally by 24 hr and at 2.5×10^{-8} M dexamethasone. Progesterone had no effect on the function of these macrophages. Thus, dexamethasone inhibits LDL receptor activity and stimulates ALDL receptor activity in macrophages, leading to the development of foam cells (89). This is remarkable evidence that a finely tuned balance of acetylated and deacetylated receptors may be modulated by GCC and may result in a critical alteration of normal function.

There is evidence that GCC inhibit both the lipooxygenase and cyclooxygenase pathways (20,64). This clearly alters the inflammatory response regulated by the lipid mediators that contribute to that response. Dexamethasone inhibits the production of thromboxane B_2 and LTB_4 by human alveolar and peritoneal macrophages in culture. Stimulation of macrophages with zymosan A enhances the release of these two factors, whereas incubation in the presence of dexamethasone inhibits release of these factors in a concentration-dependent manner (64). In addition, dexamethasone inhibits release of prostaglandins and formation of autophagic vacuoles by stimulated macrophages (19).

There is some evidence that GCC inhibit wound healing through suppression of specific prostaglandin synthesis (50). Dexamethasone and lipopolysaccharide (LPS) have opposite effects on wound healing and on the production of specific prostaglandins. Dexamethasone at pharmacologic concentrations inhibits murine macrophage production of prostaglandin E_2 (PGE_2) and 6-keto-$PGF_{1\alpha}$, and to a lesser extent $PGF_{2\alpha}$. On the other hand, LPS has the opposite effect on the production of these prostaglandins. There is evidence that GCC may suppress chronic inflammatory events that result in the degradation of connective tissue (162). Collagenase and PGE_2 are present in increased amounts at the sites of chronic inflammatory lesions in connective tissue in guinea pigs. Dexamethasone results in a dose-dependent inhibition of macrophage PGE_2 and collagenase production (162). Finally, monocyte bactericidal action is suppressed by *in vitro* GCC (140). After *in vivo* GCC administration, both bactericidal and fungicidal activities are suppressed (141). Thus, recent research has augmented our knowledge of GCC effects on cellular components of inflammation and immunity and has demonstrated an important role for GCC modulation through the monocyte/macrophage, with a diversity similar to that described for GCC effects on the polymorphonuclear leukocyte.

Eosinophils

Eosinophils, like basophils, but unlike neutrophils, are redistributed out of the circulation within 4 to 5 hr following GCC administration; recovery from this effect occurs within 72 hr (48,105). Oral administration of one dose of 60 mg of prednisone caused a 97% decrease in total blood eosinophils within 5 hr (2).

Eosinophil adherence and chemotaxis are altered by GCC and may contribute to the continued and marked peripheral eosinopenia observed during GCC therapy (2,112). This is in contrast to the case for neutrophils, which are also affected by GCC by decreased adherence and chemotaxis. In the case of neutrophils, however, increased bone marrow release and delayed migration from the intravascular space result in a net peripheral neutrophilia.

Because of the observed eosinopenic effect *in vivo,* GCC have been found to provide effective chemotherapy for many illnesses associated with peripheral or tissue eosinophilia, including the idiopathic hypereosinophilic syndrome, Addison's disease, and allergic diseases associated with eosinophilia (23,139).

Basophils

Basophils are redistributed from the circulation after *in vivo* GCC (50). The peak effect occurs at 8 hr following GCC administration, which is slightly later than the effect of GCC on lymphocytes (4–6 hr) or on other polymorphonuclear leukocytes such as eosinophils (4–5 hr). Similarly, recovery from the GCC effect on basophils occurs at 72 hr, rather than at 24 hr as reported for other redistributed cell types (48).

Basophil histamine release is inhibited by corticosteroids (147). Dose–response studies of suppression of whole-blood histamine levels and basophil counts by prednisone have shown a correlation of these parameters with dose (146). This effect of GCC is dependent on the basophil subset examined. It has been demonstrated that *in vitro* culture of human basophils for 24 hr with even physiologic concentrations of GCC leads to a pronounced inhibition of the subsequent release of histamine or leukotrienes when the cells are challenged with anti-IgE. However, both acute and chronic *in vivo* therapy with GCC fails to impair subsequent histamine release from basophils *in vitro*. When normals and patients receiving chronic GCC therapy were studied, histamine release from basophils of normals and non-steroid-dependent asthmatics was markedly inhibited after *in vitro* dexamethasone treatment, as compared with both asthmatics and patients with collagen vascular diseases receiving chronic daily prednisone therapy. These may represent functional correlates for the observed redistribution of basophils (111).

Mast Cells

Mast cells constitute a heterogeneous cell population that may be concentrated in specific organs, may have different staining characteristics, and may respond differently to factors or to other immunoregulatory cells (114). Many of the recent data concerning GCC effects on mast cell function have been obtained from mouse studies. A decrease in markers of cellular activation, diminished factor release by specific antigenic challenge, and a decrease in IgE Fc-receptor expression have been demonstrated in the presence of GCC (9,39,142).

A decrease in IgE Fc-receptor expression on mouse bone-marrow-derived mast cells (BMMC) and inhibition of platelet-activating factor (PAF-acether) formation and of β-hexosaminidase (the granule marker) release by dexamethasone in the presence of DNP-specific monoclonal-IgE-specific antigenic challenge have been demonstrated (9). By contrast, ionophore-induced PAF-acether formation and β-hexosaminidase release were unaffected by dexamethasone. In addition, specific antigen-induced increase in acetyltransferase activity, which is used as an index of cellular activation for these mast cells, was diminished by 37% after pretreatment. The number of IgE Fc receptors was decreased by 55% in treated mast cells as compared with untreated cells. To demonstrate the possible link between decreased IgE Fc-receptor expression and alteration of the secretory response and acetyltransferase activity, BMMC were incubated with IgE under conditions resulting in half-sensitization of the cells. On antigen challenge, a 10% decrease in acetyltransferase activity and a 29% decrease in PAF-acether release were observed with half-sensitized cells, demonstrating the correlation between diminished IgE Fc-receptor expression induced by dexamethasone and the consequent cellular activation events (9).

Similarly, treatment of BMMC with dexamethasone produced a decrease in IgE Fc receptors by more than 55% and was associated with inhibition of IgE-dependent release of β-hexosaminidase, as well as of LTC_4 and LTB_4 (142).

GCC do not appear to affect cutaneous mast cell histamine release, because they have no effect on immediate reactions to skin testing (156) or on nasal allergen challenge (121). However, specific IgE-mediated *in vitro* histamine release by mouse peritoneal mast cells was inhibited by GCC, as noted previously (41).

Late-phase allergic reactions characterized by mixed cellular infiltrates, with predominantly lymphocytes and, to a lesser extent, polymorphonuclear leukocytes, occur at 8 hr after the immediate allergic response in humans (135). This late-phase reaction can be evoked by components of isolated mast cell granules, indicating that the mast cell granule matrix is the source of an inflammation-inducing factor. Even though pharmacologic concentrations of GCC do not affect the immediate allergic skin-test response, they do prevent the late cutaneous allergic responses in humans induced by IgE antiserum (135), compound 48/80, or ragweed (155). Clinically, GCC are the most effective agents available for preventing or reversing late-phase reactions in skin, nose, or airway. The mechanism of action of GCC in preventing late-phase reactions is not known in humans; however, in rats, GCC inhibit mast-cell-granule-induced late-phase reactions by depleting neutrophils from the site, thereby preventing the inflammatory component of the response (102).

Platelets

Although GCC have been shown to be efficacious in autoimmune disease in which platelets play a role in the pathogenesis, no specific effect of GCC on platelet function or distribution has been demonstrated in either normal volunteers or patients on chronic therapeutic doses of prednisone. Prednisone at 20 mg/day for 11 days in normal volunteers did not alter peripheral platelet counts (96).

It was previously demonstrated that high concentrations of GCC added to platelet-rich plasma inhibited platelet aggregation, presumably by inhibiting platelet thromboxane production (99). However, therapeutic doses of GCC had no effect on the platelet function of patients treated for various connective-tissue and hematologic disorders when examined at 12 hr after administration (98).

Capillary fragility has been attributed to possible platelet dysfunction resulting from long-term GCC administration. In order to address this question, 22 patients with connective-tissue disease or hematologic disorders were studied during a 2-day-to-6-week course of oral prednisone therapy, with doses ranging from 10 to 60 mg/day. Bleeding time, capillary fragility, threshold adenosine diphosphate concentration for secondary platelet aggregation, and platelet adhesiveness were unchanged by oral prednisone at 2 days or after 6 weeks of therapy (98). Such parameters of platelet function have not been examined after longer administration of GCC.

Fibroblasts

Dexamethasone at physiologic concentrations stimulates the growth of normal bone-marrow-derived fibroblasts *in vitro*. Specific binding sites for the hormone are present in normal fibroblasts (100).

GCC inhibit mouse fibroblast arachidonic acid release, possibly through phospholipase A_2 inhibition, as previously noted (62). This effect may contribute to the reduction in availability of mediators for inflammatory and immune responses in affected organs.

Lymphocytes

The most frequently studied immunoregulatory cell is the lymphocyte, and numerous effects of GCC on lymphocyte development and function have been reported. The majority of lymphoid cells from GCC-resistant species such as humans are resistant to the *in vivo* lytic effects of pharmacologic concentrations of GCC (28,30). Furthermore, *in vitro*, GCC do not induce lysis of human mononuclear cells (49).

In humans, a single dose of GCC results in a rapid (within 4 hr) and transient lymphopenia, with a return to normal peripheral lymphocyte counts in 24 hr (54). This lymphopenia is a result of redistribution rather than of cell lysis (56,57).

The redistribution of peripheral lymphocytes was found to be most profound for T lymphocytes of the Tμ phenotype (82), although B cells were also depressed in numbers following treatment with GCC. Tγ (82) and null cells (55) were not affected by GCC treatment. More recently, these results have been refined by the demonstration that OKT4 cells are preferentially decreased over OKT8 cells (38). In another study, prednisone induced T-lymphocyte depletion in peripheral blood, increased the cytotoxic/suppressor T-cell population, inhibited Ia expression on mitogenic activation of lymphocytes, and inhibited the autologous mixed leukocyte reaction (151). Monoclonal antibodies were used to detect each of these effects in the same cell population after a single GCC dose.

The population of cells depleted from the peripheral circulation during GCC administration is that part of the intravascular pool that normally recirculates between the intravascular and extravascular compartments (56,57). This observation was made by using radioactive chromium-labeled autologous lymphocytes (150). The circulatory pattern of the nonrecirculating intravascular lymphocytes is apparently unaltered by GCC administration *in vivo*. The extravascular site of redistribution in humans is not definitively known, although other steroid-resistant species have been shown to redistribute lymphocytes to the bone marrow in response to GCC administration (54).

Redistribution of cell subtypes may well play an immunomodulatory role in GCC therapy. There is evidence of lymphocyte subset redistribution after treatment with GCC at local sites of immunologic or inflammatory reactions in disease processes. The lymphocyte profiles of a cohort of 35 patients with sarcoidosis were analyzed with monoclonal antibodies to lymphocyte subsets (25). Untreated patients had significantly higher percentages of Leu-3a$^+$ T helper-inducer cells and lower percentages of Leu-2a$^+$ cytotoxic-suppressor cells within the alveolar lymphocyte population than did normal control subjects ($p < 0.002$). These untreated sarcoidosis patients also had enrichment of Leu-3a cells in bronchial lavage lymphocytes when compared to control subjects. GCC decreased the numbers of alveolar Leu-3a cells, with a marked increase in the proportion of suppressor cells, although the total numbers of alveolar T cells were not affected by the treatment (25). Numbers of helper cells were found to correlate positively with disease activity.

Massive lysis of normal lymphoid tissue following GCC administration does not occur in humans. However, activated lymphocyte subsets, such as seen in certain lymphoid tumors, may be sensitive to the lytic effect of GCC. Furthermore, HC in physiologic concentrations lyses activated T lymphocytes in a mixed leukocyte reaction, but does not lyse resting peripheral lymphocytes, thymocytes, or mitogen-activated T cells *in vitro* (66). Activated T cells in arthritic joints are also sensitive to GCC-induced lysis (66). Thus, although large-scale lysis is not a significant immunoregulatory mechanism in humans, GCC-induced lysis of a small subset of activated human lymphoid cells may be an important mechanism in GCC immunoregulation.

Several investigators have shown that proliferation of mitogenically stimulated lymphocytes is suppressed by *in vitro* GCC. The degree and length of this suppression are dependent on the type of mitogen, the concentration of mitogen, and cell maturity or cell-cycle phase (15,138). Figure 2 depicts a proposed model of B-cell activation and the GCC effects noted on cells in different cell-cycle phases.

For T lymphocytes, concanavalin-A-induced blastogenesis is readily suppressed by *in vitro* or *in vivo* pharmacologic doses of GCC. The phytohemagglutinin response is also suppressed whether GCC are administered *in vivo* or *in vitro*, although this response is clearly dependent on the purity of the cell population and on the GCC analogue administered. Dexamethasone and high-dose methylprednisolone given in pulse form produce the most profound suppression of the phytohemagglutinin response (54,165). Compared with the phytohemagglutinin response of lymphocytes, the PWM response is only moderately sensitive to the suppressive effects of GCC administered *in vivo* or *in vitro*. Furthermore, the observed GCC-induced suppression of proliferation is related to the kinetics of the responses of the cultures (84,85) and is dose-responsive (overcome with increasing concentrations of PWM) (75).

Independent observations in studies on resting human B lymphocytes have also demonstrated distinct effects of GCC, depending on the mitogen selected. HC most completely induces suppression of the B-cell proliferative response to phorbol esters, intermediately suppresses the response to sIg-mediated mitogens, and does not suppress the B-cell proliferative response to the calcium ionophore A23187 (D. L. Bowen and A. S. Fauci, *unpublished data*). In the case of B-lymphocyte responses, a contaminating mitogen-responsive accessory cell population has been virtually excluded as an explanation for the differences in the GCC modulations of these mitogenic responses. Of more physiologic relevance is the fact that lymphocyte proliferative responses to specific antigens are remarkably suppressed by GCC both *in vivo* and *in vitro*. The proliferative responses of T cells to streptokinase-streptodornase and tetanus toxoid are markedly suppressed by *in vivo* administration of GCC, as compared with the mitogenic response of the same lymphocyte population (55). Both

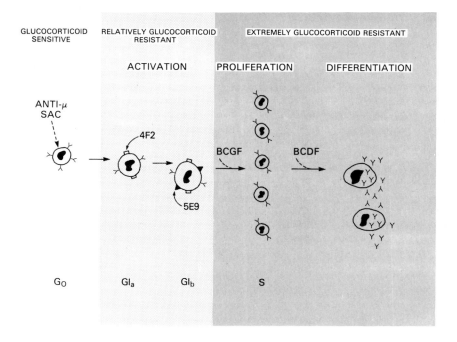

FIG. 2. Hypothetical model of B-cell activation. GCC exert the most suppressive effect on B cells that are in the G_0 phase of the cell cycle, preventing effective cycle entry in the presence of typical mitogens. Antigens that define cell-cycle entry into G_{1a} phase (4F2) and G_{1b} phase (5E9) have been shown to be diminished in expression in the presence of GCC added at the initiation of cultures. Functions of B cells that are activated *in vivo* or *in vitro* prior to GCC addition are not affected.

allogeneic and autologous MLRs are inhibited by GCC, with a striking sensitivity of the autologous MLR (94) to even physiologic concentrations of GCC. It is not known if this effect plays a role in normal immune surveillance or in the prevention of autoimmune processes.

It is clear that GCC-induced suppression of mitogenic or antigenic responses is dependent on a critically timed exposure to GCC in culture. It was found that GCC affected the proliferative response of human lymphocytes stimulated *in vitro* by a polysaccharide purified from *Candida albicans.* If dexamethasone was added at the beginning of the culture period, cell proliferation and IL-1/IL-2 synthesis was suppressed; however, if dexamethasone was added after 48 hr, enhancement of cellular proliferation was seen and was maximum at day 4 (134). These authors concluded that GCC inhibited the differentiation of T suppressor cells and that IL-2 was unable to reverse this inhibitory effect.

With regard to the effect of GCC on suppressor cell function, the suppressor cell of the PWM-stimulated anti-sheep-red-blood-cell plaque-forming cell response is sensitive to both *in vitro* and *in vivo* GCC (83). In contrast, GCC enhance the concanavalin-A-induced suppressor cell activity that affects B-cell function if added at the initiation of culture (83) and augment the concanavalin-A-induced suppressor cell function present in an MLR (90).

Thus, GCC appear to affect suppressor cell function under different culture conditions. Undoubtedly, the mechanisms of the GCC effects in these situations are different. Nevertheless, some of the observed effects may be explained by the fact that T-cell production of IL-2 is also directly suppressed by GCC at the T-cell message level as well as through suppression of the monocyte-derived, IL-1-stimulated production of IL-2 in an MLR.

The MLR response involving T-cell and macrophage cooperation is markedly inhibited by GCC, as previously stated. However, depletion of monocytes from lymphocyte cultures that are mitogenically treated results in enhanced suppression of proliferation by GCC *in vitro* (13,169), and readdition of autologous monocytes may partially correct this *in vivo* GCC-induced suppression (55).

In any case, suppressor cell regulation is not the only mechanism of GCC-induced effects on lymphocyte proliferation. We have shown that when added to cultures early, GCC suppressed the mitogenic response of highly purified resting B cells. If the cells were exposed to mitogen and allowed to stay in culture for 36 to 48 hr, GCC did not diminish the mitogenic response (15). These results suggest that the B-lymphocyte response to GCC is cell-cycle-dependent (Fig. 2).

The relationship between the binding of dexamethasone and the particular phase of the cell cycle in mouse and human lymphoid cell lines has been determined. The amount of dexamethasone bound per cell in each fraction was measured by a whole-cell binding assay. In three dexamethasone-responsive cell lines (2 mouse and 1 human) the amount of dexamethasone bound per cell increased fourfold between G_1 phase and S phase and decreased during G_2/M phase without a change in binding affinity (49). On the other hand, three dexamethasone-nonresponsive lines (1 human) did not increase the amount of dexamethasone bound per cell during S phase. Therefore, an increase in GCC binding during S phase may be required for GCC to inhibit cell growth, and failure of GCC binding to increase during S phase might represent a mechanism of GCC resistance in lymphoid cells. As mentioned previously, purified populations of human cells that vary in their stages of the cell cycle have been examined for the presence of intracytoplasmic receptors, and no relationship between GCC effects and steroid binding parameters has been defined (65,113,125). However, responses to GCC binding in cellular subsets at the same stage of the cell cycle may define populations of cells that respond similarly to GCC.

T cells with an Fc receptor for IgE have been demonstrated to be significantly depressed in the circulation following GCC administration (157). The basis of this peripheral depletion may not involve redistribution of lymphocyte subsets, because direct inhibition of expression of IgE receptors on lymphocytes bearing this phenotype has been demonstrated in rodents. Dexamethasone was also demonstrated to prevent glycosylation of IgE-binding factors derived from T cells (168). As previously noted, this effect has been attributed to the generation of a lipocortin, glycosylation-inhibiting factor (6).

GCC-induced suppression of immune-response-gene-associated antigens on murine B cells has been demonstrated after *in vivo* intravenous administration of dexamethasone. A 75% reduction in the expression of sIa that peaked within 6 hr and returned to base-line levels by 12 hr after injection was observed. The observed effect was dose-dependent. This effect was also observed after injection of dexamethasone into athymic nude mice, suggesting that the suppressive effect of dexamethasone on expression of B-cell sIa was T-cell-independent (43).

In vivo administration of GCC may result in early (4 hr) potentiation (126) and in later (24 hr) suppression of natural killer (NK) activity (31,124,128). In addition, a suppressed expression of NK cell activity has been described in the presence of *in vitro* GCC (128). In other studies, overall NK activity was suppressed by dexamethasone (17,130). This effect appears to be due to a direct developmental inhibition of NK cells by dexamethasone and to the known suppression of IL-2 production that modulates the NK activity of otherwise normally developed NK cells. Dexamethasone inhibits the recoverable number of NK cells when added to peripheral-blood mononuclear cells cultured with soluble microbial antigens such as PPD or *Candida* polysaccharide extract (133). In addition, NK cell activity against the tumor cell target K562 was suppressed by dexamethasone, but overcome by addition of IL-2 to the culture medium (159). An early (4 hr) increase in antibody-dependent cellular cytotoxicity after *in vivo* GCC probably reflects the relative enrichment of cytotoxic effector cells in the circulation resulting from the redistribution effect previously described (127).

Thus, numerous effects of GCC on lymphocytes have been described. The most significant effects, however, appear to be suppression of growth and *in vivo* differentiation of both T and B cells, redistribution of cellular subsets, and inhibition of lymphokine production.

SUMMARY

GCC affect many components of the inflammatory and immune response in humans. These effects may be separated into several categories and have been summarized in Table 1.

First, GCC affect the generation of humoral mediators of inflammation and immunity. GCC inhibit *in vivo* Ig production, and this may in part explain why they are helpful agents in certain diseases characterized by polyclonal Ig responses or in illnesses that are characterized by excess Ig production. *In vitro* Ig production is enhanced by GCC and may be related to increased BCDF production by a T4 subset or to the differential effects of GCC on cells in later stages of differentiation. We have discussed data supporting each of these hypotheses. In either case, discovery of the mechanism of this apparent paradoxical response will further explain the specific effects of GCC on the immune response.

Eicosanoid generation and release may be inhibited through phospholipase A_2 suppression, perhaps by the GCC-induced production of lipocortins. However, at this date, more evidence is needed to support this hypothesis.

Selective histamine generation and release are inhibited in basophils and in some mast cells by GCC. The IgE-mediated response is prevented by GCC, but other signals such as ionophores or phorbol esters are not regulated by GCC. The effect of GCC is most apparent after 24 hr in culture. Furthermore, this effect of GCC does not appear to be mediated through phospholipase inhibition.

Cytokine generation is generally inhibited by GCC, and cell functions regulated by these cytokines are also suppressed. An exception to this general rule appears to be the observed increased *in vitro* production of BCDF by T4 cells stimulated with mitogen or by MLR. The physiologic significance of this apparent GCC potentiation of BCDF activity is not clear at the present time.

Second, GCC affect the function of cellular components

TABLE 1. *Effects of GCC on inflammation and immunity*

Humoral mediators
  Eicosanoids: inhibit production and release
  Histamine: inhibit generation and release in basophils and mast cells
  Ig production: in vivo, inhibit polyclonal production and decreases specific IgE synthesis; in vitro, effect depends on culture conditions and assay system used
  Cytokine generation: inhibit production of IL-1, IL-2, IL-3, MAF, CSF, γ-interferon, and plasminogen activator; may selectively enhance production of BCDF and Sendai-virus-induced interferon production
Cellular components
  Phagocytic cells: alter the distribution pattern, resulting in peripheral neutrophilia and in neutropenia at inflammatory sites; deplete monocytes from peripheral blood; prevent chemotaxis directly; inhibit phagocytosis and pinocytosis; suppress oxidative antimicrobial function through diminished production of superoxide; decrease cytotoxic function; decrease cytokine production; change surface receptor characteristics and alter cellular interactions
  Eosinophils: result in peripheral eosinophil depletion; decrease adherence and chemotaxis
  Basophils/mast cells: result in peripheral basophil depletion; decrease histamine and specific granule release; deplete histamine content in cells; change cell surface marker density
  Lymphocytes: deplete peritoneal cells of the OKT4 phenotype; suppress cell-cycle progression; may alter the mitogenic response, depending on the signal given; alter Ia and activation surface marker expression in cells in the early phases of cell cycle; suppress production of most lymphokines; inhibit cell-cell interactions
  Platelets: may inhibit platelet aggregation
  Fibroblasts: inhibit arachidonic acid release; stimulate growth of bone-marrow-derived fibroblasts

of inflammation and immunity. GCC inhibit the function of phagocytic cells by altering their normal distribution patterns, by preventing chemotaxis directly, by inhibiting endocytosis, by changing surface receptor characteristics, by decreasing superoxide production, by suppressing cytokine production, and by altering immune and inflammatory cell interactions.

Basophils and mast cells are redistributed by GCC, and histamine and specific granule release is blocked by GCC. Furthermore, GCC deplete histamine content in basophils over weeks to months. In addition, mast cells are prevented by GCC from eliciting the late-phase reaction in immediate hypersensitivity responses. This makes GCC the most effective therapeutic agent for the late phase of an allergic reaction. The mechanism of this effect in humans, however, is not yet known.

Lymphocyte function is inhibited by GCC suppression of cell-cycle progression. Furthermore, the effects of GCC on lymphocytes appear to be dependent on the phase of the cycle that the cell is in at the time of exposure to GCC. Surface markers of activation and Ia expression are decreased by incubation with GCC in responsive cellular subsets. Cytokine production is generally suppressed by GCC, and this has been shown to occur at the mRNA level in T-cell clones. Cellular cooperation of lymphocytes with each other or with monocytes is also decreased in the presence of GCC.

The efficacy of GCC in chemotherapy for severe asthma is a specific example of the complex effects that GCC may have on a disease process that has known inflammatory and immunologic sequelae. The asthmatic response is complex, involving both inflammatory and immune components. The major steps involved in this response include bronchial smooth-muscle spasm, mucosal edema, increased mucus secretion with mucus plugging, mucosal inflammation with eosinophilic and neutrophilic infiltrates, shedding of airway epithelial cells, basement membrane thickening, and hyperresponsiveness of the airway persisting even after the acute phases have cleared. Specific interactions with antigen and cell surface IgE appear to trigger the initial steps in this inflammatory response. The immunologic mechanisms involved in sensitization of the mast cells or basophils that possess this specific surface IgE are not yet defined. It is apparent that GCC can affect many components of this response, and it would be misleading to emphasize the GCC effect on only selected components. Clearly, we have discussed data suggesting that the primary therapeutic effects of GCC are to redistribute the cellular components of the response (including eosinophils, basophils, and neutrophils), to diminish specific IgE synthesis *in vivo,* to inhibit mediator release by cells that results in amplification of the asthmatic response, to inhibit mucus release (120), to potentiate the effects of β-adrenergic stimulation through several mechanisms, and to significantly reduce the late-phase reaction.

The net effect of GCC on human inflammatory and immune responses is suppression. In autoimmune and acute or chronic inflammatory illnesses, GCC can be lifesaving. On the other hand, in normal individuals, or when used in excess, GCC can lead to life-threatening complications.

REFERENCES

1. Adolf, G. R., and Swetley, P. (1979): Glucocorticoid hormones inhibit DNA synthesis and enhance interferon production in a human lymphoid cell line. *Nature,* 282:736–738.
2. Altman, L. C., Hill, J. S., Hairfield, W. M., and Mullarkey, M. F. (1981): Effects of corticosteroids on eosinophil chemotaxis and adherence. *J. Clin. Invest.,* 67:28–36.
3. Arya, S. K., Wong-Staal, F., and Gallo, R. C. (1984): Dexamethasone-mediated inhibition of human T cell growth factor and gamma interferon messenger RNA. *J. Immunol.,* 133:273–276.
4. Ashman, R. F., and Young-Karlan, B. R. (1981): Inhibition of

5. antigen-induced and anti-immunoglobulin-induced capping by hydrocortisone and propranolol. *Immunopharmacology,* 3:41–47.
5. Atkinson, J. P., and Frank, M. M. (1973): Effect of cortisone therapy on serum complement components. *J. Immunol.,* 111:1061–1066.
6. Beck-Neilson, H., DePirro, R., and Pedersen, O. (1980): Prednisone increases the number of insulin receptors on monocytes from normal subjects. *J. Clin. Endocrinol. Metab.,* 50:1–4.
7. Becker, J., and Grasso, R. J. (1985): Suppression of phagocytosis by dexamethasone in macrophage cultures: Inability of arachidonic acid, indomethacin, and nordihydroguaiaretic acid to reverse the inhibitory response mediated by a steroid-inducible factor. *Int. J. Immunopharmacol.,* 7:839–847.
8. Benacerraf, B. (1978): A hypothesis to relate the specificity of T lymphocytes and the activity of I region-specific Ir genes in macrophages and B lymphocytes. *J. Immunol.,* 120:1809–1812.
9. Benhamou, M., Ninio, E., Salem, P., Hieblot, C., Bessou, G., Pitton, C., Liu, F. T., and Mencia-Huerta, J. M. (1986): Decrease in IgE Fc receptor expression on mouse bone marrow-derived mast cells and inhibition of paf-acether formation and of β-hexosaminidase release by dexamethasone. *J. Immunol.,* 136:1385–1392.
10. Bettens, F., Kristensen, F., Walker, C., Schwul'era, U., and Bonnard, G. D. (1984): Lymphokine regulation of activated lymphocytes. II. Glucocorticoid and anti-Tac-induced inhibition of human T lymphocyte proliferation. *J. Immunol.,* 132:261–265.
11. Biggar, W. D., Crawford, L., Cardella, C., Bear, R. A., and Galdman, D. (1985): Malakoplakia and immunosuppressive therapy. Reversal of clinical and leukocyte abnormalities after withdrawal of prednisone and azathioprine. *Am. J. Pathol.,* 119:5–11.
12. Blackwell, G. J., Carnuccio, R., DiRosa, M., Flower, R. J., Parenta, L., and Persico, P. (1980): Macrocortin: A polypeptide causing the antiphospholipase effect of corticosteroids. *Nature,* 287:147.
13. Blomgren, H., and Andersson, B. (1976): Steroid sensitivity of the PHA and PWM responses *in vitro. Exp. Cell Res.,* 97:233–240.
14. Blowers, L. E., Jayson, M. I., and Jasani, M. K. (1985): Effect of dexamethasone on polypeptide synthesized in polymorphonuclear leucocytes. *FEBS Lett.,* 181:362–366.
15. Bowen, D. L., and Fauci, A. S. (1984): Selective suppressive effects of glucocorticoids on the early events in the human B cell activation process. *J. Immunol.,* 133:1885–1890.
16. Bowen, D. L., and Fauci, A. S. (1986): Anti-Tac alters glucocorticoid (GC) related in vitro T cell B cell differentiation factor (BCDF) production. *Fed. Proc.,* 45:998.
17. Bray, R., Abrams, S., and Brahmi, Z. (1983): Studies on the mechanism of human natural killer cell-mediated cytolysis. I. Modulation by dexamethasone and arachidonic acid. *Cell. Immunol.,* 78:100–113.
18. Brugge, J. S. (1986): The p35/p36 substrates of protein-tyrosine kinase as inhibitors of phospholipase A_2. *Cell,* 46:149–150.
19. Brune, K., Kalin, H., Rainsford, K. D., and Wagner, K. (1980): Dexamethasone inhibits the release of prostaglandins and the formation of autophagic vacuoles from stimulated macrophages. *Adv. Prostaglandin Thromboxane Res.,* 8:1679–1684.
20. Burke, J. F., and Flower, R. J. (1979): Effects of modulators of arachidonic acid metabolism in the synthesis and release of slow-reacting substance of anaphylaxis. *Br. J. Pharmacol.,* 65:35.
21. Bush, R. K., Geller, M., Busse, W. W., Flaherty, D. K., and Dickie, H. A. (1978): Response to corticosteroids in the hypereosinophilic syndrome: Association with increased IgE levels. *Arch. Intern. Med.,* 138:1244.
22. Butler, W. T., and Rossen, R. D. (1973): Effects of corticosteroids in immunity in man. I. Decreased serum IgG concentration caused by 3 or 5 days of high doses of methylprednisolone. *J. Clin. Invest.,* 52:2629–2640.
23. Byyny, R. L. (1976). Withdrawal from glucocorticoid therapy. *N. Engl. J. Med.,* 295:30–32.
24. Orson, F. M., Flagge, F. P., and Cashaw, J. L. (1985): Steroid-dependent T cell replacing factor: A 45,000-dalton protein produced by a T4-positive T cell. *Fed. Proc.,* 44:1713.
25. Ceuppens, J. L., Lacquet, L. M., Marien, G., Demedts, M., van den Eeckhout, A., and Stevens, E. (1984): Alveolar T-cell subsets in pulmonary sarcoidosis. Correlation with diseases activity and effect of steroid treatment. *Am. Rev. Respir. Dis.,* 129:563–568.

26. Chestnut, R. W., Colon, S. M., and Grey, H. M. (1982): Antigen presentation by normal B cells, B cell tumors, and macrophages: Functional and biochemical comparison. *J. Immunol.*, 128:1784-1788.

27. Chestnut, R. W., and Grey, H. M. (1981): Studies on the capacity of B cells to serve as antigen-presenting cells. *J. Immunol.*, 126: 1075-1079.

28. Claman, H. N. (1972): Corticosteroids and lymphoid cells. *N. Engl. J. Med.*, 287:388-397.

29. Claman, H. N. (1975): How corticosteroids work. *J. Allergy Clin. Immunol.*, 55:145-151.

30. Claman, H. N., Moorehead, J. W., and Benner, W. H. (1971): Corticosteroids and lymphoid cells *in vitro*. I. Hydrocortisone lysis of human, guinea pig, and mouse thymus cells. *J. Lab. Clin. Med.*, 78:499-507.

31. Clarke, J. R., Ganon, R. F., Gotch, F. M., Heyworth, M. R., MaClennan, I. C. M., Truelove, S. C., and Waller, C. A. (1977): The effect of prednisolone on leukocyte function in man. *Clin. Exp. Immunol.*, 28:292-301.

32. Cloix, J. F., Collard, O., Rothhut, B., and Russo-Marie, F. (1983): Characterization and partial purification of 'renocortins': Two polypeptides formed in renal cells causing the anti-phospholipase-like action of glucocorticoids. *Br. J. Pharmacol.*, 79:313-321.

33. Coates, T. D., Wolach, B., Tzeng, D. Y., Higgins, C., Baehner, R. L., and Boxner, L. A. (1983): The mechanism of action of the anti-inflammatory agents dexamethasone and Auranofin in human polymorphonuclear leukocytes. *Blood*, 62:1070-1077.

34. Cooper, D. A., Ducket, M., Petts, V., and Penny, R. (1979): Corticosteroid enhancement of immunoglobulin synthesis by pokeweed mitogen-stimulated human lymphocytes. *Clin. Exp. Immunol.*, 37: 145-151.

35. Crabtree, G. R., Munck, A., and Smith, K. A. (1980): Glucocorticoids and lymphocytes. II. Cell cycle-dependent changes in glucocorticoid receptor content. *J. Immunol.*, 125:13-17.

36. Culpepper, J. A., and Lee, F. (1985): Regulation of IL-3 expression by glucocorticoids in cloned murine T lymphocytes. *J. Immunol.*, 135:3191-3197.

37. Cupps, T. R., Edgar, L. C., and Fauci, A. S. (1982): Corticosteroid-induced modulation of immunoglobulin secretion by human B lymphocytes potentiation of background mitogenic signals. *J. Immunopharmacol.*, 4:255-263.

38. Cupps, T. R., Edgar, L. C., Thomas, C. A., and Fauci, A. S. (1984): Multiple mechanisms of B cell immunoregulation in man after administration of *in vivo* corticosteroids. *J. Immunol.*, 132:170-175.

39. Daeron, M., Sterk, A. R., Hirata, F., and Ishizaka, T. (1982): Biochemical analysis of glucocorticoid-induced inhibition of IgE-mediated histamine release from mouse mast cells. *J. Immunol.*, 129: 1212-1218.

40. Dale, D. C., Fauci, A. S., Guerry, D. I. V., and Wolff, S. M. (1975): Comparison of agents producing a neutrophilic leukocytosis in man. Hydrocortisone, prednisone, endotoxin and etiocholanolone. *J. Clin. Invest.*, 56:808-813.

41. Dale, D. C., Fauci, A. S., and Wolff, S. M. (1974): Alternate-day prednisone leukocyte kinetics and susceptibility to infections. *N. Engl. J. Med.*, 291:1154-1158.

42. Davies, A. O., and Lefkowitz, R. J. (1980): Corticosteroid-induced differential regulation of β-adrenergic receptors in circulating human polymorphonuclear leukocytes and mononuclear leukocytes. *J. Clin. Endocrinol. Metab.*, 51:599-605.

43. Dennis, G. J., and Mond, J. J. (1986): Corticosteroid-induced suppression of murine B cell immune response antigens. *J. Immunol.*, 136:1600-1604.

44. DiRosa, M., Calignano, A., Carnuccio, R., Ialenti, A., and Sautebin, L. (1986): Multiple control of inflammation by glucocorticoids. *Agents Actions*, 17:284-289.

45. DiRosa, M., Flower, F. J., Hirata, F., Parente, L., and Russo-Marie, F. (1984): Nomenclature announcement. Anti-phospholipase proteins. *Prostaglandins*, 28:441-442.

46. Distelhorst, C. W., and Benutto, B. M. (1981): Glucocorticoid receptor content of T lymphocytes: Evidence for heterogeneity. *J. Immunol.*, 126:1630-1634.

47. Distelhorst, C. W., Benutto, B. M., and Bergamini, R. A. (1984): Effect of cell cycle position on dexamethasone binding by mouse and human lymphoid cell lines: Correlation between an increase in dexamethasone binding during S phase and dexamethasone sensitivity. *Blood*, 63:105-113.

48. Dunsky, E. H., Zweiman, B., Fishchler, E., and Levy, D. A. (1979): Early effects of corticosteroids on basophils, leukocyte histamine, and tissue histamine. *J. Allergy Clin. Immunol.*, 64:426-432.

49. Dupont, E., Berkenboom, G., Leempoel, M., and Potvliege, P. (1980): Failure of dexamethasone to induce *in vivo* lysis of human mononuclear cells. *Transplantation*, 30:387-389.

50. Durant, S., Homo-Delarche, F., Duval, D., Papiernik, M., Smets, P., and Zalisz, R. (1985): Opposite effects of glucocorticoid and an immunostimulating agent on prostaglandin production by two different cell types. *Int. J. Tissue React.*, 7:117-122.

51. Eichacker, P., and Lawrence, C. (1985): Steroid-induced hypersegmentation in neutrophils. *Am. J. Hematol.*, 18:41-45.

52. Errasfa, M., Rothhut, B., Fradin, A., Billardon, C., Junien, J. L., Bure, J., and Russo-Marie, F. (1985): The presence of lipocortin in human embrylonic skin fibroblasts and its regulation by anti-inflammatory steroids. *Biochim. Biophys. Acta*, 847:247-254.

53. Fauci, A. S. (1975): Mechanism of corticosteroid action on lymphocyte subpopulations. I. Redistribution of the circulating T and B lymphocytes to the bone marrow. *Immunology*, 28:669-680.

54. Fauci, A. S. (1976): Mechanisms of corticosteroid action on lymphocyte subpopulations. II. Differential effects of *in vivo* hydrocortisone, prednisone and dexamethasone on *in vitro* expression of lymphocyte function. *Clin. Exp. Immunol.*, 24:54-62.

55. Fauci, A. S., and Dale, D. C. (1974): The effect of *in vivo* hydrocortisone on subpopulations of human lymphocytes. *J. Clin. Invest.*, 53:240-246.

56. Fauci, A. S., and Dale, D. C. (1975): Alternate-day prednisone therapy and human lymphocyte subpopulations. *J. Clin. Invest.*, 55:22-32.

57. Fauci, A. S., and Dale, D. C. (1975): The effect of hydrocortisone on the kinetics of normal human lymphocytes. *Blood*, 46:235-243.

58. Fauci, A. S., Dale, D. C., and Balow, J. E. (1976): Glucocorticosteroid therapy: Mechanism of action and clinical considerations. *Ann. Intern. Med.*, 84:304-315.

59. Fauci, A. S., Murakami, T., Brandon, D. D., Loriaux, D. L., and Lipsett, M. B. (1980): Mechanism of corticosteroid action on lymphocyte subpopulations. VI. Lack of correlation between glucocorticoid receptors and the differential effects of glucocorticosteroids on T-cell subpopulations. *Cell. Immunol.*, 49:43-50.

60. Fauci, A. S., Pratt, K. R., and Whalen, G. (1977): Activation of human B lymphocytes. IV. Regulating effects of corticosteroids on the triggering signal in the plaque-forming response of human peripheral blood B lymphocytes to polyclonal activation. *J. Immunol.*, 119:598-603.

61. Flower, R. (1981): Corticosteroids, phospholipase A$_2$ and inflammation. *Trends Pharm. Sci.*, 2:186.

62. Flower, R. J. (1986): Background and discovery of lipocortins. *Agents Actions*, 17:255-262.

63. Fries, L. F., Brickman, C. M., and Frank, M. M. (1983): Monocyte receptors for the Fc portion of IgG increase in number in autoimmune hemolytic anemia and other hemolytic states and are decreased by glucocorticoid therapy. *J. Immunol.*, 131:1240-1245.

64. Fuller, R. W., Kelsey, C. R., Cole, P. J., Dollery, C. T., and MacDermot, J. (1984): Dexamethasone inhibits the production of thromboxane B$_2$ and leukotriene B$_4$ by human alveolar and peritoneal macrophages in culture. *Clin. Sci.*, 67:653-656.

65. Gailani, S., Minowada, J., Silvernail, P., Nassbaum, A., Kaiser, N., Rosen, F., and Shimaoka, K. (1973): Specific glucocorticoid binding in human hemopoietic cell lines and neoplastic tissue. *Cancer Res.*, 33:2653-2657.

66. Galini, N., Galili, U., Klein, E., Rosenthal, L., and Nordenskjold, B. (1980): Human T lymphocytes become glucocorticoid-sensitive upon immune action. *Cell. Immunol.*, 50:440-444.

67. Galindo, B. (1984): Glucocorticoid modulation of lymphokine-induced giant cell formation. *Inflammation*, 8:393-406.

68. Gallin, J. I., Durocher, J. R., and Kaplan, A. P. (1975): Interaction

of leukocyte chemotactic factors with the cell surface. I. Chemotactic factor induced changes in human granulocyte surface charge. *J. Clin. Invest.*, 55:967–974.

69. Geddes, B. A., Jones, T. R., Dvorsky, R. J., and Lefcoe, N. M. (1974): Interaction of glucocorticoids and bronchodilators on isolated guinea pig tracheal and human bronchial smooth muscle. *Am. Rev. Respir. Dis.*, 110:420–427.

70. Gerrard, T. L., Cupps, T. R., Jurgensen, C. H., and Fauci, A. S. (1984): Increased expression of HLA-DR antigens in hydrocortisone-treated monocytes. *Cell. Immunol.*, 84:311–316.

71. Gerrard, T. L., Cupps, T. R., Jurgensen, C. H., and Fauci, A. S. (1984): Hydrocortisone-mediated inhibition of monocyte antigen presentation: Dissociation of inhibitory effect and expression of DR antigens. *Cell. Immunol.*, 85:330–339.

72. Gertel, H., and Kaliner, M. (1984): The biologic activity of mast cell granules in rat skin: Effects of adrenocorticosteroids on late-phase inflammatory responses induced by mast cell granules. *J. Allergy Clin. Immunol.*, 68:228–235.

73. Gillis, S., Crabtree, G. R., and Smith, K. A. (1979): Glucocorticoid-induced inhibition of T cell growth factor production. I. The effect on mitogen-induced lymphocyte proliferation. *J. Immunol.*, 123:1624–1631.

74. Goodwin, J. S., Atluru, D., Sierakowski, S., and Lianos, E. A. (1986): Mechanism of action of glucocorticosteroids. Inhibition of T cell proliferation and interleukin 2 production by hydrocortisone is reversed by leukotriene B_4. *J. Clin. Invest.*, 77:1244–1250.

75. Gordon, D., and Nouri, A. M. E. (1981): Comparison of the inhibition by glucocorticosteroids and cyclosporin A of mitogen-stimulated human lymphocyte proliferation. *Clin. Exp. Immunol.*, 44:287–294.

76. Granelli-Piperno, A., Yassalli, J. D., and Reich, E. (1977): Secretion of plasminogen activator by human polymorphonuclear leukocytes: Modulation by glucocorticoids and other effectors. *J. Exp. Med.*, 146:1693–1706.

77. Gupta, C., and Goldman, A. S. (1985): Dexamethasone-induced phospholipase A_2-inhibitory proteins (PLIP) influenced by the H-2 histocompatibility region. *Proc. Soc. Exp. Biol. Med.*, 178:29–35.

78. Gupta, C., Katsumata, M., Goldman, A. S., Herold, R., and Piddington, R. (1984): Glucocorticoid-induced phospholipase A_2-inhibitory proteins mediate glucocorticoid teratogenicity *in vitro*. *Proc. Natl. Acad. Sci. USA*, 81:1140–1143.

79. Gurpide, E., Markiewicz, L., Schatz, F., and Hirata, F. (1986): Lipocortin output by human endometrium in vitro. *J. Clin. Endocrinol. Metab.*, 63:162–166.

80. Hahn, B. H., MacDermott, R. P., Jacobs, S. B., Pletscher, L. S., and Beale, M. G. (1980): Immunosuppressive effects of low doses of glucocorticoids: Effects on autologous and allogenic mixed leukocyte reactions. *J. Immunol.*, 124:2812–2817.

81. Hammond, C. V., Hammond, M. D., and Taylor, W. A. (1982): Selective inhibition by β-methasone of allergen-induced release of SRS-A from human lung. *Int. Arch. Allergy Appl. Immunol.*, 67:284–286.

82. Haynes, B. F., and Fauci, A. S. (1978): The differential effect of *in vivo* hydrocortisone on kinetics of subpopulations of human peripheral blood thymus-derived lymphocytes. *J. Clin. Invest.*, 61:703–707.

83. Haynes, B. F., and Fauci, A. S. (1979): Mechanisms of corticosteroid action of lymphocyte subpopulations. IV. Effects of *in vitro* hydrocortisone on naturally occurring and mitogen-induced suppressor cells in man. *Cell. Immunol.*, 44:157–168.

84. Heilman, D. H. (1972): Failure of hydrocortisone to inhibit blastogenesis by pokeweed mitogen in human leukocyte cultures. *Clin. Exp. Immunol.*, 11:393–403.

85. Heilman, D. H., Gambrill, M., and Leichner, J. P. (1973): The effect of hydrocortisone on the incorporation of tritiated thymidine by human blood lymphocytes cultured with phytohaemagglutinin and pokeweed mitogen. *Clin. Exp. Immunol.*, 15:203–212.

86. Hench, P. S., and Boland, E. W. (1949): Potential reversibility of rheumatoid arthritis. *Proc. Staff Meeting Mayo Clin.*, 24:167–168.

87. Hirata, F., and Axelrod, J. (1980): Phospholipid methylation and biological signal transmission. *Science*, 20:1082–1090.

88. Hirata, F., Schiffmann, E., Venkatasubramanian, K., Salomon, D., and Axelrod, J. (1980): A phospholipase A_2 inhibitory protein in rabbit neutrophils induced by corticosteroids. *Proc. Natl. Acad. Sci. USA*, 77:2533–2536.

89. Hirsch, L. J., and Mazzone, T. (1986): Dexamethasone modulates lipoprotein metabolism in cultured human monocyte-derived macrophages. Stimulation of scavenger receptor activity. *J. Clin. Invest.*, 77:485–490.

90. Hirschberg, T., Brandazzo, B., and Hirschberg, H. (1980): Effects of methylprednisolone on the *in vitro* induction and function of suppressor cells in man. *Scand. J. Immunol.*, 12:33–39.

91. Hokland, M., Larsen, B., Heron, I., and Plesner, T. (1981): Corticosteroids decrease the expressions of beta-2-microglobulin and histocompatibility antigens on human peripheral blood lymphocytes *in vitro*. *Clin. Exp. Immunol.*, 44:239–246.

92. Hoover, R. L., Dawidowicz, E. A., Rabinson, J. M., and Karnovsky, M. J. (1983): Role of cholesterol in the capping of surface immunoglobulin receptors on murine lymphocytes. *J. Cell Biol.*, 97:73–80.

93. Huang, K. S., Wallner, B. P., Mattaliano, R. J., Tizard, R., Burne, C., Frey, A., Hession, C., McGray, P., Sinclair, L. K., Chow, E. P., et al. (1986): Two human 35 kd inhibitors of phospholipase A_2 are related to substrates of pp60v-src and of the epidermal growth factor receptor/kinase. *Cell*, 46:191–199.

94. Ilfeld, D. N., Krakauer, R. S., and Blaese, M. (1977): Suppression of the human autologous mixed leukocyte reaction by physiologic concentrations of hydrocortisone. *J. Immunol.*, 119:428–434.

95. Indiveri, F., Scudeletti, M., Pende, D., Barabino, A., Russo, C., Pellegrino, M. A., and Ferrone, S. (1983): Inhibitory effect of a low dose of prednisone on PHA-induced Ia antigen expression by human T cells and on proliferation of T cells stimulated with autologous PHA-T cells. *Cell. Immunol.*, 80:320–328.

96. Isacson, S. (1970): Effect of prednisolone on the coagulation and fibrinolytic systems. *Scand. J. Haematol.*, 7:212–216.

97. Jardieu, P., Akasaki, M., and Ishizaka, K. (1986): Association of I-J determinants with lipomodulin/macrocortin. *Proc. Natl. Acad. Sci. USA*, 83:160–164.

98. Jorgensen, K. A., Freund, L., and Sorensen, P. (1982): The effect of prednisone on platelet function tests. *Scand. J. Haematol.*, 28:118–121.

99. Jorgensen, K. A., and Stoffersen, E. (1981): Hydrocortisone inhibits platelet prostaglandin and endothelial prostacyclin production. *Pharmacol. Res. Commun.*, 13:579–586.

100. Juneja, H. S., Minguell, J. J., Gardner, F. H., Helmer, R. E., and Lee, S. (1984): The effect of dexamethasone on the growth of bone marrow fibroblasts in aplastic anemia. *Prog. Clin. Biol. Res.*, 154:265–274.

101. Kakiuchi, T., Chestnut, R. W., and Grey, H. M. (1983): B cells as antigen-presenting cells: The requirement for B cell activation. *J. Immunol.*, 131:109–114.

102. Kaliner, M. (1985): Mechanisms of glucocorticosteroid action in bronchial asthma. *J. Allergy Clin. Immunol.*, 76:231–329.

103. Kaliner, M., and Lemanske, R. (1984): Inflammatory responses to mast cell granules. *Fed. Proc.*, 43:2845–2851.

104. Katz, P., and Fauci, A. S. (1979): Autologous and allogeneic intercellular interactions: Modulation by adherent cells, irradiation, and *in vitro* and *in vivo* corticosteroids. *J. Immunol.*, 123:2270–2277.

105. Kellgren, J. H., and Janus, O. (1951): The eosinopenic response to cortisone and ACTH in normal subjects. *Br. Med. J.*, 2:1183.

106. Kelso, A., and Munck, A. (1984): Glucocorticoid inhibition of lymphokine secretion by alloreactive T lymphocyte clones. *J. Immunol.*, 133:784–791.

107. Kristensen, T., Saris, C. J., Hunter, T., Hicks, L. J., Noonan, D. J., Glenney, J. R., Jr., and Tack, B. F. (1986): Primary structure of bovine calpactin I heavy chain (p36), a major cellular substrate for retroviral protein-tyrosine kinases: Homology with the human phospholipase A_2 inhibitor lipocortin. *Biochemistry*, 25:4497–4503.

108. Kumar, L., Newcomb, R. W., Ishizaka, K., Middleton, E., and Hornbrook, M. M. (1971): IgE levels in sera of children with asthma. *Pediatrics*, 47:848–856.

109. Kurihara, A., Ojima, F., and Tsurufuji, S. (1984): Analysis of the

effect of an anti-inflammatory steroid, dexamethasone, on neutrophil chemotaxis in the Boyden chamber with a modified ^{51}Cr-labeling method. *J. Pharmacobiodyn.*, 7:747–754.

110. Kurihara, A., Ojima, F., and Tsurufuji, S. (1984): Chemotactic factor production by rat polymorphonuclear leukocytes: Stimulation with opsonized zymosan particles and inhibition by dexamethasone. *Biochem. Biophys. Res. Commun.*, 119:720–725.

111. Lampl, K. L., Lichtenstein, L. M., and Schleimer, R. P. (1985): *In vitro* resistance to dexamethasone of basophils from patients receiving long-term steroid therapy. *Am. Rev. Respir. Dis.*, 132:1015–1018.

112. Lippman, M., and Barr, R. (1977): Glucocorticoid receptors in purified subpopulations of human peripheral blood lymphocytes. *J. Immunol.*, 118:1977–1981.

113. Lippman, M. E., Perry, S., and Thompson, E. B. (1974): Cytoplasmic glucocorticoid-binding proteins in glucocorticoid-unresponsive human and mouse leukemic cell lines. *Cancer Res.*, 34: 1572–1576.

114. Liu, A. Y. C. (1984): Modulation of the function and activity of cAMP-dependent protein kinase by steroid hormones. *Trends Pharm. Sci.*, 3:106.

115. MacDonald, R. G., and Cidlowski, J. A. (1981): Glucocorticoid-stimulated protein degradation in lymphocytes: Quantitation by sodium dodecyl sulfate-polyacrylamide gel electrophoresis. *Arch. Biochem. Biophys.*, 212:399–410.

116. MacDonald, R. G., and Cidlowski, J. A. (1982): Glucocorticoids inhibit precursor incorporation into protein in splenic lymphocytes by stimulating protein degradation and expanding intracellular amino acid pools. *Biochem. Biophys. Acta*, 717:236–247.

117. MacDonald, R. G., Martin, T. P., and Cidlowski, J. A. (1980): Glucocorticoids stimulate protein degradation in lymphocyte: A possible mechanism of steroid-induced cell death. *Endocrinology*, 107:1512–1524.

118. MacGregor, R. R., Spangnuolo, P. J., and Lentnek, A. L. (1974): Inhibition of granulocyte adherence by ethanol, prednisone and aspirin measured in an assay system. *N. Engl. J. Med.*, 291:642–646.

119. Madsen, M., Kissmeyer-Neilson, F., Rasmussen, P., and Andersen, P. (1981): Decreased expression of HLA-DR antigens on peripheral blood B lymphocytes during glucocorticoid treatment. *Tissue Antigens*, 17:195–204.

120. Marom, Z., Shelhamer, J., Alling, D., and Kaliner, M. (1984): The effects of corticosteroids on mucous glycoprotein secretion from human airways *in vitro. Am. Rev. Respir. Dis.*, 129:62–65.

121. Mygind, N., Johnson, N. J., and Thomsen, J. (1977): Intranasal allergen challenge during corticosteroid treatment. *Clin. Allergy*, 7:69–74.

122. Naccache, P. H., Showell, S. J., Becker, E. L., and Sha'afi, R. I. (1977): Changes in ionic movements across rabbit polymorphonuclear leukocyte membranes during lysosomal enzyme release. *J. Cell Biol.*, 75:635–649.

123. Nelson, D. H., Murray, D. K., and Brady, R. O. (1982): Dexamethasone-induced change in the sphingomyelin content of human polymorphonuclear leukocytes *in vitro. J. Clin. Endocrinol. Metab.*, 54:292–295.

124. Onsrud, M., and Thorsby, E. (1981): Influence of *in vivo* hydrocortisone on some human blood lymphocyte subpopulations. I. Effect on natural killer cell activity. *Scand. J. Immunol.*, 13:573–579.

125. Paavonen, T., Andersson, L. C., and Kontula, K. (1980): Lack of correlation between the glucocorticoid receptor density and the *in vivo* growth-inhibitory effect of dexamethasone in human leukemia cell lines. *J. Recept. Res.*, 1:459–472.

126. Parker, C. W., Huber, M. G., and Baumann, M. L. (1973): Alterations of the cyclic AMP metabolism in human bronchial asthma. III. Leukocyte and lymphocyte responses to steroids. *J. Clin. Invest.*, 52:1342–1348.

127. Parrillo, J. E., and Fauci, A. S. (1978): Mechanism of corticosteroid action on lymphocyte subpopulations. III. Differential effects of dexamethasone administration on subpopulations of effector cells mediating cellular cytotoxicity in man. *Clin. Exp. Immunol.*, 31: 116–125.

128. Parrillo, J. E., and Fauci, A. S. (1978): Comparison of the effector cells in human spontaneous cellular cytotoxicity and antibody-dependent cellular cytotoxicity: Differential sensitivity of effector cells to *in vivo* and *in vitro* corticosteroids. *Scand. J. Immunol.*, 8:99–107.

129. Parrillo, J. E., and Fauci, A. S. (1979): Mechanisms of glucocorticoid action on immune processes. *Annu. Rev. Pharmacol. Toxicol.*, 19: 179–201.

130. Patek, P. Q., Collins, J. L., and Cohn, M. (1982): Activity and dexamethasone sensitivity of natural cytotoxic cell subpopulations. *Cell. Immunol.*, 72:113–121.

131. Pepinsky, R. B., and Sinclair, L. K. (1986): Epidermal growth factor-dependent phosphorylation of lipocortin. *Nature*, 321:81–84.

132. Peterson, A. P., Altman, L. C., Hill, J. S., Gosney, K., and Kadin, M. E. (1981): Glucocorticoid receptors in normal human eosinophils: Comparison with neutrophils. *J. Allergy Clin. Immunol.*, 62: 212–217.

133. Piccolella, E., Lombardi, G., Vismara, D., DelGallo, F., Colizzi, V., Dolei, A., and Dianzani, F. (1986): Effects of dexamethasone on human natural killer cell cytoxicity, interferon production, and interleukin-2 receptor expression induced by microbial antigens. *Infect. Immunol.*, 51:712–714.

134. Piccolella, E., Vismara, D., Lombardi, G., Guerritore, D., Piantelli, M., and Ranelletti, F. O. (1985): Effect of glucocorticoids on the development of suppressive activity in human lymphocyte response to a polysaccharide purified from *Candida albicans. J. Immunol.*, 134:1166–1171.

135. Poothullil, J., Umemoto, L., Dolovich, J., Hargreave, F. E., and Day, R. P. (1976): Inhibition by prednisone of late cutaneous allergic responses induced by antiserum to human IgE. *J. Allergy Clin.*, 57:164–167.

136. Ramachandran, C. K., and Melnkovych, G. (1983): Transient changes in phospholipid methylation induced by dexamethasone in lymphoid cells. *Cancer Res.*, 43:4725–5728.

137. Ranelletti, F. O., Piantelli, M., Iacobelli, S., Musiani, P., Longo, P., Lauriolo, L., and Marchetti, P. (1981): Glucocorticoid receptors and *in vitro* sensitivity of peanut-positive and peanut-negative human thymocyte subpopulations. *J. Immunol.*, 127:849–855.

138. Ranelletti, F. O., Musiani, P., Maggiano, N., Lauriola, L., and Piantelli, M. (1983): Modulation of glucocorticoid inhibitory action on human lymphocyte mitogenesis: Dependence on mitogen concentration and T-cell maturity. *Cell. Immunol.*, 76:22–28.

139. Ricketti, A. J., Greenberger, P. A., and Patterson, R. (1984): Serum IgE as an important aid in management of allergic bronchopulmonary aspergillosis. *J. Allergy Clin. Immunol.*, 74:68–71.

140. Rinehart, J. J., Balcerzak, S. P., Sagone, A. L., and LoBuglio, A. F. (1975): Effects of corticosteroids on human monocyte function. *J. Clin. Invest.*, 54:1337–1343.

141. Rinehart, J. J., Sagone, A. L., Balcerzak, S. P., Ackerman, G. A., and LoBuglio, A. F. (1975): Effects of corticosteroid therapy in human monocyte function. *N. Engl. J. Med.*, 292:236–241.

142. Robin, J. L., Seldin, D. C., Austen, K. F., and Lewis, R. A. (1985): Regulation of mediatory release from mouse bone marrow-derived mast cells by glucocorticoids. *J. Immunol.*, 135:2719–2726.

143. Rose, B., and Brown, J. S. C. (1941): The effect of adrenalectomy on the histamine content of the tissues of the rat. *Am. J. Physiol.*, 131:589.

144. Rothhut, B., Russo-Marie, F., Wood, J., DiRosa, M., and Flower, R. J. (1983): Further characterization of the glucocorticoid-induced antiphospholipase protein "renocortin." *Biochem. Biophys. Res. Commun.*, 117:878–884.

145. Ruhl, H., Vogt, W., Bochert, G., Schmidt, S., Moelle, R., and Schaoua, H. (1974): Effect of L-asparaginase and hydrocortisone on human lymphocyte transformation and production of mononuclear leukocyte transformation and production of mononuclear leukocyte chemotactic factor *in vitro. Immunology*, 26:989–994.

146. Saavedra-Delgado, A. M., Mathews, K. P., Pan, P. M., Kay, D. R., and Muilenberg, M. L. (1980): Dose-response studies of the suppression of whole blood histamine and basophil counts by prednisone. *J. Allergy Clin. Immunol.*, 66:464–471.

147. Schleimer, R. P., Lichtenstein, L. M., and Gillespie, E. (1981):

Inhibition of basophil histamine release by anti-inflammatory steroids. *Nature,* 292:454–455.

148. Schleimer, R. P., Schulman, E. S., MacGlashan, D. W., Peters, S. P., Hayes, E. C., Adams, G. K., Lichtenstein, L. M., and Adkinson, N. F. (1983): Effects of DM on mediator release from human lung fragments and purified human lung mast cells. *J. Clin. Invest.,* 71:1830–1835.

149. Schreiber, A. D., Parson, J., McDermott, P., and Cooper, R. A. (1975): Effect of corticosteroids on the human monocyte IgG and complement receptors. *J. Clin. Invest.,* 56:1189–1197.

150. Scott, J. L., Davidson, J. G., Marino, J. V., and McMillian, R. (1972): Leukocyte labeling with 51 chromium. III. The kinetics of normal lymphocytes. *Blood,* 40:276–281.

151. Scudeletti, M., Pende, D., Barabino, A., Imbimbo, B., Grifoni, V., and Indiveri, F. (1984): Effect of single oral doses of prednisone and deflazacort on human lymphocyte distribution and functions. Analysis with monoclonal antibodies. *Adv. Exp. Med.,* 171:335–344.

152. Shepard, V. L., Konish, M. G., and Stahl, P. (1985): Dexamethasone increases expression of mannose receptors and decreases extracellular lysosomal enzyme accumulation in macrophages. *J. Biol. Chem.,* 260:160–164.

153. Shezen, E., Shirman, M., and Goldman, R. (1985): Opposing effects of dexamethasone on the clonal growth of granulocyte and macrophage progenitor cells and on the phagocytic capability of mononuclear phagocytes at different stages of differentiation. *J. Cell. Physiol.,* 124:545–548.

154. Slott, R. I., and Zweiman, B. (1974): A controlled study of the effect of corticosteroid on immediate skin reactivity. *J. Allergy Clin. Immunol.,* 54:229–234.

155. Slott, R. I., and Zweiman, B. (1975): Histologic studies of human skin test responses to ragweed and 48/80. *J. Allergy Clin. Immunol.,* 55:232.

156. Smith, K. A., Crabtree, G. R., Kennedy, S. J., and Munck, A. (1977): Glucocorticoid receptors and glucocorticoid sensitivity of mitogen stimulated and unstimulated human lymphocytes. *Nature,* 267:523–526.

157. Spiegelberg, H. L., O'Connor, R. D., Simon, R. A., and Mathison, D. A. (1979): Lymphocytes with immunoglobulin E Fc receptors in patients with atopic disorders. *J. Clin. Invest.,* 64:714–720.

158. Stelling, B. C., and Keats, T. E. (1984): Synovial calcifications associated with long-term steroid therapy for chronic arthritis. *South. Med. J.,* 77:1455–1457.

159. Suzuki, H., Yamashita, N., Sato, M., Iwata, M., Maruyama, M., and Yano, S. (1985): Natural killer-like activity in human cultured lymphoid cells propagated in the presence of interleukin-2: Acquired resistance to prostaglandin E_2- or dexamethasone-mediated suppression. *Experimentia,* 41:667–669.

160. Tanner, A. R., Halliday, J. W., and Powell, L. W. (1980): Effect of long-term corticosteroid therapy on monocyte chemotaxis in man. *Scand. J. Immunol.,* 11:335.

161. Tsurufuji, S., Kurihara, A., Kiso, S., Suzuki, Y., and Ohuchi, K. (1984): Dexamethasone inhibits generation in inflammatory sites of the chemotactic activity attributable to leukotriene B_4. *Biochem. Biophys. Res. Commun.,* 119:884–890.

162. Wahl, L. M., and Winter, C. C. (1984): Regulation of guinea pig macrophage collagenase production by dexamethasone and colchicine. *Arch. Biochem. Biophys.,* 230:661–667.

163. Wallner, B. P., Mattaliano, R. J., Hession, C., Cate, R. L., Tizard, R., Sinclair, L. K., Foeller, C., Chow, E. P., Browling, J. L., Ramachandran, K. L., et al. (1986): Cloning and expression of human lipocortin, a phospholipase A_2 inhibitor with potential anti-inflammatory activity. *Nature,* 320:77–81.

164. Ward, P. A. (1966): The chemosuppression of chemotaxis. *J. Exp. Med.,* 124:209–226.

165. Webel, M. L., Ritts, R. E., Taswell, H. F., Donadio, J. V., and Woods, J. E. (1974): Cellular immunity after intravenous administration of methylprednisolone. *J. Lab. Clin. Med.,* 83:383–392.

166. Werb, Z., Foley, R., and Munck, A. (1978): Interaction of glucocorticoids with macrophages. Identification of glucocorticoid receptors in monocytes and macrophages. *J. Exp. Med.,* 147:1684.

167. Williams, T. W., and Granger, G. A. (1969): Lymphocyte *in vitro* cytotoxicity correlation of depression with the release of lymphotoxin from human lymphocytes. *J. Immunol.,* 103:170–178.

168. Yodoi, J., Hirashima, M., and Ishizaka, K. (1981): Lymphocytes bearing Fc receptors for IgE. VI. Suppressive effects of glucocorticoids on the expression of Fc receptors and glycosylation of the IgE-binding factors. *J. Immunol.,* 127:471–476.

169. Yu, D. T., Clements, P. J., and Pearson, C. M. (1977): Effect of corticosteroids on exercise-induced lymphocytes. *Clin. Exp. Immunol.,* 28:326–331.

Inflammation: Basic Principles and Clinical Correlates.
Edited by J. I. Gallin, I. M. Goldstein, and R. Snyderman.
Raven Press, Ltd., New York © 1988.

CHAPTER 50

Gold, Penicillamine, and Antimalarials

Peter E. Lipsky

Gold Compounds
Historical   Perspective • Clinical   Efficacy • Toxicity •
Pharmacology • Mechanism of Action
Antimalarials
Historical   Perspective • Clinical   Efficacy • Toxicity •
Mechanism of Action

D-Penicillamine
Historical   Perspective • Clinical   Efficacy • Toxicity •
Biochemical   Properties   and   Pharmacology • Peni-
cillamine-like Drugs • Mechanism of Action
Comparative Efficacy
Conclusions
References

Several pharmacologic agents have been used in an attempt to treat rheumatoid arthritis. Because the cause of the disease is unknown, therapy has largely been directed at suppressing the inflammatory process, with the aim of diminishing symptoms and preventing damage to articular structures. One group of compounds appears to have unique therapeutic potential in rheumatoid arthritis. These agents have minimal nonspecific anti-inflammatory effects, but appear to have the potential to modify the course of the disease in some treated individuals (91,213). This activity distinguishes these disease-modifying drugs from the nonsteroidal anti-inflammatory agents and corticosteroids that decrease symptoms but have not been demonstrated to modify the course of the disease (8,29,44).

The disease-modifying drugs include gold compounds, antimalarials, D-penicillamine, and perhaps newer agents such as levamisole and sulfasalazine (Table 1). None of these compounds was developed specifically to treat rheumatoid arthritis. Rather, they were tested in an attempt to suppress a hypothetical etiologic process, or because a chance clinical observation suggested efficacy. Although clinical experience has shown these agents to be effective, the salient pharmacologic actions that facilitate their activities in rheumatoid arthritis have not been delineated. Therefore, the principles guiding the use of these agents are based on accumulated clinical experience, not knowledge of specific drug actions.

The actions of these drugs are significantly different from the effects of the nonsteroidal anti-inflammatory drugs (189), in that they exert minimal nonspecific anti-inflammatory effects. Moreover, they do not appear to induce systemic immunosuppression, and therefore their actions can be contrasted with the effects of traditional immunosuppressive drugs. These observations have suggested the hypothesis that they may exert specific actions on rheumatoid arthritis. This does not appear to be the case, however, because some have also been shown to be effective in other inflammatory conditions. Thus, for example, gold has been shown to be effective in psoriatic arthritis (41) and perhaps pemphigus vulgaris (157), the antimalarials may be effective in the treatment of psoriatic arthritis (101) and systemic lupus erythematosus (150), and D-penicillamine may be useful in the treatment of scleroderma (196). Moreover, the effectiveness of these agents in other inflammatory conditions has not been examined sufficiently to conclude that their activities are specifically directed at the rheumatoid process.

A characteristic feature of therapy with these drugs is a delayed onset of clinical effect. Gradual suppression of the signs and symptoms of inflammation may not be apparent until months after initiation of therapy and may persist for weeks or even months after the drug has been discontinued. This is to be contrasted with clinical responses to nonsteroidal anti-inflammatory drugs which, when observed, are prompt and persist only as long as the drug is continued (21,189). Suppression of disease ac-

TABLE 1. *Disease-modifying drugs*

1. Agents
   Gold compounds
   D-penicillamine
   Antimalarials
   Levamisole
   Sulfasalazine
2. Nomenclature
   Disease-modifying drugs
   Specific antirheumatoid agents
   Slow-acting antiinflammatory drugs
   Remission-inducing drugs
   Second-line drugs
3. Clinical effects
   a. Minimal nonspecific antiinflammatory effects
   b. Minimal systemic immunosuppression
   c. Delayed onset of action
   d. Disease modification
      1. Clinical
      2. Serologic
      3. Tissue-protective
   e. Toxic

tivity with disease-modifying agents is frequently accompanied by normalization of serologic correlates of disease activity, such as the erythrocyte sedimentation rate (213), whereas nonsteroidal anti-inflammatory drugs do not alter acute-phase reactants (8). In addition, therapy with some of these agents may have a tissue-protective effect and thus suppress the development of new erosive changes in periarticular bones (91). However, when the criterion of slowing of radiographic progression is applied, few studies have documented that any of the disease-modifying drugs can actually alter the course of rheumatoid arthritis (93). In view of the difficulties in attempting to evaluate an effect on erosive disease with the currently available technology, the contention that these agents slow progressive erosive disease remains unproved.

Many, but not all, patients with rheumatoid arthritis respond to therapy with disease-modifying agents. Total clinical remission as a result of therapy with one of these agents, however, remains a relatively uncommon event. More usual than remission is a temporary reduction in the rate of progression of the disease in some treated patients. As a result, a significant impact of any of these agents on the long-term outcome of rheumatoid arthritis has not been documented (184). No clinical or serologic feature has been identified that will predict whether or not an individual patient will respond to therapy with a disease-modifying agent. Moreover, it is not possible to identify patients who will develop toxicity to one of these agents. Therefore, the use of these agents is empirical, with little to guide the clinician in the decision to use one of them in the treatment of rheumatoid arthritis.

GOLD COMPOUNDS

Historical Perspective

The use of gold compounds in the treatment of rheumatoid arthritis originated with the observation of Koch in 1890 that gold cyanide inhibited the growth of *Mycobacterium tuberculosis* (107). Because of the beliefs that gold compounds possessed nonspecific antiseptic properties and that rheumatoid arthritis might be a manifestation of tuberculosis, or a related infectious process, attempts to treat the disease with gold compounds were begun. Forestier reported that 70 to 80% of 550 patients with chronic rheumatoid arthritis responded favorably to treatment with sodium aurothiopropanol (48,49). As a result, many therapeutic trials with gold compounds were undertaken, and many reports confirmed the apparent usefulness of gold therapy in rheumatoid arthritis (78,121). However, the failure to include an appropriate control group of patients made it difficult to assess the real value of gold compounds in rheumatoid arthritis.

Clinical Efficacy

Several controlled studies have confirmed that gold compounds are useful in the treatment of rheumatoid arthritis (50,163,164,187). A number of features of gold therapy became clear as a result of these trials. First, gold therapy clearly was shown to be more effective than placebo in the treatment of rheumatoid arthritis. Improvement could be demonstrated in a variety of clinical and laboratory measures of disease activity. At least 3 months and often 6 to 9 months of treatment were required before improvement became apparent. In general, one-half to two-thirds of patients improved clinically as a result of prolonged gold therapy, compared with one-quarter to one-half who improved with placebo. As many as 20% of patients experienced complete clinical remission of disease activity (163,187).

The results of these trials demonstrated that gold compounds were not curative for rheumatoid arthritis. Significant improvement resulting from gold treatment might last for as long as a year after the end of the treatment period (163). However, resumption of disease activity was eventually noted, with deterioration to the level experienced by placebo-treated patients (164). It was also noted, however, that ongoing gold therapy could maintain clinical improvement for at least 2 years (30,187). However, long-term trials have indicated that few patients will receive ongoing benefit from gold (168). As few as 15% of all patients in whom gold therapy is begun will still be receiving benefit 4 to 6 years later.

It became apparent from the initial studies that gold therapy was associated with a considerable degree to toxicity. In the Empire Rheumatism Council trial, for example, 14% of gold-treated and 4% of placebo-treated patients were withdrawn from the study because of side effects, whereas a total of 35% and 16%, respectively, of these groups experienced complications (163). A similar degree of toxicity was observed in other trials.

The final issue raised by the results of these trials related to the potential of gold compounds to retard the progression of bone erosions. Whereas the Empire Rheumatism Council trial found that gold therapy resulted in improvement in serologic correlates of disease activity, no significant effect on radiographic progression was found (163,164). By contrast, another study (187) suggested that gold therapy retarded the progression of bone erosions significantly. However, the number of patients studied was small. Moreover, progression of disease was noted in both control and gold-treated groups, with only marginal advantage noted in the latter. Because the rate of development of erosions is not constant during the course of rheumatoid arthritis (184) and accurate assessment of erosive disease is difficult, such results can only be suggestive. At present, the contention that gold therapy retards the development of bone erosions requires conclusive proof.

Several studies have attempted to identify patients most likely to respond to treatment with gold compounds. It has been claimed that treatment with gold compounds may be most effective at slowing the radiographic progression of rheumatoid arthritis when begun as early as possible in the course of disease (124). It has also been suggested that gold therapy is most effective at controlling symptoms in early nonerosive rheumatoid arthritis (25,54), especially in men with seronegative disease who receive the medication within 12 months of onset (125). However, it is also effective in ameliorating symptoms in patients with long-standing active disease with established erosions (62). A recent study confirmed that no single clinical or laboratory feature in the pretreatment assessment predicted response, but, as a group, the patients with the best responses appeared to have the mildest disease (183). In most studies, the outcome of gold therapy does not appear to be significantly influenced by any of a number of features of the patient, including age at onset of disease or at initiation of therapy (30,104,183), duration of disease (30,183), sex (183), presence of nodules (183) or rheumatoid factor (30,183), development of gold toxicity (24,165), or serum gold levels (16,59,64). Moreover, patients who fail to respond to an initial trial of gold have little likelihood of responding to a second course (46,164). A recent report has suggested that there may be a genetic component to the response to gold, in that patients who are HLA-D4-negative and HLA-A3-positive may be more likely to have favorable responses to therapy (147).

The currently employed regimen of gold therapy is rooted in tradition. Whereas many patients improve on the standard therapeutic program, optimal responses of individual patients may require deviation from this regimen. Although many patients respond within the 20-week loading period, some may require longer loading courses to achieve an optimal therapeutic response (193). Whereas most respond to 50 mg per week, some require an increased dosage (167,190). Although maintenance therapy appears to be useful, it is not uniformly valuable and may not prevent relapses in all patients (24,168). Patients who relapse after an initial response may or may not respond to a second course of gold therapy (46,63,167,172). Finally, not all patients with rheumatoid arthritis will respond to gold therapy, despite alterations in the standard therapeutic regimen. The basis for the degree of variability in patients' responses is unknown, and therefore it is impossible to predict the likelihood of a therapeutic response in an individual patient.

Toxicity

The major limitation to the use of gold therapy is toxicity. The incidence of adverse reactions ranges between 30 and 40%. Many of these reactions are mild, but variable percentages of the reactions are severe enough to necessitate cessation of therapy. Although side effects to gold therapy may occur at any time throughout the course of treatment, the incidence of toxic manifestations decreases as therapy is prolonged (102,193).

The incidence of toxicity appears to be related to the amount of drug administered (24,56,182), with the incidence of toxic side effects greater when larger doses of gold are employed (24,56). A dosage of 50 mg per week is as effective as higher dosages with respect to both degree and rapidity of therapeutic effect and causes a lower incidence of toxicity. Decreasing the weekly dose below 50 mg does not appear to decrease the incidence of side effects (182). There is no evidence that toxicity is related to the total cumulative amount of gold administered (24,102). There are no clinical parameters or laboratory tests to predict toxicity in an individual patient. Toxicity cannot be predicted from measurement of serum gold concentration or the pattern of drug excretion (64,66,68,133). Finally, it has become apparent that there is no correlation between the development of toxicity and clinical improvement (24,165).

Recent reports have suggested that the development of certain side effects from gold therapy may be more common in individuals who express particular HLA antigens.

Individuals who express the class II HLA antigen HLA-DR3 appear to have a marked increase in the likelihood of developing proteinuria, thrombocytopenia, and skin rash (10,11,14,27,128,160,177,192,212).

The major toxic manifestations of gold therapy involve the skin and mucous membranes (158), the kidney (188,202), and the hematopoietic system (27,134). The pathogenesis of these side effects is not known.

Pharmacology

A number of gold compounds are available for treatment of rheumatoid arthritis (110). In the United States, the two forms commonly used are gold sodium thiomalate (Myochrysin, Merck Sharp & Dohme), a soluble crystalline salt prepared in aqueous solution, and gold thioglucose (Solganol, Schering), which is a water-soluble organic compound prepared as a suspension in oil. Both compounds contain 50% gold and are administered intramuscularly. Gold sodium thiosulfate (Sanocrysine) contains 37% gold and may be given intravenously.

Auranofin (Ridaura, Smith Kline & French, S-triethylphosphine gold 2,3,4,6-tetra-O-acetyl-1-thio-β-D-glucopyranoside), an orally absorbable gold compound, has recently been developed for treatment of rheumatoid arthritis (26,162). Auranofin appears to possess a number of physical, chemical, and pharmacokinetic properties that differ significantly from those of the other clinically used gold compounds (26,110,162). Approximately 25% of auranofin is absorbed orally; therapeutic serum gold levels ranging between 30 and 100 μg/dl may be achieved using 2 to 9 mg per day. Additionally, auranofin has been reported to exert a variety of anti-inflammatory, antiarthritic, and immunoregulatory activities that have not been previously reported with the injectable gold preparations. In clinical trials, auranofin appears to be effective for treatment of rheumatoid arthritis, although not as active as gold sodium thiomalate (208). The most frequent side effects are diarrhea, dermatitis, proteinuria, and thrombocytopenia, occurring in approximately 32%, 4%, 1%, and 0.4%, respectively, of treated patients.

There have been a few controlled studies that have directly compared the efficacies of the various gold compounds in rheumatoid arthritis. Auranofin has been found to be somewhat less effective than gold sodium thiomalate, but to cause a lower incidence of serious adverse effects (208). Gold sodium thiomalate and aurothioglucose appear to produce comparable clinical benefits, although one prospective study has suggested that the use of gold thioglucose may result in less toxicity and a higher incidence of improvement than therapy with gold sodium thiomalate (167). It has been suggested that some of the adverse effects may result from altered gold kinetics owing to different rates of absorption, rather than actual differences in the compounds (73,109).

The metabolism, excretion, and distribution of gold in humans have been extensively evaluated (66,68,108,133). Despite the wealth of information available regarding various aspects of pharmacokinetics, it has become clear that serum levels and other pharmacologic parameters of gold do not correlate with nor permit prediction of the clinical response or development of toxicity in an individual patient.

Mechanism of Action

Despite the documentation of clinical efficacy, there is no adequate explanation for the mechanism of action of gold compounds in rheumatoid arthritis. Gold compounds have been shown to exert a number of effects in different model systems. These include inhibition of the activity of lysosomal and other cellular and extracellular enzymes (45,141), interference with complement activation (20,180), inhibition of prostaglandin biosynthesis (159,199), alterations in protein interactions (2), protection from the damaging effects of locally produced oxidizing molecules (33), and various nonspecific anti-inflammatory effects (205). Although each of these may contribute to the effectiveness of gold compounds, none appears to explain their disease-modifying capability.

The observation that gold therapy decreases immunoglobulin levels (123) and rheumatoid factor titers (67,106,163) suggests the possibility that gold compounds may suppress immune responsiveness. This contention is supported by the observations that gold therapy causes a reduction in the number of circulating lymphocytes in patients with rheumatoid arthritis (76) and a decrease in the number of circulating cells capable of making rheumatoid factor spontaneously or in response to in vitro stimulation with polyclonal B-cell activators (149).

The capacity of gold compounds to suppress immune responsiveness has been confirmed by in vitro studies. Gold sodium thiomalate and gold thioglucose were found to inhibit proliferative responses of human peripheral blood mononuclear cells stimulated with either antigens or mitogenic lectins (112). Inhibition of responsiveness was noted with concentrations of gold comparable to those achieved in the synovial tissue as a result of therapeutic administration (65). A number of other reports have confirmed that various gold compounds inhibit mitogen- and antigen-stimulated human lymphocyte proliferation in vitro (79,111), thereby supporting the idea that gold may exert an immunosuppressive action in vivo. Experiments carried out to dissect the mechanism by which antigen- and mitogen-induced responses were inhibited demonstrated that gold depressed the accessory function of monocytes, but had no inhibitory effect on the potential responsiveness of the lymphocytes (112). These data suggested the conclusion that the action of gold compounds in rheumatoid arthritis might result from the capacity of these drugs to inhibit the functional capability of mononuclear phagocytes involved in initiation of the chronic, immunologically mediated inflammatory synovitis. This conclusion is supported by the finding that gold accumulates in the lysosomes of macrophages in synovial tissue (204).

Mononuclear phagocytes are involved not only in the initiation of immune responses but also in the expression of immunologically mediated inflammatory responses by virtue of their phagocytic, degradative, and secretory capabilities. Gold compounds have been found to interfere with a number of other functional activities of mononuclear phagocytes that allow them to function as effector cells at sites of chronic inflammation, such as pinocytosis and phagocytosis (114,201). In addition, gold compounds have been found to inhibit other functions of monocytes, including their responses to chemotactic stimuli (84), their capacity to produce complement components (118), their capacity to secrete collagenase (191), and their ability to function as mediators of spontaneous cytotoxicity (119). Migration of mononuclear phagocytes into inflammatory sites *in vivo* has also been shown to be decreased as a result of gold administration (99,203).

The mechanism by which gold compounds inhibit mononuclear phagocyte function appears to involve binding of the gold moiety to surface sulfhydryl-containing compounds, followed by uptake into the cell (67,201). As a result, the functional consequences of mononuclear phagocyte exposure to gold can be prevented by sulfhydryl-containing reducing agents, including thiol compounds, which themselves are disease-modifying drugs, such as D-penicillamine (112). This may be important in understanding the effectiveness of gold compounds in patients with rheumatoid arthritis, as active disease is associated with markedly depressed levels of serum sulfhydryl-containing reducing compounds (122). The decreased levels of these modulators of the action of gold on mononuclear phagocytes may facilitate the activity of these disease-modifying drugs in patients with rheumatoid arthritis.

Auranofin exerts a number of effects not shared with injectable gold compounds, because of its triethylphosphine group (110). Thus, auranofin has antiinflammatory and immunosuppressive properties in various animal models. At concentrations of gold equivalent to those attained in the synovial fluid of treated patients ($\sim$0.3 μg/ml) (69), auranofin appears to suppress the accessory cell function of mononuclear phagocytes, while having minimal effects on other cell types (173). A number of other functions of monocytes are also inhibited by auranofin

(175). Unlike injectable gold compounds, auranofin inhibits monocyte function rapidly and at low concentrations, presumably because of the lipophilicity conveyed by the triethylphosphine group. Whereas the function of other inflammatory cells such as polymorphonuclear leukocytes is also inhibited by auranofin (72), these effects usually require higher concentrations of the drug than are likely to be attained in treated patients.

The data support the idea that a major action of gold compounds involves inhibition of various functions of mononuclear phagocytes. In view of the critical role of these cells in both the induction and expression of immunologically mediated inflammatory responses, interference with their function locally by gold compounds may well explain the suppression of rheumatoid inflammation.

ANTIMALARIALS

Historical Perspective

The impetus for the use of antimalarials in rheumatoid arthritis was the observation that polyarthritis was improved in patients with discoid lupus undergoing treatment with the antimalarial quinacrine (150). This result encouraged a number of other investigators to try a variety of antimalarial agents in an effort to treat rheumatoid arthritis (12,51,80,105). Chloroquine and hydroxychloroquine became the most frequently used antimalarials for this purpose because of their relative safety. After preliminary uncontrolled studies suggested efficacy, a number of controlled trials demonstrated the therapeutic benefit of chloroquine and hydroxychloroquine in rheumatoid arthritis (28,52,53,75,129,161).

Clinical Efficacy

The controlled trials supported the conclusion that chloroquine and hydroxychloroquine are beneficial in rheumatoid arthritis. Moreover, treatment with antimalarials shared many features with gold therapy, including the slow onset of action and the tendency to normalize serologic correlates of disease activity.

The controlled clinical trials demonstrated that antimalarials are safe and reasonably effective therapeutic agents for treatment of rheumatoid arthritis. The therapeutic effect is evidenced by improvement in both clinical and laboratory criteria of disease activity. There is no evidence that antimalarials alter the radiographic progression of the disease. However, one study suggested that patients treated with chloroquine for at least 6 months exhibited less change in the articular cartilage of the metatarsal head than did control patients, suggesting that the drug had exerted a tissue-protective effect (100). The results of the clinical trials suggest that patients with disease of short duration may respond better than individuals with disease of prolonged duration. The trials documented a low incidence of toxicity. The majority of side effects occurred during the early period of drug administration and decreased with cessation of the drug. However, all of the early trials were of relatively short duration, and therefore the question of long-term or cumulative toxicity could not be addressed. The effects of long-term drug treatment have not been systematically evaluated, although retrospective analyses have suggested that frequently therapy is terminated within 1 or 2 years of initiation because of lack of efficacy (166).

Toxicity

Antimalarials cause a number of toxic side effects in treated patients (198). The most commonly reported side effects are gastrointestinal, generally noted within 2 to 3 weeks of the onset of treatment and subsiding within a few days of treatment withdrawal. A rash and a variety of central nervous system symptoms have also been reported with antimalarial therapy. The most serious complication of antimalarial therapy is retinopathy, which varies in incidence from 0.1 to 15% (81,148,206). Retinopathy has been reported more frequently in association with chloroquine therapy (7,23,206), but hydroxychloroquine may also produce retinal toxicity (7,23,178). Although early studies suggested that there was a correlation between ocular toxicity and the cumulative dose of antimalarial (146), more recent studies have indicated that the development of retinal toxicity is not related to duration of therapy or total accumulated dose of the antimalarial (171). It appears that retinal toxicity is related to the daily dose of hydroxychloroquine and can be nearly completely avoided if the dose is maintained at less than 6.5 mg/kg/day (126,127).

Mechanism of Action

The mechanisms of action of antimalarials in rheumatoid arthritis remain unclear. Antimalarials have been shown to stabilize lysosomal membranes, interfere with sulfhydryl-disulfide interchange reactions, inhibit phospholipase A_2 activity, and trap free radicals (215). A number of observations have suggested that antimalarials may function as immunosuppressive agents. Thus, chloroquine has been shown to inhibit lymphocyte responsiveness *in vitro* (88). In addition, peripheral-blood mononuclear cells obtained from chloroquine-treated patients with rheumatoid arthritis have been shown to have reduced responsiveness to mitogens *in vitro,* as compared with cells

obtained from patients treated with salicylates (151). Moreover, administration of chloroquine has been shown to inhibit production of antirabies antibody in immunized volunteers (152).

Antimalarials may also alter monocyte/macrophage function (47,145). These findings suggest the possibility that antimalarials may be effective in rheumatoid arthritis because of their capacity to alter mononuclear phagocyte function. *In vitro* experiments have supported this point of view. Thus, chloroquine was found to inhibit human lymphocyte responsiveness by inhibiting the accessory function of monocytes (174). One particular action of chloroquine on monocyte function may be especially important in understanding the action of this agent in rheumatoid arthritis. Thus, chloroquine appears to inhibit the release of interleukin 1 by monocytes (174,176), an action that may occur with pharmacologically attainable concentrations (174). In view of the wide spectrum of activities of interleukin 1 on cells of the immune system and in promoting various aspects of the inflammatory response (37), modulation of the release of this cytokine could well explain some of the activities of the antimalarials in rheumatoid arthritis.

D-PENICILLAMINE

Historical Perspective

Penicillamine, a structural analogue of the naturally occurring amino acid cysteine, was first described in 1943 by Abraham et al. (1). It was used to treat rheumatoid arthritis because of the belief that it could dissociate IgM rheumatoid factor *in vivo* and thereby ameliorate the disease (42,70,94–96). Subsequently, a number of uncontrolled (89,98,214) and controlled trials (15,39,135,138,185) confirmed that D-penicillamine was an effective therapeutic agent in rheumatoid arthritis. Initial studies used large doses of D-penicillamine (>1 g/day), but more recent studies have used lower doses (<1 g/day), thereby reducing the incidence of toxicity without compromising efficacy.

Clinical Efficacy

All trials have found that D-penicillamine is effective in the treatment of rheumatoid arthritis. Approximately two-thirds of patients experience improvement in symptoms and signs of disease activity, whereas side effects occur in about one-third of treated patients. Although penicillamine therapy has been claimed to be useful in the treatment of extraarticular manifestations of disease, no statistically significant effects have been noted in controlled trials (138). The onset of a therapeutic response is delayed, as is also seen with gold therapy and treatment with antimalarials. Finally, there is no conclusive evidence that therapy with D-penicillamine alters the radiographic progress of the disease (39,61,130,138), although serum hemoglobin concentrations, levels of acute-phase reactants, and rheumatoid factor titers tend to be corrected. In long-term trials, few patients appear to receive lasting benefit from D-penicillamine therapy (19).

The optimal dosage regimen for administration of D-penicillamine remains a matter of controversy. A number of clinical trials have suggested that lower daily doses may be effective and perhaps less toxic. Thus, dosage regimens of 500 to 600 mg/day appear to be comparable in effectiveness to higher dosage schedules (1–2 g/day) and to be associated with a lower incidence of side effects (36,39,82,135,209). Dosage regimens of less than 500 mg/day usually are not effective, although occasionally patients may respond (144,211).

Toxicity

Most studies indicate that 30 to 65% of patients treated with D-penicillamine will experience adverse reactions (15,39,135,138,185). As many as 25 to 40% of treated patients may have to stop therapy because of the severity of the side effects. The incidence and nature of the side effects associated with D-penicillamine therapy have recently been reviewed (13). The most common adverse reactions are gastrointestinal. Aberrations of taste, which are found in about 12% of patients, usually occur in the first few months of therapy, with a return to normal at the same rate whether or not penicillamine is discontinued. Skin rashes occur in 5 to 12% of patients. The rashes that occur early during the course of therapy can be adequately managed with local steroids and antihistamines. Skin reactions occurring later in therapy usually are more serious and include pemphigus foliaceous, pemphigus vulgaris (55,131), and elastosis perforans serpiginosa (155). Proteinuria, which may occur in 6 to 9% of treated patients, usually develops late in the course of therapy (after 7–12 months), but may develop at any time (82). Penicillamine-induced nephropathy is associated with subepithelial deposits in the glomerular basement membrane containing both IgG and C3 (9). The renal lesion tends to be reversible, but proteinuria may persist for months or even years before it completely resolves. Thrombocytopenia occurs in about 4 to 7% of treated patients and usually is seen between 10 and 20 weeks of therapy (82). The platelet count most often falls progressively, not abruptly, and appears to be related to the daily dose of D-penicillamine.

Because of its capacity to inhibit collagen cross-linking (142,143,186), administration of D-penicillamine can in-

hibit wound healing (58,179). However, the increase in the time of wound healing is modest and does not pose a significant problem.

Administration of D-penicillamine has also been associated with the development of a number of side effects that appear to involve the development of autoantibodies or other autoimmune phenomena. These include myasthenia gravis (18), with antiacetylcholine receptor antibodies (57,169), pemphigus foliaceous, and pemphigus vulgaris (55,131), Goodpasture's syndrome, usually without anti-glomerular-basement-membrane antibodies (60), the drug-induced lupus syndrome (77), and polymyositis (32). The causes of these toxic reactions are not known.

The development of toxic reactions to D-penicillamine has not been found to correlate with any of a variety of characteristics of the patients treated, including sex, age, duration of disease, latex-fixation titer, antinuclear antibody (ANA) titer, complement level, serum immunoglobulin concentrations, or presence of Sjögren's syndrome (31). Recent reports suggest that the development of proteinuria during treatment with D-penicillamine is associated with the histocompatibility antigen HLA-DR3 (10,160,177,192,212).

Biochemical Properties and Pharmacology

As an amino acid, penicillamine can exist as either the D or L optical isomer. Early studies used the racemic mixture, D,L-penicillamine, but more recently only the D isomer has been used because of its decreased toxicity (6). There is considerable information available concerning the pharmacology of D-penicillamine. From a clinical point of view, it is important to realize that patients with therapeutic or toxic responses to D-penicillamine do not appear to handle the drug uniquely.

Penicillamine-like Drugs

Several penicillamine-like drugs, including 5-thiopyridoxine (92), pyrithioxine (22), 2-mercaptopropionylglycine (4,5,153,154), and captopril (132), are currently being tested in rheumatoid arthritis. These trials have yielded promising results and have suggested that these agents share properties with the other disease-modifying agents, especially D-penicillamine. The activities of these drugs in rheumatoid arthritis appear to relate to the fact that each possesses a thiol group.

Mechanism of Action

Despite its well-described clinical efficacy, the mechanism of action of D-penicillamine in rheumatoid arthritis remains unclear. D-penicillamine has been shown to decrease rheumatoid factor titers in treated patients (97,138,214). However, it is unlikely that this effect results from D-penicillamine-induced dissociation of serum or synovial fluid IgM rheumatoid factor, because the concentration of D-penicillamine attained *in vivo* is hundreds of times lower than that needed to dissociate macroglobulins (42,140,170). In addition, rheumatoid factor titers remain depressed for prolonged periods after cessation of drug therapy (97). It would thus appear that the reduction in rheumatoid factor titer is a secondary phenomenon that reflects an amelioration of the underlying inflammatory process.

A number of observations in treated patients have suggested that D-penicillamine might exert an immunosuppressive action and thus act by suppressing the ongoing immune response that underlies the chronic inflammation. In this regard, therapy with penicillamine often results in decreased rheumatoid factor titers (97,138,214), immunoglobulin levels (17,136), and concentrations of circulating immune complexes (97,136). Evidence as to whether or not penicillamine acts to suppress immune responses in laboratory animals is conflicting. Thus, various studies have indicated that it can inhibit (3,85), enhance (200), or have no effect (120,181) on the immune responses of intact animals. Hunneyball et al. (86,87) found that rabbits treated chronically with D-penicillamine exhibited depressed antibody responses to immunization with egg albumin. Concomitant with this was a more striking decline in delayed-type hypersensitivity, with no loss of nonspecific cutaneous inflammatory reactivity.

The possibility that the effectiveness of D-penicillamine in rheumatoid arthritis might result from its capacity to function as an immunosuppressive agent is supported by the *in vitro* observation that D-penicillamine inhibits mitogen- and antigen-induced human T-cell activation (113,115–117). Penicillamine-mediated inhibition of lymphocyte responsiveness specifically required the presence of copper ions. Penicillamine, however, is not unique in its ability to inhibit lymphocyte responsiveness in the presence of copper ions. Various other reduced, but not oxidized, thiols are also inhibitory in the presence of copper. Compounds that have been shown in preliminary trials to be effective for treatment of rheumatoid arthritis, such as 2-mercaptopropionylglycine, 5-thiopyridoxine, and captopril, are comparable to D-penicillamine in suppressing mitogen responsiveness in the presence of copper ions (116).

In contrast to the actions of gold and antimalarials, which inhibited the accessory cell function of mononuclear phagocytes, D-penicillamine and other thiol-containing disease-modifying drugs inhibited T-lymphocyte function directly, while causing no alteration of mononuclear phagocyte function (113). Helper T cells were particularly sensitive to the inhibitory action of D-penicillamine (115). Recent studies of the function of lymphocytes in treated patients have confirmed that administration of D-penicillamine can inhibit helper T-cell function (149).

Inhibition of lymphocyte function depends on the presence of copper ions and results from the copper-mediated oxidation of the thiol group of penicillamine, leading to the generation of hydrogen peroxide (117,194,195). Monocytes, but not other cells found in rheumatoid synovium, were able to protect T cells from inhibition by virtue of their abundant content of catalase (117). These results suggest that the functional competence of mononuclear phagocytes within the inflamed synovium may play a critical role in determining the therapeutic effectiveness of D-penicillamine and other thiol-containing disease-modifying drugs. Other features of the rheumatoid synovium may also be important in determining the effectiveness of therapy with D-penicillamine. For example, the immunosuppressive activity of D-penicillamine requires the drug to be in the reduced form; the oxidized disulfide is inactive (113). Thus, the acidic environment of the inflamed rheumatoid joint (207) would tend to favor maintenance of D-penicillamine in the reduced thiol form and thus facilitate its immunosuppressive capacity.

COMPARATIVE EFFICACY

Several trials have compared the therapeutic efficacies of the various disease-modifying drugs (15,19,34, 43,71,90,130,156,166). The three major disease-modifying drugs appear to be comparably effective for treatment of large groups of patients with rheumatoid arthritis. Despite individual physicians' preferences, there is little evidence that any of these drugs is superior to any of the others. This does not diminish the importance of the clinical observation that an individual patient may respond to one, but not another, of the disease-modifying agents and that such idiosyncratic responses are unpredictable.

Therapy with one disease-modifying drug does not appear to have an impact on the success of therapy with a second agent. When gold and antimalarials have been compared, antecedent therapy with one appeared to have no effect on the outcome of therapy with the other (166). The relationship of the outcome of D-penicillamine therapy and antecedent gold therapy is somewhat more complex. A number of studies indicated that previous gold therapy did not affect the subsequent outcome of D-penicillamine therapy (38,74,137,139,209,210). However, it was thought that D-penicillamine-induced toxicity might be more frequent in individuals who had previously taken gold (35,39,83) or who had a history of gold toxicity (40).

Subsequent studies, however, have not confirmed this finding (103,197). Thus, it appears that the disease-modifying drugs can be safely given in sequence. Antecedent therapy with one disease-modifying agent appears to have little predictable effect on the likelihood of either a therapeutic response or a toxic side effect to another agent. Moreover, it appears that the same percentage of patients will respond to treatment with a disease-modifying agent irrespective of antecedent therapy with another disease-modifying agent.

Combinations of disease-modifying drugs have generally been avoided because of the similar toxicities of the agents and the possibility of pharmacologic interaction between the drugs, which could prevent the development of a therapeutic effect to either agent. One trial compared the combination of D-penicillamine and hydroxychloroquine to either drug alone (19) and found that the combination was less effective than either drug alone. These results suggested that a pharmacologic interaction had taken place between the two agents that interfered with the efficacy of each.

CONCLUSIONS

Rheumatoid arthritis is a chronic inflammatory disease characterized by persistent immunologic activity at sites of inflammation. The immunologic activity in the synovial tissue appears to stimulate both acute and chronic inflammations in the synovial fluid and tissue, respectively. In addition, the immunologic reactivity promotes bone and cartilage loss and also may induce the systemic manifestations of disease. Disease-modifying agents exert a number of activities in patients with rheumatoid arthritis that suggest that they belong to a functionally defined class of pharmacologic agents. The evidence suggests that local immunosuppression is an action that is shared by disease-modifying agents and thus supports the view that disease modification may result from suppression of the immunologic activity that underlies rheumatoid inflammation. Despite the fact that these agents can function as immunosuppressives, each appears to have a unique site of action, specifically inhibiting the function of only one of the populations of cells likely to be involved in chronic immunologically mediated inflammation. Gold compounds and antimalarials appear to be active by virtue of their capacity to depress various functions of mononuclear phagocytes, whereas D-penicillamine and other thiol-containing agents act by inhibiting a number of the activities of T lymphocytes. The conclusion that disease-modifying agents have different sites of immunosuppressive action in rheumatoid arthritis may explain the observation that their success rates are comparable regardless of antecedent therapy with another. Unique features of

the rheumatoid synovium, such as sulfhydryl reactivity, pH, and the integrity of mononuclear phagocyte function, may influence the activities of these agents within the affected tissue. Disease-modifying agents may therefore function as regionally active immunosuppressive agents whose inhibitory capacities are predicated on the nature of rheumatoid inflammation.

REFERENCES

1. Abraham, E. P., Chain, E., Baker, W., and Robinson, R. (1943): Penicillamine, a characteristic degradation product of penicillin. *Nature (Lond.)*, 151:107.
2. Adam, M., and Kühn, K. (1968): Investigations on the reaction of metals with collagen in vivo. I. Comparison of the reaction of gold thiosulfate with collagen in vivo and in vitro. *Eur. J. Biochem.*, 3: 407–410.
3. Altman, K., and Tobin, M. S. (1965): Suppression of the primary immune response induced by D-L-penicillamine. *Proc. Soc. Exp. Biol. Med.*, 118:554–557.
4. Amor, B., Mery, C., and DeGery, A. (1980): Tiopronine. New antirheumatic slow acting drug in rheumatoid arthritis. *Rev. Rhum.*, 47:157–162.
5. Amor, B., Mery, C., and DeGery, A. (1982): Tiopronin (*N*-[2-mercaptopropionyl]-glycine) in rheumatoid arthritis. *Arthritis Rheum.*, 25:698–703.
6. Apsohian, H. V. (1971): Penicillamine and analogous chelating agents. *Ann. N.Y. Acad. Sci.*, 179:481–486.
7. Arden, G. B., and Kolb, H. (1966): Antimalarial therapy and early retinal changes in patients with rheumatoid arthritis. *Br. Med. J.*, 1:270–273.
8. Aylward, M., Maddock, J., Wheeldon, R., and Parker, R. J. (1975): A study of the influence of various antirheumatic drug regimens on serum acute-phase proteins, plasma tryptophan, and erythrocyte sedimentation rate in rheumatoid arthritis. *Rheumatol. Rehabil.*, 14:101–114.
9. Bacon, P. A., Tribe, C. R., MacKenzie, J. C., Jones, J. V., Cumming, R. H., and Amer, B. (1976): Penicillamine nephropathy in rheumatoid arthritis. A clinical, pathological and immunological study. *Q. J. Med.*, 45:661–684.
10. Bardin, R., Dryll, A., Debeyre, N., Ryckewaert, A., Legrand, L., Marcelli, A., and Dausset, J. (1982): HLA system and side effects of gold salts and D-penicillamine treatment of rheumatoid arthritis. *Ann. Rheum. Dis.*, 41:599–601.
11. Barger, B. O., Acton, R. T., Koopman, W. J., and Alarcon, G. S. (1984): DR antigens and gold toxicity in white rheumatoid arthritis patients. *Arthritis Rheum.*, 27:601–605.
12. Bartholomew, L. E., and Duff, I. F. (1963): Amopyroquin (Propoquin) in rheumatoid arthritis. *Arthritis Rheum.*, 6:356–363.
13. Baum, J. (1979): The use of penicillamine in the treatment of rheumatoid arthritis and scleroderma. *Scand. J. Rheumatol. [Suppl.]*, 28:65–70.
14. Benson, W. G., Moore, N., Tugwell, P., D'Souza, M., and Singal, D. P. (1984): HLA antigens and toxic reactions to sodium aurothiomalate in patients with rheumatoid arthritis. *J. Rheum.*, 11: 358–361.
15. Berry, J., Liyanage, S. P., Durance, R. A., Barnes, C. G., Berger, L. A., and Evans, S. (1976): Azathioprine and penicillamine in treatment of rheumatoid arthritis: A controlled trial. *Br. Med. J.*, 1:1052–1054.
16. Billings, R., Grahame, R., Marks, V., Wood, P. J., and Taylor, A. (1975): Blood and urine levels during chrysotherapy for rheumatoid arthritis. *Rheumatol. Rehabil.*, 14:13–18.
17. Bluestone, R., and Goldberg, L. S. (1973): Effect of D-penicillamine on serum immunoglobulins and rheumatoid factor. *Ann. Rheum. Dis.*, 32:50–52.
18. Bucknall, R. C., Dixon, A. St. J., Glick, E. N., Woodland, J., and Zutshi, D. W. (1975): Myasthenia gravis associated with penicillamine treatment for rheumatoid arthritis. *Br. Med. J.*, 1:600–602.

19. Bunch, T. W., O'Duffy, J. D., Tompkins, R. B., and O'Fallon, W. M. (1984): Controlled trial of hydroxychloroquine and D-penicillamine singly and in combination in the treatment of rheumatoid arthritis. *Arthritis Rheum.*, 27:267–276.

20. Burge, J. J., Fearon, D. T., and Austin, K. F. (1978): Inhibition of the alternative pathway of complement by gold sodium thiomalate in vitro. *J. Immunol.*, 120:1626–1630.

21. Calabro, J. J., and Paulus, H. E. (1970): Anti-inflammatory effect of acetylsalicylic acid in rheumatoid arthritis. *Clin. Orthop.*, 71: 124–131.

22. Camus, J.-P., Crouzet, J., Prier, A., and Bergevin, H. (1981): Pyrithioxine and tiopronine: New penicillamine-like drugs in rheumatoid arthritis. *J. Rheum. [Suppl. 7]*, 8:175–179.

23. Carr, R. E., Henkind, P., Rothfield, N., and Siegel, I. M. (1968): Ocular toxicity of antimalarial drugs: Long-term follow-up. *Am. J. Ophthalmol.*, 66:738–744.

24. Cats, A. (1976): A multicentre controlled trial of the effects of different dosages of gold followed by maintenance dosage. *Agents Actions*, 6:355–363.

25. Cecil, R. L., Kammerer, W. H., and DePrume, F. J. (1942): Gold salts in the treatment of rheumatoid arthritis. *Ann. Intern. Med.*, 16:811–827.

26. Chaffman, M., Brogden, R. N., Heel, R. C., Speight, T. M., and Avery, G. S. (1984): Auranofin. A preliminary review of its pharmacological properties and therapeutic use in rheumatoid arthritis. *Drugs*, 27:378–424.

27. Coblyn, J. S., Weinblatt, M., Holdsworth, D., and Glass, D. (1981): Gold-induced thrombocytopenia. A clinical and immunogenetic study of twenty-three patients. *Ann. Intern. Med.*, 95:178–181.

28. Cohen, A. S., and Calkins, E. (1958): A controlled study of chloroquine as an anti-rheumatic agent. *Arthritis Rheum.*, 1:297–312.

29. Cooperating Clinics Committee of the American Rheumatism Association (1967): A three-month trial of indomethacin in rheumatoid arthritis, with special reference to analysis and inference. *Clin. Pharmacol. Ther.*, 8:11–37.

30. Cooperating Clinics Committee of the American Rheumatism Association (1973): A controlled trial of gold salt therapy in rheumatoid arthritis. *Arthritis Rheum.*, 16:353–358.

31. Corke, C. F., and Huskisson, E. C. (1978): Factors affecting the development of penicillamine side-effects. *Rheumatol. Rehabil.*, 17:34–37.

32. Cucher, B. G., and Goldman, A. L. (1976): D-penicillamine-induced polymyositis in rheumatoid arthritis. *Ann. Intern. Med.*, 85:615–616.

33. Cuperus, R. A., Muijsers, A. O., and Wever, R. (1985): Antiarthritis drugs containing thiol groups scavenge hypochlorite and inhibit its formation by myeloperoxidase from human leukocytes. *Arthritis Rheum.*, 28:1228–1233.

34. Currey, H. L. F., Harris, J., Mason, R. M., Woodland, J., Beveridge, T., Roberts, C. J., Vere, D. W., Dixon, A. St. J., Davies, J., and Owen-Smith, B. (1974): Comparison of azathioprine, cyclophosphamide, and gold in treatment of rheumatoid arthritis. *Br. Med. J.*, 3:763–766.

35. Day, A. T., and Golding, J. R. (1974): Hazards of penicillamine therapy in the treatment of rheumatoid arthritis. *Postgrad. Med. J. [Suppl. 2]*, 50:71–73.

36. Day, A. T., Golding, J. R., Lee, P. N., and Butterworth, A. D. (1974): Penicillamine in rheumatoid disease: A long-term study. *Br. Med. J.*, 1:180–183.

37. Dinarello, C. A. (1984): Interleukin 1. *Rev. Infect. Dis.*, 1:51–95.

38. Dippy, J. E. (1977): Penicillamine in rheumatoid arthritis—a 2-year retrospective study in 70 patients. *Br. J. Clin. Pract.*, 31:5–11.

39. Dixon, A. St. J., Davies, J., Dormandy, T. L., Hamilton, E. B. D., Holt, P. J. L., Mason, R. M., Thompson, M., Weber, J. C. P., and Zutshi, D. W. (1975): Synthetic D-penicillamine in rheumatoid arthritis. Double-blind controlled study of a high and low dosage regimen. *Ann. Rheum. Dis.*, 34:416–421.

40. Dodd, M. J., Griffiths, I. D., and Thompson, M. (1980): Adverse reactions to D-penicillamine after gold toxicity. *Br. Med. J.*, 199:1498–1504.

41. Dorwart, B. B., Gall, E. P., Schumacher, H. R., and Krauser, R. E. (1978): Chrysotherapy in psoriatic arthritis. *Arthritis Rheum.*, 21:513–515.

42. Dresner, E., and Trombly, P. (1960): Chemical dissociation of rheumatoid factor in vitro and in vivo. *Clin. Res.*, 8:16.

43. Dwosh, I. L., Stein, H. B., Urowitz, M. D., Smythe, H. A., Hunter, T., and Ogryzlo, M. A. (1977): Azathioprine in early rheumatoid arthritis: Comparison with gold and chloroquine. *Arthritis Rheum.*, 20:685–692.

44. Empire Rheumatism Council (1957): Multi-centre controlled trial comparing cortisone acetate and acetyl salicylic acid in the long-term treatment of rheumatoid arthritis. *Ann. Rheum. Dis.*, 16:277–289.

45. Ennis, R. S., Granda, J. L., and Posner, A. S. (1968): Effect of gold salts and other drugs on the release and activity of lysosomal hydrolases. *Arthritis Rheum.*, 11:756–764.

46. Evers, A. E., and Sundstrom, W. R. (1983): Second course gold therapy in the treatment of rheumatoid arthritis. *Arthritis Rheum.*, 26:1071–1075.

47. Fedorko, M. E., Hirsch, J. G., and Cohn, Z. A. (1968): Autophagic vacuoles produced in vitro. I. Studies on cultured macrophages exposed to chloroquine. *J. Cell Biol.*, 38:377–391.

48. Forestier, J. (1932): The treatment of rheumatoid arthritis with gold salts injections. *Lancet*, 1:441–444.

49. Forestier, J. (1935): Rheumatoid arthritis and its treatment by gold salts. The results of six years' experience. *J. Lab. Clin. Med.*, 20:827–840.

50. Fraser, T. N. (1945): Gold treatment in rheumatoid arthritis. *Ann. Rheum. Dis.*, 4:71–75.

51. Freedman, A., and Bach, F. (1952): Mepacrine and rheumatoid arthritis. *Lancet*, 2:321.

52. Freedman, A. (1956): Chloroquine and rheumatoid arthritis: Short-term controlled trial. *Ann. Rheum. Dis.*, 15:251–257.

53. Freedman, A., and Steinberg, V. L. (1960): Chloroquine in rheumatoid arthritis. A double-blindfold trial of treatment for one year. *Ann. Rheum. Dis.*, 19:243–250.

54. Freyberg, R. H., Block, W. D., and Wells, G. S. (1942): Gold therapy for rheumatoid arthritis. *Clinics*, 1:537–549.

55. From, E., and Frederisken, P. (1976): Pemphigus vulgaris following D-penicillamine. *Dermatologica*, 152:358–362.

56. Furst, D. E., Levine, S., Srinivasan, R., Metzger, A. L., Bangert, R., and Paulus, H. E. (1977): A double-blind trial of high versus conventional dosages of gold salts for rheumatoid arthritis. *Arthritis Rheum.*, 20:1473–1480.

57. Garlepp, M. J., Dawkins, R. L., and Christiansen, F. T. (1983): HLA antigens and acetylcholine receptor antibodies in penicillamine-induced myasthenia gravis. *Br. Med. J.*, 286:338–340.

58. Geever, E. F., Youssef, S., Seifter, E., and Levenson, S. M. (1967): Penicillamine and wound healing in young guinea pigs. *J. Surg. Res.*, 7:160–166.

59. Gerber, R. C., Paulus, H. E., Bluestone, R., and Pearson, C. M. (1972): Clinical response and serum gold levels in chrysotherapy: Lack of correlation. *Ann. Rheum. Dis.*, 31:308–310.

60. Gibson, T., Burry, H. C., and Ogg, G. (1976): Goodpasture syndrome and D-penicillamine. *Ann. Intern. Med.*, 84:100.

61. Gibson, T., Huskisson, E. C., Wojtulewski, J. A., Scott, P. J., Balme, H. W., Burry, H. C., Grahame, R., and Hart, F. D. (1976): Evidence that D-penicillamine alters the course of rheumatoid arthritis. *Rheumatol. Rehabil.*, 15:211–215.

62. Goldlieb, N. L., and Bjelle, A. (1977): Gold compounds in rheumatoid arthritis. *Scand. J. Rheumatol.*, 6:225–230.

63. Gospe, S. R., and Spencer, E. M. (1983): Intramuscular gold in the treatment of rheumatoid arthritis. *Clin. Rheum. Pract.*, 1:173–178.

64. Gottlieb, N. L., Smith, P. M., and Smith, E. M. (1972): Gold excretion correlated with clinical course during chrysotherapy in rheumatoid arthritis. *Arthritis Rheum.*, 15:582–592.

65. Gottlieb, N. L., Smith, P. M., and Smith, E. M. (1972): Tissue gold concentration in a rheumatoid arthritis patient receiving chrysotherapy. *Arthritis Rheum.*, 15:66–72.

66. Gottlieb, N. L., Smith, P. M., and Smith, E. M. (1974): Pharmacodynamics of ^{195}Au-labeled aurothiomalate in blood. Correlation

with course of rheumatoid arthritis, gold toxicity and gold excretion. *Arthritis Rheum.*, 17:161–170.

67. Gottlieb, N. L., Kiem, I. M., Penneys, N. S., and Schultz, D. R. (1975): The influence of chrysotherapy on serum protein and immunoglobulin levels, rheumatoid factor and antiepithelial antibody titers. *J. Lab. Clin. Med.*, 86:962–972.

68. Gottlieb, N. L. (1979): Gold compounds in rheumatoid arthritis: Clinical-pharmacokinetic correlates. *J. Rheum.*, 6:51–55.

69. Gottlieb, N. L. (1982): Comparative pharmacokinetics of parenteral and oral gold compounds. *J. Rheum. [Suppl.]*, 8:99–109.

70. Griffin, S. W., Ulloa, A., Henry, M., Johnston, M. L., and Holley, H. L. (1960): In vivo effect of penicillamine on circulating rheumatoid factor. *Clin. Res.*, 8:87.

71. Haataja, M., Nissilä, M., and Ruutsalo, H.-M. (1978): Serum sulfhydryl levels in rheumatoid patients treated with gold thiomalate and penicillamine. *Scand. J. Rheumatol.*, 7:212–214.

72. Häfström, I., Seligmann, B. E., and Gallin, J. I. (1984): Auranofin affects early events in human polymorphonuclear neutrophil activation by receptor mediated stimuli. *J. Immunol.*, 132:2007–2014.

73. Halla, J. T., Hardin, J. G., and Linn, J. E. (1977): Postinjection nonvasomotor reactions during chrysotherapy. Constitutional and rheumatic symptoms following injections of gold salts. *Arthritis Rheum.*, 20:1188–1191.

74. Halla, J. T., Cassady, J., and Hardin, J. G. (1982): Sequential gold and penicillamine therapy in rheumatoid arthritis. Comparative study of effectiveness and toxicity and review of the literature. *Am. J. Med.*, 72:423–426.

75. Hamilton, E. B. D., and Scott, J. T. (1962): Hydroxychloroquine sulfate ("Plaquenil") in treatment of rheumatoid arthritis. *Arthritis Rheum.*, 5:502–512.

76. Hanly, J. G., and Bresnihan, B. (1985): Reduction of peripheral blood lymphocytes in patients receiving gold therapy for rheumatoid arthritis. *Ann. Rheum. Dis.*, 44:299–301.

77. Harpey, J. P., Caille, B., Moulias, R., and Goust, J. M. (1971): Lupus-like syndrome induced by D-penicillamine in Wilson's disease. *Lancet*, 1:292–293.

78. Hartfall, S. J., Garland, H. G., and Goldie, W. (1937): Gold treatment of arthritis. A review of 900 cases. *Lancet*, 233:838–842.

79. Harth, M., Stiller, C. R., and Sinclair, N. R. St. C. (1977): Effects of a gold salt on lymphocyte responses. *Clin. Exp. Immunol.*, 27:357–364.

80. Haydu, G. G. (1953): Rheumatoid arthritis therapy; rationale and use of chloroquine diphosphate. *Am. J. Med. Sci.*, 225:71–75.

81. Henkine, P., and Rothfield, N. F. (1963): Ocular abnormalities in patients treated with synthetic antimalarial drugs. *N. Engl. J. Med.*, 269:433–439.

82. Hill, H. F. H. (1977): Treatment of rheumatoid arthritis with penicillamine. *Semin. Arthritis Rheum.*, 6:361–388.

83. Hill, H. (1978): Penicillamine and previous treatment with gold. *Br. Med. J.*, 2:961.

84. Ho, P. P. K., Young, A. L., and Southard, G. L. (1978): Methyl ester of *N*-formylmethionyl-leucyl-phenylalanine. Chemotactic responses of human blood monocytes and inhibition of gold compounds. *Arthritis Rheum.*, 21:133–136.

85. Hubner, K. F., and Gengozian, N. (1965): Depression of the primary immune response by D-L-penicillamine. *Proc. Soc. Exp. Biol. Med.*, 118:561–565.

86. Hunneyball, I. M., Stewart, G. A., and Stanworth, D. R. (1978): The effects of oral D-penicillamine treatment on experimental arthritis and associated immune response in rabbits. I. Effect on humoral parameters. *Immunology*, 34:1053–1061.

87. Hunneyball, I. M., Stewart, G. A., and Stanworth, D. R. (1978): The effects of oral D-penicillamine treatment on experimental arthritis and associated immune response in rabbits. II. The effects on cellular parameters. *Immunology*, 35:159–166.

88. Hurvitz, D., and Hirschhorn, K. (1965): Suppression of in vitro lymphocyte responses by chloroquine. *N. Engl. J. Med.*, 283:23–26.

89. Huskisson, E. C., and Hart, F. D. (1972): Penicillamine in the treatment of rheumatoid arthritis. *Ann. Rheum. Dis.*, 31:402–404.

90. Huskisson, E. C., Gibson, R. J., Balme, H. W., Berry, H., Burry, H. C., Grahame, R., Hart, F. D., Henderson, D. R. F., and Wojtu-

kewski, J. A. (1974): Trial comparing D-penicillamine and gold in rheumatoid arthritis. Preliminary report. *Ann. Rheum. Dis.*, 33:532–535.

91. Huskisson, E. C. (1976): Specific therapy for rheumatoid arthritis. *Rheumatol. Rehabil.*, 15:133–135.

92. Huskisson, E. C., Jaffe, I. A., Scott, J., and Dieppe, P. A. (1980): 5-Thiopyridoxine in rheumatoid arthritis: Clinical and experimental studies. *Arthritis Rheum.*, 23:106–110.

93. Iannuzzi, L., Dawson, N., Zein, N., and Kushner, I. (1983): Does drug therapy slow radiographic deterioration in rheumatoid arthritis? *N. Engl. J. Med.*, 309:1023–1028.

94. Jaffe, I. A. (1962): Intra-articular dissociation of the rheumatoid factor. *J. Lab. Clin. Med.*, 60:409–421.

95. Jaffe, I. A. (1963): Comparison of the effect of plasmapheresis and penicillamine on the level of circulating rheumatoid factor. *Ann. Rheum. Dis.*, 22:71–76.

96. Jaffe, I. A. (1964): Rheumatoid arthritis with arteritis. Report of a case treated with penicillamine. *Ann. Intern. Med.*, 61:556–563.

97. Jaffe, I. A. (1965): The effect of penicillamine on the laboratory parameters in rheumatoid arthritis. *Arthritis Rheum.*, 8:1064–1079.

98. Jaffe, I. A. (1970): The treatment of rheumatoid arthritis and necrotizing vasculitis with penicillamine. *Arthritis Rheum.*, 13:436–443.

99. Jessop, J. D., Vernon-Roberts, B., and Harris, J. (1973): Effects of gold salts and prednisolone on inflammatory cells. I. Phagocytic activity of macrophages and polymorphs in inflammatory exudates studied by a "skin-window" technique in rheumatoid and control patients. *Ann. Rheum. Dis.*, 32:294–300.

100. Julkunen, H., Rokkanen, P., and Laine, H. (1976): Chloroquine treatment and bone changes in rheumatoid arthritis. *Scand. J. Rheumatol.*, 5:36–38.

101. Kammer, G. M., Soter, N. A., Gibson, D. J., and Schur, P. H. (1979): Psoriatic arthritis: A clinical immunologic and HLA study of 100 patients. *Semin. Arthritis Rheum.*, 9:75–97.

102. Kean, W. F., and Anastassiades, T. P. (1979): Long term chrysotherapy. Incidence of toxicity and efficacy during sequential time periods. *Arthritis Rheum.*, 22:495–501.

103. Kean, W. F., Lock, C. J. L., Howard-Lock, H. E., and Buchanan, W. W. (1982): Prior gold therapy does not influence the adverse effects of D-penicillamine in rheumatoid arthritis. *Arthritis Rheum.*, 25:917–922.

104. Kean, W. F., Bellamy, N., and Brook, P. M. (1983): Gold therapy in the elderly rheumatoid arthritis patient. *Arthritis Rheum.*, 26:705–711.

105. Kersley, G. D., and Palin, A. G. (1959): Amodiaquine and hydroxychloroquine in rheumatoid arthritis. *Lancet*, 2:886–888.

106. Klinefelter, H. F., and Achurra, A. (1973): Effect of gold salts and antimalarials on the rheumatoid factor in rheumatoid arthritis. *Scand. J. Rheumatol.*, 2:177–182.

107. Koch, R. (1890): Ueber bacteriologische Forschung. *Deutsch. Med. Wochenschr.*, 16:756–757.

108. Lawrence, J. S. (1961): Studies with radioactive gold. *Ann. Rheum. Dis.*, 20:341–351.

109. Lawrence, J. S. (1976): Comparative toxicity of gold preparations in treatment of rheumatoid arthritis. *Ann. Rheum. Dis.*, 35:171–174.

110. Lewis, A. J., and Walz, D. T. (1982): Immunopharmacology of gold. *Prog. Med. Chem.*, 19:1–58.

111. Lies, R. B., Cardin, C., and Paulus, H. E. (1977): Inhibition by gold of human lymphocyte stimulation. An in vitro study. *Ann. Rheum. Dis.*, 36:216–218.

112. Lipsky, P. E. and Ziff, M. (1977): Inhibition of antigen and mitogen-induced human lymphocyte proliferation by gold compounds. *J. Clin. Invest.*, 59:455–466.

113. Lipsky, P. E., and Ziff, M. (1978): The effect of D-penicillamine on mitogen-induced human lymphocyte proliferation. Synergistic inhibition by D-penicillamine and copper salts. *J. Immunol.*, 120:1006–1013.

114. Lipsky, P. E., Ugai, K., and Ziff, M. (1979): Alterations in human monocyte structure and function induced by incubation with gold sodium thiomalate. *J. Rheum. [Suppl.]*, 5:130–136.

115. Lipsky, P. E., and Ziff, M. (1980): Inhibition of human helper T

cell function in vitro by D-penicillamine and CuSO₄. *J. Clin. Invest.,* 65:1069–1076.

116. Lipsky, P. E. (1981): Modulation of lymphocyte function by copper and thiols. *Agents Actions [Suppl.],* 8:95–102.

117. Lipsky, P. E. (1984): Immunosuppression by D-penicillamine in vitro: Inhibition of human T lymphocyte proliferation by copper or ceruloplasmin-dependent generation of hydrogen peroxide and protection by monocytes. *J. Clin. Invest.,* 73:56–65.

118. Littman, B. H., and Schwartz, P. (1982): Gold inhibition of the production of the second complement component by lymphokine-stimulated human monocytes. *Arthritis Rheum.,* 25:288–296.

119. Littman, B. H., and Hall, R. E. (1985): Effects of gold sodium thiomalate on functional correlates of human monocyte maturation. *Arthritis Rheum.,* 28:1384–1392.

120. Liyanage, S. P., and Currey, H. L. F. (1972): Failure of oral D-penicillamine to modify adjuvant arthritis or immune response in the rat. *Ann. Rheum. Dis.,* 31:521.

121. Lockie, L. M., and Smith, D. M. (1985): Forty-seven years experience with gold therapy in 1,019 rheumatoid arthritis patients. *Semin. Arthritis Rheum.,* 14:238–246.

122. Lorber, A., Pearson, C. M., Meredith, W. L., and Gantz-Mandell, L. E. (1964): Serum sulfhydryl determinations and significance in connective tissue diseases. *Ann. Intern. Med.,* 61:423–434.

123. Lorber, A., Simon, T., Leeb, J., Peter, A., and Wilcox, S. (1978): Chrysotherapy. Suppression of immunoglobulin synthesis. *Arthritis Rheum.,* 21:785–791.

124. Luukkainen, R., Kajander, A., and Isomäki, H. (1977): Effect of gold on progression of erosions in rheumatoid arthritis. *Scand. J. Rheumatol.,* 6:180–192.

125. Luukkainen, R. (1980): Chrysotherapy in rheumatoid arthritis with particular emphasis on the effect of chrysotherapy on radiographical changes and on the optimal time of initiation of therapy. *Scand. J. Rheumatol. [Suppl. 34],* 9:6–56.

126. Mackenzie, A. H. (1970): An appraisal of chloroquine. *Arthritis Rheum.,* 13:280–291.

127. Mackenzie, A. H. (1983): Dose refinements in long-term therapy of rheumatoid arthritis with anti-malarials. *Am. J. Med.,* 75:40–45.

128. Madhok, R., Pullar, T., Capell, H. A., Dawood, F., Sturrock, R. D., and Dick, H. M. (1985): Chrysotherapy and thrombocytopenia. *Ann. Rheum. Dis.,* 44:589–591.

129. Mainland, D., and Sutcliffe, M. I. (1962): Hydroxychloroquine sulfate in rheumatoid arthritis, a six month, double-blind trial. *Bull. Rheum. Dis.,* 13:287–290.

130. Mäkisara, P., Nissilä, M., Kajander, A., Martio, J., von Essen, R., Anttila, P., and Mäsisara, G. L. (1978): Comparison of penicillamine and gold treatment in early rheumatoid arthritis. *Scand. J. Rheumatol.,* 7:166–170.

131. Marsden, R. A., Ryan, T. J., Vanhegan, R. I., Walshe, M., Hill, H., and Mowat, A. G. (1976): Pemphigus foliaceus induced by penicillamine. *Br. Med. J.,* 2:1423.

132. Martin, M. F. R., McKenna, F., Bird, H. A., Surrall, K. E., Dixon, J. S., and Wright, V. (1984): Captopril: A new treatment for rheumatoid arthritis. *Lancet,* 1:1325–1327.

133. Mascarhenas, B. R., Granda, J. L., and Freyberg, R. N. (1972): Gold metabolism in patients with rheumatoid arthritis treated with gold compounds—reinvestigated. *Arthritis Rheum.,* 15:391–402.

134. McCarty, D. J., Brill, J. M., and Harrop, D. (1962): Aplastic anemia secondary to gold-salt therapy: Report of a fatal case and a review of the literature. *J.A.M.A.,* 179:655–657.

135. Mery, C., Delrieu, F., Ghozlan, R., Saporta, L., Simon, F., Amor, B., Menkes, C. J., and Delbarre, F. (1976): Controlled trial of D-penicillamine in rheumatoid arthritis. *Scand. J. Rheumatol.,* 5:241–247.

136. Mohammed, I., Barraclough, D., Holborow, E. J., and Ansell, B. M. (1976): Effect of penicillamine therapy on circulating immune complexes in rheumatoid arthritis. *Ann. Rheum. Dis.,* 35:458–462.

137. Molony, J., McNamara, A., Doyle, D., Durkin, H., Murphy, J., and Prenderville, J. (1976): Clinical experiences with penicillamine in rheumatoid disease. *J. Irish Med. Assoc.,* 69:41–46.

138. Multicentre Trial Group (1973): Controlled trial of D(−)-penicillamine in severe rheumatoid arthritis. *Lancet,* 1:275–280.

139. Multicentre Trial Group (1974): Absence of toxic or therapeutic interaction between penicillamine and previously administered gold in a trial of penicillamine in rheumatoid disease. *Postgrad. Med. J. [Suppl. 2],* 50:77–78.

140. Muijsers, A. O., Van de Stadt, R. J., Henrichs, A. M., and Van der Korst, J. K. (1979): Determination of D-penicillamine in serum and urine of patients with rheumatoid arthritis. *Clin. Chim. Acta,* 94:173–180.

141. Nechay, B. R. (1980): Inhibition of adenosine triphophatases by gold. *Arthritis Rheum.,* 23:464–470.

142. Nimni, M. E., and Bavetta, L. A. (1965): Collagen defect induced by penicillamine. *Science,* 150:905–907.

143. Nimni, M. E. (1968): A defect in the intramolecular and inter-molecular cross-linking of collagen caused by penicillamine. *J. Biol. Chem.,* 243:1457–1466.

144. Nissilä, M., Nuotio, P., von Essen, R., and Mäkisara, P. (1982): Low dose penicillamine treatment of RA. Comparison of 600 mg and 300 mg regimens. *Scand. J. Rheumatol.,* 11:161–164.

145. Norris, D. A., Weston, W. L., and Sams, W. M. (1977): The effect of immunosuppressive and anti-inflammatory drugs on monocyte function in vitro. *J. Lab. Clin. Med.,* 90:569–580.

146. Nylander, U. (1966): Ocular damage in chloroquine therapy. *Acta Ophthalmol.,* 44:335–348.

147. O'Duffy, J. D., O'Fallon, W. M., Hunder, G. G., McDuffie, F. C., and Moore, S. B. (1984): An attempt to predict the response to gold therapy in rheumatoid arthritis. *Arthritis Rheum.,* 27:1210–1217.

148. Okun, G., Gouras, P., Bernstein, H., and Von Sallmann, L. (1963): Chloroquine retinopathy. *Arch. Ophthalmol.,* 69:59–71.

149. Olsen, N., Ziff, M., and Jasin, H. E. (1984): Spontaneous synthesis of IgM rheumatoid factor by blood mononuclear cells from patients with rheumatoid arthritis: Effect of treatment with gold salts or D-penicillamine. *J. Rheum.,* 11:17–21.

150. Page, F. (1951): Treatment of lupus erythematosus with mepacrine. *Lancet,* 2:755–758.

151. Panayi, G. S., Neill, W. A., Duthie, J. J. R., and McCormick, J. N. (1973): Action of chloroquine phosphate in rheumatoid arthritis. I. Immunosuppressive effect. *Ann. Rheum. Dis.,* 32:316–318.

152. Pappaioanou, M., Fishbein, D. B., Dreesen, D. W., Schwartz, I. K., Campbell, G. H., Sumner, J. W., Patchen, L. C., and Brown, W. J. (1986): Antibody response to preexposure human diploid-cell rabies vaccine given concurrently with chloroquine. *N. Engl. J. Med.,* 314:280–284.

153. Pasero, G., Pellegrini, P., Ciompi, M. L., Colamussi, V., Barbieri, P., and Mazzoni, M. R. (1980): Tiopronine: New basic treatment of rheumatoid arthritis. *Rev. Rhum.,* 47:163–168.

154. Pasero, G., Pellegrini, P., Ambanelli, U., Ciompi, M. L., Colamussi, V., Ferraccioli, G., Barbieri, P., Mazzoni, M. R., Menegale, G., and Trippi, D. (1982): Controlled multicenter trial of tiopronin and D-penicillamine for rheumatoid arthritis. *Arthritis Rheum.,* 25:923–929.

155. Pass, F., Goldfischer, S., Sternlieb, I., and Scheinberg, I. H. (1973): Elastosis perforans serpiginosa during penicillamine therapy for Wilson disease. *Arch. Dermatol.,* 108:713–715.

156. Paulus, H. E., Williams, H. J., Ward, J. R., Reading, J. C., Egger, M. J., Coleman, M. L., Samuelson, C. O., Jr., Willkens, R. F., Guttadauria, M., Alarcon, G. S., Kaplan, S. B., MacLaughlin, E. J., Weinstein, A., Wilder, R. L., Solsky, M. A., and Meenan, R. F. (1984): Azathioprine versus D-penicillamine in rheumatoid arthritis patients who have been treated unsuccessfully with gold. *Arthritis Rheum.,* 27:721–727.

157. Penneys, N. S., Eaglstein, W. H., Indgin, S., and Frost, P. (1973): Gold sodium thiomalate treatment of pemphigus. *Arch. Dermatol.,* 108:56–60.

158. Penneys, N. S., Ackerman, A. B., and Gottlieb, N. L. (1974): Gold dermatitis. *Arch. Dermatol.,* 109:372–376.

159. Penneys, N. S., Ziboh, V., Gottlieb, N. L., and Katz, S. (1974): Inhibition of prostaglandin synthesis and human epidermal enzymes by aurothiomalate in vitro: Possible actions of gold in pemphigus. *J. Invest. Dermatol.,* 63:356–361.

160. Perrier, P., Raffoux, C., Thomas, P., Tamisier, J. N., Busson, M.,

Gaucher, A., and Streiff, F. (1985): HLA antigens and toxic reactions to sodium aurothiopropanol sulphonate and D-penicillamine in patients with rheumatoid arthritis. *Ann. Rheum. Dis.*, 44:621–624.

161. Popert, A. J., Meijers, K. A. E., Sharp, J., and Bier, F. (1961): Chloroquine diphosphate in rheumatoid arthritis. *Ann. Rheum. Dis.*, 20:18–35.

162. Proceedings of the worldwide auranofin symposium (1982): Therapeutic innovation in rheumatoid arthritis. *J. Rheum. [Suppl. 8]*, 9:1–209.

163. Research Subcommittee of the Empire Rheumatism Council (1960): Gold therapy in rheumatoid arthritis. Report of a multicentre controlled trial. *Ann. Rheum. Dis.*, 19:95–119.

164. Research Subcommittee of the Empire Rheumatism Council (1961): Gold therapy in rheumatoid arthritis. Final report of a multicentre controlled trial. *Ann. Rheum. Dis.*, 20:315–334.

165. Research Subcommittee of the Empire Rheumatism Council (1961): Relation of toxic reactions in gold therapy to improvement in rheumatoid arthritis. *Ann. Rheum. Dis.*, 20:335–340.

166. Richter, J. A., Runge, L. A., Pinals, R. S., and Oates, R. P. (1980): Analysis of treatment terminations with gold and antimalarial compounds in rheumatoid arthritis. *J. Rheum.*, 7:153–159.

167. Rothermich, N. O., Philips, V. K., Bergen, W., and Thomas, M. H. (1976): Chrysotherapy. A prospective study. *Arthritis Rheum.*, 19:1321–1327.

168. Rothermich, N. O., Philips, V. K., Bergen, W., and Thomas, M. H. (1979): Followup study of chrysctherapy. *Arthritis Rheum.*, 22:423.

169. Russell, A. S., and Lindstrom, J. M. (1978): Penicillamine-induced myasthenia gravis associated with antibodies to acetylcholine receptor. *Neurology (Minneap.)*, 28:847–849.

170. Russell, A. S., Saetre, R., Davis, P., and Rabenstein, D. L. (1979): A rapid, sensitive technique to assay penicillamine levels in blood and urine. *J. Rheum.*, 6:15–19.

171. Rynes, R. O., Krohel, G., Falbo, A., Reinecke, R. D., Wolfe, B., and Bartholomew, L. E. (1979): Ophthalmologic safety of long-term hydroxychloroquine treatment. *Arthritis Rheum.*, 22:832–836.

172. Sagransky, D. M., and Greenwald, R. A. (1980): Efficacy and toxicity of retreatment with gold salts: A retrospective review of 25 cases. *J. Rheum.*, 7:474–478.

173. Salmeron, G., and Lipsky, P. E. (1982): Modulation of human immune responsiveness in vitro by auranofin. *J. Rheum. [Suppl. 8]*, 9:25–32.

174. Salmeron, G., and Lipsky, P. E. (1983): The immunosuppressive potential of antimalarials. *Am. J. Med.*, 75:19–24.

175. Scheinberg, M. A., Santos, L. M. B., and Finkelstein, A. E. (1982): The effect of auranofin and sodium aurothiomalate on peripheral blood monocytes. *J. Rheum.*, 9:366–369.

176. Scala, G., and Oppenheim, J. J. (1983): Antigen presentation by human monocytes: Evidence for stimulant processing and requirement for interleukin 1. *J. Immunol.* 131:1160–1166.

177. Scherak, O., Smolen, J. S., Mayr, W. R., Mayrhofer, F., Kolarz, G., and Thumb, N. J. (1984): HLA antigens and toxicity to gold and penicillamine in rheumatoid arthritis. *J. Rheum.*, 11:610–614.

178. Scherbel, A. L., Mackenzie, A. H., Nousek, J. E., and Atdjian, M. (1965): Ocular lesions in rheumatoid arthritis and related disorders with particular reference to retinopathy: A study of 741 patients treated with and without chloroquine drugs. *N. Engl. J. Med.*, 273: 360–366.

179. Schorn, D., and Mowat, A. G. (1977): Penicillamine in rheumatoid arthritis: Wound healing, skin thickness and osteoporosis. *Rheumatol. Rehabil.*, 16:223–230.

180. Schultz, D. R., Volanakis, J. E., Arnold, P. J., Gottlieb, N. L., Sakai, K., and Stroud, R. M. (1974): Inactivation of C1 in rheumatoid synovial fluid, purified C1 and C1 esterase by gold compounds. *Clin. Exp. Immunol.*, 187:395–406.

181. Schumacher, K., Maerker-Alzer, G., and Schaaf, W. (1975): Influence of D-penicillamine on the immune response of mice. *Arzneim. Forsch.*, 25:600–603.

182. Sharp, J. T., Lidsky, M. D., Duffy, J., Thompson, H. K., Person, B. D., Masri, A. F., and Andrianakos, A. A. (1977): Comparison of two dosage schedules of gold salts in the treatment of rheumatoid arthritis. Relationship of serum gold levels to therapeutic response. *Arthritis Rheum.*, 20:1179–1187.

183. Sharp, J. T., Lidsky, M. D., and Duffy, J. (1982): Clinical responses during gold therapy for rheumatoid arthritis. Changes in synovitis, radiologically detectable erosive lesions, serum proteins and serologic abnormalities. *Arthritis Rheum.*, 25:540–549.

184. Sherrer, Y. S., Bloch, D. A., Mitchell, D. M., Young, D. Y., and Fries, J. F. (1986): The development of disability in rheumatoid arthritis. *Arthritis Rheum.*, 29:494–500.

185. Shiokawa, Y., Horiuchi, Y., Honma, M., Kageyama, T., Okada, T., and Azuma, T. (1977): Clinical evaluation of D-penicillamine by multicentric double-blind comparative study in chronic rheumatoid arthritis. *Arthritis Rheum.*, 20:1464–1472.

186. Siegel, R. C. (1977): Collagen cross-linking. Effect of D-penicillamine on cross-linking in vitro. *J. Biol. Chem.*, 252:254–259.

187. Sigler, J. W., Bluhm, G. B., Duncan, H., Sharp, J. T., Ensign, D. C., and McCrum, W. R. (1974): Gold salts in the treatment of rheumatoid arthritis. A double-blind study. *Ann. Intern. Med.*, 80: 21–26.

188. Silverberg, D. S., Kidd, E. G., and Schnitka, T. K. (1970): Gold nephropathy. A clinical and pathologic study. *Arthritis Rheum.*, 13:812–825.

189. Simon, L. S., and Mills, J. A. (1980): Nonsteroidal anti-inflammatory drugs. *N. Engl. J. Med.*, 302:1179–1185.

190. Smith, R. T., Peak, W. P., and Kron, J. M. (1958): Increasing the effectiveness of gold therapy in rheumatoid arthritis. *J.A.M.A.*, 167: 1197–1204.

191. Spalding, D. M., Darby, W. L., III, and Heck, L. W. (1986): Alterations in macrophage collagenase secretion induced by gold sodium thiomalate. *Arthritis Rheum.*, 29:75–81.

192. Speerstra, F., Reekers, P., van de Putte, L. B. A., Vandenbroucke, J. P., Rasker, J. J., and de Rooij, D. J. R. A. M. (1983): HLA-DR antigens and proteinuria induced by aurothioglucose and D-penicillamine in patients with rheumatoid arthritis. *J. Rheum.*, 10:948–953.

193. Srinivasan, R., Miller, B. L., and Paulus, H. E. (1979): Long-term chrysotherapy in rheumatoid arthritis. *Arthritis Rheum.*, 22:105–110.

194. Staite, N. D., Messner, R. P., and Zoschke, D. C. (1985): In vitro production and scavenging of hydrogen peroxide by D-penicillamine: Relationship to copper availability. *Arthritis Rheum.*, 28: 914–921.

195. Starkebaum, G., and Root, R. K. (1985): D-penicillamine: Analysis of the mechanism of copper-catalyzed hydrogen peroxide generation. *J. Immunol.*, 134:3371–3378.

196. Steen, V. D., Medsger, T. A., and Rodnan, G. P. (1982): D-penicillamine therapy in progressive systemic sclerosis (scleroderma). *Ann. Intern. Med.*, 97:652–659.

197. Steven, M. M., Hunter, J. A., Murdoch, R. M., and Cappell, H. A. (1982): Does the order of second-line treatment of rheumatoid arthritis matter? *Br. Med. J.*, 284:79–81.

198. Stillman, J. S. (1981): Anti-malarials. In: *Textbook of Rheumatology*, edited by W. N. Kelley, E. D. Harris, S. Ruddy, and C. S. Sledge, pp. 785–795. W. B. Saunders, Philadelphia.

199. Stone, K. J., Mather, S. J., and Gibson, P. P. (1975): Selective inhibition of prostaglandin biosynthesis by gold salts and phenylbutazone. *Prostaglandins*, 10:241–251.

200. Tobin, M. S., and Altman, K. (1964): Accelerated immune response induced by D-L-penicillamine. *Proc. Soc. Exp. Biol. Med.*, 115: 225–228.

201. Ugai, K., Ziff, M., and Lipsky, P. E. (1979): Gold-induced changes in the morphology and functional capabilities of human monocytes. *Arthritis Rheum.*, 22:1352–1360.

202. Vaamonde, C. A., and Hunt, F. R. (1970): The nephrotic syndrome as a complication of gold therapy. *Arthritis Rheum.*, 13:826–834.

203. Vernon-Roberts, B., Jessop, J. D., and Dore, J. (1973): Effects of gold salts and prednisone on inflammatory cells. II. Suppression of inflammation and phagocytosis in the rat. *Ann. Rheum. Dis.*, 32:301–307.

204. Vernon-Roberts, B., Dore, J. L., Jessop, J. D., and Henderson, W. J. (1976): Selective concentration and localization of gold in

macrophages of synovial and other tissue during and after chrysotherapy in rheumatoid patients. *Ann. Rheum. Dis.*, 35:477–486.

205. Vernon-Roberts, B. (1979): Action of gold salts on the inflammatory response and inflammatory cell function. *J. Rheum. [Suppl.]*, 5: 120–129.

206. Voipio, H. (1966): Incidence of chloroquine retinopathy. *Acta Ophthalmol.*, 44:349–354.

207. Wallis, W. J., Simkin, P. A., and Nelp, W. B. (1985): Low synovial clearance of iodide provides evidence of hypoperfusion in chronic rheumatoid synovitis. *Arthritis Rheum.*, 28:1096–1104.

208. Ward, J. R., Williams, J. J., Egger, M. J., Reading, J. C., Boyce, E., Altzsmith, M., Samuelson, C. O., Jr., Willkens, R. F., Solsky, M. A., Hayes, S. P., Blocka, K. L., Weinstein, A., Meenan, R. F., Guttadauria, M., Kaplan, S. B., and Klippel, J. (1983): Comparison of auranofin, gold sodium thiomalate and placebo in the treatment of rheumatoid arthritis. *Arthritis Rheum.*, 26:1303–1315.

209. Webley, M., and Coomes, E. N. (1979): An assessment of penicillamine therapy in rheumatoid arthritis and the influence of previous gold therapy. *J. Rheum.*, 6:20–24.

210. Weiss, A. S., Markenson, J. A., Weiss, M. S., and Kammerer, W. H. (1978): Toxicity of D-penicillamine in rheumatoid arthritis. *Am. J. Med.*, 64:114–120.

211. Williams, H. J., Ward, J. R., Reading, J. C., Egger, M. J., Grandone, J. T., Samuelson, C. O., Furst, D. E., Sullivan, J. M., Watson, M. A., Guttadauria, M., Cathcart, E. S., Kaplan, S. B., Halla, J. T., Weinstein, A., and Plotz, P. (1983): Low-dose D-penicillamine therapy in rheumatoid arthritis. A controlled, double-blind clinical trial. *Arthritis Rheum.*, 26:581–592.

212. Wooley, P. H., Griffin, J., Panayi, G. S., Batchelor, J. R., Welch, K. I., and Gibson, T. J. (1980): HLA-DR antigens and toxic reactions to sodium aurothiomalate and D-penicillamine in patients with rheumatoid arthritis. *N. Engl. J. Med.*, 303:300–302.

213. Wright, V., and Amos, R. (1980): Do drugs change the course of rheumatoid arthritis? *Br. Med. J.*, 280:964–966.

214. Zuckner, J., Ramsey, R. H., Dorner, R. W., and Gantner, G. E., Jr., (1970): D-penicillamine in rheumatoid arthritis. *Arthritis Rheum.*, 13:131–138.

215. Zvaifler, N. J. (1968): Antimalarial treatment of rheumatoid arthritis. *Med. Clin. North Am.*, 52:759–764.

Inflammation: Basic Principles and Clinical Correlates.
Edited by J. I. Gallin, I. M. Goldstein, and R. Snyderman.
Raven Press, Ltd., New York © 1988.

CHAPTER 51

Immunoregulatory Agents

Michael F. Seldin and Alfred D. Steinberg

THE CONCEPT OF IMMUNE REGULATION IN TREATMENT OF NONMALIGNANT DISEASES

The use of immunosuppressive drugs in nonmalignant diseases is best understood by appreciating the history of these drugs. Immunosuppressive drugs have largely been designed as anticancer drugs. Such drugs have been used as immunosuppressive drugs in human transplantation and, with some exceptions, only subsequently have achieved widespread use in the treatment of inflammatory diseases of unknown cause. As a result, these drugs were, for the most part, not designed for the purpose of treating nonmalignant diseases. Their use in nonmalignant diseases has several underlying assumptions: (a) that the diseases are mediated by the immune system, (b) that the diseases have inflammatory components, (c) that immunosuppression will reduce the severity of disease, and (d) that killing unwanted cells (as in anticancer therapy) will be helpful. Most of these assumptions probably are reasonable in many of these diseases. Moreover, the practice of trying drugs that have been used in cancer chemotherapy has the advantage that there is already a history on which to base expectations regarding potential side

effects and toxicities. The drugs that have been available do have toxicities, and they are not uniformly effective. Thus, it is necessary to point out that current use of these drugs is occurring despite limitations. If the drugs were less toxic, more drug could be given, and diseases would be better treated without side effects. Unfortunately, the majority of drugs available, and essentially all those in current use, have therapeutic windows that are narrow. The therapeutic window concerns the dosage of drug that will be effective in most patients and yet will cause minimal toxicity in those receiving that dosage of drug. Examples of therapeutic windows are shown in Fig. 1. For many of the drugs we use, there is no window; that is, in order to suppress disease in the great majority of patients, unacceptable toxicity would occur in too many.

GENERAL PRINCIPLES OF PHARMACOLOGICAL IMMUNOREGULATION

Drugs capable of immunoregulation include both those given specifically for this purpose and others with secondary immunoregulatory effects. The latter group, which will not be considered in this chapter, includes antihis-

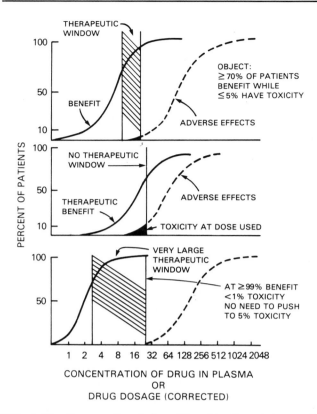

FIG. 1. The therapeutic window. The objective of therapy is to benefit the great majority of patients while limiting toxicity to a minimum number. In this theoretical example, the objective is to benefit at least 70% of patients while limiting toxicity to 5% of patients or fewer. The dosage required to achieve this objective depends on the dose–response curve of benefit, as well as the curve for toxicity. **Top:** The therapeutic window is shown by the vertical lines connected by hashed lines. This therapeutic window is rather narrow, covering only a twofold range of drug dosage; however, things could be worse. **Middle:** The therapeutic window for another drug. Here there is no therapeutic window: The dosage required to benefit at least 70% of patients is already associated with unacceptable toxicity in more than 5%. This is a typical therapeutic window for immunosuppressive drugs in inflammatory diseases of uncertain etiology. **Bottom:** An example of a wide therapeutic window. Here there is an eightfold or greater range of drug dosage within which desired levels of benefit and minimal toxicities may be expected. In fact, it may be possible to choose a drug dosage such that more than 99% of patients are benefited while less than 1% experience toxicity. This drug is desired, but is not yet available for use.

tamines, polypeptide hormones, cardiac glycosides, antiarrhythmics, food and food additives, anticonvulsants, and many other medications. Immunoregulatory drugs used specifically for these properties in inflammatory diseases were, in the past, almost exclusively developed for chemotherapy for malignant diseases and later applied in patients with nonmalignant disease. Important exceptions to this include heavy metals and adrenocorticosteroids,

both considered in other chapters. More recently, pharmacologic agents such as cyclosporin have been specifically developed for their immunoregulatory properties.

Many of the immunoregulatory drugs were originally tested in rodents, and although the observed effects are not directly applicable to humans, important insights into both the mechanisms of action and metabolism of these agents have been achieved by these investigations. Many drugs are metabolized in proportion to body surface area, which allows for rough interspecies approximations. A dosage, in milligrams per kilogram, for a full-grown mouse may be divided by 12 to give an approximate equivalent dosage for adult humans (mg/kg), because the surface-area:body-weight ratio between mouse and human is 12. The factor is approximately 6 for rat–human comparisons.

Cell Cycle

Many immunoregulatory agents are cell-cycle-specific, and hence their actions are in part dependent on the relationship of the cell cycle to target function. Modulation of lymphocyte commitment to differentiate or proliferate is determined as part of the cell cycle (Table 1). G_0-to-G_1 transition corresponds to cellular activation; RNA and new protein synthesis occur, and membrane receptors allowing proliferation or differentiation at future stages are formed. Certain cellular oncogenes such as c-*myc* are also increased during this transition from the quiescent stage. Subsequent interactions between receptors and ligands direct the cell to proceed through the cell cycle and perhaps through subsequent rounds of division or toward differ-

TABLE 1. *Immunoregulatory drugs and the cell cycle*

Phase	Cellular activation	Agents active during this phase
G_0	Interphase	All cell-cycle-nonspecific agents
G_1	Activation, mRNA synthesis, receptor formation	Vinblastine
S	DNA synthesis	Methotrexate, hydroxyurea, thioguanine, cyclophosphamide (also acts throughout the cell cycle)
G_2	Postsynthetic rest	Daunorubicin
M	Mitosis	Vincristine, vinblastine (cells must first be exposed in S phase)

entiation into effector cells. For example, interaction with antigen induces B-cell receptors for growth factors that interact with ligands, resulting in the appearance of cell surface receptors for B-cell differentiation factors. Alternatively, soluble factors can induce a resting B cell into the S phase of the cell cycle without requiring antigen. Many factors are necessary for growth or differentiation of lymphocyte or macrophage populations, including various lymphokines, such as interleukin-1 (IL-1), IL-2, IL-3, colony-stimulating factor 1 (CSF-1), and B-cell-stimulating factor 1 (BSF-1), as well as insulin and transferrin. Receptors for these growth factors, and the growth factors themselves, are potential sites for immunoregulatory therapy.

The cytotoxic and cytostatic drugs largely interfere with cellular events involved in proliferation, rather than the differentiation of a particular cell type or subset of regulatory or effector lymphocytes. Most of these drugs have been developed as antineoplastic agents that have no specificity for receptors responsible for triggering differentiation or proliferation. These drugs either kill cells or prevent their subsequent division (Table 2). Drugs such as methotrexate, which are primarily active during the S phase, kill rapidly dividing cells, with only minimal effects on resting cells. Drugs that induce nonlethal chromosomal damage in a resting cell prevent subsequent division and may also appear to have a greater effect on proliferating cells. Irradiation, methotrexate, and certain of the alkylating agents that are primarily active during the S phase of the cell cycle may be more effective when given in large doses intermittently. On the other hand, purine and pyrimidine analogues are given in repeated small doses because such a schedule allows continued access to cells in all phases of the cell cycle.

Drug Interactions

The effects of two or more drugs given together or sequentially may be difficult to judge *a priori*. Moreover, the typical hospitalized patient receives an average of more than six drugs. As a result, it is necessary to consider a great variety of drug interactions. Some of these are straightforward. For example, patients receiving standard doses of both azathioprine and allopurinol will have a marked increase in azathioprine effect and life-threatening granulocytopenia. This occurs because azathioprine is metabolized along the same purine-breakdown pathway, and allopurinol inhibits two enzymes in that pathway, so as to retard the breakdown of azathioprine. The result is a fivefold increase in effective dose of azathioprine. The two drugs synergize, if you will, with regard to immunosuppression, because allopurinol in standard doses has trivial effects. The large number of drug interactions possible has led to constructs that help to classify and quantitate such interactions in typical clinical settings. Some of these ideas are depicted in Fig. 2. There are two drugs, A and B. They have similar dose–response curves (Fig. 2B); however, drug A is effective at approximately 10% of the dose of drug B that is effective. Together, 1 mg of A and 10 mg of B reduce the response by 90%. This is not synergy, because 2 mg of A (i.e., 2 units) alone or 20 mg of B (i.e., 2 units) alone also reduce the response 90%. Three possible drug interactions are shown in Fig. 2A. One is simple addition along the dotted line. Simple addition is what is depicted in Fig. 2B; however, the lower curve of Fig. 2A shows a different interaction: synergy. In this case, a relatively small dose of A plus a relatively small dose of B give an effect that could not be achieved with the drugs given separately in appropriately increased

TABLE 2. *Mechanisms of action of immunoregulatory drugs*

Type of agent	Mechanism	Examples
Alkylating	Binding to DNA, RNA, and proteins	Nitrogen mustard, cyclophosphamide chlorambucil
Purine analogues	Inhibition of purine synthesis	Azathioprine, 6-mercaptopurine, 6-thioguanine, deoxycoformycin
Folic acid antagonists	Interfere with 1-carbon transport for purine and protein synthesis; interfere with methylation of deoxyuridylic acid	Methotrexate
Pyrimidine analogues	Inhibit ribodeoxyribonucleotide synthesis	5-Fluorouracil
Hydroxyureas	Kill cells in S phase by inhibition of ribonucleotide reductase; prevent cells from entering S phase	Hydroxyurea
Alkaloids	Inhibit mitotic spindle formation, resulting in metaphase arrest	Vinblastine, vincristine
Antibiotics	Inhibit DNA-dependent RNA polymerase and DNA synthesis	Daunorubicin, actinomycin D

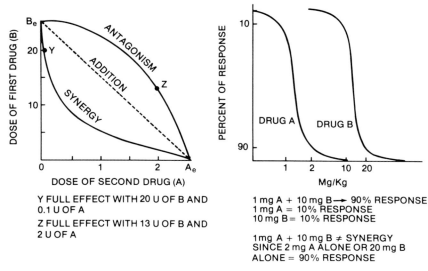

FIG. 2. Drug interactions: synergy, addition, and antagonism. Two drugs, A and B, can interact so as to bring about various outcomes on a given function. The dose–response curves shown in the right-hand panel have similar shapes, but drug A is approximately 10 times more effective on a mg/kg basis throughout the linear part of the dose–response curve. It might appear that 1 mg/kg of drug A plus 10 mg/kg of drug B (each of which produces only a 10% response) would be a synergistic interaction, because the combination produces a 90% response; however, two units of either drug separately (2 mg/kg of A or 20 mg/kg of B) will also yield a 90% response. In order to determine whether or not there is synergy, it is necessary to correct for the different effective doses of different drugs and consider units of drug rather than mg/kg. An example of such an analysis is shown in the left panel. The vertical axis gives the drug dose of drug B in units, 25 units being an effective dose (B_e). The horizontal axis gives the dose of drug A in units, with 2.5 units an effective dose (A_e). The dotted line shows the additive effect of the two drugs when there is no special interaction between the two. The upper curve (antagonism) indicates that the drugs interfere with each other's actions. The lower curve (synergy) shows what happens when the two drugs act together such that the result is greater than would be expected for the two drugs based on their individual effects. For example, point Y represents the full effect (achievable with 25 units of B or with 2.5 units of A separately) that can be achieved with 20 units of B and only 0.1 unit of A. This represents a synergistic interaction, because if the drugs were merely additive, 20 units of B and 0.5 unit of A would be necessary for a full effect.

amounts. The formula for synergistic drug interactions in mice is given in Table 3, along with several examples. The opposite effect, drug antagonism, is shown by the upper curve in Fig. 2A. In this case, disproportionately large amounts of each drug are needed to get the effect achievable by either drug separately. Examples of such interactions are given in Table 3, along with the formula for calculation.

Lymphocyte Subpopulations

The modes of action of immunoregulatory agents are, in part, determined by their effects on particular lymphocyte subpopulations in the tissues or circulation in patients with inflammatory diseases. The underlying disease, as well as the immune-modulating agents, may alter the ratios of these subpopulations, and often it is difficult to determine whether or not observed differences are caused by a direct effect of a therapeutic agent on lymphoid cells. Changes in peripheral blood, which are easiest to study, may reflect recirculation patterns and give little insight into the composition and function of lymphoid cells in lymph nodes, spleen, bone marrow, Peyer's patches, thymus, or tissue involved in a specific inflammatory disease.

Nonetheless, it is clear that different therapeutic agents do affect different lymphoid subpopulations preferentially. Cyclophosphamide, for example, appears to cause a greater reduction in small lymphocytes than in larger mononuclear cells. Chronic administration of cyclophosphamide at low dosage appears to result in selective suppression of B-cell reactivity, with a relative sparing of T-cell responses (46). Furthermore, in experimental animals, a single low dose of cyclophosphamide can result in selective inhibition of "suppressor" T cells (15,208).

TABLE 3. *Examples of synergy and antagonism in mice[a]*

	Sum of fractions[b]
Synergy	
Chlorambucil + methylprednisolone	0.25
Cyclophosphamide + methylprednisolone	0.15
Azathioprine + methylprednisolone	0.22
Cyclophosphamide + methotrexate	0.46
Cyclophosphamide + azathioprine + methylprednisolone	0.32
Cortisol + PGE$_2$	0.50
Antagonism	
Nitrogen mustard + cysteine	4
Azathioprine + bromodeoxyuridine	3
Methotrexate + 5-fluorouracil	7

[a] For most studies in mice and essentially all in humans, it is not possible to determine whether or not drug interactions have occurred.

[b] $A + B + C = S$, where A is the dose of drug A given divided by the effective dose of drug A, B is the dose of drug B given divided by the effective dose of drug B, and C is the dose of drug C given divided by the effective dose of drug C. If $S < 1$, the interaction is synergistic; if $S = 1$, it is additive; if $S > 1$, the interaction is antagonistic.

In contrast, azathioprine appears preferentially to affect monocytes, whereas adenosine deaminase inhibitors are relatively T-cell-specific (40,148), and cyclosporin A has specificity for the T helper/inducer subset (33,37,96).

Immune Suppression

Most immunoregulatory agents that have been used result in nonspecific suppression of the immune system. A variety of interventions may result in nonspecific suppression of immune responses. These include such procedures as total-body irradiation, the use of large doses of cyclophosphamide prior to bone marrow transplantation, and physical removal of lymphoid cells or organs. These methods are truly nonspecific, in that they do not selectively eliminate abnormal lymphoid cells, nor do they spare normal lymphoid cells or other components of the host defense. Strategies must therefore be applied that will balance between the desired effect of inhibiting an aberrant immune response and maintaining sufficient host defenses. In regard to cytotoxic drug therapy, regimens are designed to reduce certain immune functions without eliminating the ability of the patient to fight infections, especially through maintenance of adequate granulocyte and phagocyte function.

Splenectomy results in reduced autoantibody production in many autoimmune diseases, such as systemic lupus erythematosus, idiopathic thrombocytopenic purpura, and autoimmune hemolytic anemia. More important, this procedure has a profound effect on the mononuclear phagocyte system for removing opsonized particles. Splenectomy impairs the mononuclear phagocytic system, reducing removal of antibody-coated cells, but has little or no effect on the patient's granulocyte function. It does, however, lead to decreased ability to eliminate those bacteria that require opsonization for efficient removal. Appropriate immunization with pneumococcal vaccine may reduce the risk of pneumococcal sepsis following splenectomy.

Because pure antigen-specific immunosuppression is, at this time, largely theoretical, rather than a practical consideration, attempts to induce suppression with some specificity have combined antigen and nonspecific immunosuppressive agents. Physical (irradiation), chemical (medications), biological (antibodies), and adjuvant (BCG) agents may result in either antigen-specific or non-specific immunosuppression, depending on whether or not they are given with specific antigens. For example, large doses of cyclophosphamide given with an antigen tend to suppress the antibody response to that antigen to a greater extent than responses to other unrelated antigens. It should be noted that administration of small doses of cyclophosphamide prior to antigen can lead to an en-

hanced immune response to that antigen (217). Other attempts at introducing a degree of specificity to immunosuppressive therapy include therapeutic administration of vinblastine-coated platelets in patients with idiopathic thrombocytopenic purpura (6). This procedure, which is variably successful, probably is directed against the mononuclear phagocyte system, rather than antibody-producing cells.

Immune Stimulation

Many inflammatory conditions are characterized by both pathologic hyperactive immune features and hyporeactive immune components necessary to fight pathogens. The most striking examples are patients with acquired immune-deficiency syndrome (AIDS), who often have hypergammaglobulinemia, but are unable to mount appropriate cellular or humoral responses to a variety of viral and bacterial pathogens. Patients with various autoimmune diseases likewise may have aberrant autoantibody production, but have profound defects in their ability to mount normal immune responses. Thus, immune enhancement might be a valuable adjunct to therapy. On a more theoretical level, augmenting the function of a particular subset of regulatory cells might result in "down-modulation" of an aberrant immune response.

The use of immune adjuvants to enhance responses to antigens has been well studied in a variety of animal models. Commonly, adjuvants have been administered together with antigen. In experimental animals, Freund's adjuvant (which consists of killed mycobacteria, paraffin oil, and an emulsifying agent) is widely used to augment specific antibody production as well as delayed hypersensitivity (76); however, toxicity precludes its use clinically. More recently, muramyl peptides, and, more specifically, *N*-acetylmuramyl-L-alanyl-D-isoglutamine, have received attention as immune adjuvants with properties similar to those of Freund's adjuvant, but with apparently fewer side effects (4,16,42,115). These synthetic peptides exert their effects, at least in part, via macrophage activation and release of cytokines, including IL-1 (55); however, these peptides have somnogenic and pyrogenic activities that likely are secondary to direct nervous system effects (125). Future studies of muramyl peptide derivatives may lead to the introduction of a clinically applicable immune adjuvant.

Other nonspecific immune stimulators, such as IL-2 and γ-interferon, have shown promise as immune enhancers (175,234). Current studies with recombinant IL-2 show promise in activating lymphoid cells to kill tumor cells in animals and in preliminary studies in patients (175). γ-Interferon, which is capable of activating macrophages, inducing class II histocompatibility antigens, and activating killer cells, has in a preliminary study shown some promise in treating rheumatoid arthritis (234). Levamisole, an immune-enhancing drug that will be considered in the section on specific agents, has been used to treat patients with a large variety of autoimmune diseases (129,147,180,188,209). Thus, immune enhancers may have a role in treating diseases generally thought to involve an overactive immune system. While this may appear paradoxical, it illustrates the complexity of the immune system and its regulation, as well as our lack of knowledge concerning the details of specific pathogenetic mechanisms.

Future Considerations

At present, our use of immunoregulatory agents is more empiric than directed at particular sites, mechanisms of action, or subpopulations of cells involved in the immune response. In the future, the use of monoclonal antibodies both by themselves and coupled to cytotoxic agents may allow specific targeting of therapy to an aberrant cell population. OKT3, a murine monoclonal antibody that reacts with virtually all mature T cells, has been used with some success in renal and bone marrow transplantation (72,165). Unfortunately, formation of antimurine antibodies, some of which are specific for binding sites (antiidiotypic), causes considerable limitation in the use of OKT3. Monoclonal antibodies directed against a specific patient's tumor cells have also shown promise. Monoclonal antibodies against class II antigens have been able to arrest progression of autoimmune diseases in experimental models of systemic lupus (5) and myasthenia gravis (220). In the future, antibodies directed against human class II histocompatibility antigens, the human equivalent of murine Ia determinants, may be used in therapy for a wide range of autoimmune diseases.

Finally, cytokines, as noted earlier, have shown promise as potent therapeutic immune modulators. The rapid growth of molecular technology and resources should shortly make available a wide spectrum of recombinant cytokines. These developments may revolutionize our approach to immunoregulation of inflammatory diseases.

SPECIFIC IMMUNOREGULATORY AGENTS

Purine Analogues

Because azathioprine is converted *in vivo* to 6-mercaptopurine, which is the active drug, these two purine analogues will be considered together. 6-Mercaptopurine is the thiopurine analogue of hypoxanthine resulting from substitution of a thiol group for the 6-hydroxyl group of this base. Azathioprine has an imidazole group attached

to the sulfur atom. They are metabolized to their corresponding monophosphate ribonucleotide analogues (91,192,239), which serve as poor substrates for enzymes responsible for forming diphosphates and triphosphates and lead to their intracellular accumulation. Multiple biosynthetic pathways are subsequently affected, including feedback inhibition of phosphoribosyl pyrophosphate conversion to ribosylamine 5-phosphate, a rate limiting step in purine nucleotide synthesis. Another critical step, the conversion of inosinic acid to xanthylic acid, is also inhibited (64). In addition, the triphosphate nucleotide analogues that are formed may be incorporated into cellular DNA and lead to transcriptional errors (184).

Both drugs have plasma half-lives of 60 to 90 min after intravenous administration, resulting from cellular uptake, renal excretion, and metabolic degradation. They are commonly given orally, with about half of the administered drug being absorbed. Although drug levels vary considerably after an oral dose, absolute neutrophil counts correlate well with thioguanine metabolite levels (132). Approximately half of an absorbed oral dose is excreted in the urine during the first 24 hr. Metabolism is primarily by direct oxidation by xanthine oxidase to 6-thiouric acid and subsequent conversion to uric acid. Consequently, if allopurinol, a potent xanthine oxidase inhibitor, is given to patients being treated with these drugs, the dosage must be dramatically decreased. In contrast, 5-thioguanine is not so metabolized, and it can be given with allopurinol.

Azathioprine and 6-mercaptopurine can suppress both antibody production and cell-mediated immune function (2,94). They can cause lymphopenia of both T and B cells (240), as well as inhibit γ-globulin synthesis (133); however, standard oral doses of azathioprine result in only minor reductions of *in vitro* responses to mitogens and antigens. Both drugs can suppress induction of primary sensitization of delayed hypersensitivity, but established delayed hypersensitivity responses remain intact (140, 189). The degree of T-cell immunosuppression with these drugs is unclear, and much of the antiinflammatory activity has been attributed to inhibition of monocyte function (79,163).

The major toxicity of 6-mercaptopurine and azathioprine is an effect on bone marrow elements (177). Leukopenia is more frequent than thrombocytopenia or significant anemia. Neutropenia has been correlated with 6-mercaptopurine and 6-thioguanine levels, 2 weeks after institution of therapy (132). Sudden onset of white cell maturation arrest has been seen in an idiosyncratic fashion in some patients within 1 week after treatment has begun. Other allergic phenomena include rash, fever, and hepatitis. Gastrointestinal intolerance occurs in some individuals.

An increased incidence of malignancy, especially lymphomas, has been reported in patients given azathioprine, but appears to be more common in kidney transplant patients (99). Occurrences of lymphomas in the brain and other unusual sites have been reported. The increased incidence of tumors relates in part to underlying diseases. Cancer of the skin and uterine cervix also have been attributed to azathioprine therapy. These agents increase the risk of infection, sometimes without a major effect on neutrophil counts or function (136).

Azathioprine has been an important adjunctive treatment in preventing or diminishing organ graft rejection. Its precise role in other inflammatory conditions is under reevaluation. While many uncontrolled studies support its use as a steroid-sparing agent in systemic lupus erythromatosus, controlled studies in patients with lupus nephritis have found mixed results (34,52,58,59,88, 105,120,198,200,210). This agent has also been used in therapy for rheumatoid arthritis (3,45,47,119,219), but usually it is used only in patients in whom multiple therapeutic regimens have failed.

Alkylating Agents

Alkylating agents are drugs that contain alkylating groups capable of substituting alkyl radicals into other molecules. These drugs often contain two or more reactive groups that allow cross-linking of macromolecules such as DNA. These agents impair cell division, because cross-linked DNA cannot replicate (173). Proteins and ribonucleic acids may also be directly affected by cross-linking.

Nitrogen mustard was the first of these agents to be employed clinically, but it has been largely supplanted by other alkylating agents that have higher therapeutic indices. In this section we shall consider chlorambucil and cyclophosphamide, the latter being one of the major drugs used in treating inflammatory diseases.

Chlorambucil

Chlorambucil is a bifunctional alkylating agent structurally related to nitrogen mustard, with a methyl group being replaced by phenylbutyric acid. β-Oxidation of the butyric acid gives rise to 2-(4-*N,N*-bis-2-chloroethylaminophenyl)acetic acid, which probably is necessary for most of its cytotoxic activity (142). It has a plasma half-life of approximately 90 min, and it appears to be eliminated by metabolic transformation.

High doses of chlorambucil result in suppression of maturation of all marrow elements. At low doses, this drug exerts a stronger effect on lymphopoiesis than on granulopoiesis (205). In combination chemotherapy, it apparently synergizes with other drugs, preferentially with respect to lymphopoiesis (205). In general, it is thought to have less efficacy than cyclophosphamide in treating vasculitic diseases (103); however, it can be linked to an-

tibodies without reducing its alkylating activity and may prove to be a valuable agent in this regard (69,82).

The typical dosage is 0.1 to 0.2 mg/kg/day orally. The dosage must be adjusted according to the degree of myelosuppression, which is the most worrisome toxicity. Both leukopenia and thrombocytopenia may occur, and irreversible bone marrow suppression has been reported in several patients with autoimmune disease treated with this medication (179). Nausea, vomiting, hepatotoxicity, dermatitis, and infertility are additional side effects (128). A markedly increased incidence of leukemia has also been reported (8,36,85,87,111).

Cyclophosphamide

Cyclophosphamide is a cyclic phosphamide mustard. It requires metabolism in the liver to undergo activation, because the bis(2-chloroethyl) alkylating sites cannot ionize until the ring is cleaved at the phosphorus-nitrogen bond. Despite the requirement for hepatic metabolism for activation, the rate of renal elimination is more important in determining its biologic activity, because both unmetabolized drug and active metabolites are cleared by the kidney. Metabolites accumulate in patients with severe renal insufficiency, and drug dosage should be lowered (18,45,152). Concomitant administration of phenobarbital, adrenocorticosteroids, or other drugs that induce the hepatic mixed oxidase system leads to more complete metabolism (81).

Cyclophosphamide may be administered intravenously or orally. Its half-life in humans is approximately 5 hr (range 3–11 hr). Intravenous doses (0.5–1.5 g/m^2) every 3 to 4 weeks may increase the efficacy and reduce the toxicity of cyclophosphamide in some diseases.

Cyclophosphamide affects virtually all components of cellular and humoral immune responses. Although primarily active during the S phase, it can affect cells at all phases of the cell cycle. It causes lymphopenia of both B and T cells and can decrease serum immunoglobulin (Ig) levels (46). Its effects on B lymphocytes appear to be more profound than its effects on T-cell function. Nevertheless, delayed hypersensitivity reactions may be diminished by induction of T-cell lymphopenia (46). As noted previously, the timing of cyclophosphamide treatment with respect to immunization with antigen can dramatically alter its effect (217).

Toxicity includes bone marrow suppression, but thrombocytopenia is much less common than with other alkylating agents. Neutropenia is common, and with therapeutic dosages should be expected. Dosages should be adjusted so that the nadir of the neutrophil count is not below 1,500/mm^3. Figure 3 illustrates various leukocyte count profiles that may be obtained after bolus therapy. In general, the later the white count nadir, the more prolonged the leukopenia and concomitant increased risk of infection. Leukocyte counts should be monitored 7, 10, and 14 days after cyclophosphamide boluses, and this should be done after each treatment. In general, the leukopenia is dose-related and predictable in individual patients based on their previous responses; however, the bone marrow may lose its capacity to regenerate rapidly after multiple treatments, and careful monitoring is essential. The problem is greater with daily oral therapy than with bolus therapy. Allopurinol increases the risk of leukopenia by an unknown mechanism.

Cystitis, often hemorrhagic, is a frequent side effect (5–10%) of daily cyclophosphamide therapy, and bladder fibrosis, intractable hemorrhage, and bladder carcinoma may occur (11,106,164). These result from damage to the transitional epithelium caused by cyclophosphamide metabolites. The risk of these complications can be decreased by concurrent administration of large volumes of fluid and frequent bladder elimination or simultaneous administration of protective reducing agents. Bladder irrigation may be used in patients with limitations of bladder emptying. Intermittent boluses of large doses of cyclo-phosphamide are associated with far fewer bladder problems than daily administration. Administration of saline is useful in avoiding the complications of hyponatremia from inappropriate ADH syndrome, which can be caused by boluses of this drug (53).

Other complications include frequent nausea and vomiting and variable reversible alopecia. Massive doses can have cardiac and pulmonary toxicity, and interstitial pulmonary fibrosis may occur with chronically administered low doses (13,230). Similar to other alkylating agents, cyclophosphamide can damage the germinal epithelium and may result in azoospermia (216). It can inhibit thecal cell proliferation, preventing follicle and ovum formation (226). Premature menopause is common; the older the woman at the onset of therapy, the greater the likelihood (185,226).

Cyclophosphamide has also been associated with an increased risk of malignancy, particularly lymphomas and leukemias (110,123,166). In one series of patients with rheumatologic diseases, 19 of 2,006 patients developed leukemia (110). This rate was 20 times greater than expected and must be taken into account when recommending this agent to patients with nonmalignant disease.

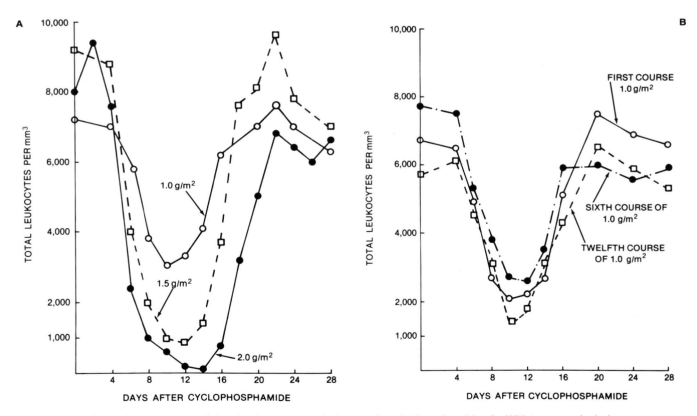

FIG. 3. Leukocyte counts following intravenous boluses of cyclophosphamide. **A:** With progressively larger doses, there is a progressively lower nadir. **B:** There is no progressive increase in leukopenia with subsequent boluses.

Folic Acid Analogue: Methotrexate

Methotrexate (amethopterin) is the only clinically important folic acid inhibitor. It is a folic acid analogue that has an affinity 10^5 times that of dihydrofolic acid for binding to dihydrofolate reductase. Methotrexate enters cells both by active transport and by a second, poorly characterized process that probably involves diffusion. The latter mechanism, which is carrier-independent, provides a rationale for clinical use of high-dose methotrexate with leucovorin rescue. The inhibition of dihyrofolate reductase results in depletion of intracellular pools of reduced folate. Thymidylate synthesis, which requires $N^{5\text{-}10}$-methylene FH_4, is particularly sensitive to folate depletion and accounts, in large part, for the antiproliferative actions of methotrexate. Methotrexate is active predominantly during the S phase of the cell cycle, as would be expected from its mechanism of action (107).

Methotrexate has been used in a variety of regimens for treating inflammatory conditions and may be administered either parenterally or orally. Approximately 60% of the drug is absorbed when given orally; larger doses (>0.1 mg/kg) are less completely absorbed (92). Approximately 50% of the circulating drug is bound to serum proteins and can be displaced by many drugs that bind to albumin, including salicylates. Increased caution must be used in the many situations in which these drugs are given concomitantly. Under normal circumstances, nearly all of the medication is excreted unchanged in the urine within 24 hr after administration. If renal excretion is inefficient, binding of methotrexate to vast extravascular protein pools occurs and leads to markedly delayed excretion and severe toxicity. The pleural or peritoneal cavities may act as storage sites if such spaces are expanded by ascites or pleural effusions. This may result in prolonged elevation of plasma concentrations and increased toxicity. With ordinary doses, very little drug is transported across the blood-brain barrier.

Methotrexate usually is administered in an intermittent fashion, to allow for maximal effects on proliferating cells in the S phase of the cell cycle and to minimize toxicity. Oral regimens usually are given in three divided doses over 36 hr, once each week, to optimize absorption. The adult oral dosage ranges from 5 to 40 mg per week; it must be lowered in patients with renal insufficiency. Methotrexate may also be given in large doses (1 g/m^2) intravenously, followed by leucovorin (N^5-formyltetrahydrofolic acid) rescue, which overcomes the metabolic block by supplying a usable form of reduced folate.

Toxicity from methotrexate therapy includes bone marrow suppression, with leukopenia and thrombocytopenia, ulcerative stomatitis, nausea, vomiting, diarrhea from loss of intestinal epithelium, dermatitis, alopecia, nephrotoxicity, pneumonia, and, with long-term therapy,

cirrhosis and pulmonary fibrosis. The drug causes abortion and teratogenesis. Defective oogenesis and spermatogenesis have also been reported.

Most treatment regimens induce little myelotoxicity. The development of cirrhosis in some patients who have received chronic methotrexate therapy is of concern, but it, too, is uncommon unless patients have preexisting liver disease or concomitant hepatotoxic exposure (e.g., alcohol). Monitoring of liver function tests and serum albumin is recommended, but the former correlates only with acute, usually transient, liver inflammation, and the latter is a late indicator of significant dysfunction. If hepatic transaminase levels are raised to 3 times normal after treatment, on more than one occasion, we would advocate a decrease in dosage. Liver biopsies can determine whether or not significant damage has occurred and have been advocated by some, after a cumulative dose of 1.5 g has been given. Increased risk of malignancy, if it occurs, is not well documented.

Methotrexate can suppress both primary and secondary antibody responses in humans (24,183,207). In experimental animals, this drug can markedly suppress delayed hypersensitivity reactions (78), but it has had little effect on established delayed hypersensitivity responses in humans (149). Clinically, it has been used extensively in severe psoriasis, psoriatic arthritis, and polymyositis and in many patients with rheumatoid arthritis in whom other treatment regimens have failed. Its utility in psoriasis and rheumatoid arthritis may be related to its effects on epithelial and synovial cell proliferation, respectively, rather than its actions as an immunosuppressive agent.

Other Cytotoxic Agents

There are many other agents that have been used in chemotherapy for malignant disease whose immunoregulatory properties have not been well studied and/or which have been applied rarely, if at all, in patients with nonmalignant disease. These include pyrimidine analogues such as 5-fluorouracil, antibiotics (actinomycin D, bleomycin, daunorubicin, and others), adenosine deaminase inhibitors, and procarbazine. Vincristine has been used to treat idiopathic thrombocytopenic purpura, as have vinblastine-coated platelets in a more novel approach (6). Hydroxyurea has been used in treatment of idiopathic hypereosinophilic syndrome (68).

Sex Hormones

Androgens are capable of suppressing immune responses in animals (63,64,198) and, given early in life, murine autoimmunity (62,143,144,170,178,201). *In vitro*, testosterone can decrease T-cell mitogen responses (238);

however, toxicities have largely precluded the use of these agents in treatment of inflammatory diseases. Danazol, an impeded androgen, has been used to treat hereditary angioneurotic edema (51,80,190,195) and autoimmune thrombocytopenia.

Dapsone

Dapsone is a sulfone (4,4′-diaminodiphenylsulfone) that has been an effective agent in treating leprosy and has been used in a variety of autoimmune-mediated skin diseases. Although the mechanism of action is unclear, it has proved effective in treating dermatitis herpetiformis (117), bullus eruptions in patients with systemic lupus erythematosus (89), which are thought to be caused by immune-complex deposition, and erythema elevatum diutinum (116), a leukocytoclastic vasculitis. It is absorbed well with oral administration (50–100 mg daily) and is acetylated in the liver and excreted primarily through the kidney. The plasma half-life is approximately 1 day, but tissue levels may remain high for weeks following cessation of therapy.

Toxic side effects limit the use of this agent. Hemolysis and methemoglobinemia are dose-dependent and relatively common. Other side effects include anorexia, nausea, vomiting, and occasionally peripheral neuropathy, nervousness, insomnia, and headache.

Ionizing Radiation

X-rays and gamma rays cause ejection of electrons from the atoms of tissues to which they are directed. The ejected electrons may then ionize surrounding atoms, resulting in the formation of reactive free radicals that can damage relevant macromolecules such as DNA. Impairment of cell division by scission of DNA is the most important biologic effect of irradiation (102). Proliferating cells are most sensitive to the effects of irradiation.

Precursor lymphoid cells are more sensitive to irradiation than mature T and B cells. Furthermore, different subpopulations of T cells and B cells are more or less sensitive to the effects of irradiation, depending on the dosage, the dosage schedule, and the field of irradiation (10,65,90,137,206). Total lymphoid irradiation (TLI), which involves irradiation of lymph nodes and spleen, results in prolonged depression of cells of the helper/inducer phenotype, relative to the suppressor/cytotoxic phenotype (65,90,122,204). In patients with Hodgkin's disease, this treatment results in decreased T-cell responses to antigens and mitogens (71,113). In mice, secondary antibody responses are impaired. This therapy has been effective in treating features of systemic lupus, both in (NZB × NZW)F$_1$ (121,193) and in MRL-*lpr/lpr* mice

(212). Adjuvant arthritis in rats has also been treated successfully with a similar approach (186).

Toxicity from TLI includes malaise, anorexia, and nausea in most people. The lungs cannot be shielded completely; so at high doses of radiation, pneumonitis can be a complication. In patients with Hodgkin's disease, about 20% have herpes zoster infections associated with this therapy, and there is increased risk for other infections, as with other immunosuppressive regimens (113). Although malignancy was a potential concern, an increased risk of second neoplasms has not been observed in patients treated with TLI alone (90).

TLI has been used in a number of small trials in patients with refractory rheumatoid arthritis (122,203,215) and a small number of patients with systemic lupus erythematosus (202). Although some patients have experienced improvement, the overall results thus far have not been dramatic. Of major concern was the occurrence of several serious infections, neutropenia, thrombocytopenia, and pericarditis in a number of patients treated with high-dose TLI. Low doses of TLI that have minimal toxicities have shown some benefit (202,203), and TLI prove to be a useful adjunct in treatment of some inflammatory diseases, perhaps in conjunction with other therapeutic modalities. At present, this treatment remains experimental in nonmalignant diseases and, in our opinion, should be undertaken only in a well-controlled, prospective study.

Therapeutic Apheresis

Therapeutic apheresis consists in removal of plasma (plasmapheresis), lymphocytes (lymphapheresis), or leukocytes (leukapheresis) from the veins of a patient, with the other blood constituents being returned to the circulation, usually with the aid of a machine designed for that purpose. Physical removal of antibody has a substantial history in the treatment of the hyperviscosity syndrome of Waldenstrom's macroglobulinemia, either by itself or as an adjunct to other treatment (27,181). With improvements in continuous-flow centrifugation and automated cell-separation techniques, this approach to therapy has been applied to many autoimmune diseases, including autoimmune thrombocytopenia, hemolytic anemia, myasthenia gravis, multiple sclerosis, systemic lupus erythematosus (SLE), Goodpasture's syndrome, severe rhesus disease, and Refsum's disease.

It is possible to carry out the procedure by drawing a 500-ml sample of blood, centrifuging it, and then returning the desired portions to the patient and repeating the procedure. This time-consuming and inefficient method has been replaced by continuous- and intermittent-flow centrifuges, which were introduced in the 1960s. Flat- and hollow-fiber filtration devices allow rapid plasma exchange, but are not useful for cytapheresis. The effectiveness of removal of unwanted material from the blood depends on the rate of production, partition in the blood, and magnitude and frequency of the removal procedure. Investigators have suggested that removal of 1.5 plasma volumes is the ideal for a single plasma-exchange treatment (191). Although relatively safe, side effects have been attributed to plasmapheresis: hematoma, paresthesias secondary to hypocalcemia from citrate anticoagulation, vasovagal reaction, local infection, transfusion-related infection, air embolus, hypovolemic reactions, bleeding due to depletion of platelets or clotting factors, respiratory distress syndrome, cardiac arrhythmias, and hypersensitivity reactions. The most severe side effects, hepatitis and allergic reactions, result from administration of fresh frozen plasma. Plasmapheresis has been used either for acute therapy (on a once or twice basis) or more chronically (3–7 times per week for up to 6 weeks). Chronic therapy may be associated with depletion of important plasma components.

Plasmapheresis may be useful in removing circulating factors that inhibit tumor rejection, in reducing immune complexes in a variety of diseases (167,135,220), and in removing specific antibodies such as antibodies to factor VIII (in hemophilia), to nuclear antigens in SLE (211), to acetylcholine receptors in myasthenia gravis (48,49, 220), or to glomerular basement membrane antigen in Goodpasture's disease (236). There is a theoretical problem of rebound hypersynthesis of the unwanted antibodies that has led some to suggest combining plasmapheresis with immunosuppressive drug therapy. Our own experience suggests that such rebound is not a uniform event.

Although plasmapheresis is the most widely used apheresis method, cytapheresis also has been employed. Based on favorable results with thoracic duct drainage in patients with rheumatoid arthritis (138,161), investigators have tried removing large numbers of leukocytes from patients with this and related disorders (21,159). As many as 10^{11} peripheral-blood leukocytes have been removed (114). The purpose of this treatment is to reduce the numbers of activated T cells and macrophages that might home to the joints or other target organs and perpetuate the inflammatory process.

Antilymphocyte Sera

Antilymphocyte sera (ALS) are prepared by injecting lymphocytes from one species into an animal of another species. The specificity of the resulting antisera depends on the types of cells used for immunization and the absorption procedures. By injecting T cells and absorbing with B cells, anti-T-cell antibodies have been obtained (ATS). Moreover, the globulin fraction of the ATS, called

ATG (or the globulin fraction of ALS, called ALG), is much less toxic in humans. Currently, ATG is prepared by immunizing animals either with human thoracic duct lymphocytes (which are highly enriched in T cells) or with human thymocytes. The resulting preparations are tested for their ability to delay skin graft rejection, as well as their ability to interfere with the ability of T cells to rosette with sheep red blood cells (227). The toxicity includes serum sickness due to production by the recipient of antibodies against the administered foreign proteins. Nearly all patients develop fever, rash, and arthralgias, and some have chills, myalgias, and hypotension. These signs and symptoms are treated with antihistamines and corticosteroids. Both anaphylaxis and death from ATG are uncommon (100). In a comparative study, ALG blocked binding of anti-HLA-DR and anti-Leu-1 to a greater extent than ATG; both effectively blocked binding of anti-Leu-2a, -3a, -4, and -5b and anti-IL-2-receptor antibodies; none blocked anti-Leu-7 binding (169). All lysed 60 to 75% of T cells; however, less active lots clinically were less lytic (169). Incompletely absorbed antibodies to nonlymphocyte cellular constituents can lead to platelet aggregation or effects on granulocytes. Sulfinpyrazone is often administered to reduce the problem of platelet aggregation, which can be very serious.

The specificity of ATG can be studied *in vitro;* however, its potency is difficult to assess *in vitro* and usually must be determined *in vivo.* The purpose of the reagent is coating of cells against which it is directed and reduction of their activity; however, all currently used preparations also directly stimulate the target T cells (169). With the development of hybridoma technology, mouse antihuman antibodies specific for T cells and T-cell subsets have been developed. Monkey antihuman antibodies also are being made, and the technology for human antihuman antibodies is available. As a result, ATG will be used less frequently in the future. At the moment, its greatest use aside from transplantation is in the treatment of aplastic anemia, a disease that, in many individuals, appears to result from a T-cell-suppressive effect on marrow stem cell activity. In many of these individuals, ATG has a salutary effect on the disease process, apparently by eliminating the suppressive effect (100); however, such patients often are faced with substantial serum sickness as a result of therapy. It is likely that future treatment of patients with less toxic anti-T-cell antibodies will obviate the use of ATG.

Levamisole

Despite the hyperimmune aspects of many autoimmune rheumatic diseases, there often coexists an immune deficiency with regard to standard antigenic challenges.

As a result, attempts to improve the immune-deficiency aspects of the disease have led to the use of immune-stimulatory agents in such disorders.

Levamisole is a drug first used as an anthelmintic, but more recently it has been tried as an immunomodulator. The drug has a molecular weight of 241 and contains three rings. It is stable in aqueous solutions in acid, but is hydrolyzed in alkaline conditions. Levamisole is absorbed readily from the gastrointestinal tract, after which peak blood levels occur at 2 hr, and the plasma half-life is approximately 4 hr (209). The drug is metabolized by the liver and excreted primarily by the kidneys. Small amounts of unmetabolized drug are found in urine, breast milk, tears, and respiratory secretions.

Nonspecific inflammation is amplified by levamisole by increasing neutrophil and monocyte chemotaxis and phagocytosis, especially when those functions are impaired (168). Despite this activity, levamisole has not been very effective in improving host defenses against infections (60,98,237). In general, the drug appears to increase resistance to secondary infections to a greater extent than to primary infections.

Levamisole also has a more direct action on T-cell function that results in increased helper, amplifier, cytotoxic, and suppressor T-cell functions (182). The drug has been shown to reverse anergy in skin testing and to increase numbers of circulating T cells in patients with decreased numbers (170). This last result occurs at the expense of circulating non-T non-B cells, suggesting possible maturation of pre-T cells. As a result of the increase in helper T-cell functions, an indirect increase in antibody production occurs (147). This effect is more dramatic when levamisole is used in patients receiving lymphocyte-depleting agents (244).

Levamisole has been used to treat a great variety of disorders, including malignancies, aphthous stomatitis, Crohn's disease, rheumatoid arthritis, and SLE. Unfortunately, in rheumatic patients, granulocytopenia appears to be an unexpectedly common side effect (147). This toxicity is especially common in individuals who are HLA-B27 (223). Corticosteroids have been recommended as protection against the agranulocytosis; however, 3 patients died with this combination (44). Additional side effects include nausea and vomiting, fatigue and drowsiness, rash, and drug fever. The drug stimulates both the sympathetic and parasympathetic systems, has positive chronotropic and inotropic effects on the heart, and inhibits alkaline phosphatase.

Cyclosporin A

A new type of immunoregulatory drug, cyclosporin A, has been developed and tested in a number of clinical situations over the last 10 years. Cyclosporin A is a cyclical hydrophobic polypeptide consisting of 11 amino acids with a molecular weight of 1,202, extracted from the fungus *Trichoderma polysporum*. It has *N*-methylated amino acids, which confer resistance to the acid environment and proteolytic enzymes of the gastrointestinal tract, and is thus effective by oral administration (28). Although initially tested as an antifungal agent, it was found to have potent immunosuppressive properties (155). It delayed skin graft rejection and graft-versus-host disease, prevented the occurrence of paralysis in rats with allergic encephalomyelitis, and was effective in preventing the development of Freund's-adjuvant-induced arthritis.

The primary mechanism of action is thought to be inhibition of "helper" T-lymphocyte activity (20,33,37, 96,126,231). It has been shown to decrease IL-2 production in T cells at the transcriptional level (124). It also appears to indirectly inhibit cytotoxic T cells (61), as well as B-cell function and early B-cell activation (153). Despite this, cyclosporin A therapy results in increased IgG concentrations (231). Cyclosporin A is not cytotoxic at therapeutic concentrations and appears to act primarily as an immune "modulator."

In experimental animal models, cyclosporin A has been found to prolong the life-span for autoimmune female (NZB × NZW)F$_1$ mice (109) and to virtually eliminate glomerulonephritis and synovitis in MRL-*lpr/lpr* mice (151). In the former study, anemia and immunoglobulin levels were not affected in treated mice, but anti-double-stranded DNA antibodies were decreased. In the latter study, autoantibody levels, circulating immune complexes, rheumatoid factor titers, and immunoglobulin levels were all unaffected. These data suggest that cyclosporin A may be able to modulate inflammatory diseases by its direct effects on T cells or their factors that are necessary for immunopathology, despite the presence of autoantibodies.

In humans, cyclosporin A has been used to prevent graft rejection after transplantations of kidney, heart, liver, lung, pancreas, and bone marrow (38,196,231). It has also been used with therapeutic success in patients with inflammatory uveitis unresponsive to corticosteroids and/or cytotoxic agents (156). Preliminary studies have also shown promise for this agent in many patients with rheumatoid arthritis (9,25,74,95,139,156,221).

The major toxicity seen with cyclosporin A is renal. Acute nephropathy is usually reversible (41,222). Recently, a study of renal biopsies revealed interstitial fibrosis and/or tubular atrophy in all patients treated with cyclosporin A (160). Nephrotoxicity usually is associated with trough levels in serum greater than 200 ng/ml (75,118). Progressive and irreversible nephropathy has also been described, but these patients initially received high doses of cyclosporin A that resulted in mean plasma levels of

300 to 350 ng/ml (154). Hepatic complications are also worrisome. Hepatoxicity is dose-dependent and is manifested by hyperbilirubinemia and elevated transaminases (175). Other reported complications include infection, hypertrichosis, gingival hyperplasia, and hypertension (127).

Malignancy has been reported primarily in transplantation patients, most of whom also were receiving other immunosuppressive drugs, with an overall incidence of 1% (162). This overall rate is similar to that seen with the use of azathioprine. The major type of malignancy seen is lymphoma. The incidence of neoplasia in transplantation patients in whom cyclosporin A is used alone is less than 0.5% (222).

Colchicine

Colchicine is a drug that was first introduced as an "antiarthritic" drug in the sixth century. Although usually it is not noted in reviews of immunoregulatory drugs, its therapeutic value in sarcoid arthropathy (112), Behçet's disease (150,171), and familial Mediterranean fever (29,56,84,237,242,243)—in addition to its classic application in gout—suggests that its properties are not limited to effects on polymorphonuclear-leukocyte-mediated inflammation. Colchicine can bind to microtubular proteins and can depolymerize mitotic spindles as well as interrupt lysosomal enzyme secretion from neutrophils and cellular motility. It is unclear whether or not its activities are related solely to its effects on microtubules, because it may also have direct effects on cell membranes independent of its effect on tubulin.

The mechanism of action of this drug in gout is thought to be suppression of synthesis and secretion of a non-complement-associated chemotactic factor produced by urate-crystal stimulation of polymorphonuclear leukocytes. How colchicine exerts its effect in other diseases is less clear. It can decrease production of the acute-phase reactants serum amyloid P component (SAP) and serum amyloid A protein (SAA) *in vitro* and secretion of SAA both *in vitro* and *in vivo;* however, its activity in preventing amyloidosis in patients with familial Mediterranean fever does not correlate precisely with this activity (241). Somewhat paradoxically, colchicine has been reported to increase production of IL-1, which may be an inducer of SAA (29). The occasional effectiveness of this agent in Behçet's disease, a vasculitic process, further indicates our lack of knowledge concerning its mechanism of action and our poor understanding of the pathogenesis of various inflammatory diseases.

Oral colchicine (1–2 mg/day) is rapidly absorbed, and peak plasma concentrations occur at 1 hr. Leukocyte concentrations, however, remain high for more than 24 hr. Most of the administered colchicine is excreted in the feces; liver metabolism is at least in part necessary, and doses must be decreased in patients with liver disease. Nausea, vomiting, diarrhea, and abdominal pain are the most common side effects and are dose-dependent. The drug may induce a temporary leukopenia and subsequent leukocytosis, often with basophilic granulocytosis. Chronic administration has infrequently been associated with aplastic anemia, peripheral neuropathy, and alopecia.

USE OF IMMUNOREGULATORY AGENTS IN SPECIFIC DISEASES

Evaluation of Clinical Data

The potential basis for therapy with immunomodulating drugs in inflammatory diseases of unknown cause is especially important, because all of these therapies have real or potential toxicities that are quite substantial. One of us (A.D.S.) has long supported the concept of therapy involving randomized trials. This view was projected to encourage physicians to start such trials early in the use of a drug for a particular disease, before it became morally difficult to "withhold a potentially life-saving treatment." Reliance on a series of patients treated in a new manner, using comparisons with historical controls, is not a good method for dictating clinical practice. This is especially a problem in situations in which disease is becoming milder, in which disease is being treated earlier because of the availability of more sensitive diagnostic tests, or in which improved adjunctive therapy is available. Many diseases illustrate this point. For example, systemic lupus nephritis, discussed in detail elsewhere (198), is diagnosed earlier, and adjunctive care (antihypertensives, antibiotics, etc.) is better, with patients appearing to live longer for reasons in part unrelated to therapy. As a result, by comparison with historical controls, any new therapy that does not worsen the outlook would appear to be an improvement. Many other problems, including central nervous system (CNS) lupus, polymyositis, and Wegener's granulomatosis, have not been subjected to similar trials. Treatment for CNS lupus has included high doses of corticosteroids and bolus cyclophosphamide. Polymyositis has been treated with methotrexate or cyclophosphamide, and Wegener's granulomatosis with cyclophosphamide. For these problems we can report what has come to be "standard practice." Moreover, we believe that the "standard practice" is often better than no treatment or better than corticosteroid therapy; however, the "standard practice" is a toxic therapy, and we cannot say that it is always superior to a less toxic immunosuppressive regimen. This problem comes from the introduction of the new therapy into general clinical practice without the benefit of comparative studies. For example, although we believe that cyclophosphamide is superior to corticosteroids alone in therapy for Wegener's granulomatosis, milder and milder forms of Wegener's granulomatosis are being appreciated, and patients are being diagnosed earlier and earlier. As a result, it is possible that the historical controls had sufficiently worse prognoses and that many of the currently treated patients are not comparable. A subset of such patients might respond very well to a less toxic regimen, such as azathioprine, as has been found, for example, for a subset of patients with lupus nephritis (39).

In this section we shall consider the experience with immunoregulatory agents in treating a number of specific diseases. For the most part, the data supporting the use of one drug rather than another often are less than convincing. In practice, our own anecdotal experiences and those of our colleagues influence our choice of agents, and we are humbled when asked to support the use of particular regimens with hard data from the literature. Familiarity with the toxicity and metabolism of these agents is critical to their proper use. Some of the diseases in which specific immunoregulatory agents have shown some efficacy are listed in Table 4. This list is not complete, nor is it a specific recommendation for treatment, but rather a summary, in part based on our own bias in addition to the supporting literature discussed in this section.

Rheumatoid Arthritis

Over the last 15 years, considerable experience has been gained using immunoregulatory drugs in the treatment of patients with rheumatoid arthritis. Azathioprine (3,45,47,119,219), cyclophosphamide (31,45,47,50,119, 219), and methotrexate (86,229,232) all compare favorably with gold in terms of therapeutic efficacy. Response rates for these different chemotherapeutic agents are approximately 50%. Chlorambucil may also be efficacious

in rheumatoid arthritis, but controlled studies have not been performed. Concern over toxicities (see earlier) has limited the use of these agents to those patients refractory to conventional therapy; currently, they tend to be largely reserved for those patients for whom gold therapy has failed (and, usually, penicillamine and/or antimalarials) or patients who have life-threatening complications such as vasculitis. This practice has been questioned (197), and early vigorous therapy is gaining in theoretical, if not practical, importance.

In one controlled study, azathioprine and cyclophosphamide were both superior, as individual agents, to gold in retarding bone erosions in patients with rheumatoid arthritis (45). In another controlled study, cyclophosphamide, but not azathioprine, was shown to retard bone destruction (50). Cyclophosphamide reduced steroid requirements in a third study (219). Uncontrolled studies also have suggested long-term efficacy for both azathioprine and cyclophosphamide.

Methotrexate has been shown to be effective in treating rheumatoid arthritis in low-dosage oral regimens (7.5–15 mg/week, 2.5–5 mg every 12 hr) in controlled studies, but drug-related toxicities were frequent (229,232). In one study, one-third of the patients were withdrawn for adverse drug reactions, most commonly elevated liver enzymes (232). In another study, only 1 of 28 patients was withdrawn (229). More recently, weekly intravenous methotrexate (10–50 mg) has been used. Eleven of 14 patients in this study had evidence of improvement within 2 months (98). At the National Institutes of Health, the use of high-dosage intravenous methotrexate, with subsequent leucovorin rescue, is being studied. The long-term efficacy of methotrexate has not been formally established, but anecdotal experience suggests that this agent can be effective for many years.

Cyclosporin A may also have value in treating rheumatoid arthritis refractory to other treatments. Ongoing studies at the National Institutes of Health and also at

TABLE 4. *Probable efficacies of cytotoxic drugs in rheumatologic diseases—a private view*

| | Azathioprine | Chlorambucil | Cyclophosphamide | | Methotrexate[c] |
			A[a]	B[b]	
Rheumatoid arthritis	++[d]	+	++	++	++
Rheumatoid vasculitis	0	+	++	++	NS
Wegener's granulomatosis	+	++	+++	NS	NS
Polyarteritis nodosa	+	NS	++	NS	NS
Polymyositis	++	NS	++	+	+++
Psoriatic arthritis	+	NS	+	NS	++
SLE	++	++	++	+++	NS

[a] A = daily p.o.
[b] B = intermittent i.v. bolus.
[c] Weekly p.o.—conventional.
[d] Degree of benefit, based on published studies and also unpublished observations in the National Institutes of Health experience: +++ = substantial; ++ = definite; + = probable; 0 = none; NS = not studied or inadequate for an opinion.

other centers have shown promising results; however, close monitoring of drug levels and side effects, especially hypertension and renal function, is necessary.

Finally, combining multiple agents that have different mechanisms of action could potentially be of great advantage. A multicenter study examining oral gold versus methotrexate versus combined oral gold and methotrexate is currently under way. Gold therapy is thought to affect primarily macrophages and their processing/presenting functions (see Chapter 49), whereas methotrexate (Table 5) is thought to exert its effects on synovial cell proliferation. That study also differs from previous trials of combination therapy in that the patients at entry have early disease.

Psoriatic Arthritis

Methotrexate and azathioprine have both shown efficacy in treatment of psoriatic arthritis (26,134,233). Methotrexate has been given both intravenously and orally in placebo-controlled trials. High-dose methotrexate (1–3 mg/kg) given intravenously every 10 days for three treatments resulted in improvement in both skin and joint manifestations in the majority of 21 patients in one study (26). Further treatment for an additional 3 weeks resulted in continued improvement. Not surprisingly, relapses occurred 1 to 4 months after cessation of therapy (26). Toxicity was considerable in this early study (1964), and two deaths were associated with this therapy (26). A more recent study using low-dosage oral therapy (2.5–5.0 mg every 12 hr for 3 doses, once a week for 12 weeks) showed no improvement over placebo except in physician overall assessment of disease activity and in the amount of skin surface area covered with psoriatic plaques (233). In 6 patients, oral azathioprine (2.5 mg/kg/day) given for 6 months resulted in significant improvement in joint and skin manifestations, as compared with placebo in a double-crossover trial (134).

Uncontrolled studies and our own anecdotal experience would favor the use of methotrexate in this disease. About two-thirds of the patients treated with oral methotrexate will have favorable responses. A typical regimen would start with 2.5 mg orally every 12 hr for three consecutive doses each week. Subsequently, doses could be increased every 4 to 6 weeks if there was no response and toxicity was not limiting. Careful use of this cytotoxic agent, including patient selection (no preexisting liver disease, no alcohol consumption) and monitoring for toxicity, is necessary (see earlier).

Polymyositis/Dermatomyositis

Although there have been no controlled studies of methotrexate in polymyositis, uncontrolled studies support the use of this drug as the treatment of choice in those patients refractory to steroids (14,35,93,146). Treatment with both intravenous methotrexate and oral methotrexate (5–50 mg each week) in combination with corticosteroids has resulted in improvement in muscle strength, muscle enzymes, and electromyography, as well as decreases in steroid requirements. Azathioprine and cyclophosphamide may also be of benefit in some patients with these diseases (22,30,32,35,77). A controlled study compared oral prednisone and placebo with oral prednisone and oral azathioprine (2 mg/kg/day) (30,32). There was no difference at 3 months of treatment, but at 1 and 3 years the azathioprine group required less steroid and had a lesser degree of disability (30,32). Uncontrolled studies suggest that oral azathioprine or oral cyclophosphamide has been beneficial when used in conjunction with oral steroids (22,35,77). A large multicenter trial examining the efficacy of cyclosporin A is in progress. At present, immunoregulatory drugs are used in polymyositis/dermatomyositis as an adjunct to corticosteroids, either to increase disease control or to reduce steroid requirements.

TABLE 5. *Effects of immunosuppressive drugs*

Drug	Dosage (mg/kg/day, except as noted)	Decreased antibody (0–5+)[a]	Decreased delayed hypersensitivity (0–5+)[a]	Toxicity (0–5+)[a]
Cyclophosphamide	0.7–1.0 p.o.	1+	1	1+
	2.0 p.o.	4+	3+	2 to 3+
Cyclosporin A	5.0–10.0 p.o.	0	3+	2 to 3+
6-Mercaptopurine	1.5 p.o.	0	2+	2+
	2.5 p.o.	3+	3+	4+
Azathioprine	1.4–2.5 p.o.	±	±	±
	3.0 p.o.	1 to 2+	2+	1 to 2+
Methotrexate	0.7–1.0 i.v. (mg/kg/week)	±	1+	1+
	0.1 i.v.	4+	2+	2 to 3+

[a] For all estimates, the range is from 0 = none to 5 = maximum.

Wegener's Granulomatosis and Polyarteritis Nodosa

Wegener's granulomatosis often is cited as the prime example of the value of cytotoxic immunoregulatory agents in nonmalignant disease. Although there have been no controlled studies, uncontrolled studies showed a favorable outcome in comparison with historical controls; prognosis with steroid treatment alone was extremely poor (approximately 10% 1-year survival); with the addition of cyclophosphamide, treatment survival was greatly improved (>80% 1-year survival) (67,104,172,235); however, historical controls were from an era in which Wegener's granulomatosis patients were sicker. Azathioprine and chlorambucil also have been reported to prolong survival (23,103,104,213). Treatment of limited forms of Wegener's granulomatosis (confined to lung involvement) is less clear, because the prognosis for these patients untreated is much better than for the full Wegener's granulomatosis syndrome. A randomized stratified trial is needed to determine relative efficacy and toxicity for azathioprine, chlorambucil, methotrexate, and cyclophosphamide in patients with severe and milder forms of Wegener's granulomatosis.

Uncontrolled studies also support the use of cytotoxic immunoregulatory drugs in polyarteritis nodosa and other necrotizing vasculitides in addition to Wegener's granulomatosis (67,117). Patients treated with oral cyclophosphamide alone in one study, and together with prednisone in another study, appeared to have good responses in life-threatening polyarteritis nodosa resistant to steroids alone (67). In practice, cyclophosphamide therapy often is initiated concomitantly with steroids in rapidly progressive vasculitic syndromes involving medium-size arteries. Some would initiate cytotoxic drugs at diagnosis; others would determine the response to steroids first.

For these necrotizing vasculitides (Wegener's granulomatosis and polyarteritis), cyclophosphamide most commonly is initiated with an oral dosage of 2 mg/kg/day. Subsequently, the dosage is increased by 25 mg every 2 weeks until a clinical response or toxicity. The cyclophosphamide is adjusted to a level that will control disease manifestations and maintain a leukocyte count greater than 3,000/mm^3. In general, treatment probably should be continued for 12 to 18 months after clinical remission is obtained; however, leukopenia usually limits the dosage of drug that can be given after the first 6 months of therapy.

Behçet's Syndrome

Behçet's syndrome is a vasculitis involving both small and large arteries and veins in which patients may have multiple manifestations, almost always including aphthous ulcers and uveitis. Chlorambucil (1,141,

158,214,218), cyclophosphamide (73,97,131,218), azathioprine (12,131), 6-mercaptopurine (218), colchicine (150,171), cyclosporin A (157), and levamisole (145) have all been used with some claims of efficacy, alone or in combination with steroids. Chlorambucil has been the most frequently used cytotoxic agent; in multiple uncontrolled studies it apparently has had beneficial effects in treatment of uveitis and preservation of vision (141,158,218). This agent also may be at least partially effective in treating meningoencephalitis (158). Cyclophosphamide, in conjunction with steroids, has been effective in controlling both ocular and extraocular manifestations of Behçet's syndrome (73,97,218). Other cytotoxic agents have not been studied extensively, but azathioprine does not appear to be as effective as the alkylating agents in treating this disease (12,131).

Colchicine is often used as the first drug in treating patients with Behçet's syndrome. It probably decreases the frequency of oral ulcers and the severity of Behçet's arthritis (150), and it may decrease the frequency of meningoencephalitic attacks; however, this agent was not effective in treating uveitis in a prospective double-blind trial (7).

Levamisole has been used in treating 11 patients with Behçet's syndrome, with 9 patients appearing to have reductions in the number and severity of oral and genital ulcers. In 3 patients, withdrawal of levamisole resulted in flares, and reintroduction was associated with improvement (145); however, it is extremely difficult to interpret this study because of the intermittent nature of this disease and the small number of patients examined. Whether or not levamisole has any effect on uveitis or other serious manifestations of Behçet's syndrome was not addressed.

Recently, cyclosporin A has been used to treat posterior uveitis in patients with Behçet's syndrome (157). Seven patients who were previously treated with steroids (40–60 mg/day) alone or in addition to chlorambucil and were considered therapeutic failures had good responses to oral cyclosporin A therapy. Patients were initially treated with cyclosporin A at 10 mg/kg/day, and then the dosage was adjusted based on toxicity and plasma cyclosporin A concentrations. The cyclosporin A treatment effectively abrogated the acute phase of ocular attacks and, subsequently, prevented or reduced the recurrence of attacks. Continued treatment was apparently required, and the effects of this agent on nonocular manifestations are unknown.

Systemic Lupus Erythematosus

Several cytotoxic immunoregulatory agents have been used to treat both the renal and extrarenal manifestations of SLE. These drugs have been used in attempts to reduce steroid requirements and to achieve a more favorable prognosis. Azathioprine and cyclophosphamide have been the most widely studied agents, although uncontrolled studies, anecdotal reports, and a single randomized trial suggest that chlorambucil may also be more effective than steroids in treating lupus nephritis and, in particular, the extrarenal manifestations of disease (194). Experience with nitrogen mustard, 6-mercaptopurine, methotrexate, and 6-thioguanine is limited and will not be discussed. Other immunoregulatory agents have also been studied, including plasmapheresis (43,101,108,225,228) and total nodal irradiation (202), but experience has been limited, and the results thus far do not justify their consideration. Controlled studies, for the most part, have been limited to lupus nephritis, but cytotoxic agents, particularly azathioprine, are commonly used in practice as steroid-sparing agents to control extrarenal manifestations of disease.

Multiple uncontrolled studies have concluded that azathioprine ($\sim$2 mg/kg/day) is beneficial in lupus nephritis, both in reducing proteinuria and in stabilizing or improving renal function. Controlled studies have either supported the conclusion that azathioprine, in conjunction with steroids, is superior to steroids alone in treating lupus nephritis (34,105,210) or have found no difference between treatment groups with and without azathioprine (52,58,59,88,120,199,200). Studies at the National Institutes of Health suggest that azathioprine may be effective in certain patients with lupus nephritis, namely, those with an intermediate severity of disease. Thus, patients with mild disease may respond well to steroids alone, and those with severe disease may not respond, even with the addition of azathioprine. Analysis of pooled data from separate studies has further suggested that patients treated with azathioprine and steroids or cyclophosphamide and steroids had fewer unfavorable outcomes than those treated with steroids alone (70).

Many controlled studies have suggested that cyclophosphamide, in conjunction with steroids, is a valuable agent in treating lupus nephritis (17,19,39,54,77,83). These studies have mostly used low-dosage oral cyclophosphamide (1–2 mg/kg/day), although our group at the National Institutes of Health has also used intermittent high-dosage intravenous boluses (1 g/m^2 every 1–3 months) (17,19,54). These reports have included data suggesting significant improvement in renal function, urinalysis, and renal histology and less frequent recurrence of active nephritis; however, many of the studies have shown rather minimal benefits over steroids alone (58). The heterogeneity of lupus nephritis and the small sizes of most studies have made drawing definitive conclusions difficult.

Recent analysis of an ongoing study at the National Institutes of Health has emphasized another critical variable: long-term monitoring (17). At 5 years, there was no statistical difference in renal function between a treatment group that received intravenous cyclophosphamide plus low-dosage prednisone and a matched high-dosage prednisone-alone group; however, analysis of the same patients at 7 years showed a statistically significant advantage for the group that had received intravenous cyclophosphamide. In this study, patients with lupus nephritis were given intravenous cyclophosphamide at 0.5 to 1.0 g/m^2 every 3 months for at least 18 months after induction of clinical remission or until approximately 4 years of protocol therapy had been completed. Figure 4 shows the probability of renal failure for different treatment groups

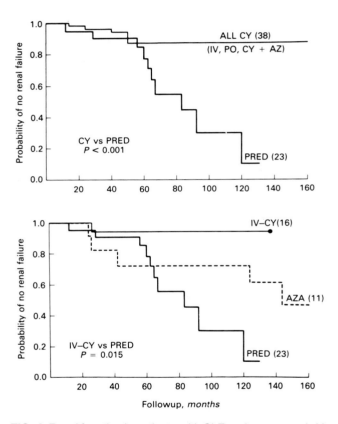

FIG. 4. Renal function in patients with SLE and severe nephritis treated with different drugs: progression to renal failure in patients treated with cyclophosphamide (CY) given orally (PO) or intravenously (IV) or orally with azathioprine (CY + AZ). **Top:** All of these groups are compared with patients randomized to receive prednisone only (PRED). The number in each group is shown in parentheses. The CY group retained renal function significantly better than did the PRED group; however, there was no difference for the first 60 months (5 years!). **Bottom:** Three individual groups: patients receiving intravenous boluses of cyclophosphamide (IV-CY), oral azathioprine (AZA), or prednisone only (PRED). In both the upper and lower panels, patients receiving the cytotoxic or cytostatic drugs also received low doses of prednisone, typically 0.25 mg/kg every other day. The prednisone-only group received at least 1 mg/kg/day for 2 to 3 months, after which the drug was tapered.

TABLE 6. Toxicity of immunosuppressive drugs

	Methotrexate	Azathioprine	Chlorambucil	Cyclophosphamide	Cyclosporin A
Infection	++[a]	++	++	++	++
Myelotoxicity	+++	+++	++++	+++	±
Pulmonary toxicity	+++	+	+	++	±
Nephrotoxicity	+	0	0	0	++++
Hepatotoxicity	++++	+	±	±	++
Allergy	0	++	0	0	0
Cystitis	0	0	0	++++	0
Pancreatitis	0	++	0	0	±
Neoplasia	±	+++	+++	+++	+
Gonadal toxicity	±	±	+++	++++	0
Fetal	++++	±	±	±	±

[a] Estimate of relative significance of toxicity: 0 = none; ± = questionable; + = definite but rare; ++ = definite; +++ = substantial; ++++ = of major clinical concern.

in the National Institutes of Health study during the course of follow-up. The advantage of intravenous cyclophosphamide over prednisone alone was most apparent in a high-risk subgroup showing chronic histologic changes on initial renal biopsy. At the National Institutes of Health, a study of the efficacy of a more intensive regimen of monthly intravenous pulse cyclophosphamide is being evaluated and is currently in its fourth year.

In summary, therapeutic use of cytotoxic drugs in SLE is beginning to be understood. Long-term follow-up of patients in current and future studies will be needed to have a firmer handle on which patients are likely to benefit from these approaches. Their toxicities are substantial (Table 6) (also see the sections on individual agents); however, the risks and complications of conventional therapy (i.e., steroids) and the natural history of the disease dictate the need for novel approaches. The available data do seem to justify our opinion that judicious use of these agents is a valuable adjunct to therapy in this disease.

GUIDELINES FOR USE OF IMMUNOREGULATORY AGENTS IN INFLAMMATORY DISEASES OF UNKNOWN CAUSE

In this chapter we have attempted to review the applications of immunoregulatory agents in "autoimmune diseases." The use of these agents is, as we have indicated, a two-edged sword. On one hand, they may have efficacy greater than that for more conventional therapy; on the other, they have toxicities that can be life-threatening. The side effects of these agents in various patient populations, as well as the severity of the disease manifestations for which treatment is being initiated, must be clearly understood by the physician and patient. In general, therapy with these agents is reserved for life-threatening or debilitating problems. We should note that a disease such

as rheumatoid arthritis, which we ordinarily do not think of as life-threatening, may in fact be associated with a prognosis no more favorable than those for certain forms of cancer.

In addition, it may be argued that the use of immunoregulatory agents early after disease onset may be more efficacious than later in the disease process; however, at present we cannot accurately determine which patients with diseases such as SLE will have a poor outcome shortly after diagnosis. Thus, we would not advocate treating pa-

TABLE 7. Guidelines for use of immunoregulatory agents in inflammatory diseases of unknown cause

1. Less toxic therapy is inadequate.
2. Disease manifestations are considered reversible.
3. The patient has no infections (if agent used suppresses host defenses).
4. Clearly defined clinical parameters are carefully monitored before, during, and after therapy to determine efficacy of treatment. Parameters include those that are subject to toxic effects of therapy.
5. If part of study, a protocol is used that is approved by peer review and includes informed consent. If very few patients with a particular disease are available, multicenter studies should be considered.
6. Before use of treatment, patients should be screened for contraindications (e.g., liver disease or alcohol intake excludes methotrexate). The ability of patients to comply with the treatment regimen in terms of their psychosocial situations should be considered.
7. The effects of withdrawal (i.e., flare-up of disease) should be anticipated if the agent needs to be discontinued because of toxicity. Alternative treatment should be planned.
8. Drug interactions need to be considered (e.g., allopurinol and azathioprine).
9. Periodic reevaluations of treatment will allow medications to be tapered or discontinued when treatment goals have been attained or when potential toxicities are more severe than potential benefits from continued treatment.

tients with recently diagnosed SLE with cytotoxic agents, because a great many of these patients will have relatively benign courses not requiring exposure to the risks associated with these agents. Current general guidelines for the commonly used immunoregulatory agents are listed in Table 7.

REFERENCES

1. Abdalla, M. I., and Bahgat, N. E. (1973): Long-lasting remission of Behçet's disease after chlorambucil therapy. *Br. J. Ophthalmol.,* 57:706–711.
2. Abdou, N. I., Sweiman, B., and Casella, S. R. (1973): Effects of azathioprine therapy on bone marrow-dependent and thymus-dependent cells in man. *Clin. Exp. Immunol.,* 13:55–64.
3. Abel, T., Urowitz, M. B., Smythe, H. A., Keystone, E. C., and Norman, C. B. (1978): Long-term effects of azathioprine in rheumatoid arthritis. *Arthritis Rheum.,* 21:539–543.
4. Adams, A., Petit, J. F., Lefrancier, P., and Lederer, E. (1981): Muramyl peptides: Chemical structure, biological activity and mechanism of action. *Mol. Cell. Biochem.,* 41:27–47.
5. Adelman, N. E., Watling, D. L., and McDevitt, H. O. (1983): Treatment of (NZB × NZW)F$_1$ disease with anti-I-A monoclonal antibodies. *J. Exp. Med.,* 158:1350–1355.
6. Ahn, Y. S., Brynes, J. J., Harrington, W. J., Cayer, M. L., Smith, D. S., Brunskill, D. E., and Pall, L. M. (1978): The treatment of idiopathic thrombocytopenia with vinblastine-loaded platelets. *N. Engl. J. Med.,* 298:1101–1107.
7. Aktulga, E., Altaç, M., Müftüoglu, A., Ozyazgan, Y., Tüzün, Y., Yalçin, B., Yacini, H., and Yurdakul, S. (1980): A double blind study of colchicine in Behçet's disease. *Haematologica (Pavia),* 65:399–402.
8. Albanin, K. S., LeBeau, M. M., Vardiman, J. W., Golomb, H. M., and Rowley, J. D. (1983): Development of dysmyelopoietic syndrome in a hairy cell leukemia patient treated with chlorambucil: Cytogenetic and morphologic evaluation. *Cytogenetics,* 8:107–115.
9. Amor, B., and Dougados, M. (1986): Ciclosporin in rheumatoid arthritis: Open trials with different dose. In: *Ciclosporin in Autoimmune Disease,* edited by R. Schindler, pp. 283–287. Springer-Verlag, Berlin.
10. Anderson, R. E., and Warner, N. L. (1976): Ionizing radiation and the immune response. *Adv. Immunol.,* 24:215–335.
11. Ansell, I. D., and Castro, J. E. (1975): Carcinoma of the bladder complicating cyclophosphamide therapy. *Br. J. Urol.,* 47:413–418.
12. Aoki, K., and Sugiura, S. (1976): Immunosuppressive treatment of Behçet's disease. *Mod. Probl. Ophthalmol.,* 16:309–313.
13. Appelbaum, F. R., Strauchen, J. A., Graw, R. G., Jr., Savage, D. D., Kent, K. M., Ferrans, U. J., and Herzig, G. P. (1976): Acute lethal carditis caused by high-dose combination chemotherapy: A unique clinical and pathological entity. *Lancet,* 1:58–62.
14. Arnett, F. C., Whelton, J. C., and Zizic, T. M. (1973): Methotrexate therapy in polymyositis. *Ann. Rheum. Dis.,* 32:536–546.
15. Askenase, P. W., Hayden, B. J., and Gershon, R. K. (1975): Augmentation of delayed-type hypersensitivity of doses of cyclophosphamide which do not effect antibody responses. *J. Exp. Med.,* 141:697–702.
16. Audibert, F., Chedid, L., Lefrancier, P., and Chory, J. (1976): Distinctive adjuvanticity of synthetic analogs of mycobacterial water-soluble components. *Cell. Immunol.,* 21:243–249.
17. Austin, H. A., Klippel, J. H., Balow, J. E., LeRiche, N. G., Steinberg, A. D., Plotz, P. H., and Decker, J. L. (1986): Therapy of lupus nephritis: Controlled trial of prednisone and cytotoxic drugs. *N. Engl. J. Med.,* 314:614–619.
18. Bagley, C. M., Jr., Bostick, F. W., and Devita, V. T. (1973): Clinical pharmacology of cyclophosphamide. *Cancer Res.,* 33:226–233.
19. Balow, J. E., Austin, H. A., III, Muenz, L. R., Joyce, K. M., Antonovych, T. T., Klippel, J. H., Steinberg, A. D., Plotz, P. H., and Decken, J. L. (1984): Effect of treatment on the evolution of renal abnormalities in lupus nephritis. *N. Engl. J. Med.,* 311:491–495.
20. Bendtzen, K., Petersen, J., and Soeberg, B. (1983): Effects of cyclosporin A (Cy-A) and methylprednisolone (MP) on the immune response. I. Further studies on the monocyte-T cell interactions leading to lymphokine production. *Acta Pathol. Microbiol. Immunol. Scand.,* 91:159–167.
21. Bennett, R. S., and Hamburger, M. I. (1982): A critical review of therapeutic apheresis in the treatment of severe rheumatoid arthritis. *Prog. Clin. Biol. Res.,* 106:33–48.
22. Benson, M. D., and Aldo, M. A. (1973): Azathioprine therapy in polymyositis. *Arch. Intern. Med.,* 132:547–551.
23. Berglund, G., Hansson, L., Persson, B., and Vikren, P. (1972): Combined chlorambucil and prednisolone treatment of five patients with Wegener's granulomatosis. *Acta Med. Scand.,* 191:5–9.
24. Berenbaum, M. C. (1962): The effect of cytotoxic agents on the production of antibody to TAB vaccine in the mouse. *Biochem. Pharmacol.,* 11:29–44.
25. Bird, H. A. (1985): Preliminary observations from a comparison of ciclosporin and azathioprine in rheumatoid arthritis. In: *Ciclosporin in Autoimmune Disease,* edited by R. Schindler, pp. 307–310. Springer-Verlag, Berlin.
26. Black, R. L., O'Brien, W. M., Van Scott, E. J., Auerbach, R., Eisen, A. Z., and Bunim, J. J. (1964): Methotrexate therapy in psoriatic arthritis. Double-blind study on 21 patients. *J.A.M.A.,* 189:743–747.
27. Bloch, K. J., and Maki, D. G. (1973): Hyperviscosity syndromes associated with immunoglobulin abnormalities. *Semin. Haematol.,* 10:113–124.
28. Borel, J. F., Feurer, C., Gubler, H. U., and Stahelin, H. (1976): Biological effects of cyclosporin A: A new antilymphocytic agent. *Agents Actions,* 6:468–475.
29. Brandwein, S. B., Sipe, J. D., Tatsuta, E., Skinner, M., and Cohen, A. S. (1983): Effect of colchicine on murine macrophage interleukin 1 mediated acute phase responses. *Clin. Res.,* 31:153A.
30. Bunch, T. W. (1981): Prednisone and azathioprine for polymyositis. Long-term follow-up. *Arthritis Rheum.,* 24:45–58.
31. Bunch, T. W., and O'Duffy, J. D. (1980): Clinical pharmacology. Series on pharmacology in practice. 6. Disease-modifying drugs for progressive rheumatoid arthritis. *Mayo Clin. Proc.,* 55:161–179.
32. Bunch, T. W., Worthington, J. W., Coombs, J. J., Ilstrup, D. M., and Engel, A. G. (1980): Azathioprine and prednisone for polymyositis: A controlled clinical trial. *Ann. Intern. Med.,* 92:365–369.
33. Bunjes, D., Hardt, C., Röllinghoff, M., and Wagner, H. (1981): Cyclosporin A mediates immunosuppression of primary cytotoxic T cell responses by impairing the release of interleukin 1 and interleukin 2. *Eur. J. Immunol.,* 11:657–661.
34. Cade, R., Spooner, G., Schlein, E., Pickering, M., De Quesada, A., Holcomb, A., Juncos, L., Richard, G., Shires, D., Levin, D., Hackett, R., Free, J., Hunt, R., and Fiegly, M. (1973): Comparison of azathioprine, prednisone and heparin alone, or combined in treating lupus nephritis. *Nephron,* 10:37–56.
35. Cairo-Glasgow Study Group (1978): Dermatomyositis: Observations on the use of immunosuppressive therapy and review of literature. *Postgrad. Med.,* 54:516–527.
36. Cameron, S. (1977): Chlorambucil and leukemia. *N. Engl. J. Med.,* 296:1065.
37. Cammisuli, S. (1981): Inhibition of a secondary humoral immune response by cyclosporin A. *Transplant. Clin. Immunol.,* 13:15.
38. Canafax, D. M., and Ascher, N. L. (1983): Cyclosporine immunosuppression. *Clin. Pharmacol.,* 2:515–524.
39. Carette, S., Klippel, J. H., Decker, J. L., Austin, H. A., III, Plotz, P. H., Steinberg, A. D., and Balow, J. E. (1983): Controlled studies of oral immunosuppressive drugs in lupus nephritis. A long-term follow-up. *Ann. Intern. Med.,* 99:1–8.
40. Carson, D. A., Kaye, J., and Seegmiller, J. E. (1978): Differential sensitivity of human leukemic T cell lines and B cell lines to growth inhibition by deoxyadenosine. *J. Immunol.,* 121:1726–1731.
41. Chapman, J. R., Griffiths, D., Harding, N. G. L., and Morris, P. J. (1985): Reversibility of cyclosporin nephrotoxicity after three months treatment. *Lancet,* 1:128–130.
42. Chedid, L., Audibert, F., Lefrancier, P., Chory, J., and Lederer, E.

(1976): Modulation of the immune response by a synthetic adjuvant and analogs. *Proc. Natl. Acad. Sci. USA*, 73:2472–2475.

43. Clark, W. F., Cattran, D. C., Balfe, J. W., Williams, W., Lindsay, R. M., and Linton, A. L. (1984): Long-term plasma exchange in patients with systemic lupus erythematosus and diffuse proliferative glomerulonephritis. *Plasma Ther. Transfus. Technol.*, 5:353–360.

44. Clara, R., and Germanes, J. (1977): Levamisole and agranulocytosis. *Lancet*, 1:47–48.

45. Cohen, J. L., Jao, J. Y., and Jusko, W. J. (1970): Pharmacokinetics of cyclophosphamide in man. *Br. J. Pharmacol.*, 43:677–680.

46. Cupps, T. R., Edgar, L. C., and Fauci, A. S. (1982): Suppression of human B lymphocyte function by cyclophosphamide. *J. Immunol.*, 128:2453–2457.

47. Currey, H. L. F., Harris, J. R. M., Mason, R. M., Woodland, J., Beveridge, T., Roberts, C. J., Vere, D. W., Dixon, A. S. J., Davies, J., and Owen-Smith, B. (1974): Comparison of azathioprine, cyclophosphamide and gold in treatment of rheumatoid arthritis. *Br. Med. J.*, 3:763–768.

48. Dau, P. C. (1982): Plasmapheresis in myasthenia gravis. *Prog. Clin. Biol. Res.*, 88:265–285.

49. Dau, P. C., Lindstrom, J. M., Cassel, C. K., Denys, E. H., Shev, E. E., and Spitler, L. E. (1977): Plasmapheresis and immunosuppressive drug therapy in myasthenia gravis. *N. Engl. J. Med.*, 297:1134–1140.

50. Davis, J. D., Muss, H. B., and Turger, R. A. (1978): Cytotoxic agents in the treatment of rheumatoid arthritis. *South. Med. J.*, 71:58–64.

51. Davis, P. J., Davis, F. B., and Charache, P. (1974): Long-term therapy of hereditary angioedema (HAE). *Johns Hopkins Med. J.*, 135:391–398.

52. Decker, J. L., Klippel, J. H., Plotz, P. H., and Steinberg, A. D. (1975): Cyclophosphamide or azathioprine in lupus glomerulonephritis. A controlled trial: Results at 28 months. *Ann. Intern. Med.*, 83:606–615.

53. De Fronzo, R. A., Braine, H., Colvin, O. M., and Davis, P. J. (1973): Water intoxication in man after cyclophosphamide therapy. Time course and relation to drug activation. *Ann. Intern. Med.*, 78:861–869.

54. Dinant, H. J., Decker, J. L., Klippel, J. H., Balow, J. E., Plotz, P. H., and Steinberg, A. D. (1982): Alternative modes of cyclophosphamide and azathioprine therapy in lupus nephritis. *Ann. Intern. Med.*, 96:728–736.

55. Dinarello, C. A., and Krueger, J. M. (1986): Induction of interleukin 1 by synthetic and naturally occurring muramyl peptides. *Fed. Proc.*, 45:2545–2548.

56. Dinarello, C. A., Wolff, S. M., Goldfinger, S. E., Dale, D. C., and Alling, D. W. (1974): Colchicine therapy for familial Mediterranean fever: A double blind trial. *N. Engl. J. Med.*, 291:934–937.

57. Donabedian, H., Alling, D. W., and Gallin, J. I. (1982): Levamisole is inferior to placebo in the hyperimmunoglobulin E recurrent-infection (Job's) syndrome. *N. Engl. J. Med.*, 307:290–292.

58. Donadio, J. V., Jr., Holley, K. E., Ferguson, R. H., and Illstrup, D. M. (1978): Treatment of diffuse proliferative lupus nephritis with prednisone and combined prednisone and cyclophosphamide. *N. Engl. J. Med.*, 299:1151–1155.

59. Donadio, J. V., Jr., Holley, K. E., and Wagoner, R. D. (1972): Treatment of lupus nephritis with prednisone and combined prednisone and azathioprine. *Ann. Intern. Med.*, 77:829–835.

60. Donadio, J. V., Holley, K. E., Wagoner, R. D., Ferguson, R. H., and McDuffie, F. C. (1974): Further observations on the treatment of lupus nephritis with prednisone and combined prednisone and azathioprine. *Arthritis Rheum.*, 17:573–581.

61. Dos Reis, G. A., and Shevach, E. M. (1982): Effect of cyclosporin A on T cell function *in vitro*: The mechanism of suppression of T cell proliferation depends on the nature of the T cell stimulus as well as the differentiation state of the responding T cell. *J. Immunol.*, 129:2360–2367.

62. Duvic, M., Steinberg, A. D., and Klassen, L. W. (1978): Effect of the anti-estrogen, Nafoxidine, on NSB/W autoimmune disease. *Arthritis Rheum.*, 21:414–417.

63. Eidinger, D., and Garrett, T. J. (1972): Studies of the regulatory effects of sex hormones on antibody formation and stem cell differentiation. *J. Exp. Med.*, 136:1098–1116.

64. Elion, G. B. (1967): Biochemistry and pharmacology of purine analogues. *Fed. Proc.*, 26:898–903.

65. Engleman, E. G., Benike, C., Hoppe, R. T., and Kaplan, H. S. (1979): Suppressor cells of mixed lymphocyte reaction in patients with Hodgkin's disease. *Transplant. Proc.*, 11:1827–1829.

66. Fauci, A. S., Harley, J. B., Roberts, W. C., Ferrans, V. J., Gralnick, H. R., and Bjornson, B. J. (1982): The idiopathic hypereosinophilic syndrome: Clinical, pathologic and therapeutic considerations. *Ann. Intern. Med.*, 97:78–92.

67. Fauci, A. S., Haynes, B. F., Katz, P., and Wolff, S. M. (1983): Wegener's granulomatosis: Prospective clinical and therapeutic experience with 85 patients for 21 years. *Ann. Intern. Med.*, 98:76–85.

68. Fauci, A. S., Katz, P., Haynes, B. F., and Wolff, S. M. (1979): Cyclophosphamide therapy of severe systemic necrotizing vasculitis. *N. Engl. J. Med.*, 301:235–238.

69. Feinerman, B., Paul, R. D., and Feinerman, G. (1983): Treatment of a murine leukemia with chlorambucil bound monoclonal antibodies. *Adv. Exp. Med. Biol.*, 166:59–66.

70. Felson, D. T., and Anderson, J. (1984): Evidence for the superiority of immunosuppressive drugs and prednisone over prednisone alone in lupus nephritis: Results of a pooled analysis. *N. Engl. J. Med.*, 311:1528–1533.

71. Ferguson, R. M., Sutherland, D. E. R., Kim, T., Simmons, R. L., and Najarian, J. S. (1981): The *in vitro* assessment of the immunosuppressive effect of fractionated total lymphoid irradiation in renal allotransplantation. *Transplant. Proc.*, 13:1673–1675.

72. Filopovich, A. H., McGlave, P. B., Ramsay, N. K. C., Goldstein, G., Warkentin, P. I., and Kersey, J. H. (1982): Pretreatment of donor bone marrow with monoclonal antibody OKT3 for prevention of acute graft-versus-host disease in allogeneic histocompatible bone marrow transplantation. *Lancet*, 1:1266–1269.

73. Firat, I. K. (1979): Immunosuppressive treatment in Behçet's disease (report of 100 cases). In: *Behçet's Disease*, edited by N. Dilsen, M. Konice, and C. Ovul, pp. 282–285. Excerpta Medica, Amsterdam.

74. Forre, O., Bjerkhoel, F., Rugstad, H. E., Berg, K. J., and Kass, E. (1986): Ciclosporin versus azathioprine in rheumatoid arthritis. In: *Ciclosporin in Autoimmune Disease*, edited by R. Schindler, pp. 302–306. Springer-Verlag, Berlin.

75. French, M. E., Thompson, J. F., Hunnisett, A. G. W., Wood, R. F. M., and Morris, P. J. (1983): Impaired function of renal allografts during treatment with cyclosporin A: Nephrotoxicity or rejection? *Transplant. Proc. [Suppl.]*, 15:485–488.

76. Freund, J. (1947): Some aspects of active immunization. *Annu. Rev. Microbiol.*, 1:291–308.

77. Fries, J. F., Sharp, G. C., McDevitt, H. O., and Holman, H. R. (1973): Cyclophosphamide therapy in systemic lupus erythematosus and polymyositis. *Arthritis Rheum.*, 16:154–162.

78. Gabrielsen, A. E., and Good, R. A. (1967): Chemical suppression of adaptive immunity. *Adv. Immunol.*, 6:91–229.

79. Gassman, A. E., and Van Furth, R. (1975): The effect of azathioprine (Imuran) on the kinetics of monocytes and macrophages during the normal steady state and an acute inflammatory reaction. *Blood*, 46:51–64.

80. Gelfand, J. A., Sherrins, R. J., Alling, D. W., and Frank, M. M. (1976): Treatment of hereditary angioedema with Danazole. Reversal of clinical and biochemical abnormalities. *N. Engl. J. Med.*, 295:1444–1448.

81. Gershwin, M. E., Goetzl, E. J., and Steinberg, A. D. (1974): Cyclophosphamide: Use in practice. *Ann. Intern. Med.*, 80:531–540.

82. Ghose, T., Norvell, S. T., Gluclu, A., Bodurtha, A., Tai, J., and MacDonald, A. S. (1977): Immunochemotherapy of malignant melanoma with chlorambucil-bound antimelanoma globulins: Preliminary results in patients with disseminated disease. *J. Natl. Cancer Inst.*, 58:845–852.

83. Ginzler, E., Diamond, H., Guttadauria, M., and Kaplan, D. (1976): Prednisone and azathioprine compared to prednisone plus low-dose azathioprine and cyclophosphamide in the treatment of diffuse lupus nephritis. *Arthritis Rheum.*, 19:693–699.

84. Goldfinger, S. E. (1972): Colchicine for familial Mediterranean fever. *N. Engl. J. Med.,* 287:1302.

85. Greene, M. H., Boice, J. D., Jr., Greer, B. E., Blessing, J. A., and Dembo, A. J. (1982): Acute nonlymphocytic leukemia after therapy with alkylating agents for ovarian cancer: A study of five randomized clinical trials. *N. Engl. J. Med.,* 307:1416–1421.

86. Groff, G. D., Shenberger, K. N., Wilke, W. S., and Taylor, T. H. (1983): Low dose oral methotrexate in rheumatoid arthritis: An uncontrolled trial and review of the literature. *Semin. Arthritis Rheum.,* 12:333–347.

87. Grunwald, H. W., and Rosner, F. (1979): Acute leukemia and immunosuppressive drug use. A review of patients undergoing immunosuppressive therapy for nonneoplastic diseases. *Arch. Intern. Med.,* 139:461–466.

88. Hahn, B. H., Kantor, O. S., and Osterland, C. K. (1975): Azathioprine plus prednisone compared with prednisone alone in the treatment of systemic lupus erythematosus. Report of a prospective controlled trial in 24 patients. *Ann. Intern. Med.,* 83:597–605.

89. Hall, R. P., Lawley, T. J., Smith, H. R., and Katz, S. (1982): Bullous eruption of systemic lupus erythematosus. *Ann. Intern. Med.,* 97:165–170.

90. Halperin, E. C. (1985): Total lymphoid irradiation as an immunosuppressive agent for transplantation and the treatment of "autoimmune" disease: A review. *Clin. Radiol.,* 36:125–130.

91. Hamilton, L., and Elion, G. B. (1954): The fate of 6-mercaptopurine in man. *Ann. N.Y. Acad. Sci.,* 60:304–314.

92. Henderson, F. S., Adamson, R. H., and Oliverio, V. T. (1965): The metabolic rate of tritiated methotrexate. II. Absorption and excretion in man. *Cancer Res.,* 25:1018–1024.

93. Hendriksson, K. G., and Sandstedt, P. (1982): Polymyositis—treatment and prognosis. A study of 107 patients. *Acta Neurol. Scand.,* 65:280–300.

94. Hersh, E. M., Carbone, P. O., and Freireich, E. J. (1966): Recovery of immune responsiveness after drug suppression in man. *J. Lab. Clin. Med.,* 67:566–572.

95. Herzog, C., and Gross, D. (1986): Low dose ciclosporin A and prednisone—a step in the direction of selective immunosuppression in rheumatoid arthritis refractory to treatment (6-month follow-up). In: *Ciclosporin in Autoimmune Disease,* edited by R. Schindler, pp. 289–296. Springer-Verlag, Berlin.

96. Hess, A. D., Tutschka, P. J., Santos, G. W., and Pu, Z. (1982): Effect of cyclosporin A on human lymphocyte responses *in vitro. J. Immunol.,* 128:355–367.

97. Hijikata, K., Ezawa, Y., Masuda, K., and Ohara, K. (1977): An evaluation of immunosuppressant therapy in Behçet's disease. In: *Behçet's Disease,* edited by N. Dilsen, M. Konice, and C. Ovul, pp. 275–278. Excerpta Medica, Amsterdam.

98. Hogan, N. A., and Hill, H. R. (1978): Enhancement of neutrophil chemotaxis and alteration of levels of cellular cyclic nucleotides by levamisole. *J. Infect. Dis.,* 138:437–444.

99. Hoover, R., and Fraumeni, J. F., Jr. (1973): Risk of cancer of renal-transplant recipients. *Lancet,* 2:55–57.

100. Hunter, R. F., and Huang, A. T. (1986): Antithymocyte globulin: A realistic approach to therapy for severe aplastic anemia. *South. Med. J.,* 79:1121–1125.

101. Huston, D. P., White, M. J., Mattioli, C., Huston, M. M., and Suki, W. N. (1983): A controlled trial of plasmapheresis and cyclophosphamide therapy of lupus nephritis. *Arthritis Rheum.,* 26:S33.

102. Hutchinson, F. (1966): The molecular basis for radiation effects on cells. *Cancer Res.,* 26:2045–2052.

103. Israel, H. L., and Patchefsky, A. S. (1975): Treatment of Wegener's granulomatosis of lung. *Am. J. Med.,* 58:671–673.

104. Israel, H. L., Patchefsky, A. S., and Saldana, M. I. (1977): Wegener's granulomatosis, lymphomatoid granulomatosis, and benign lymphocyte angiitis and granulomatosis of lung. Recognition and treatment. *Ann. Intern. Med.,* 87:691–699.

105. Ivanova, M. M., Nasonova, V. A., Solovyo, S. K., Akhnazarova, V. D., Speransky, A. I., Decker, J. L., and Steinberg, A. D. (1981): Controlled trial of cyclophosphamide, azathioprine, and chlorambucil in lupus nephritis (a double-blind trial) (in Russian). *Rheumatica,* 2:11–18.

106. Johnson, W. W., and Meadows, D. C. (1971): Urinary bladder fibrosis and telangiectasia associated with long term cyclophosphamide therapy. *N. Engl. J. Med.,* 284:290–294.

107. Jolivet, J., Cowan, K. H., Curt, G. A., Clendennin, N. J., and Chabner, B. A. (1983): The pharmacology and clinical use of methotrexate. *N. Engl. J. Med.,* 309:1094–1104.

108. Jones, J. V., Cumming, R. H., and Bucknall, R. C. (1976): Plasmapheresis in the management of acute systemic lupus erythematosus. *Lancet,* 1:709–711.

109. Jones, M. G., Harris, G., and Cowing, G. (1983): Response of murine autoimmune disease to cyclosporine and thiols. *Transplant. Proc.* [*Suppl.*], 15:2904–2908.

110. Kahn, M. F., Arlet, J., and Bloch-Michel, H. (1979): Leucémies aigues apres traitement par agents cytotoxiques en rheumatologie—19 observations chez 2006 patients. *Nouv. Presse Med.,* 8:1393–1397.

111. Kahn, M. F., and de Seze, S. (1975): Surveillance cancerologique sur long cours des patients traités par les immunodepresserus (chlorambucil) en rheumatologie. *Scand. J. Rheumatol.* [*Suppl. 8*], 4:9–23.

112. Kaplan, H. (1963): Sarcoid arthritis. *Arch. Intern. Med.,* 112:924–935.

113. Kaplan, H. S. (1980): *Hodgkin's Disease,* ed. 2. Harvard University Press, Cambridge, Mass.

114. Karsh, J., Klippel, J. H., Decker, J. L., Wright, D. G., and Flye, M. W. (1981): Lymphapheresis in rheumatoid arthritis. A randomized trial. *Arthritis Rheum.,* 24:867–873.

115. Karnovsky, M. L. (1986): Muramyl peptides in mammalian tissues and their effects at the cellular level. *Fed. Proc.,* 45:2556–2560.

116. Katz, S. I., Gallin, J. I., Hertz, K. C., Fauci, A. S., and Lawley, T. J. (1977): Erythema elevatum diutinum: Skin and systemic manifestations, immunologic studies and successful treatment with dapsone. *Medicine (Baltimore),* 56:443–455.

117. Katz, S. I., Hall, R. P., Lawley, T. J., and Strober, W. (1980): Dermatitis herpetiformis: The skin and the gut. *Ann. Intern. Med.,* 93:857–874.

118. Kennedy, M. S., Deeg, H. J., Storb, R., and Thomas, E. D. (1983): Cyclosporin in marrow transplantation: Concentration-dependent toxicity and immunosuppression *in vivo. Transplant. Proc.* [*Suppl.*], 15:471–473.

119. Klinenberg, J. R., Reichman, R., and Clements, P. J. (1984): Investigational therapy for rheumatoid arthritis. In: *Progress in Clinical Immunology, Vol. 1,* edited by A. S. Cohen, pp. 111–144. Grune & Stratton, Orlando, Fla.

120. Klippel, J. H. (1979): Studies in the treatment of lupus nephritis. *Ann. Intern. Med.,* 91:599–602.

121. Kotzin, B. L., and Strober, S. (1979): Reversal of NZB/NZW disease with total lymphoid irradiation. *J. Exp. Med.,* 150:371–378.

122. Kotzin, B. L., Strover, S., Engleman, E. G., Calin, A., Hoppe, R. T., Kansas, G. S., Terrell, C. P., and Kaplan, H. S. (1981): Arthritis with total lymphoid irradiation. *N. Engl. J. Med.,* 305:969–976.

123. Krause, J. R. (1982): Chronic idiopathic thrombocytopenic purpura (ITP): Development of acute non-lymphocytic leukemia subsequent to treatment with cyclophosphamide. *Med. Pediatr. Oncol.,* 10:61–65.

124. Krönke, M., Leonard, W. J., Depper, J. M., Arya, S. K., Wong-Staal, F., Gallo, R. C., Waldman, T. A., and Greene, W. C. (1984): Cyclosporin A inhibits T-cell growth factor gene expression at the level of mRNA transcription. *Proc. Natl. Acad. Sci. USA,* 81:5214–5218.

125. Krueger, J. M., Karaszewski, J. W., Davenne, D., and Shohan, S. (1986): Somnogenic muramyl peptides. *Fed. Proc.,* 45:2552–2555.

126. Larsson, E. L. (1980): Cyclosporin A and dexamethasone suppress T cell responses by selectively acting at distant sites of the triggering process. *J. Immunol.,* 124:2828–2833.

127. Laupacis, A. (1983): Complications of cyclosporin therapy: A comparison to azathioprine. *Transplant. Proc.,* 15:2748–2753.

128. Lazowski, Z., Janczewski, Z., and Polowiec, Z. (1982): The effect of alkylating agents on the reproductive and hormonal testicular

function in patients with rheumatoid arthritis. *Scand. J. Rheumatol.,* 11:49–54.

129. Lehner, T., Wilton, J. M. A., and Ivanyi, L. (1976): Double blind crossover trial of levamisole in recurrent aphthous ulceration. *Lancet,* 2:926–929.

130. Leib, E. S., Restivo, C., and Paulus, H. E. (1979): Immunosuppressive and corticosteroid therapy of polyarteritis nodosa. *Am. J. Med.,* 67:941–947.

131. Lessof, M. H., Jeffreys, D. B., Lehner, T., Mattock, M., and Sanders, M. D. (1979): Corticosteroids and azathiorpine: Their use in Behçet's syndrome. In: *Behçet's Syndrome,* edited by T. Lehner and C. G. Barnes, pp. 267–275. Academic Press, New York.

132. Lennard, L., Rees, C. A., Lilleyman, J. S., and Maddocks, J. L. (1983): Childhood leukaemia: A relationship between intracellular 6-mercaptopurine metabolites and neutropenia. *Br. J. Clin. Pharmacol.,* 16:359–363.

133. Levy, J., Barnett, E. V., MacDonald, N. S., Klinenberg, J. R., and Pearson, C. M. (1972): The effect of azathioprine on gammaglobulin synthesis in man. *J. Clin. Invest.,* 51:2233–2238.

134. Levy, J., Paulus, H. E., Barnett, E. V., Sokoloff, M., Bangert, R., and Pearson, C. M. (1972): A double-blind controlled evaluation of azathioprine treatment in rheumatoid arthritis and psoriatic arthritis. *Arthritis Rheum.,* 15:116–117.

135. Lockwood, C. M., Rees, A. J., Russell, B., and Peters, D. L. (1977): Experience of the use of plasma exchange in the management of glomerulonephritis and SLE. *Exp. Hematol. [Suppl.],* 5:117–136.

136. Losito, A., Williams, D. G., and Harris, L. (1978): The effects on polymorphonuclear leukocyte function of prednisolone and azathioprine *in vivo* and prednisolone, azathioprine and 6-mercaptopurine *in vitro. Clin. Exp. Immunol.,* 32:423–428.

137. Mecario, A. J. L., and Conway de Marcario, E. (1978): Enhancement and inhibition of immunological mechanisms by immunosuppressive agents. I. Dose effect on priming and generation of memory to a bacterial antigen. *Clin. Exp. Immunol.,* 31:281–290.

138. Machleder, H. I., and Paulus, H. (1978): Clinical and immunological alterations observed in patients undergoing long-term thoracic duct draining. *Surgery,* 84:157–165.

139. Madhok, R., and Capell, H. A. (1986): Ciclosporin in rheumatoid arthritis—preliminary results. In: *Ciclosporin in Autoimmune Disease,* edited by R. Schindler, pp. 297–298. Springer-Verlag, Berlin.

140. Maibach, H. I., and Epstein, W. L. (1965): Immunologic responses of healthy volunteers receiving azathioprine (Imuran). *Int. Arch. Allergy,* 27:102–109.

141. Mamo, J. G. (1976): Treatment of Behçet's disease with chlorambucil. A follow-up report. *Arch. Ophthalmol.,* 94:580–583.

142. McLean, A., Newell, D., and Baker, G. (1976): The metabolism of chlorambucil. *Biochem. Pharmacol.,* 29:2039–2047.

143. Melez, K., Reeves, J. P., and Steinberg, A. D. (1978): Modification of NZB/NZW disease by sex hormones. *J. Immunopharmacol.,* 1:27–42.

144. Melez, K., Reeves, J. P., and Steinberg, A. D. (1978): Modification of murine lupus by sex hormones. *Ann. Immunol.,* 129C:707–712.

145. Merieux, P. de, Spitler, L. E., and Paulus, H. E. (1981): Treatment of Behçet's syndrome with levamisole. *Arthritis Rheum.,* 24:64–70.

146. Metzger, A. L., Bohan, A., Goldberg, L. S., Bluestone, R., and Pearson, C. M. (1974): Polymyositis and dermatomyositis: Combined methotrexate and corticosteroid therapy. *Ann. Intern. Med.,* 81:182–189.

147. Miller, B., DeMerieux, P., and Srinivasan, R. (1980): Double-blind placebo controlled crossover evaluation of levamisole in rheumatoid arthritis. *Arthritis Rheum.,* 23:172–182.

148. Mitchell, B. S., Mejias, E., Daddona, P. E., and Kelly, W. N. (1978): Purinogenic immunodeficiency diseases: Selective toxicity of deoxyribonucleosides for T cells. *Proc. Natl. Acad. Sci. USA,* 75:5011–5014.

149. Mitchell, M. S., Wade, M. E., DeConti, R. C., Bertino, J. R., and Calabresi, P. (1969): Immunosuppressive effects of cytosine arabinoside and methotrexate in man. *Ann. Intern. Med.,* 70:535–547.

150. Mizushima, Y., Matsumura, N., Mori, M., Shimizu, T., Fukashima,

151. B., Mimura, Y., Saito, K., and Sugiura, S. (1977): Colchicine in Behçet's disease. *Lancet,* 2:1037.

151. Mountz, J. D., Smith, H. R., Wilder, R. L., Reeves, J. P., and Steinberg, A. D. (1987): CS-A therapy in MRL-lpr/lpr mice: Amelioration and immunopathology despite autoantibody production. *J. Immunol.,* 138:157–163.

152. Mouridsen, H. T., and Jacobsen, E. (1975): Pharmacokinetics of cyclophosphamide in renal failure. *Acta Pharmacol. Toxicol.,* 36:409–414.

153. Muraguchi, A., Butler, J. L., Kehrl, J. H., Falkoff, R. J., and Fauci, A. S. (1983): Selective suppression of an early step in human B cell activation by cyclosporin A. *J. Exp. Med.,* 158:690–702.

154. Myers, B. D., Ross, J., Newton, L., Lvetzcher, J., and Perloth, M. (1984): Cyclosporin-associated chronic nephropathy. *N. Engl. J. Med.,* 311:699–705.

155. Navarro, J., and Touraine, J. L. (1983): Comparative study of cycloimmune cyclosporin A on human lymphocyte proliferation *in vitro.* The lack of an immunosuppressive effect by specific clonal deletion. *Int. J. Immunopharmacol.,* 5:157–162.

156. Nussenblatt, R. B., Palestine, A. G., and Chan, C. C. (1983): Cyclosporin A therapy in the treatment of intraocular inflammatory disease resistant to systemic corticosteroids and cytotoxic agents. *Am. J. Ophthalmol.,* 96:275–283.

157. Nussenblatt, R. B., Palestine, A. G., Chan, C. C., Mochizuki, M., and Yancey, K. (1985): Effectiveness of cyclosporin therapy for Behçet's disease. *Arthritis Rheum.,* 28:671–679.

158. O'Duffy, D. J., Robertson, D. M., and Goldstein, N. P. (1984): Chlorambucil in the treatment of uveitis and meningoencephalitis of Behçet's disease. *Am. J. Med.,* 76:75–84.

159. Oon, C. J., and Hobbs, J. R. (1975): Review: Clinical application of the continuous-flow separator machine. *Clin. Exp. Immunol.,* 20:1–16.

160. Palestine, A. G., Austin, H. A., Balow, J. E., Antonovych, T. T., Sabnis, S. G., Preuss, H. G., and Nussenblatt, R. B. (1986): Renal histopathologic alterations in patients treated with cyclosporin for uveitis. *N. Engl. J. Med.,* 314:1293–1298.

161. Paulus, H. E., Machleder, H. I., Levine, S., Yu, D. T. Y., and MacDonald, N. S. (1977): Lymphocyte involvement in rheumatoid arthritis. Studies during thoracic duct drainage. *Arthritis Rheum.,* 20:1249–1262.

162. Penn, I. (1983): Lymphomas complicating organ transplantation. *Transplant. Proc.,* 15:2790–2797.

163. Phillips, S. M., and Zweiman, B. (1972): Mechanisms in the suppression of delayed hypersensitivity in the guinea pig by 6-mercaptopurine. *J. Exp. Med.,* 137:1494–1510.

164. Plotz, P. H., Klippel, J. H., Decker, J. L., Grauman, D., Wolff, B., Brown, B. L., and Rutt, G. (1979): Bladder complications in patients receiving cyclophosphamide for systemic lupus erythematosus or rheumatoid arthritis. *Ann. Intern. Med.,* 91:221–223.

165. Prentice, H. G., Blacklock, H. A., Janossy, G., Bradstock, K. F., Skeggs, D., Goldstein, G., and Hoffbrand, A. V. (1982): Use of anti-T cell monoclonal antibody OKT3 to prevent acute graft-versus-host disease in allogeneic bone-marrow transplantation for acute leukemia. *Lancet,* 1:700–703.

166. Puri, H. C., and Campbell, R. A. (1977): Cyclophosphamide and malignancy. *Lancet,* 1:1306.

167. Pusey, C. D., and Lockwood, C. M. (1982): Plasma exchange and immunosuppressive drugs in the management of severe glomerulonephritis. *Prog. Clin. Biol. Res.,* 106:91–104.

168. Rabson, A. R., Whiting, D. A., Anderson, R., Glover, A., and Koornhof, H. J. (1977): Depressed neutrophil motility in patients with recurrent herpes simplex virus infection: *In vitro* restoration with levamisole. *J. Infect. Dis.,* 135:113–116.

169. Raefsky, E. L., Gascon, P., Gratwohl, A., Speck, B., and Young, N. S. (1986): Biological and immunological characterization of ATG and ALG. *Blood,* 68:712–719.

170. Raveche, E. S., Klassen, L. W., and Steinberg, A. D. (1976): Sex differences in formation of anti-T cell antibodies. *Nature,* 263:415–416.

171. Raynor, A., and Askari, A. D. (1980): Behçet's disease and treatment with colchicine. *J. Am. Acad. Dermatol.,* 2:396–400.

172. Reza, M. J., Dornfeld, L., Goldberg, L. S., Bluestone, R., and Pearson, C. M. (1975): Wegener's granulomatosis. Long-term follow-up of patients treated with cyclophosphamide. *Arthritis Rheum.*, 18:501–506.

173. Roberts, J. J., Brent, T. P., and Crathorn, A. R. (1971): Evidence for the inactivation and repair of the mammalian DNA template after alkylation by mustard gas and half mustard gas. *Eur. J. Cancer*, 7:515–524.

174. Rodger, R. S. C., Turney, J. H., Haines, I., Michael, J., Adu, D., and McMaster, P. (1983): Cyclosporin and liver function in renal allograft recipients. *Transplant. Proc.*, 15:2754–2756.

175. Rosenberg, S. A., Lotze, M. T., Muul, L. M., Leitman, S., Cheng, A. E., Vetto, J. T., Scippe, C. A., and Simpson, C. (1986): A new approach to the therapy of cancer based on the systemic administration of autologous lymphokine activated killer cells and recombinant interleukin 2. *Surgery*, 100:262–271.

176. Rosenthal, M., Travert, U., and Mueller, W. (1976): The effect of levamisole on peripheral blood lymphocyte subpopulations in patients with rheumatoid arthritis and ankylosing spondylitis. *Clin. Exp. Immunol.*, 25:493–496.

177. Rosman, M., and Bertino, J. R. (1973): Azathioprine. *Ann. Intern. Med.*, 79:694–700.

178. Roubinian, J. R., Papoian, R., and Talal, N. (1977): Androgenic hormones modulate autoantibody responses and improve survival in murine lupus. *J. Clin. Invest.*, 59:1066–1070.

179. Rudd, P., Fried, J. F., and Epstein, W. V. (1975): Irreversible bone marrow failure with chlorambucil. *J. Rheumatol.*, 2:421–429.

180. Runge, L. A., Pinals, R. S., Lourie, S. H., and Tomar, R. H. (1977): Treatment of rheumatoid arthritis with levamisole. A controlled trial. *Arthritis Rheum.*, 20:1445–1448.

181. Russell, J. A., Toy, J. L., and Powles, R. L. (1977): Plasma exchange in malignant paraproteinanemias. *Exp. Haematol.*, [*Suppl. 1*], 5:105–109.

182. Sampson, D., and Lui, A. (1976): The effect of levamisole on cell-mediated immunity and suppressor-cell function. *Cancer Res.*, 36:952–955.

183. Santos, G. W., Owens, A. H., and Sensenbrenner, L. L. (1964): Effects of selected cytotoxic agents on antibody production in man. *Ann. N.Y. Acad. Sci.*, 114:404–423.

184. Scannel, J. P., and Hitchings, G. H. (1966): Thioguanine in deoxyribonucleic acid from tumors of 6-mercaptopurine-treated mice. *Proc. Soc. Exp. Biol. Med.*, 122:627–629.

185. Schilsky, R. L., Lewis, B. J., Sherins, R. J., and Young, R. C. (1980): Gonadal dysfunction in patients receiving chemotherapy for cancer. *Ann. Intern. Med.*, 93:109–114.

186. Schurman, D. J., Hirshman, H. P., and Strober, S. (1981): Total lymphoid and local joint irradiation in the treatment of adjuvant arthritis. *Arthritis Rheum.*, 24:38–44.

187. Scott, J., Dieppe, P. A., and Huskisson, E. C. (1978): Continuous and intermittent levamisole. *Ann. Rheum. Dis.*, 37:259–261.

188. Segal, A. W., Levi, A. J., and Loewi, G. (1977): Levamisole in the treatment of Crohn's disease. *Lancet*, 2:382–385.

189. Sharbaugh, R. J., Ainsworth, S. K., and Fitts, C. T. (1976): Lack of effect of azathioprine on phytohemagglutinin-induced lymphocyte transformation and established delayed cutaneous hypersensitivity. *Int. Arch. Allergy Appl. Immunol.*, 51:681–686.

190. Sheffer, A. L., Fearon, D. T., and Austen, K. F. (1977): Methyltestosterone therapy in hereditary angioedema. *Ann. Intern. Med.*, 86:306–308.

191. Shumak, K. H., and Rock, G. A. (1984): Therapeutic plasma exchange. *N. Engl. J. Med.*, 310:762–771.

192. Skipper, H. E. (1954): On the mechanism of action of 6-mercaptopurine. *Ann. N.Y. Acad. Sci.*, 60:315–321.

193. Slavin, S. (1979): Successful treatment of autoimmune disease in (NZB/NZW)F₁ female mice by using fractionated total lymphoid irradiation. *Proc. Natl. Acad. Sci. USA*, 76:5274–5276.

194. Snaith, M. L., Holt, J. M., and Oliver, D. O. (1973): Successful treatment of patients with systemic lupus erythematosus, including nephritis, using chlorambucil. *Ann. Rheum. Dis.*, 32:279–280.

195. Spaulding, W. B. (1960): Methyltestosterone therapy for hereditary episodic edema (hereditary angioneurotic edema). *Ann. Intern. Med.*, 53:739–744.

196. Starzl, T. E., Klintmalm, G. B. G., Weil, R., III, Porter, K. A., Watsurki, S., Schroter, G. P., Fernandez-Bueno, C., and MacHugh, N. (1981): Cyclosporin A and steroid therapy in sixty-six cadaver kidney recipients. *Surg. Gynecol. Obstet.*, 153:486–494.

197. Steinberg, A. D. (1983): On the therapy of rheumatoid arthritis. *Clin. Exp. Rheumatol.*, 1:85–86.

198. Steinberg, A. D. (1986): The treatment of lupus nephritis. *Kidney Int.*, 30:769–787.

199. Steinberg, A. D., and Decker, J. L. (1974): A double-blind controlled trial comparing cyclophosphamide, azathioprine and placebo in the treatment of lupus glomerulonephritis. *Arthritis Rheum.*, 17:923–937.

200. Steinberg, A. D., Kaltreider, H. B., Staples, P. J., Goetzl, E. J., Talal, N., and Decker, J. L. (1971): Cyclophosphamide in lupus nephritis: A controlled trial. *Ann. Intern. Med.*, 75:165–171.

201. Steinberg, A. D., Klassen, L. W., Raveche, E. S., Gerber, N. L., Reinertsen, J. L., Krakauer, R. S., Ranney, D. F., Gershwin, M. E., Kovaks, K., Williams, G. W., and Reeves, J. P. (1978): Study of the multiple factors in the pathogenesis of autoimmunity in New Zealand mice. *Arthritis Rheum.*, 21:S190–201.

202. Strober, S., Field, E., Hoppe, R. T., Kotzin, B. L., Shemesh, O., Engelman, E., Ross, J. C., and Myers, B. D. (1985): Treatment of intractable lupus nephritis with total lymphoid irradiation. *Ann. Intern. Med.*, 102:450–458.

203. Strober, S., Tanay, A., Field, E., Hoppe, R. T., Calin, A., Engleman, E. G., Kotzin, B., Brown, B. W., and Kaplan, H. S. (1985): Efficacy of total lymphoid irradiation in intractable rheumatoid arthritis. A double-blind, randomized trial. *Ann. Intern. Med.*, 102:444–449.

204. Strober, S., Slavin, S., Gottlieb, M., Zan-Bar, I., King, D. P., Hoppe, R. T., Fuks, Z., Grumet, F. C., and Kaplan, H. S. (1979): Allograft tolerance after total lymphoid irradiation (TLI). *Immunol. Rev.*, 46:87–112.

205. Stokov, A. N. (1976): Experimental study of the combined effect of leukeran, degranol, and prednisolone. *Neoplasma*, 22:181–184.

206. Sutherland, D. E. R., Ferguson, R. M., Simmons, R. L., Kim, T. H., Slavin, S., and Najarian, J. S. (1983): Total lymphoid irradiation. *Urol. Clin. North Am.*, 10:277–288.

207. Swanson, M. A., and Schwartz, R. S. (1967): Immunosuppressive therapy. The relations between clinical response and immunologic competence. *N. Engl. J. Med.*, 277:163–170.

208. Sy, M. S., Miller, S. D., and Claman, H. N. (1977): Immune suppression with supraoptimal doses of antigen in contact sensitivity. I. Demonstration of suppressor cells and their sensitivity to cyclophosphamide. *J. Immunol.*, 119:240–244.

209. Symoens, J., and Rosenthal, M. (1977): Levamisole in the modulation of the immune response: The current experimental and clinical state. *J. Reticuloendothel. Soc.*, 21:175–221.

210. Sztejnbok, M., Stewart, A., Diamond, H., and Kaplan, D. (1971): Azathioprine in the treatment of systemic lupus erythematosus. A controlled study. *Arthritis Rheum.*, 14:639–645.

211. Terman, D. S., Petty, D., and Harbeck, R. (1977): Specific removal of DNA antibody *in vivo* by extracorporeal circulation over DNA immobilized in collodion charcoal. *Clin. Immunol. Immunopathol.*, 8:90–96.

212. Theofilopoulos, A. N., Balderas, R., Shawler, D. L., Isui, S., Kotzin, B. L., Strober, S., and Dixon, F. J. (1980): Inhibition of T-cell proliferation and SLE-like syndrome of MRL/1 mice by whole body or total lymphoid irradiation. *J. Immunol.*, 125:2137–2142.

213. Thorkelsen, H., and Berdal, P. (1976): Wegener's granulomatosis, immunosuppressive therapy. *Acta Otolaryngol.*, 82:208–211.

214. Tircoulis, D. (1976): Treatment of Behçet's disease with chlorambucil. *Br. J. Ophthalmol.*, 60:55–57.

215. Trentham, D. E., Belli, J. A., Anderson, R. J., Buckley, J. A., Goetzl, E. J., David, J. R., and Austen, K. F. (1981): Clinical and immunologic effects of fractionated total lymphoid irradiation in refractory rheumatoid arthritis. *N. Engl. J. Med.*, 305:976–982.

216. Trompeter, R. S., Evans, P. R., and Barratt, T. M. (1981): Gonadal function in boys with steroid-responsive nephrotic syndrome treated with cyclophosphamide for short periods. *Lancet*, 1:1177–1179.

217. Turk, J. L., and Parker, D. (1982): Effect of cyclophosphamide on immunological control mechanisms. *Immunol. Rev.,* 65:99–113.

218. Urgancioglu, M., Saylan, T., Akarcay, K., and Sezen, T. (1979): Immunosuppressive therapy in Behçet's disease. In: *Behçet's Disease,* edited by N. Dilsen, M. Konice, and C. Ovul, pp. 282–285. Excerpta Medica, Amsterdam.

219. Urowitz, M. B. (1974): Immunosuppressive therapy in rheumatoid arthritis. *J. Rheumatol.,* 1:364–373.

220. Valbonesi, M., Garelli, S., Zerbi, D., Forlani, G., Cornelio, F., and Pelucchetti, D. (1982): Plasma exchange combined with cytotoxic drugs and lymphocytapheresis for myasthenia gravis. *Vox Sang.,* 43:142–146.

221. Van Rijthoven, A. W. A. M., Dijkmans, B. I. C., Goethe, H. S., Montnor-Beckers, Z. L. B. B., Jacobs, P. J. C., and Cats, A. (1986): Ciclosporin treatment in rheumatoid arthritis: A preliminary report of a multicenter placebo-controlled double-blind study. In: *Ciclosporin in Autoimmune Disease,* edited by R. Schindler, pp. 299–301. Springer-Verlag, Berlin.

222. Verani, R. R., Flechner, S. M., Van Buren, C. T., and Kahan, B. N. (1984): Acute cellular rejection or cyclosporin A toxicity? A review of transplant biopsies. *Am. J. Kidney Dis.,* 4:185–191.

223. Veys, E. M., Mielants, H., and Verbruggen, G. (1978): Levamisole-induced adverse reactions in HLA-B27-positive rheumatoid arthritis. *Lancet,* 1:148.

224. Waldor, M., Sriram, S., McDevitt, H. O., and Steinman, L. (1983): *In vivo* therapy with monoclonal anti-Ia antibody suppresses immune response to acetylcholine receptors. *Proc. Natl. Acad. Sci. USA,* 80:2713–2717.

225. Wallace, D. J., Goldfinger, D., and Klinenberg, J. P. (1985): Plasmapheresis in lupus nephritis: A controlled study. Preliminary results. *Arthritis Rheum.,* 28:S46.

226. Warne, G. L., Fairley, K. F., Hobbs, J. B., and Martin, F. I. R. (1973): Cyclophosphamide-induced ovarian failure. *N. Engl. J. Med.,* 289:1159–1162.

227. Wechter, W. J., Nelson, J. W., Perper, R. H., Percells, A. J., Riebe, K. W., Evans, J. S., Satoh, P. S., and Ko, H. (1979): Manufacture of antithymocyte globulin (Atgam) for clinical trials. *Transplantation,* 28:303–307.

228. Wei, N., Klippel, J. H., Huston, D. P., Hall, R. P., Lawley, T. J., Balow, J. E., Steinberg, A. D., and Decker, J. L. (1983): Randomized trial of plasma exchange in mild systemic lupus erythematosus. *Lancet,* 1:17–22.

229. Weinblatt, M. E., Coblyn, J. S., Fox, D. A., Fraser, P. A., Holdsworth, D. E., Glass, D. N., and Trentham, D. E. (1985): Efficacy of low-dose methotrexate in rheumatoid arthritis. *N. Engl. J. Med.,* 312:818–822.

230. Weiss, R. B., and Maggia, F. M. (1980): Cytotoxic drug-induced pulmonary disease: Update 1980. *Am. J. Med.,* 68:259–266.

231. White, D. J. G., and Calne, R. Y. (1982): The use of cyclosporin A immunosuppression in organ grafting. *Immunol. Rev.,* 65:115–131.

232. Williams, H. F., Willkens, R. F., Samuelson, C. O., Jr., Alarcon, G. S., Guttadauria, M., Yarboro, C., Pollison, R. P., Weiner, S. R., Luggan, M. E., Billingsley, L. M., Dahl, S. L., Egger, M. J., Reading, J. C., and Ward, J. R. (1985): Comparison of low-dose oral pulse methotrexate and placebo in the treatment of rheumatoid arthritis. A controlled clinical trial. *Arthritis Rheum.,* 28:721–730.

233. Willkins, R. F., Williams, J. H., Ward, J. R., Egger, M. J., Reading, J. C., Clements, P. J., Cathcart, E. S., Samuelson, C. O., Jr., Solsky, M. A., Kaplan, S. B., Guttadauria, M., Halla, J. T., and Weinstein, A. (1984): Randomized, double-blind, placebo controlled trial of low-dose pulse methotrexate in psoriatic arthritis. *Arthritis Rheum.,* 27:376–380.

234. Wolfe, F., Catney, M. A., Hawley, D. J., Balser, J. P., and Schnidler, J. D. (1987): Clinical trial with R-IFN-Gamma in rheumatoid arthritis. In: *Biologically Based Immunomodulators in the Therapy of Rheumatic Diseases,* edited by S. H. Pincus, D. S. Pisetsky, and L. J. Rosenwasser. Elsevier, New York (*in press*).

235. Wolff, S. M., Fauci, A. S., Horn, R. G., and Dale, D. C. (1974): Wegener's granulomatosis. *Ann. Intern. Med.,* 81:513–525.

236. Wood, L., and Jacob, P. (1983): Plasma exchange in Goodpasture's syndrome. *Plasma Ther.,* 4:175–183.

237. Wright, D. G., Kirkpatrick, C. H., and Gallin, J. I. (1977): Effects of levamisole on normal and abnormal leukocyte locomotion. *J. Clin. Invest.,* 59:941–950.

238. Wyle, F. A., and Kent, J. R. (1976): Immunosuppression by sex steroid hormones. I. The effect upon PHA and PPD stimulated lymphocytes. *Clin. Exp. Immunol.,* 27:407–415.

239. Yeh, G. C., and Phang, J. M. (1983): Pyrroline-5-carboxylate stimulates the conversion of purine antimetabolites to their nucleotide forms by a redox-dependent mechanism. *J. Biol. Chem.,* 258:9774–9779.

240. Yu, D. T., Clements, P. J., Peter, J. B., Levy, J., Paulus, H. E., and Barnett, E. V. (1974): Lymphocyte characteristics in rheumatic patients and the effect of azathioprine therapy. *Arthritis Rheum.,* 17:37–45.

241. Zemer, D., Pras, M., Sohar, E., and Gafni, J. (1976): Colchicine in familial Mediterranean fever. *N. Engl. J. Med.,* 294:170–171.

242. Zemer, D., Pras, M., Sohar, E., Modan, M., Cabili, S., and Gafni, J. (1986): Colchicine in the prevention and treatment of the amyloidosis of familial Mediterranean fever. *N. Engl. J. Med.,* 314:1001–1005.

243. Zemer, D., Revach, M., Pras, M., Modan, B., Shor, S., Sohar, E., and Gafni, J. (1974): A controlled trial of colchicine in preventing attacks of familial Mediterranean fever. *N. Engl. J. Med.,* 291:932–934.

244. Zulman, J., Michalski, J., McCombs, C., Greenspan, J., and Talal, N. (1978): Levamisole maintains cyclophosphamide-induced remission in murine lupus erythematosus. *Clin. Exp. Immunol.,* 31:321–327.

Inflammation: Basic Principles and Clinical Correlates.
Edited by J. I. Gallin, I. M. Goldstein, and R. Snyderman.
Raven Press, Ltd., New York © 1988.

CHAPTER 52

Agents that Interfere with Arachidonic Acid Metabolism

Ira M. Goldstein

Coincident with the discovery that aspirin and indomethacin inhibit conversion of arachidonic acid to biologically active prostaglandins (27,108), it was suggested that inhibition of arachidonic acid metabolism accounts for the anti-inflammatory activities of aspirin and aspirin-like drugs (122). This suggestion, which currently has assumed the status of dogma, focused attention on the roles played by products of arachidonic acid in mediating inflammation and led to intensive efforts to develop new inhibitors of arachidonic acid metabolism.

MEDIATORS OF INFLAMMATION FORMED FROM ARACHIDONIC ACID BY THE CYCLOOXYGENASE PATHWAY

Arachidonic acid (5,8,11,14-eicosatetraenoic acid) is a ubiquitous constituent of cell membrane phospholipids that can be made accessible by the actions of phospholipases to a variety of chemical transformations (35,99). In virtually all tissues that have been examined, free arachidonic acid is converted to unstable prostaglandin endoperoxides (prostaglandin G_2, prostaglandin H_2) by the

fatty acid cyclooxygenase system. It is this enzyme system that is inhibited by aspirin and by most nonsteroidal anti-inflammatory drugs (27,64,98,108). Prostaglandin G_2 and prostaglandin H_2 provoke irreversible aggregation of platelets and cause contraction of vascular smooth muscle (46). In most tissues, however, the endoperoxides are converted either to stable prostaglandins (e.g., prostaglandin E_2) or to other unstable, yet biologically active, products. In platelets, for example, the endoperoxides are converted to thromboxane A_2 (47). Thromboxane A_2 causes irreversible aggregation of platelets as well as contraction of vascular smooth muscle (vasoconstriction). In endothelial cells, on the other hand, the endoperoxides are converted to prostaglandin I_2 (prostacyclin), a potent inhibitor of platelet aggregation and a vasodilator (79). The antagonistic roles played by thromboxane A_2 and prostaglandin I_2 in modulating vascular tone and patency have received considerable attention and are discussed elsewhere in this volume (see Chapters 9, 28, and 29).

There is ample evidence that products formed from arachidonic acid by the cyclooxygenase pathway are mediators of inflammation (18,35,52,99). First, these compounds provoke many of the cardinal signs of inflammation (e.g., erythema, fever, pain, edema). Second, these compounds are synthesized by phagocytic cells and are released in large amounts during inflammatory reactions. Finally, synthesis of stable prostaglandins, thromboxane A_2, and prostaglandin I_2 is inhibited by many anti-inflammatory drugs.

Erythema, Fever, Pain, and Edema

Products of the cyclooxygenase pathway of arachidonic acid metabolism undoubtedly contribute to the erythema, local increases in temperature, and fever associated with many forms of acute and chronic inflammation. Prostaglandins I_2, E_2, D_2, and A_2, for example, dilate blood vessels and augment blood flow in the microvasculature (51,126,127).

Levels of prostaglandins are increased in the cerebrospinal fluid of animals rendered febrile by both endogenous and exogenous pyrogens (129). In addition, prostaglandins of the E series, as well as arachidonic acid, produce fever in experimental animals when injected directly into the cerebral ventricles (14). These observations, and the fact that almost all nonsteroidal anti-inflammatory drugs are antipyretic (56,83,106), suggest strongly that products of arachidonic acid formed by the cyclooxygenase pathway contribute to the development of hyperpyrexia.

The roles played by stable prostaglandins in provoking the pain and edema that accompany inflammation are complex. For example, none of the stable prostaglandins provokes pain directly (26,28). Rather, they produce the phenomenon of hyperalgesia and act synergistically with other mediators (e.g., histamine, bradykinin) to augment pain (26,29).

Prostaglandins also appear to be incapable of causing edema. They do not directly increase the permeability of small blood vessels. Prostaglandins, however, can act synergistically with other mediators to augment edema. Intradermal injections of E-type prostaglandins in rabbits, for example, produced large increases in local blood flow, with little, if any, exudation of plasma (127). Bradykinin and histamine, on the other hand, increased vascular permeability, but were far less potent with respect to their ability to increase blood flow. The ability of any individual prostaglandin to potentiate plasma exudation caused by histamine or bradykinin is directly related to its ability to enhance blood flow.

Stable prostaglandins also play a role in provoking changes in vascular permeability mediated by complement and polymorphonuclear leukocytes. For example, purified C5a-des-Arg (which lacks intrinsic anaphylatoxin activity) caused increased vascular permeability in rabbit skin only in the presence of added prostaglandins (e.g., prostaglandin E_2) and only in animals with normal numbers of circulating polymorphonuclear leukocytes (124).

Other products of the cyclooxygenase pathway may play roles in promoting vascular permeability changes. Prostaglandin I_2, for example, dilates blood vessels and augments edema provoked by other mediators (50,51). Thromboxane A_2 also may play a role in provoking some forms of vascular injury by enhancing adherence of polymorphonuclear leukocytes to endothelial surfaces (114).

Injury to Tissues

Apart from their ability to influence vascular tone and permeability, there is little evidence that prostaglandins are capable of directly causing tissue injury. Nevertheless, prostaglandin E_2 does stimulate bone resorption *in vitro* and *in vivo* (95,96,102). Robinson et al. (95) have shown that prostaglandin E_2, produced by rheumatoid synovial tissue, directly promotes resorption of bone. In addition, it has been reported that rheumatoid synovial tissue in culture produces approximately 10 times more prostaglandin E_2 than does normal synovial tissue (96). It appears likely, therefore, that prostaglandins produced by hypertrophic and hyperplastic synovial tissue contribute to the destruction of juxtaarticular bone in patients with rheumatoid arthritis.

Generation of Prostaglandins at Sites of Inflammation

Large amounts of stable prostaglandins have been detected at foci of inflammation, and it has been demonstrated that these compounds are synthesized by phagocytic cells (i.e., polymorphonuclear leukocytes, monocytes, and macrophages) (43,132). Zurier and Sayadoff (132), for example, found that appropriately stimulated human neutrophils synthesize and release prostaglandins of the E and F series. Stimulated human neutrophils also generate thromboxane A_2 (41,42).

Inhibition of Prostaglandin Biosynthesis by Anti-inflammatory Drugs

Perhaps the most compelling evidence that products formed from arachidonic acid by the cyclooxygenase pathway are mediators of inflammation has come from studies of the effects of various drugs on the biosynthesis of these compounds. Most nonsteroidal anti-inflammatory drugs, for example, as well as anti-inflammatory adrenal corticosteroids, have been found capable of inhibiting the biosynthesis of stable prostaglandins, thromboxane A_2, and prostaglandin I_2 (see following).

MEDIATORS OF INFLAMMATION FORMED FROM ARACHIDONIC ACID BY LIPOXYGENASES

In addition to being a substrate for the cyclooxygenase pathway, arachidonic acid may be acted on by various lipoxygenases to yield monohydroxyeicosatetraenoic acids and dihydroxyeicosatetraenoic acids (see Chapter 8). The profile of products formed from arachidonic acid by lipoxygenases depends on many factors, including cell type, species, and nature of the stimulus. Human platelet lipoxygenase, for example, converts arachidonic acid to 12-hydroperoxyeicosatetraenoic acid (12-HPETE), which is transformed rapidly to the stable 12-hydroxy compound (12-HETE) (85). Human polymorphonuclear leukocytes (neutrophils and eosinophils), monocytes, and some macrophages, on the other hand, contain other lipoxygenases that convert arachidonic acid to a series of monohydroxy and dihydroxy derivatives (35,75,99).

In stimulated neutrophils, eosinophils, and some macrophages, arachidonic acid released from membrane phospholipids is oxygenated by a 5-lipoxygenase to yield 5-hydroperoxyeicosatetraenoic acid (5-HPETE). This product is then converted to the highly reactive epoxide leukotriene A_4. Leukotriene A_4 either is hydrolyzed enzymatically to yield leukotriene B_4 or combines enzymatically with glutathione to yield leukotriene C_4. Leukotriene C_4 can be converted enzymatically to leukotriene D_4, and subsequently to leukotriene E_4. Leukotrienes C_4, D_4, and E_4 are potent contractile and vasoactive factors and represent the principal constituents of the slow-reacting substance of anaphylaxis (SRS-A) (35,75,99) (see Chapter 8). In addition to causing contraction of airway smooth muscle, leukotrienes C_4 and D_4 directly increase microvascular permeability (15) and increase adherence of neutrophils to surfaces (38). The 5-lipoxygenase pathway in human leukocytes also yields trihydroxy derivatives of arachidonic acid, termed "lipoxins," which stimulate some functions of neutrophils (101).

The biologic activities of products formed from arachidonic acid by lipoxygenases (particularly leukotriene B_4) appear to be particularly relevant to inflammation (Table 1). For example, although products of arachidonic acid formed by the cyclooxygenase pathway indirectly influence the ability of phagocytic cells to accumulate at sites of inflammation (by virtue of their effects on vascular tone and vascular permeability), only products formed by lipoxygenases exhibit potent chemotactic activity (36,103). The most potent of the chemotactic factors that

TABLE 1. *Biologic activities of leukotriene B_4 relevant to inflammation*

Target	Responses
Neutrophils	Chemotaxis and chemokinesis
	Degranulation
	Respiratory burst
	Aggregation
	Increased expression of C3 receptors
Lymphocytes	Enhanced suppressor activity
	Enhanced natural killer cell activity
Endothelium	Increased adherence of neutrophils
Nociceptive nerves	Hyperalgesia (neutrophil-dependent)
Fibroblasts	Chemotaxis

can be produced from arachidonic acid is leukotriene B_4. Leukotriene B_4 provokes directed migration of human neutrophils *in vitro* at concentrations less than 10 ng/ml (as compared with 1,000 ng/ml for 5-HETE and 20,000 ng/ml for 12-HETE) (36,103). At higher concentrations, leukotriene B_4 provokes selective release of granule-associated (lysosomal) enzymes from cytochalasin-B-treated neutrophils and causes these cells to aggregate (86,100). All of these actions of leukotriene B_4 appear to be mediated by binding to structurally specific cell surface receptors (40). *In vivo,* leukotriene B_4 induces adherence of neutrophils to the walls of postcapillary venules (15), neutrophil-dependent increases in vascular permeability (15,124), and accumulation of neutrophils in skin (113). In addition, leukotriene B_4 resembles prostaglandin E_2 with respect to its ability to induce the phenomenon of hyperalgesia (73). Leukotriene-B_4-induced hyperalgesia, however, is dependent on neutrophils.

Another product of arachidonic acid that possesses potent chemotactic activity for human neutrophils is 8,15-dihydroxyeicosatetraenoic acid (8,15-diHETE) (103). Formed by the 15-lipoxygenase pathway (primarily in eosinophils), 8,15-diHETE is nearly as potent as leukotriene B_4 with respect to its chemotactic activity for human neutrophils. It also resembles leukotriene B_4 with respect to its ability to stimulate random migration of neutrophils. Interestingly, 8,15-diHETE has been identified as a product formed from arachidonic acid by human tracheal epithelial cells (55) and has been implicated as being a mediator of airway inflammation.

Like stable prostaglandins, products formed from arachidonic acid by lipoxygenases have been detected at sites of inflammation. For example, Hammarstrom et al. (48) found very high levels of free arachidonic acid and 12-HETE in skin lesions of patients with psoriasis and suggested the possibility that these compounds play an important role in provoking dermal inflammation. HETEs as well as leukotrienes also have been detected in synovial fluids from patients with inflammatory arthritides (62).

NONSTEROIDAL ANTI-INFLAMMATORY DRUGS

The therapeutic efficacy of aspirin and aspirin-like compounds has been known for over 2,000 years. Indeed, well before the Christian era, physicians prepared extracts from the bark of the willow tree and used these to treat a wide variety of disorders ranging from sepsis and arthritis to toothaches and menstrual cramps. It was not until the nineteenth century, however, that the active components of willow bark were identified as salicin and salicylic acid (71,88). Acetylsalicylic acid subsequently was synthesized, named "aspirin," and proven to be useful as a therapeutic agent (20). It is quite certain that none of the chemists involved in the development of aspirin would have guessed that by the late 1970s, consumption of this drug in the United States alone would be measured in terms of millions of pounds per year.

Using aspirin as a prototype, chemists during the twentieth century developed a large number of compounds that have been proved to be clinically useful anti-inflammatory agents. These compounds, which include derivatives of indoleacetic acid and propionic acid, as well as pyrazoles, fenamates, oxicams, etc., are now referred to collectively as nonsteroidal anti-inflammatory drugs (Table 2). The pharmacology of these compounds has been studied extensively, as have their anti-inflammatory, analgesic, and antipyretic properties (reviewed in refs. 28, 56, 83, and 106).

The demonstration that aspirin and indomethacin inhibit conversion of arachidonic acid to biologically active prostaglandins in platelets and in spleen cells (27,108) led to the suggestion that such inhibition accounted for all of the anti-inflammatory properties of these drugs (122). It is now well established that despite differences with respect to potency, specificity, and mechanisms of action, nearly all of the clinically useful nonsteroidal anti-inflammatory drugs inhibit cyclooxygenase activity (28,49,56,64,98). Aspirin, for example, acetylates and irreversibly inactivates the cyclooxygenase in platelets (98). Other nonsteroidal anti-inflammatory drugs, such as indomethacin and flurbiprofen, appear to inhibit cyclooxygenase activity reversibly by binding in a stereospecific manner to one or another subunit of the enzyme (64). Yet other drugs (e.g., acetaminophenol, phenylbutazone) inhibit cyclooxygenase activity efficiently only when steady-state concentrations of lipid hydroperoxides are reduced (49). These observations, as well as differences in metabolism and bioavailability, may explain, in part, the variations in therapeutic efficacy and toxicity noted among the commonly used nonsteroidal anti-inflammatory drugs (56,83,106). It should be emphasized, however, that these variations are not great.

Alternative Actions of Nonsteroidal Anti-inflammatory Drugs

A number of observations suggest that inhibition of cyclooxygenase activity alone is insufficient to account for the anti-inflammatory activities of aspirin-like drugs. For example, concentrations of these drugs much higher than those that inhibit cyclooxygenase activity frequently are required to suppress inflammation (56,83,106). In addition, drugs that do not effectively inhibit cyclooxygenase activity, such as sodium salicylate, are anti-inflammatory (56). Finally, some products formed from arachidonic acid by the cyclooxygenase pathway have been found to be capable of exerting anti-inflammatory effects in experimental animals (*vide infra*). Consequently, the possibility that nonsteroidal anti-inflammatory drugs suppress inflammation either by interfering with various function of leukocytes or by interfering with the actions of enzymes other than cyclooxygenase has attracted a great deal of attention.

With respect to effects on leukocytes, nearly every function of human neutrophils that is relevant to inflammation has been reported to be influenced by nonsteroidal anti-inflammatory drugs. For example, human neutrophil adherence (119), aggregation (1,21,76), chemotaxis (2,37,61,76,94), phagocytosis (91,119), degranulation (21,76,78,112,119), and generation of reactive oxygen metabolites (1,21,105,121) have been reported to be inhibited by one or another nonsteroidal anti-inflammatory drug. Interestingly, aspirin is the least active of these drugs with respect to its effects on neutrophil functions. Although it is clear that nonsteroidal anti-inflammatory

---

TABLE 2. *Commonly used nonsteroidal anti-inflammatory drugs*

Salicylates	Phenylacetic acids (propionic acids)
Aspirin	Ibuprofen
Sodium salicylate	Fenoprofen
Choline salicylate	Flurbiprofen
Salicylsalicylic acid	Ketoprofen
Diflunisal	Fenamates
Indoleacetic acids	Mefenamic acid
Indomethacin	Meclofenamate
Sulindac	Oxicams
Pyrazoles	Piroxicam
Phenylbutazone	Naphthaleneacetic acids
Oxyphenbutazone	Naproxen
Pyrrolealkanoic	
acids	
Tolmetin	

drugs can inhibit functions of neutrophils independent of effects on prostaglandin biosynthesis (1), the precise way in which they influence these cells has not been elucidated. Possibilities include effects on membrane-associated or intracellular calcium (1,9,21,84), cyclic nucleotide metabolism (11,57,78), phospholipase A_2 activity (59), lysosomal membrane integrity (110), cell surface receptors (45), and ligand-receptor interactions (2,12,21,121). With respect to the latter, it is noteworthy that effects of some nonsteroidal anti-inflammatory drugs (e.g., indomethacin, piroxicam) on responses of neutrophils to the chemotactic peptide N-formyl-met-leu-phe can be explained by the ability of these compounds to interfere with binding of the peptide to its cell surface receptor (12,21,121). It also is noteworthy that inhibitory effects on neutrophil functions generally require high concentrations of nonsteroidal anti-inflammatory drugs (i.e., greater than 0.01 mM), often vary with respect to either the stimulus or the drug, and (when examined) are abrogated completely when the medium in which the cells are suspended contains more than trace amounts of protein (94,112). Consequently, it is not at all clear that the effects on neutrophils that have been demonstrated *in vitro* have any relevance to the mechanisms by which nonsteroidal anti-inflammatory drugs exert their beneficial effects *in vivo*.

Effects of Nonsteroidal Anti-inflammatory Drugs on Lipoxygenases

Considering the biologic activities of products formed from arachidonic acid by the 5-lipoxygenase pathway, it is not surprising that there is intense interest in developing clinically useful inhibitors of this pathway. With the possible exception of benoxaprofen, most nonsteroidal anti-inflammatory drugs (at relevant concentrations) do not significantly inhibit 5-lipoxygenase activity (74,107). Nevertheless, some nonsteroidal anti-inflammatory drugs (e.g., aspirin, indomethacin) interfere with peroxidase activity in platelets and thereby inhibit conversion of 12-HPETE to 12-HETE (104). Yet others (e.g., ibuprofen) stimulate 15-lipoxygenase activity in neutrophils (120). Although compounds such as sulfasalazine (116) and colchicine (93) apparently inhibit 5-lipoxygenase activity in human neutrophils *in vitro*, it is by no means clear that such inhibition accounts for the beneficial actions of these drugs *in vivo*. It remains to be determined whether or not other compounds that inhibit lipoxygenases will prove to be clinically useful as anti-inflammatory agents (5,118).

Just as inhibitors of the cyclooxygenase pathway of arachidonic acid metabolism have been found capable of suppressing functions of neutrophils *in vitro*, so, too, have inhibitors of lipoxygenases. Because some products of the 5-lipoxygenase pathway (e.g., leukotriene B_4) provoke neutrophils to degranulate (36,86,100,115), it has been suggested that these products play a physiologic role in regulating degranulation of neutrophils exposed to diverse stimuli. A number of investigators, for example, have found that inhibitors of lipoxygenase activity, such as nordihydroguaiaretic acid and eicosatetraynoic acid, inhibit degranulation of neutrophils (86,109,111,112). In addition, it has been observed that nordihydroguaiaretic acid inhibits transport of calcium into rabbit neutrophils exposed to chemotactic peptides (80). These observations, as well as the findings that lipoxygenase products per se (particularly leukotriene B_4) stimulate calcium uptake by neutrophils and translocation of intracellular calcium (100), have led to the suggestion that arachidonic acid metabolism by neutrophils is "linked" to the changes in calcium metabolism that appear to be involved in stimulus-response coupling (see Chapter 20).

Despite the observations summarized here, the precise relationship between metabolism of arachidonic acid by the 5-lipoxygenase pathway and neutrophil function remains unclear. One reason for this is the uncertain specificity of the inhibitors used in most studies. For example, like some nonsteroidal anti-inflammatory agents, eicosatetraynoic acid inhibits binding of synthetic chemotactic peptides to human neutrophils (4). In addition, inhibitors of lipoxygenases may affect other functions of neutrophils (e.g., membrane lipid composition) (115) independent of any effects they may have on the metabolism of arachidonic acid. It is interesting in this respect that eicosatetraynoic acid and nordihydroguaiaretic acid have been found capable of inhibiting degranulation of neutrophils provoked by leukotriene B_4 (86). These observations are inconsistent with the suggestion that leukotriene B_4 is a physiologically important endogenous mediator of degranulation. Finally, eicosatetraynoic acid and other putative inhibitors of 5-lipoxygenase activity inhibit degranulation of neutrophils at concentrations that do not inhibit production of 5-HETE (111). Conversely, some phenylhydrazone derivatives inhibit production of 5-HETE, but not degranulation (111). It is obvious that much more work will be required to establish the relationship, if any, between arachidonic acid metabolism by lipoxygenases and neutrophil functions.

Whereas most nonsteroidal anti-inflammatory agents effectively inhibit production by leukocytes of prostaglandins (by inhibiting cyclooxygenase activity), these agents do not significantly influence the formation of lipoxygenase products (e.g., hydroxy acids, leukotrienes). Anti-inflammatory corticosteroids, on the other hand, may act more "proximally" to suppress phospholipase activity, thereby reducing the availability of arachidonic acid as a substrate and thus limiting production of inflammatory mediators by both the cyclooxygenase and lipoxygenase pathways.

ANTI-INFLAMMATORY ADRENAL CORTICOSTEROIDS

Despite the impressive ability of adrenal corticosteroids to suppress undesirable inflammatory reactions, we still know relatively little about how these compounds exert their anti-inflammatory effects. One possibility is that adrenal corticosteroids ameliorate inflammation by interfering with the metabolism of arachidonic acid. Several investigators, for example, have reported that corticosteroids inhibit production of stable prostaglandins by inflamed synovial tissue (31,58). In addition, it has been reported that corticosteroids inhibit production by stimulated leukocytes of thromboxane A_2 and stable prostaglandins and that this inhibitory effect can be overcome by supplying the cells with exogenous arachidonic acid (19,41). It has been suggested that corticosteroids inhibit prostaglandin biosynthesis by binding to specific glucocorticoid receptors and by inducing synthesis of one or more cellular proteins that inhibit the activity of phospholipase A_2.

Working independently, three groups of investigators observed that inhibition by corticosteroids of prostaglandin production by rat renal papillae (16), perfused guinea pig lungs (32), and rat peritoneal leukocytes (a mixture of macrophages and polymorphonuclear leukocytes) (10,19) required prolonged incubations and could be prevented with agents that inhibit either DNA-directed RNA synthesis (e.g., actinomycin D) or protein synthesis (e.g., puromycin, cycloheximide). Furthermore, Carnuccio et al. (10) observed that incubation of rat peritoneal leukocytes with hydrocortisone for 90 min resulted in release into the medium surrounding the cells of a nondialyzable "factor" that inhibited production of prostaglandins by fresh leukocytes. The steroid-induced inhibitor of prostaglandin biosynthesis subsequently was identified as a polypeptide and was termed "macrocortin" (6). Macrocortin was partially purified from steroid-stimulated guinea pig lungs and rat peritoneal leukocytes and was reported to have an apparent molecular weight of either 15,000 (6) or 40,000 (7).

In 1980, Hirata et al. (53) reported that incubation of rabbit peritoneal leukocytes with adrenal corticosteroids for 16 hr resulted in inhibition of phospholipase A_2 activity *in situ* (measured by chemotactic-factor-induced release of [^{14}C]arachidonic acid previously incorporated into membrane phospholipids). The inhibitory potencies of various corticosteroids correlated well with their anti-inflammatory activities and with their abilities to bind to glucocorticoid receptors. Evidence was presented that corticosteroids induce synthesis of a 40-kd protein (termed "lipomodulin") that is expressed on the leukocyte cell surface (i.e., susceptible to digestion with pronase) and that directly inhibits the activity of porcine pancreatic phospholipase A_2 *in vitro*. Hirata et al. (54) subsequently reported that when human fibroblasts were stimulated with bradykinin in the presence of a monoclonal antibody directed against lipomodulin, the cells responded by releasing more than normal amounts of previously incorporated [^{14}C]arachidonic acid. This apparent enhancement of phospholipase activity was blocked by adding an excess of lipomodulin (partially purified from supernatants of rabbit polymorphonuclear leukocytes incubated for 16 hr with 1.0-μM fluocinolone acetonide). The activity of partially purified lipomodulin was markedly decreased after treatment with sera from patients with systemic lupus erythematosus, rheumatoid arthritis, and dermatomyositis, as well as with sera from NZB/NZW and MRL/l mice. The decrease in phospholipase A_2 inhibitory activity paralleled the amount of [^{35}S]methionine-labeled lipomodulin that was precipitated by these sera. Based on these observations, it was suggested that sera from patients with various rheumatic diseases contain "autoantibodies" directed against lipomodulin and that such "autoantibodies" facilitate activation of phospholipase A_2 *in vivo* and play a role in the pathogenesis of immunologically induced inflammation. As attractive as these suggestions may be, there is still no conclusive evidence that lipomodulin possesses anti-inflammatory activity. Furthermore, some investigators have failed to confirm that adrenal corticosteroids interfere with release of arachidonic acid from cell membrane phospholipids *in vitro* (128) or with formation of prostaglandins *in vivo* (81,92).

Lipomodulin and macrocortin appear to be identical with a protein of 35 to 40 kd (appropriately termed "lipocortin") that is found in the cytosol of a wide variety of mammalian cells and that binds to phospholipids in the presence of calcium (17,123). A very recent study has demonstrated that "inhibition" of phospholipase A_2 activity by lipocortin is due to an interaction of the protein with substrates for the enzyme (i.e., phospholipids), rather than to an interaction with the enzyme itself (17). This finding raises additional questions concerning the physiologic significance (if any) of lipocortin with respect to its putative role as a regulator of arachidonic acid metabolism in intact cells and also raises questions concerning the mechanisms by which adrenal corticosteroids interfere with arachidonic acid metabolism.

EICOSAPENTAENOIC ACID

Eicosapentaenoic acid is a 20-carbon fatty acid with five double bonds. Like arachidonic acid, which has 20 carbons and four double bonds, eicosapentaenoic acid can be metabolized by the cyclooxygenase pathway and by lipoxygenases *in vitro* (67,68,82). The products formed from eicosapentaenoic acid, however, exhibit biologic activities that are quite different from those exhibited by products formed from arachidonic acid. Thromboxane A_3, for example, does not provoke aggregation of platelets (as does thromboxane A_2) (82). Similarly, leukotriene B_5 is considerably less active than leukotriene B_4 with respect to its effects on neutrophils (39,68). In addition, eicosapentaenoic acid inhibits cyclooxygenase- and lipoxygenase-mediated metabolism of arachidonic acid *in vitro* (67,82). Thus, eicosapentaenoic acid reduces conversion of arachidonic acid into thromboxane A_2, prostaglandin E_2, and leukotriene B_4.

Eicosapentaenoic acid is found in only very small amounts in foods consumed by individuals who live in most areas of the world. Consequently, eicosapentaenoic acid usually is undetectable in extracts prepared from leukocyte or erythrocyte membrane phospholipids. In arctic regions, however, where large amounts of fish are consumed, the ratio of eicosapentaenoic acid to arachidonic acid in cell membrane phospholipids is increased significantly. Increased ratios of eicosapentaenoic acid to arachidonic acid also have been detected in phospholipid extracts prepared from blood cells of normal individuals who have enriched their diets with fish oils (30,69,87). Other effects that have been observed in studies performed *in vitro* with cells from normal individuals fed eicosapentaenoic-acid-enriched diets include decreased production of leukotriene B_4 by neutrophils and monocytes (69,87,89), increased production of leukotriene B_5 by neutrophils and monocytes (69,87,117), decreased chemotactic responses of neutrophils to leukotriene B_4 and to *N*-formyl-met-leu-phe (69,87), decreased generation of superoxide anion radicals by neutrophils exposed to opsonized zymosan (30), and decreased adherence of neutrophils to endothelial monolayers pretreated with leukotriene B_4 (69).

Considering the effects of eicosapentaenoic acid on arachidonic acid metabolism and on leukocyte functions, it is not surprising that "therapy" with this fatty acid has been examined in experimental animals and in patients with inflammatory diseases.

Female F_1 hybrids of New Zealand black (NZB) and white (NZW) mice spontaneously develop a disease that resembles systemic lupus erythematosus. The disease is associated with the appearance of circulating autoantibodies (e.g., anti-DNA antibodies) and progressive, immune-complex-mediated glomerulonephritis. Female NZB/NZW F_1 hybrid mice that were fed a diet rich in eicosapentaenoic acid did not develop proteinuria and lived longer than did similar mice fed a normal diet (90). In fact, none of the animals fed the special diet either died or exhibited proteinuria for the duration of the study (up to 13.5 months). Anti-double-strand-DNA antibodies also were reduced (approximately 50%) in treated animals.

Other beneficial effects that have been observed as a consequence of "therapy" with eicosapentaenoic acid include delayed onset of renal disease and prolonged survival in BXSB and MRL-lpr mice (other models of autoimmune disease) (60,97), decreased susceptibility to collagen-induced arthritis in mice (72), and decreased morning stiffness as well as decreased number of tender joints in patients with rheumatoid arthritis (63).

With respect to effects of dietary eicosapentaenoic acid in patients with rheumatic diseases, many controlled, prospective clinical trials are in progress. It must be emphasized, however, that until more is learned of the long-term effects of dietary eicosapentaenoic acid, this form of therapy for patients with inflammatory diseases must be considered experimental.

ANTI-INFLAMMATORY EFFECTS OF PROSTAGLANDINS

Before concluding this review of agents that interfere with the metabolism of arachidonic acid, it should be pointed out that some products of arachidonic acid have been found capable of inhibiting functions of leukocytes *in vitro* and of exerting anti-inflammatory effects in experimental animals.

Inhibition of Leukocyte Functions by Prostaglandins

Several functions of cells involved in acute and chronic inflammatory reactions (i.e., neutrophils, monocytes, macrophages, lymphocytes) can be modulated by cyclic nucleotides. For example, selective extracellular release of proinflammatory lysosomal constituents from stimulated human peripheral-blood neutrophils *in vitro* can be inhibited either by cyclic 3',5'-adenosine monophosphate (cAMP) directly or by pharmacologic agents that increase levels of this cyclic nucleotide within cells (125,131). Therefore, consistent with their ability to increase cellular levels of cAMP, some prostaglandins (e.g., prostaglandin E_2) act as "extracellular messengers" and inhibit release of mediators of inflammation from leukocytes (131). Prostaglandins of the E series, as well as prostaglandin I_2, also inhibit leukocyte chemotaxis (33), adherence to various substrates (including endothelium) (8), phagocytosis (13), and generation of oxygen-derived free radicals (70). Inhibitory effects on various functions of B and T lymphocytes also have been reported. For example, prostaglandin E_2 suppresses proliferative responses of human lymphocytes to mitogens, lymphocyte-mediated cytotoxicity, and antibody production (44). It is not surprising, therefore, that considerable attention has been focused on the potential roles played by prostaglandins in regulating inflammatory reactions as well as both humoral and cellular immune reactions. It has been suggested, for example, that by local, preferential biosynthesis of one or another of the prostaglandins, the very cells that release mediators of inflammation provide a mechanism for modulating inflammatory responses. It also is not surprising that prostaglandins that inhibit leukocyte functions *in vitro* exhibit anti-inflammatory effects *in vivo*.

Anti-inflammatory Effects of Prostaglandins in Experimental Animals

Adjuvant arthritis. Adjuvant disease in the rat includes a severe and persistent polyarthritis that appears 10 to 14 days after a single intradermal injection of complete Freund's adjuvant. Several investigators have demonstrated that prostaglandin E compounds either prevent or suppress adjuvant arthritis (3,34,130). Whereas treatment of rats with prostaglandin E compounds did not suppress delayed hypersensitivity reactions to mycobacterial antigens, there was a reduction in anti-sheep-red-blood-cell antibody titers as well as a significant reduction in the numbers of circulating lymphocytes. Despite these observations, and the observations of others concerning effects of prostaglandins on humoral and cellular immune reactivity, the mechanism whereby prostaglandin E compounds suppress adjuvant arthritis in rats is unknown.
Carrageenan-induced inflammation. Prostaglandin E compounds also suppress inflammation in rats induced with carrageenan. Administration of prostaglandin E compounds into subcutaneous air blebs at the time of carrageenan injection reduced the number of neutrophils that entered the focus of inflammation (130). Treatment of rats systemically with prostaglandin E compounds also significantly inhibited carrageenan-induced rat footpad edema (24,34).

The effects of prostaglandin E compounds on carrageenan-induced rat footpad edema are in accord with the findings that these compounds markedly reduce the increases in vascular permeability induced in rats by intradermal injections of histamine, serotonin, bradykinin, the complement-derived anaphylatoxin C3a, and compound 48/80 (22). Suppression by the prostaglandin E compounds of vascular permeability changes was associated ultrastructurally with preservation of tight junctions between endothelial cells.
Immune-complex-induced-inflammation. Vascular permeability changes following the induction of reversed passive Arthus reactions in rat skin were suppressed significantly by pretreatment with prostaglandin E compounds (65). Diminished vascular permeability in treated animals was accompanied by markedly reduced exudation of neutrophils. Neutrophils harvested from the blood of treated rats exhibited depressed chemotactic responses *in*

vitro, as well as diminished lysosomal enzyme secretion after incubation with a chemotactic peptide. Suppression of human neutrophil degranulation also has been observed following intravenous infusions of prostaglandin E$_1$ for treatment of peripheral vascular disease (23). A detailed study of this phenomenon (25) revealed evidence that administration systemically of 15-(S)-15-methyl prostaglandin E$_1$ reduces the binding affinity of the receptor on rat neutrophils for *N*-formyl-met-leu-phe. It was concluded from these studies that some of the anti-inflammatory effects observed after administration of prostaglandin E compounds may be mediated by altered functional responses of neutrophils to chemotactic peptides.

In addition to inhibiting immune-complex-induced inflammation, prostaglandin E compounds also suppress inflammation caused by antitissue antibodies. The nephrotoxicity in rats caused by single intravenous injections of antibodies directed against glomerular basement membranes was suppressed significantly by treatment with prostaglandin E$_1$ (66). Treatment reduced glomerular hypercellularity and proteinuria, but did not affect binding of the antibodies to the glomerular basement membrane.

Finally, Zurier et al. (133–135) observed that when female NZB/NZW F$_1$ hybrid mice were treated with prostaglandin E$_1$ (200 µg subcutaneously either once or twice daily) from 6 weeks through 52 weeks fo age, they not only were protected from the development of anemia and nephritis but also lived longer than untreated animals. Survival of NZB/NZW mice also was prolonged when treatment with prostaglandin E$_1$ was begun at 24 weeks, at a time when these animals begin to develop nephritis. Interestingly, although treatment with prostaglandin E$_1$ did not prevent development of antibodies to nuclear antigens (including anti-DNA antibodies), it did prevent deposition of immunoglobulins and complement in glomeruli, as well as the development of proliferative nephritis. Clearly, more work will be required to elucidate the mechanisms whereby prostaglandins modulate immune-complex-mediated inflammation and tissue injury.

REFERENCES

1. Abramson, S., Korchak, H., Ludewig, R., Edelson, H., Haines, K., Levin, R. I., Herman, R., Rider, L., Kimmel, S., and Weissmann, G. (1985): Modes of action of aspirin-like drugs. *Proc. Natl. Acad. Sci. USA*, 82:7227–7231.
2. Anderson, R., Lukey, P. T., and van Rensburg, C. E. J. (1985): Effects of benoxaprofen on the binding to and inactivation of leucoattractants by human polymorphonuclear leucocytes *in vitro*. *Agents Actions*, 16:527–534.
3. Aspinall, R. L., and Cammarata, P. S. (1969): Effect of prostaglandin E$_2$ on adjuvant arthritis. *Nature (London)*, 224:1320–1321.
4. Atkinson, J. P., Simchowitz, L., Mehta, J., and Stenson, W. F. (1982): 5,8,11,14-eicosatetraynoic acid (ETYA) inhibits binding of *N*-formyl-methionyl-leucyl-phenylalanine (FMLP) to its receptor

on human granulocytes. A note of caution. *Immunopharmacology*, 4:1–9.

5. Bach, M. K. (1984): Prospects for the inhibition of leukotriene synthesis. *Biochem. Pharmacol.*, 33:515–521.

6. Blackwell, G. J., Carnuccio, R., DiRosa, M., Flower, R. J., Parente, L., and Persico, P. (1980): Macrocortin: A polypeptide causing the anti-phospholipase effect of glucocorticoids. *Nature (London)*, 287:147–149.

7. Blackwell, G. J., Carnuccio, R., DiRosa, M., Flower, R. J., Langham, C. S. J., Parente, L., Persico, P., Russell-Smith, N. C., and Stone, D. (1982): Glucocorticoids induce the formation and release of anti-inflammatory and anti-phospholipase proteins into the peritoneal cavity of the rat. *Br. J. Pharmacol.*, 76:185–194.

8. Boxer, L. A., Allen, J. M., Schmidt, M., Yoder, M., and Baehner, R. L. (1980): Inhibition of polymorphonuclear leukocyte adhesion by prostacyclin. *J. Lab. Clin. Med.*, 95:672–678.

9. Burch, R. M., Wise, W. C., and Halushka, P. V. (1983): Prostaglandin-independent inhibition of calcium transport by nonsteroidal anti-inflammatory drugs: Differential effects of carboxylic acids and piroxicam. *J. Pharmacol. Exp. Ther.*, 227:84–91.

10. Carnuccio, R., DiRosa, M., and Persico, P. (1980): Hydrocortisone-induced inhibitor of prostaglandin biosynthesis in rat leukocytes. *Br. J. Pharmacol.*, 68:14–16.

11. Ciosek, C. P., Jr., Ortel, R. W., Thanassi, N. M., and Newcombe, D. S. (1974): Indomethacin potentiates PGE₁ stimulated cyclic AMP accumulation in human synoviocytes. *Nature (London)*, 251:148–149.

12. Cost, H., Gespach, C., and Abita, J.-P. (1981): Effect of indomethacin on the binding of the chemotactic peptide formyl-met-leu-phe on human polymorphonuclear leukocytes. *FEBS Lett.*, 132:85–88.

13. Cox, J. P., and Karnovsky, M. L. (1973): The depression of phagocytosis by exogenous cyclic nucleotides, prostaglandins and theophylline. *J. Cell Biol.*, 59:480–490.

14. Cranston, W. I. (1979): Central mechanisms of fever. *Fed. Proc.*, 38:49–51.

15. Dahlen, S.-E., Bjork, J., Hedqvist, P., Arfors, K.-E., Hammarstrom, S., Lindgren, J. A., and Samuelsson, B. (1981): Leukotrienes promote plasma leakage and leukocyte adhesion in postcapillary venules: In vivo effect with relevance to the acute inflammatory response. *Proc. Natl. Acad. Sci. USA*, 78:3887–3891.

16. Danon, A., and Assouline, G. (1978): Inhibition of prostaglandin biosynthesis by corticosteroids requires RNA and protein synthesis. *Nature (London)*, 273:552–554.

17. Davidson, F. F., Dennis, E. A., Powell, M., and Glenney, J. R., Jr. (1987): Inhibition of phospholipase A₂ by "lipocortins" and calpactins. An effect of binding to substrate phospholipids. *J. Biol. Chem.*, 262:1698–1705.

18. Davies, P., Bailey, P. J., and Goldenberg, M. M. (1984): The role of arachidonic acid oxygenation products in pain and inflammation. *Annu. Rev. Immunol.*, 2:335–357.

19. DiRosa, M., and Persico, P. (1979): Mechanism of inhibition of prostaglandin biosynthesis by hydrocortisone in rat leukocytes. *Br. J. Pharmacol.*, 66:161–163.

20. Dreser, H. (1899): Pharmacologisches über Aspirin (Acetylsalicylsäure). *Pfluegers Arch.*, 76:306–318.

21. Edelson, H. S., Kaplan, H. B., Korchak, H. M., Smolen, J. E., and Weissmann, G. (1982): Dissociation by piroxicam of degranulation and superoxide anion generation from decrements in chlortetracycline fluorescence of activated human neutrophils. *Biochem. Biophys. Res. Commun.*, 104:247–253.

22. Fantone, J. C., Kunkel, S. L., Ward, P. A., and Zurier, R. B. (1980): Suppression by prostaglandin E₁ of vascular permeability induced by vasoactive inflammatory mediators. *J. Immunol.*, 125:2591–2596.

23. Fantone, J. C., Kunkel, S. L., and Ward, P. A. (1981): Suppression of human polymorphonuclear function after intravenous infusion of prostaglandin E₁. *Prostaglandins Med.*, 7:195–198.

24. Fantone, J. C., Kunkel, S. L., and Weingarten, B. (1982): Inhibition of carrageenin-induced rat footpad edema by systemic treatment

with prostaglandins of the E series. *Biochem. Pharmacol.*, 31:1126–1128.

25. Fantone, J. C., Marasco, W. A., Elgas, L. J., and Ward, P. A. (1983): Antiinflammatory effects of prostaglandin E₁: In vivo modulation of the formyl peptide chemotactic receptor on the rat neutrophil. *J. Immunol.*, 130:1495–1497.

26. Ferreira, S. H. (1972): Prostaglandins, aspirin-like drugs and analgesia. *Nature [New Biol.]*, 240:200–203.

27. Ferreira, S. H., Moncada, S., and Vane, J. R. (1971): Indomethacin and aspirin abolish prostaglandin release from spleen. *Nature [New Biol.]*, 231:237–239.

28. Ferreira, S. H., and Vane, J. R. (1974): New aspects of the mode of action of nonsteroid anti-inflammatory drugs. *Annu. Rev. Pharmacol.*, 14:57–73.

29. Ferreira, S. H., Nakamura, M., and Castro, M. S. A. (1978): The hyperalgesic effects of prostacyclin and prostaglandin E₂. *Prostaglandins*, 16:31–37.

30. Fisher, M., Upchurch, K. S., Levine, P. H., Johnson, M. H., Vaudreuil, C. H., Natale, A., and Hoogasian, J. J. (1986): Effects of dietary fish oil supplementation on polymorphonuclear leukocyte inflammatory potential. *Inflammation*, 10:387–392.

31. Floman, Y., Floman, N., and Zor, U. (1976): Inhibition of prostaglandin E release by anti-inflammatory steroids. *Prostaglandins*, 11:591–594.

32. Flower, R. J., and Blackwell, G. J. (1979): Anti-inflammatory steroids induce biosynthesis of a phospholipase A₂ inhibitor which prevents prostaglandin generation. *Nature (London)*, 278:456–459.

33. Gallin, J. I., Sandler, J. A., Clyman, R. J., Manganiello, V. C., and Vaughan, M. (1978): Agents that increase cyclic AMP inhibit accumulation of cGMP and depress human monocyte locomotion. *J. Immunol.*, 120:492–496.

34. Glenn, E. M., and Rohloff, N. (1971): Anti-arthritic and anti-inflammatory effects of certain prostaglandins. *Proc. Soc. Exp. Biol. Med.*, 139:290–294.

35. Goetzl, E. J. (1981): Oxygenation products of arachidonic acid as mediators of hypersensitivity and inflammation. *Med. Clin. North Am.*, 65:809–828.

36. Goetzl, E. J., and Pickett, W. C. (1980): The human PMN leukocyte chemotactic activity of complex hydroxy-eicosatetraenoic acids (HETEs). *J. Immunol.*, 125:1789–1791.

37. Goetzl, E. J., and Valone, F. H. (1982): Selective immobilization of human mononuclear phagocytes by benoxaprofen. *Arthritis Rheum.*, 25:1486–1489.

38. Goetzl, E. J., Brindley, L. L., and Goldman, D. W. (1983): Enhancement of human neutrophil adherence by synthetic leukotriene constituents of the slow-reacting substance of anaphylaxis. *Immunology*, 50:35–41.

39. Goldman, D. W., Pickett, W. C., and Goetzl, E. J. (1983): Human neutrophil chemotactic and degranulating activities of leukotriene B₅ (LTB₅) derived from eicosapentaenoic acid. *Biochem. Biophys. Res. Commun.*, 117:282–288.

40. Goldman, D. W., and Goetzl, E. J. (1984): Heterogeneity of human polymorphonuclear leukocyte receptors for leukotriene B₄. Identification of a subset of high affinity receptors that transduce the chemotactic response. *J. Exp. Med.*, 159:1027–1041.

41. Goldstein, I. M., Malmsten, C. L., Samuelsson, B., and Weissmann, G. (1977): Prostaglandins, thromboxanes, and polymorphonuclear leukocytes. Mediation and modulation of inflammation. *Inflammation*, 2:309–317.

42. Goldstein, I. M., Malmsten, C. L., Kindahl, H., Kaplan, H. B., Radmark, O., Samuelsson, B., and Weissmann, G. (1978): Thromboxane generation by human peripheral blood polymorphonuclear leukocytes. *J. Exp. Med.*, 148:787–792.

43. Goldyne, M. E., and Stobo, J. D. (1979): Synthesis of prostaglandins by subpopulations of human peripheral blood monocytes. *Prostaglandins*, 18:687–694.

44. Goldyne, M. E., and Stobo, J. D. (1981): Immunoregulatory role of prostaglandins and related lipids. *Crit. Rev. Immunol.*, 2:189–223.

45. Gullner, H.-G., Kafka, M. S., and Bartter, F. C. (1980): Indo-

methacin increases leucocyte β-adrenoreceptors in man. *Clin. Sci.,* 59:397–400.

46. Hamberg, M., and Samuelsson, B. (1974): Prostaglandin endoperoxides. Novel transformations of arachidonic acid in human platelets. *Proc. Natl. Acad. Sci. USA,* 71:3400–3404.

47. Hamberg, M., Svensson, J., and Samuelsson, B. (1975): Thromboxanes: A new group of biologically active compounds derived from prostaglandin endoperoxides. *Proc. Natl. Acad. Sci. USA,* 72: 2994–2998.

48. Hammarstrom, S., Hamberg, M., Samuelsson, B., Duell, E. A., Stawiski, M., and Voorhees, J. J. (1975): Increased concentrations of nonesterified arachidonic acid, 12L-hydroxy-5,8,10,14-eicosatetraenoic acid, prostaglandin E_2, and prostaglandin $F_{2\alpha}$ in epidermis of psoriasis. *Proc. Natl. Acad. Sci. USA,* 72:5130–5134.

49. Hanel, A. M., and Lands, W. E. M. (1982): Modifications of anti-inflammatory drug effectiveness by ambient lipid peroxides. *Biochem. Pharmacol.,* 31:3307–3311.

50. Higgs, E. A., Moncada, S., and Vane, J. R. (1978): Inflammatory effects of prostacyclin (PGI_2) and 6-oxo-$PGF_{1\alpha}$ in the rat paw. *Prostaglandins,* 16:153–162.

51. Higgs, G. A., Cardinal, D. C., Moncada, S., and Vane, J. R. (1979): Microcirculatory effects of prostacyclin (PGI_2) in the hamster cheek pouch. *Microvasc. Res.,* 18:245–254.

52. Higgs, G. A., Moncada, S., and Vane, J. R. (1984): Eicosanoids in inflammation. *Ann. Clin. Sci.,* 16:287–299.

53. Hirata, F., Schiffman, E., Subramanian, V., Salomon, D., and Axelrod, J. (1980): A phospholipase A_2 inhibitory protein in rabbit neutrophils induced by glucocorticoids. *Proc. Natl. Acad. Sci. USA,* 77:2533–2536.

54. Hirata, F., Carmine, R. D., Nelson, C. A., Axelrod, J., Schiffman, E., Warabi, A., DeBlas, A., Nirenberg, M., Manganiello, V., Vaughan, M., Kumagai, S., Green, I., Decker, J. L., and Steinberg, A. D. (1981): Presence of autoantibody for phospholipase inhibitory protein, lipomodulin, in patients with rheumatic diseases. *Proc. Natl. Acad. Sci. USA,* 78:3190–3194.

55. Hunter, J. A., Finkbeiner, W. E., Nadel, J. A., Goetzl, E. J., and Holtzman, M. J. (1985): Predominant generation of 15-lipoxygenase metabolites of arachidonic acid by epithelial cells from human trachea. *Proc. Natl. Acad. Sci. USA,* 82:4633–4637.

56. Huskisson, E. C. (1977): Anti-inflammatory drugs. *Semin. Arthritis Rheum.,* 7:1–20.

57. Kantor, H. S., and Hampton, M. (1978): Indomethacin in submicromolar concentrations inhibits cyclic AMP-dependent protein kinase. *Nature (London),* 276:841–842.

58. Kantrowitz, F., Robinson, D. R., McGuire, M. B., and Levine, L. (1975): Corticosteroids inhibit prostaglandin production by rheumatoid synovia. *Nature (London),* 258:737–739.

59. Kaplan-Harris, L., and Elsbach, P. (1980): The antiinflammatory activity of analogs of indomethacin correlates with their inhibitory effects on phospholipase A_2 of rabbit polymorphonuclear leukocytes. *Biochim. Biophys. Acta,* 618:318–326.

60. Kelly, V. E., Ferretti, A., Izui, S., and Strom, T. B. (1985): A fish oil diet rich in eicosapentaenoic acid reduces cyclooxygenase metabolites and suppresses lupus in MRL-lpr mice. *J. Immunol.,* 134: 1914–1919.

61. Kemp, A. S., and Smith, J. (1982): The effect of salicylate on human leucocyte migration. *Clin. Exp. Immunol.,* 49:233–238.

62. Klickstein, L. B., Shapleigh, C., and Goetzl, E. J. (1980): Lipoxygenation of arachidonic acid as a source of polymorphonuclear leukocyte chemotactic factors in synovial fluid and tissue in rheumatoid arthritis and spondyloarthritis. *J. Clin. Invest.,* 66:1166–1170.

63. Kremer, J. M., Michalek, A. V., Lininger, L., Huyck, C., Bigauoette, J., Timchalk, M. A., Rynes, R. I., Zieminski, J., and Bartholomew, L. E. (1985): Effects of manipulation of dietary fatty acids on clinical manifestations of rheumatoid arthritis. *Lancet,* 1:184–187.

64. Kulmacz, R. J., and Lands, W. E. M. (1985): Stoichiometry and kinetics of the interactions of prostaglandin H synthase with anti-inflammatory agents. *J. Biol. Chem.,* 260:12572–12578.

65. Kunkel, S. L., Thrall, R. T., Kunkel, R. G., Ward, P. A., and Zurier, R. B. (1979): Suppression of immune complex vasculitis in rats by prostaglandin. *J. Clin. Invest.,* 64:1525–1528.

66. Kunkel, S. L., Zanetti, M., and Sapin, C. (1982): Suppression of nephrotoxic serum nephritis in rats by prostaglandin E_1. *Am. J. Pathol.,* 108:240–245.

67. Lee, T. H., Mencia-Huerta, J.-M., Shih, C., Corey, E. J., Lewis, R. A., and Austen, K. F. (1984): Effects of exogenous arachidonic, eicosapentaenoic, and docosahexaenoic acids on the generation of 5-lipoxygenase pathway products by ionophore-activated human neutrophils. *J. Clin. Invest.,* 74:1922–1933.

68. Lee, T. H., Mencia-Huerta, J.-M., Shih, C., Corey, E. J., Lewis, R. A., and Austen, K. F. (1984): Characterization and biologic properties of 5,12-dihydroxy derivatives of eicosapentaenoic acid, including leukotriene B_5 and the double lipoxygenase product. *J. Biol. Chem.,* 259:2383–2389.

69. Lee, T. H., Hoover, R. L., Williams, J. D., Sperling, R. I., Ravelese, J., Spur, B. W., Robinson, D. R., Corey, E. J., Lewis, R. A., and Austen, K. F. (1985): Effects of dietary enrichment with eicosapentaenoic and docosahexaenoic acids on in vitro neutrophil and monocyte leukotriene generation and neutrophil function. *N. Engl. J. Med.,* 312:1217–1224.

70. Lehmeyer, J. E., and Johnston, R. B. (1978): Effect of anti-inflammatory drugs and agents that elevate intracellular levels of cyclic AMP on the release of toxic oxygen metabolites by phagocytes: Studies in a model of tissue-bound IgG. *Clin. Immunol. Immunopathol.,* 9:482–490.

71. Leroux, M. (1830): Discovery of salicine. *J. Chim. Med.,* 6:341.

72. Leslie, C. A., Gonnerman, W. A., Ullman, M. D., Hayes, K. C., Franzblau, C., and Cathcart, E. S. (1985): Dietary fish oil modulates macrophage fatty acids and decreases arthritis susceptibility in mice. *J. Exp. Med.,* 162:1336–1349.

73. Levine, J. D., Lau, W., Kwait, G., and Goetzl, E. J. (1984): Leukotriene B_4 produces hyperalgesia that is dependent on polymorphonuclear leukocytes. *Science,* 225:743–745.

74. Levine, L. (1983): Inhibition of the A-23187-stimulated leukotriene and prostaglandin biosynthesis of rat basophil leukemia (RBL-1) cells by non-steroidal anti-inflammatory drugs, anti-oxidants, and calcium channel blockers. *Biochem. Pharmacol.,* 32:3023–3026.

75. Lewis, R. A., and Austen, K. F. (1984): The biologically active leukotrienes. Biosynthesis, metabolism, receptors, functions, and pharmacology. *J. Clin. Invest.,* 73:889–897.

76. Maderazo, E. G., Breaux, S. P., and Woronick, C. L. (1984): Inhibition of human polymorphonuclear leukocyte cell responses by ibuprofen. *J. Pharm. Sci.,* 73:1403–1406.

77. Metz, S. A. (1981): Anti-inflammatory agents as inhibitors of prostaglandin synthesis in man. *Med. Clin. North Am.,* 65:713–757.

78. Mikulikova, D., and Trnavsky, K. (1982): The effect of indomethacin and its ester on lysosomal enzyme release from polymorphonuclear leukocytes and intracellular levels of cAMP and cGMP after phagocytosis of urate crystals. *Biochem. Pharmacol.,* 31:460–463.

79. Moncada, S., Higgs, E. A., and Vane, J. R. (1977): Human arterial and venous tissues generate prostacyclin (prostaglandin X), a potent inhibitor of platelet aggregation. *Lancet,* 1:18–20.

80. Naccache, P. H., Showell, H. J., Becker, E. L., and Sha'afi, R. I. (1979): Arachidonic acid-induced degranulation of rabbit peritoneal neutrophils. *Biochem. Biophys. Res. Commun.,* 87:292–299.

81. Naray-Fejes-Toth, A., Fejes-Toth, G., Fischer, C., and Frolich, J. C. (1984): Effect of dexamethasone on in vivo prostanoid production in the rabbit. *J. Clin. Invest.,* 74:120–123.

82. Needleman, P., Raz, A., Minkes, M. S., Ferrendelli, J. A., and Sprecher, H. (1979): Triene prostaglandins: Prostacyclin and thromboxane biosynthesis and unique biological properties. *Proc. Natl. Acad. Sci. USA,* 76:944–948.

83. Nickander, R., McMahon, F. G., and Ridolfo, A. S. (1979): Nonsteroidal anti-inflammatory agents. *Annu. Rev. Pharmacol. Toxicol.,* 19:469–490.

84. Northover, A. M. (1985): The effects of some non-steroidal anti-

inflammatory agents on membrane-associated calcium in rabbit peritoneal neutrophils. *Biochem. Pharmacol.*, 34:3123–3129.

85. Nugteren, H. (1975): Arachidonic lipoxygenase in blood platelets. *Biochim. Biophys. Acta*, 380:299–307.

86. O'Flaherty, J. T., Wykle, R. L., Lees, C. J., Shewmake, T., McCall, C. E., and Thomas, M. J. (1981): Neutrophil degranulating action of 5,12-dihydroxy-6,8,10,14-eicosatetraenoic acid and 1-*O*-alkyl-2-*O*-acetyl-*sn*-glycero-3-phosphocholine. Comparison with other degranulating agents. *Am. J. Pathol.*, 105:264–269.

87. Payan, D. G., Wong, M. Y. S., Chernov-Rogan, T., Valone, F. H., Pickett, W. C., Blake, V. A., Gold, W. M., and Goetzl, E. J. (1986): Alterations in human leukocyte function induced by ingestion of eicosapentaenoic acid. *J. Clin. Immunol.*, 6:402–410.

88. Piria, R. (1838): Recherches sur la salicine et les produits qui en dévirent. *Ann. Chim. Phys.*, 69:281–325.

89. Prescott, S. M. (1984): The effect of eicosapentaenoic acid on leukotriene B production by human neutrophils. *J. Biol. Chem.*, 259:7615–7621.

90. Prickett, J. D., Robinson, D. R., and Steinberg, A. D. (1981): Dietary enrichment with the polyunsaturated fatty acid eicosapentaenoic acid prevents proteinuria and prolongs survival in NZB × NZW F_1 mice. *J. Clin. Invest.*, 68:556–559.

91. Pruzanski, W., Saito, S., and DeBoer, G. (1983): Modulation of phagocytosis and bactericidal activity of human polymorphonuclear and mononuclear phagocytes by antiarthritic drugs. *J. Rheumatol.*, 10:197–203.

92. Puustinen, T., Dahl, M.-L., Uotila, P., and Haataja, M. (1984): Glucocorticoids do not decrease thromboxane and prostacyclin levels in human blood. *Prostaglandins Leukotrienes Med.*, 15:409–410.

93. Reibman, J., Haines, K. A., Rich, A. M., Cristello, P., Giedd, K. N., and Weissmann, G. (1986): Colchicine inhibits ionophore-induced formation of leukotriene B_4 by human neutrophils: The role of microtubules. *J. Immunol.*, 136:1027–1032.

94. Rivkin, I. (1977): The effect of bovine serum albumin on the in vitro inhibition of chemotaxis by anti-inflammatory agents. *Agents Actions*, 7:465–468.

95. Robinson, D. R., Tashjian, A. H., Jr., and Levine, L. (1975): Prostaglandin-stimulated bone resorption by rheumatoid synovia. *J. Clin. Invest.*, 56:1181–1188.

96. Robinson, D. R., Dayer, J.-M., and Krane, S. M. (1979): Prostaglandins and their regulation in rheumatoid arthritis. *Ann. N.Y. Acad. Sci.*, 332:279–294.

97. Robinson, D. R., Prickett, J. D., Makoul, G. T., Steinberg, A. D., and Colvin, R. B. (1986): Dietary fish oil reduces progression of established renal disease in (NZB × NZW) F_1 mice and delays renal disease in BXSB and MRL/l strains. *Arthritis Rheum.*, 29:539–546.

98. Roth, G. J., Stanford, N., and Majerus, P. W. (1975): Acetylation of prostaglandin synthetase by aspirin. *Proc. Natl. Acad. Sci. USA*, 72:3073–3076.

99. Samuelsson, B. (1983): Leukotrienes: Mediators of immediate hypersensitivity reactions and inflammation. *Science*, 220:568–575.

100. Serhan, C. N., Radin, A., Smolen, J. E., Korchak, H., Samuelsson, B., and Weissmann, G. (1982): Leukotriene B_4 is a complete secretagogue in human neutrophils: A kinetic analysis. *Biochem. Biophys. Res. Commun.*, 107:1006–1012.

101. Serhan, C. N., Hamberg, M., and Samuelsson, B. (1984): Lipoxins: Novel series of biologically active compounds formed from arachidonic acid in human leukocytes. *Proc. Natl. Acad. Sci. USA*, 81:5335–5339.

102. Seyberth, H. W., Segre, G. V., Morgan, J. L., Sweetman, B. J., Potts, J. T., Jr., and Oates, J. A. (1975): Prostaglandins as mediators of hypercalcemia associated with certain types of cancer. *N. Engl. J. Med.*, 293:1278–1283.

103. Shak, S., Perez, H. D., and Goldstein, I. M. (1983): A novel dioxygenation product of arachidonic acid possesses potent chemotactic activity for human polymorphonuclear leukocytes. *J. Biol. Chem.*, 258:14948–14953.

104. Siegel, M. I., McConnell, R. T., Porter, N. A., and Cuatrecasas, P. (1980): Arachidonate metabolism via lipoxygenase and 12L-hydroperoxy-5,8,10,14-icosatetraenoic acid peroxidase sensitive to anti-inflammatory drugs. *Proc. Natl. Acad. Sci. USA*, 77:308–312.

105. Simchowitz, L., Mehta, J., and Spilberg, I. (1979): Chemotactic factor-induced generation of superoxide radicals by human neutrophils. Effect of metabolic inhibitors and antiinflammatory drugs. *Arthritis Rheum.*, 22:755–763.

106. Simon, L. S., and Mills, J. A. (1980): Drug therapy: Nonsteroidal anti-inflammatory drugs. *N. Engl. J. Med.*, 302:1179–1185, 1237–1243.

107. Sirois, P., Saura, C., Salari, H., and Borgeat, P. (1984): Comparative effects of etodolac, indomethacin, and benoxaprofen on icosanoid biosynthesis. *Inflammation*, 8:353–364.

108. Smith, J. B., and Willis, A. L. (1971): Aspirin selectively inhibits prostaglandin production in human platelets. *Nature [New Biol.]*, 231:235–237.

109. Smith, R. J. (1979): The guinea pig neutrophil calcium-dependent lysosomal enzyme secretory process. Inhibition by nonsteroid anti-inflammatory agents. *Biochem. Pharmacol.*, 28:2739–2746.

110. Smith, R. J., Sabin, C., Gilchrest, H., and Williams, S. (1976): Effect of anti-inflammatory drugs on lysosomes and lysosomal enzymes from rat liver. *Biochem. Pharmacol.*, 25:2171–2177.

111. Smith, R. J., Sun, F. F., Iden, S. S., Bowman, B. J., Sprecher, H., and McGuire, J. C. (1981): An evaluation of the relationship between arachidonic acid lipoxygenation and human neutrophil degranulation. *Clin. Immunol. Immunopathol.*, 20:157–169.

112. Smolen, J. E., and Weissmann, G. (1980): The effects of indomethacin, 5,8,11,14-eicosatetraynoic acid, and *p*-bromophenacyl bromide on lysosomal enzyme release and superoxide anion generation by human polymorphonuclear leukocytes. *Biochem. Pharmacol.*, 29:533–538.

113. Soter, N. A., Lewis, R. A., Corey, E. J., and Austen, K. F. (1983): Local effects of synthetic leukotrienes (LTC_4, LTD_4, LTE_4, and LTB_4) in human skin. *J. Invest. Dermatol.*, 80:115–119.

114. Spagnuolo, P. J., Ellner, J. J., Hassid, A., and Dunn, M. J. (1980): Thromboxane A_2 mediates augmented polymorphonuclear leukocyte adhesiveness. *J. Clin. Invest.*, 66:406–414.

115. Stenson, W. F., and Parker, C. W. (1979): Metabolism of arachidonic acid in ionophore-stimulated neutrophils. Esterification of a hydroxylated metabolite into phospholipids. *J. Clin. Invest.*, 64:1457–1465.

116. Stenson, W. F., and Lobos, E. (1982): Sulfasalazine inhibits the synthesis of chemotactic lipids by neutrophils. *J. Clin. Invest.*, 69:494–497.

117. Strasser, T., Fischer, S., and Weber, P. C. (1985): Leukotriene B_5 is formed in human neutrophils after dietary supplementation with icosapentaenoic acid. *Proc. Natl. Acad. Sci. USA*, 82:1540–1543.

118. Strasser, T., Fischer, S., and Weber, P. C. (1985): Inhibition of leukotriene B_4 formation in human neutrophils after oral nafazatrom (Bay G 6575). *Biochem. Pharmacol.*, 34:1891–1894.

119. Turner, R. A., Semble, E. L., Johnson, J. A., McCrickard, E. L., Treadway, W. J., and Kaufman, J. S. (1984): Effects of benoxaprofen on human neutrophil function. *J. Rheumatol.*, 11:265–271.

120. Vanderhoek, J. Y., and Bailey, J. M. (1984): Activation of a 15-lipoxygenase/leukotriene pathway in human polymorphonuclear leukocytes by the anti-inflammatory agent ibuprofen. *J. Biol. Chem.*, 259:6752–6756.

121. Van Dyke, K., Peden, D., Van Dyke, C., Jones, G., Castranova, V., and Ma, J. (1982): Inhibition by nonsteroidal antiinflammatory drugs of luminol-dependent human-granulocyte chemiluminescence and [³H]FMLP binding. *Inflammation*, 6:113–125.

122. Vane, J. R. (1971): Inhibition of prostaglandin synthesis as a mechanism of action for aspirin-like drugs. *Nature [New Biol.]*, 231:232–237.

123. Wallner, B. P., Mattaliano, R. J., Hession, C., Cate, R. L., Tizard, R., Sinclair, L. K., Foeller, C., Chow, E. P., Browning, J. L., Ramachandran, K. L., and Pepinsky, R. B. (1986): Cloning and

expression of human lipocortin, a phospholipase A_2 inhibitor with potential anti-inflammatory activity. *Nature (London)*, 320:77–81.

124. Wedmore, C. V., and Williams, T. J. (1981): Control of vascular permeability by polymorphonuclear leukocytes in inflammation. *Nature (London)*, 289:646–650.

125. Weissmann, G., Goldstein, I., Hoffstein, S., Chauvel, G., and Robineaux, R. (1975): Yin-yang modulation of lysosomal enzyme release from polymorphonuclear leukocytes by cyclic nucleotides. *Ann. N.Y. Acad. Sci.*, 256:222–231.

126. Williams, T. J. (1979): Prostaglandin E_2, prostaglandin I_2, and the vascular changes of inflammation. *Br. J. Pharmacol.*, 65:517–524.

127. Williams, T. J., and Peck, M. J. (1977): Role of prostaglandin-mediated vasodilation in inflammation. *Nature (London)*, 270:530–532.

128. Wood, J. N., Coote, P. R., and Rhodes, J. (1984): Hydrocortisone inhibits prostaglandin production but not arachidonic acid release from cultured macrophages. *FEBS Lett.*, 174:143–146.

129. Ziel, R., and Krupp, P. (1976): Influence of endogenous pyrogen on cerebral prostaglandin-synthetase system. *Experientia*, 32:1451–1453.

130. Zurier, R. B., Hoffstein, S., and Weissmann, G. (1973): Suppression of acute and chronic inflammation in adrenalectomized rats by pharmacologic amounts of prostaglandins. *Arthritis Rheum.*, 16:606–618.

131. Zurier, R. B., Weissmann, G., Hoffstein, S., Kammerman, S., and Tai, H.-H. (1974): Mechanisms of lysosomal enzyme release from human leukocytes. II. Effects of cAMP and cGMP, autonomic agonists, and agents which affect microtubule function. *J. Clin. Invest.*, 53:297–309.

132. Zurier, R. B., and Sayadoff, D. M. (1975): Release of prostaglandins from human polymorphonuclear leukocytes. *Inflammation*, 1:93–101.

133. Zurier, R. B., Damjanov, I., Sayadoff, D. M., and Rothfield, N. F. (1977): Prostaglandin E_1 treatment of NZB/NZW F_1 hybrid mice. II. Prevention of glomerulonephritis. *Arthritis Rheum.*, 20:1449–1456.

134. Zurier, R. B., Sayadoff, D. M., Torrey, S. B., and Rothfield, N. F. (1977): Prostaglandin E_1 treatment of NZB/NZW mice. I. Prolonged survival of female mice. *Arthritis Rheum.*, 20:723–728.

135. Zurier, R. B., Damjanov, I., Miller, P. L., and Biewer, B. F. (1978): Prostaglandin E treatment prevents progression of nephritis in murine lupus erythematosus. *J. Clin. Lab. Immunol.*, 1:95–98.

Subject Index